Michelle Mitchell

NEW Features At A Glance

- NEW! **Additional content** for **psychotropic drugs.**
- NEW! Enhanced **evidence-based content** throughout.
- NEW! **Full-color insert** on **Medication Safety Tools** in the front of the book.

otential Nursing Diagnoses
ecreased cardiac output (Indications)
effective tissue perfusion (Indications)

nplementation

- ***High Alert:*** IV vasoactive medications are potentially dangerous. Have second practitioner independently check original order, dose calculations and infusion pump settings. Do not confuse dopamine with dobutamine. If both are available as floor stock, store in separate areas.
- Correct hypovolemia with volume expanders before initiating dopamine therapy.
- Extravasation may cause severe irritation, necrosis, and sloughing of tissue. Administer into a large vein and assess administration site frequently. If extravasation occurs, affected area should be infiltrated liberally with 10–15 ml of 0.9% NaCl containing 5–10 mg of phentolamine. Reduce proportionally for pediatric patients. Infiltration within 12 hr of extravasation produces immediate hyperemic changes.

IV Administration

- **Continuous Infusion:** ***Diluent:*** Dopamine vials must be diluted before use. Dilute 200–800 mg of dopamine in 250–500 ml of 0.9% NaCl, D5W, D5/LR, D5/0.45% NaCl, D5/0.9% NaCl, or LR. Admixed solution is stable for 24 hr. Discard solutions that are cloudy, discolored or contain a precipitate. Premixed infusions are already diluted and ready to use. ***Concentration:*** 0.8–3.2 mg/ml. ***Rate:*** Based on patient's weight (see Route/Dosage section). Infusion must be administered via infusion pump to ensure precise amount delivered. Titrate to response (blood pressure, heart rate, urine output, peripheral perfusion, presence of ectopic activity, cardiac index). Decrease rate gradually when discontinuing to prevent marked decreases in blood pressure
- **Y-Site Compatibility:** amifostine, amikacin, aminophylline, amiodarone, anidulafungin, argatroban, atracurium, atropine, aztreonam, bivalirudin, bumetanide, calcium chloride, calcium gluconate, caspofungin, cefotaxime, cefoxitin, ceftazidime, ceftizoxime, ceftriaxone, cefuroxime, cimetidine, ciprofloxacin, cisatracurium, cladribine, clindamycin, cyclosporine, daptomycin, dexamethasone sodium phosphate, dexmedetomidine, digoxin, diltiazem, diphenhydramine, dobutamine, docetaxel, doxorubicin liposome, doxycycline, droperidol, enalaprilat, epinephrine, ertapenem, erythromycin, esmolol, etoposide phosphate, famotidine, fenoldopam, fentanyl, fluconazole, foscarnet, gatifloxacin, gemcitabine, gentamicin, granisetron, haloperidol, heparin, hydrocortisone sodium succinate, hydromorphone, imipenem/cilastatin, inamrinone, isoproterenol, ketorolac, labetalol, levofloxacin, lidocaine, linezolid, lorazepam, magnesium sulfate, meperidine, methylprednisolone sodium succinate, metoclopramide, metoprolol, metronidazole, micafungin, midazolam, milrinone, morphine, nafcillin, nicardipine, nitroglycerin, nitroprusside, norepinephrine, ondansetron, oxaliplatin, palonosetron, pancuronium, pantoprazole, pemetrexed, penicillin G potassium, phenylephrine, phytonadione, piperacillin/tazobactam, potassium chloride, procainamide, prochlorperazine, promethazine, propofol, propranolol, protamine, ranitidine, remifentanil, sargramostim, streptokinase, tacrolimus, theophylline, thiotepa, ticarcillin/clavulanate, tigecycline, tirofiban, tobramycin, tolazoline, vancomycin, vasopressin, vecuronium, verapamil, vitamin B complex with C, voriconazole, warfarin, zidovudine.
- **Y-Site incompatibility:** acyclovir, alteplase, amphotericin B cholesteryl sulfate, ampicillin, cefazolin, chloramphenicol, diazepam, ganciclovir, indomethacin, insulin, lansoprazole, phenytoin, thiopental, trimethoprim/sulfamethoxazole.

D

Patient/Family Teaching

- Explain to patient the rationale for instituting this medication and the need for frequent monitoring.
- Advise patient to inform nurse immediately if chest pain; dyspnea; numbness, tingling, or burning of extremities occurs.
- Instruct patient to inform nurse immediately of pain or discomfort at the site of administration.

Evaluation/Desired Outcomes

- Increase in blood pressure
- Increase in peripheral circulation.
- Increase in urine output.

♣ = Canadian drug name.
*CAPITALS indicates life-threatening; underlines indicate most frequent.

- Offers **MORE high alert coverage**—to keep patients safe.
- Features a **NEW** heading for **IV administration.**
- Uses **NEW** sub-heads for **Diluent** and **Concentration** to accompany sub-head for **Rate.**
- Offers extensive **patient/family teaching** information.

F.A. DAVIS COMPANY

EARLY MANAGEMENT OF ANAPHYLACTIC REACTIONS

1 Discontinue suspected drug.
(stop IV, tourniquet IM or subcut site).

2 Maintain airway.
Aminophylline or other bronchodilators may be required for severe respiratory distress.

3 Administer *epinephrine*.
Subcut (Adults): 0.2–0.5 mg, may repeat q 5–15 min
Subcut (Children): 0.01 mg/kg or 0.1 mg, may repeat q 5–15 min
IV (Adults): 0.3–0.5 mg over 5 min, may repeat q 15 min or 0.1 mg over 5–10 min *or* 1–4 mcg/min infusion
IV (Children): 0.01 mg/kg/dose or 0.1–0.2 mg over 5 min, may repeat q 30 min or 0.1–1.5 mcg (maxi-um)/kg/min infusion

4 Administer *antihistamines*.
May prevent recurrence and decrease intensity of reaction.
diphenyhydramine (Benadryl)
IM, IV (Adults): 50–100 mg single dose, may follow with 5 mg/kg/day in divided doses or 50 mg every 6 hr for 1–2 days
IM, IV (Children): 5 mg/kg/day in divided doses q 6–8 hr (not to exceed 300 mg/day), may follow with oral therapy for 1–2 days
cimetidine (Tagamet)
IV (Adults): 300 mg q 6 hr
IV (Children): 25–30 mg/kg/day in 6 divided doses

5 Support blood pressure.
If necessary use fluids and/or vasopressors. Patients receiving beta blockers may be resistant to the effects of vasopressors.

6 Administer *corticosteroids*
(may decrease intensity of reaction).
hydrocortisone (Solu-Cortef)
IV (Adults and Children): 100–1000 mg, may follow with 7 mg/kg/day IV or oral therapy for 1–2 days.

7 Document reaction
in medical record, inform patient/family to carry identification

Davis's

DRUG GUIDE FOR NURSES®

ELEVENTH EDITION

JUDITH HOPFER DEGLIN, PharmD
Consultant Pharmacist
Hospice of Southeastern Connecticut
Uncasville, Connecticut

APRIL HAZARD VALLERAND, PhD, RN, FAAN
Wayne State University
College of Nursing
Detroit, Michigan

F. A. DAVIS COMPANY • Philadelphia

F. A. Davis Company
1915 Arch Street
Philadelphia, PA 19103
www.fadavis.com

Printed in the United States of America

Last digit indicates print number 10 9 8 7 6 5 4 3

Editor-in-Chief, Nursing: Patti L. Cleary
Publisher, Nursing: Robert G. Martone
Acquisitions Editor: Thomas A. Ciavarella
Project Editor: Meghan K. Ziegler
Director of Production: Michael W. Bailey
Managing Editor: David Orzechowski

NOTE: As new scientific information becomes available through basic and clinical research, recommended treatments and drug therapies undergo changes. The authors and publisher have done everything possible to make this book accurate, up to date, and in accord with accepted standards at the time of publication. However, the reader is advised always to check product information (package inserts) for changes and new information regarding dose and contraindications before administering any drug. Caution is especially urged when using new or infrequently ordered drugs.

ISBN-13: 978-0-8036-1911-1 (with CD) (alk. paper)
ISBN-10: 0-8036-1911-1 (with CD) (alk. paper)

ISBN-13: 978-0-8036-1912-8 (without CD) (alk. paper)
ISBN-10: 0-8036-1912-X (without CD) (alk. paper)

Deglin, Judith Hopfer, 1950–
Davis's drug guide for nurses/Judith Hopfer Deglin, April Hazard Vallerand—11th ed. p.; cm.
Includes bibliographical references and index.
ISBN-13: 978-0-8036-1911-1 (alk. paper)
ISBN-10: 0-8036-1911-1 (alk. paper)
1. Drugs—Handbooks, manuals, etc. 2. Nursing—Handbooks, manuals, etc. 3. Clinical pharmacology—Handbooks, manuals, etc. I. Vallerand, April Hazard. II Title. III. Title: Drug guide for nurses.
[DNLM: 1. Pharmaceutical Preparations–administration & dosage–Handbooks. 2. Drug Therapy–nursing–Handbooks. 3. Pharmacology, Clinical–methods–Handbooks. QV 735 D318 2009]
RM301.12.D44 2009
615'.1'024613-dc22

2008041012
CIP

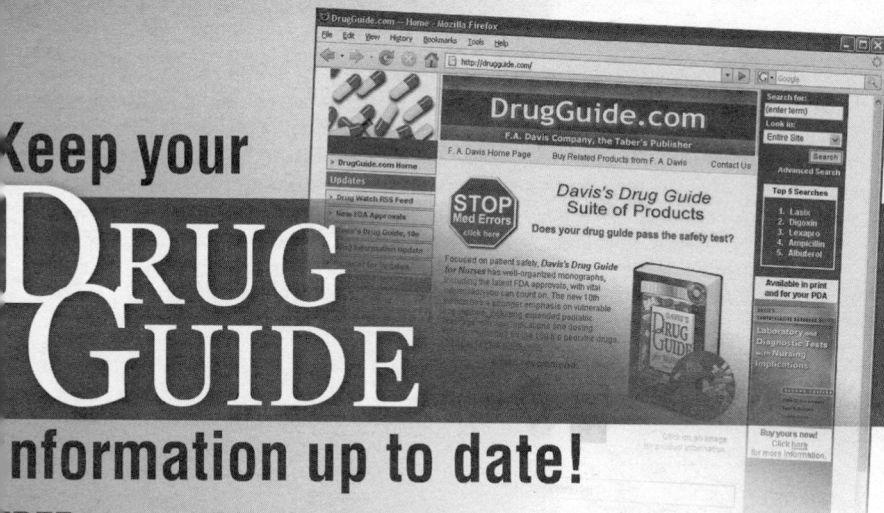

DEDICATION

In loving memory of my older children, Samantha Ann and Randy Eli, both struck and killed by a drinking driver on January 9, 1997. They remain forever in our hearts. The wonder and joy they brought to our lives continues to inspire us.

To Stu, for his continued support and love.

To my daughter Hanna, whose hard work, talent and grace never cease to amaze me.
To my son Reuben, whose smile warms my heart and whose energy is boundless.
To my parents, Charlotte and Kurt Hopfer, who continue to inspire me.

JHD

To my father, Keith Hazard, whose love and support are always there.
To my mother-in-law, Roberta, who remains a guiding presence in my life.
To my son, Ben, whose sensitivity and sense of humor make even the toughest day easier.
To my daughter, Katharine, whose fearlessness and determination in seeking her goals I admire.
To my husband, Warren, my colleague and friend, whose encouragement and love I have always cherished.

AHV

ACKNOWLEDGMENTS

We offer our thanks to the students and nurses who have used our book for over 20 years. We hope our book provides you with the current knowledge of pharmacotherapeutics you need to continue to give quality care in our rapidly changing health-care environment.

Judi and April

F. A. DAVIS PHARMACOLOGIC PUBLICATIONS ADVISORY BOARD

Grant E. Fraser, MD
President
Fraser Consulting, LLC
Bradenton, FL

Matthew Grissinger, RPh, FISMP, FASCP
Director, Error Reporting Programs
Institute for Safe Mediation Practices
Huntingdon Valley, PA

Linda G. Gooen, PharmD, MS
Certified Geriatric Pharmacist, Certified Consultant Pharmacist
Adjunct Professor, Rutgers Ernest Mario School of Pharmacy
President, Gooen Consulting, LLC
Basking Ridge, NJ

Susan M. Hasenau, PhDc, RN, CNNP
Professor
Madonna University
School of Nursing
Livonia, MI

Marilyn J. Hehr, RN, MSN
CNCC Nursing Program Director
Colorado Northwestern Community College
Craig, CO

Nadine T. James, RN, PhD
Dean and Associate Professor
Joseph and Nancy Fail School of Nursing
William Carey University
Hattiesburg, MS

Kathy Kumer, MS, CS, RN
Director of Nurses
Castle Rock Convalescent Center
Green River, WY

Stuart Levine, PharmD
Informatics Specialist
Institute for Safe Medication Practices
Huntingdon Valley, PA

Lynn R. Parker-McBride, MA, NP, CNS, RN
Holistic Nurse Practitioner
Drew University
Madison, NJ

Ginette A. Pepper, PhD, RN, FAAN
Helen Lowe Bamberger Colby Presidential Endowed Chair in Gerontological Nursing
Associate Dean for Research & PhD Programs
Salt Lake City, UT
Director
University of Utah Hartford Center of Geriatric Nursing Excellence
Salt Lake City, UT

Rosemary C. Polomano, PhD, RN, FAAN
Associate Professor of Pain Practice
University of Pennsylvania
School of Nursing
Philadelphia, PA

Alicia M. Reese, PharmD, MS, BCPS
Clinical Education Manager
Endo Pharmaceuticals
Chadds Ford, PA

Debbie Richmond, NP-C
Wayne State University
Detroit, MI

Noel Dougherty Rosner, MSN, RN, ANP-C, DNP
Nurse Practitioner
Raritan Bay Medical Center
Department of Infectious Diseases
Perth Amboy, NJ
Faculty
University of Medicine and Dentistry
Newark, NJ

Dorie Schwertz, PhD, RN, FAAN, FAHA
Associate Professor
University of Illinois-Chicago College of Nursing
Department of Medical Surgical Nursing and
Adjunct Professor of Pharmacology
Chicago, IL

Emily Karwacki-Sheff, MS, CMS, RN, FNP-BC
Lecturer and Clinical Instructor
Massachusetts General Hospital
Institute of Health Professions
Charlestown, MA
Clinical Instructor
Boston College
Chestnut Hill, MA

Sue Seckinger, BSN, RN, CWOCN
Wound Care Specialist
Lower Bucks Hospital
Bristol, PA

Kim Subasic, MSN, RN
The University of Scranton
Scranton, PA

Cynthia Ulreich, RN, BSN, OCN
P2 Chemotherapy Nurse Coordinator
Henry Ford Health System
Detroit, MI

Lisa Velazquez-Marsh, RN, BSN, OCN
Community Cancer Center of North Florida
North Florida Regional Medical Center
Gainesville, FL

Frances B. Wimbush, PhD, RN
Acute Care Nurse Practitioner and Consultant
Ocean View, DE

Kevin Zakrzewski, MD
Internal Medicine
Abington Memorial Hospital
Abington, PA

CONSULTANTS

Michelle Farkas-Cameron, APRN-PMH, BC
Clinical Nurse Specialist
Sinai-Grace Hospital
Inpatient Psychiatry
Detroit, MI

Jamie Crawley, B.Sc.N., B.A., M.B.A./H.C.M., PhD(c)
Doctoral Student
Wayne State University
Detroit, MI
Lecturer
University of Windsor
Faculty of Nursing
Windsor, ON, Canada

Deborah A. Ennis, RN, MSN, CCRN
Harrisburg Area Community College
Harrisburg, PA

Linda Felver, PhD, RN
Associate Professor
Oregon Health & Science University
School of Nursing
Portland, OR

Charlene C. Gyurko, PhD, RN, CNE
Assistant Professor
Purdue University, Calumet School of Nursing
Hammond, IN

Althea DuBose Hayes, RD
Renal Dietitian
Greenfield Health System,
a division of Henry Ford Health System
Southfield, MI

Janeen Kidd, RN, BN
Instructor/School Placement Project Coordinator
University of Victoria
School of Nursing
Victoria, BC, Canada

Wendy Neander, BS, BScN, RN, MN, PhD (student)
Assistant Professor
University of Victoria
School of Nursing
Victoria, BC, Canada
Staff Nurse
Nanaimo Regional Correctional Centre
Nanaimo, BC, Canada
Assistant Professor
Oregon Health & Science University
School of Nursing
Ashland, OR

Norma Perez, BSN, RN
Nursing Faculty & Clinical Coordinator
Ivy Tech Community College
School of Nursing
Valparaiso, IN

Gladdi Tomlinson, RN, MSN
Professor of Nursing
Harrisburg Area Community College
Harrisburg, PA

Linda S. Weglicki, RN, PhD
Assistant Professor
Wayne State University
College of Nursing
Detroit, MI

CONTENTS

HOW TO USE *DAVIS'S DRUG GUIDE FOR NURSES* 1

EVIDENCE-BASED PRACTICE AND PHARMACOTHERAPEUTICS: Implications for Nurses 5

MEDICATION ERRORS: Improving Practices and Patient Safety 8

DETECTING AND MANAGING ADVERSE DRUG REACTIONS 14

SPECIAL DOSING CONSIDERATIONS 18
- The Pediatric Patient 18
- The Geriatric Patient 18
- The Patient of Reproductive Age 19
- Renal Disease 19
- Liver Disease 19
- Heart Failure 19
- Body Size 20
- Drug Interactions 20

EDUCATING PATIENTS ABOUT SAFE MEDICATION USE 21

CLASSIFICATIONS 23
- Anti-Alzheimer's agents 23
- Antianemics 24
- Antianginals 25
- Antianxiety agents 26
- Antiarrhythmics 28
- Antiasthmatics 29
- Anticholinergics 31
- Anticoagulants 32
- Anticonvulsants 34
- Antidepressants 36
- Antidiabetics 38
- Antidiarrheals 40
- Antiemetics 41
- Antifungals 42
- Antihistamines 44
- Antihypertensives 45
- Anti-infectives 47
- Antineoplastics 50
- Antiparkinson agents 53
- Antiplatelet agents 54
- Antipsychotics 56
- Antipyretics 58
- Antiretrovirals 59
- Antirheumatics 61
- Antituberculars 62
- Antiulcer agents 63
- Antivirals 65
- Beta blockers 67

Bone resorption inhibitors 69
Bronchodilators 70
Calcium channel blockers 71
Central nervous system stimulants 73
Corticosteroids 74
Diuretics 76
Hormones 78
Immunosuppressants 80
Laxatives 82
Lipid-lowering agents 83
Minerals/electrolytes/pH modifiers 84
Natural/Herbal Products 86
Nonopioid analgesics 87
Nonsteroidal anti-inflammatory agents 88
Opioid analgesics 90
Sedative/hypnotics 92
Skeletal muscle relaxants 94
Thrombolytics 95
Vaccines/immunizing agents 97
Vascular headache suppressants 98
Vitamins 99
Weight control agents 100

DRUG MONOGRAPHS IN ALPHABETICAL ORDER BY GENERIC NAME 103–1266

LESS COMMONLY USED DRUGS 1267–1296

NATURAL/HERBAL PRODUCTS 1297–1318

APPENDICES 1319
Appendix A. Recent Drug Approvals 1321
Appendix B. Combination Drugs 1329
Appendix C. Ophthalmic Medications 1349
Appendix D. Medication Administration Techniques 1357
Appendix E. Dose Calculation Formulas 1360
Appendix F. Body Surface Area Nomograms 1363
Appendix G. Normal Values of Common Laboratory Tests 1365
Appendix H. Commonly Used Abbreviations 1368
Appendix I. Pregnancy Categories and Controlled Substance Schedules 1370
Appendix J. Equianalgesic Dosing Guidelines 1372
Appendix K. Recommendations for the Safe Handling of Hazardous Drugs 1375
Appendix L. Food Sources for Specific Nutrients 1377
Appendix M. Insulins and Insulin Therapy 1379
Appendix N. Canadian and U.S. Pharmaceutical Practices 1381
Appendix O. Routine Pediatric and Adult Immunizations 1383
Appendix P. Administering Medications to Children 1390
Appendix Q. Pediatric Dosage Calculations 1391
Appendix R. Pediatric Fluid and Electrolyte Requirements 1392

BIBLIOGRAPHY 1393

COMPREHENSIVE GENERIC/TRADE/CLASSIFICATIONS INDEX 1395

HOW TO USE *DAVIS'S DRUG GUIDE FOR NURSES*

Davis's Drug Guide for Nurses provides comprehensive, up-to-date drug information in well-organized, nursing-focused monographs. It also includes extensive supplemental material in 18 appendices and the accompanying CD-ROM, thoroughly addresses the issue of safe medication administration, and educates the reader about 50 different therapeutic classes of drugs. In this 11th edition, we have continued the tradition of focusing on safe medication administration by adding a new **Medication Safety Tools** color insert and even more information about health care's most vulnerable patients: children, the elderly, pregnant women, and breastfeeding mothers. Look for more Pedi, Geri, OB, and Lactation headings throughout the monographs. In addition, we've expanded our information relevant to Canadian students and nurses. You'll find a new appendix comparing Canadian and U.S. pharmaceutical practices, more Canada-only combination drugs in the Combination Drugs appendix, and additional Canadian brand names in the drug monographs. To help you find this information quickly, we've also added a maple leaf icon (✸) in the index next to each Canadian entry. Use this book to enhance your competence in implementing and evaluating medication therapies. The following sections describe the organization of *Davis's Drug Guide for Nurses* and explain how to quickly find the information you need.

Safe Medication Use Articles

"Medication Errors: Improving Practices and Patient Safety", "Detecting and Managing Adverse Drug Reactions", "Special Dosing Considerations", and "Educating Patients About Medication Use", comprise the safe medication use articles and provide an overview of the medication safety issues that confront practitioners and patients. Leading off this series, the medication errors article familiarizes you with the systems issues and clinical situations repeatedly implicated in medication errors and suggests practical means to avoid them. It also teaches you about *high alert* medications, which have a greater potential to cause patient harm than other medications. "Detecting and Managing Adverse Drug Reactions" explains the different types of adverse reactions and provides guidance on how to detect and manage them. "Special Dosing Considerations" identifies the patient populations, such as neonates and patients with renal impairment, who require careful dose adjustments to ensure optimal therapeutic outcomes. "Educating Patients About Medication Use" reviews the most important teaching points for nurses to discuss with their patients and their families. In addition to these safety articles, other critical information is highlighted in red throughout the drug monographs. This allows the reader to quickly identify important information and to see how nursing practice, including assessment, implementation, and patient teaching, relates to it.

Classifications Profile

Medications in the same therapeutic class often share similar mechanisms of action, assessment guidelines, precautions, and interactions. The Classifications Profile provides summaries of the major therapeutic classifications used in *Davis's Drug Guide for Nurses*. It also provides patient teaching information common to all agents within the class and a list of drugs within each class.

Medication Safety Tools

New to this edition is a color insert with tables and charts that nurses can use for a quick but thorough reference to information that will help them avoid making medication errors. It includes compatibility charts; dilution tables for pediatric medications; lists of drugs that are associated with adverse reactions and falls in the elderly; high alert drugs; sound-alike, look-alike drugs and more.

Drug Monographs

Drug monographs are organized in the following manner:

High Alert Status: Some medications, such as chemotherapeutic agents, anticoagulants, and insulins, have a greater potential for harm than others. These medications have been identified by the *Institute for Safe Medication Practices* as **high alert drugs**. *Davis's Drug Guide for Nurses* includes a high alert tab in the upper right corner of the monograph header in appropriate medications to alert the nurse to the medication's risk. The term "high alert" is used in other parts of the monograph as well, to help the nurse administer these medications safely. See the new **Medication Safety Tools** color insert for a complete list of high alert medications in *Davis's Drug Guide for Nurses*. Refer to ISMP.org for all solutions, groups, and individual high alert drugs.

Generic/Trade Name: The generic name appears first, with a pronunciation key, followed by an alphabetical list of trade names. Canadian trade names are preceded by a maple leaf (✱). Common names, abbreviations, and selected foreign names are also included.

Classification: The therapeutic classification, which categorizes drugs by the disease state they are used to treat, appears first, followed by the pharmacologic classification, which is based on the drug's mechanism of action.

Controlled Substance Schedule: All drugs regulated by federal law are placed into one of five schedules, based on the drug's medicinal value, harmfulness, and potential for abuse or addiction. Schedule I drugs, the most dangerous and having no medicinal value, are not included in *Davis's Drug Guide for Nurses*. (See Appendix I for a description of the Schedule of Controlled Substances.)

Pregnancy Category: Pregnancy categories (A, B, C, D, and X) provide a basis for determining a drug's potential for fetal harm and are included in each monograph. The designation UK is used when the pregnancy category is unknown. (See Appendix I for more information.)

Indications: Medications are approved by the FDA (Food and Drug Administration) for specific disease states. This section identifies the diseases or conditions for which the drug is commonly used and includes significant unlabeled uses as well.

Action: This section contains a concise description of how the drug produces the desired therapeutic effect.

Pharmacokinetics: Pharmacokinetics refers to the way the body processes a medication by absorption, distribution, metabolism, and excretion. This section also includes information on the drug's half-life.

Absorption: Absorption describes the process that follows drug administration and its subsequent delivery to systemic circulation. If only a small fraction is absorbed following oral administration (diminished bioavailability), then the oral dose must be much greater than the parenteral dose. Absorption into systemic circulation also follows other routes of administration such as topical, transdermal, intramuscular, subcutaneous, rectal, and ophthalmic routes. Drugs administered intravenously are usually 100% bioavailable.

Distribution: This section comments on the drug's distribution in body tissues and fluids. Distribution becomes important in choosing one drug over another, as in selecting an antibiotic that will penetrate the central nervous system to treat meningitis or in avoiding drugs that cross the placenta or concentrate in breast milk. Information on protein binding is included for drugs that are >95% bound to plasma proteins, which has implications for drug-drug interactions.

Metabolism and Excretion: Drugs are primarily eliminated from the body either by hepatic conversion to inactive compounds (metabolism or biotransformation) and subsequent excretion by the kidneys, or by renal elimination of unchanged drug. Therefore, drug metabolism and excretion information is important in determining dosage regimens and intervals for patients with impaired renal or hepatic function. The creatinine clearance (CCr) helps quantify renal function and guides dosage adjustments. Formulas to estimate CCr are included in Appendix E.

Half-Life: The half-life of a drug is the amount of time it takes for the drug level to decrease by 50% and roughly correlates with the duration of action. Half-lives are given for drugs assuming the patient has normal renal or hepatic function. Conditions that alter the half-life are noted.

Time/Action Profile: The time/action profile table provides the onset of drug action, its peak effect, and its duration of activity. This can aid in planning administration schedules and allows the reader to appreciate differences in choosing one route over another.

Contraindications and Precautions: Situations in which drug use should be avoided or alternatives strongly considered are listed as contraindications. In general, most drugs are contraindicated in pregnancy or lactation, unless the potential benefits outweigh the possible risks to the mother or baby (e.g., anticonvulsants, antihypertensives, and antiretrovirals). Contraindications may be absolute (i.e., the drug in question should be avoided completely) or relative, in which certain clinical situations may allow cautious use of the drug. The precautions portion includes disease states or clinical situations in which drug use involves particular risks or in which dosage modification may be necessary. Extreme cautions are noted separately to draw attention to conditions under which use of the drug results in serious, potentially life-threatening consequences.

Adverse Reactions and Side Effects: Although it is not possible to include all reported reactions, major side effects for all drugs are included. Life-threatening adverse reactions or side effects are **CAPITALIZED**, and the most frequent side effects are underlined. Those underlined generally have an incidence of 10% or greater. Those not underlined occur in fewer than 10% but more than 1% of patients. Although life-threatening reactions may be rare (fewer than 1%), they are included because of their significance. The following abbreviations are used for body systems:

CNS: central nervous system
EENT: eye, ear, nose, and throat
Resp: respiratory
CV: cardiovascular
GI: gastrointestinal
GU: genitourinary
Derm: dermatologic
Endo: endocrinologic
F and E: fluid and electrolyte
Hemat: hematologic
Local: local
Metab: metabolic
MS: musculoskeletal
Neuro: neurologic
Misc: miscellaneous

Interactions: Drug interactions are a significant risk for patients. As the number of medications a patient receives increases, so does the likelihood of drug-drug interactions. This section provides the most important drug-drug interactions and their physiological effects. Significant drug-food and drug-natural product interactions are also noted as are recommendations for avoiding or minimizing these interactions

Route and Dosage: Routes of administration are grouped together and include recommended doses for adults, children, and other more specific age groups (such as geriatric patients). Dosage units are expressed in the terms in which they are usually prescribed. For example, penicillin G dosage is given in units rather than in milligrams. Dosing intervals also are provided in the manner in which they are frequently ordered. If a specific clinical situation (indication) requires a different dose or interval, this is listed separately for clarity. Specific dosing regimens for hepatic or renal impairment are also included.

Availability: This section lists the strengths and concentrations of available dose forms. Such information is useful in planning more convenient regimens (fewer tablets/capsules, less injection volume) and in determining whether certain dosing forms are available (suppositories, oral concentrates, sustained- or extended-release forms). Flavors of oral liquids and chewable tablets have been included to improve compliance and adherence in pediatric patients. General availability and average wholesale prices of commonly prescribed drugs have also been added as an aid to nurses with prescriptive authority.

Nursing Implications: This section helps the nurse apply the nursing process to pharmacotherapeutics. The subsections provide a step-by-step guide to clinical assessment, implementation (drug administration), and evaluation of the outcomes of pharmacologic therapy.

Assessment: This section includes guidelines for assessing patient history and physical data before and during drug therapy. Assessments specific to the drug's various indications are also included.

The **Lab Test Considerations** section provides the nurse with information regarding which laboratory tests to monitor and how the results may be affected by the medication. **Toxicity and Overdose** alerts the nurse to therapeutic serum drug levels that must be monitored and signs and symptoms of toxicity. The antidote and treatment for toxicity or overdose of appropriate medications also are included.

Potential Nursing Diagnoses: The two or three most pertinent North American Nursing Diagnoses Association (NANDA) diagnoses that potentially apply to a patient receiving the medication are listed. Each diagnosis includes the pharmacologic effect from which the diagnosis has been derived. For instance, the patient receiving immunosuppressant drugs should be diagnosed with Risk for Infection. The diagnosis is followed by the term Side Effects in parentheses. Since patient education is fundamental to all nurse-patient interactions, the diagnosis Knowledge Deficit should be assumed to be a nursing diagnosis applicable to all drugs.

Implementation: Guidelines specific for medication administration are discussed in this subsection. **High Alert** information, i.e., information that directly relates to preventing medication errors with inherently dangerous drugs, is included first if applicable. Sound-alike look-alike name confusion alerts are also included here. Other headings in this section provide data regarding routes of administration. **PO** describes when and how to administer the drug, whether tablets may be crushed or capsules opened, and when to administer the medication in relation to food. The **IV** section includes specific information about administering the medication intravenously. It has been thoroughly updated for this edition beginning with a more prominent IV Administration heading that introduces this section. New bold, red headings have been added to highlight the recommended **diluents** and **concentrations**. These new headings complement the **Rate** heading and make this critical information easy to find. Wherever possible, new information has been added to these topics. Several subsections comprise the IV Administration section. The first section, **Direct IV**, which refers to administering medications from a syringe directly into a saline lock, Y-site of IV tubing, or a 3–way stopcock, provides details for reconstitution, concentration, dilution, and rate. **Rate** is also included in both other methods of IV administration, direct or intermittent infusion **Intermittent Infusion** and **Continuous Infusion** specify standard dilution solutions and amounts, stability information, and rates. In addition, a quick reference for information about dilution amounts in neonates and infants, who are extremely sensitive to excess fluids, is contained in the new **Medication Safety Tools** color insert. **Syringe Compatibility/Incompatibility** identifies compatibile medications when mixed in a syringe. Compatibility of medications in a syringe is usually limited to 15 minutes after mixing. **Y-Site Compatibility/Incompatibility** identifies medications compatible or incompatible with each drug when administered via Y-site injection or 3-way stopcock in IV tubing. **Additive Compatibility/Incompatibility** identifies medications compatible or incompatible when admixed in solution. Compatibility of diluted medications administered through a Y-site for continuous or intermittent infusion is usually limited to 24 hours. **Solution Compatibility/Incompatibility** identifies compatible or incompatible solutions for dilution for administration purposes. Compatibility information is compiled from Trissel's *Handbook of Injectable Drugs*, ed 14. Compatibility and incompatibility information is also located in charts contained in the **Medication Safety Tools** color insert. A printable version of syringe compatibilities is also available at www.drugguide.com.

Patient/Family Teaching: This section includes information that should be taught to patients and/or families of patients. Side effects that should be reported, information on minimizing and managing side effects, details on administration, and follow-up requirements are presented. The nurse also should refer to the **Implementation** section for specific information to teach to the patient and family about taking the medication. **Home Care Issues** discusses aspects to be considered for medications taken in the home setting.

Evaluation: Outcome criteria for determination of the effectiveness of the medication are provided.

EVIDENCE-BASED PRACTICE AND PHARMACOTHERAPEUTICS: Implications for Nurses

The purpose of evidence-based practice is to improve the outcomes of treatment for patients. How pharmacologic agents affect patients is often the subject of research; such research is required by the Food and Drug Administration (FDA) before and after drug approval. Any medication can be the subject of an evidence-based clinical review article. But what does "evidence-based" mean and how does it relate to nursing?

According to Ingersoll, "Evidence-based nursing practice is the conscientious, explicit and judicious use of theory-derived, research-based information in making decisions about care delivery to individuals or groups of patients and in consideration of individual needs and preferences" (2000, p. 152). Still subject to debate are questions about the sufficiency and quality of evidence. For example, what kind of evidence is needed? How much evidence is necessary to support, modify, or change clinical practice? And, were the studies reviewed of "good" quality and are their results valid?

In general, clinicians use **hierarchy of evidence** schemas to rank types of research reports from the most valuable and scientifically rigorous to the least useful. The hierarchy makes clear that some level of evidence about the effect of a particular treatment or condition exists, even if the evidence is considered weak. Figure 1 illustrates a hierarchy of evidence pyramid with widely accepted rankings: the most scientifically rigorous at the top, the least scientifically rigorous at the bottom. Practitioners and clinicians should look for the highest level of available evidence to answer their clinical questions.

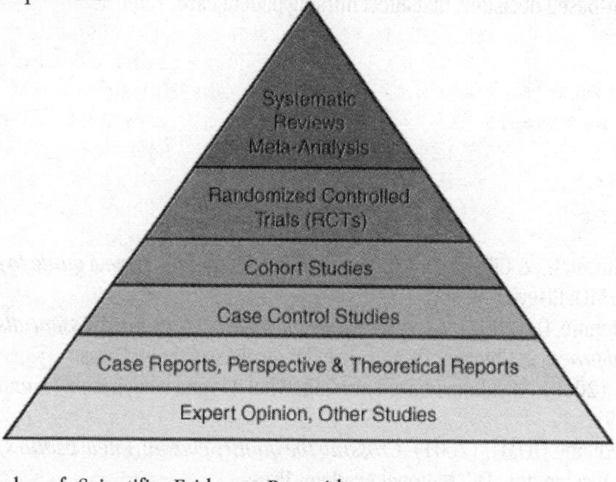

Figure 1 Hierarchy of Scientific Evidence Pyramid

Evidence-Based Practice and Its Importance in Pharmacology

Evidence-based practices in pharmacology generally are derived from well-designed randomized controlled trials (RCTs) or other experimental designs that investigate drugs' therapeutic and non-therapeutic effects. However, although FDA-approved pharmacologic agents have undergone rigorous testing through RCTs, nurses have the responsibility to evaluate the findings for the best scientific evidence available and to determine the most appropriate, safest, and efficacious drugs for their patients.

While numerous databases are available through Internet searches, two valuable and quickly accessible resources for evaluating the current highest level of pharmacologic evidence are 1) the Cochrane Database of Systematic Reviews and the Central Register of Controlled Trials and 2) the National Guidelines Clearinghouse (NGC), supported by the Agency for Healthcare Research and Quality (AHRQ). The Cochrane library and databases provide full text of high-quality, regularly updated systematic reviews, protocols, and clinical trials. The Web address is http://www.cochrane.org/reviews.clibintro.htm.

AHRQ's Evidence-Based Practice Centers (EPCs) provide evidence reports and technology assessments that can assist nurses in their efforts to provide the highest quality and safest pharmacologic health care available. The EPCs systematically review the relevant scientific literature, conduct additional analyses (when appropriate) prior to developing their reports and assessments, and provide guideline comparisons. The Web address is http://www.guideline.gov.

Evidence-based systematic reports and guidelines provide nurses with instantaneous access to the most current knowledge, enabling them to critically appraise the scientific evidence and its appropriateness to their patient population. This is especially important given the need for nurses to keep abreast of the rapidly changing pharmacologic agents in use. New drugs are approved each month, compelling nurses to know these drugs' intended uses, therapeutic effects, interactions, and adverse effects.

Evidence-based practice requires a shift from the traditional paradigm of clinical practice—grounded in intuition, clinical experience, and pathophysiologic rationale—to a paradigm in which nurses must combine clinical expertise, patient values and preferences, and clinical circumstances with the integration of the best scientific evidence in order to make conscientious, well-informed, research-based decisions that affect nursing patient care.

***

Linda S. Weglicki, PhD, RN
Wayne State University College of Nursing
Detroit, Michigan

REFERENCES

1. DiCenso, A., Guyatt, G., & Ciliska, D. (2005). *Evidence-based nursing: A guide to clinical practice*. St. Louis, MO: Elsevier Mosby.
2. Guyatt, G., & Rennie, D. (2002). *Users' guide to the medical literature: Essentials of evidence-based clinical practice*. Chicago, IL: American Medical Association Press.
3. Ingersoll, G.L. (2000). "Evidence-based nursing: What it is and what it isn't." *Nursing Outlook*. 48(4), 151-152.
4. Institute of Medicine [IOM]. (2001). *Crossing the quality chasm: A new health system for the 21st century*. Washington, DC: National Academy Press.
5. Leavitt, S.B. (2003). Evidence-based addiction medicine for practitioners: Evaluating and using research evidence in clinical practice. Addiction Treatment Forum, March. Retrieved May, 2007, from http://www.atforum.com/SiteRoot/pages/addiction_resources/EBAM_16_Pager.pdf
6. Melnyk, B.M., & Fineout-Overholt, E. (2005). *Evidence-based practice in nursing & healthcare: A guide to best practice*. Philadelphia, PA: Lippincott Williams & Wilkins.
7. Mitchell, G.J. (1999). "Evidence-based practice: Critique and alternative view." *Nursing Science Quarterly*. 12, 30-35.

8. Polit, D.F., & Beck, C.T. (2008). *Nursing research: Generating and assessing evidence for practice.* (8th ed). Philadelphia, PA: Lippincott Williams & Wilkins.
9. Sackett, D., Rosenberg, W., Gray, J., Haynes, R., & Richardson, W. (1996). "Evidence-based medicine: What it is and what it isn't." *British Medical Journal*. 312, 71-72.

Note: This content is an excerpt from an article written exclusively for the 11th edition of Davis's Drug Guide for Nurses. To access the full article, visit DavisPlus, F.A. Davis's online center for student and instructor ancillaries at http://davisplus.fadavis.com.

MEDICATION ERRORS: Improving Practices and Patient Safety

It is widely acknowledged that medication errors result in thousands of adverse drug events, preventable reactions, and deaths per year. Nurses, physicians, pharmacists, patient safety organizations, the Food and Drug Administration, the pharmaceutical industry, and other parties share in the responsibility for determining how medication errors occur and designing strategies to reduce error.

One impediment to understanding the scope and nature of the problem has been the reactive "blaming, shaming, training" culture that singled out one individual as the cause of the error. Also historically, medication errors that did not result in patient harm—near-miss situations in which an error could have but didn't happen—or errors that did not result in serious harm were not reported. In contrast, serious errors often instigated a powerful punitive response in which one or a few persons were deemed to be at fault and, as a result, lost their jobs and sometimes their licenses.

In 1999, the Institute of Medicine (IOM) published *To Err Is Human: Building a Safer Health System*, which drew attention to the problem of medication errors. It pointed out that excellent health care providers do make medication errors, that many of the traditional processes involved in the medication use system were error-prone, and that other factors, notably drug labeling and packaging, contributed to error. Furthermore, the IOM report, in conjunction with other groups such as the United States Pharmacopeia (USP) and the Institute for Safe Medication Practices (ISMP), called for the redesign of error-prone systems to include processes that anticipated the fallibility of humans working within the system. This initiative is helping shift the way the health care industry addresses medication errors from a single person/bad apple cause to a systems issue.[1]

The National Coordinating Council for Medication Error Reporting and Prevention (NCC-MERP) developed the definition of a medication error that reflects this shift and captures the scope and breadth of the issue:

> "A medication error is any preventable event that may cause or lead to inappropriate medication use or patient harm while the medication is in the control of the health care professional, patient, or consumer. Such events may be related to professional practice, health care products, procedures, and systems, including prescribing; order communication; product labeling, packaging, and nomenclature; compounding; dispensing; distribution; administration; education; monitoring; and use."[2]

Inherent in this definition's mention of related factors are the human factors that are part of the medication use system. For example, a nurse or pharmacist may automatically reach into the bin where dobutamine is usually kept, see "do" and "amine" but select dopamine instead of dobutamine. Working amidst distractions, working long hours or shorthanded, and working in a culture where perfection is expected and questioning is discouraged are other examples of the human factors and environmental conditions that contribute to error.

The goal for the design of any individual or hospital-wide medication use system is to determine where systems are likely to fail and to build in safeguards that minimize the potential for error. One way to begin that process is to become familiar with medications or practices that have historically been shown to be involved in serious errors.

High Alert Medications

Some medications, because of a narrow therapeutic range or inherent toxic nature, have a high risk of causing devastating injury or death if improperly ordered, prepared, stocked, dispensed, administered, or monitored. Although these medications may not be involved in more errors, they require special attention due to the potential for serious, possibly fatal consequences. These have been termed **high-alert medications**, to communicate the need for extra care and safeguards. Many of these drugs are used commonly in the general population or are used frequently in urgent clinical situations. The Joint Commission (JC) monitors the use of frequently prescribed high-alert medications, which include insulin, opiates and narcotics, injectable potassium chloride (or phosphate) concentrate, intravenous anticoagulants (such as heparin), sodium chloride solutions above 0.9 percent, and others. See the High Alert Drugs table in the **Medication Safety Tools** color insert, and Table 2 in this article for a complete list of the high alert meds found in *Davis's Drug Guide for Nurses*. (Visit the Institute for Safe Medication Practices at www.ismp.org for more information on high alert drugs.)

Causes of Medication Errors

Many contributing factors and discrete causes of error have been identified, including failed communication, poor drug distribution practices, dose miscalculations, drug packaging and drug-device related problems, incorrect drug administration, and lack of patient education.[3]

Failed Communication: Failed communication covers many of the errors made in the ordering phase, and although ordering is performed by the prescriber, the nurse, the clerk, and the pharmacist who interpret that order are also involved in the communication process.

- ***Poorly handwritten or verbal orders.*** Handwriting is a major source of error and has led to inaccurate interpretations of the drug intended, the route of administration, the frequency, and dose. Telephone and verbal orders are likewise prone to misinterpretation.
- ***Drugs with similar-sounding or similar-looking names.*** Similar sounding names, or names that look similar when handwritten, are frequently confused. Amiodarone and amrinone (now renamed inamrinone to help prevent confusion), or Zebeta® and Diabeta® are two examples. The United States Pharmacopoeia (USP) has identified over 700 "sound-alike, look-alike" drugs. Mix-ups are more likely when each drug has similar dose ranges and frequencies.
  Several of the sound-alike/look-alike drugs were targeted for labeling intervention by the FDA, which requested manufacturers of 33 drugs with look-alike names to voluntarily revise the appearance of the established names. The revision visually differentiates the drug names by using "tall man" letters (capitals) to highlight distinguishing syllables (ex.: acetoHEXAMIDE versus acetaZOLAMIDE or buPROPrion versus busPIRone. See the TALL MAN Lettering table in the **Medication Safety Tools** color insert for the list of the pairs of drugs that are commonly confused, often with serious consequences.
- ***Misuse of zeroes in decimal numbers.*** Massive, ten-fold overdoses are traceable to not using a leading zero (.2 mg instead of 0.2 mg) or adding an unnecessary trailing zero (2.0 mg instead of 2 mg) in decimal expressions of dose. Similar overdosages are found in decimal expressions in which the decimal point is obscured by poor handwriting, stray marks, or lined orders sheets (e.g., reading 3.1 grams as 31 grams). Underdosing also may occur by the same mechanism and prevent a desired, perhaps life-saving effect.
- ***Use of apothecary measures (grains, drams) or package units (amps, vials, tablets) instead of metric measures (grams, milligrams, milliequivalents).*** Apothecary measurements are poorly understood and their abbreviations are easily confused with other units of measurement. Use of such measures should be abandoned. Errors also occur when dosage units are used instead of metric weight. For example, orders for 2 tablets, ½ vials, or 2 ampoules can result in overdose or underdose when the medications ordered come in various strengths.
- ***Misinterpreted abbreviations.*** Abbreviations can be misinterpreted or, when used in the dosage part of the order, can result in incorrect dosage of the correct medication. For example, lower or upper case "U" for units has been read as a zero, making 10 u of insulin look like 100 units when

handwritten. The Latin abbreviation "QOD" for every other day has been misinterpreted as QID (4 times per day). See Table 2 for a list of confusing abbreviations and safer alternatives.

- ***Ambiguous or incomplete orders.*** Orders that do not clearly specify dose, route, frequency, or indication do not communicate complete information and are open to misinterpretation.

Poor Distribution Practices: Poor distribution includes error-prone storing practices such as keeping similar looking products next to each other. Dispensing multidose floor stock vials of potentially dangerous drugs instead of unit doses is also associated with error as is allowing non-pharmacists to dispense medications in the absence of the pharmacist.

Dose Miscalculations: Dose miscalculations are a prime source of medication error. Also, many medications need to be dose-adjusted for renal or hepatic impairment, age, height and weight, and body composition (i.e., correct for obesity). Complicated dosing formulas provide many opportunities to introduce error. Often vulnerable populations, such as premature infants, children, the elderly, and those with serious underlying illnesses are at greatest risk.

Drug Packaging and Drug Delivery Systems: Similar packaging or poorly designed packaging encourages error. Drug companies may use the same design for different formulations, or fail to highlight information about concentration or strength. Lettering, type size, color, and packaging methods can either help or hinder drug identification.

Drug delivery systems include infusion pumps and rate controllers. Some models do not prevent free flow of medication, leading to sudden high dose infusion of potent and dangerous medications. The lack of safeguards preventing free flow and programming errors are among the problems encountered with infusion control devices.

Incorrect Drug Administration: Incorrect drug administration covers many problems. Misidentification of a patient, incorrect route of administration, missed doses, or improper drug preparation are types of errors that occur during the administration phase.

Lack of Patient Education: Safe medication use is enhanced in the hospital and the home when the patient is well informed. The knowledgeable patient can recognize when something has changed in his or her medication regimen and can question the health care provider. At the same time, many issues related to medication errors, such as ambiguous directions, unfamiliarity with a drug, and confusing packaging, affect the patient as well as the health care provider, underscoring the need for careful education. Patient education also enhances adherence, which is a factor in proper medication use.

Prevention Strategies

Since medication use systems are complex and involve many steps and people, they are error-prone. On an individual basis, nurses can help reduce the incidence of error by implementing the following strategies:

- Clarify any order that is not obviously and clearly legible. Ask the prescriber to print orders using block style letters.
- Do not accept orders with the abbreviation "u" or "IU" for units. Clarify the dosage and ask the prescriber to write out the word units.
- Clarify any abbreviated drug name or the abbreviated dosing frequencies q.d., QD, q.o.d., QOD, and q.i.d or QID. Suggest abandoning Latin abbreviations in favor of spelling out dosing frequency.
- Do not accept doses expressed in package units or volume instead of metric weight. Clarify any order written for number of ampoules, vials, or tablets (e.g., calcium, 1 ampoule or epinephrine, 1 Bristojet).
- Decimal point errors can be hard to see. Suspect a missed decimal point and clarify any order if the dose requires more than 3 dosing units.

- If dose ordered requires use of multiple dosage units or very small fractions of a dose unit, review the dose, have another health care provider check the original order and recalculate formulas and confirm the dose with the prescriber.
- If taking a verbal order, ask prescriber to spell out the drug name and dosage to avoid sound-alike confusion (e.g., hearing Cerebyx for Celebrex, or fifty for fifteen). Read back the order to the prescriber after you have written it in the chart. Confirm and document the indication to further enhance accurate communication.
- Clarify any order that does not include metric weight, dosing frequency, or route of administration.
- Check the nurse's/clerk's transcription against the original order. Make sure stray marks or initials do not obscure the original order.
- Do not start a patient on new medication by borrowing medications from another patient. This action bypasses the double check provided by the pharmacist's review of the order.
- Always check the patient's name band before administering medications. Verbally addressing a patient by name does not provide sufficient identification.
- Use the facility's standard drug administration times to reduce the chance of an omission error.
- Be sure to fully understand any drug administration device before using it. This includes infusion pumps, inhalers, and transdermal patches.
- Have a second practitioner independently check original order, dosage calculations, and infusion pump settings for high alert medications.
- Realize that the printing on packaging boxes, vials, ampoules, pre-filled syringes, or any container in which a medication is stored can be misleading. Be sure to differentiate clearly the medication and the number of milligrams per milliliter versus the total number of milligrams contained within. Massive overdoses have been administered by assuming that the number of milligrams per ml is all that is contained within the vial or ampoule. Read the label when obtaining the medication, before preparing or pouring the medication, and after preparing or pouring the medication.
- Educate patients about the medications they take. Provide verbal and written instruction and ask the patient to restate important points. Refer to Educating Patients about Safe Medication Use on page 21 for recommendations on what patients should understand about their medications.

As stated previously, errors are a result of problems within the medication use system and cannot be eliminated by the vigilance of any one group of health care providers. System redesign involves strong leadership from administration and all involved departments. Health care facilities should consider the following when addressing the issue of medication errors:

- Do not provide unit stock of critical, high alert medications. If eliminating these medications from floor stock is not feasible, consider reducing the number available and standardizing the concentrations or forms in which the medication is available.
- Create committees that address safety issues.
- Install a computer physician order entry (CPOE) system to help reduce prescribing orders. Link order entry to pertinent lab, allergy, and medication data.
- Implement bar code technology to ensure the right drug reaches the right patient.
- Develop policies that discourage error-prone prescribing practices such as inappropriate use of verbal orders, use of confusing dosing symbols, and use of abbreviations.
- Develop policies that encourage better communication of medication information such as requiring block-style printing of medications, including indication in prescription, and using both the trade and generic name in prescriptions.
- Ensure a reasonable workload for pharmacists and nurses, and provide a well-designed work area.
- Limit the availability of varying concentrations of high alert medications.
- Provide standard concentrations and infusion rate tables.
- Supply pharmacy and patient care areas with current reference material.
- Cultivate a culture that does not assign blame when medication errors occur but looks for root causes instead.

- Encourage staff to participate in the USP-ISMP-MERP error reporting program.

REFERENCES

1. Kohn, L.T., Corrigan, J.M., and Donaldson, M.S. (eds). *To Err Is Human: Building a Safer Health System*. National Academy Press, Washington, DC (1999).
2. National Coordinating Council for Medication Error Reporting and Prevention. http://www.nccmerp.org/aboutMedErrors.html
3. Cohen, M.R. *Medication Errors: Causes, Prevention, Risk Management*. Jones and Bartlett Publishers, Sudbury (1999).
4. Branowicki P., et al. "Improving complex medication systems: an interdisciplinary approach." *J Nurs Adm*. (2003) Apr; 33(4):199-200.
5. Burke K.G. "Executive summary: the state of the science on safe medication administration symposium." *J Infus Nurs*. (2005) Mar-Apr; 28(2 Suppl):4-9.
6. McPhillips H.A., et al. "Potential medication dosing errors in outpatient pediatrics." *J Pediatr*. (2005) Dec; 147(6):727-8.
7. ISMP. "What's in a name? Ways to prevent dispensing errors linked to name confusion." *ISMP Medication Safety Alert!* 7(12) June 12 (2002). http://www.ismp.org/Newsletters/acutecare/archives/Jun02.asp
8. Santell J.P., Cousins D.D. "Medication Errors Related to Product Names." *Joint Commission J Qual Pt Safety* (2005) 31:649-54.

Table 1: High Alert Medications in Davis's Drug Guide for Nurses

aldesleukin	DOXOrubicin hydrochloride	meperidine
alemtuzumab	DOXOrubicin hydrochloride liposome	methadone
altretamine	epinephrine	methotrexate
amiodarone	epirubicin	metoprolol
arsenic trioxide	eptifibatide	midazolam
asparaginase	esmolol	milrinone
bleomycin	etoposides	morphine
buprenorphine	fentanyl (oral, transmucosal)	nalbuphine
busulfan	fentanyl (parenteral)	nesiritide
butorphanol	fentanyl (transdermal)	oxycodone compound
calcium salts	fluorouracil	oxymorphone
capecitabine	fondaparinux	pancuronium
carboplatin	gemcitabine	pentazocine
carmustine	gemtuzumab ozogamicin	potassium phosphates
chloralhydrate	heparin	potassium supplements
chlorambucil	heparins (low molecular weight)	pramlintide
cisplatin	hydrocodone	propranolol
codeine	hydromorphone	sodium chloride
colchicine	hypoglycemic agents, oral	thrombolytic agents
cyclophosphamide	imatinib	tirofiban
cytarabine	insulin mixtures	topotecan
DAUNOrubicin citrate liposome	insulins (short-acting)	trastuzumab
DAUNOrubicin hydrochloride	insulins (intermediate-acting)	vinBLAStine
decitabine	insulins (long-acting)	vinCRIStine
digoxin	insulins (rapid-acting)	vinorelbine
DOBUTamine	labetalol	warfarin
docetaxel	lidocaine	
DOPamine	magnesium sulfate (IV, parenteral)	

Table 2: Abbreviations and Symbols Associated with Medication Errors

Abbreviation/Symbol	Intended Meaning	Mistaken For	Recommendation
AZT	Zidovudine	Azathioprine	Use full drug name
CPZ	Compazine	Thorazine (chlorpromazine)	Use full drug name
HCl	Hydrochloric acid	KCl (potassium chloride)	Use full drug name
HCT	Hydrocortisone	hydrochlorothiazide	Use full drug name
$MgSO_4$*	Magnesium sulfate	Morphine sulfate	Use full drug name
MS, MSO_4*	Morphine sulfate	Magnesium sulfate	Use full drug name
MTX	Methotrexate	Mitoxantrone	Use full drug name
Nitro drip	Nitroprusside	Nitroglycerin	Use full drug name
Norflox	Norfloxacin	Norflex	Use full drug name
PCA	Procainamide	Patient controlled analgesia	Use full drug name
PIT	Pitocin	Pitressin	Use full drug name
µg†	microgram	Mg (milligram)	Use mcg
/ (slash mark)	"per"	"1" (numeral one)	Spell out per
HS or hs†	Half strength or hour of sleep	One mistaken for the other	Spell out half strength or bedtime
+	Plus sign	"4" (numeral four)	Spell out and
Zero **after** a decimal point (e.g. 1.0 mg)*	1 mg	10 mg	DO NOT USE zero after a decimal point
No zero **before** a decimal point (e.g.,. 1 mg)*	.1 mg	1 mg	ALWAYS USE zero before a decimal point
u or U*	units	0 (zero), 4 (four) or cc	Spell out unit
I.U.*	International Units	IV or 10	Spell out unit
HS*	Half strength	Hour of sleep	Write out medication strength
q.d. or QD*	Every day	q.i.d. (4 times per day)	Write out daily
q.o.d. or QOD*	Every other day	q.i.d. (4 times per day) or qd (daily)	Write out every other day
SC, SQ, sub q†	subcutaneously	SC mistaken as SL (sublingual), SQ as "5 every" or "every"	Use subcut or write out subcutaneously
AD, AS, AU†	Right ear, left ear, each ear	OD, OS, OU (right eye, left eye, each eye)	Spell out right ear, left ear, each ear
OD, OS, OU	Right eye, left eye, each eye	AD, AS, AU (right ear, left ear, each ear)	Spell out right eye, left eye, each eye
Cc†	cubic centimeters	u (units)	Use ml
@	At	2	Use at
&	And	2	Use and
+	Plus or and	4	Use and
°	hour	Zero (q 1° seen as q 10)	Use hr, h, or hour
Drug name and dose run together. Example: Inderal40 mg	Inderal 40 mg	Inderal 140 mg	Leave space between drug name, dose, and unit of measure
Numerical dose and unit of measure run together. Example: 10mg	10 mg	100 mg	Leave space between drug dose and unit of measure

*Appears on JCAHO's "Do Not Use" list of abbreviations.

†Appears on JCAHO's list of abbreviations not recommended for use.

Modified from The Institute for Safe Medication Practices Safety Alert, Vol 8: Issue 24. Nov 27, 2003.

DETECTING AND MANAGING ADVERSE DRUG REACTIONS

An *adverse drug reaction* (ADR) is any unexpected, undesired, or excessive response to a medication that results in:

- temporary or permanent serious harm or disability
- admission to a hospital, transfer to a higher level of care, or prolonged stay
- death.

Adverse drug reactions are distinguished from adverse drug events, in which causality is uncertain, and side effects, which may be bothersome to the patient and necessitate a change in therapy but are not considered serious.[1] Although some ADRs are the result of medications errors, many are not.

Types of ADRs

The Food and Drug Administration (FDA) classifies ADRs into 2 broad categories: Type A and Type B.[2] Type A reactions are predictable reactions based on the primary or secondary pharmacologic effect of the drug. Dose-related reactions and drug-drug interactions are examples of Type A reactions. Type B reactions are unpredictable, are not related to dose, and are not the result of the drug's primary or secondary pharmacologic effect. Idiosyncratic and hypersensitivity reactions are examples of Type B reactions.

Dose-Related Reactions (Toxic Reactions): In dose related reactions, the dose prescribed for the patient is excessive. Although a variety of mechanisms may interact, reasons for this type of reaction include:

- renal or hepatic impairment
- extremes in age (neonates and frail elderly)
- drug-drug or drug-food interactions
- underlying illness. Dose-related reactions are often the result of preventable errors in prescribing in which physiologic factors such as age, renal impairment, and weight were not considered sufficiently, or in inadequate therapeutic monitoring. Medications with narrow therapeutic ranges (digoxin, aminoglycosides, antiepileptic drugs) and those that require careful monitoring or laboratory testing (anticoagulants, nephrotoxic drugs) are most frequently implicated in dose-related reactions.[3,4] Dose-related reactions usually are managed successfully by temporarily discontinuing the drug and then reducing the dose or increasing the dosing interval. In some instances, the toxic effects need to be treated with another agent (e.g. Digibind for digoxin toxicity or Kayexalate for drug induced hyperkalemia). Appropriately timed therapeutic drug level monitoring, review of new drugs added to an existing regimen that may affect the drug level, and frequent assessment of relevant laboratory values are critical to safe medical management and prevention of dose-related reactions.

Drug-Drug Interactions: Drug-drug interactions occur when the pharmacokinetic or pharmacodynamic properties of an individual drug affect another drug. Pharmacokinetics refers to the way the body processes a medication (absorption, distribution, metabolism, and elimination). In a drug-drug interaction, the pharmacokinetic properties of one drug can cause a change in drug concentration of another drug and an altered response. For example, one drug may block enzymes that metabolize a second drug. The concentration of the second drug is then increased and may become toxic or cause adverse reactions. Pharmacodynamic drug-drug interactions involve the known effects and side-effects of the drugs. For example, two drugs with similar therapeutic effects may act together in a synergistic way. The increased anticoagulant effects that occur when warfarin and aspirin are taken together, or the increased CNS depression that results when two drugs with CNS depressant effects potentiate each other, are examples of pharmacodymanic drug-drug interactions. Certain classes of drugs are more likely to result in serious drug-drug interactions and patients receiving these agents should be monitored carefully. The medication classes include anticoagulants, oral hypoglycemic agents, nonsteroidal anti-inflammatory agents, MAO inhibitors, antihypertensives, antiepileptics, and antiretrovirals. In addition, specific drugs such as theophylline, cimetidine, lithium, and digoxin may result in serious ADRs.

Idiosyncratic Reactions: Idiosyncratic reactions occur without relation to dose and are unpredictable and sporadic. Reactions of this type may manifest in many different ways, including fever, blood dyscrasias, cardiovascular effects, or mental status changes. The time frame between the occurrence of a problem and initiation of therapy is sometimes the only clue linking drug to symptom. Some idiosyncratic reactions may be explained by genetic differences in drug-metabolizing enzymes.

Hypersensitivity Reactions: Hypersensitivity reactions are usually allergic responses. Manifestations of hypersensitivity reactions range from mild rashes, to nephritis, pneumonitis, hemolytic anemia, and anaphylaxis. Protein drugs (vaccines, enzymes) are frequently associated with hypersensitivity reactions. In most instances, antibody formation is involved in the process and therefore cross-sensitivity may occur. An example of this is hypersensitivity to penicillin and cross-sensitivity with other penicillins and/or cephalosporins. Documenting drugs to which the patient is allergic and the specific hypersensitivity reaction is very important. If the reaction to an agent is anaphylaxis the nurse should monitor the patient during administration of a cross-hypersensitive agent, especially during the initial dose, and ensure ready access to emergency resuscitative equipment.

Recognizing an ADR

Adverse drug reactions should be suspected whenever there is a negative change in a patient's condition, particularly when a new drug has been introduced. Strategies that can enhance recognition include knowing the side effect/adverse reaction profile of medications. Nurses should be familiar with a drug's most commonly encountered side effects and adverse reactions before administering it. (In *Davis's Drug Guide for Nurses*, side effects are underlined, and adverse reactions are CAPITALIZED and appear in second color in the **Adverse Reactions and Side Effects** section.) As always, monitoring the patient's response to a medication and ongoing assessment are key nursing actions. Learn to recognize patient findings that suggest an ADR has occurred. These include:

- rash
- change in respiratory rate, heart rate, blood pressure or mental state
- seizure
- anaphylaxis
- diarrhea
- fever.

Any of these findings can suggest an ADR and should be reported and documented promptly so that appropriate interventions, including discontinuation of suspect medications, can occur. Prompt intervention can prevent a mild adverse reaction from escalating into a serious health problem. Other steps taken by the health care team when identifying and treating an ADR include:

1. Determining that the drug ordered was the drug given and intended.
2. Determining that the drug was given in the correct dosage by the correct route.
3. Establishing the chronology of events: time drug was taken and onset of symptoms.
4. Stopping the drug and monitoring patient status for improvement (dechallenge).
5. Restarting the drug, if appropriate, and monitoring closely for adverse reactions (rechallenge).[2]

Prevention

Healthcare organizations have responded to consumer, regulator and insurer pressures by developing programs that aim to eliminate preventable ADRs. In the inpatient setting, computer systems can display the patient's age, height, weight, and creatinine clearance or serum creatinine level and send an alert to the clinician if a prescribed dose is out of range for any of the displayed parameters. Allergy alerts and drug-drug interactions can be presented to the clinician at the time an order is entered.

In the outpatient setting, strategies that increase the patient's knowledge base and access to pharmacists and nurses may help prevent adverse reactions.[5] Outpatient pharmacy computer systems that are linked within a chain of pharmacies may allow the pharmacist to view the patient's profile if the patient is filling a prescription in a pharmacy other than the usual one. Many pharmacy computers have dose limits and drug-drug reaction verfication to assist pharmacists filling orders.

Such strategies are a valuable auxiliary to, but cannot replace, conscientious history taking, careful patient assessment, and ongoing monitoring. A thorough medication history including all prescription and non-prescription drugs, all side effects and adverse reactions encountered, allergies, and all pertinent physical data should be available to the prescriber. The prescriber is responsible for reviewing this data, along with current medications, laboratory values, and any other variable that affects drug response.

It is not expected that practitioners will remember all relevant information when prescribing. In fact, reliance on memory is error-fraught and clinicians need to use available resources to verify drug interactions whenever adding a new drug to the regimen. Setting expectations that clinicians use evidence-based information rather than their memories when prescribing, dispensing, administering or monitoring patients has the potential to reduce the incidence of preventable ADRs.

Food and Drug Administration MedWatch Program

To monitor and assess the incidence of adverse reactions, the Food and Drug Administration (FDA) sponsors MedWatch, a program that allows health care practitioners and consumers the opportunity to report serious adverse reactions or product defects encountered from medications, medical devices, special nutritional products, or other FDA-regulated items. The FDA considers serious those reactions that result in death, life-threatening illness or injury, hospitalization, disability, congenital anomaly, or those that require medical/surgical intervention.

In addition to reporting serious adverse reactions, health care providers should also report problems related to suspected contamination, questionable stability, defective components, or poor packaging/labeling. Reports should be submitted even if there is some uncertainty about the cause/effect relationship or if some details are missing. This reporting form may be accessed at www.fda.gov/medwatch/report/hcp.htm. Reports also may be faxed to the FDA (1-800-FDA-0178). Reactions to vaccines should be reported to the Vaccine Adverse Event Reporting System (VAERS; 1-800-822-7967). Nurses share with other health care providers an obligation to report adverse reactions to the MedWatch program so that all significant data can be analyzed for opportunities to improve patient care.

REFERENCES

1. Lehmann, J. (2002-2003). "Adverse Events - Adverse Reactions." *Drug Intel* http://www.drugintel.com/public/medwatch/adverse_drug_events.htm (accessed 10 July 2003).
2. Goldman, S., Kennedy, D., Lieberman, R., (1995). "Clinical Therapeutics and the Recognition of Drug-Induced Disease." FDA MEDWATCH Continuing Education Article http://www.fda.gov/medwatch/articles/dig/rcontent.htm#toc (accessed 10 July 2003).
3. Daniels, C., Calis, K., (2001). "Clinical Analysis of Adverse Drug Reactions." Pharmacy Update National Institutes of Health. Sept-Oct http://www.cc.nih.gov/phar/updates/septoct01/01sept-oct.html (accessed 10 July 2003).

4. Winterstein, A., et. al. (2002). "Identifying Clinically Significant Preventable Adverse Drug Events Through a Hospital's Database of Adverse Drug Reaction Reports." *Am J Health-Syst Pharm.* 59(18):1742-1749.
5. Ghandi, T., Weingart, S., Borus J., et. al. (2003). "Adverse Drug Events in Ambulatory Care." *New England Journal of Medicine.* Volume 348:1556-1564. Number 16. April 17.
6. Bennett, C.L, et al. (2005). "The Research on Adverse Drug Events and Reports (RADAR) project." *JAMA.* May 4;293(17):2131-40.
7. Field, T.S., et al. (2005). "The costs associated with adverse drug events among older adults in the ambulatory setting." *Med Care.* Dec;43(12):1171-6.
8. Petrone, K, Katz P. (2005). "Approaches to appropriate drug prescribing for the older adult." *Prim Care.* Sep;32(3):755-75.
9. Pezalla, E. (2005). "Preventing adverse drug reactions in the general population." *Manag Care Interface.* Oct;18(10):49-52.

SPECIAL DOSING CONSIDERATIONS

For many patients the average dose range for a given drug can be toxic. The purpose of this section is to describe vulnerable patient populations for which special dosing considerations must be made to protect the patient and improve clinical outcomes.

The Pediatric Patient

Most drugs prescribed to children are not approved by the FDA for use in pediatric populations. This does not mean it's wrong to prescribe these drugs to children, rather it means that the medications were not tested in children. The lack of pediatric drug information can result in patient harm or death, such as what occurred with the drug chloramphenicol. When given to very young children, chloramphenicol caused toxicity and multiple deaths. Referred to as "gray syndrome," this toxic reaction was eventually found to be dose dependent. The FDA now requires that new drugs that may be used in children include information for safe pediatric use. For this edition of *Davis's Drug Guide for Nurses*, we have had the pediatric dosing for the top 100 drugs used in children revised and updated by a pediatric doctor of pharmacology.

The main reason for adjusting dosages in pediatric patients is body size, which is measured by body weight or body surface area (BSA). Weight-based pediatric drug dosages are expressed in number of milligrams per kilogram of body weight (mg/kg) while dosages calculated on body surface area are expressed in number of milligrams per meter squared (mg/m^2). BSA is determined using a BSA nomogram (Appendix F) or calculated by using formulas (Appendix E).

The neonate and the premature infant require additional adjustments secondary to immature function of body systems. For example, absorption may be incomplete or altered secondary to differences in gastric pH or motility. Distribution may be altered because of varying amounts of total body water, and metabolism and excretion can be delayed due to immature liver and kidney function. Furthermore, rapid weight changes and progressive maturation of hepatic and renal function require frequent monitoring and careful dosage adjustments. Gestational age, as well as weight, may be needed to properly dose some drugs in the neonate.

The Geriatric Patient

Absorption, distribution, metabolism and excretion are altered in adults over 55 years of age, putting the older patient at risk for toxic reactions. Pharmacokinetic properties in the older patient are affected by

- percentage of body fat, lean muscle mass, and total body water
- decreased plasma proteins, especially in the malnourished patient, which allows a larger proportion of free or unbound drug to circulate and exert effects
- diminished GI motility and blood flow, which delays absorption
- slower hepatic and renal function, which delays excretion.

All of these variables change with age, however, and not predictably. Older patients should be prescribed the lowest possible effective dose at the initiation of therapy followed by careful titration of doses as needed. Just as importantly, they should be monitored very carefully for signs and symptoms of adverse drug reactions.

Another concern is that many elderly patients are prescribed multiple drugs. As the number of medications a patient takes increases, so does the risk for an adverse drug reaction. One drug may negate, potentiate, or otherwise alter the effects of another drug (drug-drug interaction). This situation is compounded by concurrent use of nonprescription drugs and natural products. In general, doses of most medications (especially digoxin, sedative/hypnotics, anticoagulants, thrombolytics, nonsteroidal anti-inflammatory agents, and antihypertensives) should be decreased in the geriatric population. The Beers List/Criteria, which appears in the *Medication Safety Tools section*, is a list of drugs to be used with caution in the elderly, and is based on these concerns.

The Patient of Reproductive Age

Generally, pregnant women should avoid medications, except when absolutely necessary. Both the mother and the fetus must be considered. The placenta protects the fetus only from extremely large molecules. The fetus is particularly vulnerable during the first and the last trimesters of pregnancy. During the first trimester, vital organs are forming and ingestion of teratogenic drugs may lead to fetal malformation or miscarriage. Unfortunately, this is the time when a woman is least likely to know that she is pregnant. In the third trimester, drugs administered to the mother and transferred to the fetus may not be safely metabolized and excreted by the fetus. This is especially true of drugs administered near term. After the infant is delivered, he or she no longer has the placenta to help with drug excretion, and drugs administered before delivery may result in toxicity.

Of course, many conditions, such as asthma, diabetes, gastrointestinal disorders, and mental illness affect pregnant women and require long-term medication use. When the medications are used, whether over the counter or prescription, prescribing the lowest effective dose for the shortest period of time necessary is the rule.

The possibility of a medication altering sperm quality and quantity in a potential father also is an area of concern. Male patients should be informed of this risk when taking any medications known to have this potential.

Renal Disease

The kidneys are the major organ of drug elimination. Failure to account for decreased renal function is a preventable source of adverse drug reactions. Renal function is measured by the creatinine clearance (CCr), which can be approximated in the absence of a 24-hour urine collection (Appendix E). In addition, dosages in the renally impaired patient can be optimized by measuring medication blood levels.

Patients with underlying renal disease, premature infants with immature renal function, and elderly patients with age-related decrease in renal function require careful dose adjustments. Renal function may fluctuate over time and should be re-assessed periodically.

Liver Disease

The liver is the major organ of drug metabolism. It changes a drug from a relatively fat-soluble compound to a more water-soluble substance, which means that the drug can then be excreted by the kidneys. Liver function is not as easily quantified as renal function, and it therefore is difficult to predict the correct dosage for a patient with liver dysfunction based on laboratory tests.

A patient who is severely jaundiced or who has very low serum proteins (particularly albumin) can be expected to have some problems metabolizing drugs. In advanced liver disease, portal vascular congestion also impairs drug absorption. Examples of drugs that should be carefully dosed in patients with liver disease include theophylline, diuretics, phenytoin, and sedatives. Some drugs require the liver for activation (such as sulindac or cyclophosphamide) and should be avoided in patients with severely compromised liver function.

Heart Failure

Heart failure results in passive congestion of blood vessels in the GI tract, which impairs drug absorption. Heart failure also slows drug delivery to the liver, delaying metabolism. Renal function is frequently compromised as well, adding to delayed elimination and prolonged drug action. Dosages of drugs metabolized mainly by the liver or excreted mainly by the kidneys should be decreased in patients with congestive heart failure.

Body Size

Drug dosing is often based on total body weight. However, some drugs selectively penetrate fatty tissues. If the drug does not penetrate fatty tissues (e.g., digoxin, gentamicin), dosages for the obese patient should be determined by ideal body weight or estimated lean body mass. Ideal body weight may be determined from tables of desirable weights or may be estimated using formulas for lean body mass when the patient's height and weight are known (Appendix E). If such adjustments are not made considerable toxicity can result.

Body size is also a factor in patients who are grossly underweight. Elderly patients, chronic alcoholics, patients with AIDS, and patients who are terminally ill from cancer or other debilitating illnesses need careful attention to dosing. Patients who have had a limb amputated also need to have this change in body size taken into account.

Drug Interactions

Use of multiple drugs, especially those known to interact with other drugs, may necessitate dosage adjustments. Drugs highly bound to plasma proteins, such as warfarin and phenytoin, may be displaced by other highly protein-bound drugs. When this phenomenon occurs, the drug that has been displaced exhibits an increase in its activity because the free or unbound drug is active.

Some drugs decrease the liver's ability to metabolize other drugs. Drugs capable of doing this include cimetidine and chloramphenicol. Concurrently administered drugs that are both highly metabolized by the liver may need to be administered in decreased dosages. Other agents such as phenobarbital, other barbiturates, and rifampin are capable of stimulating the liver to metabolize drugs more rapidly, requiring larger doses to be administered.

Drugs that significantly alter urine pH can affect excretion of drugs for which the excretory process is pH dependent. Alkalinizing the urine will hasten the excretion of acidic drugs. Acidification of the urine will enhance reabsorption of acidic drugs, prolonging and enhancing drug action. In the reverse situation, drugs that acidify the urine will hasten the excretion of alkaline drugs. An example of this is administering sodium bicarbonate in cases of aspirin overdose. Alkalinizing the urine promotes renal excretion of aspirin.

Some drugs compete for enzyme systems with other drugs. Allopurinol inhibits the enzyme involved in uric acid production, but it also inhibits metabolism (inactivation) of 6-mercaptopurine, greatly increasing its toxicity. The dosage of mercaptopurine needs to be significantly reduced when coadministered with allopurinol.

The same potential for interactions exists for some foods. Dietary calcium, found in high concentrations in dairy products, combines with tetracycline and prevents its absorption. Foods high in pyridoxine (vitamin B_6) can negate the anti-Parkinson effect of levodopa. Grapefruit juice inhibits the enzyme that breaks down some drugs, and concurrent ingestion may significantly increase drug levels and the risk for toxicity. There are no general guidelines for nutritional factors. It is prudent to check whether these problems exist and to make the necessary dosage adjustments.

Many commonly taken natural products interact with pharmaceutical drugs. St. John's wort, garlic, ephedra, and other natural products can interact with medications and cause known or unpredictable reactions.

Nurses and prescribers should consult drug references and remember that the average dosing range for drugs is intended for an average patient. However, every patient is an individual with specific drug-handling capabilities. Taking these special dosing considerations into account allows for an individualized drug regimen that promotes the desired therapeutic outcome and minimizes the risk of toxicity.

EDUCATING PATIENTS ABOUT SAFE MEDICATION USE

Research has shown that patients need information about several medication-related topics, no matter what the medication. A well-informed patient and/or family can help prevent medication errors by hospital staff and is less likely to make medication errors at home. Adherence to the medication regimen is another goal achieved through patient education.

Before beginning any teaching, however, always assess the patient's current knowledge by asking if he or she is familiar with the medication, how it is taken at home, what precautions or follow-up care is required, and other questions specific to each drug. Based on the patient's current knowledge level and taking into consideration factors such as readiness to learn, environmental and social barriers to learning or adherence, and cultural factors, discuss the following:

1. **Generic and brand names of the medication.** Patients should know both the brand and generic names of each medication for two reasons. It helps them identify their medications when a generic equivalent is substituted for a brand name version and it prevents patients or health care providers from making sound-alike confusion errors when giving or documenting a medication history. An example of this is saying Celebrex but meaning or hearing Cerebyx.

2. **Purpose of the medication.** Patients have a right to know what the therapeutic benefit of the medication will be but also should be told the consequences of not taking the prescribed medication. This may enhance adherence. For example, a patient may be more likely to take blood pressure medication if told lowering high blood pressure will prevent heart attack, kidney disease, or stroke, rather than saying only that it will lower blood pressure.

3. **Dosage and how to take the medication.** To derive benefit and avoid adverse reactions or other poor outcomes, the patient must know how much of the medication to take and when to take it. Refer to dosages in metric weight (i.e., milligram, gram) rather than dosage unit (tablet) or volume (1 teaspoon). The patient must also be informed of the best time to take the medication, for example, on an empty or a full stomach, before bedtime, or with or without other medications. If possible, help the patient fit the medication schedule into his or her own schedule, so that taking the medication is not difficult or forgotten.

4. **What to do if a dose is missed.** Always explain to patients what to do if a dose is missed. Patients have been reported to take a double dose of medications when a missed dose occurs, putting themselves at risk for side effects and adverse reactions.

5. **Duration of therapy.** It is not uncommon for patients to stop taking a medication when they feel better or to discontinue a medication when they cannot perceive a benefit. For very long term, even lifelong therapy, the patient may need to be reminded that the medication helps maintain the current level of wellness. Patients may need to be reminded to finish short-term courses of medications even though they frequently will feel much better before the prescription runs out. Some medications cannot be discontinued abruptly and patients should be warned to consult a health care professional before discontinuing such agents. Patients will need to know to refill prescriptions several days before running out or to take extra medication if traveling.

6. **Minor side effects and what to do if they occur.** Inform the patient that all medications have potential side effects. Explain the most common side effects associated with the medication and how to avoid or manage them if they occur. An informed patient is less likely to stop taking a medication because of a minor and potentially avoidable side effect.

7. **Serious side effects and what to do if they occur.** Inform the patient of the possibility of serious side effects. Describe signs and symptoms associated with serious side effects, and tell the patient to immediately inform a physician or nurse should they occur. Tell the patient to call before the next dose of the medication is scheduled and to not assume that the medication is the source of the symptom and prematurely discontinue it.

8. **Medications to avoid.** Drug-drug interactions can dampen drug effects, enhance drug effects, or cause life-threatening adverse events such as cardiac dysrhythmias, hepatitis, renal failure, or internal bleeding. The patient and family need to know which other medications, including which over-the-counter medications, to avoid.

9. **Foods to avoid and other precautions.** Food-drug interactions are not uncommon and can have effects similar to drug-drug interactions. Excessive sun exposure resulting in severe dermal reactions is not uncommon and represents an environmental-drug interaction. Likewise, the patient should be informed of what activities to avoid, in case the medication affects alertness or coordination, for example.

10. **How to store the medication:** Medications must be stored properly to maintain potency. Most medications should not be stored in the bathroom medicine cabinet because of excess heat and humidity. In addition, thoughtful storage practices, such as separating two family members' medications, can prevent mix-ups and inadvertent accessibility by children (or pets). Review storage with patients and ask about current methods for storing medications.

11. **Follow-up care.** Anyone taking medication requires ongoing care to assess effectiveness and appropriateness of medications. Many medications require invasive and noninvasive testing to monitor blood levels; hematopoietic, hepatic, or renal function; or other effects on other body systems. Ongoing medical evaluation may result in dosage adjustments, change in medication, or discontinuation of medication.

12. **What not to take.** Inform patients not to take expired medications or someone else's medication. Warn them not to self-medicate with older, no-longer-used prescriptions even if the remaining supply is not expired. Tell patients to keep a current record of all medications taken and to ask health care providers if new medications are meant to replace a current medication.

As you teach, encourage the patient and the family to ask questions. Providing feedback about medication questions will increase their understanding and help you identify areas that need reinforcement. Also, ask patients to repeat what you have said and return to demonstrate application or administration techniques.

Stress the importance of concurrent therapies. Medications often are only a part of a recommended therapy. Review with the patient and family other measures that will enhance or maintain health. Always consider the cultural context in which health information is provided and plan accordingly. This might include obtaining a same-gender translator or adjusting dosing times to avoid conflict with traditional rituals.

Finally, provide written instructions in a simple and easy-to-read format. Keep in mind that most health care information is written at a 10th grade reading level, while many patients read at a 5th grade level. Tell patients to keep the written instructions, so that they can be reviewed at home, when stress levels are lower and practical difficulties in maintaining the medication plan are known.

• ANTI-ALZHEIMER'S AGENTS

PHARMACOLOGIC PROFILE

General Use
Management of Alzheimer's dementia.

General Action and Information
All agents act by increasing the amount of acetylcholine in the CNS by inhibiting cholinesterase. No agents to date can slow the progression of Alzheimer's dementia. Current agents may temporarily improve cognitive function and therefore improve quality of life.

Contraindications
Hypersensitivity. Tacrine should not be used in patients who have had previous hepatic reactions to the drug.

Precautions
Use cautiously in patients with a history of "sick sinus syndrome" or other supraventricular cardiac conduction abnormalities (may cause bradycardia). Cholingeric effects may result in adverse GI effects (nausea, vomiting, diarrhea, weight loss) and may also increase gastric acid secretion resulting in GI bleeding, especially during concurrent NSAID therapy. Other cholinergic effects may include urinary tract obstruction, seizures, or bronchospasm.

Interactions
Additive effects with other drugs having cholinergic properties. May exaggerate the effects of succinylcholine-type muscle relaxation during anesthesia. May decrease therapeutic effects of anticholinergics.

NURSING IMPLICATIONS

Assessment
- Assess cognitive function (memory, attention, reasoning, language, ability to perform simple tasks) throughout therapy.
- Monitor nausea, vomiting, anorexia, and weight loss. Notify health care professional if these side effects occur.

Potential Nursing Diagnoses
- Disturbed thought process (Indications).
- Imbalanced nutrition: less than body requirements.
- Deficient knowledge, related to disease processes and medication regimen (Patient/Family Teaching).

Patient/Family Teaching
- Instruct patient and caregiver that medication should be taken as directed.
- Advise patient and caregiver to notify health care professional if nausea, vomiting, anorexia, and weight loss occur.

Evaluation/Desired Outcomes
- Temporary improvement in cognitive function (memory, attention, reasoning, language, ability to perform simple tasks) in patients with Alzheimer's disease.

Anti-Alzheimer's agents included in *Davis's Drug Guide for Nurses*

donepezil 447
galantamine 592
memantine 783
rivastigmine 1077
tacrine 1133

• ANTIANEMICS

PHARMACOLOGIC PROFILE

General Use

Prevention and treatment of anemias.

General Action and Information

Iron (ferrous fumarate, ferrous gluconate, ferrous sulfate, iron dextran, iron sucrose, polysaccharide-iron complex, sodium ferric gluconate complex) is required for production of hemoglobin, which is necessary for oxygen transport to cells. Cyanocobalamin and hydroxocobalamin (Vitamin B_{12}) and folic acid are water-soluble vitamins that are required for red blood cell production. Darbepoetin and epoetin stimulate production of red blood cells. Nandrolone stimulates production of erythropoetin.

Contraindications

Undiagnosed anemias. Hemochromatosis, hemosiderosis, hemolytic anemia (Iron). Uncontrolled hypertension (darbepoetin, epoetin).

Precautions

Use parenteral iron (iron dextran, iron sucrose, sodium ferric gluconate complex) cautiously in patients with a history of allergy or hypersensitivity reactions.

Interactions

Oral iron can decrease the absorption of tetracyclines, fluoroquinolones, or penicillamine. Vitamin E may impair the therapeutic response to iron. Phenytoin and other anticonvulsants may decrease the absorption of folic acid. Response to Vitamin B_{12} or folic acid may be delayed by chloramphenicol. Darbepoetin and epoetin may increase the requirement for heparin during hemodialysis.

NURSING IMPLICATIONS

Assessment

- Assess patient's nutritional status and dietary history to determine possible causes for anemia and need for patient teaching.

Potential Nursing Diagnoses

- Activity intolerance (Indications).
- Imbalanced nutrition: less than body requirements (Indications).
- Deficient knowledge, related to disease processes and medication regimen (Patient/Family Teaching).

Implementation

- Available in combination with many vitamins and minerals (see Appendix B)

Patient/Family Teaching

- Encourage patients to comply with diet recommendations of health care professional. Explain that the best source of vitamins and minerals is a well-balanced diet with foods from the four basic food groups.

- Patients self-medicating with vitamin and mineral supplements should be cautioned not to exceed RDA. The effectiveness of mega doses for treatment of various medical conditions is unproven and may cause side effects.

Evaluation/Desired Outcomes

- Resolution of anemia.

Antianemics included in *Davis's Drug Guide for Nurses*

hormones
darbepoetin 377
epoetin 487
methoxypolyethylene glycol-epoetin beta 1322
nandrolone decanoate 25

iron supplements
carbonyl iron 700
ferrous fumarate 700
ferrous gluconate 700
ferrous sulfate 700
iron dextran 700
iron polysaccharide 701
iron sucrose 701
sodium ferric gluconate complex 701

vitamins
cyanocobalamin 1233
folic acid 574
hydroxocobalamin 1233

• ANTIANGINALS

PHARMACOLOGIC PROFILE

General Use

Nitrates are used to treat and prevent attacks of angina. Only nitrates (sublingual, lingual spray, or intravenous) may be used in the acute treatment of attacks of angina pectoris. Calcium channel blockers and beta blockers are used prophylactically in long-term management of angina.

General Action and Information

Several different groups of medications are used in the treatment of angina pectoris. The nitrates (isosorbide dinitrate, isosorbide mononitrate, and nitroglycerin) are available as a lingual spray, sublingual tablets, parenterals, transdermal systems, and sustained-release oral dosage forms. Nitrates dilate coronary arteries and cause systemic vasodilation (decreased preload). Calcium channel blockers dilate coronary arteries (some also slow heart rate). Beta blockers decrease myocardial oxygen consumption via a decrease in heart rate. Therapy may be combined if selection is designed to minimize side effects or adverse reactions.

Contraindications

Hypersensitivity. Avoid use of beta blockers or calcium channel blockers in advanced heart block, cardiogenic shock, or untreated CHF.

Precautions

Beta blockers should be used cautiously in patients with diabetes mellitus, pulmonary disease, or hypothyroidism.

Interactions

Nitrates, calcium channel blockers, and beta blockers may cause hypotension with other antihypertensives or acute ingestion of alcohol. Verapamil, diltiazem, and beta blockers may have additive myocardial depressant effects when used with other agents that affect cardiac function. Verapamil has a number of other significant drug-drug interactions.

NURSING IMPLICATIONS

Assessment

- Assess location, duration, intensity, and precipitating factors of patient's anginal pain.
- Monitor blood pressure and pulse periodically throughout therapy.

Potential Nursing Diagnoses

- Acute pain (Indications).
- Ineffective tissue perfusion (Indications).
- Deficient knowledge, related to disease processes and medication regimen (Patient/Family Teaching).

Implementation

- Available in various dose forms. See specific drugs for information on administration.

Patient/Family Teaching

- Instruct patient on concurrent nitrate therapy and prophylactic antianginals to continue taking both medications as ordered and to use SL nitroglycerin as needed for anginal attacks.
- Advise patient to contact health care professional immediately if chest pain does not improve; worsens after therapy; is accompanied by diaphoresis or shortness of breath; or if severe, persistent headache occurs.
- Caution patient to make position changes slowly to minimize orthostatic hypotension.
- Advise patient to avoid concurrent use of alcohol with these medications.

Evaluation/Desired Outcomes

- Decrease in frequency and severity of anginal attacks.
- Increase in activity tolerance.

Antianginals included in *Davis's Drug Guide for Nurses*

beta blockers
atenolol 197
carteolol 1273
labetalol 719
metoprolol 814
nadolol 856
propranolol 1026, 1327
calcium channel blockers
diltiazem 418
felodipine 530
isradipine 708
niCARdipine 879
NIFEdipine 884
verapamil 1224
nitrates
isosorbide dinitrate 707
isosorbide mononitrate 707
nitroglycerin 892
miscellaneous
ranolazine 1054

• ANTIANXIETY AGENTS

PHARMACOLOGIC PROFILE

General Use

Antianxiety agents are used in the management of various forms of anxiety, including generalized anxiety disorder (GAD). Some agents are more suitable for intermittent or short-term use (benzodiazepines) while others are more useful long-term (buspirone, doxepin, fluoxetine, paroxetine, sertraline, venlafaxine).

General Action and Information

Most agents cause generalized CNS depression. Benzodiazepines may produce tolerance with long-term use and have potential for psychological or physical dependence. These agents have NO analgesic properties.

Contraindications
Hypersensitivity. Should not be used in comatose patients or in those with pre-existing CNS depression. Should not be used in patients with uncontrolled severe pain. Avoid use during pregnancy or lactation.

Precautions
Use cautiously in patients with hepatic dysfunction, severe renal impairment, or severe underlying pulmonary disease (benzodiazepines only). Use with caution in patients who may be suicidal or who may have had previous drug addictions. Patients may be more sensitive to CNS depressant effects; dosage reduction may be required.

Interactions
Mainly for benzodiazepines; additive CNS depression with alcohol, antihistamines, some antidepressants, opioid analgesics, or phenothiazines may occur. Most agents should not be used with MAO inhibitors.

NURSING IMPLICATIONS

Assessment
- Monitor blood pressure, pulse, and respiratory status frequently throughout IV administration.
- Prolonged high-dose therapy may lead to psychological or physical dependence. Restrict the amount of drug available to patient, especially if patient is depressed, suicidal, or has a history of addiction.
- **Anxiety:** Assess degree of anxiety and level of sedation (ataxia, dizziness, slurred speech) before and periodically throughout therapy.

Potential Nursing Diagnoses
- Risk for injury (Side Effects).
- Deficient knowledge, related to disease processes and medication regimen (Patient/Family Teaching).

Implementation
- Patients changing to buspirone from other antianxiety agents should receive gradually decreasing doses. Buspirone will not prevent withdrawal symptoms.

Patient/Family Teaching
- May cause daytime drowsiness. Caution patient to avoid driving and other activities requiring alertness until response to medication is known.
- Advise patient to avoid the use of alcohol and other CNS depressants concurrently with these medications.
- Advise patient to inform health care professional if pregnancy is planned or suspected.

Evaluation/Desired Outcomes
- Decrease in anxiety level.

Antianxiety agents included in *Davis's Drug Guide for Nurses*

benzodiazepines
alprazolam 131
chlordiazepoxide 298
diazepam 404
lorazepam 762
midazolam 822
oxazepam 921

selective serotonin reuptake inhibitors (SSRIs)
paroxetine hydrochloride 949
paroxetine mesylate 950

miscellaneous
busPIRone 243
doxepin 452
hydrOXYzine 644
meprobamate 1282
venlafaxine 1222, 1325

• ANTIARRHYTHMICS

PHARMACOLOGIC PROFILE

General Use

Suppression of cardiac arrhythmias.

General Action and Information

Correct cardiac arrhythmias by a variety of mechanisms, depending on the group used. The therapeutic goal is decreased symptomatology and increased hemodynamic performance. Choice of agent depends on etiology of arrhythmia and individual patient characteristics. Treatable causes of arrhythmias should be corrected before therapy is initiated (e.g., electrolyte disturbances, other drugs). Antiarrhythmics are generally classified by their effects on cardiac conduction tissue (see the following table). Adenosine, atropine, and digoxin are also used as antiarrhythmics.

MECHANISM OF ACTION OF MAJOR ANTIARRHYTHMIC DRUGS

CLASS	DRUGS	MECHANISM
I	moricizine	Shares properties of IA, IB, and IC agents
IA	quinidine, procainamide, disopyramide	Depress Na conductance, increase APD and ERP, decrease membrane responsiveness
IB	tocainide, lidocaine, phenytoin, mexiletine	Increase K conductance, decrease APD and ERP
IC	flecainide, propafenone	Profound slowing of conduction, markedly depress phase O
II	acebutolol, esmolol, propranolol	Interfere with Na conductance, depress cell membrane, decrease automaticity, and increase ERP of the AV node, block excess sympathetic activity
III	amiodarone, dofetilide, ibutilide, sotalol	Interfere with norepinephrine, increase APD and ERP
IV	diltiazem, verapamil	Increase AV nodal ERP, Ca channel blocker

APD = action-potential duration; Ca = calcium; ERP = effective refractory period; K = potassium; Na = sodium.

Contraindications

Differ greatly among various agents. See individual drugs.

Precautions

Differ greatly among agents used. Appropriate dosage adjustments should be made in elderly patients and those with renal or hepatic impairment, depending on agent chosen. Correctable causes (electrolyte abnormalities, drug toxicity) should be evaluated. See individual drugs.

Interactions

Differ greatly among agents used. See individual drugs.

NURSING IMPLICATIONS

Assessment

- Monitor ECG, pulse, and blood pressure continuously throughout IV administration and periodically throughout oral administration.

Potential Nursing Diagnoses

- Decreased cardiac output (Indications).
- Deficient knowledge, related to disease processes and medication regimen (Patient/Family Teaching).

Implementation

- Take apical pulse before administration of oral doses. Withhold dose and notify physician or other health care professional if heart rate is <50 bpm.
- Administer oral doses with a full glass of water. Most sustained-release preparations should be swallowed whole. Do not crush, break, or chew tablets or open capsules, unless specifically instructed.

Patient/Family Teaching

- Instruct patient to take oral doses around the clock, as directed, even if feeling better.
- Instruct patient or family member on how to take pulse. Advise patient to report changes in pulse rate or rhythm to health care professional.
- Caution patient to avoid taking OTC medications without consulting health care professional.
- Advise patient to carry identification describing disease process and medication regimen at all times.
- Emphasize the importance of follow-up exams to monitor progress.

Evaluation/Desired Outcomes

- Resolution of cardiac arrhythmias without detrimental side effects.

Antiarrhythmics included in *Davis's Drug Guide for Nurses*

class IA
disopyramide 430
moricizine 1284
procainamide 1008
quinidine gluconate 1045
quinidine sulfate 1045

class IB
fosphenytoin 583, 1325
lidocaine 746, 1325
mexiletine 819
phenytoin 976
tocainide 29

class IC
flecainide 550
propafenone 1020

class II
acebutolol 105
esmolol 502
propranolol 1026, 1327
sotalol 1122

class III
amiodarone 145, 1326
dofetilide 443
ibutilide 657

class IV
diltiazem 418
verapamil 1224

miscellaneous
adenosine 116
atropine 202, 1353
digoxin 412
phenytoin 976

• ANTIASTHMATICS

PHARMACOLOGIC PROFILE

General Use

Management of acute and chronic episodes of reversible bronchoconstriction. Goal of therapy is to treat acute attacks (short-term control) and to decrease incidence and intensity of future attacks (long-term control). The choice of modalities depends on the continued requirement for short term control agents.

General Action and Information

Adrenergic bronchodilators and phosphodiesterase inhibitors both work by increasing intracellular levels of cyclic-3', 5'-adenosine monophsphate (cAMP); adrenergics by increasing production and phosphodiesterase inhibitors by decreasing breakdown. Increased levels of cAMP produce bronchodilation. Corticosteroids act by decreasing airway inflammation. Anticholinergics (ipratropium) produce bronchodilation by decreasing intracellular levels of cyclic guanosine monophosphate (cGMP). Leukotriene receptor antagonists and mast cell stabilizers decrease the release of substances that can contribute to bronchospasm.

Contraindications

Inhaled corticosteroids, long-acting adrenergic agents, and mast cell stabilizers should not be used during acute attacks of asthma.

Precautions

Adrenergic bronchodilators and anticholinergics should be used cautiously in patients with cardiovascular disease. Chronic use of systemic corticosteroids should be avoided in children or during pregnancy or lactation. Diabetic patients may experience loss of glycemic control during corticosteroid therapy. Corticosteroids should never be abruptly discontinued.

Interactions

Adrenergic bronchodilators and phosphodiesterase inhibitors may have additive CNS and cardiovascular effects with other adrenergic agents. Cimetidine increases theophylline levels and the risk of toxicity. Coritcosteroids may decrease the effectiveness of antidiabetics. Corticosteroids may cause hypokalemia which may be additive with potassium-losing diuretics and may also increase the risk of digoxin toxicity.

NURSING IMPLICATIONS

Assessment

- Assess lung sounds and respiratory function prior to and periodically throughout therapy.
- Assess cardiovascular status of patients taking adrenergic bronchodilators or anticholinergics. Monitor for ECG changes and chest pain.

Potential Nursing Diagnoses

- Ineffective airway clearance (Indications).
- Deficient knowledge, related to disease processes and medication regimen (Patient/Family Teaching).
- Noncompliance (Patient/Family Teaching).

Patient/Family Teaching

- Instruct patient to take antiasthmatics as directed. Do not take more than prescribed or discontinue without discussing with health care professional.
- Advise patient to avoid smoking and other respiratory irritants.
- Instruct patient in correct use of metered-dose inhaler or other administration devices (see Appendix D).
- Advise patient to contact health care professional promptly if the usual dose of medication fails to produce the desired results, if symptoms worsen after treatment, or if toxic effects occur.
- Patients using inhalation medications and bronchodilators should be advised to use the bronchodilator first and allow 5 minutes to elapse before administering other medications, unless otherwise directed by health care professional.

Evaluation/Desired Outcomes

- Prevention of and reduction in symptoms of asthma.

Antiasthmatics included in *Davis's Drug Guide for Nurses*

bronchodilators
albuterol 120
epinephrine 480, 1356
formoterol 577
levalbuterol 741, 1325
metaproterenol 1283
pirbuterol 30
salmeterol 1090
terbutaline 1148

corticosteroids
beclomethasone 343, 347
betamethasone 350, 357
budesonide 343, 347, 350
cortisone 350
dexamethasone 350, 1352
flunisolide 343, 347
fluticasone 343, 347, 358
hydrocortisone 350, 358
methylPREDNISolone 350
mometasone 343, 347, 358
prednisoLONE 350, 1353
predniSONE 350
triamcinolone 343, 347, 350, 358, 1327

leukotriene antagonists
zafirlukast 1249

mast cell stabilizers
cromolyn 773, 1354
nedocromil 773, 1354

monoclonal antibodies
omalizumab 906

• ANTICHOLINERGICS

PHARMACOLOGIC PROFILE

General Use

Atropine— Bradyarrhythmias. **Ipratropium**— bronchospasm (inhalation) and rhinorrhea (intranasal). **Scopolamine**— Nausea and vomiting related to motion sickness and vertigo. **Propantheline and glycopyrrolate**— Decreasing gastric secretory activity and increasing esophageal sphincter tone. Atropine and scopolamine are also used as ophthalmic mydriatics. Benztropine, biperidin, and trihexyphenidyl are used in the management of Parkinson's disease. Oxybutynin and tolterodine are used as urinary tract spasmodics.

General Action and Information

Competitively inhibit the action of acetylcholine. In addition, atropine, glycopyrrolate, propantheline, and scopolamine are antimuscarinic in that they inhibit the action of acetylcholine at sites innervated by postganglionic cholinergic nerves.

Contraindications

Hypersensitivity, narrow-angle glaucoma, severe hemorrhage, tachycardia (due to thyrotoxicosis or cardiac insufficiency), or myasthenia gravis.

Precautions

Geriatric and pediatric patients are more susceptible to adverse effects. Use cautiously in patients with urinary tract pathology; those at risk for GI obstruction; and those with chronic renal, hepatic, pulmonary, or cardiac disease.

Interactions

Additive anticholinergic effects (dry mouth, dry eyes, blurred vision, constipation) with other agents possessing anticholinergic activity, including antihistamines, antidepressants, quinidine, and disopyramide. May alter GI absorption of other drugs by inhibiting GI motility and increasing transit time. Antacids may decrease absorption of orally administered anticholinergics.

NURSING IMPLICATIONS

Assessment

- Assess vital signs and ECG frequently during IV drug therapy. Report any significant changes in heart rate or blood pressure or increase in ventricular ectopy or angina promptly.
- Monitor intake and output ratios in elderly or surgical patients; may cause urinary retention.
- Assess patient regularly for abdominal distention and auscultate for bowel sounds. Constipation may become a problem. Increasing fluids and adding bulk to the diet may help alleviate constipation.

C L A S S I F I C A T I O N S

Potential Nursing Diagnoses
- Decreased cardiac output (Indications).
- Impaired oral mucous membrane (Side Effects).
- Constipation (Side Effects).

Implementation
- **PO:** Administer oral doses of atropine, glycopyrrolate, propantheline, or scopolamine 30 min before meals.
- Scopolamine transdermal patch should be applied at least 4 hr before travel.

Patient/Family Teaching
- Instruct patient that frequent rinses, sugarless gum or candy, and good oral hygiene may help relieve dry mouth.
- May cause drowsiness. Caution patient to avoid driving or other activities requiring alertness until response to medication is known.
- **Ophth:** Advise patients that ophthalmic preparations may temporarily blur vision and impair ability to judge distances. Dark glasses may be needed to protect eyes from bright light.

Evaluation/Desired Outcomes
- Increase in heart rate.
- Decrease in nausea and vomiting related to motion sickness or vertigo.
- Dryness of mouth.
- Dilation of pupils.
- Decrease in GI motility.
- Resolution of signs and symptoms of Parkinson's disease.

Anticholinergics included in *Davis's Drug Guide for Nurses*

atropine 202, 1353
benztropine 218
biperiden 32
darifenacin 380
dicyclomine 410
difenoxin/atropine 427
diphenoxylate/atropine 427
glycopyrrolate 603
hyoscyamine 646
ipratropium 696
oxybutynin 924
propantheline 1290
scopolamine 1096, 1353
solifenacin 1121
tolterodine 1189
trihexyphenidyl 1295

• ANTICOAGULANTS

PHARMACOLOGIC PROFILE

General Use
Prevention and treatment of thromboembolic disorders including deep vein thrombosis, pulmonary embolism, and atrial fibrillation with embolization. Also used in the management of MI sequentially or in combination with thrombolytics and/or antiplatelet agents.

General Action and Information
Anticoagulants are used to prevent clot extension and formation. They do not dissolve clots. The two types of anticoagulants in common use are parenteral heparins and oral warfarin. Therapy is usually initiated with heparin or a heparin-like agent because of rapid onset of action, while maintenance therapy consists of warfarin. Warfarin takes several days to produce therapeutic anticoagulation. In serious or severe thromboembolic events, heparin therapy may be preceded by thrombolytic therapy. Low doses of heparin or heparin-like compounds and fondaparinux are mostly used to prevent deep vein thrombosis after certain surgical procedures and in similar si-

tuations in which prolonged bedrest increases the risk of thromboembolism. Argatroban and lepirudin are used as anticoagulation in patients who have developed thrombocytopenia during heparin therapy.

Contraindications

Underlying coagulation disorders, ulcer disease, malignancy, recent surgery, or active bleeding.

Precautions

Anticoagulation should be undertaken cautiously in any patient with a potential site for bleeding. Pregnant or lactating patients should not receive warfarin. Heparin does not cross the placenta. Heparin and heparin-like agents should be used cautiously in patients receiving epidural analgesia.

Interactions

Warfarin is highly protein bound and may displace or be displaced by other highly protein-bound drugs. The resultant interactions depend on which drug is displaced. Bleeding may be potentiated by aspirin or large doses of penicillins or penicillin-like drugs, cefotetan, cefoperazone, valproic acid, or NSAIDs.

NURSING IMPLICATIONS

Assessment

- Assess patient taking anticoagulants for signs of bleeding and hemorrhage (bleeding gums; nosebleed; unusual bruising; tarry, black stools; hematuria; fall in hematocrit or blood pressure; guaiac-positive stools; urine; or NG aspirate).
- Assess patient for evidence of additional or increased thrombosis. Symptoms will depend on area of involvement.
- **Lab Test Considerations:** Monitor prothrombin time (PT) or international normalized ratio (INR) with warfarin therapy, activated partial thromboplastin time (aPTT) with full-dose heparin therapy and hematocrit, and other clotting factors frequently during therapy.
- Monitor bleeding time throughout antiplatelet therapy. Prolonged bleeding time, which is time and dose dependent, is expected.
- **Toxicity and Overdose:** If overdose occurs or anticoagulation needs to be immediately reversed, the antidote for heparins is protamine sulfate; for warfarin, the antidote is vitamin K (phytonadione [AquaMEPHYTON]). Administration of whole blood or plasma may also be required in severe bleeding due to warfarin because of the delayed onset of vitamin K.

Potential Nursing Diagnoses

- Ineffective tissue perfusion (Indications).
- Risk for injury (Side Effects).
- Deficient knowledge, related to disease processes and medication regimen (Patient/Family Teaching).

Implementation

- Inform all health care professionals caring for patient of anticoagulant therapy. Venipunctures and injection sites require application of pressure to prevent bleeding or hematoma formation.
- Use an infusion pump with continuous infusions to ensure accurate dosage.

Patient/Family Teaching

- Caution patient to avoid activities leading to injury, to use a soft toothbrush and electric razor, and to report any symptoms of unusual bleeding or bruising to health care professional immediately.
- Instruct patient not to take OTC medications, especially those containing aspirin, NSAIDs, or alcohol, without advice of health care professional.

CLASSIFICATIONS

- Review foods high in vitamin K (see Appendix L) with patients on warfarin. Patient should have consistent limited intake of these foods, as vitamin K is the antidote for warfarin and greatly alternating intake of these foods will cause PT levels to fluctuate.
- Emphasize the importance of frequent lab tests to monitor coagulation factors.
- Instruct patient to carry identification describing medication regimen at all times and to inform all health care professionals caring for patient of anticoagulant therapy before laboratory tests, treatment, or surgery.

Evaluation/Desired Outcomes

- Prevention of undesired clotting and its sequelae without signs of hemorrhage. Prevention of stroke, MI, and death in patients at risk.

Anticoagulants included in *Davis's Drug Guide for Nurses*

active factor X inhibitors
fondaparinux 575

antithrombotics
heparin 616

coumarins
warfarin 1245

thrombin inhibitors
argatroban 189
bivalirudin 228
desirudin 393
lepirudin (rDNA) 733

heparins (low molecular weight)
dalteparin 619
enoxaparin 619
tinzaparin 619

• ANTICONVULSANTS

PHARMACOLOGIC PROFILE

General Use

Anticonvulsants are used to decrease the incidence and severity of seizures due various etiologies. Some anticonvulsants are used parenterally in the immediate treatment of seizures. It is not uncommon for patients to require more than one anticonvulsant to control seizures on a long-term basis. Many regimens are evaluated with serum level monitoring.
Several anticonvulsants are also used to treat neuropathic pain.

General Action and Information

Anticonvulsants include a variety of agents, all capable of depressing abnormal neuronal discharges in the CNS that may result in seizures. They may work by preventing the spread of seizure activity, depressing the motor cortex, raising seizure threshold, or altering levels of neurotransmitters, depending on the group. See individual drugs.

Contraindications

Previous hypersensitivity.

Precautions

Use cautiously in patients with severe hepatic or renal disease; dose adjustment may be required. Choose agents carefully in pregnant and lactating women. Fetal hydantoin syndrome may occur in offspring of patients who receive phenytoin during pregnancy.

Interactions

Barbiturates stimulate the metabolism of other drugs that are metabolized by the liver, decreasing their effectiveness. Hydantoins are highly protein-bound and may displace or be displaced by other highly protein-bound drugs. Lamotrigine, tiagabine, and topiramate are capable of interacting with several other anticonvulsants. For more specific interactions, see individual drugs.

Many drugs are capable of lowering seizure threshold and may decrease the effectiveness of anticonvulsants, including tricyclic antidepressants and phenothiazines.

NURSING IMPLICATIONS

Assessment

- Assess location, duration, and characteristics of seizure activity.
- **Toxicity and Overdose:** Monitor serum drug levels routinely throughout anticonvulsant therapy, especially when adding or discontinuing other agents.

Potential Nursing Diagnoses

- Risk for injury (Indications, Side Effects).
- Deficient knowledge, related to disease processes and medication regimen (Patient/Family Teaching).

Implementation

- Administer anticonvulsants around the clock. Abrupt discontinuation may precipitate status epilepticus.
- Implement seizure precautions.

Patient/Family Teaching

- Instruct patient to take medication every day, exactly as directed.
- May cause drowsiness. Caution patient to avoid driving or other activities requiring alertness until response to medication is known. Do not resume driving until physician gives clearance based on control of seizures.
- Advise patient to avoid taking alcohol or other CNS depressants concurrently with these medications.
- Advise patient to carry identification describing disease process and medication regimen at all times.

Evaluation/Desired Outcomes

- Decrease or cessation of seizures without excessive sedation.

Anticonvulsants included in *Davis's Drug Guide for Nurses*

barbiturates
pentobarbital 1287
phenobarbital 972

benzodiazepines
clonazepam 320
clorazepate 325
diazepam 404

hydantoins
phenytoin 976

valproates
divalproex sodium 1212
valproate sodium 1212
valproic acid 1212

miscellaneous
acetaZOLAMIDE 109
carbamazepine 263, 1326
fosphenytoin 583, 1325
gabapentin 591
lamotrigine 725
levetiracetam 742
oxcarbazepine 922
pregabalin 1005
tiagabine 1173
topiramate 1190
zonisamide 1264

CLASSIFICATIONS

• ANTIDEPRESSANTS

PHARMACOLOGIC PROFILE

General Use

Used in the treatment of various forms of endogenous depression, often in conjunction with psychotherapy. Other uses include: Treatment of anxiety (doxepin, fluoxetine, paroxetine, sertraline, venlafaxine); Enuresis (imipramine); Chronic pain syndromes (amitriptyline, doxepin, imipramine, nortriptyline); Smoking cessation (bupropion); Bulimia (fluoxetine); Obsessive-compulsive disorder (fluoxetine, fluvoxamine, paroxetine, sertraline); Social anxiety disorder (paroxetine, sertraline).

General Action and Information

Antidepressant activity is most likely due to preventing the reuptake of dopamine, norepinephrine, and serotonin by presynaptic neurons, resulting in accumulation of these neurotransmitters. The two major classes of antidepressants are the tricyclic antidepressants and the SSRIs. Most tricyclic agents possess significant anticholinergic and sedative properties, which explains many of their side effects (amitriptyline, amoxapine, doxepin, imipramine, nortriptyline). The SSRIs are more likely to cause insomnia (fluoxetine, fluvoxamine, paroxetine, sertraline).

Contraindications

Hypersensitivity. Should not be used in narrow-angle glaucoma. Should not be used in pregnancy or lactation or immediately after MI.

Precautions

Use cautiously in older patients and those with pre-existing cardiovascular disease. Elderly men with prostatic enlargement may be more susceptible to urinary retention. Anticholinergic side effects of tricyclic antidepressants (dry eyes, dry mouth, blurred vision, and constipation) may require dosage modification or drug discontinuation. Dosage requires slow titration; onset of therapeutic response may be 2-4 wk. May decrease seizure threshold, especially bupropion.

Interactions

Tricyclic antidepressants— May cause hypertension, tachycardia, and convulsions when used with MAO inhibitors. May prevent therapeutic response to some antihypertensives. Additive CNS depression with other CNS depressants. Sympathomimetic activity may be enhanced when used with other sympathomimetics. Additive anticholinergic effects with other drugs possessing anticholinergic properties. **MAO inhibitors**— Hypertensive crisis may occur with concurrent use of MAO inhibitors and amphetamines, methyldopa, levodopa, dopamine, epinephrine, norepinephrine, desipramine, imipramine, reserpine, vasoconstrictors, or ingestion of tyramine-containing foods. Hypertension or hypotension, coma, convulsions, and death may occur with meperidine or other opioid analgesics and MAO inhibitors. Additive hypotension with antihypertensives or spinal anesthesia and MAO inhibitors. Additive hypoglycemia with insulin or oral hypoglycemic agents and MAO inhibitors. SSRIs, bupropion, or venlafaxine should not be used in combination with or within weeks of MAO inhibitors (see individual monographs). Risk of adverse reactions may be increased by almotriptan, frovatriptan, rizatriptan, naratriptan, sumatriptan, or zolmitriptan.

NURSING IMPLICATIONS

Assessment

- Monitor mental status and affect. Assess for suicidal tendencies, especially during early therapy. Restrict amount of drug available to patient.
- **Toxicity and Overdose:** Concurrent ingestion of MAO inhibitors and tyramine-containing foods may lead to hypertensive crisis. Symptoms include chest pain, severe headache, nuchal

SYRINGE COMPATIBILITY CHART

C = COMPATIBLE
N = NOT COMPATIBLE
BLANK = NO DATA AVAILABLE

	atropine	buprenorphine	butorphanol	chlorpromazine	codeine	diazepam	diphenhydramine	droperidol	glycopyrrolate	haloperidol	hydromorphone	hydroxyzine	meperidine	metoclopramide	midazolam	morphine	nalbuphine	ondansetron	pentobarbitol	prochlorperazine	promethazine	scopolamine
atropine			C	C			C	C	C		C	C	C	C	C	C	C	C	N	C	C	C
buprenorphine									C	C					C							
butorphanol	C			C			C	C				C	C	C	C	C			N	C	C	C
chlorpromazine	C		C				C	C	C		C	C	C	C	C	C			N	C	C	C
codeine									C			C										
diazepam							N		N		N						N					
diphenhydramine	C		C	C		N		C	C	N	C	C	C	C	C	C	C		N	C	C	C
droperidol	C		C	C			C		C			C	C	C	C	C	C	N	N	C	C	C
glycopyrrolate	C	C		C	C	N	C	C			C	C	C		C	C	C	C	N	C	C	C
haloperidol		C					N				N	N				N						N
hydromorphone	C			C		N	C		C	N		C		C	C				C	N	C	C
hydroxyzine	C		C	C	C		C	C	C	N	C		C	C	C	C	C		N	C	C	C
meperidine	C		C	C			C	C	C			C		C	C	N		C	N	C	C	C
metoclopramide	C		C	C			C	C			C	C	C		C	C		C		C	C	C
midazolam	C	C	C	C			C	C	C		C	C	C	C		C	C	C	N	N	C	C
morphine	C		C	C			C	C	C	N		C	N	C	C			C	N	N	N	C
nalbuphine	C					N	C	C	C			C			C				N	C	N	C
ondansetron	C							N	C				C	C	C	C						
pentobarbitol	N		N	N			N	N	N		C	N	N		N	N	N			N	N	C
prochlorperazine	C		C	C			C	C	C		N	C	C	C	N	N	C		N		C	C
promethazine	C		C	C			C	C	C		C	C	C	C	C	N	N		N	C		C
scopolamine	C		C	C			C	C	C	N	C	C	C	C	C	C	C		C	C	C	

Medications combined in a syringe must be administered within 15 minutes. Recommendations may change as new scientific information becomes available.

IV COMPATIBILITY QUICK REFERENCE CHART

C = COMPATIBLE
N = NOT COMPATIBLE
BLANK = NO DATA AVAILABLE

	amiodarone HCl	calcium chloride	calcium gluconate	diltiazem HCl	dobutamine HCl	dopamine HCl	fentanyl citrate	furosemide	heparin sodium	hydromorphone	inamrinone lactate	insulin, regular	lidocane HCl	lorazepam	magnesium sulfate	meperidine HCl	midazolam	morphine sulfate	nitroglycerin	nitroprusside sodium	norepinephrine bitartrate	oxytocin	potassium chloride	sodium bicarbonate	vasopressin
acylclovir sodium				N	N	N			C	C				C	C	N		N					C	C	
amikacin sulfate	C	C	C	C	C			N	N	C			C	C	C	C	C	C			C	C		C	
amphotericin B	C			C		N			C						N										
amphotericin B cholesteryl		N	N		N	N		C		N			N	C	N	N	N	N	C					N	
ampicillin sodium		N	N	N		N	C		N	C		C		C	C	C	N	C			N	C			
ampicillin Na/sulbactam Na	N			N					C			C				C		C							
anidulafungin																							C		
atropine sulfate	C				C		C			C	C					C	C	C			N		C	N	
azithromycin							N	N		N								N				C	N		
aztreonam			C	C	C	C				C		C		N	C	C							C	C	
bumetanide				C	N							C		C		C	N	C					C		
butorphanol tartrate										C													C		
cefazolin sodium	N		C	C			C		C	C			C		C	C	C	C				C	C		
cefepime HCl																		N					N		
cefoperazone sodium				N	N			C		N					C	N		C				C	C		
cefotaxime sodium							C			C				C	C	C	N	C				C	C		
cefotetan disodium				C		C		C	N			C				C		C				C	C		
cefoxitin sodium										C			C		C	C		C				C	C		
ceftazidime	N								N							C	N	C					C	N	
ceftizoxime sodium	N									C			C			C		C					C		
ceftriaxone sodium	N								C				C			C		C					C		
cefuroxime sodium	N						C		C	C						C	N	C					C		
chlorpromazine HCl									C	C			C		N	C		N				C	C	N	
chlorthiazide												N	C					N			N				
ciprofloxacin	C		C		C	C		N	N				C	C	N		C						C	N	
clindamycin phosphate	C		N				C		C	C					C	C	C	C				C	C		
co-trimoxazole				C						C				C	C	C	N	C				C	N		
daptomycin						C			C				C												
dexamethasone			C				C		C	N			C	N		C	C	C					C		
diazepam					N			N					N			N					N	N	N	N	
digoxin	N			C	N		C				C	N	C			C	C	C					C		
diltiazem HCl					C	C		N				N	C	C		C			C	C	C		C	N	C
diphenhydramine HCl			C					N		C			C	N		C		C					C		
doxycycline hyclate	C			C		N				C			C		C	C		C				C	C	N	
droperidol								N								C	C						C		
drotrecogin alfa	N				N	N		N				N			N		N			N			C		
enalaprilat			C		C	C	C						C		C			C		C			C		
erythromycin gluceptate			C						C															C	
erythromycin lactobionate	C			C					N	C			C	C	C	C	C	C				C		C	
famotidine	C		C		C	C		N		C	C	C	C	C	C	C	C	C	C	C	C		C	C	
fentanyl citrate	C		C		C	C		C		C				C			C		C				C	C	
filgrastim			C					N	N	C				C		C		C					C	C	
fluconazole	C		N	C	C	C		N						C		C	C	C	C				C		
furosemide	N			N	N		C	C			N			C		N	N	N	N	C			C	C	
ganciclovir																							C		
gatifloxacin		C	C		C	C	C	N		C			C	C	C	C	C	C	C				C	C	
gentamicin sulfate	C			C		N	C	N		C		C		C	C	C	C	C				C	C		
glycopyrrolate										C			C			C	C	C					C	N	
granisetron HCl			C		C	C		C		C				C		C		C					C	C	
haloperidol					C	C				N			C	C	N		C	N	C	N	C		N		

IV COMPATIBILITY QUICK REFERENCE CHART

C = COMPATIBLE
N = NOT COMPATIBLE
BLANK = NO DATA AVAILABLE

	amiodarone HCl	calcium chloride	calcium gluconate	diltiazem HCl	dobutamine HCl	dopamine HCl	fentanyl citrate	furosemide	heparin sodium	hydromorphone	inamrinone lactate	insulin, regular	lidocane HCl	lorazepam	magnesium sulfate	meperidine HCl	midazolam	morphine sulfate	nitroglycerin	nitroprusside sodium	norepinephrine bitartrate	oxytocin	potassium chloride	sodium bicarbonate	vasopressin
heparin sodium			C	N	N	C	C	C		N		C	C	C	C	C	C	C	N	C	N	C	C	C	C
hydralazine HCl					C			N	C						N				N						
hydrocortisone		C	N	N		C	C	C			C	C	C	C	C	C	N	C			C	C		C	
hydromorphone HCl							C						C	C	C		C						C	N	
imipenem/cilastatin	N			C								C		N		N	N						C		
insulin, regular	C			N	N	N							C		C	C	C	C	C	C	N	C	C	C	
ketorolac										N				C		C		C					C		
labetalol HCl	C		C		C	C	C	N				N	C		C	C	C	C	C	C	C		C	N	
levofloxacin					C	C	C	N				N	C	C				C	N	N			C	C	
levothyroxine																							N		
linezolid					C	C	C	C		C			C	C	C	C	C	C	C				C	C	
lorazepam	C			C			C	C		C				C									C		
magnesium sulfate					C				C	C		C			C	C		C					C		
mannitol						C		N															C	C	
meperidine HCl				C	C	C		N				C	C		C	C	C	N				C	C	N	
methicillin sodium		N	C													N		N			N		C	C	
methylprednisolone	C		C			C					C		N			C	N	C			C				
metoclopramide HCl			N					N				C	C	N	C	C		C					C	N	
metoprolol tartrate																C		C					C		
metronidazole HCl	C					N	C		C	C				C	C	C	C	C				C			
mezlocillin sodium	N									C						N		C					C		
midazolam HCl	C		C		N	C	C	N		C		C				C	C	C	C	C	C		C	N	
minocycline HCl										N					C	N		N					C		
morphine sulfate	C	C			C	C		N				C	C	C	C	N	C	C		C	C	C	C	C	
moxifloxacin																									
mycafungin																									
nafcillin sodium					N		C			N		C	C		C	N	N	N			N	C	C	C	
nalbuphine HCl																	C						C	N	
ondansetron HCl						C	C	N		C				N	C	C	C	C					C	N	
oxacillin sodium			N	C		C				C					C	C		C			N	C	C		
pantoprazole																							C		
penicillin G potassium	C	C	C	C		C				C		N	C		N	C		C			N	C	C	N	
phenobarbital sodium		C	C									N				N		N			N		C	N	
phenylephrine HCl	C		C		C				C		C		C								C		C		C
phenytoin			N	N								N	N			N		N	N		N		N		
piperacillin sodium	N			C						C			C	C	C	C	C	C				C	C	C	
piperacillin/tazobactam	N		C		N	C		C		C				C	C	C		C					C	C	
potassium chloride	C		C	C	C	C	C	C	C	C		C	C	C	C	C	C	C			C	C	C	C	
potassium phosphate	N		N		N										N					C			N		
prednisolone			N																		C		C		
prochlorperazine		N	N							N			C		N	C		N				N	C		
promethazine HCl						C		N		C						C	C	C					C	N	
sodium bicarbonate	N	N	N	N	N	N	C	C		N	C	C			N	N	N	C			N		C	C	
ticarcillin disodium				C						C		C			C	C		C				C	C		
ticarcillin/clavulanate				C								C				C		C					C		
tigecycline					C	C							C										C		
tobramycin sulfate	C		C	C			C	C		C		C			C	C	C	C				C	C		
vancomycin HCl	C	N	C	C			C			C		C		C	C	C	C	C				C	C	N	
verapamil HCl	C	C	C		C	C		C		C	C	C	C		C	C		C	C	C	C	C	C	C	C
voriconazole																							C		

Be aware: New studies may alter the information on this chart.

PEDIATRIC INTRAVENOUS MEDICATION QUICK REFERENCE CHART

Risk of fluid overload in infants and children is always a consideration when administering IV medications. The following table provides maximum concentrations—the smallest amount of fluid necessary for diluting specific medications—and the maximum rate at which the medications can be given.

Drug	Maximum Concentration	Maximum Rate
acetazolamide	100 mg/ml	500 mg/min
acyclovir	10 mg/ml	Give over 1 hr
adenosine	3 mg/ml	Give over 1-2 sec
allopurinol	6 mg/ml	Give over 15-20 min
amikacin	10 mg/ml	Give over 30 min
aminocaproic acid	20 mg/ml	Give over 1 hr
aminophylline	25 mg/ml	25 mg/min
amphotericin B	0.1 mg/ml (peripherally) 0.5 mg/ml (centrally)	Give over 2-6 hr
amphotericin B liposomal	2 mg/ml	Give over 2 hr
ampicillin	100 mg/ml	10 mg/kg/min
ampicillin/sulbactam	45 mg/ml	Give over 15-30 min
atropine	1 mg/ml	Give over 1 min
azithromycin	2 mg/ml	Give over 1 hr
bumetanide	0.25 mg/ml	Give over 1-2 min
calcitriol	2 mcg/ml	Give over 15 sec
calcium chloride	100 mg/ml	100 mg/min
calcium gluconate	100 mg/ml	100 mg/min
cefazolin	138 mg/ml (IVP) 20 mg/ml (Intermittent infusion)	Give over 3-5 min Give over 10-60 min
cefepime	160 mg/ml	Give over 30 min
cefotaxime	< 200 mg/ml (IVP) 60 mg/ml (Intermittent infusion)	Give over 3-5 min Give over 10-30 min
cefoxitin	180 mg/ml (IVP) 40 mg/ml (Intermittent infusion)	Give over 3-5 min Give over 15-40 min
ceftazidime	200 mg/ml (IVP) 40 mg/ml (Intermittent infusion)	Give over 3-5 min Give over 10-30 min
ceftriaxone	40 mg/ml	Give over 10-30 min
cefuroxime	100 mg/ml (IVP) 30 mg/ml (Intermittent infusion)	Give over 3-5 min Give over 15-60 min
chlorpromazine	1 mg/ml	0.5 mg/min
ciprofloxacin	2 mg/ml	Give over 60 min
clindamycin	18 mg/ml	30 mg/min
cyclosporine	2.5 mg/ml	Give over 2-8 hr
dexamethasone	10 mg/ml	Doses <10 mg: Give over 1-4 min Doses >10 mg: Give over 10-20 min
diazepam	5 mg/ml	2 mg/min
diazoxide	15 mg/ml	Give over 30-60 min
digoxin	100 mcg/ml	Give over 5 min
diphenhydramine	50 mg/ml	25 mg/min
doxycycline	1 mg/ml	Give over 1 hr
enalaprilat	1.25 mg/ml	Give over 5 min
erythromycin	5 mg/ml	Give over 20-120 min
famotidine	4 mg/ml	Give over 2-10 min
fentanyl	50 mcg/ml	Give over 1-3 min
fluconazole	2 mg/ml	Give over 1-2 hr
flumazenil	0.1 mg/ml	Give over 15-30 sec
fosphenytoin	25 mg/ml	3 mg/kg/min
furosemide	10 mg/ml	0.5 mg/kg/min
ganciclovir	10 mg/ml	Give over 1 hr
gentamicin	40 mg/ml	Give over 30 min
glycopyrrolate	0.2 mg/ml	Give over 5-10 sec
granisetron	50 mcg/ml	Give over 2-60 min
hydralazine	20 mg/ml	5 mg/min or 0.2 mg/kg/min

Drug	Maximum Concentration	Maximum Rate
hydrocortisone	50 mg/ml (IVP) 5 mg/ml (Intermittent infusion)	Give over 1-10 min Give over 20-30 min
imipenem/cilastatin	7 mg/ml	Give over 20-60 min
inamrinone	5 mg/ml	Give over 2-3 min
indomethacin	1 mg/ml	Give over 20-35 min
kanamycin	6 mg/ml	Give over 30-60 min
ketamine	50 mg/ml (IVP) 2 mg/ml (Intermittent infusion)	2 mg/min or 0.5 mg/kg/min 2 mg/min or 0.5 mg/kg/min
ketorolac	30 mg/ml	Give over 1-5 min
labetalol	5 mg/ml	2 mg/min
levocarnitine	200 mg/ml	Give over 2-3 min
levothyroxine	100 mcg/ml	Give over 2-3 min
lorazepam	4 mg/ml	2 mg/min or 0.05 mg/kg over 2-5 min
magnesium sulfate	60 mg/ml	1 mEq/kg/hr (125 mg/kg/hr)
meperidine	10 mg/ml	Give over 5 min
meropenem	50 mg/ml	Give over 15-30 min
methylprednisolone	125 mg/ml (IVP) 2.5 mg/ml (Intermittent infusion)	Give over 1-30 min Give over 20-60 min
metoclopramide	5 mg/ml	Give over 1-2 min
metronidazole	8 mg/ml	Give over 1 hr
midazolam	5 mg/ml	Give over 20-30 sec (5 min in neonates)
milrinone	1 mg/ml	Give over 10 min
morphine	5 mg/ml	Give over 4-5 min
nafcillin	100 mg/ml	Give over 15-60 min
naloxone	1 mg/ml	Give over 30 sec
ondansetron	2 mg/ml	Give over 2-15 min
oxacillin	100 mg/ml (IVP) 40 mg/ml (Intermittent infusion)	Give over 10 min Give over 15-30 min
pancuronium	2 mg/ml	Give over seconds
penicillin g	50,000 units/ml (neonates/infants) 500,000 units/ml (children)	Give over 15-30 min
pentamidine	2.5 mg/ml	Give over 1-2 hr
pentobarbital	50 mg/ml	Give over 10-30 min
phenobarbital	130 mg/ml	2 mg/kg/min
phenytoin	50 mg/ml	3 mg/kg/min
phytonadione	10 mg/ml	Give over 15-30 min
piperacillin	200 mg/ml (IVP) 20 mg/ml (Intermittent infusion)	Give over 3-5 min Give over 20-60 min
piperacillin/tazobactam	20 mg/ml	Give over 30 min
potassium chloride	80 mEq/L (peripherally) 200 mEq/L (centrally)	1 mEq/kg/hr
promethazine	25 mg/ml	< 25 mg/min
propranolol	1 mg/ml	Give over 10-15 min
protamine	10 mg/ml	5 mg/min
ranitidine	2.5 mg/ml	10 mg/min
rifampin	6 mg/ml	Give over 30 min
tacrolimus	0.02 mg/ml	Give over 4-24 hr
terbutaline	1 mg/ml	Give over 5-10 min
ticarcillin	100 mg/ml	Give over 10-120 min
ticarcillin/clavulanate	100 mg/ml	Give over 10-60 min
tobramycin	40 mg/ml	Give over 30 min
trimethoprim/sulfamethoxazole	1 ml drug per 10 ml diluent	Give over 1-1.5 hr
valproate sodium	50 mg/ml	2-6 mg/kg/min
vancomycin	5 mg/ml	Give over 60 min
vasopressin	1 unit/ml	Give over 5-30 min
verapamil	2.5 mg/ml	Give over 30-60 sec
zidovudine	4 mg/ml	Give over 30-60 min

Adapted from Phelps SJ and Hak EB: Pediatric Injectable Drugs, 7th Edition. American Society of Heath-System Pharmacists, Bethesda, MD 2004.

BEERS CRITERIA

The Beers criteria for potentially inappropriate medication use in adults 65 years and older in the United States is a compilation of drugs and drug classes found to increase the risk of adverse events in older adults. Frequently, older adults are more sensitive to the medications or their side effects. The potential for adverse events can be minimized by prescribing safer alternatives or prescribing at the lowest effective dose.

alprazolam (Xanax)	fluoxetine (Prozac)
amiodarone (Cordarone)	flurazepam (Dalmane)
amitriptyline (Elavil)	guanadrel (Hylorel)
amphetamines	halazepam (Paxipam)
anorexic agents	halazepam (Paxipam)
barbiturates	hydroxyzine (Vistaril, Atarax)
belladonna alkaloids (Donnatal)	hyoscyamine (Levsin, Levsinex)
bisacodyl (Dulcolax)	meperidine (Demerol)
carisoprodol (Soma)	meprobamate (Miltown, Equanil)
cascara sagrada	mesoridazine (Serentil)
castor oil (Neoloid)	metaxalone (Skelaxin)
chlordiazepoxide (Librium, Mitran)	methocarbamol (Robaxin)
chlordiazepoxide-amitriptyline (Limbitrol)	methyldopa (Aldomet)
chlorpheniramine (Chlor-Trimeton)	methyldopa-hydrochlorothiazide (Aldoril)
chlorpropamide (Diabinese)	methyltestosterone (Android, Virilon, Testrad)
chlorzoxazone (Paraflex)	mineral oil
cimetidine (Tagamet)	naproxen (Naprosyn, Avaprox, Aleve)
clidinium-chlordiazepoxide (Librax)	nifedipine (Procardia, Adalat)
clonidine (Catapres)	nitrofurantoin (Microdantin)
clorazepate (Tranxene)	orphenadrine (Norflex)
cyclandelate (Cyclospasmol)	oxaprozin (Daypro)
cyclobenzaprine (Flexeril)	oxazepam (Serax)
cyproheptadine (Periactin)	oxybutynin (Ditropan)
dessicated thyroid	pentazocine (Talwin)
dexchlorpheniramine (Polaramine)	perphenazine-amitriptyline (Triavil)
diazepam (Valium)	piroxicam (Feldene)
dicyclomine (Bentyl)	promethazine (Phenergan)
digoxin (Lanoxin)	propantheline (Pro-Banthine)
diphenhydramine (Benadryl)	propoxyphene (Darvon) and combination products
dipyridamole (Persantine)	quazepam (Doral)
disopyramide (Norpace, Norpace CR)	reserpine (Serpalan, Serpasil)
doxazosin (Cardura)	temazepam (Restoril)
doxepin (Sinequan)	thioridazine (Mellaril)
ergot mesyloids (Hydergine)	ticlopidine (Ticlid)
estrogens	triazolam (Halcion)
ethacrynic acid (Edecrin)	trimethobenzamide (Tigan)
ferrous sulfate (iron, Feosol)	tripelennamine

Adapted from Frick DM, et al. Potentially Inappropriate Medications for Use in Older Adults (Beers List. Updating the Beers criteria for potentially inappropriate medication use in older adults: results of a US consensus panel of experts. Arch Intern Med. 2003;163:2716-2724.)

DRUGS ASSOCIATED WITH INCREASED RISK OF FALLS IN THE ELDERLY

Many factors are associated with falls in the elderly, including frailty, disease, vision, polypharmacy, and certain medications. Below is a list of drugs associated with falls. Assess geriatric patients on these medications for fall risk, and implement fall reduction strategies.

ACE Inhibitors

benazepril (Lotensin)
captopril (Capoten, Zestril)
cilazapril (Inhibace)
enalapril (Vasotec)
fosinopril (Monopril)
lisinopril (Prinivil)
perindopril (Coversyl)
quinapril (Accupril)
ramipril (Altace)

Angiotensin II Receptor Antagonists

candesartan (Atacand)
eprosartan (Teveten)
irbesartan (Avapro)
losartan (Cozaar)
telmisartan (Micardis)
valsartan (Diovan)

Anti-Alzheimer's Agents

donepezil (Aricept)
galantamine (Reminyl)
rivastigmine (Exelon)

Anticonvulsants

carbamazepine (Tegretol)
gabapentin (Neurontin)
lamotrigine (Lamictal)
phenobarbital (Luminal)
phenytoin (Dilantin)
topiramate (Topamax)
valproate (Depakene)
vigabatrin (Sabril)

Antidepressants

amitriptyline (Elavil)
bupropion (Wellbutrin)
citalopram (Celexa)
clomipramine (Anafranil)
desipramine (Norpramin)
doxepin (Sinequan)
fluoxetine (Prozac)
fluvoxamine (Luvox)
imipramine (Tofranil)
mirtazapine (Remeron)
moclobemide (Manerix)
nortriptyline (Aventyl)
paroxetine (Paxil)
sertraline (Zoloft)
trazodone (Desyrel)
venlafaxine (Effexor)

Antihistamines/Antinauseants

dimenhydrinate (Dramamine, Gravol)
diphenhydramine (Benadryl)
meclizine (Bonamine)
metoclopramide (Maxeran, Reglan)
prochlorperazine (Compazine, Stemetil)
promethazine (Phenergan)
scopolamine patch (Transderm Scop, Transderm V)

Antiparkinsonian Agents

amantadine (Symmetrel)
bromocriptine (Parlodel)
entacapone (Comtan)
levodopa/benserazide (Prolopa)
levodopa/carbidopa (Sinemet)
pramipexole (Mirapex)
selegiline (Eldepryl)

Antipsychotics (Atypical)

clozapine (Clozaril)
olanzapine (Zyprexa)
quetiapine (Seroquel)

Antipsychotics (Neuroleptics)

chlorpromazine (Largactil, Thorazine)
haloperidol (Haldol)
hydroxyzine (Atarax)
lithium loxapine (Loxapac)
methotrimeprazine (Nozinan)
perphenazine (Trilafon)
prochlorperazine (Compazine, Stemetil)
risperidone (Risperdal)
thioridazine (Mellaril)
trifluoperazine (Stelazine)

Benzodiazepines (Intermediate Acting)

alprazolam (Xanax)
lorazepam (Ativan)
nitrazepam (Mogadon)
oxazepam (Serax)
temazepam (Restoril)

Benzodiazepines (Long Acting)

chlordiazepoxide (Librium)
clonazepam (Klonopin, Rivotril)
diazepam (Valium)
flurazepam (Dalmane)

Benzodiazepines (Short Acting)

midazolam (Versed)
triazolam (Halcion)

Beta Blockers

acebutolol (Sectral)
atenolol (Tenormin)
bisoprolol (Monocor)
carvedilol (Coreg)
labetalol (Normodyne, Trandate)
metoprolol (Lopressor)
propranolol (Inderal)
sotalol (Betapace, Sotacor)
timolol (Blocadren)

Calcium Channel Blockers

amlodipine (Norvasc)
diltiazem (Cardizem)
felodipine (Plendil)
nifedipine (Adalat)
verapamil (Calan, Isoptin)

Diuretics

amiloride/HCTZ (Moduretic)
furosemide (Lasix)
hydrochlorothiazide
triamterene/HCTZ (Dyazide)

Opioid Analgesics

acetaminophen-Codeine (Tylenol #1, #2, #3)
codeine
fentanyl (Sublimaze, Duragesic)
hydromorphone (Dilaudid, Hydromorph Contin)
meperidine (Demerol)
morphine (MOS, MS Contin, M-Eslon, Roxanol)
oxycodone (Percocet/Percodan, OxyContin)
pentazocine (Talwin)

Over the Counter (OTC) Medications

allergy medicines
analgesics
antiemetics
cold remedies
cough preparations
muscle relaxants
sleeping pills

Vasodilators

hydralazine (Apresoline)
isosorbide (Isordil)
nitroglycerin (Nitro-Dur)
terazosin (Hytrin)

Adapted from American Geriatrics Society (AGS) Panel on Falls in Older Persons, Guideline for the Prevention of Falls in Older Persons. JAGS 49:664–672, 2001.
Keys PA. Preventing Falls in the Elderly: The Role of the Pharmacist. J Pharm Pract. 17(2):149-152, 2004.

LOOK-ALIKE, SOUND-ALIKE (LASA) DRUG NAMES

The Joint Commission established a National Patient Safety Goal that requires accredited organizations to identify a list of look-alike or sound-alike drugs used in their organization and, at a minimum, to review the list annually and take action to prevent errors involving the use of these drugs. Organizations must list at least 10 drug combinations from the Joint Commission's list of LASA drugs.

The following are drug pairs that the Joint Commission and others have rated as most problematic. Names in ALL CAPITALS are brand names; those in lowercase are generic names.

ABELCET	amphotericin B
acetazolamide	acetohexamide
acetohexamide	acetohexamide
AMARYL	REMINYL
AMBISOME	amphotericin B
amphotericin B	ABELCET
amphotericin B	AMBISOME
AVANDIA	COUMADIN
AVINZA	EVISTA
carboplatin	cisplatin
CELEXA	CEREBYX
CELEXA	CELEBREX
CELEBREX	CELEXA
CEREBYX	CELEXA
cisplatin	carboplatin
COUMADIN	AVANDIA
daunorubicin	idarubicin
daunorubicin	daunorubicin citrate liposomal
DIABETA	ZEBET A
doxorubicin hydrochloride	doxorubicin liposomal
ephedrine	epinephrine
EVISTA	AVINZA
fentanyl	sufentanil
folic acid	folinic acid (leucovorin calcium)
folinic acid (leucovorin calcium)	folic acid
heparin	HESPAN
HESPAN	heparin
HUMALOG	HUMULIN
HUMALOG MIX	HUMULIN
HUMULIN	HUMALOG
HUMULIN	HUMALOG MIX
hydromorphone	morphine
idarubicin	daunorubicin
LAMICTAL	LAMISIL
LAMISIL	LAMICTAL
LANTUS	LENTE
LENTE	LANTUS
leucovorin calcium	LEUKERAN
LEUKERAN	leucovorin calcium
morphine	hydromorphone
morphine oral liquid **concentrate**	morphine **non-concentrated** oral liquid
NOVOLIN	NOVOLOG MIX
NOVOLOG MIX	NOVOLIN
REMINYL	AMARYL
RETROVIR	ritonavir
ritonavir	RETROVIR
SEROQUEL	SERZONE
SERZONE	SEROQUEL
sufentanil	fentanyl
TAXOL	TAXOTERE
TAXOTERE	TAXOL
tiagabine	tizanidine
tizanidine	tiagabine
vinblastine	vincristine
vincristine	vinblastine
WELLBUTRIN SR	WELLBUTRIN XL
WELLBUTRIN XL	WELLBUTRIN SR
ZANTAC	ZYRTEC
ZEBET A	DIABETA
ZYPREXA	ZYRTEC
ZYRTEC	ZYPREXA
ZYRTEC	ZANTAC

Adapted from Joint Commission. Look-alike/Sound-alike Drug Lists.
Available at: http://www.jointcommission.org
Accessed November 30, 2007.

Joint Commission. 2008 National Patient Safety Goals.
Available at: http://www.jointcommission.org
Accessed November 30, 2007.

HIGH ALERT MEDICATIONS

High alert medications are those drugs that have the highest potential for harm when prescribed or administered inappropriately. Below is a complete list of high alert medications found in *Davis's Drug Guide for Nurses*. The list may change based on new research; refer to *Medication Errors: Improving Practices and Patient Safety* on page 8 for additional information.

aldesleukin	DOXOrubicin hydrochloride	magnesium sulfate (IV, parenteral)
alemtuzumab	DOXOrubicin hydrochloride liposome	meperidine
altretamine	epinephrine	methadone
amiodarone	epirubicin	methotrexate
arsenic trioxide	eptifibatide	metoprolol
asparaginase	esmolol	midazolam
bleomycin	etoposides	milrinone
buprenorphine	fentanyl (oral, transmucosal)	morphine
busulfan	fentanyl (parenteral)	nalbuphine
butorphanol	fentanyl (transdermal)	nesiritide
calcium salts	fluorouracil	oxycodone compound
capecitabine	fondaparinux	oxymorphone
carboplatin	gemcitabine	pancuronium
carmustine	gemtuzumab ozogamicin	pentazocine
chloralhydrate	heparin	potassium phosphates
chlorambucil	heparins (low molecular weight)	potassium supplements
cisplatin	hydrocodone	pramlintide
codeine	hydromorphone	propranolol
colchicine	hypoglycemic agents, oral	sodium chloride
cyclophosphamide	imatinib	thrombolytic agents
cytarabine	insulin mixtures	tirofiban
DAUNOrubicin citrate liposome	insulins (short-acting)	topotecan
DAUNOrubicin hydrochloride	insulins (intermediate-acting)	trastuzumab
decitabine	insulins (long-acting)	vinBLAStine
digoxin	insulins (rapid-acting)	vinCRIStine
DOBUTamine	labetalol	vinorelbine
docetaxel	lidocaine	warfarin
DOPamine		

TALL MAN LETTERING CHANGES

The Food and Drug Administration has asked manufacturers to update the appearance of 33 look-alike drug names. The changes involve using capital letters ("Tall Man") to minimize medication errors resulting from look-alike confusion.

Acetohexamide Acetazolamide	AcetoHEXAMIDE AcetaZOLAMIDE
Bupropion Buspirone	BuPROPion BusPIRone
Chlorpromazine Chlorpropamide	ChlorproMAZINE ChlorproPAMIDE
Clomiphene Clomipramine	ClomiPHENE ClomiPRAMINE
Cyclosporine Cycloserine	CycloSPORINE CycloSERINE
Daunorubicin Doxorubicin	DAUNOrubicin DOXOrubicin
Dimenhydrinate Diphenhydramine	DimenhyDRINATE DiphenhydrAMINE
Dobutamine Dopamine	DOBUTamine DOPamine
Glipizide Glyburide	GlipiZIDE GlyBURIDE
Hydralazine Hydroxyzine	HydrALAZINE HydrOXYzine
Medroxyprogesterone Methylprednisolone Methyltestosterone	MedroxyPROGESTERone MethylPREDNISolone MethylTESTOSTERone
Nicardipine Nifedipine	NiCARdipine NIFEdipine
Prednisone Prednisolone	PredniSONE PrednisoLONE
Sulfadiazine Sulfisoxazole	SulfADIAZINE SulfiSOXAZOLE
Tolazamide Tolbutamide	TOLAZamide TOLBUTamide
Vinblastine Vincristine	VinBLAStine VinCRIStine

Adapted from U.S. Food and Drug Administration Center for Drug Evaluation and Research. Available at: http://www.fda.gov/cder/index.html.

TALL MAN List

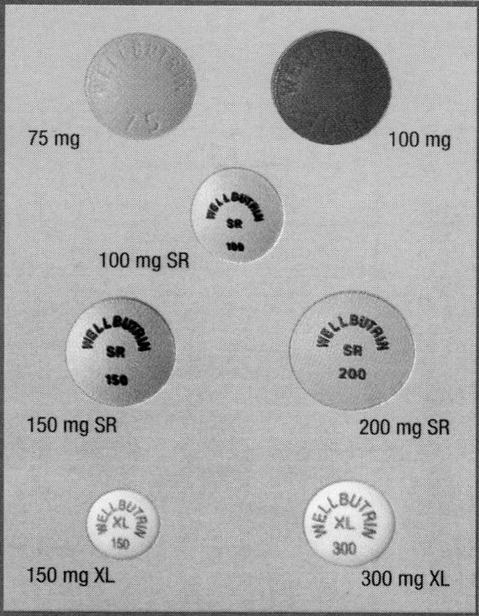

BuPROPion (Wellbutrin®)

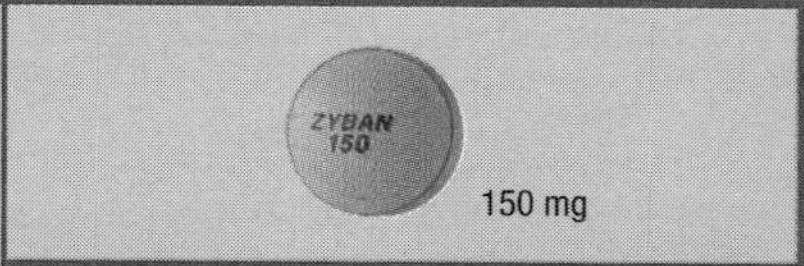

BuPROPion (Zyban®)

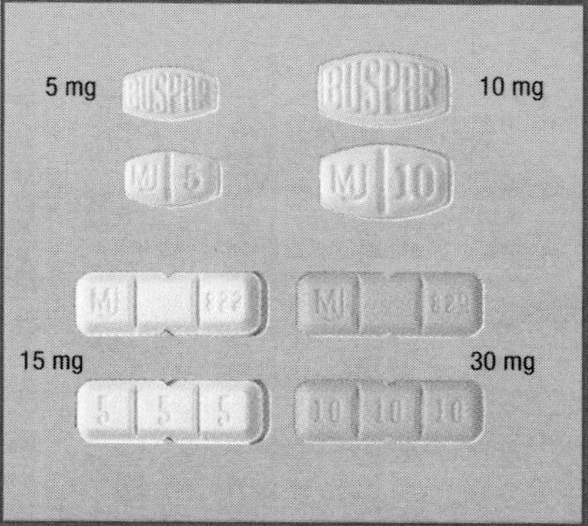

BusPIRone (Buspar®)

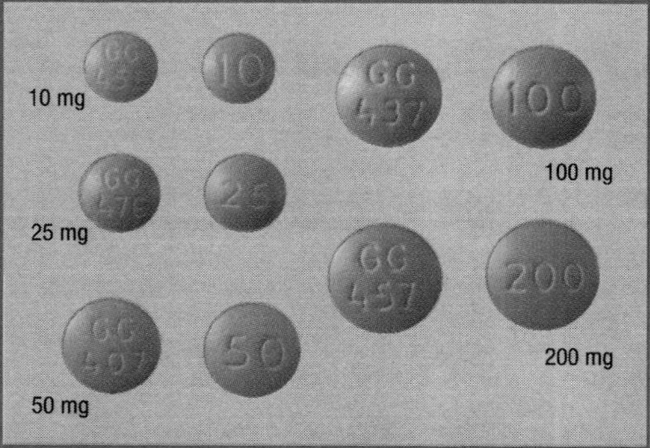

ChlorproMAZINE

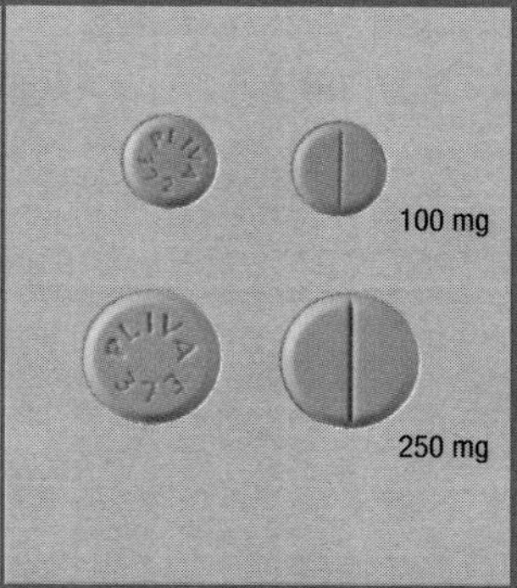

ChlorproPAMIDE

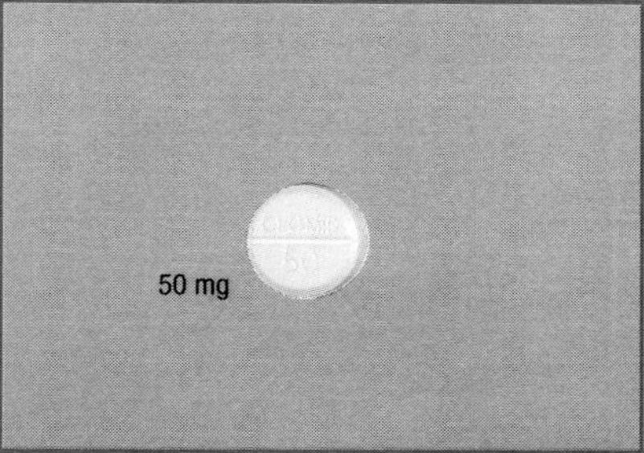

ClomiPHENE

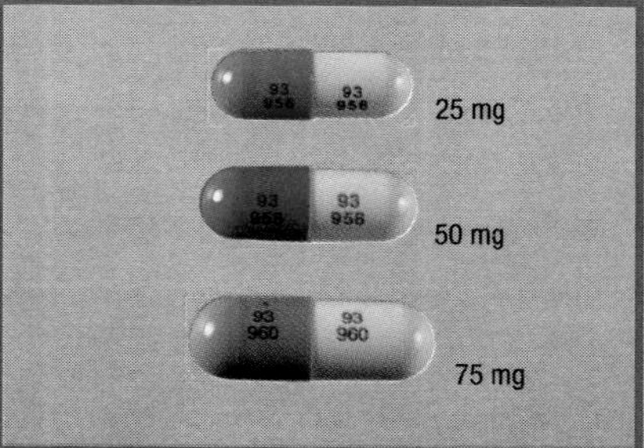

ClomiPRAMINE

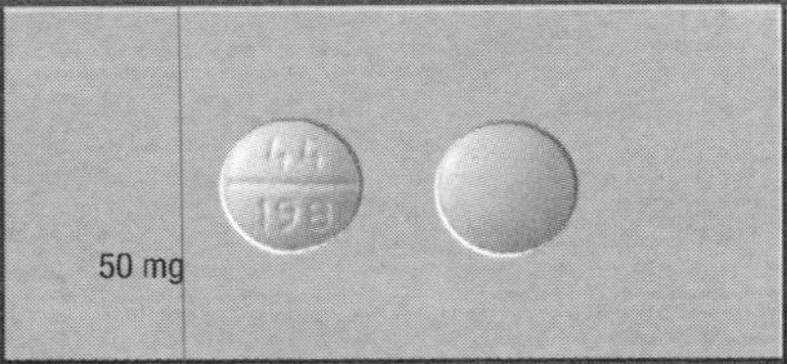

DimenhyDRINATE

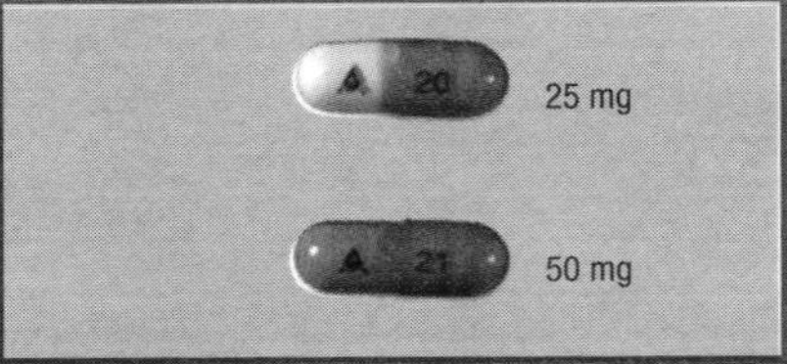

DyphenhydrAMINE

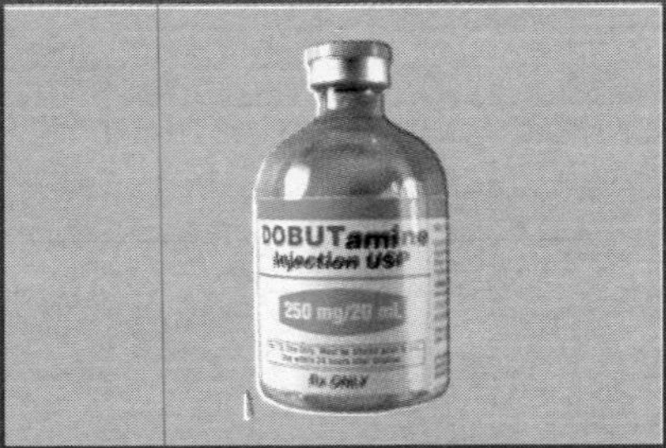

DOBUTamine

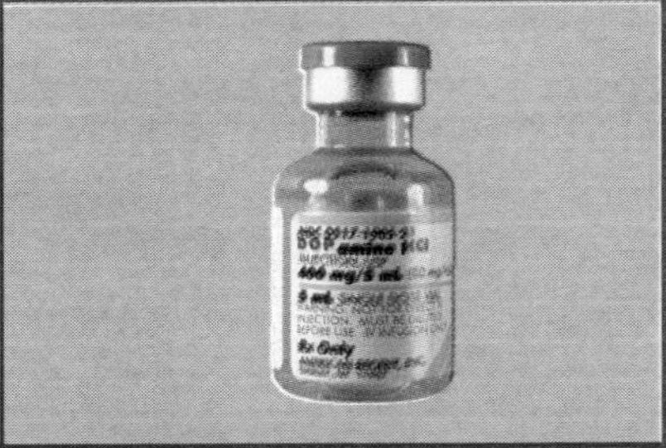

DOPamine

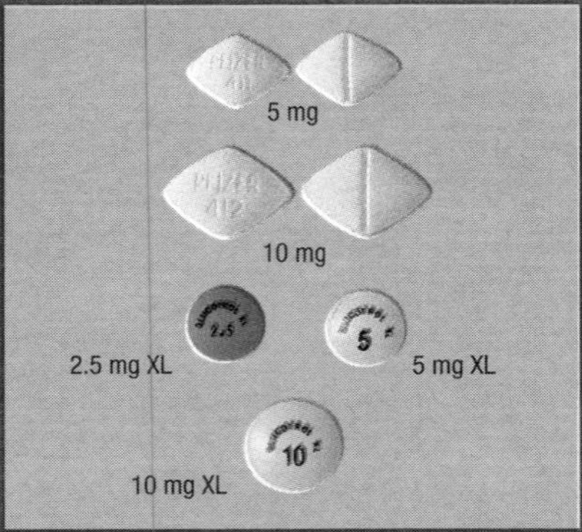

GlipiZIDE (Glucotrol®)

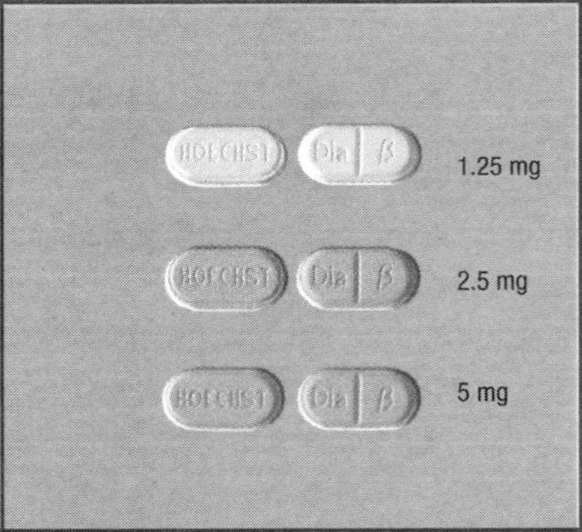

GlyBURIDE (DiaBeta®)

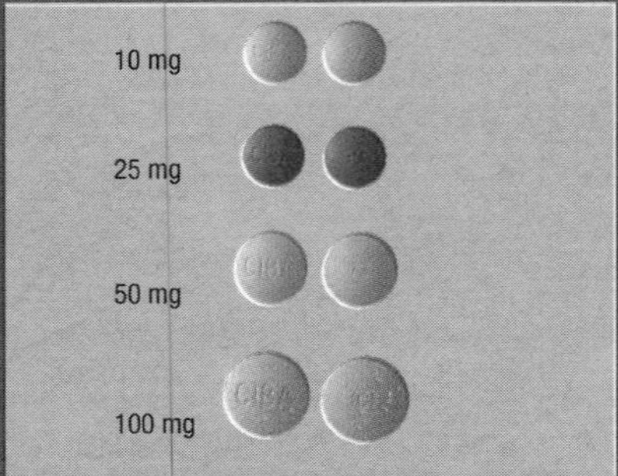

HydrALAZINE

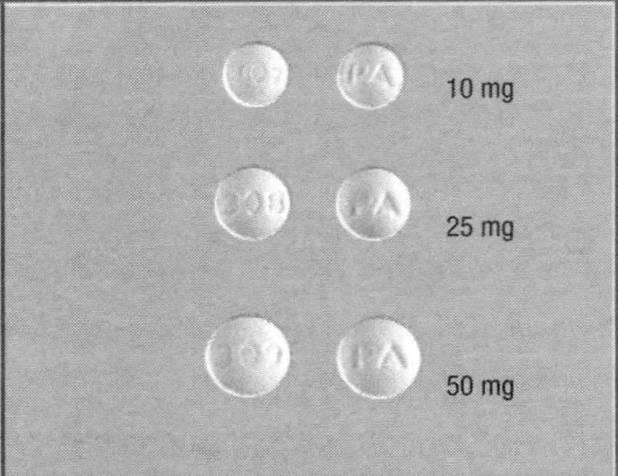

HydrOXYzine

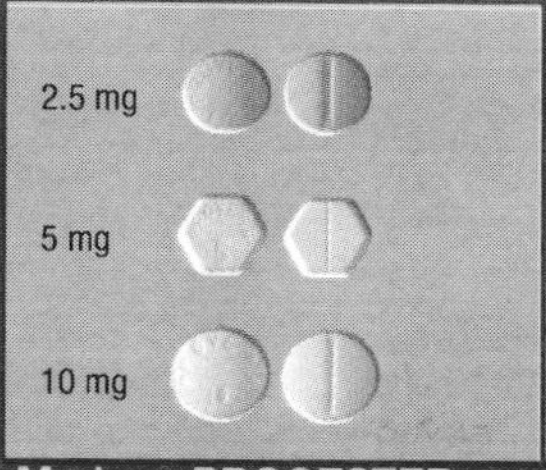

MedroxyPROGESTERone (Provera®)

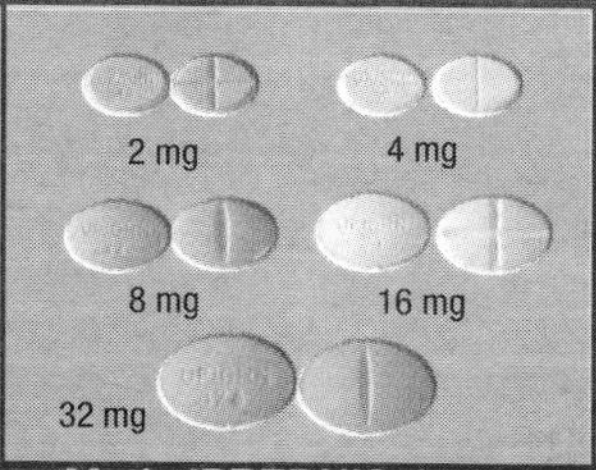

MethylPREDNISolone (Medrol®)

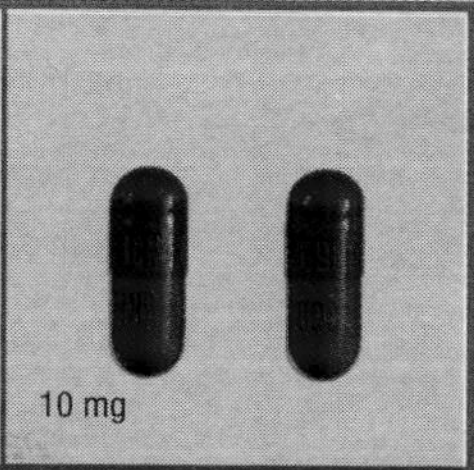

MethylTESTOSTERone

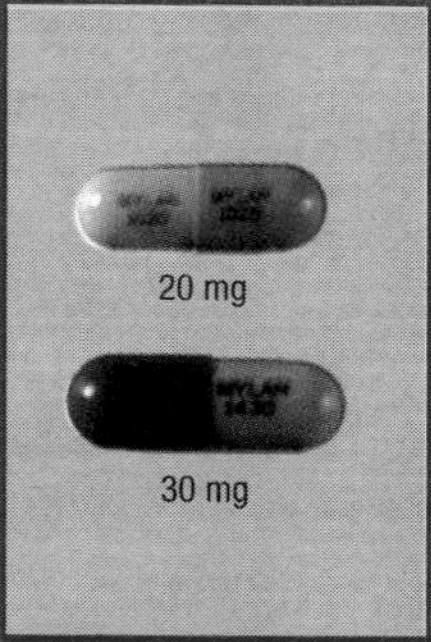

NiCARdipine

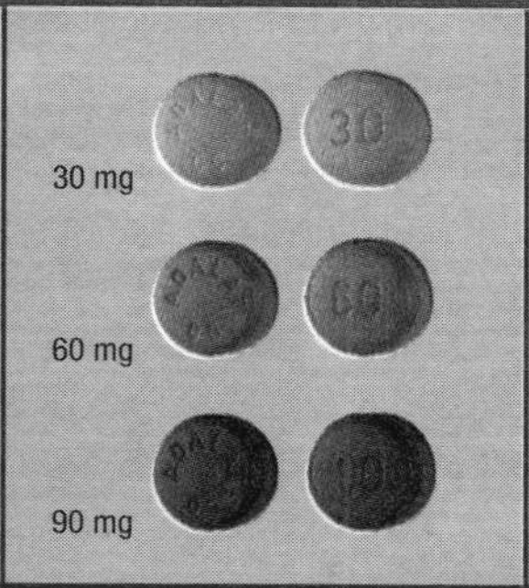

NIFEdipine (Adalat® CC)

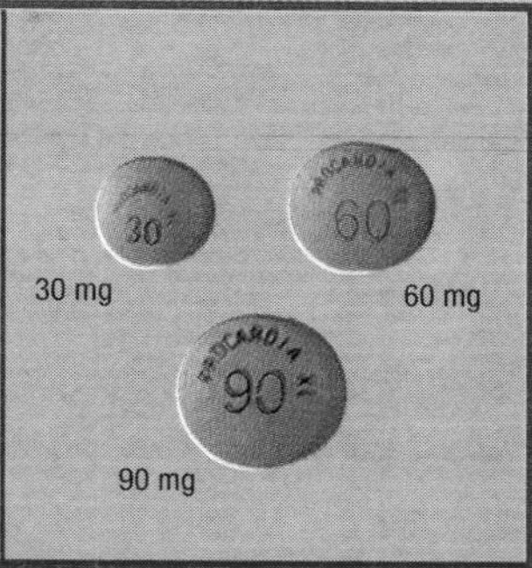

NIFEdipine (Procardia-XL®)

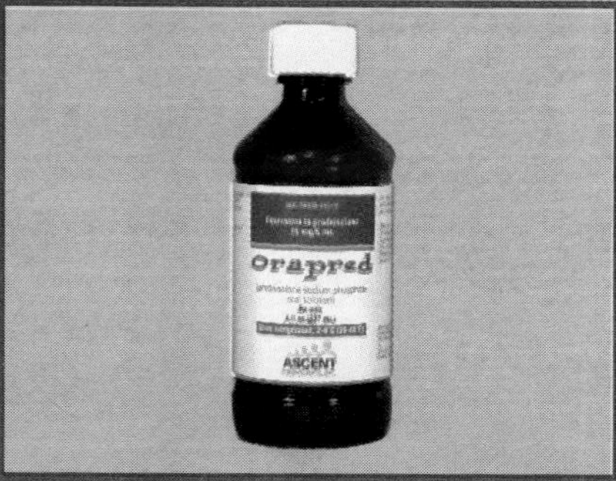

PrednisoLONE (Orapred®)

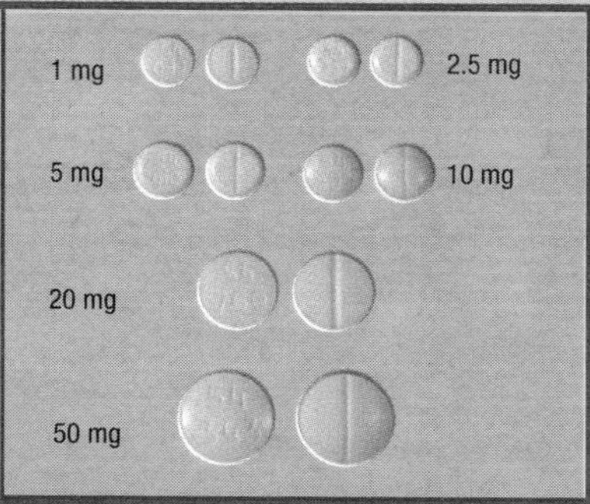

PredniSONE

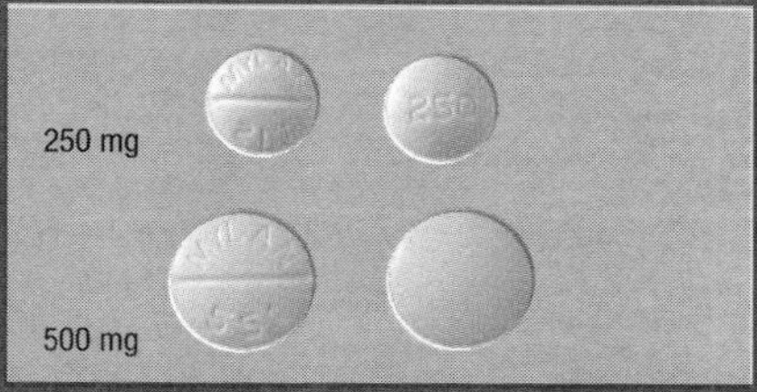

TOLAZamide

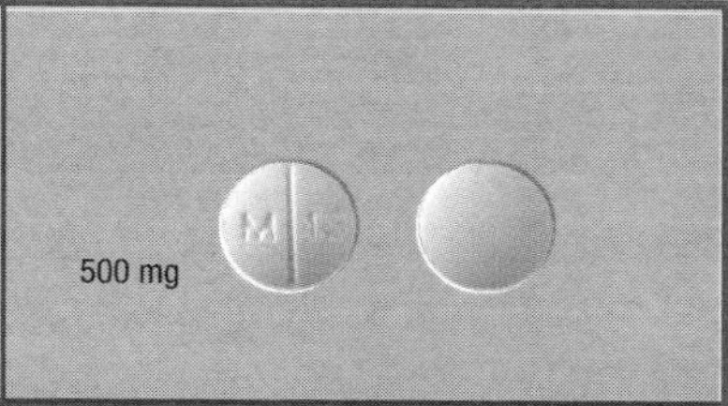

TOLBUTamide

Additional Drugs

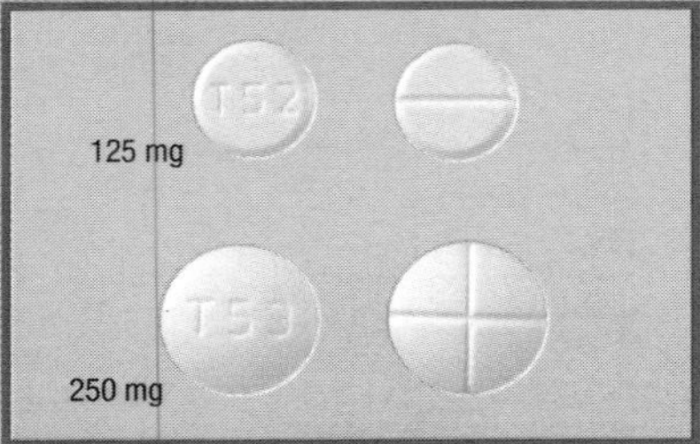

AcetaZOLAMIDE

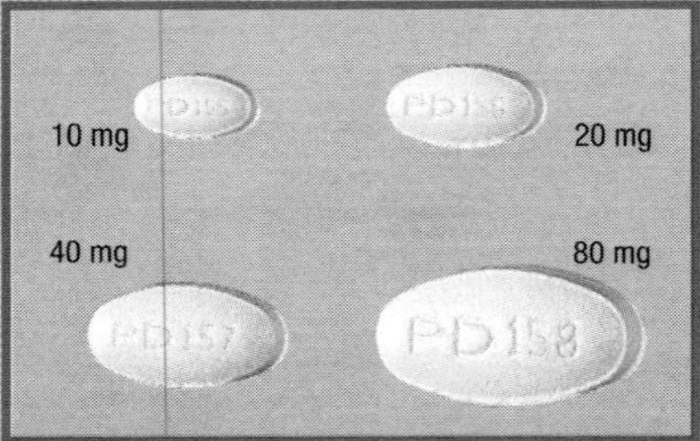

Atorvastatin (Lipitor®)

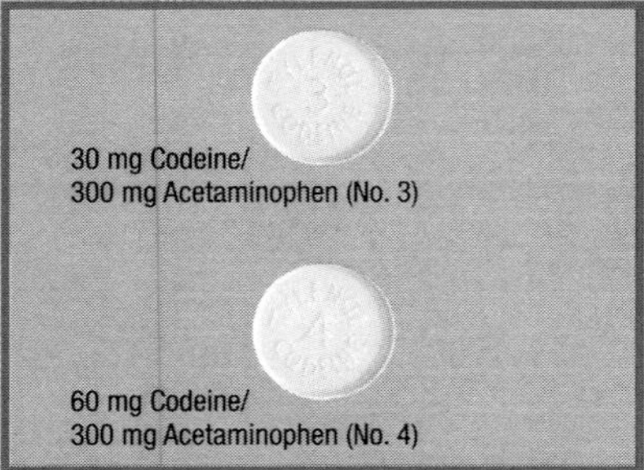

Codeine/Acetaminophen (Tylenol® with Codeine)

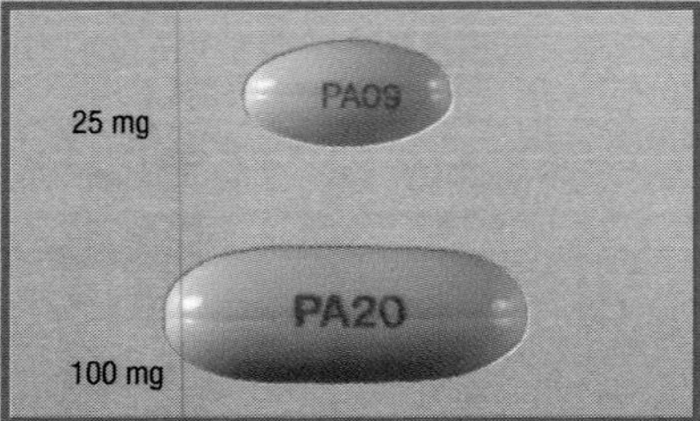

CycloSPORINE

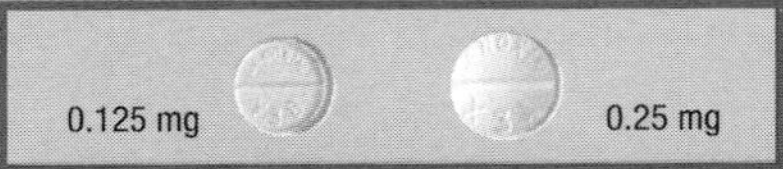

Digoxin (Lanoxin®)

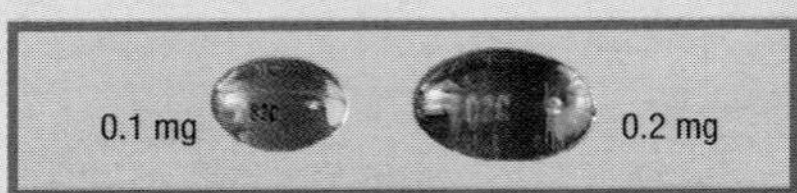

Digoxin (Lanoxicaps®)

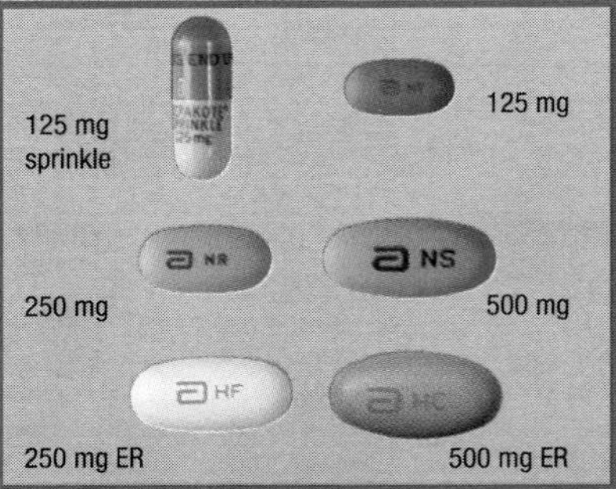

Divalproex (Depakote®)

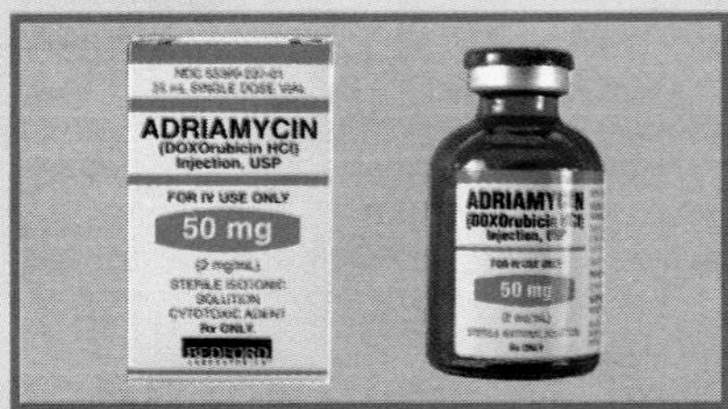

DOXOrubicin (Adriamycin®)

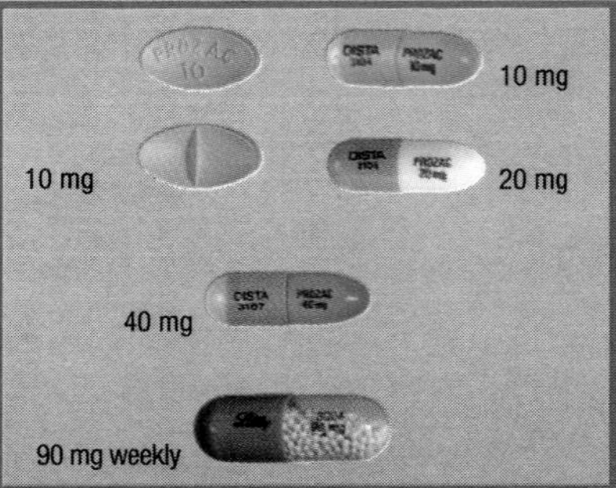

Fluoxetine (Prozac®)

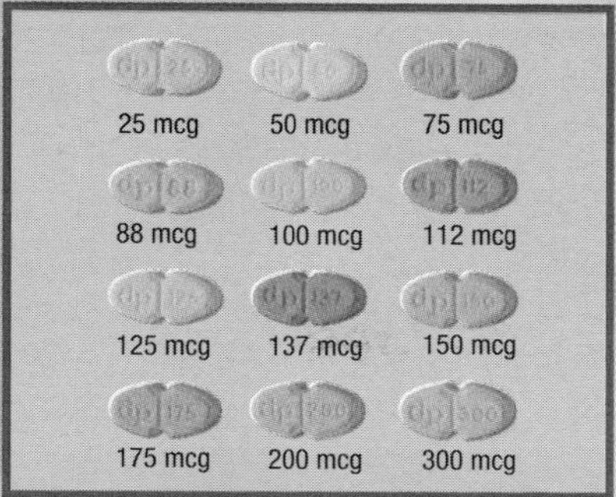

Levothyroxine (Levoxyl®)

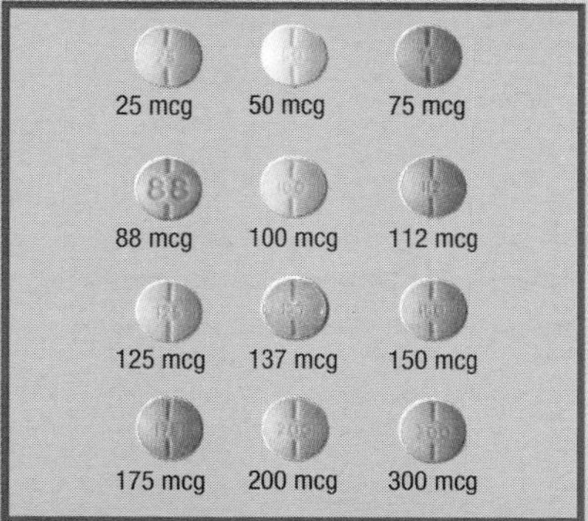

Levothyroxine (Synthroid®)

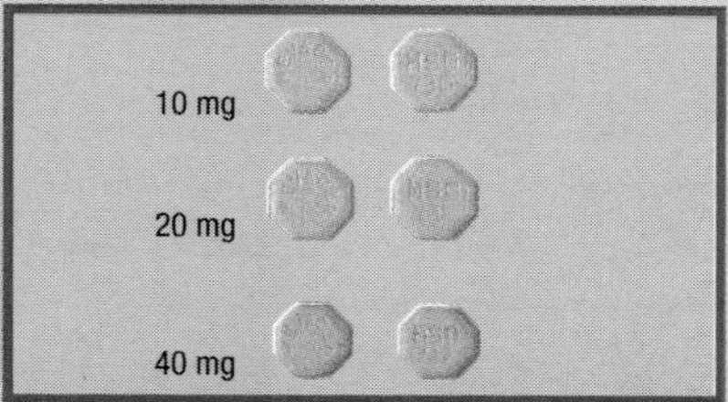

Lovastatin (Mevacor®)

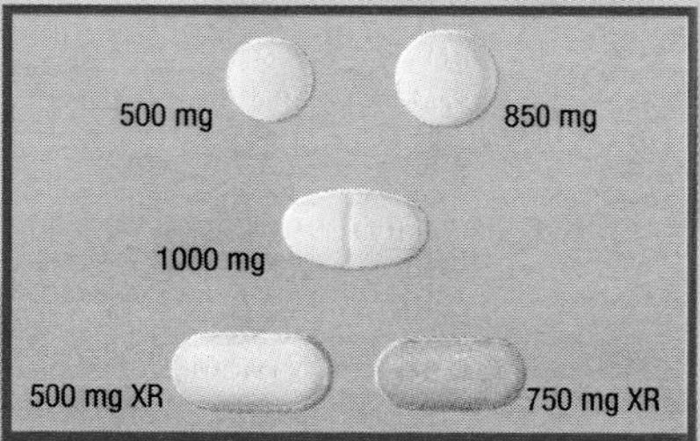

Metformin (Glucophage®)

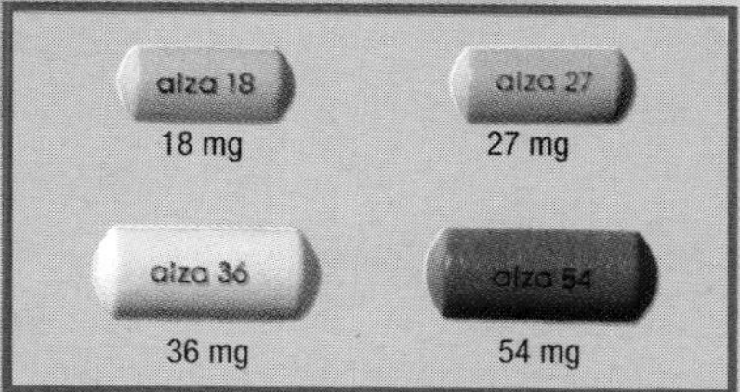

Methylphenidate (Concerta®)

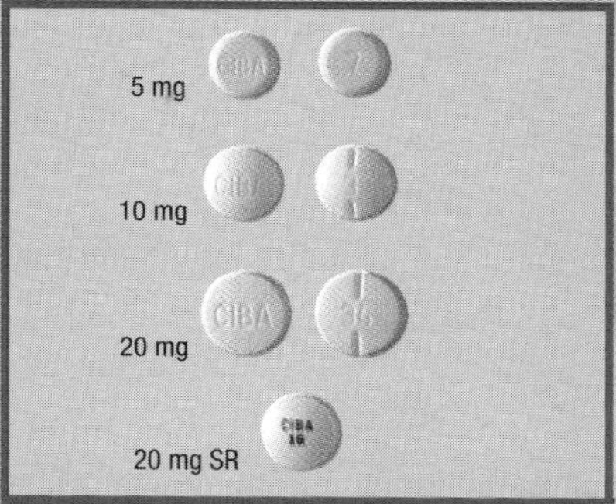

Methylphenidate (Ritalin®)

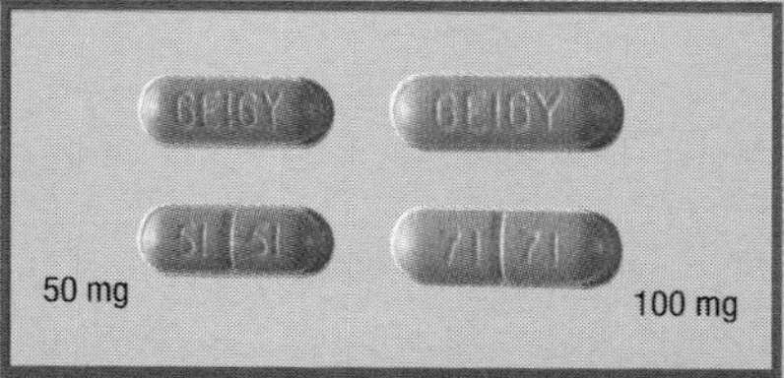

Metoprolol (Toprol XL®)

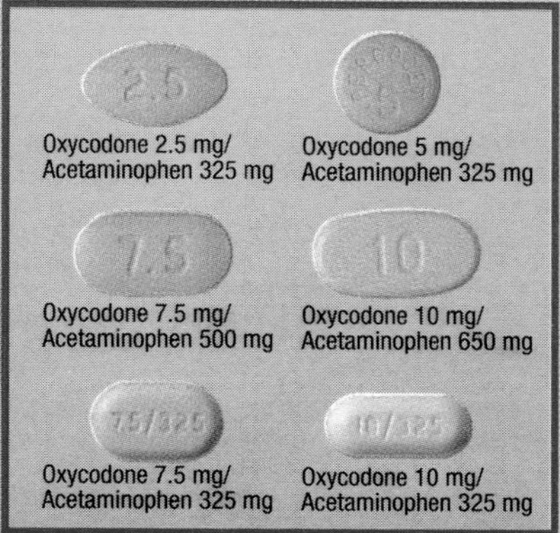

Oxycodone/Acetaminophen (Percocet®)

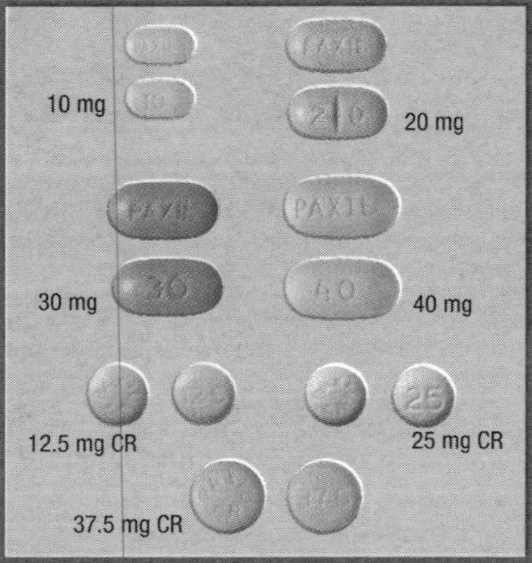

Paroxetine (Paxil®)

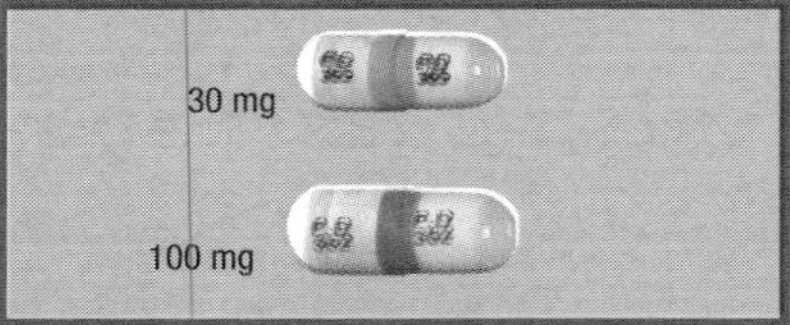

Phenytoin extended (Dilantin® Kapseals®)

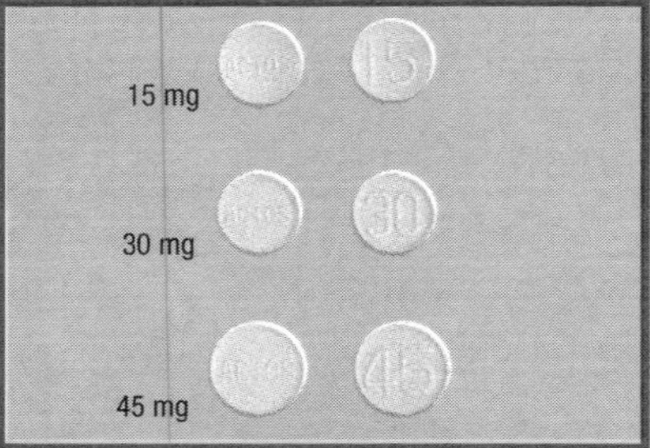

Pioglitazone (Actos®)

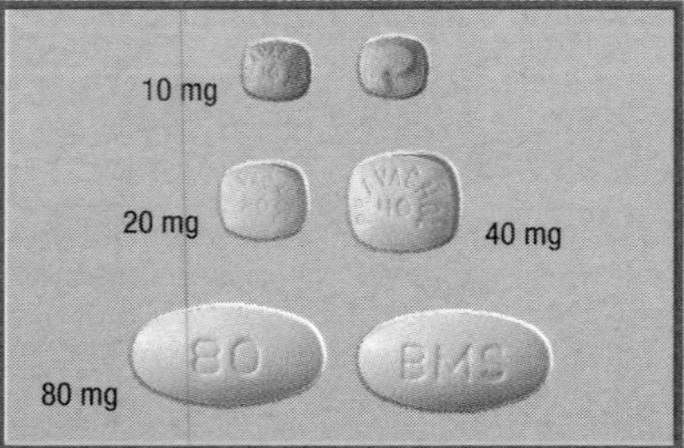

Pravastatin (Pravachol®)

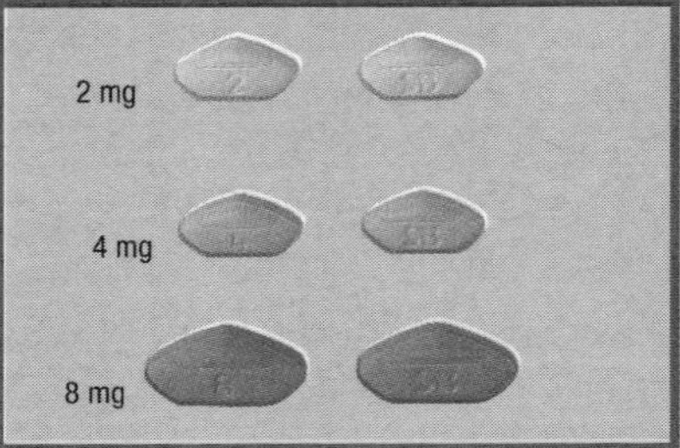

Rosiglitazone (Avandia®)

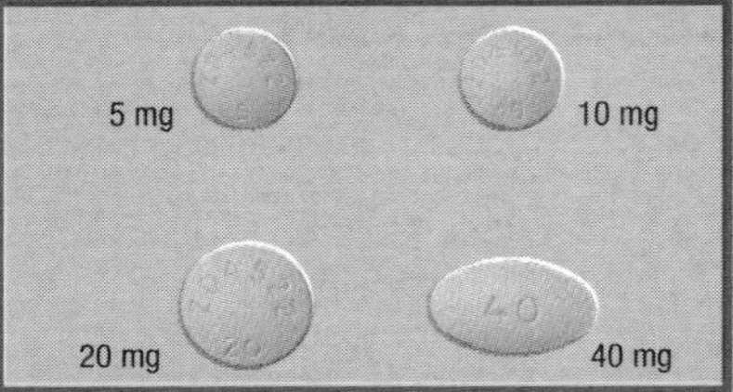

Rosuvastatin (Crestor®)

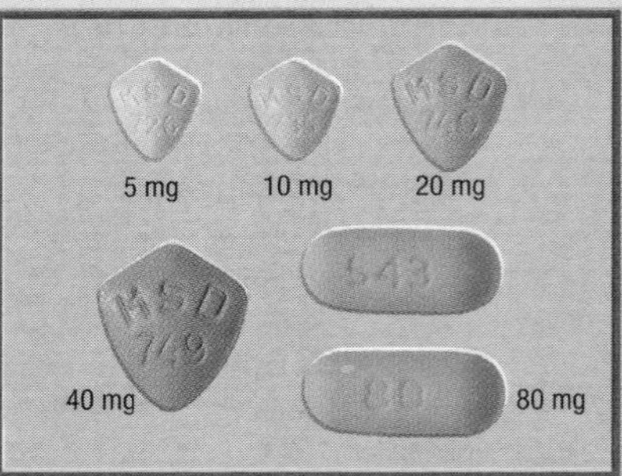

Simvastatin (Zocor®)

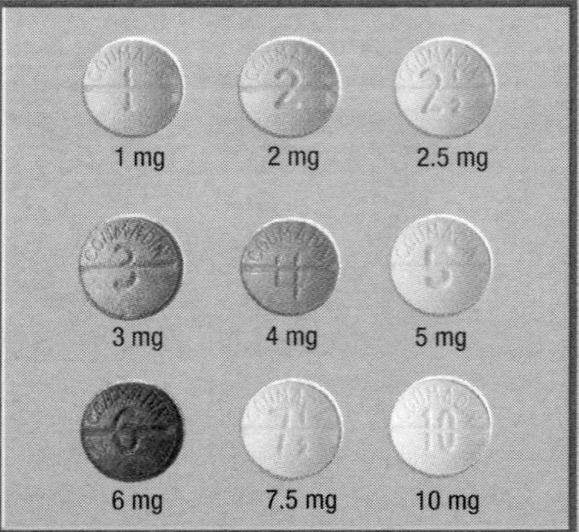

Warfarin (Coumadin®)

rigidity, nausea and vomiting, photosensitivity, and enlarged pupils. Treatment includes IV phentolamine.

Potential Nursing Diagnoses

- Ineffective coping (Indications).
- Risk for injury (Side Effects).
- Deficient knowledge, related to disease processes and medication regimen (Patient/Family Teaching).

Implementation

- Administer drugs that are sedating at bedtime to avoid excessive drowsiness during waking hours, and administer drugs that cause insomnia (fluoxetine, fluvoxamine, paroxetine, sertraline, MAO inhibitors) in the morning.

Patient/Family Teaching

- Caution patient to avoid alcohol and other CNS depressants. Patients receiving MAO inhibitors should also avoid OTC drugs and foods or beverages containing tyramine (see Appendix L) during and for at least 2 wk after therapy has been discontinued, as they may precipitate a hypertensive crisis. Health care professional should be contacted immediately if symptoms of hypertensive crisis develop.
- Inform patient that dizziness or drowsiness may occur. Caution patient to avoid driving and other activities requiring alertness until response to the drug is known.
- Caution patient to make position changes slowly to minimize orthostatic hypotension.
- Advise patient to notify health care professional if dry mouth, urinary retention, or constipation occurs. Frequent rinses, good oral hygiene, and sugarless candy or gum may diminish dry mouth. An increase in fluid intake, fiber, and exercise may prevent constipation.
- Advise patient to notify health care professional of medication regimen and any herbal alternative therapies before treatment or surgery. MAO inhibitor therapy usually needs to be withdrawn at least 2 wk before use of anesthetic agents.
- Emphasize the importance of participation in psychotherapy and follow-up exams to evaluate progress.

Evaluation/Desired Outcomes

- Resolution of depression.
- Decrease in anxiety.
- Control of bedwetting in children over 6 yr of age.
- Management of chronic neurogenic pain.

Antidepressants included in *Davis's Drug Guide for Nurses*

selective serotonin reuptake inhibitors (SSRIs)

citalopram 313
duloxetine 464, 1326
escitalopram 501
fluoxetine 565, 1326
fluvoxamine 572
paroxetine hydrochloride 949
paroxetine mesylate 950
sertraline 1103, 1327

tetracyclic antidepressants

mirtazapine 830

tricyclic antidepressants

amitriptyline 149
desipramine 391
doxepin 452
imipramine 666
nortriptyline 897

monamine oxidase (MAO) inhibitors

isocarboxazid 838
phenelzine 839
tranylcypromine 839

miscellaneous

amoxapine 1270
buPROPion 241
nefazodone 869
selegiline transdermal 1099
trazodone 1200
venlafaxine 1222, 1325

CLASSIFICATIONS

CLASSIFICATIONS

• ANTIDIABETICS

PHARMACOLOGIC PROFILE

General Use

Insulin is used in the management of type 1 diabetes mellitus. It may also be used in type 2 diabetes mellitus when diet and/or oral medications fail to adequately control blood sugar. The choice of insulin preparation (rapid-acting, intermediate-acting, long-acting) and source (semisynthetic, human recombinant DNA) depend on the degree of control desired, daily blood glucose fluctuations, and history of previous reactions. Oral agents are used primarily in type 2 diabetes mellitus. Oral agents are used when diet therapy alone fails to control blood glucose or symptoms or when patients are not amenable to using insulin. Some oral agents may be used with insulin.

General Action and Information

Insulin, a hormone produced by the pancreas, lowers blood glucose by increasing transport of glucose into cells and promotes the conversion of glucose to glycogen. It also promotes the conversion of amino acids to proteins in muscle, stimulates triglyceride formation, and inhibits the release of free fatty acids. Sulfonylureas, nateglinide, repaglinide, and metformin lower blood glucose by stimulating endogenous insulin secretion by beta cells of the pancreas and by increasing sensitivity to insulin at intracellular receptor sites. Intact pancreatic function is required. Miglitol delays digestion of ingested carbohydrates, thus lowering blood glucose, especially after meals. It may be combined with sulfonylureas. Pioglitazone and rosiglitazone increase insulin sensitivity.

Contraindications

Insulin— Hypoglycemia. **Oral hypoglycemic agents—** Hypersensitivity (cross-sensitivity with other sulfonylureas and sulfonamides may exist). Hypoglycemia. Type 1 diabetes. Avoid use in patients with severe kidney, liver, thyroid, and other endocrine dysfunction. Should not be used in pregnancy or lactation.

Precautions

Insulin— Infection, stress, or changes in diet may alter requirements. **Oral hypoglycemic agents—** Use cautiously in geriatric patients. Dose reduction may be necessary. Infection, stress, or changes in diet may alter requirements. Use with sulfonylureas with caution in patients with a history of cardiovascular disease. Metformin may cause lactic acidosis.

Interactions

Insulin— Additive hypoglycemic effects with oral hypoglycemic agents. **Oral hypoglycemic agents—** Ingestion of alcohol may result in disulfiram-like reaction with some agents. Alcohol, corticosteroids, rifampin, glucagon, and thiazide diuretics may decrease effectiveness. Anabolic steroids, chloramphenicol, clofibrate, MAO inhibitors, most NSAIDs, salicylates, sulfonamides, and warfarin may increase hypoglycemic effect. Beta blockers may produce hypoglycemia and mask signs and symptoms.

NURSING IMPLICATIONS

Assessment

- Observe patient for signs and symptoms of hypoglycemic reactions.
- Acarbose, miglitol, and pioglitazone do not cause hypoglycemia when taken alone but may increase the hypoglycemic effect of other hypoglycemic agents.
- Patients who have been well controlled on metformin but develop illness or laboratory abnormalities should be assessed for ketoacidosis or lactic acidosis. Assess serum electrolytes, ketones, glucose, and, if indicated, blood pH, lactate, pyruvate, and metformin levels. If either form of acidosis is present, discontinue metformin immediately and treat acidosis.

- **Lab Test Considerations:** Serum glucose and glycosylated hemoglobin should be monitored periodically throughout therapy to evaluate effectiveness of treatment.

Potential Nursing Diagnoses

- Imbalanced nutrition: more than body requirements (Indications).
- Deficient knowledge, related to medication regimen (Patient/Family Teaching).
- Noncompliance (Patient/Family Teaching).

Implementation

- Patients stabilized on a diabetic regimen who are exposed to stress, fever, trauma, infection, or surgery may require sliding scale insulin. Withhold oral hypoglycemic agents and reinstitute after resolution of acute episode.
- Patients switching from daily insulin dose may require gradual conversion to oral hypoglycemics.
- **Insulin:** Available in different types and strengths and from different species. Check type, species, source, dose, and expiration date with another licensed nurse. Do not interchange insulins without physician's order. Use only insulin syringes to draw up dose. Use only U100 syringes to draw up insulin lispro dose.

Patient/Family Teaching

- Explain to patient that medication controls hyperglycemia but does not cure diabetes. Therapy is long-term.
- Review signs of hypoglycemia and hyperglycemia with patient. If hypoglycemia occurs, advise patient to take a glass of orange juice or 2–3 tsp of sugar, honey, or corn syrup dissolved in water (glucose, not table sugar, if taking miglitol), and notify health care professional.
- Encourage patient to follow prescribed diet, medication, and exercise regimen to prevent hypoglycemic or hyperglycemic episodes.
- Instruct patient in proper testing of serum glucose and ketones.
- Advise patient to notify health care professional if nausea, vomiting, or fever develops; if unable to eat usual diet; or if blood glucose levels are not controlled.
- Advise patient to carry sugar or a form of glucose and identification describing medication regimen at all times.
- Insulin is the recommended method of controlling blood glucose during pregnancy. Counsel female patients to use a form of contraception other than oral contraceptives and to notify health care professional promptly if pregnancy is planned or suspected.
- **Insulin:** Instruct patient on proper technique for administration; include type of insulin, equipment (syringe and cartridge pens), storage, and syringe disposal. Discuss the importance of not changing brands of insulin or syringes, selection and rotation of injection sites, and compliance with therapeutic regimen.
- **Sulfonylureas:** Advise patient that concurrent use of alcohol may cause a disulfiram-like reaction (abdominal cramps, nausea, flushing, headache, and hypoglycemia).
- **Metformin:** Explain to patient the risk of lactic acidosis and the potential need for discontinuation of metformin therapy if a severe infection, dehydration, or severe or continuing diarrhea occurs or if medical tests or surgery is required.

Evaluation/Desired Outcomes

- Control of blood glucose levels without the appearance of hypoglycemic or hyperglycemic episodes.

Antidiabetics included in *Davis's Drug Guide for Nurses*

alpha-glucosidase inhibitors
acarbose 104
miglitol 827

biguanides
metformin 793

enzyme inhibitors
sitagliptin 1112, 1327

hormone
pramlintide 1001
incretrin mimetic agent
exenatide 525
insulins
concentrated regular insulin 40
insulin aspart protamine suspension/insulin aspart solution mixtures, rDNA origin 678, 1380
insulin aspart, rDNA origin 670, 1380
insulin detemir 685, 1380
insulin glargine 685, 1380
insulin glulisine 670, 1380
insulin lispro protamine suspension/insulin lispro solution mixtures, rDNA origin 678
insulin lispro, rDNA origin 670, 1380
insulin lispro/protamine insulin lispro mixture, rDNA origin 40
insulin, regular (injection, concentrated) 681
NPH insulin (isophane insulin suspension) 683, 1380
NPH/regular insulin mixtures 678, 1380
regular insulin (insulin injection) 40, 1380
meglitinides
nateglinide 868
repaglinide 1058
sulfonylureas
glimepiride 648
glipiZIDE 648
glyBURIDE 648
thiazolidinediones
pioglitazone 986
rosiglitazone 1082

• ANTIDIARRHEALS

PHARMACOLOGIC PROFILE

General Use
For the control and symptomatic relief of acute and chronic nonspecific diarrhea.

General Action and Information
Diphenoxylate/atropine, difenoxin/atropine, and loperamide slow intestinal motility and propulsion. Kaolin/pectin and bismuth subsalicylate affect fluid content of the stool. Bismuth subsalicylate is also used a part of the management of ulcer disease due to *Helicobacter pylori*. Polycarbophil acts as an antidiarrheal by taking on water within the bowel lumen to create a formed stool. Polycarbophil may also be used to treat constipation. Octreotide is used specifically for diarrhea associated with GI endocrine tumors.

Contraindications
Previous hypersensitivity. Severe abdominal pain of unknown cause, especially when associated with fever.

Precautions
Use cautiously in patients with severe liver disease or inflammatory bowel disease. Safety in pregnancy and lactation not established (diphenoxylate/atropine and loperamide). Octreotide may aggravate gallbladder disease.

Interactions
Kaolin may decrease absorption of digoxin. Polycarbophil decreases the absorption of tetracycline. Octreotide may alter the response to insulin or oral hypoglycemic agents.

NURSING IMPLICATIONS

Assessment
- Assess the frequency and consistency of stools and bowel sounds before and throughout therapy.
- Assess patient's fluid and electrolyte status and skin turgor for dehydration.

Potential Nursing Diagnoses
- Diarrhea (Indications).
- Constipation (Side Effects).
- Deficient knowledge, related to disease processes and medication regimen (Patient/Family Teaching).

Implementation
- Shake liquid preparations before administration.

Patient/Family Teaching
- Instruct patient to notify health care professional if diarrhea persists; or if fever, abdominal pain, or palpitations occur.

Evaluation/Desired Outcomes
- Decrease in diarrhea.

Antidiarrheals included in *Davis's Drug Guide for Nurses*

bismuth subsalicylate 225
difenoxin/atropine 427
diphenoxylate/atropine 427
loperamide 756
octreotide 901, 1326
polycarbophil 1289

• ANTIEMETICS

PHARMACOLOGIC PROFILE

General Use
Phenothiazines, dolasetron, granisetron, metoclopramide, and ondansetron are used to manage nausea and vomiting of many causes, including surgery, anesthesia, and antineoplastic and radiation therapy. Palonosetron and aprepitant are used specifically with emetogenic chemotherapy. Dimenhydrinate, scopolamine, and meclizine are used almost exclusively to prevent motion sickness.

General Action and Information
Phenothiazines act on the chemoreceptor trigger zone to inhibit nausea and vomiting. Dimenhydrinate, scopolamine, and meclizine act as antiemetics mainly by diminishing motion sickness. Metoclopramide decreases nausea and vomiting by its effects on gastric emptying. Dolasetron, granisetron, palonosetron, and ondansetron block the effects of serotonin at 5-HT_3 receptor sites.

Contraindications
Previous hypersensitivity.

Precautions
Use phenothiazines cautiously in children who may have viral illnesses. Choose agents carefully in pregnant patients (no agents are approved for safe use).

Interactions
Additive CNS depression with other CNS depressants including antidepressants, antihistamines, opioid analgesics, and sedative/hypnotics. Phenothiazines may produce hypotension when used with antihypertensives, nitrates, or acute ingestion of alcohol.

NURSING IMPLICATIONS

Assessment
- Assess nausea, vomiting, bowel sounds, and abdominal pain before and following administration.

- Monitor hydration status and intake and output. Patients with severe nausea and vomiting may require IV fluids in addition to antiemetics.

Potential Nursing Diagnoses

- Deficient fluid volume (Indications).
- Imbalanced nutrition: less than body requirements (Indications).
- Risk for injury (Side Effects).

Implementation

- For prophylactic administration, follow directions for specific drugs so that peak effect corresponds to time of anticipated nausea.
- Phenothiazines should be discontinued 48 hr before and not resumed for 24 hr following myelography, as they lower seizure threshold.

Patient/Family Teaching

- Advise patient and family to use general measures to decrease nausea (begin with sips of liquids and small, nongreasy meals; provide oral hygiene; and remove noxious stimuli from environment).
- May cause drowsiness. Advise patient to call for assistance when ambulating and to avoid driving or other activities requiring alertness until response to medication is known.
- Advise patient to make position changes slowly to minimize orthostatic hypotension.

Evaluation/Desired Outcomes

- Prevention of, or decrease in, nausea and vomiting.

Antiemetics included in *Davis's Drug Guide for Nurses*

5-HT$_3$ antagonists
dolasetron 445
granisetron 605
ondansetron 910
palonosetron 941, 1327
phenothiazines
chlorproMAZINE 301
prochlorperazine 1012
promethazine 1017
thiethylperazine 1293
miscellaneous
aprepitant 187
dimenhyDRINATE 420
meclizine 775
metoclopramide 810
scopolamine 1096, 1353

• ANTIFUNGALS

PHARMACOLOGIC PROFILE

General Use

Treatment of fungal infections. Infections of skin or mucous membranes may be treated with topical or vaginal preparations. Deep-seated or systemic infections require oral or parenteral therapy. New parenteral formulations of amphotericin employ lipid encapsulation technology designed to decrease toxicity.

General Action and Information

Kill (fungicidal) or stop growth of (fungistatic) susceptible fungi by affecting the permeability of the fungal cell membrane or protein synthesis within the fungal cell itself.

Contraindications

Previous hypersensitivity.

Precautions

Because most systemic antifungals may have adverse effects on bone marrow function, use cautiously in patients with depressed bone marrow reserve. Amphotericin B commonly causes renal impairment. Fluconazole requires dosage adjustment in the presence of renal impairment. Adverse reactions to fluconazole may be more severe in HIV-positive patients.

Interactions

Differ greatly among various agents. See individual drugs.

NURSING IMPLICATIONS

Assessment

- Assess patient for signs of infection and assess involved areas of skin and mucous membranes before and throughout therapy. Increased skin irritation may indicate need to discontinue medication.

Potential Nursing Diagnoses

- Risk for infection (Indications).
- Impaired skin integrity (Indications).
- Deficient knowledge, related to disease processes and medication regimen (Patient/Family Teaching).

Implementation

- Available in various dosage forms. Refer to specific drugs for directions for administration.
- **Topical:** Consult physician or other health care professional for cleansing technique before applying medication. Wear gloves during application. Do not use occlusive dressings unless specified by physician or other health care professional.

Patient/Family Teaching

- Instruct patient on proper use of medication form.
- Instruct patient to continue medication as directed for full course of therapy, even if feeling better.
- Advise patient to report increased skin irritation or lack of therapeutic response to health care professional.

Evaluation/Desired Outcomes

- Resolution of signs and symptoms of infection. Length of time for complete resolution depends on organism and site of infection. Deep-seated fungal infections may require prolonged therapy (weeks–months). Recurrent fungal infections may be a sign of serious systemic illness.

Antifungals included in *Davis's Drug Guide for Nurses*

echinocandins
anidulafungin 180
caspofungin 273
micafungin 821

systemic
amphotericin B cholesteryl sulfate 160
amphotericin B deoxycholate 160
amphotericin B lipid complex 160
amphotericin B liposome 43
fluconazole 552
itraconazole 710
ketoconazole (systemic) 713
posaconazole 993
terbinafine 181, 1147, 1325
voriconazole 1241, 1325, 1327

topical/local
butenafine 181
butoconazole 184
ciclopirox 181
clotrimazole 181, 184
econazole 181
ketoconazole 181
miconazole 181, 184
naftifine 181
nystatin 181, 184, 899
oxiconazole 181
sertaconazole 1102
sulconazole 181
terbinafine 181, 1147, 1325
terconazole 184
tioconazole 184
tolnaftate 181

CLASSIFICATIONS

• ANTIHISTAMINES

PHARMACOLOGIC PROFILE

General Use

Relief of symptoms associated with allergies, including rhinitis, urticaria, and angioedema, and as adjunctive therapy in anaphylactic reactions. Topical and ophthalmic antihistamines may immunize systemic side effects. Some antihistamines are used to treat motion sickness (dimenhydrinate and meclizine), insomnia (diphenhydramine), Parkinson-like reactions (diphenhydramine), and other nonallergic conditions.

General Action and Information

Antihistamines block the effects of histamine at the H_1 receptor. They do not block histamine release, antibody production, or antigen-antibody reactions. Most antihistamines have anticholinergic properties and may cause constipation, dry eyes, dry mouth, and blurred vision. In addition, many antihistamines cause sedation. Some phenothiazines have strong antihistaminic properties (hydroxyzine and promethazine).

Contraindications

Hypersensitivity and angle-closure glaucoma. Should not be used in premature or newborn infants.

Precautions

Elderly patients may be more susceptible to adverse anticholinergic effects of antihistamines. Use cautiously in patients with pyloric obstruction, prostatic hypertrophy, hyperthyroidism, cardiovascular disease, or severe liver disease. Use cautiously in pregnancy and lactation.

Interactions

Additive sedation when used with other CNS depressants, including alcohol, antidepressants, opioid analgesics, and sedative/hypnotics. MAO inhibitors prolong and intensify the anticholinergic properties of antihistamines.

NURSING IMPLICATIONS

Assessment

- Assess allergy symptoms (rhinitis, conjunctivitis, hives) before and periodically throughout therapy.
- Monitor pulse and blood pressure before initiating and throughout IV therapy.
- Assess lung sounds and character of bronchial secretions. Maintain fluid intake of 1500–2000 ml/day to decrease viscosity of secretions.
- **Nausea and Vomiting:** Assess degree of nausea and frequency and amount of emesis when administering for nausea and vomiting.
- **Anxiety:** Assess mental status, mood, and behavior when administering for anxiety.
- **Pruritus:** Observe the character, location, and size of affected area when administering for pruritic skin conditions.

Potential Nursing Diagnoses

- Ineffective airway clearance (Indications).
- Risk for injury (Adverse Reactions).
- Deficient knowledge, related to disease processes and medication regimen (Patient/Family Teaching).

Implementation

- When used for prophylaxis of motion sickness, administer at least 30 min and preferably 1–2 hr before exposure to conditions that may precipitate motion sickness.

- When administering concurrently with opioid analgesics (hydroxyzine, promethazine), supervise ambulation closely to prevent injury secondary to increased sedation.

Patient/Family Teaching

- Inform patient that drowsiness may occur. Avoid driving or other activities requiring alertness until response to drug is known.
- Caution patient to avoid using concurrent alcohol or CNS depressants.
- Advise patient that good oral hygiene, frequent rinsing of mouth with water, and sugarless gum or candy may help relieve dryness of mouth.
- Instruct patient to contact health care professional if symptoms persist.

Evaluation/Desired Outcomes

- Decrease in allergic symptoms.
- Prevention or decreased severity of nausea and vomiting.
- Decrease in anxiety.
- Relief of pruritus.
- Sedation when used as a hypnotic.

Antihistamines included in *Davis's Drug Guide for Nurses*

systemic
azatadine 45
brompheniramine 1273
cetirizine 293
chlorpheniramine 300
cyproheptadine 367
desloratadine 395
dimenhyDRINATE 420
diphenhydrAMINE 424
fexofenadine 545
hydrOXYzine 644
loratadine 760
meclizine 775
promethazine 1017

ophthalmic antihistamines
azelastine 1349
emedastine 1349
epinastine 1349
levocabastine 45
olopatadine 1349

topical
doxepin 452

• ANTIHYPERTENSIVES

PHARMACOLOGIC PROFILE

General Use

Treatment of hypertension of many causes, most commonly essential hypertension. Parenteral products are used in the treatment of hypertensive emergencies. Oral treatment should be initiated as soon as possible and individualized to ensure adherence and compliance for long-term therapy. Therapy is initiated with agents having minimal side effects. When such therapy fails, more potent drugs with different side effects are added in an effort to control blood pressure while causing minimal patient discomfort.

General Action and Information

As a group, the antihypertensives are used to lower blood pressure to a normal level (<90 mm Hg diastolic) or to the lowest level tolerated. The goal of antihypertensive therapy is prevention of end-organ damage. Antihypertensives are classified into groups according to their site of action. These include peripherally-acting antiadrenergics; centrally-acting alpha-adrenergics; beta blockers; vasodilators; ACE inhibitors; angiotensin II antagonists; calcium channel blockers; and diuretics. Hypertensive emergencies may be managed with parenteral agents, such as enalaprilat or fenoldopam.

CLASSIFICATIONS

Contraindications

Hypersensitivity to individual agents.

Precautions

Choose agents carefully in pregnancy, during lactation, or in patients receiving digoxin. ACE inhibitors and angiotensin II antagonists should be avoided during pregnancy. Alpha-adrenergic agonists and beta blockers should be used only in patients who will comply, because abrupt discontinuation of these agents may result in rapid and excessive rise in blood pressure (rebound phenomenon). Thiazide diuretics may increase the requirement for treatment of diabetics. Vasodilators may cause tachycardia if used alone and are commonly used in combination with beta blockers. Some antihypertensives cause sodium and water retention and are usually combined with a diuretic.

Interactions

Many drugs can negate the therapeutic effectiveness of antihypertensives, including antihistamines, NSAIDs, sympathomimetic bronchodilators, decongestants, appetite suppressants, antidepressants, and MAO inhibitors. Hypokalemia from diuretics may increase the risk of digoxin toxicity. Potassium supplements and potassium-sparing diuretics may cause hyperkalemia when used with ACE inhibitors.

NURSING IMPLICATIONS

Assessment

- Monitor blood pressure and pulse frequently during dosage adjustment and periodically throughout therapy.
- Monitor intake and output ratios and daily weight.
- Monitor frequency of prescription refills to determine compliance.

Potential Nursing Diagnoses

- Ineffective tissue perfusion (Indications).
- Deficient knowledge, related to disease processes and medication regimen (Patient/Family Teaching).
- Noncompliance (Patient/Family Teaching).

Implementation

- Many antihypertensives are available as combination products to enhance compliance (see Appendix B).

Patient/Family Teaching

- Instruct patient to continue taking medication, even if feeling well. Abrupt withdrawal may cause rebound hypertension. Medication controls, but does not cure, hypertension.
- Encourage patient to comply with additional interventions for hypertension (weight reduction, low-sodium diet, regular exercise, discontinuation of smoking, moderation of alcohol consumption, and stress management).
- Instruct patient and family on proper technique for monitoring blood pressure. Advise them to check blood pressure weekly and report significant changes.
- Caution patient to make position changes slowly to minimize orthostatic hypotension. Advise patient that exercise or hot weather may enhance hypotensive effects.
- Advise patient to consult health care professional before taking any OTC medications, especially cold remedies.
- Advise patient to inform health care professional of medication regimen before treatment or surgery.
- Patients taking ACE inhibitors or angiotensin II antagonists should notify health care professional if pregnancy is planned or suspected.
- Emphasize the importance of follow-up exams to monitor progress.

Evaluation/Desired Outcomes

- Decrease in blood pressure.

Antihypertensives included in *Davis's Drug Guide for Nurses*

adrenergics
clonidine 321
aldosterone antagonists
eplerenone 486
ACE inhibitors
benazepril 170
captopril 170
enalapril/enalaprilat 170
fosinopril 170
lisinopril 170
moexipril 170
perindopril 170
quinapril 170
ramipril 170
trandolapril 170
angiotensin II receptor antagonists
candesartan 177
eprosartan 177
irbesartan 177
losartan 177
olmesartan 177
telmisartan 177
valsartan 177, 1327
beta blockers (nonselective)
carteolol 1273
carvedilol 271
labetalol 719
nadolol 856
penbutolol 47
pindolol 1288
propranolol 1026, 1327
timolol 1179, 1352
beta blockers (selective)
acebutolol 105
atenolol 197
betaxolol 219, 1351
bisoprolol 226
metoprolol 814
nebivolol 1323
calcium channel blockers
amlodipine 151
diltiazem 418
felodipine 530
isradipine 708
niCARdipine 879
NIFEdipine 884
nisoldipine 889, 1325
verapamil 1224
centrally acting antiadrenergics
guanfacine 47
methyldopa 804
loop diuretics
torsemide 1194
peripherally acting antiadrenergics
doxazosin 450
prazosin 1003
terazosin 1145
thiazide diuretics
chlorothiazide 434
chlorthalidone (thiazide–like) 434
hydrochlorothiazide 434
thiazide-like diuretics
indapamide 672
metolazone 812
vasodilators
fenoldopam 534
hydrALAZINE 633
minoxidil (systemic) 1284
nitroprusside 895

• ANTI-INFECTIVES

PHARMACOLOGIC PROFILE

General Use

Treatment and prophylaxis of various bacterial infections. See specific drugs for spectrum and indications. Some infections may require additional surgical intervention and supportive therapy.

CLASSIFICATIONS

General Action and Information

Kill (bactericidal) or inhibit the growth of (bacteriostatic) susceptible pathogenic bacteria. Not active against viruses or fungi. Anti-infectives are subdivided into categories depending on chemical similarities and antimicrobial spectrum.

Contraindications

Known hypersensitivity to individual agents. Cross-sensitivity among related agents may occur.

Precautions

Culture and susceptibility testing are desirable to optimize therapy. Dosage modification may be required in patients with hepatic or renal insufficiency. Use cautiously in pregnant and lactating women. Prolonged inappropriate use of broad spectrum anti-infective agents may lead to superinfection with fungi or resistant bacteria.

Interactions

Penicillins and aminoglycosides chemically inactivate each other and should not be physically admixed. Erythromycins may decrease hepatic metabolism of other drugs. Probenecid increases serum levels of penicillins and related compounds. Highly protein-bound anti-infectives such as sulfonamides may displace or be displaced by other highly bound drugs. See individual drugs. Extended-spectrum penicillins (ticarcillin, piperacillin) and some cephalosporins (cefoperazone, cefotetan) may increase the risk of bleeding with anticoagulants, thrombolytic agents, antiplatelet agents, or NSAIDs. Fluoroquinolone absorption is decreased by antacids, bismuth subsalicylate, iron salts, sucralfate, and zinc salts.

NURSING IMPLICATIONS

Assessment

- Assess patient for signs and symptoms of infection prior to and throughout therapy.
- Determine previous hypersensitivities in patients receiving penicillins or cephalosporins.
- Obtain specimens for culture and sensitivity prior to initiating therapy. First dose may be given before receiving results.

Potential Nursing Diagnoses

- Risk for infection (Indications).
- Deficient knowledge, related to disease processes and medication regimen (Patient/Family Teaching).
- Noncompliance (Patient/Family Teaching).

Implementation

- Most anti-infectives should be administered around the clock to maintain therapeutic serum drug levels.

Patient/Family Teaching

- Instruct patient to continue taking medication around the clock until finished completely, even if feeling better.
- Advise patient to report the signs of superinfection (black, furry overgrowth on the tongue; vaginal itching or discharge; loose or foul-smelling stools) and allergy to health care professional.
- Instruct patient to notify health care professional if fever and diarrhea develop, especially if stool contains pus, blood, or mucus. Advise patient not to treat diarrhea without consulting health care professional.
- Instruct patient to notify health care professional if symptoms do not improve.

Evaluation/Desired Outcomes

- Resolution of the signs and symptoms of infection. Length of time for complete resolution depends on organism and site of infection.

Anti-infectives included in *Davis's Drug Guide for Nurses*

aminoglycosides
amikacin 140
gentamicin 140, 1350
kanamycin 140
neomycin 140
streptomycin 140
tobramycin 140, 1351

carbapenems
doripenem 1321
ertapenem 496
imipenem/cilastatin 664
meropenem 787, 1326

first-generation cephalosporins
cefadroxil 279
cefazolin 279
cephalexin 279
cephradine 279

second-generation cephalosporins
cefaclor 282
cefotetan 282
cefoxitin 282
cefprozil 282
cefuroxime 282

third-generation cephalosporins
cefdinir 286
cefditoren 287
cefixime 287
cefoperazone 287
cefotaxime 287
cefpodoxime 287
ceftazidime 287
ceftibuten 287
ceftizoxime 287
ceftriaxone 287

extended spectrum penicillins
piperacillin 49
piperacillin/tazobactam 987
ticarcillin 49
ticarcillin/clavulanate 1174

fluoroquinolones
ciprofloxacin 557, 1350
gemifloxacin 557
levofloxacin 557, 1350
moxifloxacin 557, 1326, 1350
norfloxacin 557, 1350
ofloxacin 558, 1350

macrolides
azithromycin 208, 1325–1326, 1349
clarithromycin 315
erythromycin 498, 1326, 1350

penicillins
amoxicillin 153, 1325
amoxicillin/clavulanate 155
ampicillin 164
ampicillin/sulbactam 166
benzathine penicillin G 958
cloxacillin 961
dicloxacillin 961
nafcillin 961
oxacillin 961
penicillin G 958
penicillin V 958
procaine penicillin G 958

doxycycline 1155, 1325
minocycline 1155
tetracycline 1155
tetracyclines 1155

miscellaneous
trimethoprim/sulfamethoxazole 1205
cefepime 275
clindamycin 317
daptomycin 376
drotrecogin 463
linezolid 752
metronidazole 817
mupirocin 847
nitrofurantoin 890
quinupristin/dalfopristin 1049
rifaximin 1068
telithromycin 1141
tigecycline 1177
trimethoprim 1203
vancomycin 1215

• ANTINEOPLASTICS

PHARMACOLOGIC PROFILE

General Use

Used in the treatment of various solid tumors, lymphomas, and leukemias. Also used in some autoimmune disorders such as rheumatoid arthritis (cyclophosphamide, methotrexate). Often used in combinations to minimize individual toxicities and increase response. Chemotherapy may be combined with other treatment modalities such as surgery and radiation therapy. Dosages vary greatly, depending on extent of disease, other agents used, and patient's condition. Some new formulations (daunorubicin, doxorubicin) encapsulated in a lipid membrane have less toxicity with greater efficacy.

General Action and Information

Act by many different mechanisms (see the following table). Many affect DNA synthesis or function; others alter immune function or affect hormonal status of sensitive tumors. Action may not be limited to neoplastic cells.

MECHANISM OF ACTION OF VARIOUS ANTINEOPLASTICS

MECHANISM OF ACTION	AGENT	EFFECTS ON CELL CYCLE
ALKYLATING AGENTS	busulfan	Cell cycle–nonspecific
Cause cross-linking of DNA	carboplatin	
	chlorambucil	
	cisplatin	
	cyclophosphamide	
	ifosfamide	
	mechlorethamine	
	melphalan	
	procarbazine	
	temozolamide	
ANTHRACYCLINES	daunorubicin	Cell cycle–nonspecific
Interfere with DNA and RNA synthesis	doxorubicin	
	epirubicin	
	idarubicin	
ANTITUMOR ANTIBIOTIC	bleomycin	Cell cycle–nonspecific (except bleomycin)
Interfere with DNA and RNA synthesis	mitomycin	
	mitoxantrone	
ANTIMETABOLITES	cytarabine	Cell cycle–specific, work mostly in S phase (DNA synthesis)
Take the place of normal proteins	fluorouracil	
	hydroxyurea	
	methotrexate	
ENZYMES	asparaginase	Cell-cycle phase–specific
Deplete asparagine	pegaspargase	
ENZYME INHIBITORS	irinotecan	Cell-cycle phase–specific
Inhibits topoisomerase	topotecan	
Inhibits kinase	imatinib	Unknown
HORMONAL AGENTS	bicalutamide	Unknown
Alter hormonal status in tumors that are sensitive	estramustine	
	flutamide	
	leuprolide	
	megestrol	
	nilutamide	
	tamoxifen	
	testosterone (androgens)	
	triptorelin	
HORMONAL AGENTS—AROMATASE INHIBITORS	anastrazole	Unknown
Inhibit enzyme responsible for activating estrogen	letrozole	
IMMUNE MODULATORS	aldesleukin	Unknown
	alemtuzumab	
	gemtuzumab	

MECHANISM OF ACTION	AGENT	EFFECTS ON CELL CYCLE
	toremifene	
	trastuzumab	
PODOPHYLLOTOXIN DERIVATIVES Damages DNA before mitosis	etoposide	Cell-cycle phase–specific
TAXOIDS Interupt interphase and mitosis	docetaxel paclitaxel	Cell-cycle phase–specific
VINCA ALKALOIDS Interfere with mitosis	vinblastine vinCRIStine vinorelbine	Cell cycle–specific, work during M phase (mitosis)
MISCELLANEOUS	aldesleukin	Unknown
	altretamine	Unknown

Contraindications

Previous bone marrow depression or hypersensitivity. Contraindicated in pregnancy and lactation.

Precautions

Use cautiously in patients with active infections, decreased bone marrow reserve, radiation therapy, or other debilitating illnesses. Use cautiously in patients with childbearing potential.

Interactions

Allopurinol decreases metabolism of mercaptopurine. Toxicity from methotrexate may be increased by other nephrotoxic drugs or larger doses of aspirin or NSAIDs. Bone marrow depression is additive. See individual drugs.

NURSING IMPLICATIONS

Assessment

- Monitor for bone marrow depression. Assess for bleeding (bleeding gums, bruising, petechiae, guaiac stools, urine, and emesis) and avoid IM injections and rectal temperatures if platelet count is low. Apply pressure to venipuncture sites for 10 min. Assess for signs of infection during neutropenia. Anemia may occur. Monitor for increased fatigue, dyspnea, and orthostatic hypotension.
- Monitor intake and output ratios, appetite, and nutritional intake. Prophylactic antiemetics may be used. Adjusting diet as tolerated may help maintain fluid and electrolyte balance and nutritional status.
- Monitor IV site carefully and ensure patency. Discontinue infusion immediately if discomfort, erythema along vein, or infiltration occurs. Tissue ulceration and necrosis may result from infiltration.
- Monitor for symptoms of gout (increased uric acid, joint pain, and edema). Encourage patient to drink at least 2 L of fluid each day. Allopurinol may be given to decrease uric acid levels. Alkalinization of urine may be ordered to increase excretion of uric acid.

Potential Nursing Diagnoses

- Risk for infection (Side Effects).
- Imbalanced nutrition: less than body requirements (Adverse Reactions).
- Deficient knowledge, related to disease processes and medication regimen (Patient/Family Teaching).

Implementation

- Solutions for injection should be prepared in a biologic cabinet. Wear gloves, gown, and mask while handling medication. Discard equipment in designated containers (see Appendix K).
- Check dose carefully. Fatalities have resulted from dosing errors.

CLASSIFICATIONS

Patient/Family Teaching

- Caution patient to avoid crowds and persons with known infections. Health care professional should be informed immediately if symptoms of infection occur.
- Instruct patient to report unusual bleeding. Advise patient of thrombocytopenia precautions.
- These drugs may cause gonadal suppression; however, patient should still use birth control, as most antineoplastics are teratogenic. Advise patient to inform health care professional immediately if pregnancy is suspected.
- Discuss with patient the possibility of hair loss. Explore methods of coping.
- Instruct patient to inspect oral mucosa for erythema and ulceration. If ulceration occurs, advise patient to use sponge brush and to rinse mouth with water after eating and drinking. Topical agents may be used if mouth pain interferes with eating. Stomatitis pain may require treatment with opioid analgesics.
- Instruct patient not to receive any vaccinations without advice of health care professional. Antineoplastics may decrease antibody response and increase risk of adverse reactions.
- Advise patient of need for medical follow-up and frequent lab tests.

Evaluation/Desired Outcomes

- Decrease in size and spread of tumor.
- Improvement in hematologic status in patients with leukemia.

Antineoplastics included in *Davis's Drug Guide for Nurses*

alkylating agents
busulfan 245
carboplatin 265
carmustine 269
chlorambucil 1274
cisplatin 310
cyclophosphamide 361
ifosfamide 660
mechlorethamine 52
melphalan 781
procarbazine 1010
temozolomide 1292

anthracyclines
DAUNOrubicin citrate liposome 383
DAUNOrubicin hydrochloride 385
DOXOrubicin hydrochloride 454
DOXOrubicin hydrochloride liposome 457
epirubicin 484
idarubicin 658

antiandrogens
bicalutamide 222
flutamide 1280
nilutamide 887

antiestrogens
tamoxifen 1138
toremifene 1294

antimetabolites
capecitabine 259
clofarabine 1275
cytarabine 368
fluorouracil 563
gemcitabine 597
hydroxyurea 1281
methotrexate 801
pemetrexed 955

antitumor antibiotics
bleomycin 230
gemtuzumab ozogamicin 1280
mitomycin 833
mitoxantrone 835

aromatase inhibitors
anastrazole 169
letrozole 735

enzyme inhibitors
erlotinib 495
gefitinib 596
imatinib 662, 1326
irinotecan 698
lapatinib 730
nilotinib 1323
temsirolimus 1324
topotecan 1192

enzymes
asparaginase 193
pegaspargase 952

hormones
goserelin 1280
leuprolide 738
medroxyPROGESTERone 337, 776
triptorelin 1296

monoclonal antibodies
alemtuzumab 122

bevacizumab 221, 1326
cetuximab 294
gemtuzumab ozogamicin 1280
rituximab 1075
trastuzumab 1198

podophyllotoxin derivatives
etoposide 522
etoposide phosphate 523

progestins
megestrol 778

taxoids
docetaxel 439
paclitaxel 935

vinca alkaloids
vinBLAStine 1227
vinCRIStine 1229
vinorelbine 1231

miscellaneous
abarelix 1267
aldesleukin 1268
alitretinoin 1269
altretamine 1269
arsenic trioxide 1270
azacitidine 204
ixabepilone 1322
methylaminolevulinate 53
oxaliplatin 917

C L A S S I F I C A T I O N S

• ANTIPARKINSON AGENTS

PHARMACOLOGIC PROFILE

General Use

Used in the treatment of parkinsonism of various causes: degenerative, toxic, infective, neoplastic, or drug-induced.

General Action and Information

Drugs used in the treatment of the parkinsonian syndrome and other dyskinesias are aimed at restoring the natural balance of two major neurotransmitters in the CNS: acetylcholine and dopamine. The imbalance is a deficiency in dopamine that results in excessive cholinergic activity. Drugs used are either anticholinergics (benztropine, biperiden, and trihexyphenidyl) or dopaminergic agonists (bromocriptine, levodopa). Pramipexole and ropinerole are two new nonergot dopamine agonists. Entacapone inhibits the enzyme that breaks down levodopa, thereby enhancing its effects.

Contraindications

Anticholinergics should be avoided in patients with angle-closure glaucoma.

Precautions

Use cautiously in patients with severe cardiac disease, pyloric obstruction, or prostatic enlargement.

Interactions

Pyridoxine, MAO inhibitors, benzodiazepines, phenytoin, phenothiazines, and haloperidol may antagonize the effects of levodopa. Agents that antagonize dopamine (phenothiazines, metoclopramide) may decrease effectiveness of dopamine agonists.

NURSING IMPLICATIONS

Assessment

- Assess parkinsonian and extrapyramidal symptoms (akinesia, rigidity, tremors, pill rolling, mask facies, shuffling gait, muscle spasms, twisting motions, and drooling) before and throughout course of therapy. On-off phenomenon may cause symptoms to appear or improve suddenly.
- Monitor blood pressure frequently during therapy. Instruct patient to remain supine during and for several hours after first dose of bromocriptine, as severe hypotension may occur.

CLASSIFICATIONS

Potential Nursing Diagnoses

- Impaired physical mobility (Indications).
- Risk for injury (Indications).
- Deficient knowledge, related to disease processes and medication regimen (Patient/Family Teaching).

Implementation

- In the carbidopa/levodopa combination, the number following the drug name represents the milligram of each respective drug.

Patient/Family Teaching

- May cause drowsiness or dizziness. Advise patient to avoid driving or other activities that require alertness until response to medication is known.
- Caution patient to make position changes slowly to minimize orthostatic hypotension.
- Instruct patient that frequent rinsing of mouth, good oral hygiene, and sugarless gum or candy may decrease dry mouth. Patient should notify health care professional if dryness persists (saliva substitutes may be used). Also notify the dentist if dryness interferes with use of dentures.
- Advise patient to confer with health care professional before taking OTC medications, especially cold remedies, or drinking alcoholic beverages. Patients receiving levodopa should avoid multivitamins. Vitamin B_6 (pyridoxine) may interfere with levodopa's action.
- Caution patient that decreased perspiration may occur. Overheating may occur during hot weather. Patients should remain indoors in an air-conditioned environment during hot weather.
- Advise patient to increase activity, bulk, and fluid in diet to minimize constipating effects of medication.
- Advise patient to notify health care professional if confusion, rash, urinary retention, severe constipation, visual changes, or worsening of parkinsonian symptoms occur.

Evaluation/Desired Outcomes

- Resolution of parkinsonian signs and symptoms.
- Resolution of drug-induced extrapyramidal symptoms.

Antiparkinson agents included in *Davis's Drug Guide for Nurses*

anticholinergics
benztropine 218
biperiden 32
trihexyphenidyl 1295

antiviral
amantadine 135

catechol-O-methyltransferase inhibitors
entacapone 475
tolcapone 1188

dopamine agonists
apomorphine 186
bromocriptine 1272
carbidopa/levodopa 743
levodopa 743
pramipexole 1000
ropinirole 1081
rotigotine transdermal system 1084

monoamine oxidase type B inhibitors
selegiline 1098

• ANTIPLATELET AGENTS

PHARMACOLOGIC PROFILE

General Use

Antiplatelet agents are used to treat and prevent thromboembolic events such as stroke and MI. Dipyridamole is commonly used after cardiac surgery.

General Action and Information

Inhibit platelet aggregation, prolongs bleeding time, and are used to prevent MI or stroke (aspirin, clopidogrel, dipyridamole, ticlopidine). Eptifibatide and tirofiban are used in the management of various acute coronary syndromes. These agents have been used concurrently/sequentially with anticoagulants and thrombolytics.

Contraindications

Hypersensitivity, ulcer disease, active bleeding, and recent surgery.

Precautions

Use cautiously in patients at risk for bleeding (trauma, surgery). History of GI bleeding or ulcer disease. Safety not established in pregnancy, lactation, or children.

Interactions

Concurrent use with NSAIDs, heparin, thrombolytics, or warfarin may increase the risk of bleeding.

NURSING IMPLICATIONS

Assessment

- Assess patient for evidence of additional or increased thrombosis. Symptoms will depend on area of involvement.
- Assess patient taking antiplatelet agents for symptoms of stroke, peripheral vascular disease, or MI periodically throughout therapy.
- **Lab Test Considerations:** Monitor bleeding time throughout antiplatelet therapy. Prolonged bleeding time, which is time- and dose-dependent, is expected.

Potential Nursing Diagnoses

- Ineffective tissue perfusion (Indications).
- Risk for injury (Side Effects).
- Deficient knowledge, related to disease processes and medication regimen (Patient/Family Teaching).

Implementation

- Use an infusion pump with continuous infusions to ensure accurate dosage.

Patient/Family Teaching

- Instruct patient to notify health care professional immediately if any bleeding is noted.

Evaluation/Desired Outcomes

- Prevention of stroke, MI, and vascular death in patients at risk.

Antiplatelet agents included in *Davis's Drug Guide for Nurses*

glycoprotein IIb/IIIa inhibitors

eptifibatide 490
tirofiban 1185

platelet adhesion inhibitors

dipyridamole 428

platelet aggregation inhibitors

cilostazol 309, 1326
clopidogrel 324
ticlopidine 1176

• ANTIPSYCHOTICS

PHARMACOLOGIC PROFILE

General Use
Treatment of acute and chronic psychoses, particularly when accompanied by increased psychomotor activity. Use of clozapine is limited to schizophrenia unresponsive to conventional therapy. Selected agents are also used as antihistamines or antiemetics. Chlorpromazine is also used in the treatment of intractable hiccups.

General Action and Information
Block dopamine receptors in the brain; also alter dopamine release and turnover. Peripheral effects include anticholinergic properties and alpha-adrenergic blockade. Most antipsychotics are phenothiazines except for haloperidol, which is a butyrophenone, and clozapine, which is a miscellaneous compound. Newer "atypical" agents such as olanzapine, quetiapine, and risperidone may have fewer adverse reactions. Phenothiazines differ in their ability to produce sedation (greatest with chlorpromazine and thioridazine), extrapyramidal reactions (greatest with prochlorperazine and trifluoperazine), and anticholinergic effects (greatest with chlorpromazine).

Contraindications
Hypersensitivity. Cross-sensitivity may exist among phenothiazines. Should not be used in angle-closure glaucoma. Should not be used in patients who have CNS depression.

Precautions
Safety in pregnancy and lactation not established. Use cautiously in patients with symptomatic cardiac disease. Avoid exposure to extremes in temperature. Use cautiously in severely ill or debilitated patients, diabetic patients, and patients with respiratory insufficiency, prostatic hypertrophy, or intestinal obstruction. May lower seizure threshold. Clozapine may cause agranulocytosis. Most agents are capable of causing neuroleptic malignant syndrome. Should not be used routinely for anxiety or agitation not related to psychoses.

Interactions
Additive hypotension with acute ingestion of alcohol, antihypertensives, or nitrates. Antacids may decrease absorption. Phenobarbital may increase metabolism and decrease effectiveness. Additive CNS depression with other CNS depressants, including alcohol, antihistamines, antidepressants, opioid analgesics, or sedative/hypnotics. Lithium may decrease blood levels and effectiveness of phenothiazines. May decrease the therapeutic response to levodopa. May increase the risk of agranulocytosis with antithyroid agents.

NURSING IMPLICATIONS

Assessment
- Assess patient's mental status (orientation, mood, behavior) before and periodically throughout therapy.
- Monitor blood pressure (sitting, standing, lying), pulse, and respiratory rate before and frequently during the period of dosage adjustment.
- Observe patient carefully when administering medication to ensure medication is actually taken and not hoarded.
- Monitor patient for onset of *akathisia*—restlessness or desire to keep moving—and extrapyramidal side effects; *parkinsonian*—difficulty speaking or swallowing, loss of balance control, pill rolling, mask-like face, shuffling gait, rigidity, tremors; and *dystonia*—muscle spasms, twisting motions, twitching, inability to move eyes, weakness of arms or legs—every 2 mo during therapy and 8–12 wk after therapy has been discontinued. Parkinsonian effects are more common in geriatric patients and dystonias are more common in younger patients. Notify health care professional if these symptoms occur, as reduction in dosage or discontinuation

of medication may be necessary. Trihexyphenidyl or diphenhydramine may be used to control these symptoms.

- Monitor for *tardive dyskinesia*—uncontrolled rhythmic movement of mouth, face, and extremities; lip smacking or puckering; puffing of cheeks; uncontrolled chewing; rapid or worm-like movements of tongue. Notify health care professional immediately if these symptoms occur; these side effects may be irreversible.
- Monitor for development of *neuroleptic malignant syndrome*—fever, respiratory distress, tachycardia, convulsions, diaphoresis, hypertension or hypotension, pallor, tiredness, severe muscle stiffness, loss of bladder control. Notify health care professional immediately if these symptoms occur.

Potential Nursing Diagnoses

- Disturbed thought process (Indications).
- Deficient knowledge, related to disease processes and medication regimen (Patient/Family Teaching).
- Noncompliance (Patient/Family Teaching).

Implementation

- Keep patient recumbent for at least 30 min following parenteral administration to minimize hypotensive effects.
- To prevent contact dermatitis, avoid getting solution on hands.
- Phenothiazines should be discontinued 48 hr before and not resumed for 24 hr following myelography, as they lower the seizure threshold.
- **PO:** Administer with **food, milk,** or a full glass of **water** to minimize gastric irritation.
- Dilute most concentrates in 120 ml of distilled or acidified tap water or **fruit juice** just before administration.

Patient/Family Teaching

- Advise patient to take medication exactly as directed and not to skip doses or double up on missed doses. Abrupt withdrawal may lead to gastritis, nausea, vomiting, dizziness, headache, tachycardia, and insomnia.
- Advise patient to make position changes slowly to minimize orthostatic hypotension.
- Medication may cause drowsiness. Caution patient to avoid driving or other activities requiring alertness until response to the medication is known.
- Caution patient to avoid taking alcohol or other CNS depressants concurrently with this medication.
- Advise patient to use sunscreen and protective clothing when exposed to the sun to prevent photosensitivity reactions. Extremes of temperature should also be avoided, as these drugs impair body temperature regulation.
- Advise patient that increasing activity, bulk, and fluids in the diet helps minimize the constipating effects of this medication.
- Instruct patient to use frequent mouth rinses, good oral hygiene, and sugarless gum or candy to minimize dry mouth.
- Advise patient to notify health care professional of medication regimen before treatment or surgery.
- Emphasize the importance of routine follow-up exams and continued participation in psychotherapy as indicated.

Evaluation/Desired Outcomes

- Decrease in excitable, paranoic, or withdrawn behavior. Relief of nausea and vomiting. Relief of intractable hiccups.

Antipsychotics included in *Davis's Drug Guide for Nurses*

phenothiazines
chlorproMAZINE 301
fluphenazine 568
prochlorperazine 1012
thioridazine 1162
trifluoperazine 1295
miscellaneous
aripiprazole 191, 1326
clozapine 327
haloperidol 613
olanzapine 902
paliperidone 939
quetiapine 1043, 1327
risperidone 1070
ziprasidone 1257

• ANTIPYRETICS

PHARMACOLOGIC PROFILE

General Use

Used to lower fever of many causes (infection, inflammation, and neoplasms).

General Action and Information

Antipyretics lower fever by affecting thermoregulation in the CNS and by inhibiting the action of prostaglandins peripherally. Many antipyretics affect platelet function; of these, aspirin has the most profound effect as compared with other salicylates, ibuprofen, or ketoprofen.

Contraindications

Avoid aspirin, ibuprofen, or ketoprofen in patients with bleeding disorders (risk of bleeding is less with other salicylates). Aspirin and other salicylates should be avoided in children and adolescents.

Precautions

Use aspirin, ibuprofen, or ketoprofen cautiously in patients with ulcer disease. Avoid chronic use of large doses of acetaminophen.

Interactions

Large doses of aspirin may displace other highly protein-bound drugs. Additive GI irritation with aspirin, ibuprofen, ketoprofen, and other NSAIDs or corticosteroids. Aspirin, ibuprofen, ketoprofen, or naproxen may increase the risk of bleeding with other agents affecting hemostasis (anticoagulants, thrombolytic agents, antineoplastics, and certain anti-infectives).

NURSING IMPLICATIONS

Assessment

- Assess fever; note presence of associated symptoms (diaphoresis, tachycardia, and malaise).

Potential Nursing Diagnoses

- Risk for imbalanced body temperature (Indications).
- Deficient knowledge, related to disease processes and medication regimen (Patient/Family Teaching).

Implementation

- Administration with food or antacids may minimize GI irritation (aspirin, ibuprofen, ketoprofen, naproxen).
- Available in oral and rectal dosage forms and in combination with other drugs.

Patient/Family Teaching

- Advise patient to consult health care professional if fever is not relieved by routine doses or if greater than 39.5°C (103°F) or lasts longer than 3 days.
- Centers for Disease Control and Prevention warns against giving aspirin to children or adolescents with varicella (chickenpox) or influenza-like or viral illnesses because of a possible association with Reye's syndrome.

Evaluation/Desired Outcomes

- Reduction of fever.

Antipyretics included in *Davis's Drug Guide for Nurses*

acetaminophen 107
aspirin 1087
choline and magnesium salicylates 1087
choline salicylate 1087
ibuprofen, oral 654
ketoprofen 714
magnesium salicylate 1087
naproxen 864
salsalate 1087
sodium salicylate 1087

• ANTIRETROVIRALS

PHARMACOLOGIC PROFILE

General Use

The goal of antiretroviral therapy in the management of HIV infection is to improve CD4 cell counts and decrease viral load. If accomplished, this generally results in slowed progression of the disease, improved quality of life, and decreased opportunistic infections. Perinatal use of agents also prevents transmission of the virus to the fetus. Post-exposure prophylaxis with antiretrovirals is also recommended.

General Action and Information

Because of the rapid emergence of resistance and toxicities of individual agents, HIV infection is almost always managed by a combination of agents. Selections and doses are based on individual toxicities, underlying organ system disease, concurrent drug therapy, and severity of illness. Various combinations are used; up to 4 agents may be used simultaneously. More than 100 agents are currently being tested in addition to those already approved by the FDA.

Contraindications

Hypersensitivity. Because of highly varying toxicities among agents, see individual monographs for more specific information.

Precautions

Many agents require modification for renal impairment. Protease inhibitors may cause hyperglycemia and should be used cautiously in patients with diabetes. Hemophiliacs may also be at risk of bleeding when taking protease inhibitors. See individual monographs for specific information.

Interactions

There are many significant and potentially serious drug-drug interactions among the antiretrovirals. They are affected by drugs that alter metabolism; some agents themselves affect metabolism. See individual agents.

NURSING IMPLICATIONS

Assessment

- Assess patient for change in severity of symptoms of HIV and for symptoms of opportunistic infections throughout therapy.

- **Lab Test Considerations:** Monitor viral load and CD4 counts prior to and periodically during therapy.

Potential Nursing Diagnoses

- Risk for infection (Indications).
- Deficient knowledge, related to disease processes and medication regimen (Patient/Family Teaching).
- Noncompliance (Patient/Family Teaching).

Implementation

- Administer doses around the clock.

Patient/Family Teaching

- Instruct patient to take medication exactly as directed, around the clock, even if sleep is interrupted. Emphasize the importance of complying with therapy, not taking more than prescribed amount, and not discontinuing without consulting health care professional. Missed doses should be taken as soon as remembered unless almost time for next dose; patient should not double doses. Inform patient that long-term effects are unknown at this time.
- Instruct patient that antiretrovirals should not be shared with others.
- Inform patient that antiretroviral therapy does not cure HIV and does not reduce the risk of transmission of HIV to others through sexual contact or blood contamination. Caution patient to use a condom during sexual contact and to avoid sharing needles or donating blood to prevent spreading the AIDS virus to others.
- Advise patient to avoid taking any Rx, OTC, or herbal products without consulting health care professional.
- Emphasize the importance of regular follow-up exams and blood counts to determine progress and to monitor for side effects.

Evaluation/Desired Outcomes

- Decrease in viral load and increase in CD4 counts in patients with HIV.

Antiretrovirals included in *Davis's Drug Guide for Nurses*

CCR5 co-receptor antagonists
maraviroc 772
fusion inhibitors
enfuvirtide 473
metabolic inhibitors
lopinavir/ritonavir 758
non-nucleoside reverse transcriptase inhibitors
delavirdine 1276
efavirenz 469
etravirine 1321
nevirapine 875
nucleoside reverse transcriptase inhibitors
abacavir 103
didanosine 1277
emtricitabine 472
lamivudine 723, 1325
stavudine 1292
tenofovir disoproxil fumarate 1144
zidovudine 1253
protease inhibitors
atazanavir 195, 1325
darunavir 381, 1326
fosamprenavir calcium 580
indinavir 1282
lopinavir/ritonavir 758
nelfinavir 1285
ritonavir 1073
saquinavir 1092
tipranavir 1183
integrase strand transfer inhibitor (INSTI)
raltegravir 1324

C L A S S I F I C A T I O N S

• ANTIRHEUMATICS

PHARMACOLOGIC PROFILE

General Use

Antirheumatics are used to manage symptoms of rheumatoid arthritis (pain, swelling) and in more severe cases to slow down joint destruction and preserve joint function. NSAIDs, aspirin, and other salicylates are used to manage symptoms such as pain and swelling, allowing continued motility and improved quality of life. Corticosteroids are reserved for more advanced swelling and discomfort, primarily because of their increased side effects, especially with chronic use. They can be used to control acute flares of disease. Neither NSAIDs nor corticosteroids prevent disease progression or joint destruction. Disease-modifying antirheumatics drugs (DMARDs, sometimes called slow-acting agents) slow the progression of rheumatoid arthritis and delay joint destruction. DMARDs are reserved for severe cases because of their toxicity. Several months of therapy may be required before benefit is noted and maintained. Serious and frequent adverse reactions may require discontinuation of therapy, despite initial benefit.

General Action and Information

Both NSAIDs and corticosteroids have potent anti-inflammatory properties. DMARDs work by a variety of mechanisms. See individual agents, but most work by suppressing the auto-immune response thought to be responsible for joint destruction.

Contraindications

Hypersensitivity. Patients who are allergic to aspirin should not receive other NSAIDs. Corticosteroids should not be used in patients with active untreated infections.

Precautions

NSAIDs and corticosteroids should be used cautiously in patients with a history of GI bleeding. Corticosteroids should be used with caution in diabetic patients. Many DMARDs have immunosuppressive properties and should be avoided in patients for whom immunosuppression poses a serious risk, including patients with active infections, underlying malignancy, and uncontrolled diabetes mellitus.

Interactions

NSAIDs may diminish the response to diuretics and antihypertensives. Corticosteroids may augment hypokalemia from other medications and increase the risk of digoxin toxicity. DMARDs increase the risk of serious immunosuppression with other immunosuppressants.

NURSING IMPLICATIONS

Assessment

- Assess patient monthly for pain, swelling, and range of motion.

Potential Nursing Diagnoses

- Chronic pain (Indications).
- Deficient knowledge, related to disease processes and medication regimen.

Implementation

- Most agents require regular administration to obtain maximum effects.

Patient/Family Teaching

- Instruct patient to contact health care professional if no improvement is noticed within a few days.

Evaluation/Desired Outcomes

- Improvement in signs and symptoms of rheumatoid arthritis.

Antirheumatics included in *Davis's Drug Guide for Nurses*

corticosteroids
betamethasone 350, 357
cortisone 350
dexamethasone 350, 1352
hydrocortisone 350, 358
methylprednisolone 350
prednisolone 350, 1353
prednisone 350
triamcinolone 343, 347, 350, 358, 1327

DMARDs
adalimumab 114
anakinra 168
etanercept 516
hydroxychloroquine 642
infliximab 676
leflunomide 731
methotrexate 801
penicillamine 1286

NSAIDs
celecoxib 278, 1326
flurbiprofen 1279, 1354
ibuprofen 62
indomethacin 674
ketoprofen 714
nabumetone 855
oxaprozin 919
piroxicam 989
sulindac 1128
tolmetin 1294

miscellaneous
cycloSPORINE 364, 1354
sulfasalazine 1126

• ANTITUBERCULARS

PHARMACOLOGIC PROFILE

General Use
Used in the treatment and prevention of tuberculosis. Combinations are used in the treatment of active disease tuberculosis to rapidly decrease the infectious state and delay or prevent the emergence of resistant strains. In selected situations, intermittent (twice weekly) regimens may be employed. Streptomycin is also used as an antitubercular. Rifampin is used in the prevention of meningococcal meningitis and *Haemophilus influenzae* type b disease.

General Action and Information
Kill (tuberculocidal) or inhibit the growth of (tuberculostatic) mycobacteria responsible for causing tuberculosis. Combination therapy with two or more agents is required, unless used as prophylaxis (isoniazid alone).

Contraindications
Hypersensitivity. Severe liver disease.

Precautions
Use cautiously in patients with a history of liver disease or in elderly or debilitated patients. Ethambutol requires ophthalmologic follow-up. Safety in pregnancy and lactation not established, although selected agents have been used without adverse effects on the fetus. Compliance is required for optimal response.

Interactions
Isoniazid inhibits the metabolism of phenytoin. Rifampin significantly decreases saquinavir levels (combination should be avoided).

NURSING IMPLICATIONS

Assessment
- Mycobacterial studies and susceptibility tests should be performed prior to and periodically throughout therapy to detect possible resistance.
- Assess lung sounds and character and amount of sputum periodically throughout therapy.

Potential Nursing Diagnoses
- Risk for infection (Indications).
- Deficient knowledge, related to disease processes and medication regimen (Patient/Family Teaching).
- Noncompliance (Patient/Family Teaching).

Implementation
- Most medications can be administered with food or antacids if GI irritation occurs.

Patient/Family Teaching
- Advise patient of the importance of continuing therapy even after symptoms have subsided.
- Emphasize the importance of regular follow-up exams to monitor progress and check for side effects.
- Inform patients taking rifampin that saliva, sputum, sweat, tears, urine, and feces may become red-orange to red-brown and that soft contact lenses may become permanently discolored.

Evaluation/Desired Outcomes
- Resolution of the signs and symptoms of tuberculosis. Negative sputum cultures.

Antituberculars included in *Davis's Drug Guide for Nurses*

ethambutol 517
isoniazid 705
pyrazinamide 1036
rifampin 1066
rifapentine 1291

• ANTIULCER AGENTS

PHARMACOLOGIC PROFILE

General Use
Treatment and prophylaxis of peptic ulcer and gastric hypersecretory conditions such as Zollinger-Ellison syndrome. Histamine H_2-receptor antagonists (blockers) and proton pump inhibitors are also used in the management of GERD.

General Action and Information
Because a great majority of peptic ulcer disease may be traced to GI infection with the organism *Helicobacter pylori*, eradication of the organism decreases symptomatology and recurrence. Anti-infectives with significant activity against the organism include amoxicillin, clarithromycin, metronidazole, and tetracycline. Bismuth also has anti-infective activity against *H. pylori*. Regimens usually include: a histamine H_2-receptor antagonist or a proton pump inhibitor and 2 anti-infectives with or without bismuth subsalicylate for 1-14 days.
Other medications used in the management of gastric/duodenal ulcer disease are aimed at neutralizing gastric acid (antacids), decreasing acid secretion (histamine H_2 antagonists, proton pump inhibitors, misoprostol), or protecting the ulcer surface from further damage (misoprostol, sucralfate). Histamine H_2-receptor antagonists competitively inhibit the action of histamine at the H_2 receptor, located primarily in gastric parietal cells, resulting in inhibition of gastric acid secretion. Misoprostol decreases gastric acid secretion and increases production of protective mucus. Proton pump inhibitors prevent the transport of hydrogen ions into the gastric lumen.

Contraindications
Hypersensitivity.
Pregnancy.

Precautions

Most histamine H_2 antagonists require dose reduction in renal impairment and in elderly patients. Magnesium-containing antacids should be used cautiously in patients with renal impairment. Misoprostol should be used cautiously in women with childbearing potential.

Interactions

Calcium- and magnesium-containing antacids decrease the absorption of tetracycline and fluoroquinolones. Cimetidine inhibits the ability of the liver to metabolize several drugs, increasing the risk of toxicity from warfarin, tricyclic antidepressants, theophylline, metoprolol, phenytoin, propranolol, and lidocaine. Omeprazole decreases metabolism of phenytoin, diazepam, and warfarin. All agents that increase gastric pH will decrease the absorption of ketoconazole.

NURSING IMPLICATIONS

Assessment

- Assess patient routinely for epigastric or abdominal pain and frank or occult blood in the stool, emesis, or gastric aspirate.
- **Antacids:** Assess for heartburn and indigestion as well as the location, duration, character, and precipitating factors of gastric pain.
- **Histamine H_2 Antagonists:** Assess elderly and severely ill patients for confusion routinely. Notify health care professional promptly should this occur.
- **Misoprostol:** Assess women of childbearing age for pregnancy. Medication is usually begun on 2nd or 3rd day of menstrual period following a negative serum pregnancy test within 2 wk of beginning therapy.
- **Lab Test Considerations:** Histamine H_2 antagonists antagonize the effects of pentagastrin and histamine during gastric acid secretion test. Avoid administration during the 24 hr preceding the test.
- May cause false-negative results in skin tests using allergen extracts. These drugs should be discontinued 24 hr prior to the test.

Potential Nursing Diagnoses

- Acute pain (Indications).
- Deficient knowledge, related to disease processes and medication regimen (Patient/Family Teaching).

Implementation

- **Antacids:** Antacids cause premature dissolution and absorption of enteric-coated tablets and may interfere with absorption of other oral medications. Separate administration of antacids and other oral medications by at least 1 hr.
- Shake liquid preparations well before pouring. Follow administration with water to ensure passage to stomach. Liquid and powder dosage forms are considered to be more effective than chewable tablets.
- Chewable tablets must be chewed thoroughly before swallowing. Follow with half a glass of water.
- Administer 1 and 3 hr after meals and at bedtime for maximum antacid effect.
- **Misoprostol:** Administer with meals and at bedtime to reduce the severity of diarrhea.
- **Proton pump inhibitors:** Administer before meals, preferably in the morning. Capsules should be swallowed whole; do not open, crush, or chew.
- May be administered concurrently with antacids.
- **Sucralfate:** Administer on an empty stomach 1 hr before meals and at bedtime. Do not crush or chew tablets. Shake suspension well prior to administration. If nasogastric administration is required, consult pharmacist, as protein-binding properties of sucralfate have resulted in formation of a bezoar when administered with enteral feedings and other medications.

Patient/Family Teaching

- Instruct patient to take medication as directed for the full course of therapy, even if feeling better. If a dose is missed, it should be taken as soon as remembered but not if almost time for next dose. Do not double doses.
- Advise patient to avoid alcohol, products containing aspirin, NSAIDs, and foods that may cause an increase in GI irritation.
- Advise patient to report onset of black, tarry stools to health care professional promptly.
- Inform patient that cessation of smoking may help prevent the recurrence of duodenal ulcers.
- **Antacids:** Caution patient to consult health care professional before taking antacids for more than 2 wk or if problem is recurring. Advise patient to consult health care professional if relief is not obtained or if symptoms of gastric bleeding (black, tarry stools; coffee-ground emesis) occur.
- **Misoprostol:** Emphasize that sharing of this medication may be dangerous.
- Inform patient that misoprostol may cause spontaneous abortion. Women of childbearing age must be informed of this effect through verbal and written information and must use contraception throughout therapy. If pregnancy is suspected, the woman should stop taking misoprostol and immediately notify her health care professional.
- **Sucralfate:** Advise patient to continue with course of therapy for 4–8 wk, even if feeling better, to ensure ulcer healing.
- Advise patient that an increase in fluid intake, dietary bulk, and exercise may prevent drug-induced constipation.

Evaluation/Desired Outcomes

- Decrease in GI pain and irritation. Prevention of gastric irritation and bleeding. Healing of duodenal ulcers can be seen by x-rays or endoscopy. Therapy with histamine H_2 antagonists is continued for at least 6 wk after initial episode. Decreased symptoms of GERD. Increase in the pH of gastric secretions (antacids). Prevention of gastric ulcers in patients receiving chronic NSAID therapy (misoprostol only).

Antiulcer agents included in *Davis's Drug Guide for Nurses*

antacids
aluminum hydroxide 133
magaldrate 765
magnesium hydroxide/aluminum hydroxide 765

histamine H_2 antagonists
cimetidine 623, 1325
famotidine 623
nizatidine 623
ranitidine 623

proton-pump inhibitors
esomeprazole 505, 1325
lansoprazole 727
omeprazole 908
pantoprazole 948, 1325
rabeprazole 1051

miscellaneous
amoxicillin 153, 1325
bismuth subsalicylate 225
clarithromycin 315
metronidazole 817
misoprostol 832
propantheline 1290
sodium bicarbonate 1114
sucralfate 1124

• ANTIVIRALS

PHARMACOLOGIC PROFILE

General Use

Acyclovir, famciclovir, and valacyclovir are used in the management of herpes virus infections. Acyclovir also is used in the management of chickenpox. Oseltamivir and zanamivir are used primarily in the prevention of influenza A viral infections. Cidofovir, ganciclovir, valganciclovir, and foscarnet are used in the treatment of cytomegalovirus (CMV) retinitis. Vidarabine is used only to treat ophthalmic viral infections. Penciclovir and docosanol are used in the treatment and prevention of oral-facial herpes simplex.

General Action and Information

Most agents inhibit viral replication.

Contraindications

Previous hypersensitivity.

Precautions

All except zanamivir require dose adjustment in renal impairment. Acyclovir may cause renal impairment. Acyclovir may cause CNS toxicity. Foscarnet increases risk of seizures.

Interactions

Acyclovir may have additive CNS and nephrotoxicity with drugs causing similar adverse reactions.

NURSING IMPLICATIONS

Assessment

- Assess patient for signs and symptoms of infection before and throughout therapy.
- **Ophth:** Assess eye lesions before and daily during therapy.
- **Topical:** Assess lesions before and daily during therapy.

Potential Nursing Diagnoses

- Risk for infection (Indications).
- Impaired skin integrity (Indications).
- Deficient knowledge, related to disease processes and medication regimen (Patient/Family Teaching).

Implementation

- Most systemic antiviral agents should be administered around the clock to maintain therapeutic serum drug levels.

Patient/Family Teaching

- Instruct patient to continue taking medication around the clock for full course of therapy, even if feeling better.
- Advise patient that antivirals and antiretrovirals do not prevent transmission to others. Precautions should be taken to prevent spread of virus.
- Instruct patient in correct technique for topical or ophthalmic preparations.
- Instruct patient to notify health care professional if symptoms do not improve.

Evaluation/Desired Outcomes

- Prevention or resolution of the signs and symptoms of viral infection. Length of time for complete resolution depends on organism and site of infection.

Antivirals included in *Davis's Drug Guide for Nurses*

acyclovir 111
amantadine 135
cidofovir 308
docosanol 441
entecavir 476
famciclovir 529
foscarnet 582
ganciclovir 594
imiquimod 669
lamivudine 723, 1325
oseltamivir 916
penciclovir 957
ribavirin 1062
valacyclovir 1209
valganciclovir 1210
zanamivir 1251

• BETA BLOCKERS

PHARMACOLOGIC PROFILE

General Use

Management of hypertension, angina pectoris, tachyarrhythmias, hypertrophic subaortic stenosis, migraine headache (prophylaxis), MI (prevention), glaucoma (ophthalmic use), CHF (carvedilol and sustained-release metoprolol only) and hyperthyroidism (management of symptoms only).

General Action and Information

Beta blockers compete with adrenergic (sympathetic) neurotransmitters (epinephrine and norepinephrine) for adrenergic receptor sites. $Beta_1$-adrenergic receptor sites are located chiefly in the heart where stimulation results in increased heart rate, contractility, and AV conduction. $Beta_2$-adrenergic receptors are found mainly in bronchial and vascular smooth muscle and the uterus. Stimulation of $beta_2$-adrenergic receptors produces vasodilation, bronchodilation, and uterine relaxation. Blockade of these receptors antagonizes the effects of the neurotransmitters. Beta blockers may be relatively selective for $beta_1$-adrenergic receptors (acebutolol, atenolol, betaxolol, esmolol, and metoprolol) or nonselective (carteolol, carvedilol, labetalol, levobunolol, nadolol, penbutolol, pindolol, propranolol, sotalol, and timolol) blocking both $beta_1$- and $beta_2$-adrenergic receptors. Carvedilol and labetalol have additional alpha-adrenergic blocking properties. Acebutolol, carvedilol, penbutolol, and pindolol possess intrinsic sympathomimetic action (ISA) that may result in less bradycardia than other agents. Ophthalmic beta blockers decrease production of aqueous humor.

Contraindications

Uncompensated CHF (most beta blockers), acute bronchospasm, some forms of valvular heart disease, bradyarrhythmias, and heart block.

Precautions

Use cautiously in pregnant and lactating women (may cause fetal bradycardia and hypoglycemia). Use cautiously in any form of lung disease or underlying compensated CHF (most agents). Use with caution in diabetics and patients with severe liver disease. Beta blockers should not be abruptly discontinued in patients with cardiovascular disease.

Interactions

May cause additive myocardial depression and bradycardia when used with other agents having these effects (digoxin and some antiarrhythmics). May antagonize the therapeutic effects of bronchodilators. May alter the requirements for insulin or hypoglyemic agents in diabetics. Cimetidine may decrease the metabolism and increase the effects of some beta blockers.

NURSING IMPLICATIONS

Assessment

- Monitor blood pressure and pulse frequently during dosage adjustment and periodically throughout therapy.
- Monitor intake and output ratios and daily weight. Assess patient routinely for signs and symptoms of CHF (dyspnea, rales/crackles, weight gain, peripheral edema, jugular venous distention).
- **Angina:** Assess frequency and severity of episodes of chest pain periodically throughout therapy.
- **Migraine prophylaxis:** Assess frequency and severity of migraine headaches periodically throughout therapy.

Potential Nursing Diagnoses

- Ineffective tissue perfusion (Indications).

- Deficient knowledge, related to disease processes and medication regimen (Patient/Family Teaching).
- Noncompliance (Patient/Family Teaching).

Implementation

- Take apical pulse prior to administering. If heart rate is <50 bpm or if arrhythmias occur, hold medication and notify health care professional.
- Many beta blockers are available in combination products to enhance compliance (see Appendix B).

Patient/Family Teaching

- Instruct patient to continue taking medication, even if feeling well. Abrupt withdrawal may cause life-threatening arrhythmias, hypertension, or myocardial ischemia. Medication controls, but does not cure, hypertension.
- Encourage patient to comply with additional interventions for hypertension (weight reduction, low-sodium diet, regular exercise, smoking cessation, moderation of alcohol consumption, and stress management).
- Instruct patient and family on proper technique for monitoring blood pressure. Advise them to check blood pressure weekly and report significant changes to health care professional.
- Caution patient to make position changes slowly to minimize orthostatic hypotension. Advise patient that exercising or hot weather may enhance hypotensive effects.
- Advise patient to consult health care professional before taking any OTC medications or herbal/alternative therapies, especially cold remedies.
- Caution patient that these medications may cause increased sensitivity to cold.
- Diabetics should monitor blood glucose closely, especially if weakness, malaise, irritability, or fatigue occurs.
- Advise patient to advise health care professional of medication regimen prior to treatment or surgery.
- Advise patient to carry identification describing disease process and medication regimen at all times.
- Emphasize the importance of follow-up exams to monitor progress.
- **Ophth:** Instruct patient in correct technique for administration of ophthalmic preparations.

Evaluation/Desired Outcomes

- Decrease in blood pressure.
- Decrease in frequency and severity of anginal attacks.
- Control of arrhythmias.
- Prevention of myocardial reinfarction.
- Prevention of migraine headaches.
- Decrease in tremors.
- Lowering of intraocular pressure.

Beta blockers included in *Davis's Drug Guide for Nurses*

beta blockers (nonselective)

carteolol 1273
carvedilol 271
labetalol 719
nadolol 856
penbutolol 47
pindolol 1288
propranolol 1026, 1327
sotalol 1122
timolol 1179, 1352

beta blockers (selective)

acebutolol 105
atenolol 197
betaxolol 219, 1351
bisoprolol 226
esmolol 502
metoprolol 814

ophthalmic beta blockers

betaxolol 219, 1351
carteolol 1273
levobetaxolol 1351
levobunolol 1351
metipranolol 1351
timolol 1179, 1352

• BONE RESORPTION INHIBITORS

PHARMACOLOGIC PROFILE

General Use

Bone resorption inhibitors are primarily used to treat and prevent osteoporosis in postmenopausal women. Other uses include treatment of osteoporosis due to other causes, including corticosteroid therapy, treatment of Paget's disease of the bone, and management of hypercalcemia.

General Action and Information

Biphosphonates (alendronate, etidronate, risedronate, and tiludronate) inhibit resorption of bone by inhibiting hydroxyapatite crystal dissolution and osteoclast activity. Raloxifene binds to estrogen receptors, producing estrogen-like effects on bone including decreased bone resorption and decreased bone turnover.

Contraindications

Hypersensitivity. Biphosphonates should not be used in patients with hypocalcemia. Raloxifene should not be used in women with childbearing potential or a history of thromboembolic disease.

Precautions

Use cautiously in patients with renal impairment; some agents should be avoided in moderate to severe renal impairment.

Interactions

Calcium supplements decrease absorption of biphosphonates. Tilundronate's effects may be altered by aspirin or other NSAIDs. Aspirin may increase GI adverse reactions with alendronate. Cholestyramine decreases absorption of raloxifene (concurrent use is contraindicated).

NURSING IMPLICATIONS

Assessment

- Assess patients for low bone density before and periodically during therapy.
- Assess for symptoms of Paget's disease (bone pain, headache, decreased visual and auditory acuity, increased skull size).
- **Lab Test Considerations:** Monitor serum calcium in patients with osteoporosis. Monitor alkaline phosphatase in patients with Paget's disease.

Potential Nursing Diagnoses

- Risk for injury (Indications).
- Deficient knowledge, related to disease processes and medication regimen (Patient/Family Teaching).

Patient/Family Teaching

- Instruct patient to take medication exactly as directed.
- Encourage patient to participate in regular exercise and to modify behaviors that increase the risk of osteoporosis.

Evaluation/Desired Outcomes

- Prevention of, or decrease in, the progression of osteoporosis in postmenopausal women. Decrease in the progression of Paget's disease.

Bone resorption inhibitors included in *Davis's Drug Guide for Nurses*

biphosphonates
alendronate 124
etidronate 519
ibandronate 653
pamidronate 942
risedronate 1069, 1325
tiludronate 1293
zoledronic acid 1259

selective estrogen receptor modulators
raloxifene 1052

• BRONCHODILATORS

PHARMACOLOGIC PROFILE

General Use

Used in the treatment of reversible airway obstruction due to asthma or COPD. Recently revised recommendations for management of asthma recommend that rapid-acting inhaled beta-agonist bronchodilators (not salmeterol) be reserved as acute relievers of bronchospasm; repeated or chronic use indicates the need for additional long-term control agents, including inhaled corticosteroids, mast cell stabilizers, and long-acting bronchodilators (oral theophylline or beta-agonists) and leukotriene modifiers (montelukast, zafirlukast).

General Action and Information

Beta-adrenergic agonists (albuterol, epinephrine, isoproterenol, metaproterenol, pirbuterol, and terbutaline) produce bronchodilation by stimulating the production of cyclic adenosine monophosphate (cAMP). Newer agents (albuterol, metaproterenol, pirbuterol, and terbutaline) are relatively selective for pulmonary (beta$_2$) receptors, whereas older agents produce cardiac stimulation (beta$_1$-adrenergic effects) in addition to bronchodilation. Onset of action allows use in management of acute attacks except for salmeterol, which has delayed onset. Phosphodiesterase inhibitors (aminophylline and theophylline) inhibit the breakdown of cAMP. Ipratropium is an anticholinergic compound that produces bronchodilation by blocking the action of acetylcholine in the respiratory tract. Montelukast, zafirlukast, and zileuton are leukotriene modifiers. Leukotrienes are components of slow-reacting substance of anaphylaxis A (SRS-A), which may be a cause of bronchospasm.

Contraindications

Hypersensitivity to agents, preservatives (bisulfites), or propellants used in their formulation. Avoid use in uncontrolled cardiac arrhythmias.

Precautions

Use cautiously in patients with diabetes, cardiovascular disease, or hyperthyroidism.

Interactions

Therapeutic effectiveness may be antagonized by concurrent use of beta blockers. Additive sympathomimetic effects with other adrenergic (sympathetic) drugs, including vasopressors and decongestants. Cardiovascular effects may be potentiated by antidepressants and MAO inhibitors.

NURSING IMPLICATIONS

Assessment

- Assess blood pressure, pulse, respiration, lung sounds, and character of secretions before and throughout therapy.
- Patients with a history of cardiovascular problems should be monitored for ECG changes and chest pain.

Potential Nursing Diagnoses
- Ineffective airway clearance (Indications).
- Activity intolerance (Indications).
- Deficient knowledge, related to disease processes and medication regimen (Patient/Family Teaching).

Implementation
- Administer around the clock to maintain therapeutic plasma levels.

Patient/Family Teaching
- Emphasize the importance of taking only the prescribed dose at the prescribed time intervals.
- Encourage the patient to drink adequate liquids (2000 ml/day minimum) to decrease the viscosity of the airway secretions.
- Advise patient to avoid OTC cough, cold, or breathing preparations without consulting health care professional and to minimize intake of xanthine-containing foods or beverages (colas, coffee, and chocolate), as these may increase side effects and cause arrhythmias.
- Caution patient to avoid smoking and other respiratory irritants.
- Instruct patient on proper use of metered-dose inhaler (see Appendix D).
- Advise patient to contact health care professional promptly if the usual dose of medication fails to produce the desired results, symptoms worsen after treatment, or toxic effects occur.
- Patients using other inhalation medications and bronchodilators should be advised to use bronchodilator first and allow 5 min to elapse before administering the other medication, unless otherwise directed by health care professional.

Evaluation/Desired Outcomes
- Decreased bronchospasm. Increased ease of breathing.

Bronchodilators included in *Davis's Drug Guide for Nurses*

adrenergics
albuterol 120
epinephrine 480, 1356
formoterol 577
levalbuterol 741, 1325
metaproterenol 1283
pirbuterol 30
salmeterol 1090
terbutaline 1148

anticholinergics
ipratropium 696
tiotropium 1182, 1327

leukotriene antagonists
montelukast 841
zafirlukast 1249
zileuton 1296

xanthines
aminophylline 232
theophylline 232

• CALCIUM CHANNEL BLOCKERS

PHARMACOLOGIC PROFILE

General Use
Used in the treatment of hypertension (amlodipine, diltiazem, felodipine, isradipine, nicardipine, nifedipine, nisoldipine, verapamil) or in the treatment and prophylaxis of angina pectoris or coronary artery spasm (amlodipine, diltiazem, felodipine, nicardipine, verapamil). Verapamil and diltiazem are also used as antiarrhythmics. Nimodipine is used to prevent neurologic damage due to certain types of cerebral vasospasm.

General Action and Information
Block calcium entry into cells of vascular smooth muscle and myocardium. Dilate coronary arteries in both normal and ischemic myocardium and inhibit coronary artery spasm. Diltiazem and

verapamil decrease AV conduction. Nimodipine has a relatively selective effect on cerebral blood vessels.

Contraindications

Hypersensitivity. Contraindicated in bradycardia, 2nd- or 3rd-degree heart block, or uncompensated CHF (verapamil).

Precautions

Safety in pregnancy and lactation not established. Use cautiously in patients with liver disease or uncontrolled arrhythmias.

Interactions

Additive myocardial depression with beta blockers and disopyramide (diltiazem and verapamil). Effectiveness may be decreased by phenobarbital or phenytoin and increased by propranolol or cimetidine. Verapamil and diltiazem may increase serum digoxin levels and cause toxicity.

NURSING IMPLICATIONS

Assessment

- Monitor blood pressure and pulse frequently during dosage adjustment and periodically throughout therapy.
- Monitor intake and output ratios and daily weight. Assess patient routinely for signs and symptoms of CHF (dyspnea, rales/crackles, weight gain, peripheral edema, jugular venous distention).
- **Angina:** Assess frequency and severity of episodes of chest pain periodically throughout therapy.
- **Arrhythmias:** ECG should be monitored continuously during IV therapy and periodically during long-term therapy with verapamil.
- **Cerebral vasospasm:** Assess patient's neurological status (level of consciousness, movement) before and periodically during therapy with nimodipine.

Potential Nursing Diagnoses

- Ineffective tissue perfusion (Indications).
- Acute pain (Indications).
- Deficient knowledge, related to disease processes and medication regimen (Patient/Family Teaching).

Implementation

- May be administered without regard to meals.
- Do not open, crush, or chew sustained-release capsules.

Patient/Family Teaching

- Instruct patient to continue taking medication, even if feeling well.
- Caution patient to make position changes slowly to minimize orthostatic hypotension. Advise patient that exercising or hot weather may enhance hypotensive effects.
- Instruct patient on the importance of maintaining good dental hygiene and seeing dentist frequently for teeth cleaning to prevent tenderness, bleeding, and gingival hyperplasia (gum enlargement).
- Advise patient to consult health care professional before taking any OTC medications or herbal/alternative therapies, especially cold remedies.
- Advise patient to advise health care professional of medication regimen prior to treatment or surgery.
- Advise patient to carry identification describing disease process and medication regimen at all times.
- Emphasize the importance of follow-up exams to monitor progress.

- **Angina:** Instruct patients on concurrent nitrate therapy to continue taking both medications as directed and using SL nitroglycerin as needed for anginal attacks. Advise patient to contact health care professional if chest pain worsens or does not improve after therapy, or is accompanied by diaphoresis or shortness of breath, or if severe, persistent headache occurs. Caution patient to discuss exercise precautions with health care professional prior to exertion.
- **Hypertension:** Encourage patient to comply with additional interventions for hypertension (weight reduction, low-sodium diet, regular exercise, smoking cessation, moderation of alcohol consumption, and stress management). Medication controls, but does not cure, hypertension.
- Instruct patient and family on proper technique for monitoring blood pressure. Advise them to check blood pressure weekly and report significant changes to health care professional.

Evaluation/Desired Outcomes

- Decrease in blood pressure.
- Decrease in frequency and severity of anginal attacks.
- Decrease need for nitrate therapy.
- Increase in activity tolerance and sense of well-being.
- Suppression and prevention of supraventricular tachyarrhythmias.
- Improvement in neurological deficits due to vasospasm following subarachnoid hemorrhage.

Calcium channel blockers included in *Davis's Drug Guide for Nurses*

amlodipine 151
diltiazem 418
felodipine 530
isradipine 708
niCARdipine 879
NIFEdipine 884
nimodipine 888
nisoldipine 889, 1325
verapamil 1224

• CENTRAL NERVOUS SYSTEM STIMULANTS

PHARMACOLOGIC PROFILE

General Use

Used in the treatment of narcolepsy and as adjunctive treatment in the management of ADHD.

General Action and Information

Produce CNS stimulation by increasing levels of neurotransmitters in the CNS. Produce CNS and respiratory stimulation, dilated pupils, increased motor activity and mental alertness, and a diminished sense of fatigue. In children with ADHD these agents decrease restlessness and increase attention span.

Contraindications

Hypersensitivity. Should not be used in pregnant or lactating women. Should not be used in hyperexcitable states. Avoid using in patients with psychotic personalities or suicidal/homicidal tendencies. Contraindicated in glaucoma and severe cardiovascular disease.

Precautions

Use cautiously in patients with a history of cardiovascular disease, hypertension, diabetes mellitus, or in elderly or debilitated patients. Continual use may result in psychological dependence or addiction.

Interactions

Additive sympathomimetic (adrenergic effects). Use with MAO inhibitors can result in hypertensive crises. Alkalinizing the urine (sodium bicarbonate, acetazolamide) decreases excretion and enhances effects of amphetamines. Acidification of the urine (ammonium chloride, large doses of ascorbic acid) decreases effect of amphetamines. Phenothiazines may also decrease effects. Methylphenidate may decrease the metabolism and increase effects of other drugs (warfarin, anticonvulsants, tricyclic antidepressants).

NURSING IMPLICATIONS

Assessment

- Monitor blood pressure, pulse, and respiration before administering and periodically during therapy.
- Monitor weight biweekly and inform health care professional of significant loss.
- Monitor height periodically in children; inform health care professional if growth inhibition occurs.
- May produce false sense of euphoria and well-being. Provide frequent rest periods and observe patient for rebound depression after the effects of the medication have worn off.
- **ADHD:** Assess attention span, impulse control, and interactions with others in children. Therapy may be interrupted at intervals to determine if symptoms are sufficient to warrant continued therapy.
- **Narcolepsy:** Observe and document frequency of episodes.

Potential Nursing Diagnoses

- Disturbed thought process (Side Effects).
- Deficient knowledge, related to disease processes and medication regimen (Patient/Family Teaching).

Patient/Family Teaching

- Instruct patient not to alter dose without consulting health care professional. These medications have high dependence and abuse potential. Abrupt cessation with high doses may cause extreme fatigue and mental depression.
- Advise patient to avoid intake of large amounts of caffeine.
- Medication may impair judgment. Caution patient to avoid driving or other activities requiring judgment until response to medication is known.
- Inform patient that periodic holidays from the drug may be used to assess progress and decrease dependence.

Evaluation/Desired Outcomes

- Decreased frequency of narcoleptic episodes.
- Improved attention span and social interactions.

Central nervous system stimulants included in *Davis's Drug Guide for Nurses*

amphetamine mixtures 158
dexmethylphenidate 398
dextroamphetamine 401, 1325
methylphenidate 808, 1325
modafinil 837

• CORTICOSTEROIDS

PHARMACOLOGIC PROFILE

General Use

Used in replacement doses (20 mg of hydrocortisone or equivalent) systemically to treat adrenocortical insufficiency. Larger doses are usually used for their antiinflammatory, immunosuppressive, or antineoplastic activity. Used adjunctively in many other situations, including hypercalcemia and autoimmune diseases. Topical corticosteroids are used in a variety of inflammatory and allergic conditions. Inhalant corticosteroids are used in the chronic management of reversible airway disease (asthma); intranasal and ophthalmic corticosteroids are used in the management of chronic allergic and inflammatory conditions.

General Action and Information

Produce profound and varied metabolic effects, in addition to modifying the normal immune response and suppressing inflammation. Available in a variety of dosage forms, including oral, injectable, topical, and inhalation. Prolonged used of large amounts of topical or inhaled agent may result in systemic absorption and/or adrenal suppression.

Contraindications

Serious infections (except for certain forms of meningitis). Do not administer live vaccines to patients on larger doses.

Precautions

Prolonged treatment will result in adrenal suppression. Do not discontinue abruptly. Additional doses may be needed during stress (surgery and infection). Safety in pregnancy and lactation not established. Long-term use in children will result in decreased growth. May mask signs of infection. Use lowest dose possible for shortest time possible. Alternate-day therapy is preferable during long-term treatment.

Interactions

Additive hypokalemia with amphotericin B and potassium-losing diuretics. Hypokalemia may increase the risk of digoxin toxicity. May increase requirements for insulin or oral hypoglycemic agents. Phenytoin, phenobarbital, and rifampin stimulate metabolism and may decrease effectiveness. Oral contraceptives may block metabolism. Cholestyramine and colestipol may decrease absorption.

NURSING IMPLICATIONS

Assessment

- These drugs are indicated for many conditions. Assess involved systems prior to and periodically throughout course of therapy.
- Assess patient for signs of adrenal insufficiency (hypotension, weight loss, weakness, nausea, vomiting, anorexia, lethargy, confusion, restlessness) prior to and periodically throughout course of therapy.
- Children should have periodic evaluations of growth.

Potential Nursing Diagnoses

- Risk for infection (Side Effects).
- Deficient knowledge, related to disease processes and medication regimen (Patient/Family Teaching).
- Disturbed body image (Side Effects).

Implementation

- If dose is ordered daily or every other day, administer in the morning to coincide with the body's normal secretion of cortisol.
- **PO:** Administer with meals to minimize gastric irritation.

Patient/Family Teaching

- Emphasize need to take medication exactly as directed. Review symptoms of adrenal insufficiency that may occur when stopping the medication and that may be life-threatening.
- Encourage patients on long-term therapy to eat a diet high in protein, calcium, and potassium and low in sodium and carbohydrates.
- These drugs cause immunosuppression and may mask symptoms of infection. Instruct patient to avoid people with known contagious illnesses and to report possible infections. Advise patient to consult health care professional before receiving any vaccinations.

- Discuss possible effects on body image. Explore coping mechanisms.
- Advise patient to carry identification in the event of an emergency in which patient cannot relate medical history.

Evaluation/Desired Outcomes

- Suppression of the inflammatory and immune responses in autoimmune disorders, allergic reactions, and organ transplants.
- Replacement therapy in adrenal insufficiency.
- Resolution of skin inflammation, pruritus, or other dermatologic conditions.

Corticosteroids included in *Davis's Drug Guide for Nurses*

corticosteroids, inhalation
beclomethasone 343, 347
budesonide 343, 347, 350
flunisolide 343, 347
fluticasone 343, 347, 358
triamcinolone 343, 347, 350, 358, 1327

corticosteroids, nasal
beclomethasone 343, 347
budesonide 343, 347, 350
flunisolide 343, 347
fluticasone 343, 347, 358
mometasone 343, 347, 358
triamcinolone 343, 347, 350, 358, 1327

corticosteroids, ophthalmic
dexamethasone 350, 1352
fluorometholone 1352
loteprednol 1353
medrysone 76
prednisoLONE 350, 1353
rimexolone 1353

corticosteroids, systemic (short-acting)
cortisone 350
hydrocortisone 350, 358

corticosteroids, systemic (intermediate-acting)
methylPREDNISolone 350
prednisoLONE 350, 1353
predniSONE 350
triamcinolone 343, 347, 350, 358, 1327

corticosteroids, systemic (long-acting)
betamethasone 350, 357
budesonide 343, 347, 350
dexamethasone 350, 1352

corticosteroids, topical/local
alclometasone 357
amcinonide 357
betamethasone 350, 357
clobetasol 357
clocortolone 357
desonide 357
desoximetasone 357
dexamethasone 350, 1352
diflorasone 357
fluocinolone 357
fluocinonide 358
flurandrenolide 358
fluticasone 343, 347, 358
halcinonide 358
halobetasol 358
hydrocortisone 350, 358
methylPREDNISolone 350
mometasone 343, 347, 358
prednicarbate 358
triamcinolone 343, 347, 350, 358, 1327

• DIURETICS

PHARMACOLOGIC PROFILE

General Use

Thiazide diuretics and loop diuretics are used alone or in combination in the treatment of hypertension or edema due to CHF or other causes. Potassium-sparing diuretics have weak diuretic and antihypertensive properties and are used mainly to conserve potassium in patients receiving thiazide or loop diuretics. Osmotic diuretics are often used in the management of cerebral edema.

General Action and Information

Enhance the selective excretion of various electrolytes and water by affecting renal mechanisms for tubular secretion and reabsorption. Groups commonly used are thiazide diuretics and thiazide-like diuretics (chlorothiazide, chlorthalidone, hydrochlorothiazide, indapamide, and metolazone), loop diuretics (bumetanide, furosemide, and torsemide), potassium-sparing diuretics (amiloride, spironolactone, and triamterene), and osmotic diuretics (mannitol). Mechanisms vary, depending on agent.

Contraindications

Hypersensitivity. Thiazide diuretics may exhibit cross-sensitivity with other sulfonamides.

Precautions

Use with caution in patients with renal or hepatic disease. Safety in pregnancy and lactation not established.

Interactions

Additive hypokalemia with corticosteroids, amphotericin B, piperacillin, or ticarcillin. Hypokalemia enhances digitalis glycoside toxicity. Potassium-losing diuretics decrease lithium excretion and may cause toxicity. Additive hypotension with other antihypertensives or nitrates. Potassium-sparing diuretics may cause hyperkalemia when used with potassium supplements or ACE inhibitors.

NURSING IMPLICATIONS

Assessment

- Assess fluid status throughout therapy. Monitor daily weight, intake and output ratios, amount and location of edema, lung sounds, skin turgor, and mucous membranes.
- Assess patient for anorexia, muscle weakness, numbness, tingling, paresthesia, confusion, and excessive thirst. Notify health care professional promptly if these signs of electrolyte imbalance occur.
- **Hypertension:** Monitor blood pressure and pulse before and during administration. Monitor frequency of prescription refills to determine compliance in patients treated for hypertension.
- **Increased Intracranial Pressure:** Monitor neurologic status and intracranial pressure readings in patients receiving osmotic diuretics to decrease cerebral edema.
- **Increased Intraocular Pressure:** Monitor for persistent or increased eye pain or decreased visual acuity.
- **Lab Test Considerations:** Monitor electrolytes (especially potassium), blood glucose, BUN, and serum uric acid levels before and periodically throughout course of therapy.
- Thiazide diuretics may cause increased serum cholesterol, low-density lipoprotein (LDL), and triglyceride concentrations.

Potential Nursing Diagnoses

- Excess fluid volume (Indications).
- Deficient knowledge, related to disease processes and medication regimen (Patient/Family Teaching).

Implementation

- Administer oral diuretics in the morning to prevent disruption of sleep cycle.
- Many diuretics are available in combination with antihypertensives or potassium-sparing diuretics.

Patient/Family Teaching

- Instruct patient to take medication exactly as directed. Advise patients on antihypertensive regimen to continue taking medication, even if feeling better. Medication controls, but does not cure, hypertension.

- Caution patient to make position changes slowly to minimize orthostatic hypotension. Caution patient that the use of alcohol, exercise during hot weather, or standing for long periods during therapy may enhance orthostatic hypotension.
- Instruct patient to consult health care professional regarding dietary potassium guidelines.
- Instruct patient to monitor weight weekly and report significant changes.
- Caution patient to use sunscreen and protective clothing to prevent photosensitivity reactions.
- Advise patient to consult health care professional before taking OTC medication concurrently with this therapy.
- Instruct patient to notify health care professional of medication regimen before treatment or surgery.
- Advise patient to contact health care professional immediately if muscle weakness, cramps, nausea, dizziness, or numbness or tingling of extremities occurs.
- Emphasize the importance of routine follow-up.
- **Hypertension:** Reinforce the need to continue additional therapies for hypertension (weight loss, regular exercise, restricted sodium intake, stress reduction, moderation of alcohol consumption, and cessation of smoking).
- Instruct patients with hypertension in the correct technique for monitoring weekly blood pressure.

Evaluation/Desired Outcomes

- Decreased blood pressure.
- Increased urine output.
- Decreased edema.
- Reduced intracranial pressure.
- Prevention of hypokalemia in patients taking diuretics.
- Treatment of hyperaldosteronism.

Diuretics included in *Davis's Drug Guide for Nurses*

carbonic anhydrase inhibitors
acetaZOLAMIDE 109, 9

loop diuretics
bumetanide 236
furosemide 587
torsemide 1194

osmotic diuretics
mannitol 770

potassium-sparing diuretics
amiloride 432
spironolactone 432
triamterene 432

thiazide diuretics
chlorothiazide 434
chlorthalidone (thiazide-like) 78
hydrochlorothiazide 434

thiazide-like diuretics
indapamide 672
metolazone 812

• HORMONES

PHARMACOLOGIC PROFILE

General Use

Used in the treatment of deficiency states including diabetes (insulin), diabetes insipidus (desmopressin), hypothyroidism (thyroid hormones), and menopause (estrogens or estrogens/progestins). Estrogenic and progestational hormones are used as contraceptive agents in various combinations and sequences. Hormones may be used to treat hormonally sensitive tumors (androgens, estrogens) and in other selected situations. See individual drugs.

General Action and Information
Natural or synthetic substances that have a specific effect on target tissue. Differ greatly in their effects, depending on individual agent and function of target tissue.

Contraindications
Differ greatly among individual agents; see individual entries.

Precautions
Differ greatly among individual agents; see individual entries.

Interactions
Differ greatly among individual agents; see individual entries.

NURSING IMPLICATIONS

Assessment
- Monitor patient for symptoms of hormonal excess or insufficiency.
- **Sex Hormones:** Blood pressure and hepatic function tests should be monitored periodically throughout therapy.

Potential Nursing Diagnoses
- Sexual dysfunction (Indications).
- Disturbed body image (Indications, Side Effects).
- Deficient knowledge, related to disease processes and medication regimen (Patient/Family Teaching).

Implementation
- **Sex Hormones:** During hospitalization, continue to administer according to schedule followed prior to hospitalization.

Patient/Family Teaching
- Explain dose schedule (and withdrawal bleeding with female sex hormones).
- Emphasize the importance of follow-up exams to monitor effectiveness of therapy and to ensure proper development of children and early detection of possible side effects.
- **Female Sex Hormones:** Advise patient to report signs and symptoms of fluid retention, thromboembolic disorders, mental depression, or hepatic dysfunction to health care professional.

Evaluation/Desired Outcomes
- Resolution of clinical symptoms of hormone imbalance including menopause symptoms and contraception.
- Correction of fluid and electrolyte imbalances.
- Control of the spread of advanced metastatic breast or prostate cancer.
- Slowed progression of postmenopausal osteoporosis.

Hormones included in *Davis's Drug Guide for Nurses*

hormones

calcitonin (salmon) 254
danazol 1276
darbepoetin 377
desmopressin 396, 1326
epoetin 487
estrogens, conjugated (equine) 510
estrogens, conjugated (synthetic, A) 510
estrogens, conjugated (synthetic, B) 510
estropipate 512
fludrocortisone 554
glucagon 601
goserelin 1280
leuprolide 738
levothyroxine 1169, 1325
liothyronine 1169
liotrix 1169
medroxyPROGESTERone 337, 776
megestrol 778
nafarelin 858

nandrolone decanoate 25
octreotide 901, 1326
oxytocin 931
pramlintide 1001
progesterone 1015
somatrem (recombinant) 80
somatropin (recombinant) 607
teriparatide 1151, 1327
testosterone buccal system, mucoadhesive 1152
testosterone cypionate 1152
testosterone enanthate 1152
testosterone pellets 1152
testosterone transdermal 1152
thyroid 1169
triptorelin 1296
vasopressin 1220

insulins

insulin aspart protamine suspension/insulin aspart solution mixtures, rDNA origin 678, 1380
insulin aspart, rDNA origin 670, 1380
insulin detemir 685, 1380
insulin glargine 685, 1380
insulin glulisine 670, 1380
insulin lispro protamine suspension/insulin lispro solution mixtures, rDNA origin 678
insulin lispro, rDNA origin 670, 1380
insulin, regular (injection, concentrated) 681
NPH insulin (isophane insulin suspension) 683, 1380
NPH/regular insulin mixtures 678, 1380

contraceptive hormones

estradiol acetate 506
estradiol cypionate 506
estradiol cypionate/medroxyprogesterone acetate 80
estradiol topical emulsion 507
estradiol topical gel 507
estradiol transdermal spray 507
estradiol transdermal system 507
estradiol vaginal ring 507
estradiol vaginal tablet 507
estradiol valerate 507
ethinyl estradiol/desogestrel 336
ethinyl estradiol/drospirenone 336
ethinyl estradiol/ethynodiol 336
ethinyl estradiol/etonogestrel 337
ethinyl estradiol/levonergestrel 80
ethinyl estradiol/norelgestromin 337
ethinyl estradiol/norethindrone 336–337
ethinyl estradiol/norgestimate 336–337
ethinyl estradiol/norgestrel 336
levonorgestrel 337
levonorgestrel/ethinyl estradiol 80
medroxyprogesterone 337, 776
mestranol/norethindrone 336
norethindrone 337
norethindrone/ethinyl acetate 337
norgestimate/ethinyl estradiol 80
norgestrel 80

• IMMUNOSUPPRESSANTS

PHARMACOLOGIC PROFILE

General Use

Azathioprine, basiliximab, cyclosporine, daclizumab, mycophenolate, sirolimus, and tacrolimus are used with corticosteroids in the prevention of transplantation rejection reactions. Muromonab-CD3 is used to manage rejection reactions not controlled by other agents. Azathioprine, cyclophosphamide, and methotrexate are used in the management of selected autoimmune diseases (nephrotic syndrome of childhood and severe rheumatoid arthritis).

General Action and Information

Inhibit cell-mediated immune responses by different mechanisms. In addition to azathioprine and cyclosporine, which are used primarily for their immunomodulating properties, cyclophosphamide and methotrexate are used to suppress the immune responses in certain disease states (nephrotic syndrome of childhood and severe rheumatoid arthritis). Muromonab-CD3 is a recombinant immunoglobulin antibody that alters T-cell function. Basiliximab and daclizumab are monoclonal antibodies.

Contraindications

Hypersensitivity to drug or vehicle.

Precautions

Use cautiously in patients with infections. Safety in pregnancy and lactation not established.

Interactions

Allopurinol inhibits the metabolism of azathioprine. Drugs that alter liver-metabolizing processes may change the effect of cyclosporine. The risk to toxicity of methotrexate may be increased by other nephrotoxic drugs, large doses of aspirin, or NSAIDs. Muromonab-CD3 has additive immunosuppressive properties; concurrent immunosuppressive doses should be decreased or eliminated.

NURSING IMPLICATIONS

Assessment

- Monitor for infection (vital signs, sputum, urine, stool, WBC). Notify physician or other health care professional immediately if symptoms occur.
- **Organ Transplant:** Assess for symptoms of organ rejection throughout therapy.
- **Lab Test Consideration:** Monitor CBC and differential throughout therapy.

Potential Nursing Diagnoses

- Risk for infection (Side Effects).
- Deficient knowledge, related to disease processes and medication regimen (Patient/Family Teaching).

Implementation

- Protect transplant patients from staff and visitors who may carry infection.
- Maintain protective isolation as indicated.

Patient/Family Teaching

- Reinforce the need for lifelong therapy to prevent transplant rejection. Review symptoms of rejection for transplanted organ and stress need to notify health care professional immediately if they occur.
- Advise patient to avoid contact with contagious persons and those who have recently taken oral polio virus vaccine. Patients should not receive vaccinations without first consulting with health care professional.
- Emphasize the importance of follow-up exams and lab tests.

Evaluation/Desired Outcomes

- Prevention or reversal of rejection of organ transplants or decrease in symptoms of autoimmune disorders.

Immunosuppressants included in *Davis's Drug Guide for Nurses*

azathioprine 206
basiliximab 215
chlorambucil 1274
cyclophosphamide 361
cycloSPORINE 364, 1354
daclizumab 373
methotrexate 801
muromonab-CD3 849
mycophenolate mofetil 850
mycophenolic acid 850
pimecrolimus 985
sirolimus 1110, 1327
tacrolimus (oral, IV) 1134
tacrolimus (topical) 1134
thalidomide 1158

CLASSIFICATIONS

• LAXATIVES

PHARMACOLOGIC PROFILE

General Use

Used to treat or prevent constipation or to prepare the bowel for radiologic or endoscopic procedures.

General Action and Information

Induce one or more bowel movements per day. Groups include stimulants (bisacodyl, sennosides), saline laxatives (magnesium salts and phosphates), stool softeners (docusate), bulk-forming agents (polycarbophil and psyllium), and osmotic cathartics (lactulose, polyethylene glycol/electrolyte). Increasing fluid intake, exercising, and adding more dietary fiber are also useful in the management of chronic constipation.

Contraindications

Hypersensitivity. Contraindicated in persistent abdominal pain, nausea, or vomiting of unknown cause, especially if accompanied by fever or other signs of an acute abdomen.

Precautions

Excessive or prolonged use may lead to dependence. Should not be used in children unless advised by a physician or other health care professional.

Interactions

Theoretically may decrease the absorption of other orally administered drugs by decreasing transit time.

NURSING IMPLICATIONS

Assessment

- Assess patient for abdominal distention, presence of bowel sounds, and usual pattern of bowel function.
- Assess color, consistency, and amount of stool produced.

Potential Nursing Diagnoses

- Constipation (Indications).
- Deficient knowledge, related to disease processes and medication regimen (Patient/Family Teaching).

Implementation

- Many laxatives may be administered at bedtime for morning results.
- Taking oral doses on an empty stomach will usually produce more rapid results.
- Do not crush or chew enteric-coated tablets. Take with a full glass of water or juice.
- Stool softeners and bulk laxatives may take several days for results.

Patient/Family Teaching

- Advise patients, other than those with spinal cord injuries, that laxatives should be used only for short-term therapy. Long-term therapy may cause electrolyte imbalance and dependence.
- Advise patient to increase fluid intake to a minimum of 1500–2000 ml/day during therapy to prevent dehydration.
- Encourage patients to use other forms of bowel regulation: increasing bulk in the diet, increasing fluid intake, and increasing mobility. Normal bowel habits are individualized and may vary from 3 times/day to 3 times/wk.
- Instruct patients with cardiac disease to avoid straining during bowel movements (Valsalva maneuver).
- Advise patient that laxatives should not be used when constipation is accompanied by abdominal pain, fever, nausea, or vomiting.

Evaluation/Desired Outcomes

- A soft, formed bowel movement.
- Evacuation of the colon.

Laxatives included in *Davis's Drug Guide for Nurses*

bulk-forming agents
polycarbophil 1289
psyllium 1035
osmotics
lactulose 721
polyethylene glycol/electrolyte 992
polyethylene glycol 991
salines
magnesium chloride 766
magnesium citrate 766
magnesium gluconate 766
magnesium hydroxide 766
magnesium oxide 766
phosphate/biphosphate 980
stimulant laxatives
bisacodyl 223
sennosides 1101
stool softeners
docusate calcium 442
docusate sodium 442

• LIPID-LOWERING AGENTS

PHARMACOLOGIC PROFILE

General Use

Used as a part of a total plan including diet and exercise to reduce blood lipids in an effort to reduce the morbidity and mortality of atherosclerotic cardiovascular disease and its sequelae.

General Action and Information

HMG-CoA reductase inhibitors (atorvastatin, fluvastatin, lovastatin, pravastatin, simvastatin) inhibit an enzyme involved in cholesterol synthesis. Bile acid sequestrants (cholestyramine, colestipol, colesevelam) bind cholesterol in the GI tract. Fenofibrate, niacin, and gemfibrozil act by other mechanisms (see individual monographs).

Contraindications

Hypersensitivity.

Precautions

Safety in pregnancy, lactation, and children not established. See individual drugs. Dietary therapy should be given a 2–3 mo trial before drug therapy is initiated.

Interactions

Bile acid sequestrants (cholestyramine and colestipol) may bind lipid-soluble vitamins (A, D, E, and K) and other concurrently administered drugs in the GI tract. The risk of myopathy from HMG-CoA reductase inhibitors is increased by niacin, erythromycin, gemfibrozil, and cyclosporine.

NURSING IMPLICATIONS

Assessment

- Obtain a diet history, especially in regard to **fat** and alcohol consumption.
- **Lab Test Considerations:** Serum cholesterol and triglyceride levels should be evaluated before initiating and periodically throughout therapy. Medication should be discontinued if paradoxical increase in cholesterol level occurs.
- Liver function tests should be assessed before and periodically throughout therapy. May cause an increase in levels.

CLASSIFICATIONS

Potential Nursing Diagnoses

- Deficient knowledge, related to disease processes and medication regimen (Patient/Family Teaching).
- Noncompliance (Patient/Family Teaching).

Implementation

- See specific medications to determine timing of doses in relation to meals.

Patient/Family Teaching

- Advise patient that these medications should be used in conjunction with diet restrictions (**fat, cholesterol, carbohydrates,** and alcohol), exercise, and cessation of smoking.

Evaluation/Desired Outcomes

- Decreased serum triglyceride and LDL **cholesterol** levels and improved HDL cholesterol ratios. Therapy is usually discontinued if the clinical response is not evident after 3 mo of therapy.

Lipid-lowering agents included in *Davis's Drug Guide for Nurses*

bile acid sequestrants
cholestyramine 306
colesevelam 333, 1326
colestipol 334
HMG-CoA reductase inhibitors
atorvastatin 629
fluvastatin 629
lovastatin 629
pravastatin 629
rosuvastatin 629
simvastatin 629
miscellaneous
ezetimibe 527
fenofibrate 532
gemfibrozil 599
niacin 877
niacinamide 877
omega-3 acid ethyl esters 84

• MINERALS/ELECTROLYTES/PH MODIFIERS

PHARMACOLOGIC PROFILE

General Use

Prevention and treatment of deficiencies or excesses of electrolytes and maintenance of optimal acid/base balance for homeostasis. Acidifiers and alkalinizers are also used to promote urinary excretion of substances that accumulate in certain disease states (kidney stones, uric acid).

General Action and Information

Electrolytes and minerals are necessary for many body processes. Maintenance of electrolyte levels within normal limits is required for many physiological processes such as cardiac, nerve, and muscle function; bone growth and stability; and a number of other activities. Minerals and electrolytes may also serve as catalysts in many enzymatic reactions. Acid/base balance allows for normal transfer of substances at the cellular and intracellular level.

Contraindications

Contraindicated in situations in which replacement would cause excess or when risk factors for retention are present.

Precautions

Use cautiously in disease states in which electrolyte imbalances are common such as significant hepatic or renal disease, adrenal or pituitary disorders.

Interactions

Depend on individual agents. Alkalinizers and acidifiers can alter the excretion of drugs for which elimination is pH dependent. See specific entries.

NURSING IMPLICATIONS

Assessment

- Observe patient carefully for evidence of electrolyte excess or insufficiency. Monitor lab values before and periodically throughout therapy.

Potential Nursing Diagnoses

- Imbalanced nutrition: less than body requirements (Indications).
- Deficient knowledge, related to medication regimen (Patient/Family Teaching).

Implementation

- **Potassium Chloride:** Do not administer potassium chloride undiluted.

Patient/Family Teaching

- Review diet modifications with patients with chronic electrolyte disturbances.

Evaluation/Desired Outcomes

- Return to normal serum electrolyte concentrations and resolution of clinical symptoms of electrolyte imbalance.
- Changes in pH or composition of urine, which prevent formation of renal calculi.

Minerals/Electrolytes/pH Modifiers included in *Davis's Drug Guide for Nurses*

alkalinizing agents
sodium bicarbonate 1114
sodium citrate and citric acid 1118

calcium salts
calcium acetate (25% Ca or 12.6 mEq/g) 85
calcium carbonate (40% Ca or 20 mEq/g) 85
calcium chloride (27% Ca or 13.6 mEq/g) 85
calcium citrate (21% Ca or 12 mEq/g) 85
calcium gluconate (9% Ca or 4.5 mEq/g) 85
calcium lactate (13% Ca or 6.5 mEq/g) 85
tricalcium phosphate (39% Ca or 19.5 mEq/g) 85

magnesium salts
magnesium chloride (12% Mg; 9.8 mEq Mg/g) 85
magnesium citrate (16.2% Mg; 4.4 mEq Mg/g) 85
magnesium gluconate (5.4 % Mg; 4.4 mEq/g) 85
magnesium hydroxide (41.7% Mg; 34.3 mEq Mg/g) 85
magnesium oxide (60.3% Mg; 49.6 mEq Mg/g) 85
magnesium sulfate (IV, parenteral) 768

phosphate supplements
sodium phosphate 1291

potassium and sodium phosphates
monobasic potassium phosphate 1289
monobasic potassium and sodium phosphates 85
potassium phosphates 1289
potassium and sodium phosphates 994

potassium phosphates
monobasic potassium phosphate 1289
potassium phosphates 1289

potassium salts
potassium acetate 996
potassium bicarbonate 996
potassium bicarbonate/potassium chloride 996
potassium bicarbonate/potassium citrate 996
potassium chloride 996
potassium chloride/potassium bicarbonate/potassium citrate 996
potassium gluconate 996
potassium gluconate/potassium chloride 996
potassium gluconate/potassium citrate 996

miscellaneous
sodium chloride 12
sodium phosphate 1291
zinc sulfate 1256

• NATURAL/HERBAL PRODUCTS

PHARMACOLOGIC PROFILE

General Use
These remedies are used for a wide variety of conditions. Prescriptions are not required and consumers have the choice of many products.

General Action and Information
Use of these agents is based on historical and sometimes anecdotal evidence. The FDA has little control over these agents, so currently there is little standardization among products.

Contraindications
Hypersensitivity. Most products are plant extracts that may contain a variety of impurities.

Precautions
Elderly, pediatric, and pregnant or lactating patients should be aware that these agents carry many of the same risks as prescription medications. Patients with serious chronic medical conditions should consult their health care professional before use.

Interactions
These agents have the ability to interact with prescription medications and may prevent or augment a desired therapeutic outcome. St. John's wort and kava-kava have the greatest risk for serious interactions.

NURSING IMPLICATIONS

Assessment
- Assess the condition for which the patient is taking the product.

Potential Nursing Diagnoses
- Deficient knowledge, related to disease processes and medication regimen (Patient/Family Teaching).

Patient/Family Teaching
- Discuss with patient the reason for using the product. Encourage patient to choose products with USP label, if possible, to guarantee content and purity of medication.
- Inform patient of known side effects and interactions with other medications.

Evaluation/Desired Outcomes
- Improvement in condition for which medication was taken.

Natural/Herbal Products included in *Davis's Drug Guide for Nurses*

arnica 1297
black cohosh 1298
chondroitin 1299
dong quai 1300
echinacea 1301
feverfew 1303
garlic 1304
ginger 1305
ginkgo 1306
ginseng 1308
glucosamine 1309
hawthorne 1310
kava-kava 1312
milk thistle 1313
SAMe 1314
saw palmetto 1315
St. John's wort 1316
valerian 1317

• NONOPIOID ANALGESICS

PHARMACOLOGIC PROFILE

General Use

Used to control mild to moderate pain and/or fever. Phenazopyridine is used only to treat urinary tract pain, and capsaicin is used topically for a variety of painful syndromes.

General Action and Information

Most nonopioid analgesics inhibit prostaglandin synthesis peripherally for analgesic effect and centrally for antipyretic effect. Tramadol is a centrally acting agent.

Contraindications

Hypersensitivity and cross-sensitivity among NSAIDs may occur.

Precautions

Use cautiously in patients with severe hepatic or renal disease, chronic alcohol use/abuse, or malnutrition. Tramadol has CNS depressant properties.

Interactions

Long-term use of acetaminophen with NSAIDs may increase the risk of adverse renal effects. Prolonged high-dose acetaminophen may increase the risk of bleeding with warfarin. Hepatotoxicity may be additive with other hepatotoxic agents, including alcohol. NSAIDs increase the risk of bleeding with warfarin, thrombolytic agents, antiplatelet agents, some cephalosporins, and valproates (effect is greatest with aspirin). NSAIDs may also decrease the effectiveness of diuretics and antihypertensives. The risk of CNS depression with tramadol is increased by concurrent use of other CNS depressants, including alcohol, antihistamines, sedative/hypnotics, and some antidepressants.

NURSING IMPLICATIONS

Assessment

- Patients who have asthma, allergies, and nasal polyps or who are allergic to tartrazine are at an increased risk for developing hypersensitivity reactions.
- **Pain:** Assess pain and limitation of movement; note type, location, and intensity prior to and at the peak (see Time/Action Profile) following administration.
- **Fever:** Assess fever and note associated signs (diaphoresis, tachycardia, malaise, chills).
- **Lab Test Considerations:** Hepatic, hematologic, and renal function should be evaluated periodically throughout prolonged high-dose therapy. Aspirin and most NSAIDs prolong bleeding time due to suppressed platelet aggregation and, in large doses, may cause prolonged prothrombin time. Monitor hematocrit periodically in prolonged high-dose therapy to assess for GI blood loss.

Potential Nursing Diagnoses

- Acute pain (Indications).
- Risk for imbalanced body temperature (Indications).
- Deficient knowledge, related to disease processes and medication regimen (Patient/Family Teaching).

Implementation

- **PO:** Administer salicylates and NSAIDs after meals or with food or an antacid to minimize gastric irritation.

Patient/Family Teaching

- Instruct patient to take salicylates and NSAIDs with a full glass of water and to remain in an upright position for 15–30 min after administration.
- Adults should not take acetaminophen longer than 10 days and children not longer than 5 days unless directed by health care professional. Short-term doses of acetaminophen with salicylates or NSAIDs should not exceed the recommended daily dose of either drug alone.
- Caution patient to avoid concurrent use of alcohol with this medication to minimize possible gastric irritation; 3 or more glasses of alcohol per day may increase the risk of GI bleeding with salicylates or NSAIDs. Caution patient to avoid taking acetaminophen, salicylates, or NSAIDs concurrently for more than a few days, unless directed by health care professional to prevent analgesic nephropathy.
- Advise patients on long-term therapy to inform health care professional of medication regimen prior to surgery. Aspirin, salicylates, and NSAIDs may need to be withheld prior to surgery.

Evaluation/Desired Outcomes

- Relief of mild to moderate discomfort.
- Reduction of fever.

Nonopioid analgesics included in *Davis's Drug Guide for Nurses*

nonsteroidal anti-inflammatory agents

diclofenac potassium 408
diclofenac sodium 408
diclofenac topical 408
etodolac 521
ibuprofen, oral 654
ketoprofen 714
ketorolac 716, 1326, 1354
meloxicam 779
naproxen 864

salicylates

aspirin 1087
choline and magnesium salicylates 1087
choline salicylate 1087
magnesium salicylate 1087
salsalate 1087
sodium salicylate 1087

miscellaneous

acetaminophen 107
butalbital compounds 88
capsaicin 261
flavocoxid 550
phenazopyridine 971

• NONSTEROIDAL ANTI-INFLAMMATORY AGENTS

PHARMACOLOGIC PROFILE

General Use

NSAIDs are used to control mild to moderate pain, fever, and various inflammatory conditions, such as rheumatoid arthritis and osteoarthritis. Ophthalmic NSAIDs are used to decrease postoperative ocular inflammation, to inhibit perioperative miosis, and to decrease inflammation due to allergies.

General Action and Information

NSAIDs have analgesic, antipyretic, and anti-inflammatory properties. Analgesic and anti-inflammatory effects are due to inhibition of prostaglandin synthesis. Antipyretic action is due to vasodilation and inhibition of prostaglandin synthesis in the CNS. COX-2 inhibitors (celecoxib) may cause less GI bleeding.

Contraindications

Hypersensitivity to aspirin is a contraindication for the whole group of NSAIDs. Cross-sensitivity may occur.

Precautions

Use cautiously in patients with a history of bleeding disorders, GI bleeding, and severe hepatic, renal, or cardiovascular disease. Safe use in pregnancy is not established and, in general, should be avoided during the second half of pregnancy.

Interactions

NSAIDs prolong bleeding time and potentiate the effect of warfarin, thrombolytic agents, some cephalosporins, antiplatelet agents, and valproates. Prolonged use with aspirin may result in increased GI side effects and decreased effectiveness. NSAIDs may also decrease response to diuretics or antihypertensive therapy. Ibuprofen negates the cardioprotective benefits of low-dose aspirin. COX-2 inhibitors do not negate the cardioprotective effect of low-dose aspirin.

NURSING IMPLICATIONS

Assessment

- Patients who have asthma, allergies, and nasal polyps or who are allergic to tartrazine are at an increased risk for developing hypersensitivity reactions.
- **Pain:** Assess pain and limitation of movement; note type, location, and intensity prior to and at the peak (see Time/Action Profile) following administration.
- **Fever:** Assess fever and note associated signs (diaphoresis, tachycardia, malaise, chills).
- **Lab Test Considerations:** Most NSAIDs prolong bleeding time due to suppressed platelet aggregation and, in large doses, may cause prolonged PT. Monitor periodically in prolonged high-dose therapy to assess for GI blood loss.

Potential Nursing Diagnoses

- Acute pain (Indications).
- Risk for imbalanced body temperature (Indications).
- Deficient knowledge, related to disease processes and medication regimen (Patient/Family Teaching).

Implementation

- **PO:** Administer NSAIDs after meals or with food or an antacid to minimize gastric irritation.

Patient/Family Teaching

- Instruct patient to take NSAIDs with a full glass of water and to remain in an upright position for 15–30 min after administration.
- Caution patient to avoid concurrent use of alcohol with this medication to minimize possible gastric irritation; 3 or more glasses of alcohol per day may increase the risk of GI bleeding with salicylates or NSAIDs. Caution patient to avoid taking acetaminophen, salicylates, or NSAIDs concurrently for more than a few days, unless directed by health care professional to prevent analgesic nephropathy.
- Advise patient on long-term therapy to inform health care professional of medication regimen prior to surgery. NSAIDs may need to be withheld prior to surgery.

Evaluation/Desired Outcomes

- Relief of mild to moderate discomfort.
- Reduction of fever.

Nonsteroidal anti-inflammatory agents included in *Davis's Drug Guide for Nurses*

nonsteroidal anti-inflammatory agents

celecoxib 278, 1326
diclofenac potassium 408
diclofenac sodium 408
dicofenac topical 89
diclofenac (topical patch) 1321
flurbiprofen 1279, 1354
ibuprofen, oral 654
indomethacin 674

CLASSIFICATIONS

ketoprofen 714
ketorolac 716, 1326, 1354
meloxicam 779
nabumetone 855
naproxen 864
oxaprozin 919
piroxicam 989
sulindac 1128
tolmetin 1294

ophthalmic NSAIDs

bromfenac 1273, 1354
diclofenac 408, 1354
flurbiprofen 1279, 1354
ketorolac 716, 1326, 1354
nepafenac 1355
suprofen 90

• OPIOID ANALGESICS

PHARMACOLOGIC PROFILE

General Use

Management of moderate to severe pain. Fentanyl is also used as a general anesthetic adjunct.

General Action and Information

Opioids bind to opiate receptors in the CNS, where they act as agonists of endogenously occurring opioid peptides (eukephalins and endorphins). The result is alteration to the perception of and response to pain.

Contraindications

Hypersensitivity to individual agents.

Precautions

Use cautiously in patients with undiagnosed abdominal pain, head trauma or pathology, liver disease, or history of addiction to opioids. Use smaller doses initially in the elderly and those with respiratory diseases. Prolonged use may result in tolerance and the need for larger doses to relieve pain. Psychological or physical dependence may occur.

Interactions

Increases the CNS depressant properties of other drugs, including alcohol, antihistamines, antidepressants, sedative/hypnotics, phenothiazines, and MAO inhibitors. Use of partial-antagonist opioid analgesics (buprenorphine, butorphanol, nalbuphine, and pentazocine) may precipitate opioid withdrawal in physically dependent patients. Use with MAO inhibitors or procarbazine may result in severe paradoxical reactions (especially with meperidine). Nalbuphine or pentazocine may decrease the analgesic effects of other concurrently administered opioid analgesics.

NURSING IMPLICATIONS

Assessment

- Assess type, location, and intensity of pain prior to and at peak following administration. When titrating opioid doses, increases of 25–50% should be administered until there is either a 50% reduction in the patient's pain rating on a numerical or visual analogue scale or the patient reports satisfactory pain relief. A repeat dose can be safely administered at the time of the peak if previous dose is ineffective and side effects are minimal. Patients requiring higher doses of opioid agonist-antagonists should be converted to an opioid agonist.
- Opioid agonist-antagonists are not recommended for prolonged use or as first-line therapy for acute or cancer pain.
- An equianalgesic chart (see Appendix J) should be used when changing routes or when changing from one opioid to another.
- Assess blood pressure, pulse, and respirations before and periodically during administration. If respiratory rate is <10/min, assess level of sedation. Physical stimulation may be sufficient

to prevent significant hypoventilation. Dose may need to be decreased by 25–50%. Initial drowsiness will diminish with continued use.

- Assess prior analgesic history. Antagonistic properties of agonist-antagonists may induce withdrawal symptoms (vomiting, restlessness, abdominal cramps, and increased blood pressure and temperature) in patients physically dependent on opioids.
- Prolonged use may lead to physical and psychological dependence and tolerance. This should not prevent patient from receiving adequate analgesia. Most patients who receive opioid analgesics for pain do not develop psychological dependence. Progressively higher doses may be required to relieve pain with chronic therapy.
- Assess bowel function routinely. Prevention of constipation should be instituted with increased intake of fluids and bulk, stool softeners, and laxatives to minimize constipating effects. Stimulant laxatives should be administered routinely if opioid use exceeds 2–3 days, unless contraindicated.
- Monitor intake and output ratios. If significant discrepancies occur, assess for urinary retention and inform physician or other health care professional.
- **Toxicity and Overdose:** If an opioid antagonist is required to reverse respiratory depression or coma, naloxone (Narcan) is the antidote. Dilute the 0.4-mg ampule of naloxone in 10 ml of 0.9% NaCl and administer 0.5 ml (0.02 mg) by direct IV push every 2 min. For children and patients weighing <40 kg, dilute 0.1 mg of naloxone in 10 ml of 0.9% NaCl for a concentration of 10 mcg/ml and administer 0.5 mcg/kg every 1–2 min. Titrate dose to avoid withdrawal, seizures, and severe pain.

Potential Nursing Diagnoses

- Acute pain (Indications).
- Disturbed sensory perception (auditory, visual) (Side Effects).
- Risk for injury (Side Effects).
- Deficient knowledge, related to disease processes and medication regimen (Patient/Family Teaching).

Implementation

- Do not confuse morphine with hydromorphone or meperidine; errors have resulted in fatalities.
- Explain therapeutic value of medication before administration to enhance the analgesic effect.
- Regularly administered doses may be more effective than prn administration. Analgesic is more effective if given before pain becomes severe.
- Coadministration with nonopioid analgesics may have additive analgesic effects and may permit lower doses.
- Medication should be discontinued gradually after long-term use to prevent withdrawal symptoms.

Patient/Family Teaching

- Instruct patient on how and when to ask for pain medication.
- Medication may cause drowsiness or dizziness. Caution patient to call for assistance when ambulating or smoking and to avoid driving or other activities requiring alertness until response to medication is known.
- Advise patient to make position changes slowly to minimize orthostatic hypotension.
- Caution patient to avoid concurrent use of alcohol or other CNS depressants with this medication.
- Encourage patient to turn, cough, and breathe deeply every 2 hr to prevent atelectasis.

Evaluation/Desired Outcomes

- Decreased severity of pain without a significant alteration in level of consciousness or respiratory status.

Opioid analgesics included in *Davis's Drug Guide for Nurses*

opioid agonists/antagonists
buprenorphine 238, 1373
butorphanol 249, 1373
pentazocine 966, 1373

opioid agonists
codeine 330
fentanyl (oral transmucosal) 538
fentanyl (parenteral) 540
fentanyl (transdermal) 542
hydrocodone 637
hydromorphone 640, 1372, 1374
meperidine 784, 1373
methadone 795, 1372
morphine 843, 1372–1374
nalbuphine 860, 1373
oxycodone 926, 1372
oxymorphone 929, 1372
propoxyphene 1024

• SEDATIVE/HYPNOTICS

PHARMACOLOGIC PROFILE

General Use

Sedatives are used to provide sedation, usually prior to procedures. Hypnotics are used to manage insomnia. Selected agents are useful as anticonvulsants (clorazepate, diazepam, phenobarbital), skeletal muscle relaxants (diazepam), adjuncts in the management of alcohol withdrawal syndrome (chlordiazepoxide, diazepam, oxazepam), as adjuncts in general anesthesia (droperidol) or amnestics (midazolam, diazepam).

General Action and Information

Cause generalized CNS depression. May produce tolerance with chronic use and have potential for psychological or physical dependence. These agents have NO analgesic properties.

Contraindications

Hypersensitivity. Should not be used in comatose patients nor in those with pre-existing CNS depression. Should not be used in patients with uncontrolled severe pain. Avoid use during pregnancy or lactation.

Precautions

Use cautiously in patients with hepatic dysfunction, severe renal impairment, or severe underlying pulmonary disease. Use with caution in patients who may be suicidal or who may have had previous drug addictions. Hypnotic use should be short-term. Geriatric patients may be more sensitive to CNS depressant effects; dosage reduction may be required.

Interactions

Additive CNS depression with alcohol, antihistamines, some antidepressants, opioid analgesics, or phenothiazines. Barbiturates induce hepatic drug-metabolizing enzymes and can decrease the effectiveness of drugs metabolized by the liver, including oral contraceptives. Should not be used with MAO inhibitors.

NURSING IMPLICATIONS

Assessment

- Monitor blood pressure, pulse, and respiratory status frequently throughout IV administration. Prolonged high-dose therapy may lead to psychological or physical dependence. Restrict the amount of drug available to patient, especially if patient is depressed, suicidal, or has a history of addiction.
- **Insomnia:** Assess sleep patterns before and periodically throughout course of therapy.
- **Seizures:** Observe and record intensity, duration, and characteristics of seizure activity. Institute seizure precautions.

- **Muscle Spasms:** Assess muscle spasms, associated pain, and limitation of movement before and throughout therapy.
- **Alcohol Withdrawal:** Assess patient experiencing alcohol withdrawal for tremors, agitation, delirium, and hallucinations. Protect patient from injury.

Potential Nursing Diagnoses

- Imsomnia (Indications).
- Risk for injury (Side Effects).
- Deficient knowledge, related to disease processes and medication regimen (Patient/Family Teaching).

Implementation

- Supervise ambulation and transfer of patients following administration of hypnotic doses. Remove cigarettes. Side rails should be raised and call bell within reach at all times. Keep bed in low position.

Patient/Family Teaching

- Discuss the importance of preparing the environment for sleep (dark room, quiet, avoidance of nicotine and caffeine). If less effective after a few weeks, consult health care professional; do not increase dose. Gradual withdrawal may be required to prevent reactions following prolonged therapy.
- May cause daytime drowsiness. Caution patient to avoid driving and other activities requiring alertness until response to medication is known.
- Advise patient to avoid the use of alcohol and other CNS depressants concurrently with these medications.
- Advise patient to inform health care professional if pregnancy is planned or suspected.

Evaluation/Desired Outcomes

- Improvement in sleep patterns.
- Control of seizures.
- Decrease in muscle spasms.
- Decreased tremulousness.
- More rational ideation when used for alcohol withdrawal.

Sedative/hypnotics included in *Davis's Drug Guide for Nurses*

barbiturates
phenobarbital 972

benzodiazepines
chlordiazepoxide 298
clorazepate 325
diazepam 404
flurazepam 571
lorazepam 762
midazolam 822
oxazepam 921
temazepam 1143
triazolam 1202

miscellaneous
chloral hydrate 296
dexmedetomidine 1277
droperidol 461
eszopiclone 514, 1326
hydrOXYzine 644
promethazine 1017
ramelteon 1053
zaleplon 1250
zolpidem 1262

• SKELETAL MUSCLE RELAXANTS

PHARMACOLOGIC PROFILE

General Use
Two major uses are spasticity associated with spinal cord diseases or lesions (baclofen and dantrolene) or adjunctive therapy in the symptomatic relief of acute painful musculoskeletal conditions (cyclobenzaprine, diazepam, and methocarbamol). IV dantrolene is also used to treat and prevent malignant hyperthermia.

General Action and Information
Act either centrally (baclofen, carisoprodol, cyclobenzaprine, diazepam, and methocarbamol) or directly (dantrolene).

Contraindications
Baclofen and oral dantrolene should not be used in patients in whom spasticity is used to maintain posture and balance.

Precautions
Safety in pregnancy and lactation not established. Use cautiously in patients with a history of previous liver disease.

Interactions
Additive CNS depression with other CNS depressants, including alcohol, antihistamines, antidepressants, opioid analgesics, and sedative/hypnotics.

NURSING IMPLICATIONS

Assessment
- Assess patient for pain, muscle stiffness, and range of motion before and periodically throughout therapy.

Potential Nursing Diagnoses
- Acute pain (Indications).
- Impaired physical mobility (Indications).
- Risk for injury (Side Effects).

Implementation
- Provide safety measures as indicated. Supervise ambulation and transfer of patients.

Patient/Family Teaching
- Encourage patient to comply with additional therapies prescribed for muscle spasm (rest, physical therapy, heat).
- Medication may cause drowsiness. Caution patient to avoid driving or other activities requiring alertness until response to drug is known.
- Advise patient to avoid concurrent use of alcohol or other CNS depressants with these medications.

Evaluation/Desired Outcomes
- Decreased musculoskeletal pain.
- Decreased muscle spasticity.
- Increased range of motion.
- Prevention or decrease in temperature and skeletal rigidity in malignant hyperthermia.

Skeletal muscle relaxants included in *Davis's Drug Guide for Nurses*

centrally-acting
baclofen 213
carisoprodol 268
chlorzoxazone 305
cyclobenzaprine 360, 1325
diazepam 404
metaxalone 792
methocarbamol 799
orphenadrine 915

direct-acting
dantrolene 374

• THROMBOLYTICS

PHARMACOLOGIC PROFILE

General Use

Acute management of coronary thrombosis (MI). Streptokinase and urokinase are used in the management of massive pulmonary emboli, deep vein thrombosis, and arterial thromboembolism. Alteplase is used in the management of acute ischemic stroke.

General Action and Information

Converts plasminogen to plasmin, which then degrades fibrin in clots. Alteplase, reteplase, and urokinase directly activate plasminogen. Streptokinase binds with plasminogen to form activator complexes, which then convert plasminogen to plasmin. Results in lysis of thrombi in coronary arteries, pulmonary emboli, or deep vein thrombosis, or clearing of clots in cannulae/catheters.

Contraindications

Hypersensitivity. Cross-sensitivity with streptokinase may occur. Contraindicated in active internal bleeding, history of cerebrovascular accident, recent CNS trauma or surgery, neoplasm, or arteriovenous malformation. Severe uncontrolled hypertension and known bleeding tendencies.

Precautions

Recent (within 10 days) major surgery, trauma, GI or GU bleeding. Severe hepatic or renal disease. Subacute bacterial endocarditis or acute pericarditis. Use cautiously in geriatric patients. Safety not established in pregnancy, lactation, or children.

Interactions

Concurrent use with aspirin, NSAIDs, warfarin, heparins, ticlopidine, or dipyridamole may increase the risk of bleeding, although these agents are frequently used together or in sequence. Risk of bleeding may also be increased by concurrent use with cefotetan, cefoperazone, and valproic acid.

NURSING IMPLICATIONS

Assessment

- Begin therapy as soon as possible after the onset of symptoms.
- Monitor vital signs, including temperature, continuously for coronary thrombosis and at least every 4 hr during therapy for other indications. Do not use lower extremities to monitor blood pressure.
- Assess patient carefully for bleeding every 15 min during the 1st hr of therapy, every 15–30 min during the next 8 hr, and at least every 4 hr for the duration of therapy. Frank bleeding may occur from sites of invasive procedures or from body orifices. Internal bleeding may also occur (decreased neurologic status; abdominal pain with coffee-ground emesis or black, tarry stools; hematuria; joint pain). If uncontrolled bleeding occurs, stop medication and notify physician immediately.
- Inquire about previous reaction to streptokinase therapy. Assess patient for hypersensitivity reaction (rash, dyspnea, fever, changes in facial color, swelling around the eyes, wheezing). If

these occur, inform physician promptly. Keep epinephrine, an antihistamine, and resuscitation equipment close by in the event of an anaphylactic reaction.

- Inquire about recent streptococcal infection. Streptokinase may be less effective if administered between 5 days and 6 mo of a streptococcal infection.
- Assess neurologic status throughout therapy.
- Altered sensorium or neurologic changes may be indicative of intracranial bleeding.
- **Coronary Thrombosis:** Monitor ECG continuously. Notify physician if significant arrhythmias occur. IV lidocaine or procainamide (Pronestyl) may be ordered prophylactically. Cardiac enzymes should be monitored. Radionuclide myocardial scanning and/or coronary angiography may be ordered 7–10 days following therapy to monitor effectiveness of therapy.
- Monitor heart sounds and breath sounds frequently. Inform physician if signs of CHF occur (rales/crackles, dyspnea, S3 heart sound, jugular venous distention, relieved CVP).
- **Pulmonary Embolism:** Monitor pulse, blood pressure, hemodynamics, and respiratory status (rate, degree of dyspnea, arterial blood gases).
- **Deep Vein Thrombosis/Acute Arterial Occlusion:** Observe extremities and palpate pulses of affected extremities every hour. Notify physician immediately if circulatory impairment occurs. Computed tomography, impedance plethysmography, quantitative Doppler effect determination, and/or angiography or venography may be used to determine restoration of blood flow and duration of therapy; however, repeated venograms are not recommended.
- **Cannula/Catheter Occlusion:** Monitor ability to aspirate blood as indicator of patency. Ensure that patient exhales and holds breath when connecting and disconnecting IV syringe to prevent air embolism.
- **Acute Ischemic Stroke:** Assess neurologic status. Determine time of onset of stroke symptoms. Alteplase must be administered within 3 hr of onset.
- **Lab Test Considerations:** Hematocrit, hemoglobin, platelet count, fibrin/fibrin degradation product (FDP/fdp) titer, fibrinogen concentration, prothrombin time, thrombin time, and activated partial thromboplastin time may be evaluated prior to and frequently throughout therapy. Bleeding time may be assessed prior to therapy if patient has received platelet aggregation inhibitors. Obtain type and cross match and have blood available at all times in case of hemorrhage. Stools should be tested for occult blood loss and urine for hematuria periodically during therapy.
- **Toxicity and Overdose:** If local bleeding occurs, apply pressure to site. If severe or internal bleeding occurs, discontinue infusion. Clotting factors and/or blood volume may be restored through infusions of whole blood, packed RBCs, fresh frozen plasma, or cryoprecipitate. Do not administer dextran, as it has antiplatelet activity. Aminocaproic acid (Amicar) may be used as an antidote.

Potential Nursing Diagnoses

- Ineffective tissue perfusion (Indications).
- Risk for injury (Side Effects).
- Deficient knowledge, related to disease processes and medication regimen (Patient/Family Teaching).

Implementation

- This medication should be used only in settings in which hematologic function and clinical response can be adequately monitored.
- Starting two IV lines prior to therapy is recommended: one for the thrombolytic agent, the other for any additional infusions.
- Avoid invasive procedures, such as IM injections or arterial punctures, with this therapy. If such procedures must be performed, apply pressure to all arterial and venous puncture sites for at least 30 min. Avoid venipunctures at noncompressible sites (jugular vein, subclavian site).
- Systemic anticoagulation with heparin is usually begun several hours after the completion of thrombolytic therapy.

- Acetaminophen may be ordered to control fever.

Patient/Family Teaching

- Explain purpose of medication and the need for close monitoring to patient and family. Instruct patient to report hypersensitivity reactions (rash, dyspnea) and bleeding or bruising.
- Explain need for bedrest and minimal handling during therapy to avoid injury. Avoid all unnecessary procedures such as shaving and vigorous tooth brushing.

Evaluation/Desired Outcomes

- Lysis of thrombi and restoration of blood flow.
- Prevention of neurologic sequelae in acute ischemic stroke.
- Cannula or catheter patency.

Thrombolytics included in *Davis's Drug Guide for Nurses*

alteplase 1164
reteplase 1164
streptokinase 1164
tenecteplase 1164
urokinase 1164

• VACCINES/IMMUNIZING AGENTS

PHARMACOLOGIC PROFILE

General Use

Immune globulins provide passive immunization to infectious diseases by providing antibodies. Immunization with vaccines and toxoids containing bacterial or viral antigenic material results in endogenous production of antibodies.

General Action and Information

Immunity from immune globulins is rapid, but short-lived (up to 3 months). Active immunization with vaccine or toxoids produces prolonged immunity (years).

Contraindications

Hypersensitivity to product, preservatives, or other additives. Some products contain thimerisol, neomycin, and/or **egg protein.**

Precautions

Severe bleeding problems (IM injections).

Interactions

Decreased antibody response to vaccine/toxoids and increased risk of adverse reactions in patients receiving concurrent antineoplastic, immunosuppressive, or radiation therapy.

NURSING IMPLICATIONS

Assessment

- Assess previous immunization history and history of hypersensitivity.

Potential Nursing Diagnoses

- Risk for infection (Indications).
- Deficient knowledge, related to disease processes and medication regimen (Patient/Family Teaching).

Implementation

- Measles, mumps, and rubella vaccine, trivalent oral polio virus vaccine, and diptheria toxoid, tetanus toxoid, and pertussis vaccine may be given concurrently.
- Administer each immunization by appropriate route.

Patient/Family Teaching

- Inform patient/parent of potential and reportable side effects of immunization. Health care professional should be notified if patient develops fever over 39.4°C (103°F); difficulty breathing; hives; itching; swelling of the eyes, face, or inside of nose; sudden severe tiredness or weakness; or convulsions occur.
- Review next scheduled immunization with parent. Emphasize the importance of keeping a record of immunizations and dates given.

Evaluation/Desired Outcomes

- Prevention of diseases through active immunity.

Vaccines/immunizing agents included in *Davis's Drug Guide for Nurses*

immune globulins

botulism immune globulin 1272
cytomegalovirus immune globulin 1276
Rh_0(D) immune globulin standard dose IM 1060
Rh_0(D) globulin IV 98
Rh_0(D) globulin microdose IM 98

miscellaneous

quadravalent human papillomavirus (types 6, 11, 16, 18) recombinant vaccine 98
zoster vaccine, live 1265

• VASCULAR HEADACHE SUPPRESSANTS

PHARMACOLOGIC PROFILE

General Use

Used for acute treatment of vascular headaches (migraine, cluster headaches, migraine variants). Other agents such as some beta blockers and some calcum channel blockers are used for suppression of frequently occurring vascular headaches.

General Action and Information

Ergot derivatives (ergotamine, dihydroergotamine) directly stimulate alpha-adrenergic and serotonergic receptors, producing vascular smooth muscle vasoconstriction. Almotriptan, frovatriptan, naratriptan, rizatriptan, sumatriptan, and zolmitriptan produce vasoconstriction by acting as serotonin ($5\text{-}HT_1$) agonists.

Contraindications

Avoid using these agents in patients with ischemic cardiovascular disease.

Precautions

Use cautiously in patients with a history of or risk for cardiovascular disease.

Interactions

Avoid concurrent use of ergot derivative agents with serotonin agonist agents; see also individual agents.

NURSING IMPLICATIONS

Assessment

- Assess pain location, intensity, duration, and associated symptoms (photophobia, phonophobia, nausea, vomiting) during migraine attack and frequency of attacks.

Potential Nursing Diagnoses

- Acute pain (Indications).
- Deficient knowledge, related to disease processes and medication regimen (Patient/Family Teaching).

Implementation

- Medication should be administered at the first sign of a headache.

Patient/Family Teaching

- Inform patient that medication should be used only during a migraine attack. It is meant to be used for relief of migraine attacks but not to prevent or reduce the number of attacks.
- Advise patient that lying down in a darkened room following medication administration may further help relieve headache.
- May cause dizziness or drowsiness. Caution patient to avoid driving or other activities requiring alertness until response to medication is known.
- Advise patient to avoid alcohol, which aggravates headaches.

Evaluation/Desired Outcomes

- Relief of migraine attack.

Vascular headache suppressants included in *Davis's Drug Guide for Nurses*

alpha-adrenergic blockers

dihydroergotamine 493
ergotamine 493

beta blockers

propranolol 1026, 1327
timolol 1179, 1352

5-HT$_1$ agonists

almotriptan 130
eletriptan 470
frovatriptan 586
naratriptan 866
rizatriptan 1079
sumatriptan 1129
zolmitriptan 1261

miscellaneous

divalproex sodium 1212
valproate sodium 1212
valproic acid 1212
verapamil 1224

• VITAMINS

PHARMACOLOGIC PROFILE

General Use

Used in the prevention and treatment of vitamin deficiencies and as supplements in various metabolic disorders.

General Action and Information

Serve as components of enzyme systems that catalyze numerous varied metabolic reactions. Necessary for homeostasis. Water-soluble vitamins (B-vitamins and vitamin C) rarely cause toxicity. Fat-soluble vitamins (vitamins D and E) may accumulate and cause toxicity.

Contraindications

Hypersensitivity to additives, preservatives, or colorants.

Precautions

Dose should be adjusted to avoid toxicity, especially for fat-soluble vitamins.

Interactions

Pyridoxine in large amounts may interfere with the effectiveness of levodopa. Cholestyramine, colestipol, and mineral oil decrease absorption of fat-soluble vitamins.

NURSING IMPLICATIONS

Assessment

- Assess patient for signs of vitamin deficiency before and periodically throughout therapy.

- Assess nutritional status through 24-hr diet recall. Determine frequency of consumption of vitamin-rich foods.

Potential Nursing Diagnoses

- Imbalanced nutrition: less than body requirements (Indications).
- Deficient knowledge, related to disease processes and medication regimen (Patient/Family Teaching).

Implementation

- Because of infrequency of single vitamin deficiencies, combinations are commonly administered.

Patient/Family Teaching

- Encourage patients to comply with diet recommendations of physician or other health care professional. Explain that the best source of vitamins is a well-balanced diet with foods from the four basic food groups.
- Patients self-medicating with vitamin supplements should be cautioned not to exceed RDAs. The effectiveness of megadoses for treatment of various medical conditions is unproved and may cause side effects and toxicity.

Evaluation/Desired Outcomes

- Prevention of or decrease in the symptoms of vitamin deficiencies.

Vitamins included in *Davis's Drug Guide for Nurses*

fat-soluble vitamins
calcitriol 1236
doxercalciferol 1236
ergocalciferol 1236
paricalcitol 1236
phytonadione 982
vitamin E 1240

water soluble vitamins
ascorbic acid 1271
cyanocobalamin 1233
folic acid 574
leucovorin calcium 736
niacin 877
niacinamide 877
pyridoxine 1039
riboflavin 1291
thiamine 1160
hydroxocobalamin 1233

• WEIGHT CONTROL AGENTS

PHARMACOLOGIC PROFILE

General Use

These agents are used in the management of exogenous obesity as part of a regimen including a reduced-calorie diet. They are especially useful in the presence of other risk factors including hypertension, diabetes or dyslipidemias.

General Action and Information

Phentermine and sibutramine are anorexiants that are designed to decrease appetite via their action in the CNS. Orlistat is a lipase inhibitor that decreases absorption of dietary fat.

Contraindications

None of these agents should be used during pregnancy or lactation. Phentermine and sibutramine should not be used in patients with severe hepatic or renal disease, uncontrolled hypertension, known CHF, or cardiovascular disease. Orlistat should not be used in patients with chronic malabsorption.

Precautions

Phentermine and sibutramine should be used cautiously in patients with a history of seizures, or angle-closure glaucoma and in geriatric patients.

Interactions

Phentermine and sibutramine may have additive, adverse effects with CNS stimulants, some vascular headache suppressants, MAO inhibitors, and some opioids (concurrent use should be avoided). Orlistat reduces absorption of some fat-soluble vitamins and beta-carotene.

NURSING IMPLICATIONS

Assessment

- Monitor weight and dietary intake prior to and periodically during therapy. Adjust concurrent medications (antihypertensives, antidiabetics, lipid-lowering agents) as needed.

Potential Nursing Diagnoses

- Disturbed body image (Indications).
- Imbalanced nutrition: more than body requirements (Indications).
- Deficient knowledge, related to medication regimen (Patient/Family Teaching).

Patient/Family Teaching

- Advise patient that regular physical activity, approved by healthcare professional, should be used in conjunction with medication and diet.

Evaluation/Desired Outcomes

- Slow, consistent weight loss when combined with a reduced-calorie diet.

Weight control agents included in *Davis's Drug Guide for Nurses*

orlistat 913, 1325
phentermine 1288

A

abacavir (ah-**back**-ah-veer)
Ziagen

Classification
Therapeutic: antiretrovirals
Pharmacologic: nucleoside reverse transcriptase inhibitors

Pregnancy Category C

Indications
Management of HIV infection (AIDS) in combination with other antiretrovirals (not with lamivudine and/or tenofovir).

Action
Converted inside cells to carbovir triphosphate, its active metabolite. Carbovir triphosphate inhibits the activity of HIV-1 reverse transcriptase, which in turn terminates viral DNA growth.
Therapeutic Effects: Slows the progression of HIV infection and decreases the occurrence of its sequelae. Increases CD4 cell counts and decreases viral load.

Pharmacokinetics
Absorption: Rapidly and extensively (83%) absorbed.
Distribution: Distributes into extravascular space and readily distributes into erythrocytes.
Metabolism and Excretion: Mostly metabolized by the liver; 1.2% excreted unchanged in urine.
Half-life: 1.5 hr.

TIME/ACTION PROFILE (blood levels)

ROUTE	ONSET	PEAK	DURATION
PO	unknown	unknown	unknown

Contraindications/Precautions
Contraindicated in: Hypersensitivity (rechallenge may be fatal); Lactation: Breastfeeding not recommended for HIV-infected patients.
Use Cautiously in: OB: Safety not established; Pedi: Safety not established in children <3 mo.

Adverse Reactions/Side Effects
CNS: headache, insomnia. **GI:** HEPATOTOXICITY, diarrhea, nausea, vomiting, anorexia. **Derm:** rashes. **F and E:** LACTIC ACIDOSIS. **Misc:** HYPERSENSITIVITY REACTIONS.

Interactions
Drug-Drug: Alcohol increases blood levels. May increase **methadone** metabolism in some patients; slight increase in **methadone** dosing may be needed.

Route/Dosage
PO (Adults): 300 mg twice daily.
PO (Children 3 mo–16 yr): 8 mg/kg twice daily (not to exceed 300 mg twice daily).

Availability
Tablets: 300 mg. **Oral solution (strawberry/banana flavor):** 20 mg/ml in 240-ml bottles. ***In combination with:*** lamivudine and zidovudine (Trizivir). See Appendix B.

NURSING IMPLICATIONS

Assessment
- Assess patient for change in severity of HIV symptoms and for symptoms of opportunistic infections throughout therapy.
- Assess for signs of hypersensitivity reactions (fever; rash; gastrointestinal—nausea, vomiting, diarrhea, abdominal pain; constitutional—malaise, fatigue, achiness; respiratory—dyspnea, cough, pharyngitis). May also cause elevated liver function tests, increased creatine phosphokinase or creatinine, and lymphopenia. Discontinue abacavir at the first sign of hypersensitivity reaction. Do not restart abacavir following reaction; more severe symptoms may occur within hours and may include life-threatening hypotension and death. Symptoms usually resolve upon discontinuation.
- May cause lactic acidosis and severe hepatomegaly with steatosis. Monitor patient for signs (increased serum lactate levels, elevated liver enzymes, liver enlargement on palpation). Therapy should be suspended if clinical or laboratory signs occur.
- ***Lab Test Considerations:*** Monitor viral load and CD4 cell count regularly during therapy.
- May cause ↑ serum glucose and triglyceride levels.

Potential Nursing Diagnoses
Risk for infection (Indications)
Noncompliance (Patient/Family Teaching)

Implementation
- **PO:** May be administered with or without food. Oral solution may be stored at room temperature or refrigerated; do not freeze.

♣ = Canadian drug name.
* CAPITALS indicates life-threatening; underlines indicate most frequent.

Patient/Family Teaching

- Emphasize the importance of taking abacavir as directed. Must always be used in combination with other antiretroviral drugs. Do not take more than prescribed amount and do not stop taking without consulting health care professional. Take missed doses as soon as remembered; do not double doses.
- Instruct patient not to share abacavir with others.
- Inform patient that abacavir does not cure AIDS or prevent associated or opportunistic infections. Abacavir does not reduce the risk of transmission of HIV to others through sexual contact or blood contamination. Caution patient to use a condom, and avoid sharing needles or donating blood to prevent spreading the AIDS virus to others. Advise patient that the long-term effects of abacavir are unknown at this time.
- Advise patient of potential for hypersensitivity reactions that may result in death. Instruct patient to discontinue abacavir and notify health care professional immediately if symptoms of hypersensitivity occur. Medication guide for patients should be dispensed with prescription. Advise patient to read it thoroughly with each refill. A warning card summarizing symptoms of abacavir hypersensitivity should be provided with each prescription; instruct patient to carry card at all times.
- Emphasize the importance of regular follow-up exams and blood counts to determine progress and monitor for side effects.

Evaluation/Desired Outcomes

- Delayed progression of AIDS, and decreased opportunistic infections in patients with HIV.
- Decrease in viral load and increase in CD4 cell counts.

acarbose (aye-**kar**-bose)

Precose

Classification
Therapeutic: antidiabetics
Pharmacologic: alpha-glucosidase inhibitors

Pregnancy Category B

Indications

Management of type 1 diabetes in conjunction with dietary therapy; may be used with insulin or other hypoglycemic agents.

Action

Lowers blood glucose by inhibiting the enzyme alpha-glucosidase in the GI tract. Delays and reduces glucose absorption. **Therapeutic Effects:** Lowering of blood glucose in diabetic patients, especially postprandial hyperglycemia.

Pharmacokinetics

Absorption: <2% systemically absorbed; action is primarily local (in the GI tract).
Distribution: Unknown.
Metabolism and Excretion: Minimal amounts absorbed are excreted by the kidneys.
Half-life: 2 hr.

TIME/ACTION PROFILE (effect on blood glucose)

ROUTE	ONSET	PEAK	DURATION
PO	unknown	1 hr	unknown

Contraindications/Precautions

Contraindicated in: Hypersensitivity; Diabetic ketoacidosis; Cirrhosis; Serum creatinine >2 mg/dl; OB, Lactation, Pedi: Safety not established.
Use Cautiously in: Presence of fever, infection, trauma, stress (may cause hyperglycemia, requiring alternative therapy).

Adverse Reactions/Side Effects

GI: abdominal pain, diarrhea, flatulence, ↑ transaminases.

Interactions

Drug-Drug: Thiazide diuretics and **loop diuretics**, **corticosteroids**, **phenothiazines**, **thyroid preparations**, **estrogens (conjugated)**, **progestins**, **hormonal contraceptives**, **phenytoin**, **niacin**, **sympathomimetics**, **calcium channel blockers**, and **isoniazid** may ↑ glucose levels in diabetic patients and lead to ↓ control of blood glucose. Effects are ↓ by **intestinal adsorbents**, including **activated charcoal** and **digestive enzyme preparations (amylase, pancreatin)**; avoid concurrent use. ↑ effects of **sulfonylurea hypoglycemic agents**. May ↓ absorption of **digoxin**; may require dosage adjustment.
Drug-Natural Products: Glucosamine may worsen blood glucose control. **Chromium** and **coenzyme Q-10** may ↑ hypoglycemic effects.

Route/Dosage

PO (Adults): 25 mg 3 times daily; may be increased q 4–8 wk as needed/tolerated (range 50–100 mg 3 times daily; not to exceed 50 mg 3 times daily in patients ≤60 kg or 100 mg 3 times daily in patients >60 kg).

Availability

Tablets: 25 mg, 50 mg, 100 mg.

NURSING IMPLICATIONS

Assessment

- Observe patient for signs and symptoms of hypoglycemia (sweating, hunger, weakness, dizziness, tremor, tachycardia, anxiety) when taking concurrently with other oral hypoglycemic agents.
- ***Lab Test Considerations:*** Monitor serum glucose and glycosylated hemoglobin periodically during therapy to evaluate effectiveness.
- Monitor AST and ALT every 3 mo for the 1st yr and then periodically. Elevated levels may require dosage reduction or discontinuation of acarbose. Elevations occur more commonly in patients taking more than 300 mg/day and in female patients. Levels usually return to normal without other evidence of liver injury after discontinuation.
- ***Toxicity and Overdose:*** Symptoms of overdose are transient increase in flatulence, diarrhea, and abdominal discomfort. Acarbose alone does not cause hypoglycemia; however, other concurrently administered hypoglycemic agents may produce hypoglycemia requiring treatment.

Potential Nursing Diagnoses

Imbalanced nutrition: more than body requirements (Indications)
Noncompliance (Patient/Family Teaching)

Implementation

- Patients stabilized on a diabetic regimen who are exposed to stress, fever, trauma, infection, or surgery may require administration of insulin.
- Does not cause hypoglycemia when taken while fasting, but may increase hypoglycemic effect of other hypoglycemic agents.
- **PO:** Administer with first bite of each meal 3 times/day.

Patient/Family Teaching

- Instruct patient to take acarbose at same time each day. If a dose is missed and the meal is completed without taking the dose, skip missed dose and take next dose with the next meal. Do not double doses.
- Explain to patient that acarbose controls hyperglycemia but does not cure diabetes. Therapy is longterm.
- Review signs of hypoglycemia and hyperglycemia (blurred vision; drowsiness; dry mouth; flushed, dry skin; fruit-like breath odor; increased urination; ketones in urine; loss of appetite; stomachache; nausea or vomiting; tiredness; rapid, deep breathing; unusual thirst; unconsciousness) with patient. If hypoglycemia occurs, advise patient to take a form of oral glucose (e.g., glucose tablets, liquid gel glucose) rather than sugar (absorption of sugar is blocked by acarbose) and notify health care professional.
- Encourage patient to follow prescribed diet, medication, and exercise regimen to prevent hypoglycemic or hyperglycemic episodes.
- Instruct patient in proper testing of serum glucose and urine ketones. Monitor closely during periods of stress or illness. Notify health care professional if significant changes occur.
- Caution patient to avoid using other medications without consulting health care professional.
- Advise patient to inform health care professional of medication regimen before treatment or surgery.
- Advise patient to carry a form of oral glucose and identification describing disease process and medication regimen at all times.
- Emphasize the importance of routine follow-up examinations.

Evaluation/Desired Outcomes

- Control of blood glucose levels without the appearance of hypoglycemic or hyperglycemic episodes.

acebutolol

(a-se-**byoo**-toe-lole)
✤Monitan, Sectral

Classification
Therapeutic: antiarrhythmics (class II), antihypertensives
Pharmacologic: beta blockers

Pregnancy Category B

Indications
Treatment of hypertension (single agent or with other antihypertensives). Treatment of ventricular tachyarrhythmias. **Unlabeled uses:** Prophylaxis of MI, treatment of angina pectoris, management of anxiety, tremors, thyrotoxicosis, mitral valve prolapse, idiopathic hypertrophic subaortic stenosis.

Action
Blocks stimulation of $beta_1$–(myocardial)-adrenergic receptors. Does not usually affect $beta_2$ (pulmonary, vascular, or uterine) receptor sites. Mild intrinsic sympathomimetic activity (ISA). **Therapeutic Effects:** Decreased heart rate. Decreased AV conduction. Decreased blood pressure.

Pharmacokinetics
Absorption: Well absorbed following oral administration but rapidly undergoes metabolism.
Distribution: Minimal penetration of the CNS. Crosses the placenta and enters breast milk in small amounts.
Metabolism and Excretion: Mostly metabolized to diacetolol, which is also a beta blocker.
Half-life: 3–4 hr (8–13 hr for diacetolol).

TIME/ACTION PROFILE

ROUTE	ONSET	PEAK	DURATION
PO (effect on BP)	1–1.5 hr	2–8 hr	12–24 hr
PO (antiarrhythmic)	1 hr	4–6 hr	up to 10 hr

Contraindications/Precautions
Contraindicated in: Uncompensated CHF; Pulmonary edema; Cardiogenic shock; Bradycardia or heart block; Obstructive airway disease including asthma.
Use Cautiously in: Renal or hepatic impairment (dosage reduction recommended if CCr <50 ml/min/1.73 m^2); Geri: Increased sensitivity; Thyrotoxicosis (may mask symptoms); Diabetes mellitus (may mask symptoms of hypoglycemia); History of severe allergic reactions (intensity of reactions may be increased); OB, Lactation, Pedi: Safety not established; neonatal bradycardia, hypotension, hypoglycemia, and respiratory depression may occur rarely.

Adverse Reactions/Side Effects
CNS: fatigue, weakness, anxiety, depression, dizziness, drowsiness, insomnia, memory loss, nervousness, nightmares. **EENT:** blurred vision, stuffy nose. **Resp:** bronchospasm, wheezing. **CV:** BRADYCARDIA, CHF, PULMONARY EDEMA, hypotension, peripheral vasoconstriction. **GI:** constipation, diarrhea, nausea, vomiting. **GU:** erectile dysfunction, diminished libido, urinary frequency. **Derm:** rashes. **Endo:** hyperglycemia, hypoglycemia. **MS:** arthralgia, joint pain. **Misc:** drug-induced lupus syndrome.

Interactions
Drug-Drug: General anesthetics, **IV phenytoin**, and **verapamil** may cause additive myocardial depression. Concurrent use with **digoxin** may increase bradycardia.
Antihypertensives, acute ingestion of **alcohol**, or **nitrates** may cause additive hypotension. Use with **epinephrine** may result in unopposed alpha-adrenergic stimulation. Concurrent use with **thyroid preparations** may decrease effectiveness. Concurrent use with **insulin** may result in prolonged hypoglycemia. May decrease effectiveness of **theophylline**.

Route/Dosage
PO (Adults): 400–800 mg/day—single dose or twice daily (up to 1200 mg/day or 800 mg/day in geriatric patients).

Renal Impairment
PO (Adults): If CCr <50 ml/min/1.73 m^2, use 50% of normal dose. If CCr <25 ml/min/1.73 m^2, use 25% of normal dose.

Availability (generic available)
Capsules: 200 mg, 400 mg. **Tablets:** ✤ 100 mg, ✤ 200 mg, ✤ 400 mg.

NURSING IMPLICATIONS

Assessment
- Monitor blood pressure, ECG, and pulse frequently during dosage adjustment period and periodically throughout therapy.
- Monitor intake and output ratios and daily weights. Assess routinely for signs and symptoms of CHF (dyspnea, rales/crackles, weight gain, peripheral edema, jugular venous distention).
- Monitor frequency of prescription refills to determine compliance.
- ***Lab Test Considerations:*** May cause increased BUN, serum lipoprotein, potassium, triglyceride, and uric acid levels.
- May cause increased serum alkaline phosphatase, LDH, AST, and ALT levels.
- May cause increased ANA titers.
- May cause increase in blood glucose levels.

Potential Nursing Diagnoses
Decreased cardiac output (Side Effects)

Noncompliance, related to medication regimen (Patient/Family Teaching)

Implementation

- **PO:** Take apical pulse prior to administering. If <50 bpm or if arrhythmia occurs, withhold medication and notify physician or other health care professional.
- May be administered with food or on an empty stomach.

Patient/Family Teaching

- Instruct patient to take medication exactly as directed, at the same time each day, even if feeling well; do not skip or double up on missed doses. If a dose is missed, it should be taken as soon as possible up to 4 hr before next dose. Abrupt withdrawal may precipitate life-threatening arrhythmias, hypertension, or myocardial ischemia.
- Advise patient to make sure enough medication is available for weekends, holidays, and vacations. A written prescription may be kept in wallet in case of emergency.
- Teach patient and family how to check pulse and blood pressure. Instruct them to check pulse daily and blood pressure biweekly and to report significant changes to health care professional.
- May cause drowsiness or dizziness. Caution patients to avoid driving or other activities that require alertness until response to the drug is known.
- Caution patient that this medication may increase sensitivity to cold.
- Instruct patient to consult health care professional before taking any OTC medications, especially cold preparations, concurrently with this medication.
- Diabetic patients should closely monitor blood glucose, especially if weakness, malaise, irritability, or fatigue occurs. May mask tachycardia and blood pressure changes as signs of hypoglycemia, but dizziness and sweating may still occur.
- Advise patient to notify health care professional if slow pulse, difficulty breathing, wheezing, cold hands and feet, dizziness, light-headedness, confusion, depression, rash, fever, sore throat, unusual bleeding, or bruising occurs.
- Instruct patient to inform health care professional of medication regimen prior to treatment or surgery.
- Advise patient to carry identification describing disease process and medication regimen at all times.
- **Hypertension:** Reinforce the need to continue additional therapies for hypertension (weight loss, sodium restriction, stress reduction, regular exercise, moderation of alcohol consumption, and smoking cessation). Acebutolol controls, but does not cure, hypertension.

Evaluation/Desired Outcomes

- Decrease in blood pressure.
- Control of arrhythmias without appearance of detrimental side effects.

acetaminophen

(a-seet-a-**min**-oh-fen)

✤Abenol, Acephen, Aceta, Aminofen, Apacet, APAP, ✤Apo-Acetaminophen, Aspirin Free Anacin, Aspirin Free Pain Relief, Children's Pain Reliever, Dapacin, Feverall, Extra Strength Dynafed E.X., Extra Strength Dynafed (Billups, P.J.), Genapap, Genebs, Halenol, Infant's Pain Reliever, Liquiprin, Mapap, Maranox, Meda, Neopap, ✤Novo-Gesic, Oraphen-PD, Panadol, paracetamol, Redutemp, Ridenol, Silapap, Tapanol, Tempra, Tylenol, Uni-Ace

Classification

Therapeutic: antipyretics, nonopioid analgesics

Pregnancy Category B

Indications

Mild pain. Fever.

Action

Inhibits the synthesis of prostaglandins that may serve as mediators of pain and fever, primarily in the CNS. Has no significant anti-inflammatory properties or GI toxicity. **Therapeutic Effects:** Analgesia. Antipyresis.

✤ = Canadian drug name.

* CAPITALS indicates life-threatening; underlines indicate most frequent.

Pharmacokinetics

Absorption: Well absorbed following oral administration. Rectal absorption is variable.
Distribution: Widely distributed. Crosses the placenta; enters breast milk in low concentrations.
Metabolism and Excretion: 85–95% metabolized by the liver. Metabolites may be toxic in overdose situation. Metabolites excreted by the kidneys.
Half-life: Neonates: 2–5 hr. Adults: 1–3 hr.

TIME/ACTION PROFILE (analgesia and antipyresis)

ROUTE	ONSET	PEAK	DURATION
PO	0.5–1 hr	1–3 hr	3–8 hr†
Rect	0.5–1 hr	1–3 hr	3–4 hr

†Depends on dose

Contraindications/Precautions

Contraindicated in: Previous hypersensitivity; Products containing alcohol, aspartame, saccharin, sugar, or tartrazine (FDC yellow dye #5) should be avoided in patients who have hypersensitivity or intolerance to these compounds.
Use Cautiously in: Hepatic disease/renal disease (lower chronic doses recommended); Chronic alcohol use/abuse; Malnutrition.

Adverse Reactions/Side Effects

GI: HEPATIC FAILURE, HEPATOTOXICITY (overdose). **GU:** renal failure (high doses/chronic use). **Hemat:** neutropenia, pancytopenia, leukopenia. **Derm:** rash, urticaria.

Interactions

Drug-Drug: Chronic high-dose acetaminophen (>2 g/day) may ↑ risk of bleeding with **warfarin** (PT should be monitored regularly and INR should not exceed 4). Hepatotoxicity is additive with other **hepatotoxic substances**, including **alcohol**. Concurrent use of **sulfinpyrazone**, **isoniazid**, **rifampin**, **rifabutin**, **phenytoin**, **barbiturates**, and **carbamazepine** may ↑ the risk of acetaminophen-induced liver damage (limit self-medication); these agents will also ↓ therapeutic effects of acetaminophen. Concurrent **NSAIDs** ↑ the risk of adverse renal effects (avoid chronic concurrent use). **Propranolol** ↓ metabolism and may ↑ effects. May ↓ effects of **lamotrigine** and **zidovudine**.

Route/Dosage

Children ≤12 yr should not receive >5 doses/24 hr without notifying physician or other health care professional.

PO (Adults and Children >12 yr): 325–650 mg q 4–6 hr or 1 g 3–4 times daily or 1300 mg q 8 hr (not to exceed 4 g or 2.5 g/24 hr in patients with hepatic/renal impairment).
PO (Children 1–12 yr): 10–15 mg/kg/dose q 4–6 hr as needed (not to exceed 5 doses/24 hr).
PO (Infants): 10–15 mg/kg/dose q 4–6 hr as needed (not to exceed 5 doses/24 hr).
PO (Neonates): 10–15 mg/kg/dose q 6–8 hr as needed.
Rect (Adults and Children >12 yr): 325–650 mg q 4–6 hr as needed or 1 g 3–4 times/day (not to exceed 4 g/24 hr).
Rect (Children 1–12 yr): 10–20 mg/kg/dose q 4–6 hr as needed.
Rect (Infants): 10–20 mg/kg/dose q 4–6 hr as needed.
Rect (Neonates): 10–15 mg/kg/dose q 6–8 hr as needed.

Availability (generic available)

Chewable tablets (fruit, bubblegum, or grape flavor): 80 mg^OTC, 160 mg^OTC. **Tablets:** 160 mg^OTC, 325 mg^OTC, 500 mg^OTC, 650 mg^OTC. **Caplets:** 325 mg^OTC, 500 mg^OTC. **Solution (berry, fruit, and grape flavor):** 100 mg/ml^OTC. **Liquid (mint):** 160 mg/5 ml^OTC, 500 mg/15 ml^OTC. **Elixir (grape and cherry flavor):** 160 mg/5 ml^OTC. **Drops:** 100 mg/ml^OTC. **Suspension:** ✤100 mg/ml^OTC, ✤160 mg/5 ml^OTC. **Syrup:** 160 mg/5 ml^OTC. **Suppositories:** 80 mg^OTC, 120 mg^OTC, 325 mg^OTC, 650 mg^OTC. ***In combination with:*** many other medications. See Appendix B.

NURSING IMPLICATIONS

Assessment

- Assess overall health status and alcohol usage before administering acetaminophen. Patients who are malnourished or chronically abuse alcohol are at higher risk of developing hepatotoxicity with chronic use of usual doses of this drug.
- Assess amount, frequency, and type of drugs taken in patients self-medicating, especially with OTC drugs. Prolonged use of acetaminophen increases the risk of adverse renal effects. For short-term use, combined doses of acetaminophen and salicylates should not exceed the recommended dose of either drug given alone.
- **Pain:** Assess type, location, and intensity prior to and 30–60 min following administration.

- **Fever:** Assess fever; note presence of associated signs (diaphoresis, tachycardia, and malaise).
- ***Lab Test Considerations:*** Evaluate hepatic, hematologic, and renal function periodically during prolonged, high-dose therapy.
- May alter results of blood glucose monitoring. May cause falsely ↓ values when measured with glucose oxidase/peroxidase method, but probably not with hexokinase/G6PD method. May also cause falsely ↑ values with certain instruments; see manufacturer's instruction manual.
- Increased serum bilirubin, LDH, AST, ALT, and prothrombin time may indicate hepatotoxicity.
- ***Toxicity and Overdose:*** If overdose occurs, **acetylcysteine** (Acetadote) is the antidote.

Potential Nursing Diagnoses

Acute pain (Indications)
Risk for imbalanced body temperature (Indications)

Implementation

- When combined with opioids do not exceed the maximum recommended daily dose of acetaminophen.
- **PO:** Administer with a full glass of water.
- May be taken with food or on an empty stomach.

Patient/Family Teaching

- Advise patient to take medication exactly as directed and not to take more than the recommended amount. Chronic excessive use of >4 g/day (2 g in chronic alcoholics) may lead to hepatotoxicity, renal or cardiac damage. Adults should not take acetaminophen longer than 10 days and children not longer than 5 days unless directed by health care professional. Short-term doses of acetaminophen with salicylates or NSAIDs should not exceed the recommended daily dose of either drug alone.
- Advise patient to avoid alcohol (3 or more glasses per day increase the risk of liver damage) if taking more than an occasional 1–2 doses and to avoid taking concurrently with salicylates or NSAIDs for more than a few days, unless directed by health care professional.
- Pedi: Advise parents or caregivers to check concentrations of liquid preparations. Errors have resulted in serious liver damage. Have parents or caregivers determine the correct formulation and dose for their child (based on the child's age/weight), and demonstrate how to measure it using an appropriate measuring device.
- Inform patients with diabetes that acetaminophen may alter results of blood glucose monitoring. Advise patient to notify health care professional if changes are noted.
- Caution patient to check labels on all OTC products. Advise patients to avoid taking more than one product containing acetaminophen at a time to prevent toxicity.
- Advise patient to consult health care professional if discomfort or fever is not relieved by routine doses of this drug or if fever is greater than 39.5°C (103°F) or lasts longer than 3 days.

Evaluation/Desired Outcomes

- Relief of mild pain.
- Reduction of fever.

acetaZOLAMIDE

(a-set-a-**zole**-a-mide)
✤Acetazolam, AK-Zol, ✤Apo-Acetazolamide, Dazamide, Diamox, Diamox Sequels, Storzolamide

Classification
Therapeutic: anticonvulsants, antiglaucoma agents, diuretics, ocular hypotensive agents
Pharmacologic: carbonic anhydrase inhibitors

Pregnancy Category C

Indications

Lowering of intraocular pressure in the treatment of glaucoma. Management of acute altitude sickness. **Unlabeled uses:** Diuretic. Adjunct to the treatment of refractory seizures. Reduce cerebrospinal fluid production in hydrocephalus. Prevention of renal calculi composed of uric acid or cystine.

Action

Inhibition of carbonic anhydrase in the eye results in decreased secretion of aqueous humor.

Inhibition of renal carbonic anhydrase, resulting in self-limiting urinary excretion of sodium, potassium, bicarbonate, and water. CNS inhibition of carbonic anhydrase and resultant diuresis may decrease abnormal neuronal firing. Alkaline diuresis prevents precipitation of uric acid or cystine in the urinary tract. **Therapeutic Effects:** Lowering of intraocular pressure. Control of some types of seizures. Prevention and treatment of acute altitude sickness. Prevention of uric acid or cystine renal calculi.

Pharmacokinetics

Absorption: Dose dependent; erratic with doses >10 mg/kg/day.
Distribution: Crosses the placenta and blood-brain barrier; enters breast milk.
Protein Binding: 95%.
Metabolism and Excretion: Excreted mostly unchanged in urine.
Half-life: 2.4–5.8 hr.

TIME/ACTION PROFILE (lowering of intraocular pressure)

ROUTE	ONSET	PEAK	DURATION
PO	1–1.5 hr	2–4 hr	8–12 hr
PO-ER	2 hr	8–18 hr	18–24 hr
IV	2 min	15 min	4–5 hr

Contraindications/Precautions

Contraindicated in: Hypersensitivity or cross-sensitivity with sulfonamides may occur; Hepatic disease or insufficiency; Concurrent use with ophthalmic carbonic anhydrase inhibitors (brinzolamide, dorzolamide) is not recommended; OB: Avoid during first trimester of pregnancy.
Use Cautiously in: Chronic respiratory disease; Electrolyte abnormalities; Gout; Renal disease (dosage reduction necessary for ClCr <50 ml/min); Diabetes mellitus; OB: Use with caution during second or third trimester of pregnancy; Lactation: Safety not established.

Adverse Reactions/Side Effects

CNS: depression, tiredness, weakness, drowsiness. **EENT:** transient nearsightedness. **GI:** anorexia, metallic taste, nausea, vomiting, melena. **GU:** crystalluria, renal calculi. **Derm:** STEVENS-JOHNSON SYNDROME, rashes. **Endo:** hyperglycemia. **F and E:** hyperchloremic acidosis, hypokalemia, growth retardation (in children receiving chronic therapy). **Hemat:** APLASTIC ANEMIA, HEMOLYTIC ANEMIA, LEUKOPENIA. **Metab:** weight loss, hyperuricemia. **Neuro:** paresthesias. **Misc:** allergic reactions including ANAPHLYAXIS.

Interactions

Drug-Drug: Excretion of **barbiturates**, **aspirin**, and **lithium** is ↑ and may lead to ↓ effectiveness. Excretion of **amphetamine**, **quinidine**, **procainamide**, and possibly **tricyclic antidepressants** is ↓ and may lead to toxicity. May ↑ **cyclosporine** levels.

Route/Dosage

PO (Adults): *Glaucoma (open angle)*—250–1000 mg/day in 1–4 divided doses (up to 250 mg q 4 hr) or 500-mg extended-release capsules twice daily. *Epilepsy*—4–16 mg/kg/day in 1–4 divided doses (maximum 30 mg/kg/day or 1 g/day). *Altitude sickness*—250 mg 2–4 times daily started 24–48 hr before ascent, continued for 48 hr or longer to control symptoms. *Antiurolithic*—250 mg at bedtime. *Edema*—250–375 mg/day. *Urine alkalinization*—5 mg/kg/dose repeated 2–3 times over 24 hrs.
PO (Children): *Glaucoma*—8–30 mg/kg (300–900 mg/m²/day) in 3 divided doses (usual range 10–15 mg/kg/day). *Edema*—5 mg/kg/dose once daily. *Epilepsy*—4–16 mg/kg/day in 1–4 divided doses (maximum 30 mg/kg/day or 1 g/day).
PO (Neonates): *Hydrocephalus*—5 mg/kg/dose q 6 hrs increased by 25 mg/kg/day up to a maximum of 100 mg/kg/day.
IV (Adults): *Glaucoma (closed angle)*—250–500 mg, may repeat in 2–4 hr to a maximum of 1 g/day. *Edema*—250–375 mg/day.
IV (Children): *Glaucoma*—5–10 mg/kg q 6 hr, not to exceed 1 g/day. *Edema*—5 mg/kg/dose once daily.
IV (Neonates): *Hydrocephalus*—5 mg/kg/dose q 6 hrs increased by 25 mg/kg/day up to a maximum of 100 mg/kg/day.

Availability

Tablets: 125 mg, 250 mg. **Extended-release capsules:** 500 mg. **Injection:** 500 mg/vial.

NURSING IMPLICATIONS

Assessment

- Observe for signs of hypokalemia (muscle weakness, malaise, fatigue, ECG changes, vomiting).
- Assess for allergy to sulfonamides.
- **Intraocular Pressure:** Assess for eye discomfort or decrease in visual acuity.
- **Seizures:** Monitor neurologic status in patients receiving acetazolamide for seizures. Initiate seizure precautions.

- **Altitude Sickness:** Monitor for decrease in severity of symptoms (headache, nausea, vomiting, fatigue, dizziness, drowsiness, shortness of breath). Notify health care professional immediately if neurologic symptoms worsen or if patient becomes more dyspneic and rales or crackles develop.
- ***Lab Test Considerations:*** Serum electrolytes, complete blood counts, and platelet counts should be evaluated initially and periodically throughout prolonged therapy. May cause ↓ potassium, bicarbonate, WBCs, and RBCs. May cause ↑ serum chloride.
- May cause ↑ in serum and urine glucose; monitor serum and urine glucose carefully in diabetic patients.
- May cause false-positive results for urine protein and 17-hydroxysteroid tests.
- May cause ↑ blood ammonia, bilirubin, uric acid, urine urobilinogen, and calcium. May ↓ urine citrate.

Potential Nursing Diagnoses

Disturbed sensory perception (visual) (Indications)

Implementation

- Do not confuse acetazolamide with acetohexamide.
- Encourage fluids to 2000–3000 ml/day, unless contraindicated, to prevent crystalluria and stone formation.
- A potassium supplement without chloride should be administered concurrently with acetazolamide.
- **PO:** Give with food to minimize GI irritation. Tablets may be crushed and mixed with fruit-flavored syrup to minimize bitter taste for patients with difficulty swallowing. Extended-release capsules may be opened and sprinkled on soft food, but do not crush, chew, or swallow contents dry. Extended-release capsules are only indicated for glaucoma and altitude sickness; do not use for epilepsy or diuresis.
- **IM:** Extremely painful; avoid if possible.
- **Direct IV:** Dilute 500 mg of acetazolamide in at least 5 ml of sterile water for injection for a concentration of 100 mg/ml. Use reconstituted solution within 24 hr. ***Rate:*** Not to exceed 500 mg/min.
- **Intermittent Infusion:** Further dilute in D5W, D10W, 0.45% NaCl, 0.9% NaCl, Ringer's or lactated Ringer's solution, or combinations of dextrose and saline or dextrose and Ringer's solution. ***Rate:*** Infuse over 4–8 hr.
- **Additive Compatibility:** cimetidine, ranitidine.
- **Additive Incompatibility:** multiple parenteral multivitamins.

Patient/Family Teaching

- Instruct patient to take as directed. Take missed doses as soon as possible unless almost time for next dose. Do not double doses. Patients on anticonvulsant therapy may need to gradually withdraw medication.
- Advise patient to report numbness or tingling of extremities, weakness, rash, sore throat, unusual bleeding or bruising, or fever to health care professional. If hematopoietic reactions, fever, rash, or renal problems occur, carbonic anhydrase inhibitor therapy should be discontinued.
- May occasionally cause drowsiness. Caution patient to avoid driving and other activities that require alertness until response to the drug is known.
- Caution patient to use sunscreen and wear protective clothing to prevent photosensitivity reactions.
- **Intraocular Pressure:** Advise patient of the need for periodic ophthalmologic exams; loss of vision may be gradual and painless.

Evaluation/Desired Outcomes

- Decrease in intraocular pressure when used for glaucoma. If therapy is not effective or patient is unable to tolerate one carbonic anhydrase inhibitor, using another may be effective and more tolerable.
- Decrease in the frequency of seizures.
- Prevention of altitude sickness.
- Prevention of uric acid or cystine stones in the urinary tract.

acyclovir (ay-**sye**-kloe-veer)

♣Avirax, Zovirax

Classification

Therapeutic: antivirals

Pharmacologic: purine analogues

Pregnancy Category B (PO, IV), C (topical)

Indications

PO: Recurrent genital herpes infections. Localized cutaneous herpes zoster infections (shingles) and chickenpox (varicella). **IV:** Severe initial episodes of genital herpes in nonimmunosuppressed patients. Mucosal or cutaneous herpes simplex infections or herpes zoster infections (shingles) in immunosuppressed patients. Herpes simplex encephalitis. **Topical:** *Cream*—Recurrent herpes labialis (cold sores). *Ointment*—Treatment of limited non–life-threatening herpes simplex infections in immunocompromised patients (systemic treatment is preferred).

Action

Interferes with viral DNA synthesis. **Therapeutic Effects:** Inhibition of viral replication, decreased viral shedding, and reduced time for healing of lesions.

Pharmacokinetics

Absorption: Despite poor absorption (15–30%), therapeutic blood levels are achieved.
Distribution: Widely distributed. CSF concentrations are 50% of plasma. Crosses placenta; enters breast milk.
Protein Binding: <30%.
Metabolism and Excretion: >90% eliminated unchanged by kidneys; remainder metabolized by liver.
Half-life: Neonates: 4 hr; Children 1–12 yr: 2–3 hr; Adults: 2–3.5 hr (↑ in renal failure).

TIME/ACTION PROFILE (antiviral blood levels)

ROUTE	ONSET	PEAK	DURATION
PO	unknown	1.5–2.5 hr	4 hr
IV	prompt	end of infusion	8 hr

Contraindications/Precautions

Contraindicated in: Hypersensitivity to acyclovir or valacyclovir.
Use Cautiously in: Pre-existing serious neurologic, hepatic, pulmonary, or fluid and electrolyte abnormalities; Renal impairment (dose alteration recommended if CCr <50 ml/min); Geriatric patients (due to age related ↓ in renal function); Obese patients (dose should be based on ideal body weight); Patients with hypoxia; OB, Lactation: Safety not established.

Adverse Reactions/Side Effects

CNS: SEIZURES, dizziness, headache, hallucinations, trembling. **GI:** diarrhea, nausea, vomiting, elevated liver enzymes, hyperbilirubinemia, abdominal pain, anorexia. **GU:** RENAL FAILURE, crystalluria, hematuria. **Derm:** acne, hives, skin rashes, unusual sweating, Stevens-Johnson syndrome. **Endo:** changes in menstrual cycle. **Hemat:** THROMBOTIC THROMBOCYTOPENIC PURPURA/HEMOLYTIC UREMIC SYNDROME (high doses in immunosuppressed patients). **Local:** pain, phlebitis, local irritation. **MS:** joint pain. **Misc:** polydipsia.

Interactions

Drug-Drug: Probenecid ↑ blood levels of acyclovir. ↑ blood levels and risk of toxicity from **theophylline**; dose adjustment may be necessary. ↓ blood levels and may ↓ effectiveness of **valproic acid** or **hydantoins**. Concurrent use of other **nephrotoxic drugs** ↑ risk of adverse renal effects. **Zidovudine** and IT **methotrexate** may ↑ risk of CNS side effects.

Route/Dosage

Initial Genital Herpes

PO (Adults and Children): 200 mg q 4 hr while awake (5 times/day) for 7–10 days or 400 mg q 8 hr for 7–10 days; maximum dose in children: 80 mg/kg/day in 3–5 divided doses.
IV (Adults and Children): 5 mg/kg q 8 hr or 750 mg/m^2/day divided q 8 hr for 5–7 days.

Chronic Suppressive Therapy for Recurrent Genital Herpes

PO (Adults and Children): 400 mg twice daily or 200 mg 3–5 times/day for up to 12 mo. Maximum dose in children: 80 mg/kg/day in 2–5 divided doses.

Intermittent Therapy for Recurrent Genital Herpes

PO (Adults and Children): 200 mg q 4 hr while awake (5 times/day) or 400 mg q 8 hr or 800 mg q 12 hr for 5 days, start at first sign of symptoms. Maximum dose in children: 80 mg/kg/day in 2–5 divided doses.

Acute Treatment of Herpes Zoster in Immunosuppressed Patients

PO (Adults): 800 mg q 4 hr while awake (5 times/day) for 7–10 days. *Prophylaxis*—400 mg 5 times/day.
PO (Children): 250–600 mg/m^2/dose 4–5 times/day.

Herpes Zoster in Immunocompetent Patients

PO (Adults and Children): 4000 mg/day in 5 divided doses for 5–7 days, maximum dose in children: 80 mg/kg/day in 5 divided doses.

Chickenpox

PO (Adults and Children): 20 mg/kg (not to exceed 800 mg/dose) qid for 5 days. Start within 24 hr of rash onset.

Mucosal and Cutaneous Herpes Simplex Infections in Immunosuppressed Patients

IV (Adults and Children >12 yr): 5 mg/kg q 8 hr for 7 days.
IV (Children <12 yr): 10 mg/kg q 8 hr for 7 days.
Topical (Adults): 0.5 in. ribbon of 5% *ointment* for every 4-square-in. area q 3 hr (6 times/day) for 7 days.

Herpes Simplex Encephalitis

IV (Adults): 10 mg/kg q 8 hr for 14–21 days.
IV (Children 3 mo–12 yr): 10 mg/kg q 8 hr for 14–21 days.
IV (Children birth–3 mo): 20 mg/kg q 8 hr for 14–21 days.
IV (Neonates, premature): 10 mg/kg q 12 hr for 14–21 days.

Varicella Zoster Infections in Immunosuppressed Patients

IV (Adults): 10 mg/kg q 8 hr for 7–10 days.
IV (Children <12 yr): 10 mg/kg q 8 hr for 7–10 days.

Renal Impairment

PO, IV (Adults and Children): *CCr >50 ml/min/1.73 m²*—no dosage adjustment needed; *CCr 25–50 ml/min/1.73 m²*—administer normal dose q 12 hr; *CCr 10–25 ml/min/1.73 m²*—administer normal dose q 24 hr; *CCr 0–10 ml/min/1.73 m²*—50% of dose q 24 hr.
IV (Neonates): *SCr 0.8–1.1 mg/dl:* Administer 20 mg/kg/dose q 12 hr; *SCr 1.2–1.5 mg/dl:* Administer 20 mg/kg/dose q 24 hr; *SCr >1.5 mg/dl:* Administer 10 mg/kg/dose q 24 hr.

Herpes labialis

Topical (Adults and Children >12 yr): Apply 5 times/day for 4 days; start at first symptoms.

Availability (generic available)

Capsules: 200 mg. **Cost:** *Generic*—$12.99/30. **Tablets:** 400 mg, 800 mg. **Cost:** *Generic*—400 mg $14.50/30, 800 mg $24.99/30. **Suspension (banana flavor):** 200 mg/5 ml. **Cost:** $123.97/473 ml. **Powder for injection:** 500 mg/vial, 1000 mg/vial. **Solution for injection:** 25 mg/ml in 20-ml and 40-ml vials, 50 mg/ml in 10-ml and 20-ml vials. **Cream:** 5% in 2-g and 5-g tubes. **Cost:** $51.36/2-g tube, $115.99/5-g tube. **Ointment:** 5% in 15-g tubes. **Cost:** $129.99/15-g tube.

NURSING IMPLICATIONS

Assessment

- Assess lesions before and daily during therapy.
- Monitor neurologic status in patients with herpes encephalitis.
- ***Lab Test Considerations:*** Monitor BUN, serum creatinine, and CCr before and during therapy. ↑ BUN and serum creatinine levels or ↓ CCr may indicate renal failure.

Potential Nursing Diagnoses

Risk for impaired skin integrity (Indications)
Risk for infection (Patient/Family Teaching)

Implementation

- Acyclovir treatment should be started as soon as possible after herpes simplex symptoms appear and within 24 hr of a herpes zoster outbreak.
- **PO:** Acyclovir may be administered with food or on an empty stomach, with a full glass of water.
- Shake oral suspension well before administration.

IV Administration

- **IV:** Maintain adequate hydration (2000–3000 ml/day), especially during first 2 hr after IV infusion, to prevent crystalluria.
- Observe infusion site for phlebitis. Rotate infusion site to prevent phlebitis.
- Acyclovir injectable should not be administered topically, IM, subcut, PO, or in the eye.
- **Intermittent Infusion:** ***Diluent:*** Reconstitute 500-mg or 1-g vial with 10 ml or 20 ml, respectively, of sterile water for injection. Do not reconstitute with bacteriostatic water with benzyl alcohol or parabens. Shake well to dissolve completely. Further dilute in at least 100 ml of D5W, 0.9% NaCl, dextrose/saline combinations or LR. ***Concentration:*** 7 mg/ml. Patients requiring fluid restriction: 10 mg/ml. ***Rate:*** Administer via infusion pump over 1 hr to minimize renal tubular damage. Use reconstituted solution within 12 hr. Once diluted for infusion, the solution should be used within 24 hr. Refrigeration results in

precipitation, which dissolves at room temperature.

- **Y-Site Compatibility:** allopurinol, amikacin, amphotericin B cholesteryl sulfate, ampicillin, anidulafungin, cefazolin, cefotaxime, cefoxitin, ceftazidime, ceftizoxime, ceftriaxone, cefuroxime, chloramphenicol, cimetidine, clindamycin, dexamethasone sodium phosphate, dimenhydrinate, diphenhydramine, docetaxel, doxorubicin liposome, doxycycline, erythromycin lactobionate, etoposide phosphate, famotidine, filgrastim, fluconazole, gentamicin, granisetron, heparin, hydrocortisone sodium succinate, hydromorphone, imipenem/cilastatin, lansoprazole, linezolid, lorazepam, magnesium sulfate, melphalan, methylprednisolone sodium succinate, metoclopramide, metronidazole, milrinone, multivitamin infusion, nafcillin, oxacillin, paclitaxel, pemetrexed, penicillin G potassium, pentobarbital, perphenazine, piperacillin, potassium chloride, propofol, ranitidine, remifentanil, sodium bicarbonate, teniposide, theophylline, thiotepa, tobramycin, trimethoprim/sulfamethoxazole, vancomycin, zidovudine.
- **Y-Site Incompatibility:** amifostine, aztreonam, cefepime, dobutamine, dopamine, fludarabine, foscarnet, gemcitabine, idarubicin, levofloxacin, ondansetron, piperacillin/tazobactam, sargramostim, tacrolimus, vinorelbine.
- **Additive Compatibility:** fluconazole.
- **Additive Incompatibility:** blood products, pantoprazole, protein-containing solutions.
- **Topical:** Apply to skin lesions only; do not use in the eye.

Patient/Family Teaching

- Advise patient to take medication as directed for the full course of therapy. Take missed doses as soon as possible but not just before next dose is due; do not double doses. Acyclovir should not be used more frequently or longer than prescribed.
- Advise patients that the additional use of OTC creams, lotions, and ointments may delay healing and may cause spreading of lesions.
- Inform patient that acyclovir is not a cure. The virus lies dormant in the ganglia, and acyclovir will not prevent the spread of infection to others.
- Advise patient that condoms should be used during sexual contact and that no sexual contact should be made while lesions are present.
- Patient should consult health care professional if symptoms are not relieved after 7 days of topical therapy or if oral acyclovir does not decrease the frequency and severity of recurrences. Immunocompromised patients may require a longer time, usually 2 weeks, for crusting over of lesions.
- Instruct women with genital herpes to have yearly Papanicolaou smears because they may be more likely to develop cervical cancer.
- **Topical:** Instruct patient to apply ointment in sufficient quantity to cover all lesions every 3 hr, 6 times/day for 7 days. 0.5-in. ribbon of ointment covers approximately 4 square in. Use a finger cot or glove when applying to prevent inoculation of other areas or spread to other people. Keep affected areas clean and dry. Loose-fitting clothing should be worn to prevent irritation.
- Avoid drug contact in or around eyes. Report any unexplained eye symptoms to health care professional immediately; ocular herpetic infection can lead to blindness.

Evaluation/Desired Outcomes

- Crusting over and healing of skin lesions.
- Decrease in frequency and severity of recurrences.
- Acceleration of complete healing and cessation of pain in herpes zoster.
- Decrease in intensity of chickenpox.

adalimumab (a-da-li-**mu**-mab)
Humira

Classification
Therapeutic: antirheumatics
Pharmacologic: DMARDs, monoclonal antibodies

Pregnancy Category B

Indications

Treatment of moderately to severely active rheumatoid arthritis in patients who have responded inadequately to other DMARDs; may be used with methotrexate or other DMARDs. Psoriatic arthritis. Active ankylosing spondylitis. Crohn's disease.

Action

Neutralizes and prevents the action of tumor necrosis factor (TNF), resulting in anti-inflammatory and antiproliferative activity. **Therapeutic Effects:** Decreased pain and swelling with decreased rate of joint destruction in patients with rheumatoid arthritis, psoriatic arthritis, and ankylosing spondylitis. Reduced signs and symptoms of Crohn's disease.

Pharmacokinetics

Absorption: 64% absorbed after subcut administration.
Distribution: Synovial fluid concentrations are 31–96% of serum.
Metabolism and Excretion: Unknown.
Half-life: 14 days (range 10–20 days).

TIME/ACTION PROFILE (improvement)

ROUTE	ONSET	PEAK	DURATION
Subcut	8–26 wk	131 hr*	2 wk†

*Blood level
†Following discontinuation

Contraindications/Precautions

Contraindicated in: Hypersensitivity; Concurrent use of anakinra; Active infection (including chronic or localized); Lactation: Potential for serious side effects in the infant; discontinue drug or provide formula.
Use Cautiously in: History of recurrent infection or underlying illness/treatment predisposing to infection; Patients residing, or who have resided, where tuberculosis or histoplasmosis is endemic; Pre-existing or recent onset CNS demyelinating disorders; History of lymphoma; Geri: ↑ risk of infection/malignancy; OB: Use only if clearly needed; Pedi: Safety not established.

Adverse Reactions/Side Effects

CNS: headache. **CV:** hypertension. **GI:** abdominal pain, nausea. **GU:** hematuria. **Derm:** rash. **Hemat:** neutropenia, thrombocytopenia. **Local:** injection site reactions. **Metab:** hypercholesterolemia, hyperlipidemia. **MS:** back pain. **Misc:** allergic reactions including ANAPHYLAXIS, INFECTIONS (including reactivation tuberculosis).

Interactions

Drug-Drug: Concurrent use with **anakinra** or other **TNF blocking agents** ↑ risk of serious infections and is contraindicated. **Live vaccinations** should not be given concurrently.

Route/Dosage

Rheumatoid Arthritis, Ankylosing Spondylitis, and Psoriatic Arthritis

Subcut (Adults): 40-mg every other week; patients not receiving concurrent methotrexate may receive additional benefit by increasing dose to 40-mg once weekly.

Crohn's Disease

Subcut (Adults): 160 mg initially on Day 1 (given as four 40-mg injections in one day or as two 40-mg injections given in two consecutive days), followed by 80 mg 2 wks later on Day 15. Two wks later (Day 29) begin maintenance dose of 40 mg every other wk. Aminosalicylates, corticosteroids, and/or immunomodulatory agents may be continued during therapy.

Availability

Solution for subcut injection (pre-filled syringes): 40 mg/0.8 ml. **Pen:** Single use pre-filled glass syringe containing 40 mg (0.8 mL).

NURSING IMPLICATIONS

Assessment

- Assess pain and range of motion before and periodically during therapy.
- Assess for signs of infection (fever, dyspnea, flu-like symptoms, frequent or painful urination, redness or swelling at the site of a wound), including tuberculosis, prior to injection. Adalimumab is contraindicated in patients with active infection. New infections should be monitored closely; most common are upper respiratory tract infections, bronchitis, and urinary tract infections. Infections may be fatal, especially in patients taking immunosuppressive therapy.
- Monitor for injection site reactions (redness and/or itching, rash, hemorrhage, bruising, pain, or swelling). Rash will usually disappear within a few days. Application of a towel soaked in cold water may relieve pain or swelling.
- Assess patient for latex allergy. Needle cover of syringe contains latex and should not be handled by persons sensitive to latex.
- Monitor patient for signs of anaphylaxis (urticaria, dyspnea, facial edema) following injection. Medications (antihistamines, corticosteroids, epinephrine) and equipment should be readily available in the event of a severe re-

action. Discontinue adalimumab immediately if anaphylaxis or other severe allergic reaction occurs.
- Assess patient for latent tuberculosis with a tuberculin skin test prior to initiation of therapy. Treatment of latent tuberculosis should be started before therapy with adalimumab.
- ***Lab Test Considerations:*** May cause agranulocytosis, granulocytopenia, leukopenia, pancytopenia, and polycythemia.

Potential Nursing Diagnoses
Acute pain (Indications)
Risk for infection (Side Effects)

Implementation
- Administer a tuberculin skin test prior to administration of adalimumab. Patients with active latent TB should be treated for TB prior to therapy.
- Administer initial injection under supervision of a health care professional.
- Do not administer solutions that are discolored or contain particulate matter. Discard unused solution.
- Other DMARDs should be continued during adalimumab therapy.
- **Subcut:** Administer at a 45° angle in upper thighs or abdomen, avoiding the 2 inches around the navel. Put pressure on injection site for 10 sec, do not rub. Rotate injection sites; avoid areas that are tender, bruised, hard, or red.

Patient/Family Teaching
- Instruct patient on the correct technique for administering adalimumab. Review patient information sheet, preparation of dose, administration sites and technique, and disposal of equipment into a puncture-resistant container.
- Advise patient to use calendar stickers provided to by manufacturer to assist in remembering when dose is due. If a dose is missed, instruct patient to administer as soon as possible, then take next dose according to regular schedule. If more than prescribed dose is taken, caution patient to consult health care professional or the HUMIRA Patient Resource Center at 1-800-4HUMIRA (448-6472).
- Caution patient to notify health care professional immediately if signs of infection, severe rash, swollen face, or difficulty breathing occurs while taking adalimumab.
- Advise patient to consult health care professional before taking other Rx or OTC medications or herbal products.
- Instruct patient to notify health care professional of medication regimen prior to treatment or surgery.
- **Pen:** Clean area for injection with alcohol swab. Hold pen with gray cap pointing up. Check solution through window; if discolored, cloudy, or contains flakes, discard solution. Turn pen over and point cap down to make sure solution reaches fill line; if not, do not use and contact pharmacist. Remove gray cap exposing the needle and the plum cap exposing the button; removing the plum cap activates the pen. Pinch skin and place pen, with window visible, against skin at a 90° angle and press button until a click is heard. Hold pen in place until all solution is injected (10 seconds) and yellow marker is visible in window and has stopped moving. Continue to pinch skin throughout injection. Remove needle and press with a gauze pad or cotton ball for 10 seconds. Do not rub injection site. Dispose of pen into a puncture-resistant container.

Evaluation/Desired Outcomes
- Decreased pain and swelling with decreased rate of joint destruction in patients with rheumatoid arthritis.
- Decreased signs and symptoms, slowed progression of joint destruction, and improved physical function in patients with psoriatic arthritis.
- Reduced signs and symptoms of ankylosing spondylitis.
- Decreased signs and symptoms and maintenance of remission in patients with Crohn's disease.

adenosine (a-**den**-oh-seen)
Adenocard, Adenoscan

Classification
Therapeutic: antiarrhythmics

Pregnancy Category C

Indications
Conversion of paroxysmal supraventricular tachycardia (PSVT) to normal sinus rhythm when vagal maneuvers are unsuccessful. As a diagnostic agent (with noninvasive techniques) to assess myocardial perfusion defects occur-

ring as a consequence of coronary artery disease.

Action

Restores normal sinus rhythm by interrupting re-entrant pathways in the AV node. Slows conduction time through the AV node. Also produces coronary artery vasodilation. **Therapeutic Effects:** Restoration of normal sinus rhythm.

Pharmacokinetics

Absorption: Following IV administration, absorption is complete.
Distribution: Taken up by erythrocytes and vascular endothelium.
Metabolism and Excretion: Rapidly converted to inosine and adenosine monophosphate.
Half-life: <10 sec.

TIME/ACTION PROFILE (antiarrhythmic effect)

ROUTE	ONSET	PEAK	DURATION
IV	immediate	unknown	1–2 min

Contraindications/Precautions

Contraindicated in: Hypersensitivity; 2nd- or 3rd-degree AV block or sick sinus syndrome, unless a functional artificial pacemaker is present.
Use Cautiously in: Patients with a history of asthma (may induce bronchospasm); Unstable angina; OB, Lactation: Safety not established.

Adverse Reactions/Side Effects

CNS: apprehension, dizziness, headache, head pressure, light-headedness. **EENT:** blurred vision, throat tightness. **Resp:** shortness of breath, chest pressure, hyperventilation. **CV:** facial flushing, transient arrhythmias, chest pain, hypotension, palpitations. **GI:** metallic taste, nausea. **Derm:** burning sensation, facial flushing, sweating. **MS:** neck and back pain. **Neuro:** numbness, tingling. **Misc:** heaviness in arms, pressure sensation in groin.

Interactions

Drug-Drug: Carbamazepine may ↑ risk of progressive heart block. **Dipyridamole** ↑ effects of adenosine (dosage reduction of adenosine recommended). Effects of adenosine ↑ by **theophylline** or **caffeine** (larger doses of adenosine may be required). Concurrent use with **digoxin** may ↑ risk of ventricular fibrillation.

Route/Dosage

IV (Adults and Children >50 kg): *Antiarrhythmic*—6 mg by rapid IV bolus; if no results, repeat 1–2 min later as 12-mg rapid bolus. This dose may be repeated (single dose not to exceed 12 mg). *Diagnostic use*—140 mcg/kg/min for 6 min (0.84 mg/kg total).
IV (Children <50 kg): *Antiarrhythmic*—0.05–0.1 mg/kg as a rapid bolus, may repeat in 1–2 min; if response is inadequate, may increase by 0.05–0.1 mg/kg until sinus rhythm is established or maximum dose of 0.3 mg/kg is used.

Availability (generic available)

Injection: 6 mg/2-ml vial (Adenocard), 3 mg/1 ml in 30-ml vial (Adenoscan).

NURSING IMPLICATIONS

Assessment

- Monitor heart rate frequently (every 15–30 sec) and ECG continuously during therapy. A short, transient period of 1st-, 2nd-, or 3rd-degree heart block or asystole may occur following injection; usually resolves quickly due to short duration of adenosine. Once conversion to normal sinus rhythm is achieved, transient arrhythmias (premature ventricular contractions, atrial premature contractions, sinus tachycardia, sinus bradycardia, skipped beats, AV nodal block) may occur, but generally last a few seconds.
- Monitor blood pressure during therapy.
- Assess respiratory status (breath sounds, rate) following administration. Patients with history of asthma may experience bronchospasm.

Potential Nursing Diagnoses

Decreased cardiac output (Indications)

Implementation

- Do not confuse adenosine (Adenocard) with adenosine phosphate.

IV Administration

- **IV:** Crystals may occur if adenosine is refrigerated. Warm to room temperature to dissolve crystals. Solution must be clear before use. Do not administer solutions that are discolored or contain particulate matter. Discard unused portions.
- **Direct IV:** ***Diluent:*** Administer undiluted. ***Concentration:*** 3 mg/ml. ***Rate:*** Adminis-

ter over 1–2 seconds via peripheral IV as proximal as possible to trunk. Slow administration may cause increased heart rate in response to vasodilation. Follow each dose with 20 ml rapid saline flush to ensure injection reaches systemic circulation.

- **Intermittent Infusion:** (for use in diagnostic testing) ***Diluent:*** Administer 30-ml vial undiluted. ***Concentration:*** 3 mg/ml. ***Rate:*** Administer at a rate of 140 mcg/kg/min over 6 min for a total dose of 0.84 mg/kg. Thallium-201 should be injected as close to the venous access as possible at the midpoint (after 3 min) of the infusion.
- **Y-Site Compatibility:** abciximab, Thallium-201.

Patient/Family Teaching

- Caution patient to change positions slowly to minimize orthostatic hypotension. Doses >12 mg decrease blood pressure by decreasing peripheral vascular resistance.
- Instruct patient to report facial flushing, shortness of breath, or dizziness.

Evaluation/Desired Outcomes

- Conversion of supraventricular tachycardia to normal sinus rhythm.
- Diagnosis of myocardial perfusion defects.

albumin (human)

(al-**byoo**-min)

Albuminar, Albutein, Buminate, normal human serum albumin, Plasbumin

Classification

Therapeutic: volume expanders

Pharmacologic: blood products, colloids

Pregnancy Category C

Indications

Expansion of plasma volume and maintenance of cardiac output in situations associated with fluid volume deficit, including shock, hemorrhage, and burns. Temporary replacement of albumin in diseases associated with low levels of plasma proteins, such as nephrotic syndrome or end-stage liver disease, resulting in relief or reduction of associated edema.

Action

Provides colloidal oncotic pressure, which serves to mobilize fluid from extravascular tissues back into the intravascular space. Requires concurrent administration of appropriate crystalloid. **Therapeutic Effects:** Increase in intravascular fluid volume.

Pharmacokinetics

Absorption: Following IV administration, absorption is essentially complete.

Distribution: Confined to the intravascular space, unless capillary permeability is increased.

Metabolism and Excretion: Probably degraded by the liver.

Half-life: 2–3 wk.

TIME/ACTION PROFILE (oncotic effect)

ROUTE	ONSET	PEAK	DURATION
IV	15–30 min	unknown	24 hrs

Contraindications/Precautions

Contraindicated in: Allergic reactions to albumin; Severe anemia; CHF; Normal or increased intravascular volume.

Use Cautiously in: Severe hepatic or renal disease; Dehydration (additional fluids may be required); Patients requiring sodium restriction; Preterm neonates (infuse slowly due to increased risk of intravascular hemorrhage).

Adverse Reactions/Side Effects

CNS: headache. **CV:** PULMONARY EDEMA, fluid overload, hypertension, hypotension, tachycardia. **GI:** increased salivation, nausea, vomiting. **Derm:** rash, urticaria. **MS:** back pain. **Misc:** chills, fever, flushing.

Interactions

Drug-Drug: None significant.

Route/Dosage

Dose is highly individualized and depends on condition being treated.

Hypovolemic shock—5% Albumin

IV (Adults): 25 g (500 ml), may be repeated within 30 min.

IV (Children): 0.5–1 g/kg/dose (10–20 mL/kg/dose) may repeat as needed (maximum 6 g/kg/day).

IV (Infants and Neonates): 0.25–0.5 g/kg/dose (5–10 ml/kg/dose).

Hypoproteinemia—25% Albumin

IV (Adults): 50–75 g.

IV (Children, Infants, and Neonates): 0.5–1 g/kg/dose, may repeat every 1–2 days; doses up to 1.5 g/kg/day have been added to hyperalimentation solutions and given over 24 hrs.

Nephrotic Syndrome—25% Albumin
IV (Adults): 12.5–50 g/day in 3–4 divided doses.
IV (Children and Infants): 0.25–1 g/kg/dose.

Availability
Injection: 5% (50 mg/mL), 25% (250 mg/mL).

NURSING IMPLICATIONS

Assessment
- Monitor vital signs, CVP, and intake and output before and frequently throughout therapy. If fever, tachycardia, or hypotension occurs, stop infusion and notify physician immediately. Antihistamines may be required to suppress this hypersensitivity response. Hypotension may also result from infusing too rapidly. May be given without regard to patient's blood group.
- Assess for signs of vascular overload (elevated CVP, rales/crackles, dyspnea, hypertension, jugular venous distention) during and after administration.
- **Surgical Patients:** Assess for increased bleeding after administration caused by increased blood pressure and circulating blood volume. Albumin does not contain clotting factors.
- ***Lab Test Considerations:*** Serum albumin levels should increase with albumin therapy.
- Monitor serum sodium levels; may cause ↑ concentrations.
- Infusions of normal serum albumin may cause false ↑ of alkaline phosphatase levels.
- Hemorrhage: Monitor hemoglobin and hematocrit levels. These values may ↓ because of hemodilution.

Potential Nursing Diagnoses
Decreased cardiac output (Indications)
Deficient fluid volume (Indications)
Excess fluid volume (Side Effects)

Implementation
- Follow manufacturer's recommendations for administration. Administer through a large-gauge (at least 20-gauge) needle or catheter. Record lot number in patient record.
- Solution should be clear amber; 25% albumin solution is equal to 5 times the osmotic value of plasma. Do not administer solutions that are discolored or contain particulate matter. Each liter of both 5% and 25% albumin contains 130–160 mEq of sodium and is thus no longer labeled "salt-poor" albumin.
- Administration of large quantities of normal serum albumin may need to be supplemented with whole blood to prevent anemia. If more than 1000 ml of 5% normal serum albumin is given or if hemorrhage has occurred, the administration of whole blood or packed RBCs may be needed. Hydration status should be monitored and maintained with additional fluids.

IV Administration
- **Intermittent Infusion:** ***Diluent:*** Administer 5% normal serum albumin undiluted. Normal serum albumin 25% may be administered undiluted or diluted in 0.9% NaCl, D5W, or sodium lactate injection; do not dilute in sterile water (may result in hypotonic-associated hemolysis which may be fatal). Infusion must be completed within 4 hr. ***Concentration:*** 5%: 50 mg/ml undiluted. 25%: 250 mg/ml undiluted. ***Rate:*** Rate of administration is determined by concentration of solution, blood volume, indication, and patient response (usual rate over 30–60 min). In patients with normal blood volume, rate of 5% and 25% solutions should not exceed 2–4 ml/min and 1 ml/min, respectively for both adults and children.
- **Hypovolemia:** 5% or 25% normal serum albumin may be administered as rapidly as tolerated and repeated in 15–30 min if necessary.
- **Burns:** Rate after the first 24 hr should be set to maintain a plasma albumin level of 2.5 g/100 ml or a total serum protein level of 5.2 g/100 ml.
- **Hypoproteinemia:** Normal serum albumin 25% is the preferred solution because of the increased concentration of protein. The rate should not exceed 2–3 ml/min of 25% or 5–10 ml/min of 5% solution to prevent circulatory overload and pulmonary edema. This treatment provides a temporary rise in plasma protein until the hypoproteinemia is corrected.
- **Y-Site Compatibility:** diltiazem, lorazepam.
- **Y-Site Incompatibility:** fat emulsion, midazolam, vancomycin, verapamil.

- **Solution Compatibility:** 0.9% NaCl, D5W, D5/0.9% NaCl, D5/0.45% NaCl, sodium lactate ⅙M, D5/LR, and LR.

Patient/Family Teaching
- Explain the purpose of this solution to the patient.
- Instruct patient to report signs and symptoms of hypersensitivity reaction.

Evaluation/Desired Outcomes
- Increase in blood pressure and blood volume when used to treat shock and burns.
- Increased urinary output reflects the mobilization of fluid from extravascular tissues.
- Elevated serum plasma protein in patients with hypoproteinemia.

albuterol (al-byoo-ter-ole)
Airet, ✱Apo-Salvent, ✱Gen-Salbutamol, ✱Novo-Salmol, Proventil, Proventil HFA, salbutamol, ✱Ventodisk, Ventolin, Ventolin HFA, ✱Ventolin nebules, Ventolin rotacaps

Classification
Therapeutic: bronchodilators
Pharmacologic: adrenergics

Pregnancy Category C

Indications
Used as a bronchodilator to control and prevent reversible airway obstruction caused by asthma or COPD. **Inhaln:** Used as a quick-relief agent for acute bronchospasm and for prevention of exercise-induced bronchospasm. **PO:** Used as a long-term control agent in patients with chronic/persistent bronchospasm.

Action
Binds to beta$_2$-adrenergic receptors in airway smooth muscle, leading to activation of adenyl cyclase and increased levels of cyclic-3′, 5′-adenosine monophosphate (cAMP). Increases in cAMP activate kinases, which inhibit the phosphorylation of myosin and decrease intracellular calcium. Decreased intracellular calcium relaxes smooth muscle airways. Relaxation of airway smooth muscle with subsequent bronchodilation. Relatively selective for beta$_2$ (pulmonary) receptors. **Therapeutic Effects:** Bronchodilation.

Pharmacokinetics
Absorption: Well absorbed after oral administration but rapidly undergoes extensive metabolism.
Distribution: Small amounts appear in breast milk.
Metabolism and Excretion: Extensively metabolized by the liver and other tissues.
Half-life: Oral 2.7–5 hr; Inhalation: 3.8 hr.

TIME/ACTION PROFILE (bronchodilation)

ROUTE	ONSET	PEAK	DURATION
PO	15–30 min	2–3 hr	4–6 hr or more
PO–ER	30 min	2–3 hr	12 hr
Inhaln	5–15 min	60–90 min	3–6 hr

Contraindications/Precautions
Contraindicated in: Hypersensitivity to adrenergic amines; Hypersensitivity to fluorocarbons (some inhalers).
Use Cautiously in: Cardiac disease; Hypertension; Hyperthyroidism; Diabetes; Glaucoma; Seizure disorders; Excess inhaler use may lead to tolerance and paradoxical bronchospasm; OB, Lactation, Pedi: Safety not established for pregnant women near term, breastfeeding women, and children <2 yr; Geri: Increased risk adverse reactions; may require dosage reduction.

Adverse Reactions/Side Effects
CNS: nervousness, restlessness, tremor, headache, insomnia (Pedi: occurs more frequently in young children than adults), hyperactivity in children. **CV:** chest pain, palpitations, angina, arrhythmias, hypertension. **GI:** nausea, vomiting. **Endo:** hyperglycemia. **F and E:** hypokalemia. **Neuro:** tremor.

Interactions
Drug-Drug: Concurrent use with other **adrenergic agents** will have ↑ adrenergic side effects. Use with **MAO inhibitors** may lead to hypertensive crisis. **Beta blockers** may negate therapeutic effect. May decrease serum **digoxin** levels. Cardiovascular effects are potentiated in patients receiving **tricyclic antidepressants**. Risk of hypokalemia ↑ concurrent use of **potassium-losing diuretics**. Hypokalemia ↑ the risk of **digoxin** toxicity.
Drug-Natural Products: Use with caffeine-containing herbs (**cola nut**, **guarana**, **tea**, **coffee**) ↑ stimulant effect.

Route/Dosage
PO (Adults and Children ≥12 yr): 2–4 mg 3–4 times daily (not to exceed 32 mg/day) or 4–8 mg of extended-release tablets twice daily.

PO (Geriatric Patients): Initial dose should not exceed 2 mg 3–4 times daily, may be increased carefully (up to 32 mg/day).
PO (Children 6–12 yr): 2 mg 3–4 times daily or 0.3–0.6 mg/kg/day as extended-release tablets divided twice daily; may be carefully increased as needed (not to exceed 8 mg/day).
PO (Children 2–6 yr): 0.1 mg/kg 3 times daily (not to exceed 2 mg 3 times daily initially); may be carefully increased to 0.2 mg/kg 3 times daily (not to exceed 4 mg 3 times daily).
Inhaln (Adults and Children ≥4 yr): *Via metered-dose inhaler*—2 inhalations q 4–6 hr or 2 inhalations 15 min before exercise (90 mcg/spray); some patients may respond to 1 inhalation. *NIH Guidelines for acute asthma exacerbation: Children*—4–8 puffs q 20 min for 3 doses then q 1–4 hr; *Adults*—4–8 puffs q 20 min for up to 4 hr then q 1–4 hr prn.
Inhaln (Adults and Children >12 yr): *NIH Guidelines for acute asthma exacerbation via nebulization or IPPB*—2.5–5 mg q 20 min for 3 doses then 2.5–10 mg q 1–4 hr prn; *Continuous nebulization*—10–15 mg/hr.
Inhaln (Children 2–12 yr): *NIH Guidelines for acute asthma exacerbation via nebulization or IPPB*—0.15 mg/kg/dose (minimum dose 2.5 mg) q 20 min for 3 doses then 0.15–0.3 mg/kg (not to exceed 10 mg) q 1–4 hr prn *or* 1.25 mg 3–4 times daily for children 10–15 kg *or* 2.5 mg 3–4 times daily for children >15 kg; *Continuous nebulization*—0.5–3 mg/kg/hr.
Inhaln (Adults and Children ≥4 yr): *Via Rotahaler inhalation device*—200 mcg (as Ventolin Rotacaps) q 4–6 hr (up to 400 mcg q 4–6 hr). May also be given 15 min before exercise.

Availability (generic available)

Tablets: 2 mg, 4 mg. **Cost:** *Generic*—2 mg $62.96/270, 4 mg $49.49/270. **Extended-release tablets:** 4 mg, 8 mg. **Cost:** 4 mg $265.43/180, 8 mg $488.93/180. **Oral syrup (strawberry-flavored):** 2 mg/5 ml. **Cost:** *Generic*—$11.42/480 ml. **Metered-dose aerosol:** 90 mcg/inhalation in 6.7-g, 8.5-g, 17-g, and 18-g canisters (200 metered inhalations), ✤100 mcg/spray. **Cost:** *Proair HFA*—$35.99/8.5-g canister; *Proventil HFA*—$45.99/6.7-g canister; *Ventolin HFA*—$37.99/18-g canister. **Inhalation solution:** 0.63 mg/3 ml, 1.25 mg/3 ml, 0.83 mg/ml in vials and 3 ml unit dose, ✤1 mg/ml, ✤2 mg/ml, 5 mg/ml. **Cost:** *Generic*—5 mg/ml $15.99/20 ml, 0.63 mg/ml $8.99/3 ml, 0.83 mg/ml $18.99/3 ml (25 vials). **Powder for inhalation (Ventodisk):** ✤200 mcg, ✤400 mcg. ***In combination with:*** ipratropium (Combivent, DuoNeb). See Appendix B.

NURSING IMPLICATIONS

Assessment

- Assess lung sounds, pulse, and blood pressure before administration and during peak of medication. Note amount, color, and character of sputum produced.
- Monitor pulmonary function tests before initiating therapy and periodically during therapy to determine effectiveness of medication.
- Observe for paradoxical bronchospasm (wheezing). If condition occurs, withhold medication and notify physician or other health care professional immediately.
- ***Lab Test Considerations:*** May cause transient ↓ in serum potassium concentrations with nebulization or higher-than-recommended doses.

Potential Nursing Diagnoses

Ineffective airway clearance (Indications)

Implementation

- Do not confuse Salbutamol (albuterol) with Salmeterol.
- **PO:** Administer oral medication with meals to minimize gastric irritation.
- Extended-release tablets should be swallowed whole; do not break, crush, or chew.
  Inhaln: Shake inhaler well, and allow at least 1 min between inhalations of aerosol medication. Prime the inhaler before first use by releasing 4 test sprays into the air away from the face. Pedi: Use spacer for children <8 years of age.
- For nebulization or IPPB, the 0.5-, 0.83-, 1-, and 2-mg/ml solutions do not require dilution before administration. The 5 mg/ml (0.5%) solution must be diluted with 1–2.5 ml of 0.9% NaCl for inhalation. Diluted solutions are stable for 24 hr at room temperature or 48 hr if refrigerated.
- For nebulizer, compressed air or oxygen flow should be 6–10 L/min; a single treatment of 3 ml lasts about 10 min.
- IPPB usually lasts 5–20 min.

Patient/Family Teaching

- Instruct patient to take albuterol as directed. If on a scheduled dosing regimen, take missed dose as soon as remembered, spacing remaining doses at regular intervals. Do not double doses or increase the dose or frequency of doses. Caution patient not to exceed recommended dose; may cause adverse effects, paradoxical bronchospasm (more likely with first dose from new cannister), or loss of effectiveness of medication.
- Instruct patient to contact health care professional immediately if shortness of breath is not relieved by medication or is accompanied by diaphoresis, dizziness, palpitations, or chest pain.
- Instruct patient to prime unit with 4 sprays before using and to discard cannister after 200 sprays. Actuators should not be changed among products.
- Inform patient that these products contain hydrofluoralkane (HFA) and the propellant and are described as non-CFC or CFC-free (contain no chlorofluorocarbons).
- Advise patient to consult health care professional before taking any OTC medications, natural/herbal products, or alcohol concurrently with this therapy. Caution patient also to avoid smoking and other respiratory irritants.
- Inform patient that albuterol may cause an unusual or bad taste.
- **Inhaln:** Instruct patient in the proper use of the metered-dose inhaler, Rotahaler, or nebulizer (see Appendix D).
- Advise patients to use albuterol first if using other inhalation medications and allow 5 min to elapse before administering other inhalant medications unless otherwise directed.
- Advise patient to rinse mouth with water after each inhalation dose to minimize dry mouth.
- Instruct patient to notify health care professional if no response to the usual dose of albuterol or if contents of one canister are used in less than 2 wk.
- Pedi: Caution adolescents and their parents about overuse of inhalers, which can cause heart damage and life-threatening arrhythmias.

Evaluation/Desired Outcomes

- Prevention or relief of bronchospasm.

---

alclometasone, **See CORTICOSTEROIDS (TOPICAL/LOCAL).**

HIGH ALERT

alemtuzumab

(a-lem-**too**-zoo-mab)

Campath

Classification

Therapeutic: antineoplastics

Pharmacologic: monoclonal antibodies

Pregnancy Category C

Indications

Treatment of B-cell chronic lymphocytic leukemia in patients who have been treated with alkylating agents and in which fludarabine therapy has failed.

Action

Binds to the CD52 antigen found on the surface of B- and T-lymphocytes and other white blood cells; resulting in lysis. **Therapeutic Effects:** Lysis of leukemic cells with eventual improvement in hematologic parameters.

Pharmacokinetics

Absorption: IV administration results in complete bioavailability.

Distribution: Binds to CD52 receptors.

Metabolism and Excretion: Unknown.

Half-life: 12 days.

TIME/ACTION PROFILE (hematologic parameters)

ROUTE	ONSET	PEAK	DURATION
IV	unknown	2–4 mos‡	7–11 mos‡‡

‡Median time to response

‡‡Duration of response

Contraindications/Precautions

Contraindicated in: Hypersensitivity; Systemic infections; Underlying immunodeficiency, including HIV infection; Lactation: Discontinue breast-feeding during and for 3 mos following last dose of alemtuzumab.

Use Cautiously in: Patients with ischemic heart disease or in patients on antihypertensive medications; Women and men with reproduction potential should use contraception during treatment and for 6 mos after therapy; OB: Should be administered only if clearly needed.

Adverse Reactions/Side Effects

CNS: depression, dizziness, drowsiness, fatigue, headache, weakness. **Resp:** bronchospasm, cough, dyspnea. **CV:** hypertension, hypotension, tachycardia. **GI:** abdominal pain, anorexia, constipation, stomatitis. **Derm:** rash, sweating. **F and E:** edema. **Hemat:** NEUTROPENIA, PANCYTOPENIA/MARROW HYPOPLASIA, anemia, lymphopenia, thrombocytopenia. **MS:** back pain, skeletal pain. **Misc:** infusion-related events, infection, sepsis.

Interactions

Drug-Drug: Additive bone marrow depression with other **antineoplastics** or **radiation therapy**. May ↓ antibody response to and increase the risk of adverse reactions to **live-virus vaccines**.

Route/Dosage

IV (Adults): 3 mg/day initially, as tolerated increase dose to 10 mg/day and then 30 mg/day given three times weekly for up to 12 weeks; single doses should not exceed 30 mg or more than 90 mg/wk.

Availability

Solution for injection (requires further dilution): 30 mg/3 ml in single-use ampules.

NURSING IMPLICATIONS

Assessment

- Monitor for infusion reactions (hypotension, rigors, fever, shortness of breath, bronchospasm, chills, rash). Premedicate with an oral antihistamine and acetaminophen 30 min prior to initial dose, dose increases, and as clinically indicated. Monitor blood pressure and hypotensive symptoms in patients with ischemic heart disease with extra care. Antihistamines, acetaminophen, antiemetics, meperidine, corticosteroids, and incremental dose escalation have been used to prevent and treat infusion-related reactions. Initiate therapy at lowest dose and increase gradually. If therapy is interrupted for 7 or more days, reinstitute with gradual dose escalation.
- ***Lab Test Considerations:*** Obtain CBC and platelet counts weekly during therapy and more frequently if worsening anemia, neutropenia, or thrombocytopenia is observed. For first occurrence of ANC<250 cells/mm^3 and/or platelet count <25,000 cells/mm^3, withhold alemtuzumab therapy. When ANC >500 cells/mm^3 and platelet count is >50,000 cells/mm^3, resume at same dose. If delay of 7 days or more occurred initiate therapy at 3 mg and escalate to 10 mg and then to 30 mg as tolerated. For second occurrence of ANC <250 cells/mm^3 and/or platelet count <25,000 cells/mm^3, withhold alemtuzumab. When ANC >500 cells/mm^3 and platelet count >50,000 cells/mm^3, resume therapy at 10 mg. If delay is 7 days or more, initiate therapy at 3 mg and escalate to 10 mg only. For third occurrence of ANC <250 cells/mm^3 and/or platelet count <25,000 cells/mm^3, discontinue alemtuzumab therapy permanently. For a decrease of ANC and/or platelet count of 50% of baseline value in patients initiating therapy with a baseline ANC of <500 cells/mm^3 and/or a baseline platelet count of 25,000 cells/mm^3, withhold therapy. When baseline levels return, resume therapy. If delay is 7 days or more, initiate therapy at 3 mg and escalate to 10 mg and 30 mg as tolerated.
- Assess CD4 counts after treatment until recovery to ≥200 cells cells/mm^3.

Potential Nursing Diagnoses

Risk for infection (Side Effects)
Risk for injury (Adverse Reactions)

Implementation

- ***High Alert:*** Fatalities have occurred with chemotherapeutic agents. Before administering, clarify all ambiguous orders; double-check single, daily, and course-of-therapy dose limits; have second practitioner independently double-check original order, calculations, and infusion pump settings. Alemtuzumab should only be administered under the supervision of a physician experienced in the use antineoplastic therapy.
- Administer via IV only. Inspect solution for particulate matter or discoloration. Do not administer solutions that contain particulate matter or are discolored.

IV Administration

- Withdraw necessary amount from ampule into syringe. Filter with a sterile low-protein binding, non-fiber releasing 5 micron filter prior to dilution.
- **Intermittent Infusion:** ***Diluent:*** Dilute with 100 ml of 0.9% NaCl or D5W. Gently invert bag to mix. Dispose of syringe and unused drug product according to institutional

guidelines. Use within 8 hr of dilution. Store at room temperature or in refrigerator. Protect solution from light. ***Rate:*** Administer over 2 hr.

- **Y-Site Incompatibility:** No data is available regarding mixing with other solutions and medications. Do not add to or infuse simultaneously with other solutions or medications.

Patient/Family Teaching

- Inform patient and family of purpose of alemtuzumab.
- Caution patient to avoid immunizations with a live virus due to immunosuppression.

Evaluation/Desired Outcomes

- Improvement in hematologic parameters in patients with B-cell chronic lymphocytic leukemia.

alendronate (a-**len**-drone-ate)

Fosamax

Classification
Therapeutic: bone resorption inhibitors
Pharmacologic: biphosphonates

Pregnancy Category C

Indications

Treatment and prevention of postmenopausal osteoporosis. Treatment of osteoporosis in men. Treatment of Paget's disease of the bone. Treatment of corticosteroid-induced osteoporosis in patients (men and women) who are receiving ≥7.5 mg of prednisone/day (or equivalent) with evidence of decreased bone mineral density.

Action

Inhibits resorption of bone by inhibiting osteoclast activity. **Therapeutic Effects:** Reversal of the progression of osteoporosis with decreased fractures. Decreased progression of Paget's disease.

Pharmacokinetics

Absorption: Poorly absorbed (0.6–0.8%) after oral administration.
Distribution: Transiently distributes to soft tissue, then distributes to bone.
Metabolism and Excretion: Excreted in urine.
Half-life: 10 yr (reflects release of drug from skeleton).

TIME/ACTION PROFILE (inhibition of bone resorption)

ROUTE	ONSET	PEAK	DURATION
PO	1 mo	3–6 mo	3 wk–7 mo†

†After discontinuation of alendronate

Contraindications/Precautions

Contraindicated in: Renal insufficiency (CCr <35 ml/min); OB, Lactation: Safety not established.
Use Cautiously in: Patients with active GI pathology (dysphagia, esophageal disease, gastritis, duodenitis, ulcers); Pre-existing hypocalcemia or vitamin D deficiency.

Adverse Reactions/Side Effects

CNS: headache. **EENT:** blurred vision, conjunctivitis, eye pain/inflammation. **GI:** abdominal distention, abdominal pain, acid regurgitation, constipation, diarrhea, dyspepsia, dysphagia, esophageal ulcer, flatulence, gastritis, nausea, taste perversion, vomiting. **Derm:** erythema, photosensitivity, rash. **MS:** musculoskeletal pain.

Interactions

Drug-Drug: Calcium supplements, **antacids**, and **other oral medications** ↓ the absorption of alendronate. Doses >10 mg/day ↑ risk of adverse GI events when used with **NSAIDs**. IV **ranitidine** ↑ blood levels.
Drug-Food: Food significantly ↓ absorption. **Caffeine (coffee, tea, cola)**, **mineral water**, and **orange juice** also ↓ absorption.

Route/Dosage

PO (Adults): *Treatment of osteoporosis*—10 mg once daily or 70 mg once weekly. *Prevention of osteoporosis*—5 mg once daily or 35 mg once weekly. *Paget's disease*—40 mg once daily for 6 mo. Re-treatment may be considered for patients who relapse. *Treatment of corticosteroid-induced osteoporosis in men and premenopausal women*—5 mg once daily. *Treatment of corticosteroid-induced osteoporosis in postmenopausal women not receiving estrogen*—10 mg once daily.

Availability

Tablets: 5 mg, 10 mg, 35 mg, 40 mg, 70 mg. **Cost:** 5 mg $248.19/90, 10 mg $240.97/90, 35 mg $235.97/12, 40 mg $177.89/30, 70 mg $239.96/12. **Oral solution (raspberry flavor):** 70 mg/75 ml. **Cost:** $27.99/75 ml. ***In combination with:*** Cholecalciferol (Fosamax plus D) See Appendix B.

NURSING IMPLICATIONS

Assessment

- **Osteoporosis:** Assess patients for low bone mass before and periodically during therapy.
- **Paget's Disease:** Assess for symptoms of Paget's disease (bone pain, headache, decreased visual and auditory acuity, increased skull size).
- ***Lab Test Considerations:*** *Osteoporosis:* Assess serum calcium before and periodically during therapy. Hypocalcemia and vitamin D deficiency should be treated before initiating alendronate therapy. May cause mild, transient elevations of calcium and phosphate.
- **Paget's Disease:** Monitor alkaline phosphatase before and periodically during therapy. Alendronate is indicated for patients with alkaline phosphatase twice the upper limit of normal.

Potential Nursing Diagnoses

Risk for injury (Indications)

Implementation

- Do not confuse Fosamax (alendronate) with Flomax (tamsulosin).
- **PO:** Administer first thing in the morning with 6–8 oz plain water 30 min before other medications, beverages, or food.

Patient/Family Teaching

- Instruct patient on the importance of taking exactly as directed, first thing in the morning, 30 min before other medications, beverages, or food. Waiting longer than 30 min will improve absorption. Alendronate should be taken with 6–8 oz plain water (mineral water, orange juice, coffee, and other beverages decrease absorption). If a dose is missed, skip dose and resume the next morning; do not double doses or take later in the day. If a weekly dose is missed, take the morning after remembered and resume the following week on the chosen day. Do not take 2 tablets on the same day. Do not discontinue without consulting health care professional.
- Caution patient to remain upright for 30 min following dose to facilitate passage to stomach and minimize risk of esophageal irritation. Advise patient to discontinue alendronate and notify health care provider if pain or difficulty swallowing, retrosternal pain, or new/worsening heartburn occur.
- Advise patient to eat a balanced diet and consult health care professional about the need for supplemental calcium and vitamin D.
- Encourage patient to participate in regular exercise and to modify behaviors that increase the risk of osteoporosis (stop smoking, reduce alcohol consumption).
- Caution patient to use sunscreen and protective clothing to prevent photosensitivity reactions.
- Advise patient to notify health care professional if blurred vision, eye pain or inflammation occur.
- Advise female patient to notify health care professional if pregnancy is planned or suspected or if she is breastfeeding.

Evaluation/Desired Outcomes

- Prevention of or decrease in the progression of osteoporosis in postmenopausal women.
- Treatment of osteoporosis in men.
- Decrease in the progression of Paget's disease.
- Treatment of corticosteroid-induced osteoporosis.

alfuzosin (al-**fyoo**-zo-sin)

Uroxatral

Classification

Therapeutic: urinary tract antispasmodics

Pharmacologic: peripherally acting antiadrenergics

Pregnancy Category B

Indications

Management of symptomatic benign prostatic hyperplasia (BPH).

Action

Selectively blocks $alpha_1$-adrenergic receptors in the lower urinary tract to relax smooth muscle in the bladder neck and prostate. **Therapeutic Effects:** Increased urine flow and decreased symptoms of BPH.

Pharmacokinetics

Absorption: 49% absorbed following oral administration; food enhances absorption.

Distribution: Unknown.

Metabolism and Excretion: Mostly metabolized by the liver (CYP3A4 enzyme system); 69% eliminated in feces, 24% in urine.

Half-life: 10 hr.

TIME/ACTION PROFILE

ROUTE	ONSET	PEAK	DURATION
PO-ER	within hr	8 hr	24 hr

Contraindications/Precautions

Contraindicated in: Hypersensitivity; Moderate to severe hepatic impairment; Potent inhibitors of the CYP3A4 enzyme system; Concurrent use of other alpha-adrenergic blocking agents; Severe renal impairment; OB, Pedi: No indications for women and children.

Use Cautiously in: Congenital or acquired QTc prolongation or concurrent use of other drugs known to prolong QTc; Mild hepatic impairment; Geri: Consider age-related changes in body mass, cardiac, renal and hepatic function when prescribing.

Adverse Reactions/Side Effects

CNS: dizziness, fatigue, headache. **Resp:** bronchitis, sinusitis, pharyngitis. **CV:** postural hypotension. **GI:** abdominal pain, constipation, dyspepsia, nausea. **GU:** erectile dysfunction.

Interactions

Drug-Drug: Ketoconazole, **itraconazole**, and **ritonavir** ↓ metabolism and significantly ↑ levels and effects (concurrent use in contraindicated). Levels are also ↑ by **cimetidine**, **atenolol**, and **diltiazem**. Alfuzosin ↑ levels and may ↑ effects of **atenolol** and **diltiazem** (monitor blood pressure and heart rate). ↑ risk of hypotension with **antihypertensives**, **nitrates**, and acute ingestion of **alcohol**.

Route/Dosage

PO (Adults): 10 mg once daily.

Availability

Extended-release tablets: 10 mg. **Cost:** $229.96/90.

NURSING IMPLICATIONS

Assessment

- Assess patient for symptoms of benign prostatic hyperplasia (urinary hesitancy, feeling of incomplete bladder emptying, interruption of urinary stream, impairment of size and force of urinary stream, terminal urinary dribbling, straining to start flow, dysuria, urgency) before and periodically during therapy.
- Assess patient for orthostatic reaction and syncope. Monitor BP (lying and standing) and pulse frequently during initial dose adjustment and periodically thereafter. May occur within a few hrs after initial doses and occasionally thereafter.
- Rule out prostatic carcinoma before therapy; symptoms are similar.

Potential Nursing Diagnoses

Risk for injury (Side Effects)
Noncompliance (Patient/Family Teaching)

Implementation

- **PO:** Administer with food at the same meal each day. Tablets must be swallowed whole; do not crush, break, or chew.

Patient/Family Teaching

- Instruct patient to take medication with the same meal each day. Take missed doses as soon as remembered. If not remembered until next day, omit; do not double doses.
- May cause dizziness or drowsiness. Advise patient to avoid driving or other activities requiring alertness until response to the medication is known.
- Caution patient to avoid sudden changes in position to decrease orthostatic hypotension.
- Advise patient to consult health care professional before taking any cough, cold, or allergy remedies.
- Instruct patient to notify health care professional of medication regimen before any surgery.
- Advise patient to notify health care professional if frequent dizziness or fainting occurs.
- Emphasize the importance of follow-up exams to evaluate effectiveness of medication.
- Geri: Assess risk for falls; implement fall prevention program and instruct patient and family in preventing falls at home.

Evaluation/Desired Outcomes

- Decreased symptoms of benign prostatic hyperplasia.

aliskiren (a-lis-ki-ren)

Tekturna

Classification

Therapeutic: antihypertensives
Pharmacologic: renin inhibitors

Pregnancy Category C

Indications

Treatment of hypertension (alone or with other agents).

Action
Inhibition of renin results in decreased formation of angiotensin II, a powerful vasoconstrictor. **Therapeutic Effects:** Decreased blood pressure.

Pharmacokinetics
Absorption: Poorly absorbed (bioavailability 2.5%).
Distribution: Unknown.
Metabolism and Excretion: 2% excreted unchanged in urine, remainder is probably metabolized (CYP3A4 enzyme system).
Half-life: 24 hr.

TIME/ACTION PROFILE (antihypertensive effect)

ROUTE	ONSET	PEAK	DURATION
PO	unknown	2 wk	24 hr

Contraindications/Precautions
Contraindicated in: Hypersensitivity; OB: Known or suspected pregnancy (may cause fetal injury or death).
Use Cautiously in: Salt or volume depletion (correct before use); Severe renal impairment; Pedi: Safe use not established.

Adverse Reactions/Side Effects
Resp: cough. **GI:** abdominal pain, diarrhea (↑ in females and elderly), dyspepsia, reflux. **Misc:** ANGIOEDEMA.

Interactions
Drug-Drug: Blood levels are ↓ by **irbesartan**. Blood levels are ↑ by **atorvastatin** and **ketoconazole**. ↓ blood levels and may ↓ effects of **furosemide**. Antihypertensive effects may be ↑ by other **antihypertensives**, **diuretics**, and **nitrates**. ↑ risk of hyperkalemia with **ACE inhibitors** in diabetic patients.
Drug-Food: High fat meals significantly ↓ absorption.

Route/Dosage
PO (Adults): 150 mg/day initially; may be increased to 300 mg/day.

Availability
Tablets: 150 mg, 300 mg.

NURSING IMPLICATIONS

Assessment
- Monitor blood pressure and pulse frequently during initial dose adjustment and periodically during therapy. Notify health care professional of significant changes. If an excessive fall in BP occurs, place patient in a supine position and administer IV 0.9% NaCl, if necessary. A transient hypotensive response does not contraindicate further therapy.
- Monitor frequency of prescription refills to determine adherence.
- ***Lab Test Considerations:*** May cause minor ↑ in BUN, serum creatinine, potassium, uric acid, and creatine kinase.
- May cause small ↓ in hemoglobin and hematocrit.

Potential Nursing Diagnoses
Noncompliance (Patient/Family Teaching)

Implementation
- Correct volume or sodium depletion prior to initiating therapy.
- **PO:** Administer at the same time each day without regard to meals.

Patient/Family Teaching
- Instruct patient to take aliskiren as directed at the same time each day, even if feeling better. Take missed doses as soon as remembered, but not if almost time for next dose. Do not double doses. Do not share medication with others, even with same condition; may be harmful.
- May cause dizziness. Caution patient to lie down and notify health care professional. Also, avoid driving and other activities requiring alertness until response to aliskiren is known.
- Advise patient to report signs and symptoms of angioedema (swelling of face, extremities, eyes, lips, tongue, difficulty swallowing or breathing) to health care professional immediately.
- Instruct patient to notify health care professional prior to taking other Rx, OTC, or herbal products.
- Advise female patients to notify health care professional if pregnancy is planned or suspected or if breastfeeding. If pregnancy is detected, discontinue aliskiren as soon as possible.

Evaluation/Desired Outcomes
- Decrease in blood pressure without appearance of side effects. Antihypertensive effect is 90% attained by 2 wks.

allopurinol (al-oh-**pure**-i-nole)

Alloprim, ✤Apo-Allopurinol, Lopurin, ✤Purinol, Zyloprim

Classification

Therapeutic: antigout agents, antihyperuricemics

Pharmacologic: xanthine oxidase inhibitors

Pregnancy Category C

Indications

PO: Prevention of attack of gouty arthritis and nephropathy. **PO, IV:** Treatment of secondary hyperuricemia, which may occur during treatment of tumors or leukemias.

Action

Inhibits the production of uric acid by inhibiting the action of xanthine oxidase. **Therapeutic Effects:** Lowering of serum uric acid levels.

Pharmacokinetics

Absorption: Well absorbed (80%) following oral administration.

Distribution: Widely distributed in tissue and breast milk.

Protein Binding: <1%.

Metabolism and Excretion: Metabolized to oxypurinol, an active compound with a long half-life. 12% excreted unchanged, 76% excreted as oxypurinol.

Half-life: 1–3 hr (oxypurinol 18–30 hr).

TIME/ACTION PROFILE (hypouricemic effect)

ROUTE	ONSET	PEAK	DURATION
PO, IV	1–2 days	1–2 wk	1–3 wk

†Duration after discontinuation of allopurinol

Contraindications/Precautions

Contraindicated in: Hypersensitivity.

Use Cautiously in: Acute attacks of gout; Renal insufficiency (dose reduction required if CCr <20 ml/min); Dehydration (adequate hydration necessary); OB, Lactation: Rarely used; Geri: Begin at lower end of dosage range.

Adverse Reactions/Side Effects

CV: hypotension, flushing, hypertension, bradycardia, and heart failure (reported with IV administration).

CNS: drowsiness. **GI:** diarrhea, hepatitis, nausea, vomiting. **GU:** renal failure, hematuria.

Derm: rash (discontinue drug at first sign of rash), urticaria. **Hemat:** bone marrow depression. **Misc:** hypersensitivity reactions.

Interactions

Drug-Drug: Use with **mercaptopurine** and **azathioprine** ↑ bone marrow depressant properties—doses of these drugs should be ↓. Use with **ampicillin** or **amoxicillin** ↑ risk of rash. Use with **oral hypoglycemic agents** and **warfarin** ↑ effects of these drugs. Use with **thiazide diuretics** or **ACE inhibitors** ↑ risk of hypersensitivity reactions. Large doses of allopurinol may ↑ risk of **theophylline** toxicity. May ↑ **cyclosporine** levels.

Route/Dosage

Management of Gout

PO (Adults and Children >10 yr): *Initially*—100 mg/day; increase at weekly intervals based on serum uric acid (not to exceed 800 mg/day). Doses >300 mg/day should be given in divided doses. *Maintenance dose*—100–200 mg 2–3 times daily. Doses of ≤300 mg may be given as a single daily dose.

Management of Secondary Hyperuricemia

PO (Adults and Children >10 yr): 600–800 mg/day in 2–3 divided doses starting 1–2 days before chemotherapy or radiation.

PO (Children 6–10 yr): 10 mg/kg/day in 2–3 divided doses (maximum 800 mg/day) or 300 mg daily in 2–3 divided doses.

PO (Children <6 yr): 10 mg/kg/day in 2–3 divided doses (maximum 800 mg/day) or 150 mg daily in 3 divided doses.

IV (Adults and Children >10 yr): 200–400 mg/m^2/day (up to 600 mg/day) as a single daily dose or in divided doses q 8–24 hr.

IV (Children <10 yr): 200 mg/m^2/day initially as a single daily dose or in divided doses q 8–24 hr (maximum dose 600 mg/day).

Renal Impairment

(Adults and Children): *CCr >50 ml/min*—No dosage change; *CCr 10–50 ml/min*—Reduce dosage to 50% of recommended; *CCr <10 ml/min*—Reduce dosage to 30% of recommended.

Availability (generic available)

Tablets: 100 mg, 300 mg. **Cost:** *Generic*—100 mg $12.99/100, 300 mg $22.99/100. **Injection:** 500 mg/vial.

NURSING IMPLICATIONS

Assessment

- Monitor intake and output ratios. Decreased kidney function can cause drug accumulation and toxic effects. Ensure that patient maintains adequate fluid intake (minimum 2500–3000 ml/day) to minimize risk of kidney stone formation.

- Assess patient for rash or more severe hypersensitivity reactions. Discontinue allopurinol immediately if rash occurs. Therapy should be discontinued permanently if reaction is severe. Therapy may be reinstated after a mild reaction has subsided, at a lower dose (50 mg/day with very gradual titration). If skin rash recurs, discontinue permanently.
- **Gout:** Monitor for joint pain and swelling. Addition of colchicine or NSAIDs may be necessary for acute attacks. Prophylactic doses of colchicine or an NSAID should be administered concurrently during the first 3–6 mo of therapy because of an increased frequency of acute attacks of gouty arthritis during early therapy.
- ***Lab Test Considerations:*** Serum and urine uric acid levels usually begin to ↓ 2–3 days after initiation of oral therapy.
- Monitor blood glucose in patients receiving oral hypoglycemic agents. May cause hypoglycemia.
- Monitor hematologic, renal, and liver function tests before and periodically during therapy, especially during the first few months. May cause ↑ serum alkaline phosphatase, bilirubin, AST, and ALT levels. ↓ CBC and platelets may indicate bone marrow depression. ↑ BUN, serum creatinine, and CCr may indicate nephrotoxicity. These are usually reversed with discontinuation of therapy.

Potential Nursing Diagnoses

Acute pain (Indications)

Implementation

- **PO:** May be administered after milk or meals to minimize gastric irritation; give with plenty of fluid. May be crushed and given with fluid or mixed with food for patients who have difficulty swallowing.

IV Administration

- **Intermittent Infusion:** ***Diluent:*** Reconstitute each 500 mg vial with 25 ml of sterile water for injection. Solution should be clear and almost colorless with only slight opalescence. Dilute to desired concentration with 0.9% NaCl or D5W. Administer within 10 hr of reconstitution; do not refrigerate. Do not administer solutions that are discolored or contain particulate matter. ***Concentration:*** Not >6 mg/ml. ***Rate:*** Infusion should be initiated 24–48 hr before start of chemotherapy known to cause tumor cell lysis. Rate of infusion depends on volume of infusate (100–300 mg doses may be infused over 30 minutes). May be administered as a single infusion or equally divided infusions at 6-, 8-, or 12-hr intervals.
- **Y-Site Compatibility:** acyclovir, aminophylline, aztreonam, bleomycin, bumetanide, buprenorphine, butorphanol, calcium gluconate, carboplatin, cefazolin, cefotetan, ceftazidime, ceftizoxime, ceftriaxone, cefuroxime, cisplatin, cyclophosphamide, dactinomycin, dexamethasone sodium phosphate, doxorubicin liposome, enalaprilat, etoposide, famotidine, filgrastim, fluconazole, fludarabine, fluorouracil, furosemide, ganciclovir, granisetron, heparin, hydrocortisone, hydromorphone, ifosfamide, lorazepam, mannitol, mesna, methotrexate, metronidazole, mitoxandrone, morphine, piperacillin, potassium chloride, ranitidine, teniposide, thiotepa, ticarcillin/clavulanate, trimethoprim/sulfamethoxazole, vancomycin, vinblastine, vincristine, zidovudine.
- **Y-Site Incompatibility:** amikacin, amphotericin B, carmustine, cefotaxime, chlorpromazine, cimetidine, clindamycin, cytarabine, dacarbazine, daunorubicin, diphenhydramine, doxorubicin, doxycycline, droperidol, floxuridine, gentamicin, haloperidol, idarubicin, imipenem/cilastatin, mechlorethamine, meperidine, methylprednisolone sodium succinate, metoclopramide, minocycline, nalbuphine, ondansetron, prochlorperazine, promethazine, sodium bicarbonate, streptozocin, tobramycin, vinorelbine.

Patient/Family Teaching

- Instruct patient to take allopurinol as directed. Take missed doses as soon as remembered. If dosing schedule is once daily, do not take if remembered the next day. If dosing schedule is more than once a day, take up to 300 mg for the next dose.
- Instruct patient to continue taking allopurinol along with an NSAID or colchicine during an acute attack of gout. Allopurinol helps prevent, but does not relieve, acute gout attacks.

- Alkaline diet may be ordered. Urinary acidification with large doses of vitamin C or other acids may increase kidney stone formation (see Appendix L). Advise patient of need for increased fluid intake.
- May occasionally cause drowsiness. Caution patient to avoid driving or other activities requiring alertness until response to drug is known.
- Instruct patient to report skin rash, blood in urine, or influenza symptoms (chills, fever, muscle aches and pains, nausea, or vomiting) to health care professional immediately; skin rash may indicate hypersensitivity.
- Advise patient that large amounts of alcohol increase uric acid concentrations and may decrease the effectiveness of allopurinol.
- Emphasize the importance of follow-up exams to monitor effectiveness and side effects.

Evaluation/Desired Outcomes

- Decreased serum and urinary uric acid levels. May take 2–6 wk to observe clinical improvement in patients treated for gout.

almotriptan (al-moe-**trip**-tan)

Axert

Classification

Therapeutic: vascular headache suppressants

Pharmacologic: 5-HT_1 agonists

Pregnancy Category C

Indications

Acute treatment of migraine headache.

Action

Acts as an agonist at specific 5-HT_1 receptor sites in intracranial blood vessels and sensory trigeminal nerves. **Therapeutic Effects:** Cranial vessel vasoconstriction with associated decrease in release of neuropetides and resultant decrease in migraine headache.

Pharmacokinetics

Absorption: Well absorbed following oral administration (70%).

Distribution: Unknown.

Metabolism and Excretion: 40% excreted unchanged in urine; 27% metabolized by monoamine oxidase-A (MAO-A); 12% metabolized by cytochrome P450 hepatic enzymes (3A4 and 2D6); 13% excreted in feces as unchanged and metabolized drug.

Half-life: 3–4 hr.

TIME/ACTION PROFILE (Blood levels)

ROUTE	ONSET	PEAK	DURATION
PO	unknown	1–3 hr	unknown

Contraindications/Precautions

Contraindicated in: Hypersensitivity; Ischemic cardiovascular, cerebrovascular, or peripheral vascular syndromes; History of significant cardiovascular disease; Uncontrolled hypertension; Should not be used within 24 hr of other 5-HT_1 agonists or ergot-type compounds (dihydroergotamine); Basilar or hemiplegic migraine; Concurrent MAO-A inhibitor therapy or within 2 wk of discontinuing MAO-A inhibitor therapy.

Use Cautiously in: Cardiovascular risk factors (hypertension, hypercholesterolemia, cigarette smoking, obesity, diabetes, strong family history, menopausal women or men >40 yr); use only if cardiovascular status has been evaluated and determined to be safe and first dose is administered under supervision; Impaired hepatic or renal function; OB, Lactation, Pedi: Safety not established.

Adverse Reactions/Side Effects

CNS: drowsiness, headache. **CV:** CORONARY ARTERY VASOSPASM, MI, myocardial ischemia, VENTRICULAR FIBRILLATION, VENTRICULAR TACHYCARDIA. **GI:** dry mouth, nausea. **Neuro:** paresthesia.

Interactions

Drug-Drug: Concurrent use with **MAO-A inhibitors** increases blood levels and the risk of adverse reactions (concurrent use or use within 2 wk or MAO inhibitor is contraindicated). Concurrent use with other **5-HT_1 agonists** or **ergot-type compounds (dihydroergotamine)** may result in additive vasoactive properties (avoid use within 24 hr of each other). Concurrent use with **SSRI antidepressants** may result in weakness, hyperreflexia, and incoordination. Blood levels and effects may be increased by **ketoconazole**, **itraconazole**, **ritonavir**, and **erythromycin** (inhibitors of CYP3A4 enzymes).

Route/Dosage

PO (Adults): 6.25–12.5 mg initially, may repeat in 2 hr; not to exceed 2 doses per 24-hr period.

Hepatic/Renal Impairment
PO (Adults): 6.25 mg initially, may repeat in 2 hr; not to exceed 2 doses per 24-hr period.

Availability
Tablets: 6.25 mg, 12.5 mg.

NURSING IMPLICATIONS

Assessment
- Assess pain location, character, intensity, and duration and associated symptoms (photophobia, phonophobia, nausea, vomiting) during migraine attack.

Potential Nursing Diagnoses
Acute pain (Indications)

Implementation
- **PO:** Tablets should be swallowed whole with liquid.

Patient/Family Teaching
- Inform patient that almotriptan should only be used during a migraine attack. It is meant to be used for relief of migraine attacks but not to prevent or reduce the number of attacks.
- Instruct patient to administer almotriptan as soon as symptoms of a migraine attack appear, but it may be administered any time during an attack. If migraine symptoms return, a second dose may be used. Allow at least 2 hr between doses, and do not use more than 2 doses in any 24-hr period.
- If first dose does not relieve headache, additional almotriptan doses are not likely to be effective; notify health care professional.
- Caution patient not to take almotriptan within 24 hr of another vascular headache suppressant.
- Advise patient that lying down in a darkened room following almotriptan administration may further help relieve headache.
- Caution patient not to use almotriptan if she is pregnant, suspects she is pregnant, plans to become pregnant, or is breastfeeding. Adequate contraception should be used during therapy.
- Advise patient to notify health care professional prior to next dose of almotriptan if pain or tightness in the chest occurs during use. If pain is severe or does not subside, notify health care professional immediately. If feelings of tingling, heat, flushing, heaviness, pressure, drowsiness, dizziness, tiredness, or sickness develop discuss with health care professional at next visit.
- May cause dizziness or drowsiness. Caution patient to avoid driving or other activities requiring alertness until response to medication is known.
- Advise patient to avoid alcohol, which aggravates headaches, during almotriptan use.
- Instruct patient to consult health care professional before taking other prescription or OTC or herbal/alternative preparations.

Evaluation/Desired Outcomes
- Relief of migraine attack.

alprazolam (al-**pray**-zoe-lam)
✤ Apo-Alpraz, ✤ Novo-Alprazol, Niravam, ✤ Nu-Alpraz, Xanax, Xanax XR

Classification
Therapeutic: antianxiety agents
Pharmacologic: benzodiazepines

Schedule IV

Pregnancy Category D

Indications
Treatment of Generalized Anxiety Disorder (GAD). Panic Disorder. Management of anxiety associated with depression. **Unlabeled uses:** Management of symptoms of premenstrual syndrome (PMS). Insomnia, irritable bowel syndrome (IBS) and other somatic symptoms associated with anxiety. Used as an adjunct with acute mania, acute psychosis.

Action
Acts at many levels in the CNS to produce anxiolytic effect. May produce CNS depression. Effects may be mediated by GABA, an inhibitory neurotransmitter. **Therapeutic Effects:** Relief of anxiety.

Pharmacokinetics
Absorption: Well absorbed (90%) from the GI tract; absorption is slower with extended-release tablets.
Distribution: Widely distributed, crosses blood-brain barrier. Probably crosses the placenta and enters breast milk. Accumulation is minimal.

Metabolism and Excretion: Metabolized by the liver (CYP3A4 enzyme system) to an active compound that is subsequently rapidly metabolized.
Half-life: 12–15 hr.

TIME/ACTION PROFILE (sedation)

ROUTE	ONSET	PEAK	DURATION
PO	1–2 hr	1–2 hr	up to 24 hr

Contraindications/Precautions

Contraindicated in: Hypersensitivity; Cross-sensitivity with other benzodiazepines may exist; Pre-existing CNS depression; Severe uncontrolled pain; Angle-closure glaucoma, obstructive sleep apnea, pulmonary disease; Pregnancy and lactation; Concurrent itraconazole or ketoconazole; OB, Lactation: Use in pregnancy or lactation may cause CNS depression, flaccidity, feeding difficulties, and seizures in infant.
Use Cautiously in: Renal Impairment, Hepatic dysfunction (↓ dose required); Concurrent use with nefazodone, fluvoxamine, cimetidine, fluoxetine, hormonal contraceptives, propoxyphene, diltiazem, isoniazid, erythromycin, clarithromycin, grapefruit juice (↓ dose may be necessary); History of suicide attempt or alcohol/drug dependence, debilitated patients (↓ dose required); Pedi: Safety and efficacy not established. Decreased dosage and frequent monitoring required; Geri: Elderly patients have increased sensitivity to benzodiazepines. Appears on Beers list and is associated with increased risk of falls (↓ dose required) and excessive CNS effects.

Adverse Reactions/Side Effects

CNS: <u>dizziness</u>, <u>drowsiness</u>, <u>lethargy</u>, confusion, hangover, headache, mental depression, paradoxical excitation. **EENT:** blurred vision. **GI:** constipation, diarrhea, nausea, vomiting, weight gain. **Derm:** rashes. **Misc:** physical dependence, psychological dependence, tolerance.

Interactions

Drug-Drug: Alcohol, antidepressants, other **benzodiazepines, antihistamines**, and **opioid analgesics**—concurrent use results in ↑ CNS depression. **Hormonal contraceptives, disulfiram, fluoxetine, isoniazid, metoprolol, propoxyphene, propranolol, valproic acid, CYP3A4 inhibitors (erythromycin, ketoconazole, itraconazole, fluvoxamine, cimetidine, nefazodone)** ↓ metabolism of alprazolam, ↑ blood levels and ↑ its actions (dose adjustments may be necessary). May ↓ efficacy of **levodopa. CYP3A4 inducers (rifampin, carbamazepine**, or **barbiturates)** ↑ metabolism and ↓ effects of alprazolam. Sedative effects may be ↓ by **theophylline. Cigarette smoking** ↓ blood levels and effects.
Drug-Natural Products: Kava kava, valerian, or chamomile can ↑ CNS depression.
Drug-Food: Concurrent ingestion of **grapefruit juice** ↑ blood levels.

Route/Dosage

Anxiety

PO (Adults): 0.25–0.5 mg 2–3 times daily (not >4 mg/day; begin with 0.25 mg 2–3 times daily in geriatric/debilitated patients).

Panic Attacks

PO (Adults): 0.5 mg 3 times daily; may be increased by 1 mg or less every 3–4 days as needed (not >10 mg/day). *Extended-release tablets (Xanax XR)*—0.5–1 mg once daily in the morning, may be increased every 3–4 days by not more than 1 mg/day; up to 10 mg/day (usual range 3–6 mg/day).

Availability (generic available)

Tablets: 0.25 mg, 0.5 mg, 1 mg, 2 mg. **Cost:** 0.25 mg $98.21/100, 0.5 mg $122.35/100, 1 mg $163.25/100, 2 mg $277.56/100. **Extended-release tablets:** 0.5 mg, 1 mg, 2 mg, 3 mg. **Orally disintegrating tablets (orange):** 0.25 mg, 0.5 mg, 1 mg, 2 mg.

NURSING IMPLICATIONS

Assessment

- Assess degree and manifestations of anxiety and mental status (orientation, mood, behavior) prior to and periodically during therapy.
- Assess patient for drowsiness, light-headedness, and dizziness. These symptoms usually disappear as therapy progresses. Dose should be reduced if these symptoms persist.
- Geri: Assess CNS effects and risk of falls. Institute falls prevention strategies.
- Prolonged high-dose therapy may lead to psychological or physical dependence. Risk is greater in patients taking >4 mg/day. Restrict the amount of drug available to patient. Assess regularly for continued need for treatment.
- ***Lab Test Considerations:*** Monitor CBC and liver and renal function periodically dur-

ing long-term therapy. May cause ↓ hematocrit and neutropenia.

- ***Toxicity and Overdose:*** Flumazenil is the antidote for alprazolam toxicity or overdose. (Flumazenil may induce seizures in patients with a history of seizures disorder or who are on tricyclic antidepressants.)

Potential Nursing Diagnoses

Anxiety (Indications)
Risk for injury (Side Effects)
Risk for falls (Side Effects)

Implementation

- Do not confuse Xanax (alprazolam) with Zantac (ranitidine).
- If early morning anxiety or anxiety between doses occurs, the same total daily dose should be divided into more frequent intervals.
- **PO:** May be administered with food if GI upset occurs. Administer greatest dose at bedtime to avoid daytime sedation.
- Tablets may be crushed and taken with food or fluids if patient has difficulty swallowing. Do not crush, break, or chew extended-release tablets.
- Taper by 0.5 mg q 3 days to prevent withdrawal. Some patients may require longer tapering period (months).
- For *orally disintegrating tablets:* Remove tablet from bottle with dry hands just prior to taking medication. Place tablet on tongue. Tablet will dissolve with saliva; may also be taken with water. Remove cotton from bottle and reseal tightly to prevent moisture from entering bottle. If only ½ tablet taken, discard unused portion immediately; may not remain stable.

Patient/Family Teaching

- Instruct patient to take medication exactly as directed; do not skip or double up on missed doses. If a dose is missed, take within 1 hr; otherwise, skip the dose and return to regular schedule. If medication is less effective after a few weeks, check with health care professional; do not increase dose. Abrupt withdrawal may cause sweating, vomiting, muscle cramps, tremors, and seizures.
- May cause drowsiness or dizziness. Caution patient to avoid driving and other activities requiring alertness until response to the medication is known. Geri: Instruct patient and family how to reduce falls risk at home.
- Advise patient to avoid drinking grapefruit juice during therapy.
- Advise patient to avoid the use of alcohol or other CNS depressants concurrently with alprazolam. Instruct patient to consult health care professional before taking Rx, OTC, or herbal products concurrently with this medication.
- Inform patient that benzodiazepines are usually prescribed for short-term use and do not cure underlying problems.
- Teach other methods to decrease anxiety (exercise, support group, relaxation techniques).
- Advise patient to not share medication with anyone.

Evaluation/Desired Outcomes

- Decreased sense of anxiety without CNS side effects.
- Decreased frequency and severity of panic attacks.
- Decreased symptoms of premenstrual syndrome.

alteplase, **See THROMBOLYTIC AGENTS.**

aluminum hydroxide

AlternaGEL, Alu-Cap, ✤Alugel, Aluminet, Alu-Tab, Amphojel, Basalgel, Dialume

Classification
Therapeutic: antiulcer agents, hypophosphatemics
Pharmacologic: antacids, phosphate binders

Pregnancy Category UK

Indications

Lowering of phosphate levels in patients with chronic renal failure. Adjunctive therapy in the treatment of peptic, duodenal, and gastric ulcers. Hyperacidity, indigestion, reflux esophagitis.

Action

Binds phosphate in the GI tract. Neutralizes gastric acid and inactivates pepsin. **Therapeutic**

✤ = Canadian drug name.
* CAPITALS indicates life-threatening; underlines indicate most frequent.

Effects: Lowering of serum phosphate levels. Healing of ulcers and decreased pain associated with ulcers or gastric hyperacidity. Constipation limits use alone in the treatment of ulcer disease. Frequently found in combination with magnesium-containing compounds.

Pharmacokinetics

Absorption: With chronic use, small amounts of aluminum are systemically absorbed.
Distribution: If absorbed, aluminum distributes widely, crosses the placenta, and enters breast milk. Concentrates in the CNS with chronic use.
Metabolism and Excretion: Mostly excreted in feces. Small amounts absorbed are excreted by the kidneys.
Half-life: Unknown.

TIME/ACTION PROFILE

ROUTE	ONSET	PEAK	DURATION
PO†	hr–days	days–wk	days
PO‡	15–30 min	30 min	30 min–3 hr

†Hypophosphatemic effect
‡Antacid effect

Contraindications/Precautions

Contraindicated in: Severe abdominal pain of unknown cause.
Use Cautiously in: Hypercalcemia; Hypophosphatemia; OB: Generally considered safe; chronic high-dose therapy should be avoided.

Adverse Reactions/Side Effects

GI: constipation. **F and E:** hypophosphatemia.

Interactions

Drug-Drug: Absorption of **tetracyclines**, **chlorpromazine**, **iron salts**, **isoniazid**, **digoxin**, or **fluoroquinolones** may be decreased. **Salicylate** blood levels may be decreased. **Quinidine**, **mexiletine**, and **amphetamine** levels may be increased if enough antacid is ingested such that urine pH is increased.

Route/Dosage

Hypophosphatemia

PO (Adults): 1.9–4.8 g (30–40 ml of regular suspension or 15–20 ml of concentrated suspension) 3–4 times daily.
PO (Children): 50–150 mg/kg/24 hr in 4–6 divided doses; titrate to normal serum phosphate levels.

Antacid

PO (Adults): 500–1500 mg (5–30 ml) 3–6 times daily.

Availability (generic available)

Capsules: 475 mg[OTC], 500 mg[OTC]. **Tablets:** 300 mg[OTC], 500 mg[OTC], 600 mg[OTC]. **Suspension:** 320 mg/5 ml[OTC], 450 mg/5 ml[OTC], 600 mg/5 ml[OTC], 675 mg/5 ml[OTC]. ***In combination with:*** magnesium carbonate, calcium carbonate, simethicone, and mineral oil. See Appendix B.

NURSING IMPLICATIONS

Assessment

- Assess location, duration, character, and precipitating factors of gastric pain.
- ***Lab Test Considerations:*** Monitor serum phosphate and calcium levels periodically during chronic use of aluminum hydroxide.
- May cause increased serum gastrin and decreased serum phosphate concentrations.
- In treatment of severe ulcer disease, guaiac stools, and emesis, monitor pH of gastric secretions.

Potential Nursing Diagnoses

Acute pain (Indications)
Constipation (Side Effects)

Implementation

- Antacids cause premature dissolution and absorption of enteric-coated tablets and may interfere with absorption of other oral medications. Separate administration of aluminum hydroxide and oral medications by at least 1–2 hr.
- Tablets must be chewed thoroughly before swallowing to prevent their entering small intestine in undissolved form. Follow with a glass of water.
- Shake liquid preparations well before pouring. Follow administration with water to ensure passage into stomach.
- Liquid dosage forms are considered more effective than tablets.
- **Hypophosphatemic:** For phosphate lowering, follow dose with full glass of water or fruit juice.
- **Antacid:** May be given in conjunction with magnesium-containing antacids to minimize constipation, except in patients with renal failure. Administer 1 and 3 hr after meals and at bedtime for maximum antacid effect.
- For treatment of peptic ulcer, aluminum hydroxide may be administered every 1–2 hr while the patient is awake or diluted with 2–3

parts water and administered intragastrically every 30 min for 12 or more hr per day. Physician may order NG tube clamped after administration.

- For reflux esophagitis, administer 15 ml 20–40 min after meals and at bedtime.

Patient/Family Teaching

- Instruct patient to take aluminum hydroxide exactly as directed. If on a regular dosing schedule and a dose is missed, take as soon as remembered if not almost time for next dose; do not double doses.
- Advise patient not to take aluminum hydroxide within 1–2 hr of other medications without consulting health care professional.
- Advise patients to check label for sodium content. Patients with CHF or hypertension, or those on sodium restriction, should use low-sodium preparations.
- Inform patients of potential for constipation from aluminum hydroxide.
- **Hypophosphatemia:** Patients taking aluminum hydroxide for hyperphosphatemia should be taught the importance of a low-phosphate diet.
- **Antacid:** Caution patient to consult health care professional before taking antacids for more than 2 wk if problem is recurring, if taking other medications, if relief is not obtained, or if symptoms of gastric bleeding (black tarry stools, coffee-ground emesis) occur.

Evaluation/Desired Outcomes

- Decrease in serum phosphate levels.
- Decrease in GI pain and irritation.
- Increase in the pH of gastric secretions. In treatment of peptic ulcer, antacid therapy should be continued for at least 4–6 wk after symptoms have disappeared because there is no correlation between disappearance of symptoms and healing of ulcers.

amantadine (a-**man**-ta-deen)

Symmetrel

Classification

Therapeutic: antiparkinson agents, antivirals

Pregnancy Category C

Indications

Symptomatic initial and adjunct treatment of Parkinson's disease. Prophylaxis and treatment of influenza A viral infections.

Action

Potentiates the action of dopamine in the CNS. Prevents penetration of influenza A virus into host cell. **Therapeutic Effects:** Relief of Parkinson's symptoms. Prevention and decreased symptoms of influenza A viral infection.

Pharmacokinetics

Absorption: Well absorbed from the GI tract.
Distribution: Distributed to various body tissues and fluids. Crosses blood-brain barrier and enters breast milk.
Metabolism and Excretion: Excreted unchanged in the urine.
Half-life: 10–28 hr.

TIME/ACTION PROFILE (antiparkinson effect)

ROUTE	ONSET	PEAK	DURATION
PO	within 48 hr	up to 2 wk	unknown

Contraindications/Precautions

Contraindicated in: Hypersensitivity.
Use Cautiously in: Seizure disorders; Liver disease; Psychiatric problems; Congestive heart failure; Renal impairment (dosage reduction/increased dosing interval required if CCr ≤50 ml/min); May increase susceptibility to rubella infections; OB, Lactation: Safety not established; Geri: Increased sensitivity to adverse effects.

Adverse Reactions/Side Effects

CNS: ataxia, dizziness, insomnia, anxiety, confusion, depression, drowsiness, psychosis, seizures. **GI:** nausea, vomiting, anorexia, constipation. **EENT:** blurred vision, dry mouth. **Resp:** dyspnea. **CV:** hypotension, CHF, edema. **GU:** urinary retention. **Derm:** mottling, livedo reticularis, rashes. **Hemat:** leukopenia, neutropenia.

Interactions

Drug-Drug: Concurrent use of **antihistamines**, **phenothiazines**, **quinidine**, **disopyramide**, and **tricyclic antidepressants** may increase anticholinergic effects (dry mouth, blurred vision, constipation). Increased risk of adverse CNS reactions with **alcohol**. Increased risk of CNS stimulation with other **CNS stimulants**.

Route/Dosage

Parkinson's Disease

PO (Adults): 100 mg 1–2 times daily (up to 400 mg/day).

Influenza A Viral Infection

PO (Adults and Children >12 yr): *Treatment*—200 mg/day as a single dose or 100 mg bid (not >100 mg/day in geriatric patients); *Prophylaxis*—100 mg/day in 1–2 divided doses.

PO (Children 10–12 yr): 100 mg q 12 hr *or* 5 mg/kg/day in 1–2 divided doses; not to exceed 200 mg/day.

PO (Children 1–9 yr): 5 mg/kg/day in 1–2 divided doses; not to exceed 150 mg/day.

Renal Impairment

PO (Adults): *CCr 30–50 ml/min*—200 mg on the first day, then 100 mg once daily; *CCr 15–29 ml/min*—200 mg on the first day, then 100 mg every other day; *<15 ml/min or hemodialysis patients*—200 mg once every 7 days.

Availability (generic available)

Liquid-filled capsules: 100 mg. **Tablets:** 100 mg. **Syrup (raspberry flavor):** 50 mg/5 ml.

NURSING IMPLICATIONS

Assessment

- Monitor blood pressure periodically. Assess patient for drug-induced orthostatic hypotension.
- Monitor vital signs and mental status periodically during first few days of dosage adjustment in patients receiving >200 mg daily; side effects are more likely.
- Assess for CHF (peripheral edema, weight gain, dyspnea, rales/crackles, jugular venous distention), especially in patients on chronic therapy or with a history of CHF.
- Assess patient for the appearance of a diffuse red mottling of the skin (livedo reticularis), especially in the lower extremities or on exposure to cold. Disappears with continued therapy but may not completely resolve until 2–12 wk after therapy has been discontinued.
- Geri: Monitor intake and output closely in geriatric patients. May cause urinary retention. Report significant discrepancy or bladder distention.
- **Parkinson's Disease:** Assess akinesia, rigidity, tremors, and gait disturbances before and throughout therapy.
- **Influenza Prophylaxis or Treatment:** Monitor respiratory status (rate, breath sounds, sputum) and temperature periodically. Supportive treatment is indicated if symptoms occur.
- ***Toxicity and Overdose:*** Symptoms of toxicity include CNS stimulation (confusion, mood changes, tremors, seizures, arrhythmias, and hypotension). There is no specific antidote, although physostigmine has been used to reverse CNS effects.

Potential Nursing Diagnoses

Impaired physical mobility
Risk for infection (Indications)

Implementation

- Do not confuse amantadine with rimantidine or ranitidine.
- **PO:** Do not administer last dose of medication near bedtime; may produce insomnia in some patients.
- Administering amantadine in divided doses may decrease CNS side effects.
- The contents of capsules may be mixed with food or fluids if the patient has difficulty swallowing.
- **Antiviral Prophylaxis:** Treatment should be started in anticipation of contact or as soon as possible after exposure and continue for at least 10 days following exposure. Infectious period is just before onset of symptoms to up to 1 wk after. If vaccine is unavailable or contraindicated, may be administered up to 90 days to protect from repeated exposures.
- May be used with inactivated influenza A virus vaccine until protective antibody response develops. Administer for 2–3 wk after vaccine has been given.
- **Antiviral Treatment:** Administer as soon as possible after onset of symptoms and continue for 24–48 hr after symptoms disappear.

Patient/Family Teaching

- Advise patient to take medication around the clock as directed and not to skip doses or double up on missed doses. If a dose is missed, do not take within 4 hr of the next dose.
- May cause dizziness or blurred vision. Advise patient to avoid driving or other activities that require alertness until response to the drug is known.

- Advise patient to make position changes slowly to minimize orthostatic hypotension.
- Inform patient that frequent mouth rinses, good oral hygiene, and sugarless gum or candy may decrease dry mouth. Consult health care professional if dry mouth persists for >2 wk.
- Advise patient to confer with health care professional before taking OTC medications, especially cold remedies, or drinking alcoholic beverages.
- Instruct patient to notify health care professional if confusion, mood changes, difficulty with urination, edema and shortness of breath, or worsening of Parkinson's disease symptoms occurs.
- **Antiviral:** Instruct patient and family to notify health care professional if influenza symptoms occur when amantadine is used as prophylaxis or if symptoms do not improve in a few days when product is used for treatment.
- **Parkinson's Disease:** Advise patient that up to 2 wk of therapy may be needed for full benefit of medication. Notify health care professional if medication gradually loses its effectiveness. Amantadine should be tapered gradually; abrupt withdrawal may precipitate a parkinsonian crisis.

Evaluation/Desired Outcomes

- Decrease in akinesia and rigidity. Full therapeutic effects may require 2 wk of therapy.
- Absence or reduction of influenza A symptoms.

---

amcinonide, See CORTICOSTEROIDS (TOPICAL/LOCAL).

---

amifostine (a-mi-**fos**-teen)

Ethyol

Classification

Therapeutic: cytoprotective agents

Pregnancy Category C

Indications

Reduces renal toxicity from cisplatin. Reduces the incidence of moderate to severe xerostomia from postoperative radiation for head and neck cancer in which the radiation port includes a large portion of the parotid glands.

Action

Converted by alkaline phosphatase in tissue to a free thiol compound that binds and detoxifies damaging metabolites of cisplatin and reactive oxygen species generated by radiation. **Therapeutic Effects:** Decreased renal damage from cisplatin. Decreased severity of xerostomia following radiation for head and neck cancer.

Pharmacokinetics

Absorption: IV administration results in complete bioavailability.
Distribution: Unknown.
Metabolism and Excretion: Rapidly cleared from plasma; converted to cytoprotective compounds by alkaline phosphatase in tissues.
Half-life: 8 min.

TIME/ACTION PROFILE

ROUTE	ONSET	PEAK	DURATION
IV	unknown	unknown	unknown

Contraindications/Precautions

Contraindicated in: Known sensitivity to aminothiol compounds; Hypotension or dehydration; Lactation: Use an alternative to breast milk; Concurrent antineoplastic therapy for other tumors (especially malignancies of germ cell origin).
Use Cautiously in: OB, Pedi: Safety not established; Geri: Geriatric patients or patients with cardiovascular disease have increased risk of adverse reactions.

Adverse Reactions/Side Effects

CNS: dizziness, somnolence. **EENT:** sneezing. **CV:** hypotension. **GI:** hiccups, nausea, vomiting. **Derm:** flushing. **F and E:** hypocalcemia. **Misc:** allergic reactions including ANAPHYLAXIS, STEVENS-JOHNSON SYNDROME, TOXIC EPIDERMAL NECROLYSIS, TOXODERMA, ERYTHEMA MULTIFORMA, EXFOLIATIVE DERMATITIS (↑ when used as a radioprotectant), chills.

Interactions

Drug-Drug: Concurrent use of **antihypertensives** ↑ risk of hypotension.

Route/Dosage

Reduction of Renal Damage with Cisplatin

IV (Adults): 910 mg/m² once daily, within 30 min before chemotherapy; if full dose is poorly tolerated, subsequent doses should be decreased to 740 mg/m².

Reduction of Xerostomia from Radiation

IV (Adults): 200 mg/m² once daily, as a 3-minute infusion starting 15–30 min before standard fraction radiation therapy.

Availability

Powder for injection: 500 mg/vial.

NURSING IMPLICATIONS

Assessment

- Monitor blood pressure before and every 5 min during infusion. Discontinue antihypertensives 24 hr prior to treatment. If significant hypotension requiring interruption of therapy occurs, place patient in Trendelenburg position and administer an infusion of 0.9% NaCl using a separate IV line. If blood pressure returns to normal in 5 min and patient is asymptomatic, infusion may be resumed so that full dose may be given.
- Assess fluid status before administration. Correct dehydration before instituting therapy. Nausea and vomiting are frequent and may be severe. Prophylactic antiemetics including dexamethasone 20 mg IV and a serotonin-antagonist antiemetic (ondansetron, dolasetron, granisetron, palonosetron) should be administered before and during infusion. Monitor fluid status closely.
- Observe patient for signs and symptoms of anaphylaxis (rash, pruritus, laryngeal edema, wheezing). Discontinue the drug and notify physician or other health care professional immediately if these problems occur. Keep epinephrine, an antihistamine, and resuscitation equipment close by in case of an anaphylactic reaction.
- **Xerostomia:** Assess patient for dry mouth and mouth sores periodically during therapy.
- ***Lab Test Considerations:*** Monitor serum calcium concentrations before and periodically during therapy. May cause hypocalcemia. Calcium supplements may be necessary.

Potential Nursing Diagnoses

Risk for injury (Indications)

Implementation

IV Administration

- **Intermittent Infusion:** ***Diluent:*** Reconstitute with 9.7 ml of sterile 0.9% NaCl. Dilute further with 0.9% NaCl. Do not administer solutions that are discolored or contain particulate matter. Solution is stable for 5 hr at room temperature or 24 hr if refrigerated. ***Concentration:*** Adults: dilute dose to a final volume of 50 ml; Children: 5–40 mg/ml. ***Rate:*** *For renal toxicity:* Administer over 15 min within 30 min before chemotherapy administration. Longer infusion times are not as well tolerated. *For xerostomia:* Administer over 3 min starting 15–30 min prior to radiation therapy.
- **Y-Site Compatibility:** amikacin, aminophylline, ampicillin, ampicillin/sulbactam, aztreonam, bleomycin, bumetanide, buprenorphine, butorphanol, calcium gluconate, carboplatin, carmustine, cefazolin, cefotaxime, cefotetan, cefoxitin, ceftazidime, ceftizoxime, ceftriaxone, cefuroxime, cimetidine, ciprofloxacin, clindamycin, cyclophosphamide, cytarabine, dacarbazine, dactinomycin, daunorubicin, diphenhydramine, dobutamine, docetaxel, dopamine, doxorubicin, doxycycline, droperidol, enalaprilat, etoposide, famotidine, floxuridine, fluconazole, fludarabine, fluorouracil, furosemide, gentamicin, gemcitabine, granisetron, haloperidol, heparin, hydrocortisone, hydromorphone, idarubicin, ifosfamide, imipenem/cilastatin, leucovorin, lorazepam, magnesium sulfate, mannitol, mechlorethamine, meperidine, mesna, methotrexate, methylprednisolone, metoclopramide, metronidazole, mitomycin, mitoxantrone, morphine, nalbuphine, ondansetron, pemetrexed, piperacillin, potassium chloride, promethazine, ranitidine, sodium bicarbonate, streptozocin, teniposide, thiotepa, ticarcillin/clavulanate, tobramycin, trimethoprim/sulfamethoxazole, trimetrexate, vancomycin, vinblastine, vincristine, zidovudine.
- **Y-Site Incompatibility:** acyclovir, amphotericin B, cefoperazone, chlorpromazine, cisplatin, ganciclovir, prochlorperazine.
- **Additive Incompatibility:** Do not mix with other solutions or medications.

Patient/Family Teaching

- Explain the purpose of amifostine infusion to patient.
- Inform patient that amifostine may cause hypotension, nausea, vomiting, flushing, chills, dizziness, somnolence, hiccups, and sneezing.

Evaluation/Desired Outcomes

- Prevention of renal toxicity associated with repeated administration of cisplatin in patients with ovarian cancer.

- Decreased severity of xerostomia from radiation treatment of head and neck cancer.

amikacin, See AMINOGLYCOSIDES.

amiloride, See DIURETICS (POTASSIUM-SPARING).

aminocaproic acid

(a-mee-noe-ka-**pro**-ik)
Amicar, epsilon aminocaproic acid

Classification
Therapeutic: hemostatic agents
Pharmacologic: fibrinolysis inhibitors

Pregnancy Category C

Indications

Management of acute, life-threatening hemorrhage due to systemic hyperfibrinolysis or urinary fibrinolysis. **Unlabeled uses:** Prevention of recurrent subarachnoid hemorrhage. Prevention of bleeding following oral surgery in hemophiliacs. Management of severe hemorrhage caused by thrombolytic agents.

Action

Inhibits activation of plasminogen. **Therapeutic Effects:** Inhibition of fibrinolysis. Stabilization of clot formation.

Pharmacokinetics

Absorption: Rapidly absorbed following oral administration.
Distribution: Widely distributed.
Metabolism and Excretion: Mostly eliminated unchanged by the kidneys.
Half-life: Unknown.

TIME/ACTION PROFILE (peak blood levels)

ROUTE	ONSET	PEAK	DURATION
PO	unknown	2 hr	N/A
IV	unknown	2 hr	N/A

Contraindications/Precautions

Contraindicated in: Active intravascular clotting.
Use Cautiously in: Upper urinary tract bleeding; Cardiac, renal, or liver disease (dosage reduction may be required); Disseminated intravascular coagulation (should be used concurrently with heparin); OB, Lactation: Safety not established; Pedi: Do not use products containing benzyl alcohol with neonates.

Adverse Reactions/Side Effects

CNS: dizziness, malaise. **EENT:** nasal stuffiness, tinnitus. **CV:** arrhythmias, hypotension (IV only). **GI:** anorexia, bloating, cramping, diarrhea, nausea. **GU:** diuresis, renal failure. **MS:** myopathy.

Interactions

Drug-Drug: Concurrent use with **estrogens, conjugated** may result in a hypercoagulable state. Concurrent use with **clotting factors** may ↑ risk of thromboses.

Route/Dosage

Acute Bleeding Syndromes due to Elevated Fibrinolytic Activity

PO (Adults): 5 g 1st hr, followed by 1–1.25 g q hr for 8 hr or until hemorrhage is controlled; or 6 g over 24 hr after prostate surgery (not >30 g/day).
IV (Adults): 4–5 g over 1st hr, followed by 1 g/hr for 8 hr or until hemorrhage is controlled; or 6 g over 24 hr after prostate surgery (not >30 g/day).
PO, IV (Children): 100 mg/kg or 3 g/m^2 over 1st hr, followed by continuous infusion of 33.3 mg/kg/hr; or 1 g/m^2/hr (total dosage not >18 g/m^2/24 hr).

Subarachnoid Hemorrhage

PO (Adults): *To follow IV*—3 g q 2 hr (36 g/day). If no surgery is performed, continue for 21 days after bleeding stops, then decrease to 2 g q 2 hr (24 g/day) for 3 days, then 1 g q 2 hr (12 g/day) for 3 days.
IV (Adults): 36 g/day for 10 days followed by PO.

Prevention of Bleeding Following Oral Surgery in Hemophiliacs

PO (Adults): 75 mg/kg (up to 6 g) immediately after procedure, then q 6 hr for 7–10 days; syrup may also be used as an oral rinse of 1.25 g (5 ml) 4 times a day for 7–10 days.
IV, PO (Children): *Also for epistaxis*—50–100 mg/kg/dose administered IV every 6 hr for 2–3 days starting 4 hr before the procedure. After completion of IV therapy, aminocaproic acid

should be given as 50–100 mg/kg/dose orally every 6 hr for 5–7 days.

Availability

Tablets: 500 mg. **Syrup (raspberry flavor):** 1.25 g/5 ml. **Injection:** 250 mg/ml.

NURSING IMPLICATIONS

Assessment

- Monitor blood pressure, pulse, and respiratory status as indicated by severity of bleeding.
- Monitor for overt bleeding every 15–30 min.
- Monitor neurologic status (pupils, level of consciousness, motor activity) in patients with subarachnoid hemorrhage.
- Monitor intake and output ratios frequently; notify physician if significant discrepancies occur.
- Assess for thromboembolic complications (especially in patients with history). Notify physician of positive Homans' sign, leg pain and edema, hemoptysis, dyspnea, or chest pain.
- ***Lab Test Considerations:*** Monitor platelet count and clotting factors prior to and periodically throughout therapy in patients with systemic fibrinolysis.
- ↑ CPK, AST, and serum aldolase may indicate myopathy.
- May ↑ serum potassium.

Potential Nursing Diagnoses

Ineffective tissue perfusion (Indications)
Risk for injury (Indications, Side Effects)

Implementation

- Do not confuse Amicar (aminocaproic acid) with Amikin (amikacin).
- **PO:** Syrup may be used as an oral rinse, swished for 30 sec 4 times/day for 7–10 days for the control of bleeding during dental and oral surgery in hemophilic patients. Small amounts may be swallowed, except during 1st and 2nd trimesters of pregnancy. Syrup may be applied with an applicator in children or unconscious patients.

IV Administration

- **IV:** Stabilize IV catheter to minimize thrombophlebitis. Monitor site closely.
- **Intermittent Infusion:** ***Diluent:*** Do not administer undiluted. Dilute initial 4–5 g dose in 250 ml of sterile water for injection, 0.9% NaCl, D5W, or LR. Do not dilute with sterile water in patients with subarachnoid hemorrhage. ***Concentration:*** 20 mg/ml. ***Rate:*** Single doses: Administer over 1 hr. Rapid infusion rate may cause hypotension, bradycardia, or other arrhythmias.
- **Continuous Infusion:** Administer IV solution using infusion pump to ensure accurate dose. Administer via slow IV infusion. ***Rate:*** Initial dose may be followed by a continuous infusion of 1–1.25 g/hr in adults or 33.3 mg/kg/hr in children.
- **Additive Incompatibility:** Do not admix with other medications.

Patient/Family Teaching

- Instruct patient to notify the nurse immediately if bleeding recurs or if thromboembolic symptoms develop.
- **IV:** Caution patient to make position changes slowly to avoid orthostatic hypotension.

Evaluation/Desired Outcomes

- Cessation of bleeding.
- Prevention of rebleeding in subarachnoid hemorrhage without occurrence of undesired clotting.

AMINOGLYCOSIDES

amikacin (am-i-**kay**-sin)
Amikin

gentamicin† (jen-ta-**mye**-sin)
✤Cidomycin, Garamycin, G-Mycin, Jenamicin

kanamycin (kan-a-**mye**-sin)
Kantrex

neomycin (neo-oh-**mye**-sin)
Neo-Fradin

streptomycin (strep-toe-**mye**-sin)

tobramycin† (toe-bra-**mye**-sin)
Nebcin, TOBI

Classification
Therapeutic: anti-infectives
Pharmacologic: aminoglycosides

Pregnancy Category C (gentamicin, topical use of others), D (amikacin, kanamycin, neomycin, streptomycin, tobramycin)

†See Appendix C for ophthalmic use

Indications

Amikacin, gentamicin, kanamycin, and tobramycin: Treatment of serious gram-negative bacillary infections and infections caused by staphylococci when penicillins or other less toxic drugs are contraindicated. **Streptomycin:** In combination with other agents in the management of active tuberculosis. **Neomycin:** Used orally to prepare the GI tract for surgery, to decrease the number of ammonia-producing bacteria in the gut as part of the management of hepatic encephalopathy, and to treat diarrhea caused by *Escherichia coli*. **Tobramycin by inhalation:** Management of *Pseudomonas aeruginosa* in cystic fibrosis patients. **Gentamicin, streptomycin:** In combination with other agents in the management of serious enterococcal infections. **Gentamicin IV:** Prevention of infective endocarditis. **Gentamicin (topical), tobramycin (ophthalmic):** Treatment of localized infections caused by susceptible organisms. **Unlabeled uses:** Amikacin: In combination with other agents in the management of *Mycobacterium avium* complex infections.

Action

Inhibits protein synthesis in bacteria at level of 30S ribosome. **Therapeutic Effects:** Bactericidal action. **Spectrum:** Most aminoglycosides notable for activity against *P. aeruginosa*, *Klebsiella pneumoniae*, *E. coli*, *Proteus*, *Serratia*, *Acinetobacter*, *Staphylococcus aureus*. In treatment of enterococcal infections, synergy with a penicillin is required. Streptomycin and amikacin also active against *Mycobacterium*.

Pharmacokinetics

Absorption: Well absorbed after IM administration. IV administration results in complete bioavailability. Some absorption follows administration by other routes. Minimal systemic absorption with neomycin (may accumulate in patients with renal failure).
Distribution: Widely distributed throughout extracellular fluid; cross the placenta; small amounts enter breast milk. Poor penetration into CSF (↑ when meninges are inflammed).
Metabolism and Excretion: Excretion is >90% renal.
Half-life: 2–4 hr (increased in renal impairment).

TIME/ACTION PROFILE (blood levels*)

ROUTE	ONSET	PEAK	DURATION
PO (neomycin)	rapid	1–4 hr	N/A
IM	rapid	30–90 min	6–24 hr
IV	rapid	15–30 min†	6–24 hr

*All parenterally administered aminoglycosides
†Postdistribution peak occurs 30 min after the end of a 30-min infusion and 15 min after the end of a 1-hr infusion

Contraindications/Precautions

Contraindicated in: Hypersensitivity to aminoglycosides; Most parenteral products contain bisulfites and should be avoided in patients with known intolerance; Products containing benzyl alcohol should be avoided in neonates; Intestinal obstruction (neomycin only).
Use Cautiously in: Renal impairment (dose adjustments necessary; blood level monitoring useful in preventing ototoxicity and nephrotoxicity); Hearing impairment; Neuromuscular diseases such as myasthenia gravis; Obese patients (dose should be based on ideal body weight); OB: Tobramycin and streptomycin may cause congenital deafness; Lactation: Safety not established; Pedi: Neonates have increased risk of neuromuscular blockade; cautious use due to difficulty in assessing auditory and vestibular function and immature renal function; Geri: Cautious use in geriatric patients due to difficulty in assessing auditory and vestibular function and age-related renal impairment.

Adverse Reactions/Side Effects

CNS: ataxia, vertigo. **EENT:** ototoxicity (vestibular and cochlear). **GU:** nephrotoxicity. **GI:** *Neomycin*— diarrhea, nausea, vomiting. **F and E:** hypomagnesemia. **MS:** muscle paralysis (high parenteral doses). **Neuro:** ↑ neuromuscular blockade. **Resp:** apnea. **Misc:** hypersensitivity reactions.

Interactions

Drug-Drug: Inactivated by **penicillins** and **cephalosporins** when coadministered to patients with renal insufficiency. Possible respiratory paralysis after **inhalation anesthetics** or **neuromuscular blocking agents**. ↑ incidence of ototoxicity with **loop diuretics**. ↑ incidence of nephrotoxicity with other **nephrotoxic drugs**. Neomycin may ↑ anticoagulant effects of **warfarin**. Neomycin may ↓ absorption of **digoxin** and **methotrexate**.

Route/Dosage

Amikacin

IM, IV (Adults and Children): 5 mg/kg q 8 hr or 7.5 mg/kg q 12 hr (not to exceed 1.5 g/day).

M. avium complex—7.5–15 mg/kg/day divided q 12–24 hr.
IM, IV (Neonates): *Loading dose* –10 mg/kg; *Maintenance dose*—7.5 mg/kg q 12 hr.

Renal Impairment

IM, IV (Adults): *Loading dose* –7.5 mg/kg, further dosing based on blood level monitoring and renal function assessment.

Gentamicin

Many regimens are used; most involve dosing adjusted on the basis of blood level monitoring and assessment of renal function.
IM, IV (Adults): 1–2 mg/kg q 8 hr (up to 6 mg/kg/day in 3 divided doses); *Once-daily dosing (unlabeled)*—4–7 mg/kg q 24 hr.
IM, IV (Children >5 yr): 2–2.5 mg/kg/dose q 8 hr. *Once daily*—5–7.5 mg/kg/dose q 24 hr. *Cystic fibrosis*—2.5–3.3 mg/kg/dose q 6–8 hr. *Hemodialysis*—1.25–1.75 mg/kg/dose postdialysis.
IM, IV (Children 1 mo-5 yr): 2.5 mg/kg/dose q 8 hr. *Once daily*—5–7.5 mg/kg/dose q 24 hr. *Cystic fibrosis*—2.5–3.3 mg/kg/dose q 6–8 hr. *Hemodialysis*—1.25–1.75 mg/kg/dose postdialysis.
IM, IV (Neonates full term and/or >1 wk): *Weight <1200 g*—2.5 mg/kg/dose q 18–24 hr. *Weight 1200–2000 g*—2.5 mg/kg/dose q 8–12 hr. *Weight >2000 g*—2.5 mg/kg/dose q 8 hr. *ECMO*—2.5 mg/kg/dose q 18 hr, subsequent doses based on serum concentrations. *Once daily*—3.5–5 mg/kg/dose q 24 hr.
IM, IV (Neonates premature and/or ≤1 wk): *Weight <1000 g*—3.5 mg/kg/dose q 24 hr. *Weight 1000–1200 g*—2.5 mg/kg/dose q 18–24 hr. *Weight >1200 g*—2.5 mg/kg/dose q 12 hr. *Once daily*—3.5–4 mg/kg/dose q 24 hr.
IT (Adults): 4–8 mg/day.
IT (Infants >3 months and Children): 1–2 mg/day.
IT (Neonates): 1 mg/day.
Topical (Adults and Children >1 month): Apply cream or ointment 3–4 times daily.

Renal Impairment

IM, IV (Adults): Initial dose of 2 mg/kg. Subsequent doses/intervals based on blood level monitoring and renal function assessment.

Kanamycin

IM, IV (Adults and Children and Infants): 5 mg/kg q 8 hr *or* 7.5 mg/kg q 12 hr (not to exceed 15 mg/kg/day).
Inhaln (Adults): 250 mg 2–4 times daily.

Renal Impairment

IM, IV (Adults): 7.5 mg/kg; further dosing and intervals determined by blood level monitoring and assessment of renal function.

Neomycin

PO (Adults): *Preoperative intestinal antisepsis*—1 g q hr for 4 doses, then 1 g q 4 hr for 5 doses *or* 1 g at 1 PM, 2 PM, and 11 PM on day before surgery; *Hepatic encephalopathy*—1–3 g q 6 hr for 5–6 days; may be followed by 4 g/day chronically.
PO (Children): *Preoperative intestinal antisepsis*—15 mg/kg q 4 hr for 2 days *or* 25 mg/kg at 1 PM, 2 PM, and 11 PM on day before surgery; *Hepatic encephalopathy*—12.5–25 mg/kg q 6 hr for 5–6 days (maximum dose = 12 g/day).

Streptomycin

IM (Adults): *Tuberculosis*—1 g/day initially, decreased to 1 g 2–3 times weekly; *Other infections*—250 mg–1 g q 6 hr *or* 500 mg–2 g q 12 hr.
IM (Children): *Tuberculosis*—20 mg/kg/day (not to exceed 1 g/day); *Other infections*—5–10 mg/kg q 6 hr *or* 10–20 mg/kg q 12 hr.

Renal Impairment

IM (Adults): 1 g initially, further dosing determined by blood level monitoring and assessment of renal function.

Tobramycin

IM, IV (Adults): 1–2 mg/kg q 8 hr *or* 4–6.6 mg/kg/day q 24 hr.
IM, IV (Adults): 3–6 mg/kg/day in 3 divided doses, or 4–6.6 mg/kg once daily.
IM, IV (Children >5 yr): 6–7.5 mg/kg/day divided q 8 hr, up to 13 mg/kg/day divided q 6–8 hr in cystic fibrosis patients (dosing interval may vary from q 6 hr–q 24 hr, depending on clinical situation).
IM, IV (Children 1 month-5 yr): 7.5 mg/kg/day divided q 8 hr, up to 13 mg/kg/day divided q 6–8 hr in cystic fibrosis.
IM, IV (Neonates): *Preterm <1000 g*—3.5 mg/kg/dose q 24 hr. *0–4 weeks, <1200 g*—2.5 mg/kg/dose q 18 hr. *Postnatal age <7 days*—2.5 mg/kg/dose q 12 hr. *Postnatal age >7 days, 1200–2000 g*—2.5 mg/kg/dose q 8–12 hr. *Postnatal age >7 days, >2000 g*—2.5 mg/kg/dose q 8 hr.
Inhaln (Adults and Children): Standard dose: 40–80 mg 2–3 times/day; High dose: 300 mg twice daily for 28 days, then off for 28 days, then repeat cycle.

Ophth (Adults and Children >2 months): Apply 0.5" ribbon into the affected eye 2–3 times/day; for severe infections, apply q 3–4 hr.

Renal Impairment

IM, IV (Adults): 1 mg/kg initially, further dosing determined by blood level monitoring and assessment of renal function.

Availability

Amikacin

Injection: 50 mg/ml, 62.5 mg/ml, 250 mg/ml.

Gentamicin

Injection: 10 mg/ml, 40 mg/ml. **Premixed injection:** 40 mg/50 ml, 60 mg/50 ml, 60 mg/100 ml, 70 mg/50 ml, 80 mg/50 ml, 80 mg/100 ml, 90 mg/100 ml, 100 mg/50 ml, 100 mg/100 ml, 120 mg/100 ml. **Topical cream:** 0.1%. **Topical ointment:** 0.1%.

Kanamycin

Injection: 37.5 mg/ml, 250 mg/ml, 333.3 mg/ml.

Neomycin

Oral solution: 125 mg/5 ml. **Tablets:** 500 mg. ***In combination with:*** other topical antibiotics or anti-inflammatory agents for skin, ear, and eye infections. See Appendix B.

Streptomycin

Injection: ✱500 mg/ml, 1 g.

Tobramycin

Injection: 10 mg/ml, 40 mg/ml, 1.2-g vial. **Nebulizer solution:** 300 mg/5 ml in 5-ml ampules. **Ophthalmic solution:** 3 mg/ml in 5-ml container. **Ophthalmic ointment:** 3 mg/g in 3.5-g tube.

NURSING IMPLICATIONS

Assessment

- Assess patient for infection (vital signs, wound appearance, sputum, urine, stool, WBC) at beginning of and throughout therapy.
- Obtain specimens for culture and sensitivity before initiating therapy. First dose may be given before receiving results.
- Evaluate eighth cranial nerve function by audiometry before and throughout therapy. Hearing loss is usually in the high-frequency range. Prompt recognition and intervention are essential in preventing permanent damage. Also monitor for vestibular dysfunction (vertigo, ataxia, nausea, vomiting). Eighth cranial nerve dysfunction is associated with persistently elevated peak aminoglycoside levels. Discontinue aminoglycosides if tinnitus or subjective hearing loss occurs.
- Monitor intake and output and daily weight to assess hydration status and renal function.
- Assess patient for signs of superinfection (fever, upper respiratory infection, vaginal itching or discharge, increasing malaise, diarrhea). Report to physician or other health care professional.
- **Hepatic Encephalopathy:** Monitor neurologic status. Before administering oral medication, assess patient's ability to swallow.
- ***Lab Test Considerations:*** Monitor renal function by urinalysis, specific gravity, BUN, creatinine, and CCr before and during therapy.
- May cause ↑ BUN, AST, ALT, serum alkaline phosphatase, bilirubin, creatinine, and LDH concentrations.
- May cause ↓ serum calcium, magnesium, potassium, and sodium concentrations (streptomycin and tobramycin).
- ***Toxicity and Overdose:*** Monitor blood levels periodically during therapy. Timing of blood levels is important in interpreting results. Draw blood for peak levels 1 hr after IM injection and 30 min after a 30-min IV infusion is completed. Draw trough levels just before next dose. Peak level for **amikacin** and **kanamycin** is 20–30 mcg/ml; trough level should be <10 mcg/ml. Peak level for **gentamicin** and **tobramycin** should not exceed 10 mcg/ml; trough level should not exceed 2 mcg/ml. Peak level for **streptomycin** should not exceed 25 mcg/ml.

Potential Nursing Diagnoses

Risk for infection (Indications)

Disturbed sensory perception (auditory) (Side Effects)

Implementation

- Do not confuse Amikin (amikacin) with Amicar (aminocaproic acid).
- Keep patient well hydrated (1500–2000 ml/day) during therapy.
- **Preoperative Bowel Prep:** Neomycin is usually used in conjunction with erythromycin, a low-residue diet, and a cathartic or enema.

- **PO:** Neomycin may be administered without regard to meals.
- **IM:** IM administration should be deep into a well-developed muscle. Alternate injection sites.

Amikacin

IV Administration

- **Intermittent Infusion:** ***Diluent:*** Dilute with D5W, D10W, 0.9% NaCl, dextrose/saline combinations, or LR. Solution may be pale yellow without decreased potency. Stable for 24 hr at room temperature. ***Concentration:*** 10 mg/ml. ***Rate:*** Infuse over 30–60 min for adults and children and over 1–2 hr in infants.
- **Syringe Incompatibility:** heparin, pantoprazole.
- **Y-Site Compatibility:** acyclovir, aldesleukin, amifostine, amiodarone, amsacrine, anidulafungin, aztreonam, bivalirudin, cefepime, ceftazidime, cisatracurium, cyclophosphamide, dexamethasone sodium phosphate, dexmedetomidate, diltiazem, docetaxel, enalaprilat, esmolol, etoposide, fenoldopam, filgrastim, fluconazole, fludarabine, foscarnet, furosemide, gemcitabine, granisetron, hydromorphone, idarubicin, labetalol, lansoprazole, levofloxacin, linezolid, lorazepam, magnesium sulfate, melphalan, meperidine, midazolam, milrinone, morphine, nicardipine, ondansetron, paclitaxel, pemetrexed, perphenazine, remifentanil, sargramostim, teniposide, thiotepa, vinorelbine, warfarin, zidovudine.
- **Y-Site Incompatibility:** allopurinol sodium, amphotericin B cholesteryl sulfate, azithromycin, hetastarch, propofol. If aminoglycosides and penicillins or cephalosporins must be administered concurrently, administer in separate sites, at least 1 hr apart.
- **Additive Incompatibility:** Manufacturer does not recommend admixing.

Gentamicin

IV Administration

- **Intermittent Infusion:** ***Diluent:*** Dilute each dose with D5W, 0.9% NaCl, or LR. Also available in commercially mixed piggyback injections. Do not use solutions that are discolored or that contain a precipitate. ***Concentration:*** 10 mg/ml. ***Rate:*** Infuse slowly over 30 min–2 hr.
- **Syringe Incompatibility:** ampicillin, heparin, pantoprazole.
- **Y-Site Compatibility:** acyclovir, aldesleukin, amifostine, amiodarone, amsacrine, atracurium, aztreonam, bivalirudin, cefepime, ceftazidime, ciprofloxacin, cisatracurium, cyclophosphamide, cytarabine, daptomycin, dexmedetomidate, diltiazem, docetaxel, doxapram, doxorubicin liposome, enalaprilat, esmolol, etoposide, famotidine, fenoldopam, fluconazole, fludarabine, foscarnet, gemcitabine, granisetron, hydromorphone, insulin, labetalol, lansoprazle, levofloxacin, linezolid, lorazepam, magnesium sulfate, melphalan, meperidine, meropenem, midazolam, milrinone, morphine, multivitamins, nicardipine, ondansetron, paclitaxel, pancuronium, perphenazine, remifentanil, sargramostim, tacrolimus, teniposide, theophylline, thiotepa, tolazoline, vecuronium, vinorelbine, vitamin B complex with C, zidovudine.
- **Y-Site Incompatibility:** allopurinol, amphotericin B cholesteryl sulfate, azithromycin, drotrecogin, furosemide, heparin, idarubicin, indomethacin, pemetrexed, propofol, warfarin.
- **Additive Compatibility:** atracurium, aztreonam, bleomycin, cimetidine, ciprofloxacin, metronidazole, ofloxacin, ranitidine.
- **Additive Incompatibility:** amphotericin B, heparin.

Kanamycin

IV Administration

- **Intermittent Infusion:** ***Diluent:*** Dilute each 500 mg in 100–200 ml or each 1 g in 200–400 ml of D5W, D10W, D5/0.9% NaCl, 0.9% NaCl, or LR. Dilute in a proportionately smaller volume for pediatric patients. Darkening of solution does not alter potency. ***Concentration:*** 2.5–5 mg/ml. ***Rate:*** Infuse slowly over 30–60 min.
- **Syringe Incompatibility:** heparin.
- **Y-Site Compatibility:** cyclophosphamide, furosemide, hydromorphone, magnesium sulfate, meperidine, morphine, perphenazine, potassium chloride, vitamin B complex with C.
- **Additive Incompatibility:** Manufacturer does not recommend admixing with other antibacterial agents.

Tobramycin

IV Administration

- **Intermittent Infusion:** ***Diluent:*** Dilute each dose in 50–100 ml of D5W, D10W, D5/

0.9% NaCl, 0.9% NaCl, Ringer's, or LR. Stable for 24 hr at room temperature, 96 hr if refrigerated. Also available in commercially mixed piggyback injections. ***Concentration:*** 10 mg/ml. ***Rate:*** Infuse slowly over 30–60 min in both adult and pediatric patients.

- **Syringe Incompatibility:** clindamycin, heparin, pantoprazole.
- **Y-Site Compatibility:** acyclovir, aldesleukin, amifostine, amiodarone, amsacrine, aztreonam, bivalirudin, cefepime, ceftazidime, ciprofloxacin, cisatracurium, cyclophosphamide, dexmedetomidine, diltiazem, docetaxel, doxorubicin liposome, enalaprilat, esmolol, etoposide, fenoldopam, filgrastim, fluconazole, fludarabine, foscarnet, furosemide, gemcitabine, granisetron, hydromorphone, insulin, labetalol, linezolid, magnesium sulfate, melphalan, meperidine, midazolam, milrinone, morphine, nicardipine, perphenazine, remifentanil, tacrolimus, teniposide, theophylline, thiotepa, tolazoline, vinorelbine, zidovudine.
- **Y-Site Incompatibility:** allopurinol, amphotericin B cholesteryl sulfate, azithromycin, drotrecogin, heparin, hetastarch, indomethacin, lansoprazole, pemetrexed, propofol, sargramostim.
- **Additive Incompatibility:** Manufacturer recommends administering separately; do not admix.
- **Topical:** Cleanse skin before application. Wear gloves during application.

Patient/Family Teaching

- Instruct patient to report signs of hypersensitivity, tinnitus, vertigo, hearing loss, rash, dizziness, or difficulty urinating.
- Advise patient of the importance of drinking plenty of liquids.
- Teach patients with a history of rheumatic heart disease or valve replacement the importance of using antimicrobial prophylaxis before invasive medical or dental procedures.
- **PO:** Instruct patient to take neomycin as directed for full course of therapy. Take missed doses as soon as possible if not almost time for next dose; do not take double doses.
- Caution patient that neomycin may cause nausea, vomiting, or diarrhea.
- **Topical:** Instruct patient to wash affected skin gently and pat dry. Apply a thin film of ointment. Apply occlusive dressing only if directed by health care professional. Patient should assess skin and inform health care professional if skin irritation develops or infection worsens.
- **Inhaln:** Instruct patient to take inhalation twice daily as close to 12 hr apart as possible; not <6 hr apart. Administer over 10–15 min period using a hand-held PARI LC PLUS reusable nebulizer with a *DeVilbiss Pulmo-Aide* compressor. Do not mix with dornase alpha in nebulizer. Instruct patient on multiple therapies to take others first and use tobramycin last. Tobramycin-induced bronchospasm may be reduced if tobramycin is administered after bronchodilators. Instruct patient to sit or stand upright during inhalation and breathe normally through mouthpiece of nebulizer. Nose clips may help patient breath through mouth.

Evaluation/Desired Outcomes

- Resolution of the signs and symptoms of infection. If no response is seen within 3–5 days, new cultures should be taken.
- Prevention of infection in intestinal surgery (neomycin).
- Improved neurologic status in hepatic encephalopathy (neomycin).
- Endocarditis prophylaxis (gentamicin).

aminophylline, See BRONCHODILATORS (XANTHINES).

HIGH ALERT

amiodarone

(am-ee-**oh**-da-rone)
Cordarone, Pacerone

Classification
Therapeutic: antiarrhythmics (class III)

Pregnancy Category D

Indications

Life-threatening ventricular arrhythmias unresponsive to less toxic agents. **Unlabeled uses: PO:** Management of supraventricular tachyarrhythmias. **IV:** As part of the Advanced Cardiac Life Support (ACLS) and Pediatric Advanced Life Support (PALS) guidelines for the management of ventricular fibrillation/pulseless ventricular tachycardia after cardiopulmonary resuscitation and defibrillation have failed; also for other life-threatening tachyarrhythmias.

Action

Prolongs action potential and refractory period. Inhibits adrenergic stimulation. Slows the sinus rate, increases PR and QT intervals, and decreases peripheral vascular resistance (vasodilation). **Therapeutic Effects:** Suppression of arrhythmias.

Pharmacokinetics

Absorption: IV administration results in complete bioavailability. Slowly and variably absorbed from the GI tract (35–65%).
Distribution: Distributed to and accumulates slowly in body tissues. Reaches high levels in fat, muscle, liver, lungs, and spleen. Crosses the placenta and enters breast milk.
Protein Binding: 96% bound to plasma proteins.
Metabolism and Excretion: Metabolized by the liver, excreted into bile. Minimal renal excretion. One metabolite has antiarrhythmic activity.
Half-life: 13–107 days.

TIME/ACTION PROFILE (suppression of ventricular arrhythmias)

ROUTE	ONSET	PEAK	DURATION
PO	2–3 days (up to 2–3 mos)	3–7 hr	wks–mos
IV	2 hr	3–7 hr	unknown

Contraindications/Precautions

Contraindicated in: Patients with cardiogenic shock; Severe sinus node dysfunction; 2nd- and 3rd-degree AV block; Bradycardia (has caused syncope unless a pacemaker is in place); Hypersensitivity to amiodarone or iodine; OB: Can cause fetal hypo- or hyperthyroidism; Lactation: Enters breast milk and can cause harm to the neonate; use an alternative to breast milk; Pedi: Safety not established; products containing benzyl alcohol should not be used in neonates.
Use Cautiously in: History of CHF; Thyroid disorders; Corneal refractive laser surgery; Severe pulmonary or liver disease; Geri: Appears on Beers list. Potential to affect QT interval and cause torsades de pointes. Initiate therapy at the low end of the dosing range due to decreased hepatic, renal, or cardiac function; comorbid disease; or other drug therapy.

Adverse Reactions/Side Effects

CNS: confusional states, disorientation, hallucinations, dizziness, fatigue, malaise, headache, insomnia. **EENT:** corneal microdeposits, abnormal sense of smell, dry eyes, optic neuritis, optic neuropathy, photophobia. **Resp:** ADULT RESPIRATORY DISTRESS SYNDROME (ARDS), PULMONARY FIBROSIS, PULMONARY TOXICITY. **CV:** CHF, WORSENING OF ARRHYTHMIAS, bradycardia, hypotension. **GI:** LIVER FUNCTION ABNORMALITIES, anorexia, constipation, nausea, vomiting, abdominal pain, abnormal sense of taste. **GU:** decreased libido, epididymitis. **Derm:** TOXIC EPIDERMAL NECROLYSIS (rare), photosensitivity, blue discoloration. **Endo:** hypothyroidism, hyperthyroidism. **Neuro:** ataxia, involuntary movement, paresthesia, peripheral neuropathy, poor coordination, tremor.

Interactions

Drug-Drug: Increased risk of QT prolongations with **fluoroquinolones**, **macrolides**, and **azole antifungals** (undertake concurrent use with caution). ↑ blood levels and may lead to toxicity from **digoxin** (↓ dose of digoxin by 50%). ↑ blood levels and may lead to toxicity from other **class I antiarrhythmics (quinidine**, **procainamide**, **mexiletine**, **lidocaine**, or **flecainide**— ↓ doses of other drugs by 30–50%). ↑ blood levels of **cyclosporine**, **dextromethorphan**, **methotrexate**, **phenytoin**, and **theophylline**. **Phenytoin** ↓ amiodarone blood levels. ↑ activity of **warfarin** (↓ dose of warfarin by 33–50%). ↑ risk of bradyarrhythmias, sinus arrest, or AV heart block with **beta blockers** or **calcium channel blockers**. **Cholestyramine** may ↓ amiodarone blood levels. **Cimetidine** and **ritonavir** ↑ amiodarone blood levels. Risk of myocardial depression is ↑ by **volatile anesthetics**.
Drug-Natural Products: St. John's wort induces enzymes that metabolize amiodarone; may ↓ levels and effectiveness. Avoid concurrent use.
Drug-Food: Grapefruit juice inhibits enzymes in the GI tract that metabolize amiodarone resulting in ↑ levels and risk of toxicity; avoid concurrent use.

Route/Dosage

Ventricular Arrhythmias

PO (Adults): 800–1600-mg/day in 1–2 doses for 1–3 wk, then 600–800 mg/day in 1–2 doses for 1 mo, then 400 mg/day maintenance dose.
PO (Children): 10 mg/kg/day (800 mg/1.72 m^2/day) for 10 days or until response or adverse

reaction occurs, then 5 mg/kg/day (400 mg/ 1.72 m^2/day) for several weeks, then decreased to 2.5 mg/kg/day (200 mg/1.72 m^2/day) or lowest effective maintenance dose.
IV (Adults): 150 mg over 10 min, followed by 360 mg over the next 6 hr and then 540 mg over the next 18 hr. Continue infusion at 0.5 mg/min until oral therapy is initiated. If arrhythmia recurs, a small loading infusion of 150 mg over 10 min should be given; in addition, the rate of the maintenance infusion may be increased. *Conversion to initial oral therapy*—If duration of IV infusion was <1 wk, oral dose should be 800–1600 mg/day; if IV infusion was 1–3 wk, oral dose should be 600–800 mg/day; if IV infusion was >3 wk, oral dose should be 400 mg/ day. *ACLS guidelines for pulseless VFib/ VTach*—300 mg IV push, may repeat once after 3–5 min with 150 mg IV push (maximum cumulative dose 2.2 g/24 hr; unlabeled).
IV: Intraosseous **(Children and infants):** *PALS guidelines for pulseless VFib/VTach* 5 mg/kg as a bolus; *perfusion tachycardia*—5 mg/kg loading dose over 20–60 min (maximum of 15 mg/kg/day; unlabeled).

Supraventricular Tachycardia
PO (Adults): 600–800 mg/day for 1 wk or until desired response occurs or side effects develop, then decrease to 400 mg/day for 3 wk, then maintenance dose of 200–400 mg/day.
PO (Children): 10 mg/kg/day (800 mg/1.72 m^2/day) for 10 days or until response or side effects occur, then 5 mg/kg/day (400 mg/1.72 m^2/ day) for several weeks, then decreased to 2.5 mg/kg/day (200 mg/1.72 m^2/day) or lowest effective maintenance dose.

Availability (generic available)
Tablets: 200 mg, 400 mg. **Cost:** 200 mg $235.39/60. **Injection:** 50 mg/ml in 3-, 9-, and 18-ml vials. **Cost:** 50 mg $1057.13/10 ampules.

NURSING IMPLICATIONS

Assessment
- Monitor ECG continuously during IV therapy or initiation of oral therapy. Monitor heart rate and rhythm throughout therapy; PR prolongation, slight QRS widening, T-wave amplitude reduction with T-wave widening and bifurcation, and U waves may occur. QT prolongation may be associated with worsening of arrhythmias and should be monitored closely during IV therapy. Report bradycardia or increase in arrhythmias promptly; patients receiving IV therapy may require slowing rate, discontinuing infusion, or inserting a temporary pacemaker.
- Assess for signs of pulmonary toxicity (rales/ crackles, decreased breath sounds, pleuritic friction rub, fatigue, dyspnea, cough, wheezing, pleuritic pain, fever, hemoptysis, hypoxia). Chest x-ray and pulmonary function tests are recommended before therapy. Monitor chest x-ray every 3–6 mo during therapy to detect diffuse interstitial changes or alveolar infiltrates. Bronchoscopy or gallium radionuclide scan may also be used for diagnosis. Usually reversible after withdrawal, but fatalities have occurred.
- **IV:** Assess for signs and symptoms of ARDS throughout therapy. Report dyspnea, tachypnea, or rales/crackles promptly. Bilateral, diffuse pulmonary infiltrates are seen on chest x-ray.
- Monitor blood pressure frequently. Hypotension usually occurs during first several hours of therapy and is related to rate of infusion. If hypotension occurs, slow rate.
- **PO:** Assess for neurotoxicity (ataxia, proximal muscle weakness, tingling or numbness in fingers or toes, uncontrolled movements, tremors); common during initial therapy, but may occur within 1 wk to several months of initiation of therapy and may persist for more than 1 yr after withdrawal. Dose reduction is recommended. Assist patient during ambulation to prevent falls.
- Ophthalmic exams should be performed before and regularly during therapy and whenever visual changes (photophobia, halos around lights, decreased acuity) occur. May cause permanent loss of vision.
- Assess for signs of thyroid dysfunction, especially during initial therapy. Lethargy; weight gain; edema of the hands, feet, and periorbital region; and cool, pale skin suggest hypothyroidism and may require decrease in dose or discontinuation of therapy and thyroid supplementation. Tachycardia; weight loss; nervousness; sensitivity to heat; insomnia; and warm, flushed, moist skin suggest hyperthyroidism and may require discontinuation of therapy and treatment with antithyroid agents.

- ***Lab Test Considerations:*** Monitor liver and thyroid functions before and periodically throughout therapy. Drug effects persist long after discontinuation. Thyroid function abnormalities are common, but clinical thyroid dysfunction is uncommon.
- Monitor AST, ALT, and alkaline phosphatase at regular intervals during therapy, especially in patients receiving high maintenance dose. If liver function studies are 3 times normal or double in patients with elevated baseline levels or if hepatomegaly occurs, dose should be reduced.
- May cause asymptomatic elevations in ANA titer concentrations.

Potential Nursing Diagnoses

Decreased cardiac output (Indications)
Impaired gas exchange (Side Effects)

Implementation

- ***High Alert:*** IV vasoactive medications are inherently dangerous; fatalities have occurred from medication errors involving amiodarone. Before administering, have second practitioner check original order, dose calculations, and infusion pump settings. Patients should be hospitalized and monitored closely during IV therapy and initiation of oral therapy. IV therapy should be administered only by physicians experienced in treating life-threatening arrhythmias. Do not confuse amiodarone with inamrinone, formerly called amrinone.
- Hypokalemia and hypomagnesemia may decrease effectiveness or cause additional arrhythmias; correct before therapy.
- Monitor closely when converting from IV to oral therapy, especially in geriatric patients.
- **PO:** May be administered with meals and in divided doses if GI intolerance occurs or if daily dose exceeds 1000 mg.

IV Administration

- **IV:** Administer via volumetric pump; drop size may be reduced, causing altered dosing with drop counter infusion sets.
- Administer through an in-line filter.
- Infusions exceeding 2 hr must be administered in glass or polyolefin bottles to prevent adsorption. However, polyvinyl chloride (PVC) tubing must be used during administration because concentrations and infusion rate recommendations have been based on PVC tubing.
- **Direct IV:** ***Diluent:*** Administer undiluted. May also be diluted in 20–30 ml of D5W or 0.9% NaCl. ***Concentration:*** 50 mg/ml. ***Rate:*** Administer IV push.
- **Intermittent Infusion:** ***Diluent:*** Dilute 150 mg of amiodarone in 100 ml of D5W. Infusion stable for 2 hr in PVC bag. ***Concentration:*** 1.5 mg/ml. ***Rate:*** Infuse over 10 min. Do not administer IV push.
- **Continuous Infusion:** ***Diluent:*** Dilute 900 mg (18 ml) of amiodarone in 500 ml of D5W. Infusion stable for 24 hr in glass or polyolefin bottle. ***Concentration:*** Solution above: 1.8 mg/ml. Concentration may range from 1–6 mg/ml (concentrations >2 mg/ml must be administered via central venous catheter). ***Rate:*** Infuse at a rate of 1 mg/min for the first 6 hr, then decrease infusion rate to 0.5 mg/min and continue until oral therapy initiated.
- **Y-Site Compatibility:** amikacin, amphotericin B, atracurium, atropine, bumetanide, calcium chloride, calcium gluconate, caspofungin, ceftizoxime, ceftriaxone, cefuroxime, ciprofloxacin, clindamycin, daptomycin, dexmedetomidine, diltiazem, dobutamine, dopamine, doxycycline, epinephrine, eptifibatide, erythromycin lactobionate, esmolol, famotidine, fenoldopam, fentanyl, fluconazole, gentamicin, granisetron, insulin, isoproterenol, labetalol, lepirudin, lidocaine, linezolid, lorazepam, methylprednisolone, metronidazole, midazolam, milrinone, morphine, nesiritide, nitroglycerin, norepinephrine, palonosetron, penicillin G potassium, phenylephrine, potassium chloride, procainamide, quinupristin/dalfopristin, rifampin, tacrolimus, tirofiban, tobramycin, vancomycin, vasopressin, vecuronium, voriconazole.
- **Y-Site Incompatibility:** aminophylline, bivalirudin, ceftazidime, digoxin, ertapenem, heparin, imipenem-cilastatin, levofloxacin, micafungin, piperacillin/tazobactam, potassium phosphates, sodium bicarbonate.
- **Additive Incompatibility:** aminophylline, heparin, sodium bicarbonate.

Patient/Family Teaching

- Instruct patient to take amiodarone as directed. Patient should read the *Medication Guide* prior to first dose and with each Rx refill. If a dose is missed, do not take at all. Consult health care professional if more than two doses are missed.
- Advise patient to avoid drinking grapefruit juice during therapy.

- Inform patient that side effects may not appear until several days, weeks, or years after initiation of therapy and may persist for several months after withdrawal.
- Teach patients to monitor pulse daily and report abnormalities.
- Advise patients that photosensitivity reactions may occur through window glass, thin clothing, and sunscreens. Protective clothing and sunblock are recommended during and for 4 months after therapy. If photosensitivity occurs, dosage reduction may be useful.
- Inform patients that bluish discoloration of the face, neck, and arms is a possible side effect of this drug after prolonged use. This is usually reversible and will fade over several months. Notify health care professional if this occurs.
- Instruct male patients to notify health care professional if signs of epididymitis (pain and swelling in scrotum) occur. May require reduction in dose.
- Instruct patient to notify health care professional of medication regimen before treatment or surgery.
- Emphasize the importance of follow-up exams, including chest x-ray and pulmonary function tests every 3–6 mo and ophthalmic exams after 6 mo of therapy, and then annually.

Evaluation/Desired Outcomes

- Cessation of life-threatening ventricular arrhythmias. Adverse effects may take up to 4 months to resolve.

amitriptyline

(a-mee-**trip**-ti-leen)

✦Apo-Amitriptyline, Elavil, ✦Levate, ✦Novotriptyn

Classification

Therapeutic: antidepressants

Pharmacologic: tricyclic antidepressants

Pregnancy Category C

Indications

Depression. **Unlabeled uses:** Anxiety, insomnia, treatment-resistant depression. Chronic pain syndromes (i.e., fibromyalgia, neuropathic pain/chronic pain, headache, low back pain).

Action

Potentiates the effect of serotonin and norepinephrine in the CNS. Has significant anticholinergic properties. **Therapeutic Effects:** Antidepressant action.

Pharmacokinetics

Absorption: Well absorbed from the GI tract.
Distribution: Widely distributed.
Protein Binding: 95% bound to plasma proteins.
Metabolism and Excretion: Extensively metabolized by the liver. Some metabolites have antidepressant activity. Undergoes enterohepatic recirculation and secretion into gastric juices. Probably crosses the placenta and enters breast milk.
Half-life: 10–50 hr.

TIME/ACTION PROFILE (antidepressant effect)

ROUTE	ONSET	PEAK	DURATION
PO	2–3 wk (up to 30 days)	2–6 wk	days–wks
IM	2–3 wk	2–6 wk	days–wks

Contraindications/Precautions

Contraindicated in: Angle-closure glaucoma; Known history of QTc prolongation, recent MI, heart failure.
Use Cautiously in: May ↑ risk of suicide attempt/ideation especially during dose early treatment or dose adjustment; risk may be greater in children or adolescents; Patients with pre-existing cardiovascular disease; Prostatic hyperplasia (increased risk of urinary retention); History of seizures (threshold may be ↓); OB: Use only if clearly needed and maternal benefits outweigh risk to fetus Lactation: May cause sedation in infant; Pedi: Safety not established in children <12 yr; Geri: Appears on Beers list. Geriatric patients are at increased risk of adverse reactions including falls secondary to sedative and anticholinergic effects.

Adverse Reactions/Side Effects

CNS: <u>lethargy</u>, <u>sedation</u>. **EENT:** <u>blurred vision</u>, <u>dry eyes</u>, <u>dry mouth</u>. **CV:** ARRHYTHMIAS, <u>hypotension</u>, ECG changes. **GI:** <u>constipation</u>, hepatitis, paralytic ileus, increased appetite, weight gain. **GU:** urinary retention, ↓ libido. **Derm:** photosensitivity. **Endo:** changes in blood glucose, gynecomastia. **Hemat:** blood dyscrasias.

✦ = Canadian drug name.

* CAPITALS indicates life-threatening; <u>underlines</u> indicate most frequent.

Interactions

Drug-Drug: Amitriptyline is metabolized in the liver by the cytochrome P450 2D6 enzyme, and its action may be affected by drugs that compete for metabolism by this enzyme, including other **antidepressants**, **phenothiazines**, **carbamazepine**, **class 1C antiarrhythmics** including **propafenone**, and **flecainide**; when these drugs are used concurrently with amitriptyline, dosage ↓ of one or the other or both may be necessary. Concurrent use of other drugs that inhibit the activity of the enzyme, including **cimetidine**, **quinidine**, **amiodarone**, and **ritonavir**, may result in ↑ effects of amitriptyline. May cause hypotension, tachycardia, and potentially fatal reactions when used with **MAO inhibitors** (avoid concurrent use—discontinue 2 wk before starting amitriptyline). Concurrent use with **SSRI antidepressants** may result in ↑ toxicity and should be avoided (**fluoxetine** should be stopped 5 wk before starting amitriptyline). Concurrent use with **clonidine** may result in hypertensive crisis and should be avoided. Concurrent use with **levodopa** may result in delayed or ↓ absorption of levodopa or hypertension. Blood levels and effects may be ↓ by **rifamycins** (**rifampin**, **rifapentine**, and **rifabutin**). Concurrent use with **moxifloxacin** ↑ risk of adverse cardiovascular reactions. ↑ CNS depression with other **CNS depressants** including **alcohol**, **antihistamines**, **clonidine**, **opioids**, and **sedative/hypnotics**. **Barbiturates** may alter blood levels and effects. **Adrenergic** and **anticholinergic** side effects may be ↑ with other agents having **anticholinergic** properties. **Phenothiazines** or **oral contraceptives** ↑ levels and may cause toxicity. **Nicotine** may ↑ metabolism and alter effects.

Drug-Natural Products: St. John's wort may decrease serum concentrations and efficacy. Concomitant use of **kava kava**, **valerian**, or **chamomile** can increase CNS depression. Increased anticholinergic effects with **jimson weed** and **scopolia**.

Route/Dosage

PO (Adults): 75 mg/day in divided doses; may be increased up to 150 mg/day *or* 50–100 mg at bedtime, may increase by 25–50 mg up to 150 mg (in hospitalized patients, may initiate with 100 mg/day, increasing total daily dose up to 300 mg).

PO (Geriatric Patients and Adolescents): 10 mg tid and 20 mg at bedtime *or* 25 mg at bedtime initially, slowly increased to 100 mg/day as a single bedtime dose or divided doses.

Availability (generic available)

Tablets: 10 mg, 25 mg, 50 mg, 75 mg, 100 mg, 150 mg. **Cost:** *Generic*—10 mg $13.32/100, 25 mg $12.22/100, 50 mg $14.20/100, 75 mg $12.21/100, 100 mg $12.21/100, 150 mg $24.42/100. **Syrup:** 10 mg/5 ml.

NURSING IMPLICATIONS

Assessment

- Obtain weight and BMI initially and periodically throughout treatment.
- Assess fasting glucose and cholesterol levels in overweight/obese individuals.
- Monitor blood pressure and pulse before and during initial therapy. Notify physician or other health care professional of decreases in blood pressure (10–20 mm Hg) or sudden increase in pulse rate. Patients taking high doses or with a history of cardiovascular disease should have ECG monitored before and periodically during therapy.
- **Depression:** Monitor mental status (orientation, mood behavior) frequently. Assess for suicidal tendencies, especially during early therapy. Restrict amount of drug available to patient.
- **Pain:** Assess intensity, quality, and location of pain periodically during therapy. May require several weeks for effects to be seen. Use pain scale to monitor effectiveness of medication. Assess for sexual dysfunction (decreased libido; erectile dysfunction). Geri: Geriatric patients started on amitriptyline may be at an increased risk for falls; start with low dose and monitor closely. Assess for anticholinergic effects (weakness and sedation).
- ***Lab Test Considerations:*** Assess leukocyte and differential blood counts, liver function, and serum glucose before and periodically during therapy. May cause an ↑ serum bilirubin and alkaline phosphatase. May cause bone marrow depression. Serum glucose may be ↑ or ↓.

Potential Nursing Diagnoses

Ineffective coping (Indications)
Chronic pain (Indications)
Risk for injury (Side Effects)

Implementation

- Do not confuse Elavil (amitriptyline) with Oruvail (ketoprofen).

- Dose increases should be made at bedtime because of sedation. Dose titration is a slow process; may take weeks to months. May give entire dose at bedtime. Sedative effect may be apparent before antidepressant effect is noted. May require tapering to avoid withdrawal effects.
- **PO:** Administer medication with or immediately after a meal to minimize gastric upset. Tablet may be crushed and given with food or fluids.

Patient/Family Teaching

- Instruct patient to take medication exactly as directed. If a dose is missed, take as soon as possible unless almost time for next dose; if regimen is a single dose at bedtime, do not take in the morning because of side effects. Advise patient that drug effects may not be noticed for at least 2 wk. Abrupt discontinuation may cause nausea, vomiting, diarrhea, headache, trouble sleeping with vivid dreams, and irritability.
- May cause drowsiness and blurred vision. Caution patient to avoid driving and other activities requiring alertness until response to drug is known.
- Orthostatic hypotension, sedation, and confusion are common during early therapy, especially in geriatric patients. Protect patient from falls and advise patient to make position changes slowly. Institute fall precautions. Advise patient to make position changes slowly. Refer as appropriate for nutrition/weight management and medical management.
- Advise patient to avoid alcohol or other CNS depressant drugs during and for 3–7 days after therapy has been discontinued.
- Instruct patient to notify health care professional if urinary retention, dry mouth, or constipation persists. Sugarless candy or gum may diminish dry mouth, and an increase in fluid intake or bulk may prevent constipation. If symptoms persist, dose reduction or discontinuation may be necessary. Consult health care professional if dry mouth persists for >2 wk.
- Caution patient to use sunscreen and protective clothing to prevent photosensitivity reactions. Alert patient that medication may turn urine blue-green in color.
- Inform patient of need to monitor dietary intake. Increase in appetite may lead to undesired weight gain.
- Advise patient to notify health care professional if pregnancy is planned or suspected or if breastfeeding.
- Advise patient to notify health care professional of medication regimen before treatment or surgery. Medication should be discontinued as long as possible before surgery.
- Therapy for depression is usually prolonged and should be continued for at least 3 months to prevent relapse. Emphasize the importance of follow-up exams to monitor effectiveness, side effects, and improve coping skills. Advise patient and family that treatment is not a cure and symptoms can recur after discontinuation of medication. Refer patient to local support group.

Evaluation/Desired Outcomes

- Increased sense of well-being.
- Renewed interest in surroundings.
- Increased appetite.
- Improved energy level.
- Improved sleep.
- Decrease in chronic pain symptoms.
- Full therapeutic effects may be seen 2–6 wk after initiating therapy.

amlodipine (am-**loe**-di-peen)
Norvasc

Classification
Therapeutic: antihypertensives
Pharmacologic: calcium channel blockers

Pregnancy Category C

Indications

Alone or with other agents in the management of hypertension, angina pectoris, and vasospastic (Prinzmetal's) angina.

Action

Inhibits the transport of calcium into myocardial and vascular smooth muscle cells, resulting in inhibition of excitation-contraction coupling and subsequent contraction. **Therapeutic Effects:** Systemic vasodilation resulting in decreased blood pressure. Coronary vasodilation resulting in decreased frequency and severity of attacks of angina.

Pharmacokinetics

Absorption: Well absorbed after oral administration (64–90%).
Distribution: Probably crosses the placenta.
Protein Binding: 95–98%.
Metabolism and Excretion: Mostly metabolized by the liver.
Half-life: 30–50 hr (↑ in geriatric patients and patients with hepatic impairment).

TIME/ACTION PROFILE (cardiovascular effects)

ROUTE	ONSET	PEAK	DURATION
PO	unknown	6–9	24 hr

Contraindications/Precautions

Contraindicated in: Hypersensitivity; Blood pressure <90 mm Hg.
Use Cautiously in: Severe hepatic impairment (dosage reduction recommended); Aortic stenosis; History of CHF; OB, Lactation, Pedi: Safety not established; Geri: Dose reduction recommended; increased risk of hypotension.

Adverse Reactions/Side Effects

CNS: headache, dizziness, fatigue. **CV:** peripheral edema, angina, bradycardia, hypotension, palpitations. **GI:** gingival hyperplasia, nausea. **Derm:** flushing.

Interactions

Drug-Drug: Additive hypotension may occur when used concurrently with **fentanyl**, other **antihypertensives**, **nitrates**, acute ingestion of **alcohol**, or **quinidine**. Antihypertensive effects may be ↓ by concurrent use of **nonsteroidal anti-inflammatory agents**. May ↑ risk of neurotoxicity with **lithium**.
Drug-Food: **Grapefruit juice** ↑ serum levels and effect.

Route/Dosage

PO (Adults): 5–10 mg once daily; *antihypertensive in fragile or small patients or patients already receiving other antihypertensives*—initiate at 2.5 mg/day, increase as required/tolerated (up to 10 mg/day) as an antihypertensive therapy with 2.5 mg/day in patients with hepatic insufficiency.
PO (Geriatric Patients): *Antihypertensive*—Initiate therapy at 2.5 mg/day, increase as required/tolerated (up to 10 mg/day); *antianginal*—initiate therapy at 5 mg/day, increase as required/tolerated (up to 10 mg/day).

Hepatic Impairment

PO (Adults): *Antihypertensive*—Initiate therapy at 2.5 mg/day, increase as required/tolerated (up to 10 mg/day); *antianginal*—initiate therapy at 5 mg/day, increase as required/tolerated (up to 10 mg/day).

Availability (generic available)

Tablets: 2.5 mg, 5 mg, 10 mg. **Cost:** *Generic*—2.5 mg $99.97/90, 5 mg $105.97/90, 10 mg $135.96/90. ***In combination with:*** atorvastatin (Caduet), benazepril (Lotrel), olmesartan (Azor), and valsartan (Exforge). See Appendix B.

NURSING IMPLICATIONS

Assessment

- Monitor blood pressure and pulse before therapy, during dose titration, and periodically during therapy. Monitor ECG periodically during prolonged therapy.
- Monitor intake and output ratios and daily weight. Assess for signs of CHF (peripheral edema, rales/crackles, dyspnea, weight gain, jugular venous distention).
- **Angina:** Assess location, duration, intensity, and precipitating factors of patient's anginal pain.
- ***Lab Test Considerations:*** Total serum calcium concentrations are not affected by calcium channel blockers.

Potential Nursing Diagnoses

Ineffective tissue perfusion (Indications)
Acute pain (Indications)

Implementation

- **PO:** May be administered without regard to meals.

Patient/Family Teaching

- Advise patient to take medication as directed, even if feeling well. Take missed doses as soon as possible unless almost time for next dose; do not double doses. May need to be discontinued gradually.
- Advise patient to avoid large amounts (6–8 glasses of grapefruit juice/day) during therapy.
- Instruct patient on correct technique for monitoring pulse. Instruct patient to contact health care professional if heart rate is <50 bpm.
- Caution patient to change positions slowly to minimize orthostatic hypotension.

- May cause drowsiness or dizziness. Advise patient to avoid driving or other activities requiring alertness until response to the medication is known.
- Instruct patient on importance of maintaining good dental hygiene and seeing dentist frequently for teeth cleaning to prevent tenderness, bleeding, and gingival hyperplasia (gum enlargement).
- Instruct patient to avoid concurrent use of alcohol or OTC medications, especially cold preparations, without consulting health care professional.
- Advise patient to notify health care professional if irregular heartbeats, dyspnea, swelling of hands and feet, pronounced dizziness, nausea, constipation, or hypotension occurs or if headache is severe or persistent.
- Caution patient to wear protective clothing and use sunscreen to prevent photosensitivity reactions.
- Advise patient to inform health care professional of medication regimen before treatment or surgery.
- **Angina:** Instruct patient on concurrent nitrate or beta-blocker therapy to continue taking both medications as directed and to use SL nitroglycerin as needed for anginal attacks.
- Advise patient to contact health care professional if chest pain does not improve or worsens after therapy, if it occurs with diaphoresis, if shortness of breath occurs, or if severe, persistent headache occurs.
- Caution patient to discuss exercise restrictions with health care professional before exertion.
- **Hypertension:** Encourage patient to comply with other interventions for hypertension (weight reduction, low-sodium diet, smoking cessation, moderation of alcohol consumption, regular exercise, and stress management). Medication controls but does not cure hypertension.
- Instruct patient and family in proper technique for monitoring blood pressure. Advise patient to take blood pressure weekly and to report significant changes to health care professional.

Evaluation/Desired Outcomes

- Decrease in blood pressure.
- Decrease in frequency and severity of anginal attacks.
- Decrease in need for nitrate therapy.
- Increase in activity tolerance and sense of well-being.

---

amoxicillin (a-mox-i-**sil**-in)

Amoxil, ✤Apo-Amoxi, DisperMox, ✤Novamoxin, ✤Nu-Amoxi, Trimox, Wymox

Classification

Therapeutic: anti-infectives, antiulcer agents

Pharmacologic: aminopenicillins

Pregnancy Category B

Indications

Treatment of: Skin and skin structure infections, Otitis media, Sinusitis, Respiratory infections, Genitourinary infections. Endocarditis prophylaxis. Postexposure inhalational anthrax prophylaxis. Management of ulcer disease due to *Helicobacter pylori*. **Unlabeled uses:** Lyme disease in children <8 years.

Action

Binds to bacterial cell wall, causing cell death. **Therapeutic Effects:** Bactericidal action; spectrum is broader than penicillins. **Spectrum:** Active against: Streptococci, Pneumococci, Enterococci, *Haemophilus influenzae*, *Escherichia coli*, *Proteus mirabilis*, *Neisseria meningitidis*, *Neisseria gonorrhoeae*, *Shigella*, *Chlamydia trachomatis*, *Salmonella*, *Borrelia burgdorferi*, *H. pylori*.

Pharmacokinetics

Absorption: Well absorbed from duodenum (75–90%). More resistant to acid inactivation than other penicillins.

Distribution: Diffuses readily into most body tissues and fluids. CSF penetration increased when meninges are inflamed. Crosses placenta; enters breast milk in small amounts.

Metabolism and Excretion: 70% excreted unchanged in the urine; 30% metabolized by the liver.

Half-life: Neonates: 3.7 hr; Infants and Children: 1–2 hr; Adults: 0.7–1.4 hr.

TIME/ACTION PROFILE (blood levels)

ROUTE	ONSET	PEAK	DURATION
PO	30 min	1–2 hr	8–12 hr

Contraindications/Precautions

Contraindicated in: Hypersensitivity to penicillins; Tablets for oral suspension (DisperMox) contain aspartame; avoid in patients with phenylketonuria.
Use Cautiously in: Severe renal insufficiency (↓ dose if CCr <30 ml/min); Infectious mononucleosis, acute lymphocytic leukemia, or cytomegalovirus infection (↑ risk of rash); Patients with a history of cephalosporin allergy; OB, Lactation: Has been used safely in pregnant and breastfeeding women.

Adverse Reactions/Side Effects

CNS: SEIZURES (high doses). **GI:** PSEUDOMEMBRANOUS COLITIS, diarrhea, nausea, vomiting, elevated liver enzymes. **Derm:** rashes, urticaria. **Hemat:** blood dyscrasias. **Misc:** allergic reactions including ANAPHYLAXIS, SERUM SICKNESS, superinfection.

Interactions

Drug-Drug: Probenecid ↓ renal excretion and ↑ blood levels of amoxicillin—therapy may be combined for this purpose. May ↑ effect of **warfarin**. May ↓ effectiveness of **oral contraceptives**. **Allopurinol** may ↑ frequency of rash.

Route/Dosage

Most Infections

PO (Adults): 250–500 mg q 8 hr *or* 500–875 mg q 12 hr (not to exceed 2–3 g/day).
PO (Children >3 mo): 25–50 mg/kg/day in divided doses q 8 hr *or* 25–50 mg/kg/day individual doses q 12 hr. *Acute otitis media due to highly resistant strains of S. pneumoniae*: 80–90 mg/kg/day divided q 12 hr. *Postexposure inhalational anthrax prophylaxis:* <40 kg: 45 mg/kg/day in divided doses q 8 hr; >40 kg: 500 mg q 8 hr.
PO (Infants ≤3 mo and neonates): 20–30 mg/kg/day in divided doses q 12 hr.

H. Pylori

PO (Adults): *Triple therapy*—1000 mg amoxicillin twice daily with lansoprazole 30 mg twice daily and clarithromycin 500 mg twice daily for 14 days *or* 1000 mg amoxicillin twice daily with omeprazole 20 mg twice daily and clarithromycin 500 mg twice daily for 14 days *or* amoxicillin 1000 mg twice daily with esomeprazole 40 mg daily and clarithromycin 500 mg twice daily for 10 days. *Dual therapy*—1000 mg amoxicillin three times daily with lansoprazole 30 mg three times daily for 14 days.

Endocarditis Prophylaxis

PO (Adults): 2 g 1 hr prior to procedure.
PO (Children): 50 mg/kg 1 hr prior to procedure (not to exceed adult dose).

Gonorrhea

PO (Adults and Children ≥40 kg): single 3 g dose.
PO (Children >2 yr and <40 kg): 50 mg/kg with probenecid 25 mg/kg as a single dose.

Renal Impairment

PO (Adults CCr 10–30 ml/min): 250–500 mg q 12 hr.

Renal Impairment

PO (Adults CCr <10 ml/min): 250–500 mg q 24 hr.

Availability (generic available)

Chewable tablets (cherry, banana, peppermint flavors): 125 mg, 200 mg, 250 mg, 400 mg. **Cost:** *Generic*—125 mg $17.13/30, 200 mg $16.99/20, 250 mg $13.99/30, 400 mg $16.36/30. **Tablets:** 500 mg, 875 mg. **Cost:** *Generic*—500 mg $12.80/21, 875 mg $24.99/30. **Capsules:** 250 mg, 500 mg. **Cost:** *Generic*—250 mg $7.99/30, 500 mg $7.99/30. **Suspension (pediatric drops) (bubblegum flavor):** 50 mg/ml in 30-ml bottles. **Cost:** *Generic*—$7.99/30 ml. **Suspension (strawberry [125 mg/5 ml] and bubblegum [200 mg/5 ml, 250 mg/5 ml, 400 mg/5 ml] flavors):** 125 mg/5 ml, 200 mg/5 ml, 250 mg/5 ml, 400 mg/5 ml. **Cost:** *Generic*—125 mg/5 ml $11.25/100 ml, 200 mg/5 ml $16.92/100 ml, 250 mg/5 ml $7.99/150 ml, 400 mg/5 ml $17.47/100 ml. **Tablets for oral suspension (strawberry):** 200 mg, 400 mg. ***In combination with:*** clarithromycin and lansoprazole in a compliance package (Prevpac). See Appendix B.

NURSING IMPLICATIONS

Assessment

- Assess for infection (vital signs; appearance of wound, sputum, urine, and stool; WBC) at beginning of and throughout therapy.
- Obtain a history before initiating therapy to determine previous use of and reactions to penicillins or cephalosporins. Persons with a negative history of penicillin sensitivity may still have an allergic response.

- Observe for signs and symptoms of anaphylaxis (rash, pruritus, laryngeal edema, wheezing). Notify the physician or other health care professional immediately if these occur.
- Obtain specimens for culture and sensitivity prior to therapy. First dose may be given before receiving results.
- Monitor bowel function. Diarrhea, abdominal cramping, fever, and bloody stools should be reported to health care professional promptly as a sign of pseudomembranous colitis. May begin up to several weeks following cessation of therapy.
- ***Lab Test Considerations:*** May cause ↑ serum alkaline phosphatase, LDH, AST, and ALT concentrations.
- May cause false-positive direct Coombs' test result.

Potential Nursing Diagnoses

Risk for infection (Indications, Side Effects)
Noncompliance (Patient/Family Teaching)

Implementation

- **PO:** Administer around the clock. May be given without regard to meals or with meals to decrease GI side effects. Capsule contents may be emptied and swallowed with liquids. Chewable tablets should be crushed or chewed before swallowing with liquids.
- Shake oral suspension before administering. Suspension may be given straight or mixed in formula, milk, fruit juice, water, or ginger ale. Administer immediately after mixing. Discard refrigerated reconstituted suspension after 10 days.
- Mix each *tablet for oral suspension (DisperMox)* in 2 tsp of water. Patient should drink entire mixture, rinse container with a small amount of water and drink to make sure entire dose is taken. Do not chew or swallow tablet. Tablets will not dissolve in mouth. Use only water to dissolve tablets, other liquids are not recommended. Store tablets at room temperature.

Patient/Family Teaching

- Instruct patients to take medication around the clock and to finish the drug completely as directed, even if feeling better. Advise patients that sharing of this medication may be dangerous.
- Review use and preparation of *tablets for oral suspension (DisperMox)*.
- Instruct female patients taking oral contraceptives to use an alternate or additional nonhormonal method of contraception during therapy with amoxicillin and until next menstrual period.
- Advise patient to report the signs of superinfection (furry overgrowth on the tongue, vaginal itching or discharge, loose or foul-smelling stools) and allergy.
- Instruct patient to notify health care professional immediately if diarrhea, abdominal cramping, fever, or bloody stools occur and not to treat with antidiarrheals without consulting health care professionals.
- Instruct the patient to notify health care professional if symptoms do not improve.
- Teach patients with a history of rheumatic heart disease or valve replacement the importance of using antimicrobial prophylaxis before invasive medical or dental procedures.
- Pedi: Teach parents or caregivers to calculate and measure doses accurately. Reinforce importance of using measuring device supplied by pharmacy or with product, not household items.

Evaluation/Desired Outcomes

- Resolution of the signs and symptoms of infection. Length of time for complete resolution depends on the organism and site of infection.
- Endocarditis prophylaxis.
- Eradication of *H. pylori* with resolution of ulcer symptoms.

amoxicillin/clavulanate

(a-mox-i-**sill**-in/klav-yoo-**lan**-ate)
Augmentin, Augmentin ES, Augmentin XR, ✤Clavulin

Classification
Therapeutic: anti-infectives
Pharmacologic: aminopenicillins/beta lactamase inhibitors

Pregnancy Category B

Indications

Treatment of a variety of infections including: Skin and skin structure infections, Otitis media,

Sinusitis, Respiratory tract infections, Genitourinary tract infections.

Action

Binds to bacterial cell wall, causing cell death; spectrum of amoxicillin is broader than penicillin. Clavulanate resists action of beta-lactamase, an enzyme produced by bacteria that is capable of inactivating some penicillins. **Therapeutic Effects:** Bactericidal action against susceptible bacteria. **Spectrum:** Active against: Streptococci, Pneumococci, Enterococci, *Haemophilus influenzae*, *Escherichia coli*, *Proteus mirabilis*, *Neisseria meningitidis*, *Neisseria gonorrhoeae*, *S. aureus*, *Klebsiella pneumoniae*, *Shigella*, *Salmonella*, *Moraxella catarrhalis*.

Pharmacokinetics

Absorption: Well absorbed from the duodenum (75–90%). More resistant to acid inactivation than other penicillins.
Distribution: Diffuses readily into most body tissues and fluids. Does not readily enter brain/CSF; CSF penetration is increased in the presence of inflamed meninges. Crosses the placenta and enters breast milk in small amounts.
Metabolism and Excretion: 70% excreted unchanged in the urine; 30% metabolized by the liver.
Half-life: 1–1.3 hr.

TIME/ACTION PROFILE (peak blood levels)

ROUTE	ONSET	PEAK	DURATION
PO	30 min	1–2 hr	8—12 hrhr

Contraindications/Precautions

Contraindicated in: Hypersensitivity to penicillins; Hypersensitivity to clavulanate; Suspension and chewable tablets contain aspartame and should be avoided in phenylketonurics; History of amoxicillin/clavulanate-associated cholestatic jaundice.
Use Cautiously in: Severe renal insufficiency (dose reduction necessary); Infectious mononucleosis (increased incidence of rash); Hepatic impairment (dose cautiously, monitor liver function).

Adverse Reactions/Side Effects

CNS: SEIZURES (high doses). **GI:** PSEUDOMEMBRANOUS COLITIS, diarrhea, hepatic dysfunction, nausea, vomiting. **GU:** vaginal candidiasis. **Derm:** rashes, urticaria. **Hemat:** blood dyscrasias. **Misc:** allergic reactions including ANAPHYLAXIS and SERUM SICKNESS, superinfection.

Interactions

Drug-Drug: Probenecid ↓ renal excretion and ↑ blood levels of amoxicillin—therapy may be combined for this purpose. May potentiate the effect of **warfarin**. Concurrent **allopurinol** therapy ↑ risk of rash. May decrease the effectiveness of **hormonal contraceptives**.
Drug-Food: Clavulanate absorption is decreased by a **high fat** meal.

Route/Dosage

Most Infections (Dosing based on amoxicillin component)

PO (Adults and Children >40 kg): 250 mg q 8 hr or 500 mg q 12 hr.

Serious Infections and Respiratory Tract Infections

PO (Adults and Children >40 kg): 875 mg q 12 hr *or* 500 mg q 8 hr; *Acute bacterial sinusitis*—2000 mg q 12 hr for 10 days as extended release (XR) product; *Community-acquired pneumonia*—2000 mg every 12 hr for 7–10 days as extended release (XR) product.

Recurrent/persistent acute otitis media due to Multidrug-resistant *S. pneumonia, H. influenzae,* or *M. catarrhalis*

PO (Children <40 kg): 80–90 mg/kg/day in divided doses q 12 hr for 10 days (as ES formulation only).

Renal Impairment

PO (Adults): *CCr 10–30 ml/min*—250–500 mg q 12 hr (do not use 875 mg tablet); *CCr <10 ml/min*—250–500 mg q 24 hr.

Otitis Media, Sinusitis, Lower Respiratory Tract Infections, Serious Infections

PO (Children ≥3 mo): *200 mg/5 ml or 400 mg/5 ml suspension*—45 mg/kg/day divided q 12 hr; *125 mg/5 ml or 250 mg/5 ml suspension*—40 mg/kg/day divided q 8 hr.

Less Serious Infections

PO (Children ≥3 mo): *200 mg/5 ml or 400 mg/5 ml suspension*—25 mg/kg/day divided q 12 hr *or* 20 mg/kg/day divided q 8 hr (as 125 mg/5 ml or 250 mg/5 ml suspension).
PO (Children <3 mo): 15 mg/kg q 12 hr (125 mg/ml suspension recommended).

Availability (generic available)

Tablets: 250 mg amoxicillin with 125 mg clavulanate, 500 mg amoxicillin with 125 mg clavulanate, 875 mg amoxicillin with 125 mg clavulanate. **Cost:** *Generic*—250 mg $97.19/30, 500 mg $45.99/20, 875 mg $83.99/20. **Chewable tablets (125 mg and 250 mg are lemon-**

lime flavor; 200 mg and 400 mg are cherry-banana flavor): 125 mg amoxicillin with 31.25 mg clavulanate, 200 mg amoxicillin with 28.5 mg clavulanate, 250 mg amoxicillin with 62.5 mg clavulanate, 400 mg amoxicillin with 57 mg clavulanate. **Cost:** *Generic*—125 mg $39.88/30, 200 mg $36.90/20, 250 mg $76.06/30, 400 mg $63.79/20. **Extended-release tablets (scored):** 1000 mg amoxicillin with 62.5 mg clavulanate. **Cost:** 1000 mg $101.53/28. **Suspension (125 mg/5 ml and 250 mg/5 ml are orange flavor; 200 mg/5 ml, 400 mg/5 ml and 600 mg/5 ml are orange-raspberry flavor):** 125 mg amoxicillin with 31.25 mg clavulanate/5 ml, 200 mg amoxicillin with 28.5 mg clavulanate/5 ml, 250 mg amoxicillin with 62.5 mg clavulanate/5 ml, 400 mg amoxicillin with 57 mg clavulanate/5 ml, 600 mg amoxicillin with 42.9 mg clavulanate/5 ml (ES formulation). **Cost:** *Generic*—125 mg $27.11/100 ml, 200 mg $40.85/100 ml, 250 mg $51.77/100 ml, 400 mg $69.21/100 ml, 600 mg $35.99/75 ml.

NURSING IMPLICATIONS

Assessment

- Assess for infection (vital signs; appearance of wound, sputum, urine, and stool; WBC) at beginning of and throughout therapy.
- Obtain a history before initiating therapy to determine previous use of and reactions to penicillins or cephalosporins. Persons with a negative history of penicillin sensitivity may still have an allergic response.
- Observe for signs and symptoms of anaphylaxis (rash, pruritus, laryngeal edema, wheezing). Notify the physician or other health care professional immediately if these occur.
- Obtain specimens for culture and sensitivity prior to therapy. First dose may be given before receiving results.
- Monitor bowel function. Diarrhea, abdominal cramping, fever, and bloody stools should be reported to health care professional promptly as a sign of pseudomembranous colitis. May begin up to several weeks following cessation of therapy.
- ***Lab Test Considerations:*** May cause ↑ serum alkaline phosphatase, LDH, AST, and ALT concentrations. Elderly men and patients receiving prolonged treatment are at ↑ risk for hepatic dysfunction.
- May cause false-positive direct Coombs' test result.

Potential Nursing Diagnoses

Risk for infection (Indications, Side Effects)
Noncompliance (Patient/Family Teaching)

Implementation

- **PO:** Administer around the clock. Administer at the start of a meal to enhance absorption and to decrease GI side effects. Do not administer with high fat meals; clavulanate absorption is decreased. XR tablet is scored and can be broken for ease of administration. Capsule contents may be emptied and swallowed with liquids. Chewable tablets should be crushed or chewed before swallowing with liquids. Shake oral suspension before administering. Refrigerated reconstituted suspension should be discarded after 10 days.
- Two 250-mg tablets are not bioequivalent to one 500-mg tablet; 250-mg tablets and 250-mg chewable tablets are also not interchangeable. Two 500-mg tablets are not interchangeable with one 1000-mg XR tablet; amounts of clavulanic acid and durations of action are different. Augmentin ES-600 (600 mg/5-ml) does not contain the same amount of clavulanic acid as any of the other Augmentin suspensions. Suspensions are not interchangeable.
- Pedi: Do not administer 250-mg chewable tablets to children <40 kg due to clavulanate content. Children <3 months should receive the 125-mg/5-ml oral solution.

Patient/Family Teaching

- Instruct patients to take medication around the clock and to finish the drug completely as directed, even if feeling better. Advise patients that sharing of this medication may be dangerous.
- Instruct female patients taking oral contraceptives to use an alternate or additional method of contraception during therapy and until next menstrual period.
- Advise patient to report the signs of superinfection (furry overgrowth on the tongue, vaginal itching or discharge, loose or foul-smelling stools) and allergy.
- Instruct patient to notify health care professional immediately if diarrhea, abdominal

cramping, fever, or bloody stools occur and not to treat with antidiarrheals without consulting health care professionals.

- Instruct the patient to notify health care professional if symptoms do not improve or if nausea or diarrhea persists when drug is administered with food.
- Pedi: Teach parents or caregivers to calculate and measure doses accurately. Reinforce importance of using measuring device supplied by pharmacy or with product, not household items.

Evaluation/Desired Outcomes

- Resolution of the signs and symptoms of infection. Length of time for complete resolution depends on the organism and site of infection.

amphetamine mixtures

(am-**fet**-a-meen)
Amphetamine Salt, Adderall, Adderall XR

Classification
Therapeutic: central nervous system stimulants

Schedule II

Pregnancy Category C

Indications

Narcolepsy, ADHD.

Action

Causes release of norepinephrine from nerve endings. Pharmacologic effects are: CNS and respiratory stimulation, Vasoconstriction, Mydriasis (pupillary dilation). **Therapeutic Effects:** Increased motor activity, mental alertness, and decreased fatigue in narcoleptic patients. Increased attention span in ADHD.

Pharmacokinetics

Absorption: Well absorbed after oral administration.
Distribution: Widely distributed in body tissues, with high concentrations in the brain and CSF. Crosses placenta and enters breast milk.
Metabolism and Excretion: Some metabolism by the liver. Urinary excretion is pH-dependent. Alkaline urine promotes reabsorption and prolongs action.
Half-life: Children 6–12 yrs: 9–11 hr; Adults: 10–13 hr (depends on urine pH).

TIME/ACTION PROFILE (CNS stimulation)

ROUTE	ONSET	PEAK	DURATION
PO	tablet: 0.5–1 hr	tablet: 3 hr capsule: 7 hr	4–6 hr

Contraindications/Precautions

Contraindicated in: Hyperexcitable states including hyperthyroidism; Psychotic personalities; Suicidal or homicidal tendencies; Chemical dependence; Glaucoma; Structural cardiac abnormalities (may increase the risk of sudden death); OB, Pedi: Potentially embryotoxic.
Use Cautiously in: Cardiovascular disease (sudden death has occurred in children with structural cardiac abnormalities or other serious heart problems); History of substance abuse (misuse may result in serious cardiovascular events/sudden death); Hypertension; Diabetes mellitus; Tourette's syndrome (may exacerbate tics); Geri: Geriatric or debilitated patients may be more susceptible to side effects.

Adverse Reactions/Side Effects

CNS: <u>hyperactivity</u>, <u>insomnia</u>, irritability, <u>restlessness</u>, <u>tremor</u>, dizziness, headache. **CV:** <u>palpitations</u>, <u>tachycardia</u>, cardiomyopathy (increased with prolonged use, high doses), hypertension, hypotension. **GI:** <u>anorexia</u>, constipation, cramps, diarrhea, dry mouth, metallic taste, nausea, vomiting. **GU:** erectile dysfunction, increased libido. **Derm:** urticaria. **Endo:** growth inhibition (with long term use in children). **Misc:** psychological dependence.

Interactions

Drug-Drug: Use with **MAO inhibitors** or **meperidine** can result in hypertensive crisis. ↑ adrenergic effects with other **adrenergics** or **thyroid preparations**. **Drugs that alkalinize urine** (**sodium bicarbonate**, **acetazolamide**) ↓ excretion, ↑ effects. **Drugs that acidify urine** (**ammonium chloride**, large doses of **ascorbic acid**) ↑ excretion, ↓ effects. ↑ risk of hypertension and bradycardia with **beta blockers**. ↑ risk of arrhythmias with **digoxin**. **Tricyclic antidepressants** may ↑ effect of amphetamine but may ↑ risk of arrhythmias, hypertension, or hyperpyrexia.
Drug-Natural Products: Use with **St. John's wort may increase serious side effects (avoid concurrent use).**
Drug-Food: Foods that alkalinize the urine (fruit juices) can ↑ effect of amphetamine.

Route/Dosage

Dose is expressed in total amphetamine content (amphetamine + dextroamphetamine).

Narcolepsy

PO (Adults and Children ≥12 yr): 10–60 mg/day in divided doses; start with 10 mg/day, increase by 10 mg/day at weekly intervals. Sustained-release capsules can be given once daily, tablets every 8–12 hr.

PO (Children 6–12 yr): 5 mg once daily; may increase by 5 mg/day at weekly intervals to a maximum of 60 mg/day.

ADHD

PO (Children ≥6 yr): 5 mg/day 1–2 times daily; increase daily dose by 5 mg at weekly intervals. Sustained-release capsules can be given once daily, tablets every 8–12 hr. If starting therapy with extended release capsules, start with 10 mg once daily and increase by 10 mg/day at weekly intervals (up to 40 mg/day).

PO (Adults): 20 mg/day initially (as extended-release product).

PO (Children 3–5 yr): 2.5 mg/day in the morning; increase daily dose by 2.5 mg at weekly intervals not to exceed 40 mg/day.

Availability (generic available)

Amount is expressed in total amphetamine content (amphetamine + dextroamphetamine. **Tablets:** 5 mg, 7.5 mg, 10 mg, 12.5 mg, 15 mg, 20 mg, 30 mg. **Extended-release capsules:** 5 mg, 10 mg, 15 mg, 20 mg, 25 mg, 30 mg.

NURSING IMPLICATIONS

Assessment

- Monitor blood pressure, pulse, and respiration before and periodically during therapy.
- May produce a false sense of euphoria and well-being. Provide frequent rest periods and observe patient for rebound depression after the effects of the medication have worn off.
- Has high dependence and abuse potential. Tolerance to medication occurs rapidly; do not increase dose.
- **ADHD:** Monitor weight biweekly and inform physician of significant loss. Pedi: Monitor height periodically in children; inform physician of growth inhibition.
- Assess attention span, impulse control, motor and vocal tics, and interactions with others in children with ADHDs.
- **Narcolepsy:** Observe and document frequency of narcoleptic episodes.
- ***Lab Test Considerations:*** May interfere with urinary steroid determinations.
- May cause ↑ plasma corticosteroid concentrations; greatest in evening.

Potential Nursing Diagnoses

Disturbed thought process (Side Effects)

Implementation

- **PO:** Use the lowest effective dose.
- May be taken without regard to food.
- Extended-release capsules may be swallowed whole or opened and sprinkled on applesauce; swallow contents without chewing. Applesauce should be swallowed immediately; do not store. Do not divide contents of capsule; entire contents of capsule should be taken.
- **ADHD:** Pedi: When symptoms are controlled, dose reduction or interruption of therapy may be possible during summer months or may be given on each of the 5 school days, with medication-free weekends and holidays.

Patient/Family Teaching

- Instruct patient to take medication at least 6 hr before bedtime to avoid sleep disturbances. Missed doses should be taken as soon as remembered up to 6 hr before bedtime. With extended release capsule, avoid afternoon doses to prevent insomnia. Do not double doses. Advise patient and parents to read the Medication Guide prior to starting therapy and with each Rx refill. Instruct patient not to alter dose without consulting physician. Abrupt cessation of high doses may cause extreme fatigue and mental depression.
- Inform patient that the effects of drug-induced dry mouth can be minimized by rinsing frequently with water or chewing sugarless gum or candies.
- Advise patient to limit caffeine intake.
- May impair judgment. Advise patient to use caution when driving or during other activities requiring alertness.
- Inform patient that periodic holidays from the drug may be used to assess progress and decrease dependence. Pedi: Children should be given a drug-free holiday each year to reassess symptoms and treatment. Doses will change as children age due to pharmacoki-

netic changes such as slower hepatic metabolism.

- Advise patient to notify physician if nervousness, restlessness, insomnia, dizziness, anorexia, or dry mouth becomes severe. Pedi: If reduced appetite and weight loss are a problem, advise parents to provide high calorie meals when drug levels are low (at breakfast and or bedtime).

Evaluation/Desired Outcomes

- Improved attention span.
- Decrease in narcoleptic symptoms.

amphotericin B deoxycholate
(am-foe-**ter**-i-sin)
✤Fungizone
amphotericin B cholesteryl sulfate
Amphotec
amphotericin B lipid complex
Abelcet
amphotericin B liposome
AmBisome

Classification
Therapeutic: antifungals

Pregnancy Category B

Indications

IV: Treatment of progressive, potentially fatal fungal infections. The cholesteryl sulfate, lipid complex, and liposome formulations should be considered for patients who are intolerant (e.g., renal dysfunction) or refractory to amphotericin B dexycholate. **Amphotericin B liposome:** Management of suspected fungal infections in febrile neutropenic patients: Treatment of visceral leishmaniasis, Treatment of crytococcal meningitis in HIV patients.

Action

Binds to fungal cell membrane, allowing leakage of cellular contents. Toxicity (especially acute infusion reactions and nephrotoxicity) is less with lipid formulations. **Therapeutic Effects:** Can be fungistatic or fungicidal (depends on concentration achieved and susceptibility of organism). **Spectrum:** Active against: Aspergillosis, Blastomycosis, Candidiasis, Coccidioidomycosis, Cryptococcosis, Histoplasmosis, Leishmaniasis (liposomal formulation only), Mucormycosis.

Pharmacokinetics

Absorption: Not absorbed orally.
Distribution: Extensively distributed to body tissues and fluids. Poor penetration into CSF.
Metabolism and Excretion: Elimination is very prolonged. Detectable in urine up to 7 wk after discontinuation.
Half-life: Biphasic—initial phase, 24–48 hr; terminal phase, 15 days. *Cholesteryl sulfate*—28 hr. *Lipid complex*—174 hr. *Liposomal*—100–153 hr.

TIME/ACTION PROFILE (blood levels)

ROUTE	ONSET	PEAK	DURATION
IV	rapid	end of infusion	24 hr

Contraindications/Precautions

Contraindicated in: Hypersensitivity; Lactation: Potential for distribution into breast milk and toxicity in infant; discontinue nursing.
Use Cautiously in: Renal impairment or electrolyte abnormalities; Patients receiving concurrent leukocyte transfusions (increased risk of pulmonary toxicity); OB: Has been used safely.

Adverse Reactions/Side Effects

CNS: anxiety, confusion, headache, insomnia. **Resp:** dyspnea, hypoxia, wheezing. **CV:** chest pain, hypotension, tachycardia, edema, hypertension. **GI:** diarrhea, hyperbilirubinemia, liver enzyme elevation, nausea, vomiting, abdominal pain. **GU:** nephrotoxicity, hematuria. **F and E:** hyperglycemia, hypocalcemia, hypokalemia, hypomagnesemia. **Hemat:** anemia, leukopenia, thrombocytopenia. **Derm:** pruritis, rashes. **Local:** phlebitis. **MS:** arthralgia, myalgia. **Misc:** HYPERSENSITIVITY REACTIONS, chills, fever, acute infusion reactions.

Interactions

Drug-Drug: Increased risk of renal toxicity, bronchospasm, and hypotension with **antineoplastics**. Concurrent use with **corticosteroids** ↑ risk of hypokalemia. Concurrent use with **zidovudine** may increase the risk of myelotoxicity and nephrotoxicity. Combined use with **flucytosine** ↑ antifungal activity but may ↑ the risk of toxicity from flucytosine. Combined use with **azole antifungals** may induce fungal resistance. Increased risk of nephrotoxicity with other **nephrotoxic agents** such as **aminoglycosides**, **cyclosporine**, or **tacrolimus**.

Hypokalemia from amphotericin ↑ the risk of **digoxin** toxicity. Hypokalemia may enhance the curariform effects of **neuromuscular blocking agents**.

Route/Dosage

Specific dosage and duration of therapy depend on nature of infection being treated.

Amphotericin Deoxycholate

IV (Adults): Give test dose of 1 mg. If test dose tolerated, initiate therapy with 0.25 mg/kg/day (doses up to 1.5 mg/kg/day may be used, depending on type of infection) (alternate-day dosing may also be used); *Bladder irrigation*—Instill 50 mcg/ml solution into bladder daily for 5–10 days.

IV (Infants and Children): Give test dose of 0.1 mg/kg (maximum dose 1 mg) or may administer initial dose of 0.25–1 mg/kg/day over 6 hr (without test dose) (some infections may require 1.5 mg/kg/day; alternate-day dosing may be used).

IT (Adults): 25–300 mcg q 48–72 hr, ↑ to 500 mcg—1 mg as tolerated (maximum total dose = 15 mg).

IT (Children): 25–100 mcg q 48–72 hr; ↑ to 500 mcg as tolerated.

Amphotericin B Cholesteryl Sulfate (Amphotec)

IV (Adults and Children): 3–4 mg/kg q 24 hr (no test dose needed).

Amphotericin B Lipid Complex (Abelcet)

IV (Adults and Children): 5 mg/kg q 24 hr (no test dose needed).

Amphotericin B Liposome (AmBisome)

IV (Adults and Children): *Empiric therapy*—3 mg/kg q 24 hr; *Documented infections*—3–5 mg/kg q 24 hr; *Visceral leishmaniasis (immunocompetent patients)*—3 mg/kg q 24 hr on days 1–5, then 3 mg/kg q 24 hr on days 14 and 21; *Visceral leishmaniasis (immunosuppressed patients)*—4 mg/kg q 24 hr on days 1–5, then 4 mg/kg q 24 hr on days 10, 17, 24, 31, and 38; *Cryptococcal meningitis in HIV patients*—6 mg/kg q 24 hr.

Availability

Amphotericin Deoxycholate

Powder for injection: 50 mg/vial.

Amphotericin B Cholesteryl Sulfate

Powder for injection: 50 mg/vial, 100 mg/vial.

Amphotericin B Lipid Complex

Suspension for injection: 100 mg/20-ml vial.

Amphotericin B Liposome

Powder for injection: 50 mg/vial.

NURSING IMPLICATIONS

Assessment

- Monitor patient closely during test dose and the first 1–2 hr of each dose for fever, chills, headache, anorexia, nausea, or vomiting. Premedicating with antipyretics, corticosteroids, antihistamines, meperidine, and antiemetics may decrease these reactions. Febrile reaction usually subsides within 4 hr after the infusion is completed.
- Assess injection site frequently for thrombophlebitis or leakage. Drug is very irritating to tissues.
- Monitor vital signs every 15 min during test dose and every 30 min for 2–4 hr after administration. Meperidine and dantrolene have been used to prevent and treat rigors. Assess respiratory status (lung sounds, dyspnea) daily. Notify physician of changes. If respiratory distress occurs, discontinue infusion immediately; anaphylaxis may occur. Equipment for cardiopulmonary resuscitation should be readily available.
- Monitor intake and output and weigh daily. Adequate hydration (2000–3000 ml/day) and maintaining sodium balance may minimize nephrotoxicity.
- ***Lab Test Considerations:*** Monitor CBC, BUN and serum creatinine, and potassium and magnesium levels daily. If BUN and serum creatinine ↑ significantly, may need to discontinue or consider switching to cholesteryl sulfate, lipid complex, or liposomal formulation.

Potential Nursing Diagnoses

Risk for infection (Indications)

Implementation

- Do not confuse amphotericin B cholesteryl sulfate (Amphotec) with amphotericin deoxycholate, amphotericin B lipid complex (Abelcet), or amphotericin B liposome (AmBisome); they are not interchangeable.

- This drug should be administered IV only to hospitalized patients or those under close supervision. Diagnosis should be confirmed before administration.

Amphotericin B Deoxycholate

IV Administration

- Test dose: ***Diluent:*** Reconstitute 50-mg vial with 10 ml of sterile water for injection to achieve a concentration of 5 mg/ml. Reconstituted vial stable for 24 hr at room temperature or 1 wk if refrigerated. Further dilute with 500 ml of D5W. May be diluted in 250 ml of D5W if being administered via a central venous catheter. Protect infusion from light. Infusion stable for 24 hr at room temperature or 2 days if refrigerated. To obtain test dose, withdraw 1 mg (10 ml) from 500 ml infusion and further dilute with D5W to a total volume of 20 ml. ***Concentration:*** 0.05 mg/ml. ***Rate:*** Infuse over 10–30 min to determine patient tolerance. Pedi: Infuse over 30–60 min.
- **Intermittent Infusion: *Diluent:*** Reconstitute and dilute 50-mg vial as per the directions above. ***Concentration:*** Final concentration of infusion should not exceed 0.1 mg/ml for peripheral infusion or 0.25 mg/ml for central line administration. ***Rate:*** Infuse slowly over 4–6 hr.
- **Y-Site Compatibility:** amiodarone, diltiazem, hydromorphone, lorazepam, tacrolimus.
- **Y-Site Incompatibility:** acyclovir, amikacin, ampicillin, ampicillin/sulbactam, anidulafungin, atropine, aztreonam, bivalirudin, bumetanide, calcium chloride, calcium gluconate, caspofungin, cefepime, ceftizoxime, chloramphenicol, cimetidine, clindamycin, daptomycin, dexamethasone sodium phosphate, diazepam, digoxin, diphenhydramine, dobutamine, dopamine, doxycycline, ertapenem, erythromycin, esmolol, famotidine, fenoldopam, filgrastim, fluconazole, ganciclovir, gentamicin, granisetron, haloperidol, hydralazine, hydrocortisone sodium succinate, hydroxyzine, isoproterenol, ketorolac, labetalol, lansoprazole, levofloxacin, lidocaine, linezolid, meperidine, meropenem, methylprednisolone sodium succinate, metoclopramide, metoprolol, metronidazole, midazolam, morphine, nafcillin, nitroprusside, norepinephrine, ondansetron, palonosetron, pantoprazole, penicillin G potassium, phenylephrine, phenytoin, piperacillin/tazobactam, potassium chloride, prochlorperazine, promethazine, propofol, propranolol, protamine, quinupristin/dalfopristin, sodium bicarbonate, tigecycline, tirofiban, tobramycin, trimethoprim/sulfamethoxazole, vancomycin, vasopressin, verapamil, voriconazole.
- **Solution Incompatibility:** LR injection, saline solutions.

Amphotericin B Cholesteryl Sulfate

IV Administration

- Test Dose: ***Diluent:*** Reconstitute 50-mg vial with 10 ml and 100-mg vial with 20 ml of sterile water for injection to achieve a concentration of 5 mg/ml. Reconstituted vials are stable for 24 hr if refrigerated. Further dilute with D5W to achieve concentration below. Do not use other diluents. Infusion stable for 24 hr if refrigerated. Protect from light. To obtain test dose, withdraw 10 ml from final preparation. ***Concentration:*** Final concentration of infusion should be approximately 0.6 mg/ml (range 0.16–0.83 mg/ml). ***Rate:*** Infuse over 15–30 min.
- **Intermittent Infusion: *Diluent:*** Prepare infusion according to directions above. ***Concentration:*** Final concentration of infusion should be approximately 0.6 mg/ml (range 0.16–0.83 mg/ml). ***Rate:*** Infuse at a rate of 1 mg/kg/hr. If patient tolerates infusion without adverse reactions, infusion time may be shortened to a minimum of 2 hr. If reactions occur or patient cannot tolerate volume, infusion time may be extended. Rapid infusions may cause hypotension, hypokalemia, arrhythmias, and shock.
- **Y-Site Compatibility:** acyclovir, aminophylline, cefoxitin, ceftizoxime, clindamycin, dexamethasone sodium phosphate, fentanyl, furosemide, ganciclovir, granisetron, hydrocortisone, lorazepam, methylprednisolone, nitroglycerin, trimethoprim/sulfamethoxazole.
- **Y-Site Incompatibility:** amikacin, ampicillin, ampicillin/sulbactam, aztreonam, calcium chloride, calcium gluconate, cefazolin, cefepime, ceftazidime, ceftriaxone, cimetidine, cisatracurium, cyclosporine, diazepam, digoxin, diphenhydramine, dobutamine, dopamine, droperidol, enalaprilat, esmolol, famotidine, fluconazole, gentamicin, haloperidol, heparin, hydromorphone, hydroxyzine, imipenem/cilastatin, labetalol, lidocaine, magnesium sulfate, meperidine, metoclopramide, metoprolol, metronidazole, midazolam, morphine, ondansetron, pheny-

toin, piperacillin/tazobactam, potassium chloride, prochlorperazine, promethazine, propranolol, ranitidine, sodium bicarbonate, ticarcillin-clavulanate, tobramycin, vancomycin, vecuronium, verapamil.

- **Solution Incompatibility:** saline solutions.

Amphotericin B Lipid Complex

IV Administration

- **Intermittent Infusion:** ***Diluent:*** Shake vial gently until yellow sediment at bottom has dissolved. Withdraw dose from required number of vials with 18-gauge needle. Replace needle from syringe filled with amphotericin B lipid complex with 5-micron filter needle. Each filter needle may be used to filter the contents of no more than 4 vials. Insert filter needle of syringe into IV bag of D5W and empty contents of syringe into bag. Protect from light. Infusion is stable for 6 hr at room temperature or 48 hr if refrigerated. ***Concentration:*** Final concentration of infusion should be 1 mg/ml; a concentration of 2 mg/ml can be used for pediatric patients or patients who cannot tolerate large volumes of fluid. ***Rate:*** Do not use an in-line filter. Infuse at a rate of 2.5 mg/kg/hr via infusion pump. If infusion exceeds 2 hr, mix contents by shaking infusion bag every 2 hr. If administering through an existing line, flush line with D5W before infusion or use a separate line.
- **Y-Site Compatibility:** anidulafungin, ertapenem.
- **Y-Site Incompatibility:** daptomycin, tigecycline, tirofiban.
- **Solution Incompatibility:** saline solutions.

Amphotericin B Liposome

IV Administration

- **Intermittent Infusion:** ***Diluent:*** Reconstitute each 50-mg vial with 12 ml of sterile water for injection to achieve concentration of 4 mg/ml. Immediately shake vial vigorously for at least 30 seconds until all particulate matter is completely dispersed. Reconstituted vials are stable for 24 hr if refrigerated. Withdraw appropriate volume for dilution into a syringe. Attach the 5-micron filter to the syringe and inject syringe contents into an appropriate volume of D5W. Infusion should be administered within 6 hr of dilution. ***Concentration:*** Final concentration of infusion should be 1–2 mg/ml; a lower concentration (0.2–0.5 mg/ml) may be used for infants and small children. ***Rate:*** Infuse over 2 hr. Infusion time may be shortened to 1 hr if patient tolerates infusion without any adverse reactions. If discomfort occurs during infusion, duration of infusion may be increased. May be administered through an in-line filter with pore diameter of at least 1 micron. If administering through an existing line, flush line with D5W before infusion or use a separate line.
- **Y-Site Compatibility:** acyclovir, anidulafungin, atropine, azithromycin, bumetanide, cefazolin, cefoxitin, ceftizoxime, ceftriaxone, cefuroxime, cimetidine, clindamycin, daptomycin, dexamethasone sodium phosphate, diphenhydramine, enalaprilat, epinephrine, ertapenem, esmolol, famotidine, fenoldopam, fentanyl, furosemide, haloperidol, heparin, hydrocortisone sodium succinate, hydromorphone, isoproterenol, ketorolac, lidocaine, linezolid, methylprednisolone sodium succinate, metoprolol, milrinone, nitroglycerin, nitroprusside, palonosetron, pantoprazole, phenylephrine, piperacillin/tazobactam, potassium chloride, procainamide, ranitidine, tacrolimus, ticarcillin/clavulanate, trimethoprim/sulfamethoxazole, voriconazole.
- **Y-Site Incompatibility:** amikacin, ampicillin, ampicillin/sulbactam, aztreonam, calcium chloride, calcium gluconate, caspofungin, cefepime, cefotaxime, ceftazidime, ciprofloxacin, cyclosporine, diazepam, digoxin, diltiazem, dobutamine, dolasetron, dopamine, doxycycline, droperidol, erythromycin, gentamicin, hydroxyzine, imipenem/cilastatin, labetalol, lorazepam, magnesium sulfate, meperidine, meropenem, metoclopramide, metronidazole, midazolam, morphine, nicardipine, ondansetron, phenytoin, potassium phosphate, prochlorperazine, promethazine, propranolol, quinupristin/dalfopristin, sodium bicarbonate, tobramycin, vancomycin, verapamil.
- **Solution Incompatibility:** Do not dilute or admix with saline solutions, other medications, or solutions containing a bacteriostatic agent.

Patient/Family Teaching

- Explain need for long duration of IV or topical therapy.
- **IV:** Inform patient of potential side effects and discomfort at IV site. Advise patient to notify health care professional if side effects occur.
- **Home Care Issue:** Instruct family or caregiver on dilution, rate, and administration of drug and proper care of IV equipment.

Evaluation/Desired Outcomes

- Resolution of signs and symptoms of infection. Several weeks to months of therapy may be required to prevent relapse.

ampicillin (am-pi-**sil**-in)

✦Ampicin, ✦Apo-Ampi, Marcillin, ✦Nu-Ampi, ✦Novo-Ampicillin, Omnipen, Penbritin, Principen, Polycillin, Totacillin

Classification
Therapeutic: anti-infectives
Pharmacologic: aminopenicillins

Pregnancy Category B

Indications

Treatment of the following infections: Skin and skin structure infections, Soft-tissue infections, Otitis media, Sinusitis, Respiratory infections, Genitourinary infections, Meningitis, Septicemia. Endocarditis prophylaxis. **Unlabeled uses:** Prevention of infection in certain high-risk patients undergoing cesarean section.

Action

Binds to bacterial cell wall, resulting in cell death. **Therapeutic Effects:** Bactericidal action; spectrum is broader than penicillin. **Spectrum:** Active against: Streptococci, nonpenicillinase-producing staphylococci, *Listeria*, Pneumococci, Enterococci, *Haemophilus influenzae*, *Escherichia coli*, *Enterobacter*, *Klebsiella*, *Proteus mirabilis*, *Neisseria meningitidis*, *N. gonorrhoeae*, *Shigella*, *Salmonella*.

Pharmacokinetics

Absorption: Moderately absorbed from the duodenum (30–50%).
Distribution: Diffuses readily into body tissues and fluids. CSF penetration is increased in the presence of inflamed meninges. Crosses the placenta; enters breast milk in small amounts.
Metabolism and Excretion: Variably metabolized by the liver (12–50%). Renal excretion is variable (25–60% after oral dosing; 50–85% after IM administration).
Half-life: Neonates: 1.7–4 hr; Children and Adults: 1–1.5 hr (increased in renal impairment).

TIME/ACTION PROFILE (blood levels)

ROUTE	ONSET	PEAK	DURATION
PO	rapid	1.5–2 hr	4–6 hr
IM	rapid	1 hr	4–6 hr
IV	rapid	end of infusion	4–6 hr

Contraindications/Precautions

Contraindicated in: Hypersensitivity to penicillins.
Use Cautiously in: Severe renal insufficiency (dosage reduction required if CCr <10 ml/min); Infectious mononucleosis, acute lymphocytic leukemia or cytomegalovirus infection (increased incidence of rash); Patients allergic to cephalosporins; OB: Has been used during pregnancy; Lactation: Is distributed into breast milk. Can cause rash, diarrhea, and sensitization in the infant.

Adverse Reactions/Side Effects

CNS: SEIZURES (high doses). **GI:** PSEUDOMEMBRANOUS COLITIS, diarrhea, nausea, vomiting. **Derm:** rashes, urticaria. **Hemat:** blood dyscrasias. **Misc:** allergic reactions including ANAPHYLAXIS and SERUM SICKNESS, superinfection.

Interactions

Drug-Drug: Probenecid decreases renal excretion and increases blood levels of ampicillin—therapy may be combined for this purpose. Large doses may increase the risk of bleeding with **warfarin**. Incidence of rash increases with concurrent **allopurinol** therapy. May decrease the effectiveness of oral **hormonal contraceptives**.

Route/Dosage

Respiratory and Soft-Tissue Infections

PO (Adults and Children ≥20 kg): 250–500 mg q 6 hr.
PO (Children <20 kg): 50–100 mg/kg/day in divided doses q 6–8 hr (not to exceed 2–3 g/day).
IM, IV (Adults and Children ≥40 kg): 500 mg to 3 g q 6 hr (not to exceed 14 g/day).

IM, IV (Children <40 kg): 100–200 mg/kg/day in divided doses q 6–8 hr (not to exceed 12 g/day).

Bacterial Meningitis Caused by *H. influenzae, Streptococcus pneumoniae*, Group B streptococcus or *N. meningitidis* or Septicemia

IM, IV (Adults): 500 mg to 3 g q 6 hr (not to exceed 14 g/day).

IM, IV (Children >1 mo): 200–400 mg/kg/day in divided doses q 6 hr (not to exceed 12 g/day).

IM, IV (Neonates ≤7 days): 200 mg/kg/day divided q 8 hr.

IM, IV (Neonates >7 days): 300 mg/kg/day divided q 6 hr.

GI/GU Infections Other Than *N. gonorrhoeae*

PO (Adults and Children >20 kg): 250–500 mg q 6 hr (larger doses for more serious/chronic infections).

PO (Children ≤20 kg): 50–100 mg/kg/day in divided doses q 6 hr.

N. gonorrhoeae

PO (Adults): 3 g with 1 g probenecid.

IM, IV (Adults and Children ≥40 kg): 500 mg q 6 hr.

IM, IV (Children <40 kg): 100–200 mg/kg/day in divided doses q 6–8 hr.

Urethritis Caused by *N. gonorrhoeae* in Men

IM, IV (Adults and Children ≥40 kg): 500 mg, repeated 8–12 hr later; additional doses may be necessary for more complicated infections (prostatitis, epididymitis).

Prevention of Bacterial Endocarditis

IM, IV (Adults): 2 g 30 min before procedure (gentamicin may be added for high-risk patients); additional 1 g may be given 6 hr later for high-risk patients.

IM, IV (Children): 50 mg/kg (not to exceed 2 g) 30 min before procedure (gentamicin may be added for high-risk patients); additional 25 mg/kg may be given 6 hr later for high-risk patients.

Renal Impairment

(Adults and Children): CCr ≤10 ml/min—Increase dosing interval to q 12 hr.

Availability

Capsules: 250 mg, 500 mg. **Suspension (wild cherry flavor):** 125 mg/5 ml, 250 mg/5 ml. **Powder for injection:** 125 mg, 250 mg, 500 mg[Rx], 1 g, 2 g, 10 g.

NURSING IMPLICATIONS

Assessment

- Assess patient for infection (vital signs, wound appearance, sputum, urine, stool, and WBC) at beginning of and throughout therapy.
- Obtain a history before initiating therapy to determine previous use and reactions to penicillins or cephalosporins. Persons with a negative history of penicillin sensitivity may still have an allergic response.
- Obtain specimens for culture and sensitivity before therapy. First dose may be given before receiving results.
- Observe patient for signs and symptoms of anaphylaxis (rash, pruritus, laryngeal edema, wheezing). Discontinue the drug and notify the physician or other health care professional immediately if these occur. Keep epinephrine, an antihistamine, and resuscitation equipment close by in the event of an anaphylactic reaction.
- Assess skin for "ampicillin rash," a nonallergic, dull red, macular or maculopapular, mildly pruritic rash.
- ***Lab Test Considerations:*** May cause increased AST and ALT.
- May cause transient decreases in estradiol, total conjugated estriol, estriol-glucuronide, or conjugated estrone in pregnant women.
- May cause a false-positive direct Coombs' test result.
- May cause a false-positive urinary glucose.

Potential Nursing Diagnoses

Risk for infection (Indications, Side Effects)
Noncompliance (Patient/Family Teaching)

Implementation

- Do not confuse with omnipen with imipenem.
- Reserve IM or IV route for moderately severe or severe infections or patients unable to take oral medication. Change to PO as soon as possible.
- **PO:** Administer around the clock on an empty stomach at least 1 hr before or 2 hr after meals with a full glass of water. Capsules may be opened and mixed with water. Reconstituted oral suspensions retain potency for 7 days at room temperature and 14 days if re-

frigerated. Combination with probenecid should be used immediately after reconstitution.

- **IM:** Reconstitute for IM or IV use by adding sterile water for injection 0.9–1.2 ml to the 125-mg vial, 0.9–1.9 ml to the 250-mg vial, 1.2–1.8 ml to the 500-mg vial, 2.4–7.4 ml to the 1-g vial, and 6.8 ml to the 2-g vial.

IV Administration

- **Direct IV:** ***Diluent:*** Add 5 ml of sterile water for injection to each 125-, 250-, or 500-mg vial or at least 7.4–10 ml of diluent to each 1- or 2-g vial. Solution should be used within 1 hr of reconstitution. ***Rate:*** Doses of 125–500 mg may be given over 3–5 min (not to exceed 100 mg/min). Rapid administration may cause seizures.
- **Intermittent Infusion:** ***Diluent:*** Reconstitute vials as per the directions above. Further dilute in 50 ml or more of 0.9% NaCl, D5W, D5/0.45% NaCl, or LR. Administer within 4 hr (more stable in NaCl). ***Concentration:*** Final concentration of infusion should not exceed 30 mg/ml. ***Rate:*** Infuse over 10–15 min.
- **Y-Site Compatibility:** acyclovir, anidulafungin, bivalirudin, daptomycin, filgrastim, granisetron, heparin, levofloxacin, linezolid, milrinone, palonosetron, pantoprazole, propofol, tacrolimus, voriconazole.
- **Y-Site Incompatibility:** If aminoglycosides and penicillins must be administered concurrently, administer in separate sites at least 1 hr apart, aminophylline, amphotericin B, caspofungin, diazepam, diphenhydramine, dobutamine, dopamine, doxycycline, fenoldopam, fluconazole, ganciclovir, haloperidol, hydroxyzine, lansoprazole, lorazepam, midazolam, nafcillin, nicardipine, nitroprusside, ondansetron, penicillin G potassium, phenytoin, prochlorperazine, promethazine, protamine, quinupristin/dalfopristin, sodium bicarbonate, trimethoprim/sulfamethoxazole, verapamil.

Patient/Family Teaching

- Instruct patient to take medication around the clock and to finish the drug completely as directed, even if feeling better. Advise patients that sharing of this medication can be dangerous. Pedi: Instruct parents and caregivers not to save or use this medication for other infections.
- Advise patient to report the signs of superinfection (furry overgrowth on the tongue, vaginal itching or discharge, loose or foul-smelling stools) and allergy.
- Advise patients taking oral contraceptives to use an alternate or additional nonhormonal method of contraception while taking ampicillin and until next menstrual period.
- Caution patient to notify health care professional if fever and diarrhea occur, especially if stool contains blood, pus, or mucus. Advise patient not to treat diarrhea without consulting health care professional. May occur up to several weeks after discontinuation of medication.
- Instruct the patient to notify health care professional if symptoms do not improve.
- Patients with a history of rheumatic heart disease or valve replacement need to be taught the importance of using antimicrobial prophylaxis before invasive medical or dental procedures.
- Lactation: Small amounts of ampicillin in breast milk can cause sensitization and alter intestinal flora of the infant. Instruct patient to monitor infant for reactions and discuss with health care provider possible need to temporarily avoid breastfeeding.

Evaluation/Desired Outcomes

- Resolution of the signs and symptoms of infection. Length of time for complete resolution depends on the organism and site of infection.
- Endocarditis prophylaxis.

ampicillin/sulbactam

(am-pi-**sil**-in/sul-**bak**-tam)
Unasyn

Classification
Therapeutic: anti-infectives
Pharmacologic: aminopenicillins/beta lactamase inhibitors

Pregnancy Category B

Indications

Treatment of the following infections: Skin and skin structure infections, soft-tissue infections, Otitis media, Intra-abdominal infections, Sinusitis, Respiratory infections, Genitourinary infections, Meningitis, Septicemia.

Action

Binds to bacterial cell wall, resulting in cell death; spectrum is broader than that of penicillin. Addition of sulbactam increases resistance to beta-lactamases, enzymes produced by bacteria that may inactivate ampicillin. **Therapeutic Effects:** Bactericidal action. **Spectrum:** Active against: Streptococci, Pneumococci, Enterococci, *Haemophilus influenzae*, *Escherichia coli*, *Proteus mirabilis*, *Neisseria meningitidis*, *N. gonorrhoeae*, *Shigella*, *Salmonella*, *Bacteroides fragilis*, *Moraxella catarrhalis*. Use should be reserved for infections caused by beta-lactamase–producing strains.

Pharmacokinetics

Absorption: Well absorbed from IM sites.
Distribution: Ampicillin diffuses readily into bile, blister and tissue fluids. Poor CSF penetration unless meninges are inflamed. Crosses the placenta; enters breast milk in small amounts.
Metabolism and Excretion: Ampicillin is variably metabolized by the liver (12–50%). Renal excretion is also variable. Sulbactam is eliminated unchanged in urine.
Protein Binding: *Ampicillin*—28%; *sulbactam*—38%.
Half-life: *Ampicillin*—1–1.8 hr; *sulbactam*—1–1.3 hr.

TIME/ACTION PROFILE (blood levels)

ROUTE	ONSET	PEAK	DURATION
IM	rapid	1 hr	6–8 hr
IV	immediate	end of infusion	6–8 hr

Contraindications/Precautions

Contraindicated in: Hypersensitivity to penicillins or sulbactam.
Use Cautiously in: Severe renal insufficiency (dosage reduction required if CCr <30 ml/min); Epstein-Barr virus infection, acute lymphocytic leukemia, or cytomegalovirus infection (increased incidence of rash).

Adverse Reactions/Side Effects

CNS: SEIZURES (high doses). **GI:** PSEUDOMEMBRANOUS COLITIS, diarrhea, nausea, vomiting. **Derm:** rashes, urticaria. **Hemat:** blood dyscrasias. **Local:** pain at IM site, pain at IV site. **Misc:** allergic reactions including ANAPHYLAXIS and SERUM SICKNESS, superinfection, elevated liver enzymes.

Interactions

Drug-Drug: Probenecid decreases renal excretion and increases blood levels of ampicillin—therapy may be combined for this purpose. May potentiate the effect of **warfarin**. Concurrent **allopurinol** therapy (increased incidence of rash). May decrease the effectiveness of **hormonal contraceptives**.

Route/Dosage

Dosage based on ampicillin component.
IM, IV (Adults and Children ≥40 kg): 1–2 g ampicillin q 6–8 hr (not to exceed 12 g ampicillin/day).
IM, IV (Children ≥1 yr): 100–200 mg ampicillin/kg/day divided q 6 hr; *Meningitis*—200–400 mg ampicillin/kg/day divided every 6 hr; maximum dose: 8 g ampicillin/day.
IM, IV (Infants >1 month): 100–150 mg ampicillin/kg/day divided q 6 hr.

Renal Impairment

IM, IV (Adults, Children, and Infants): *CCr 15–29 ml/min*—Administer q 12 hr; *CCr 5–14*—Administer q 24 hr.

Availability

Powder for injection: 1.5 g (1 g ampicillin with 500 mg sulbactam), 3 g (2 g ampicillin with 1 g sulbactam), 15 g (10 g ampicillin with 5 g sulbactam).

NURSING IMPLICATIONS

Assessment

- Assess patient for infection (vital signs, wound appearance, sputum, urine, stool, and WBCs) at beginning and throughout therapy.
- Obtain a history before initiating therapy to determine previous use of, and reactions to, penicillins or cephalosporins. Persons with a negative history of penicillin sensitivity may still have an allergic response.
- Obtain specimens for culture and sensitivity before therapy. First dose may be given before receiving results.
- Observe patient for signs and symptoms of anaphylaxis (rash, pruritus, laryngeal edema, wheezing). Discontinue the drug and notify the physician or other health care professional immediately if these occur. Keep epinephrine, an antihistamine, and resuscitation equipment close by in the event of an anaphylactic reaction.
- ***Lab Test Considerations:*** May cause increased AST, ALT, LDH, bilirubin, alkaline phosphatase, BUN, and creatinine.

- May cause decreased hemoglobin, hematocrit, RBC, WBC, neutrophils, and lymphocytes.
- May cause transient decreases in estradiol, total conjugated estriol, estriol-glucuronide, or conjugated estrone in pregnant women.
- May cause a false-positive Coombs' test result.

Potential Nursing Diagnosis

Risk for infection (Indications, Side Effects)

Implementation

- **IM:** Reconstitute for IM use by adding 3.2 ml of sterile water or 0.5% or 2% lidocaine HCl to the 1.5-g vial or 6.4 ml to the 3-g vial. Administer within 1 hr of preparation, deep IM into well-developed muscle.

IV Administration

- **Direct IV:** ***Diluent:*** Reconstitute 1.5-g vial with 3.2 ml of sterile water for injection and the 3-g vial with 6.4 ml. ***Concentration:*** 375 mg ampicillin/sulbactam per ml. ***Rate:*** Administer over at least 10–15 min within 1 hr of reconstitution. More rapid administration may cause seizures.
- **Intermittent Infusion:** ***Diluent:*** Reconstitute vials as per the directions above. Further dilute in 50–100 ml of 0.9% NaCl, D5W, D5/0.45% NaCl, or LR. Stability of solution varies from 2–8 hr at room temperature or 3–72 hr if refrigerated, depending on concentration and diluent. ***Concentration:*** Final concentration of infusion should be 3–45 mg of ampicillin/sulbactam per ml. ***Rate:*** Infuse over 15–30 min.
- **Y-Site Compatibility:** anidulafungin, bivalirudin, daptomycin, fenoldopam, filgrastim, fluconazole, granisetron, hydromorphone, levofloxacin, linezolid, palonosetron, pantoprazole, tacrolimus, tirofiban, voriconazole.
- **Y-Site Incompatibility:** acyclovir, amiodarone, amphotericin B cholesteryl sulfate, caspofungin, cefotaxime, cefoxitin, ciprofloxacin, diazepam, dobutamine, doxycycline, ganciclovir, haloperidol, hydralazine, hydroxyzine, lansoprazole, lorazepam, methylprednisolone sodium succinate, midazolam, nicardipine, ondansetron, phenytoin, prochlorperazine, promethazine, protamine, quinupristin/dalfopristin, trimethoprim/sulfamethoxazole, verapamil. If aminoglycosides and penicillins must be given concurrently, administer in separate sites at least 1 hr apart.

Patient/Family Teaching

- Advise patient to report signs of superinfection (furry overgrowth on the tongue, vaginal itching or discharge, loose or foul-smelling stools) and allergy.
- Advise patients taking oral contraceptives to use an alternative or additional nonhormonal method of contraception while taking ampicillin/sulbactam and until next menstrual period.
- Caution patient to notify health care professional if fever and diarrhea occur, especially if stool contains blood, pus, or mucus. Advise patient not to treat diarrhea without consulting health care professional. May occur up to several weeks after discontinuation of medication.
- Instruct the patient to notify health care professional if symptoms do not improve.

Evaluation/Desired Outcomes

- Resolution of signs and symptoms of infection. Length of time for complete resolution depends on the organism and site of infection.

anakinra (a-na-**kin**-ra)

Kineret

Classification

Therapeutic: antirheumatics (DMARD)
Pharmacologic: interleukin antagonists

Pregnancy Category B

Indications

Reduction of the signs and symptoms of moderately to severely active rheumatoid arthritis in patients who have failed other DMARDs (may be used in combination with other DMARDs other than tumor necrosis factor [TNF] blocking agents).

Action

Blocks the destructive effects of interleukin-1 on cartilage and bone resorption by inhibiting its binding at specific tissue receptor sites. **Therapeutic Effects:** Slowed progression of rheumatoid arthritis.

Pharmacokinetics

Absorption: Well absorbed (95%) following subcut administration.
Distribution: Unknown.
Metabolism and Excretion: Unknown.
Half-life: 4–6 hr.

TIME/ACTION PROFILE (clinical response)

ROUTE	ONSET	PEAK	DURATION
Subcut	within 12 wk	unknown	unknown

Contraindications/Precautions

Contraindicated in: Active infections; Hypersensitivity; Hypersensitivity to other *Escherichia coli*-derived products.
Use Cautiously in: Other chronic debilitating illness; Underlying immunosuppression; Renal impairment; OB, Lactation, Pedi: Safety not established; Geri: May be more sensitive to toxicity due to age-related decline in renal function; increased incidence of infection in geriatric population.
Exercise Extreme Caution in: Concurrent use of TNF blocking agents such as etanercept (higher risk of serious infections).

Adverse Reactions/Side Effects

CNS: headache. **GI:** diarrhea, nausea. **Hemat:** neutropenia. **Local:** injection site reactions. **Misc:** INFECTIONS, hypersensitivity reactions (rare).

Interactions

Drug-Drug: ↑ risk of serious infection with **TNF blocking agents**, such as **etanercept**. May ↓ antibody response to and increase the risk of adverse reactions from **vaccines**; avoid concurrent administration of **live vaccines**.

Route/Dosage

Subcut (Adults ≥18 yr): 100 mg/day.

Availability

Solution for injection: 100 mg/ml in 1-ml prefilled glass syringes.

NURSING IMPLICATIONS

Assessment

- Assess patient's range of motion and degree of swelling and pain in affected joints before and periodically during therapy.
- Assess for signs and symptoms of infection (fever, elevated WBC) prior to and periodically during therapy. Anakinra should not be instituted in patients with active infections and should be discontinued if patient develops a serious infection.
- Observe patient for hypersensitivity reactions (urticaria, dyspnea, hypotension). Discontinue anakinra if severe reaction occurs. Medications (antihistamines, acetaminophen, corticosteroids, epinephrine) and equipment should be readily available in the event of a severe reaction.
- ***Lab Test Considerations:*** Monitor neutrophil count prior to and during therapy, then monthly for 3 mo and quarterly thereafter for up to 1 yr.

Potential Nursing Diagnoses

Impaired physical mobility (Indications)
Acute pain (Indications)

Implementation

- Administration of higher than recommended doses did not result in higher responses.
- **Subcut:** Administer 1 dose/day. Do not administer solutions that are discolored or contain particulate matter. Provided in single-use 1-ml prefilled glass syringes.

Patient/Family Teaching

- Inform patient of the signs and symptoms of hypersensitivity reactions and other adverse reactions. Advise patient of appropriate actions if reactions occur.
- Advise patients not to receive live vaccines during therapy with anakinra without consulting health care professional.
- **Home Care Issues:** Instruct patient and family on preparation and correct technique for administration of injection and care and disposal of equipment. Caution patients and caregivers not to reuse needles, syringes, or drug product.

Evaluation/Desired Outcomes

- Reduction of signs and symptoms and slowed progression of moderate to severe active rheumatoid arthritis.

anastrazole (a-**nass**-stra-zole)

Arimidex

Classification
Therapeutic: antineoplastics
Pharmacologic: aromatase inhibitors

Pregnancy Category D

Indications

Postmenopausal hormone receptor-positive or unknown, locally advanced, or metastatic breast cancer. Advanced postmenopausal breast cancer in with disease progression despite tamoxifen therapy.

Action
Inhibits the enzyme aromatase, which is partially responsible for conversion of precursors to estrogen. **Therapeutic Effects:** Lowers levels of circulating estrogen, which may halt progression of estrogen-sensitive breast cancer.

Pharmacokinetics
Absorption: 83–85% absorbed following oral administration.
Distribution: Unknown.
Metabolism and Excretion: 85% metabolized by the liver; 11% excreted renally.
Half-life: 50 hr.

TIME/ACTION PROFILE (lowering of serum estradiol)

ROUTE	ONSET	PEAK	DURATION
PO	within 24 hr	14 days	6 days†

†Following cessation of therapy

Contraindications/Precautions
Contraindicated in: OB: Potential harm to fetus or spontaneous abortion.
Use Cautiously in: Women with childbearing potential; Lactation, Pedi: Safety not established.

Adverse Reactions/Side Effects
CNS: headache, weakness, dizziness. **EENT:** pharyngitis. **Resp:** dyspnea, increased cough. **CV:** peripheral edema. **GI:** nausea, abdominal pain, anorexia, constipation, diarrhea, dry mouth, vomiting. **GU:** pelvic pain, vaginal bleeding, vaginal dryness. **Derm:** rash, including mucocutaneous disorders, sweating. **Metab:** weight gain. **MS:** back pain, bone pain. **Neuro:** paresthesia. **Misc:** allergic reactions including ANGIOEDEMA, URTICARIA, and ANAPHYLAXIS, hot flashes, pain.

Interactions
Drug-Drug: None significant.

Route/Dosage
PO (Adults): 1 mg daily.

Availability
Tablets: 1 mg. **Cost:** $795.94/90.

NURSING IMPLICATIONS

Assessment
- Assess patient for pain and other side effects periodically during therapy.
- ***Lab Test Considerations:*** May cause ↑ GTT, AST, ALT, alkaline phosphatase, total cholesterol, and LDL cholesterol levels.

Potential Nursing Diagnoses
Acute pain (Side Effects)

Implementation
- **PO:** Take medication consistently with regard to food.

Patient/Family Teaching
- Instruct patient to take medication as directed.
- Inform patient of potential for adverse reactions and advise her to notify health care professional if side effects are problematic.
- Advise patient that vaginal bleeding may occur during first few weeks after changing over from other hormonal therapy. Continued bleeding should be evaluated.
- Teach patient to report increase in pain so treatment can be initiated.

Evaluation/Desired Outcomes
- Slowing of disease progression in women with advanced breast cancer.

ANGIOTENSIN-CONVERTING ENZYME (ACE) INHIBITORS

benazepril (ben-**aye**-ze-pril)
Lotensin

captopril (**kap**-toe-pril)
Capoten

enalapril/enalaprilat
(e-**nal**-a-pril/e-**nal**-a-pril-at)
Vasotec, Vasotec IV

fosinopril (foe-**sin**-oh-pril)
Monopril

lisinopril (lyse-**in**-oh-pril)
Prinivil, Zestril

moexipril (moe-**eks**-i-pril)
Univasc

perindopril (pe-**rin**-do-pril)
Aceon, ✤Coversyl

quinapril (**kwin**-a-pril)
Accupril

ramipril (ra-**mi**-pril)
Altace

trandolapril (tran-**doe**-la-pril)
Mavik

Classification
Therapeutic: antihypertensives
Pharmacologic: ACE inhibitors

Pregnancy Category C (first trimester), D (second and third trimesters)

Indications
Alone or with other agents in the management of hypertension. **Captopril, enalapril, fosinopril, lisinopril, quinapril, ramipril, trandolapril:** Management of CHF. **Captopril, lisinopril, ramipril, trandolapril:** Reduction of risk of death or development of CHF following MI. **Enalapril:** Slowed progression of left ventricular dysfunction into overt heart failure. **Ramipril:** Reduction of the risk of MI, stroke, and death from cardiovascular disease in patients at risk (>55 years old with a history of CAD, stroke, peripheral vascular disease, or diabetes with another cardiovascular risk factor). **Captopril:** Decreased progression of diabetic nephropathy. **Perindopril:** Reduction of risk of death from cardiovascular causes or non-fatal MI in patients with stable CAD.

Action
ACE inhibitors block the conversion of angiotensin I to the vasoconstrictor angiotensin II. ACE inhibitors also prevent the degradation of bradykinin and other vasodilatory prostaglandins. ACE inhibitors also increase plasma renin levels and reduce aldosterone levels. Net result is systemic vasodilation. **Therapeutic Effects:** Lowering of blood pressure in hypertensive patients. Improved symptoms in patients with CHF (selected agents only). Decreased development of overt heart failure (enalapril only). Improved survival and reduced development of overt CHF after MI (selected agents only). Decreased risk of death from cardiovascular causes or MI in patients with stable CAD (perindopril only). Decreased risk of MI, stroke, or death from cardiovascular causes in high-risk patients (ramipril only). Decreased progression of diabetic nephropathy (captopril only).

Pharmacokinetics
Absorption: *Benazepril*—37% absorbed after oral administration. *Captopril*—60–75% absorbed after oral administration (↓ by food). *Enalapril*—55–75% absorbed after oral administration. *Enalaprilat*—IV administration results in complete bioavailability. *Fosinopril*—36% absorbed after oral administration. *Lisinopril*—25% absorbed after oral administration (much variability). *Moexipril*—13% bioavailability as moexiprilat after oral administration (↓ by food). *Perindopril*—25% bioavailability as perindoprilat after oral administration. *Quinapril*—60% absorbed after oral administration (high-fat meal may ↓ absorption). *Ramipril*—50–60% absorbed after oral administration. *Trandolapril*—70% bioavailability as trandolaprilat after oral administration.
Distribution: All ACE inhibitors cross the placenta. *Benazepril, captopril, enalapril, fosinopril, quinapril,* and *trandolapril*—Enter breast milk. *Lisinopril*—Minimal penetration of CNS. *Ramipril*—Probably does not enter breast milk. *Trandolapril*—Enters breast milk.
Protein Binding: *Benazepril*—95%, *Fosinopril*—99.4%, *Moexipril*—90%, *Quinapril*—97%.
Metabolism and Excretion: *Benazepril*—Converted by the liver to benazeprilat, the active metabolite. 20% excreted by kidneys; 11–12% nonrenal (biliary elimination). *Captopril*—50% metabolized by the liver to inactive compounds, 50% excreted unchanged by the kidneys. *Enalapril, enalaprilat*—Enalapril is converted by the liver to enalaprilat, the active metabolite; primarily eliminated by the kidneys. *Fosinopril*—Converted by the liver and GI mucosa to fosinoprilat, the active metabolite—50% excreted in urine, 50% in feces. *Lisinopril*—100% eliminated by the kidneys. *Moexipril*—Converted by liver and GI mucosa to moexiprilat, the active metabolite; 13% excreted in urine, 53% in feces. *Perindopril*—Converted by the liver to perindoprilat, the active metabolite; primarily excreted in urine. *Quinapril*—Converted by the liver, GI mucosa, and tissue to quinaprilat, the active metabolite: 96% eliminated by the kidneys. *Ramipril*—Converted by the liver to ramiprilat, the active metabolite; 60% excreted in urine, 40% in feces. *Trandolapril*—Converted by the liver to trandolaprilat, the active metabolite; 33% excreted in urine, 66% in feces.
Half-life: *Benazeprilat*—10–11 hr. *Captopril*—2 hr (increased in renal impairment). *Enalapril*—2 hr (increased in renal impairment). *Enalaprilat*—35–38 hr (increased in

renal impairment). *Fosinoprilat*—12 hr. *Lisinopril*—12 hr (increased in renal impairment). *Moexiprilat*—2–9 hr (increased in renal impairment). *Perindoprilat*—3–10 hr (increased in renal impairment). *Quinaprilat*—3 hr (increased in renal impairment). *Ramiprilat*—13–17 hr (increased in renal impairment). *Trandolaprilat*—10 hr (increased in renal impairment).

TIME/ACTION PROFILE (effect on blood pressure—single dose†)

ROUTE	ONSET	PEAK	DURATION
Benazepril	within 1 hr	2–4 hr	24 hr
Captopril	15–60 min	60–90 min	6–12 hr
Enalapril PO	1 hr	4–8 hr	12–24 hr
Enalapril IV	15 min	1–4 hr	4–6 hr
Fosinopril	within 1 hr	2–6 hr	24 hr
Lisinopril	1 hr	6 hr	24 hr
Moexipril	within 1 hr	3–6 hr	up to 24 hr
Perindoprilat	within 1–2 hr	3–7 hr	up to 24 hr
Quinapril	within 1 hr	2–4 hr	up to 24 hr
Ramipril	within 1–2 hr	3–6 hr	24 hr
Trandolapril	within 1–2 hr	4–10 hr	up to 24 hr

†Full effects may not be noted for several weeks

Contraindications/Precautions

Contraindicated in: Hypersensitivity; History of angioedema with previous use of ACE inhibitors; OB: Can cause injury or death of fetus; Lactation: Certain ACE inhibitors appear in breast milk; discontinue drug or use formula.

Use Cautiously in: Renal impairment, hepatic impairment, hypovolemia, hyponatremia, concurrent diuretic therapy; Black patients with hypertension (monotherapy less effective, may require additional therapy; higher risk of angioedema); Women of childbearing potential; Surgery/anesthesia (hypotension may be exaggerated); Pedi: Safety not established for most agents; benazepril, fosinopril, and lisinopril may be used in children ≥6 yr (captopril and enalapril may be used in children of all ages); Geri: Initial dosage reduction recommended for most agents due to age-related decline in renal function.

Exercise Extreme Caution in: Family history of angioedema.

Adverse Reactions/Side Effects

CNS: dizziness, drowsiness, fatigue, headache, insomnia, vertigo, weakness. **Resp:** cough, dyspnea. **CV:** hypotension, chest pain, edema, tachycardia. **Endo:** hyperuricemia. **GI:** taste disturbances, abdominal pain, anorexia, constipation, diarrhea, nausea, vomiting. **GU:** erectile dysfunction, proteinuria, renal dysfunction, renal failure. **Derm:** flushing, pruritis, rashes. **F and E:** hyperkalemia. **Hemat:** AGRANULOCYTOSIS, neutropenia (captopril only). **MS:** back pain, muscle cramps, myalgia. **Misc:** ANGIOEDEMA, fever.

Interactions

Drug-Drug: Excessive hypotension may occur with concurrent use of **diuretics** and other **antihypertensives**. ↑ risk of hyperkalemia with concurrent use of **potassium supplements**, **potassium-sparing diuretics**, **potassium-containing salt substitutes**, or **angiotensin II receptor antagonists**. Antihypertensive response may be ↓ by **NSAIDs**. Absorption of fosinopril may be ↓ by **antacids** (separate administration by 1–2 hr). ↑ levels and may ↑ risk of **lithium** toxicity. Quinapril may ↓ absorption of **tetracycline**, **doxycycline**, and **fluoroquinolones** (because of magnesium in tablets).

Drug-Food: Food significantly ↓ absorption of captopril and moexipril (administer drugs 1 hr before meals).

Route/Dosage

Benazepril

PO (Adults): 10 mg once daily; increase gradually to maintenance dose of 20–40 mg/day in 1–2 divided doses (begin with 5 mg/day in patients receiving diuretics).

PO (Children ≥6 yr): 0.2 mg/kg once daily; may be titrated up to 0.6 mg/kg/day (or 40 mg/day).

Renal Impairment

PO (Adults): *CCr <30 ml/min*—Initiate therapy with 5 mg once daily.

Renal Impairment

PO (Children ≥6 yr): *CCr <30 ml/min*—Contraindicated.

Captopril

PO (Adults): *Hypertension*—12.5–25 mg 2–3 times daily, may be increased at 1–2 wk intervals up to 150 mg 3 times daily (begin with 6.25–12.5 mg 2–3 times daily in patients receiving diuretics) (maximum dose = 450 mg/day). *CHF*—25 mg 3 times daily (6.25–12.5 mg 3 times daily in patients who have been vigorously diuresed); titrated up to target dose of 50 mg 3 times daily. *Post-MI*—6.25-mg test dose, followed by 12.5 mg 3 times daily, may be increased up to 50 mg 3 times daily. *Diabetic nephropathy*—25 mg 3 times daily.

PO (Children): *CHF*—0.3 mg/kg–0.5 mg/kg/dose 3 times daily, titrate up to a maximum of 6 mg/kg/day in 2–4 divided doses; *Older Children:* 6.25–12.5 mg/dose q 12–24 hr, titrate up to a maximum of 6 mg/kg/day in 2–4 divided doses.
PO (Infants): *CHF*—0.15–0.3 mg/kg/dose; titrate up to a maximum of 6 mg/kg/day in 1–4 divided doses.
PO (Neonates): *CHF*—0.05–0.1 mg/kg/dose q 8–24 hr; may increase as needed up to 0.5 mg/kg q 6–24 hr; *Premature neonates:* 0.01 mg/kg/dose q 8–12 hr.

Renal Impairment
PO (Adults): *CCr 10–50 ml/min*—Administer 75% of dose; *CCr <10 ml/min*—Administer 50% of dose.

Enalapril/Enalaprilat

PO (Adults): *Hypertension*—2.5–5 mg once daily, increase as required up to 40 mg/day in 1–2 divided doses (initiate therapy at 2.5 mg once daily in patients receiving diuretics). *CHF*—2.5 mg 1–2 times daily, titrated up to target dose of 10 mg twice daily; begin with 2.5 mg once daily in patients with hyponatremia (serum sodium <130 mEq/L). *Asymptomatic left ventricular dysfunction*—2.5 mg twice daily, titrated up to a target dose of 10 mg twice daily.
PO (Children and Neonates): *Hypertension*—0.1 mg/kg/day q 12–24 hr (once a day in neonates); may be slowly titrated up to a maximum of 0.5 mg/kg/day.
IV (Adults): *Hypertension*—0.625–1.25 mg (0.625 mg if receiving diuretics) q 6 hr; can be titrated up to 5 mg q 6 hr.
IV (Children and Neonates): *Hypertension*—5–10 mcg/kg/dose given q 8–24 hr.

Renal Impairment
PO, IV (Adults): *Hypertension CCr 10–50 ml/min*—Administer 75% of dose; *CCr <10 ml/min*—Administer 50% of dose.

Renal Impairment
PO, IV (Children and Neonates): *CCr <30 ml/min*—Contraindicated.

Fosinopril

PO (Adults): *Hypertension*—10 mg once daily, may be increased as required up to 80 mg/day. *CHF*—10 mg once daily (5 mg once daily in patients who have been vigorously diuresed); may be increased over several weeks up to 40 mg/day.
PO (Children ≥6 yr and >50 kg): *Hypertension*—5–10 mg once daily.

Lisinopril

PO (Adults): *Hypertension*—10 mg once daily, can be increased up to 20–40 mg/day (initiate therapy at 5 mg/day in patients receiving diuretics). *CHF*—5 mg once daily; may be titrated every 2 wk up to 40 mg/day; begin with 2.5 mg once daily in patients with hyponatremia (serum sodium <130 mEq/L). *Post-MI*—5 mg once daily for 2 days, then 10 mg daily.
PO (Children ≥6 yr): *Hypertension*—0.07 mg/kg once daily (up to 5 mg/day), may be titrated every 1–2 wk up to 0.6 mg/kg/day (or 40 mg/day).

Renal Impairment
PO (Adults): *CCr 10–30 ml/min*—Begin with 5 mg once daily; may be slowly titrated up to 40 mg/day; *CCr <10ml/min*—Begin with 2.5 mg once daily; may be slowly titrated up to 40 mg/day.

Renal Impairment
(Children ≥6 yr): *CCr <30 ml/min*—Contraindicated.

Moexipril

PO (Adults): 7.5 mg once daily, may be increased up to 30 mg/day in 1–2 divided doses (begin with 3.75 mg/day in patients receiving diuretics).

Renal Impairment
PO (Adults): *CCr ≤40 ml/min*—Initiate therapy at 3.75 mg once daily, may be titrated upward carefully to 15 mg/day.

Perindopril

PO (Adults): *Hypertension*—4 mg once daily, may be slowly titrated up to 16 mg/day in 1–2 divided doses (should not exceed 8 mg/day in elderly patients) (begin with 2–4 mg/day in 1–2 divided doses in patients receiving diuretics); *Stable CAD*—4 mg once daily for 2 weeks; may be increased, if tolerated, to 8 mg once daily; for elderly patients, begin with 2 mg once daily for 1 week (may be increased, if tolerated, to 4 mg once daily for 1 week, then, increase as tolerated to 8 mg once daily).

Renal Impairment

PO (Adults): *CCr 30–60 ml/min*—2 mg/day initially; may be slowly titrated up to 8 mg/day in 1–2 divided doses.

Quinapril

PO (Adults): *Hypertension*—10–20 mg once daily initially, may be titrated q 2 wk up to 80 mg/day in 1–2 divided doses (initiate therapy at 5 mg/day in patients receiving diuretics). *CHF*—5 mg twice daily initially; may be titrated at weekly intervals up to 20 mg twice daily.

Renal Impairment

PO (Adults): *CCr >60 ml/min*—Initiate therapy at 10 mg/day; *CCr 30–60 ml/min*—Initiate therapy at 5 mg/day; *CCr 10–30 ml/min*—Initiate therapy at 2.5 mg/day.

Ramipril

PO (Adults): *Hypertension*—2.5 mg once daily; may be increased slowly up to 20 mg/day in 1–2 divided doses (initiate therapy at 1.25 mg/day in patients receiving diuretics). *CHF post-MI*—1.25–2.5 mg twice daily initially; may be increased slowly up to 5 mg twice daily. *Reduction in risk of MI, stroke, and death from cardiovascular causes*—2.5 mg once daily for 1 wk, then 5 mg once daily for 3 wk, then increased as tolerated to 10 mg once daily (can also be given in 2 divided doses).

Renal Impairment

PO (Adults): *CCr <40 ml/min*—Initiate therapy at 1.25 mg once daily; may be slowly titrated up to 5 mg/day in 1–2 divided doses.

Trandolapril

PO (Adults): *Hypertension*—1 mg once daily (2 mg once daily in black patients); *CHF post-MI*—Initiate therapy at 1 mg once daily, titrate up to 4 mg once daily if possible.

Renal Impairment

PO (Adults): *CCr <30 ml/min*—Initiate therapy at 0.5 mg once daily; may be slowly titrated upward (maximum dose = 4 mg/day).

Hepatic Impairment

PO (Adults): Initiate therapy at 0.5 mg once daily; may be slowly titrated upward (maximum dose = 4 mg/day).

Availability

Benazepril

Tablets: 5 mg, 10 mg, 20 mg, 40 mg. ***In combination with:*** amlodipine (Lotrel) and hydrochlorothiazide (Lotensin HCT). See Appendix B.

Captopril

Tablets: 12.5 mg, 25 mg, 50 mg, 100 mg. ***In combination with:*** hydrochlorothiazide (Capozide). See Appendix B.

Enalapril

Tablets: 2.5 mg, 5 mg, 10 mg, 20 mg. ***In combination with:*** felodipine (Lexxel), hydrochlorothiazide (Vaseretic). See Appendix B.

Enalaprilat

Injection: 1.25 mg/ml.

Fosinopril

Tablets: 10 mg, 20 mg, 40 mg. ***In combination with:*** hydrochlorothiazide (Monopril-HCT). See Appendix B.

Lisinopril

Tablets: 2.5 mg, 5 mg, 10 mg, 20 mg, 30 mg, 40 mg. ***In combination with:*** hydrochlorothiazide (Prinzide, Zestoretic). See Appendix B.

Moexipril

Tablets: 7.5 mg, 15 mg. ***In combination with:*** hydrochlorothiazide (Uniretic).

Perindopril

Tablets: 2 mg, 4 mg, 8 mg.

Quinapril

Tablets: 5 mg, 10 mg, 20 mg, 40 mg. ***In combination with:*** hydrochlorothiazide (Accuretic, Quinaretic). See Appendix B.

Ramipril

Capsules: 1.25 mg, 2.5 mg, 5 mg, 10 mg. **Cost:** 1.25 mg $133.41/90, 2.5 mg $165.97/90, 5 mg $175.98/90, 10 mg $195.97/90.

Trandolapril

Tablets: 1 mg, 2 mg, 4 mg. ***In combination with:*** verapamil (Tarka). See Appendix B.

NURSING IMPLICATIONS

Assessment

- **Hypertension:** Monitor blood pressure and pulse frequently during initial dose adjustment and periodically during therapy. Notify health care professional of significant changes.
- Monitor frequency of prescription refills to determine adherence.
- Assess patient for signs of angioedema (dyspnea, facial swelling).
- **CHF:** Monitor weight and assess patient routinely for resolution of fluid overload (peripheral edema, rales/crackles, dyspnea, weight gain, jugular venous distention).
- ***Lab Test Considerations:*** Monitor BUN, creatinine, and electrolyte levels periodically.

Serum potassium, BUN, and creatinine may be ↑, whereas sodium levels may be ↓. If ↑ BUN or serum creatinine concentrations occur, dose reduction or withdrawal may be required.

- Monitor CBC periodically during therapy. Certain drugs may rarely cause slight ↓ in hemoglobin and hematocrit, leukopenia, and eosinophilia.
- May cause ↑ AST, ALT, alkaline phosphatase, serum bilirubin, uric acid, and glucose.
- Assess urine protein prior to and periodically during therapy for up to 1 yr in patients with renal impairment or in those receiving >150 mg/day of captopril. If excessive or ↑ proteinuria occurs, re-evaluate ACE inhibitor therapy.
- *Captopril:* May cause positive ANA titer.
- *Captopril:* May cause false-positive test results for urine acetone.
- *Captopril:* Monitor CBC with differential prior to initiation of therapy, every 2 wk for the first 3 mo, and periodically for up to 1 yr in patients at risk for neutropenia (patients with renal impairment or collagen-vascular disease) or at first sign of infection. Discontinue therapy if neutrophil count is <1000/mm³.

Potential Nursing Diagnoses

Decreased cardiac output (Indications, Side Effects)
Noncompliance (Patient/Family Teaching)

Implementation

- Do not confuse Lotensin (benazepril) with Loniten (minoxidil) or lovastatin. Do not confuse enalapril with Eldepryl (seligiline). Do not confuse Monopril (fosinopril) with Accupril (quinapril), minoxidil, or Monoket (isosorbide mononitrate). Do not confuse Prinivil (lisinopril) with Plendil (felodipine) or Prilosec (omeprazole). Do not confuse Accupril (quinapril) with Accutane (isotretinoin). Do not confuse Altace (ramipril) with Artane (trihexyphenidyl).
- Correct volume depletion, if possible, before initiation of therapy.
- **PO:** Precipitous drop in blood pressure during first 1–3 hr after first dose may require volume expansion with normal saline but is not normally considered an indication for stopping therapy. Discontinuing diuretic therapy or cautiously increasing salt intake 2–3 days before initiation may decrease risk of hypotension. Monitor closely for at least 1 hr after blood pressure has stabilized. Resume diuretics if blood pressure is not controlled.

Benazepril

- **PO:** For patients with difficulty swallowing tablets, pharmacist may compound oral suspension; stable for 30 days if refrigerated. Shake suspension before each use.

Captopril

- **PO:** Administer 1 hr before or 2 hr after meals. May be crushed if patient has difficulty swallowing. Tablets may have a sulfurous odor.
- An oral solution may be prepared by crushing a 25-mg tablet and dissolving it in 25–100 ml of water. Shake for at least 5 min and administer within 30 min.

Enalapril

- **PO:** For patients with difficulty swallowing tablets, pharmacist may compound oral suspension. Shake suspension before each use.

Enalaprilat

IV Administration

- **Direct IV:** ***Diluent:*** May be administered undiluted. ***Concentration:*** 1.25 mg/ml. ***Rate:*** Administer over at least 5 min.
- **Intermittent Infusion:** ***Diluent:*** Dilute in up to 50 ml of D5W, 0.9% NaCl, D5/0.9% NaCl, or D5/LR. Diluted solution is stable for 24 hr. ***Rate:*** Administer as a slow infusion over at least 5 min.
- **Y-Site Compatibility:** allopurinol, amifostine, amikacin, aminophylline, ampicillin, ampicillin/sulbactam, aztreonam, bivalirudin, butorphanol, calcium gluconate, cefazolin, cefoperazone, ceftazidime, ceftizoxime, chloramphenicol, cimetidine, cisatracurium, cladribine, clindamycin, dexmedetomidine, dextran 40, dobutamine, docetaxel, dopamine, doxorubicin liposome, erythromycin lactobionate, esmolol, etoposide phosphate, famotidine, fenoldopam, fentanyl, filgrastim, ganciclovir, gemcitabine, gentamicin, granisetron, heparin, hetastarch, hydrocortisone sodium succinate, labetalol, lidocaine, linezolid, magnesium sulfate, melphalan, meropenem, methylprednisolone sodium succinate, metronidazole, morphine, nafcillin,

nicardipine, nitroprusside, oxaliplatin, pemetrexed, penicillin G potassium, phenobarbital, piperacillin, piperacillin/tazobactam, potassium chloride, potassium phosphate, propofol, ranitidine, remifentanil, sodium acetate, teniposide, thiotepa, tobramycin, trimethoprim/sulfamethoxazole, vancomycin, vinorelbine.

- **Y-Site Incompatibility:** amphotericin B, amphotericin B cholesteryl sulfate, cefepime, lansoprazole, phenytoin.
- **Additive Compatibility:** dobutamine, dopamine, heparin, meropenem, nitroglycerin, nitroprusside, potassium chloride.

Lisinopril

- **PO:** For patients with difficulty swallowing tablets, pharmacist may compound oral suspension; stable at room temperature for 4 wk. Shake suspension before each use.

Moexipril

- **PO:** Administer moexipril on an empty stomach, 1 hr before a meal.

Ramipril

- **PO:** Capsules may be opened and sprinkled on applesauce, or dissolved in 4 oz water or apple juice for patients with difficulty swallowing. Effectiveness is same as capsule. Prepared mixtures can be stored for up to 24 hrs at room temperature or up to 48 hrs if refrigerated.

Patient/Family Teaching

- Instruct patient to take medication as directed at the same time each day, even if feeling well. Take missed doses as soon as possible but not if almost time for next dose. Do not double doses. Warn patient not to discontinue ACE inhibitor therapy unless directed by health care professional.
- Caution patient to avoid salt substitutes or foods containing high levels of potassium or sodium unless directed by health care professional (see Appendix L).
- Caution patient to change positions slowly to minimize hypotension. Use of alcohol, standing for long periods, exercising, and hot weather may ↑ orthostatic hypotension.
- Advise patient to consult health care professional before taking any OTC cough, cold, or allergy remedies, or other medications or herbal products.
- May cause dizziness. Caution patient to avoid driving and other activities requiring alertness until response to medication is known.
- Advise patient to inform health care professional of medication regimen prior to treatment or surgery.
- Advise patient that medication may cause impairment of taste that generally resolves within 8–12 wk, even with continued therapy.
- Instruct patient to notify health care professional if rash; mouth sores; sore throat; fever; swelling of hands or feet; irregular heart beat; chest pain; dry cough; hoarseness; swelling of face, eyes, lips, or tongue; difficulty swallowing or breathing occur; or if taste impairment or skin rash persists. Persistent dry cough may occur and may not subside until medication is discontinued. Consult health care professional if cough becomes bothersome. Also notify health care professional if nausea, vomiting, or diarrhea occurs and continues.
- Emphasize the importance of follow-up examinations to monitor progress.
- OB: Advise women of childbearing age to use contraception and notify health care professional if pregnancy is planned or suspected. If pregnancy is detected, discontinue medication as soon as possible.
- **Hypertension:** Encourage patient to comply with additional interventions for hypertension (weight reduction, low sodium diet, discontinuation of smoking, moderation of alcohol consumption, regular exercise, and stress management). Medication controls but does not cure hypertension.
- Instruct patient and family on correct technique for monitoring blood pressure. Advise them to check blood pressure at least weekly and to report significant changes to health care professional.

Evaluation/Desired Outcomes

- Decrease in blood pressure without appearance of excessive side effects.
- Decrease in signs and symptoms of CHF (some drugs may also improve survival).
- Decrease in development of overt CHF (enalapril).
- Reduction of risk of death or development of CHF following MI.
- Reduction of risk of death from cardiovascular causes and MI in patients with stable CAD (perindopril).
- Reduction of risk of MI, stroke, or death from cardiovascular causes in patients at high-risk for these events (ramipril).
- Decrease in progression of diabetic nephropathy (captopril).

ANGIOTENSIN II RECEPTOR ANTAGONISTS

candesartan (can-de-**sar**-tan)
Atacand

eprosartan (ep-roe-**sar**-tan)
Teveten

irbesartan (ir-be-**sar**-tan)
Avapro

losartan (loe-**sar**-tan)
Cozaar

olmesartan (ole-me-**sar**-tan)
Benicar

telmisartan (tel-mi-**sar**-tan)
Micardis

valsartan (val-**sar**-tan)
Diovan

Classification
Therapeutic: antihypertensives
Pharmacologic: angiotensin II receptor antagonists

Pregnancy Category C (first trimester), D (second and third trimesters)

Indications

Alone or with other agents in the management of hypertension. Treatment of diabetic nephropathy in patients with type 2 diabetes and hypertension (irbesartan and losartan only). Management of CHF (New York Heart Association class II-IV) in patients who cannot tolerate ACE inhibitors (candesartan and valsartan only) or in combination with an ACE inhibitor and beta-blocker (candesartan only). Prevention of stroke in patients with hypertension and left ventricular hypertrophy (losartan only). Reduction of risk of death from cardiovascular causes in patients with left ventricular systolic dysfunction after MI (valsartan only).

Action

Blocks vasoconstrictor and aldosterone-producing effects of angiotensin II at receptor sites, including vascular smooth muscle and the adrenal glands. **Therapeutic Effects:** Lowering of blood pressure. Slowed progression of diabetic nephropathy (irbesartan and losartan only). Reduced cardiovascular death and hospitalizations due to CHF in patients with CHF (candesartan and valsartan only). Decreased risk of cardiovascular death in patients with left ventricular systolic dysfunction who are post-MI (valsartan only). Decreased risk of stroke in patients with hypertension and left ventricular hypertrophy (effect may be less in black patients) (losartan only).

Pharmacokinetics

Absorption: *Candesartan*—Candesartan cilexetil is converted to candesartan, the active component; 15% bioavailability of candesartan; *Eprosartan*—13% absorbed after oral administration; *Irbesartan*—60–80% absorbed after oral administration; *Losartan*—well absorbed, with extensive first-pass hepatic metabolism, resulting in 33% bioavailability; *Olmesartan*—Olmesartan medoxomil is converted to olmesartan, the active component; 26% bioavailability of olmesartan; *Telmisartan*—42–58% absorbed following oral administration (bioavailability ↑ in patients with hepatic impairment); *Valsartan*—10–35% absorbed following oral administration.

Distribution: All angiotensin receptor blockers (ARBs) cross the placenta; *Candesartan*—enters breast milk.

Protein Binding: All ARBs are >90% protein-bound.

Metabolism and Excretion: *Candesartan*—Minor metabolism by the liver; 33% excreted in urine, 67% in feces (via bile); *Eprosartan*—Excreted primarily unchanged in feces via biliary excretion; *Irbesartan*—Some hepatic metabolism; 20% excreted in urine, 80% in feces; *Losartan*—Undergoes extensive first-pass hepatic metabolism; 14% is converted to an active metabolite. 4% excreted unchanged in urine; 6% excreted in urine as active metabolite; some biliary elimination; *Olmesartan*—30–50% excreted unchanged in urine, remainder eliminated in feces via bile; *Telmisartan*—Excreted mostly unchanged in feces via biliary excretion; *Valsartan*—Minor metabolism by the liver; 13% excreted in urine, 83% in feces.

Half-life: *Candesartan*—9 hr; *Eprosartan*—20 hr; *Irbesartan*—11–15 hr; *Losartan*—2 hr (6–9 hr for metabolite); *Olmesartan*—13 hr; *Telmisartan*—24 hr; *Valsartan*—6 hr.

TIME/ACTION PROFILE (antihypertensive effect with chronic dosing)

ROUTE	ONSET	PEAK	DURATION
Candesartan	2–4 hr	4 wk	24 hr
Eprosartan	1–2 hr	2–3 wk	12–24 hr
Irbesartan	within 2 hr	2 wk	24 hr
Losartan	6 hr	3–6 wk	24 hr
Olmesartan	within 1 wk	2 wk	24 hr
Telmisartan	within 3 hr	4 wk	24 hr
Valsartan	within 2 hr	4 wk	24 hr

Contraindications/Precautions

Contraindicated in: Hypersensitivity; OB: Can cause injury or death of fetus; Lactation: Discontinue drug or provide formula.

Use Cautiously in: CHF (may result in azotemia, oliguria, acute renal failure, and/or death); Volume- or salt-depleted patients or patients receiving high doses of diuretics (correct deficits before initiating therapy or initiate at lower doses); Black patients (may not be effective); Impaired renal function due to primary renal disease or CHF (may worsen renal function); Obstructive biliary disorders (telmisartan) or hepatic impairment (candesartan, losartan, or telmisartan); Women of childbearing potential; Pedi: Safety not established in children <18 yr (<6 yr for losartan).

Adverse Reactions/Side Effects

CNS: dizziness, anxiety, depression, fatigue, headache, insomnia, weakness. **CV:** hypotension, chest pain, edema, tachycardia. **Derm:** rashes. **EENT:** nasal congestion, pharyngitis, rhinitis, sinusitis. **GI:** abdominal pain, diarrhea, drug-induced hepatitis, dyspepsia, nausea, vomiting. **GU:** impaired renal function. **F and E:** hyperkalemia. **MS:** arthralgia, back pain, myalgia. **Misc:** ANGIOEDEMA.

Interactions

Drug-Drug: Antihypertensive effect may be blunted by **NSAIDs**. ↑ antihypertensive effects with other **antihypertensives** and **diuretics**. Telmisartan may ↑ serum **digoxin** levels. Concurrent use of **potassium-sparing diuretics**, **potassium-containing salt substitutes**, **angiotensin-converting enzyme inhibitors**, or **potassium supplements** may ↑ risk of hyperkalemia. Candesartan may ↑ serum **lithium** levels. Irbesartan and losartan may ↑ effects of **amiodarone**, **fluoxetine**, **glimepiride**, **glipizide**, **phenytoin**, **rosiglitazone**, and **warfarin**. **Rifampin** may ↓ effects of losartan.

Route/Dosage

Candesartan

PO (Adults): *Hypertension*—16 mg once daily; may be ↑ up to 32 mg/day in 1–2 divided doses (begin therapy at a lower dose in patients who are receiving diuretics or are volume depleted). *CHF*—4 mg once daily initially, dose may be doubled at 2-wk intervals up to target dose of 32 mg once daily.

Hepatic Impairment

PO (Adults): *Moderate hepatic impairment*—Initiate at a lower dose.

Eprosartan

PO (Adults): 600 mg once daily; may be ↑ to 800 mg/day (in 1–2 divided doses) (usual range 400–800 mg/day).

Renal Impairment

PO (Adults): *CCr <60 ml/min* —Do not exceed 600 mg/day.

Irbesartan

PO (Adults): *Hypertension*—150 mg once daily; may be increased to 300 mg once daily. Initiate therapy at 75 mg once daily in patients who are receiving diuretics or are volume depleted. *Type 2 diabetic nephropathy*—300 mg once daily.

Losartan

PO (Adults): *Hypertension*—50 mg once daily initially (range 25–100 mg/day as a single daily dose or 2 divided doses) (initiate therapy at 25 mg once daily in patients who are receiving diuretics or are volume depleted). *Prevention of stroke in patients with hypertension and left ventricular hypertrophy*—50 mg once daily initially; hydrochlorothiazide 12.5 mg once daily should be added and/or dose of losartan increased to 100 mg once daily followed by an increase in hydrochlorothiazide to 25 mg once daily based on blood pressure response. *Type 2 diabetic nephropathy*—50 mg once daily; may increase to 100 mg once daily; depending on blood pressure response.

Hepatic Impairment

PO (Adults): 25 mg once daily initially; may be increased as tolerated.

PO (Children >6 yr): *Hypertension*—0.7 mg/kg once daily (up to 50 mg/day); may be titrated up to 1.4 mg/kg/day (or 100 mg/day).

Renal Impairment

PO (Children >6 yr): *CCr <30 ml/min* —Contraindicated.

Olmesartan

PO (Adults): 20 mg once daily; may be ↑ up to 40 mg once daily (patients who are receiving diuretics or are volume-depleted should be started on lower doses).

Telmisartan

PO (Adults): 40 mg once daily (volume-depleted patients should start with 20 mg once daily); may be titrated up to 80 mg/day.

Valsartan

PO (Adults): *Hypertension*—80 mg or 160 mg once daily initially in patients who are not volume-depleted; may be increased to 320 mg once daily; *CHF*–40 mg twice daily, may be titrated up to target dose of 160 mg twice daily as tolerated; *Post-MI*—20 mg twice daily (may be initiated ≥12 hr after MI); dose may be titrated up to target dose of 160 mg twice daily, as tolerated.

Availability

Candesartan

Tablets: 4 mg, 8 mg, 16 mg, 32 mg. **Cost:** 4 mg \$154.54/90, 8 mg \$155.97/90, 16 mg \$155.97/90, 32 mg \$215.96/90. ***In combination with:*** hydrochlorothiazide (Atacand HCT; see Appendix B).

Eprosartan

Tablets: 400 mg, 600 mg. ***In combination with:*** hydrochlorothiazide (Teveten HCT; see Appendix B).

Irbesartan

Tablets: 75 mg, 150 mg, 300 mg. **Cost:** 75 mg \$149.97/90, 150 mg \$165.97/90, 300 mg \$199.97/90. ***In combination with:*** hydrochlorothiazide (Avalide; see Appendix B).

Losartan

Tablets: 25 mg, 50 mg, 100 mg. **Cost:** 25 mg \$157.96/90, 50 mg \$162.98/90, 100 mg \$219.97/90. ***In combination with:*** hydrochlorothiazide (Hyzaar; see Appendix B).

Olmesartan

Tablets: 5 mg, 20 mg, 40 mg. **Cost:** 5 mg \$149.97/90, 20 mg \$153.50/90, 40 mg \$179.96/90. ***In combination with:*** hydrochlorothiazide (Benicar HCT; see Appendix B).

Telmisartan

Tablets: 20 mg, 40 mg, 80 mg. **Cost:** 20 mg \$50.32/28, 40 mg \$58.99/30, 80 mg \$65.99/30. ***In combination with:*** hydrochlorothiazide (Micardis HCT; see Appendix B).

Valsartan

Tablets: 40 mg, 80 mg, 160 mg, 320 mg. **Cost:** 40 mg \$151.97/90, 80 mg \$179.97/90, 160 mg \$179.97/90, 320 mg \$261.95/90. ***In combination with:*** amlodipine (Exforge); hydrochlorothiazide (Diovan HCT; See Appendix B).

NURSING IMPLICATIONS

Assessment

- Assess blood pressure (lying, sitting, standing) and pulse periodically during therapy. Notify health care professional of significant changes.
- Monitor frequency of prescription refills to determine adherence.
- Assess patient for signs of angioedema (dyspnea, facial swelling). May rarely cause angioedema.
- **CHF:** Monitor daily weight and assess patient routinely for resolution of fluid overload (peripheral edema, rales/crackles, dyspnea, weight gain, jugular venous distention).
- ***Lab Test Considerations:*** Monitor renal function and electrolyte levels periodically. Serum potassium, BUN, and serum creatinine may be ↑.
- May cause ↑ AST, ALT, and serum bilirubin (candesartan and olmesartan only).
- May cause ↑ uric acid, slight ↓ in hemoglobin and hematocrit, neutropenia, and thrombocytopenia.

Potential Nursing Diagnoses

Risk for injury (Adverse Reactions)
Noncompliance (Patient/Family Teaching)

Implementation

- Do not confuse valsartan with losartan.
- Correct volume depletion, if possible, prior to initiation of therapy.
- **PO:** May be administered without regard to meals.

Losartan

- **PO:** For patients with difficulty swallowing tablets, pharmacist can compound oral suspension; stable for 4 wk if refrigerated. Shake suspension before each use.

Patient/Family Teaching

- Emphasize the importance of continuing to take as directed, even if feeling well. Take

missed doses as soon as remembered if not almost time for next dose; do not double doses. Instruct patient to take medication at the same time each day. Warn patient not to discontinue therapy unless directed by health care professional.
- Caution patient to avoid salt substitutes containing potassium or food containing high levels of potassium or sodium unless directed by health care professional. See Appendix L.
- Caution patient to avoid sudden changes in position to decrease orthostatic hypotension. Use of alcohol, standing for long periods, exercising, and hot weather may increase orthostatic hypotension.
- Advise women of childbearing age to use contraception and notify health care professional if pregnancy is suspected or planned. If pregnancy is detected, discontinue medication as soon as possible.
- May cause dizziness. Caution patient to avoid driving or other activities requiring alertness until response to medication is known.
- Advise patient to consult health care professional before taking any OTC or herbal cough, cold, or allergy remedies or other medications.
- Instruct patient to notify health care professional of medication regimen prior to treatment or surgery.
- Instruct patient to notify health care professional if swelling of face, eyes, lips, or tongue occurs, or if difficulty swallowing or breathing occurs.
- Emphasize the importance of follow-up exams to evaluate effectiveness of medication.
- **Hypertension:** Encourage patient to comply with additional interventions for hypertension (weight reduction, low-sodium diet, discontinuation of smoking, moderation of alcohol consumption, regular exercise, stress management). Medication controls, but does not cure, hypertension.
- Instruct patient and family on proper technique for monitoring blood pressure. Advise them to check blood pressure at least weekly and to report significant changes.

Evaluation/Desired Outcomes
- Decrease in blood pressure without appearance of excessive side effects.
- Slowed progression of diabetic nephropathy (irbesartan, losartan).
- Decreased cardiovascular death and CHF-related hospitalizations in patients with CHF (candesartan).
- Decreased hospitalizations in patients with CHF (valsartan).
- Decreased risk of cardiovascular death in patients with left ventricular systolic dysfunction after MI (valsartan).
- Reduced risk of stroke in patients with hypertension and left ventricular hypertrophy (losartan).

anidulafungin
(a-**ni**-du-la-fun-gin)
Eraxis

Classification
Therapeutic: antifungals
Pharmacologic: echinocandins

Pregnancy Category C

Indications
Candidemia and other serious candidal infections including intra-abdominal abscess, peritonitis. Esophageal candidiasis.

Action
Inhibits the synthesis of fungal cell wall. **Therapeutic Effects:** Death of susceptible fungi. **Spectrum:** Active against *Candida albicans*, *Candida glabrata*, *Candida parapsilosis*, and *Candida tropicalis*.

Pharmacokinetics
Absorption: IV administration results in complete bioavailability.
Distribution: Crosses the placenta.
Metabolism and Excretion: Undergoes chemical degradation without hepatic metabolism; <1% excreted in urine.
Half-life: 40–50 hr.

TIME/ACTION PROFILE (blood levels)

ROUTE	ONSET	PEAK	DURATION
IV	rapid	end of infusion	24 hr

Contraindications/Precautions
Contraindicated in: Hypersensitivity.
Use Cautiously in: Underlying liver disease (may worsen); OB: Pregnancy or lactation (use only if benefits outweigh potential risk; Pedi: Safe use in children not established.

Adverse Reactions/Side Effects

Resp: dyspnea. **CV:** hypotension. **GI:** diarrhea, ↑ liver enzymes. **Derm:** flushing, rash, urticaria. **F and E:** hypokalemia.

Interactions

Drug-Drug: None noted.

Route/Dosage

IV (Adults): *Esophageal candidiasis*—100 mg loading dose on day 1, then 50 mg daily. *Candidemia and other candidal infections*—200 mg loading dose on day 1, then 100 mg daily.

Availability

Lyophilized powder for IV use (requires reconsitution): 50 mg/vial.

NURSING IMPLICATIONS

Assessment

- Assess infected area and monitor cultures before and periodically during therapy.
- Specimens for culture should be taken before instituting therapy. Therapy may be started before results are obtained.
- ***Lab Test Considerations:*** May cause ↑ ALT, AST, alkaline phosphatase, and hepatic enzymes.
- May cause hypokalemia.
- May cause neutropenia and leukopenia.

Potential Nursing Diagnoses

Risk for infection (Indications)

Implementation

- **Intermittent Infusion:** Reconstitute each 50 mg vial with 15 mL of companion diluent (20% Dehydrated Alcohol in Water for injection) for a concentration of 3.33 mg/mL. Store reconstituted solution at room temperature; do not freeze. Further dilute within 24 hr by transferring contents of reconstituted vial into IV bag containing D5W or 0.9% NaCl to provide a concentration of 0.5 mg/mL. For the 50 mg dose, dilute with 85 mL for an infusion volume of 100 mL. For the 100 mg dose, dilute with 170 mL for an infusion volume of 200 mL. For the 200 mg dose, dilute with 340 mL for a total infusion volume of 400 mL. Do not administer solutions that are discolored or contain particulate matter. ***Rate:*** Administer at a rate not to exceed 1.1 mg/min.

Patient/Family Teaching

- Explain purpose of medication to patient.
- Instruct patient to notify health care professional if diarrhea becomes pronounced.

Evaluation/Desired Outcomes

- Resolution of clinical and laboratory indications of fungal infections. Duration of therapy should be based on the patient's clinical response. Therapy should be continued for at least 14 days after the last positive culture. For esophageal candidiasis, treatment should continue for at least 7 days following resolution of symptoms.

ANTIFUNGALS (TOPICAL)

butenafine (byoo-**ten**-a-feen)
Lotrimin Ultra, Mentax

ciclopirox (sye-kloe-**peer**-ox)
Loprox, Penlac, ✤Stieprox

clotrimazole (kloe-**trye**-ma-zole)
✤Canesten, ✤Clotrimaderm, Cruex, Lotrimin, ✤Lotriderm

econazole (ee-**kon**-a-zole)
Spectazole

ketoconazole (kee-toe-**kon**-a-zole)
Extina, Nizoral, Nizoral A-D

miconazole (mye-**kon**-a-zole)
Fungoid, Lotrimin AF, ✤Micozole, Monistat-Derm, Ony-Clear, Zeasorb-AF

naftifine (**naff**-ti-feen)
Naftin

nystatin (nye-**stat**-in)
Mycostatin, ✤Nadostine, ✤Nyaderm, Nystop

oxiconazole (ox-i-**kon**-a-zole)
Oxistat

sulconazole (sul-**kon**-a-zole)
Exelderm

terbinafine (ter-**bin**-a-feen)
Lamisil AT

tolnaftate (tol-**naff**-tate)
✤Pitrex, Podactin, Q-Naftate, Tinactin, Ting

Classification
Therapeutic: antifungals (topical)

Pregnancy Category B (butenafine, ciclopirox, clotrimazole, naftifine, oxiconazole, terbinafine), C (econazole, ketoconazole, miconazole, sulconazole, tolnaftate), UK (nystatin)

Indications
Treatment of a variety of cutaneous fungal infections, including cutaneous candidiasis, tinea pedis (athlete's foot), tinea cruris (jock itch), tinea corporis (ringworm), tinea versicolor, seborrheic dermatitis, dandruff, and onychomycosis of fingernails and toes.

Action
Butenafine, nystatin, clotrimazole, econazole, ketoconazole, miconazole, naftifine, oxiconazole, sulconazole, and terbinafine affect the synthesis of the fungal cell wall, allowing leakage of cellular contents. Tolnaftate distorts the hyphae and stunts mycelial growth in fungi. Ciclopirox inhibits the transport of essential elements in the fungal cell, disrupting the synthesis of DNA, RNA, and protein. **Therapeutic Effects:** Decrease in symptoms of fungal infection.

Pharmacokinetics
Absorption: Absorption through intact skin is minimal.
Distribution: Distribution after topical administration is primarily local.
Metabolism and Excretion: Metabolism and excretion not known following local application.
Half-life: *Butenafine*—35 hr; *Ciclopirox*—5.5 hr (gel); *Terbinafine* —21 hr.

TIME/ACTION PROFILE (resolution of symptoms/lesions†)

ROUTE	ONSET	PEAK	DURATION
Butenafine	unknown	up to 4 wk	unknown
Tolnaftate	24–72 hr	unknown	unknown

† Only the drugs with known information included in this table

Contraindications/Precautions
Contraindicated in: Hypersensitivity to active ingredients, additives, preservatives, or bases; Some products contain alcohol or bisulfites and should be avoided in patients with known intolerance.
Use Cautiously in: Nail and scalp infections (may require additional systemic therapy); OB, Lactation: Safety not established.

Adverse Reactions/Side Effects
Local: burning, itching, local hypersensitivity reactions, redness, stinging.

Interactions
Drug-Drug: Either not known or insignificant.

Route/Dosage
Butenafine
Topical (Adults and Children >12 yr): Apply once daily for 2 wk for tinea corporis, tinea cruris, or tinea versicolor. Apply once daily for 4 wk or once daily for 7 days for tinea pedis.

Ciclopirox
Topical (Adults and Children >10 yr): *Cream/lotion*—Apply twice daily for 2–4 wk; *Topical solution (nail lacquer)*—Apply to nails at bedtime or 8 hr prior to bathing for up to 48 wk. Each daily application should be made over the previous coat and then removed with alcohol every 7 days; *Gel*—Apply twice daily for 4 wk; *Shampoo*—5–10 ml applied to scalp, lather and leave on for 3 min, rinse; repeat twice weekly for 4 wk (at least 3 days between applications).

Clotrimazole
Topical (Adults and Children >3 yr): Apply twice daily for 1–4 wk.

Econazole
Topical (Adults and Children): Apply once daily for tinea pedis (for 4 wk), tinea cruris (for 2 wk), tinea corporis (for 2 wk), or tinea versicolor (for 2 wk). Apply twice daily for cutaneous candidiasis (for 2 wk).

Ketoconazole
Topical (Adults): Apply cream once daily for cutaneous candidiasis (for 2 wk), tinea corporis (for 2 wk), tinea cruris (for 2 wk), tinea pedis (for 6 wk), or tinea versicolor (for 2 wk). Apply cream twice daily for seborrheic dermatitis (for 4 wk). For dandruff, use shampoo twice weekly (wait 3–4 days between treatments) for 4 wk, then intermittently.

Miconazole
Topical (Adults and Children >2 yr): Apply twice daily. Treat tinea cruris for 2 wk and tinea pedis or tinea corporis for 4 wk.

Naftifine
Topical (Adults): Apply cream once daily for up to 4 wk. Apply gel twice daily for up to 4 wk.

Nystatin
Topical (Adults and Children): Apply 2–3 times daily until healing is complete.

Oxiconazole
Topical (Adults and Children): Apply cream or lotion 1–2 times daily for tinea pedis (for 4 wk), tinea corporis (for 2 wk), or tinea cruris (for 2 wk). Apply cream once daily for tinea versicolor (for 2 wk).

Sulconazole
Topical (Adults): Apply 1–2 times daily (twice daily for tinea pedis). Treat tinea corporis, tinea cruris, or tinea versicolor for 3 wk, and tinea pedis for 4 wk.

Terbinafine
Topical (Adults): Apply twice daily for tinea pedis (for 1 wk) or daily for tinea cruris or tinea corporis for 1 wk.

Tolnaftate
Topical (Adults): Apply twice daily for tinea cruris (for 2 wk), tinea pedis (for 4 wk), or tinea corporis (for 4 wk).

Availability

Butenafine
Cream: 1%$^{Rx, OTC}$.

Ciclopirox
Cream: 0.77%. **Lotion:** 0.77%. **Nail lacquer:** 8%. **Shampoo:** 1%.

Clotrimazole
Cream: 1%^{OTC}. **Solution:** 1%^{OTC}. ***In combination with:*** betamethasone (Lotrisone). See Appendix B.

Econazole
Cream: 1%.

Ketoconazole
Cream: 2%. **Shampoo:** 1%^{OTC}. **Foam:** 2%.

Miconazole
Cream: 2%$^{Rx, OTC}$. **Lotion powder:** 2%^{OTC}. **Ointment:** 2%^{OTC}. **Powder:** 2%^{OTC}. **Spray powder:** 2%^{OTC}. **Spray liquid:** 2%^{OTC}. **Solution:** 2%^{OTC}. **Tincture:** 2%^{OTC}. ***In combination with:*** zinc oxide (Vusion). See Appendix B.

Naftifine
Cream: 1%$^{Rx, OTC}$. **Gel:** 1%^{OTC}.

Nystatin
Cream: 100,000 units/g$^{Rx, OTC}$. **Ointment:** 100,000 units/g$^{Rx, OTC}$. **Powder:** 100,000 units/g$^{Rx, OTC}$. ***In combination with:*** triamcinolone. See Appendix B.

Oxiconazole
Cream: 1%. **Lotion:** 1%.

Sulconazole
Cream: 1%. **Solution:** 1%.

Terbinafine
Cream: 1%^{OTC}. **Spray liquid:** 1%^{OTC}.

Tolnaftate
Cream: 1%^{OTC}. **Solution:** 1%^{OTC}. **Powder:** 1%^{OTC}. **Spray powder:** 1%^{OTC}. **Spray liquid:** 1%^{OTC}.

NURSING IMPLICATIONS

Assessment

- Inspect involved areas of skin and mucous membranes before and frequently during therapy. Increased skin irritation may indicate need to discontinue medication.

Potential Nursing Diagnoses

Risk for impaired skin integrity (Indications)
Risk for infection (Indications)

Implementation

- Do not confuse Lotrimin (clotrimazole) with Lotrisone (betamethasone/clotrimazole).
- Consult physician or other health care professional for proper cleansing technique before applying medication.
- Choice of vehicle is based on use. Ointments, creams, and liquids are used as primary therapy. Lotion is usually preferred in intertriginous areas; if cream is used, apply sparingly to avoid maceration. Powders are usually used as adjunctive therapy but may be used as primary therapy for mild conditions (especially for moist lesions).
- **Topical:** Apply small amount to cover affected area completely. Avoid the use of occlusive wrappings or dressings unless directed by physician or other health care professional.
- **Nail lacquer:** Avoid contact with skin other than skin immediately surrounding treated nail. Avoid contact with eyes or mucous membranes. Removal of unattached, infected nail, as frequently as monthly, by health care professional is needed with use of this medication. Up to 48 wk of daily application and pro-

fessional removal may be required to achieve clear or almost clear nail. Six months of treatment may be required before results are noticed.

- **Ciclopirox or Ketoconazole shampoo:** Moisten hair and scalp thoroughly with water. Apply sufficient shampoo to produce enough lather to wash scalp and hair and gently massage it over the entire scalp area for approximately 1 min. Rinse hair thoroughly with warm water. Repeat process, leaving shampoo on hair for an additional 3 min. After the 2nd shampoo, rinse and dry hair with towel or warm air flow. Shampoo twice a week for 4 wk with at least 3 days between each shampooing and then intermittently as needed to maintain control.
- **Ketoconazole foam:** Hold container upright and dispense foam into cap of can or other smooth surface; dispensing directly on to hand is not recommended as the foam begins to melt immediately on contact with warm skin. Pick up small amounts with fingertips and gently massage into affected areas until absorbed. Move hair to allow direct application to skin.

Patient/Family Teaching

- Instruct patient to apply medication as directed for full course of therapy, even if feeling better. Emphasize the importance of avoiding the eyes.
- Caution patient that some products may stain fabric, skin, or hair. Check label information. Fabrics stained from cream or lotion can usually be cleaned by handwashing with soap and warm water; stains from ointments can usually be removed with standard cleaning fluids.
- Patients with athlete's foot should be taught to wear well-fitting, ventilated shoes, to wash affected areas thoroughly, and to change shoes and socks at least once a day.
- Advise patient to report increased skin irritation or lack of response to therapy to health care professional.
- **Nail lacquer:** File away loose nail and trim nails every 7 days after solution is removed with alcohol. Do not use nail polish on treated nails. Inform health care professional if patient has diabetes mellitus before using.

Evaluation/Desired Outcomes

- Decrease in skin irritation and resolution of infection. Early relief of symptoms may be seen in 2–3 days. For *Candida,* tinea cruris, and tinea corporis, 2 wk are needed, and for tinea pedis, therapeutic response may take 3–4 wk. Recurrent fungal infections may be a sign of systemic illness.

ANTIFUNGALS (VAGINAL)

butoconazole
(byoo-toe-**kon**-a-zole)
Gynezole-1, Mycelex-3

clotrimazole (kloe-**trye**-ma-zole)
✤Canesten, ✤Clotrimaderm, Gyne-Lotrimin-3, Mycelex-7, ✤Trivagizole-3

miconazole (mye-**kon**-a-zole)
Monistat-1, Monistat-3, Monistat-7, Vagistat-3

nystatin (nye-**stat**-in)
Mycostatin

terconazole (ter-**kon**-a-zole)
Terazol-3, Terazol-7

tioconazole (tye-oh-**kon**-a-zole)
1–Day, Vagistat-1

Classification
Therapeutic: antifungals (vaginal)

Pregnancy Category A (nystatin), B (clotrimazole), C (butoconazole, miconazole, terconazole, tioconazole)

Indications

Treatment of vulvovaginal candidiasis.

Action

Affects the permeability of the fungal cell wall, allowing leakage of cellular contents. Not active against bacteria. **Therapeutic Effects:** Inhibited growth and death of susceptible *Candida*, with decrease in accompanying symptoms of vulvovaginitis (vaginal burning, itching, discharge).

Pharmacokinetics

Absorption: Absorption through intact skin is minimal.
Distribution: Unknown. Action is primarily local.
Metabolism and Excretion: Negligible with local application.
Half-life: Not applicable.

TIME/ACTION PROFILE

ROUTE	ONSET	PEAK	DURATION
All agents	rapid	unknown	24 hr

Contraindications/Precautions

Contraindicated in: Hypersensitivity to active ingredients, additives, or preservatives; OB: Safety not established; Lactation: Safety not established.

Use Cautiously in: None noted.

Adverse Reactions/Side Effects

GU: itching, pelvic pain, vulvovaginal burning.

Interactions

Drug-Drug: Concurrent use of vaginal miconazole with **warfarin** ↑ risk of bleeding/bruising (appropriate monitoring recommended).

Route/Dosage

Butoconazole

Vag (Adults and Children ≥12 yr): 1 applicatorful (5 g) at bedtime for 3 days (Mycelex-3) *or* one applicatorful single dose (Gynezole•1).

Clotrimazole

Vag (Adults and Children >12 yr): *Vaginal tablets*—100 mg at bedtime for 7 nights (preferred regimen for pregnancy) *or* 200 mg at bedtime for 3 nights. *Vaginal cream*—1 applicatorful (5 g) of 1% cream at bedtime for 7 days *or* 1 applicatorful (5 g) of 2% cream at bedtime for 3 days.

Miconazole

Vag (Adults and Children ≥12 yr): *Vaginal suppositories*—one 100-mg suppository at bedtime for 7 days *or* one 200-mg suppository at bedtime for 3 days *or* one 1200-mg suppository as a single dose. *Vaginal cream*—1 applicatorful of 2% cream at bedtime for 7 days *or* 1 applicatorful of 4% cream at bedtime for 3 days. *Combination packages*—contain a cream or suppositories as well as an external vaginal cream (may be used twice daily for up to 7 days, as needed, for symptomatic management of itching).

Nystatin

Vag (Adults): 100,000 units (1 tablet) daily for 2 wk.

Terconazole

Vag (Adults): *Vaginal cream*—1 applicatorful (5 g) of 0.4% cream at bedtime for 7 days *or* 1 applicatorful (5 g) of 0.8% cream at bedtime for 3 days. *Vaginal suppositories*—1 suppository (80 mg) at bedtime for 3 days.

Tioconazole

Vag (Adults and Children ≥12 yr): 1 applicatorful (4.6 g) at bedtime as a single dose.

Availability

Butoconazole

Vaginal cream: 2%Rx, OTC.

Clotrimazole

Vaginal tablets: 100 mgOTC, 200 mgOTC. **Vaginal cream:** 1%OTC, 2%OTC.

Miconazole

Vaginal cream: 2%OTC, 4%OTC. **Vaginal suppositories:** 100 mgOTC, 200 mgRx, OTC. ***In combination with:*** combination package of 3 200-mg suppositories and 2% external creamOTC; one 1200-mg suppository and 2% external creamOTC; 4% vaginal cream and 2% external creamOTC; 7 100-mg suppositories and 2% external creamOTC; 2% vaginal cream and 2% external creamOTC.

Nystatin

Vaginal tablets: 100,000 units.

Terconazole

Vaginal cream: 0.4%, 0.8%. **Vaginal suppositories:** 80 mg.

Tioconazole

Vaginal ointment: 6.5%OTC.

NURSING IMPLICATIONS

Assessment

- Inspect involved areas of skin and mucous membranes before and frequently during therapy. Increased skin irritation may indicate need to discontinue medication.

Potential Nursing Diagnoses

Risk for infection (Indications)
Risk for impaired skin integrity (Indications)

Implementation

- Consult physician or other health care professional for proper cleansing technique before applying medication.
- Nystatin vaginal tablets should be refrigerated.
- **Vag:** Applicators are supplied for vaginal administration.

Patient/Family Teaching

- Instruct patient to apply medication as directed for full course of therapy, even if feeling better. Therapy should be continued during menstrual period.
- Instruct patient on proper use of vaginal applicator. Medication should be inserted high into the vagina at bedtime. Instruct patient to remain recumbent for at least 30 min after insertion. Advise use of sanitary napkins to prevent staining of clothing or bedding.
- Advise patient to avoid using tampons while using this product.
- Advise patient to consult health care professional regarding intercourse during therapy. Vaginal medication may cause minor skin irritation in sexual partner. Advise patient to refrain from sexual contact during therapy or have male partner wear a condom. Some products may weaken latex contraceptive devices. Another method of contraception should be used during treatment.
- Advise patient to report to health care professional increased skin irritation or lack of response to therapy. A second course may be necessary if symptoms persist.
- Advise patient to dispose of applicator after each use (except for terconazole).

Evaluation/Desired Outcomes

- Decrease in skin irritation and vaginal discomfort. Therapeutic response is usually seen after 1 wk. Diagnosis should be reconfirmed with smears or cultures before a second course of therapy to rule out other pathogens associated with vulvovaginitis. Recurrent vaginal infections may be a sign of systemic illness.

apomorphine (a-po-**mor**-feen)

Apokyn

Classification
Therapeutic: antiparkinson agents
Pharmacologic: dopamine agonists

Pregnancy Category C

Indications

Acute, intermittent treatment of hypomotility, "off" episodes due to advanced Parkinson's disease.

Action

Stimulation of specific dopamine receptors improves motor function. **Therapeutic Effects:** Improved motor function.

Pharmacokinetics

Absorption: Well absorbed (100%) following subcut administration.
Distribution: Enters CSF.
Metabolism and Excretion: Unknown.
Half-life: 40 min.

TIME/ACTION PROFILE (blood levels)

ROUTE	ONSET	PEAK	DURATION
subcut	rapid	10–60 min	2 hr

Contraindications/Precautions

Contraindicated in: Hypersensitivity to apomorphine or bisulfites; Concurrent use of 5-HT_3 antagonists (granisetron, ondansetron, palonosetron, alosetron, dolasetron); Lactation: May appear in human milk; discontinue medication or discontinue breast-feeding.
Use Cautiously in: Hypokalemia, hypomagnesemia, bradycardia, congenital QTc prolongation or concurrent use of drugs causing QTc prolongation (↑ risk of serious arrhythmias); Mild to moderate renal impairment (↓ starting dose); Mild to moderate hepatic impairment; OB: Use only if clearly needed; Pedi: Safety not established; Geri: Increased risk of confusion/hallucinations, falls, and cardiac, respiratory, and gastrointestinal events.
Exercise Extreme Caution in: Cardiovascular or cerebrovascular disease (may exacerbate condition).

Adverse Reactions/Side Effects

CNS: dizziness, hallucinations, somnolence, confusion, sudden drowsiness, headache. **EENT:** rhinorrhea. **CV:** CARDIAC ARREST, chest pain, hypotension, angina, CHF, QTc prolongation. **GI:** nausea, vomiting. **GU:** priapism. **Derm:** flushing, pallor, sweating. **Local:** injection site pain. **MS:** arthralgia, back pain, limb pain. **Neuro:** aggravation of Parkinson's disease, dyskinesia. **Misc:** yawning.

Interactions

Drug-Drug: Profound hypotension, loss of consciousness occurs with **5-HT_3 antagonists.** ↑ risk of hypotension with **alcohol**, **antihypertensives**, **vasodilators**, especially **nitrates**.

Route/Dosage

Subcut (Adults): *Test dose*—0.2 mL (2 mg); with further assessment and monitoring, doses should be titrated at 0.1 mL (1 mg) less than highest tolerated dose. Doses may be increased by 0.1 mL (1 mg) every few days as an outpatient or no more frequently than every 2 hours in a supervised setting. Only single doses should be used during a particular off period. If more than one week passes between doses, titration should be restarted at the 0.2 mL (2 mg) level. Doses should not exceed 0.6 mL (6 mg).

Availability

Solution for injection (contains bisulfites): 10 mg/mL in 2 mL ampules and 3 mL glass cartridges.

NURSING IMPLICATIONS

Assessment

- Assess for nausea and vomiting; severe with recommended doses. Premedicate with trimethobenzamide or another antiemetic prior to and for at least the first 2 mo of therapy. Do not administer 5-HT_3 antagonist; results in profound hypotension and loss of consciousness.
- Monitor blood pressure standing and lying during dose titration. Orthostatic hypotension may occur any time during therapy but occurs more frequently during initial therapy or with a dose increase.

Potential Nursing Diagnoses

Risk for injury (Adverse Reactions)

Implementation

- Always prime the APOKYN pen before every injection and after loading a new cartridge.
- Never dial the dose or attempt to correct a dialing error with the BD pen needle in the skin, as this may result in an incorrect dose.
- Do not store or carry APOKYN pen with a pen needle attached. Use a new sterile BD pen needle with each injection.
- **Subcut:** Administer subcutaneously into stomach, upper arm, or upper leg. Pinch skin with finger and thumb and insert needle all the way into pinched skin. Push the injection button until a clicking sound is heard, and hold button for 5 min and gently rub injection site. Rotate site with each injection. Do not inject into skin that is red, sore, infected, or damaged. Solution should be clear and colorless; do not administer solution that is cloudy, green, or contains particles. Do not administer IV.
- Store apomorphine at room temperature. Syringes can be filled from ampules the night before and stored in the refrigerator until next day.

Patient/Family Teaching

- Provide patient and caregiver with detailed instructions on preparation and injection of dose, use of dosing pen, storage, and disposal of equipment. Advise patient to read the Patient Package Insert and Directions for Use. Medication is dosed in mL, not mg. A dose of 1 mg is represented on dosing pen as 0.1 mL (1.0 mL equals 10 mg). Caution patient that apomorphine is not used to prevent "off" episodes and does not take the place of other medications for Parkinson's disease.
- Advise patient to change positions slowly to prevent orthostatic hypotension. Caution patient to avoid drinking alcohol; will increase hypotensive effects of apomorphine.
- May cause sudden bouts of falling asleep during activities of daily living. Advise patient to notify health care professional if daytime sleepiness occurs and to avoid other medications that cause drowsiness. May require discontinuation of apomorphine. Caution patients to avoid other medications that cause sedation and to avoid driving and other activities requiring alertness until response to medication is known.
- Caution patients that hallucinations may occur.
- Advise patients to notify health care professional if pregnancy is planned or suspected or if breast feeding.

Evaluation/Desired Outcomes

- Improvement in ability to control movements when used during an "off" episode of Parkinson's disease. May improve ability to walk, talk, or move around.

aprepitant (a-prep-i-tant)

Emend

Classification

Therapeutic: antiemetics

Pharmacologic: neurokinin antagonists

Pregnancy Category B

Indications

Prevention of acute and delayed nausea and vomiting caused by initial/repeat treatment with highly emetogenic chemotherapy (with other antiemetics). Prevention of postoperative nausea and vomiting.

Action

Acts as a selective antagonist at substance P/neurokinin 1 (NK_1) receptors in the brain. **Therapeutic Effects:** Decreased nausea and vomiting associated with chemotherapy. Augments the antiemetic effects of dexamethasone and 5-HT_3 antagonists (ondansetron).

Pharmacokinetics

Absorption: 60–65% absorbed following oral administration.
Distribution: Crosses the blood brain barrier; remainder of distribution unknown.
Metabolism and Excretion: Mostly metabolized by the liver (CYP3A4 enzyme system); not renally excreted.
Half-life: 9–13 hr.

TIME/ACTION PROFILE (antiemetic effect)

ROUTE	ONSET	PEAK	DURATION
PO	1 hr	4 hr*	24 hr

*Blood level

Contraindications/Precautions

Contraindicated in: Hypersensitivity; Concurrent use with pimozide (risk of life-threatening adverse cardiovascular reactions); Lactation: May cause unwanted effects in nursing infants.
Use Cautiously in: Concurrent use with any agents metabolized by CYP3A4 (see Drug-Drug Interactions); OB: Use only if clearly needed; Pedi: Safety not established.

Adverse Reactions/Side Effects

CV: dizziness, fatigue, weakness. **GI:** diarrhea. **Misc:** hiccups.

Interactions

Drug-Drug: Aprepitant inhibits, induces, and is metabolized by the CYP3A4 enzyme system; it also induces the CYP2C9 system. Concurrent use with other medications that are metabolized by CYP3A4 may result in increased toxicity from these agents including **docetaxel**, **paclitaxel**, **etoposide**, **irinotecan**, **ifosfamide**, **imatinib**, **vinorelbine**, **vinblastine**, **vincristine**, **midazolam**, **triazolam**, and **alprazolam**; concurrent use should be undertaken with caution. Concurrent use with **drugs that significantly inhibit the CYP3A4 enzyme system** including (**ketoconazole**, **itraconazole**, **nefazodone**, **clarithromycin**, **ritonavir**, **nelfinavir**, and **diltiazem**) may ↑ blood levels and effects of aprepitant. Concurrent use with **drugs that induce the CYP3A4 enzyme system** including **rifampin**, **carbamazepine**, and **phenytoin** may ↓ blood levels and effects of aprepitant. ↑ blood levels and effects of **dexamethasone** (regimen reflects a 50% dose reduction); a similar effect occurs with **methylprednisolone** (↓ IV dose by 25%, ↓ PO dose by 50% when used concurrently). May ↓ the effects of **warfarin** (careful monitoring for 2 wk recommended), **oral contraceptives** (use alternate method), **tolbutamide**, and **phenytoin**.

Route/Dosage

PO (Adults): *Chemotherapy*—125 mg 1 hr prior to chemotherapy, then 80 mg once daily for 2 days (with dexamethasone 12 mg PO 30 min prior to chemotherapy, then 8 mg once daily for 3 days and ondansetron 32 mg IV 30 min prior to chemotherapy); *Postoperative*—40 mg given within 3 hrs prior to induction of anesthesia.

Availability

Capsules: 40 mg, 80 mg, 125 mg.

NURSING IMPLICATIONS

Assessment

- Assess nausea, vomiting, appetite, bowel sounds, and abdominal pain prior to and following administration.
- Monitor hydration, nutritional status, and intake and output. Patients with severe nausea and vomiting may require IV fluids in addition to antiemetics.
- ***Lab Test Considerations:*** Monitor clotting status closely during the 2 wk period, especially at 7–10 days, following aprepitant therapy in patients on chronic warfarin therapy.
- May cause mild, transient ↑ in AST and ALT.

Potential Nursing Diagnoses

Risk for deficient fluid volume (Indications)
Imbalanced nutrition: less than body requirements (Indications)

Implementation

- Aprepitant is given as part of a regimen that includes a corticosteroid and a 5-HT_3 antagonist (see Route/Dosage).
- **PO:** Administer daily for 3 days. *Day 1*—administer 125 mg 1 hr prior to chemotherapy. *Days 2 and 3*—administer 80 mg once in

the morning. May be administered without regard to food.

Patient/Family Teaching

- Instruct patient to take aprepitant as directed. Direct patient to read the patient package insert before starting therapy and to reread it each time the prescription is renewed.
- Advise patient to notify health care professional prior to taking any other Rx, OTC, or herbal products.
- Caution patient that aprepitant may decrease the effectiveness of oral contraceptives. Advise patient to use alternate nonhormonal methods of contraception.
- Advise patient and family to use general measures to decrease nausea (begin with sips of liquids and small, nongreasy meals; provide oral hygiene; remove noxious stimuli from environment).

Evaluation/Desired Outcomes

- Decreased nausea and vomiting associated with chemotherapy.
- Prevention of postoperative nausea and vomiting.

argatroban (ar-gat-tro-ban)

Argatroban

Classification

Therapeutic: anticoagulants
Pharmacologic: thrombin inhibitors

Pregnancy Category B

Indications

Prophylaxis or treatment of thrombosis in patients with heparin-induced thrombocytopenia. As an anticoagulant in patients with or at risk for heparin-induced thrombocytopenia who are undergoing percutaneous coronary intervention (PCI).

Action

Inhibits thrombin by binding to its receptor sites. Inhibition of thrombin prevents activation of factors V, VIII, and XII; the conversion of fibrinogen to fibrin; platelet adhesion and aggregation. **Therapeutic Effects:** Decreased thrombus formation and extension with decreased sequelae of thrombosis (emboli, postphlebitic syndromes).

Pharmacokinetics

Absorption: IV administration results in complete bioavailability.
Distribution: Unknown.
Metabolism and Excretion: Mostly metabolized by the liver; excreted primarily in feces via biliary excretion. 16% excreted unchanged in urine, 14% excreted unchanged in feces.
Half-life: 39–51 min (increased in hepatic impairment).

TIME/ACTION PROFILE (anticoagulant effect)

ROUTE	ONSET	PEAK	DURATION
IV	immediate	1–3 hr	2–4 hr

Contraindications/Precautions

Contraindicated in: Major bleeding; Hypersensitivity; Lactation.
Use Cautiously in: Hepatic impairment (↓ initial infusion rate recommended); OB: Use only if clearly needed; Pedi: Safety not established in children <18 yr.

Adverse Reactions/Side Effects

CV: hypotens. **GI:** diarrhea, nausea, vomiting. **Hemat:** BLEEDING. **Misc:** allergic reactions including ANAPHYLAXIS, fever.

Interactions

Drug-Drug: Risk of bleeding may be ↑ by concurrent use of **antiplatelet agents, thrombolytic agents**, or **other anticoagulants**.
Drug-Natural Products: ↑ bleeding risk with **anise, arnica, chamomile, clove, feverfew, garlic, ginger, ginkgo, Panax ginseng**, and others.

Route/Dosage

IV (Adults): 2 mcg/kg/min as a continuous infusion; adjust infusion rate on the basis of activated partial thromboplastin time (aPTT). *Patients undergoing PCI*—350 mcg/kg bolus followed by infusion at 25 mcg/kg/min, activated clotting time (ACT) should be assessed 5–10 min later. If ACT is 300–450 sec, procedure may be started. If ACT <300 sec, give additional bolus of 150 mcg/kg and increase infusion rate to 30 mg/kg/min. If ACT is >450 sec infusion rate should be decreased to 15 mcg/kg/min and ACT rechecked after 5–10 min. If thrombotic complications occur or ACT drops to <300 sec, an additional bolus of 150 mcg/kg may be given and the infusion rate increased to 40 mcg followed by ACT monitoring. If anticoagulation is required after surgery, lower infusion rates should be used.

Hepatic Impairment

IV (Adults): 0.5 mcg/kg/min as a continuous infusion; adjust infusion rate on the basis of aPTT.

Availability

Solution for injection (must be diluted 100-fold): 250 mg/2.5 ml vial.

NURSING IMPLICATIONS

Assessment

- Monitor vital signs periodically during therapy. Unexplained decreases in blood pressure may indicate hemorrhage. Assess patient for bleeding. Arterial and venous punctures, IM injections, and use of urinary catheters, nasotracheal intubation, and nasogastric tubes should be minimized. Noncompressible sites for IV access should be avoided. Monitor for blood in urine, lower back pain, pain or burning on urination. If bleeding cannot be controlled with pressure, decrease dose or discontinue argatroban immediately.
- Monitor for signs of anaphylaxis (rash, coughing, dyspnea) throughout therapy.
- ***Lab Test Considerations:*** Monitor aPTT prior to initiation of continuous infusion, 2 hours after initiation of therapy, and periodically during therapy to confirm aPTT is within desired therapeutic range.
- For patients undergoing PCI, monitor ACT as described in Route and Dose section.
- Assess hemoglobin, hematocrit, and platelet count prior to, and periodically during, argatroban therapy. May cause ↓ hemoglobin and hematocrit. Unexplained ↓ hematocrit may indicate hemorrhage.
- Use of argatroban concurrently with multiple doses of warfarin will result in more prolonged prothrombin time and international normalized ratio (INR) (although there is not an ↑ in vitamin K-dependent factor X_a activity) than when warfarin is used alone. Monitor INR daily during concomitant therapy. Repeat INR 4–6 hr after argatroban is discontinued. If the repeat value is below the desired therapeutic value for warfarin alone, restart argatroban therapy and continue until the desired therapeutic range for warfarin alone is reached. To obtain the INR for warfarin alone when the dose of argatroban is >2 mcg/kg/min the argatroban dose should be temporarily reduced to 2 mcg/kg/min; the INR for combined therapy may then be obtained 4–6 hr after argatroban dose was redeuced.
- ***Toxicity and Overdose:*** There is no specific antidote for argatroban. If overdose occurs, discontinue argatroban. Anticoagulation parameters usually return to baseline within 2–4 hr after discontinuation.

Potential Nursing Diagnoses

Ineffective tissue perfusion (Indications)

Implementation

- All parenteral anticoagulants should be discontinued before argatroban therapy is initiated. Oral anticoagulation may be initiated with maintenance dose of warfarin; do not administer loading dose. Discontinue argatroban therapy when INR for combined therapy is >4.

IV Administration

- **IV:** Solution is slightly viscous, clear, and colorless to pale yellow. Do not administer solutions that are cloudy or contain particulate matter. Discard unused portion
- **Direct IV:** ***Diluent:*** Bolus dose of 350 mcg/kg should be given prior to continuous infusion in patients undergoing PCI. For Diluent information, see Continuous Infusion section below. ***Rate:*** Administer bolus over 3–5 min.
- **Continuous Infusion:** ***Diluent:*** Dilute each 2.5 ml vial in 250 ml of 0.9% NaCl, D5W, or LR. Mix by repeated inversion for 1 min. Solution may show a slight haziness that disappears upon mixing. ***Concentration:*** 1 mg/ml. ***Rate:*** Based on patient's weight (See Route/Dosage section). Dose adjustment may be made 2 hr after starting infusion or changing dose until steady-state aPTT is 1.5–3 times the initial baseline value (not to exceed 100 sec).
- **Y-Site Compatibility:** atropine, diltiazem, diphenhydramine, dobutamine, dopamine, fenoldopam, fentanyl, furosemide, hydrocortisone sodium succinate, hydromorphone, lidocaine, metoprolol, midazolam, milrinone, morphine, nesiritide, nitroglycerin, nitroprusside, norepinephrine, phenylephrine, vasopressin, verapamil.
- **Y-Site Incompatibility:** amiodarone.

Patient/Family Teaching

- Inform patient of the purpose of argatroban.

- Instruct patient to notify health care professional immediately if any bleeding is noted.

Evaluation/Desired Outcomes

- Decreased thrombus formation and extension.
- Decreased sequelae of thrombosis (emboli, post-phlebitic syndromes).

aripiprazole (a-ri-**pip**-ra-zole)

Abilify

Classification

Therapeutic: antipsychotics, mood stabilizers

Pharmacologic: dihydrocarbostyril

Pregnancy Category C

Indications

Schizophrenia. Acute mania, mixed mania. Maintenance of mood stability in patients with bipolar disorder. Adjunct treatment of depression in adults.

Action

Psychotropic activity may be due to agonist activity at dopamine D_2 and serotonin 5-HT_{1A} receptors and antagonist activity at the 5-HT_{2A} receptor. Also has $alpha_1$ adrenergic blocking activity. **Therapeutic Effects:** Decreased manifestations of schizophrenia. Decreased mania in bipolar patients.

Pharmacokinetics

Absorption: Well absorbed (87%) following oral administration; 100% following IM injection.

Distribution: Extensive extravascular distribution.

Protein Binding: *aripiprazole and dehydro-aripiprazole*—>99%.

Metabolism and Excretion: Mostly metabolized by the liver (CYP3A4 and CYP2D6 enzymes); one metabolite (dehydro-aripiprazole) has antipsychotic activity. 18% excreted unchanged in feces; <1% excreted unchanged in urine. A small percentage of patients are poor metabolizers and may need smaller doses.

Half-life: *Aripiprazole*—75 hr; *dehydro-aripiprazole—94 hr.*

TIME/ACTION PROFILE (antipsychotic effect)

ROUTE	ONSET	PEAK	DURATION
PO	unknown	2 wk	unknown
IM	unk	1–3 hrs	unk

Contraindications/Precautions

Contraindicated in: Hypersensitivity; Lactation: Presumed to be excreted in breast milk; discontinue drug or bottle feed.

Use Cautiously in: Known cardiovascular or cerebrovascular disease; Conditions which cause hypotension (dehydration, treatment with antihypertensives or diuretics); Concurrent ketoconazole or other potential CYP3A4 inhibitors (reduce aripiprazole dose by 50%); Concurrent quinidine, fluoxetine, paroxetine, or other potential CYP2D6 inhibitors; Concurrent carbamazepine or other potential CYP3A4 inducers; OB: Use only if benefit outweighs risk to fetus; Pedi: Safety not established; Geri: Inappropriate use in elderly patients with dementia is associated with increased mortality.

Adverse Reactions/Side Effects

CNS: akathisia, confusion, depression, drowsiness, extrapyramidal reactions, fatigue, hostility, insomnia, lightheadedness, manic reactions, impaired cognitive function, nervousness, restlessness, seizures, suicidal thoughts, tardive dyskinesia. **Resp:** dyspnea. **CV:** bradycardia, chest pain, edema, hypertension, orthostatic hypotension, tachycardia. **EENT:** blurred vision, conjunctivitis, ear pain. **GI:** constipation, anorexia, ↑ salivation, nausea, vomiting, weight loss. **GU:** urinary incontinence. **Hemat:** anemia. **Derm:** dry skin, ecchymosis, skin ulcer, sweating. **MS:** muscle cramps, neck pain. **Neuro:** abnormal gait, tremor. **Misc:** NEUROLEPTIC MALIGNANT SYNDROME, ↓ heat regulation.

Interactions

Drug-Drug: Ketoconazole or **other potential CYP3A4 inhibitors** decrease metabolism and increase effects (reduce aripiprazole dose by 50%). **Quinidine, fluoxetine, paroxetine,** or **other potential CYP2D6 inhibitors** decrease metabolism and increase effects (reduce aripiprazole dose by at least 50%). Concurrent **carbamazepine** or **other potential CYP3A4 inducers** (double aripiprazole dose; then decrease to 10–15 mg/day when interfering drug is withdrawn).

Route/Dosage

Schizophrenia

PO (Adults): *Starting and target dose*—10 or 15 mg/day as a single dose, doses up to 30 mg/day have been used; increments in dosing should not be made before 2 wk at a given dose.
PO (Adults and Children 13–17 yrs): *Starting and target dose*—2 mg/day as a single dose, then titrated up for 5 days to a target dose of 10 mg/day.
IM (Adults): 9.75 mg/day, may use a dose of 5.25 mg based on clinical situation. May give additional doses up to 30 mg if needed for agitation.

Bipolar mania

PO (Adults): 30 mg once daily, some patients may require 15 mg/day if 30 mg/day is not tolerated.
IM (Adults): 9.75 mg/day, may use a dose of 5.25 mg based on clinical situation. May give additional doses up to 30 mg if needed for agitation.

Depression

PO, IM (Adults): 2–5 mg/day, may titrate upward at 1-wk intervals to 5–10 mg/day; not to exceed 15 mg/day.

Availability

Tablets: 2 mg, 5 mg, 10 mg, 15 mg, 20 mg, 30 mg. **Cost:** 2 mg $999.90/90, 5 mg $999.90/90, 10 mg $1,035.88/90, 15 mg $999.88/90, 20 mg $1,375.83/90, 30 mg $1,375.83/90. **Tablets, orally disintegrating:** 10 mg, 15 mg. **Oral solution (orange cream):** 1 mg/ml. **Injection:** 7.5 mg/ml in ready-to-use vials.

NURSING IMPLICATIONS

Assessment

- Assess patient's mental status (orientation, mood, behavior) before and periodically during therapy. Assess for suicidal tendencies, especially during early therapy for depression. Restrict amount of drug available to patient.
- Assess weight and BMI initially and throughout therapy.
- Obtain fasting blood glucose and cholesterol levels initially and periodically throughout therapy.
- Monitor blood pressure (sitting, standing, lying), pulse, and respiratory rate before and periodically during therapy.
- Observe patient carefully when administering medication to ensure that medication is actually taken and not hoarded or cheeked.
- Monitor patient for onset of akathisia (restlessness or desire to keep moving) and extrapyramidal side effects (*parkinsonian*—difficulty speaking or swallowing, loss of balance control, pill rolling of hands, mask-like face, shuffling gait, rigidity, tremors; and *dystonic*—muscle spasms, twisting motions, twitching, inability to move eyes, weakness of arms or legs) periodically throughout therapy. Report these symptoms.
- Monitor for tardive dyskinesia (uncontrolled rhythmic movement of mouth, face, and extremities; lip smacking or puckering; puffing of cheeks; uncontrolled chewing; rapid or worm-like movements of tongue). Notify health care professional immediately if these symptoms occur, as these side effects may be irreversible.
- Monitor for development of neuroleptic malignant syndrome (fever, muscle rigidity, altered mental status, respiratory distress, tachycardia, seizures, diaphoresis, hypertension or hypotension, pallor, tiredness, loss of bladder control). Notify health care professional immediately if these symptoms occur.
- ***Lab Test Considerations:*** May cause ↑ creatinine phosphokinase.

Potential Nursing Diagnoses

Disturbed thought process (Indications)
Imbalanced nutrition: risk for more than body requirements (Side Effects)

Implementation

- **PO:** Administer once daily without regard to meals.
- Do not open the blister until ready to administer. For single tablet removal, open the package and peel back the foil on the blister to expose the tablet. Do not push the tablet through the foil; may damage tablet. Immediately upon opening the blister, using dry hands, remove the tablet and place the entire orally disintegrating tablet on the tongue. Tablet disintegration occurs rapidly in saliva. Take tablet without liquid; but if needed, it can be taken with liquid. Do not attempt to split the tablet.
- **IM:** IM route should be used for agitation. Convert to oral dose as soon as possible. Administer IM; for dose of 5.25 mg use 0.7 mL, 9.75 mg use 1.3 mL, and 15 mg use 2 mL of aripiprazole solution. Solution should be

clear and colorless; do not administer solutions that are discolored or contain a precipitate.

Patient/Family Teaching

- Advise patient to take medication as directed and not to skip doses or double up on missed doses. Take missed doses as soon as remembered unless almost time for the next dose.
- Inform patient of possibility of extrapyramidal symptoms and tardive dyskinesia. Instruct patient to report these symptoms immediately.
- Advise patient to make position changes slowly to minimize orthostatic hypotension.
- Medication may cause drowsiness and lightheadedness. Caution patient to avoid driving or other activities requiring alertness until response to medication is known.
- Caution patient to avoid taking alcohol or other CNS depressants concurrently with this medication.
- Advise patient that extremes in temperature should be avoided, because this drug impairs body temperature regulation.
- Advise patient to notify health care professional of medication regimen prior to treatment or surgery.
- Emphasize the importance of routine follow-up exams and continued participation in psychotherapy as indicated.

Evaluation/Desired Outcomes

- Decrease in excitable, paranoic, or withdrawn behavior.
- Decrease incidence of mood swings in patients with bipolar disorders.
- Increased sense of well-being in patients with depression.

HIGH ALERT

asparaginase

(a-**spare**-a-ji-nase)

Elspar, ✤Kidrolase

Classification

Therapeutic: antineoplastics

Pharmacologic: enzymes

Pregnancy Category C

Indications

Part of combination chemotherapy in the treatment of acute lymphocytic leukemia (ALL).

Action

Catalyst in the conversion of asparagine (an amino acid) to aspartic acid and ammonia. Depletes asparagine in leukemic cells. **Therapeutic Effects:** Death of leukemic cells.

Pharmacokinetics

Absorption: Is absorbed from IM sites.

Distribution: Remains in the intravascular space. Poor penetration into the CSF.

Metabolism and Excretion: Slowly sequestered in the reticuloendothelial system.

Half-life: IV: 8–30 hr; IM: 39–49 hr.

TIME/ACTION PROFILE (depletion of asparagine)

ROUTE	ONSET	PEAK†	DURATION
IM	immediate	14–24 hr	23–33 days
IV	immediate	unknown	23–33 days

†Plasma levels of asparaginase

Contraindications/Precautions

Contraindicated in: Previous hypersensitivity; Lactation: May cause unwanted effects in the nursing infant.

Use Cautiously in: History of hypersensitivity reactions; Severe liver disease; Renal or pancreatic disease; CNS depression; Clotting abnormalities; Chronic debilitating illnesses; OB: Use only if the potential benefit justifies the potential risk to the fetus.

Adverse Reactions/Side Effects

CNS: SEIZURES, agitation, coma, confusion, depression, dizziness, fatigue, hallucinations, headache, irritability, somnolence. **GI:** nausea, vomiting, anorexia, cramps, hepatotoxicity, pancreatitis, weight loss. **Derm:** rashes, urticaria. **Endo:** hyperglycemia. **Hemat:** coagulation abnormalities, transient bone marrow depression. **Metab:** hyperammonemia, hyperuricemia. **Misc:** hypersensitivity reactions including ANAPHYLAXIS.

Interactions

Drug-Drug: May negate the antineoplastic activity of **methotrexate**. May enhance the hepatotoxicity of other **hepatotoxic drugs**. Concurrent IV use with or immediately preceding **vincristine** and **prednisone** may result in ↑ neurotoxicity and hyperglycemia. May alter the response to **live vaccines** (↓ antibody response, ↑ risk of adverse reactions).

✤ = Canadian drug name.

*CAPITALS indicates life-threatening; underlines indicate most frequent.

Route/Dosage

Various other regimens may be used.

Multiple-Agent Induction Regimen (in Combination with Vincristine and Prednisone)

IV (Children): 1000 IU/kg/day for 10 successive days beginning on day 22 of regimen.
IM (Children): 6000 IU/m^2 on days 4, 7, 10, 13, 16, 19, 22, 25, 28.

Single-Agent Therapy for Acute Lymphocytic Leukemia

IV (Adults and Children): 200 IU/kg daily for 28 days.

Desensitization Regimen

IV (Adults and Children): Administer 1 IU, then double dose every 10 min until total dose for that day has been given or reaction occurs.

Test Dose

Intradermal (Adults and Children): 2 IU.

Availability

Injection: 10,000-IU vial (with mannitol).

NURSING IMPLICATIONS

Assessment

- Monitor vital signs before and frequently during therapy. Inform physician if fever or chills occur.
- Monitor intake and output. Notify physician of significant discrepancies. Encourage patient to drink 2000–3000 ml/day to promote excretion of uric acid. Allopurinol and alkalinization of the urine may be used to prevent urate stone formation.
- Monitor for hypersensitivity reaction (urticaria, diaphoresis, facial swelling, joint pain, hypotension, bronchospasm). Epinephrine and resuscitation equipment should be readily available. Reaction may occur up to 2 hr after administration. If patient requires continued therapy, pegaspargase is an alternative.
- Assess nausea, vomiting, and appetite. Weigh weekly. An antiemetic may be given before administration.
- Monitor affect and neurologic status. Notify physician if depression, drowsiness, or hallucinations occur. Symptoms usually resolve 2–3 days after drug is discontinued.
- ***Lab Test Considerations:*** Monitor CBC before and periodically throughout therapy. May alter coagulation studies. Platelets, PT, PTT, and thrombin time may be ↑. May cause ↑ BUN.
- Hepatotoxicity may be manifested by ↑ AST, ALT, alkaline phosphatase, bilirubin, or cholesterol. Liver function test results usually return to normal after therapy. May cause pancreatitis; monitor frequently for ↑ amylase or glucose.
- Monitor blood glucose during therapy. May cause hyperglycemia treatable with fluids and insulin. May be fatal.
- May cause ↑ serum and urine uric acid concentrations.
- May interfere with thyroid function tests.

Potential Nursing Diagnoses

Risk for injury (Side Effects)
Risk for infection (Side Effects)

Implementation

- ***High Alert:*** Fatalities have occurred with chemotherapeutic agents. Before administering, clarify all ambiguous orders; double-check single, daily, and course-of-therapy dose limits; have second practitioner independently double-check original order and dose calculations. Do not confuse asparaginase with pegaspargase.
- Solution should be prepared in a biologic cabinet. Wear gloves, gown, and mask while handling medication. Discard equipment in specially designated containers. See Appendix K.
- If coagulopathy develops, apply pressure to venipuncture sites; avoid IM injections.
- **Test Dose:** Intradermal test dose must be performed before initial dose; doses must be separated by more than 1 wk. Reconstitute vial with 5 ml of sterile water for injection or 0.9% NaCl for injection (without preservatives). Add 0.1 ml of this 2000-IU/ml solution to 9.9 ml additional diluent to yield a 20-IU/ml solution. Inject 0.1 ml (2 IU) intradermally. Observe site for 1 hr for formation of wheal. Wheal is indicative of a positive reaction.
- **Desensitization Therapy:** Begin by administering 1 IU intravenously. Double dose every 10 min if hypersensitivity does not occur until full daily dose is administered.
- **IM:** Prepare for IM dose by adding 2 ml of 0.9% NaCl for injection (without preservatives) to the 10,000-IU vial. Shake vial gently. Administer no more than 2 ml per injection site.

IV Administration

- **Direct IV:** ***Diluent:*** Prepare *Elspar* IV dose by diluting 10,000-IU vial with 5 ml of sterile water for injection or 0.9% NaCl (without preservatives). If gelatinous fibers are present, administration through a 5-micron filter will not alter potency. Administration through a 0.2-micron filter may cause loss of potency. Solution should be clear after reconstitution. Discard if cloudy. Stable for 8 hr if refrigerated. Prepare *Kidrolase* for IM or IV administration by adding 4 ml sterile water to 10,000 IU vial and rotate gently to dissolve. Unused reconstituted solution is stable for 14 days if refrigerated. May be further diluted with 0.9% NaCl or D5W. ***Concentration:*** Dilute doses in 50–250 ml of diluent. ***Rate:*** Administer through Y-site of rapidly flowing IV of D5W or 0.9% NaCl over 30–60 min. Maintain IV infusion for 2 hr after dose.
- **Y-Site Compatibility:** methotrexate, sodium bicarbonate.
- **Additive Incompatibility:** Information unavailable. Do not admix with other drugs.

Patient/Family Teaching

- Instruct patient to notify health care professional if abdominal pain, severe nausea and vomiting, jaundice, fever, chills, sore throat, bleeding or bruising, excess thirst or urination, or mouth sores occur. Caution patient to avoid crowds and persons with known infections. Instruct patient to use soft toothbrush and electric razor, and to be especially careful to avoid falls. Patients should also be cautioned not to drink alcoholic beverages or take medication containing aspirin or NSAIDs because these may precipitate gastric bleeding.
- Advise both men and women not to conceive a child while taking asparaginase. Barrier methods of contraception are recommended.
- Instruct patient not to receive any vaccinations without advice of health care professional. Advise parents that this may alter immunization schedule.
- Emphasize need for periodic lab tests to monitor for side effects.

Evaluation/Desired Outcomes

- Improvement of hematologic status in patients with leukemia.

aspirin, See SALICYLATES.

atazanavir (a-ta-**zan**-a-vir)

Reyataz

Classification

Therapeutic: antiretrovirals
Pharmacologic: protease inhibitors

Pregnancy Category B

Indications

HIV infection (with other antiretrovirals).

Action

Inhibits the action of HIV protease, preventing maturation of virions. **Therapeutic Effects:** ↑ CD4 cell counts and ↓ viral load with subsequent slowed progression of HIV and its sequelae.

Pharmacokinetics

Absorption: Rapidly absorbed (↑ by food).
Distribution: Enters cerebrospinal fluid and semen.
Metabolism and Excretion: 80% metabolized (CYP3A); 13% excreted unchanged in urine.
Half-life: 7 hr.

TIME/ACTION PROFILE (blood levels)

ROUTE	ONSET	PEAK	DURATION
PO	rapid	2.5 hr	24 hr

Contraindications/Precautions

Contraindicated in: Hypersensitivity; Severe hepatic impairment; Concurrent use of ergotamine, ergonovine, dihydroergotamine, methylergonovine, midazolam, pimozide, or triazolam (potential for life-threatening toxicity); Concurrent use of rifampin, irinotecan, lovastatin, simvastatin, indinavir, proton-pump inhibitors, or St. John's wort; Pedi: ↑ risk of kernicterus in infants <3 mo.
Use Cautiously in: Mild to moderate hepatic impairment; Pre-existing conduction system disease (marked first-degree AV block or second- or third-degree AV block) or concurrent use of other drugs that increase the PR interval (especially those metabolized by CYP3A4 including verapamil or diltiazem); Diabetes melli-

tus; Hemophilia (↑ risk of bleeding); OB: Use only if clearly needed; Breastfeeding is not recommended if HIV-infected.

Adverse Reactions/Side Effects

When used in combination with other antiretrovirals.

CNS: headache, depression, dizziness, insomnia. **CV:** ↑ PR interval. **GI:** nausea, abdominal pain, ↑ bilirubin, diarrhea, jaundice, vomiting, ↑ transaminases. **Derm:** rash. **Endo:** hyperglycemia. **Metab:** fat redistribution. **MS:** myalgia. **Misc:** fever.

Interactions

Drug-Drug: Atazanavir is an inhibitor of CYP3A and UGT1A1 enzyme systems. It is also a substrate of CYP3A. ↑ levels of **ergotamine**, **ergonovine**, **dihydroergotamine**, **methylergonovine**, **midazolam**, **bepridol**, **pimozide**, **triazolam**, **lovastatin**, **simvastatin**, and **irinotecan**; concurrent use may result in life-threatening CNS, cardiovascular, hematologic or musculoskeletal toxicity and is contraindicated. Combination therapy with **tenofovir** may lead to ↓ virologic response and possible resistance (100 mg **ritonavir** should be added to boost blood levels and dose of atazanavir ↓ to 300 mg/day). Levels are significantly ↓ by **rifampin**, **proton-pump inhibitors**, and **St. John's wort**; may promote viral resistance, avoid concurrent use. Concurrent use with **indinavir** may ↑ risk of hyperbilirubinemia and should be avoided. Concurrent use with **didanosine** buffered tablets will ↓ absorption and levels; give atazanavir with food 2 hr before or 1 hr after **didanosine**. **Efavirenz** decreases levels and may promote viral resistance; 600 mg efavirenz should be given with 100 mg ritonavir to counteract this effect and ↓ dose of azatanavir to 300 mg/day. ↑ **saquinavir** levels. Levels are ↑ by **ritonavir**; ↓ atazanavir dose to 300 mg/day. **Nevirapine** may ↓ levels; avoid concurrent use. **Antacids** or **buffered medications** will ↓ absorption; atazanavir should be given 2 hr before or 1 hr after. ↑ levels of **lidocaine**, **amiodarone**, or **quinidine**; blood level monitoring is recommended. ↑ risk of bleeding with **warfarin**. ↑ of **tricyclic antidepressants**; blood level monitoring is recommended. ↑ levels of **rifabutin**; ↓ rifabutin dose by 75% (150 mg every other day or 3 times weekly). ↑ levels of **diltiazem** and its active metabolite; ↓ diltiazem dose by 50% and ECG monitoring recommended. Similar precautions may be needed with **felodipine**, **nifedipine**, **nicardipine**, and **verapamil**. ↑ levels of **fluticasone**; consider alternative therapy; should not be used when atazanavir is used with ritonavir. ↓ levels of **voriconazole** when atazanavir is used with ritonavir; avoid concurrent use. **Voriconazole** may also ↑ levels of atazanavir (when used without ritonavir). ↑ levels of **ketoconazole** or **itraconazole** when atazanavir is used with ritonavir. ↑ levels of **trazodone**; ↓ dose of trazodone. ↑ levels of **sildenafil**, **vardenafil**, and **tadalafil**; ↓ **sildenafil** dose to 25 mg every 48 hr; ↓ **vardenafil** dose to 2.5 mg every 72 hr; ↓ **tadalafil** dose to 10 mg every 72 hr. Exercise caution and monitor for hypertension, visual changes, and priapism. ↑ risk of myopathy with **atorvastatin**. Levels may be ↓ by **histamine H_2 antagonists**, promoting viral resistance; separate doses by at least 12 hr. ↑ levels of **cyclosporine**, **sirolimus**, and **tacrolimus**; monitor immunosuppressant blood levels. ↑ levels of **clarithromycin**; ↓ clarithromycin dose by 50% or consider alternative therapy. May ↓ levels of some **estrogens** found in **hormonal contraceptives**; use alternative non-hormonal method of contraception. Concurrent use of other **drugs known to ↑ PR interval**.

Route/Dosage

PO (Adults): *Therapy-naive*—400 mg once daily with food. *Therapy-experienced with prior virologic failure*—300 mg once daily with ritonavir 100 mg once daily with food *With efavirenz*—atazanavir 300 mg with ritonavir 100 mg and efavirenz 600 mg (all as single daily dose with food). *With tenofovir*—atazanavir 300 mg with ritonavir 100 mg and tenofovir 300 mg (all as single daily dose with food).

Hepatic Impairment

(Adults): 300 mg once daily.

Availability

Capsules: 100 mg, 150 mg, 200 mg.

NURSING IMPLICATIONS

Assessment

- Assess for change in severity of HIV symptoms and for symptoms of opportunistic infections throughout therapy.
- May also cause elevated liver function tests, increased creatine kinase or glucose, and neutropenia.
- Assess for rash which can occur within initial 8 wk of therapy. Usually resolves within 2 weeks without altering therapy.

A

- If pregnant patient is exposed to atazanavir, register patient in Antiretroviral Pregnancy Registry by calling 1-800-258-4263.
- ***Lab Test Considerations:*** Monitor viral load and CD4 cell count regularly during therapy.
- May cause ↑ serum amylase and lipase.
- May ↑ liver enzymes.
- May ↑ creatine kinase.
- May cause ↓ hemoglobin, neutrophils, and platelets.
- May cause ↑ in unconjugated bilirubin; reversible on discontinuation.

Potential Nursing Diagnoses

Risk for infection (Indications)
Noncompliance (Patient/Family Teaching)

Implementation

- **PO:** Administer daily with food to enhance absorption. Capsules should be swallowed whole; do not open.
- If administered with ritonavir and efavirenz, administer as one daily dose with food. Do not administer with efavirenz without also using ritonavir.
- If administered with ritonavir and tenofovir, administer as one daily dose with food. Do not administer with tenofovir without also using ritonavir.
- If administered with didanosine buffered formulations, administer atazanavir with food 2 hr before or 1 hr after didanosine.

Patient/Family Teaching

- Emphasize the importance of taking atazanavir with food as directed. Advise patient to read the Patient Information that comes with the medication each time the Rx is refilled. Atazanavir must always be used in combination with other antiretroviral drugs. Do not take more than prescribed amount and do not stop taking without consulting health care professional. Take missed doses as soon as remembered, then return to regular dose schedule. If within 6 hr of next dose, omit dose and take next dose at regular time. Do not double doses.
- Instruct patient that atazanavir should not be shared with others.
- Inform patient that atazanavir does not cure HIV or prevent associated or opportunistic infections. Atazanavir does not reduce the risk of transmission of HIV to others through sexual contact or blood contamination. Caution patient to use a condom and to avoid sharing needles or donating blood to prevent spreading the HIV virus to others. Advise patient that atazanavir may cause lipodystrophy (redistribution or accumulation of body fat) and the long-term effects of atazanavir are unknown at this time.
- Instruct patient to consult health care professional before taking other Rx, OTC, or herbal products, especially St. John's wort; interactions may be fatal.
- May cause dizziness. Caution patient to notify health care professional if this occurs and to avoid driving and other activities requiring alertness until response to medication is known.
- Notify health care professional immediately if yellowing of eyes, change in heart rhythm, or high blood sugar occur.
- Emphasize the importance of regular follow-up exams and blood counts to determine progress and monitor for side effects.
- Instruct females using hormonal contraceptives to use an alternative non-hormonal method of contraception.
- OB, Lactation: Advise patient to notify health care professional if pregnancy is planned or suspected or if breastfeeding.

Evaluation/Desired Outcomes

- Delayed progression of HIV and decreased opportunistic infections in patients with HIV.
- Decrease in viral load and increase in CD4 cell counts.

atenolol (a-**ten**-oh-lole)

✤Apo-Atenolol, ✤Novo-Atenolol, Tenormin

Classification

Therapeutic: antianginals, antihypertensives

Pharmacologic: beta blockers

Pregnancy Category D

Indications

Management of hypertension. Management of angina pectoris. Prevention of MI.

Action

Blocks stimulation of $beta_1$ (myocardial)-adrenergic receptors. Does not usually affect

$beta_2$ (pulmonary, vascular, uterine)-receptor sites. **Therapeutic Effects:** Decreased blood pressure and heart rate. Decreased frequency of attacks of angina pectoris. Prevention of MI.

Pharmacokinetics

Absorption: 50–60% absorbed after oral administration.

Distribution: Minimal penetration of CNS. Crosses the placenta and enters breast milk.

Metabolism and Excretion: 40–50% excreted unchanged by the kidneys; remainder excreted in feces as unabsorbed drug.

Half-life: 6–9 hr.

TIME/ACTION PROFILE (cardiovascular effects)

ROUTE	ONSET	PEAK	DURATION
PO	1 hr	2–4 hr	24 hr
IV	rapid	5 min	unknown

Contraindications/Precautions

Contraindicated in: Uncompensated CHF; Pulmonary edema; Cardiogenic shock; Bradycardia or heart block.

Use Cautiously in: Renal impairment (dosage reduction recommended if CCr ≤35 ml/min); Hepatic impairment; Geriatric patients (increased sensitivity to beta blockers; initial dosage reduction recommended); Pulmonary disease (including asthma; beta selectivity may be lost at higher doses); Diabetes mellitus (may mask signs of hypoglycemia); Thyrotoxicosis (may mask symptoms); Patients with a history of severe allergic reactions (intensity of reactions may be increased); OB: Crosses the placenta and may cause fetal/neonatal bradycardia, hypotension, hypoglycemia, or respiratory depression; Lactation, Pedi: Safety not established.

Adverse Reactions/Side Effects

CNS: fatigue, weakness, anxiety, depression, dizziness, drowsiness, insomnia, memory loss, mental status changes, nervousness, nightmares. **EENT:** blurred vision, stuffy nose. **Resp:** bronchospasm, wheezing. **CV:** BRADYCARDIA, CHF, PULMONARY EDEMA, hypotension, peripheral vasoconstriction. **GI:** constipation, diarrhea, liver function abnormalities, nausea, vomiting. **GU:** erectile dysfunction, decreased libido, urinary frequency. **Derm:** rashes. **Endo:** hyperglycemia, hypoglycemia. **MS:** arthralgia, back pain, joint pain. **Misc:** drug-induced lupus syndrome.

Interactions

Drug-Drug: General anesthesia, **IV phenytoin** and **verapamil** may cause additive myocardial depression. Additive bradycardia may occur with **digoxin**. Additive hypotension may occur with other **antihypertensives**, acute ingestion of **alcohol**, or **nitrates**. Concurrent use with **amphetamine**, **cocaine**, **ephedrine**, **epinephrine**, **norepinephrine**, **phenylephrine**, or **pseudoephedrine** may result in unopposed alpha-adrenergic stimulation (excessive hypertension, bradycardia). Concurrent **thyroid** administration may decrease effectiveness. May alter the effectiveness of **insulins** or **oral hypoglycemic agents** (dosage adjustments may be necessary). May decrease the effectiveness of **theophylline**. May decrease the beneficial $beta_1$-cardiovascular effects of **dopamine** or **dobutamine**. Use cautiously within 14 days of **MAO inhibitor** therapy (may result in hypertension).

Route/Dosage

PO (Adults): *Antianginal*—50 mg once daily; may be increased after 1 wk to 100 mg/day (up to 200 mg/day). *Antihypertensive*—25–50 mg once daily; may be increased after 2 wk to 50–100 mg once daily. *MI*—50 mg (given 10 min after last IV dose), then 50 mg 12 hr later, then 100 mg/day as a single dose or in 2 divided doses for 6–9 days or until hospital discharge.

Renal Impairment

PO (Adults): *CCr 15–35 ml/min*—dosage should not exceed 50 mg/day; *CCr <15 ml/min*—dosage should not exceed 50 mg every other day.

IV (Adults): *MI*—5 mg, followed by another 5 mg after 10 min; after 10 more min follow with oral dosing.

Availability (generic available)

Tablets: 25 mg, 50 mg, 100 mg. **Cost:** *Generic*—25 mg $11.99/90, 50 mg $12.99/90, 100 mg $15.89/90. **Injection:** 0.5 mg/ml. ***In combination with:*** chlorthalidone (Tenoretic). See Appendix B.

NURSING IMPLICATIONS

Assessment

- Monitor blood pressure, ECG, and pulse frequently during dosage adjustment period and periodically throughout therapy.
- Monitor intake and output ratios and daily weights. Assess routinely for CHF (dyspnea,

rales/crackles, weight gain, peripheral edema, jugular venous distention).

- Monitor frequency of prescription refills to determine adherence.
- **Angina:** Assess frequency and characteristics of angina periodically throughout therapy.
- ***Lab Test Considerations:*** May cause ↑ BUN, serum lipoprotein, potassium, triglyceride, and uric acid levels.
- May cause ↑ ANA titers.
- May cause ↑ in blood glucose levels.
- ***Toxicity and Overdose:*** Monitor patients receiving beta blockers for signs of overdose (bradycardia, severe dizziness or fainting, severe drowsiness, dyspnea, bluish fingernails or palms, seizures). Notify physician immediately if these signs occur.

Potential Nursing Diagnoses

Decreased cardiac output (Side Effects)
Noncompliance (Patient/Family Teaching)

Implementation

- **PO:** Take apical pulse before administering drug. If <50 bpm or if arrhythmia occurs, withhold medication and notify physician or other health care professional.

IV Administration

- **Direct IV:** ***Diluent:*** May be administered undiluted. May also be diluted in D5W, 0.9% NaCl, or D5/0.9% NaCl. Diluted solution stable for 48 hr. ***Concentration:*** 0.5 mg/ml. ***Rate:*** Administer at a rate of 1 mg/min.
- **Y-Site Compatibility:** acyclovir, amphotericin B liposome, daptomycin, diltiazem, ertapenem, granisetron, hydromorphone, linezolid, lorazepam, meperidine, meropenem, morphine, ondansetron, palonosetron, piperacillin/tazobactam, tacrolimus, tirofiban, voriconazole.
- **Y-Site Incompatibility:** amphotericin B cholesteryl sulfate, caspofungin, pantoprazole.

Patient/Family Teaching

- Instruct patient to take atenolol as directed at the same time each day, even if feeling well; do not skip or double up on missed doses. Take missed doses as soon as possible up to 8 hr before next dose. Abrupt withdrawal may cause life-threatening arrhythmias, hypertension, or myocardial ischemia.
- Advise patient to make sure enough medication is available for weekends, holidays, and vacations. A written prescription may be kept in wallet in case of emergency.
- Teach patient and family how to check pulse and blood pressure. Instruct them to check pulse daily and blood pressure biweekly and to report significant changes.
- May cause drowsiness or dizziness. Caution patients to avoid driving or other activities that require alertness until response to the drug is known.
- Advise patients to change positions slowly to minimize orthostatic hypotension.
- Caution patient that atenolol may increase sensitivity to cold.
- Instruct patient to consult health care professional before taking any OTC medications, especially cold preparations, concurrently with this medication.
- Patients with diabetes should closely monitor blood glucose, especially if weakness, malaise, irritability, or fatigue occurs. Medication does not block sweating as a sign of hypoglycemia.
- Advise patient to notify health care professional if slow pulse, difficulty breathing, wheezing, cold hands and feet, dizziness, light-headedness, confusion, depression, rash, fever, sore throat, unusual bleeding, or bruising occurs.
- Instruct patient to inform health care professional of medication regimen before treatment or surgery.
- Advise patient to carry identification describing disease process and medication regimen at all times.
- **Hypertension:** Reinforce the need to continue additional therapies for hypertension (weight loss, sodium restriction, stress reduction, regular exercise, moderation of alcohol consumption, and smoking cessation). Medication controls, but does not cure, hypertension.

Evaluation/Desired Outcomes

- Decrease in blood pressure.
- Reduction in frequency of angina
- Increase in activity tolerance.
- Prevention of MI.

atomoxetine
(a-to-**mox**-e-teen)
Strattera

Classification
Therapeutic: agents for attention deficit disorder
Pharmacologic: selective norepinephrine reuptake inhibitors

Pregnancy Category C

Indications
Attention-Deficit/Hyperactivity Disorder (ADHD).

Action
Selectively inhibits the presynaptic transporter of norepinephrine. **Therapeutic Effects:** Increased attention span.

Pharmacokinetics
Absorption: Well absorbed following oral administration.
Distribution: Unknown.
Protein Binding: 98%.
Metabolism and Excretion: Mostly metabolized by the liver (CYP2D6 enzyme pathway). A small percentage of the population are poor metabolizers and will have higher blood levels with increased effects).
Half-life: 5 hr.

TIME/ACTION PROFILE

ROUTE	ONSET	PEAK	DURATION
PO	unknown	1–2 hr	12–24 hr

Contraindications/Precautions
Contraindicated in: Concurrent or within 2 wk therapy with MAO inhibitors; Angle-closure glaucoma.
Use Cautiously in: Hypertension, tachycardia, cardiovascular or cerebrovascular disease; Preexisting psychiatric illness; May ↑ risk of suicide attempt/ideation especially during dose early treatment or dose adjustment; risk may be greater in children or adolescents; Concurrent albuterol or vasopressors (increases risk of adverse cardiovascular reactions); OB: Use only if benefits outweigh risks to fetus; Lactation, Pedi: Safety not established.

Adverse Reactions/Side Effects
CNS: dizziness, fatigue, mood swings; *Adults*— insomnia. **CV:** hypertension, orthostatic hypotension, tachycardia. **GI:** dyspepsia, severe liver injury (rare), nausea, vomiting; *Adults*— dry mouth, constipation. **Derm:** rash, urticaria. **GU:** *Adults*— dysmenorrhea, ejaculatory problems, ↓ libido, erectile dysfunction, urinary hesitation, urinary retention. **Metab:** decreased appetite, weight/growth loss. **Misc:** allergic reactions including ANGIONEUROTIC EDEMA.

Interactions
Drug-Drug: Concurrent use with **MAO inhibitors** may result in serious, potentially fatal reactions (do not use within 2 wk of each other). Increased risk of cardiovascular effects with **albuterol** or **vasopressors** (use cautiously). **Drugs which inhibit the CYP2D6 enzyme pathway (quinidine, fluoxetine, paroxetine)** will increase blood levels and effects, dose ↓ recommended.

Route/Dosage
PO (Children and adolescents <70 kg): 0.5 mg/kg/day initially, may be increased every 3 days to a daily target dose of 1.2 mg/kg, given as a single dose in the morning or evenly divided doses in the morning and late afternoon/early evening (not to exceed 1.4 mg/kg/day or 100 mg/day whichever is less). *If taking concurrent CYP2D6 inhibitor (quinidine, fluoxetine, paroxetine)*—0.5 mg/kg/day initially, may increase if needed to 1.2 mg/kg/day after 4 wk.
PO (Adults, adolescents, and children >70 kg): 40 mg/day initially, may be increased every 3 days to a daily target dose of 80 mg/day given as a single dose in the morning or evenly divided doses in the morning and late afternoon/early evening; may be further increased after 2–4 wk up to 100 mg/day. *If taking concurrent CYP2D6 inhibitor (quinidine, fluoxetine, paroxetine)*—40 mg/day initially, may increase if needed to 80 mg/day after 4 wk.

Hepatic Impairment
PO (Adults and Children): *Moderate hepatic impairment (Child-Pugh Class B)*—decrease initial and target dose by 50%; *Severe hepatic impairment (Child-Pugh Class C)*—decrease initial and target dose to 25% of normal.

Availability
Capsules: 10 mg, 18 mg, 25 mg, 40 mg, 60 mg, 80 mg, 100 mg. **Cost:** 10 mg $368.58/90, 18 mg $433.13/90, 25 mg $369.98/90, 40 mg $389.95/90, 60 mg $389.95/90, 80 mg $435.93/90, 100 mg $439.96/90.

NURSING IMPLICATIONS

Assessment

- Assess attention span, impulse control, and interactions with others.
- Monitor blood pressure and pulse periodically during therapy.
- Monitor growth, body height, and weight in children.
- Assess for signs of liver injury (pruritus, dark urine, jaundice, right upper quadrant tenderness, unexplained "flu-like" symptoms) during therapy. Monitor liver function tests at first sign of liver injury. Discontinue and do not restart atomoxetine in patients with jaundice if laboratory evidence of liver injury.

Potential Nursing Diagnoses

Disturbed thought process (Indications)
Impaired social interaction (Indications)

Implementation

- **PO:** Administer without regard to food.

Patient/Family Teaching

- Instruct patient to take medication as directed. Take missed doses as soon as possible, but should not take more than the total daily amount in any 24-hr period. Advise patient and parents to read the Medication Guide prior to starting therapy and with each Rx refill.
- Advise patient to notify health care professional immediately if signs of liver injury occur.
- Caution patient to consult health care professional prior to taking other prescription, OTC, dietary supplements, or herbal products.
- May cause dizziness. Caution patient to avoid driving or other activities requiring alertness until response to medication is known.
- OB, Lactation: Advise female patients to notify health care professional if pregnancy is planned or suspected or if they are breastfeeding.
- Pedi: Advise parents to notify school nurse of medication regimen.

Evaluation/Desired Outcomes

- Improved attention span and social interactions in ADHD.

atorvastatin, See HMG-CoA REDUCTASE INHIBITORS (statins).

atovaquone (a-toe-va-kwone)

Mepron

Classification
Therapeutic: antiprotozoals

Pregnancy Category C

Indications

Treatment of mild to moderate *Pneumocystis carinii* pneumonia (PCP) in patients who are unable to tolerate trimethoprim/sulfamethoxazole. Prophylaxis of *PCP*.

Action

Inhibits the action of enzymes necessary to nucleic acid and ATP synthesis in protozoa. **Therapeutic Effects:** Antiprotozoal action against *P. carinii*.

Pharmacokinetics

Absorption: Absorption is poor but is increased by food, particularly fat.
Distribution: Enters CSF in very low concentrations (<1% of plasma levels).
Protein Binding: >99.9%.
Metabolism and Excretion: Undergoes enterohepatic recycling; elimination occurs in feces.
Half-life: 2.2–2.9 days.

TIME/ACTION PROFILE (blood levels)

ROUTE	ONSET	PEAK	DURATION
PO	unknown	1–8 hr; 24–96 hr†	12 hr

†Two peaks are due to enterohepatic recycling

Contraindications/Precautions

Contraindicated in: Hypersensitivity; Lactation: May appear in breast milk.
Use Cautiously in: Decreased hepatic, renal, or cardiac function (dosage modification may be necessary); GI disorders (absorption may be limited); OB: Safety not established; Pedi: Safety not established.

Adverse Reactions/Side Effects

CNS: headache, insomnia. **Resp:** cough. **GI:** diarrhea, nausea, vomiting. **Derm:** rash. **Misc:** fever.

Interactions

Drug-Drug: May interact with **drugs that are highly bound to plasma proteins** (does not appear to interact with phenytoin).

Drug-Food: Food enhances absorption.

Route/Dosage

Treatment

PO (Adults): 750 mg twice daily for 21 days.
PO (Children): 40 mg/kg/day (unlabeled).

Prevention

PO (Adults and Adolescents 13–16 yr): 1500 mg once daily.

Availability

Suspension: 750 mg/5 ml.

NURSING IMPLICATIONS

Assessment

- Assess patient for signs of *PCP* (vital signs, lung sounds, sputum, WBCs) at beginning of and throughout therapy.
- Obtain specimens prior to initiating therapy. First dose may be given before receiving results.
- ***Lab Test Considerations:*** Monitor hematologic and hepatic functions. May cause mild, transient anemia and neutropenia. May also cause elevated serum amylase, AST, ALT, and alkaline phosphatase.
- Monitor electrolytes. May cause hyponatremia.

Potential Nursing Diagnoses

Risk for infection (Indications, Side Effects)
Deficient knowledge, related to medication regimen (Patient/Family Teaching)

Implementation

- **PO:** Administer with food twice daily for 21 days for treatment and once daily for prevention.

Patient/Family Teaching

- Instruct patient to take atovaquone exactly as directed around the clock for the full course of therapy, even if feeling better. Emphasize the importance of taking atovaquone with food, especially foods high in fat; taking without food may decrease plasma concentrations and effectiveness.
- Advise patient to notify health care professional if rash occurs.

Evaluation/Desired Outcomes

- Resolution of the signs and symptoms of *PCP*.

atropine† (at-ro-peen)

AtroPen

Classification
Therapeutic: antiarrhythmics
Pharmacologic: anticholinergics, antimuscarinics

Pregnancy Category C

†See Appendix C for ophthalmic use

Indications

IM: Given preoperatively to decrease oral and respiratory secretions. **IV:** Treatment of sinus bradycardia and heart block. **PO:** Adjunctive therapy in the management of peptic ulcer and irritable bowel syndrome. **IV:** Reversal of adverse muscarinic effects of anticholinesterase agents (neostigmine, physostigmine, or pyridostigmine). **IM, IV:** Treatment of anticholinesterase (organophosphate pesticide) poisoning. **Inhaln:** Treatment of exercise-induced bronchospasm.

Action

Inhibits the action of acetylcholine at postganglionic sites located in: Smooth muscle, Secretory glands, CNS (antimuscarinic activity). Low doses decrease: Sweating, Salivation, Respiratory secretions. Intermediate doses result in: Mydriasis (pupillary dilation), Cycloplegia (loss of visual accommodation), Increased heart rate. GI and GU tract motility are decreased at larger doses. **Therapeutic Effects:** Increased heart rate. Decreased GI and respiratory secretions. Reversal of muscarinic effects. May have a spasmolytic action on the biliary and genitourinary tracts.

Pharmacokinetics

Absorption: Well absorbed following oral, subcut, or IM administration.
Distribution: Readily crosses the blood-brain barrier. Crosses the placenta and enters breast milk.
Metabolism and Excretion: Mostly metabolized by the liver; 30–50% excreted unchanged by the kidneys.
Half-life: Children <2 yr: 4–10 hr; Children >2 yr: 1.5–3.5 hr; Adults: 4–5 hr.

TIME/ACTION PROFILE (inhibition of salivation)

ROUTE	ONSET	PEAK	DURATION
PO	30 min	30–60 min	4–6 hr
IM, subcut	rapid	15–50 min	4–6 hr

IV	immediate	2–4 min	4–6 hr

Contraindications/Precautions

Contraindicated in: Hypersensitivity; Angle-closure glaucoma; Acute hemorrhage; Tachycardia secondary to cardiac insufficiency or thyrotoxicosis; Obstructive disease of the GI tract.
Use Cautiously in: Intra-abdominal infections; Prostatic hyperplasia; Chronic renal, hepatic, pulmonary, or cardiac disease; OB, Lactation: Safety not established; IV administration may produce fetal tachycardia; Pedi: Infants with Down's syndrome have increased sensitivity to cardiac effects and mydriasis. Children may have increased susceptibility to adverse reactions. Exercise care when prescribing to children with spastic paralysis or brain damage; Geri: Increased susceptibility to adverse reactions.

Adverse Reactions/Side Effects

CNS: <u>drowsiness</u>, confusion, hyperpyrexia. **EENT:** <u>blurred vision</u>, cycloplegia, photophobia, dry eyes, mydriasis. **CV:** <u>tachycardia</u>, palpitations, arrhythmias. **GI:** <u>dry mouth</u>, constipation, impaired GI motility. **GU:** <u>urinary hesitancy</u>, retention, impotency. **Resp:** tachypnea, pulmonary edema. **Misc:** flushing, decreased sweating.

Interactions

Drug-Drug: ↑ anticholinergic effects with other **anticholinergics**, including **antihistamines**, **tricyclic antidepressants**, **quinidine**, and **disopyramide**. Anticholinergics may alter the absorption of other **orally administered drugs** by slowing motility of the GI tract. **Antacids** ↓ absorption of **anticholinergics**. May ↑ GI mucosal lesions in patients taking oral **potassium chloride** tablets. May alter response to **beta-blockers**.

Route/Dosage

Preanesthesia (To Decrease Salivation/Secretions)

IM, IV, Subcut, PO (Adults): 0.4–0.6 mg 30–60 min pre-op.
IM, IV, Subcut, PO (Children >5 kg): 0.01–0.02 mg/kg/dose 30–60 min preop to a maximum of 0.4 mg/dose; minimum: 0.1 mg/dose.
IM, IV, Subcut, PO (Children <5 kg): 0.02 mg/kg/dose 30–60 min preop then q 4–6 hr as needed.

Bradycardia

IV (Adults): 0.5–1 mg; may repeat as needed q 5 min, not to exceed a total of 2 mg (q 3–5 min in Advanced Cardiac Life Support guidelines) or 0.04 mg/kg (total vagolytic dose).
IV (Children): 0.02 mg/kg (maximum single dose is 0.5 mg in children and 1 mg in adolescents); may repeat q 5 min up to a total dose of 1 mg in children (2 mg in adolescents).
Endotracheal (Children): use the IV dose and dilute before administration.

Reversal of Adverse Muscarinic Effects of Anticholinesterases

IV (Adults): 0.6–12 mg for each 0.5–2.5 mg of neostigmine methylsulfate or 10–20 mg of pyridostigmine bromide concurrently with anticholinesterase.

Organophosphate Poisoning

IM (Adults): 2 mg initially, then 2 mg q 10 min as needed up to 3 times total.
IV (Adults): 1–2 mg/dose q 10–20 min until atropinic effects observed then q 1–4 hr for 24 hr; up to 50 mg in first 24 hr and 2 g over several days may be given in severe intoxication.
IM (Children >10 yr >90 lbs): 2 mg.
IM (Children 4–10 yr 40–90 lbs): 1 mg.
IM (Children 6 mo–4 yr 15–40 lbs): 0.5 mg.
IV (Children): 0.02–0.05 mg/kg q 10–20 min until atropinic effects observed then q 1–4 hr for 24 hr.

Bronchospasm

Inhaln (Adults): 0.025–0.05 mg/kg/dose q 4–6 hr as needed; maximum 2.5 mg/dose.
Inhaln (Children): 0.03–0.05 mg/kg/dose 3–4 times/day; maximum 2.5 mg/dose.

Availability (generic available)

Tablets: 0.4 mg. ***In combination with:*** phenobarbital oral solution (Antrocol). See Appendix B. **Injection:** 0.05 mg/ml, 0.1 mg/ml, 0.4 mg/ml, 1 mg/ml, 0.5 mg/0.7 ml Auto-injector, 1 mg/0.7 ml Auto-injector, 2 mg/0.7 ml Auto-injector.

NURSING IMPLICATIONS

Assessment

- Assess vital signs and ECG tracings frequently during IV drug therapy. Report any significant changes in heart rate or blood pressure, or

increased ventricular ectopy or angina to physician promptly.
- Monitor intake and output ratios in elderly or surgical patients because atropine may cause urinary retention.
- Assess patients routinely for abdominal distention and auscultate for bowel sounds. If constipation becomes a problem, increasing fluids and adding bulk to the diet may help alleviate constipation.
- ***Toxicity and Overdose:*** If overdose occurs, physostigmine is the antidote.

Potential Nursing Diagnoses

Decreased cardiac output (Indications)
Impaired oral mucous membrane (Side Effects)
Constipation (Side Effects)

Implementation

- **PO:** Oral doses of atropine may be given without regard to food.
- **IM:** Intense flushing of the face and trunk may occur 15–20 min following IM administration. In children, this response is called "atropine flush" and is not harmful.

IV Administration

- **Direct IV:** ***Diluent:*** Administer undiluted. ***Rate:*** Administer over 1 min; more rapid administration may be used during cardiac resuscitation (follow with 20 ml saline flush). Slow administration (over >1 min) may cause a paradoxical bradycardia (usually resolved in approximately 2 min).
- **Y-Site Compatibility:** abciximab, amikacin, aminophylline, amiodarone, argatroban, buprenorphine, butorphanol, etomidate, famotidine, fenoldopam, fentanyl, heparin, hydrocortisone sodium succinate, hydromorphone, inamrinone, meropenem, methadone, morphine, nafcillin, potassium chloride, sufentanil, tirofiban, vitamin B complex with C.
- **Y-Site Incompatibility:** thiopental.
- **Endotracheal:** Dilute with 5–10 ml of 0.9% NaCl. ***Rate:*** Inject directly into the endotracheal tube followed by several positive pressure ventilations.

Patient/Family Teaching

- Instruct patient to take as directed. Take missed doses as soon as remembered unless almost time for next dose. Do not double doses.
- May cause drowsiness. Caution patients to avoid driving or other activities requiring alertness until response to medication is known.
- Instruct patient that oral rinses, sugarless gum or candy, and frequent oral hygiene may help relieve dry mouth.
- Caution patients that atropine impairs heat regulation. Strenuous activity in a hot environment may cause heat stroke.
- Instruct patient to consult health care professional before taking any OTC medications or herbal products concurrently with atropine.
- Pedi: Instruct parents or caregivers that medication may cause fever and to notify health care professional before administering to a febrile child.
- Geri: Inform male patients with benign prostatic hyperplasia that atropine may cause urinary hesitancy and retention. Changes in urinary stream should be reported to health care professional.

Evaluation/Desired Outcomes

- Increase in heart rate.
- Dryness of mouth.
- Reversal of muscarinic effects.

azacitidine (a-za-**sye**-ti-deen)
Vidaza

Classification
Therapeutic: antineoplastics
Pharmacologic: nucleoside analogues

Pregnancy Category D

Indications

Myelodysplastic syndromes including: some refractory anemias, chronic myelomonocytic leukemia.

Action

Inhibits DNS synthesis. **Therapeutic Effects:** Death of rapidly replicating cells, particularly malignant ones.

Pharmacokinetics

Absorption: Rapidly absorbed following subcutaneous administration; 89% bioavailable.
Distribution: Unknown.
Metabolism and Excretion: 85% excreted in urine; some hepatic metabolism may occur. Less than 1% fecal elimination.
Half-life: 4 hr.

TIME/ACTION PROFILE (effects on bone marrow)

ROUTE	ONSET	PEAK	DURATION
Subcut	unknown	unknown	unknown

Contraindications/Precautions

Contraindicated in: Hypersensitivity; Advanced malignant hepatic tumors; OB: Potential for congenital anomalies; Lactation: Potential for serious side effects in infants.

Use Cautiously in: Renal impairment; Liver disease; OB: Patients with child-bearing potential (male and female) due to potential fetal harm; Pedi: Safety not established.

Adverse Reactions/Side Effects

CNS: fatigue. **GI:** HEPATOTOXICITY, constipation, diarrhea, nausea. **GU:** nephrotoxicity, renal tubular acidosis. **Derm:** ecchymosis. **F and E:** hypokalemia. **Hemat:** anemia, neutropenia, thrombocytopenia. **Local:** injection site erythema. **Misc:** allergic reactions including ANAPHYLAXIS, fever.

Interactions

Drug-Drug: Additive bone marrow depression may occur with other **antineoplastics**.

Route/Dosage

Subcut, IV (Adults): 75 mg/m²/day for 7 days every 4 weeks; may be increased to 100 mg/m²/day for 7 days every 4 wks if no beneficial effect occurs after 2 cycles. Continue for as long as patient benefits.

Availability

Suspension for injection (requires reconstitution): 100 mg/vial.

NURSING IMPLICATIONS

Assessment

- Monitor for bone marrow depression. Assess for bleeding (bleeding gums, bruising, petechiae, stools, urine, and emesis) and avoid IM injections and taking rectal temperatures if platelet count is low. Apply pressure to venipuncture sites for 10 min. Assess for signs of infection during neutropenia. Anemia may occur. Monitor for increased fatigue, dyspnea, and orthostatic hypotension.
- Assess patient for nausea and vomiting during therapy. Premedicate patient before each dose.
- Monitor for signs of anaphylaxis (facial edema, wheezing, dizziness, fainting, tachycardia, hypotension). Discontinue medication immediately and report symptoms. Epinephrine and resuscitation equipment should be readily available.
- ***Lab Test Considerations:*** Monitor CBC with differential and platelet count prior to each dosing cycle. If baseline WBC is more than 3×10^9 /L, ANC is more than 1.5×10^9 /L, and platelets are more than 75×10^9 /L, then dose is adjusted based on nadir counts for each cycle. If ANC is less than 0.5×10^9 and platelets are less than 25×10^9 then decrease dose by 50%. If ANC is 0.5–1.5×10^9 and platelets are 25–50×10^9 then decrease dose to 67% in next course. If ANC is greater than 1.5×10^9 and platelets are greater than 50, then 100% of dose can be given in subsequent cycle.
- Obtain liver chemistries and serum creatinine prior to initiation of therapy.
- Monitor renal function during therapy. If serum bicarbonate is less than 20 mEq/L, reduce dose by 50% in next course. If unexplained ↑ in BUN or serum creatinine occur, delay next cycle until values return to normal or baseline and decrease dose by 50% in next course.
- May cause hypokalemia.

Potential Nursing Diagnoses

Risk for infection (Adverse Reactions)
Risk for injury (Adverse Reactions)

Implementation

- Solution should be prepared in a biologic cabinet. Wear gloves, gown, and mask while handling medication. If powder or solution comes in contact with skin or mucosa, wash thoroughly with soap and water. Discard equipment in specially designated containers (see Appendix K).
- **Subcut:** Reconstitute by adding 4 mL of sterile water for injection slowly into the azacitadine vial for a concentration of 25 mg/mL. Invert vial 2–3 times and rotate gently until suspension is uniform. Suspension will be cloudy. Stable for up to 1 hr at room temperature; must be administered within 1 hr of reconstitution. Suspension may also be refrigerated for up to 8 hr; may be allowed to equilibrate to room temperature for up to 30

min. Invert syringe 2–3 times and roll syringe gently between palms immediately prior to administration to mix suspension.

- Divide doses greater than 4 mL equally into 2 syringes and administer into separate sites. Rotate sites (thigh, abdomen, upper arm) with new injections at least one inch from old site. Do not use site that is bruised, tender, red, or hard.

IV Administration

- **Intermittent Infusion:** ***Diluent:*** Reconstitute each vial with 10 mL sterile water for injection. Shake vigorously or roll vial until all solids are dissolved. Solution should be clear; do not administer solutions that are not clear or contain particulate matter. ***Concentration:*** 10 mg/mL. Withdraw solution from required number of vials and inject into 50–100 mL of 0.9% NaCl or LR. Solution is stable for 1 hr at room temperature. ***Rate:*** Infuse over 10–40 min. Infusion must be completed within 1 hr of reconstitution.
- **Solution Incompatibility:** 5% dextrose, hespan, solutions containing bicarbonate.

Patient/Family Teaching

- Instruct patient to notify health care professional promptly if fever; chills; cough; hoarseness; sore throat; signs of infection; lower back or side pain; painful or difficult urination; bleeding gums; bruising; petechiae; blood in stools, urine, or emesis; increased fatigue; dyspnea; or orthostatic hypotension occurs. Caution patient to avoid crowds and persons with known infections. Instruct patient to use soft toothbrush and electric razor and to avoid falls. Caution patient not to drink alcoholic beverages or take medication containing aspirin or NSAIDs; may precipitate gastric bleeding.
- May cause dizziness. Caution patient to avoid driving or other activities requiring alertness until response to medication is known.
- Advise patient to notify health care professional if they have underlying liver or renal disease.
- OB: Advise both male and female patients of the need for contraception during therapy.

Evaluation/Desired Outcomes

- Improved bone marrow and blood counts.

azathioprine

(ay-za-**thye**-oh-preen)
Azasan, Imuran

Classification
Therapeutic: immunosuppressants
Pharmacologic: purine antagonists

Pregnancy Category D

Indications

Prevention of renal transplant rejection (with corticosteroids, local radiation, or other cytotoxic agents). Treatment of severe, active, erosive rheumatoid arthritis unresponsive to more conventional therapy. **Unlabeled uses:** Management of Crohn's disease.

Action

Antagonizes purine metabolism with subsequent inhibition of DNA and RNA synthesis. **Therapeutic Effects:** Suppression of cell-mediated immunity and altered antibody formation.

Pharmacokinetics

Absorption: Readily absorbed after oral administration.
Distribution: Crosses the placenta. Enters breast milk in low concentrations.
Metabolism and Excretion: Metabolized to mercaptopurine, which is further metabolized. Minimal renal excretion of unchanged drug.
Half-life: 3 hr.

TIME/ACTION PROFILE

ROUTE	ONSET	PEAK	DURATION
PO (anti-inflammatory)	6–8 wk	12 wk	unknown
IV (immunosuppression)	days–wk	unknown	days–wk

Contraindications/Precautions

Contraindicated in: Hypersensitivity; Concurrent use of mycophenolate; OB: Has been shown to cause fetal harm; Lactation: Appears in breast milk.
Use Cautiously in: Infections; Malignancies; Decreased bone marrow reserve; Previous or concurrent radiation therapy; Other chronic debilitating illnesses; Severe renal impairment/oliguria (increased sensitivity); OB: Patients with childbearing potential.

Adverse Reactions/Side Effects

EENT: retinopathy. **Resp:** pulmonary edema. **GI:** anorexia, hepatotoxicity, nausea, vomiting, diarrhea, mucositis, pancreatitis. **Derm:** alopecia, rash. **Hemat:** anemia, leukopenia, pancytopenia, thrombocytopenia. **MS:** arthralgia.

A

Misc: SERUM SICKNESS, chills, fever, Raynaud's phenomenon, retinopathy.

Interactions

Drug-Drug: Additive myelosuppression with **antineoplastics**, **cyclosporine**, and **myelosuppressive agents**. **Allopurinol** inhibits the metabolism of azathioprine, increasing toxicity. Dose of azathioprine should be decreased by 25–33% with concurrent allopurinol. May ↓ antibody response to **live-virus vaccines** and ↑ the risk of adverse reactions.
Drug-Natural Products: Concommitant use with **echinacea** and **melatonin** may interfere with immunosuppression.

Route/Dosage

Renal Allograft Rejection Prevention

PO, IV (Adults and Children): 3–5 mg/kg/day initially; maintenance dose 1–3 mg/kg/day.

Rheumatoid Arthritis

PO (Adults and Children): 1 mg/kg/day for 6–8 wk, increase by 0.5 mg/kg/day q 4 wk until response or up to 2.5 mg/kg/day, then decrease by 0.5 mg/kg/day q 4–8 wk to minimal effective dose.

Availability (generic available)

Tablets: 50 mg, 75 mg, 100 mg. **Injection:** 100-mg vial.

NURSING IMPLICATIONS

Assessment

- Assess for infection (vital signs, sputum, urine, stool, WBC) during therapy.
- Monitor intake and output and daily weight. Decreased urine output may lead to toxicity with this medication.
- **Rheumatoid Arthritis:** Assess range of motion; degree of swelling, pain, and strength in affected joints; and ability to perform activities of daily living before and periodically during therapy.
- ***Lab Test Considerations:*** Monitor renal, hepatic, and hematologic functions before beginning therapy, weekly during the 1st mo, bimonthly for the next 2–3 mo, and monthly thereafter.
- Leukocyte count of <3000 or platelet count of <100,000/mm^3 may necessitate a reduction in dosage or temporary discontinuation.
- A ↓ in hemoglobin may indicate bone marrow suppression.
- Hepatotoxicity may be manifested by ↑ alkaline phosphatase, bilirubin, AST, ALT, and amylase concentrations. Usually occurs within 6 mo of transplant, rarely with rheumatoid arthritis, and is reversible on discontinuation of azathioprine.
- May ↓ serum and urine uric acid and plasma albumin.

Potential Nursing Diagnoses

Risk for infection (Indications)

Implementation

- Do not confuse Imuran (azathioprine) with IMDUR (isosorbide mononitrate).
- Protect transplant patients from staff members and visitors who may carry infection. Maintain protective isolation as indicated.
- **PO:** May be administered with or after meals or in divided doses to minimize nausea.

IV Administration

- **IV:** Reconstitute 100 mg with 10 ml of sterile water for injection. Swirl vial gently until completely dissolved. Reconstituted solution may be administered up to 24 hr after preparation.
- Solution should be prepared in a biologic cabinet. Wear gloves, gown, and mask while handling medication. Discard equipment in specially designated containers (see Appendix K).
- **Direct IV:** ***Diluent:*** 0.9% NaCl, 0.45% NaCl, or D5W. ***Concentration:*** 10 mg/ml. ***Rate:*** Give over 5 min.
- **Intermittent Infusion:** ***Diluent:*** Solution may be further diluted in 50 mL with 0.9% NaCl, 0.45% NaCl, or D5W. Do not admix. ***Rate:*** Usually infused over 30–60 min; may range 5 min–8 hr.

Patient/Family Teaching

- Instruct patient to take azathioprine exactly as directed. If a dose is missed on a once-daily regimen, omit dose; if on several-times-a-day dosing, take as soon as possible or double next dose. Consult health care professional if more than 1 dose is missed or if vomiting occurs shortly after dose is taken. Do not discontinue without consulting health care professional.

- Advise patient to report unusual tiredness or weakness; cough or hoarseness; fever or chills; lower back or side pain; painful or difficult urination; severe diarrhea; black, tarry stools; blood in urine; or transplant rejection to health care professional immediately.
- Reinforce the need for lifelong therapy to prevent transplant rejection.
- Instruct the patient to consult health care professional before taking any OTC medications or natural/herbal products, or receiving any vaccinations while taking this medication.
- Advise patient to avoid contact with persons with contagious diseases and persons who have recently taken oral poliovirus vaccine.
- This drug may have teratogenic properties. Advise patient to use contraception during and for at least 4 mo after therapy is completed.
- Emphasize the importance of follow-up exams and lab tests.
- **Rheumatoid Arthritis:** Concurrent therapy with salicylates, NSAIDs, or corticosteroids may be necessary. Patient should continue physical therapy and adequate rest. Explain that joint damage will not be reversed; goal is to slow or stop disease process.

Evaluation/Desired Outcomes

- Prevention of transplant rejection.
- Decreased stiffness, pain, and swelling in affected joints in 6–8 wk in rheumatoid arthritis. Therapy is discontinued if no improvement in 12 wk.

azithromycin

(aye-**zith**-row-my-sin)
Zithromax, Zmax

Classification
Therapeutic: agents for atypical mycobacterium, anti-infectives
Pharmacologic: macrolides

Pregnancy Category B

Indications

Treatment of the following infections due to susceptible organisms: Upper respiratory tract infections, including streptococcal pharyngitis, acute bacterial exacerbations of chronic bronchitis and tonsillitis, Lower respiratory tract infections, including bronchitis and pneumonia, Acute otitis media, Skin and skin structure infections, Nongonococcal urethritis, cervicitis, gonorrhea, and chancroid. Prevention of disseminated *Mycobacterium avium* complex (MAC) infection in patients with advanced HIV infection. *Extended-release suspension (ZMax)* Acute bacterial sinusitis and community-acquired pneumonia in adults. **Unlabeled uses:** Prevention of bacterial endocarditis. Treatment of cystic fibrosis lung disease.

Action

Inhibits protein synthesis at the level of the 50S bacterial ribosome. **Therapeutic Effects:** Bacteriostatic action against susceptible bacteria. **Spectrum:** Active against the following gram-positive aerobic bacteria: *Staphylococcus aureus*, *Streptococcus pneumoniae*, *Streptococcus pyogenes* (group A strep). Active against these gram-negative aerobic bacteria: *Haemophilus influenzae*, *Moraxella catarrhalis*, *Neisseria gonorrhoeae*. Also active against: *Mycoplasma*, *Legionella*, *Chlamydia pneumoniae*, *Ureaplasma urealyticum*, *Borrelia burgdorferi*, *M. avium*. Not active against methicillin-resistant *S. aureus*.

Pharmacokinetics

Absorption: Rapidly absorbed (40%) after oral administration. IV administration results in complete bioavailability.
Distribution: Widely distributed to body tissues and fluids. Intracellular and tissue levels exceed those in serum; low CSF levels.
Metabolism and Excretion: Mostly excreted unchanged in bile; 4.5% excreted unchanged in urine.
Half-life: 11–14 hr after single dose; 2–4 days after several doses; 59 hr after extended release suspension.

TIME/ACTION PROFILE (serum)

ROUTE	ONSET	PEAK	DURATION
PO	rapid	2.5–3.2 hr	24 hr
IV	rapid	end of infusion	24 hr

Contraindications/Precautions

Contraindicated in: Hypersensitivity to azithromycin, erythromycin, or other macrolide anti-infectives.
Use Cautiously in: Severe liver impairment (dosage adjustment may be required); Severe renal impairment (CCr <10 ml/min); OB, Lactation: Safety not established; Pedi: Safety not established in children <5 yr.

Adverse Reactions/Side Effects

CNS: dizziness, seizures, drowsiness, fatigue, headache. **CV:** chest pain, hypotension, palpitations, QT prolongation (rare). **GI:** PSEUDOMEMBRANOUS COLITIS, abdominal pain, diarrhea, nausea, cholestatic jaundice, elevated liver enzymes, dyspepsia, flatulence, melena, oral candidiasis. **GU:** nephritis, vaginitis. **Hemat:** anemia, leukopenia, thrombocytopenia. **Derm:** photosensitivity, Stevens-Johnson syndrome, rashes. **EENT:** ototoxicity. **F and E:** hyperkalemia. **Misc:** ANGIOEDEMA.

Interactions

Drug-Drug: Aluminum- and **magnesium-containing antacids** decrease peak serum levels. **Nelfinavir** increases serum levels (monitor carefully). Other macrolide anti-infectives have been known to increase serum levels and effects of **digoxin**, **theophylline**, **ergotamine**, **dihydroergotamine**, **triazolam**, **carbamazepine**, **cyclosporine**, **tacrolimus**, and **phenytoin**; careful monitoring of concurrent use is recommended.

Route/Dosage

Most Respiratory and Skin Infections

PO (Adults): 500 mg on 1st day, then 250 mg/day for 4 more days (total dose of 1.5 g); *Acute bacterial sinusitis*—500 mg once daily for 3 days or single 2-g dose of extended-release suspension (Zmax).

PO (Children ≥6 months): 10 mg/kg (not >500 mg/dose) on 1st day, then 5 mg/kg (not >250 mg/dose) for 4 more days. *Pharyngitis/tonsilitis*—12 mg/kg once daily for 5 days (not >500 mg/dose); *Acute bacterial sinusitis*—10 mg/kg/day for three days.

Otitis media

PO (Children ≥6 mo): 30 mg/kg single dose (not >1500 mg/dose) *or* 10 mg/kg/day as a single dose (not >500 mg/dose) for 3 days *or* 10 mg/kg as a single dose (not >500 mg/dose) on 1st day, then 5 mg/kg as a single dose (not >250 mg/dose) daily for 4 more days.

Acute bacterial exacerbations of chronic bronchitis

PO (Adults): 500 mg on 1st day, then 250 mg/day for 4 more days (total dose of 1.5 g) *or* 500 mg daily for 3 days.

Community-Acquired Pneumonia

IV, PO (Adults): *More severe*—500 mg IV q 24 hr for at least 2 doses, then 500 mg PO q 24 hr for a total of 7–10 days; *less severe*—500 mg PO, then 250 mg/day PO for 4 more days or 2 g single dose as extended-release suspension (Zmax).

PO (Children >6 mo): 10 mg/kg on 1st day, then 5 mg/kg for 4 more days.

Pelvic Inflammatory Disease

IV, PO (Adults): 500 mg IV q 24 hr for 1–2 days, then 250 mg PO q 24 hr for a total of 7 days.

Endocarditis Prophylaxis

PO (Adults): 500 mg 1 hr before procedure.

PO (Children): 15 mg/kg 1 hr before procedure.

Nongonococcal Urethritis, Cervicitis, Chancroid, Chlamydia

PO (Adults): Single 1-g dose.

PO (Children): *Chancroid:* Single 20 mg/kg dose (not >1000 mg/dose). *Urethritis or cervicitis:* Single 10 mg/kg dose (not >1000 mg/dose).

Gonorrhea

PO (Adults): Single 2-g dose.

Prevention of Disseminated MAC Infection

PO (Adults): 1.2 g once weekly (alone or with rifabutin).

PO (Children): 5 mg/kg once daily (not >250 mg/dose) or 20 mg/kg (not >1200 mg/dose) once weekly (alone or with rifabutin).

Cystic Fibrosis

PO (Children ≥6 yrs, weight ≥25 kg to <40 kg): 250 mg q MWF. ≥40 kg: 500 mg q MWF.

Availability (generic available)

Tablets: 250 mg, 500 mg, 600 mg. **Cost:** *Generic*—250 mg $15.99/6, 500 mg $44.32/3, 600 mg $399.99/30. **Powder for oral suspension (cherry, creme de vanilla, and banana flavor):** 1 g/pkt. **Cost:** $93.99/3 packets. **Powder for oral suspension (cherry, creme de vanilla, and banana flavor):** 100 mg/5 ml in 15-ml bottles, 200 mg/5 ml in 15-ml, 22.5-ml, and 30-ml bottles. **Cost:** *Zithromax*—100 mg/5 ml $44.99/15 ml, 200 mg/5 ml $43.99/22.5 ml, 200 mg/5 ml $43.99/30 ml; *Generic*—200 mg/5 ml $32.27/15 ml. **Extended-release**

oral suspension (ZMax) (cherry-banana): 2-g single-dose bottle. **Powder for injection:** 500 mg/vial.

NURSING IMPLICATIONS

Assessment

- Assess patient for infection (vital signs; appearance of wound, sputum, urine, and stool; WBC) at beginning of and throughout therapy.
- Obtain specimens for culture and sensitivity before initiating therapy. First dose may be given before receiving results.
- Observe for signs and symptoms of anaphylaxis (rash, pruritus, laryngeal edema, wheezing). Notify the physician or other health care professional immediately if these occur.
- ***Lab Test Considerations:*** May cause ↑ serum bilirubin, AST, ALT, LDH, and alkaline phosphatase concentrations.
- May cause ↑ creatine phosphokinase, potassium, prothrombin time, BUN, serum creatinine, and blood glucose concentrations.
- May occasionally cause ↓ WBC and platelet count.

Potential Nursing Diagnoses

Risk for infection (Indications, Side Effects)
Noncompliance (Patient/Family Teaching)

Implementation

- Do not confuse azithromycin with erythromycin.
- *Zmax extended release oral suspension* is not bioequivalent or interchangeable with azithromycin oral suspension.
- **PO:** Administer 1 hr before or 2 hr after meals.
- For administration of single 1-g packet, thoroughly mix entire contents of packet with 2 oz (60 ml) of water. Drink entire contents immediately; add an additional 2 oz of water, mix and drink to assure complete consumption of dose. Do not use the single packet to administer doses other than 1000 mg of azithromycin. Pedi: 1-g packet is not for pediatric use.
- For *Zmax* shake suspension well and drink entire contents of bottle. Use within 12 hrs of reconstitution. If patient vomits within 1 hr of administration, contact prescriber for instructions. *Zmax* may be taken without regard to antacids containing magnesium or aluminum hydroxide.

IV Administration

- **Intermittent Infusion:** ***Diluent:*** Reconstitute each 500-mg vial with 4.8 ml of sterile water for injection to achieve a concentration of 100 mg/ml. Reconstituted solution is stable for 24 hr at room temperature. Further dilute the 500-mg dose in 250 ml or 500 ml of 0.9% NaCl, 0.45% NaCl, D5W, LR, D5/0.45% NaCl, or D5/LR. Infusion is stable for 24 hr at room temperature or for 7 days if refrigerated. ***Concentration:*** Final concentration of infusion is 1–2 mg/ml. ***Rate:*** Administer the 1 mg/ml solution over 3 hr or the 2 mg/ml solution over 1 hr. Do not administer as a bolus.
- **Y-Site Compatibility:** amphotericin B liposome, bivalirudin, daptomycin, diphenhydramine, dolasetron, droperidol, ertapenem, fenoldopam, palonosetron, pantoprazole, tigecycline, tirofiban, voriconazole.
- **Y-Site Incompatibility:** amikacin, aztreonam, caspofungin, cefotaxime, ceftazidime, ceftriaxone, cefuroxime, ciprofloxacin, clindamycin, famotidine, fentanyl, furosemide, gentamicin, imipenem-cilastatin, ketorolac, morphine, ondansetron, piperacillin-tazobactam, potassium chloride, quinupristin/dalfopristin, ticarcillin-clavulanate, tobramycin.

Patient/Family Teaching

- Instruct patients to take medication as directed and to finish the drug completely, even if they are feeling better. Tell patient to take missed doses as soon as possible unless almost time for next dose; do not double doses. Advise patients that sharing of this medication may be dangerous.
- Instruct patient not to take azithromycin with food or antacids.
- May cause drowsiness and dizziness. Caution patient to avoid driving or other activities requiring alertness until response to medication is known.
- Advise patient to use sunscreen and protective clothing to prevent photosensitivity reactions.
- Advise patient to report symptoms of chest pain, palpitations, yellowing of skin or eyes, or signs of superinfection (black, furry overgrowth on the tongue; vaginal itching or discharge; loose or foul-smelling stools).
- Instruct patient to notify health care professional if fever and diarrhea develop, especially if stool contains blood, pus, or mucus. Ad-

vise patient not to treat diarrhea without advice of health care professional.

- Advise patients being treated for nongonococcal urethritis or cervicitis that sexual partners should also be treated.
- Instruct parents, caregivers, or patient to notify health care professional if symptoms do not improve.
- Pedi: Tell parents or caregivers that medication is generally well tolerated in children. Most common side effects in children are mild diarrhea and rash. Tell parents to notify health care practitioner if these occur.

Evaluation/Desired Outcomes

- Resolution of the signs and symptoms of infection. Length of time for complete resolution depends on the organism and site of infection.

baclofen (bak-loe-fen)
Kemstro, Lioresal

Classification
Therapeutic: antispasticity agents, skeletal muscle relaxants (centrally acting)

Pregnancy Category C

Indications
PO: Treatment of reversible spasticity due to multiple sclerosis or spinal cord lesions.
IT: Treatment of severe spasticity originating in the spinal cord. **Unlabeled uses:** Management of pain in trigeminal neuralgia.

Action
Inhibits reflexes at the spinal level. **Therapeutic Effects:** Decreased muscle spasticity; bowel and bladder function may also be improved.

Pharmacokinetics
Absorption: Well absorbed after oral administration.
Distribution: Widely distributed; crosses the placenta.
Metabolism and Excretion: 70–80% eliminated unchanged by the kidneys.
Half-life: 2.5–4 hr.

TIME/ACTION PROFILE (effects on spasticity)

ROUTE	ONSET	PEAK	DURATION
PO	hrs–wks	unknown	unknown
IT	0.5–1 hr	4 hr	4–8 hr

Contraindications/Precautions
Contraindicated in: Hypersensitivity; Orally-disintegrating tablets contain aspartame and should not be used in patients with phenylketonuria.
Use Cautiously in: Patients in whom spasticity maintains posture and balance; Patients with epilepsy (may ↓ seizure threshold); Renal impairment (↓ dose may be required); OB, Lactation, Pedi: Safety not established; Geri: Geriatric patients are at ↑ risk of CNS side effects.

Adverse Reactions/Side Effects
CNS: SEIZURES (IT), dizziness, drowsiness, fatigue, weakness, confusion, depression, headache, insomnia. **EENT:** nasal congestion, tinnitus. **CV:** edema, hypotension. **GI:** nausea, constipation. **GU:** frequency. **Derm:** pruritus, rash. **Metab:** hyperglycemia, weight gain. **Neuro:** ataxia. **Misc:** hypersensitivity reactions, sweating.

Interactions
Drug-Drug: ↑ CNS depression with other **CNS depressants** including **alcohol**, **antihistamines**, **opioid analgesics**, and **sedative/hypnotics**. Use with **MAO inhibitors** may lead to ↑ CNS depression or hypotension.
Drug-Natural Products: Concomitant use of **kava kava, valerian, or chamomile can ↑ CNS depression.**

Route/Dosage
PO (Adults): 5 mg 3 times daily. May increase q 3 days by 5 mg/dose up to 80 mg/day (some patients may have a better response to 4 divided doses).
IT (Adults): 100–800 mcg/day infusion; dose is determined by response during screening phase.
IT (Children): 25–1200 mcg/day infusion (average 275 mcg/day); dose is determined by response during screening phase.

Availability (generic available)
Tablets: 10 mg, 20 mg. **Cost:** *Generic*—10 mg $78.16/270, 20 mg $137.92/270. **Orally-disintegrating tablets (Kemstro) (orange):** 10 mg, 20 mg. **Intrathecal injection:** 50 mcg/ml, 500 mcg/ml, 2000 mcg/ml.

NURSING IMPLICATIONS

Assessment
- Assess muscle spasticity before and periodically during therapy.
- Observe patient for drowsiness, dizziness, or ataxia. May be alleviated by a change in dose.
- **IT:** Monitor patient closely during test dose and titration. Resuscitative equipment should be immediately available for life-threatening or intolerable side effects.
- ***Lab Test Considerations:*** May cause ↑ in serum glucose, alkaline phosphatase, AST, and ALT levels.

Potential Nursing Diagnoses
Impaired wheelchair mobility (Indications)
Risk for injury (Adverse Reactions)

Implementation
- **PO:** Administer with milk or food to minimize gastric irritation.
- For *orally disintegrating tablets,* just prior to administration place tablet on tongue with

dry hands. Tablet will disintegrate, then swallow with saliva or water. Administration with liquid is not necessary. **IT:** For *screening phase,* dilute for a concentration of 50 mcg/ml with sterile preservative-free NaCl for injection. Test dose should be administered over at least 1 min. Observe patient for a significant decrease in muscle tone or frequency or severity of spasm. If response is inadequate, 2 additional test doses, each 24 hr apart, 75 mcg/1.5 ml and 100 mcg/2 ml respectively, may be administered. Patients with an inadequate response should not receive chronic IT therapy.

- Dose titration for implantable IT pumps is based on patient response. If no substantive response after dose increase, check pump function and catheter patency.

Patient/Family Teaching

- Instruct patient to take baclofen as directed. Take a missed dose within 1 hr; do not double doses. Caution patient to avoid abrupt withdrawal of this medication because it may precipitate an acute withdrawal reaction (hallucinations, increased spasticity, seizures, mental changes, restlessness). Discontinue baclofen gradually over 2 wk or more.
- May cause dizziness and drowsiness. Advise patient to avoid driving or other activities requiring alertness until response to drug is known.
- Instruct patient to change positions slowly to minimize orthostatic hypotension.
- Advise patient to avoid concurrent use of alcohol or other CNS depressants while taking this medication.
- Instruct patient to notify health care professional if frequent urge to urinate or painful urination, constipation, nausea, headache, insomnia, tinnitus, depression, or confusion persists. Geri: Geriatric patients are at greater risk for these side effects.
- Advise patient to report signs and symptoms of hypersensitivity (rash, itching) promptly.
- **IT:** Caution patient and caregiver to not discontinue IT therapy abruptly. May result in fever, mental status changes, exaggerated rebound spasticity, and muscle rigidity. Advise patient not to miss scheduled refill appointments and to notify health care professional promptly if signs of withdrawal occur.

Evaluation/Desired Outcomes

- Decrease in muscle spasticity and associated musculoskeletal pain with an increased ability to perform activities of daily living.
- Decreased pain in patients with trigeminal neuralgia. May take weeks to obtain optimal effect.

balsalazide (ba-**sal**-a-zide)

Colazal

Classification

Therapeutic: gastrointestinal anti-inflammatories—therapeutic

Pregnancy Category B

Indications

Treatment of mild to moderately active ulcerative colitis.

Action

Drug is metabolized in the colon to mesalamine (5-aminosalicylic acid), which is a local anti-inflammatory. **Therapeutic Effects:** Reduction in the symptoms of ulcerative colitis.

Pharmacokinetics

Absorption: Absorption is low and variable; drug is delivered intact to the colon.

Distribution: Mostly delivered intact to the colon; remainder of distribution unknown.

Protein Binding: ≥99%.

Metabolism and Excretion: Following delivery to the colon, bacteria break balsalazide down into mesalamine (5-aminosalicylic acid) and an inactive metabolite; mostly excreted in feces.

Half-life: *Mesalamine*—12 hr (range 2–15 hr).

TIME/ACTION PROFILE (decreased symptoms)

ROUTE	ONSET	PEAK	DURATION
PO	unknown	up to 8 wk	unknown

Contraindications/Precautions

Contraindicated in: Hypersensitivity to salicylates or other metabolites.

Use Cautiously in: Pyloric stenosis (may have prolonged gastric retention of capsules); OB: Use only if clearly needed; Lactation, Pedi: Safety not established.

Adverse Reactions/Side Effects

GI: abdominal pain, diarrhea.

Interactions

Drug-Drug: None known.

B

Route/Dosage
PO (Adults): three 750-mg capsules three times daily for 8–12 wks.
PO (Children 5–17 yrs): three 750-mg capsules three times daily for up to 8 wks *or* one 750-mg capsule three times daily for up to 8 wks.

Availability
Capsules: 750 mg.

NURSING IMPLICATIONS

Assessment
- Assess abdominal pain and frequency, quantity, and consistency of stools at the beginning of and throughout therapy.
- Assess patient for allergy to salicylates.
- ***Lab Test Considerations:*** May cause elevated AST, ALT, serum alkaline phosphatase, gamma glutamyl transpepsidase (GGT), LDH, and bilirubin.

Potential Nursing Diagnoses
Acute pain (Indications)
Diarrhea (Indications)

Implementation
- **PO:** Administer capsules three times a day. Capsules may be opened and sprinkled on applesauce and taken immediately; do not store mixture. Color of powder inside of capsules may range from yellow to orange. Teeth or tongue staining may occur when powder is sprinkled on applesauce and swallowed.

Patient/Family Teaching
- Instruct patient on the correct method of administration. Advise patient to take medication as directed, even if feeling better. If a dose is missed, it should be taken as soon as remembered unless almost time for next dose.
- Advise patient to notify health care professional if skin rash, difficulty breathing, or hives occur.
- Instruct patient to notify health care professional if symptoms do not improve after 1–2 mo of therapy.

Evaluation/Desired Outcomes
- Decrease in diarrhea and abdominal pain in patients with ulcerative colitis.

basiliximab (ba-sil-**ix**-i-mab)
Simulect

Classification
Therapeutic: immunosuppressants
Pharmacologic: monoclonal antibodies

Pregnancy Category B

Indications
Prevention of acute organ rejection in patients undergoing renal transplantation; used with corticosteroids and cyclosporine.

Action
Binds to and blocks specific interleukin-2 (IL-2) receptor sites on activated T lymphocytes. **Therapeutic Effects:** Prevention of acute organ rejection following renal transplantation.

Pharmacokinetics
Absorption: IV administration results in complete bioavailability.
Distribution: Unknown.
Metabolism and Excretion: Unknown.
Half-life: 7.2 days.

TIME/ACTION PROFILE (effect on immune function)

ROUTE	ONSET	PEAK	DURATION
IV	2 hr	unknown	36 days

Contraindications/Precautions
Contraindicated in: Hypersensitivity; OB: May affect fetal developing immune system; Lactation: Make enter breast milk.
Use Cautiously in: Women with childbearing potential; Geri: Due to greater incidence of infection.

Adverse Reactions/Side Effects
Noted for patients receiving corticosteroids and cyclosporine in addition to basiliximab.
CNS: dizziness, headache, insomnia, weakness. **EENT:** abnormal vision, cataracts. **Resp:** coughing. **CV:** HEART FAILURE, edema, hypertension, angina, arrhythmias, hypotension. **GI:** abdominal pain, constipation, diarrhea, dyspepsia, moniliasis, nausea, vomiting, GI bleeding, gingival hyperplasia, stomatitis. **Derm:** acne, wound complications, hypertrichosis, pruritus. **Endo:** hyperglycemia, hypoglycemia. **F and E:** acidosis, hypercholesterolemia, hyperkalemia, hyperuricemia, hypocalcemia, hypokalemia, hypophosphatemia. **Hemat:** bleeding, coagulation abnormalities. **MS:** back pain, leg pain.

Neuro: tremor, neuropathy, paresthesia. **Misc:** hypersensitivity reactions including ANAPHYLAXIS, infection, weight gain, chills.

Interactions

Drug-Drug: Immunosuppression may be ↑ with other **immunosuppressants**.
Drug-Natural Products: Concommitant use with **echinacea** and **melatonin** may interfere with immunosuppression.

Route/Dosage

IV (Adults and Children ≥35 kg): 20 mg given 2 hr before transplantation; repeated 4 days after transplantation. Second dose should be withheld if complications or graft loss occurs.
IV (Children <35 kg): 10 mg given 2 hr before transplantation; repeated 4 days after transplantation. Second dose should be withheld if complications or graft loss occurs.

Availability

Powder for reconstitution: 20 mg/vial, 10 mg/vial.

NURSING IMPLICATIONS

Assessment

- Monitor for signs of anaphylactic or hypersensitivity reactions (hypotension, tachycardia, cardiac failure, dyspnea, wheezing, bronchospasm, pulmonary edema, respiratory failure, urticaria, rash, pruritus, sneezing) at each dose. Onset of symptoms is usually within 24 hr. Resuscitation equipment and medications for treatment of severe hypersensitivity should be readily available. If a severe hypersensitivity reaction occurs, basiliximab therapy should be permanently discontinued. Patients who have previously received basiliximab should only receive subsequent therapy with extreme caution.
- Monitor for infection (fever, chills, rash, sore throat, purulent discharge, dysuria). Notify physician immediately if these symptoms occur; may necessitate discontinuation of therapy.
- ***Lab Test Considerations:*** May cause ↑ or ↓ hemoglobin, hematocrit, serum glucose, potassium, and calcium concentrations.
- May cause ↑ serum cholesterol levels.
- May cause ↑ BUN, serum creatinine, and uric acid concentrations.
- May cause ↓ serum magnesium, phosphate, and platelet levels.

Potential Nursing Diagnoses

Risk for infection (Side Effects)

Implementation

IV Administration

- Basiliximab is usually administered concurrently with cyclosporine and corticosteroids
- Reconstitute with 2.5 ml or 5 ml of sterile water for injection for the 10 mg or 20 mg vial, respectively. Shake gently to dissolve powder.
- **Direct IV:** ***Diluent:*** May be administered undiluted. Bolus administration may be associated with nausea, vomiting, and local reactions (pain). ***Concentration:*** 4 mg/ml. ***Rate:*** Administer over 20–30 min via peripheral or central line.
- **Intermittent Infusion:** ***Diluent:*** Dilute further with 25–50 ml of 0.9% NaCl or D5W. Gently invert bag to mix; do not shake, to avoid foaming. Solution is clear to opalescent and colorless; do not administer solutions that are discolored or contain particulate matter. Discard unused portion. Administer within 4 hr or may be refrigerated for up to 24 hr. Discard after 24 hr. ***Concentration:*** 0.08–0.16 mg/ml. ***Rate:*** Administer over 20–30 min via peripheral or central line. **Compatibility:** Do not admix; do not administer in IV line containing other medications.

Patient/Family Teaching

- Explain purpose of medication to patient. Explain that patient will need to resume lifelong therapy with other immunosuppressive drugs after completion of basiliximab course.
- May cause dizziness. Caution patient to avoid driving or other activities requiring alertness until response is known.
- Instruct patient to continue to avoid crowds and persons with known infections, because basiliximab also suppresses the immune system.

Evaluation/Desired Outcomes

- Prevention of acute organ rejection in patients receiving renal transplantation.

---

beclomethasone, See CORTICOSTEROIDS (INHALATION), CORTICOSTEROIDS (NASAL).

---

benazepril, See ANGIOTENSIN-CONVERTING ENZYME (ACE) INHIBITORS.

benzathine penicillin G, See PENICILLINS.

benzonatate (ben-zoe-na-tate)
Tessalon

Classification
Therapeutic: allergy, cold, and cough remedies, antitussives (local anesthetic)

Pregnancy Category C

Indications
Relief of nonproductive cough due to minor throat or bronchial irritation from inhaled irritants or colds.

Action
Anesthetizes cough or stretch receptors in vagal nerve afferent fibers found in lungs, pleura, and respiratory passages. May also decrease transmission of the cough reflex centrally. **Therapeutic Effects:** Decrease in cough.

Pharmacokinetics
Absorption: Unknown.
Distribution: Unknown.
Metabolism and Excretion: Unknown.
Half-life: Unknown.

TIME/ACTION PROFILE (antitussive effect)

ROUTE	ONSET	PEAK	DURATION
PO	15–20 min	unknown	3–8 hr

Contraindications/Precautions
Contraindicated in: Hypersensitivity to benzonatate. Cross-sensitivity with other ester-type local anesthetics (tetracaine, procaine, and others) may occur.
Use Cautiously in: OB, Lactation: Safety not established; Pedi: Safety not established in children <10 yr.

Adverse Reactions/Side Effects
CNS: headache, mild dizziness, sedation. **EENT:** burning sensation in eyes, nasal congestion. **GI:** constipation, GI upset, nausea. **Derm:** pruritus, skin eruptions. **Misc:** chest numbness, chilly sensation, hypersensitivity reactions.

Interactions
Drug-Drug: Additive CNS depression may occur with **antihistamines**, **alcohol**, **opioids**, and **sedative/hypnotics**.

Route/Dosage
PO (Adults and Children ≥10 yr): 100 mg 3 times daily (up to 600 mg/day).

Availability (generic available)
Capsules: 100 mg.

NURSING IMPLICATIONS

Assessment
- Assess frequency and nature of cough, lung sounds, and amount and type of sputum produced. Unless contraindicated, maintain fluid intake of 1500–2000 ml to decrease viscosity of bronchial secretions.

Potential Nursing Diagnoses
Ineffective airway clearance (Indications)

Implementation
- Capsules should be swallowed whole. Do not chew, because release of benzonatate from capsules may cause local anesthetic effect and choking.

Patient/Family Teaching
- Instruct patient to take exactly as directed. If a dose is missed, take as soon as possible unless almost time for next dose. Do not double doses.
- Caution patient not to chew capsules.
- Instruct patient to cough effectively: Sit upright and take several deep breaths before attempting to cough.
- Advise patient to minimize cough by avoiding irritants, such as cigarette smoke, fumes, and dust. Humidification of environmental air, frequent sips of water, and sugarless hard candy may also decrease the frequency of dry, irritating cough.
- Caution patient to avoid taking alcohol or other CNS depressants concurrently with this medication.
- May occasionally cause dizziness or drowsiness. Caution patient to avoid driving or other activities requiring alertness until response to the medication is known.
- Advise patient that any cough lasting more than 1 wk or accompanied by fever, chest pain, persistent headache, or skin rash warrants medical attention.
- Advise patient to notify health care professional if symptoms of overdose (seizures, restlessness, trembling) occur.

Evaluation/Desired Outcomes

- Decrease in frequency and intensity of cough without eliminating patient's cough reflex.

benztropine (benz-troe-peen)

Apo-Benztropine, Cogentin

Classification

Therapeutic: antiparkinson agents
Pharmacologic: anticholinergics

Pregnancy Category C

Indications

Adjunctive treatment of all forms of Parkinson's disease, including drug-induced extrapyramidal effects and acute dystonic reactions.

Action

Blocks cholinergic activity in the CNS, which is partially responsible for the symptoms of Parkinson's disease. Restores the natural balance of neurotransmitters in the CNS. **Therapeutic Effects:** Reduction of rigidity and tremors.

Pharmacokinetics

Absorption: Well absorbed following PO and IM administration.
Distribution: Unknown.
Metabolism and Excretion: Unknown.
Half-life: Unknown.

TIME/ACTION PROFILE (antidyskinetic activity)

ROUTE	ONSET	PEAK	DURATION
PO	1–2 hr	several days	24 hr
IM, IV	within min	unknown	24 hr

Contraindications/Precautions

Contraindicated in: Hypersensitivity; Children <3 yr; Angle-closure glaucoma; Tardive dyskinesia.
Use Cautiously in: Prostatic hyperplasia; Seizure disorders; Cardiac arrhythmias; OB, Lactation: Safety not established; Geri: Increased risk of adverse reactions.

Adverse Reactions/Side Effects

CNS: confusion, depression, dizziness, hallucinations, headache, sedation, weakness. **EENT:** blurred vision, dry eyes, mydriasis. **CV:** arrhythmias, hypotension, palpitations, tachycardia. **GI:** constipation, dry mouth, ileus, nausea. **GU:** hesitancy, urinary retention. **Misc:** decreased sweating.

Interactions

Drug-Drug: Additive anticholinergic effects with **drugs sharing anticholinergic properties**, such as **antihistamines**, **phenothiazines**, **quinidine**, **disopyramide**, and **tricyclic antidepressants**. Counteracts the cholinergic effects of **bethanechol**. **Antacids** and **antidiarrheals** may ↓ absorption.
Drug-Natural Products: ↑ anticholinergic effect with **angel's trumpet**, **jimson weed**, and **scopolia**.

Route/Dosage

Parkinsonism

PO (Adults): 1–2 mg/day in 1–2 divided doses (range 0.5–6 mg/day).

Acute Dystonic Reactions

IM, IV (Adults): 1–2 mg, then 1–2 mg PO twice daily.

Drug-Induced Extrapyramidal Reactions

PO, IM, IV (Adults): 1–4 mg given once or twice daily (1–2 mg 2–3 times daily may also be used PO).

Availability (generic available)

Tablets: 0.5 mg, 1 mg, 2 mg. **Injection:** 1 mg/ml.

NURSING IMPLICATIONS

Assessment

- Assess parkinsonian and extrapyramidal symptoms (restlessness or desire to keep moving, rigidity, tremors, pill rolling, mask-like face, shuffling gait, muscle spasms, twisting motions, difficulty speaking or swallowing, loss of balance control) before and throughout therapy.
- Assess bowel function daily. Monitor for constipation, abdominal pain, distention, or absence of bowel sounds.
- Monitor intake and output ratios and assess patient for urinary retention (dysuria, distended abdomen, infrequent voiding of small amounts, overflow incontinence).
- Patients with mental illness are at risk of developing exaggerated symptoms of their disorder during early therapy with benztropine. Withhold drug and notify physician or other health care professional if significant behavioral changes occur.
- **IM/IV:** Monitor pulse and blood pressure closely and maintain bedrest for 1 hr after administration. Advise patients to change posi-

tions slowly to minimize orthostatic hypotension.

Potential Nursing Diagnoses

Impaired physical mobility (Indications)
Risk for injury (Indications)

Implementation

- **PO:** Administer with food or immediately after meals to minimize gastric irritation. May be crushed and administered with food if patient has difficulty swallowing.
- **IM:** Parenteral route is used only for dystonic reactions.

IV Administration

- **Direct IV:** IV route is rarely used because onset is same as with IM route. ***Rate:*** Administer at a rate of 1 mg over 1 min.
- **Syringe Compatibility:** metoclopramide, perphenazine.
- **Y-Site Compatibility:** fluconazole, tacrolimus.

Patient/Family Teaching

- Encourage patient to take benztropine as directed. Take missed doses as soon as possible, up to 2 hr before the next dose. Taper gradually when discontinuing or a withdrawal reaction may occur (anxiety, tachycardia, insomnia, return of parkinsonian or extrapyramidal symptoms).
- May cause drowsiness or dizziness. Advise patient to avoid driving or other activities that require alertness until response to the drug is known.
- Instruct patient that frequent rinsing of mouth, good oral hygiene, and sugarless gum or candy may decrease dry mouth. Patient should notify health care professional if dryness persists (saliva substitutes may be used). Also, notify the dentist if dryness interferes with use of dentures.
- Caution patient to change positions slowly to minimize orthostatic hypotension.
- Instruct patient to notify health care professional if difficulty with urination, constipation, abdominal discomfort, rapid or pounding heartbeat, confusion, eye pain, or rash occurs.
- Advise patient to confer with health care professional before taking OTC medications, especially cold remedies, or drinking alcoholic beverages.
- Caution patient that this medication decreases perspiration. Overheating may occur during hot weather. Patient should notify health care professional if unable to remain indoors in an air-conditioned environment during hot weather.
- Advise patient to avoid taking antacids or antidiarrheals within 1–2 hr of this medication.
- Emphasize the importance of routine follow-up exams.

Evaluation/Desired Outcomes

- Decrease in tremors and rigidity and an improvement in gait and balance. Therapeutic effects are usually seen 2–3 days after the initiation of therapy.

betamethasone, See CORTICOSTEROIDS (SYSTEMIC), CORTICOSTEROIDS (TOPICAL/LOCAL).

betaxolol† (be-**tax**-oh-lol)

Kerlone

Classification
Therapeutic: antihypertensives
Pharmacologic: beta blockers

Pregnancy Category C

†See Appendix C for ophthalmic use

Indications

Management of hypertension.

Action

Blocks stimulation of $beta_1$ (myocardial)-adrenergic receptors. Does not usually affect $beta_2$ (pulmonary, vascular, uterine) receptor sites. **Therapeutic Effects:** Decreased blood pressure and heart rate.

Pharmacokinetics

Absorption: Well absorbed after oral administration.
Distribution: Widely distributed.
Metabolism and Excretion: Mostly metabolized by the liver, 20% excreted unchanged by the kidneys.
Half-life: 15–20 hr.

TIME/ACTION PROFILE (antihypertensive effect)

ROUTE	ONSET	PEAK	DURATION
PO	3–4 hr	3–4 hr	24 hr

Contraindications/Precautions

Contraindicated in: Uncompensated CHF; Pulmonary edema; Cardiogenic shock; Bradycardia or heart block.

Use Cautiously in: Renal or hepatic impairment; Pulmonary disease (including asthma; $beta_1$ selectivity may be lost at higher doses); avoid use if possible; Diabetes mellitus; Thyrotoxicosis; Patients with a history of severe allergic reactions (intensity of reactions may be increased); OB, Lactation, Pedi: Safety not established; all agents cross the placenta and may cause fetal/neonatal bradycardia, hypotension, hypoglycemia, or respiratory depression; Geri: Increased sensitivity to beta blockers; initial dosage reduction recommended.

Adverse Reactions/Side Effects

CNS: fatigue, weakness, anxiety, depression, dizziness, drowsiness, insomnia, memory loss, mental status changes, nightmares. **EENT:** blurred vision, stuffy nose. **Resp:** bronchospasm, wheezing. **CV:** BRADYCARDIA, CHF, PULMONARY EDEMA, hypotension, peripheral vasoconstriction. **GI:** constipation, diarrhea, liver function abnormalities, nausea, vomiting. **GU:** erectile dysfunction, decreased libido, urinary frequency. **Derm:** rashes. **Endo:** hyperglycemia, hypoglycemia. **MS:** arthralgia, back pain, joint pain. **Misc:** drug-induced lupus syndrome.

Interactions

Drug-Drug: General anesthetics, **IV phenytoin**, and **verapamil** may cause additive myocardial depression. Additive bradycardia may occur with **digoxin**. Additive hypotension may occur with other **antihypertensives**, acute ingestion of **alcohol**, or **nitrates**. Concurrent use with **amphetamine**, **cocaine**, **ephedrine**, **epinephrine**, **norepinephrine**, **phenylephrine**, or **pseudoephedrine** may result in unopposed alpha-adrenergic stimulation (excessive hypertension, bradycardia). Concurrent **thyroid preparation** administration may decrease effectiveness. May alter the effectiveness of **insulins** or **oral hypoglycemic agents** (dosage adjustments may be necessary). May decrease the effectiveness of **theophylline**. May decrease the beneficial $beta_1$-cardiovascular effects of **dopamine** or **dobutamine**. Use cautiously within 14 days of **MAO inhibitor** therapy (may result in hypertension).

Route/Dosage

PO (Adults): 10 mg once daily, may be increased to 20 mg after 7 days; start with 5 mg in geriatric patients.

Renal Impairment

PO (Adults): start with 5 mg once daily.

Availability

Tablets: 10 mg, 20 mg. **Cost:** 10 mg $82.63/100, 20 mg $123.95/100.

NURSING IMPLICATIONS

Assessment

- Monitor blood pressure, ECG, and pulse frequently during dose adjustment and periodically during therapy.
- Monitor intake and output ratios and daily weights. Assess routinely for signs and symptoms of congestive heart failure (dyspnea, rales/crackles, weight gain, peripheral edema, jugular venous distention).
- **Angina:** Assess frequency and characteristics of angina periodically during therapy.
- ***Lab Test Considerations:*** May cause increased BUN, serum lipoprotein, potassium, triglyceride, and uric acid levels.
- May cause increased ANA titers.
- May cause increase in blood glucose levels.
- ***Toxicity and Overdose:*** Monitor patients receiving beta blockers for signs of overdose (bradycardia, severe dizziness or fainting, severe drowsiness, dyspnea, bluish fingernails or palms, seizures). Notify physician or health care professional immediately if these signs occur: Glucagon has been used to treat bradycardia and hypotension.

Potential Nursing Diagnoses

Decreased cardiac output (Side Effects)
Noncompliance (Patient/Family Teaching)

Implementation

- **PO:** Take apical pulse before administering. If <50 bpm or if arrhythmia occurs, withhold medication and notify physician or other health care professional.
- May be administered without regard to food.

Patient/Family Teaching

- Instruct patient to take medication exactly as directed, at the same time each day, even if feeling well; do not skip or double up on missed doses. Take missed doses as soon as possible up to 4 hr before next dose. Abrupt withdrawal may precipitate life-threatening arrhythmias, hypertension, or myocardial ischemia.

- Advise patient to make sure enough medication is available for weekends, holidays, and vacations. A written prescription may be kept in wallet in case of emergency.
- Teach patient and family how to check pulse and blood pressure. Instruct them to check pulse daily and blood pressure biweekly and to report significant changes.
- May cause drowsiness or dizziness. Caution patients to avoid driving or other activities that require alertness until response to the drug is known.
- Advise patients to change positions slowly to minimize orthostatic hypotension.
- Caution patient that this medication may increase sensitivity to cold.
- Instruct patient to consult health care professional before taking any OTC medications, especially cold preparations, concurrently with this medication.
- Patients with diabetes should closely monitor blood glucose, especially if weakness, malaise, irritability, or fatigue occurs. Betaxolol may mask some signs of hypoglycemia, but sweating and dizziness may occur.
- Advise patient to notify health care professional if slow pulse, difficulty breathing, wheezing, cold hands and feet, dizziness, confusion, depression, rash, fever, sore throat, unusual bleeding, or bruising occurs.
- Instruct patient to inform health care professional of medication regimen before treatment or surgery.
- Advise patient to carry identification describing disease process and medication regimen at all times.
- **Hypertension:** Reinforce the need to continue additional therapies for hypertension (weight loss, sodium restriction, stress reduction, regular exercise, moderation of alcohol consumption, and smoking cessation). Medication controls but does not cure hypertension.

Evaluation/Desired Outcomes

- Decrease in blood pressure without appearance of detrimental side effects.

B

bevacizumab

(be-va-**kiz**-oo-mab)
Avastin

Classification
Therapeutic: antineoplastics
Pharmacologic: monoclonal antibodies

Pregnancy Category C

Indications

Metastatic colon or rectal carcinoma (with IV 5–fluorouracil). First line treatment of patients with unresectable, locally advanced, recurrent or metastatic non-squamous, non-small cell lung cancer with carboplatin and paclitaxel.

Action

A monoclonal antibody that binds to vascular endothelial growth factor (VEGF), preventing its attachment to binding sites on vascular endothelium, thereby inhibiting growth of new blood vessels (angiogenesis). **Therapeutic Effects:** Decreased metastatic disease progression and microvascular growth.

Pharmacokinetics

Absorption: IV administration results in complete bioavailability.
Distribution: Unknown.
Metabolism and Excretion: Unknown.
Half-life: 20 days (range 11–50 days).

TIME/ACTION PROFILE

ROUTE	ONSET	PEAK	DURATION
IV	rapid	end of infusion	14 days

Contraindications/Precautions

Contraindicated in: Hypersensitivity; Recent hemoptysis or other serious recent bleeding episode; First 28 days after major surgery; OB: Angiogenesis is critical to the developing fetus. Contraindicated unless benefit to mother outweighs potential fetal harm. Lactation: Discontinue nursing during treatment and, due to long half-life, for several weeks following treatment.
Use Cautiously in: Cardiovascular disease; Pedi: Safety not established; Geri: ↑ risk of serious adverse reactions including arterial thromboembolic events.

Adverse Reactions/Side Effects

CNS: reversible posterior leukoencephalopathy syndrome (RPLS). **CV:** ARTERIAL THROMBOEMBOLIC

EVENTS, CHF, hypertension, hypotension. **Resp:** HEMOPTYSIS, non-gastrointestinal fistulas, nasal septum perforation. **GI:** GI PERFORATION. **GU:** nephrotic syndrome, proteinuria. **Hemat:** BLEEDING. **Misc:** WOUND DEHISCENCE, impaired wound healing, infusion reactions.

Interactions

Drug-Drug: ↑ blood levels of SN 38 (the active metabolite of **irinotecan**); significance is not known.

Route/Dosage

Colon Cancer

IV (Adults): 5 mg/kg infusion every 14 days.

Lung Cancer

IV (Adults): 15 mg/kg infusion every 3 wks.

Availability

Solution for injection (requires dilution): 100 mg/4 ml vial, 400 mg/16 ml vial.

NURSING IMPLICATIONS

Assessment

- Assess for signs of GI perforation (abdominal pain associated with constipation and vomiting), fistula formation, and wound dehiscence during therapy; therapy should be discontined.
- Assess for signs of hemorrhage (epistaxis, hemoptysis, bleeding) and thromboembolic events (stroke, MI, deep vein thrombosis) during therapy; may require discontinuation.
- Monitor BP every 2–3 wk during therapy. Temporarily suspend therapy during severe hypertension not controlled with medical management; permanently discontinue if hypertensive crisis occurs.
- Assess for infusion reactions (stridor, wheezing) during therapy.
- Assess for signs of CHF (dyspnea, peripheral edema, rales/crackles, jugular venous distension) during therapy.
- Monitor for signs of RPLS (headache, seizure, lethargy, confusion, blindness). Hypertension may or may not be present. May occur within 16 hrs to 1 yr of initiation of therapy. Treat hypertension if present and discontinue bevacizumab therapy. Symptoms usually resolve within days.
- ***Lab Test Considerations:*** Monitor serial urinalysis for proteinuria during therapy. Patients with a 2+ or greater urine dipstick require further testing with a 24–hr urine collection.
- May cause leukopenia, thrombocytopenia, hypokalemia, and bilirubinemia.

Potential Nursing Diagnoses

Ineffective tissue perfusion (Adverse Reactions)

Implementation

- Avoid administration for at least 28 days following major surgery; surgical incision should be fully healed due to potential for impaired wound healing.
- **Intermittent Infusion:** ***Diluent:*** Dilute by withdrawing necessary amount of bevacizumab for a dose of 5 mg/kg and dilute in total volume of 100 ml of 0.9% NaCl. Do not shake. Discard unused portions. Do not administer solution that is discolored or contains particulate matter. Stable if refrigerated for up to 8 hr. ***Rate:*** Administer initial dose over 90 min. If well tolerated, second infusion may be administered over 60 min. If well tolerated, all subsequent infusions may be administered over 30 min. **Do not administer as an IV push or bolus**.
- **Additive Incompatibility:** Do not mix or administer with dextrose solutions.

Patient/Family Teaching

- Inform patient of purpose of medication.
- Advise patient to report any signs of bleeding immediately to health care professional.

Evaluation/Desired Outcomes

- Decreased metastatic disease progression and microvascular growth.

bicalutamide

(bye-ka-**loot**-a-mide)
Casodex

Classification
Therapeutic: antineoplastics
Pharmacologic: antiandrogens

Pregnancy Category X

Indications

Treatment of metastatic prostate carcinoma in conjunction with luteinizing hormone–releasing hormone (LHRH) analogues (goserelin, leuprolide).

Action

Antagonizes the effects of androgen at the cellular level. **Therapeutic Effects:** Decreased spread of prostate carcinoma.

B

Pharmacokinetics

Absorption: Well absorbed after oral administration.
Distribution: Unknown.
Protein Binding: 96%.
Metabolism and Excretion: Mostly metabolized by the liver.
Half-life: 5.8 days.

TIME/ACTION PROFILE (blood levels)

ROUTE	ONSET	PEAK	DURATION
PO	unknown	31.3 hr	unknown

Contraindications/Precautions

Contraindicated in: Hypersensitivity; OB: Not for use in women.
Use Cautiously in: Moderate to severe liver impairment; Patients with childbearing potential; Lactation: Not for use in women; Pedi: Safety not established.

Adverse Reactions/Side Effects

CNS: weakness, dizziness, headache, insomnia. **Resp:** dyspnea. **CV:** chest pain, hypertension, peripheral edema. **GI:** constipation, diarrhea, nausea, abdominal pain, increased liver enzymes, vomiting. **GU:** hematuria, erectile dysfunction, incontinence, nocturia, urinary tract infections. **Derm:** alopecia, rashes, sweating. **Endo:** breast pain, gynecomastia. **Hemat:** anemia. **Metab:** hyperglycemia, weight loss. **MS:** back pain, pelvic pain, bone pain. **Neuro:** paresthesia. **Misc:** generalized pain, hot flashes, flu-like syndrome, infection.

Interactions

Drug-Drug: May increase the effect of **warfarin**.

Route/Dosage

PO (Adults): 50 mg once daily (must be given concurrently with LHRH analogue or following surgical castration).

Availability

Tablets: 50 mg.

NURSING IMPLICATIONS

Assessment

- Assess patient for adverse GI effects. Diarrhea is the most common cause of discontinuation of therapy.
- ***Lab Test Considerations:*** Monitor serum prostate-specific antigen (PSA) periodically to determine response to therapy. If levels rise, assess patient for disease progression. May require periodic LHRH analogue administration without bicalutamide.
- Monitor liver function tests before and periodically during therapy. May cause elevated serum alkaline phosphatase, AST, ALT, and bilirubin concentrations. If transaminases increase >2 times normal, bicalutamide should be discontinued; levels usually return to normal after discontinuation.
- May cause increased BUN and serum creatinine, and decreased hemoglobin and WBCs.

Potential Nursing Diagnoses

Diarrhea (Adverse Reactions)

Implementation

- Start treatment with bicalutamide at the same time as LHRH analogue.
- **PO:** May be administered in the morning or evening, without regard to food.

Patient/Family Teaching

- Instruct patient to take bicalutamide exactly as directed at the same time each day. Do not discontinue without consulting health care professional.
- Advise patient not to take other medications without consulting health care professional.
- Instruct patient to report severe or persistent diarrhea.
- Discuss with patient the possibility of hair loss. Explore methods of coping.
- Emphasize the importance of regular follow-up exams and blood tests to determine progress; monitor for side effects.

Evaluation/Desired Outcomes

- Decreased spread of prostate carcinoma.

bisacodyl (bis-a-**koe**-dill)
Bisac-Evac, ✤Bisaco-Lax, ✤Bisacolax, Caroid, Carter's Little Pills, Dacodyl, Deficol, Dulcagen, Dulcolax, Feen-a-Mint, Fleet Laxative, ✤Laxit, Modane, Reliable Gentle Laxative, Theralax, Women's Gentle Laxative

Classification
Therapeutic: laxatives
Pharmacologic: stimulant laxatives

Pregnancy Category UK

Indications
Treatment of constipation. Evacuation of the bowel before radiologic studies or surgery. Part of a bowel regimen in spinal cord injury patients.

Action
Stimulates peristalsis. Alters fluid and electrolyte transport, producing fluid accumulation in the colon. **Therapeutic Effects:** Evacuation of the colon.

Pharmacokinetics
Absorption: Variable absorption follows oral administration; rectal absorption is minimal; action is local in the colon.
Distribution: Small amounts of metabolites excreted in breast milk.
Metabolism and Excretion: Small amounts absorbed are metabolized by the liver.
Half-life: Unknown.

TIME/ACTION PROFILE (evacuation of bowel)

ROUTE	ONSET	PEAK	DURATION
PO	6–12 hr	unknown	unknown
Rectal	15–60 min	unknown	unknown

Contraindications/Precautions
Contraindicated in: Hypersensitivity; Abdominal pain; Obstruction; Nausea or vomiting (especially with fever or other signs of an acute abdomen).
Use Cautiously in: Severe cardiovascular disease; Anal or rectal fissures; Excess or prolonged use (may result in dependence); Products containing tannic acid (Clysodrast) should not be used as multiple enemas (increased risk of hepatotoxicity); May be used during pregnancy and lactation.

Adverse Reactions/Side Effects
GI: abdominal cramps, nausea, diarrhea, rectal burning. **F and E:** hypokalemia (with chronic use). **MS:** muscle weakness (with chronic use). **Misc:** protein-losing enteropathy, tetany (with chronic use).

Interactions
Drug-Drug: Antacids, histamine H_2-receptor antagonists, and **gastric acid–pump inhibitors** may remove enteric coating of tablets resulting in gastric irritation/dyspepsia. May decrease the absorption of other **orally administered drugs** because of increased motility and decreased transit time.
Drug-Food: Milk may remove enteric coating of tablets, resulting in gastric irritation/dyspepsia.

Route/Dosage
PO (Adults and Children ≥12 yr): 5–15 mg (up to 30 mg/day) as a single dose.
PO (Children 3–11 yr): 5–10 mg (0.3 mg/kg) as a single dose.
Rect (Adults and Children ≥12 yr): 10 mg single dose.
Rect (Children 2–11 yr): 5–10 mg single dose.
Rect (Children <2 yr): 5 mg single dose.

Availability (generic available)
Enteric-coated tablets: 5 mg^{OTC}. **Enteric coated and delayed release:** 5 mg^{OTC}. **Suppositories:** 5 mg^{OTC}, 10 mg^{OTC}. **Rectal suspension:** 10 mg/30 ml^{OTC}. ***In combination with:*** tannic acid (Clysodrast^{OTC}), docusate (Dulcodos^{OTC}), hydroxypropyl methylcellulose (Fleet Bisacodyl Prep^{OTC}). Also in Bowel Preparation kits with Magnesium citrate (Evac-Q-Kwik^{OTC}, EZ-EM Prep Kit^{OTC}, LiquiPrep Bowel Evacuant^{OTC}, Tridate Bowel Cleansing Kit^{OTC}), Phosphate/biphosphate (Fleet Prep Kit. No. 1^{OTC}, Fleet Prep Kit No. 2^{OTC}, Fleet Prep Kit No. 3^{OTC}), sennosides (X-Prep Bowel Evacuant Kit #1^{OTC}), sennosides, magnesium citrate, magnesium sulfate (X-Prep Bowel Evacuant Kit #2^{OTC}). See Appendix B.

NURSING IMPLICATIONS

Assessment
- Assess patient for abdominal distention, presence of bowel sounds, and usual pattern of bowel function.
- Assess color, consistency, and amount of stool produced.

Potential Nursing Diagnoses
Constipation (Indications)

Implementation
- May be administered at bedtime for morning results.
- **PO:** Taking on an empty stomach will produce more rapid results.
- Do not crush or chew enteric-coated tablets. Take with a full glass of water or juice.

- Do not administer oral doses within 1 hr of milk or antacids; this may lead to premature dissolution of tablet and gastric or duodenal irritation.
- **Rect:** Suppository or enema can be given at the time a bowel movement is desired. Lubricate suppositories with water or water-soluble lubricant before insertion. Encourage patient to retain the suppository or enema 15–30 min before expelling.

Patient/Family Teaching

- Advise patients, other than those with spinal cord injuries, that laxatives should be used only for short-term therapy. Prolonged therapy may cause electrolyte imbalance and dependence.
- Advise patient to increase fluid intake to at least 1500–2000 ml/day during therapy to prevent dehydration.
- Encourage patients to use other forms of bowel regulation (increasing bulk in the diet, increasing fluid intake, or increasing mobility). Normal bowel habits may vary from 3 times/day to 3 times/wk.
- Instruct patients with cardiac disease to avoid straining during bowel movements (Valsalva maneuver).
- Advise patient that bisacodyl should not be used when constipation is accompanied by abdominal pain, fever, nausea, or vomiting.

Evaluation/Desired Outcomes

- The patient's having a soft, formed bowel movement when used for constipation.
- Evacuation of colon before surgery or radiologic studies, or for patients with spinal cord injury.

bismuth subsalicylate

(**biz**-muth sub-sa-**lis**-i-late)
Bismatrol, Bismed, Kaopectate, Kapectolin, Kao-Tin, K-Pek, Peptic Relief, Pepto-Bismol, Pink Bismuth, ✤PMS-Bismuth Subsalicylate

Classification
Therapeutic: antidiarrheals, antiulcer agents
Pharmacologic: adsorbents

Pregnancy Category C

Indications

Mild to moderate diarrhea. Nausea, abdominal cramping, heartburn, and indigestion that may accompany diarrheal illnesses. Treatment of ulcer disease associated with *Helicobacter pylori* (with anti-infectives). Treatment/prevention of traveler's (enterotoxigenic *Escherichia coli*) diarrhea. **Unlabeled uses:** Chronic infantile diarrhea.

Action

Promotes intestinal adsorption of fluids and electrolytes. Decreases synthesis of intestinal prostaglandins. **Therapeutic Effects:** Relief of diarrhea. Eradication of *H. pylori* with decreased recurrence of ulcer disease (with other agents).

Pharmacokinetics

Absorption: Bismuth is not absorbed; salicylate split from parent compound is >90% absorbed from the small intestine. Salicylate is highly bound to albumin.
Distribution: Salicylate crosses the placenta and enters breast milk.
Metabolism and Excretion: Bismuth is excreted unchanged in the feces. Salicylate undergoes extensive hepatic metabolism.
Half-life: Salicylate—2–3 hr for low doses; 15–30 hr with larger doses.

TIME/ACTION PROFILE (relief of diarrhea and other GI symptoms)

ROUTE	ONSET	PEAK	DURATION
PO	within 24 hr	unknown	unknown

Contraindications/Precautions

Contraindicated in: Aspirin hypersensitivity; cross-sensitivity with NSAIDs or oil of wintergreen may occur; Pedi: During or after recovery from chickenpox or flu-like illness (contains salicylate, which can cause Reye's syndrome); Geri: Geriatric patients who may have fecal impaction.
Use Cautiously in: Patients undergoing radiologic examination of the GI tract (bismuth is ra-

diopaque); Diabetes mellitus; Gout; OB, Lactation: Safety not established; avoid chronic use of large doses; Pedi, Geri: Potential for impaction.

Adverse Reactions/Side Effects

GI: constipation, gray-black stools, impaction (infants, debilitated patients).

Interactions

Drug-Drug: If taken with **aspirin**, may ↑ the risk of salicylate toxicity. May ↓ absorption of **tetracycline**. May ↓ effectiveness of **probenecid** (large doses).

Route/Dosage

PO (Adults): *Antidiarrheal*—2 tablets or 30 ml (15 ml of extra/maximum strength) q 30 min *or* 2 tablets q 60 min as needed (not to exceed 4.2 g/24 hr). *Antiulcer*—524 mg 4 times daily (as 2 tablets, 30 ml of regular strenth suspension or 15 ml of extra/maximum strength).

PO (Children 9–12 yr): 1 tablet or 15 ml (7.5 ml of extra/maximum strength) q 30–60 min (not to exceed 2.1 g/24 hr).

PO (Children 6–9 yr): 10 ml (5 ml of extra/maximum strength) q 30–60 min (not to exceed 1.4 g/24 hr).

PO (Children 3–6 yr): 5 ml (2.5 ml of extra/maximum strength) q 30–60 min (not to exceed 704 mg/24 hr).

Availability (generic available)

Tablets: 262 mg^{OTC}. **Chewable tablets (cherry and other flavors):** 262 mg (contain calcium carbonate)^{OTC}, ♣ 300 mg^{OTC}. **Liquid (cherry, caramel, peppermint, and other flavors):** 262 mg/15 ml^{OTC}, ♣ 264 mg/15 ml^{OTC}, 525 mg/15 ml^{OTC}. ***In combination with:*** kaolin/pectin (Kaodene Non-Narcotic)^{OTC}, in a convenience package with metronidazole and tetracycline (Helidac). See Appendix B.

NURSING IMPLICATIONS

Assessment

- **Diarrhea:** Assess the frequency and consistency of stools, presence of nausea and indigestion, and bowel sounds before and during therapy.
- Assess fluid and electrolyte balance and skin turgor for dehydration if diarrhea is prolonged.
- **Ulcers:** Assess for epigastric or abdominal pain and frank or occult blood in the stool, emesis, or gastric aspirate.
- ***Lab Test Considerations:*** Chronic high doses may cause falsely ↑ uric acid levels with colorimetric assay.
- May interfere with radiologic examination of the GI tract.
- May cause abnormal results with alkaline phosphatase, AST, and ALT tests.
- May cause ↓ potassium levels and serum T_3 and T_4 concentrations.
- Large doses of salicylates may also cause prolonged prothrombin time (PT).
- For additional lab test considerations related to salicylate content, see salicylates monograph.

Potential Nursing Diagnoses

Diarrhea (Indications)
Constipation (Side Effects)

Implementation

- **PO:** Shake liquid before using. Chewable tablets may be chewed or allowed to dissolve before swallowing.

Patient/Family Teaching

- Instruct patient to take medication exactly as directed.
- Inform patient that medication may temporarily cause stools and tongue to appear gray-black.
- Instruct patient that this medication contains aspirin. Advise patient taking concurrent aspirin products to discontinue bismuth subsalicylate if tinnitus, ringing in the ears occurs.
- **Diarrhea:** Instruct patient to notify health care professional if diarrhea persists for more than 2 days or if accompanied by a high fever.
- U.S. Centers for Disease Control and Prevention warn against giving salicylates to children or adolescents with varicella (chickenpox) or influenza-like or viral illnesses because of a possible association with Reye's syndrome.
- **Ulcers:** Advise patient to consult health care professional before taking other OTC ulcer remedies concurrently with bismuth subsalicylate.

Evaluation/Desired Outcomes

- Decrease in diarrhea.
- Decrease in symptoms of indigestion.
- Prevention of traveler's diarrhea.
- Treatment of ulcers.

bisoprolol (bis-**oh**-proe-lol)

Monocor, Zebeta

B

Classification
Therapeutic: antihypertensives
Pharmacologic: beta blockers

Pregnancy Category C

Indications

Management of hypertension.

Action

Blocks stimulation of $beta_1$ (myocardial)-adrenergic receptors. Does not usually affect $beta_2$ (pulmonary, vascular, uterine)-receptor sites. **Therapeutic Effects:** Decreased blood pressure and heart rate.

Pharmacokinetics

Absorption: Well absorbed after oral administration, but 20% undergoes first-pass hepatic metabolism.
Distribution: Unknown.
Metabolism and Excretion: 50% excreted unchanged by the kidneys; remainder renally excreted as metabolites; 2% excreted in feces.
Half-life: 9–12 hr.

TIME/ACTION PROFILE (antihypertensive effect)

ROUTE	ONSET	PEAK	DURATION
PO	unknown	1–4 hr	24 hr

Contraindications/Precautions

Contraindicated in: Uncompensated CHF; Pulmonary edema; Cardiogenic shock; Bradycardia or heart block.
Use Cautiously in: Renal impairment (dosage reduction recommended); Hepatic impairment (dosage reduction recommended); Pulmonary disease (including asthma; $beta_1$ selectivity may be lost at higher doses); avoid use if possible; Diabetes mellitus (may mask signs of hypoglycemia); Thyrotoxicosis (may mask symptoms); Patients with a history of severe allergic reactions (intensity of reactions may be increased); OB, Lactation, Pedi: Safety not established; crosses the placenta and may cause fetal/neonatal bradycardia, hypotension, hypoglycemia, or respiratory depression; Geri: Increased sensitivity to beta blockers; initial dosage reduction recommended.

Adverse Reactions/Side Effects

CNS: fatigue, weakness, anxiety, depression, dizziness, drowsiness, insomnia, memory loss, mental status changes, nervousness, nightmares. **EENT:** blurred vision, stuffy nose. **Resp:** bronchospasm, wheezing. **CV:** BRADYCARDIA, CHF, PULMONARY EDEMA, hypotension, peripheral vasoconstriction. **GI:** constipation, diarrhea, liver function abnormalities, nausea, vomiting. **GU:** erectile dysfunction, decreased libido, urinary frequency. **Derm:** rashes. **Endo:** hyperglycemia, hypoglycemia. **MS:** arthralgia, back pain, joint pain. **Misc:** drug-induced lupus syndrome.

Interactions

Drug-Drug: General anesthetics, IV phenytoin, and **verapamil** may cause additive myocardial depression. Additive bradycardia may occur with **digoxin**. Additive hypotension may occur with other **antihypertensives**, acute ingestion of **alcohol**, or **nitrates**. Concurrent use with **amphetamine**, **cocaine**, **ephedrine**, **epinephrine**, **norepinephrine**, **phenylephrine**, or **pseudoephedrine** may result in unopposed alpha-adrenergic stimulation (excessive hypertension, bradycardia). Concurrent thyroid preparation administration may decrease effectiveness. May alter the effectiveness of **insulins** or **oral hypoglycemic agents** (dosage adjustments may be necessary). May decrease the effectiveness of **theophylline**. May decrease the beneficial $beta_1$-cardiovascular effects of **dopamine** or **dobutamine**. Use cautiously within 14 days of **MAO inhibitor** therapy (may result in hypertension).

Route/Dosage

PO (Adults): 5 mg once daily, may be increased to 10 mg once daily (range 2.5–20 mg/day).

Renal Impairment

Hepatic Impairment

PO (Adults): *CCr <40 ml/min*—Initiate therapy with 2.5 mg/day, titrate cautiously.

Availability (generic available)

Tablets: 5 mg, 10 mg. **Cost:** 5-mg and 10-mg tablets $35.75/30 tablets. ***In combination with:*** hydrochlorothiazide (Ziac). See Appendix B.

NURSING IMPLICATIONS

Assessment

- Monitor blood pressure, ECG, and pulse frequently during dosage adjustment period and periodically throughout therapy.

- Monitor intake and output ratios and daily weights. Assess routinely for signs and symptoms of CHF (dyspnea, rales/crackles, weight gain, peripheral edema, jugular venous distention).
- Monitor frequency of prescription refills to determine adherence.
- ***Lab Test Considerations:*** May cause increased BUN, serum lipoprotein, potassium, triglyceride, and uric acid levels.
- May cause increased ANA titers.
- May cause increase in blood glucose levels.

Potential Nursing Diagnoses
Decreased cardiac output (Side Effects)
Noncompliance (Patient/Family Teaching)

Implementation
- **PO:** Take apical pulse before administering. If <50 bpm or if arrhythmia occurs, withhold medication and notify physician or other health care professional.
- May be administered without regard to meals.

Patient/Family Teaching
- Instruct patient to take medication exactly as directed, at the same time each day, even if feeling well; do not skip or double up on missed doses. If a dose is missed, it should be taken as soon as possible up to 4 hr before next dose. Abrupt withdrawal may precipitate life-threatening arrhythmias, hypertension, or myocardial ischemia.
- Teach patient and family how to check pulse and blood pressure. Instruct them to check pulse daily and blood pressure biweekly and to report significant changes to health care professional.
- May cause drowsiness. Caution patients to avoid driving or other activities that require alertness until response to the drug is known.
- Advise patients to change positions slowly to minimize orthostatic hypotension.
- Caution patient that this medication may increase sensitivity to cold.
- Instruct patient to consult health care professional before taking any OTC medications, especially cold preparations, concurrently with this medication. Patients on antihypertensive therapy should also avoid excessive amounts of coffee, tea, and cola.
- Diabetics should closely monitor blood glucose, especially if weakness, malaise, irritability, or fatigue occurs. Medication does not block dizziness or sweating as signs of hypoglycemia.
- Advise patient to notify health care professional if slow pulse, difficulty breathing, wheezing, cold hands and feet, dizziness, light-headedness, confusion, depression, rash, fever, sore throat, unusual bleeding, or bruising occurs.
- Instruct patient to inform health care professional of medication regimen before treatment or surgery.
- Advise patient to carry identification describing disease process and medication regimen at all times.
- **Hypertension:** Reinforce the need to continue additional therapies for hypertension (weight loss, sodium restriction, stress reduction, regular exercise, moderation of alcohol consumption, and smoking cessation). Medication controls, but does not cure, hypertension.

Evaluation/Desired Outcomes
- Decrease in blood pressure.

bivalirudin (bi-val-i-**roo**-din)
Angiomax

Classification
Therapeutic: anticoagulants
Pharmacologic: thrombin inhibitors

Pregnancy Category B

Indications
Used in conjunction with aspirin to reduce the risk of acute ischemic complications in patients with unstable angina who are undergoing percutaneous transluminal angioplasty (PCTA) or percutaneous coronary intervention (PCI). Patients with or at risk of heparin-induced thrombocytopenia (HIT) and thrombosis syndrome (HITTS) who are undergoing PCI.

Action
Specifically and reversibly inhibits thrombin by binding to its receptor sites. Inhibition of thrombin prevents activation of factors V, VIII, and XII; the conversion of fibrinogen to fibrin; platelet adhesion and aggregation. **Therapeutic Effects:** Decreased acute ischemic complications in patients with unstable angina (death, MI, or the urgent need for revascularization procedures).

Pharmacokinetics
Absorption: IV administration results in complete bioavailability.

Distribution: Unknown.
Metabolism and Excretion: Cleared from plasma by a combination of renal mechanisms and proteolytic breakdown.
Half-life: 25 min (increased in renal impairment).

TIME/ACTION PROFILE (anticoagulant effect)

ROUTE	ONSET	PEAK	DURATION
IV	immediate	unknown	1–2 hr

Contraindications/Precautions

Contraindicated in: Active major bleeding; Hypersensitivity.
Use Cautiously in: Any disease state associated with an increased risk of bleeding; Heparin-induced thrombocytopenia or heparin-induced thrombocytopenia-thrombosis syndrome; Patients with unstable angina not undergoing PCTA; Patients with other acute coronary syndromes; Concurrent use with other platelet aggregation inhibitors (safety not established); Renal impairment (infusion rate reduction recommended if GFR <60 ml/min); Lactation, Pedi: Safety not established; OB: Use only if clearly needed.

Adverse Reactions/Side Effects

CNS: headache, anxiety, insomnia, nervousness. **CV:** hypotension, bradycardia, hypertension. **GI:** nausea, abdominal pain, dyspepsia, vomiting. **Hemat:** BLEEDING. **Local:** injection site pain. **MS:** back pain. **Misc:** pain, fever, pelvic pain.

Interactions

Drug-Drug: Risk of bleeding may be ↑ by concurrent use of **abciximab**, **heparin**, **low molecular weight heparins/heparinoids**, **ticlopidine**, **thrombolytics**, or any other **drugs that inhibit coagulation**.
Drug-Natural Products: ↑ risk of bleeding with **arnica, chamomile, clove, dong quai, feverfew, garlic, ginger, gingko, Panax ginseng, and others.**

Route/Dosage

IV (Adults): 0.75 mg/kg as a bolus injection, followed by a an infusion at a rate of 1.75 mg/kg/hr for the duration of the PCI procedure. An activated clotting time (ACT) should be performed 5 min after bolus dose and an additional bolus dose of 0.3 mg/kg may be administered if needed. Continuation of the infusion (at a rate of 1.75 mg/kg/hr) for up to 4 hr post-procedure is optional. If needed, the infusion may be continued beyond this initial 4 hr at a rate of 0.2 mg/kg/hr for up to 20 hr. Therapy should be initiated prior to the procedure and given in conjunction with aspirin.

Renal Impairment

IV (Adults): No reduction in the bolus dose is needed in any patient with renal impairment. *GFR 10–29 ml/min*—Reduce infusion rate to 1 mg/kg/hr; *Dialysis-dependent patients (off dialysis)*—Reduce infusion rate to 0.25 mg/kg/hr. ACT should be monitored in all patients with renal impairment.

Availability

Powder for injection: 250 mg/vial.

NURSING IMPLICATIONS

Assessment

- Assess for bleeding. Most common is oozing from the arterial access site for cardiac catheterization. Arterial and venous punctures, IM injections, and use of urinary catheters, nasotracheal intubation, and nasogastric tubes should be minimized. Noncompressible sites for IV access should be avoided. If bleeding cannot be controlled with pressure, discontinue bivalirudin immediately.
- Monitor vital signs. May cause bradycardia, hypertension, or hypotension. An unexplained decrease in blood pressure may indicate hemorrhage.
- ***Lab Test Considerations:*** Assess hemoglobin, hematocrit, and platelet count prior to bivalirudin therapy and periodically during therapy. May cause ↓ hemoglobin and hematocrit. An unexplained ↓ in hematocrit may indicate hemorrhage.
- Monitor ACT periodically in patients with renal dysfunction.

Potential Nursing Diagnoses

Ineffective tissue perfusion (Indications)

Implementation

- Administer IV just prior to PTCA, in conjunction with aspirin 300 mg to 325 mg/day. Do not administer IM.

IV Administration

- **Direct IV:** (for bolus dose). ***Diluent:*** Reconstitute each 250-mg vial with 5 ml of sterile water for injection. Reconstituted vials are stable for 24 hr if refrigerated. Further dilute in 50 ml of D5W or 0.9% NaCl. Withdraw bolus dose out of bag. Infusion is stable for 24 hr at room temperature. ***Concentration:*** Final concentration of infusion is 5 mg/ml. ***Rate:*** Administer as a bolus injection.

- **Intermittent Infusion:** ***Diluent:*** Reconstitute each 250-mg vial as per the above directions. Further dilute in 50 ml of D5W or 0.9% NaCl. If infusion is to be continued after 4 hr (at a rate of 0.2 mg/kg/hr), reconstituted vial should be diluted in 500 ml of D5W or 0.9% NaCl. Infusion is stable for 24 hr at room temperature. ***Concentration:*** 5 mg/ml (for infusion rate of 1.75 mg/kg/hr); 0.5 mg/ml (for infusion rate of 0.2 mg/kg/hr). ***Rate:*** Based on patient's weight (see Route/Dosage section).
- **Y-Site Compatibility:** abciximab, amikacin, aminophylline, ampicillin, ampicillin-sulbactam, atropine, azithromycin, aztreonam, bumetanide, calcium gluconate, cefazolin, cefepime, cefoperazone, cefotaxime, cefoxitin, ceftazidime, ceftozoxime, ceftriaxone, cefuroxime, cimetidine, ciprofloxacin, clindamycin, dexamethasone sodium phosphate, digoxin, diltiazem, diphenhydramine, dopamine, doxycycline, droperidol, enaprilat, epinephrine, epoprostenol, eptifibatide, erythromycin, esmolol, famotidine, fentanyl, fluconazole, furosemide, gentamicin, haloperidol, heparin, hydrocortisone, hydromorphone, isoproterenol, labetalol, levofloxacin, lidocaine, lorazepam, magnesium sulfate, meperidine, methylprednisolone, metoclopramide, metoprolol, metronidazole, midazolam, milrinone, morphine, nitroglycerin, nitroprusside, norepinephrine, phenylephrine, piperacillin-tazobactam, potassium chloride, procainamide, promethazine, ranitidine, sodium bicarbonate, theophylline, ticarcillin-clavulanate, tirofiban, tobramycin, trimethoprim/sulfamethoxazole, verapamil.
- **Y-Site Incompatibility:** alteplase, amiodarone, amphotericin B, diazepam, prochlorperazine, reteplase, vancomycin.

Patient/Family Teaching

- Inform patient of the purpose of bivalirudin.
- Instruct patient to notify health care professional immediately if any bleeding is noted.

Evaluation/Desired Outcomes

- Decreased acute ischemic complications in patients with unstable angina (death, MI, or the urgent need for revascularization procedures).

HIGH ALERT

bleomycin (blee-oh-**mye**-sin)

Blenoxane

Classification

Therapeutic: antineoplastics

Pharmacologic: antitumor antibiotics

Pregnancy Category D

Indications

Treatment of: Lymphomas, Squamous cell carcinoma, Testicular embryonal cell carcinoma, Choriocarcinoma, Teratocarcinoma. Intrapleural administration to prevent the reaccumulation of malignant effusions.

Action

Inhibits DNA and RNA synthesis. **Therapeutic Effects:** Death of rapidly replicating cells, particularly malignant ones.

Pharmacokinetics

Absorption: Well absorbed from IM and subcut sites. Absorption follows intrapleural and intraperitoneal administration.

Distribution: Widely distributed, concentrates in skin, lungs, peritoneum, kidneys, and lymphatics.

Metabolism and Excretion: 60–70% excreted unchanged by the kidneys.

Half-life: 2 hr (increased in renal impairment).

TIME/ACTION PROFILE (tumor response)

ROUTE	ONSET	PEAK	DURATION
IV, IM, Subcut	2–3 wk	unknown	unknown

Contraindications/Precautions

Contraindicated in: Hypersensitivity; OB, Lactation: Potential for fetal, infant harm.

Use Cautiously in: Renal impairment (dosage reduction required if <35 ml/min); Pulmonary impairment; Nonmalignant chronic debilitating illness; Patients with childbearing potential; Geri: Increased risk of pulmonary toxicity and related decrease in renal function.

Adverse Reactions/Side Effects

CNS: aggressive behavior, disorientation, weakness. **Resp:** PULMONARY FIBROSIS, pneumonitis. **CV:** hypotension, peripheral vaso-

B

constriction. **GI:** anorexia, nausea, stomatitis, vomiting. **Derm:** hyperpigmentation, mucocutaneous toxicity, alopecia, erythema, rashes, urticaria, vesiculation. **Hemat:** anemia, leukopenia, thrombocytopenia. **Local:** pain at tumor site, phlebitis at IV site. **Metab:** weight loss. **Misc:** ANAPHYLACTOID REACTIONS, chills, fever.

Interactions

Drug-Drug: Hematologic toxicity ↑ with concurrent use of **radiation therapy** and other **antineoplastics**. Concurrent use with **cisplatin** ↓ elimination of bleomycin and may ↑ toxicity. ↑ risk of pulmonary toxicity with other **antineoplastics** or thoracic **radiation therapy**. **General anesthesia** ↑ the risk of pulmonary toxicity. ↑ risk of Raynaud's syndrome when used with **vinblastine**.

Route/Dosage

Lymphoma patients should receive initial test doses of 2 units or less for the first 2 doses.

IV, IM, Subcut (Adults and Children): 0.25–0.5 unit/kg (10–20 units/m^2) weekly or twice weekly initially. If favorable response, lower maintenance doses given (1 unit/day or 5 units/wk IM or IV). May also be given as continuous IV infusion at 0.25 unit/kg or 15 units/m^2/day for 4–5 days.

Intrapleural (Adults): 15–20 units instilled for 4 hr, then removed.

Availability

Injection: 15 units/vial, 30 units vial/.

NURSING IMPLICATIONS

Assessment

- Monitor vital signs before and frequently during therapy.
- Assess for fever and chills. May occur 3–6 hr after administration and last 4–12 hr.
- Monitor for anaphylactic (fever, chills, hypotension, wheezing) and idiosyncratic (confusion, hypotension, fever, chills, wheezing) reactions. Keep resuscitation equipment and medications on hand. Lymphoma patients are at particular risk for idiosyncratic reactions that may occur immediately or several hours after therapy, usually after the first or second dose.
- Assess respiratory status for dyspnea and rales/crackles. Monitor chest x-ray before and periodically during therapy. Pulmonary toxicity occurs primarily in geriatric patients (age 70 or older) who have received 400 or more units or at lower doses in patients who received other antineoplastics or thoracic radiation. May occur 4–10 wk after therapy. Discontinue and do not resume bleomycin if pulmonary toxicity occurs.
- Assess nausea, vomiting, and appetite. Weigh weekly. Modify diet as tolerated. Antiemetics may be given before administration.
- ***Lab Test Considerations:*** Monitor CBC before and periodically during therapy. May cause thrombocytopenia and leukopenia (nadir occurs in 12 days and usually returns to pretreatment levels by day 17).
- Monitor baseline and periodic renal and hepatic function.

Potential Nursing Diagnoses

Risk for injury (Side Effects)
Disturbed body image (Side Effects)

Implementation

- ***High Alert:*** Fatalities have occurred with chemotherapeutic agents. Before administering, clarify all ambiguous orders; double-check single, daily, and course-of-therapy dose limits; have second practitioner independently double-check original order and dose calculations.
- Solution should be prepared in a biologic cabinet. Wear gloves, gown, and mask while handling medication. Discard equipment in specially designated containers.
- Lymphoma patients should receive a 1- or 2-unit test dose 2–4 hrs before initiation of therapy. Monitor closely for anaphylactic reaction. May not detect reactors.
- Premedication with acetaminophen, corticosteroids, and diphenhydramine may reduce drug fever and risk of anaphylaxis.
- Reconstituted solution is stable for 24 hr at room temperature and for 14 days if refrigerated.
- **IM, Subcut: *Diluent:*** Reconstitute vial with 1–5 ml of sterile water for injection, 0.9% NaCl, or bacteriostatic water for injection. Do not reconstitute with diluents containing benzyl alcohol when used for neonates.

IV Administration

- **Direct IV: *Diluent:*** Prepare IV doses by diluting 15-unit vial with at least 5 ml of 0.9% NaCl. ***Concentration:*** Further dilute dose in 50 to 1000 ml of D5W or 0.9% NaCl. ***Rate:*** Administer slowly over 10 min.

- **Syringe Compatibility:** cisplatin, cyclophosphamide, doxorubicin, droperidol, fluorouracil, furosemide, heparin, leucovorin calcium, methotrexate, metoclopramide, mitomycin, vinblastine, vincristine.
- **Y-Site Compatibility:** allopurinol, amifostine, aztreonam, cefepime, cisplatin, cyclophosphamide, doxorubicin, doxorubicin liposome, droperidol, etoposide phosphate, filgrastim, fludarabine, fluorouracil, gemcitabine, granisetron, heparin, leucovorin calcium, melphalan, methotrexate, metoclopramide, mitomycin, ondansetron, paclitaxel, piperacillin/tazobactam, sargramostim, teniposide, thiotepa, vinblastine, vincristine, vinorelbine.
- **Intrapleural:** Dissolve 60 units in 50–100 ml of 0.9% NaCl.
- May be administered through thoracotomy tube by physician. Position patient as directed.

Patient/Family Teaching

- Instruct patient to notify health care professional if fever, chills, wheezing, faintness, diaphoresis, shortness of breath, prolonged nausea and vomiting, or mouth sores occur.
- Encourage patient not to smoke because this may worsen pulmonary toxicity.
- Explain to the patient that skin toxicity may manifest itself as skin sensitivity, hyperpigmentation (especially at skin folds and points of skin irritation), and skin rashes and thickening.
- Instruct patient to inspect oral mucosa for erythema and ulceration. If ulceration occurs, advise patient to use sponge brush and rinse mouth with water after eating and drinking. Opioid analgesics may be required if pain interferes with eating.
- Discuss with patient the possibility of hair loss. Explore coping strategies.
- Advise patient of the need for contraception.
- Instruct patient not to receive any vaccinations without advice of health care professional.
- Emphasize need for periodic lab tests to monitor for side effects.

Evaluation/Desired Outcomes

- Decrease in tumor size without evidence of hypersensitivity or pulmonary toxicity.

BRONCHODILATORS (XANTHINES)

aminophylline (am-in-**off**-i-lin)
✤Phyllocontin, Truphylline

theophylline (thee-**off**-i-lin)
✤Apo-Theo LA, ✤Novo-Theophyl SR, ✤PMS-Theophylline, ✤Pulmophylline, Quibron-T, Theochron, Theo-24, Uniphyl

Classification
Therapeutic: bronchodilators
Pharmacologic: xanthines

Pregnancy Category C

Indications

Long-term control of reversible airway obstruction caused by asthma or COPD. Increases diaphragmatic contractility (aminophylline). **Unlabeled uses:** Respiratory and myocardial stimulant in premature infant apnea (apnea of prematurity) (aminophylline).

Action

Inhibit phosphodiesterase, producing increased tissue concentrations of cyclic adenosine monophosphate (cAMP). Increased levels of cAMP result in: Bronchodilation, CNS stimulation, Positive inotropic and chronotropic effects, Diuresis, Gastric acid secretion. **Therapeutic Effects:** Bronchodilation.

Pharmacokinetics

Absorption: Aminophylline releases theophylline after administration. Well absorbed from oral dosage forms; absorption from extended-release dosage forms is slow but complete.
Distribution: Widely distributed; crosses the placenta; breast milk concentrations are 70% of plasma levels; not distributed into adipose tissue.
Metabolism and Excretion: Aminophylline is converted to theophylline; theophylline is 90% metabolized by the liver to several metabolites (including the active metabolites, caffeine and 3–methylxanthine) which may accumulate in neonates; metabolites are renally excreted; 10% excreted unchanged by the kidneys.
Half-life: *Theophylline*—Premature infants: 20–30 hr; Term infants: 11–25 hr; Children 1–4 yr: 3.4 hr; Children 6–17 yr: 3.7 hr; Adults: 9–10 hr (increased in patients >60 yr, patients with CHF or liver disease; decreased in cigarette smokers).

TIME/ACTION PROFILE (bronchodilation)

ROUTE	ONSET†	PEAK	DURATION
Aminophylline PO	15–60 min	1–2 hr	6–8 hr
Aminophylline PO–ER	unknown	4–7 hr	8–12 hr
Aminophylline IV	rapid	end of infusion	6–8 hr
Theophylline PO	rapid	1–2 hr	6 hr
Theophylline PO–ER	delayed	4–8 hr	8–24 hr
Theophylline IV	rapid	end of infusion	6–8 hr

†Provided that a loading dose has been given and steady-state blood levels exist

Contraindications/Precautions

Contraindicated in: Hypersensitivity to aminophylline or theophylline.

Use Cautiously in: CHF, liver disease, or hypothyroidism (dosage reduction required); Cardiac arrhythmias; Peptic ulcer disease; Seizure disorder; OB: Has been used safely; Lactation: Safety not established; Pedi: Dosage reduction required in children <1 yr; Geri, OB: Dosage reduction required due to enhanced potential for adverse reaction.

Adverse Reactions/Side Effects

CNS: SEIZURES, anxiety, headache, insomnia, irritability. **CV:** ARRHYTHMIAS, tachycardia, angina, palpitations. **GI:** nausea, vomiting, anorexia. **Neuro:** tremor. **Derm:** rashes.

Interactions

Drug-Drug: Additive CV and CNS side effects with **adrenergics (sympathomimetic)**. May ↓ the therapeutic effect of **lithium** and **phenytoin**. **Nicotine** (cigarettes, gum, transdermal patches), **barbiturates**, **phenytoin**, **nevirapine** and **rifampin** may ↑ metabolism and may ↓ effectiveness. **Erythromycin**, **beta blockers**, **clarithromycin**, **calcium channel blockers**, **cimetidine**, **doxycycline**, **estrogens**, **hormonal contraceptives**, **disulfiram**, **fluvoxamine**, **isoniazid**, **ketoconazole**, **mexiletine**, **nefazodone**, **protease inhibitors**, **quinidine**, some **fluoroquinolones**, and large doses of **allopurinol** ↓ metabolism and may lead to toxicity.

Drug-Natural Products: Caffeine-containing herbs (**cola nut**, **guarana**, **mate**, **tea**, **coffee**) may ↑ serum levels and risk of CNS and cardiovascular side effects. ↓ serum levels and effectiveness with **St. John's wort**.

Drug-Food: Excessive regular intake of **charcoal-broiled foods** may ↓ effectiveness.

Route/Dosage

Dose should be determined by theophylline serum level monitoring. Loading dose should be decreased or eliminated if theophylline preparation has been used in preceding 24 hr. Aminophylline is 80% theophylline (100 mg aminophylline = 80 mg theophylline). Extended-release (controlled-release, sustained-release) products may be given q 8–24 hr, depending upon the formulation.

Aminophylline

PO (Adults and Children): See theophylline for oral doses.

IV (Adults): *Loading dose*—6 mg/kg (4.7 mg/kg of theophylline) given over 20–30 min, followed by 0.7 mg/kg/hr (0.56 mg/kg/hr of theophylline) via continuous infusion (non-smokers); an infusion rate of 0.9 mg/kg/hr (0.72 mg/kg/hr of theophylline) should be used for smokers.

IV (Geriatric Patients and Adult Patients with Cor Pulmonale): *Loading dose*—6 mg/kg (4.7 mg/kg of theophylline) given over 20–30 min, followed by 0.6 mg/kg/hr (0.47 mg/kg/hr of theophylline) via continuous infusion.

IV (Adults with CHF or Liver Failure): *Loading dose*—6 mg/kg (4.7 mg/kg of theophylline) given over 20–30 min, followed by 0.5 mg/kg/hr (0.39 mg/kg/hr of theophylline) via continuous infusion.

IV (Children 12–16 yr): *Loading dose:* 6 mg/kg (4.7 mg/kg of theophylline) given over 20–30 min, followed by 0.7 mg/kg/hr (0.56 mg/kg/hr of theophylline) via continuous infusion.

IV (Children 9–12 yr): *Loading dose:* 6 mg/kg (4.7 mg/kg of theophylline) given over 20–30 min, followed by 0.9 mg/kg/hr (0.72 mg/kg/hr of theophylline) via continuous infusion.

IV (Children 1–9 yr): *Loading dose:* 6 mg/kg (4.7 mg/kg of theophylline) given over 20–30 min, followed by 1–1.2 mg/kg/hr (0.8–0.96 mg/kg/hr of theophyllne) via continuous infusion.

IV (Children 6 mo–1 yr): *Loading dose:* 6 mg/kg (4.7 mg/kg of theophylline) given over 20–30 min, followed by 0.6–0.7 mg/kg/hr

(0.48–0.56 mg/kg/hr of theophylline) via continuous infusion.
IV (Infants 6 wk–6 mo): *Loading dose*—6 mg/kg (4.7 mg/kg of theophylline) given over 20–30 min, followed by 0.5 mg/kg/hr (0.4 mg/kg/hr of theophylline) via continuous infusion.

Theophylline

PO (Adults Healthy, Non-smoking): *Loading dose*—5 mg/kg, followed by 10 mg/kg/day divided q 8–12 hr (not to exceed 900 mg/day).
PO (Adults with CHF, Cor Pulmonale, or Liver Dysfunction): *Loading dose*—5 mg/kg, followed by 5 mg/kg/day divided q 8–12 hr (not to exceed 400 mg/day).
PO (Children 12–16 yr, Non-smoking): *Loading dose*—5 mg/kg, followed by 13 mg/kg/day divided q 8–12 hr.
PO (Children 9–12 yr, adolescent and adult smokers <50 yr): *Loading dose*—5 mg/kg, followed by 16 mg/kg/day divided q 8–12 hr.
PO (Children 1–9 yr): *Loading dose*—5 mg/kg, followed by 20–24 mg/kg/day divided q 8–12 hr.
PO (Infants 6 mo–1 yr): *Loading dose*—5 mg/kg, followed by 12–18 mg/kg/day divided q 6–8 hr.
PO (Infants 6 wk–6 mo): *Loading dose*—5 mg/kg, followed by 10 mg/kg/day divided q 6–8 hr.
PO (Neonates up to 6 wks): *Loading dose*—4 mg/kg, followed by 4 mg/kg/day divided q 12 hr.
IV (Adults and Children): See aminophylline for IV doses.

Availability

Aminophylline

Tablets: 100 mg, 200 mg. **Extended-release tablets:** ♣225 mg, ♣350 mg. **Oral solution:** 105 mg/5 ml. **Suppositories:** 250 mg, 500 mg. **Injection:** 25 mg/ml.

Theophylline

Sustained-release tablets (8–12 hr): 300 mg. **Extended-release tablets (12–24 hr):** 100 mg, 200 mg, 300 mg, 450 mg. **Controlled-release tablets (24 hr):** 400 mg, 600 mg. **Extended-release capsules (12 hr):** 125 mg, 200 mg, 300 mg. **Extended-release capsules (24 hr):** 100 mg, 200 mg, 300 mg, 400 mg. **Elixir (orange/raspberry, mixed fruit, and other flavors):** 80 mg/15 ml. **Injection (with dextrose):** 0.8 mg/ml, 1.6 mg/ml, 2 mg/ml, 3.2 mg/ml, 4 mg/ml.

NURSING IMPLICATIONS

Assessment

- Assess blood pressure, pulse, respiratory status (rate, lung sounds, use of accessory muscles, number and severity of apnea spells in infants) before and throughout therapy. Ensure that oxygen therapy is correctly instituted during acute asthma attacks.
- Monitor intake and output ratios for an increase in diuresis or fluid overload.
- Patients with a history of cardiovascular problems should be monitored for chest pain and ECG changes (PACs, supraventricular tachycardia, PVCs, ventricular tachycardia). Resuscitative equipment should be readily available.
- Monitor pulmonary function tests before and periodically during therapy to determine therapeutic efficacy in patients with chronic bronchitis or emphysema.
- ***Lab Test Considerations:*** Monitor ABGs, acid-base, and fluid and electrolyte balance in patients receiving parenteral therapy or whenever required by patient's condition.
- ***Toxicity and Overdose:*** Monitor drug levels routinely, especially in patients requiring high doses or during prolonged intensive therapy. Serum sample should be obtained at time of peak absorption. Peak levels should be evaluated 30 min after a 30 min IV loading dose, 12–24 hr after initiation of a continuous infusion, 1–2 hr after rapid-acting oral forms, and 4–12 hr after extended-release oral forms. Therapeutic plasma levels range from 10–15 mcg/ml for asthma and 6–14 mcg/ml for apnea of prematurity. Drug levels in excess of 20 mcg/ml are associated with toxicity. Caffeine ingestion may falsely elevate drug concentration levels: Observe patient for symptoms of drug toxicity (anorexia, nausea, vomiting, stomach cramps, diarrhea, confusion, headache, restlessness, flushing, increased urination, insomnia, tachycardia, arrhythmias, seizures). Notify physician or other health care professional immediately if these occur. Tachycardia, ventricular arrhythmias, or seizures may be the first sign of toxicity. Geri: Patients over 60 yr have increased risk of toxicity and sensitivity to toxic effects due to age-related pharmacodynamic and pharmacokinetic changes. Theophylline doses should not exceed 400 mg/d. Assess frequently.

Potential Nursing Diagnoses

Ineffective airway clearance (Indications)
Activity intolerance (Indications)

Implementation

- Administer around the clock to maintain therapeutic plasma levels. Once-a-day doses should be administered in the morning.
- Do not refrigerate elixirs; crystals may form. Crystals should dissolve when liquid is warmed to room temperature.
- Wait at least 4–6 hr after stopping IV therapy to begin immediate-release oral dosage; for extended-release oral dosage form, give first oral dose at time of IV discontinuation.
- **PO:** Administer oral preparations with food or a full glass of water to minimize GI irritation. Food slows, but does not reduce, the extent of absorption. May be administered 1 hr before or 2 hr after meals for more rapid absorption. Swallow tablets whole; do not crush, break, or chew enteric-coated or extended-release tablets (extended-release tablets may be broken if scored). Pedi: Use calibrated measuring device to ensure accurate dose of liquid preparations.

Aminophylline

IV Administration

- **IV:** ***Diluent:*** May be diluted in D5W, D10W, D20W, 0.9% NaCl, 0.45% NaCl, D5/0.9% NaCl, D5/0.45% NaCl, D5/0.25% NaCl, or LR. ***Concentration:*** 1 mg/ml (maximum 25 mg/ml). Mixture is stable for 24 hr if refrigerated.
- Do not administer discolored or precipitated solution. Flush main IV line before administration.
- If extravasation occurs, local injection of 1% procaine and application of heat may relieve pain and promote vasodilation. Loading Dose. Administer over 20–30 min. ***Rate:*** Do not exceed 20–25 mg/min in adults or 0.36 mg/kg/min in children. Administer via infusion pump to ensure accurate dosage. Rapid administration may cause chest pain, dizziness, hypotension, tachypnea, flushing, arrhythmias, or a reaction to the solution or administration technique (chills; fever; redness, pain, or swelling at injection site).
- **Continuous Infusion:** Usually given as a loading dose in a small volume followed by continuous infusion in larger volume. ***Rate:*** See Route and Dosage section for rates.
- **Syringe Compatibility:** heparin, metoclopramide.
- **Syringe Incompatibility:** doxapram.
- **Y-Site Compatibility:** allopurinol, amifostine, amphotericin B cholesteryl sulfate complex, ceftazidime, cimetidine, cladribine, docetaxel, doxorubicin liposome, enalaprilat, esmolol, etoposide, famotidine, filgrastim, fluconazole, fludarabine, foscarnet, gemcitabine, granisetron, inamrinone, labetalol, melphalan, meropenem, morphine, paclitaxel, pancuronium, piperacillin/tazobactam, potassium chloride, propofol, ranitidine, remifentanil, sargramostim, tacrolimus, teniposide, thiotepa, tolazoline, vecuronium, vitamin B complex with vitamin C.
- **Y-Site Incompatibility:** amiodarone, ciprofloxacin, dobutamine, hydralazine, ondansetron, vinorelbine, warfarin.
- **Additive Incompatibility:** Admixing is not recommended because of dose titration and incompatibilities.

Theophylline

IV Administration

- **Continuous Infusion:** Premixed IV theophylline and 5% dextrose are packed in a moisture-barrier overwrap. Remove immediately before administration and squeeze bag to check for leaks. Discard if solution is not clear.
- **Loading Dose:** Administer over 20–30 min. If patient has had another form of theophylline before loading dose, serum theophylline level should be obtained and loading dose proportionately reduced. ***Rate:*** Do not exceed 20–25 mg/min. Rapid administration may cause chest pain, dizziness, hypotension, tachypnea, flushing, arrhythmias, or a reaction to the solution or administration technique (chills; fever; redness, pain, or swelling at injection site). Infusion rate may be increased after 12 hr. Administer via infusion pump to ensure accurate dosage. Monitor ECG continuously; tachyarrhythmias may occur.
- **Y-Site Compatibility:** acyclovir, ampicillin, ampicillin/sulbactam, aztreonam, cefazolin, cefotetan, ceftazidime, ceftriaxone, cimetidine, cisatracurium, clindamycin, diltiazem,

dobutamine, dopamine, doxycycline, erythromycin lactobionate, famotidine, fluconazole, gentamicin, haloperidol, heparin, hydrocortisone sodium succinate, lidocaine, methyldopate, methylprednisolone sodium succinate, metronidazole, midazolam, milrinone, nafcillin, nitroglycerin, nitroprusside, penicillin G potassium, piperacillin, potassium chloride, ranitidine, remifentanil, ticarcillin, ticarcillin/clavulanate, tobramycin, vancomycin.

- **Y-Site Incompatibility:** hetastarch, phenytoin.
- **Additive Incompatibility:** Admixing is not recommended because of dose titration and incompatibilities.

Patient/Family Teaching

- Emphasize the importance of taking only the prescribed dose at the prescribed time intervals. Missed doses should be taken as soon as possible or omitted if close to next dose.
- Encourage the patient to drink adequate liquids (2000 ml/day minimum) to decrease the viscosity of the airway secretions.
- Advise patient to avoid OTC cough, cold, or breathing preparations without consulting health care professional. These medications may increase side effects and cause arrhythmias.
- Encourage patients not to smoke. A change in smoking habits may necessitate a change in dosage.
- Advise patient to minimize intake of xanthine-containing foods or beverages (colas, coffee, chocolate) and not to eat charcoal-broiled foods daily.
- Instruct patient not to change brands without consulting health care professional.
- Advise patient to contact health care professional promptly if the usual dose of medication fails to produce the desired results, symptoms worsen after treatment, or toxic effects occur.
- Emphasize the importance of having serum levels routinely tested every 6–12 mo.

Evaluation/Desired Outcomes

- Increased ease in breathing.
- Clearing of lung fields on auscultation.
- Respiratory and myocardial stimulation in apnea of infancy (aminophylline).

budesonide, See CORTICOSTEROIDS (INHALATION), CORTICOSTEROIDS (NASAL), CORTICOSTEROIDS (SYSTEMIC).

bumetanide

(byoo-**met**-a-nide)
Bumex, ✤Burinex

Classification
Therapeutic: diuretics
Pharmacologic: loop diuretics

Pregnancy Category C

Indications

Edema due to heart failure, hepatic disease, or renal impairment.

Action

Inhibits the reabsorption of sodium and chloride from the loop of Henle and distal renal tubule. Increases renal excretion of water, sodium chloride, magnesium, potassium, and calcium. Effectiveness persists in impaired renal function. **Therapeutic Effects:** Diuresis and subsequent mobilization of excess fluid (edema, pleural effusions).

Pharmacokinetics

Absorption: Well absorbed after oral or IM administration.
Distribution: Widely distributed.
Protein Binding: 72–96%.
Metabolism and Excretion: Partially metabolized by liver; 50% eliminated unchanged by kidneys and 20% excreted in feces.
Half-life: 60–90 min (6 hr in neonates).

TIME/ACTION PROFILE (diuretic effect)

ROUTE	ONSET	PEAK	DURATION
PO	30–60 min	1–2 hr	4–6 hr
IM	30–60 min	1–2 hr	4–6 hr
IV	2–3min	15–45 min	2–3 hr

Contraindications/Precautions

Contraindicated in: Hypersensitivity; Cross-sensitivity with thiazides and sulfonamides may occur; Hepatic coma or anuria.
Use Cautiously in: Severe liver disease (may precipitate hepatic coma; concurrent use with potassium-sparing diuretics may be necessary); Electrolyte depletion; Diabetes mellitus; Increasing azotemia; Lactation, Pedi: Safety not established; bumetanide is a potent displacer of bilirubin and should be used cautiously in critically ill or jaundiced neonates because of risk of kernicterus. Injection contains benzyl alcohol, which may cause gasping syndrome in neonates; Geri: May have increased risk of side ef-

B

fects, especially hypotension and electrolyte imbalance, at usual doses.

Adverse Reactions/Side Effects

CNS: dizziness, encephalopathy, headache. **EENT:** hearing loss, tinnitus. **CV:** hypotension. **GI:** diarrhea, dry mouth, nausea, vomiting. **GU:** excessive urination. **Derm:** photosensitivity, pruritis, rash. **Endo:** hyperglycemia, hyperuricemia. **F and E:** dehydration, hypocalcemia, hypochloremia, hypokalemia, hypomagnesemia, hyponatremia, hypovolemia, metabolic alkalosis. **MS:** arthralgia, muscle cramps, myalgia. **Misc:** increased BUN.

Interactions

Drug-Drug: ↑ hypotension with **antihypertensives**, **nitrates**, or acute ingestion of **alcohol**. ↑ risk of hypokalemia with other **diuretics**, **amphotericin B**, **stimulant laxatives**, and **corticosteroids**. Hypokalemia may ↑ risk of **digoxin** toxicity and ↑ risk of arrhythmia in patients taking drugs that prolong the QT interval. ↓ **lithium** excretion, may cause **lithium** toxicity. ↑ risk of ototoxicity with **aminoglycosides**. **NSAIDS** ↓ effects of bumetanide.

Route/Dosage

PO (Adults): 0.5–2 mg/day given in 1–2 doses; titrate to desired response (maximum daily dose = 10 mg/day).

IM, IV (Adults): 0.5–1 mg/dose, may repeat q 2–3 hr as needed (up to 10 mg/day).

Availability (generic available)

Tablets: 0.5 mg, 1 mg, 2 mg, ✤5 mg. **Cost:** *Generic*—0.5 mg $37.32/100, 1 mg $31.31/100, 2 mg $49.97/100. **Injection:** 0.25 mg/ml.

NURSING IMPLICATIONS

Assessment

- Assess fluid status during therapy. Monitor daily weight, intake and output ratios, amount and location of edema, lung sounds, skin turgor, and mucous membranes. Notify physician or other health care professional if thirst, dry mouth, lethargy, weakness, hypotension, or oliguria occurs.
- Monitor blood pressure and pulse before and during administration. Monitor frequency of prescription refills to determine compliance.
- Assess patients receiving digoxin for anorexia, nausea, vomiting, muscle cramps, paresthesia, and confusion. ↑ risk of digoxin toxicity due to potassium-depleting effect of diuretic. Potassium supplements or potassium-sparing diuretics may be used concurrently to prevent hypokalemia.
- Assess patient for tinnitus and hearing loss. Audiometry is recommended for patients receiving prolonged high-dose IV therapy. Hearing loss is most common after rapid or high-dose IV administration in patients with decreased renal function or those taking other ototoxic drugs.
- Assess for allergy to sulfonamides.
- Geri: Diuretic use is associated with increased risk for falls in older adults. Assess falls risk and implement fall prevention strategies.
- ***Lab Test Considerations:*** Monitor electrolytes, renal and hepatic function, serum glucose, and uric acid levels before and periodically during therapy. May cause ↓ serum sodium, potassium, calcium, and magnesium concentrations. May also cause ↑ BUN, serum glucose, creatinine, and uric acid levels.

Potential Nursing Diagnoses

Excess fluid volume (Indications)
Risk for deficient fluid volume (Side Effects)

Implementation

- Do not confuse Bumex (bumetanide) with Buprenex (buprenorphine).
- If administering twice daily, give last dose no later than 5pm to minimize disruption of sleep cycle.
- IV is preferred over IM for parenteral administration.
- **PO:** May be taken with food to minimize gastric irritation.

IV Administration

- **Direct IV:** ***Diluent:*** Administer undiluted. ***Concentration:*** 0.25 mg/ml. ***Rate:*** Administer slowly over 1–2 min.
- **Continuous Infusion:** ***Diluent:*** May dilute in D5W or 0.9% NaCl. May also administer as undiluted drug. Protect from light. ***Concentration:*** Not to exceed 0.25 mg/ml. ***Rate:*** Infuse over 5 min. May be administered over 12 hr for patients with renal impairment.
- **Y-Site Compatibility:** acyclovir, amikacin, aminophylline, amiodarone, atropine, aztreonam, bivalirudin, calcium chloride, calcium gluconate, caspofungin, cefazolin, cefepime, cefotaxime, cefoxitin, ceftazidime,

ceftizoxime, ceftriaxone, cefuroxime, chloramphenicol, cimetidine, cisatracurium, clindamycin, cyclosporine, daptomycin, dexamethasone, dexmedetomidate, digoxin, diltiazem, diphenhydramine, dobutamine, dopamine, doxycycline, enalaprilat, epinephrine, ertapenem, erythromycin, esmolol, famotidine, fentanyl, filgrastim, fluconazole, gentamicin, granisetron, heparin, hydrocortisone sodium succinate, hydromorphone, imipenem, insulin, isoproterenol, ketorolac, labetalol, levofloxacin, lidocaine, linezolid, lorazepam, magnesium sulfate, meperidine, methylprednisolone sodium succinate, metoclopramide, metoprolol, metronidazole, micafungin, milrinone, morphine, nafcillin, nitroglycerin, nitroprusside, norepinephrine, ondansetron, palonosetron, pantoprazole, penicillin G potassium, phenylephrine, phytonadione, piperacillin/tazobactam, potassium chloride, procainamide, promethazine, propofol, propranolol, protamine, ranitidine, rifampin, sodium bicarbonate, tacrolimus, ticarcillin/clavulanate, tirofiban, tobramycin, vancomycin, vasopressin, verapamil, voriconazole.

- **Y-Site Incompatibility:** diazepam, fenoldopam, ganciclovir, haloperidol, nesiritide, phenytoin, quinupristin/dalfopristin, sulfamethoxazole/trimethoprim.

Patient/Family Teaching

- Instruct patient to take bumetanide as directed. Take missed doses as soon as possible; do not double doses.
- Caution patient to change positions slowly to minimize orthostatic hypotension. Caution patient that drinking alcohol, exercising during hot weather, or standing for long periods may enhance orthostatic hypotension.
- Instruct patient to consult health care professional regarding a diet high in potassium. See Appendix L.
- Advise patient to contact health care professional of gain more than 3 lbs in one day.
- Advise patient to consult health care professional before taking Rx, OTC, or herbal products concurrently with therapy.
- Instruct patient to notify health care professional of medication regimen before treatment or surgery.
- Caution patient to use sunscreen and protective clothing to prevent photosensitivity reactions.
- Advise patient to contact health care professional immediately if muscle weakness, cramps, nausea, dizziness, numbness, or tingling of extremities occurs.
- Advise patients with diabetes to monitor blood glucose closely; may cause increased levels.
- Emphasize the importance of routine follow-up examinations.
- Geri: Caution older patients or their caregivers about increased risk for falls. Suggest strategies for fall prevention.

Evaluation/Desired Outcomes

- Decrease in edema.
- Decrease in abdominal girth and weight.
- Increase in urinary output.

---

bupivacaine, See EPIDURAL LOCAL ANESTHETICS.

HIGH ALERT

buprenorphine

(byoo-pre-**nor**-feen)
Buprenex, Subutex

Classification
Therapeutic: opioid analgesics
Pharmacologic: opioid agonists/antagonists

Schedule III

Pregnancy Category C

Indications

IM, IV: Management of moderate to severe acute pain. **SL:** Treatment of opioid dependence; suppresses withdrawal symptoms in opioid detoxification.

Action

Binds to opiate receptors in the CNS. Alters the perception of and response to painful stimuli while producing generalized CNS depression. Has partial antagonist properties that may result in opioid withdrawal in physically dependent patients when used as an analgesic. **Therapeutic Effects: IM, IV: Decreased severity of pain. SL:** Suppression of withdrawal symptoms during detoxification and maintenance from heroin or other opioids. Produces a relatively mild withdrawal compared to other agents.

Pharmacokinetics

Absorption: Well absorbed after IM and SL use; IV administration results in complete bioavailability.

Distribution: Crosses the placenta; enters breast milk. CNS concentration is 15–25% of plasma.

Protein Binding: 96%.

Metabolism and Excretion: Metabolized by the liver mostly via the CYP3A4 enzyme system; one metabolite is active.

Half-life: 2–3 hr (parenteral).

TIME/ACTION PROFILE (analgesia)

ROUTE	ONSET	PEAK	DURATION
IM	15 min	60 min	6 hr†
IV	rapid	less than 60 min	6 hr†

†4–5 hr in children

Contraindications/Precautions

Contraindicated in: Hypersensitivity; Lactation: Enters breast milk; avoid use or discontinue nursing.

Use Cautiously in: Increased intracranial pressure; Severe renal, hepatic, or pulmonary disease; Hypothyroidism; Adrenal insufficiency; Alcoholism; Debilitated patients (dose reduction required); Undiagnosed abdominal pain; Prostatic hyperplasia; OB: Safety not established; neonatal withdrawal may occur in infants born to patients receiving SL buprenorphine during pregnancy; Geri: Dose reduction required.

Adverse Reactions/Side Effects

CNS: <u>confusion</u>, <u>dysphoria</u>, <u>hallucinations</u>, <u>sedation</u>, dizziness, euphoria, floating feeling, headache, unusual dreams. **EENT:** blurred vision, diplopia, miosis (high doses). **Resp:** respiratory depression. **CV:** hypertension, hypotension, palpitations. **GI:** <u>nausea</u>, constipation, dry mouth, ileus, vomiting. **GU:** urinary retention. **Derm:** <u>sweating</u>, clammy feeling. **Misc:** physical dependence, psychological dependence, tolerance.

Interactions

Drug-Drug: Use with extreme caution in patients receiving **MAO inhibitors** (↑ CNS and respiratory depression and hypotension ↓ buprenorphine dose by 50%; may need to ↓ **MAO inhibitor** dose). ↑ CNS depression with **alcohol**, **antihistamines**, **antidepressants**, and **sedative/hypnotics**. May ↓ effectiveness of other **opioid analgesics**. Inhibitors of the CYP3A4 enzyme system including **azole antifungals (itraconazole, ketoconazole)**, **erythromycin protease inhibitor antiretrovirals (ritonavir, indinavir, saquinavir)** ↑ blood levels and effects; dose reduction may be necessary during concurrent use. Inducers of the CYP3A4 enzyme system including **carbamazepine**, **rifampin**, or **phenytoin** ↓ blood levels and effects; dose modification may be necessary during concurrent use. Concurrent abuse of IV buprenorphine and **benzodiazepines** may result in coma and death.

Drug-Natural Products: Concomitant use of **kava kava, valerian, chamomile**, or **hops can ↑ CNS depression.**

Route/Dosage

Analgesia

IM, IV (Adults): 0.3 mg q 4–6 hr as needed. May repeat initial dose after 30 min (up to 0.3 mg q 4 hr or 0.6 mg q 6 hr); 0.6-mg doses should be given only IM.

IM, IV (Children 2–12 yr): 2–6 mcg (0.002–0.006 mg)/kg q 4–6 hr.

Treatment of opioid dependence

SL (Adults): 12–16 mg/day as a single dose.

Availability

Sublingual tablets: 2 mg, 8 mg. ***In combination with:*** naloxone (Suboxone). See Appendix B. **Injection:** 300 mcg (0.3 mg)/ml.

NURSING IMPLICATIONS

Assessment

- **Pain:** Assess type, location, and intensity of pain before and 1 hr after IM and 5 min (peak) after IV administration. When titrating opioid doses, increases of 25–50% should be administered until there is either a 50% reduction in the patient's pain rating on a numerical or visual analogue scale or the patient reports satisfactory pain relief. A repeat dose can be safely administered at the time of the peak if previous dose is ineffective and side effects are minimal. Single doses of 600 mcg (0.6 mg) should be administered IM. Patients requiring doses higher than 600 mcg (0.6 mg) should be converted to an opioid agonist. Buprenorphine is not recommended for prolonged use or as first-line therapy for acute or cancer pain.

- An equianalgesic chart (see Appendix J) should be used when changing routes or when changing from one opioid to another.
- Assess level of consciousness, blood pressure, pulse, and respirations before and periodically during administration. If respiratory rate is <10/min, assess level of sedation. Dose may need to be decreased by 25–50%. Buprenorphine 0.3–0.4 mg has approximately equal analgesic and respiratory depressant effects to morphine 10 mg.
- Assess previous analgesic history. Antagonistic properties may induce withdrawal symptoms (vomiting, restlessness, abdominal cramps, increased blood pressure and temperature) in patients who are physically dependent on opioid agonists. Symptoms may occur up to 15 days after discontinuation and persist for 1–2 wk.
- Buprenorphine has a lower potential for dependence than other opioids; however, prolonged use may lead to physical and psychological dependence and tolerance. This should not prevent patient from receiving adequate analgesia. Most patients receiving buprenorphine for pain do not develop psychological dependence. If tolerance develops, changing to an opioid agonist may be required to relieve pain.
- **Opioid Dependence:** Assess patient for signs and symptoms of opioid withdrawal before and during therapy.
- ***Lab Test Considerations:*** May cause ↑ serum amylase and lipase levels.
- Monitor liver function tests prior to and periodically during therapy for opioid dependence.
- ***Toxicity and Overdose:*** If an opioid antagonist is required to reverse respiratory depression or coma, naloxone (Narcan) is the antidote. Dilute the 0.4-mg ampule of naloxone in 10 ml of 0.9% NaCl and administer 0.5 ml (0.02 mg) by direct IV push every 2 min. For children and patients weighing <40 kg, dilute 0.1 mg of naloxone in 10 ml of 0.9% NaCl for a concentration of 10 mcg/ml and administer 0.5 mcg/kg every 1–2 min. Titrate dose to avoid withdrawal, seizures, and severe pain. Naloxone may not completely reverse respiratory depressant effects of buprenorphine; may require mechanical ventilation, oxygen, IV fluids, and vasopressors.

Potential Nursing Diagnoses

Acute pain (Indications)
Risk for injury (Side Effects)
Ineffective coping (Indications)

Implementation

- ***High Alert:*** Accidental overdosage of opioid analgesics has resulted in fatalities. Before administering, clarify all ambiguous orders; have second practitioner independently check original order, dose calculations, route of administration, and infusion pump programming. Do not confuse Buprenex (buprenorphine) with Bumex (bumetanide).
- **Pain:** Explain therapeutic value of medication before administration to enhance the analgesic effect.
- Regularly administered doses may be more effective than prn administration. Analgesic is more effective if given before pain becomes severe.
- Coadministration with nonopioid analgesics has additive effects and may permit lower opioid doses. **SL:** Administer sublingually. Usually takes 2–10 min for tablets to dissolve. If more than one tablet is prescribed, place multiple tablets under the tongue or 2 at a time until all tablets are dissolved. Do not chew or swallow; decreases amount of medication absorbed.
- **IM:** Administer IM injections deep into well-developed muscle. Rotate sites of injections.

IV Administration

- **Direct IV:** May give IV undiluted. ***High Alert:*** Administer slowly. Rapid administration may cause respiratory depression, hypotension, and cardiac arrest. ***Rate:*** Give over at least 2 minutes.
- **Syringe Compatibility:** glycopyrrolate, heparin, midazolam.
- **Y-Site Compatibility:** allopurinol, amifostine, aztreonam, cefipime, cisatracurium, cladribine, docetaxel, etoposide phosphate, filgrastim, granisetron, linezolid, melphalan, oxaliplatin, pemetrexed, piperacillin/tazobactam, propofol, remifentanil, teniposide, thiotepa, vinorelbine.
- **Y-Site Incompatibility:** amphotericin B cholesteryl sulfate, doxorubicin liposome, lansoprazole.
- **Solution Compatibility:** 0.9% NaCl, D5W, D5/0.9% NaCl, lactated Ringer's injection,

Ringer's injection. Opioid Dependence. Must be prescribed by health care professional with special training. Induction is usually started with buprenorphine (Subutex) over 3–4 days. Initial dose should be administered at least 4 hr after last opioid dose and preferably when early signs of opioid whitdrawal appear. Once patient is on a stable dose, maintenance therapy with buprenorphine/naloxone (Suboxone) is preferred for continued, unsupervised treatment.

Patient/Family Teaching

- Medication may cause drowsiness or dizziness. Advise patient to call for assistance when ambulating and to avoid driving or other activities requiring alertness until response to medication is known.
- Advise patient to avoid concurrent use of alcohol or other CNS depressants.
- Advise patient to notify health care professional before taking other Rx or OTC medication or herbal products.
- **Pain:** Instruct patient on how and when to ask for pain medication.
- Encourage patients on bedrest to turn, cough, and deep-breathe every 2 hr to prevent atelectasis.
- Instruct patient to change positions slowly to minimize orthostatic hypotension.
- Advise patient that good oral hygiene, frequent mouth rinses, and sugarless gum or candy may decrease dry mouth.
- **Opioid Dependence:** Instruct patient in the correct use of medication; directions for use must be followed exactly. Medication must be used regularly, not occasionally. Take missed doses as soon as remembered; if almost time for next dose, skip missed dose and return to regular dosing schedule. Do not take 2 doses at once unless directed by health care professional. Do not discontinue use without consulting health care professional; abrupt discontinuation may cause withdrawal symptoms. If medication is discontinued, flush unused tablets down the toilet.
- Caution patient that buprenorphine may be a target for people who abuse drugs; store medications in a safe place to protect them from theft. Selling or giving this medication to others is against the law.
- Caution patient that injection of Suboxone can lead to bad withdrawal symptoms.
- Advise patient if admitted to the emergency room to inform treating physician and emergency room staff of physical dependence on opioids and of treatment regimen.
- Advise patient to notify health care professional promptly if faintness, dizziness, confusion, slowed breathing, skin or whites of eyes turn yellow, urine turns dark, light colored stools, decreased appetite, nausea, or abdominal pain occur.

Evaluation/Desired Outcomes

- Decrease in severity of pain without a significant alteration in level of consciousness or respiratory status.
- Suppression of withdrawal symptoms during detoxification and maintenance from heroin or other opioids.

buPROPion

(byoo-**proe**-pee-on)
Wellbutrin, Wellbutrin SR, Wellbutrin XL, Zyban

Classification
Therapeutic: antidepressants
Pharmacologic: aminoketones

Pregnancy Category B

Indications

Treatment of depression (with psychotherapy). Depression in patient with seasonal affective disorder (XL only). Smoking cessation (Zyban only). **Unlabeled uses:** Treatment of ADHD in adults (SR only). To increase sexual desire in women.

Action

Decreases neuronal reuptake of dopamine in the CNS. Diminished neuronal uptake of serotonin and norepinephrine (less than tricyclic antidepressants). **Therapeutic Effects:** Diminished depression. Decreased craving for cigarettes.

Pharmacokinetics

Absorption: Although well absorbed, rapidly and extensively metabolized by the liver.
Distribution: Unknown.

Metabolism and Excretion: Extensively metabolized by the liver. Some conversion to active metabolites.
Half-life: 14 hr (active metabolites may have longer half-lives).

TIME/ACTION PROFILE (antidepressant effect)

ROUTE	ONSET	PEAK	DURATION
PO	1–3 wk	unknown	unknown

Contraindications/Precautions

Contraindicated in: Hypersensitivity; History of bulimia, and anorexia nervosa; Concurrent MAO inhibitor or ritonavir therapy; Lactation: Secreted in breast milk; potential for serious adverse reactions in nursing infants. Discontinue nursing or discontinue drug.
Use Cautiously in: Renal/hepatic impairment (↓ dose recommended); Recent history of MI; History of suicide attempt; Unstable cardiovascular status; May ↑ risk of suicide attempt/ideation especially during early treatment or dose adjustment; this risk appears to be greater in adolescents or children; OB: Use only if benefit to patient outweighs potential risk to fetus; Geri: Increased risk of drug accumulation; increased sensitivity to effects.
Exercise Extreme Caution in: History of seizures, head trauma or concurrent medications that ↓ seizure threshold (theophylline, antipsychotics, antidepressants, systemic corticosteroids); Severe hepatic cirrhosis (↓ dose required). Pedi: Increased risk of suicidal thinking and behavior. Observe carefully, especially at initiation of therapy and during increases or decreases in dose.

Adverse Reactions/Side Effects

CNS: SEIZURES, agitation, headache, insomnia, mania, psychoses. **GI:** dry mouth, nausea, vomiting, change in appetite, weight gain, weight loss. **Derm:** photosensitivity. **Endo:** hyperglycemia, hypoglycemia, syndrome of inappropriate ADH secretion. **Neuro:** tremor.

Interactions

Drug-Drug: ↑ risk of adverse reactions when used with **amantadine**, **levodopa**, or **MAO inhibitors** (concurrent use of MAO inhibitors is contraindicated). ↑ risk of seizures with **phenothiazines**, **antidepressants**, **theophylline**, **corticosteroids**, **OTC stimulants/anorectics**, or cessation of **alcohol** or **benzodiazepines** (avoid or minimize alcohol use). Blood levels ↑ by **ritonavir** (avoid concurrent use). **Carbamazepine** may ↓ blood levels and effectiveness. Concurrent use with **nicotine** replacement may cause hypertension. ↑ risk of bleeding with **warfarin**. Bupropion and one of its metabolites inhibit the CYP2D6 enzyme system and may ↑ levels and risk of toxicity from **antidepressants** (SSRIs and tricyclic), some **beta blockers**, **antiarrhythmics**, and **antipsychotics**.

Route/Dosage

Depression

PO (Adults): *Immediate-release*—100 mg twice daily initially; after 3 days may increase to 100 mg 3 times daily; after at least 4 wk of therapy, may increase up to 450 mg/day in divided doses (not to exceed 150 mg/dose; wait at least 6 hr between doses at the 300 mg/day dose or at least 4 hr between doses at the 450 mg/day dose). *Sustained-release*—150 mg once daily in the morning; after 3 days, may increase to 150 mg twice daily with at least 8 hr between doses; after at least 4 wk of therapy, may increase to a maximum daily dose of 400 mg given as 200 mg twice daily. *Extended-release*—150 mg once daily in the morning, may be increased after 4 days to 300 mg once daily; some patients may require up to 450 mg/day as a single daily dose.

Seasonal Affective Disorder

PO (Adults): 150 mg/day in the morning; if dose is well tolerated, increase to 300 mg/day in one wk. Doses should be tapered to 150 mg/day for 2 wks before discontinuing.

Smoking cessation

PO (Adults): *Zyban*—150 mg once daily for 3 days, then 150 mg twice daily for 7–12 wk (doses should be at least 8 hr apart).

Availability (generic available)

Tablets: 75 mg, 100 mg. **Cost:** *Generic*—75 mg $54.99/90, 100 mg $66.99/90. **Sustained-release tablets:** 100 mg, 150 mg, 200 mg. **Cost:** *Generic*—100 mg $189.97/180, 150 mg $163.93/180, 200 mg $334.96/180. **Extended-release tablets:** 150 mg, 300 mg. **Cost:** *Generic*—150 mg $367.97/90, 300 mg $365.96/90.

NURSING IMPLICATIONS

Assessment

- Monitor mood changes. Inform physician or other health care professional if patient dem-

B

onstrates significant increase in anxiety, nervousness, or insomnia.

- Assess for suicidal tendencies, especially during early therapy. Restrict amount of drug available to patient.
- ***Lab Test Considerations:*** Monitor hepatic and renal function closely in patients with kidney or liver impairment to prevent ↑ serum and tissue bupropion concentrations.

Potential Nursing Diagnoses

Ineffective coping (Indications)

Implementation

- Do not confuse bupropion with buspirone. Do not confuse Zyban (bupropion) with Zagam (Sparfloxacin). Do not administer bupropion (Wellbutrin) with Zyban, which contains the same ingredients.
- Administer doses in equally spaced time increments during day to minimize the risk of seizures. Risk of seizures increases fourfold in doses greater than 450 mg per day.
- May be initially administered concurrently with sedatives to minimize agitation. This is not usually required after the 1st wk of therapy.
- Insomnia may be decreased by avoiding bedtime doses. May require treatment during 1st wk of therapy.
- May be administered with food to lessen GI irritation.
- Nicotine patches, gum, inhalers, and spray may be used concurrently with bupropion.
- **PO:** Sustained-release (SR or XL) tablets should be swallowed whole; do not break, crush, or chew.
- **Seasonal Affective Disorder:** Begin administration in autumn prior to the onset of depressive symptoms. Continue therapy through winter and begin to taper and discontinue in early spring.

Patient/Family Teaching

- Instruct patient to take bupropion as directed. Take missed doses as soon as possible and space day's remaining doses evenly at not less than 4-hr intervals. Missed doses for smoking cessation should be omitted. Do not double doses or take more than prescribed. May require 4 wk or longer for full effects. Do not discontinue without consulting health care professional. May require gradual reduction before discontinuation.
- Bupropion may impair judgment or motor and cognitive skills. Caution patient to avoid driving and other activities requiring alertness until response to medication is known.
- Advise patient to avoid alcohol during therapy and to consult with health care professional before taking other medications with bupropion, such as Zyban.
- Inform patient that frequent mouth rinses, good oral hygiene, and sugarless gum or candy may minimize dry mouth. If dry mouth persists for more than 2 wk, consult health care professional regarding use of saliva substitute.
- Advise patient to notify health care professional if rash or other troublesome side effects occur.
- Inform patient that unused shell of XL tablets may appear in stool; this is normal.
- Advise patient to use sunscreen and protective clothing to prevent photosensitivity reactions.
- Instruct female patients to inform health care professional if pregnancy is planned or suspected.
- Advise patient to notify health care professional of medication regimen before treatment or surgery.
- Emphasize the importance of follow-up exams to monitor progress. Encourage patient participation in psychotherapy.
- **Smoking Cessation:** Smoking should be stopped during the 2nd week of therapy to allow for the onset of bupropion and to maximize the chances of quitting.

Evaluation/Desired Outcomes

- Increased sense of well-being.
- Renewed interest in surroundings. Acute episodes of depression may require several months of treatment.
- Cessation of smoking.

busPIRone (byoo-**spye**-rone)

BuSpar

Classification

Therapeutic: antianxiety agents

Pregnancy Category B

Indications
Management of anxiety.

Action
Binds to serotonin and dopamine receptors in the brain. Increases norepinephrine metabolism in the brain. **Therapeutic Effects:** Relief of anxiety.

Pharmacokinetics
Absorption: Rapidly absorbed.
Distribution: Unknown.
Protein Binding: 95% bound to plasma proteins.
Metabolism and Excretion: Extensively metabolized by the liver (CYP3A4 enzyme system); 20–40% excreted in feces.
Half-life: 2–3 hr.

TIME/ACTION PROFILE (relief of anxiety)

ROUTE	ONSET	PEAK	DURATION
PO	7–10 days	3–4 wk	unknown

Contraindications/Precautions
Contraindicated in: Hypersensitivity; Severe hepatic or renal impairment; Concurrent use of MAO inhibitors; Ingestion of large amounts of grapefruit juice.
Use Cautiously in: Patients receiving other antianxiety agents (other agents should be slowly withdrawn to prevent withdrawal or rebound phenomenon); Patients receiving other psychotropics; Lactation, OB, Pedi: Safety not established.

Adverse Reactions/Side Effects
CNS: dizziness, drowsiness, excitement, fatigue, headache, insomnia, nervousness, weakness, personality changes. **EENT:** blurred vision, nasal congestion, sore throat, tinnitus, altered taste or smell, conjunctivitis. **Resp:** chest congestion, hyperventilation, shortness of breath. **CV:** chest pain, palpitations, tachycardia, hypertension, hypotension, syncope. **GI:** nausea, abdominal pain, constipation, diarrhea, dry mouth, vomiting. **GU:** changes in libido, dysuria, urinary frequency, urinary hesitancy. **Derm:** rashes, alopecia, blisters, dry skin, easy bruising, edema, flushing, pruritus. **Endo:** irregular menses. **MS:** myalgia. **Neuro:** incoordination, numbness, paresthesia, tremor. **Misc:** clamminess, sweating, fever.

Interactions
Drug-Drug: Use with **MAO inhibitors** may result in hypertension and is not recommended. **Erythromycin**, **nefazodone**, **ketoconazole**, **itraconazole**, **ritonavir**, and other **inhibitors of CYP3A4** ↑ blood levels and effects of buspirone; dose reduction is recommended (decrease to 2.5 mg twice daily with erythromycin, decrease to 2.5 mg once daily with nefazodone). **Rifampin**, **dexamethasone**, **phenytoin**, **phenobarbital**, **carbamazepine**, and other **inducers of CYP3A4** ↓ blood levels and effects of buspirone; dose adjustment may be necessary. Avoid concurrent use with **alcohol**.
Drug-Natural Products: Concomitant use of **kava kava**, **valerian**, or **chamomile** can ↑ CNS depression.
Drug-Food: Grapefruit juice ↑ serum levels and effect; ingestion of large amounts of grapefruit juice is not recommended.

Route/Dosage
PO (Adults): 7.5 mg twice daily; increase by 5 mg/day q 2–4 days as needed (not to exceed 60 mg/day). Usual dose is 20–30 mg/day (in 2 divided doses).

Availability (generic available)
Tablets: 5 mg, 7.5 mg, 10 mg, 15 mg, 30 mg. **Cost:** *Generic*—5 mg $79.97/180, 7.5 mg $110.97/180, 10 mg $128.99/180, 15 mg $129.40/180, 30 mg $267.93/180.

NURSING IMPLICATIONS

Assessment
- Assess degree and manifestations of anxiety before and periodically during therapy.
- Buspirone does not appear to cause physical or psychological dependence or tolerance. However, patients with a history of drug abuse should be assessed for tolerance or dependence. Restrict amount of drug available to these patients.

Potential Nursing Diagnoses
Anxiety (Indications)
Risk for injury (Side Effects)

Implementation
- Do not confuse buspirone with bupropion.
- Patients changing from other antianxiety agents should receive gradually decreasing doses. Buspirone will not prevent withdrawal symptoms.
- **PO:** May be administered with food to minimize gastric irritation. Food slows but does not alter extent of absorption.

Patient/Family Teaching
- Instruct patient to take buspirone exactly as directed. Take missed doses as soon as possi-

ble if not just before next dose; do not double doses. Do not take more than amount prescribed.

- May cause dizziness or drowsiness. Caution patient to avoid driving or other activities requiring alertness until response to the medication is known.
- Advise patient to avoid concurrent use of alcohol or other CNS depressants.
- Advise patient to consult health care professional before taking OTC medications or herbal products with this drug.
- Instruct patient to notify health care professional if any chronic abnormal movements occur (dystonia, motor restlessness, involuntary movements of facial or cervical muscles) or if pregnancy is suspected.
- Emphasize the importance of follow-up exams to determine effectiveness of medication.

Evaluation/Desired Outcomes

- Increase in sense of well-being.
- Decrease in subjective feelings of anxiety. Some improvement may be seen in 7–10 days. Optimal results take 3–4 wk of therapy. Buspirone is usually used for short-term therapy (3–4 wk). If prescribed for long-term therapy, efficacy should be periodically assessed.

HIGH ALERT

busulfan (byoo-sul-fan)

Busulfex, Myleran

Classification
Therapeutic: antineoplastics
Pharmacologic: alkylating agents

Pregnancy Category D

Indications

PO: Treatment of chronic myelogenous leukemia (CML) and bone marrow disorders. **IV:** With cyclophosphamide as a conditioning regimen before allogenic hematopoietic progenitor cell transplantation for CML.

Action

Disrupts nucleic acid function and protein synthesis (cell-cycle phase–nonspecific). **Therapeutic Effects:** Death of rapidly growing cells, especially malignant ones.

Pharmacokinetics

Absorption: Rapidly absorbed from the GI tract.
Distribution: Unknown.
Metabolism and Excretion: Extensively metabolized by the liver.
Half-life: 2.5 hr.

TIME/ACTION PROFILE (effects on blood counts)

ROUTE	ONSET	PEAK	DURATION
PO	1–2 wk	weeks	up to 1 mo†
IV	unknown	unknown	13 days‡

†Complete recovery may take up to 20 mo
‡After administration of last dose

Contraindications/Precautions

Contraindicated in: Hypersensitivity; Failure to respond to previous courses; OB, Lactation: Potential for serious side effects in fetus or infant.
Use Cautiously in: Active infections; Decreased bone marrow reserve; Obese patients (base dose on ideal body weight); Other chronic debilitating diseases; Patients with childbearing potential; Geri: Begin therapy at lower end of dose range due to increased frequency of impaired cardiac, hepatic, or renal function.

Adverse Reactions/Side Effects

Incidence and severity of adverse reactions and side effects are increased with IV use.
CNS: *IV*— SEIZURES, CEREBRAL HEMORRHAGE/COMA, anxiety, confusion, depression, dizziness, headache, encephalopathy, mental status changes, weakness. **EENT:** *PO*— cataracts; *IV*— epistaxis, pharyngitis, ear disorders. **CV:** hepatic veno-oclusive disease (↑ allogenic transplantation). **Resp:** *PO*— PULMONARY FIBROSIS; *IV*— alveolar hemorrhage, asthma, atelectasis, cough, hemoptysis, hypoxia, pleural effusion, pneumonia, rhinitis, sinusitis. **CV:** *PO*— CARDIAC TAMPONADE (WITH HIGH-DOSE CYCLOPHOSPHAMIDE); *IV*— chest pain, hypotension, tachycardia, thrombosis, arrhythmias, atrial fibrillation, cardiomegaly, ECG changes, edema, heart block, hypertension, left-sided heart failure, pericardial effusion, ventricular extrasystoles. **GI:** *PO*— drug-induced hepatitis, nausea, vomiting; *IV*— abdominal enlargement, anorexia, constipation, diarrhea, dry mouth, hematemesis, nausea, rectal discomfort, vomiting, abdominal pain, dyspepsia,

hepatomegaly, pancreatitis, stomatitis. **GU:** oliguria, dysuria, hematuria. **Derm:** *PO*— itching, rashes, acne, alopecia, erythema nodosum, exfoliative dermatitis, hyperpigmentation. **Endo:** *PO*— sterility, gynecomastia. **F and E:** hypokalemia, hypomagnesemia, hypophosphatemia. **Hemat:** BONE MARROW DEPRESSION. **Local:** inflammation/pain at injection site. **Metab:** *PO and IV*— hyperuricemia; *IV*— hyperglycemia. **MS:** arthralgia, myalgia, back pain. **Misc:** allergic reactions, chills, fever, infection.

Interactions

Drug-Drug: Concurrent or previous (within 72 hr) use of **acetaminophen** may ↓ elimination and ↑ toxicity. Concurrent use with high-dose **cyclophosphamide** in patients with thalassemia may result in cardiac tamponade. Concurrent use with **itraconazole** or **phenytoin** ↓ blood level effectiveness. Long-term continuous therapy with **thioguanine** may ↑ risk of hepatic toxicity. ↑ bone marrow suppression with other **antineoplastics** or **radiation therapy**. May ↓ the antibody response to and ↑ risk of adverse reactions from **live-virus vaccines**.

Route/Dosage

Many other regimens are used. See current protocols for up-to-date dosage.

PO (Adults): *Induction*—1.8 mg/m²/day or 60 mcg (0.06 mg)/kg/day until WBCs <15,000/mm³. Usual dose is 4–8 mg/day (range 1–12 mg/day). *Maintenance*—1–3 mg/day.

PO (Children): 0.06–0.12 mg/kg/day or 1.8–4.6 mg/m²/day initially. Titrate dose to maintain WBC of approximately 20,000/mm³.

IV (Adults): 0.8 mg/kg q 6 hr (dose based on ideal body weight or actual weight, whichever is less; in obese patients, dosage should be based on adjusted ideal body weight) for 4 days (total of 16 doses); given in combination with cyclophosphamide.

Availability

Tablets: 2 mg. **Solution for injection:** 6 mg/ml in 10 ml ampules (60 mg).

NURSING IMPLICATIONS

Assessment

- ***High Alert:*** Monitor for bone marrow depression. Assess for bleeding (bleeding gums, bruising, petechiae, guaiac stools, urine, emesis) and avoid IM injections and taking rectal temperatures. Apply pressure to venipuncture sites for at least 10 min. Assess for signs of infection (fever, chills, sore throat, cough, hoarseness, lower back or side pain, difficult or painful urination) during neutropenia. Anemia may occur. Monitor for increased fatigue, dyspnea, and orthostatic hypotension. Notify physician if these symptoms occur.
- Monitor intake and output ratios and daily weights. Report significant changes in totals.
- Monitor for symptoms of gout (increased uric acid, joint pain, lower back or side pain, swelling of feet or lower legs). Encourage patient to drink at least 2 L of fluid each day. Allopurinol may be given to decrease uric acid levels. Alkalinization of urine may be ordered to increase excretion of uric acid.
- Assess for pulmonary fibrosis (fever, cough, shortness of breath) periodically during and after therapy. Discontinue therapy at the first sign of pulmonary fibrosis. Usually occurs 8 mo–10 yr (average 4 yr) after initiation of therapy.
- **IV:** Premedicate patient with phenytoin before IV administration to minimize the risk of seizures.
- Administer antiemetics before IV administration and on a fixed schedule throughout IV administration.
- ***Lab Test Considerations:*** Monitor CBC with differential and platelet count before and weekly during therapy. The nadir of leukopenia occurs within 10–15 days and the nadir of WBC at 11–30 days. Recovery usually occurs within 12–20 wk. Notify physician if WBC is <15,000/mm³ or if a precipitous drop occurs. Institute thrombocytopenia precautions if platelet count is <150,000/mm³. Bone marrow depression may be severe and progressive, with recovery taking 1 mo–2 yr after discontinuation of therapy.
- Monitor serum ALT, bilirubin, alkaline phosphatase, and uric acid before and periodically during therapy. May cause ↑ uric acid levels.
- May cause false-positive cytology results of breast, bladder, cervix, and lung tissues.

Potential Nursing Diagnoses

Disturbed body image (Side Effects)
Risk for injury (Side Effects)
Risk for infection (Side Effects)

Implementation

- ***High Alert:*** Fatalities have occurred with chemotherapeutic agents. Before administering, clarify all ambiguous orders; double-

check single, daily, and course-of-therapy dose limits; have second practitioner independently double-check original order, calculations, and infusion pump settings.
- **PO:** Administer at the same time each day. Administer on an empty stomach to decrease nausea and vomiting.

IV Administration

- **IV:** Solution for IV administration should be prepared in a biologic cabinet. Wear gloves, gown, and mask while handling IV medication. Discard IV equipment in specially designated containers.
- **Intermittent Infusion:** ***Diluent:*** Dilute with 10 times the volume of busulfan using 0.9% NaCl or D5W. ***Concentration:*** ≥0.5 mg/ml. When drawing busulfan from vial, use needle with 5-micron nylon filter provided, remove calculated volume from vial, remove needle and filter, replace needle and inject busulfan into diluent. Do not use polycarbonate syringes with busulfan. Only use filters provided with busulfan. Always add busulfan to diluent, not diluent to busulfan. Solution diluted with 0.9% NaCl or D5W is stable for 8 hr at room temperature and solution diluted with 0.9% NaCl is stable for 12 hr if refrigerated. Administration must be completed during this time. ***Rate:*** Administer via central venous catheter over 2 hr every 6 hr for 4 days for a total of 16 doses. Use infusion pump to administer entire dose over 2 hr.
- **Y-Site Incompatibility:** Do not administer with other solutions. Flush catheter with 0.9% NaCl or D5W before and after administration.

Patient/Family Teaching

- Instruct patient to take medication as directed, at the same time each day, even if nausea and vomiting are a problem. Consult health care professional if vomiting occurs shortly after dose is taken. If a dose is missed, do not take at all; do not double doses.
- Advise patient to notify health care professional if fever; sore throat; signs of infection; lower back or side pain; difficult or painful urination; sores in the mouth or on the lips; chills; dyspnea; persistent cough; bleeding gums; bruising; petechiae; or blood in urine, stool, or emesis occurs. Instruct patient to use soft toothbrush and electric razor. Caution patient not to drink alcoholic beverages or take products containing aspirin or NSAIDs.
- Caution patient to avoid crowds and persons with known infections. Health care professional should be informed immediately if symptoms of infection occur.
- Discuss with patient the possibility of hair loss. Explore methods of coping.
- Review with patient the need for contraception during therapy. Women need to use contraception even if amenorrhea occurs.
- Instruct patient not to receive any vaccinations without advice of health care professional.
- Advise patient to notify health care professional if unusual bleeding; bruising; or flank, stomach, or joint pain occurs. Advise patients on long-term therapy to notify health care professional immediately if cough, shortness of breath, and fever occur or if darkening of skin, diarrhea, dizziness, fatigue, anorexia, confusion, or nausea and vomiting become pronounced.
- Inform patient of increased risk of a second malignancy with busulfan.

Evaluation/Desired Outcomes

- Decrease in leukocyte count to within normal limits.
- Decreased night sweats.
- Increase in appetite.
- Increased sense of well-being. Therapy is resumed when leukocyte count reaches 50,000/mm³.

BUTALBITAL COMPOUND

(byoo-**tal**-bi-tal)

butalbital, acetaminophen†

Axocet, Bucet, Bupap, Butex Forte, Dolgic, Marten-Tab, Phrenilin, Phrenilin Forte, Repap CF, Sedapap, Tencon, Triaprin

butalbital, acetaminophen, caffeine†

Endolor, Esgic, Esgic-Plus, Fioricet, Margesic, Medigesic, Repan, Triad

butalbital, aspirin, caffeine‡

Fiorinal, Fiortal, ♣Tecnal

Classification
Therapeutic: nonopioid analgesics (combination with barbiturate)
Pharmacologic: barbiturates

Schedule III (products with aspirin only)

Pregnancy Category D

†For information on acetaminophen component in formulation, see acetaminophen monograph

‡For information on aspirin component in formulation, see salicylates monograph

Indications
Management of mild to moderate pain.

Action
Contain an analgesic (aspirin or acetaminophen) for relief of pain, a barbiturate (butalbital) for its sedative effect, and some contain caffeine, which may be of benefit in vascular headaches. **Therapeutic Effects:** Decreased severity of pain with some sedation.

Pharmacokinetics
Absorption: Well absorbed.
Distribution: Widely distributed; cross the placenta and enter breast milk.
Metabolism and Excretion: Mostly metabolized by the liver.
Half-life: 35 hr.

TIME/ACTION PROFILE

ROUTE	ONSET	PEAK	DURATION
PO	15–30 min	1–2 hr	2–6 hr

Contraindications/Precautions
Contraindicated in: Hypersensitivity to individual components; Cross-sensitivity may occur; Comatose patients or those with pre-existing CNS depression; Uncontrolled severe pain; Aspirin should be avoided in patients with bleeding disorders or thrombocytopenia; Acetaminophen should be avoided in patients with severe hepatic or renal disease; Caffeine should be avoided in patients with severe cardiovascular disease; Pregnancy or lactation; Porphyria.
Use Cautiously in: History of suicide attempt or drug addiction; Chronic alcohol use/abuse (for aspirin and acetaminophen content); Geri: Appears on Beers list. Geriatric patients are at increased risk for side effects (dosage reduction recommended); Use should be short-term only; Children (safety not established).

Adverse Reactions/Side Effects
CNS: *caffeine*— drowsiness, hangover, delirium, depression, excitation, headache (with chronic use), insomnia, irritability, lethargy, nervousness, vertigo. **Resp:** respiratory depression. **CV:** *caffeine*— palpitations, tachycardia. **GI:** *caffeine*— constipation, diarrhea, epigastric distress, heartburn, nausea, vomiting. **Derm:** dermatitis, rash. **Misc:** hypersensitivity reactions including ANGIOEDEMA and SERUM SICKNESS, physical dependence, psychological dependence, tolerance.

Interactions
Drug-Drug: Additive CNS depression with other **CNS depressants**, including **alcohol**, **antihistamines**, **antidepressants**, **opioid analgesics**, and **sedative/hypnotics**. May increase the liver metabolism and decrease the effectiveness of other drugs including **hormonal contraceptives**, **chloramphenicol**, **acebutolol**, **propranolol**, **metoprolol**, **timolol**, **doxycycline**, **corticosteroids**, **tricyclic antidepressants**, **phenothiazines**, **phenylbutazone**, and **quinidine**. **MAO inhibitors**, **primidone**, and **valproic acid** may prevent metabolism and increase the effectiveness of butalbital. May enhance the hematologic toxicity of **cyclophosphamide**.
Drug-Natural Products: St. John's wort may decrease barbiturate effect. Concurrent use of **kava kava, valerian, skullcap, chamomile, or hops** can increase CNS depression.

Route/Dosage
PO (Adults): 1–2 capsules or tablets (50–100 mg butalbital) every 4 hr as needed for pain (not to exceed 4 g acetaminophen or aspirin/24 hr).

Availability (generic available)
Tablets and capsules: 50 mg. ***In combination with:*** aspirin, acetaminophen, caffeine, and codeine Rx. See Appendix B.

NURSING IMPLICATIONS

Assessment
- Assess type, location, and intensity of pain before and 60 min following administration.
- Prolonged use may lead to physical and psychological dependence and tolerance. This should not prevent patient from receiving adequate analgesia. Most patients who receive butalbital compound for pain do not develop psychological dependence.

- Assess frequency of use. Frequent, chronic use may lead to daily headaches in headache-prone individuals because of physical dependence on caffeine and other components. Chronic headaches from overmedication are difficult to treat and may require hospitalization for treatment and prophylaxis.

Potential Nursing Diagnosis

Acute pain (Indications)
Risk for injury (Side Effects)

Implementation

- Do not confuse Fiorinal with Fioricet.
- Explain therapeutic value of medication before administration to enhance the analgesic effect.
- Regularly administered doses may be more effective than prn administration. Analgesic is more effective if given before pain becomes severe.
- Medication should be discontinued gradually after long-term use to prevent withdrawal symptoms.
- **PO:** Oral doses should be administered with food, milk, or a full glass of water to minimize GI irritation.

Patient/Family Teaching

- Instruct patient to take medication exactly as directed. Do not increase dose because of the habit-forming potential of butalbital. If medication appears less effective after a few weeks, consult health care professional. Doses of acetaminophen or aspirin should not exceed the maximum recommended daily dose. Chronic excessive use of >4 g/day (2 g in chronic alcoholism) may lead to hepatotoxicity, renal or cardiac damage.
- Advise patients with vascular headaches to take medication at first sign of headache. Lying down in a quiet, dark room may also be helpful. Medications taken for prophylaxis should be continued.
- May cause drowsiness or dizziness. Advise patient to avoid driving and other activities requiring alertness until response to medication is known.
- Caution patient to avoid concurrent use of alcohol or other CNS depressants.
- Advise patient to use an additional nonhormonal method of contraception while taking butalbital compound.

Evaluation/Desired Outcomes

- Decrease in severity of pain without a significant alteration in level of consciousness.

butenafine, See ANTIFUNGALS (TOPICAL).

butoconazole, See ANTIFUNGALS (VAGINAL).

HIGH ALERT

butorphanol (byoo-**tor**-fa-nole)

Stadol, Stadol NS

Classification
Therapeutic: opioid analgesics
Pharmacologic: opioid agonists/antagonists

Schedule IV

Pregnancy Category C

Indications

Management of moderate to severe pain. Analgesia during labor. Sedation before surgery. Supplement in balanced anesthesia.

Action

Binds to opiate receptors in the CNS. Alters the perception of and response to painful stimuli while producing generalized CNS depression. Has partial antagonist properties that may result in opioid withdrawal in physically dependent patients. **Therapeutic Effects:** Decreased severity of pain.

Pharmacokinetics

Absorption: Well absorbed from IM sites and nasal mucosa.
Distribution: Crosses the placenta and enters breast milk.
Metabolism and Excretion: Mostly metabolized by the liver; 11–14% excreted in the feces. Minimal renal excretion.
Half-life: 3–4 hr.

TIME/ACTION PROFILE (analgesia)

ROUTE	ONSET	PEAK	DURATION
IM	within 15 min	30–60 min	3–4 hr
IV	within mins	4–5 min	2–4 hr
Intranasal	within 15 min	1–2 hr	4–5 hr

Contraindications/Precautions

Contraindicated in: Hypersensitivity; Patients physically dependent on opioids (may precipitate withdrawal).

Use Cautiously in: Head trauma; Increased intracranial pressure; Severe renal, hepatic, or pulmonary disease (increase interval to q 6–8 hr initially in hepatic/renal impairment); Hypothyroidism; Adrenal insufficiency; Alcoholism; Undiagnosed abdominal pain; Prostatic hyperplasia; OB, Lactation, Pedi: Safety not established but has been used during labor (may cause respiratory depression in the newborn); Geri: Decrease usual dose by 50%; give at twice the usual interval initially.

Adverse Reactions/Side Effects

CNS: confusion, dysphoria, hallucinations, sedation, euphoria, floating feeling, headache, unusual dreams. **EENT:** blurred vision, diplopia, miosis (high doses). **Resp:** respiratory depression. **CV:** hypertension, hypotension, palpitations. **GI:** nausea, constipation, dry mouth, ileus, vomiting. **GU:** urinary retention. **Derm:** sweating, clammy feeling. **Misc:** physical dependence, psychological dependence, tolerance.

Interactions

Drug-Drug: Use with extreme caution in patients receiving **MAO inhibitors** (may produce severe, potentially fatal reactions—reduce initial dose of butorphanol to 25% of usual dose). Additive CNS depression with **alcohol**, **antidepressants**, **antihistamines**, and **sedative/hypnotics**. May precipitate withdrawal in patients who are physically dependent on **opioids** and have not been detoxified. May ↓ effects of concurrently administered **opioids**.

Drug-Natural Products: Concomitant use of **kava kava**, **valerian**, **chamomile**, or **hops** can ↑ CNS depression.

Route/Dosage

IM (Adults): 2 mg q 3–4 hr as needed (range 1–4 mg).

IV (Adults): 1 mg q 3–4 hr as needed (range 0.5–2 mg).

IM, IV (Geriatric Patients): 1 mg q 4–6 hr, increased as necessary.

Intranasal (Adults): 1 mg (1 spray in 1 nostril) initially. An additional dose may be given 60–90 min later. This sequence may be repeated in 3–4 hr. If pain is severe, an initial dose of 2 mg (1 spray in each nostril) may be given. May be repeated in 3–4 hr.

Intranasal (Geriatric Patients): 1 mg (1 spray in 1 nostril) initially. An additional dose may be given 90–120 min later. This sequence may be repeated in 3–4 hr.

Availability (generic available)

Injection: 1 mg/ml, 2 mg/ml. **Intranasal solution:** 10 mg/ml, in 2.5-ml metered-dose spray pump (14–15 doses; 1 mg/spray).

NURSING IMPLICATIONS

Assessment

- Assess type, location, and intensity of pain before and 30–60 min after IM, 5 min after IV, and 60–90 min after intranasal administration. When titrating opioid doses, increases of 25–50% should be administered until there is either a 50% reduction in the patient's pain rating on a numerical or visual analogue scale or the patient reports satisfactory pain relief. A repeat dose can be safely administered at the time of the peak if previous dose is ineffective and side effects are minimal. Patients requiring doses higher than 4 mg should be converted to an opioid agonist. Butorphanol is not recommended for prolonged use or as first-line therapy for acute or cancer pain.
- An equianalgesic chart (see Appendix J) should be used when changing routes or when changing from one opioid to another.
- Assess blood pressure, pulse, and respirations before and periodically during administration. If respiratory rate is <10/min, assess level of sedation. Dose may need to be decreased by 25–50%. Respiratory depression does not increase in severity, only in duration, with increased dosage.
- Assess previous analgesic history. Antagonistic properties may induce withdrawal symptoms (vomiting, restlessness, abdominal cramps, increased blood pressure and temperature) in patients who are physically dependent on opioid agonists.
- Butorphanol has a lower potential for dependence than other opioids; however, prolonged use may lead to physical and psychological dependence and tolerance. This should not prevent the patient from receiving adequate analgesia. Most patients receiving butorphanol for pain do not develop psychological dependence. If tolerance develops, changing to an opioid agonist may be required to relieve pain.

B

- ***Lab Test Considerations:*** May cause ↑ serum amylase and lipase levels.
- ***Toxicity and Overdose:*** If an opioid antagonist is required to reverse respiratory depression or coma, naloxone (Narcan) is the antidote. Dilute the 0.4-mg ampule of naloxone in 10 ml of 0.9% NaCl and administer 0.5 ml (0.02 mg) by direct IV push every 2 min. For children and patients weighing <40 kg, dilute 0.1 mg of naloxone in 10 ml of 0.9% NaCl for a concentration of 10 mcg/ml and administer 0.5 mcg/kg every 1–2 min. Titrate dose to avoid withdrawal, seizures, and severe pain.

Potential Nursing Diagnoses

Acute pain (Indications)
Risk for injury (Side Effects)
Disturbed sensory perception (visual, auditory) (Side Effects)

Implementation

- ***High Alert:*** Accidental overdosage of opioid analgesics has resulted in fatalities. Before administering, clarify all ambiguous orders; have second practitioner independently check original order, dose calculations, route of administration, and infusion pump programming. Do not confuse Stadol with Haldol.
- Explain therapeutic value of medication before administration to enhance the analgesic effect.
- Regularly administered doses may be more effective than prn administration. Analgesic is more effective if given before pain becomes severe.
- Coadministration with nonopioid analgesics may have additive analgesic effects and permit lower opioid doses.
- **IM:** Administer IM injections deep into well-developed muscle. Rotate sites of injections.

IV Administration

- **Direct IV:** ***Diluent:*** May give IV undiluted. ***Concentration:*** 1–2 mg/ml. ***Rate:*** Administer over 3–5 min. ***High Alert:*** Rapid administration may cause respiratory depression, hypotension, and cardiac arrest.
- **Syringe Compatibility:** atropine, chlorpromazine, cimetidine, diphenhydramine, droperidol, fentanyl, hydroxyzine, meperidine, metoclopramide, midazolam, morphine, pentazocine, perphenazine, prochlorperazine, promethazine, scopolamine, thiethylperazine.
- **Syringe Incompatibility:** dimenhydrinate, pentobarbital.
- **Y-Site Compatibility:** allopurinol sodium, amifostine, aztreonam, bivalirudin, cefepime, cisatracurium, cladribine, dexmedetomidine, docetaxel, doxorubicin liposome, enalaprilat, esmolol, etoposide phosphate, fenoldopam, filgrastim, fludarabine, gemcitabine, granisetron, labetalol, linezolid, melphalan, nicardipine, oxaliplatin, paclitaxel, pemetrexed, piperacillin/tazobactam, propofol, remifentanil, sargramostim, teniposide, thiotepa, vinorelbine.
- **Y-Site Incompatibility:** amphotericin B cholesteryl sulfate complex, lansoprazole, midazolam. **Intranasal:** Administer 1 spray in 1 nostril.

Patient/Family Teaching

- Instruct patient on how and when to ask for pain medication.
- Medication may cause drowsiness or dizziness. Advise patient to call for assistance when ambulating and to avoid driving or other activities requiring alertness until response to the medication is known.
- Encourage patients on bedrest to turn, cough, and deep-breathe every 2 hr to prevent atelectasis.
- Instruct patient to change positions slowly to minimize orthostatic hypotension.
- Caution patient to avoid concurrent use of alcohol or other CNS depressants with this medication.
- Advise patient that good oral hygiene, frequent mouth rinses, and sugarless gum or candy may decrease dry mouth.
- **Intranasal:** Instruct patient on proper use of nasal spray. See package insert for detailed instructions. Instruct patient to replace protective clip and clear cover after use and to store the unit in the child resistant container. Caution patient that medication should not be used by anyone other than the person for whom it was prescribed. Excess medication should be disposed of as soon as it is no longer needed. To dispose of, unscrew cap, rinse bottle and pump with water, and dispose of in waste can.

- If 2-mg dose is prescribed, administer additional spray in other nostril. May cause dizziness and dysphoria. Patient should remain recumbent after administration of 2-mg dose until response to medication is known.

Evaluation/Desired Outcomes

- Decrease in severity of pain without a significant alteration in level of consciousness or respiratory status.

cabergoline (ka-**ber**-goe-leen)
Dostinex

Classification
Therapeutic: antihyperprolactinemics
Pharmacologic: dopamine agonists

Pregnancy Category C

Indications

Treatment of hyperprolactinemia (idiopathic or pituitary in origin). **Unlabeled uses:** Adjunctive treatment of Parkinson's disease.

Action

Inhibits secretion of prolactin by acting as a dopamine agonist. In Parkinson's, dopamine agonists directly stimulate neural dopamine receptors. **Therapeutic Effects:** Decreased secretion of prolactin in hyperprolactinemia. Reduced involuntary movements associated with Parkinson's disease.

Pharmacokinetics

Absorption: Well absorbed but undergoes extensive first-pass hepatic metabolism.
Distribution: Widely distributed; concentrates in pituitary.
Metabolism and Excretion: Extensively metabolized by the liver; <4% excreted unchanged in urine.
Protein Binding: 40–42%.
Half-life: 63–69 hr.

TIME/ACTION PROFILE (effect on serum prolactin levels)

ROUTE	ONSET	PEAK	DURATION
PO	unknown	2–3 hrs	unknown

Contraindications/Precautions

Contraindicated in: Hypersensitivity to cabergoline or ergot alkaloids; Uncontrolled hypertension; Coadministration with potent inhibitors of CYP3A4 (**protease inhibitors**, **azole antifungals**, **clarithromycin**, and **telithromycin**; OB, Lactation: Has been associated with hypertension, stroke, and seizures. Not to be used for suppression of physiologic lactation.
Use Cautiously in: Hepatic impairment; Lactation: Will interfere with breast milk production; Pedi: Safety not established.

Adverse Reactions/Side Effects

CNS: dizziness, headache, depression, drowsiness, fatigue, nervousness, vertigo, weakness. **EENT:** abnormal vision. **CV:** postural hypotension, hot flashes. **GI:** constipation, nausea, abdominal pain, dyspepsia, vomiting. **GU:** dysmenorrhea. **Endo:** breast pain. **Neuro:** paresthesia.

Interactions

Drug-Drug: Increased risk of hypotension with **antihypertensives**. May increase the effects of **sibutramine**, **SSRIs**, and other **serotonin agonists** (induces serotonin syndrome). Effectiveness may be decreased by **phenothiazines**, **butyrophenones (haloperidol)**, **thioxanthenes**, or **metoclopramide** (avoid concurrent use).

Route/Dosage

PO (Adults): 0.25 mg twice weekly; may be increased at 4-wk intervals up to 1 mg twice weekly.

Availability

Tablets: 0.5 mg.

NURSING IMPLICATIONS

Assessment

- Monitor blood pressure before and frequently during initial therapy. Initial doses >1 mg may cause orthostatic hypotension. Use with caution when administering concurrently with other medications that lower blood pressure. Supervise ambulation and transfer during initial dosing to prevent injury from hypotension.
- **Parkinson's Disease:** Assess symptoms (restlessness or desire to keep moving, rigidity, tremors, pill rolling, masklike face, shuffling gait, muscle spasms, twisting motions, difficulty speaking or swallowing, loss of balance control) before and throughout therapy.
- ***Lab Test Considerations:*** Serum prolactin concentrations should be measured monthly until normalized (<20 mcg/liter in women and <15 mcg/liter in men).

Potential Nursing Diagnoses

Risk for injury (Side Effects)
Impaired physical mobility (Indications)

Implementation

- **PO:** May be taken without regard to food.

Patient/Family Teaching

- Instruct patient to take medication exactly as directed. If a dose is missed, take as soon as possible within 1 or 2 days. If not remembered until time of next dose, double dose. If nausea occurs, discuss with health care professional.
- May cause drowsiness and dizziness. Caution patient to avoid driving and other activities requiring alertness until response to medication is known.
- Advise patient to change positions slowly to minimize orthostatic hypotension.
- Caution patient to avoid concurrent use of alcohol during the course of therapy.
- Advise women to consult with health care professional regarding a nonhormonal method of birth control. Women should contact health care professional promptly if pregnancy is planned or suspected.
- Instruct patients taking cabergoline for pituitary tumors to inform health care professional immediately if signs of tumor enlargement occur (blurred vision, sudden headache, severe nausea, and vomiting).
- Emphasize the importance of regular follow-up exams to determine effectiveness and monitor side effects.

Evaluation/Desired Outcomes

- Decrease in galactorrhea in patients with hyperprolactinemia.
- After a normal serum prolactin level has been maintained for more than 6 mo, cabergoline may be discontinued. Serum prolactin levels should be monitored periodically to determine necessity of reinstituting cabergoline.
- Decrease in tremor, rigidity, and bradykinesia.
- Improvement in balance and gait in patients with Parkinson's disease.

CALCITONIN

calcitonin (salmon)
(kal-si-**toe**-nin)
Miacalcin

calcitonin (rDNA)
Fortical

Classification
Therapeutic: hypocalcemics
Pharmacologic: hormones

Pregnancy Category C

Indications

IM, Subcut Treatment of Paget's disease of bone. Adjunctive therapy for hypercalcemia. **IM, Subcut, Intranasal:** Management of postmenopausal osteoporosis.

Action

Inhibits osteoclastic bone resorption and promotes renal excretion of calcium. **Therapeutic Effects:** Decreased rate of bone turnover. Lowering of serum calcium.

Pharmacokinetics

Absorption: Completely absorbed from IM and subcut sites. Rapidly absorbed from nasal mucosa; absorption is 3% compared with parenteral administration.
Distribution: Unknown.
Metabolism and Excretion: Rapidly metabolized in kidneys, blood, and tissues.
Half-life: 40–90 min.

TIME/ACTION PROFILE

ROUTE	ONSET	PEAK	DURATION
IM, subcut†	Unknown	2 hr	6–8 hr
Intranasal‡	rapid	31–39 min	Unknown

†Effects on serum calcium; effects on serum alkaline phosphates and urinary hydroxyproline in Paget's disease may require 6–24 months of continuous treatment
‡Serum levels of administered calcitonin

Contraindications/Precautions

Contraindicated in: Hypersensitivity to calcitonin, salmon protein, or gelatin diluent (in some products); OB, Lactation: Use is not recommended.
Use Cautiously in: Pedi: Safety not established.

Adverse Reactions/Side Effects

CNS: *nasal only*— headaches. **EENT:** *nasal only*— rhinitis, epistaxis, nasal irritation. **GI:** *IM, subcut*— nausea, vomiting. **GU:** *IM, subcut*— urinary frequency. **Derm:** rashes. **Local:** injection site reactions. **MS:** *nasal*— arthralgia, back pain. **Misc:** allergic reactions including ANAPHYLAXIS, facial flushing, swelling.

Interactions

Drug-Drug: Previous bisphosphonate therapy, including **alendronate**, **risedronate**, **etidronate**, **ibandronate**, or **pamidronate**, may ↓ response to calcitonin.

Route/Dosage

Postmenopausal osteoporosis

IM, Subcut (Adults): 100 IU every other day.

Intranasal (Adults): 1 spray (200 IU)/day in alternating nostrils.

Paget's disease

IM, Subcut (Adults): 100 IU/day initially, after titration, maintenance dose is usually 50 IU/day or every other day.

Hypercalcemia

IM, Subcut (Adults): 4 IU/kg q 12 hr; if adequate response not achieved, may increase dose after 1–2 days to 8 IU/kg q 12 hr, and if necessary after 2 more days may be increased to 8 IU/kg q 6 hr.

Availability

Injection: 200 IU/ml in 2-ml vials. **Cost:** $50.89/vial. **Nasal spray:** 200 IU/actuation in 3.7-ml bottles. **Cost:** *Miacalcin*—$112.22/bottle.

NURSING IMPLICATIONS

Assessment

- Observe patient for signs of hypersensitivity (skin rash, fever, hives, anaphylaxis, serum sickness). Keep epinephrine, antihistamines, and oxygen nearby in the event of a reaction.
- Assess patient for signs of hypocalcemic tetany (nervousness, irritability, paresthesia, muscle twitching, tetanic spasms, seizures) during the first several doses of calcitonin. Parenteral calcium, such as calcium gluconate, should be available in case of this event.
- **Intranasal:** Assess nasal mucosa, septum, turbinates, and mucosal blood vessels periodically during therapy. If severe ulceration occurs, drug should be discontinued.
- ***Lab Test Considerations:*** Monitor serum calcium and alkaline phosphatase periodically during therapy. Levels should normalize within a few months of initiation of therapy.
- Urine hydroxyproline (24 hr) may be monitored periodically in patients with Paget's disease.

Potential Nursing Diagnoses

Acute pain (Indications)
Risk for injury (Indications, Side Effects)

Implementation

- In patients with suspected sensitivity to calcitonin, skin test should be considered before starting therapy. Test dose is prepared in a dilution of 10 IU/ml by withdrawing 0.05 ml in a tuberculin syringe and filling to 1 ml with 0.9% NaCl for injection. Mix well and discard 0.9 ml. Administer 0.1 ml intradermally on inner aspect of forearm and observe site for 15 min. More than mild erythema or wheal constitutes positive response.
- Store injection and unopened nasal spray bottle in refrigerator. Nasal spray bottle in use can be stored at room temperature.
- **IM, Subcut:** Inspect injection site for the appearance of redness, swelling, or pain. Rotate injection sites. Subcut is the preferred route. Use IM route if dose exceeds 2 ml in volume. Use multiple sites to minimize inflammatory reaction.

Patient/Family Teaching

- Advise patient to take medication exactly as directed. If dose is missed and medication is scheduled for twice a day, take only if possible within 2 hr of correct time. If scheduled for daily dose, take only if remembered that day. If scheduled for every other day, take when remembered and restart alternate day schedule. If taking 1 dose 3 times weekly (Mon, Wed, Fri), take missed dose the next day and set each injection back 1 day; resume regular schedule the following week. Do not double doses.
- Instruct patient in the proper method of self-injection and care and disposal of equipment.
- Advise patient to report signs of hypercalcemic relapse (deep bone or flank pain, renal calculi, anorexia, nausea, vomiting, thirst, lethargy) or allergic response promptly.
- Reassure patient that flushing and warmth following injection are transient and usually last about 1 hr.
- Explain that nausea following injection tends to decrease even with continued therapy.
- Instruct patient to follow low-calcium diet if recommended by health care professional (see Appendix L). Women with postmenopausal osteoporosis should adhere to a diet high in calcium and vitamin D.
- **Osteoporosis:** Advise patients receiving calcitonin for the treatment of osteoporosis that exercise has been found to arrest and reverse bone loss. The patient should discuss any exercise limitations with health care professional before beginning program.

- **Intranasal:** Instruct patient on correct use of nasal spray. Demonstrate procedure for use. Before first use, activate pump by holding upright and depressing white side arms down toward bottle 5 times until a full spray is emitted. Following activation, place nozzle firmly in nostril with head in an upright position and depress the pump toward the bottle. The pump should NOT be primed before each daily use. Discard bottle 30 days after first use.
- Advise patient to notify health care professional if significant nasal irritation occurs.

Evaluation/Desired Outcomes

- Lowered serum calcium levels.
- Decreased bone pain.
- Slowed progression of postmenopausal osteoporosis. Significant increases in bone marrow density may be seen as early as 6 months after initiation of therapy.

calcitriol, See VITAMIN D COMPOUNDS.

HIGH ALERT

CALCIUM SALTS

calcium acetate (25% Ca or 12.6 mEq/g)
(**kal**-see-um **ass**-e-tate)
Calphron, PhosLo

calcium carbonate (40% Ca or 20 mEq/g)
(**kal**-see-um **kar**-bo-nate)
Alka-Mints, Amitone, ✤Apo-Cal, BioCal, Calcarb, Calci-Chew, Calciday, Calcilac, Calci-Mix, ✤Calcite, ✤Calglycine, Cal-Plus, ✤Calsan, Caltrate, Chooz, Dicarbosil, Equilet, Gencalc, Liqui-Cal, Liquid Cal-600, Maalox Antacid Caplets, Mallamint, ✤Mylanta Lozenges, Nephro-Calci, ✤Nu-Cal, Os-Cal, Oysco, Oyst-Cal, Oystercal, Rolaids Calcium Rich, Surpass, Surpass Extra Strength, Titralac, Tums, Tums E-X

calcium chloride (27% Ca or 13.6 mEq/g)
(**kal**-see-um **kloh**-ride)

calcium citrate (21% Ca or 12 mEq/g) (**kal**-see-um **si**-trate)
Cal-Citrate 250, Citrical, Citrical Liquitab

calcium gluconate (9% Ca or 4.5 mEq/g)
(**kal**-see-um **gloo**-koh-nate)
Kalcinate

calcium lactate (13% Ca or 6.5 mEq/g) (**kal**-see-um **lak**-tate)
Cal-Lac

tricalcium phosphate (39% Ca or 19.5 mEq/g)
Posture

Classification
Therapeutic: mineral and electrolyte replacements/supplements

Pregnancy Category C (calcium acetate, calcium chloride, calcium gluconate injections), UK (calcium carbonate, calcium citrate, calcium lactate, tricalcium phosphate)

Indications

PO, IV: Treatment and prevention of hypocalcemia. **PO:** Adjunct in the prevention of postmenopausal osteoporosis. **IV:** Emergency treatment of hyperkalemia and hypermagnesemia and adjunct in cardiac arrest or calcium channel blocking agent toxicity (calcium chloride, calcium gluconate). **Calcium carbonate:** May be used as an antacid. **Calcium acetate:** Control of hyperphosphatemia in end-stage renal disease.

Action

Essential for nervous, muscular, and skeletal systems. Maintain cell membrane and capillary permeability. Act as an activator in the transmission of nerve impulses and contraction of cardiac, skeletal, and smooth muscle. Essential for bone formation and blood coagulation. **Therapeutic Effects:** Replacement of calcium in deficiency states. Control of hyperphosphatemia in end-stage renal disease without promoting aluminum absorption (calcium acetate).

C

Pharmacokinetics

Absorption: Absorption from the GI tract requires vitamin D. IV administration results in complete bioavailability.
Distribution: Readily enters extracellular fluid. Crosses the placenta and enters breast milk.
Metabolism and Excretion: Excreted mostly in the feces; 20% eliminated by the kidneys.
Half-life: Unknown.

TIME/ACTION PROFILE (effects on serum calcium)

ROUTE	ONSET	PEAK	DURATION
PO	unknown	unknown	unknown
IV	immediate	immediate	0.5–2 hr

Contraindications/Precautions

Contraindicated in: Hypercalcemia; Renal calculi; Ventricular fibrillation.
Use Cautiously in: Patients receiving digitalis glycosides; Severe respiratory insufficiency; Renal disease; Cardiac disease.

Adverse Reactions/Side Effects

CNS: syncope (IV only), tingling. **CV:** CARDIAC ARREST (IV only), arrhythmias, bradycardia. **GI:** constipation, nausea, vomiting. **GU:** calculi, hypercalciuria. **Local:** phlebitis (IV ONLY).

Interactions

Drug-Drug: Hypercalcemia increases the risk of **digoxin** toxicity. Chronic use with **antacids** in renal insufficiency may lead to milk-alkali syndrome. Ingestion by mouth decreases the absorption of orally administered **tetracyclines**, **fluoroquinolones**, **phenytoin**, and **iron salts**. Excessive amounts may decrease the effects of **calcium channel blockers**. Decreases absorption of **etidronate** and **risedronate** (do not take within 2 hr of calcium supplements). May decrease the effectiveness of **atenolol**. Concurrent use with **diuretics (thiazide)** may result in hypercalcemia. May decrease the ability of **sodium polystyrene sulfonate** to decrease serum potassium.
Drug-Food: Cereals, **spinach**, or **rhubarb** may decrease the absorption of calcium supplements. Calcium acetate should not be given concurrently with other calcium supplements.

Route/Dosage

Doses are expressed in mg, g, or mEq of calcium.

PO (Adults): *Prevention of hypocalcemia, treatment of depletion, osteoporosis*—1–2 g/day. *Antacid*—0.5–1.5 g as needed (calcium carbonate only). *Hyperphosphatemia in end-stage renal disease (calcium acetate only)*—Amount necessary to control serum phosphate and calcium.
PO (Children): *Supplementation*—45–65 mg/kg/day.
PO (Infants): *Neonatal hypocalcemia*—50–150 mg/kg (not to exceed 1 g).
IV (Adults): *Emergency treatment of hypocalcemia, cardiac standstill*—7–14 mEq. *Hypocalcemic tetany*—4.5–16 mEq; repeat until symptoms are controlled. *Hyperkalemia with cardiac toxicity*—2.25–14 mEq; may repeat in 1–2 min. *Hypermagnesemia*—7 mEq.
IV (Children): *Emergency treatment of hypocalcemia*—1–7 mEq. *Hypocalcemic tetany*—0.5–0.7 mEq/kg 3–4 times daily.
IV (Infants): *Emergency treatment of hypocalcemia*—<1 mEq. *Hypocalcemic tetany*—2.4 mEq/kg/day in divided doses.

Availability (generic available)

Calcium Acetate

Tablets: 250 mg (65 mg Ca)[OTC], 667 mg (169 mg Ca)[OTC], 668 mg (169 mg Ca)[OTC], 1 g (250 mg Ca)[OTC]. **Capsules:** 500 mg (125 mg Ca)[OTC].

Calcium Carbonate

Tablets: 500 mg (200 mg Ca)[OTC], 600 mg (240 mg Ca)[OTC], 650 mg (260 mg Ca)[OTC], 667 mg (266.8 mg Ca)[OTC], 1 g (400 mg Ca)[OTC], 1.25 g (500 mg Ca)[OTC], 1.5 g (600 mg Ca)[OTC]. **Chewable tablets:** 350 mg (300 mg Ca)[OTC], 420 mg (168 mg Ca)[OTC], 450 mg[OTC], 500 mg (200 mg Ca)[OTC], 750 mg (300 mg Ca)[OTC], 1 g (400 mg Ca)[OTC], 1.25 g (500 mg Ca)[OTC]. **Gum tablets:** 300 mg[OTC], 450 mg[OTC], 500 mg (200 mg Ca)[OTC]. **Capsules:** 1.25 g (500 mg Ca)[OTC]. **Lozenges:** 600 mg (240 mg Ca)[OTC]. **Oral suspension:** 1.25 g (500 mg Ca)/5 ml[OTC]. **Powder:** 6.5 g (2400 mg Ca)/packet[OTC].

Calcium Chloride

Injection: 10% (1.36 mEq/ml).

Calcium Citrate

Tablets: 250 mg[OTC].

Calcium Gluconate

Tablets: 500 mg (45 mg Ca)[OTC], 650 mg (58.5 mg Ca)[OTC], 975 mg (87.75 mg Ca)[OTC], 1 g (90 mg Ca)[OTC]. **Injection:** 10% (0.45 mEq/ml).

Calcium Lactate

Tablets: 325 mg (42.45 mg Ca)[OTC], 500 mg[OTC], 650 mg (84.5 mg Ca)[OTC].

NURSING IMPLICATIONS

Assessment

- **Calcium Supplement/Replacement:** Observe patient closely for symptoms of hypocalcemia (paresthesia, muscle twitching, laryngospasm, colic, cardiac arrhythmias, Chvostek's or Trousseau's sign). Notify physician or other health care professional if these occur. Protect symptomatic patients by elevating and padding siderails and keeping bed in low position.
- Monitor blood pressure, pulse, and ECG frequently throughout parenteral therapy. May cause vasodilation with resulting hypotension, bradycardia, arrhythmias, and cardiac arrest. Transient increases in blood pressure may occur during IV administration, especially in geriatric patients or in patients with hypertension.
- Assess IV site for patency. Extravasation may cause cellulitis, necrosis, and sloughing.
- Monitor patient on digitalis glycosides for signs of toxicity.
- **Antacid:** When used as an antacid, assess for heartburn, indigestion, and abdominal pain. Inspect abdomen; auscultate bowel sounds.
- ***Lab Test Considerations:*** Monitor serum calcium or ionized calcium chloride, sodium, potassium, magnesium, albumin, and parathyroid hormone (PTH) concentrations before and periodically during therapy for treatment of hypocalcemia.
- May cause decreased serum phosphate concentrations with excessive and prolonged use. When used to treat hyperphosphatemia in renal failure patients, monitor phosphate levels.
- ***Toxicity and Overdose:*** Assess patient for nausea, vomiting, anorexia, thirst, severe constipation, paralytic ileus, and bradycardia. Contact physician or other health care professional immediately if these signs of hypercalcemia occur.

Potential Nursing Diagnoses

Imbalanced nutrition: less than body requirements (Indications)

Risk for injury, related to osteoporosis or electrolyte imbalance (Indications)

Implementation

- ***High Alert:*** Errors with IV calcium gluconate and chloride have occurred secondary to confusion over which salt is ordered. Clarify incomplete orders. Confusion has occurred with milligram doses of calcium chloride and calcium gluconate, which are not equal. Chloride and gluconate forms are routinely available on most hospital crash carts; physician should specify form of calcium desired. Doses should be expressed in mEq.
- Do not confuse Os-Cal (calcium carbonate) with Asacol (mesalamine).
- In arrest situations, the use of calcium chloride is now limited to patients with hyperkalemia, hypocalcemia, and calcium channel blocker toxicity.
- **PO:** Administer calcium carbonate or phosphate 1–1.5 hr after meals and at bedtime. Chewable tablets should be well chewed before swallowing. Dissolve effervescent tablets in glass of water. Follow oral doses with a full glass of water, except when using calcium carbonate as a phosphate binder in renal dialysis. Administer on an empty stomach before meals to optimize effectiveness in patients with hyperphosphatemia.
- **IM:** IM administration of calcium salts can cause severe necrosis and tissue sloughing. Do not administer IM.

IV Administration

- **IV:** IV solution should be warmed to body temperature and given through a small-bore needle in a large vein to minimize phlebitis. Do not administer through a scalp vein. May cause cutaneous burning sensation, peripheral vasodilation, and drop in blood pressure. Patient should remain recumbent for 30–60 min after IV administration.
- If infiltration occurs, discontinue IV. May be treated with application of heat, elevation, and local infiltration of normal saline, 1% procaine HCl, or hyaluronidase.
- ***High Alert:*** Administer slowly. High concentrations may cause cardiac arrest. Rapid administration may cause tingling, sensation of warmth, and a metallic taste. Halt infusion if these symptoms occur, and resume infusion at a slower rate when they subside.
- Do not administer solutions that are not clear or that contain a precipitate.

Calcium Chloride

IV Administration

- **Direct IV:** May be administered undiluted by IV push. **Intermittent/Continuous Infusion:** May be diluted with D5W, D10W, 0.9% NaCl, D5/0.25% NaCl, D5/0.45% NaCl, D5/0.9% NaCl, or D5/LR. ***Rate:*** Maximum rate for adults is 0.7–1.4 mEq/min (0.5–1 ml of 10% solution); for children, 0.5 ml/min.
- **Syringe Compatibility:** milrinone.
- **Y-Site Compatibility:** amiodarone, dobutamine, doxapram, epinephrine, esmolol, inamrinone, milrinone, morphine, nitroprusside, paclitaxel.
- **Y-Site Incompatibility:** amphotericin B cholesteryl sulfate, propofol, sodium bicarbonate.

Calcium Gluconate

IV Administration

- **Direct IV:** Administer slowly by direct IV push. ***Rate:*** Maximum administration rate for adults is 1.5–2 ml/min.
- **Continuous Infusion:** May be further diluted in 1000 ml of D5W, D10W, D20W, D5/0.9% NaCl, 0.9% NaCl, D5/LR, or LR. ***Rate:*** Administer at a rate not to exceed 200 mg/min over 12–24 hr.
- **Syringe Incompatibility:** metoclopramide.
- **Y-Site Compatibility:** aldesleukin, allopurinol, amifostine, amiodarone, aztreonam, bivalirudin, cefazolin, cefepime, ciprofloxacin, cisatracurium, cladribine, dexmedetomidate, dobutamine, docetaxel, doxapram, doxorubicin liposome, enalaprilat, epinephrine, etoposide, famotidine, fenoldopam, filgrastim, gemcitabine, granisetron, labetalol, linezolid, melphalan, midazolam, milrinone, piperacillin/tazobactam, potassium chloride, prochlorperazine edisylate, propofol, remifentanil, sargramostim, tacrolimus, teniposide, thiotepa, tolazoline, vinorelbine, vitamin B complex with C.
- **Y-Site Incompatibility:** amphotericin B cholesteryl sulfate, fluconazole, indomethacin.

Patient/Family Teaching

- Instruct patient not to take enteric-coated tablets within 1 hr of calcium carbonate; this will result in premature dissolution of the tablets.
- Do not administer concurrently with foods containing large amounts of oxalic acid (spinach, rhubarb), phytic acid (brans, cereals), or phosphorus (milk or dairy products). Administration with milk products may lead to milk-alkali syndrome (nausea, vomiting, confusion, headache). Do not take within 1–2 hr of other medications if possible.
- Instruct patients on a regular schedule to take missed doses as soon as possible, then go back to regular schedule.
- Advise patient that calcium carbonate may cause constipation. Review methods of preventing constipation (increasing bulk in diet, increasing fluid intake, increasing mobility) and using laxatives. Severe constipation may indicate toxicity.
- Advise patient to avoid excessive use of tobacco or beverages containing alcohol or caffeine.
- **Calcium Supplement:** Encourage patients to maintain a diet adequate in vitamin D (see Appendix L).
- **Osteoporosis:** Advise patients that exercise has been found to arrest and reverse bone loss. Patient should discuss any exercise limitations with health care professional before beginning program.

Evaluation/Desired Outcomes

- Increase in serum calcium levels.
- Decrease in the signs and symptoms of hypocalcemia.
- Resolution of indigestion.
- Control of hyperphosphatemia in patients with renal failure (calcium acetate only).

candesartan, See ANGIOTENSIN II RECEPTOR ANTAGONISTS.

HIGH ALERT

capecitabine

(kap-pe-**site**-a-been)
Xeloda

Classification
Therapeutic: antineoplastics
Pharmacologic: antimetabolites

Pregnancy Category D

Indications

Metastatic colorectal cancer. Adjuvant treatment for Dukes' C colon cancer following primary resection. Metastatic breast cancer that has worsened despite prior therapy with anthracycline (daunorubicin, doxorubicin, idarubicin) (to be used in combination with docetaxel). Metastatic breast cancer that is resistant to both paclitaxel and an anthracycline (daunorubicin, doxorubicin, idarubicin) or is resistant to paclitaxel and further anthracycline therapy is contraindicated.

Action

Converted in tissue to 5-fluorouracil (5-FU), which inhibits DNA and RNA synthesis by preventing thymidine production. The enzyme responsible for the final step in the conversion to 5-FU may be found in higher concentrations in some tumors. **Therapeutic Effects:** Death of rapidly replicating cells, particularly malignant ones.

Pharmacokinetics

Absorption: Well absorbed after oral administration.
Distribution: Unknown.
Metabolism and Excretion: Metabolized mostly in tissue and by the liver; inactive metabolites are excreted primarily in urine.
Half-life: 45 min.

TIME/ACTION PROFILE (blood levels)

ROUTE	ONSET	PEAK	DURATION
PO	unknown†	1.5 hr (2 hr for 5-FU)‡	unknown

†Onset of antineoplastic effect is 6 wk
‡Peak 5-FU levels occur at 2 hr

Contraindications/Precautions

Contraindicated in: Hypersensitivity to capecitabine or 5-FU; Dihydropyrimidine dehydrogenase deficiency (enzyme metabolizes 5-FU to nontoxic compounds); Severe renal impairment (CCr <30 ml/min); OB: Potential for fetal harm or death; Lactation: Potential for serious adverse effects in nursing infants.
Use Cautiously in: Mild-moderate renal impairment (decrease starting dose to 75% in patients with CCr 30–50 ml/min); Hepatic dysfunction; Coronary artery disease; Pedi: Safety not established; Geri: Increased risk of severe diarrhea in patients ≥80 yr.

Adverse Reactions/Side Effects

CNS: fatigue, headache, dizziness, insomnia. **EENT:** eye irritation, epistaxis, rhinorrhea. **CV:** edema, chest pain. **GI:** DIARRHEA, NECROTIZING ENTEROCOLITIS, abdominal pain, anorexia, constipation, dysgeusia, hyperbilirubinemia, nausea, stomatitis, vomiting, dyspepsia, xerostomia. **Derm:** dermatitis, hand-and-foot syndrome, nail disorder, alopecia, erythema, rashes. **F and E:** dehydration. **Hemat:** anemia, leukopenia, thrombocytopenia. **MS:** arthralgia, myalgia. **Neuro:** peripheral neuropathy. **Resp:** cough, dyspnea. **Misc:** fever.

Interactions

Drug-Drug: May ↑ risk of bleeding with **warfarin** (frequent monitoring of PT/INR recommended). Toxicity ↑ by concurrent **leucovorin**. **Antacids** may ↑ absorption. May ↑ blood levels and risk of toxicity from **phenytoin** (may need to decrease phenytoin dose).
Drug-Food: Food ↑ absorption, although capecitabine should be given within 30 min after a meal.

Route/Dosage

PO (Adults): 1250 mg/m² twice daily for 14 days, followed by 7-day rest period; given as 3-wk cycles.

Renal Impairment

PO (Adults CCr 30-50 ml/min): Decrease initial dose to 75% of usual.

Availability

Tablets: 150 mg, 500 mg.

NURSING IMPLICATIONS

Assessment

- Assess mucous membranes, number and consistency of stools, and frequency of vomiting. Assess for signs of infection (fever, chills, sore throat, cough, hoarseness, pain in lower back or side, difficult or painful urination). Assess for bleeding (bleeding gums; bruising; petechiae; and guaiac-test stools, urine, and emesis). Avoid IM injections and taking rectal temperatures. Apply pressure to venipuncture sites for 10 min. Anemia may occur. Monitor for increased fatigue, dyspnea, and orthostatic hypotension.
- ***High Alert:*** Notify physician if symptoms of toxicity (stomatitis, uncontrollable vomiting, diarrhea, fever) occur; drug may need to be discontinued or dose decreased. Patients with severe diarrhea should be monitored

carefully and given fluid and electrolyte replacement if they become dehydrated.

- Assess patient for hand-and-foot syndrome. Symptoms include numbness, dysesthesia or paresthesia, tingling, painless or painful swelling, erythema, desquamation, blistering, and severe pain.
- ***Lab Test Considerations:*** Monitor hepatic (serum alkaline phosphatase, AST, ALT, and bilirubin), renal, and hematologic (hematocrit, hemoglobin, leukocyte, platelet count) function before and periodically during therapy. May cause leukopenia, anemia, and thrombocytopenia. Leukopenia may require discontinuation of therapy. Therapy should be interrupted if serum bilirubin ↑ to 1.5 times normal or greater; may be reinstituted after bilirubin returns to normal.
- ***Lab Test Considerations: High Alert:*** Monitor PT or INR frequently in patients receiving warfarin and capecitabine to adjust warfarin dose. May cause ↑ bleeding within a few days of initiation of therapy to 1 mo following discontinuation of therapy. Risk is greater in patients over 60 years.

Potential Nursing Diagnoses

Risk for infection (Side Effects)
Imbalanced nutrition: less than body requirements (Side Effects)

Implementation

- ***High Alert:*** Fatalities have occurred with chemotherapeutic agents. Before administering, clarify all ambiguous orders; double-check single, daily, and course-of-therapy dose limits; have second practitioner independently double-check original order and dose calculations. Do not confuse capecitabine (Xeloda) with orlistat (Xenical).
- Dose modifications are based on degree of toxicity encountered. Once a dose has been reduced because of toxicity, it should not be increased at a later time. See manufacturer's recommendations.
- **PO:** Administer every 12 hr for 2 wk, followed by a 1-wk rest period. Tablets should be taken with water within 30 min after a meal.

Patient/Family Teaching

- Instruct patient to take medication every 12 hr with water within 30 min after a meal. Missed doses should be omitted; continue regular schedule. Do not double dose.
- Inform patient of the most common side effects. Instruct patient to notify health care provider immediately if any of the following occur: diarrhea (>4 bowel movements in a day or any diarrhea at night), vomiting (more than once in 24 hr), nausea (loss of appetite and significant decrease in daily food intake), stomatitis (pain, redness, swelling, or sore in mouth), hand-and-foot syndrome (pain, swelling, or redness of hands and/or feet), fever or infection (temperature of ≥100.5° F or other signs of infection).
- Instruct patient to notify health care professional if he or she is taking folic acid.
- Instruct patient to notify health care professional if fever; chills; sore throat; signs of infection; yellowing of skin or eyes; abdominal pain; joint or flank pain; swelling of feet or legs; bleeding gums; bruising; petechiae; or blood in urine, stool, or emesis occurs. Caution patient to avoid crowds and persons with known infections. Instruct patient to use soft toothbrush and electric razor. Patients should be cautioned not to drink alcoholic beverages or take products containing aspirin or NSAIDs.
- Advise patient to rinse mouth with clear water after eating and drinking and to avoid flossing to minimize stomatitis. Viscous lidocaine may be used if mouth pain interferes with eating. Stomatitis pain may require treatment with opioid analgesics.
- Review with patient the need for contraception during therapy.
- Emphasize the importance of routine follow-up lab tests to monitor progress and to check for side effects.

Evaluation/Desired Outcomes

- Tumor regression.

capsaicin (kap-**say**-sin)

✤Axsam, Capsin, Capzasin-P, Dolorac, No Pain-HP, Pain Doctor, Pain-X, R-Gel, Rid•a•Pain•HP, Zostrix, Zostrix-HP

✤ = Canadian drug name.

*CAPITALS indicates life-threatening; underlines indicate most frequent.

Classification
Therapeutic: nonopioid analgesics (topical)

Pregnancy Category UK

Indications
Temporary management of pain due to rheumatoid arthritis and osteoarthritis. Treatment of pain associated with postherpetic neuralgia or diabetic neuropathy. **Unlabeled uses:** Treatment of postmastectomy pain syndrome. Treatment of complex regional pain syndrome.

Action
May deplete and prevent the reaccumulation of a chemical (substance P) responsible for transmitting painful impulses from peripheral sites to the CNS. **Therapeutic Effects:** Relief of discomfort associated with painful peripheral syndromes.

Pharmacokinetics
Absorption: Unknown.
Distribution: Unknown.
Metabolism and Excretion: Unknown.
Half-life: Unknown.

TIME/ACTION PROFILE

ROUTE	ONSET	PEAK	DURATION
topical	1–2 wk	2–4 wk†	unknown

†May take up to 6 wk for head and neck neuralgias

Contraindications/Precautions
Contraindicated in: Hypersensitivity to capsaicin or hot peppers; Not for use near eyes or on open or broken skin.
Use Cautiously in: OB, Lactation, Pedi: Safety not established for pregnant women, breastfeeding infants, or children <2 yr.

Adverse Reactions/Side Effects
Resp: cough. **Derm:** transient burning.

Interactions
Drug-Drug: None significant.

Route/Dosage
Topical (Adults and Children ≥2 yr): Apply to affected areas 3–4 times daily.

Availability
Cream: 0.025%^{OTC}, 0.075%^{OTC}. **Gel:** 0.05%^{OTC}. **Lotion:** 0.025%^{OTC}. **Roll-on:** 0.075%^{OTC}. ***In combination with:*** methyl salicylate (Ziks^{OTC}). See Appendix B.

NURSING IMPLICATIONS

Assessment
- Assess pain intensity and location before and periodically throughout therapy.

Potential Nursing Diagnoses
Chronic pain (Indications)
Noncompliance (Patient/Family Teaching)

Implementation
- **Topical:** Apply to affected area not more than 3–4 times daily. Avoid getting medication into eyes or on broken or irritated skin. Do not bandage tightly.
- Topical lidocaine may be applied during the first 1–2 wk of treatment to reduce initial discomfort.

Patient/Family Teaching
- Instruct patient on the correct method for application of capsaicin. Rub cream into affected area well so that little or no cream is left on the surface. Gloves should be worn during application or hands should be washed immediately after application. If application is to hands for arthritis, do not wash hands for at least 30 min after application.
- Advise patient to apply missed doses as soon as possible unless almost time for next dose. Pain relief lasts only as long as capsaicin is used regularly.
- Advise patient that transient burning may occur with application, especially if applied fewer than 3–4 times daily. Burning usually disappears after the first few days but may continue for 2–4 wk or longer. Burning is increased by heat, sweating, bathing in warm water, humidity, and clothing. Burning usually decreases in frequency and intensity the longer capsaicin is used. Decreasing number of daily doses will not lessen burning but may decrease amount of pain relief and may prolong period of burning.
- Caution patient to flush area with water if capsaicin gets into eyes and to wash with warm, but not hot, soapy water if capsaicin gets on other sensitive areas of the body.
- Instruct patient with herpes zoster (shingles) not to apply capsaicin cream until lesions have healed completely.
- Advise patient to discontinue use and notify health care professional if pain persists longer than 1 month, worsens, or if signs of infection are present.

Evaluation/Desired Outcomes

- Decrease in discomfort associated with: Postherpetic neuropathy, Diabetic neuropathy, Rheumatoid arthritis, Osteoarthritis. Pain relief usually begins within 1–2 wk with arthritis, 2–4 wk with neuralgias, and 4–6 wk with neuralgias of the head and neck.

captopril, See ANGIOTENSIN-CONVERTING ENZYME (ACE) INHIBITORS.

carbamazepine

(kar-ba-**maz**-e-peen)
♣Apo-Carbamazepine, Carbatrol, Epitol, Equetro, ♣Novo-Carbamaz, Tegretol, ♣Tegretol CR, Tegretol-XR, Teril

Classification
Therapeutic: anticonvulsants, mood stabilizers

Pregnancy Category D

Indications

Treatment of tonic-clonic, mixed, and complex-partial seizures. Management of pain in trigeminal neuralgia or diabetic neuropathy. **Equetro only:** Acute mania and mixed mania. **Unlabeled uses:** Other forms of neurogenic pain.

Action

Decreases synaptic transmission in the CNS by affecting sodium channels in neurons. **Therapeutic Effects:** Prevention of seizures. Relief of pain in trigeminal neuralgia. Decreased mania.

Pharmacokinetics

Absorption: Absorption is slow but complete. Suspension produces earlier, higher peak and lower trough levels.
Distribution: Widely distributed. Crosses the blood-brain barrier. Crosses the placenta rapidly and enters breast milk in high concentrations.
Protein Binding: *Carbamazepine*—75–90%; *epoxide*—50%.
Metabolism and Excretion: Extensively metabolized in the liver by cytochrome P450 3A4 to active epoxide metabolite; epoxide metabolite has anticonvulsant and antineuralgic activity.
Half-life: *Carbamazapine*—single dose—25–65 hr, chronic dosing— *Children*—8–14 hr; *Adults*—12–17 hr; *epoxide*—34±9hr.

TIME/ACTION PROFILE (anticonvulsant activity)

ROUTE	ONSET	PEAK	DURATION
PO	up to one month†	4–5 hr‡	6–12 hr
PO-ER	up to one month†	2–3–12 hr‡	12 hr

†Onset of antineuralgic activity is 8–72 hr
‡Listed for tablets; peak level occurs 1.5 hr after a chronic dose of suspension

Contraindications/Precautions

Contraindicated in: Hypersensitivity; Bone marrow suppression; Concomitant use or use within 14 days of MAO inhibitors; OB: Use only during pregnancy if potential benefits outweigh risks to the fetus; additional vitamin K during last weeks of pregnancy has been recommended; Lactation: Discontinue drug or bottle feed.
Use Cautiously in: Cardiac or hepatic disease; renal failure (dosing adjustment required for ClCr <10 ml/min; Increased intraocular pressure; Geri: Older men with prostatic hyperplasia may be at increased risk for acute urinary retention or difficulty initiating stream.

Adverse Reactions/Side Effects

CNS: ataxia, drowsiness, fatigue, psychosis, sedation, vertigo. **EENT:** blurred vision, nystagmus, corneal opacities. **Resp:** pneumonitis. **CV:** CHF, edema, hypertension, hypotension, syncope. **GI:** hepatitis, pancreatitis, weight gain. **GU:** hesitancy, urinary retention. **Derm:** photosensitivity, rashes, Stevens-Johnson syndrome, toxic epidermal necrolysis, urticaria. **Endo:** syndrome of inappropriate antidiuretic hormone (SIADH), hyponatremia. **Hemat:** AGRANULOCYTOSIS, APLASTIC ANEMIA, THROMBOCYTOPENIA, eosinophilia, leukopenia. **Misc:** chills, fever, lymphadenopathy, elevated liver enzymes, multi-organ hypersensitivity reactions, hepatic failure (rare).

Interactions

Drug-Drug: May ↑ metabolism of and therefore ↓ levels/effectiveness of **corticosteroids**, **doxycycline**, **felbamate**, **quinidine**, **warfarin**, **estrogen-containing contraceptives**, **barbiturates**, **cyclosporine**, **benzodiaze-**

♣ = Canadian drug name.
* CAPITALS indicates life-threatening; underlines indicate most frequent.

pines, **theophylline**, **lamotrigine**, **phenytoin**, **topiramate**, **valproic acid**, **bupropion**, and **haloperidol**. **Danazol** ↑ blood levels (avoid concurrent use if possible). Concurrent use (within 2 wk) of **MAO inhibitors** may result in hyperpyrexia, hypertension, seizures, and death. **Verapamil**, **diltiazem**, **propoxyphene**, **itraconazole**, **ketoconazole**, **erythromycin**, **clarithromycin**, **SSRIs**, **antidepressants**, or **cimetidine** may inhibit the hepatic metabolism or carbamazepine and ↑ levels; may cause toxicity. Enzyme inducers such as **rifampin**, **phenobarbital**, **phenytoin**, **primidone**, and **methosuximide** may ↓ serum concentration of carbamazepine. May ↑ risk of hepatotoxicity from **isoniazid**. **Felbamate** ↓ carbamazepine levels but ↑ levels of active metabolite. May ↓ effectiveness and ↑ risk of toxicity from **acetaminophen**. May ↑ risk of CNS toxicity from **lithium**. May ↓ duration of action of **nondepolarizing neuromuscular blocking agents**.
Drug-Food: Grapefruit juice ↑ serum levels and oral bioavailability by 40% and therefore may ↑ effects.

Route/Dosage

PO (Adults): *Anticonvulsant*—200 mg twice daily (tablets) or 100 mg 4 times daily (suspension); increase by 200 mg/day q 7 days until therapeutic levels are achieved (range is 600–1200 mg/day in divided doses q 6–8 hr; not to exceed 1 g/day in 12–15-yr-olds. Extended-release products are given twice daily (XR, CR). *Antineuralgic*—100 mg twice daily or 50 mg 4 times daily (suspension); increase by up to 200 mg/day until pain is relieved, then maintenance dose of 200–1200 mg/day in divided doses (usual range, 400–800 mg/day).
PO (Children 6–12 yr): 100 mg twice daily (tablets) or 50 mg 4 times daily (suspension) increased by 100 mg weekly until therapeutic levels are obtained (usual range 400–800 mg/day; not to exceed 1 g/day). Extended-release products (XR, CR) are given twice daily.
PO (Children <6 yr): 10–20 mg/kg/day in 2–3 divided doses; may be increased at weekly intervals until optimal response and therapeutic levels are acheived. Usual maintenance dose is 250–350 mg/day (not to exceed 35 mg/kg/day).

Availability (generic available)

Tablets: 200 mg. **Cost:** *Generic*—$25.97/180. **Chewable tablets:** 100 mg, ✱200 mg. **Cost:** *Generic*—100 mg $21.98/180. **Extended-release capsules:** 100 mg, 200 mg, 300 mg. **Cost:** 100 mg $235.66/180, 200 mg $226.49/180, 300 mg $216.88/180. **Extended-release tablets:** 100 mg, 200 mg, 400 mg. **Cost:** 100 mg $83.93/180, 200 mg $143.93/180, 400 mg $279.94/180. **Oral suspension (citrus/vanilla flavor):** 100 mg/5 ml. **Cost:** *Generic*—$28.26/450 ml.

NURSING IMPLICATIONS

Assessment

- **Seizures:** Assess frequency, location, duration, and characteristics of seizure activity.
- **Trigeminal Neuralgia:** Assess for facial pain (location, intensity, duration). Ask patient to identify stimuli that may precipitate facial pain (hot or cold foods, bedclothes, touching face).
- **Bipolar Disorder:** Assess mental status (mood, orientation, behavior) and cognitive abilities before and periodically during therapy.
- ***Lab Test Considerations:*** Monitor CBC, including platelet count, reticulocyte count, and serum iron, weekly during the first 2 mo and yearly thereafter for evidence of potentially fatal blood cell abnormalities. Medication should be discontinued if bone marrow depression occurs.
- Liver function tests, urinalysis, and BUN should be routinely performed. May cause ↑ AST, ALT, serum alkaline phosphatase, bilirubin, BUN, urine protein, and urine glucose levels.
- Monitor serum ionized calcium levels every 6 mo or if seizure frequency increases. Thyroid function tests and ionized serum calcium concentrations may be ↓; hypocalcemia decreases seizure threshold.
- Monitor ECG and serum electrolytes before and periodically during therapy. May cause hyponatremia.
- May occasionally cause ↑ serum cholesterol, high-density lipoprotein, and triglyceride concentrations.
- May cause false-negative pregnancy test results with tests that determine human chorionic gonadotropin.
- ***Toxicity and Overdose:*** Serum blood levels should be routinely monitored during therapy. Therapeutic levels range from 4–12 mcg/ml.

Potential Nursing Diagnoses

Risk for injury (Indications, Side Effects)

Chronic pain (Indications)
Disturbed thought process (Indications)

Implementation

- Implement seizure precautions as indicated.
- **PO:** Administer medication with food to minimize gastric irritation. May take at bedtime to reduce daytime sedation. Tablets may be crushed if patient has difficulty swallowing. Do not crush or chew extended-release tablets. Extended-release capsules may be opened and the contents sprinkled on applesauce or other similar foods.
- Do not administer suspension simultaneously with other liquid medications or diluents; mixture produces an orange rubbery mass.

Patient/Family Teaching

- Instruct patient to take carbamazepine around the clock, as directed. Take missed doses as soon as possible but not just before next dose; do not double doses. Notify health care professional if more than one dose is missed. Medication should be gradually discontinued to prevent seizures.
- May cause dizziness or drowsiness. Advise patients to avoid driving or other activities requiring alertness until response to medication is known.
- Instruct patients that fever, sore throat, mouth ulcers, easy bruising, petechiae, unusual bleeding, abdominal pain, chills, rash, pale stools, dark urine, or jaundice should be reported to health care professional immediately.
- Inform patient that coating of *Tegretol XR* is not absorbed, but is excreted in feces and may be visible in stool.
- Advise patient not to take alcohol or other CNS depressants concurrently with this medication.
- Caution patients to use sunscreen and protective clothing to prevent photosensitivity reactions.
- Inform patient that frequent mouth rinses, good oral hygiene, and sugarless gum or candy may help reduce dry mouth. Saliva substitute may be used. Consult dentist if dry mouth persists >2 wk.
- Advise female patients to use a nonhormonal form of contraception while taking carbamazepine.
- Instruct patient to notify health care professional of medication regimen before treatment or surgery.
- Emphasize the importance of follow-up lab tests and eye exams to monitor for side effects.
- Inform patient and family that the Manic-Depressive and Depressive Association can offer support for mania.
- **Seizures:** Advise patients to carry identification describing disease and medication regimen at all times.

Evaluation/Desired Outcomes

- Absence or reduction of seizure activity.
- Decrease in trigeminal neuralgia pain. Patients with trigeminal neuralgia who are pain-free should be re-evaluated every 3 mo to determine minimum effective dose.
- Decreased mania and depressive symptoms in Bipolar I disorder.

carbonyl iron, See IRON SUPPLEMENTS.

HIGH ALERT

carboplatin (kar-boe-**pla**-tin)

Paraplatin, ✤Paraplatin-AQ

Classification
Therapeutic: antineoplastics
Pharmacologic: alkylating agents

Pregnancy Category D

Indications

Advanced ovarian carcinoma (with other agents). Palliative treatment of ovarian carcinoma unresponsive to other modalities.

Action

Inhibits DNA synthesis by producing cross-linking of parent DNA strands (cell-cycle phase–nonspecific). **Therapeutic Effects:** Death of rapidly replicating cells, particularly malignant ones.

Pharmacokinetics

Absorption: IV administration results in complete bioavailability.
Distribution: Unknown.
Protein Binding: Platinum is irreversibly bound to plasma proteins.

Metabolism and Excretion: Excreted mostly by the kidneys.
Half-life: *Carboplatin*—2.6–5.9 hr (increased in renal impairment); *platinum*—5 days.

TIME/ACTION PROFILE (effects on blood counts)

ROUTE	ONSET	PEAK	DURATION
IV	unknown	21 days	28 days

Contraindications/Precautions

Contraindicated in: Hypersensitivity to carboplatin, cisplatin, or mannitol; OB: Pregnancy or lactation.
Use Cautiously in: Hearing loss; Electrolyte abnormalities; Renal impairment (dose reduction recommended if creatinine <60 ml/min); Active infections; Diminished bone marrow reserve (dose reduction recommended); Other chronic debilitating illnesses; Geri: ↑ risk of thrombocytopenia, consider renal function in dose determination; Patients with childbearing potential; Pedi: Safe use in children not established.

Adverse Reactions/Side Effects

CNS: weakness. **EENT:** ototoxicity. **GI:** abdominal pain, nausea, vomiting, constipation, diarrhea, hepatitis, stomatitis. **GU:** gonadal suppression, nephrotoxicity. **Derm:** alopecia, rash. **F and E:** hypocalcemia, hypokalemia, hypomagnesemia, hyponatremia. **Hemat:** ANEMIA, LEUKOPENIA, THROMBOCYTOPENIA. **Metab:** hyperuricemia. **Neuro:** peripheral neuropathy. **Misc:** hypersensitivity reactions including ANAPHYLACTIC-LIKE REACTIONS.

Interactions

Drug-Drug: ↑ nephrotoxicity and ototoxicity with other **nephrotoxic** and **ototoxic drugs (aminoglycosides, loop diuretics)**. ↑ bone marrow depression with other **bone marrow–depressing drugs** or **radiation therapy**. May ↓ antibody response to **live-virus vaccines** and ↑ risk of adverse reactions.

Route/Dosage

Other dosing formulas are used.
IV (Adults): *Initial treatment*—300 mg/m² with cyclophosphamide at 4-wk intervals. *Treatment of refractory tumors*—360 mg/m² as a single dose; may be repeated at 4-wk intervals, depending on response.

Renal Impairment

IV (Adults): *CCr 41–59 ml/min*—initial dose 250 mg/m²; *CCr 16–40 ml/min*—initial dose 200 mg/m².

Availability (generic available)

Lyophilized powder for injection: 50-mg vials, 150-mg vials, 450-mg vials. **Aqueous solution for injection:** 50 mg/5-ml vial, 150-mg/15-ml vial, 450-mg/45-ml vial, 600 mg/60-ml vial.

NURSING IMPLICATIONS

Assessment

- Assess for nausea and vomiting; often occur 6–12 hr after therapy (1–4 hr for aqueous solution) and may persist for 24 hr. Prophylactic antiemetics may be used. Adjust diet as tolerated to maintain fluid and electrolyte balance and ensure adequate nutritional intake. May require discontinuation of therapy.
- Assess patients receiving *Paraplatin-AQ* for neurotoxicity (paresthesias in a stocking—glove distribution, areflexia, loss of proprioception and vibratory sensations). Discontinue therapy when symptoms are first observed. May progress further even after stopping therapy. May be irreversible.
- Monitor for bone marrow depression. Assess for bleeding (bleeding gums, bruising, petechiae, guaiac stools, urine, and emesis) and avoid IM injections and rectal temperatures if platelet count is low. Apply pressure to venipuncture sites for 10 min. Assess for signs of infection during neutropenia. Anemia may occur and may be cumulative; transfusions are frequently required. Monitor for increased fatigue, dyspnea, and orthostatic hypotension.
- Monitor for signs of anaphylaxis (rash, urticaria, pruritus, facial swelling, wheezing, tachycardia, hypotension). Discontinue medication immediately and notify physician if these occur. Epinephrine and resuscitation equipment should be readily available.
- Audiometry is recommended before initiation of therapy and subsequent doses. Ototoxicity manifests as tinnitus and unilateral or bilateral hearing loss in high frequencies and becomes more frequent and severe with repeated doses. Ototoxicity is more pronounced in children.
- ***Lab Test Considerations:*** Monitor CBC, differential, and clotting studies before and weekly during therapy. For *Paraplatin:* The

nadirs of thrombocytopenia and leukopenia occur after 21 days and recover by 30 days after a dose. Nadir of granulocyte counts usually occurs after 21–28 days and recovers by day 35. Withhold subsequent doses until neutrophil count is >2000/mm³ and platelet count is >100,000/mm³. For *Paraplatin-AQ:* The nadirs of thrombocytopenia and leukopenia occur between days 18 and 23 and recover by day 39. Anemia also occurs with the same frequency and timing as thrombocytopenia and leukopenia.

- Monitor renal function and serum electrolytes before initiation of therapy and before each course of carboplatin. Nephrotoxicity with *Paraplatin-AQ* is cumulative and is potentiated by aminoglycoside antibiotics. Monitor serum creatinine, BUN, creatinine clearance, and magnesium, sodium, potassium, and calcium levels prior to initiating therapy and before each subsequent dose. May cause ↑ BUN and serum creatinine concentrations and ↓ CCr. May cause ↓ serum potassium, calcium, magnesium, and sodium concentrations. Renal function must return to normal before each dose of *Paraplatin-AQ* is given.
- Monitor hepatic function before and periodically during therapy. May cause ↑ serum bilirubin, alkaline phosphatase, and AST concentrations.
- *Paraplatin-AQ* may cause hyperuricemia, usually occurring 3–5 days after therapy. Allopurinol may be used to ↓ uric acid levels.
- *Paraplatin-AQ* may cause ↑ serum amylase levels.

Potential Nursing Diagnoses

Risk for infection (Adverse Reactions)
Risk for injury (Side Effects)

Implementation

- ***High Alert:*** Fatalities have occurred with chemotherapeutic agents. Before administering, clarify all ambiguous orders; double-check single, daily, and course-of-therapy dose limits; have second practitioner independently double-check original order, calculations, and infusion pump settings.
- ***High Alert:*** Do not confuse carboplatin with cisplatin. Do not confuse Paraplatin (carboplatin) with Platinol (cisplatin).
- ***High Alert:*** Carboplatin should be administered in a monitored setting under the supervision of a physician experienced in cancer chemotherapy.

IV Administration

- Solution should be prepared in a biologic cabinet. Wear gloves, gown, and mask while handling medication. Discard equipment in specially designated containers.
- Do not use aluminum needles or equipment during preparation or administration; aluminum reacts with the drug.

Paraplatin

- **Intermittent Infusion:** Reconstitute to a concentration of 10 mg/ml with sterile water for injection, D5W, or 0.9% NaCl for injection. ***Diluent:*** May be further diluted in D5W or 0.9% NaCl. ***Concentration:*** 0.5 mg/ml. Stable for 8 hr at room temperature.
- May also be administered over 24 hr or by dividing total dose into 5 consecutive pulse doses; may decrease nausea and vomiting but does not decrease nephrotoxicity or ototoxicity. ***Rate:*** Administer over 15–60 min.
- **Y-Site Compatibility:** allopurinol, amifostine, anidlafungin, aztreonam, cefepime, cladribine, doxorubicin liposome, etoposide phosphate, filgrastim, fludarabine, gemcitabine, granisetron, linezolid, melphalan, ondansetron, oxaliplatin, paclitaxel, palonosetron, pemetrexed, piperacillin/tazobactam, propofol, sargramostim, teniposide, thiotepa, topotecan, vinorelbine.
- **Y-Site Incompatibility:** amphotericin B cholesteryl sulfate complex, lansoprazole.

Paraplatin-AQ

- Hydrate patient with 1–2 liters of fluid infused over 8–12 hr prior to therapy. Adequate hydration and urinary output must be maintained for 24 hr following infusion
- **Intermittent Infusion:** ***Diluent:*** Dilute Paraplatin-AQ with 2 liters of D5/0.45% NaCl containing 37.5 g of mannitol. Do not dilute with D5W. If diluted solution is not to be used within 6 hrs, protect solution from light. Do not refrigerate.

Patient/Family Teaching

- Instruct patient to notify health care professional promptly if fever; chills; sore throat; signs of infection; lower back or side pain; difficult or painful urination; bleeding gums; bruising; pinpoint red spots on skin; blood in

stools, urine, or emesis; increased fatigue, dyspnea, or orthostatic hypotension occurs.
- Caution patient to avoid crowds and persons with known infections. Instruct patient to use soft toothbrush and electric razor and to avoid falls. Caution patients not to drink alcoholic beverages or take medication containing aspirin or NSAIDs because they may precipitate gastric bleeding.
- Instruct patient to promptly report any numbness or tingling in extremities or face, decreased coordination, difficulty with hearing or ringing in the ears, unusual swelling, or weight gain to health care professional.
- Instruct patient not to receive any vaccinations without advice of health care professional and to avoid contact with persons who have received oral polio vaccine within the past several months.
- Advise patient of the need for contraception (if patient is not infertile as a result of surgical or radiation therapy).
- Instruct patient to inspect oral mucosa for erythema and ulceration. If ulceration occurs, advise patient to notify health care professional, rinse mouth with water after eating, and use sponge brush. Mouth pain may require treatment with opioids.
- Discuss with patient the possibility of hair loss. Explore methods of coping.
- Emphasize the need for periodic lab tests to monitor for side effects.

Evaluation/Desired Outcomes
- Decrease in size or spread of ovarian carcinoma.

carisoprodol
(kar-i-**sop**-roe-dole)
Soma, Vanadom

Classification
Therapeutic: skeletal muscle relaxants (centrally acting)

Pregnancy Category UK

Indications
Adjunct to rest and physical therapy in the treatment of muscle spasm associated with acute painful musculoskeletal conditions.

Action
Skeletal muscle relaxation, probably due to CNS depression. **Therapeutic Effects:** Skeletal muscle relaxation.

Pharmacokinetics
Absorption: Well absorbed after oral administration.
Distribution: Crosses the placenta; high concentrations in breast milk.
Metabolism and Excretion: Mostly metabolized by the liver.
Half-life: 8 hr.

TIME/ACTION PROFILE (skeletal muscle relaxation)

ROUTE	ONSET	PEAK	DURATION
PO	30 min	unknown	4–6 hr

Contraindications/Precautions
Contraindicated in: Hypersensitivity to carisoprodol or to meprobamate; Porphyria or suspected porphyria.
Use Cautiously in: Severe liver or kidney disease; OB, Lactation, Pedi: Safety not established for pregnant women, breastfeeding infants, or children <16 yr; Geri: Poorly tolerated due to anticholinergic effects. Appears on Beers list.

Adverse Reactions/Side Effects
CNS: dizziness, drowsiness, agitation, ataxia, depression, headache, insomnia, irritability, syncope. **Resp:** asthma attacks. **CV:** hypotension, tachycardia. **GI:** epigastric distress, hiccups, nausea, vomiting. **Derm:** flushing, rashes. **Hemat:** eosinophilia, leukopenia. **Misc:** ANAPHYLACTIC SHOCK, fever, psychological dependence, severe idiosyncratic reaction.

Interactions
Drug-Drug: Additive CNS depression with other **CNS depressants** including **alcohol**, **antihistamines**, **opioid analgesics**, and **sedative/hypnotics**.
Drug-Natural Products: Concomitant use of **kava kava**, **valerian**, **skullcap**, **chamomile**, or **hops** can increase CNS depression.

Route/Dosage
PO (Adults ≥16 yrs): 250–350 mg 4 times daily for no >2–3 wks.

Availability (generic available)
Tablets: 250 mg, 350 mg. ***In combination with:*** aspirin (Soma compound) and codeine. See Appendix B.

NURSING IMPLICATIONS

Assessment
- Assess patient for pain, muscle stiffness, and range of motion before and periodically throughout therapy.

- Observe patient for idiosyncratic symptoms that may appear within minutes or hours of administration during the first dose. Symptoms include extreme weakness, quadriplegia, dizziness, ataxia, dysarthria, visual disturbances, agitation, euphoria, confusion, and disorientation. Usually subsides over several hours.
- Geri: Assess geriatric patients for anticholinergic effects (sedation and weakness).

Potential Nursing Diagnoses
Acute pain (Indications)
Impaired bed mobility (Indications)
Risk for injury (Side Effects)

Implementation
- Do not confuse Soma with Soma Compound.
- Provide safety measures as indicated. Supervise ambulation and transfer of patients.
- **PO:** Administer with food to minimize GI irritation. Give dose at bedtime.

Patient/Family Teaching
- Instruct patient to take medication as directed. Missed doses should be taken within 1 hr; if not, omit and return to regular dosing schedule. Do not double doses.
- Encourage patient to comply with additional therapies prescribed for muscle spasm (rest, physical therapy, heat, etc.).
- May cause dizziness or drowsiness. Advise patient to avoid driving or other activities requiring alertness until response to drug is known.
- Instruct patient to change positions slowly to minimize orthostatic hypotension.
- Advise patient to avoid concurrent use of alcohol and other CNS depressants while taking this medication.
- Instruct patient to notify health care professional if signs of allergy (rash, hives, swelling of tongue or lips, dyspnea) or idiosyncratic reaction occur.

Evaluation/Desired Outcomes
- Decreased musculoskeletal pain and muscle spasticity.
- Increased range of motion.

HIGH ALERT

carmustine (kar-mus-teen)
BCNU, BiCNU, Gliadel

Classification
Therapeutic: antineoplastics
Pharmacologic: alkylating agents

Pregnancy Category D

Indications
Alone or with other treatments (surgery, radiation) in the management of: Brain tumors, Multiple myeloma, Hodgkin's disease, Other lymphomas.

Action
Inhibits DNA and RNA synthesis (cell-cycle phase–nonspecific). **Therapeutic Effects:** Death of rapidly replicating cells, especially malignant ones.

Pharmacokinetics
Absorption: Following IV administration, absorption is complete. Following implantation, action is primarily local.
Distribution: Highly lipid soluble; readily penetrates CSF. Enters breast milk.
Metabolism and Excretion: Rapidly metabolized. Some metabolites have antineoplastic activity.
Half-life: *Biologic*—15–30 min; *chemical*—5 min.

TIME/ACTION PROFILE (effect on platelet counts)

ROUTE	ONSET	PEAK	DURATION
IV	days	4–5 wk	6 wk

Contraindications/Precautions
Contraindicated in: Hypersensitivity; Pregnancy or lactation.
Use Cautiously in: Infections; Depressed bone marrow reserve; Geriatric patients (consider age related decrease in body mass, renal/hepatic/cardiovascular function, concurrent medications and chronic illnesses); Impaired pulmonary, hepatic, or renal function; Other chronic debilitating illnesses; Patients with childbearing potential.

Adverse Reactions/Side Effects
Resp: PULMONARY FIBROSIS, pulmonary infiltrates. **GI:** hepatotoxicity, nausea, vomiting, anorexia, diarrhea, esophagitis. **GU:** renal failure. **Derm:** alopecia. **Hemat:** LEUKOPENIA, THROMBOCYTOPENIA, anemia. **Local:** pain at IV site.

Interactions

Drug-Drug: ↑ bone marrow depression with other **antineoplastics** or **radiation therapy**. **Smoking** ↑ risk of pulmonary toxicity. May ↓ antibody response to **live-virus vaccines** and ↑ risk of adverse reactions. Myelosuppression may be ↑ by **cimetidine**.

Route/Dosage

IV (Adults and Children): 150–200 mg/m^2 single dose every 6–8 wk *or* 75–100 mg/m^2/day for 2 days q 6 wk *or* 40 mg/m^2/day for 5 days q 6 wk.

Intracavitary (Adults): Up to 61.6 mg (8 implants) placed in cavity created during surgical resection of brain tumor.

Availability

Injection: 100-mg vial. **Intracavitary wafer:** 7.7 mg in packages of 8.

NURSING IMPLICATIONS

Assessment

- Monitor vital signs before and frequently during therapy.
- Monitor for bone marrow depression. Assess for bleeding (bleeding gums, bruising, petechiae, guaiac stools, urine, and emesis) and avoid IM injections and taking rectal temperatures if platelet count is low. Apply pressure to venipuncture sites for 10 min. Assess for signs of infection during neutropenia. Anemia may occur; monitor for increased fatigue, dyspnea, and orthostatic hypotension.
- Assess respiratory status for dyspnea or cough. Pulmonary toxicity usually occurs after high cumulative doses or several courses of therapy but may also occur following 1–2 courses of low doses. Symptoms may be rapid or gradual in onset; damage may be reversible or irreversible. Delayed pulmonary fibrosis may occur years after therapy. Notify physician promptly if symptoms occur.
- Monitor IV site closely. Carmustine is an irritant. Instruct patient to notify nurse immediately if discomfort occurs at IV site. Discontinue IV immediately if infiltration occurs. Ice may be applied to site. May cause hyperpigmentation of skin along vein.
- Monitor intake and output, appetite, and nutritional intake. Assess for nausea and vomiting, which occur within 2 hr of administration and persist for 4–6 hr. Administration of an antiemetic before and during therapy and adjusting diet as tolerated may help maintain fluid and electrolyte balance and nutritional status.
- ***Lab Test Considerations:*** Monitor CBC with differential and platelet count before and throughout therapy. The nadir of thrombocytopenia occurs in 4–5 wk; the nadir of leukopenia in 5–6 wk. Recovery usually occurs in 6–7 wk but may take 10–12 wk after prolonged therapy. Withhold dose and notify physician if platelet count is <100,000/mm^3 or leukocyte count is <4000/mm^3. Anemia is usually mild.
- Monitor serum bilirubin, AST, ALT, and LDH before and periodically during therapy. May cause mild, reversible ↑ in AST, alkaline phosphatase, and bilirubin.
- Monitor BUN, serum creatinine, and uric acid before and periodically during therapy. Notify physician if BUN is elevated.

Potential Nursing Diagnoses

Risk for injury (Side Effects)
Disturbed body image (Side Effects)

Implementation

- ***High Alert:*** Fatalities have occurred with chemotherapeutic agents. Before administering, clarify all ambiguous orders; double-check single, daily, and course-of-therapy dose limits; have second practitioner independently double-check original order, calculations, and infusion pump settings.

IV Administration

- Solution should be prepared in a biologic cabinet. Wear gloves, gown, and mask while handling medication. Discard equipment in designated containers. Contact with skin may cause transient hyperpigmentation.
- **Intermittent Infusion:** Dilute contents of each 100-mg vial with 3 ml of absolute ethyl alcohol provided as a diluent. Dilute this solution with 27 ml of sterile water for injection. ***Concentration:*** 3.3 mg/ml. ***Diluent:*** May be further diluted with 500 ml of D5W or 0.9% NaCl in a glass container.
- Solution is clear and colorless. Do not use vials that contain an oily film, which indicates decomposition. Reconstituted solution is stable for 24 hr when refrigerated and protected from light. Solution contains no preservatives; do not use as a multidose vial.
- IV lines may be flushed with 5–10 ml of 0.9% NaCl before and after carmustine infusion to minimize irritation at the injection site. ***Rate:*** Administer dose over 1–2 hr at rate of <3

mg/ml/min. Rapid infusion rate may cause local pain, burning at site, and flushing. Facial flushing occurs within 2 hr and may persist for 4 hr.

- **Y-Site Compatibility:** amifostine, aztreonam, cefepime, etoposide, filgrastim, fludarabine, gemcitabine, granisetron, melphalan, ondansetron, piperacillin/tazobactam, sargramostim, teniposide, thiotepa, vinorelbine.
- **Additive Incompatibility:** allopurinol, sodium bicarbonate.

Patient/Family Teaching

- Instruct patient to notify health care professional if fever; chills; sore throat; signs of infection; lower back or side pain; difficult or painful urination; bleeding gums; bruising; petechiae; or blood in urine, stool, or emesis occurs. Caution patient to avoid crowds and persons with known infections. Instruct patient to use soft toothbrush and electric razor. Patients should be cautioned not to drink alcoholic beverages or to take products containing aspirin or NSAIDs.
- Instruct patient to notify health care professional if shortness of breath or increased cough occurs. Encourage patient not to smoke, because smokers are at greater risk for pulmonary toxicity.
- Instruct patient to inspect oral mucosa for redness and ulceration. If mouth sores occur, advise patient to use sponge brush and rinse mouth with water after eating and drinking. Stomatitis may require treatment with opioid analgesics.
- Discuss with patient the possibility of hair loss. Explore coping strategies.
- Advise patient of the need for contraception.
- Instruct patient not to receive any vaccinations without advice of health care professional.
- Emphasize need for periodic lab tests to monitor for side effects.

Evaluation/Desired Outcomes

- Decrease in size and spread of tumor.
- Improvement in hematologic parameters in nonsolid cancers.

carvedilol (kar-**ve**-dil-ole)

Coreg, Coreg CR

Classification
Therapeutic: antihypertensives
Pharmacologic: beta blockers

Pregnancy Category C

Indications

Hypertension. CHF (ischemic or cardiomyopathic) with digoxin, diuretics, and ACE inhibitors. Left ventricular dysfunction after myocardial infarction.

Action

Blocks stimulation of $beta_1$ (myocardial) and $beta_2$ (pulmonary, vascular, and uterine)-adrenergic receptor sites. Also has $alpha_1$ blocking activity, which may result in orthostatic hypotension. **Therapeutic Effects:** Decreased heart rate and blood pressure. Improved cardiac output, slowing of the progression of CHF and decreased risk of death.

Pharmacokinetics

Absorption: Well absorbed but rapidly undergoes extensive first-pass hepatic metabolism, resulting in 25–35% bioavailability. Food slows absorption.
Distribution: Unknown.
Protein Binding: 98%.
Metabolism and Excretion: Extensively metabolized, excreted in feces via bile, <2% excreted unchanged in urine.
Half-life: 7–10 hr.

TIME/ACTION PROFILE (cardiovascular effects)

ROUTE	ONSET	PEAK	DURATION
PO	within 1 hr	1–2 hr	12 hr
PO-CR	unknown	5 hr	24 hr

Contraindications/Precautions

Contraindicated in: Pulmonary edema; Cardiogenic shock; Bradycardia, heart block, or sick sinus syndrome (unless a pacemaker is in place); Uncompensated CHF requiring IV inotropic agents (wean before starting carvedilol); Severe hepatic impairment; Asthma or other bronchospastic disorders.
Use Cautiously in: CHF (condition may deteriorate during initial therapy); Renal impairment; Hepatic impairment; Diabetes mellitus (may mask signs of hypoglycemia); Thyrotoxicosis (may mask symptoms); Peripheral vascular dis-

ease; History of severe allergic reactions (intensity of reactions may be increased); OB: Crosses placenta and may cause fetal/neonatal bradycardia, hypotension, hypoglycemia, or respiratory depression; Lactation, Pedi: Safety not established; Geri: Increased sensitivity to beta blockers; initial dosage reduction recommended.

Adverse Reactions/Side Effects

CNS: dizziness, fatigue, weakness, anxiety, depression, drowsiness, insomnia, memory loss, mental status changes, nervousness, nightmares. **EENT:** blurred vision, dry eyes, nasal stuffiness. **Resp:** bronchospasm, wheezing. **CV:** BRADYCARDIA, CHF, PULMONARY EDEMA. **GI:** diarrhea, constipation, nausea. **GU:** erectile dysfunction, decreased libido. **Derm:** itching, rashes. **Endo:** hyperglycemia, hypoglycemia. **MS:** arthralgia, back pain, muscle cramps. **Neuro:** paresthesia. **Misc:** drug-induced lupus syndrome.

Interactions

Drug-Drug: General anesthetics, **IV phenytoin**, **diltiazem**, and **verapamil** may cause ↑ myocardial depression. ↑ risk of bradycardia with **digoxin**. ↑ hypotension may occur with other **antihypertensives**, acute ingestion of **alcohol**, or **nitrates**. Concurrent use with **clonidine** ↑ hypotension and bradycardia. May ↑ withdrawal phenomenon from **clonidine** (discontinue carvedilol first). Concurrent administration of **thyroid preparations** may ↓ effectiveness. May alter the effectiveness of **insulins** or **oral hypoglycemic agents** (dose adjustments may be necessary). May ↓ effectiveness of **theophylline**. May ↓ beneficial $beta_1$-cardiovascular effects of **dopamine** or **dobutamine**. Use cautiously within 14 days of **MAO inhibitor** therapy (may result in hypotension/bradycardia). **Cimetidine** may ↑ toxicity from carvedilol. Concurrent **NSAIDs** may ↓ antihypertensive action. Effectiveness may be ↓ by **rifampin**. May ↑ serum **digoxin** levels. May ↑ blood levels of **cyclosporine** (monitor blood levels).

Route/Dosage

PO (Adults): *Hypertension*—6.25 mg twice daily, may be increased q 7–14 days up to 25 mg twice daily or Extended-release-20 mg once daily, dose may be doubled every 7–14 days up to 80 mg once daily; *CHF*—3.125 mg twice daily for 2 wk; may be increased to 6.25 mg twice daily. Dose may be doubled q 2 wk as tolerated (not to exceed 25 mg twice daily in patients <85 kg or 50 mg twice daily in patients >85 kg *or* Extended-release-10 mg once daily, dose may be doubled every 2 wks as tolerated up to 80 mg once daily; *Left ventricular dysfunction after MI*—6.25 mg twice daily, increase after 3–10 days to 12.5 twice daily then to target dose of 25 mg twice daily; some patients may require lower initial doses and slower titration *or* Extended-release-20 mg once daily, dose may be doubled every 3–10 days up to 80 mg once daily.

Availability (generic available)

Tablets: 3.125 mg, 6.25 mg, 12.5 mg, 25 mg. **Cost:** *Generic*—3.125 mg $89.95/180, 6.25 mg $79.94/180, 12.5 mg $79.94/180, 25 mg $89.93/180. **Extended-release capsules:** 10 mg, 20 mg, 40 mg, 80 mg. **Cost:** all strengths $333.97/90.

NURSING IMPLICATIONS

Assessment

- Monitor blood pressure and pulse frequently during dose adjustment period and periodically during therapy. Assess for orthostatic hypotension when assisting patient up from supine position.
- Monitor intake and output ratios and daily weight. Assess patient routinely for evidence of fluid overload (peripheral edema, dyspnea, rales/crackles, fatigue, weight gain, jugular venous distention). Patients may experience worsening of symptoms during initiation of therapy for CHF.
- **Hypertension:** Check frequency of refills to determine adherence.
- ***Lab Test Considerations:*** May cause ↑ BUN, serum lipoprotein, potassium, triglyceride, and uric acid levels.
- May cause ↑ ANA titers.
- May cause ↑ in blood glucose levels.
- ***Toxicity and Overdose:*** Monitor patients receiving beta blockers for signs of overdose (bradycardia, severe dizziness or fainting, severe drowsiness, dyspnea, bluish fingernails or palms, seizures). Notify physician or other health care professional immediately if these signs occur.

Potential Nursing Diagnoses

Decreased cardiac output (Side Effects)
Noncompliance (Patient/Family Teaching)

Implementation

- Do not confuse carvedilol with captopril or carteolol.

- Discontinuation of concurrent clonidine should be gradual, with carvedilol discontinued first over 1-2 week with limitation of physical activity; then, after several days, discontinue clonidine.
- **PO:** Take apical pulse before administering. If <50 bpm or if arrhythmia occurs, withhold medication and notify physician or other health care professional.
- Administer with food to minimize orthostatic hypotension.
- Extended-release capsules should be taken in the morning and swallowed whole, do not crush, break, or chew. Extended-release capsules may be opened and sprinkled on cold applesauce and take immediately; do not store mixture.
- To convert from immediate-release to extended-release product, doses of 3.125 mg twice daily can be converted to 10 mg daily; doses of 6.25 mg twice daily can be converted to 20 mg daily; doses of 12.5 mg twice daily can be converted to 40 mg daily; and doses of 25 mg twice daily can be converted to 80 mg daily.

Patient/Family Teaching

- Instruct patient to take medication as directed, at the same time each day, even if feeling well. Do not skip or double up on missed doses. Take missed doses as soon as possible up to 4 hr before next dose. Abrupt withdrawal may precipitate life-threatening arrhythmias, hypertension, or myocardial ischemia.
- Advise patient to make sure enough medication is available for weekends, holidays, and vacations. A written prescription may be kept in wallet in case of emergency.
- Teach patient and family how to check pulse and blood pressure. Instruct them to check pulse daily and blood pressure biweekly. Advise patient to hold dose and contact health care professional if pulse is <50 bpm or blood pressure changes significantly.
- May cause drowsiness or dizziness. Caution patients to avoid driving or other activities that require alertness until response to the drug is known.
- Advise patient to change positions slowly to minimize orthostatic hypotension, especially during initiation of therapy or when dose is increased.
- Caution patient that this medication may increase sensitivity to cold.
- Instruct patient to consult health care professional before taking any Rx, OTC, or herbal products, especially cold preparations, concurrently with this medication.
- Patients with diabetes should closely monitor blood glucose, especially if weakness, malaise, irritability, or fatigue occurs. Medication may mask some signs of hypoglycemia, but dizziness and sweating may still occur.
- Advise patient to notify health care professional if slow pulse, difficulty breathing, wheezing, cold hands and feet, dizziness, confusion, depression, rash, fever, sore throat, unusual bleeding, or bruising occurs.
- Instruct patient to inform health care professional of medication regimen before treatment or surgery.
- Advise patient to carry identification describing disease process and medication regimen at all times.
- **Hypertension:** Reinforce the need to continue additional therapies for hypertension (weight loss, sodium restriction, stress reduction, regular exercise, moderation of alcohol consumption, and smoking cessation). Medication controls but does not cure hypertension.

Evaluation/Desired Outcomes

- Decrease in blood pressure without appearance of detrimental side effects.
- Decrease in severity of CHF.

caspofungin (kas-po-**fun**-gin)

Cancidas

Classification

Therapeutic: antifungals (systemic)
Pharmacologic: echinocandins

Pregnancy Category C

Indications

Invasive aspergillosis refractory to, or intolerant of, other therapies. Candidemia and associated serious infections (intra-abdominal abscesses, peritonitis, pleural space infections). Esophageal candidiasis. Suspected fungal infections in febrile neutropenic patients.

Action

Inhibits the synthesis of β (1, 3)-D-glucan, a necessary component of the fungal cell wall.
Therapeutic Effects: Death of susceptible fungi.

Pharmacokinetics

Absorption: IV administration results in complete bioavailability.
Distribution: Widely distributed to tissues.
Protein Binding: 97%.
Metabolism and Excretion: Slowly and extensively metabolized; <1.5% excreted unchanged in urine.
Half-life: Polyphasic: β *phase*—9–11 hr; ξ *phase*—40–50 hr.

TIME/ACTION PROFILE

ROUTE	ONSET	PEAK	DURATION
IV	unknown	end of infusion	24 hr

Contraindications/Precautions

Contraindicated in: Hypersensitivity; Concurrent use with cyclosporine.
Use Cautiously in: Moderate hepatic impairment (decreased maintenance dose recommended); Pedi: Children <18 yr (safety not established).

Adverse Reactions/Side Effects

CNS: headache. **GI:** diarrhea, nausea, vomiting. **Derm:** flushing. **Local:** venous irritation at injection site. **Misc:** allergic reactions including ANAPHYLAXIS, fever.

Interactions

Drug-Drug: Concurrent use with **cyclosporine** is not recommended due to ↑ risk of hepatic toxicity. May ↓ blood levels and effects of **tacrolimus**. Blood levels and effectiveness may be ↓ by **rifampin**; maintenance dose should be ↑ to 70 mg (in patients with normal liver function). Blood levels and effectiveness may be also be ↓ by **efavirenz**, **nelfinavir**, **nevirapine**, **phenytoin**, **dexamethasone**, or **carbamazepine** an ↑ in the maintenance dose to 70 mg should be considered in patients who are not clinically responding.

Route/Dosage

IV (Adults): 70 mg initially followed by 50 mg daily, duration determined by clinical situation and response; *Esophageal candidiasis*—50 mg daily, duration determined by clinical situation and response.

Moderate Hepatic Impairment (Child-Pugh Score 5–6)

IV (Adults): 70 mg initially followed by 35 mg daily, duration determined by clinical situation and response.

Availability

Powder for injection: 50 mg/vial, 70 mg/vial.

NURSING IMPLICATIONS

Assessment

- Assess patient for signs and symptoms of fungal infections prior to and periodically during therapy.
- Monitor patient for signs of anaphylaxis (rash, dyspnea, stridor) during therapy.
- ***Lab Test Considerations:*** May cause ↑ serum alkaline phosphatase, AST, ALT, eosinophils, and urine protein and RBCs. May also cause ↓ serum potassium, hemoglobin, hematocrit, and WBCs.

Potential Nursing Diagnoses

Risk for infection (Indications)

Implementation

IV Administration

- **Intermittent Infusion: *Diluent:*** Allow refrigerated vial to reach room temperature. *For 75-mg or 50-mg dose*—Reconstitute vials with 10.5 ml of 0.9% NaCl or sterile water for injection. Reconstituted solution is stable for 1 hr at room temperature. Withdraw 10 ml from vial and add to 250 ml of 0.9% NaCl, 0.45% NaCl, 0.225% NaCl, or LR. The 50-mg dose can also be diluted in 100 ml when volume restriction is necessary. Infusion is stable for 24 hr at room temperature or 48 hr if refrigerated. *For 35-mg dose*—Reconstitute a 50-mg vial as per the directions above. Withdraw 7 ml from vial and add to 250 ml of appropriate diluent. May also be diluted in 100 ml if volume restriction is necessary. White cake should dissolve completely. Mix gently until a clear solution is obtained. Do not use a solution that is cloudy, discolored, or contains precipitates. ***Concentration:*** 0.14–0.47 mg/ml. ***Rate:*** Infuse over 1 hr.
- **Y-Site Compatibility:** acyclovir, amikacin, aminophylline, amiodarone, aztreonam, bumetanide, calcium chloride, calcium gluconate, ceftizoxime, cimetidine, ciprofloxacin, cisatracurium, cyclosporine, daptomycin, diltiazem, diphenhydramine, dobutamine,

dolasetron, **dopamine, doxycycline, droperidol**, epinephrine, erythromycin, esmolol, famotidine, fenoldopam, fentanyl, fluconazole, ganciclovir, gentamicin, granisetron, haloperidol, hydrocortisone sodium succinate, hydromorphone, imipenem/cilastatin, insulin, isoproterenol, labetalol, levofloxacin, linezolid, magnesium sulfate, meperidine, meropenem, metoclopramide, metoprolol, midazolam, milrinone, morphine, moxifloxacin, nicardipine, nitroglycerin, norepinephrine, ondansetron, palonosetron, phenylephrine, procainamide, prochlorperazine, promethazine, propranolol, quinupristin/dalfopristin, tacrolimus, tirofiban, tobramycin, vancomycin, vasopressin, vecuronium, verapamil.
- **Y-Site Incompatibility:** amphotericin B, ampicillin, ampicillin/sulbactam, azithromycin, cefazolin, cefepime, cefotaxime, cefoxitin, ceftazidime, ceftriaxone, cefuroxime, chloramphenicol, clindamycin, dexamethasone sodium phosphate, diazepam, digoxin, enalaprilat, ertapenem, furosemide, heparin, hydralazine, ketorolac, lidocaine, lorazepam, methylprednisolone sodium succinate, metronidazole, nafcillin, nitroprusside, pamidronate, pancuronium, pantoprazole, phenytoin, piperacillin/tazobactam, potassium chloride, potassium phosphate, ranitidine, sodium bicarbonate, ticarcillin/clavulanate, trimethoprim/sulfamethoxazole.
- **Solution Incompatibility:** Solutions containing dextrose.

Patient/Family Teaching
- Explain the purpose of caspofungin to patient and family.

Evaluation/Desired Outcomes
- Decrease in signs and symptoms of fungal infections. Duration of therapy is determined based on severity of underlying disease, recovery from immunosuppression, and clinical response.

cefaclor, See CEPHALOSPORINS—SECOND GENERATION.

cefadroxil, See CEPHALOSPORINS—FIRST GENERATION.

cefazolin, See CEPHALOSPORINS—FIRST GENERATION.

cefdinir, See CEPHALOSPORINS—THIRD GENERATION.

cefditoren, See CEPHALOSPORINS—THIRD GENERATION.

cefepime (seff-e-peem)
Maxipime

Classification
Therapeutic: anti-infectives
Pharmacologic: fourth-generation cephalosporins

Pregnancy Category B

Indications
Treatment of the following infections caused by susceptible organisms: Uncomplicated skin and skin structure infections, Bone and joint infections, Uncomplicated and complicated urinary tract infections, Respiratory tract infections, Complicated intra-abdominal infections (with metronidazole), Septicemia. Empiric treatment of febrile neutropenic patients.

Action
Binds to the bacterial cell wall membrane, causing cell death. **Therapeutic Effects:** Bactericidal action against susceptible bacteria. **Spectrum:** Similar to that of second-, and third-generation cephalosporins, but activity against staphylococci is less, whereas activity against gram-negative pathogens is greater, even for organisms resistant to first-, second- and third-generation agents. Notable is increased action against: *Enterobacter*, *Haemophilus influenzae* (including β-lactamase-producing strains), *Escherichia coli*, *Klebsiella pneumoniae*, *Neisseria*, *Proteus*, *Providencia*, *Pseudomonas aeruginosa*, *Serratia*, *Moraxella catarrhalis* (including β-lactamase-producing strains). Not active against methicillin-resistant staphylococci or enterococci.

Pharmacokinetics

Absorption: Well absorbed after IM administration; IV administration results in complete bioavailability.

Distribution: Widely distributed. Crosses the placenta; enters breast milk in low concentrations. Some CSF penetration.

Metabolism and Excretion: 85% excreted unchanged in urine.

Half-life: 2 hr (increased in renal impairment).

TIME/ACTION PROFILE

ROUTE	ONSET	PEAK	DURATION
IM	rapid	1–2 hr	12 hr
IV	rapid	end of infusion	12 hr

Contraindications/Precautions

Contraindicated in: Hypersensitivity to cephalosporins; Serious hypersensitivity to penicillins.

Use Cautiously in: Renal impairment (decreased dosing/increased dosing interval recommended if CCr ≤60 ml/min); History of GI disease, especially colitis; Patients with hepatic dysfunction or poor nutritional status (may be at increased risk of bleeding); Geriatric patients (dosage adjustment due to age-related decrease in renal function may be necessary); Pregnancy, lactation, and children <2 mo (safety not established).

Adverse Reactions/Side Effects

CNS: SEIZURES (high doses in patients with renal impairment), encephalopathy, headache. **GI:** PSEUDOMEMBRANOUS COLITIS, diarrhea, nausea, vomiting. **Derm:** rashes, pruritis, urticaria. **Hemat:** bleeding, eosinophilia, hemolytic anemia, neutropenia, thrombocytopenia. **Local:** pain at IM site, phlebitis AT IV SITE. **Misc:** allergic reactions including ANAPHYLAXIS, superinfection, fever.

Interactions

Drug-Drug: Probenecid decreases excretion and increases blood levels. Concurrent use of **loop diuretics** or **aminoglycosides** may increase the risk of nephrotoxicity.

Route/Dosage

IM (Adults): *Mild-to-moderate uncomplicated or complicated urinary tract infections due to E. coli*–0.5–1 g every 12 hr.

IV (Adults): *Moderate-to-severe pneumonia*—1–2 g every 12 hr. *Mild-to-moderate uncomplicated or complicated urinary tract infections* 0.5–1 g every 12 hr. *Severe uncomplicated or complicated urinary tract infections, moderate-to-severe uncomplicated skin and skin structure infections, complicated intra-abdominal infections*—2 g every 12 hr. *Empiric treatment of febrile neutropenia*—2 g every 8 hr.

IV (Children 2 mo–16 yr): *Uncomplicated and complicated urinary tract infections, uncomplicated skin and skin structure infections, pneumonia*—50 mg/kg every 12 hr (not to exceed 2 g/dose). *Febrile neutropenia*—50 mg/kg every 8 hr (not to exceed 2 g/dose).

Renal Impairment

IM, IV (Adults): (See Manufacturer's specific recommendations) *CCr 30–60 ml/min*—0.5–1 g every 24 hr or 2 g every 12–24 hr; *CCr 11–29 ml/min*—0.5–2 g every 24 hr; *CCr <11 ml/min*—250 mg–1 g every 24 hr.

Availability

Powder for injection: 500 mg, 1 g, 2 g.

NURSING IMPLICATIONS

Assessment

- Assess patient for infection (vital signs; appearance of wound, sputum, urine, and stool; WBC) at beginning of and throughout therapy.
- Before initiating therapy, obtain a history to determine previous use of and reactions to penicillins or cephalosporins. Persons with a negative history of penicillin sensitivity may still have an allergic response.
- Obtain specimens for culture and sensitivity before initiating therapy. First dose may be given before receiving results.
- Observe patient for signs and symptoms of anaphylaxis (rash, pruritus, laryngeal edema, wheezing). Discontinue the drug and notify the physician or other health care professional immediately if these symptoms occur. Keep epinephrine, an antihistamine, and resuscitation equipment close by in the event of an anaphylactic reaction.
- ***Lab Test Considerations:*** May cause positive results for Coombs' test in patients receiving high doses or in neonates whose mothers were given cephalosporins before delivery.
- May cause increased serum AST, ALT, bilirubin, BUN, and creatinine.
- May rarely cause leukopenia, neutropenia, thrombocytopenia, and eosinophilia.

C

Potential Nursing Diagnoses

Risk for infection (Indications, Side Effects)
Diarrhea (Adverse Reactions)
Deficient knowledge, related to medication regimen (Patient/Family Teaching)

Implementation

- **IM:** Reconstitute IM doses with sterile or bacteriostatic water for injection, 0.9% NaCl, or D5W. May be diluted with lidocaine to minimize injection discomfort.
- Inject deep into a well-developed muscle mass; massage well.
- IM route should only be used for treatment of mild-to-moderate uncomplicated or complicated urinary tract infections due to *Escherichia coli*.
- **IV:** Monitor injection site frequently for phlebitis (pain, redness, swelling). Change sites every 48–72 hr to prevent phlebitis.
- If aminoglycosides are administered concurrently, administer in separate sites, if possible, at least 1 hr apart. If second site is unavailable, flush lines between medications.
- **Intermittent Infusion:** Reconstitute with 5 ml sterile water, 0.9% NaCl, or D5W for the 500-mg vial, or 10 ml for the 1-g or 2-g vials. Reconstituted solution should be further diluted in 50–100 ml of D5W, 0.9% NaCl, D10W, D5/0.9% NaCl, or D5/LR.
- Solution is stable for 24 hr at room temperature and 7 days if refrigerated. ***Rate:*** Administer over 30 min.
- **Y-Site Compatibility:** ampicillin-sulbactam, aztreonam, bleomycin, bumetanide, buprenorphine, butorphanol, calcium gluconate, carboplatin, carmustine, cyclophosphamide, cytarabine, dactinomycin, dexamethasone sodium phosphate, docetaxel, fluconazole, fludarabine, fluorouracil, furosemide, granisetron, hydrocortisone sodium phosphate, hydrocortisone sodium succinate, hydromorphone, imipenem-cilastatin, leukcovorin, lorazepam, melphalan, mesna, methotrexate, methylprednisolone sodium succinate, metronidazole, paclitaxel, piperacillin-tazobactam, ranitidine, sargramostim, sodium bicarbonate, thiotepa, ticarcillin-clavulanate, trimethoprim/sulfamethoxazole, zidovudine.
- **Y-Site Incompatibility:** acyclovir, amphotericin B, chlordiazepoxide, chlorpromazine, cimetidine, ciprofloxacin, cisplatin, dacarbazine, daunorubicin, diazepam, diphenhydramine, dobutamine, dopamine, doxorubicin, droperidol, enalaprilat, etoposide, famotidine, filgrastim, floxuridine, ganciclovir, haloperidol, hydroxyzine, idarubicin, ifosfamide, magnesium sulfate, mannitol, mechlorethamine, meperidine, metoclopramide, mitomycin, mitoxantrone, morphine, nalbuphine, ondansetron, prochlorperazine, promethazine, streptozocin, vancomycin, vinblastine, vincristine.

Patient/Family Teaching

- Advise patient to report signs of superinfection (furry overgrowth on the tongue, vaginal itching or discharge, loose or foul-smelling stools) and allergy.
- Instruct patient to notify health care professional if fever and diarrhea develop, especially if stool contains blood, pus, or mucus. Advise patient not to treat diarrhea without consulting health care professional.

Evaluation/Desired Outcomes

- Resolution of the signs and symptoms of infection. Length of time for complete resolution depends on the organism and site of infection.

---

cefixime, See CEPHALOSPORINS—THIRD GENERATION.

---

cefoperazone, See CEPHALOSPORINS—THIRD GENERATION.

---

cefotaxime, See CEPHALOSPORINS—THIRD GENERATION.

---

cefotetan, See CEPHALOSPORINS—SECOND GENERATION.

---

cefoxitin, See CEPHALOSPORINS—SECOND GENERATION.

---

cefpodoxime, See CEPHALOSPORINS—THIRD GENERATION.

cefprozil, See CEPHALOSPORINS—SECOND GENERATION.

ceftazidime, See CEPHALOSPORINS—THIRD GENERATION.

ceftibuten, See CEPHALOSPORINS—THIRD GENERATION.

ceftizoxime, See CEPHALOSPORINS—THIRD GENERATION.

ceftriaxone, See CEPHALOSPORINS—THIRD GENERATION.

cefuroxime, See CEPHALOSPORINS—SECOND GENERATION.

celecoxib (sel-e-**kox**-ib)

Celebrex

Classification

Therapeutic: antirheumatics, nonsteroidal anti-inflammatory agents

Pharmacologic: COX-2 inhibitors

Pregnancy Category C

Indications

Relief of signs and symptoms of osteoarthritis, rheumatoid arthritis, ankylosing spondylitis, and juvenile rheumatoid arthritis. Reduction of the number of adenomatous colorectal polyps in familial adenomatous polyposis (FAP), as an adjunct to usual care (endoscopic surveillance, surgery). Management of acute pain including primary dysmenorrhea.

Action

Inhibits the enzyme COX-2. This enzyme is required for the synthesis of prostaglandins. Has analgesic, anti-inflammatory, and antipyretic properties. **Therapeutic Effects:** Decreased pain and inflammation caused by arthritis or spondylitis. Decreased number of colorectal polyps. Decreased pain.

Pharmacokinetics

Absorption: Bioavailability unknown.

Distribution: 97% bound to plasma proteins; extensive tissue distribution.

Metabolism and Excretion: Mostly metabolized by the liver; <3% excreted unchanged in urine and feces.

Half-life: 11 hr.

TIME/ACTION PROFILE (pain reduction)

ROUTE	ONSET	PEAK	DURATION
PO	24–48 hr	unknown	12–24 hr†

†After discontinuation

Contraindications/Precautions

Contraindicated in: Hypersensitivity; Cross-sensitivity may exist with other NSAIDs, including aspirin; History of allergic-type reactions to sulfonamides; History of asthma, urticaria, or allergic-type reactions to aspirin or other NSAIDs, including the aspirin triad (asthma, nasal polyps, and severe hypersensitivity reactions to aspirin); Advanced renal disease; Peri-operative pain from coronary artery bypass graft (CABG) surgery; OB: Should not be used in late pregnancy (may cause premature closure of the ductus arteriosus). Lactation: Potential for serious neonatal adverse effects. Discontinue drug or bottle feed.

Use Cautiously in: Cardiovascular disease or risk factors for cardiovascular disease (may ↑ risk of serious cardiovascular thrombotic events, myocardial infarction, and stroke, especially with prolonged use); Pre-existing renal disease, heart failure, liver dysfunction, concurrent diuretic or ACE inhibitor therapy (increased risk of renal impairment); Hypertension or fluid retention; Renal insufficiency (may precipitate acute renal failure); Serious dehydration (correct deficits before administering); Pre-existing asthma; Pedi: Safety not established in children <2 yrs or for longer than 6 mos; Geri: Concurrent therapy with corticosteroids or anticoagulants, long duration of NSAID therapy, history of smoking, alcoholism, geriatric patients, or poor general health status (increased risk of GI bleeding).

Exercise Extreme Caution in: History of ulcer disease or GI bleeding.

Adverse Reactions/Side Effects

CNS: dizziness, headache, insomnia. **CV:** edema. **GI:** GI BLEEDING, abdominal pain, diarrhea, dyspepsia, flatulence, nausea. **Derm:** EXFOLIATIVE DERMATITIS, STEVENS-JOHNSON SYNDROME, TOXIC EPIDERMAL NECROLYSIS, rash.

C

Interactions

Drug-Drug: Significant interactions may occur when celecoxib is coadministered with other drugs that inhibit the CYP450 2C9 enzyme system. May ↓ effectiveness of **ACE inhibitors**, **thiazide diuretics**, and **furosemide**. **Fluconazole** ↑ celecoxib blood levels (dosage reduction recommended). May ↑ risk of bleeding with **warfarin**. May ↑ serum **lithium** levels. Does not inhibit the cardioprotective effect of low-dose **aspirin**.

Route/Dosage

PO (Adults): *Osteoarthritis*—200 mg/day as a single dose *or* 100 mg twice daily. *Rheumatoid arthritis*—100–200 mg twice daily. *Ankylosing spondylitis*—200 mg once daily *or* 100 mg twice daily; dose may be increased after 6 wk to 400 mg daily. *Familial adenomatous polyposis*—400 mg twice daily. *Acute pain, including dysmenorrhea*—400 mg initially, then a 200 mg dose if needed on the first day; then 200 mg twice daily as needed.
PO (Children 2 yrs and older, ≥10 kg–≤25 kg): 50-mg capsule twice daily.
PO (Children 2 yrs and older, >25 kg): 100-mg capsule twice daily.

Availability

Capsules: 50 mg, 100 mg, 200 mg, 400 mg. **Cost:** 100 mg $213.29/100, 200 mg $362.17/100, 400 mg $524.26/100.

NURSING IMPLICATIONS

Assessment

- Assess range of motion, degree of swelling, and pain in affected joints before and periodically throughout therapy.
- Assess patient for allergy to sulfonamides, aspirin, or NSAIDs. Patients with these allergies should not receive celecoxib.
- ***Lab Test Considerations:*** May cause ↑ AST and ALT levels.
- May cause hypophosphatemia and ↑ BUN.

Potential Nursing Diagnoses

Impaired physical mobility (Indications)
Acute pain (Indications)

Implementation

- Do not confuse with Celexa (citalopram) or Cerebyx (fosphenytoin).
- **PO:** May be administered without regard to meals. Capsules may be opened and sprinkled on applesauce and ingested immediately with water. Mixture may be stored in the refrigerator for up to 6 hrs.

Patient/Family Teaching

- Instruct patient to take celecoxib exactly as directed. Do not take more than prescribed dose. Increasing doses does not appear to increase effectiveness. Use lowest effective dose for shortest period of time.
- Advise patient to notify health care professional promptly if signs or symptoms of GI toxicity (abdominal pain, black stools), skin rash, unexplained weight gain, or edema occurs. Patients should discontinue celecoxib and notify health care professional if signs and symptoms of hepatotoxicity (nausea, fatigue, lethargy, pruritus, jaundice, upper right quadrant tenderness, flu-like symptoms) occur.
- Advise patient to notify health care professional if pregnancy is planned or suspected.
- Advise patients with FAP to continue routine surveillance procedures.

Evaluation/Desired Outcomes

- Reduction in joint pain in patients with osteoarthritis.
- Reduction in joint tenderness, pain, and joint swelling in patients with rheumatoid arthritis and juvenile rheumatoid arthritis.
- Decreased number of colonic polyps in patients with FAP.

CEPHALOSPORINS—FIRST GENERATION

cefadroxil (sef-a-**drox**-ill)
Duricef

cefazolin (sef-**a**-zoe-lin)
Ancef

cephalexin (sef-a-**lex**-in)
✤Apo-Cephalex, ✤DOM-Cephalexin, Keflex, ✤Nu-Cephalex, Panixine, ✤PMS-Cephalexin

cephradine (**sef**-re-deen)
Velosef

Classification
Therapeutic: anti-infectives
Pharmacologic: first-generation cephalosporins

Pregnancy Category B

Indications

Treatment of the following infections caused by susceptible organisms: Skin and skin structure infections (including burn wounds), Pneumonia, Urinary tract infections, Bone and joint infections, Septicemia. Not suitable for the treatment of meningitis. **Cefadroxil:** Pharyngitis and/or tonsillitis. **Cefazolin:** Perioperative prophylaxis, biliary tract infections, genital infections, bacterial endocarditis prophylaxis for dental and upper respiratory tract procedures. **Cephalexin and cephradine:** Otitis media.

Action

Bind to bacterial cell wall membrane, causing cell death. **Therapeutic Effects:** Bactericidal action against susceptible bacteria. **Spectrum:** Active against many gram-positive cocci including: *Streptococcus pneumoniae*, Group A beta-hemolytic streptococci, Penicillinase-producing staphylococci. Not active against: Methicillin-resistant staphylococci, *Bacteroides fragilis*, *Enterococcus*. Active against some gram-negative rods including: *Klebsiella pneumoniae*, *Proteus mirabilis*, *Escherichia coli*.

Pharmacokinetics

Absorption: *Cefadroxil, cephalexin,* and *cephradine* are well absorbed following oral administration. *Cefazolin* is well absorbed following IM administration.
Distribution: Widely distributed. Cefazolin penetrates bone and synovial fluid well. All cross the placenta and enter breast milk in low concentrations. Minimal CSF penetration.
Metabolism and Excretion: Excreted almost entirely unchanged by the kidneys.
Half-life: *Cefadroxil*—60–120 min; *cefazolin*—90–150 min; *cephalexin*—50–80 min; *cephradine*—60–120 min (all are increased in renal impairment).

TIME/ACTION PROFILE (blood levels)

ROUTE	ONSET	PEAK	DURATION
Cefadroxil PO	rapid	1.5–2 hr	12–24 hr
Cefazolin IM	rapid	0.5–2 hr	6–12 hr
Cefazolin IV	rapid	5 min	6–12 hr
Cephalexin PO	rapid	1 hr	6–12 hr
Cephradine PO	rapid	1–2 hr	6–12 hr

Contraindications/Precautions

Contraindicated in: Hypersensitivity to cephalosporins; Serious hypersensitivity to penicillins.
Use Cautiously in: Renal impairment (dosage reduction and/or increased dosing interval recommended for: *cefadroxil, cephradine, and cephalexin*, if CCr ≤50 ml/min, and *cefazolin*, if CCr <30 ml/min; History of GI disease, especially colitis; Geri: Dosage adjustment due to age-related decrease in renal function may be necessary; OB: Pregnancy or lactation (half-life is shorter and blood levels lower during pregnancy; have been used safely).

Adverse Reactions/Side Effects

CNS: SEIZURES (high doses). **GI:** PSEUDOMEMBRANOUS COLITIS, diarrhea, nausea, vomiting, cramps. **Derm:** rashes, pruritis, urticaria. **Hemat:** agranulocytosis, eosinophilia, hemolytic anemia, neutropenia, thrombocytopenia. **Local:** pain at IM site, phlebitis AT IV SITE. **Misc:** allergic reactions including ANAPHYLAXIS and SERUM SICKNESS, superinfection.

Interactions

Drug-Drug: Probenecid ↓ excretion and ↑ blood levels of renally excreted cephalosporins. Concurrent use of **loop diuretics** or **aminoglycosides** may ↑ risk of renal toxicity.

Route/Dosage

Cefadroxil

PO (Adults): *Pharyngitis and tonsillitis*—500 mg q 12 hr or 1 g q 24 hr for 10 days. *Skin and soft-tissue infections*—500 mg q 12 hr or 1 g q 24 hr. *Urinary tract infections*—500 mg–1 g q 12 hr or 1–2 g q 24 hr.
PO (Children): *Pharyngitis, tonsillitis, or impetigo*—15 mg/kg q 12 hr or 30 mg/kg q 24 hr for 10 days. *Skin and soft-tissue infections*—15 mg/kg q 12 hr. *Urinary tract infections*—15 mg/kg q 12 hr.

Renal Impairment

PO (Adults): *CCr 25–50 ml/min*—500 mg q 12 hr; *CCr 10–25 ml/min*—500 mg q 24 hr; *CCr <10 ml/min*—500 mg q 36 hr.

Cefazolin

IM, IV (Adults): *Moderate to severe infections*—500 mg–2 g q 6–8 hr (maximum 12 g/day). *Mild infections with gram-positive coc-*

ci—250–500 mg q 8 hr. *Uncomplicated urinary tract infections*—1 g q 12 hr. *Pneumococcal pneumonia*—500 mg q 12 hr. *Infective endocarditis or septicemia*—1–1.5 g q 6 hr. *Perioperative prophylaxis*—1 g given 30–60 min prior to incision. Additional 500 mg–1 g should be given for surgeries ≥2 hr. 500 mg–1 g should then be given for all surgeries q 6–8 hr for 24 hr postoperatively.

IM, IV (Children and Infants >1 mo): 16.7–33.3 mg/kg q 8 hr (maximum 6 g/day); *Bacterial endocarditis prophylaxis in penicillin-allergic patients:* 25 mg/kg 30 minutes prior to procedure (maximum dose = 1 g).

IM, IV (Neonates ≤7 days): 40 mg/kg/day divided q 12 hr.

IM, IV (Neonates >7 days and ≤2 kg): 40 mg/kg/day divided q 12 hr.

IM, IV (Neonates >7 days and >2 kg): 60 mg/kg/day divided q 8 hr.

Renal Impairment

IM, IV (Adults): *CCr 10–30 ml/min*—Administer q 12 hr; *CCr ≤10 ml/min*—Administer q 24 hr.

Cephalexin

PO (Adults): *Most infections*—250–500 mg q 6 hr. *Uncomplicated cystitis, skin and soft-tissue infections, streptococcal pharyngitis*—500 mg q 12 hr.

PO (Children): *Most infections*—25–50 mg/kg/day divided q 6–8 hr (can be administered q 12 hr in skin/skin structure infections or streptococcal pharyngitis). *Otitis media*—18.75—25 mg/kg q 6 hr (maximum = 4 g/day).

Renal Impairment

PO (Adults): *CCr 10–50 ml/min*—500 mg q 8–12 hr; *CCr <10 ml/min*—250–500 mg q 12–24 hr.

Cephradine

PO (Adults): *Most infections*—250–500 mg q 6–12 hr.

PO (Children ≥9 mo): *Most infections*—6.25–12.5 mg/kg q 6 hr; *Otitis media*—18.75–25 mg/kg q 6 hr *or* 37.5–50 mg/kg q 12 hr.

Renal Impairment

PO (Adults): *CCr 10–50 ml/min*—Decrease dose by 50%; *CCr <10 ml/min*—Decrease dose by 75%.

Availability

Cefadroxil

Capsules: 500 mg. **Tablets:** 1 g. **Oral suspension (orange-pineapple flavor):** 250 mg/5 ml, 500 mg/5 ml.

Cefazolin

Powder for injection: 500 mg, 1 g, 10 g, 20 g. **Premixed containers:** 500 mg/50 ml D5W, 1 g/50 ml D5W.

Cephalexin

Capsules: 250 mg, 333 mg, 500 mg, 750 mg. **Tablets:** 250 mg, 500 mg. **Oral suspension:** 100 mg/ml, 125 mg/5 ml, 250 mg/5 ml.

Cephradine

Capsules: 250 mg. **Oral suspension (fruit flavored):** 250 mg/5 ml.

NURSING IMPLICATIONS

Assessment

- Assess for infection (vital signs; appearance of wound, sputum, urine, and stool; WBC) at beginning and during therapy.
- Before initiating therapy, obtain a history to determine previous use of and reactions to penicillins or cephalosporins. Persons with a negative history of penicillin sensitivity may still have an allergic response.
- Obtain specimens for culture and sensitivity before initiating therapy. First dose may be given before receiving results.
- Observe patient for signs and symptoms of anaphylaxis (rash, pruritus, laryngeal edema, wheezing). Discontinue drug and notify physician or other health care professional immediately if these problems occur. Keep epinephrine, an antihistamine, and resuscitation equipment close by in case of an anaphylactic reaction.
- ***Lab Test Considerations:*** May cause positive results for Coombs' test in patients receiving high doses or in neonates whose mothers were given cephalosporins before delivery.
- May cause ↑ serum AST, ALT, alkaline phosphatase, bilirubin, LDH, BUN, creatinine.
- May rarely cause leukopenia, neutropenia, agranulocytosis, thrombocytopenia, or eosinophilia.

Potential Nursing Diagnoses

Risk for infection (Indications, Side Effects)

Diarrhea (Adverse Reactions)

Implementation

- **PO:** Administer around the clock. May be administered on full or empty stomach. Administration with food may minimize GI irritation. Shake oral suspension well before administering. Refrigerate oral suspensions.

Cefazolin

- **IM:** Reconstitute IM doses with 2 ml or 2.5 ml of cefazolin with sterile water for injection to achieve a final concentration of 225–330 mg/mL.
- Inject deep into a well-developed muscle mass; massage well.

IV Administration

- **Direct IV:** ***Diluent:*** 0.9% NaCl, D5W, D10W, dextrose/saline combinations, D5/LR. ***Concentration:*** 100 mg/ml. May use up to 138 mg/ml in fluid-restricted patients. ***Rate:*** May administer over 3–5 min.
- **Intermittent Infusion:** ***Diluent:*** Reconstituted 500-mg or 1-g solution may be diluted in 50–100 ml of 0.9% NaCl, D5W, D10W, dextrose/saline combinations, D5/LR. Solution is stable for 24 hr at room temperature and 10 days if refrigerated. ***Concentration:*** 20 mg/ml. ***Rate:*** Administer over 10–60 min.
- **Y-Site Compatibility:** acyclovir, allopurinol, amifostine, anidulafungin, atracurium, aztreonam, bivalirudin, calcium gluconate, cyclophosphamide, dexmedetomidine, diltiazem, docetaxel, doxapram, doxorubicin liposome, enalaprilat, esmolol, etoposide, famotidine, fenoldopma, filgrastim, fluconazole, fludarabine, foscarnet, gemcitabine, granisetron, heparin, insulin, labetalol, lidocaine, linezolid, magnesium sulfate, melphalan, meperidine, midazolam, milrinone, morphine, multivitamins, nicardipine, ondansetron, pancuronium, pantoprazole, perphenazine, propofol, ranitidine, remifentanil, sargramostim, tacrolimus, teniposide, theophylline, thiotepa, vecuronium, vitamin B complex with C, warfarin.
- **Y-Site Incompatibility:** amphotericin B cholesteryl sulfate, idarubicin, lansoprazole, pemetrexed, pentamidine, vinorelbine.

Patient/Family Teaching

- Instruct patient to take medication around the clock at evenly spaced times and to finish the medication completely as directed, even if feeling better. Take missed doses as soon as possible unless almost time for next dose; do not double doses. Instruct patient to use calibrated measuring device with liquid preparations. Advise patient that sharing this medication may be dangerous.
- Pedi: Instruct parents or caregivers to use calibrated measuring device with liquid preparations.
- Advise patient to report signs of superinfection (furry overgrowth on the tongue, vaginal itching or discharge, loose or foul-smelling stools) and allergy.
- Instruct patient to notify health care professional if fever and diarrhea develop, especially if diarrhea contains blood, mucus, or pus. Advise patient not to treat diarrhea without consulting health care professional.

Evaluation/Desired Outcomes

- Resolution of signs and symptoms of infection. Length of time for complete resolution depends on the organism and site of infection.
- Decreased incidence of infection when used for prophylaxis.

cephalexin, See CEPHALOSPORINS—FIRST GENERATION.

CEPHALOSPORINS—SECOND GENERATION

cefaclor (**sef**-a-klor)
✤Ceclor, Raniclor

cefotetan (sef-oh-**tee**-tan)
Cefotan

cefoxitin (se-**fox**-i-tin)
Mefoxin

cefprozil (sef-**proe**-zil)
Cefzil

cefuroxime (se-fyoor-**ox**-eem)
Ceftin, Zinacef

Classification
Therapeutic: anti-infectives
Pharmacologic: second-generation cephalosporins

Pregnancy Category B

Indications

Treatment of the following infections caused by susceptible organisms: Respiratory tract infections, Skin and skin structure infections, Bone and joint infections (not cefaclor or cefprozil), Urinary tract infections (not cefprozil). **Cefotetan and cefoxitin:** Intra-abdominal and gynecologic infections. **Cefuroxime:** Meningitis, gynecologic infections, and Lyme disease. **Cefaclor, cefprozil, cefuroxime:** Otitis media. **Cefoxitin and cefuroxime:** Septicemia. **Cefotetan, cefoxitin, cefuroxime:** Perioperative prophylaxis.

Action

Bind to bacterial cell wall membrane, causing cell death. **Therapeutic Effects:** Bactericidal action against susceptible bacteria. **Spectrum:** Similar to that of first-generation cephalosporins but have ↑ activity against several other gram-negative pathogens including: *Haemophilus influenzae*, *Escherichia coli*, *Klebsiella pneumoniae*, *Morganella morganii*, *Neisseria gonorrhoeae* (including penicillinase-producing strains), *Proteus*, *Providencia*, *Serratia marcescens*, *Moraxella catarrhalis*. Not active against methicillin-resistant staphylococci or enterococci. **Cefuroxime:** Active against *Borrelia burgdorferi*. **Cefotetan and cefoxitin:** Active against *Bacteroides fragilis*.

Pharmacokinetics

Absorption: *Cefotetan, cefoxitin,* and *cefuroxime*—well absorbed following IM administration. *Cefaclor, cefprozil,* and *cefuroxime*—well absorbed following oral administration.
Distribution: Widely distributed. Penetration into CSF is poor, but adequate for cefuroxime (IV) to be used in treating meningitis. All cross the placenta and enter breast milk in low concentrations.
Metabolism and Excretion: Excreted primarily unchanged by the kidneys.
Half-life: *Cefaclor*—30–60 min; *cefotetan*—3–4.6 hr; *cefoxitin*—40–60 min; *cefprozil*—90 min; *cefuroxime*—60–120 min; (all are increased in renal impairment).

TIME/ACTION PROFILE

ROUTE	ONSET	PEAK	DURATION
Cefaclor PO	rapid	30–60 min	6–12 hr
Cefaclor PO-CD	unknown	unknown	12 hr
Cefotetan IM	rapid	1–3 hr	12 hr
Cefotetan IV	rapid	end of infusion	12 hr
Cefoxitin IM	rapid	30 min	4–8 hr
Cefoxitin IV	rapid	end of infusion	4–8 hr
Cefprozil PO	unknown	1–2 hr	12–24 hr
Cefuroxime PO	unknown	2–3 hr	8–12 hr
Cefuroxime IM	rapid	15–60 min	6–12 hr
Cefuroxime IV	rapid	end of infusion	6–12 hr

Contraindications/Precautions

Contraindicated in: Hypersensitivity to cephalosporins; Serious hypersensitivity to penicillins.
Use Cautiously in: Renal impairment (↓ dose/ ↑ dosing interval recommended for: *cefotetan* if CCr ≤30 ml/min, *cefoxitin* if CCr ≤50 ml/min, *cefprozil* if CCr <30 ml/min, *cefuroxime* if CCr ≤20 ml/min); **Cefotetan and cefoxitin:** Patients with hepatic dysfunction, poor nutritional state, or cancer may be at ↑ risk for bleeding; History of GI disease, especially colitis; *Cefprozil (oral suspension)* contains aspartame and should be avoided in patients with phenylketonuria; Geri: Dosage adjustment due to age-related ↓ in renal function may be necessary; may also be at ↑ risk for bleeding with *cefotetan* or *cefoxitin*; OB: Pregnancy and lactation (have been used safely).

Adverse Reactions/Side Effects

CNS: SEIZURES (high doses). **GI:** PSEUDOMEMBRANOUS COLITIS, diarrhea, cramps, nausea, vomiting. **Derm:** rashes, urticaria. **Hemat:** agranulocytosis, bleeding (↑ with cefotetan and cefoxitin), eosinophilia, hemolytic anemia, neutropenia, thrombocytopenia. **Local:** pain at IM site, phlebitis AT IV SITE. **Misc:** allergic reactions including ANAPHYLAXIS and SERUM SICKNESS, superinfection.

Interactions

Drug-Drug: Probenecid ↓ excretion and ↑ blood levels. If **alcohol** is ingested within 48–72 hr of cefotetan, a disulfiram-like reaction may occur. Cefotetan may ↑ risk of bleeding with **anticoagulants**, **antiplatelet agents**, **thrombolytics**, and **NSAIDs. Antacids** ↓ absorption of cefaclor. Concurrent use of **aminoglycosides** or **loop diuretics** may ↑ risk of nephrotoxicity.

Route/Dosage

Cefaclor

PO (Adults): 250–500 mg q 8 hr or 375–500 mg q 12 hr as extended-release tablets.

PO (Children >1 mo): 6.7–13.4 mg/kg q 8 hr or 10–20 mg/kg q 12 hr (up to 1 g/day).

Cefotetan

IM, IV (Adults): *Most infections*—1–2 g q 12 hr. *Severe/life-threatening infections*—2–3 g q 12 hr. *Urinary tract infections*—500 mg–2 g q 12 hr *or* 1–2 g q 24 hr. *Perioperative prophylaxis* —1–2 g 30–60 min before initial incision (one-time dose).

Renal Impairment

IM, IV (Adults): *CCr 10–30 ml/min*—Usual adult dose q 24 hr *or* ½ usual adult dose q 12 hr; *<CCr 10 ml/min*—Usual adult dose q 48 hr *or* ¼ usual adult dose q 12 hr.

Cefoxitin

IM, IV (Adults): *Most infections*—1 g q 6–8 hr. *Severe infections*—1 g q 4 hr *or* 2 g q 6–8 hr. *Life-threatening infections*—2 g q 4 hr *or* 3 g q 6 hr. *Perioperative prophylaxis*—2 g 30–60 min before initial incision, then 2 g q 6 hr for up to 24 hr.

IM, IV (Children and Infants >3 mo): *Most infections*—13.3–26.7 mg/kg q 4 hr *or* 20–40 mg/kg q 6 hr. *Perioperative prophylaxis* — 30–40 mg/kg within 60 min of initial incision, then 30–40 mg/kg q 6 hr for up to 24 hr.

Renal Impairment

IM, IV (Adults): *CCr 30–50 ml/min*—1–2 g q 8–12 hr; *CCr 10–29 ml/min*—1–2 g q 12–24 hr; *CCr 5–9 ml/min*—0.5–1 g q 12–24 hr; *CCr <5 ml/min*—0.5–1 g q 24–48 hr.

Cefprozil

PO (Adults): *Most infections*—250–500 mg q 12 hr *or* 500 mg q 24 hr.

PO (Children 6 mo–12 yr): *Otitis media*—15 mg/kg q 12 hr. *Acute sinusitis* —7.5–15 mg/kg q 12 hr (higher dose should be used for moderate-to-severe infections).

PO (Children 2–12 yr): *Pharyngitis/tonsillitis*—7.5 mg/kg q 12 hr. *Skin/skin structure infections*—20 mg/kg q 24 hr.

Renal Impairment

PO (Adults and Children ≥6 mo): *CCr <30 ml/min*—½ of usual dose at normal dosing interval.

Cefuroxime

Cefuroxime oral tablets and oral suspension are not bioequivalent and are not substitutable on a mg-to-mg basis.

PO (Adults and Children >12 yr): *Pharyngitis/tonsillitis, maxillary sinusitis, uncomplicated UTIs*—250 mg q 12 hr. *Bronchitis, uncomplicated skin/skin structure infections*—250–500 mg q 12 hr. *Gonorrhea* —1 g (single dose). *Lyme disease*—500 mg q 12 hr for 20 days.

PO (Children 3 mo–12 yr): *Otitis media, acute bacterial maxillary sinusitis, impetigo*—15 mg/kg q 12 hr as oral suspension (not to exceed 1 g/day) *or* 250 mg q 12 hr as tablets. *Pharyngitis/tonsillitis*—10 mg/kg q 12 hr as oral suspension (not to exceed 500 mg/day).

IM, IV (Adults): *Uncomplicated urinary tract infections, skin/skin structure infections, disseminated gonococcal infections, uncomplicated pneumonia* —750 mg every 8 hr. *Bone/joint infections, severe or complicated infections*—1.5 g every 8 hr. *Life-threatening infections* —1.5 g every 6 hr. *Meningitis* —3 g every 8 hr. *Perioperative prophylaxis* —1.5 g IV 30–60 min before initial incision; 750 mg IM/IV every 8 hr can be given when procedure prolonged. *Prophylaxis during open-heart surgery* —1.5 g IV at induction of anesthesia and then every 12 hr for 3 additional doses. *Gonorrhea*—1.5 g IM (750 mg in two sites) with 1 g probenecid PO.

IM, IV (Children and Infants >3 mo): *Most infections*—12.5–25 mg/kg q 6 hr *or* 16.7–33.3 mg/kg q 8 hr (maximum dose = 6 g/day). *Bone and joint infections*—50 mg/kg q 8 hr (maximum dose = 6 g/day). *Bacterial meningitis*—50–60 mg/kg q 6 hr *or* 66.7–80 mg/kg q 8 hr.

Renal Impairment

IM, IV (Adults): *CCr 10–20 ml/min*—750 mg q 12 hr; *CCr <10 ml/min*—750 mg q 24 hr.

Availability

Cefaclor

Capsules: 250 mg, 500 mg. **Chewable tablets (fruity):** 125 mg, 187 mg, 250 mg, 375 mg. **Extended-release tablets (CD):** 375 mg, 500 mg. **Oral suspension (strawberry):** 125 mg/5 ml, 187 mg/5 ml, 250 mg/5 ml, 375 mg/5 ml.

Cefotetan

Powder for injection: 1 g, 2 g, 10 g. **Premixed containers:** 1 g/50 ml, 2 g/50 ml.

Cefoxitin

Powder for injection: 1 g, 2 g, 10 g. **Premixed containers:** 1 g/50 ml D5W, 2 g/50 ml D5W.

Cefprozil

Tablets: 250 mg, 500 mg. **Oral suspension (bubblegum flavor):** 125 mg/5 ml, 250 mg/5 ml.

Cefuroxime

Tablets: 250 mg, 500 mg. **Oral suspension (tutti-frutti flavor):** 125 mg/5 ml, 250 mg/5 ml. **Powder for injection:** 750 mg, 1.5 g, 7.5 g. **Premixed containers:** 750 mg/50 ml, 1.5 g/ 50 ml.

NURSING IMPLICATIONS

Assessment

- Assess for infection (vital signs; appearance of wound, sputum, urine, and stool; WBC) at beginning and during therapy.
- Before initiating therapy, obtain a history to determine previous use of and reactions to penicillins or cephalosporins. Persons with a negative history of penicillin sensitivity may still have an allergic response.
- Obtain specimens for culture and sensitivity before initiating therapy. First dose may be given before receiving results.
- Observe patient for signs and symptoms of anaphylaxis (rash, pruritus, laryngeal edema, wheezing). Discontinue the drug and notify physician or other health care professional immediately if these symptoms occur. Keep epinephrine, an antihistamine, and resuscitation equipment close by in the event of an anaphylactic reaction.
- ***Lab Test Considerations:*** May cause positive results for Coombs' test in patients receiving high doses or in neonates whose mothers were given cephalosporins before delivery.
- *Cefotetan*—monitor prothrombin time and assess patient for bleeding (guaiac stools; check for hematuria, bleeding gums, ecchymosis) daily in high-risk patients; may cause hypoprothrombinemia.
- May cause ↑ serum AST, ALT, alkaline phosphatase, bilirubin, LDH, BUN, and creatinine.
- *Cefoxitin* may cause falsely ↑ test results for serum and urine creatinine; do not obtain serum samples within 2 hr of administration.
- May rarely cause leukopenia, neutropenia, agranulocytosis, thrombocytopenia, and eosinophilia.

Potential Nursing Diagnoses

Risk for infection (Indications, Side Effects)
Diarrhea (Adverse Reactions)
Deficient knowledge, related to medication regimen (Patient/Family Teaching)

Implementation

- **PO:** Administer around the clock. May be administered on full or empty stomach. Administration with food may minimize GI irritation. Shake oral suspension well before administering.
- Administer cefaclor extended-release tablets with food; do not crush, break, or chew.
- Do not administer cefaclor within 1 hr of antacids.
- *Cefuroxime* tablets should be swallowed whole, not crushed; crushed tablets have a strong, persistent bitter taste. Tablets may be taken without regard to meals. Suspension must be taken with food. Shake well each time before using. Tablets and suspension are not interchangeable.
- **IM:** Reconstitute IM doses with sterile or bacteriostatic water for injection or 0.9% NaCl for injection. May be diluted with lidocaine to minimize injection discomfort.
- Inject deep into a well-developed muscle mass; massage well.
- **IV:** Change sites every 48–72 hr to prevent phlebitis. Monitor site frequently for thrombophlebitis (pain, redness, swelling).
- If aminoglycosides are administered concurrently, administer in separate sites if possible, at least 1 hr apart. If second site is unavailable, flush line between medications.

IV Administration

- **Direct IV:** Dilute each cephalosporin in at least 1 g/10 ml. Do not use preparations containing benzyl alcohol for neonates. ***Rate:*** Administer slowly over 3–5 min.

Cefotetan

IV Administration

- **Intermittent Infusion: *Diluent:*** Reconstituted solution may be further diluted in 50–100 ml of D5W or 0.9% NaCl. Solution may be colorless or yellow. Solution is stable for 24 hr at room temperature or 96 hr if refrigerated. ***Concentration:*** 10–40 mg/ml. ***Rate:*** Administer over 20–30 min.
- **Y-Site Compatibility:** allopurinol, amifostine, aztreonam, bivalirudin, dexmedetomi-

date, diltiazem, docetaxel, etoposide phosphate, famotidine, fenoldopam, filgrastim, fluconazole, fludarabine, gemcitabine, granisetron, heparin, insulin, lansoprazole, linezolid, melphalan, meperidine, morphine, paclitaxel, pemetrexed, propofol, remifentanil, sargramostim, tacrolimus, teniposide, theophylline, thiotepa.

- **Y-Site Incompatibility:** pemetrexed, promethazine, vinorelbine.

Cefoxitin

IV Administration

- **Intermittent Infusion:** ***Diluent:*** Reconstituted solution may be further diluted in 50–100 ml of D5W, D10W, 0.9% NaCl, dextrose/saline combinations, D5/LR, Ringer's, or LR. Stable for 24 hr at room temperature and 1 wk if refrigerated. Darkening of powder does not alter potency. ***Concentration:*** 40 mg/ml. ***Rate:*** Administer over 10–60 min.
- **Continuous Infusion:** May be diluted in 500–1000 ml for continuous infusion.
- **Syringe Compatibility:** heparin.
- **Y-Site Compatibility:** acyclovir, amifostine, amphotericin B cholesteryl sulfate, anidulafungin, aztreonam, bivalirudin, cyclophosphamide, dexmedetomidine, diltiazem, docetaxel, doxorubicin liposome, etoposide phosphate, famotidine, fluconazole, foscarnet, gemcitabine, granisetron, hydromorphone, linezolid, magnesium sulfate, meperidine, morphine, ondansetrol, perphenazine, propofol, ranitidine, remifentanil, teniposide, thiotepa.
- **Y-Site Incompatibility:** Manufacturer recommends stopping other medications during infusion, fenoldopam, filgrastim, lansoprazole, pemetrexed, pentamidine.

Cefuroxime

IV Administration

- **Intermittent Infusion:** ***Diluent:*** Solution may be further diluted in 100 ml of 0.9% NaCl, D5W, D10W, or dextrose/saline combinations. Stable for 24 hr at room temperature and 1 wk if refrigerated. ***Concentration:*** 30 mg/ml. ***Rate:*** Administer over 15–60 min.
- **Continuous Infusion:** May also be diluted in 500–1000 ml for continuous infusion.
- **Y-Site Compatibility:** acyclovir, allopurinol, amifostine, amiodarone, anidulafungin, atracurium, aztreonam, bivalirudin, cyclophosphamide, dexmedetomidine, diltiazem, docetaxel, etoposide phosphate, famotidine, fenoldopam, fludarabine, foscarnet, gemcitabine, granisetron, hydromorphone, linezolid, melphalan, meperidine, milrinone, morphine, ondansetron, pancuronium, pemetrexed, perphenazine, propofol, remifentanil, sargramostim, tacrolimus, teniposide, thiotepa, vecuronium.
- **Y-Site Incompatibility:** Manufacturer recommends temporarily discontinuing primary solution when administering cefuroxime via Y-site, azithromycin, filgrastim, fluconazole, midazolam, vinorelbine.

Patient/Family Teaching

- Instruct patient to take medication around the clock at evenly spaced times and to finish the medication completely, even if feeling better. Take missed doses as soon as possible unless almost time for next dose; do not double doses. Advise patient that sharing of this medication may be dangerous.
- Pedi: Instruct parents or caregivers to use calibrated measuring device with liquid preparations.
- Advise patient to report signs of superinfection (furry overgrowth on the tongue, vaginal itching or discharge, loose or foul-smelling stools) and allergy.
- Caution patients that concurrent use of alcohol with *cefotetan* may cause a disulfiram-like reaction (abdominal cramps, nausea, vomiting, headache, hypotension, palpitations, dyspnea, tachycardia, sweating, flushing). Alcohol and alcohol-containing medications should be avoided during and for several days after therapy.
- Instruct patient to notify health care professional if fever and diarrhea develop, especially if stool contains blood, pus, or mucus. Advise patient not to treat diarrhea without consulting health care professional.

Evaluation/Desired Outcomes

- Resolution of signs and symptoms of infection. Length of time for complete resolution depends on the organism and site of infection.
- Decreased incidence of infection when used for prophylaxis.

CEPHALOSPORINS—THIRD GENERATION

cefdinir (**sef**-di-nir)
Omnicef

cefditoren (sef-dye-**tor**-en)
Spectracef

cefixime (sef-**ik**-seem)
Suprax

cefoperazone
(sef-oh-**per**-a-zone)
Cefobid

cefotaxime (sef-oh-**taks**-eem)
Claforan

cefpodoxime (sef-poe-**dox**-eem)
Vantin

ceftazidime (sef-**tay**-zi-deem)
Fortaz, Tazicef

ceftibuten (sef-tye-**byoo**-ten)
Cedax

ceftizoxime (sef-ti-**zox**-eem)
Cefizox

ceftriaxone (sef-try-**ax**-one)
Rocephin

Classification
Therapeutic: anti-infectives
Pharmacologic: third-generation cephalosporins

Pregnancy Category B

Indications

Treatment of the following infections caused by susceptible organisms: Skin and skin structure infections (not cefixime), Urinary and gynecologic infections (not cefdinir, cefditoren, or ceftibuten), Respiratory tract infections (not cefdinir, cefditoren, or ceftibuten). **Cefotaxime, ceftazidime, ceftizoxime, ceftriaxone:** Meningitis and bone/joint infections. **Cefoperazone, cefotaxime, ceftazidime, ceftizoxime, ceftriaxone:** Intra-abdominal infections and septicemia. **Cefdinir, cefixime, cefpodoxime, ceftibuten, ceftriaxone:** Otitis media. **Cefotaxime and ceftriaxone:** Perioperative prophylaxis. **Ceftazidime:** Febrile neutropenia. **Cefotaxime, ceftriaxone:** Lyme disease.

Action

Bind to the bacterial cell wall membrane, causing cell death. **Therapeutic Effects:** Bactericidal action against susceptible bacteria. **Spectrum:** Similar to that of second-generation cephalosporins, but activity against staphylococci is less, whereas activity against gram-negative pathogens is greater, even for organisms resistant to first- and second-generation agents. Notable is increased action against: *Enterobacter, Haemophilus influenzae, Escherichia coli, Klebsiella pneumoniae, Neisseria gonorrhea, Citrobacter, Morganella, Proteus, Providencia, Serratia, Moraxella catarrhalis, Borrelia burgdorferi.* Some agents have activity against *Neisseria meningitidis* (cefotaxime, ceftazidime, ceftizoxime, ceftriaxone). Some agents have enhanced activity against *Pseudomonas aeruginosa* (ceftazidime, cefoperazone). Not active against methicillin-resistance staphylococci or enterococci. Some agents have activity against anaerobes, including *Bacteroides fragilis* (cefoperazone, cefotaxime, ceftizoxime, ceftriaxone).

Pharmacokinetics

Absorption: *Cefoperazone, cefotaxime, ceftazidime, ceftizoxime,* and *ceftriaxone* are well absorbed after IM administration. *Ceftibuten* is well absorbed after oral administration; *cefixime* 40–50% absorbed after oral administration (oral suspension); *cefdinir* 16–25% absorbed after oral administration. *Cefditoren pivoxil* and *cefpodoxime proxetil* are prodrugs that are converted to their active components in GI tract during absorption (*cefditoren*—14% absorbed [↑ by high-fat meal]; *cefpodoxime*—50% absorbed).
Distribution: Widely distributed. Cross the placenta; enter breast milk in low concentrations. CSF penetration better than with first- and second-generation agents.
Protein Binding: *Cefoperazone* and *ceftriaxone* ≥90%.
Metabolism and Excretion: *Cefdinir, ceftazidime, cefditoren,* and *ceftizoxime*—>85% excreted in urine. *Cefpodoxime* —30% excreted in urine. *Cefoperazone*—excreted in the bile. *Ceftibuten, ceftriaxone,* and *cefotaxime*—partly metabolized and partly excreted in the urine. *Cefixime*—50% excreted unchanged in urine, ≥10% in bile.
Half-life: *Cefdinir*—1.7 hr; *cefditoren*—1.6 hr; *cefixime*—3–4 hr; *cefoperazone*—2 hr; *cefotaxime*—1–1.5 hr; *cefpodoxime*—2–3 hr; *ceftazidime*—2 hr; *ceftibuten*—2 hr;

ceftizoxime—1.4–1.9 hr; *ceftriaxone*—6–9 hr (all except *cefoperazone* and *ceftriaxone* are increased in renal impairment).

TIME/ACTION PROFILE

ROUTE	ONSET	PEAK	DURATION
Cefdinir PO	rapid	2–4 hr	12–24 hr
Cefditoren PO	rapid	1.5–3 hr	12 hr
Cefixime PO	rapid	2–6 hr	24 hr
Cefoperazone IM	rapid	1–2 hr	12 hr
Cefoperazone IV	rapid	end of infusion	12 hr
Cefotaxime IM	rapid	0.5 hr	4–12 hr
Cefotaxime IV	rapid	end of infusion	4–12 hr
Cefpodoxime PO	unknown	2–3 hr	12 hr
Ceftazidime IM	rapid	1 hr	6–12 hr
Ceftazidime IV	rapid	end of infusion	6–12 hr
Ceftibuten PO	rapid	3 hr	24 hr
Ceftizoxime IM	rapid	0.5–1.5 hr	6–12 hr
Ceftizoxime IV	rapid	end of infusion	6–12 hr
Ceftriaxone IM	rapid	1–2 hr	12–24 hr
Ceftriaxone IV	rapid	end of infusion	12–24 hr

Contraindications/Precautions

Contraindicated in: Hypersensitivity to cephalosporins; Serious hypersensitivity to penicillins; Hyperbilirubinemic neonates (ceftriaxone only; may lead to kernicterus); Carnitine deficiency or inborn errors of metabolism (cefditoren only); Hypersensitivity to milk protein (ceftidoren only; contains sodium caseinate).
Use Cautiously in: Renal impairment (decreased dosing/increased dosing interval recommended for: *Cefdinir* if CCr <30 ml/min, *cefixime* if CCr ≤60 ml/min, *cefotaxime* if CCr <20 ml/min, *cefpodoxime* if CCr <30 ml/min, *ceftazidime* if CCr ≤50 ml/min, *ceftibuten* and *cefditoren* if CCr <50 ml/min, *ceftizoxime* if CCr ≤80 ml/min); Hepatic/biliary impairment or combined hepatic/biliary/renal impairment (dosage reduction/increased dosing interval recommended for *cefoperazone*); Combined severe hepatic and renal impairment (dosage reduction/increased dosing interval recommended for *ceftriaxone*); Diabetes (*ceftibuten* and *cefdinir* suspensions contain sucrose); History of GI disease, especially colitis; Patients with poor nutritional status, malabsorption states, or alcoholism may be at ↑ risk for bleeding with *cefoperazone*; Geri: Dosage adjustment due to age-related ↓ in renal function may be necessary; Pregnancy and lactation (have been used safely).

Adverse Reactions/Side Effects

CNS: SEIZURES (high doses), headache. **GI:** PSEUDOMEMBRANOUS COLITIS, diarrhea, nausea, vomiting, cholelithiasis (ceftriaxone), cramps. **Derm:** rashes, urticaria. **Hemat:** agranulocytosis, bleeding (↑ with cefoperazone), eosinophilia, hemolytic anemia, lymphocytosis, neutropenia, thrombocytopenia, thrombocytosis. **GU:** hematuria, vaginal moniliasis. **Local:** pain at IM site, phlebitis AT IV SITE. **Misc:** allergic reactions including ANAPHYLAXIS and SERUM SICKNESS, superinfection.

Interactions

Drug-Drug: Probenecid ↓ excretion and ↑ serum levels (cefdinir, cefditoren, cefixime, cefotaxime, cefpodoxime, ceftizoxime, ceftriaxone). Ingestion of **alcohol** within 48–72 hr of cefoperazone may result in a disulfiram-like reaction. Cefoperazone may ↑ risk of bleeding with **anticoagulants**, **antiplatelet agents**, **thrombolytic agents**, and **NSAIDS**. Concurrent use of **loop diuretics** or **nephrotoxic agents** including **aminoglycosides** may ↑ risk of nephrotoxicity. **Antacids** ↓ absorption of cefdinir, cefditoren, and cefpodoxime. **Iron supplements** ↓ absorption of cefdinir. **H_2-receptor antagonists** ↓ absorption of cefditoren and cefpodoxime. Cefixime may ↑ **carbamazepine** levels.

Route/Dosage

Cefdinir

PO (Adults ≥13 yr): 300 mg q 12 hr *or* 600 mg q 24 hr (use q 12 hr dosing only for community-acquired pneumonia or skin and skin structure infections).
PO (Children 6 mo–12 yr): 7 mg/kg q 12 hr (use only for skin/skin structure infections) *or* 14 mg/kg q 24 hr; dose should not exceed 600 mg/day.

Renal Impairment

PO (Adults and Children ≥13 yr): *CCr <30 ml/min*—300 mg q 24 hr.

Renal Impairment

PO (Children 6 mo–12 yr): *CCr <30 ml/min*—7 mg/kg q 24 hr.

Cefditoren

PO (Adults and Children ≥12 yr): *Pharyngitis/tonsillitis, skin/skin structure infections*—200 mg twice daily; *Acute bacterial exacerbation of chronic bronchitis or community acquired pneumonia*—400 mg twice daily.

Renal Impairment
PO (Adults): *CCr 30–49 ml/min*—dose should not exceed 200 mg twice daily; *CCr <30 ml/min*—dose should not exceed 200 mg once daily.

Cefixime

PO (Adults and Children >12 yr or >50 kg): *Most infections*—400 mg once daily; *Gonorrhea*— 400 mg single dose.
PO (Children): 8 mg/kg once daily *or* 4 mg/kg q 12 h
Renal Impairment
PO (Adults): *CCr 21–60 ml/min*— 75% of standard dose once daily; *CCr ≤20 ml/min*— 50% of standard dose once daily.

Cefoperazone

IM, IV (Adults): *Mild to moderate infections*—1–2 g q 12 hr. *Severe infections*—2–4 g q 8 hr *or* 1.5–3 g q 6 hr.
Hepatic/Renal Impairment
IM, IV (Adults): *Impaired hepatic function/biliary obstruction*—daily dose should not exceed 4 g; *combined hepatic and renal impairment*—daily dose should not exceed 1–2 g.

Cefotaxime

IM, IV (Adults and Children >12 yr): *Most uncomplicated infections*—1 g q 12 hr. *Moderate or severe infections*—1–2 g q 6–8 hr. *Life-threatening infections*—2 g q 4 hr (maximum dose = 12 g/day). *Gonococcal urethritis/cervicitis or rectal gonorrhea in females*—500 mg IM (single dose). *Rectal gonorrhea in males* —1 g IM (single dose). *Perioperative prophylaxis* —1 g 30–90 min before initial incision (one-time dose).
IM, IV (Children 1 mo–12 yr): *<50 kg*— 100–200 mg/kg/day divided q 6–8 hr. *Meningitis* —200 mg/kg/day divided q 6 hr. *Invasive pneumococcal meningitis*—225–300 mg/kg/day divided q 6–8 hr. *≥50 kg*—see adult dosing.
IV (Neonates 1–4 wk): 50 mg/kg q 6–8 hr.
IV (Neonates ≤1 wk): 50 mg/kg q 8–12 hr.
Renal Impairment
(Adults): *CCr <20 ml/min*— ↓ dose by 50%.

Cefpodoxime

PO (Adults): *Most infections*—200 mg q 12 hr. *Skin and skin structure infections*—400 mg q 12 hr. *Urinary tract infections/pharyngitis*—100 mg q 12 hr. *Gonorrhea*—200 mg single dose.
PO (Children 2 mo–12 yr): *Pharyngitis/tonsillitis/otitis media/acute maxillary sinusitis*—5 mg/kg q 12 hr (not to exceed 200 mg/dose).
Renal Impairment
PO (Adults): *CCr <30 ml/min*— ↑ dosing interval to q 24 hr.

Ceftazidime

IM, IV (Adults and Children ≥12 yr): *Pneumonia and skin/skin structure infections*— 500 mg–1 g q 8 hr. *Bone and joint infections*—2 g q 12 hr. *Severe and life-threatening infections*—2 g q 8 hr. *Complicated urinary tract infections*—500 mg q 8–12 hr. *Uncomplicated urinary tract infections*— 250 mg q 12 hr. *Cystic fibrosis lung infection caused by Pseudomonas aeruginosa* —30–50 mg/kg q 8 hr (maximum dose = 6 g/day).
IM, IV (Children 1 mo–12 yr): 33.3–50 mg/kg q 8 hr (maximum dose = 6 g/day).
IM, IV (Neonates ≤4 wk): 50 mg/kg q 8–12 hr.
Renal Impairment
IM, IV (Adults): *CCr 31–50 ml/min*—1 g q 12 hr; *CCr 16–30 ml/min*—1 g q 24 hr; *CCr 6–15 ml/min*—500 mg q 24 hr; *CCr <5 ml/min*—500 mg q 48 hr.

Ceftibuten

PO (Adults and Children ≥12 yr): 400 mg q 24 hr for 10 days.
PO (Children 6 mo–12 yr): 9 mg/kg q 24 hr for 10 days (maximum dose = 400 mg/day).
Renal Impairment
PO (Adults): *CCr 30–49 ml/min*—200 mg q 24 hr as capsules *or* 4.5 mg/kg q 24 hr as suspension; *CCr 5–29 ml/min*—100 mg q 24 hr as capsules *or* 2.25 mg/kg q 24 hr as suspension.

Ceftizoxime

IM, IV (Adults): *Severe infections*—1–2 g q 8–12 hr. *Life-threatening infections*—3–4 g q 8 hr. *Uncomplicated urinary tract infections*—500 mg q 12 hr. *Gonococcal urethritis/cervicitis* —1 g IM (single dose).
IM, IV (Children >6 mo): 50 mg/kg q 6–8 hr (not to exceed 200 mg/kg/day).

Renal Impairment

IM, IV (Adults): *CCr 50–79 ml/min*—500 mg–1.5 g q 8 hr; *CCr 5–49 ml/min*—250 mg–1 g q 12 hr; *CCr 0–4 ml/min*—500 mg–1 g q 48 hr *or* 250–500 mg q 24 hr.

Ceftriaxone

IM, IV (Adults): *Most infections*—1–2 g q 12–24 hr. *Gonorrhea*—250 mg IM (single dose). *Meningitis*—2 g q 12 hr. *Perioperative prophylaxis* —1 g 30–120 min before initial incision (single dose).

IM, IV (Children): *Most infections*—25–37.5 mg/kg q 12 hr *or* 50–75 mg/kg q 24 hr; dose should not exceed 2 g/day. *Meningitis*—100 mg/kg q 24 hr *or* 50 mg/kg q 12 hr; dose should not exceed 4 g/day. *Acute otitis media*—50 mg/kg IM single dose; dose should not exceed 1 g. *Uncomplicated gonorrhea* —125 mg IM (single dose).

Availability

Cefdinir

Oral suspension (strawberry): 125 mg/5 ml, 250 mg/5 ml. **Cost:** *Generic*—125 mg/5 ml $73.40/100 ml, 250 mg/5 ml $83.87/60 ml. **Capsules:** 300 mg. **Cost:** $104.99/20.

Cefditoren

Tablets: 200 mg.

Cefixime

Oral suspension (strawberry): 100 mg/5 ml.

Cefoperazone

Powder for injection: 1 g, 2 g, 10 g. **Premixed containers:** 1 g/50 ml, 2 g/50 ml.

Cefotaxime

Powder for injection: 500 mg, 1 g, 2 g, 10 g, 20 g. **Premixed containers:** 1 g/50 ml, 2 g/50 ml.

Cefpodoxime

Tablets: 100 mg, 200 mg. **Oral suspension (lemon creme):** 50 mg/5 ml, 100 mg/5 ml.

Ceftazidime

Powder for injection: 500 mg, 1 g, 2 g, 6 g. **Premixed containers:** 1 g/50 ml, 2 g/50 ml.

Ceftibuten

Capsules: 400 mg. **Oral suspension (cherry):** 90 mg/5 ml.

Ceftizoxime

Powder for injection: 1 g, 2 g, 10 g. **Premixed containers:** 1 g/50 ml, 2 g/50 ml.

Ceftriaxone

Powder for injection: 250 mg, 500 mg, 1 g, 2 g, 10 g. **Premixed containers:** 1 g/50 ml, 2 g/50 ml.

NURSING IMPLICATIONS

Assessment

- Assess for infection (vital signs; appearance of wound, sputum, urine, and stool; WBC) at beginning of and throughout therapy.
- Before initiating therapy, obtain a history to determine previous use of and reactions to penicillins or cephalosporins. Persons with a negative history of penicillin sensitivity may still have an allergic response.
- Obtain specimens for culture and sensitivity before initiating therapy. First dose may be given before receiving results.
- Observe patient for signs and symptoms of anaphylaxis (rash, pruritus, laryngeal edema, wheezing). Discontinue drug and notify physician or other health care professional immediately if these symptoms occur. Keep epinephrine, an antihistamine, and resuscitation equipment close by in the event of an anaphylactic reaction.
- Pedi: Assess newborns for jaundice and hyperbilirubinemia before making decision to use ceftriaxone (should not be used in jaundiced or hyperbilirubinemic neonates).
- ***Lab Test Considerations:*** May cause positive results for Coombs' test in patients receiving high doses or in neonates whose mothers were given cephalosporins before delivery.
- Monitor prothrombin time and assess patient for bleeding (guaiac stools; check for hematuria, bleeding gums, ecchymosis) daily in patients receiving *cefoperazone* or *cefditoren*, as this agent may cause hypoprothrombinemia.
- May cause ↑ serum AST, ALT, alkaline phosphatase, bilirubin, LDH, BUN, and creatinine.
- May rarely cause leukopenia, neutropenia, agranulocytosis, thrombocytopenia, eosinophilia, lymphocytosis, and thrombocytosis.

Potential Nursing Diagnoses

Risk for infection (Indications, Side Effects)
Diarrhea (Adverse Reactions)
Deficient knowledge, related to medication regimen (Patient/Family Teaching)

C

Implementation

- Cefditoren is not recommended for prolonged use since other piralate-containing compounds have caused clinical manifestations of carnitine deficiency when used over a period of months.
- **PO:** Administer around the clock. May be administered on full or empty stomach. Administration with food may minimize GI irritation. Shake oral suspension well before administering. *Cefditoren* should be administered with meals to enhance absorption. *Cefpodoxime tablets* should be administered with meals to enhance absorption (the suspension may be administered without regard to meals. *Ceftibuten* should be administered at least 1 hr before or 2 hr after meals.
- *Cefixime oral suspension* should be used to treat otitis media (results in higher peak concentrations than tablets).
- Do not administer cefdinir or cefpodoxime within 2 hr before or after an antacid. Do not administer cefpodoxime within 2 hr before or after an H_2 receptor antagonist. Do not administer cefdinir within 2 hr before or after iron supplements. Do not administer cefditoren concomitantly with antacids.
- **IM:** Reconstitute IM doses with sterile or bacteriostatic water for injection or 0.9% NaCl for injection. May be diluted with lidocaine to minimize injection discomfort.
- Inject deep into a well-developed muscle mass; massage well.
- **IV:** Monitor injection site frequently for phlebitis (pain, redness, swelling). Change sites every 48–72 hr to prevent phlebitis.
- If aminoglycosides are administered concurrently, administer in separate sites, if possible, at least 1 hr apart. If second site is unavailable, flush lines between medications.

IV Administration

- **Direct IV:** Dilute cephalosporins in at least 1 g/10 ml. Avoid direct IV administration of *cefoperazone* and *ceftriaxone*. Do not use preparations containing benzyl alcohol for neonates. ***Rate:*** Administer slowly over 3–5 min.

Cefoperazone

IV Administration

- **Intermittent Infusion: *Diluent:*** Reconstitute each gram with at least 2.8 ml of sterile or bacteriostatic water for injection or 0.9% NaCl. Shake vigorously and allow to stand for visualization and clarity. Solution may be colorless to straw colored. Each gram in solution should be further diluted in 20–40 ml of 0.9% NaCl, D5W, D10W, dextrose/saline combinations, D5/LR, or LR. ***Concentration:*** 25–50 mg/mlSolution is stable for 24 hr at room temperature and 5 days if refrigerated. ***Rate:*** Administer over 15–30 min.
- **Continuous Infusion:** For continuous infusion, concentration should be 2–25 mg/ml.
- **Syringe Compatibility:** heparin.
- **Y-Site Compatibility:** acyclovir, allopurinol, aztreonam, cyclophosphamide, docetaxel, enalaprilat, esmolol, etoposide, famotidine, fludarabine, foscarnet, granisetron, hydromorphone, linezolid, magnesium sulfate, melphalan, morphine, propofol, ranitidine, teniposide, thiotepa.
- **Y-Site Incompatibility:** amifostine, amphotericin B cholesteryl sulfate, cisatracurium, doxorubicin liposome, filgrastim, gemcitabine, labetalol, meperidine, ondansetron, pentamidine, perphenazine, promethazine, sargramostim, vinorelbine.

Cefotaxime

IV Administration

- **Intermittent Infusion: *Diluent:*** Reconstituted solution may be further diluted in 50–100 ml of D5W, D10W, LR, dextrose/saline combinations, or 0.9% NaCl. Solution may appear light yellow to amber. Solution is stable for 24 hr at room temperature and 5 days if refrigerated. ***Concentration:*** 20–60 mg/ml. ***Rate:*** Administer over 20–30 min.
- **Syringe Compatibility:** heparin.
- **Y-Site Compatibility:** acyclovir, amifostine, aztreonam, bivalirudin, cyclophosphamide, dexmedetomidine, diltiazem, docetaxel, etoposide phosphate, famotidine, fenoldopam, fludarabine, granisetron, hydromorphone, levofloxacin, lorazepam, magnesium sulfate, melphalan, meperidine, midazolam, milrinone, morphine, ondansetron, perphenazine, propofol, remifentanil, sargramostim, teniposide, thiotepa, tolazoline, vinorelbine.
- **Y-Site Incompatibility:** allopurinol, azithromycin, filgrastim, fluconazole, gemcitabine, pemetrexed, pentamidine.

Ceftazidime

IV Administration

- **Intermittent Infusion:** ***Diluent:*** Reconstituted solution may be further diluted in at least 1 g/10 ml of 0.9% NaCl, D5W, D10W, dextrose/saline combinations, or LR. Dilution causes CO_2 to form inside vial, resulting in positive pressure; vial may require venting after dissolution to preserve sterility of vial. Not required with L-arginine formulation (Ceptaz). Solution may appear yellow to amber; darkening does not alter potency. Solution is stable for 18 hr at room temperature and 7 days if refrigerated. ***Concentration:*** 40 mg/ml. ***Rate:*** Administer over 15–30 min.
- **Syringe Compatibility:** hydromorphone.
- **Y-Site Compatibility:** acyclovir, allopurinol, amifostine, aminophylline, anidulafungin, aztreonam, bivalirudin, ciprofloxacin, dexmedetomidine, diltiazem, docetaxel, dopamine, doxapram, enalaprilat, epinephrine, esmolol, etoposide phosphate, famotidine, fenoldopam, filgrastim, fludarabine, foscarnet, furosemide, gemcitabine, granisetron, heparin, hydromorphone, insulin, ketamine, labetalol, linezolid, melphalan, meperidine, milrinone, morphine, ondansetron, paclitaxel, ranitidine, remifentanil, sufentanil, tacrolimus, teniposide, theophylline, thiotepa, tobramycin, vinorelbine, zidovudine.
- **Y-Site Incompatibility:** amiodarone, amphotericin B cholesteryl sulfate, amsacrine, azithromycin, doxorubicin liposome, erythromycin, fluconazole, idarubicin, lansoprazole, midazolam, pemetrexed, pentamidine, phenytoin, warfarin.

Ceftizoxime

IV Administration

- **Intermittent Infusion:** ***Diluent:*** Reconstituted solution may be further diluted in 50–100 ml of D5W, D10W, 0.9% NaCl, dextrose/saline combinations, or LR. Solution is stable for 8 hr at room temperature and 48 hr if refrigerated. ***Concentration:*** 20 mg/ml. ***Rate:*** Administer over 15–30 min.
- **Y-Site Compatibility:** acyclovir, allopurinol, amifostine, amiodarone, amphotericin B cholesteryl sulfate, anidulafungin, aztreonam, bivalirudin, dexmedetomidine, docetaxel, doxorubicin liposome, enalaprilat, esmolol, etoposide phosphate, famotidine, fenoldopam, fludarabine, foscarnet, gemcitabine, granisetron, hydromorphone, labetalol, linezolid, melphalan, meperidine, morphine, nicardipine, ondansetron, pemetrexed, propofol, ranitidine, remifentanil, sargramostim, teniposide, thiotepa, vinorelbine.
- **Y-Site Incompatibility:** filgrastim, lansoprazole.

Ceftriaxone

IV Administration

- **Intermittent Infusion:** Reconstitute each 250-mg vial with 2.4 ml, each 500-mg vial with 4.8 ml, each 1-g vial with 9.6 ml, and each 2-g vial with 19.2 ml of sterile water for injection, 0.9% NaCl, or D5W for a concentration of 100 mg/ml. ***Diluent:*** Solution may be further diluted in 50–100 ml of 0.9% NaCl, D5W, D10W, D5/0.45% NaCl, or LR. Solution may appear light yellow to amber. Solution is stable for 3 days at room temperature. ***Concentration:*** 40 mg/ml. ***Rate:*** Administer over 10–30 min.
- **Y-Site Compatibility:** acyclovir, allopurinol, amifostine, amiodarone, anidulafungin, aztreonam, bivalirudin, cisatracurium, daptomycin, dexmedetomidine, diltiazem, docetaxel, doxorubicin liposome, drotrecogin, etoposide phosphate, famotidine, fenoldopam, fludarabine, foscarnet, gemcitabine, granisetron, heparin, lansoprazole, linezolid, melphalan, meperidine, methotrexate, morphine, paclitaxel, pantoprazole, pemetrexed, propofol, remifentanil, sargramostim, sodium bicarbonate, tacrolimus, teniposide, theophylline, thiotepa, warfarin, zidovudine.
- **Y-Site Incompatibility:** amphotericin B cholesteryl sulfate, amsacrine, azithromycin, filgrastim, fluconazole, labetalol, pentamidine, vinorelbine.

Patient/Family Teaching

- Instruct patient to take medication around the clock and to finish the medication completely, even if feeling better. Take missed doses as soon as possible unless almost time for next dose; do not double doses. Advise patient that sharing of this medication may be dangerous.
- Pedi: Instruct parents or caregivers to use calibrated measuring device with liquid preparations.
- Advise patient to report signs of superinfection (furry overgrowth on the tongue, vaginal itching or discharge, loose or foul-smelling stools) and allergy.

- Caution patients that concurrent use of alcohol with *cefoperazone* may cause a disulfiram-like reaction (abdominal cramps, nausea, vomiting, headache, hypotension, palpitations, dyspnea, tachycardia, sweating, flushing). Alcohol and alcohol-containing medications should be avoided during and for several days after therapy.
- Instruct patient to notify health care professional if fever and diarrhea develop, especially if stool contains blood, pus, or mucus. Advise patient not to treat diarrhea without consulting health care professional.

Evaluation/Desired Outcomes

- Resolution of the signs and symptoms of infection. Length of time for complete resolution depends on the organism and site of infection.
- Decreased incidence of infection when used for prophylaxis.

cephradine, See CEPHALOSPORINS—FIRST GENERATION.

cetirizine (se-ti-ra-zeen)

Zyrtec

Classification

Therapeutic: allergy, cold, and cough remedies, antihistamines
Pharmacologic: piperazines (peripherally selective)

Pregnancy Category B

Indications

Relief of allergic symptoms caused by histamine release including: Seasonal and perennial allergic rhinitis, Chronic urticaria.

Action

Antagonizes the effects of histamine at H_1-receptor sites; does not bind to or inactivate histamine. Anticholinergic effects are minimal and sedation is dose related. **Therapeutic Effects:** Decreased symptoms of histamine excess (sneezing, rhinorrhea, ocular tearing and redness, pruritus).

Pharmacokinetics

Absorption: Well absorbed following oral administration.
Distribution: Unknown.
Protein Binding: 93%.
Metabolism and Excretion: Excreted primarily unchanged by the kidneys.
Half-life: 7.4–9 hr (decreased in children to 6.2 hr, increased in renal impairment up to 19–21 hr).

TIME/ACTION PROFILE (antihistaminic effects)

ROUTE	ONSET	PEAK	DURATION
PO	30 min	4–8 hr	24 hr

Contraindications/Precautions

Contraindicated in: Hypersensitivity to cetirizine, hydroxyzine, or any component; Lactation: Excreted in breast milk; not recommended for use.
Use Cautiously in: Patients with hepatic or renal impairment (dosage reduction recommended if CCr ≤31 ml/min or hepatic function is impaired); OB, Pedi: Safety not established for pregnant women or children <6 mo; Geri: Initiate at lower doses.

Adverse Reactions/Side Effects

CNS: dizziness, drowsiness (significant with doses >10 mg/day), fatigue. **EENT:** pharyngitis. **GI:** dry mouth.

Interactions

Drug-Drug: Additive CNS depression may occur with **alcohol**, **opioid analgesics**, or **sedative/hypnotics**. **Theophylline** may decrease clearance and increase toxicity.

Route/Dosage

PO (Adults and Children >6 yr): 5–10 mg given once or divided twice daily.
PO (Children 2–5 yr): 2.5 mg once daily initially, may be increased to 5 mg once daily or 2.5 mg every 12 hr.
PO (Children 1–2 yr): 2.5 mg once daily; may be increased to 2.5 mg every 12 hr.
PO (Children 6–12 mo): 2.5 once daily.

Renal/Hepatic Impairment

PO (Adults and Children >12 yr): *CCr ≤31 ml/min, hepatic impairment or hemodialysis*—5 mg once daily.
PO (Children 6–11 yr): start therapy at <2.5 mg/day.
PO (Children <6 yr): use not recommended.

Availability

Tablets: 5 mg, 10 mg. **Cost:** 5 mg $76.99/30, 10 mg $75.99/30. **Chewable tablets (grape):** 5 mg, 10 mg. **Cost:** 5 mg $75.99/30, 10 mg $75.99/30. **Syrup (banana-grape flavor):** 1 mg/ml in 120-ml and 480-ml bottles. **Cost:** $41.99/120 ml, $145.97/480 ml. ***In combination with:*** pseudoephedrine (Zyrtec-D 12 Hour) (See Appendix B).

NURSING IMPLICATIONS

Assessment

- Assess allergy symptoms (rhinitis, conjunctivitis, hives) before and periodically during therapy.
- Assess lung sounds and character of bronchial secretions. Maintain fluid intake of 1500–2000 ml/day to decrease viscosity of secretions.
- ***Lab Test Considerations:*** May cause false-negative result in allergy skin testing.

Potential Nursing Diagnoses

Ineffective airway clearance (Indications)
Risk for injury (Adverse Reactions)

Implementation

- Do not confuse Zyrtec (cetirizine) with Zantac (ranitidine) or Zyprexa (olanzapine).
- **PO:** Administer once daily without regard to food.

Patient/Family Teaching

- Instruct patient to take medication as directed.
- May cause dizziness and drowsiness. Caution patient to avoid driving or other activities requiring alertness until response to medication is known.
- Advise patient to avoid taking alcohol or other CNS depressants concurrently with this drug.
- Advise patient that good oral hygiene, frequent rinsing of mouth with water, and sugarless gum or candy may minimize dry mouth. Patient should notify dentist if dry mouth persists >2 wk.
- Instruct patient to contact health care professional if dizziness occurs or if symptoms persist.

Evaluation/Desired Outcomes

- Decrease in allergic symptoms.

cetuximab (se-**tux**-i-mab)
Erbitux

Classification
Therapeutic: antineoplastics
Pharmacologic: monoclonal antibodies

Pregnancy Category C

Indications

Locally or regionally advanced squamous cell carcinoma of the head and neck with radiation. Recurrent or metastatic squamous cell carcinoma of the head and neck progressing after platinum-based therapy. EGFR expressing metastatic colorectal cancer in patients who have not responded to irinotecan and oxaliplatin. Metastatic colorectal cancer (with irinotecan) when tumors express the epidermal growth factor receptor (EGFR) and have not responded or are intolerant to irinotecan alone.

Action

Binds specifically to EGFR thereby preventing the binding of endogenous epidermal growth factor (EGF). This prevents cell growth and differentiation processes. Combination with irinotecan enhances antitumor effects of irinotecan. **Therapeutic Effects:** Decreased tumor growth and spread.

Pharmacokinetics

Absorption: IV administration results in complete bioavailability.
Distribution: Unknown.
Metabolism and Excretion: Unknown.
Half-life: 97–114 hr.

TIME/ACTION PROFILE

ROUTE	ONSET	PEAK	DURATION
IV	unknown	unknown	unknown

Contraindications/Precautions

Contraindicated in: Hypersensitivity to cetuximab or murine (mouse) proteins; OB: Pregnancy or lactation.
Use Cautiously in: Exposure to sunlight (may exacerbate dermatologic toxicity); Pedi: Children (safety not established).

Adverse Reactions/Side Effects

Most adverse reactions reflect combination therapy with irinotecan. **CNS:** malaise, depression, headache, insomnia. **EENT:** conjunctivitis. **Resp:** dyspnea, ↑ cough, interstitial lung disease. **CV:** PULMONARY EMBOLISM. **GI:** abdominal pain, constipation, diarrhea, nausea, vomiting, anorexia, stomatitis. **GU:** renal failure. **Derm:** acneform dermatitis, alopecia, nail disorder, pruritus, skin desquamation. **F and E:** dehydration, hypomagnesemia, peripheral edema. **Hemat:** anemia, leukopenia. **MS:** back pain. **Metab:** weight loss. **Misc:** INFUSION REACTIONS, fever, desquamation of mucosal epithelium.

Interactions

Drug-Drug: None noted.

Route/Dosage

Head & Neck Cancer with Radiation

IV (Adults): 400 mg/m² administered 1 wk prior to initiation of radiation therapy, followed by weekly maintenance doses of 250 mg/m² for the duration of radiation therapy. Complete infusion 1 hr prior to radiation therapy; dose modification recommended for dermatologic toxicity.

Head and Neck Cancer Monotherapy

IV (Adults): 400 mg/m² initial loading dose, followed by weekly maintenance doses of 250 mg/m² until disease progression or unacceptable toxicity; dose modification recommended for dermatologic toxicity.

Colorectal Cancer

IV (Adults): 400 mg/m² initial loading dose, followed by weekly maintenance doses of 250 mg/m²; dose modification recommended for dermatologic toxicity.

Availability

Solution for injection: 2 mg/ml in 50 ml vials.

NURSING IMPLICATIONS

Assessment

- Assess for infusion reaction (rapid onset of airway obstruction [bronchospasm, stridor, hoarseness], urticaria, hypotension) for at least 1 hr following infusion. Longer observation periods may be required for those who experience infusion reactions. Most reactions occur during first dose, but may also occur in later doses. For severe reactions, immediately stop infusion and discontinue cetuximab permanently. Epinephrine, corticosteroids, IV antihistamines, bronchodilators, and oxygen should be available for reactions. Mild to moderate reactions (chills, fever, dyspnea) may be managed by slowing rate of infusion and administration of antihistamines.
- Assess for onset or worsening of pulmonary symptoms. Interrupt therapy to determine nature of symptoms. If interstitial lung disease is confirmed, discontinue cetuximab and treat appropriately.
- Assess for dermatologic toxicities (acneform rash, skin drying and fissuring, inflammatory and infectious sequelae [blepharitis, cheilitis, cellulitis, cyst]). Treat symptomatically. If acneform rash occurs, modify dose of future infusions.
- ***Lab Test Considerations:*** May cause anemia and leukopenia.
- Monitor serum electrolytes periodically during and for at least 8 wks following infusion. May cause hypomagnesemia, hypocalcemia, and hypokalemia; may occur from days to months after initiation of therapy. May require electrolyte replacement.

Potential Nursing Diagnoses

Ineffective breathing pattern (Adverse Reactions)

Impaired skin integrity (Adverse Reactions)

Implementation

- Premedicate with histamine$_1$ antagonist (diphenhydramine 50 mg) 30–60 min prior to first dose; base subsequent administration on presence and severity of infusion reactions.
- Administer through a low protein binding 0.22-micrometer in-line filter placed as proximal to patient as possible. Solution should be clear and colorless and may contain a small amount of white amorphous cetuximab particles. Do not shake or dilute.
- Can be administered via infusion pump or syringe pump. Cetuximab should be piggybacked to the patient's infusion line.
- Observe patient for 1 hr following infusion.

IV Administration

- **Intermittent Infusion:** *For administration via infusion pump:* Draw up volume of a vial using vented spike needle or other transfer device. Transfer to a sterile evacuated container or bag. Repeat with new needle for each vial until calculated volume is in container. Affix infusion line and prime with cetuximab before starting infusion.
- *For administration via syringe pump:* Draw up volume of a vial using sterile syringe attached to an appropriate vented spike needle. Place syringe into syringe driver of a syringe pump and set rate. Connect infusion line and prime with cetuximab. Use a new needle and filter for each vial. ***Diluent:*** Do not dilute.

Concentration: 2 mg/ml. *Rate:* Administer over 2 hr at a rate not to exceed 10 ml/min. Use 0.9% NaCl to flush line at end of infusion.

Patient/Family Teaching

- Explain purpose of cetuximab and potential side effects to patient. Advise patient to report dermatologic changes promptly.
- Caution patient to wear sunscreen and hats and limit sun exposure during therapy.

Evaluation/Desired Outcomes

- Decreased tumor growth and spread.

HIGH ALERT

chloral hydrate

(**klor**-al **hye**-drate)

Aquachloral, ✤Novo-Chlorhydrate, ✤PMS-Chloral Hydrate

Classification

Therapeutic: sedative/hypnotics

Schedule IV

Pregnancy Category C

Indications

Short-term sedative and hypnotic (effectiveness decreases after 2 wk of use). Sedation or reduction of anxiety preoperatively (anesthetic adjunct) or prior to diagnostic procedures.

Action

Converted to trichloroethanol, which is the active drug. Has generalized CNS depressant properties. **Therapeutic Effects:** Sedation or induction of sleep.

Pharmacokinetics

Absorption: Well absorbed following oral or rectal administration.

Distribution: Widely distributed. Crosses the placenta and enters breast milk in low concentrations.

Metabolism and Excretion: Converted by liver to trichloroethanol, which is active. Trichloroethanol is, in turn, metabolized by the liver and kidneys to inactive compounds.

Half-life: *Chloral hydrate*—Infants: 1 hr. *Trichloroethanol*—Neonates: 8.5–66 hr; Children: 10 hr; Adults: 8–11 hr.

TIME/ACTION PROFILE (sedation)

ROUTE	ONSET	PEAK	DURATION
PO	30 min	1 hr	4–8 hr
Rectal	0.5–1 hr	1 hr	4–8 hr

Contraindications/Precautions

Contraindicated in: Hypersensitivity; Severe cardiac disease; Severe renal impairment (ClCr <50 ml/min); Coma or pre-existing CNS depression; Uncontrolled severe pain; OB: Crosses placenta; chronic use during pregnancy may cause withdrawal symptoms in the neonate. Lactation: Excreted in human milk, use by nursing mothers may cause sedation in the infant; Esophagitis, gastritis, or ulcer disease; Proctitis (rectal use); Tartrazine hypersensitivity (some rectal products); Impaired respiratory function; Sleep apnea.

Use Cautiously in: Hepatic dysfunction; History of suicide attempt or substance abuse; Obstructive sleep apnea; Pedi: May cause direct hyperbilirubinemia in neonates; Geri, Pedi: Dosage reduction recommended.

Adverse Reactions/Side Effects

CNS: excess sedation, disorientation, dizziness, hangover, headache, incoordination, irritability, paradoxical excitation (children). **Resp:** respiratory depression. **GI:** diarrhea, nausea, vomiting, flatulence. **Derm:** rashes. **Misc:** tolerance, physical dependence, psychological dependence.

Interactions

Drug-Drug: Additive CNS depression with other **CNS depressants**, including **alcohol**, **antihistamines**, **antidepressants**, **sedative/hypnotics**, and **opioid analgesics**. May potentiate **warfarin**. When given within 24 hr of IV **furosemide**, may cause diaphoresis, changes in blood pressure, and flushing. May increase metabolism and decrease effects of **phenytoin**. May increase toxicity of **ifosfamide** and **cyclophoshamide**.

Drug-Natural Products: Concomitant use of **kava kava**, **valerian**, **skullcap**, **chamomile**, or **hops** can increase CNS depression.

Route/Dosage

PO (Adults): *Hypnotic*—500–1000 mg 15–30 min before bedtime. *Preoperative sedation*—500 mg–1000 mg 30 min before surgery. *Daytime sedation*—250 mg 3 times daily. Single dose/daily dose should not >2 g.

PO (Geriatric Patients): *Hypnotic*—250 mg 15–30 min before bedtime.

Rect (Adults): *Sedation*—325 mg 3 times daily. *Hypnotic*—500–1000 mg. Single dose/daily dose should not >2 g.

PO, Rect (Children >1 month): *Pre-electroencephalogram sedation*—20–25 mg/kg 30–

60 min prior. *Sedation prior to dental/medical procedures*—50–75 mg/kg 30–60 min prior; may repeat within 30 min if needed; single dose should not exceed 1 g total for infants or 2 g total for children). *Hypnotic*—50 mg/kg; maximum 2 g/day. *Sedation/anxiety:* 25–50 mg/kg/day divided q 6–8 hr; maximum 500 mg/dose.

PO, Rect (Neonates): 25 mg/kg/dose prior to a procedure.

Availability (generic available)

Capsules: 500 mg. **Syrup:** 500 mg/5 ml. **Suppositories:** 325 mg, 500 mg.

NURSING IMPLICATIONS

Assessment

- Assess mental status (orientation, mood, behavior) and potential for abuse prior to administering this medication. Prolonged use may lead to physical and psychological dependence. Limit amount of drug available to the patient.
- Assess sleep pattern before and periodically throughout therapy.
- Geri: Assess CNS effects and risk for falls. Institute fall prevention strategies.
- Assess level of consciousness at time of peak effect. Notify physician or other health care professional if desired sedation does not occur or if paradoxical reaction occurs.
- ***Lab Test Considerations:*** Interferes with tests for urinary 17-hydroxycorticosteroids and urinary catecholamines.

Potential Nursing Diagnoses

Insomnia (Indications)
Anxiety (Indications)
Risk for injury (Side Effects)
Ineffective coping (Indications)
Sleep deprivation (Indications)
Risk for falls (Side Effects)
Acute confusion (Side Effects)

Implementation

- ***High Alert:*** **Pedi:** Chloral hydrate overdosage has resulted in fatalities in children. Only accept orders written in milligrams, not volume (teaspoons) or concentration. Chloral hydrate should be administered to children only by trained staff in the health care setting. When administered to children for sedation before outpatient procedures, administer at the facility where procedure is to be performed. Repeated doses should be used with great caution in neonates, as drug and metabolites accumulate and may lead to toxicity. Continue monitoring until level of consciousness is safe for discharge.
- Before administering, reduce external stimuli and provide comfort measures to increase effectiveness of medication.
- Refer for psychotherapy if ineffective coping is basis for sleep pattern disturbance.
- Protect patient from injury. Place bed-side rails up. Assist with ambulation. Remove cigarettes from patients receiving hypnotic dose.
- **PO:** Capsules should be swallowed whole with a full glass of water or juice to minimize gastric irritation; do not chew. Dilute syrup in a half glass of water, juice, ginger ale, or formula to mask taste.
- **Rect:** If suppository is too soft for insertion, chill in refrigerator for 30 min or run under cold water before removing foil wrapper.

Patient/Family Teaching

- Instruct patient to take chloral hydrate exactly as directed. Missed doses should be omitted; do not double doses. If used for 2 wk or longer, abrupt withdrawal may result in CNS excitement, tremor, anxiety, hallucinations, and delirium.
- Chloral hydrate causes drowsiness and dizziness. Caution patient to avoid driving or other activities requiring alertness until response to medication is known.
- Caution patient that concurrent alcohol use may create an additive effect that results in tachycardia, vasodilation, flushing, headache, hypotension, and pronounced CNS depression. Alcohol and other CNS depressants should be avoided while taking chloral hydrate.
- Advise patient to discontinue use and notify health care professional if skin rash, dizziness, irritability, impaired thought processes, headache, or motor incoordination occurs.
- Teach sleep hygiene techniques (dark room, quiet, bedtime ritual, limit daytime napping, avoid nicotine and caffeine).

Evaluation/Desired Outcomes

- Sedation.
- Improvement in sleep pattern.

chlordiazepoxide

(klor-dye-az-e-**pox**-ide)
✤Apo-Chlordiazepoxide, Libritabs, Librium, ✤Mitran, ✤Novopoxide, ✤Poxi

Classification
Therapeutic: antianxiety agents, sedative/hypnotics
Pharmacologic: benzodiazepines

Schedule IV

Pregnancy Category D

Indications
Adjunct management of anxiety. Treatment of alcohol withdrawal. Adjunct management of anxiety associated with acute myocardial infarction.

Action
Acts at many levels of the CNS to produce anxiolytic effect. Depresses the CNS, probably by potentiating GABA, an inhibitory neurotransmitter. **Therapeutic Effects:** Sedation. Relief of anxiety.

Pharmacokinetics
Absorption: Well absorbed from the GI tract. IM absorption may be slow and unpredictable.
Distribution: Widely distributed. Crosses the blood-brain barrier. Crosses the placenta; enters breast milk. Recommend to discontinue drug or bottle feed.
Metabolism and Excretion: Highly metabolized by the liver. Some products of metabolism are active as CNS depressants.
Half-life: 5–30 hr.

TIME/ACTION PROFILE (sedation)

ROUTE	ONSET	PEAK	DURATION
PO	1–2 hr	0.5–4 hr	up to 24 hr
IM	15–30 min	unknown	unknown
IV	1–5 min	unknown	0.25–1 hr

Contraindications/Precautions
Contraindicated in: Hypersensitivity; Some products contain tartrazine and should be avoided in patients with known intolerance; Cross-sensitivity with other benzodiazepines may occur; Comatose patients or those with pre-existing CNS depression; Uncontrolled severe pain; Pulmonary disease; Angle-closure glaucoma; Porphyria; OB, Lactation: May cause CNS depression, flaccidity, feeding difficulties, and weight loss in infants; Pedi: Not for use in children ≤6 yr.
Use Cautiously in: Hepatic dysfunction; Severe renal impairment; History of suicide attempt or substance abuse; Geri: Long-acting benzodiazepines cause prolonged sedation in the elderly. Appears on Beers list and is associated with increased risk of falls (↓ dose required or consider short-acting benzodiazepine); Debilitated patients (initial dose reduction required).

Adverse Reactions/Side Effects
CNS: dizziness, drowsiness, hangover, headache, mental depression, paradoxical excitation, sedation. **EENT:** blurred vision. **GI:** constipation, diarrhea, nausea, vomiting, weight gain. **Derm:** rashes. **Local:** pain at IM site. **Misc:** physical dependence, psychological dependence, tolerance.

Interactions
Drug-Drug: Alcohol, **antidepressants**, **antihistamines**, and **opioid analgesics**—concurrent use results in additive CNS depression. **Cimetidine**, **oral contraceptives**, **disulfiram**, **fluoxetine**, **isoniazid**, **ketoconazole**, **metoprolol**, **propoxyphene**, **propranolol**, or **valproic acid** may enhance effects. May ↓ efficacy of **levodopa**. **Rifampin** or **barbiturates** may ↓ effectiveness of chlordiazepoxide. Sedative effects may be ↓ by **theophylline**.
Drug-Natural Products: Concomitant use of **kava kava**, **valerian**, **chamomile**, or **hops** can ↑ CNS depression.

Route/Dosage
PO (Adults): *Alcohol withdrawal*—50–100 mg, repeated until agitation is controlled (up to 400 mg/day). *Anxiety*—5–25 mg 3–4 times daily.
PO (Geriatric Patients or Debilitated Patients): *Anxiety*—5 mg 2–4 times daily initially, increased as needed.
PO (Children >6 yr): *Anxiety*—5 mg 2–4 times daily, up to 10 mg 2–3 times daily.
IM, IV (Adults): *Alcohol withdrawal*—50–100 mg initially; may be repeated in 2–4 hr. *Anxiety*—50–100 mg initially, then 25–50 mg 3–4 times daily as required (25–50 mg initially in geriatric patients). *Preoperative sedation*—50–100 mg 1 hr preop.
IM, IV (Geriatric Patients or Debilitated Patients): *Anxiety/sedation*—25–50 mg/dose.
IM, IV (Children >12 yr): *Anxiety/sedation*—25–50 mg/dose.

Availability (generic available)

Capsules: 5 mg, 10 mg, 25 mg. **Tablets:** 5 mg, 10 mg, 25 mg. **Injection:** 100-mg ampule. ***In combination with:*** amitriptyline (Limbitrol DS), clidinium (Librax). See Appendix B.

NURSING IMPLICATIONS

Assessment

- Assess for anxiety and level of sedation (ataxia, dizziness, slurred speech) periodically during therapy.
- Assess degree and manifestations of anxiety and mental status (orientation, mood, behavior) prior to and periodically during therapy.
- Monitor blood pressure, heart rate, and respiratory rate frequently when administering parenterally. Report significant changes immediately.
- Prolonged high-dose therapy may lead to psychological or physical dependence. Restrict the amount of drug available to patient.
- Geri: Assess risk of falls and institute fall prevention strategies.
- **Alcohol Withdrawal:** Assess for tremors, agitation, delirium, and hallucinations. Protect patient from injury. Institute seizure precautions.
- Geri: Assess risk of falls and institute fall prevention strategies.
- ***Lab Test Considerations:*** Patients on prolonged therapy should have CBC and liver function tests evaluated periodically. May cause ↑ in serum bilirubin, AST, and ALT.
- May alter results of urine 17-ketosteroids and 17-ketogenic steroids. May cause ↓ response on metyrapone tests and decreased thyroidal uptake of ^{123}I and ^{131}I.
- ***Toxicity and Overdose:*** Flumazenil reverses sedation caused by chlordiazepoxide toxicity or overdose (flumazenil may induce seizures in patients with a history of seizures disorder or who are on tricyclic antidepressants).

Potential Nursing Diagnoses

Anxiety (Indications)
Risk for injury (Side Effects)
Ineffective coping
Dysfunctional family processes: alcoholism

Implementation

- Do not confuse Librium with Librax.
- IV administration is usually the preferred route for parenteral administration because of the slow, erratic absorption after IM administration.
- After parenteral administration, have patient remain recumbent and observe for 3–8 hr or longer, depending on patient's response.
- Equipment to maintain a patent airway should be immediately available when chlordiazepoxide is administered intravenously.
- Use parenteral solution immediately after reconstitution and discard any unused portion.
- **PO:** Administer after meals or with milk to minimize GI irritation. Tablets may be crushed and taken with food or fluids if patient has difficulty swallowing. Administer greater dose at bedtime to avoid daytime sedation. Do not discontinue abruptly; taper by 10 mg every 3 days to reduce chance of withdrawal effects. Some patients may require longer taper period (months). Monitor patients closely with seizure disorder as abrupt withdrawal may precipitate seizures.
- **IM:** Reconstitute only with 2 ml of diluent provided by manufacturer. Do not use solution if opalescent or hazy. Agitate gently to minimize bubbling. Administer slowly, deep into a well-developed muscle mass to minimize pain at injection site. Solution reconstituted with IM diluent should not be given IV.

IV Administration

- **Direct IV:** ***Diluent:*** Reconstitute 100 mg in 5 ml of 0.9% NaCl or sterile water for injection. Do not use IM diluent. ***Concentration:*** 20 mg/ml. ***Rate:*** Administer prescribed dose slowly over at least 1 min. Rapid administration may cause apnea, hypotension, bradycardia, or cardiac arrest.
- **Y-Site Compatibility:** heparin, hydrocortisone sodium succinate, potassium chloride, vitamin B complex with C.

Patient/Family Teaching

- Instruct patient to take chlordiazepoxide as directed. If medication is less effective after a few weeks, check with health care professional; do not increase dose. Medication should be tapered at the completion of long-term therapy. Sudden cessation of medication may lead to withdrawal (insomnia, irritability, nervousness, tremors).

- May cause drowsiness or dizziness. Caution patient to avoid driving or other activities requiring alertness until response to medication is known. Geri: Instruct patient and family how to reduce falls risk at home.
- Advise patient to avoid the use of alcohol and other CNS depressants concurrently with this medication.
- Instruct patient to consult health care professional before taking OTC medications.
- Instruct patient to notify health care professional if pregnancy is planned or suspected.
- Advise patient that benzodiazepines do not cure underlying problems. Psychotherapy is beneficial in addressing source of anxiety and improve coping skills.
- Teach other methods to decrease anxiety, such as: exercise, use of support group (e.g., Alcoholics Anonymous), or relaxation techniques.
- Teach patient not to share medication with anyone.

Evaluation/Desired Outcomes

- Decreased sense of anxiety.
- Increased ability to cope.
- Decreased delirium tremens and more rational ideation when used for alcohol withdrawal.

chlorothiazide, See DIURETICS (THIAZIDE).

chlorpheniramine

(klor-fen-**ir**-a-meen)
Aller-Chlor, Allergy, Chlo-Amine, Chlorate, Chlor-Trimeton, Chlor-Trimeton Allergy 4 Hour, Chlor-Trimeton Allergy 8 Hour, Chlor-Trimeton Allergy 12 Hour, ✤Chlor-Tripolon, ✤Novo-Pheniram, PediaCare Allergy Formula, Phenetron, Telechlor, Teldrin

Classification
Therapeutic: allergy, cold, and cough remedies, antihistamines

Pregnancy Category B

Indications

Relief of allergic symptoms caused by histamine release, including: Nasal allergies, Allergic dermatoses. Management of severe allergic or hypersensitivity reactions, including anaphylaxis and transfusion reactions.

Action

Antagonizes the effects of histamine at H_1-receptor sites; does not bind to or inactivate histamine. **Therapeutic Effects:** Decreased symptoms of histamine excess (sneezing, rhinorrhea, nasal and ocular pruritus, ocular tearing, and redness).

Pharmacokinetics

Absorption: Well absorbed following oral and parenteral administration.
Distribution: Widely distributed. Minimal amounts excreted in breast milk. Crosses the blood-brain barrier.
Metabolism and Excretion: Extensively metabolized by the liver.
Half-life: 12–15 hr.

TIME/ACTION PROFILE (antihistaminic effects)

ROUTE	ONSET	PEAK	DURATION
PO	15–30 min	6 hr	4–12 hr
PO–ER	unknown	unknown	8–24 hr
Subcut	unknown	unknown	4–12 hr
IM	unknown	unknown	4–12 hr
IV	rapid	unknown	4–12 hr

Contraindications/Precautions

Contraindicated in: Hypersensitivity; Acute attacks of asthma; Lactation: Avoid use or use alternative feeding method; Known alcohol intolerance (some liquid forms).
Use Cautiously in: Angle-closure glaucoma; Liver disease; Geri: Appears on Beers list. Geriatric patients are more susceptible to adverse reactions due to anticholinergic effects; OB: Pregnancy (safety not established).

Adverse Reactions/Side Effects

CNS: drowsiness, dizziness, excitation (in children). **EENT:** blurred vision. **CV:** hypertension, arrhythmias, hypotension, palpitations. **GI:** dry mouth, constipation, obstruction. **GU:** retention, urinary hesitancy.

Interactions

Drug-Drug: ↑ CNS depression with other **CNS depressants**, including **alcohol**, **opioid analgesics**, and **sedative/hypnotics**. **MAO inhibitors** intensify and prolong anticholinergic effects of antihistamines. ↑ anticholinergic effects with other **drugs possessing anticholinergic properties**, including **antidepres-**

sants, **atropine**, **haloperidol**, **phenothiazines**, **quinidine**, and **disopyramide**.

Route/Dosage

PO (Adults): 4 mg q 4–6 hr *or* 8–12 mg of extended-release formulation q 8–12 hr (not to exceed 24 mg/day).
PO (Geriatric Patients): 4 mg twice daily *or* 8 mg of extended-release formulation at bedtime.
PO (Children 6–12 yr): 2 mg 3–4 times daily (not to exceed 12 mg/day).

Injectable formulation is available only in Canada

Subcut, IM, IV (Adults): 5–40-mg single dose (not to exceed 40 mg/day).
Subcut (Children): 87.5 mcg (0.0875 mg)/kg or 2.5 mg/m^2 q 6 hr as needed.

Availability (generic available)

Tablets: 4 mg$^{Rx, OTC}$, 8 mg$^{Rx, OTC}$, 12 mg$^{Rx, OTC}$. **Chewable tablets (orange flavor):** 2 mg$^{Rx, OTC}$. **Timed-release tablets:** 8 mg$^{Rx, OTC}$, 12 mg$^{Rx, OTC}$. **Timed-release capsules:** 8 mg$^{Rx, OTC}$, 12 mg$^{Rx, OTC}$. **Syrup:** 1 mg/5 ml$^{Rx, OTC}$, 2 mg/5 ml$^{Rx, OTC}$, ✤2.5 mg/5 ml$^{Rx, OTC}$. **Injection:** 10 mg/ml, 100 mg/ml. ***In combination with:*** Codeine (Codeprex), pseudoephedrine (Advil), and decongestants$^{Rx, OTC}$. See Appendix B.

NURSING IMPLICATIONS

Assessment

- Assess allergy symptoms (rhinitis, conjunctivitis, hives) prior to and periodically during therapy.
- Monitor pulse and blood pressure before initiating and throughout IV therapy.
- Geri: Assess for adverse anticholinergic effects (delirium, acute confusion, dizziness, dry mouth, blurred vision, urinary retention, constipation, tachycardia).
- Assess lung sounds and character of bronchial secretions. Maintain fluid intake of 1500–2000 ml/day to decrease viscosity of secretions.
- ***Lab Test Considerations:*** May cause false-negative reactions on allergy skin tests; discontinue 4 days prior to testing.

Potential Nursing Diagnoses

Ineffective airway clearance (Indications)
Risk for injury (Adverse Reactions)

Implementation

- **PO:** Administer oral doses with food or milk to decrease GI irritation. Extended-release tablets and capsules should be swallowed whole; do not crush, break, or chew. Chewable tablets should not be swallowed whole; chew well before swallowing.
- **Subcut, IM:** The 100-mg/ml solution is recommended for IM or subcut routes only. The 10-mg/ml solution may be used for IM, subcut, or IV.

IV Administration

- **Direct IV:** ***Diluent:*** May be given undiluted. Use only the 10 mg/ml strength for IV administration. ***Concentration:*** 10 mg/ml. ***Rate:*** Administer each 10-mg dose over at least 1 min.

Patient/Family Teaching

- Instruct patient to take chlorpheniramine as directed.
- Geri: Teach patient and family about anticholinergic effects and to contact a health care professional if such effects persist.
- May cause drowsiness. Caution patient to avoid driving or other activities requiring alertness until response to drug is known.
- Caution patient to avoid using alcohol or other CNS depressants concurrently with this drug.
- Advise patient that good oral hygiene, frequent rinsing of mouth with water, and sugarless gum or candy may help relieve dryness of mouth.
- Instruct patient to contact health care professional if symptoms persist.

Evaluation/Desired Outcomes

- Decrease in allergic symptoms.

chlorproMAZINE

(klor-**proe**-ma-zeen)
✤Chlorpromanyl, ✤Largactil, ✤Novo-Chlorpromazine, Thorazine, Thor-Prom

Classification
Therapeutic: antiemetics, antipsychotics
Pharmacologic: phenothiazines

Pregnancy Category UK

Indications

Second-line treatment for schizophrenia and psychoses after failure with atypical antipsychotics. Hyperexcitable, combative behavior in children. Nausea and vomiting. Intractable hiccups. Preoperative sedation. Acute intermittent porphyria. **Unlabeled uses:** Vascular headache. Bipolar disorder.

Action

Alters the effects of dopamine in the CNS. Has significant anticholinergic/alpha-adrenergic blocking activity. **Therapeutic Effects:** Diminished signs/symptoms of psychosis. Relief of nausea/vomiting/intractable hiccups. Decreased symptoms of porphyria.

Pharmacokinetics

Absorption: Variable absorption from tablets/suppositories; better with oral liquid formulations. Well absorbed following IM administration.
Distribution: Widely distributed; high CNS concentrations. Crosses the placenta; enters breast milk.
Protein Binding: ≥90%.
Metabolism and Excretion: Highly metabolized by the liver and GI mucosa. Some metabolites are active.
Half-life: 30 hr.

TIME/ACTION PROFILE (antipsychotic activity, antiemetic activity, sedation)

ROUTE	ONSET	PEAK	DURATION
PO	30–60 min	unknown	4–6 hr
PO–ER	30–60 min	unknown	10–12 hr
Rectal	1–2 hr	unknown	3–4 hr
IM	unknown	unknown	4–8 hr
IV	rapid	unknown	unknown

Contraindications/Precautions

Contraindicated in: Hypersensitivity; Hypersensitivity to sulfites (injectable) or benzyl alcohol (sustained-release capsules); Cross-sensitivity with other phenothiazines may occur; Angle-closure glaucoma; Bone marrow depression; Severe liver/cardiovascular disease; Concurrent pimozide use.
Use Cautiously in: Geriatric/debilitated patients (decrease initial dose); Diabetes; Respiratory disease; Prostatic hyperplasia; CNS tumors; Epilepsy; Intestinal obstruction; OB: Lactation Safety not established. Discontinue drug or bottle feed. Pedi: Children with acute illnesses, infections, gastroenteritis, or dehydration (increased risk of extrapyramidal reactions).

Adverse Reactions/Side Effects

CNS: NEUROLEPTIC MALIGNANT SYNDROME, sedation, extrapyramidal reactions, tardive dyskinesia. **EENT:** blurred vision, dry eyes, lens opacities. **CV:** hypotension (↑ with IM, IV), tachycardia. **GI:** constipation, dry mouth, anorexia, hepatitis, ileus, priapism. **GU:** urinary retention. **Derm:** photosensitivity, pigment changes, rashes. **Endo:** galactorrhea, amenorrhea. **Hemat:** AGRANULOCYTOSIS, leukopenia. **Metab:** hyperthermia. **Misc:** allergic reactions.

Interactions

Drug-Drug: Concurrent use with **pimozide** ↑ the risk of potentially serious cardiovascular reactions. May alter serum **phenytoin** levels. ↓ pressor effect of **norepinephrine** and eliminates bradycardia. Antagonizes peripheral vasoconstriction from **epinephrine** and may reverse some of its actions. May ↓ elimination and ↑ effects of **valproic acid**. May ↓ the pharmacologic effects of **amphetamine** and **related compounds**. May ↓ the effectiveness of **bromocriptine**. May ↑ blood levels and effects of **tricyclic antidepressants**. **Antacids** or **adsorbent antidiarrheals** may ↓ adsorption; administer 1 hr before or 2 hr after chlorpromazine. **Activated charcoal** ↓ absorption. ↑ risk of anticholinergic effects with **antihistamines**, **tricyclic antidepressants**, **quinidine**, or **disopyramide**. Premedication with chlorpromazine ↑ the risk of neuromuscular excitation and hypotension when followed by **barbiturate** anesthesia. **Barbiturates** may ↑ metabolism and ↓ effectiveness. Chlorpromazine may ↓ **barbiturate** blood levels. Additive hypotension with **antihypertensives**. Additive CNS depression with **alcohol**, **antidepressants**, **antihistamines**, **MAO inhibitors**, **opioid analgesics**, **sedative/hypnotics**, or **general anesthetics**. Concurrent use with **lithium** may produce disorientation, unconsciousness, or extrapyramidal symptoms. Concurrent use with **meperidine** may produce excessive sedation and hypotension. May ↑ the risk of seizures with subarachnoid **metrizamide**. Concurrent use with **propranolol** ↑ blood levels of both drugs.
Drug-Natural Products: Concomitant use of **kava kava, valerian, chamomile, or hops can ↑ CNS depression. ↑ anticholinergic effects with angel's trumpet, jimson weed, and scopolia.**

Route/Dosage

PO (Adults): *Psychoses*—10–25 mg 2–4 times daily; may increase every 3–4 days (usual dose is 200 mg/day; up to 1 g/day) *or* 30–300 mg 1–3 times daily as extended-release capsules. *Nausea and vomiting*—10–25 mg q 4 hr as needed. *Preoperative sedation*—25–50 mg 2–3 hr before surgery. *Hiccups/porphyria*—25–50 mg 3–4 times daily.
PO (Children): *Psychoses/nausea and vomiting*—0.55 mg/kg (15 mg/m^2) q 4–6 hr as needed. *Preoperative sedation*—0.55 mg/kg (15 mg/m^2) 2–3 hr before surgery.
Rect (Adults): *Nausea/vomiting*—50–100 mg q 6–8 hr as needed.
Rect (Children >6 mo): 1 mg/kg q 6–8 hr as needed.
IM (Adults): *Severe psychoses*—25–50 mg initially, may be repeated in 1 hr; increase to maximum of 400 mg q 3–12 hr if needed (up to 1 g/day). *Nausea/vomiting*— 25 mg initially, may repeat with 25–50 mg q 3–4 hr as needed. *Nausea/vomiting during surgery*—12.5 mg, may be repeated in 30 min as needed. *Preoperative sedation*—12.5–25 mg 1–2 hr prior to surgery. *Hiccups/tetanus*—25–50 mg 3–4 times daily. *Porphyria*—25 mg q 6–8 hr until patient can take PO.
IM (Children >6 mo): *Psychoses/nausea and vomiting*—0.55 mg/kg (15 mg/m^2) q 6–8 hr (not to exceed 40 mg/day in children 6 mo–5 yr, or 75 mg/day in children 5–12 yr). *Nausea/vomiting during surgery*—0.275 mg/kg, may repeat in 30 min as needed. *Preoperative sedation*—0.55 mg/kg 1–2 hr prior to surgery. *Tetanus*—0.55 mg/kg q 6–8 hr.
IV (Adults): *Nausea/vomiting during surgery*—up to 25 mg. *Hiccups/tetanus*—25–50 mg. *Porphyria*—25 mg q 8 hr.
IV (Children): *Nausea/vomiting during surgery*—0.275 mg/kg. *Tetanus*—0.55 mg/kg.

Availability (generic available)

Tablets: 10 mg, 25 mg, 50 mg, 100 mg, 200 mg. **Sustained-release capsules:** 30 mg, 75 mg, 150 mg, 200 mg, 300 mg. **Syrup (orange custard flavor):** 10 mg/5 ml, ♣25 mg/5 ml, ♣100 mg/5 ml. **Oral concentrate (custard flavor):** 30 mg/ml, ♣40 mg/ml, 100 mg/ml. **Suppositories:** 25 mg, 100 mg. **Injection:** 25 mg/ml.

NURSING IMPLICATIONS

Assessment

- Assess mental status (orientation, mood, behavior) prior to and periodically during therapy.
- Assess weight and BMI initially and throughout therapy.
- Assess fasting blood glucose and cholesterol levels initially and periodically throughout therapy. Refer as appropriate for nutritional/weight and medical management.
- Assess positive (hallucinations, delusions, agitation) and negative (social withdrawal) symptoms of schizophrenia.
- Monitor blood pressure (sitting, standing, lying), pulse, and respiratory rate prior to and frequently during the period of dose adjustment.
- Observe patient carefully when administering medication to ensure medication is actually taken and not hoarded.
- Assess fluid intake and bowel function. Increased bulk and fluids in the diet may help minimize constipation.
- Monitor patient for onset of akathisia (restlessness or desire to keep moving) and extrapyramidal side effects (*parkinsonian*—difficulty speaking or swallowing, loss of balance control, pill rolling of hands, mask-like face, shuffling gait, rigidity, tremors; and *dystonic*—muscle spasms, twisting motions, twitching, inability to move eyes, weakness of arms or legs) every 2 mo during therapy and 8–12 wk after therapy has been discontinued. Notify health care professional if these symptoms occur; reduction in dose or discontinuation may be necessary. Trihexyphenidyl, diphenhydramine, or Benzotropine may be used to control these symptoms. Benzodiazepines may alleviate symptoms of akathisia.
- Monitor for tardive dyskinesia (uncontrolled rhythmic movement of mouth, face, and extremities; lip smacking or puckering; puffing of cheeks; uncontrolled chewing; rapid or worm-like movements of tongue, excessive eye blinking). Report these symptoms immediately; may be irreversible.
- Monitor for development of neuroleptic malignant syndrome (fever, respiratory distress, tachycardia, convulsions, diaphoresis, hypertension or hypotension, pallor, tiredness, se-

vere muscle stiffness, loss of bladder control). Report these symptoms immediately.

- **Preoperative Sedation:** Assess level of anxiety prior to and following administration.
- **Vascular Headache:** Assess type, location, intensity, and duration of pain and accompanying symptoms.
- ***Lab Test Considerations:*** Monitor CBC, liver function tests, and ocular exams periodically throughout therapy. May cause ↓ hematocrit, hemoglobin, leukocytes, granulocytes, platelets. May cause ↑ bilirubin, AST, ALT, and alkaline phosphatase. Agranulocytosis occurs 4–10 wk after initiation of therapy, with recovery 1–2 wk following discontinuation. May recur if medication is restarted. Liver function abnormalities may require discontinuation of therapy. May cause false-positive or false-negative pregnancy tests and false-positive urine bilirubin test results.

Potential Nursing Diagnoses

Disturbed thought process (Indications)
Imbalanced nutrition: risk for more than body requirements (Side Effects)

Implementation

- Do not confuse chlorpromazine with chlorpropamide or prochlorperazine.
- Keep patient recumbent for at least 30 min following parenteral administration to minimize hypotensive effects.
- To prevent contact dermatitis, avoid getting solution on hands.
- Phenothiazines should be discontinued 48 hr before and not resumed for 24 hr following metrizamide myelography, because they lower the seizure threshold.
- **Hiccups:** Initial treatment is with oral doses. If hiccups persist 2–3 days, IM injection may be used, followed by IV infusion.
- **PO:** Administer oral doses with food, milk, or a full glass of water to minimize gastric irritation. Tablets may be crushed. Do not open capsules; swallow whole. Sustained-release capsules may be opened but contents should not be chewed. Dilute concentrate just prior to administration in 120 ml of coffee, tea, tomato or fruit juice, milk, water, soup, or carbonated beverages.
- **Rect:** If suppository is too soft for insertion, chill in refrigerator for 30 min or run under cold water before removing foil wrapper.
- **IM:** Do not inject subcut. Inject slowly into deep, well-developed muscle. May be diluted with 0.9% NaCl or 2% procaine. Lemon-yellow color does not alter potency of solution. Do not administer solution that is markedly discolored or contains a precipitate.

IV Administration

- **Direct IV:** ***Diluent:*** Dilute with 0.9% NaCl. ***Concentration:*** Do not exceed 1 mg/ml. ***Rate:*** Inject slowly at a rate of at least 1 mg/min for adults and 0.5 mg/min for children.
- **Continuous Infusion:** ***Diluent:*** May further dilute 25–50 mg in 500–1000 ml of D5W, D10W, 0.45% NaCl, 0.9% NaCl, Ringer's or lactated Ringer's injection, dextrose/Ringer's or dextrose/lactated Ringer's combinations.
- **Syringe Compatibility:** atropine, benztropine, butorphanol, diphenhydramine, doxapram, droperidol, fentanyl, glycopyrrolate, hydromorphone, hydroxyzine, meperidine, metoclopramide, midazolam, morphine, pentazocine, scopolamine.
- **Syringe Incompatibility:** cimetidine, heparin, pantoprazole, pentobarbital, thiopental.
- **Y-Site Compatibility:** Amsacrine, cisatracurium, cisplatin, cladribine, cyclophosphamide, cytarabine, dexmedetomidine, docetaxel, doxorubicin, doxorubicin liposome, famotidine, filgrastim, fluconazole, gemcitabine, granisetron, heparin, hydrocortisone sodium succinate, ondansetron, oxaliplatin, potassium chloride, propofol, teniposide, thiotepa, vinorelbine, vitamin B complex with C.
- **Y-Site Incompatibility:** allopurinol, amifostine, amphotericin B cholesteryl sulfate complex, aztreonam, bivalirudin, cefepime, etoposide phosphate, fludarabine, furosemide, lansoprazole, linezolid, melphalan, methotrexate, paclitaxel, pemetrexed, piperacillin/tazobactam, sargramostim.

Patient/Family Teaching

- Advise patient to take medication as directed and not to skip doses or double up on missed doses. If a dose is missed, take within 1 hr or omit dose and return to regular schedule. Abrupt withdrawal may lead to gastritis, nausea, vomiting, dizziness, headache, tachycardia, and insomnia.
- Inform patient of possibility of extrapyramidal symptoms and tardive dyskinesia. Instruct patient to report these symptoms immediately to health care professional.
- Advise patient to change positions slowly to minimize orthostatic hypotension.
- Medication may cause drowsiness. Caution patient to avoid driving or other activities re-

quiring alertness until response to the medication is known.
- Caution patient to avoid taking alcohol or other CNS depressants concurrently with this medication.
- Advise patient to use sunscreen and protective clothing when exposed to the sun. Exposed surfaces may develop a temporary pigment change (ranging from yellow-brown to grayish purple). Extremes of temperature (exercise, hot weather, hot baths or showers) should also be avoided, because this drug impairs body temperature regulation.
- Instruct patient to use frequent mouth rinses, good oral hygiene, and sugarless gum or candy to minimize dry mouth. Consult health care professional if dry mouth continues for >2 wk.
- Advise patient not to take chlorpromazine within 2 hr of antacids or antidiarrheal medication.
- Inform patient that this medication may turn urine a pink-to-reddish-brown color.
- Advise patient to notify health care professional of medication regimen prior to treatment or surgery.
- Instruct patient to notify health care professional promptly if sore throat, fever, unusual bleeding or bruising, rash, weakness, tremors, visual disturbances, dark-colored urine, or clay-colored stools occur.
- Emphasize the importance of routine follow-up exams to monitor response to medication and detect side effects. Encourage continued participation in psychotherapy as indicated.
- Treatment is not a cure since symptoms can recur after discontinuation of medication.

Evaluation/Desired Outcomes
- Decrease in excitable, manic behavior. Therapeutic effects may not be seen for 7–8 wk.
- Relief of nausea and vomiting.
- Relief of hiccups.
- Preoperative sedation.
- Management of porphyria.
- Relief of vascular headache.
- Decrease in positive (hallucinations, delusions, agitation) symptoms of schizophrenia.

chlorthalidone, See DIURETICS (THIAZIDE).

C

chlorzoxazone
(klor-**zox**-a-zohn)
EZE-DS, Paraflex, Parafon Forte DSC, Relaxazone, Remular, Remular-S, Strifon Forte DSC

Classification
Therapeutic: skeletal muscle relaxants (centrally acting)

Pregnancy Category UK

Indications
Adjunct to rest and physical therapy in the treatment of muscle spasm associated with acute painful musculoskeletal conditions.

Action
Skeletal muscle relaxation, probably due to CNS depression. **Therapeutic Effects:** Skeletal muscle relaxation with decreased discomfort.

Pharmacokinetics
Absorption: Readily absorbed after oral administration.
Distribution: Unknown.
Metabolism and Excretion: Mostly metabolized by the liver; <1% excreted unchanged in urine.
Half-life: 1.1 hr.

TIME/ACTION PROFILE (skeletal muscle effects)

ROUTE	ONSET	PEAK	DURATION
PO	within 1 hr	1–2 hr	3–4 hr

Contraindications/Precautions
Contraindicated in: Hypersensitivity; Porphyria.
Use Cautiously in: Underlying cardiovascular disease; Impaired renal or hepatic function; OB, Lactation, Pedi: Safety not established; Geri: Appears on Beers list. Poorly tolerated due to anticholinergic effects.

Adverse Reactions/Side Effects
CNS: dizziness, drowsiness. **GI:** GI BLEEDING, constipation, diarrhea, heartburn, nausea, vomiting. **Derm:** allergic dermatitis. **Hemat:** AGRANULOCYTOSIS, anemia. **Misc:** allergic reactions including ANGIOEDEMA.

Interactions
Drug-Drug: Increased risk of CNS depression with other **CNS depressants**, including **alco-**

hol, **antihistamines**, **antidepressants**, **sedative/hypnotics**, or **opioid analgesics**.
Drug-Natural Products: Concomitant use of **kava kava**, **valerian**, **skullcap**, **chamomile**, or **hops** can increase CNS depression.

Route/Dosage

PO (Adults): 250–750 mg 3–4 times daily.
PO (Children): 20 mg/kg or 600 mg/m²/day in 3–4 divided doses.

Availability (generic available)

Tablets: 250 mg, 500 mg. **Cost:** *250-mg generic*—$29.86/100; *500 mg Parafon Forte DSC*—$126.84/100; *generic*—$102.96/100.

NURSING IMPLICATIONS

Assessment

- Assess patient for pain, muscle stiffness, and range of motion before and periodically throughout therapy.
- Geri: Assess geriatric patients for anticholinergic effects (sedation and weakness).

Potential Nursing Diagnoses

Acute pain (Indications)
Impaired physical mobility (Indications)
Risk for injury (Side Effects)

Implementation

- **PO:** May be administered with meals to minimize gastric irritation. Tablets may be crushed and mixed with food or liquid for ease of administration.

Patient/Family Teaching

- Instruct patient to take medication exactly as directed; do not take more than the prescribed amount. Missed doses should be taken within 1 hr of time ordered; otherwise, omit and return to normal dosage schedule. Do not double doses.
- Medication may cause drowsiness and dizziness. Caution patient to avoid driving or other activities requiring alertness until response to drug is known.
- Advise patient to avoid concurrent use of alcohol or other CNS depressants with this medication.
- If constipation becomes a problem, advise patient that increasing fluid intake and bulk in diet and stool softeners may alleviate this condition.

Evaluation/Desired Outcomes

- Relief of muscular spasm in acute skeletal muscle conditions.

cholecalciferol, See VITAMIN D COMPOUNDS.

cholestyramine

(koe-less-**tear**-a-meen)
LoCHOLEST, LoCHOLEST Light, Prevalite, Questran, Questran Light

Classification
Therapeutic: lipid-lowering agents
Pharmacologic: bile acid sequestrants

Pregnancy Category C

Indications

Management of primary hypercholesterolemia. Pruritus associated with elevated levels of bile acids. **Unlabeled uses:** Diarrhea associated with excess bile acids.

Action

Bind bile acids in the GI tract, forming an insoluble complex. Result is increased clearance of cholesterol. **Therapeutic Effects:** Decreased plasma cholesterol and low-density lipoproteins (LDLs). Decreased pruritus.

Pharmacokinetics

Absorption: Action takes place in the GI tract. No absorption occurs.
Distribution: No distribution.
Metabolism and Excretion: After binding bile acids, insoluble complex is eliminated in the feces.
Half-life: Unknown.

TIME/ACTION PROFILE (hypocholesterolemic effects)

ROUTE	ONSET	PEAK	DURATION
PO	24–48 hr	1–3 wk	2–4 wk

Contraindications/Precautions

Contraindicated in: Hypersensitivity; Complete biliary obstruction; Some products contain aspartame and should be avoided in patients with phenylketonuria.
Use Cautiously in: History of constipation.
Exercise Extreme Caution in: Children (may cause intestinal obstruction; deaths have occurred).

Adverse Reactions/Side Effects

EENT: irritation of the tongue. **GI:** abdominal discomfort, constipation, nausea, fecal impaction, flatulence, hemorrhoids, perianal irritation, steatorrhea, vomiting. **Derm:** irritation, rashes. **F and E:** hyperchloremic acidosis. **Metab:** vitamin A, D, and K deficiency.

Interactions

Drug-Drug: May decrease absorption/effects of orally administered **acetaminophen**, **amiodarone**, **clindamycin**, **clofibrate**, **digoxin**, **diuretics**, **gemfibrozil**, **glipizide**, **corticosteroids**, **imipramine**, **mycophenolate**, **methotrexate**, **methyldopa**, **niacin**, **NSAIDs**, **penicillin**, **phenytoin**, **phosphates**, **propranolol**, **tetracyclines**, **tolbutamide**, **thyroid preparations**, **ursodiol**, **warfarin**, and **fat-soluble vitamins (A, D, E, and K)**. May decrease absorption of other **orally administered medications**.

Route/Dosage

PO (Adults): 4 g 1–2 times daily (initially, may be increased as needed/tolerated up to 24 g/day in 6 divided doses).
PO (Children): 240 mg/kg/day in 2–3 divided doses (not >8 g/day).

Availability (generic available)

Powder for suspension with aspartame (strawberry flavor [LoCHOLEST], unflavored [Prevalite, Questran Light]): 4 g cholestyramine/packet or scoop. **Powder for suspension (strawberry flavor [LoCHOLEST], unflavored [Questran, generic]):** 4 g cholestyramine/packet or scoop.

NURSING IMPLICATIONS

Assessment

- **Hypercholesterolemia:** Obtain a diet history, especially in regard to fat consumption.
- **Pruritus:** Assess severity of itching and skin integrity. Dose may be decreased when relief of pruritus occurs.
- **Diarrhea:** Assess frequency, amount, and consistency of stools.
- ***Lab Test Considerations:*** Serum cholesterol and triglyceride levels should be evaluated before initiating, frequently during first few months and periodically throughout therapy. Discontinue medication if paradoxical increase in cholesterol level occurs.
- May cause an increase in AST, ALT, phosphorus, chloride, and alkaline phosphatase and a decrease in serum calcium, sodium, and potassium levels.
- May also cause prolonged prothrombin times.

Potential Nursing Diagnoses

Constipation (Side Effects)
Noncompliance (Patient/Family Teaching)

Implementation

- Parenteral or water-miscible forms of fat-soluble vitamins (A, D, and K) and folic acid may be ordered for patients on chronic therapy.
- **PO:** Administer before meals.
- Scoops for powdered preparations may not be exchangable between products.
- Administer other medications 1 hr before or 4–6 hr after the administration of this medication.

Patient/Family Teaching

- Instruct patient to take medication exactly as directed; do not skip doses or double up on missed doses.
- Instruct patient to take medication before meals. Mix cholestyramine with 4–6 oz water, milk, fruit juice, or other noncarbonated beverages. Shake vigorously. Slowly stir in a large glass. Rinse glass with small amount of additional beverage to ensure all medication is taken. May also mix with highly fluid soups, cereals, or pulpy fruits (applesauce, crushed pineapple). Allow powder to sit on fluid and hydrate for 1–2 min before mixing. Do not take dry. Variations in the color of cholestyramine do not alter stability.
- Advise patient that this medication should be used in conjunction with dietary restrictions (fat, cholesterol, carbohydrates, alcohol), exercise, and cessation of smoking.
- Explain that constipation may occur. Increase in fluids and bulk in diet, exercise, stool softeners, and laxatives may be required to minimize the constipating effects. Instruct patient to notify health care professional if constipation, nausea, flatulence, and heartburn persist or if stools become frothy and foul smelling.
- Advise patient to notify health care professional if unusual bleeding or bruising; petechiae; or black, tarry stools occur. Treatment with vitamin K may be necessary.

Evaluation/Desired Outcomes

- Decrease in serum low-density lipoprotein cholesterol levels. Therapy is usually discontinued if the clinical response remains poor after 3 mo of therapy.
- Decrease in severity of pruritus. Relief usually occurs 1–3 wk after therapy is initiated.
- Decrease in frequency and severity of diarrhea.

choline, See SALICYLATES.

ciclesonide, See CORTICOSTEROIDS (NASAL).

ciclopirox, See ANTIFUNGALS (TOPICAL).

cidofovir (sye-doe-**foe**-veer)

Vistide

Classification
Therapeutic: antivirals

Pregnancy Category C

Indications

Management of cytomegalovirus (CMV) retinitis in HIV-infected patients (with probenecid).

Action

Suppresses replication of CMV by inhibiting viral DNA synthesis. **Therapeutic Effects:** Slows progression of CMV retinitis; may not be curative.

Pharmacokinetics

Absorption: IV administration results in complete bioavailability.
Distribution: Unknown.
Metabolism and Excretion: Excreted mostly unchanged by the kidneys.
Half-life: Unknown.

TIME/ACTION PROFILE

ROUTE	ONSET	PEAK	DURATION
IV	rapid	end of infusion	unknown

Contraindications/Precautions

Contraindicated in: Hypersensitivity to cidofovir, probenecid, or sulfonamides; Serum Cr >1.5 mg/dl, CCr ≤55 ml/min, or urine protein ≥100 mg/dl (≥2+ proteinuria); Concurrent use of foscarnet, amphotericin B, aminoglycoside anti-infectives, NSAIDs, or IV pentamidine.
Use Cautiously in: Pregnancy or children (safety not established); breastfeeding is not recommended in HIV-positive patients.
Exercise Extreme Caution in: Any condition or medication that increases the risk of dehydration.

Adverse Reactions/Side Effects

CNS: headache, weakness. **EENT:** decreased intraocular pressure, hearing loss, iritis, ocular hypotony, uveitis. **Resp:** dyspnea, pneumonia. **GI:** HEPATIC DYSFUNCTION, PANCREATITIS, abdominal pain, nausea, vomiting, anorexia, diarrhea. **GU:** RENAL FAILURE, proteinuria. **Derm:** alopecia, rash. **F and E:** decreased serum bicarbonate. **Hemat:** neutropenia, anemia. **Metab:** METABOLIC ACIDOSIS. **Misc:** chills, fever, infection.

Interactions

Drug-Drug: ↑ risk of nephrotoxicity with **aminoglycosides**, **amphotericin B**, **foscarnet**, and **pentamidine** and should be avoided; wait 7 days after giving other nephrotoxic agents. **Probenecid**, which is required concurrently, may interact with **acetaminophen**, **acyclovir**, **ACE inhibitors**, **barbiturates**, **benzodiazepines**, **bumetanide**, **methotrexate**, **famotidine**, **furosemide**, **NSAIDs**, **theophylline**, and **zidovudine**.

Route/Dosage

IV (Adults): 5 mg/kg once weekly for 2 wk, followed by 5 mg/kg every 2 wk (must be given with probenecid).

Renal Impairment

IV (Adults): *Increase in serum creatinine of 0.3–0.4 mg/dL*—decrease dose to 3 mg/kg; discontinue if serum creatinine increases ≥0.5 mg/dL over baseline.

Availability

Solution for injection: 75 mg/ml in 5-ml ampules.

NURSING IMPLICATIONS

Assessment

- Monitor vision for progression of CMV retinitis. Monitor ocular symptoms, intraocular pressure, and visual acuity periodically.
- Antiemetics and administration after a meal may minimize nausea and vomiting associated with probenecid. If allergic reactions occur in association with probenecid, pretreat-

ment with antihistamines or acetaminophen should be considered.

- Monitor vital signs periodically. May cause fever, hypotension, and tachycardia. Monitor patients for early signs and symptoms of infection.
- ***Lab Test Considerations:*** Renal function, measured by serum Cr and urine protein, must be monitored within 48 hr before each dose and throughout cidofovir therapy. In patients with proteinuria, administer IV hydration and repeat urine protein test. If renal function deteriorates, dose modification or temporary discontinuation should be considered.
- Monitor WBC before each dose. Granulocytopenia may occur.
- May cause hyperglycemia, hyperlipemia, hypocalcemia, hypokalemia, and elevated alkaline phosphatase, AST, and ALT.

Potential Nursing Diagnoses

Risk for infection (Indications)

Implementation

- Probenecid and saline prehydration must be given with cidofovir to minimize renal toxicity. *Probenecid* must be administered 2 g orally given 3 hr before, then 1 g given 2 hr and 8 hr after completion of cidofovir infusion. *Saline prehydration* with 1 L of 0.9% NaCl must be given over 1–2 hr before cidofovir. A second liter over 1–3 hr is recommended concurrently with or after cidofovir.
- Patients receiving foscarnet, amphotericin B, aminoglycoside, NSAIDs, or IV pentamidine should wait at least 7 days after these agents to begin cidofovir.

IV Administration

- **Intermittent Infusion:** ***Diluent:*** Dilute in 100 mL of 0.9% NaCl. Solution is stable for 24 hr if refrigerated. Allow refrigerated solution to return to room temperature before administration. ***Rate:*** Administer over 1 hr.
- **Additive Incompatibility:** Information unavailable. Do not admix with other solutions or medications.

Patient/Family Teaching

- Inform patient that cidofovir is not a cure for CMV retinitis and that retinitis may continue to progress during and after therapy.
- Inform patient that concurrent antiretroviral therapy may be continued. However, zidovudine therapy should be temporarily discontinued or decreased by 50% on the days of cidofovir therapy because of the effects of probenecid on zidovudine.
- Advise patient of the possibility of renal toxicity from cidofovir. Emphasize the importance of routine lab tests to monitor renal function.
- Inform patient that cidofovir may have teratogenic effects. Women should use contraception during and for 1 mo after therapy. Men should use barrier contraception during and for 3 mo after therapy.
- Discuss with patient the possibility of hair loss. Explore coping strategies.
- Advise patients to have routine ophthalmologic exams after cidofovir therapy.

Evaluation/Desired Outcomes

- Decrease in symptoms and arrest of progression of CMV retinitis in HIV-infected patients.

cilostazol (sil-**os**-tah-zol)

Pletal

Classification

Therapeutic: antiplatelet agents

Pharmacologic: platelet aggregation inhibitors

Pregnancy Category C

Indications

Reduction of the symptoms of intermittent claudication as measured by increased walking distance.

Action

Inhibits the enzyme cyclic adenosine monophosphate (cAMP) phosphodiesterase III (PDE III), which results in increased cAMP in platelets and blood vessels, producing inhibition of platelet aggregation and vasodilation. **Therapeutic Effects:** Reduced symptoms of intermittent claudication with improved walking distance.

Pharmacokinetics

Absorption: Slowly absorbed after oral administration.

Distribution: Unknown.

Protein Binding: 95–98% bound to plasma proteins; one active metabolite is 97.4% bound, the other is 66% bound.
Metabolism and Excretion: Extensively metabolized by the liver, two metabolites have platelet aggregation inhibitory activity; metabolites are mostly excreted by the kidneys.
Half-life: *Cilostazol and its active metabolites*—11–13 hr.

TIME/ACTION PROFILE (symptom reduction)

ROUTE	ONSET	PEAK	DURATION
PO	2–4 wk	up to 12 wk	unknown

Contraindications/Precautions
Contraindicated in: Hypersensitivity; CHF; OB: Potential for congenital defects, stillbirth, and low birth weight; Lactation: Potential risk to nursing infants; discontinue or bottle feed.
Use Cautiously in: Pedi: Safety not established.

Adverse Reactions/Side Effects
CNS: headache, dizziness. **CV:** palpitations, tachycardia. **GI:** diarrhea.

Interactions
Drug-Drug: Concurrent administration of **ketoconazole**, **itraconazole**, **erythromycin**, **diltiazem**, **fluconazole**, **miconazole**, **fluvoxamine**, **fluoxetine**, **nefazodone**, **sertraline**, or **omeprazole** decreases metabolism and increases levels and activity of cilostazol (use lower doses). Concurrent use with **aspirin** has additive effects on platelet function.
Drug-Food: Grapefruit juice inhibits metabolism and increases effects; concurrent use should be avoided.

Route/Dosage
PO (Adults): 100 mg twice daily (50 mg twice daily if receiving inhibitors of cilostazol metabolism).

Availability (generic available)
Tablets: 50 mg, 100 mg.

NURSING IMPLICATIONS

Assessment
- Assess patient for intermittent claudication before and periodically during therapy.
- ***Lab Test Considerations:*** May occasionally cause anemia, hyperlipemia, hyperuricemia, and albuminuria. May prolong bleeding time.

Potential Nursing Diagnoses
Activity intolerance (Indications)

Implementation
- **PO:** Administer on an empty stomach, 1 hr before or 2 hr after meals.
- Do not administer with grapefruit juice. May increase cilostazol levels.

Patient/Family Teaching
- Instruct patient to take cilostazol on an empty stomach, exactly as directed.
- May cause dizziness. Caution patient to avoid driving or other activities requiring alertness until response to medication is known.
- Advise patient to avoid smoking; nicotine constricts blood vessels.

Evaluation/Desired Outcomes
- Relief from cramping in calf muscles, buttocks, thighs, and feet during exercise.
- Improvement in walking endurance. Therapeutic effects may be seen in 2–4 wk.

cimetidine, See HISTAMINE H_2 ANTAGONISTS.

ciprofloxacin, See FLUOROQUINOLONES.

HIGH ALERT

cisplatin (sis-pla-tin)
♣Platinol, Platinol-AQ

Classification
Therapeutic: antineoplastics
Pharmacologic: alkylating agents

Pregnancy Category D

Indications
Metastatic testicular and ovarian carcinoma. Advanced bladder cancer. Head and neck cancer. Cervical cancer. Lung cancer. Other tumors.

Action
Inhibits DNA synthesis by producing cross-linking of parent DNA strands (cell-cycle phase–nonspecific). **Therapeutic Effects:** Death of rapidly replicating cells, particularly malignant ones.

Pharmacokinetics
Absorption: IV administration results in complete bioavailability.
Distribution: Widely distributed; accumulates for months; enters breast milk.

Metabolism and Excretion: Excreted mainly by the kidneys.
Half-life: 30–100 hr.

TIME/ACTION PROFILE (effects on blood counts)

ROUTE	ONSET	PEAK	DURATION
IV	unknown	18–23 days	39 days

Contraindications/Precautions

Contraindicated in: Hypersensitivity; Pregnancy or lactation.
Use Cautiously in: Hearing loss; Renal impairment (dosage ↓ recommended); CHF; Electrolyte abnormalities; Active infections; Bone marrow depression; Geriatric patients (↑ risk of nephrotoxicity, peripheral neuropathy); Chronic debilitating illnesses; Patients with childbearing potential.

Adverse Reactions/Side Effects

CNS: SEIZURES, malaise, weakness. **EENT:** ototoxicity, tinnitus. **GI:** severe nausea, vomiting, diarrhea, hepatotoxicity. **GU:** nephrotoxicity, sterility. **Derm:** alopecia. **F and E:** hypocalcemia, hypokalemia, hypomagnesemia. **Hemat:** LEUKOPENIA, THROMBOCYTOPENIA, anemia. **Local:** phlebitis at IV site. **Metab:** hyperuricemia. **Neuro:** peripheral neuropathy. **Misc:** anaphylactoid reactions.

Interactions

Drug-Drug: ↑ nephrotoxicity and ototoxicity with other **nephrotoxic** and **ototoxic drugs (aminoglycosides, loop diuretics)**. ↑ risk of hypokalemia and hypomagnesemia with **loop diuretics** and **amphotericin B**. May ↓ **phenytoin** levels. ↑ bone marrow depression with other **antineoplastics** or **radiation therapy**. May ↓ antibody response to **live-virus vaccines** and ↑ adverse reactions.

Route/Dosage

Other regimens are used.
IV (Adults): *Metastatic testicular tumors*—20 mg/m^2 daily for 5 days repeated q 3–4 wk. *Metastatic ovarian cancer*—75–100 mg/m^2, repeat q 4 wk in combination with cyclophosphamide *or* 100 mg/m^2 q 3 wk if used as a single agent. *Advanced bladder cancer*—50–70 mg/m^2 q 3–4 wk as a single agent.

Availability (generic available)

Powder for injection: 10-mg, 50-mg vials.
Injection: 1 mg/ml in 50- and 100-mg vials.

NURSING IMPLICATIONS

Assessment

- Monitor vital signs frequently during administration. Report significant changes.
- Monitor intake and output and specific gravity frequently during therapy. Report discrepancies immediately. To reduce the risk of nephrotoxicity, maintain a urinary output of at least 100 ml/hr for 4 hr before initiating and for at least 24 hr after administration.
- Encourage patient to drink 2000–3000 ml/day to promote excretion of uric acid. Allopurinol and alkalinization of the urine may be used to help prevent uric acid nephropathy.
- Assess patency of IV site frequently during therapy. Cisplatin may cause severe irritation and necrosis of tissue if extravasation occurs. If a large amount of highly concentrated cisplatin solution extravasates, mix 4 ml of 10% sodium thiosulfate with 6 ml of sterile water or 1.6 ml of 25% sodium thiosulfate with 8.4 ml of sterile water and inject 1–4 ml (1 ml for each ml extravasated) through existing line or cannula. Inject subcut if needle has been removed. Sodium thiosulfate inactivates cisplatin.
- Severe and protracted nausea and vomiting usually occur 1–4 hr after a dose; vomiting may last for 24 hr. Administer parenteral antiemetic agents 30–45 min before therapy and routinely around the clock for the next 24 hr. Monitor amount of emesis and notify health care professional if emesis exceeds guidelines to prevent dehydration. Nausea and anorexia may persist for up to 1 wk.
- Monitor for bone marrow depression. Assess for bleeding (bleeding gums, bruising, petechiae, stools, urine, and emesis) and avoid IM injections and taking rectal temperatures if platelet count is low. Apply pressure to venipuncture sites for 10 min. Assess for signs of infection during neutropenia. Anemia may occur. Monitor for increased fatigue, dyspnea, and orthostatic hypotension.
- Monitor for signs of anaphylaxis (facial edema, wheezing, dizziness, fainting, tachycardia, hypotension). Discontinue medication

immediately and report symptoms. Epinephrine and resuscitation equipment should be readily available.

- Medication may cause ototoxicity and neurotoxicity. Assess patient frequently for dizziness, tinnitus, hearing loss, loss of coordination, loss of taste, or numbness and tingling of extremities; may be irreversible. Notify health care professional promptly if these occur. Audiometry should be performed before initiation of therapy and before subsequent doses. Hearing loss is more frequent with children and usually occurs first with high frequencies and may be unilateral or bilateral.
- Monitor for inadvertent cisplatin overdose. Doses >100 mg/m²/cycle once every 3–4 wk are rarely used. Differentiate daily doses from total dose/cycle. Symptoms of high cumulative doses include muscle cramps (localized, painful involuntary skeletal muscle contractions of sudden onset and short duration) and are usually associated with advanced stages of peripheral neuropathy.
- ***Lab Test Considerations:*** Monitor CBC with differential and platelet count before and routinely throughout therapy. The nadir of leukopenia, thrombocytopenia, and anemia occurs within 18–23 days and recovery 39 days after a dose. Withhold further doses until WBC is >4000/mm³ and platelet count is >100,000/mm³.
- Monitor BUN, serum creatinine, and CCr before initiation of therapy and before each course of cisplatin to detect nephrotoxicity. May cause ↑ BUN and creatinine and ↓ calcium, magnesium, phosphate, sodium, and potassium levels that usually occur the 2nd wk after a dose. Do not administer additional doses until BUN is <25 mg/100 ml and serum creatinine is <1.5 mg/100 ml. May cause ↑ uric acid level, which usually peaks 3–5 days after a dose.
- May cause transiently ↑ serum bilirubin and AST concentrations.
- May cause positive Coombs' test result.

Potential Nursing Diagnoses

Risk for infection (Adverse Reactions)
Risk for injury (Side Effects)

Implementation

- ***High Alert:*** Fatalities have occurred with chemotherapeutic agents. Before administering, clarify all ambiguous orders; double-check single, daily, and course-of-therapy dose limits; have second practitioner independently double-check original order, calculations, and infusion pump settings. Do not confuse with carboplatin. To prevent confusion, orders should include generic and brand names. Administer under the supervision of a physician experienced in the use of cancer chemotherapeutic agents.
- Solution should be prepared in a biologic cabinet. Wear gloves, gown, and mask while handling medication. If powder or solution comes in contact with skin or mucosa, wash thoroughly with soap and water. Discard equipment in specially designated containers (see Appendix K).
- Hydrate patient with at least 1–2 L of IV fluid 8–12 hr before initiating therapy with cisplatin. Amifostine may be administered to minimize nephrotoxicity.
- Do not use aluminum needles or equipment during preparation or administration. Aluminum reacts with this drug, forms a black or brown precipitate, and renders the drug ineffective.
- Unopened vials of powder and constituted solution must not be refrigerated.

IV Administration

- **Intermittent Infusion:** Reconstitute 10-mg vials with 10 ml of sterile water for injection and 50-mg vial with 50 ml. Stable for 20 hr if reconstituted with sterile water, for 72 hr with bacteriostatic water. Do not refrigerate, because crystals will form. Solution should be clear and colorless; discard if turbid or if it contains precipitates
- ***Diluent:*** Dilution in 2 L of 5% dextrose in 0.3% or 0.45% NaCl containing 37.5 g of mannitol is recommended. ***Concentration:*** Keep under 0.5 mg/ml to prevent tissue necrosis. ***Rate:*** Variable. Maximum rate 1 mg/min.
- **Continuous Infusion:** Has been administered as continuous infusion over 24 hr to 5 days with resultant decrease in nausea and vomiting. ***High Alert:*** Clarify dose to ensure cumulative dosage is not confused with daily dose; errors may be fatal.
- **Syringe Compatibility:** bleomycin, cyclophosphamide, doxapram, doxorubicin, droperidol, fluorouracil, furosemide, heparin, leucovorin calcium, methotrexate, metoclopramide, mitomycin, vinblastine, vincristine.
- **Y-Site Compatibility:** allopurinol, aztreonam, bleomycin, chlorpromazine, cimeti-

dine, cladribine, cyclophosphamide, dexamethasone, diphenhydramine, doxorubicin, doxorubicin liposome, droperidol, etoposide, famotidine, filgrastim, fludarabine, fluorouracil, furosemide, ganciclovir, gemcitabine, granisetron, heparin, hydromorphone, leucovorin calcium, linezolid, lorazepam, melphalan, methotrexate, methylprednisolone, metoclopramide, mitomycin, morphine, ondansetron, paclitaxel, palonosetron, pemetrexed, prochlorperazine edisylate, promethazine, propofol, ranitidine, sargramostim, teniposide, topotecan, vinblastine, vincristine, vinorelbine.

- **Y-Site Incompatibility:** amifostine, amphotericin B cholesteryl sulfate, cefepime, lansoprazole, piperacillin/tazobactam, thiotepa.
- **Additive Compatibility:** etoposide, floxuridine, ifosfamide, leucovorin calcium, magnesium sulfate, mannitol, ondansetron, 0.9% NaCl, D5/0.9% NaCl.
- **Additive Incompatibility:** fluorouracil, mesna, thiotepa.

Patient/Family Teaching

- Instruct patient to report pain at injection site immediately.
- Instruct patient to notify health care professional promptly if fever; chills; cough; hoarseness; sore throat; signs of infection; lower back or side pain; painful or difficult urination; bleeding gums; bruising; petechiae; blood in stools, urine, or emesis; increased fatigue; dyspnea; or orthostatic hypotension occurs. Caution patient to avoid crowds and persons with known infections. Instruct patient to use soft toothbrush and electric razor and to avoid falls. Caution patient not to drink alcoholic beverages or take medication containing aspirin or NSAIDs; may precipitate gastric bleeding.
- Instruct patient to report promptly any numbness or tingling in extremities or face, difficulty with hearing or tinnitus, unusual swelling, or joint pain.
- Instruct patient not to receive any vaccinations without advice of health care professional.
- Advise patient of the need for contraception, although cisplatin may cause infertility.
- Emphasize the need for periodic lab tests to monitor for side effects.

Evaluation/Desired Outcomes

- Decrease in size or spread of malignancies. Therapy should not be administered more frequently than every 3–4 wk, and only if lab values are within acceptable parameters and patient is not exhibiting signs of ototoxicity or other serious adverse effects.

C

citalopram (si-**tal**-oh-pram)

Celexa

Classification

Therapeutic: antidepressants

Pharmacologic: selective serotonin reuptake inhibitors (SSRIs)

Pregnancy Category C

Indications

Depression. **Unlabeled uses:** Premenstrual dysphoric disorder (PMDD). Obsessive-compulsive discorder (OCD). Panic disorder. Generalized anxiety disorder (GAD). Post-traumatic stress disorder (PTSD). Social anxiety disorder (social phobia).

Action

Selectively inhibits the reuptake of serotonin in the CNS. **Therapeutic Effects:** Antidepressant action.

Pharmacokinetics

Absorption: 80% absorbed after oral administration.

Distribution: Enters breast milk.

Metabolism and Excretion: Mostly metabolized by the liver (10% by CYP3A4 and 2C19 enzymes); excreted unchanged in urine.

Half-life: 35 hr.

TIME/ACTION PROFILE (antidepressant effect)

ROUTE	ONSET	PEAK	DURATION
PO	1–4 wk	unknown	unknown

Contraindications/Precautions

Contraindicated in: Hypersensitivity; Concurrent MAO inhibitor or pimozide therapy.

Use Cautiously in: History of mania; History of suicide attempt/ideation (↑ risk during early therapy and during dose adjustment); History of seizure disorder; Illnesses or conditions that are likely to result in altered metabolism or hemodynamic responses; Severe renal or hepatic impairment; OB: Use during third trimester may result in neonatal serotonin syndrome requiring prolonged hospitalization, respiratory and nutritional support; Lactation: Citalopram is present in breast milk and may result in lethargy with ↓ feeding in infants; weigh risk/benefits; Pedi: May ↑ risk of suicide attempt/ideation especially during early treatment or dose adjustment in children/adolescents (unlabeled for pediatric use); Geri: ↓ doses recommended.

Adverse Reactions/Side Effects

CNS: apathy, confusion, drowsiness, insomnia, weakness, agitation, amnesia, anxiety, decreased libido, dizziness, fatigue, impaired concentration, increased depression, migraine headache, suicide attempt. **EENT:** abnormal accommodation. **Resp:** cough. **CV:** postural hypotension, tachycardia. **GI:** abdominal pain, anorexia, diarrhea, dry mouth, dyspepsia, flatulence, increased saliva, nausea, altered taste, increased appetite, vomiting. **GU:** amenorrhea, dysmenorrhea, ejaculatory delay, erectile dysfunction, polyuria. **Derm:** increased sweating, photosensitivity, pruritus, rash. **Metab:** decreased weight, increased weight. **MS:** arthralgia, myalgia. **Neuro:** tremor, paresthesia. **Misc:** fever, yawning.

Interactions

Drug-Drug: May cause serious, potentially fatal reactions when used with **MAO inhibitors**; allow at least 14 days between citalopram and **MAO inhibitors**. Concurrent use with **pimozide** may result in prolongation of the QTc interval and is contraindicated. Use cautiously with other **centrally acting drugs** (including **alcohol**, **antihistamines**, **opioid analgesics**, and **sedative/hypnotics**; concurrent use with **alcohol** is not recommended). **Cimetidine** ↑ blood levels of citalopram. Serotonergic effects may be ↑ by **lithium** (concurrent use should be carefully monitored). **Ketoconazole**, **itraconazole**, **erythromycin**, and **omeprazole** may ↑ blood levels. **Carbamazepine** may ↓ blood levels. May ↑ blood levels of **metoprolol**. Concurrent use with **tricyclic antidepressants** should be undertaken with caution because of altered pharmacokinetics. Concurrent use with **5-HT$_1$ agonists** used for migraine headaches may ↑ risk of adverse reactions (weakness, hyperreflexia, incoordination). Use cautiously with **tricyclic antidepressants** due to unpredictable effects on serotonin and norepinephrine reuptake. Risk of bleeding may be ↑ with **aspirin**, **NSAIDs**, **warfarin**, **thrombolytics**, and other **agents affecting coagulation and platelet function**.

Drug-Natural Products: ↑ risk of serotonergic side effects including serotonin syndrome with **St. John's wort** and **SAMe**.

Route/Dosage

PO (Adults): 20 mg once daily initially, may be increased by 20 mg/day at weekly intervals, up to 60 mg/day (usual dose is 40 mg/day).

PO (Geriatric Patients): 20 mg once daily initially, may be increased to 40 mg/day only in nonresponding patients.

Hepatic Impairment

PO (Adults): 20 mg once daily initially, may be increased to 40 mg/day only in nonresponding patients.

Availability (generic available)

Tablets: 10 mg, 20 mg, 40 mg. **Cost:** *Generic*—10 mg $89.97/90, 20 mg $89.97/90, 40 mg $89.97/90. **Oral solution (peppermint flavor):** 10 mg/5 ml. **Cost:** *Generic*—10 mg/5 ml $114.00/240 ml.

NURSING IMPLICATIONS

Assessment

- Monitor mood changes during therapy.
- Assess for suicidal tendencies, especially during early therapy and dose changes. Restrict amount of drug available to patient.
- Assess for sexual dysfunction (erectile dysfunction; decreased libido).

Potential Nursing Diagnoses

Ineffective coping (Indications)
Risk for injury (Side Effects)

Implementation

- Do not confuse with Celebrex (celecoxib), Cerebyx (fosphenytoin), Zyprexa (olanzapine), or Lexapro (escitalopram).
- **PO:** Administer as a single dose in the morning or evening without regard to food.

Patient/Family Teaching

- Instruct patient to take citalopram as directed.
- May cause drowsiness, dizziness, impaired concentration, and blurred vision. Caution patient to avoid driving and other activities requiring alertness until response to the drug is known.
- Advise patient to avoid alcohol or other CNS depressant drugs during therapy and to con-

sult health care professional before taking other medications with citalopram.

- Caution patient to change positions slowly to minimize dizziness.
- Advise patient to use sunscreen and wear protective clothing to prevent photosensitivity reactions.
- Inform patient that frequent mouth rinses, good oral hygiene, and sugarless gum or candy may minimize dry mouth. If dry mouth persists for more than 2 wk, consult health care professional regarding use of saliva substitute.
- Instruct female patients to inform health care professional if pregnancy is planned or suspected, or if they plan to breastfeed an infant. If used during pregnancy should be tapered during third trimester to avoid neontal serotinin syndrome.
- Caution patients that citalopram should not be used for at least 14 days after discontinuing MAO inhibitors, and at least 14 days should be allowed after stopping citalopram before starting an MAO inhibitor.
- Emphasize the importance of follow-up exams to monitor progress. Encourage patient participation in psychotherapy to improve coping skills.
- Refer patient/family to local support group.

Evaluation/Desired Outcomes

- Increased sense of well-being.
- Renewed interest in surroundings. May require 1–4 wk of therapy to obtain antidepressant effects.

clarithromycin

(kla-**rith**-roe-mye-sin)
Biaxin, Biaxin XL

Classification
Therapeutic: agents for atypical mycobacterium, anti-infectives, antiulcer agents
Pharmacologic: macrolides

Pregnancy Category C

Indications

Respiratory tract infections including streptococcal pharyngitis, sinusitis, bronchitis, and pneumonia. Treatment (with ethambutol) and prevention of disseminated *Mycobacterium avium* complex (MAC). Treatment of following pediatric infections: Otitis media, Sinusitis, Pharyngitis, Skin/skin structure infections. Part of a combination regimen for ulcer disease due to *Helicobacter pylori*. Endocarditis prophylaxis.

Action

Inhibits protein synthesis at the level of the 50S bacterial ribosome. **Therapeutic Effects:** Bacteriostatic action. **Spectrum:** Active against these gram-positive aerobic bacteria: *Staphylococcus aureus*, *Streptococcus pneumoniae*, *Streptococcus pyogenes* (group A strep). Active against these gram-negative aerobic bacteria: *Haemophilus influenzae*, *Moraxella catarrhalis*. Also active against: *Mycoplasma*, *Legionella*, *H. pylori*, *M. avium*.

Pharmacokinetics

Absorption: Rapidly absorbed (50%) after oral administration.
Distribution: Widely distributed; tissue levels may exceed those in serum.
Protein Binding: 65–70%.
Metabolism and Excretion: 10–15% converted by the liver to 14-hydroxyclarithromycin, which has anti-infective activity; 20–30% excreted unchanged in urine. Metabolized by and also inhibits the CYP3A enzyme system.
Half-life: Dose-dependent and prolonged with renal dysfunction *250-mg dose*—3–4 hr; *500-mg dose*—5–7 hr.

TIME/ACTION PROFILE (serum levels)

ROUTE	ONSET	PEAK	DURATION
PO	unknown	2 hr	12 hr
PO-XL	unknown	4 hr	24 hr

Contraindications/Precautions

Contraindicated in: Hypersensitivity to clarithromycin, erythromycin, or other macrolide anti-infectives; Concurrent use of pimozide; OB: Avoid use during pregnancy unless no alternatives are available; Lactation: Not recommended for breastfeeding women.
Use Cautiously in: Severe liver or renal impairment (dose adjustment required if CCr <30 ml/min).

Adverse Reactions/Side Effects

CNS: headache. **Derm:** pruritus, rash, Stevens-Johnson syndrome. **GI:** PSEUDOMEMBRANOUS COLITIS, abdominal pain/discomfort, abnormal taste, diarrhea, dyspepsia, nausea.

Interactions

Drug-Drug: Clarithromycin is an inhibitor of the CYP3A enzyme system. Concurrent use with other agents metabolized by this system can ↑ levels and risk of toxicity. May prolong the QT interval and ↑ risk of arrhythmias with **pimozide**; concurrent use is contraindicated. Similar effects may occur with antiarrhythmics; ECG should be monitored for QTc prolongation and serum levels monitored. May ↑ serum levels and the risk of toxicity from **carbamazepine**, some **benzodiazepines (midazolam, triazolam, alprazolam)**, **cyclosporine**, **buspirone**, **disopyramide**, **ergot alkaloids**, **felodipine**, **omeprazole**, **tacrolimus**, **digoxin**, or **theophylline**. **Ritonavir** ↑ increases blood levels (↓ clarithromycin dose in patients with CC <60 ml/min). ↑ levels of **HMG-CoA reductase inhibitors** and may ↑ risk of rhabdomyolysis. May ↑ effect of **warfarin** and **sildenafil** (dose reduction may be warranted). May ↑ or ↓ effects of **zidovudine**. Blood levels are ↑ by **delavirdine** and **fluconazole**. Blood levels may be ↓ by **rifampin** and **rifabutin**. ↑ risk of colchicine toxicity when administered with **colchicine**, especially in the elderly.

Route/Dosage

PO (Adults): *Pharyngitis/tonsillitis*—250 mg q 12 hr for 10 days; *Acute maxillary sinusitis*—500 mg q 12 hr for 14 days or 1000 mg once daily for 14 days as XL tablets; *Acute exacerbation of chronic bronchitis*—250–500 mg q 12 hr for 7–14 days or 1000 mg once daily for 7 days as XL tablets; *Community-Acquired pneumonia*—250 mg q 12 hr for 7–14 days or 1000 mg once daily for 7 days as XL tablets; *skin/skin structure infections*—250 mg q 12 hr for 7–14 days; *H. pylori*—500 mg 2–3 times daily with a proton pump inhibitor (lansoprazole or omeprazole) or ranitidine with or without amoxicillin for 10–14 days; *Endocarditis prophylaxis*—500 mg 1 hr before procedure; *MAC prophylaxis/treatment*—500 mg twice daily, for active infection another antimycobacterial is required.

PO (Children): *Most infections*—15 mg/kg/day divided q 12 hr for 7–14 days (up to 500 mg/dose for MAC). *Endocarditis prophylaxis*—15 mg/kg 1 hr before procedure.

Renal Impairment

PO (Adults): *CCr <30 ml/min*—250 mg 1-2 times daily, a 500-mg initial dose may be used.

PO (Children): *CCr <30 ml/min*—decrease dose by 50% or double dosing interval.

Availability (generic available)

Tablets: 250 mg, 500 mg. **Cost:** *Generic*—250 mg $73.32/20, 500 mg $73.32/20. **Extended-release tablets:** 500 mg. **Cost:** $109.99/20. **Oral suspension (fruit punch and vanilla flavors):** 125 mg/5 ml, 250 mg/5 ml. **Cost:** *Generic*—125 mg/5 ml $39.98/100 ml, 250 mg/5 ml $71.38/100 ml. ***In combination with:*** amoxicillin and lansoprazole as part of a compliance package (Prevpac); See Appendix B.

NURSING IMPLICATIONS

Assessment

- Assess patient for infection (vital signs; appearance of wound, sputum, urine, and stool; WBC) at beginning of and during therapy.
- Obtain specimens for culture and sensitivity before initiating therapy. First dose may be given before receiving results.
- **Ulcers:** Assess patient for epigastric or abdominal pain and frank or occult blood in the stool, emesis, or gastric aspirate.
- ***Lab Test Considerations:*** May rarely cause ↑ serum AST, ALT, and alkaline phosphatase concentrations.
- May occasionally cause ↑ BUN.

Potential Nursing Diagnoses

Risk for infection (Indications, Side Effects)
Noncompliance (Patient/Family Teaching)

Implementation

- **PO:** Administer around the clock, without regard to meals. Food slows but does not decrease the extent of absorption.
- Administer XL tablets with food or milk; do not crush, break, or chew.
- Shake suspension well before administration. Store suspension at room temperature; do not refrigerate.
- Do not administer within 4 hr of zidovudine.

Patient/Family Teaching

- Instruct patient to take medication around the clock and to finish the drug completely as directed, even if feeling better. Take missed doses as soon as possible, unless almost time for next dose. Do not double doses. Advise

patient that sharing of this medication may be dangerous.
- Advise patient to report the signs of superinfection (black, furry overgrowth on the tongue; vaginal itching or discharge; loose or foul-smelling stools).
- Instruct patient to notify health care professional if fever and diarrhea develop, especially if stool contains blood, pus, or mucus. Advise patient not to treat diarrhea without consulting health care professional.
- Caution patients taking zidovudine that clarithromycin and zidovudine must be taken at least 4 hr apart.
- Advise patient to notify health care professional if pregnancy is planned or suspected.
- Instruct the patient to notify health care professional if symptoms do not improve within a few days.

Evaluation/Desired Outcomes
- Resolution of the signs and symptoms of infection. Length of time for complete resolution depends on the organism and site of infection.
- Treatment of ulcers.
- Endocarditis prophylaxis.

clindamycin (klin-da-**mye**-sin)
Cleocin, Cleocin T, Clinda-Derm, Clindagel, Clindesse, ClindaMax, Clindets, C/T/S, ♣Dalacin C, ♣Dalacin T, Evoclin

Classification
Therapeutic: anti-infectives

Pregnancy Category B

Indications
PO, IM, IV: Treatment of: Skin and skin structure infections, Respiratory tract infections, Septicemia, Intra-abdominal infections, Gynecologic infections, Osteomyelitis, Endocarditis prophylaxis. **Topical:** Severe acne. **Vag:** Bacterial vaginosis. **Unlabeled uses: PO, IM, IV:** Treatment of *Pneumocystis carinii* pneumonia, CNS toxoplasmosis, and babesiosis.

Action
Inhibits protein synthesis in susceptible bacteria at the level of the 50S ribosome. **Therapeutic Effects:** Bactericidal or bacteriostatic, depending on susceptibility and concentration. **Spectrum:** Active against most gram-positive aerobic cocci, including: Staphylococci, *Streptococcus pneumoniae*, Other streptococci, but not enterococci. Has good activity against those anaerobic bacteria that cause bacterial vaginosis, including *Bacteroides fragilis*, *Gardnerella vaginalis*, *Mobiluncus* spp, *Mycoplasma hominis*, and *Corynebacterium*. Also active against *P. carinii* and *Toxoplasma gondii*.

Pharmacokinetics
Absorption: Well absorbed following PO/IM administration. Minimal absorption following topical/vaginal use.
Distribution: Widely distributed. Does not significantly cross blood-brain barrier. Crosses the placenta; enters breast milk.
Protein Binding: 94%.
Metabolism and Excretion: Mostly metabolized by the liver.
Half-life: Neonates: 3.6–8.7 hr; Infants up to 1 yr: 3 hr; Children and adults: 2–3 hr.

TIME/ACTION PROFILE (blood levels)

ROUTE	ONSET	PEAK	DURATION
PO	rapid	60 min	6–8 hr
IM	rapid	1–3 hr	6–8 hr
IV	rapid	end of infusion	6–8 hr

Contraindications/Precautions
Contraindicated in: Hypersensitivity; Previous pseudomembranous colitis; Severe liver impairment; Diarrhea; Known alcohol intolerance (topical solution, suspension).
Use Cautiously in: OB: Safety not established for systemic and topical; vaginal approved for use in 3rd trimester of pregnancy. Lactation: Has been used safely but does appear in breast milk and exposes infant to drug and its side effects.

Adverse Reactions/Side Effects
CNS: dizziness, headache, vertigo. **CV:** arrhythmias, hypotension. **GI:** PSEUDOMEMBRANOUS COLITIS, diarrhea, bitter taste (IV only), nausea, vomiting. **Derm:** rashes. **Local:** phlebitis at IV site.

Interactions
Drug-Drug: Kaolin/pectin may ↓ GI absorption. May enhance the neuromuscular blocking action of other **neuromuscular blocking agents**. **Topical:** Concurrent use

♣ = Canadian drug name.
*CAPITALS indicates life-threatening; underlines indicate most frequent.

with **irritants**, **abrasives**, or **desquamating agents** may result in additive irritation.

Route/Dosage

PO (Adults): *Most infections*—150–450 mg q 6 hr. *P. carinii pneumonia*—1200–1800 mg/day in divided doses with 15–30 mg primaquine/day (unlabeled). *CNS toxoplasmosis*—1200–2400 mg/day in divided doses with pyrimethamine 50–100 mg/day (unlabeled); *Bacterial endocarditis prophylaxis*—600 mg 1 hr before procedure.

PO (Children >1 mo): 10–30 mg/kg/day divided q 6–8 hr; maximum dose 1.8 g/day. *Bacterial endocarditis prophylaxis*—20 mg/kg 1 hr before procedure.

IM, IV (Adults): *Most infections*—300–600 mg q 6–8 hr *or* 900 mg q 8 hr (up to 4.8 g/day IV has been used; single IM doses of >600 mg are not recommended). *P. carinii pneumonia*—2400–2700 mg/day in divided doses with primaquine (unlabeled). *Toxoplasmosis*—1200–4800 mg/day in divided doses with pyrimethamine. *Bacterial endocarditis prophylaxis*—600 mg 30 min before procedure.

IM, IV (Children >1 mo): 25–40 mg/kg/day divided q 6–8 hr; maximum dose: 4.8 g/day. *Bacterial endocarditis prophylaxis*—20 mg/kg 30 min before procedure; maximum dose: 600 mg.

IM, IV (Infants <1 mo and <2 kg): 5 mg/kg q 8–12 hr *≥2 kg*—20–30 mg/kg/day divided q 6–8 hr.

Vag (Adults and Adolescents): *Cleocin, Clindamax*— 1 applicatorful (5 g) q hs for 3 or 7 days (7 days in pregnant patients); *Clindesse*— one applicatorful (5 g) single dose *or* 1 suppository (100 mg) at bedtime for 3 nights.

Topical (Adults and Adolescents): *Solution*—1% solution/suspension applied twice daily (range 1–4 times daily). *Foam, gel*—1% foam or gel applied once daily.

Availability (generic available)

Capsules: 75 mg, 150 mg, 300 mg. **Oral suspension:** 75 mg/5 ml. **Injection:** 150 mg/ml. **Premixed infusion:** 300 mg/50 ml, 600 mg/50 ml, 900 mg/50 ml. **Topical:** 1% lotion, gel, foam, solution, suspension, single-use applicators. ***In combination with:*** benzoyl peroxide (BenzaClin); (see Appendix B). **Vaginal cream:** 2% cream. **Vaginal suppositories (ovules):** 100 mg. ***In combination with:*** tretinoin (Ziana); (see Appendix B).

NURSING IMPLICATIONS

Assessment

- Assess for infection (vital signs; appearance of wound, sputum, urine, and stool; WBC) at beginning of and during therapy.
- Obtain specimens for culture and sensitivity prior to initiating therapy. First dose may be given before receiving results.
- Monitor bowel elimination. Diarrhea, abdominal cramping, fever, and bloody stools should be reported to health care professional promptly as a sign of pseudomembranous colitis. This may begin up to several weeks following the cessation of therapy.
- Assess patient for hypersensitivity (skin rash, urticaria).
- ***Lab Test Considerations:*** Monitor CBC; may cause transient ↓ in leukocytes, eosinophils, and platelets.
- May cause ↑ alkaline phosphatase, bilirubin, CPK, AST, and ALT concentrations.

Potential Nursing Diagnoses

Risk for infection (Indications, Side Effects)
Diarrhea (Side Effects)

Implementation

- **PO:** Administer with a full glass of water. May be given with or without meals. Shake liquid preparations well. Do not refrigerate. Stable for 14 days at room temperature.
- **IM:** Do not administer >600 mg in a single IM injection.

IV Administration

- **Intermittent Infusion:** ***Diluent:*** Vials must be diluted before use. Dilute a dose of 300 mg or 600 mg in 50 ml and a dose of 900 mg or 1200 mg in 100 ml. Compatible diluents include D5W, 0.9% NaCl, D5/0.9% NaCl, D5/0.45% NaCl, or LR. Admixed solution stable for 16 days at room temperature. Premixed infusion is already diluted and ready to use. ***Concentration:*** Not to exceed 18 mg/ml. ***Rate:*** Not to exceed 30 mg/min. Hypotension and cardiopulmonary arrest have been reported following rapid IV administration.
- **Y-Site Compatibility:** acyclovir, amifostine, amikacin, aminophylline, amiodarone, amphotericin B cholesteryl sulfate, amsacrine, anakinra, anidulafungin, atropine, aztreonam, bumetanide, bivalirudin, calcium chloride, calcium gluconate, cefazolin, cefotaxime, cefoxitin, ceftazidime, ceftizoxime, cefuroxime, chloramphenicol, cimetidine,

cisatracurium, cyclosporine, daptomycin, dexamethasone sodium phosphate, dexmedetomidine, digoxin, diltiazem, diphenhydramine, docetaxel, dopamine, doxorubicin liposome, doxycycline, enalaprilat, epinephrine, esmolol, etoposide phosphate, famotidine, fenoldopam, fentanyl, fludarabine, foscarnet, furosemide, gentamicin, granisetron, heparin, hydrocortisone sodium succinate, hydromorphone, imipenem/cilastatin, insulin, isoproterenol, ketorolac, labetalol, levofloxacin, lidocaine, linezolid, lorazepam, magnesium sulfate, melphalan, meperidine, methylprednisolone sodium succinate, metoclopramide, metoprolol, metronidazole, midazolam, milrinone, morphine, multivitamins, nafcillin, nicardipine, nitroglycerin, nitroprusside, norepinephrine, ondansetron, palonosetron, pantoprazole, pemetrexed, penicillin G potassium, perphenazine, phenylephrine, phytonadione, piperacillin/tazobactam, potassium chloride, procainamide, propofol, propranolol, protamine, ranitidine, remifentanil, sargramostim, sodium bicarbonate, tacrolimus, teniposide, theophylline, thiotepa, ticarcillin/clavulanate, tirofiban, tobramycin, vancomycin, vasopressin, verapamil, vinorelbine, vitamin B complex with C, voriconazole, zidovudine.

- **Y-Site Incompatibility:** allopurinol, azithromycin, caspofungin, ceftriaxone, diazepam, filgrastim, fluconazole, ganciclovir, haloperidol, hydroxyzine, idarubicin, lansoprazole, phenytoin, prochlorperazine, promethazine, quinupristin/dalfopristin, trimethoprim/sulfamethoxazole.
- **Vag:** Applicators are supplied for vaginal administration. When treating bacterial vaginosis, concurrent treatment of male partner is not usually necessary.
- **Topical:** Contact with eyes, mucous membranes, and open cuts should be avoided during topical application. If accidental contact occurs, rinse with copious amounts of cool water.
- Wash affected areas with warm water and soap, rinse, and pat dry prior to application. Apply to entire affected area.

Patient/Family Teaching

- Instruct patient to take medication around the clock at evenly spaced times and to finish the drug completely as directed, even if feeling better. Take missed doses as soon as possible unless almost time for next dose. Do not double doses. Advise patient that sharing of this medication may be dangerous.
- Instruct patient to notify health care professional immediately if diarrhea, abdominal cramping, fever, or bloody stools occur and not to treat with antidiarrheals without consulting health care professional.
- Advise patient to report signs of superinfection (furry overgrowth on the tongue, vaginal or anal itching or discharge).
- Notify health care professional if no improvement within a few days.
- Patients with a history of rheumatic heart disease or valve replacement need to be taught the importance of antimicrobial prophylaxis before invasive medical or dental procedures.
- **IV:** Inform patient that bitter taste occurring with IV administration is not clinically significant.
- **Vag:** Instruct patient on proper use of vaginal applicator. Insert high into vagina at bedtime. Instruct patient to remain recumbent for at least 30 min following insertion. Advise patient to use sanitary napkin to prevent staining of clothing or bedding. Continue therapy during menstrual period.
- Advise patient to refrain from vaginal sexual intercourse during treatment.
- Caution patient that mineral oil in clindamycin cream may weaken latex or rubber contraceptive devices. Such products should not be used within 72 hr of vaginal cream.
- **Topical:** Caution patient applying topical clindamycin that solution is flammable (vehicle is isopropyl alcohol). Avoid application while smoking or near heat or flame.
- Advise patient to notify health care professional if excessive drying of skin occurs.
- Advise patient to wait 30 min after washing or shaving area before applying.

Evaluation/Desired Outcomes

- Resolution of the signs and symptoms of infection. Length of time for complete resolution depends on the organism and site of infection.
- Endocarditis prophylaxis.

- Improvement in acne vulgaris lesions. Improvement should be seen in 6 wk but may take 8–12 wk for maximum benefit.

clobetasol, See CORTICOSTEROIDS (TOPICAL/LOCAL).

clocortolone, See CORTICOSTEROIDS (TOPICAL/LOCAL).

clonazepam (kloe-na-ze-pam)

Klonopin, ✤Rivotril, ✤Syn-Clonazepam

Classification
Therapeutic: anticonvulsants
Pharmacologic: benzodiazepines

Schedule IV

Pregnancy Category C

Indications

Prophylaxis of: Petit mal, Petit mal variant, Akinetic, Myoclonic seizures. Panic disorder with or without agoraphobia. **Unlabeled uses:** Uncontrolled leg movements during sleep. Neuralgias. Sedation. Adjunct management of acute mania, acute psychosis, or insomnia.

Action

Anticonvulsant effects may be due to presynaptic inhibition. Produces sedative effects in the CNS, probably by stimulating inhibitory GABA receptors. **Therapeutic Effects:** Prevention of seizures. Decreased manifestations of panic disorder.

Pharmacokinetics

Absorption: Well absorbed from the GI tract.
Distribution: Probably crosses the blood-brain barrier and the placenta.
Metabolism and Excretion: Mostly metabolized by the liver.
Half-life: 18–50 hr.

TIME/ACTION PROFILE (anticonvulsant activity)

ROUTE	ONSET	PEAK	DURATION
PO	20–60 min	1–2 hr	6–12 hr

Contraindications/Precautions

Contraindicated in: Hypersensitivity to clonazepam or other benzodiazepines; Severe liver disease.

Use Cautiously in: Angle-closure glaucoma; Obstructive sleep apnea; Chronic respiratory disease; History of porphyria; Do not discontinue abruptly; OB: Safety not established; chronic use during pregnancy may result in withdrawal in the neonate; Lactation: May enter breast milk; discontinue drug or bottle feed; Pedi: Safety not established; Geri: May experience excessive sedation at usual doses; decreased dosage recommended.

Adverse Reactions/Side Effects

CNS: behavioral changes, drowsiness, fatigue, slurred speech, ataxia, sedation, abnormal eye movements, diplopia, nystagmus. **Resp:** increased secretions. **CV:** palpitations. **GI:** constipation, diarrhea, hepatitis, weight gain. **GU:** dysuria, nocturia, urinary retention. **Hemat:** anemia, eosinophilia, leukopenia, thrombocytopenia. **Neuro:** ataxia, hypotonia. **Misc:** fever, physical dependence, psychological dependence, tolerance.

Interactions

Drug-Drug: Alcohol, **antidepressants**, **antihistamines**, other **benzodiazepines**, and **opioid analgesics**—concurrent use results in ↑ CNS depression. **Cimetidine**, **hormonal contraceptives**, **disulfiram**, **fluoxetine**, **isoniazid**, **ketoconazole**, **metoprolol**, **propoxyphene**, **propranolol**, or **valproic acid** may ↓ metabolism of clonazepam, ↑ its actions. May ↓ efficacy of **levodopa**. **Rifampin** or **barbiturates** may ↑ metabolism and ↓ effectiveness of clonazepam. Sedative effects may be ↓ by **theophylline**. May ↑ serum **phenytoin** levels. **Phenytoin** may ↓ serum clonazepam levels.
Drug-Natural Products: Concomitant use of **kava kava**, **valerian**, or **chamomile** can increase CNS depression.

Route/Dosage

PO (Adults): 0.5 mg 3 times daily; may increase by 0.5–1 mg q 3rd day. Total daily maintenance dose not to exceed 20 mg. *Panic disorder*—0.125 mg twice daily; increase after 3 days toward target dose of 1 mg/day (some patients may require up to 4 mg/day).
PO (Children <10 yr or 30 kg): Initial daily dose 0.01–0.03 mg/kg/day (not to exceed 0.05 mg/kg/day) given in 2–3 equally divided doses; increase by no more than 0.25–0.5 mg q 3rd day until therapeutic blood levels are reached (not to exceed 0.2 mg/kg/day).

Availability (generic available)

Tablets: 0.5 mg, 1 mg, 2 mg. **Cost:** *Generic*—0.5 mg $29.99/100, 1 mg $29.99/100, 2 mg $26.66/100. **Orally-disintegrating tablets:** 0.125 mg, 0.25 mg, 0.5 mg, 1 mg, 2 mg. **Cost:** *Generic*—0.125 mg $69.99/60, 0.25 mg $72.99/60, 0.5 mg $70.99/60, 2 mg $100.00/60.

NURSING IMPLICATIONS

Assessment

- Observe and record intensity, duration, and location of seizure activity.
- Assess degree and manifestations of anxiety and mental status (orientation, mood, behavior) prior to and periodically during therapy.
- Assess need for continued treatment regularly.
- Assess patient for drowsiness, unsteadiness, and clumsiness. These symptoms are dose related and most severe during initial therapy; may decrease in severity or disappear with continued or long-term therapy.
- ***Lab Test Considerations:*** Patients on prolonged therapy should have CBC and liver function test results evaluated periodically. May cause an ↑ in serum bilirubin, AST, and ALT.
- May cause ↓ thyroidal uptake of sodium iodide, ^{123}I, and ^{131}I.
- ***Toxicity and Overdose:*** Therapeutic serum concentrations are 20–80 mg/ml. Flumazenil antagonizes clonazepam toxicity or overdose (may induce seizures in patients with history of seizure disorder or who are on tricyclic antidepressants).

Potential Nursing Diagnoses

Risk for injury (Indications, Side Effects)

Implementation

- Do not confuse clonazepam with clonidine or clorazepate.
- Institute seizure precautions for patients on initial therapy or undergoing dose manipulations.
- **PO:** Administer with food to minimize gastric irritation. Tablets may be crushed if patient has difficulty swallowing. Administer largest dose at bedtime to avoid daytime sedation. Taper by 0.25 mg every 3 days to decrease signs and symptoms of withdrawal. Some patients may require longer taper period (months).

Patient/Family Teaching

- Instruct patient to take medication exactly as directed. Take missed doses within 1 hr or omit; do not double doses. Abrupt withdrawal of clonazepam may cause status epilepticus, tremors, nausea, vomiting, and abdominal and muscle cramps.
- Medication may cause drowsiness or dizziness. Advise patient to avoid driving or other activities requiring alertness until response to drug is known.
- Caution patient to avoid taking alcohol or other CNS depressants concurrently with this medication.
- Advise patient to notify health care professional of medication regimen prior to treatment or surgery.
- Instruct patient and family to notify health care professional of unusual tiredness, bleeding, sore throat, fever, clay-colored stools, yellowing of skin, or behavioral changes.
- Patient on anticonvulsant therapy should carry identification at all times describing disease process and medication regimen.
- Emphasize the importance of follow-up exams to determine effectiveness of the medication.
- Advise patient that clonazepam is usually prescribed for short-term use and does not cure underlying problems.
- Advise patient to participate in psychotherapy to address anxiety and improve coping skills.
- Teach other methods to decrease anxiety, such as exercise, support groups, relaxation techniques.
- Advise patient to not share medication with others.

Evaluation/Desired Outcomes

- Decrease or cessation of seizure activity without undue sedation. Dose adjustments may be required after several months of therapy.
- Decrease in frequency and severity of panic attacks.
- Relief of leg movements during sleep.
- Decrease in pain from neuralgia.

clonidine (klon-i-deen)

Catapres, Catapres-TTS, ✤Dixarit, Duraclon

Classification
Therapeutic: antihypertensives
Pharmacologic: adrenergics (centrally acting)

Pregnancy Category C

Indications

PO, Transdermal: Management of mild to moderate hypertension. **Epidural:** Management of cancer pain unresponsive to opioids alone. **Unlabeled uses:** Management of opioid withdrawal.

Action

Stimulates alpha-adrenergic receptors in the CNS; which results in decreased sympathetic outflow inhibiting cardioacceleration and vasoconstriction centers. Prevents pain signal transmission to the CNS by stimulating alpha-adrenergic receptors in the spinal cord. **Therapeutic Effects:** Decreased blood pressure. Decreased pain.

Pharmacokinetics

Absorption: Well absorbed from the GI tract and skin. Enters systemic circulation following epidural use. Some absorption follows sublingual administration.
Distribution: Widely distributed; enters CNS. Crosses the placenta readily; enters breast milk in high concentrations.
Metabolism and Excretion: Mostly metabolized by the liver; 40–50% eliminated unchanged in urine.
Half-life: *Plasma*—12–22 hr; *CNS*—1.3 hr.

TIME/ACTION PROFILE (PO, TD = antihypertensive effect; epidural = analgesia)

ROUTE	ONSET	PEAK	DURATION
PO	30–60 min	2–4 hr	8–12 hr
Transdermal	2–3 days	unknown	7 days†
Epidural	unknown	unknown	unknown

†8 hr following removal of patch

Contraindications/Precautions

Contraindicated in: Hypersensitivity; *Epidural*—injection site infection, anticoagulant therapy, or bleeding problems.
Use Cautiously in: Serious cardiac or cerebrovascular disease; Renal insufficiency; Geri: Appear on Beers list due to increased risk of orthostatic hypotension and adverse CNS effects in geriatric patients (↓ dose recommended); Pregnancy or lactation (safety not established).

Adverse Reactions/Side Effects

CNS: drowsiness, depression, dizziness, nervousness, nightmares. **CV:** bradycardia, hypotension (increased with epidural), palpitations. **GI:** dry mouth, constipation, nausea, vomiting. **GU:** erectile dysfunction. **Derm:** rash, sweating. **F and E:** sodium retention. **Metab:** weight gain. **Misc:** withdrawal phenomenon.

Interactions

Drug-Drug: Additive sedation with **CNS depressants**, including **alcohol**, **antihistamines**, **opioid analgesics**, and **sedative/hypnotics**. Additive hypotension with other **antihypertensives** and **nitrates**. Additive bradycardia with **myocardial depressants**, including **beta blockers**. **MAO inhibitors**, **amphetamines**, **beta blockers**, **prazosin**, or **tricyclic antidepressants** may decrease antihypertensive effect. Withdrawal phenomenon may be increased by discontinuation of **beta blockers**. Epidural clonidine prolongs the effects of epidurally administered **local anesthetics**. May decrease effectiveness of **levodopa**. Increased risk of adverse cardiovascular reactions with **verapamil**.

Route/Dosage

PO (Adults): *Hypertension (initial dose)*—100 mcg (0.1 mg) bid, increase by 100–200 mcg (0.1–0.2 mg)/day q 2–4 days. *Usual maintenance dose* is 200–600 mcg (0.2–0.6 mg)/day in 2–3 divided doses (up to 2.4 mg/day). *Urgent treatment*—200 mcg (0.2 mg) loading dose, then 100 mcg (0.1 mg) q hr until blood pressure is controlled or 800 mcg (0.8 mg) total has been administered; follow with maintenance dosing. *Opioid withdrawal*—300 mcg (0.3 mg)–1.2 mg/day, may be decreased by 50%/day for 3 days, then discontinued or decreased by 100–200 mcg (0.1–0.2 mg)/day.
PO (Geriatric Patients): 100 mcg (0.1 mg) at bedtime initially, increased as needed.
PO (Children): 50–400 mcg (0.05–0.4 mg) twice daily.
Transdermal (Adults): *Hypertension*—Transdermal system delivering 100–300 mcg (0.1–0.3 mg)/24 hr applied every 7 days. Initiate with 100 mcg (0.1 mg)/24 hr system; dosage increments may be made q 1–2 wk when system is changed.
Epidural: (Adults): 30 mcg/hr initially; titrated according to need.
Epidural: (Children): 0.5 mcg/kg/hr initially; titrated according to need.

Availability (generic available)

Tablets: ✤25 mcg (0.025 mg), 100 mcg (0.1 mg), 200 mcg (0.2 mg), 300 mcg (0.3 mg). **Cost:** *Generic*—0.1 mg $21.65/100, 0.2 mg $12.21/100, 0.3 mg $26.65/100. **Transdermal systems:** Catapres-TTS 1, releases 0.1 mg/24 hr, Catapres-TTS 2, releases 0.2 mg/24 hr, Catapres-TTS 3, releases 0.3 mg/24 hr. **Cost:** Catapres-TTS 1 $85.99/4 patches, Catapres-TTS 2 $139.97/4 patches, Catapres-TTS 3 $194.97/4 patches. **Solution for epidural injection:** 100 mcg/ml in 10-ml vials, 500 mcg/ml in 10-ml vials. ***In combination with:*** chlorthalidone (Clorpres). See Appendix B.

NURSING IMPLICATIONS

Assessment

- Monitor intake and output ratios and daily weight, and assess for edema daily, especially at beginning of therapy.
- Monitor blood pressure and pulse frequently during initial dosage adjustment and periodically throughout therapy. Report significant changes.
- **Pain:** Assess location, character, and intensity of pain prior to, frequently during first few days, and routinely throughout administration.
- Monitor for fever as potential sign of catheter infection.
- **Opioid Withdrawal:** Monitor patient for signs and symptoms of opioid withdrawal (tachycardia, fever, runny nose, diarrhea, sweating, nausea, vomiting, irritability, stomach cramps, shivering, unusually large pupils, weakness, difficulty sleeping, gooseflesh).
- ***Lab Test Considerations:*** May cause transient increase in blood glucose levels.
- May cause decreased urinary catecholamine and vanillylmandelic acid (VMA) concentrations; these may increase on abrupt withdrawal.
- May cause weakly positive Coombs' test result.

Potential Nursing Diagnoses

Acute pain (Indications)
Risk for injury (Side Effects)

Implementation

- Do not confuse Catapres (clonidine) with Cataflam (diclofenac).
- Do not confuse clonidine with clonazepam (Klonopin).
- In the perioperative setting, continue clonidine up to 4 hr prior to surgery and resume as soon as possible thereafter. Do not interrupt *transdermal clonidine* during surgery. Monitor blood pressure carefully.
- **PO:** Administer last dose of the day at bedtime. **Transdermal:** Transdermal system should be applied once every 7 days. May be applied to any hairless site; avoid cuts or calluses. Absorption is greater when placed on chest or upper arm and decreased when placed on thigh. Rotate sites. Wash area with soap and water; dry thoroughly before application. Apply firm pressure over patch to ensure contact with skin, especially around edges. Remove old system and discard. System includes a protective adhesive overlay to be applied over medication patch to ensure adhesion, should medication patch loosen.

Patient/Family Teaching

- Instruct patient to take clonidine at the same time each day, even if feeling well. If a dose is missed, take as soon as remembered. If more than 1 oral dose in a row is missed or if transdermal system is late in being changed by 3 or more days, consult health care professional. All routes of clonidine should be gradually discontinued over 2–4 days to prevent rebound hypertension.
- Advise patient to make sure enough medication is available for weekends, holidays, and vacations. A written prescription may be kept in wallet in case of emergency.
- Clonidine may cause drowsiness, which usually diminishes with continued use. Advise patient to avoid driving or other activities requiring alertness until response to medication is known.
- Caution patient to avoid sudden changes in position to decrease orthostatic hypotension. Use of alcohol, standing for long periods, exercising, and hot weather may increase orthostatic hypotension.
- If dry mouth occurs, frequent mouth rinses, good oral hygiene, and sugarless gum or candy may decrease effect. If dry mouth continues for more than 2 wk, consult health care professional.

- Caution patient to avoid concurrent use of alcohol or other CNS depressants with this medication.
- Advise patient to consult health care professional before taking any OTC cough, cold, or allergy remedies.
- Advise patient to notify health care professional of medication regimen prior to treatment or surgery.
- Advise patient to notify health care professional if itching or redness of skin (with transdermal patch), mental depression, swelling of feet and lower legs, paleness or cold feeling in fingertips or toes, or vivid dreams or nightmares occur. May require discontinuation of therapy, especially with depression.
- **Hypertension:** Encourage patient to comply with additional interventions for hypertension (weight reduction, low-sodium diet, discontinuation of smoking, moderation of alcohol consumption, regular exercise, and stress management). Medication helps control, but does not cure, hypertension.
- Instruct patient and family on proper technique for blood pressure monitoring. Advise them to check blood pressure at least weekly and report significant changes.
- **Transdermal:** Instruct patient on proper application of transdermal system. Do not cut or trim unit. Transdermal system can remain in place during bathing or swimming.

Evaluation/Desired Outcomes

- Decrease in blood pressure.
- Decrease in severity of pain.
- Decrease in the signs and symptoms of opioid withdrawal.

clopidogrel (kloh-**pid**-oh-grel)

Plavix

Classification

Therapeutic: antiplatelet agents

Pharmacologic: platelet aggregation inhibitors

Pregnancy Category B

Indications

Reduction of atherosclerotic events (MI, stroke, vascular death) in patients at risk for such events including recent MI, acute coronary syndrome (unstable angina/non–Q-wave MI), stroke, or peripheral vascular disease.

Action

Inhibits platelet aggregation by irreversibly inhibiting the binding of ATP to platelet receptors. **Therapeutic Effects:** Decreased occurrence of atherosclerotic events in patients at risk.

Pharmacokinetics

Absorption: Well absorbed following oral administration; rapidly metabolized to an active antiplatelet compound. Parent drug has no antiplatelet activity.

Distribution: Unknown.

Protein Binding: *Clopidogrel*—98%; *active metabolite*—94%.

Metabolism and Excretion: Rapidly and extensively converted by the liver to its active metabolite, which is then eliminated 50% in urine and 45% in feces.

Half-life: 8 hr (active metabolite).

TIME/ACTION PROFILE (effects on platelet function)

ROUTE	ONSET	PEAK	DURATION
PO	within 24 hr	3–7 days	5 days†

†Following discontinuation

Contraindications/Precautions

Contraindicated in: Hypersensitivity; Pathologic bleeding (peptic ulcer, intracranial hemorrhage); Lactation.

Use Cautiously in: Patients at risk for bleeding (trauma, surgery, or other pathologic conditions); History of GI bleeding/ulcer disease; Severe hepatic impairment; OB, Lactation, Pedi: Safety not established; use in pregnancy only if clearly indicated.

Adverse Reactions/Side Effects

Incidence of adverse reactions similar to that of aspirin.

CNS: depression, dizziness, fatigue, headache. **EENT:** epistaxis. **Resp:** cough, dyspnea. **CV:** chest pain, edema, hypertension. **GI:** GI BLEEDING, abdominal pain, diarrhea, dyspepsia, gastritis. **Derm:** pruritus, purpura, rash. **Hemat:** BLEEDING, NEUTROPENIA, THROMBOTIC THROMBOCYTOPENIC PURPURA. **Metab:** hypercholesterolemia. **MS:** arthralgia, back pain. **Misc:** fever, hypersensitivity reactions.

Interactions

Drug-Drug: Concurrent **abciximab**, **eptifibatide**, **tirofiban**, **aspirin**, **NSAIDs**, **heparin**, **heparanoids**, **thrombolytic agents**, **ticlopidine**, or **warfarin** may ↑ risk of bleeding. May ↓ metabolism and ↑ effects of **phenytoin**, **tolbutamide**, **tamoxifen**, **torsemide**, **fluvastatin**, and many **NSAIDs**.

Drug-Natural Products: ↑ bleeding risk with **anise, arnica, chamomile, clove, fenugreek, feverfew, garlic, ginger, ginkgo, Panax ginseng, and others.**

Route/Dosage

Recent MI, Stroke, or Peripheral Vascular Disease

PO (Adults): 75 mg once daily.

Acute Coronary Syndrome

PO (Adults): 300 mg initially, then 75 mg once daily; aspirin 75–325 mg once daily should be given concurrently.

Availability

Tablets: 75 mg, 300 mg. **Cost:** $389.68/90.

NURSING IMPLICATIONS

Assessment

- Assess patient for symptoms of stroke, peripheral vascular disease, or MI periodically during therapy.
- Monitor patient for signs of thrombotic thrombocytic purpura (thrombocytopenia, microangiopathic hemolytic anemia, neurologic findings, renal dysfunction, fever). May rarely occur, even after short exposure (<2 wk). Requires prompt treatment.
- ***Lab Test Considerations:*** Monitor bleeding time during therapy. Prolonged bleeding time, which is time- and dose-dependent, is expected.
- Monitor CBC with differential and platelet count periodically during therapy. Neutropenia and thrombocytopenia may rarely occur.
- May cause ↑ serum bilirubin, hepatic enzymes, total cholesterol, nonprotein nitrogen (NPN), and uric acid concentrations.

Potential Nursing Diagnoses

Risk for injury (Indications, Side Effects)

Implementation

- Discontinue clopidogrel 5–7 days before planned surgical procedures.
- **PO:** Administer once daily without regard to food.

Patient/Family Teaching

- Instruct patient to take medication exactly as directed. Take missed doses as soon as possible unless almost time for next dose; do not double doses.
- Advise patient to notify health care professional promptly if fever, chills, sore throat, or unusual bleeding or bruising occurs.
- Advise patient to notify health care professional of medication regimen prior to treatment or surgery.
- Instruct patient to avoid taking OTC medications containing aspirin or NSAIDs without consulting health care professional.

Evaluation/Desired Outcomes

- Prevention of stroke, MI, and vascular death in patients at risk.

---

clorazepate (klor-**az**-e-pate)
✤Apo-Clorazepate, Gen-XENE, ✤Novo-Clopate, Tranxene, Tranxene-SD

Classification
Therapeutic: anticonvulsants, sedative/hypnotics
Pharmacologic: benzodiazepines

Schedule IV

Pregnancy Category UK

Indications

Management of simple partial seizures. Anxiety disorder, symptoms of anxiety. Acute alcohol withdrawl. **Unlabeled uses:** Anxiety associated with acute myocardial infarction.

Action

Acts at many levels in the CNS to produce anxiolytic effect and CNS depression (by stimulating inhibitory GABA receptors). Produces skeletal muscle relaxation (by inhibiting spinal polysynaptic afferent pathways). Also has anticonvulsant effect (enhances presynaptic inhibition). **Therapeutic Effects:** Relief of anxiety. Sedation. Prevention of seizures.

Pharmacokinetics

Absorption: Well absorbed from the GI tract as desmethyldiazepam.
Distribution: Widely distributed. Crosses the placenta; enters breast milk.
Metabolism and Excretion: Metabolized by the liver; some conversion to active compounds.
Half-life: 48 hr.

✤ = Canadian drug name.
* CAPITALS indicates life-threatening; underlines indicate most frequent.

TIME/ACTION PROFILE (sedation)

ROUTE	ONSET	PEAK	DURATION
PO	1–2 hr	1–2 hr	up to 24 hr†

†May last longer in geriatric patients

Contraindications/Precautions

Contraindicated in: Hypersensitivity; Cross-sensitivity with other benzodiazepines may occur; Pre-existing CNS depression; Severe uncontrolled pain; Angle-closure glaucoma; OB, Lactation: May cause CNS depression, flaccidity, feeding difficulties, and seizures in infant. In lactation discontinue drug or bottle-feed.

Use Cautiously in: Pre-existing hepatic dysfunction; Patients who may be suicidal or have been addicted to drugs in the past; Debilitated patients (dosage reduction required); Severe pulmonary disease; Geri: Long-acting benzodiazepines cause prolonged sedation in the elderly. Appears on Beers list and is associated with increased risk of falls (↓ dose required or consider short-acting benzodiazepine).

Adverse Reactions/Side Effects

CNS: dizziness, drowsiness, lethargy, hangover, headache, mental depression, slurred speech, ataxia, paradoxical excitation. **EENT:** blurred vision. **Resp:** respiratory depression. **GI:** constipation, diarrhea, nausea, vomiting, weight gain (unusual). **Derm:** rashes. **Misc:** physical dependence, psychological dependence, tolerance.

Interactions

Drug-Drug: Alcohol, **antidepressants**, **antihistamines**, and **opioid analgesics**—concurrent use results in ↑ CNS depression. **Cimetidine**, **hormonal contraceptives**, **disulfiram**, **fluoxetine**, **isoniazid**, **ketoconazole**, **metoprolol**, **propoxyphene**, **propranolol**, or **valproic acid** may ↓ the metabolism of clorazepate, ↑ its actions. May ↓ efficacy of **levodopa**. **Rifampin** or **barbiturates** may ↓ the metabolism and ↓ effectiveness of clorazepate. Sedative effects may be ↓ by **theophylline**.

Drug-Natural Products: Concomitant use of **kava kava**, **valerian**, or **chamomile** ↑ CNS depression.

Route/Dosage

Prescribe largest dose at bedtime to avoid daytime sedation. Can be used on prn basis for anxiety.

PO (Adults): *Anxiety*—7.5–15 mg 2–4 times daily *or* 15 mg at bedtime initially. May also be given in a single dose of 11.25–22.5 mg at bedtime. *Alcohol withdrawal*—30 mg initially, then 15 mg 2–4 times daily on 1st day, then gradually decreased over subsequent days. *Anticonvulsant*—7.5 mg 3 times daily; can increase by no more than 7.5 mg/day at weekly intervals (daily dose not to exceed 90 mg).

PO (Geriatric Patients or Debilitated Patients): *Anxiety*—3.75–15 mg/day, may be increased.

PO (Children 9–12 yr): *Anticonvulsant*—7.5 mg twice daily initially, may increase by 7.5 mg/wk (not to exceed 60 mg/day).

Availability

Tablets: 3.75 mg, 7.5 mg, 11.25 mg, 15 mg, 22.5 mg. **Capsules:** 3.75 mg, 7.5 mg, 15 mg.

NURSING IMPLICATIONS

Assessment

- Assess for drowsiness, unsteadiness, and clumsiness. Symptoms are dose related and most severe during initial therapy; may decrease in severity or disappear with continued or long-term therapy.
- Prolonged high-dose therapy may lead to psychological or physical dependence. Restrict amount of drug available to patient.
- Conduct regular assessment for continued need for treatment.
- **Anxiety:** Assess degree and manifestations of anxiety and mental status (orientation, mood, behavior) prior to and periodically during therapy.
- **Alcohol Withdrawal:** Assess patient experiencing alcohol withdrawal for tremors, agitation, delirium, and hallucinations. Protect from injury. Institute seizure precautions.
- **Seizures:** Observe and record intensity, duration, and location of seizure activity.
- Geri: Assess risk of falls and institute fall prevention strategies.
- ***Lab Test Considerations:*** Patients on prolonged therapy should have CBC and liver function tests evaluated periodically. May cause an ↑ in serum bilirubin, AST, and ALT.
- May cause ↓ thyroidal uptake of sodium iodide ^{123}I and ^{131}I.
- ***Toxicity and Overdose:*** Flumazenil is the antidote for alprazolam toxicity or overdose (flumazenil may induce seizures in patients with a history of seizures disorder or who are on tricyclic antidepressants).

C

Potential Nursing Diagnoses
Anxiety (Indications)
Risk for injury (Indications, Side Effects)
Risk for falls (Side Effects)

Implementation
- Do not confuse clorazepate with clonazepam.
- **PO:** If gastric irritation is a problem, may be administered with food or fluids. Capsule should be swallowed whole; do not open.
- Avoid administration of antacids within 1 hr of medication, because absorption of clorazepate may be delayed.

Patient/Family Teaching
- Instruct patient to take medication as directed, not to skip or double up on missed doses. Abrupt withdrawal may cause status epilepticus, tremors, nausea, vomiting, and abdominal and muscle cramps.
- May cause drowsiness or dizziness. Advise patient to avoid driving or other activities requiring alertness until response to drug is known. Geri: Instruct patient and family how to reduce falls risk at home.
- Caution patient to avoid alcohol or other CNS depressants concurrently with this medication.
- Instruct patient to contact health care professional immediately if pregnancy is suspected.
- Advise patient to notify health care professional of medication regimen prior to treatment or surgery.
- Instruct patient and family to notify health care professional of unusual tiredness, bleeding, sore throat, fever, clay-colored stools, yellowing of skin, or behavioral changes.
- Emphasize the importance of follow-up exams to determine effectiveness of the medication.
- Use lowest effective dose for shortest period of time. Taper by 0.5 mg q 3 days to prevent withdrawal. Some patients may require longer tapering period (months).
- **Seizures:** Patients on anticonvulsant therapy should carry identification describing disease process and medication regimen at all times.

Evaluation/Desired Outcomes
- Increase in sense of well-being.
- Decrease in subjective feelings of anxiety.
- Control of acute alcohol withdrawal.
- Decrease or cessation of seizure activity without undue sedation.

clotrimazole, See ANTIFUNGALS (TOPICAL).

clotrimazole, See ANTIFUNGALS (VAGINAL).

cloxacillin, See PENICILLINS, PENICILLINASE RESISTANT.

clozapine (kloe-za-peen)
Clozaril, FazaClo

Classification
Therapeutic: antipsychotics

Pregnancy Category B

Indications
Schizoprenia unresponsive to or intolerant of standard therapy with other antipsychotics (treatment refractory). To reduce recurrent suicidal behavior in schizophrenic patients.

Action
Binds to dopamine receptors in the CNS. Also has anticholinergic and alpha-adrenergic blocking activity. Produces fewer extrapyramidal reactions and less tardive dyskinesia than standard antipsychotics but carries high risk of hematologic abnormalities. **Therapeutic Effects:** Diminished schizophrenic behavior. Diminished suicidal behavior.

Pharmacokinetics
Absorption: Well absorbed after oral administration.
Distribution: Rapid and extensive distribution; crosses blood-brain barrier and placenta.
Protein Binding: 95%.
Metabolism and Excretion: Mostly metabolized on first pass through the liver.
Half-life: 8–12 hr.

TIME/ACTION PROFILE (antipsychotic effect)

ROUTE	ONSET	PEAK	DURATION
PO	unknown	wks	4–12 hr

Contraindications/Precautions
Contraindicated in: Hypersensitivity; Bone marrow depression; Severe CNS depression/

coma; Uncontrolled epilepsy; Granulocytopenia; Lactation: Discontinue drug or bottle-feed.
Use Cautiously in: Prostatic enlargement; Angle-closure glaucoma; Malnourished patients or patients with cardiovascular, hepatic, or renal disease (use lower initial dose, titrate more slowly); Diabetes; Seizure disorder; Pedi: Safety not established in children <16 yr; Geri: Increased risk of death of elderly patients with dementia-related psychosis.

Adverse Reactions/Side Effects

CNS: NEUROLEPTIC MALIGNANT SYNDROME, SEIZURES, dizziness, sedation. **EENT:** visual disturbances. **CV:** MYOCARDITIS, hypotension, tachycardia, ECG changes, hypertension. **GI:** constipation, abdominal discomfort, dry mouth, increased salivation, nausea, vomiting, weight gain. **Derm:** rash, sweating. **Endo:** hyperglycemia. **Hemat:** AGRANULOCYTOSIS, LEUKOPENIA. **Neuro:** extrapyramidal reactions. **Misc:** fever.

Interactions

Drug-Drug: ↑ anticholinergic effects with other **agents having anticholinergic properties**, including **antihistamines**, **quinidine**, **disopyramide**, and **antidepressants**. Concurrent use with **SSRI antidepressants** ↑ blood levels and risk of toxicity (especially **fluvoxamine**). ↑ CNS depression with **alcohol**, **antidepressants**, **antihistamines**, **opioid analgesics**, or **sedative/hypnotics**. ↑ hypotension with **nitrates**, acute ingestion of **alcohol**, or **antihypertensives**. ↑ risk of bone marrow suppression with **antihypertensives** or **radiation therapy**. Use with **lithium** ↑ risk of adverse CNS reactions, including seizures.
Drug-Natural Products: Caffeine-containing herbs (**cola nut**, **tea**, **coffee**) may increase serum levels and side effects. **St. John's wort** may decrease blood levels and efficacy.

Route/Dosage

PO (Adults): 25 mg 1–2 times daily initially; increase by 25–50 mg/day over a period of 2 wk up to target dose of 300–450 mg/day. May increase by up to 100 mg/day once or twice further (not to exceed 900 mg/day). Treatment should be continued for at least 2 yr in patients with suicidal behavior.

Availability (generic available)

Tablets: 25 mg, 100 mg. **Orally-disintegrating tablets (mint):** 25 mg, 100 mg.

NURSING IMPLICATIONS

Assessment

- Monitor patient's mental status (orientation, mood, behavior) before and periodically during therapy.
- Monitor blood pressure (sitting, standing, lying) and pulse rate before and frequently during initial dose titration.
- Assess weight and BMI initially and throughout therapy.
- Assess fasting blood glucose and cholesterol levels initially and throughout therapy. Refer as appropriate for nutritional/weight management and medical management.
- Observe patient carefully when administering medication to ensure that medication is actually taken and not hoarded or cheeked.
- Monitor for signs of myocarditis (unexplained fatigue, dyspnea, tachypnea, fever, chest pain, palpitations, other signs and symptoms of heart failure, ECG changes, such as ST-T wave abnormalities, arrhythmias, or tachycardia during first month of therapy). If these occur, clozapine should be discontinued and not restarted.
- Monitor patient for onset of akathisia (restlessness or desire to keep moving) and extrapyramidal side effects (*parkinsonian*—difficulty speaking or swallowing, loss of balance control, pill-rolling motion of hands, mask-like face, shuffling gait, rigidity, tremors and dystonic muscle spasms, twisting motions, twitching, inability to move eyes, weakness of arms or legs) every 2 mo during therapy and 8–12 wk after therapy has been discontinued. Notify health care professional if these symptoms occur; reduction in dose or discontinuation of medication may be necessary. Trihexyphenidyl or benzotropine may be used to control these symptoms.
- Although not yet reported for clozapine, monitor for possible tardive dyskinesia (uncontrolled rhythmic movement of mouth, face, and extremities, lip smacking or puckering, puffing of cheeks, uncontrolled chewing, rapid or worm-like movements of tongue). Report these symptoms immediately; may be irreversible.
- Monitor frequency and consistency of bowel movements. Increasing bulk and fluids in the diet may help to minimize constipation.
- Clozapine lowers the seizure threshold. Institute seizure precautions for patients with history of seizure disorder.

- Transient fevers may occur, especially during first 3 wk of therapy. Fever is usually self-limiting but may require discontinuation of medication. Also, monitor for development of neuroleptic malignant syndrome (fever, respiratory distress, tachycardia, seizures, diaphoresis, hypertension or hypotension, pallor, tiredness). Notify health care professional immediately if these symptoms occur.
- ***Lab Test Considerations:*** Monitor WBC, absolute neutrophil count (ANC), and differential count before initiation of therapy and WBC and ANC weekly for the first 6 months, then biweekly during therapy and weekly for 4 wk after discontinuation of clozapine. Because of the risk of agranulocytosis, clozapine is available only in a 1-wk supply through the **Clozaril Patient Management System,** which combines WBC testing, patient monitoring, and controlled distribution through participating pharmacies. If WBC is <3000 mm^3 or granulocyte count is <1500 mm^3, withhold clozapine, increase frequency of WBC monitoring according to management system guidelines, and monitor patient for signs and symptoms of infection. If acceptable WBC and ANC levels were maintained during first 6 months of continuous therapy, monitoring may decrease to every 2 wks. If levels are maintained for second 6 months, WBC and ANC may be monitored every 4 wks thereafter.
- ***Toxicity and Overdose:*** Overdose is treated with activated charcoal and supportive therapy. Monitor patient for several days because of risk of delayed effects: Avoid use of epinephrine and its derivatives when treating hypotension, and avoid quinidine and procainamide when treating arrhythmias.

Potential Nursing Diagnoses

Risk for other-directed violence (Indications)
Disturbed thought process (Indications)
Risk for injury (Side Effects)

Implementation

- **PO:** Administer capsules with food or milk to decrease gastric irritation.
- Leave oral disintegrating tablet in blister until time of use. Do not push tablet through foil. Just before use, peel foil and gently remove disintegrating tablet. Immediately place tablet in mouth and allow to disintegrate and swallow with saliva. If ½ tablet dose used, destroy other half of tablet.

Patient/Family Teaching

- Instruct patient to take medication exactly as directed. Patients on long-term therapy may need to discontinue gradually over 1–2 wk.
- Inform patient of possibility of extrapyramidal symptoms. Instruct patient to report these symptoms immediately.
- Inform patient that cigarette smoking can decrease clozapine levels. Risk for relapse increases if patient begins or increases smoking.
- Advise patient to change positions slowly to minimize orthostatic hypotension.
- May cause seizures and drowsiness. Caution patient to avoid driving or other activities requiring alertness while taking clozapine.
- Caution patient to avoid concurrent use of alcohol, other CNS depressants, and OTC medications without consulting health care professional.
- Instruct patient to use frequent mouth rinses, good oral hygiene, and sugarless gum or candy to minimize dry mouth.
- Advise patient to notify health care professional of medication regimen before treatment or surgery.
- Instruct patient to notify health care professional promptly if unexplained fatigue, dyspnea, tachypnea, chest pain, palpitations, sore throat, fever, lethargy, weakness, malaise, or flu-like symptoms occur or if pregnancy is planned or suspected.
- Advise patient of need for continued medical follow-up for psychotherapy, eye exams, and laboratory tests.
- Advise female patients to notify health care professional if pregnancy is planned or suspected, or if breast-feeding or planning to breast-feed.
- Refer to local support group.

Evaluation/Desired Outcomes

- Decreased positive symptoms (delusions, hallucinations) of schizophrenia.
- Decrease in negative symptoms (social withdrawal, flat, blunt affect) of schizophrenia.

HIGH ALERT

codeine (koe-deen)

Paveral

Classification

Therapeutic: allergy, cold, and cough remedies, antitussives, opioid analgesics

Pharmacologic: opioid agonists

Schedule II, III, IV, V (depends on content)

Pregnancy Category C

Indications

Management of mild to moderate pain. Antitussive (in smaller doses). **Unlabeled uses:** Management of diarrhea.

Action

Binds to opiate receptors in the CNS. Alters the perception of and response to painful stimuli while producing generalized CNS depression. Decreases cough reflex. Decreases GI motility. **Therapeutic Effects:** Decreased severity of pain. Suppression of the cough reflex. Relief of diarrhea.

Pharmacokinetics

Absorption: 50% absorbed from the GI tract. Completely absorbed from IM sites. Oral and parenteral doses are not equal.

Distribution: Widely distributed. Crosses the placenta; enters breast milk.

Metabolism and Excretion: Mostly metabolized by the liver; 10% converted to morphine, 5–15% excreted unchanged in urine.

Half-life: 2.5–4 hr.

TIME/ACTION PROFILE (analgesia)

ROUTE	ONSET	PEAK	DURATION
PO	30–45 min	60–120 min	4 hr
IM	10–30 min	30–60 min	4 hr
Subcut	10–30 min	unknown	4 hr

Contraindications/Precautions

Contraindicated in: Hypersensitivity.

Use Cautiously in: Head trauma; Increased intracranial pressure; Severe renal, hepatic, or pulmonary disease; Hypothyroidism; Adrenal insufficiency; Alcoholism; Geri: Geriatric or debilitated patients (dose reduction required; more susceptible to CNS depression, constipation); Undiagnosed abdominal pain; Geri: Prostatic hyperplasia; OB: Has been used during labor; respiratory depression may occur in the newborn; OB: Pregnancy or lactation (avoid chronic use).

Adverse Reactions/Side Effects

CNS: <u>confusion</u>, <u>sedation</u>, dysphoria, euphoria, floating feeling, hallucinations, headache, unusual dreams. **EENT:** blurred vision, diplopia, miosis. **Resp:** respiratory depression. **CV:** <u>hypotension</u>, bradycardia. **GI:** <u>constipation</u>, <u>nausea</u>, <u>vomiting</u>. **GU:** urinary retention. **Derm:** flushing, sweating. **Misc:** physical dependence, psychological dependence, tolerance.

Interactions

Drug-Drug: Use with extreme caution in patients receiving **MAO inhibitors** (reduce initial dose to 25% of usual dose). Additive CNS depression with **alcohol**, **antidepressants**, **antihistamines**, and **sedative/hypnotics**. Administration of **partial antagonists (buprenorphine**, **butorphanol**, **nalbuphine**, or **pentazocine)** may precipitate opioid withdrawal in physically dependent patients. **Nalbuphine** or **pentazocine** may decrease analgesia.

Drug-Natural Products: Concomitant use of **kava kava**, **valerian**, **skullcap**, **chamomile**, or **hops** can increase CNS depression.

Route/Dosage

PO (Adults): *Analgesic*—15–60 mg q 3–6 hr as needed. *Antitussive*—10–20 mg q 4–6 hr as needed (not to exceed 120 mg/day). *Antidiarrheal*—30 mg up to 4 times daily.

PO (Children 6–12 yr): *Analgesic*—0.5 mg/kg (15 mg/m^2) q 4–6 hr (up to 4 times daily) as needed. *Antitussive*—5–10 mg q 4–6 hr as needed (not to exceed 60 mg/day). *Antidiarrheal*—0.5 mg/kg up to 4 times daily.

PO (Children 2–5 yr): *Analgesic*—0.5 mg/kg (15 mg/m^2) q 4–6 hr (up to 4 times daily) as needed. *Antitussive*—0.25 mg/kg up to 4 times daily. *Antidiarrheal*—0.5 mg/kg up to 4 times daily.

IM, IV, Subcut (Adults): *Analgesic*—15–60 mg q 4–6 hr as needed.

IM, IV, Subcut (Infants and Children): *Analgesic*—0.5 mg/kg (15 mg/m^2) q 4–6 hr as needed.

Availability (generic available)

Tablets: 15 mg, 30 mg, 60 mg. **Oral solution:** 10 mg/5 ml, 15 mg/5 ml. **Injection:** 30 mg/ml, 60 mg/ml. ***In combination with:*** antihistamines, decongestants, antipyretics, caffeine, butalbital, and nonopioid analgesics. See Appendix B.

NURSING IMPLICATIONS

Assessment

- Assess blood pressure, pulse, and respirations before and periodically during administration. If respiratory rate is <10/min, assess level of sedation. Physical stimulation may be sufficient to prevent significant hypoventilation. Dose may need to be decreased by 25–50%. Initial drowsiness will diminish with continued use.
- Assess bowel function routinely. Prevention of constipation should be instituted with increased intake of fluids, bulk, and laxatives to minimize constipating effects. Stimulant laxatives should be administered routinely if opioid use exceeds 2–3 days, unless contraindicated.
- **Pain:** Assess type, location, and intensity of pain before and 1 hr (peak) after administration. When titrating opioid doses, increases of 25–50% should be administered until there is either a 50% reduction in the patient's pain rating on a numerical or visual analogue scale or the patient reports satisfactory pain relief. A repeat dose can be safely administered at the time of the peak if previous dose is ineffective and side effects are minimal.
- An equianalgesic chart (see Appendix J) should be used when changing routes or when changing from one opioid to another.
- Prolonged use may lead to physical and psychological dependence and tolerance. This should not prevent patient from receiving adequate analgesia. Most patients who receive codeine for pain do not develop psychological dependence. If progressively higher doses are required, consider conversion to a stronger opioid.
- **Cough:** Assess cough and lung sounds during antitussive use.
- ***Lab Test Considerations:*** May cause ↑ plasma amylase and lipase concentrations.
- ***Toxicity and Overdose:*** If an opioid antagonist is required to reverse respiratory depression or coma, naloxone (Narcan) is the antidote. Dilute the 0.4-mg ampule of naloxone in 10 ml of 0.9% NaCl and administer 0.5 ml (0.02 mg) by direct IV push every 2 min. For children and patients weighing <40 kg, dilute 0.1 mg of naloxone in 10 ml of 0.9% NaCl for a concentration of 10 mcg/ml and administer 0.5 mcg/kg every 2 min. Titrate dose to avoid withdrawal, seizures, and severe pain.

Potential Nursing Diagnoses

Acute pain (Indications)
Disturbed sensory perception (visual, auditory) (Side Effects)
Risk for injury (Side Effects)

Implementation

- ***High Alert:*** Accidental overdosage of opioid analgesics has resulted in fatalities. Before administering, clarify all ambiguous orders; have second practitioner independently check dose calculations and route of administration.
- ***High Alert:*** Do not confuse codeine with Cardene (nicardipine) or Lodine (etodolac).
- Explain therapeutic value of medication before administration to enhance the analgesic effect.
- Regularly administered doses may be more effective than prn administration. Analgesic is more effective if given before pain becomes severe.
- Coadministration with nonopioid analgesics may have additive analgesic effects and permit lower doses.
- Medications should be discontinued gradually after long-term use to prevent withdrawal symptoms.
- When combined with nonopioid analgesics (aspirin, acetaminophen) #2 = 15 mg, #3 = 30 mg, #4 = 60 mg codeine. Codeine as an individual drug is a Schedule II substance. In combination with other drugs, tablet form is Schedule III, liquid is Schedule IV, and elixir or cough suppressant is Schedule V (see Appendix I).
- **PO:** Oral doses may be administered with food or milk to minimize GI irritation.
- **IM, Subcut:** Do not administer solution that is more than slightly discolored or contains a precipitate.

IV Administration

- **Direct IV:** Codeine is usually administered IM or subcut, but slow IV injection has been used.
- **Syringe Compatibility:** dimenhydrinate, glycopyrrolate, hydroxyzine.

Patient/Family Teaching

- Instruct patient on how and when to ask for pain medication.
- Codeine may cause drowsiness or dizziness. Advise patient to call for assistance when ambulating or smoking. Caution ambulatory patient to avoid driving or other activities requiring alertness until response to medication is known.
- Advise patient to change positions slowly to minimize orthostatic hypotension.
- Caution patient to avoid concurrent use of alcohol or other CNS depressants with this medication.
- Encourage patient to turn, cough, and breathe deeply every 2 hr to prevent atelectasis.
- Advise patient that good oral hygiene, frequent mouth rinses, and sugarless gum or candy may decrease dry mouth.

Evaluation/Desired Outcomes

- Decrease in severity of pain without a significant alteration in level of consciousness or respiratory status.
- Suppression of cough.
- Control of diarrhea.

HIGH ALERT

colchicine (kol-chi-seen)

Classification
Therapeutic: antigout agents

Pregnancy Category D

Indications

Acute attacks of gouty arthritis (larger doses). Prevention of recurrences of gout (smaller doses). **Unlabeled uses:** Treatment of hepatic cirrhosis and familial Mediterranean fever.

Action

Interferes with the functions of WBCs in initiating and perpetuating the inflammatory response to monosodium urate crystals. **Therapeutic Effects:** Decreased pain and inflammation in acute attacks of gout. Prevention of recurrent attacks of gout.

Pharmacokinetics

Absorption: Absorbed from the GI tract, then re-enters GI tract from biliary secretions, when more absorption may occur.
Distribution: Concentrates in WBCs.
Metabolism and Excretion: Partially metabolized by the liver. Secreted in bile back into GI tract; eliminated in the feces. Small amount excreted in the urine.
Half-life: 20 min (plasma), 60 hr (WBCs).

TIME/ACTION PROFILE (anti-inflammatory activity)

ROUTE	ONSET	PEAK	DURATION
PO	12 hr	24–72 hr	unknown
IV	within 6–12 hr	unknown	unknown

Contraindications/Precautions

Contraindicated in: Hypersensitivity; Pregnancy; Severe renal (CCr <10 ml/min) or GI disease.
Use Cautiously in: Elderly or debilitated patients (toxicity may be cumulative); Renal impairment (dose reduction suggested if CCr <50 ml/min; total IV dose not >2 mg); Lactation or children (safety not established).

Adverse Reactions/Side Effects

GI: diarrhea, nausea, vomiting, abdominal pain. **GU:** anuria, hematuria, renal damage. **Derm:** alopecia. **Hemat:** AGRANULOCYTOSIS, APLASTIC ANEMIA, leukopenia, thrombocytopenia. **Local:** phlebitis at IV site. **Neuro:** peripheral neuritis.

Interactions

Drug-Drug: Additive bone marrow depression may occur with **bone marrow depressants** or **radiation therapy**. Additive adverse GI effects with **NSAIDs**. May cause reversible malabsorption of **vitamin B_{12}**. ↑ toxicity with **clarithromycin**, especially in the elderly.

Route/Dosage

PO (Adults): *Treatment of acute attacks*—0.6–1.2 mg, then 0.6 mg q 1–2 hr *or* 1–1.2 mg q 2 hr until relief, GI side effects, or a total cumulative dose of 8 mg is achieved. *Prophylaxis*—0.6 mg daily (may be used up to 3 times daily or as little as 1–4 times weekly). If surgery is planned, give 3 times daily for 3 days before and 3 days after procedure.
IV (Adults): *Treatment of acute attack*—2 mg initially, then 0.5 mg q 6 hr *or* 1 mg q 6–12 hr, until relief or cumulative dose of 4 mg has been given. Other regimens may use lower doses. *Prophylaxis*—0.5–1 mg 1–2 times daily. Other regimens may use lower doses.

Availability (generic available)

Tablets: 0.6 mg, ✤ 1 mg. **Cost:** *Generic*—$18.12/90. **Injection:** 0.5 mg/ml in 2-ml ampules.

NURSING IMPLICATIONS

Assessment

- ***High Alert:*** Assess patient for toxicity (weakness, abdominal discomfort, nausea, vomiting, diarrhea, delirium, seizures, sense of suffocation, dilated pupils, difficulty swallowing, ascending paralysis, oliguria), withhold drug and report symptoms immediately.
- Assess involved joints for pain, mobility, and edema throughout therapy. During initiation of therapy, monitor for drug response every 1–2 hr.
- Monitor intake and output ratios. Fluids should be encouraged to promote a urinary output of at least 2000 ml/day.
- ***Lab Test Considerations:*** In patients receiving prolonged therapy, monitor baseline and periodic CBC; report significant ↓ in values. May cause ↓ platelet count, leukopenia, aplastic anemia, and agranulocytosis.
- May cause ↑ in AST and alkaline phosphatase.
- May cause false-positive results for urine hemoglobin.
- May interfere with results of urinary 17-hydroxycorticosteroid concentrations.
- ***Toxicity and Overdose:*** Assess patient for toxicity (weakness, abdominal discomfort, nausea, vomiting, diarrhea). If these symptoms occur, discontinue medication and notify physician or other health care professional. Opioids may be needed to treat diarrhea.

Potential Nursing Diagnoses

Acute pain (Indications)
Impaired walking (Indications)

Implementation

- ***High Alert:*** Colchicine overdose can be fatal. Cumulative dose by any route should not exceed 4 mg. Limit IV doses to a maximum of 1-2 mg in patients who have recently received oral colchicine. Cumulative dose should not exceed 2 mg in geriatric and renal patients. After dosing limit has been reached, do not administer any additional colchicine by any route for 21 days. Do not administer oral and IV colchicine concurrently.
- Intermittent therapy with 3 days between courses may be used to decrease risk of toxicity.
- **PO:** Administer oral doses with food to minimize gastric irritation. Oral route is preferred.

IV Administration

- **IV:** Avoid extravasation; may cause necrosis of skin and soft tissue.
- **Direct IV:** ***Diluent:*** May be administered undiluted. If a lower concentration is desired, may dilute to a volume of 10–20 ml with sterile water or 0.9% NaCl for injection. Do not administer solutions that are turbid. ***Concentration:*** 0.5 mg/ml. ***Rate:*** Administer slowly over 2–10 min. Rapid administration may cause cardiac arrhythmias.
- **Y-Site Incompatibility:** Do not dilute colchicine with or inject into IV tubing containing D5W, solutions containing a bacteriostatic agent, or any other solution that might change the pH of the colchicine solution because precipitation will occur.

Patient/Family Teaching

- Review medication administration schedule. If dose is missed, take as soon as remembered unless almost time for next dose. Do not double doses.
- Instruct patients taking prophylactic doses not to increase to therapeutic doses during an acute attack to prevent toxicity. An NSAID or corticosteroid, preferably via intrasynovial injection, should be used to treat acute attacks.
- Advise patient to follow recommendations of health care professional regarding weight loss, diet, and alcohol consumption.
- Instruct patient to report nausea, vomiting, abdominal pain, diarrhea, unusual bleeding, bruising, sore throat, fatigue, malaise, or rash promptly. Medication should be withheld if gastric symptoms indicative of toxicity occur.
- Surgery may precipitate an acute attack of gout. Advise patient to confer with health care professional regarding dose 3 days before surgical or dental procedures.

Evaluation/Desired Outcomes

- Decrease in pain and swelling in affected joints within 12 hr.
- Relief of symptoms within 24–48 hr.
- Prevention of acute gout attacks.

colesevelam

(koe-le-**sev**-e-lam)
Welchol

Classification
Therapeutic: lipid-lowering agents
Pharmacologic: bile acid sequestrants

Pregnancy Category B

Indications
Adjunctive therapy to diet and exercise for the reduction of LDL cholesterol in patients with primary hypercholesterolemia; may be used alone or in combination with hepatic hydroxymethylglutaryl coenzyme A (HMG-CoA) reductase inhibitor.

Action
Binds bile acids in the GI tract. Result in increased clearance of cholesterol. **Therapeutic Effects:** Decreased cholesterol.

Pharmacokinetics
Absorption: Not absorbed; action is primarily local in the GI tract.
Distribution: Unknown.
Metabolism and Excretion: Unknown.
Half-life: Unknown.

TIME/ACTION PROFILE (cholesterol-lowering effect)

ROUTE	ONSET	PEAK	DURATION
PO	24–48 hr	2 wk	unknown

Contraindications/Precautions
Contraindicated in: Hypersensitivity; Bowel obstruction.
Use Cautiously in: Triglycerides >300 mg/dl; Dysphagia, swallowing disorders, severe GI motility disorders, or major GI tract surgery; Pregnancy, lactation, or children (safety not established).

Adverse Reactions/Side Effects
GI: constipation, dyspepsia.

Interactions
Drug-Drug: May decrease blood levels of sustained-release form of **verapamil**. May cause ↑ thyroid stimulating hormone (TSH) levels in patients receiving **thyroid hormone replacement therapy**.

Route/Dosage
PO (Adults): 3 tablets twice daily or 6 tablets once daily; may be increased to 7 tablets daily.

Availability
Tablets: 625 mg.

NURSING IMPLICATIONS

Assessment
- Obtain a diet history, especially in regard to fat consumption.
- ***Lab Test Considerations:*** Monitor serum total cholesterol, LDL, and triglyceride levels before initiating, and periodically throughout, therapy.

Potential Nursing Diagnoses
Constipation (Side Effects)
Noncompliance (Patient/Family Teaching)

Implementation
- **PO:** Administer once or twice daily with meals. Colesevelam should be taken with a liquid.

Patient/Family Teaching
- Instruct patient to take medication exactly as directed; do not skip doses or double up on missed doses.
- Advise patient that this medication should be used in conjunction with diet restrictions (fat, cholesterol, carbohydrates, alcohol), exercise, and cessation of smoking.

Evaluation/Desired Outcomes
- Decrease in serum total choesterol, LDL cholesterol, and apolipoprotein levels.

colestipol (koe-**les**-ti-pole)
Colestid

Classification
Therapeutic: lipid-lowering agents
Pharmacologic: bile acid sequestrants

Pregnancy Category UK

Indications
Management of primary hypercholesterolemia. Pruritus associated with elevated levels of bile acids. **Unlabeled uses:** Diarrhea associated with excess bile acids.

Action
Binds bile acids in the GI tract, forming an insoluble complex. Result is increased clearance of cholesterol. **Therapeutic Effects:** Decreased plasma cholesterol and LDL. Decreased pruritus.

Pharmacokinetics
Absorption: Action takes place in the GI tract. No absorption occurs.
Distribution: No distribution.

Metabolism and Excretion: After binding bile acids, insoluble complex is eliminated in the feces.
Half-life: Unknown.

TIME/ACTION PROFILE (hypocholesterolemic effects)

ROUTE	ONSET	PEAK	DURATION
PO	24–48 hr	1 mo	1 mo

Contraindications/Precautions

Contraindicated in: Hypersensitivity; Complete biliary obstruction; Some products contain aspartame and should be avoided in patients with phenylketonuria.
Use Cautiously in: History of constipation.
Exercise Extreme Caution in: Pedi: May cause potentially fatal intestinal obstruction in children.

Adverse Reactions/Side Effects

EENT: irritation of the tongue. **GI:** abdominal discomfort, constipation, nausea, fecal impaction, flatulence, hemorrhoids, perianal irritation, steatorrhea, vomiting. **Derm:** irritation, rashes. **F and E:** hyperchloremic acidosis. **Metab:** vitamin A, D, and K deficiency.

Interactions

Drug-Drug: May decrease absorption/effects of orally administered **acetaminophen**, **amiodarone**, **clindamycin**, **clofibrate**, **digoxin**, **diuretics**, **gemfibrozil**, **glipizide**, **corticosteroids**, **imipramine**, **mycophenolate**, **methotrexate**, **methyldopa**, **niacin**, **NSAIDs**, **penicillin**, **phenytoin**, **phosphates**, **propranolol**, **tetracyclines**, **tolbutamide**, **thyroid preparations**, **ursodiol**, **warfarin**, and **fat-soluble vitamins (A, D, E,** and **K)**. May decrease absorption of other **orally administered medications**.

Route/Dosage

PO (Adults): *Granules*—5 g 1–2 times daily, may be increased q 1–2 mo up to 30 g/day in 1–2 doses. *Tablets*—2 g 1–2 times daily, may be increased q 1–2 mo up to 16 g/day in 1–2 doses.

Availability

Granules for suspension (unflavored): 5 g/packet or scoop. **Flavored granules for suspension with aspartame (orange flavor):** 5 g/packet or scoop. **Tablets:** 1 g.

NURSING IMPLICATIONS

Assessment

- **Hypercholesterolemia:** Obtain a diet history, especially in regard to fat consumption.
- **Pruritus:** Assess severity of itching and skin integrity. Dose may be decreased when relief of pruritus occurs.
- **Diarrhea:** Assess frequency, amount, and consistency of stools.
- ***Lab Test Considerations:*** Serum cholesterol and triglyceride levels should be evaluated before initiating, frequently during first few months and periodically throughout therapy. Discontinue medication if paradoxical increase in cholesterol level occurs.
- May cause an increase in AST, ALT, phosphorus, chloride, and alkaline phosphatase and a decrease in serum calcium, sodium, and potassium levels.
- May also cause prolonged PT.

Potential Nursing Diagnoses

Constipation (Side Effects)
Noncompliance (Patient/Family Teaching)

Implementation

- Parenteral or water-miscible forms of fat-soluble vitamins (A, D, K) and folic acid may be ordered for patients on chronic therapy.
- **PO:** Administer before meals.
- Scoops for powdered preparations may not be exchangable between products.
- Administer other medications 1 hr before or 4–6 hr after the administration of this medication.
- Colestipol tablets should be swallowed whole; do not crush, break, or chew.

Patient/Family Teaching

- Instruct patient to take medication exactly as directed; do not skip doses or double up on missed doses.
- Instruct patient to take medication before meals. Colestipol can be mixed with water, juice, or carbonated beverages. Slowly stir in a large glass. Rinse glass with small amount of additional beverage to ensure all medication is taken. May also mix with highly fluid soups, cereals, or pulpy fruits (applesauce, crushed pineapple). Allow powder to sit on fluid and hydrate for 1–2 min before mixing. Do not take dry.

- Advise patient that this medication should be used in conjunction with diet restrictions (fat, cholesterol, carbohydrates, alcohol), exercise, and cessation of smoking.
- Explain that constipation may occur. Increase in fluids and bulk in diet, exercise, stool softeners, and laxatives may be required to minimize the constipating effects. Instruct patient to notify health care professional if constipation, nausea, flatulence, and heartburn persist or if stools become frothy and foul smelling.
- Advise patient to notify health care professional if unusual bleeding or bruising; petechiae; or black, tarry stools occur. Treatment with vitamin K may be necessary.

Evaluation/Desired Outcomes

- Decrease in serum LDL cholesterol levels. Therapy is usually discontinued if the clinical response remains poor after 3 mo of therapy.
- Decrease in severity of pruritus. Relief usually occurs 1–3 wk after therapy is initiated.
- Decrease in frequency and severity of diarrhea.

CONTRACEPTIVES, HORMONAL

MONOPHASIC ORAL CONTRACEPTIVES

ethinyl estradiol/desogestrel
(**eth**-in-il es-tra-**dye**-ole/dess-oh-**jes**-trel)
Apri 28, Desogen, Ortho-Cept, Reclipsen, Solia

ethinyl estradiol/drospirenone
(**eth**-in-il es-tra-**dye**-ole/droe-**spy**-re-nown)
Yasmin, Yaz

ethinyl estradiol/ethynodiol
(**eth**-in-il es-tra-**dye**-ole/e-thye-noe-**dye**-ole)
Kelnor 1/35, Zovia 1/35, Zovia 1/50

ethinyl estradiol/levonorgestrel
(**eth**-in-il es-tra-**dye**-ole/lee-voe-nor-**jes**-trel)
Alesse-28, Aviane-28, Lessina-28, Levlen-28, Levlite-28, Levora-28, Lutera, Nordette-28, Portia-28, Sronyx

ethinyl estradiol/norethindrone
(**eth**-in-il es-tra-**dye**-ole/nor-eth-**in**-drone)
Balziva, Brevicon, Femcon Fe, Junel 21 1/20, Junel 21 1.5/20, Junel Fe 1/20, Junel Fe 1.5/30, Loestrin 21 1/20, Loestrin 21 1.5/30, Loestrin Fe 1/20, Loestrin Fe 1.5/30, Microgestin Fe 1/20, Modicon, Necon 0.5/35, Necon 1/35, Norethin 1/35E, Norinyl 1+35, Nortrel 0.5/35, Nortrel 1/35, Ortho-Novum 1/35, Ovcon 35, Ovcon 50, Zenchant

ethinyl estradiol/norgestimate
(**eth**-in-il es-tra-**dye**-ole/nor-**jest**-i-mate)
MonoNessa, Ortho-Cyclen, Previfem, Sprintec

ethinyl estradiol/norgestrel
(**eth**-in-il es-tra-**dye**-ole/nor-**jess**-trel)
Cryselle, Lo/Ovral 28, Low-Ogestrel 28, Ogestrel 28

mestranol/norethindrone
(**mes**-tre-nole/nor-eth-**in**-drone)
Necon 1/50, Norethin 1/50M, Norinyl 1+50, Ortho-Novum 1/50

BIPHASIC ORAL CONTRACEPTIVES

ethinyl estradiol/desogestrel
(**eth**-in-il es-tra-**dye**-ole/dess-oh-**jes**-trel)
Kariva, Mircette

ethinyl estradiol/norethindrone
(**eth**-in-il es-tra-**dye**-ole/nor-eth-**in**-drone)
Necon 10/11, Ortho-Novum 10/11

TRIPHASIC ORAL CONTRACEPTIVES

ethinyl estradiol/desogestrel
(**eth**-in-il es-tra-**dye**-ole/dess-oh-**jes**-trel)
Cesia, Cyclessa, Velivet

C

ethinyl estradiol/levonorgestrel
(**eth**-in-il ess-tra-**dye**-ole/lee-voe-nor-**jes**-trel)
Enpresse, Tri-Levlen, Triphasil 28, Trivora 28

ethinyl estradiol/norethindrone
(**eth**-in-il es-tra-**dye**-ole/nor-eth-**in**-drone)
Aranelle, Leena, Necon 7/7/7, Nortrel 7/7/7, Ortho-Novum 7/7/7, Tri-Norinyl

ethinyl estradiol/norgestimate
(**eth**-in-il es-tra-**dye**-ole/nor-**jes**-ti-mate)
Ortho Tri-Cyclen, Ortho Tri-Cyclen Lo, Tri-Nessa, Tri-Previfem, Tri-Sprintec

EXTENDED-CYCLE ORAL CONTRACEPTIVE

ethinyl estradiol/levonorgestrel
(**eth**-in-il ess-tra-**dye**-ole/lee-voe-nor-**jess**-trel)
Lybrel, Seasonale, Seasonique

PROGESTIN-ONLY ORAL CONTRACEPTIVES

norethindrone (nor-eth-**in**-drone)
Errin, Camila, Jolivette, Micronor, Nor-Q D

PROGRESSIVE ESTROGEN ORAL CONTRACEPTIVES

norethindrone/ethinyl acetate
(nor-eth-**in**-drone/**eth**-in-il **a**-se-tate)
Estrostep, Estrostep Fe

CONTRACEPTIVE IMPLANT

etonorgestrel
(e-toe-nor-**jess**-trel)
Implanon

EMERGENCY CONTRACEPTIVE

levonorgestrel
(**lee**-voe-nor-jes-trel)
Plan B

INJECTABLE CONTRACEPTIVE

medroxyprogesterone
(me-**drox**-ee-proe-jess-te-rone)
Depo-Provera, Depo-subQ Provera 104

INTRAUTERINECONTRACEPTIVE

levonorgestrel
(**lee**-voe-nor-jess-trel)
Mirena

Vaginal Ring Contraceptive

ethinyl estradiol/etonogestrel
(**eth**-in-il ess-tra-**dye**-ole/e-toe-noe-**jess**-trel)
NuvaRing

Transdermal Contraceptive

ethinyl estradiol/norelgestromin
(**eth**-in-il ess-tra-**dye**-ole/nor-el-**jess**-troe-min)
Ortho Evra

Classification
Therapeutic: contraceptive hormones

Pregnancy Category X

Indications

Prevention of pregnancy. Regulation of menstrual cycle. Emergency contraception (some products). Treatment of premenstrual dysphoric disorder (Yaz, Yasmin). Management of acne in women >14 yr who desire contraception, have no health problems, and have failed topical treatment.

Action

Monophasic Oral Contraceptives: Provide a fixed dosage of estrogen/progestin over a 21-day cycle. Ovulation is inhibited by suppression of follicle-stimulating hormone (FSH) and luteinizing hormone (LH). May alter cervical mucus and the endometrial environment, preventing penetration by sperm and implantation of the egg. **Biphasic Oral Contraceptives:** Ovulation is inhibited by suppression of FSH and LH. May alter cervical mucus and the endometrial environment, preventing penetration by sperm and implantation of the egg. In addition, smaller dose of progestin in phase 1 allows for proliferation of endometrium. Larger amount in phase 2 allows for adequate secretory development.

Triphasic Oral Contraceptives: Ovulation is inhibited by suppression of FSH and LH. May alter cervical mucus and the endometrial environment, preventing penetration by sperm and implantation of the egg. Varying doses of estrogen/progestin may more closely mimic natural hormonal fluctuations. **Extended-cycle Oral Contraceptives:** Provides continuous estrogen/progestin for 84 days (365 days for Lybrel), then off for 7 days, resulting in 4 menstrual periods/year (no periods/year for Lybrel). **Progressive Estrogen Oral Contraceptives:** Contains constant amount of progestin with 3 progressive doses of estrogen. **Progestin-Only Contraceptives/Contraceptive Implant/Intrauterine Levonorgestrel/Medroxyprogesterone Injection** Mechanism not clearly known. May alter cervical mucus and the endometrial environment, preventing penetration by sperm and implantation of the egg. Ovulation may also be suppressed. **Emergency Contraceptive Pills (ECPs):** Inhibit ovulation/fertilization; may also alter tubal transport of sperm/egg and prevent implantation. **Vaginal Ring, Transdermal Patch:** Inhibits ovulation, decreases sperm entry into uterus, and decreases likelihood of implantation. Anti-acne effect Combination of estrogen/progestin may increase sex hormone binding globulin (SHBG) resulting in decreased unbound testosterone, which may be a cause of acne. **Therapeutic Effects:** Prevention of pregnancy. Decreased severity of acne. Decrease in premenstrual disphoric disorder.

Pharmacokinetics

Absorption: *Ethinyl estradiol*—rapidly absorbed; *norethindrone*—65% absorbed; *Desogesrtrel and levonorgestrel*—100% absorbed. Others are well absorbed after oral administration. Slowly absorbed from implant, subcutaneous, or IM injection. Some absorption follows intrauterine implantation.
Distribution: Unknown.
Protein Binding: *Ethinyl estradiol*—97–98%. *Drospirenone*—97%.
Metabolism and Excretion: *Ethinyl estradiol and norethindrone*—undergo extensive first-pass hepatic metabolism. *Mestranol*—is rapidly converted to ethinyl estradol. *Desogestrel*—is rapidly metabolized to 3-keto-desogestgrel, the active metabolite. Most agents are metabolized by the liver.
Half-life: *Ethinyl estradiol*—6–20 hr; *Levonorgestrel*—45 hr; *Norethindrone*—5–14 hr; *Desogestrel (metabolite)*—38 ± 20 hr; *Drospirenone* —30 hr; *Norgestimate (metabolite)—12–20 hr;* others—unknown.

TIME/ACTION PROFILE (prevention of pregnancy)

ROUTE	ONSET	PEAK	DURATION
PO	1 mo	1 mo	1 mo†
Implant	1 mo	1 mo	5 yr
Intrauterine system	1 mo	1 mo	3 yr
IM	1 mo	1 mo	3 mo
SC	Unk	1 wk	3 mo

†Only during month of taking contraceptive

Contraindications/Precautions

Contraindicated in: Pregnancy; History of thromboembolic disease (e.g., DVT, PE, MI, stroke); Valvular heart disease; Major surgery with extended periods of immobility; Diabetes with vascular involvement; Headache with focal neurological symptoms; Uncontrolled hypertension; History of breast, endometrial, or estrogen-dependent cancer; Abnormal genital bleeding; Liver disease; Hypersensitivity to parabens (injectable only); *Intrauterine levonorgestrel only*—Intrauterine anomaly, postpartum endometriosis, multiple sexual partners, pelvic inflammatory disease, liver disease, genital actinomycosis, immunosuppression, IV drug abuse, untreated genitourinary infection, history of ectopic pregnancy; Some products contain tartrazine and should be avoided in patients with known hypersensitivity intolerance; Lactation: Avoid use.
Use Cautiously in: History of cigarette smoking or age >30–35 yr (increased risk of cardiovascular or thromboembolic phenomenon); Presence of other cardiovascular risk factors (obesity, hyperglycemia, elevated lipids, hypertension); History of diabetes mellitus, bleeding disorders, concurrent anticoagulant therapy or headaches; Pedi: Should not be used before menarche.

Adverse Reactions/Side Effects

CNS: depression, migraine headache. **EENT:** contact lens intolerance, optic neuritis, retinal thrombosis. **CV:** CEREBRAL HEMORRHAGE, CEREBRAL THROMBOSIS, CORONARY THROMBOSIS, PULMONARY EMBOLISM, edema, hypertension, Raynaud's phenomenon, thromboembolic phenomena, thrombophlebitis. **GI:** abdominal cramps, bloating, cholestatic jaundice, gallbladder disease, liver tumors, nausea, vomiting. **GU:** amenorrhea, breakthrough bleeding, dysmenorrhea, spotting. *Intrauterine levonorgestrel only*—uterine imbedment/uterine rupture. **Derm:** melasma, rash. **Endo:** hyperglycemia. **MS:** *Injectable medroxyprogesterone only*—bone loss. **Misc:** weight change.

Interactions

Drug-Drug: Oral contraceptive efficacy may be ↓ by **penicillins**, **chloramphenicol**, **barbiturates**, chronic **alcohol** use, **carbamazepine oxcarbazepine**, **felbamate**, systemic **corticosteroids**, **phenytoin**, **topiramate**, **primidone**, **modafinil**, **rifampin**, **rifabutin**, some **protease inhibitor antiretrovirals** (including **ritonavir**), or **tetracyclines**. May ↑ effects/risk of toxicity of some **benzodiazepines**, **beta blockers**, **corticosteroids**, **cyclosporine**, and **theophylline**. ↑ risk of hepatic toxicity with **dantrolene** (estrogen only). **Indinavir**, **itraconazole**, **ketoconazole**, **fluconazole**, and **atorvastatin** may ↑ effects/risk of toxicity. **Smoking** ↑ risk of thromboembolic phenomena (estrogen only). May ↓ levels of **acetaminophen**, **temazepam**, **lamotrigine**, **lorazepam**, **oxazepam**, or **morphine**. *Drosperinone—containing products only*—concurrent use with **NSAIDs**, **potassium-sparing diuretics**, **potasssium supplements**, **ACE inhibitors**, or **angiotensin II receptor antagonists** may result in hyperkalemia.
Drug-Natural Products: Concomitant use with **St. John's wort** may ↓ contraceptive efficacy and cause breakthrough bleeding and irregular menses.

Route/Dosage

Monophasic Oral Contraceptives

PO (Adults): On 21-day regimen, take first tablet on first Sunday after menses begins (take on Sunday if menses begins on Sunday) for 21 days, then skip 7 days and begin again. Regimen may also be started on first day of menses, continue for 21 days, then skip 7 days and begin again. Some regimens contain 7 placebo tablets, so that 1 tablet is taken every day for 28 days.

Biphasic Oral Contraceptives

PO (Adults): Given in 2 phases. First phase is 10 days of smaller amount of progestin. Second phase is larger amount of progestin. Amount of estrogen remains constant for same length of time (total of 21 days), then skip 7 days and begin again. Some regimens contain 7 placebo tablets for 28-day regimen.

Triphasic Oral Contraceptives

PO (Adults): Progestin amount varies throughout 21-day cycle. Estrogen component stays the same or may vary. Some regimens contain 7 placebo tablets for 28-day regimen.

Extended-cycle Contraceptive

PO (Adults): *Seasonale and Seasonique* Start taking first active pill on first Sunday after menses start (if first day is Sunday, start then), continue for 84 days of active pill, followed by 7 days of placebo tablets, then resume 84/7 cycle again. For *Lybrel*, begin taking the first pill during the first day of the menstrual cycle and start the next pack the day after the previous pack ends.

Progestin-Only Oral Contraceptives

PO (Adults): Start on first day of menses. Taken daily and continuously.

Progressive Estrogen Oral Contraceptives

PO (Adults): Estrogen amount increases q 7 days throughout 21-day cycle. Progestin component stays the same. Some regimens contain 7 placebo tablets for 28-day regimen.

Emergency Contraceptive

PO (Adults and Adolescents): Given within 72 hr of unprotected intercourse and repeated 12 hr later. *Plan B*—1 tablet followed by 1 more tablet 12 hr later; *Ovral*—2 white tablets followed by 2 more white tablets 12 hr later; *Lo/Ovral*—4 white tablets followed by 4 more white tablets 12 hr later; *Levlen, Nordette*—4 light orange tablets followed by 4 more light orange tablets 12 hr later; *Triphasil, Tri-Levlen*—4 yellow tablets followed by 4 more yellow tablets 12 hr later.

Injectable Contraceptive

medroxyprogesterone (Depo-Provera)

IM (Adults): 150 mg within first 5 days of menses or within 5 days postpartum, if not breastfeeding. If breastfeeding, give 6 wk postpartum; repeat q 3 mo.

medroxyprogesterone (Depo-Sub Q Provera 104)

Subcut (Adults): 104 mg within first 5 days of menses or within 5 days postpartum, if not breastfeeding. If breastfeeding, give 6 wk postpartum; repeat q 12–14 wk.

Vaginal Ring Contraceptive

Vag (Adults): One ring inserted on or prior to day 5 of menstrual cycle. Ring is left in place for 3 wk, then removed for 1 wk, then a new ring is inserted.

Transdermal Patch

Transdermal (Adults): Patch is applied on day 1 of menstrual cycle (or convenient day in first week), changed weekly thereafter for 3 weeks. Week 4 is patch-free. Cycle is then repeated.

Acne

PO (Adults): Ortho Tri-Cyclen only, taken daily for 21 days, off for 7 days.

Availability

Combination Estrogen/Progestin Oral Contraceptives

Oral contraceptive tablets: Usually in monthly packs with enough (21) active tablets to complete a 28-day cycle. Some contain 7 inert tablets to complete the cycle with or without supplemental iron. **Cost:** *Apri*—$179.93/6 cycles; *Estrostep Fe*—$354.26/6 cycles; *Femcon Fe*—$338.97/6 cycles; *Kariva*—$239.94/6 cycles; *Levora*—$151.94/6 cycles; *Low-Ogestrel*—$151.94/6 cycles; *Necon 0.5/35*—$125.95/6 cycles; *Ovcon 35*—$322.44/6 cycles; *Sprintec*—$143.10/6 cycles; *Tri-Nessa*—$137.94/6 cycles; *Trivora-28*—$139.94/6 cycles; *Yasmin*—$299.90/6 cycles; *Yaz*—$307.96/6 cycles.

Extended-cycle Contraceptive

Tablets: Seasonale– 84 active tablets containing 0.03 mg ethinyl estradiol and 0.15 mg levonorgestrel and 7 inactive tablets, Seasonique-active tablets containing 0.03 mg ethinly estradiol, 0.15 mg levonorgestrel, and 7 inactive tablets containing 0.01 mg ethinyl estradiol, Lybrel—28 active tablets containing 0.09 mg levonorgestrel and 0.02 mg ethinyl estradiol. **Cost:** *Lybrel*—$49.99/28 tablets; *Seasonale*—$181.98/91 tablets; *Seasonique*—$165.98/91 tablets.

Levonorgestrel

Emergency contraceptives: 2 tablets containing 0.75 mg levonorgestrel (Plan B). **Implant:** Rod contains 68 mg etonogestrel. **Intrauterine system:** contains 52 mg levonorgestrel (releases 20 mcg/day).

Medroxyprogesterone

Injectable IM: 150 mg/ml. **Injectable Subcutaneous:** 104 mg/0.65 ml (in pre-filled syringes).

Vaginal Ring Contraceptive

Ring: delivers 0.015 mg ethinyl estradiol and 0.120 mg etonogestrel/day. **Cost:** $289.95/6 rings.

Transdermal Patch

Patch: contains 0.75 mg ethinyl estradiol and 6 mg of norelgestromin; releases 20 mg ethinyl estradiol/150 mg norelgestromin per 24 hr. **Cost:** $299.95/18 patches.

NURSING IMPLICATIONS

Assessment

- Assess blood pressure before and periodically during therapy.
- **Acne:** Assess skin lesion before and periodically during therapy.
- ***Lab Test Considerations:*** Monitor hepatic function periodically during therapy.
- *Estrogens only*—May cause ↑ serum glucose, sodium, triglyceride, VHDL, total cholesterol, prothrombin, and factors VII, VIII, IX, and X levels. May cause ↓ LDL and antithrombin III levels.
- May cause false interpretations of thyroid function tests.
- *Progestins only*—May cause ↑ LDL concentrations. May cause ↓ serum alkaline phosphatase and HDL concentrations.

Potential Nursing Diagnoses

Noncompliance (Patient/Family Teaching)

Implementation

- **PO:** Oral doses may be administered with or immediately after food to reduce nausea. Chewable tablets may be swallowed whole or chewed; if chewed follow with 8 ounces of liquid.
- For extended-cycle tablets, *Seasonale or Seasonique*—take active tablets for 84 days and followed by the placebo tablets for 7 days; for *Lybrel*—Take 1 pill each day for 28 days, then start the next set of pills daily for the next 28 days.
- **Subcut:** Shake vigorously before use to form a uniform suspension. Inject slowly (over 5–7 seconds) at a 45° angle into fatty area of anterior thigh or abdomen every 12 to 14 wks. If more than 14 wks elapse between injections, rule out pregnancy prior to administration. **Do not rub area after injection**.

- When switching from other hormonal contraceptives, administer within dosing period (7 days after taking last active pill, removing patch or ring, or within the dosing period for IM injection).
- **IM:** Shake vial vigorously just before use to ensure uniform suspension. Administer deep IM into gluteal or deltoid muscle. If period between injections is >14 wk, determine that patient is not pregnant before administering the drug.
- Injectable medroxyprogesterone may lead to bone loss, especially in women younger than 21 years. Injectable medroxyprogesterone should be used for >2 years only if other methods of contraception are inadequate. If used long term, women should use supplemental calcium and vitamin D, and monitor bone mineral density.

Patient/Family Teaching

- Instruct patient to take oral medication as directed at the same time each day. Pills should be taken in proper sequence and kept in the original container. Advise patient not to skip pills even if not having sex very often.
- *If single daily dose is missed:* Take as soon as remembered; if not until next day, take 2 tablets and continue on regular dosing schedule. *If 2 days in a row are missed:* Take 2 tablets a day for the next 2 days and continue on regular dosing schedule, using a second method of birth control for the remaining cycle. *If 3 days in a row are missed:* Discontinue medication and use another form of birth control until period begins or pregnancy is ruled out; then begin a new cycle of tablets. *For 28-day dosing schedule:* If schedule is followed for first 21 days and 1 dose is missed of the last 7 tablets, it is important to take the 1st tablet of next month's cycle on the regularly scheduled day.
- Advise patient taking *Seasonale or Sesonique extended-cycle tablets* that withdrawal bleeding should occur during the 7 days following discontinuation of the active tablets. If withdrawal bleeding does not occur, notify health care professional. Advise patient taking *Lybrel* that no withdrawal bleeding should occur.
- For initial use of *Seasonale or Seasonique extended cycle tablets*, caution patient to use a nonhormonal method of contraception until she has taken the first 7 days of active tablets. Each 91-day cycle should start on the same day of the week. If started later than the proper day or 2 or more days are missed, a second nonhormonal method of contraception should be used until she has taken the pink tablet for 7 days. Transient spotting or bleeding may occur. If bleeding is persistent or prolonged, notify health care professional.
- Advise patient taking extended cycle tablets that spotting or light bleeding may occur, especially during first 3 months. Continue medication; notify health care professional if bleeding lasts >7 days.
- Advise patient of the need to use another form of contraception for the first 3 wk when beginning to use *oral contraceptives*.
- Advise patient that a second method of birth control also should be used during each cycle in which any of the following are used: *Oral contraceptives*—ampicillin, corticosteroids, antiretroviral protease inhibitors, barbiturates, carbamazepine, chloramphenicol, dihydroergotamine, corticosteroids (systemic), mineral oil, oral neomycin, oxcarbazapine, penicillin V, phenylbutazone, primidone, rifampin, sulfonamides, tetracyclines, topiramate, or valproic acid.
- Explain dose schedule and maintenance routine. Discontinuing medication suddenly may cause withdrawal bleeding.
- If nausea becomes a problem, advise patient that eating solid food often provides relief. If nausea persists or vomiting or diarrhea occur, use a nonhormonal method of contraception and notify health care professional.
- Advise patient to report signs and symptoms of fluid retention (swelling of ankles and feet, weight gain), thromboembolic disorders (pain, swelling, tenderness in extremities, headache, chest pain, blurred vision), mental depression, hepatic dysfunction (yellowed skin or eyes, pruritus, dark urine, light-colored stools), or abnormal vaginal bleeding. Women with a strong family history of breast cancer, fibrocystic breast disease, abnormal mammograms or cervical dysplasia should be monitored for breast cancer at least yearly.
- Instruct patient to stop taking medication and notify health care professional if pregnancy is suspected.

- Caution patient that cigarette smoking during estrogen therapy may increase risk of serious side effects, especially for women over age 35.
- Caution patients to use sunscreen and protective clothing to prevent increased pigmentation.
- Caution patient that oral contraceptives do not protect against HIV or other sexually transmitted diseases.
- Advise patient to notify health care professional of medication regimen before treatment or surgery.
- Emphasize the importance of routine follow-up physical exams including blood pressure; breast, abdomen, and pelvic examinations; and Papanicolaou smears every 6–12 mo.
- **IM, Subcut** Advise patient to maintain adequate amounts of dietary calcium and vitamin D to help prevent bone loss.
- **Transdermal:** Instruct patient on application of patch. First patch should be applied within 24 hrs of menstrual period. If applied after day 1 of menstrual period, a nonhormonal method of contraception should be used for the next 7 days. Day of application becomes *Patch Change Day*. Patches are worn for 1 wk and changed on the same day of each wk for 3 wks. Week 4 is patch-free. Withdrawal bleeding is expected during this time.
- Apply patch to clean, dry, intact, healthy skin on buttock, abdomen, upper outer arm, or upper torso in a place where it won't be rubbed by tight clothing. Do not place on skin that is red, irritated, or cut, and do not place on breasts. Do not apply make-up, creams, lotions, powders, or other topical products to area of patch application.
- To apply patch open foil pouch by tearing along edge using fingers. Peel pouch apart and open flat. Grasp a corner of the patch firmly and remove gently from foil pouch. Use fingernail to lift one corner of the patch and peel patch **and** the plastic liner off the foil liner. Do not remove clear liner as patch is removed. Peel away half of the clear liner without touching sticky surface. Apply the sticky surface and remove the rest of the liner. Press down firmly with palm of hand for 10 seconds; make sure the edges stick well.
- On *Patch Change Day* remove patch and apply new one immediately. Used patch still contains some active hormones; fold in half so it sticks to itself and throw away. Apply new patches to a new spot to prevent skin irritation; may be applied in same anatomic area.
- Following patch-free week, apply a new patch on *Patch Change Day*, the day after Day 28, no matter when the menstrual cycle begins.
- If patch becomes partially or completely detached for less than 1 day, reapply patch or apply new patch. If patch is detached for more than 1 day, apply a new patch immediately and use a nonhormonal form of contraception for the next 7 days. Cycle will now start over with a new *Patch Change Day*. If patch is no longer sticky, apply a new patch; do not use tape or wraps to keep patch in place.
- If patch is not changed on *Patch Change Day* in the first week of the cycle, apply new patch immediately upon remembering and use a nonhormonal method of contraception for next 7 days. If patch change is missed in for 1 or 2 days during Week 2 or 3, apply new patch immediately and apply next patch on usual *Patch Change Day*. No backup contraception is needed. If patch change is missed for more than 2 days during Week 2 or 3, stop the cycle and start a new 4-wk contraceptive cycle by applying new patch immediately and using a nonhormonal method of contraception for the next 7 days. If patch is not removed on *Patch Change Day* in Week 4, remove as soon as remembered and start next cycle on usual *Patch Change Day*. No additional contraception is needed.
- **NuvaRing:** *If a hormonal contraceptive was not used in the past month*, insert *NuvaRing* between Days 1 and 5 of the menstrual cycle (Day 1 = first day of menstrual period), even if bleeding has not finished. Use a nonhormonal method of birth control other than a diaphragm during the first 7 days of ring use. *If switching from a combination estrogen/progesterone oral contraceptive*, insert *NuvaRing* any time during first 7 days after last tablet and no later than the day a new pill cycle would have started. No extra birth control is needed. *If switching from a mini-pill*, start using *NuvaRing* on any day of the month; do not skip days between last pill and first day of *NuvaRing* use. *If switching from an implant*, start using *NuvaRing* on same day implant is removed. *If switching from an injectable contraceptive*, start using *NuvaRing* on the day when next injection

is due. *If switching from a progestin-containing IUD*, start using *NuvaRing* on the same day as IUD is removed. A nonhormonal method of contraception, other than the diaphragm, should be used for the first 7 days of *NuvaRing* use when switching from the minipill, implant, injectable contraceptive, or IUD.

- *NuvaRing* comes in a reclosable foil pouch. Instruct patient to wash hands, then remove *NuvaRing* from pouch; keep pouch for ring disposal. Using the position of comfort (lying down, squatting, or standing with one leg up), hold *NuvaRing* between thumb and index finger and press opposite sides of the ring together. Gently push folded ring into vagina. Exact position is not important for function of *NuvaRing*. Most women do not feel *NuvaRing* once it is in place. If discomfort is felt, *NuvaRing* may not be inserted far enough into vagina; use finger to push further into vagina. *There is no danger of NuvaRing being pushed in too far or getting lost*. Once inserted, leave *NuvaRing* in place for 3 wks.
- Remove ring 3 wks after insertion on same day and time of insertion. Remove by hooking finger under forward rim or by holding ring between index and middle finger and pulling out. Place ring in foil pouch and dispose; do not throw in toilet. Menstrual period will usually start 2–3 days after ring is removed and may not have finished before next ring is inserted. To continue contraceptive protection, new ring must be inserted 1 wk after last one was removed, even if menstrual period has not stopped.
- If *NuvaRing* slips out of vagina and has been out less than 3 hrs, contraceptive protection is still in place. *NuvaRing* can be rinsed in cool to tepid water and should be reinserted as soon as possible. If ring is lost, insert a new ring and continue same schedule as lost ring. If *NuvaRing* has been out of vagina for more than 3 hrs, a nonhormonal method of contraception, other than a diaphragm, should be used for the next 7 days.
- *If NuvaRing has been left in for an extra wk or less (4 wks total or less)*, remove and insert a new ring after a 1-wk ring-free break. If *NuvaRing* has been left in place for more than 4 wks, woman should check to be sure she is not pregnant. A nonhormonal method of contraception, other than a diaphragm, must be used for the next 7 days.

Evaluation/Desired Outcomes

- Prevention of pregnancy.
- Regulation of the menstrual cycle.
- Decrease in acne.
- Decrease in symptoms of premenstrual dysphoric disorder.

CORTICOSTEROIDS (INHALATION)

beclomethasone
(be-kloe-**meth**-a-sone)
QVAR

budesonide (byoo-**dess**-oh-nide)
Pulmicort

flunisolide (floo-**niss**-oh-lide)
AeroBid, Aerospan

fluticasone (floo-**ti**-ka-sone)
Flovent, Flovent HFA

mometasone (mo-**met**-a-sone)
Asmanex

triamcinolone
(trye-am-**sin**-oh-lone)
Azmacort

Classification
Therapeutic: antiasthmatics, corticosteroids
Pharmacologic: corticosteroids (inhalation)

Pregnancy Category B (budesonide), C (all others)

Indications

Maintenance treatment of asthma as prophylactic therapy. May decrease the need for or eliminate use of systemic corticosteroids in patients with asthma.

Action

Potent, locally acting anti-inflammatory and immune modifier. **Therapeutic Effects:** Decreased frequency and severity of asthma attacks. Improves asthma symptoms.

Pharmacokinetics

Absorption: *Beclomethasone*—20%; *budesonide*—39% (Turbuhaler), 6–13% (Flexhal-

er), 6% (Respules); *flunisolide*—40%; *fluticasone*—<7% (aerosol), 18% (powder); *mometasone*—<1%; *triamcinolone*—25%. Action is primarily local after inhalation.
Distribution: 10–25% is deposited in airways if a spacer device is not used. All cross the placenta and enter breast milk in small amounts.
Metabolism and Excretion: *Beclomethasone*—after inhalation, beclomethasone dipropionate is converted to beclomethasone monopropionate, an active metabolite that adds to its potency, primarily excreted in feces (<10% excreted in urine; *budenoside, flunisolide, fluticasone, mometasone*, and *triamcinolone*—metabolized by the liver after absorption from lungs. *Budenoside*—60% excreted in urine, 40% in feces; *flunisolide*—50% excreted in urine, 50% in feces; *fluticasone*—primarily excreted in feces (<5% excreted in urine); *mometasone*—75% excreted in feces; *triamcinolone*—40% excreted in urine, 60% in feces.
Half-life: *Beclomethasone*—2.8 hr; *budesonide*—2–3.6 hr; *flunisolide*—1.8 hr; *fluticasone*—7.8 hr; *mometasone*—5 hr; *triamcinolone*—88 min.

TIME/ACTION PROFILE (improvement in symptoms)

ROUTE	ONSET	PEAK	DURATION
Inhalation	within 24 hr‡	1–4 wk†	unknown

†Improvement in pulmonary function; decreased airway responsiveness may take longer
‡2-8 days for budesonide Respule

Contraindications/Precautions

Contraindicated in: Some products contain chlorofluorocarbon (CFC) propellants, alcohol, or lactose and should be avoided in patients with known hypersensitivity or intolerance; Acute attack of asthma/status asthmaticus.
Use Cautiously in: Active untreated infections; Diabetes or glaucoma; Underlying immunosuppression (due to disease or concurrent therapy); Systemic corticosteroid therapy (should not be abruptly discontinued when inhalation therapy is started; additional corticosteroids needed in stress or trauma); Hepatic dysfunction (fluticasone); OB, Lactation: Safety not established; Pedi: Children (prolonged or high-dose therapy may lead to complications).

Adverse Reactions/Side Effects

CNS: headache, agitation, depression, dizziness, fatigue, insomnia, restlessness. **EENT:** dysphonia, hoarseness, cataracts, nasal congestion, pharyngitis, sinusitis. **Resp:** bronchospasm, cough, wheezing. **GI:** diarrhea, dry mouth, dyspepsia, esophageal candidiasis, taste disturbances, nausea. **Endo:** adrenal suppression (increased dose, long-term therapy only), decreased growth (children). **MS:** back pain. **Misc:** CHURG-STRAUSS SYNDROME.

Interactions

Drug-Drug: Ketoconazole ↑ levels of budesonide, fluticasone, and mometasone. **Ritonavir** ↑ levels of budesonide and fluticasone; avoid using with fluticasone. **Itraconazole**, **clarithromycin**, and **erythromycin** ↑ levels of budesonide.

Route/Dosage

Beclomethasone

Inhaln (Adults and Children ≥12 yr): *Previously on bronchodilators alone*—40–80 mcg twice daily (not to exceed 320 mcg twice daily); *Previously on inhaled corticosteroids*—40–160 mcg twice daily (not to exceed 320 mcg twice daily).
Inhaln (Children 5–11 yr): *Previously on bronchodilators alone*—40 mcg twice daily (not to exceed 80 mcg twice daily); *Previously on inhaled corticosteroids*—40 mcg twice daily (not to exceed 80 mcg twice daily).

Budesonide (Pulmicort Turbuhaler)

Inhaln (Adults): *Previously on bronchodilators alone*—200–400 mcg (1–2 inhalations) twice daily (not to exceed 2 inhalations twice daily); *Previously on other inhaled corticosteroids*—200–400 mcg (1–2 inhalations) twice daily (not to exceed 4 inhalations twice daily); *Previously on oral corticosteroids*—400–800 mcg (2–4 inhalations) twice daily (not to exceed 4 inhalations twice daily).
Inhaln (Children ≥6 yr): *Previously on bronchodilators alone*—200 mcg (1 inhalation) twice daily (not to exceed 2 inhalations twice daily); *Previously on other inhaled corticosteroids*—200 mcg (1 inhalation) twice daily (not to exceed 2 inhalations twice daily); *Previously on oral corticosteroids*—Not to exceed 400 mcg (2 inhalations) twice daily.

Budesonide (Pulmicort Flexhaler)

Inhaln (Adults): 180–360 mcg twice daily (not to exceed 720 mcg twice daily).
Inhaln (Children 6–17 yr): 180–360 mcg twice daily (not to exceed 360 mcg twice daily).

Budesonide (Pulmicort Respules)

Inhaln (Children 1–8 yr): *—Previously on bronchodilators alone*—0.5 mg once daily or 0.25 mg twice daily (not to exceed 0.5 mg/day); *Previously on other inhaled corticosteroids*—0.5 mg once daily or 0.25 mg twice daily (not to exceed 1 mg/day); *Previously on oral corticosteroids*—1 mg once daily or 0.5 mg twice daily (not to exceed 1 mg/day).

Flunisolide

Aerobid and Aerospan inhalers are not interchangeable; the dosage changes when switching from one product to another

Inhaln (Adults and Children >15 yr [Aerobid/Aerobid-M Inhaler]): 500 mcg (2 inhalations) twice daily (not to exceed 4 inhalations twice daily).

Inhaln (Adults and Children ≥12 yr [Aerospan Inhaler]): 160 mcg (2 inhalations) twice daily (not to exceed 4 inhalations twice daily).

Inhaln (Children 6–15 yr [Aerobid/Aerobid-M Inhaler]): 500 mcg (2 inhalations) twice daily (not to exceed 2 inhalations twice daily).

Inhaln (Children 6–11 yr [Aerospan Inhaler]): 80 mcg (1 inhalation) twice daily (not to exceed 2 inhalations twice daily).

Fluticasone (Aerosol Inhaler)

Inhaln (Adults and Children ≥12 yr): *Previously on bronchodilators alone*—88 mcg twice daily initially, may be ↑ up to 440 mcg twice daily; *Previously on other inhaled corticosteroids*—88–220 mcg twice daily initially, may be ↑ up to 440 mcg twice daily; *Previously on oral corticosteroids*—440 mcg twice daily initially, may be ↑ up to 880 mcg twice daily.

Inhaln (Children 4–11 yr): 88 mcg twice daily (not to exceed 88 mcg twice daily).

Fluticasone (Dry Powder Inhaler)

Inhaln (Adults and Children ≥12 yr): *Previously on bronchodilators alone*—100 mcg twice daily initially, may be ↑ up to 500 mcg twice daily; *Previously on other inhaled corticosteroids*—100–250 mcg twice daily initially, may be ↑ up to 500 mcg twice daily; *Previously on oral corticosteroids*—500–1000 mcg twice daily.

Inhaln (Children 4–11 yr): *Previously on bronchodilators alone*—50 mcg twice daily initially, may be ↑ up to 100 mcg twice daily; *Previously on other inhaled corticosteroids*—50 mcg twice daily, may be ↑ up to 100 mcg twice daily.

Mometasone

Inhaln (Adults and Children >12 yr): *Previously on bronchodilators or other inhaled corticosteroids*—220 mcg (1 inhalation) once daily, up to 440 mcg/day as a single dose or 2 divided doses; *Previously on oral corticosteroids*—440 mcg (2 inhalations) twice daily (not to exceed 880 mcg/day).

Triamcinolone

Inhaln (Adults and Children >12 yr): 200 mcg (2 inhalations) 3–4 times daily *or* 400 mcg (4 inhalations) twice daily (not to exceed 16 inhalations/day).

Inhaln (Children 6–12 yr): 100–200 mcg (1–2 inhalations) 3–4 times daily *or* 200–400 mcg (2–4 inhalations) twice daily (not to exceed 12 inhalations/day).

Availability

Beclomethasone

Inhalation aerosol: 40 mcg/metered inhalation in 7.3-g canister (delivers 100 metered inhalations), 80 mcg/metered inhalation in 7.3-g canister (delivers 100 metered inhalations). **Cost:** 40 mcg/metered inhalation $41.32/7.3-g canister; 80 mcg metered inhalation $52.04/7.3-g canister.

Budesonide

Inhalation powder (Turbuhaler): 200 mcg/metered inhalation (delivers 200 metered inhalations). **Inhalation powder (Flexhaler):** 90 mcg/metered inhalation (delivers 60 metered inhalations), 180 mcg/metered inhalation (delivers 120 metered inhalations). **Inhalation suspension (Respules):** 0.25 mg/2 ml in single-dose ampules (5 ampules/envelope), 0.5 mg/2 ml in single-dose ampules (5 ampules/envelope). **Cost:** 0.25 mg/2 ml $158.99/20 ampules, 0.5 mg/2 ml $187.00/30 ampules.

Flunisolide

Inhalation aerosol (Aerobid): 250 mcg/metered inhalation in 7-g canisters (delivers 100 metered inhalations). **Inhalation aerosol-menthol (Aerobid-M):** 250 mcg/metered inhalation in 7-g canisters (delivers 100 metered inhalations). **Inhalation aerosol (Aerospan):** 80 mcg/metered inhalation in 5.1-g canisters (delivers 60 metered inhalations) or 8.9-g canisters (delivers 120 metered inhalations).

Fluticasone

Inhalation aerosol (Flovent-HFA): 44 mcg/metered inhalation in 10.6-g canisters (delivers 120 metered inhalations), 110 mcg/metered inhalation in 12-g canisters (delivers 120 metered inhalations), 220 mcg/metered inhalation in 12-g canisters (delivers 120 metered inhalations). **Cost:** 44 mcg/inhalation $90.00/inhaler, 110 mcg/inhalation $118.99/inhaler, 220 mcg/inhalation $193.52/inhaler. **Powder for inhalation (Flovent Diskus):** 50 mcg, 100 mcg, 250 mcg. ***In combination with:*** salmeterol (Advair). See Appendix B.

Mometasone

Powder for inhalation (Twisthaler): 220 mcg units in packages of 14, 30, 60 and 120 inhalation units.

Triamcinolone

Inhalation aerosol: 100 mcg/metered inhalation in 20-g canister (delivers 240 metered inhalations).

NURSING IMPLICATIONS

Assessment

- Monitor respiratory status and lung sounds. Pulmonary function tests may be assessed periodically during and for several months after a transfer from systemic to inhalation corticosteroids.
- Assess patients changing from systemic corticosteroids to inhalation corticosteroids for signs of adrenal insufficiency (anorexia, nausea, weakness, fatigue, hypotension, hypoglycemia) during initial therapy and periods of stress. If these signs appear, notify physician or other health care professional immediately; condition may be life-threatening.
- Monitor for withdrawal symptoms (joint or muscular pain, lassitude, depression) during withdrawal from oral corticosteroids.
- Monitor growth rate in children receiving chronic therapy; use lowest possible dose.
- ***Lab Test Considerations:*** Periodic adrenal function tests may be ordered to assess degree of hypothalamic-pituitary-adrenal (HPA) axis suppression in chronic therapy. Children and patients using higher than recommended doses are at highest risk for HPA suppression.
- May cause ↑ serum and urine glucose concentrations if significant absorption occurs.

Potential Nursing Diagnoses

Ineffective airway clearance (Indications)
Risk for infection (Side Effects)
Deficient knowledge, related to medication regimen (Patient/Family Teaching)

Implementation

- After the desired clinical effect has been obtained, attempts should be made to decrease dose to lowest amount required to control symptoms. Gradually decrease dose every 2–4 wk as long as desired effect is maintained. If symptoms return, dose may briefly return to starting dose. **Inhaln:** Allow at least 1 min between inhalations.

Patient/Family Teaching

- Advise patient to take medication as directed. Take missed doses as soon as remembered unless almost time for next dose. Advise patient not to discontinue medication without consulting health care professional; gradual decrease is required.
- Advise patients using inhalation corticosteroids and bronchodilator to use bronchodilator first and to allow 5 min to elapse before administering the corticosteroid, unless otherwise directed by health care professional.
- Advise patient that inhalation corticosteroids should not be used to treat an acute asthma attack but should be continued even if other inhalation agents are used.
- Patients using inhalation corticosteroids to control asthma may require systemic corticosteroids for acute attacks. Advise patient to use regular peak flow monitoring to determine respiratory status.
- Caution patient to avoid smoking, known allergens, and other respiratory irritants.
- Advise patient to notify physician if sore throat or sore mouth occurs.
- Instruct patient whose systemic corticosteroids have been recently reduced or withdrawn to carry a warning card indicating the need for supplemental systemic corticosteroids in the event of stress or severe asthma attack unresponsive to bronchodilators.
- **Metered-Dose Inhaler:** Instruct patient in the proper use of the metered-dose inhaler. Most inhalers require priming before first use. Shake inhaler well. Exhale completely, and then close lips firmly around mouthpiece. While breathing in deeply and slowly, press down on canister. Hold breath for as long as possible to ensure deep instillation of medication. Remove inhaler from mouth and

breathe out gently. Allow 1–2 min between inhalations. Rinse mouth with water or mouthwash after each use to minimize fungal infections, dry mouth, and hoarseness. Clean the mouthpiece weekly with clean, dry tissue or cloth. Do not place in water (see Appendix D).

- **Pulmicort Turbuhaler and Flexhaler:** Advise patient to follow instructions supplied. Before first-time use, prime unit by turning cover and lifting off; hold upright with mouthpiece up and twist brown grip fully to right, then fully to left until it clicks. To administer dose, hold upright, twist brown grip fully to right, then fully to left until it clicks. Turn head away from inhaler and exhale (do not blow into inhaler). Do not shake inhaler. Place mouthpiece between lips and inhale deeply and forcefully. Remove inhaler from mouth and exhale (do not exhale into mouthpiece). Repeat procedure if 2nd dose required. Replace cover; rinse mouth with water (do not swallow).
- **Pulmicort Respules:** Administer with a jet nebulizer connected to adequate air flow, equipped with a mouthpiece or face mask. Adjust face mask to avoid exposing eyes to nebulized medication. Wash face after use of face mask. Ultrasonic nebulizers are not adequate for administration and not recommended. Store respules upright, away from heat and protected from light. Do not refrigerate or freeze. Respules are stable for 2 wks at room temperature after opening aluminum foil envelope. Open respules must be used promptly. Unused respules should be returned to aluminum foil envelope.
- **Flovent Diskus:** Do not use with a spacer. Exhale completely and then close lips firmly around mouthpiece. While breathing in deeply and slowly, press down on canister. Hold breath for as long as possible to ensure deep instillation of medication. Remover inhaler from mouth and breathe out gently. Allow 1–2 min between inhalations. After inhalation, rinse mouth with water and spit out (see Appendix D). Never wash the mouthpiece or any part of the Diskus inhaler. Discard Diskus inhaler device 6 wks (50-mcg strength) or 2 mo (100-mcg and 250-mcg strengths) after removal from protective foil overwrap pouch or after all blisters have been used (whichever comes first).
- **Asmanex Twisthaler:** Advise patient to remove cap while device is in upright position. To administer dose, exhale fully, then place mouthpiece between lips and inhale deeply and forcefully. Remove device from mouth and hold breath for 10 sec before exhaling (do not exhale into mouthpiece). Wipe the mouthpiece dry, if necessary, and replace the cap on the device. Rinse mouth with water. Advise patient to discard twisthaler 45 days from opening or when dose counter reads "00", whichever comes first.

Evaluation/Desired Outcomes

- Management of the symptoms of chronic asthma.
- Improvement in symptoms of asthma.

CORTICOSTEROIDS (NASAL)

beclomethasone
(be-kloe-**meth**-a-sone)
Beconase AQ, ✤Rivanase AQ

budesonide (byoo-**dess**-oh-nide)
Rhinocort Aqua

ciclesonide (sye-**kles**-oh-nide)
Omnaris

flunisolide (floo-**niss**-oh-lide)
Nasarel, ✤Rhinalar

fluticasone (floo-**ti**-ka-sone)
Flonase, Veramyst

mometasone (moe-**met**-a-sone)
Nasonex

triamcinolone
(trye-am-**sin**-oh-lone)
Nasacort AQ

Classification
Therapeutic: corticosteroids
Pharmacologic: corticosteroids (nasal)

Pregnancy Category B (budesonide), C (all others)

Indications

Seasonal or perennial allergic rhinitis. Nonallergic rhinitis (fluticasone). Treatment of nasal polyps.

Action

Potent, locally acting anti-inflammatory and immune modifier. **Therapeutic Effects:** ↓ in symptoms of allergic or nonallergic rhinitis. ↓ in symptoms of nasal polyps.

Pharmacokinetics

Absorption: *Beclomethasone*—44% absorbed; *budesonide*—34% absorbed; *flunisolide*—50% absorbed; *ciclesonide, fluticasone, mometasone*—-negligible absorption. Action of all agents is primarily local following nasal use.

Distribution: All agents cross the placenta and enter breast milk in small amounts.

Metabolism and Excretion: Following absorption from nasal mucosa, corticosteroids are rapidly and extensively metabolized by the liver.

Half-life: *Beclomethasone*—2.7 hr; *budesonide*—2–3 hr; *ciclesonide*—unknown; *flunisolide*—1–2 hr; *fluticasone*—7.8 hr; *mometasone*—5.8 hr; *triamcinolone*—3–5.4 hr.

TIME/ACTION PROFILE (improvement in symptoms)

ROUTE	ONSET	PEAK	DURATION
Beclomethasone	1–3 days	up to 2 wk	unknown
Budesonide	1–2 days	2 wk	unknown
Ciclesonide	1–2 days	2–5 wk	unknown
Flunisolide	few days	up to 3 wk	unknown
Fluticasone	few days	unknown	unknown
Mometasone	within 2 days	1–2 wk	unknown
Triamcinolone	few days	3–4 days	unknown

Contraindications/Precautions

Contraindicated in: Some products contain alcohol, propylene, or polyethylene glycol and should be avoided in patients with known hypersensitivity or intolerance.

Use Cautiously in: Active untreated infections; Diabetes or glaucoma; Underlying immunosuppression (due to disease or concurrent therapy); Systemic corticosteroid therapy (should not be abruptly discontinued when intranasal therapy is started); Recent nasal trauma, septal ulcers, or surgery (wound healing may be impaired by nasal corticosteroids); OB: Pregnancy or lactation (safety not established; prolonged or high-dose therapy may lead to complications); Pedi: Children (safety not established; prolonged or high-dose therapy may lead to complications).

Adverse Reactions/Side Effects

CNS: dizziness, headache. **EENT:** epistaxis, nasal burning, nasal irritation, nasal congestion, pharyngitis, rhinorrhea, sneezing, tearing eyes. **GI:** dry mouth, esophageal candidiasis, nausea, vomiting. **Endo:** adrenal suppression (increased dose, long-term therapy only), growth suppression (children). **Resp:** bronchospasm, cough.

Interactions

Drug-Drug: Ketoconazole ↑ effects of budesonide, ciclesonide, and fluticasone. **Ritonavir** ↑ effects of fluticasone (concomitant use not recommended).

Route/Dosage

Beclomethasone

Intranasal (Adults and Children ≥12 yr): 1–2 sprays in each nostril twice daily (not to exceed 2 sprays in each nostril twice daily).

Intranasal (Children 6–12 yr): 1–2 metered sprays in each nostril twice daily; once adequate control achieved, ↓ dose to 1 spray in each nostril twice daily.

Budesonide

Intranasal (Adults and Children ≥12 yr): 1 spray in each nostril once daily (not to exceed 4 sprays in each nostril once daily).

Intranasal (Children 6–11 yr): 1 spray in each nostril once daily (not to exceed 2 sprays in each nostril once daily).

Ciclesonide

Intranasal (Adults and Children ≥12 yr): 2 sprays in each nostril once daily (not to exceed 2 sprays in each nostril/day).

Flunisolide

Intranasal (Adults and Children >14 yr): 2 sprays in each nostril twice daily, may be ↑ to 2 sprays in each nostril 3 times daily if greater effect needed after 4–7 days (not to exceed 8 sprays in each nostril/day).

Intranasal (Children 6–14 yr): 1 spray in each nostril 3 times daily or 2 sprays in each nostril twice daily (not to exceed 4 sprays in each nostril/day).

Fluticasone

Intranasal (Adults and Children ≥12 yrs): 2 sprays in each nostril once daily or 1 spray in each nostril twice daily; after several days, attempt to ↓ dose to 1 spray in each nostril once daily. Patients ≥12 yr with seasonal allergic rhi-

nitis may also use 2 sprays in each nostril once daily on an as-needed basis.
Intranasal (Children >4 yr): *Flonase*—1 spray in each nostril once daily (not to exceed 2 sprays in each nostril/day).
Intranasal (Children 2–11 yrs): *Veramyst*—1 spray in each nostril daily; may increase to 2 sprays if no response. Once symptoms are controlled, attempt to ↓ dose to 1 spray/day.

Mometasone

Intranasal (Adults and Children >12 yr): *Treatment of seasonal and perennial allergic rhinitis*—2 sprays in each nostril once daily (not to exceed 2 sprays in each nostril once daily).
Intranasal (Adults): *Nasal polyps*—2 sprays in each nostril twice daily (not to exceed 2 sprays in each nostril twice daily).
Intranasal (Children 2–11 yr): *Treatment of seasonal and perennial allergic rhinitis* –1 spray in each nostril once daily.

Triamcinolone

Intranasal (Adults and Children >12 yr): 2 sprays in each nostril once daily.
Intranasal (Children 6–11 yr): 1 spray in each nostil once daily (not to exceed 2 sprays in each nostril/day).

Availability

Beclomethasone

Nasal spray: 42 mcg/metered spray in 25-g bottles (delivers 180 metered sprays), ✤50 mcg/metered spray in 25-g bottles (delivers 200 metered sprays), 84 mcg/metered spray in 25-g bottles (200 metered sprays).

Budesonide

Nasal spray: 32 mcg/metered spray in 8.6-g canister (delivers 120 metered sprays). **Cost:** $92.99/bottle.

Ciclesonide

Nasal spray: 50 mcg/metered spray in 12.5-g bottle (delivers 120 metered sprays).

Flunisolide

Nasal solution: 25 mcg/metered spray in 25-ml bottle (delivers 200 metered sprays).

Fluticasone

Nasal spray (Flonase): 50 mcg/metered spray in 16-g bottle (delivers 120 metered sprays). **Cost:** *Generic*—$59.99/bottle. **Nasal spray (Veramyst):** 55 mcg/spray in a 1-g bottle (delivers 120 sprays).

Mometasone

Nasal spray (scent-free): 50 mcg/metered spray in 17-g bottle (delivers 120 metered sprays). **Cost:** $89.24/bottle.

Triamcinolone

Nasal spray: 55 mcg/metered spray in 6.5-g bottle (delivers 30 metered sprays) and 16.5-g bottle (delivers 120 metered sprays). **Cost:** $89.99/16.5-g bottle.

NURSING IMPLICATIONS

Assessment

- Monitor degree of nasal stuffiness, amount and color of nasal discharge, and frequency of sneezing.
- Patients on long-term therapy should have periodic otolaryngologic examinations to monitor nasal mucosa and passages for infection or ulceration.
- Monitor growth rate in children receiving chronic therapy; use lowest possible dose.
- ***Lab Test Considerations:*** Periodic adrenal function tests may be ordered to assess degree of hypothalamic-pituitary-adrenal (HPA) axis suppression in chronic therapy. Children and patients using higher than recommended doses are at highest risk for HPA suppression.

Potential Nursing Diagnoses

Ineffective airway clearance (Indications)
Risk for infection (Side Effects)
Deficient knowledge, related to medication regimen (Patient/Family Teaching)

Implementation

- After the desired clinical effect has been obtained, attempts should be made to decrease dose to lowest amount. Gradually decrease dose every 2–4 wk as long as desired effect is maintained. If symptoms return, dose may briefly return to starting dose.
- **Intranasal:** Patients also using a nasal decongestant should be given decongestant 5–15 min before corticosteroid nasal spray. If patient is unable to breathe freely through nasal passages, instruct patient to blow nose gently in advance of medication administration.

C

Patient/Family Teaching

- Advise patient to take medication as directed. If a dose is missed, take as soon as remembered unless almost time for next dose.
- Caution patient not to exceed maximal daily dose of nasal spray.
- Instruct patient in correct technique for administering nasal spray (see Appendix D). Most nasal sprays include directions with pictures. Instruct patient to read patient information sheet prior to use. Shake well before use. Warn patient that temporary nasal stinging may occur.
- Instruct patient to gently blow nose to clear nostrils prior to administering dose.
- Instruct patient to notify health care professional if symptoms do not improve within 1 month, if symptoms worsen, or or if sneezing or nasal irritation occur.

Evaluation/Desired Outcomes

- Resolution of nasal stuffiness, discharge, and sneezing in seasonal or perennial allergic rhinitis or nonallergic rhinitis.
- Reduction in symptoms of nasal polyps.

CORTICOSTEROIDS (SYSTEMIC)

short-acting corticosteroids

cortisone (**kor**-ti-sone)
✤Cortone

hydrocortisone
(hye-droe-**kor**-ti-sone)
A-hydroCort, Cortef, Solu-Cortef

intermediate-acting corticosteroids

methylPREDNISolone
(meth-ill-pred-**niss**-oh-lone)
A-Methapred, Depo-Medrol, Medrol, Solu-Medrol

prednisoLONE
(pred-**niss**-oh-lone)
Orapred, Pediapred, Prelone

predniSONE (**pred**-ni-sone)
Sterapred

triamcinolone
(trye-am-**sin**-oh-lone)
Aristospan, Kenalog

long-acting corticosteroids

betamethasone
(bay-ta-**meth**-a-sone)
✤Betnelan, ✤Betnesol, Celestone, ✤Selestoject

budesonide (byoo-**des**-oh-nide)
Entocort EC

dexamethasone
(dex-a-**meth**-a-sone)
DexPak

Classification
Therapeutic: antiasthmatics, corticosteroids
Pharmacologic: corticosteroids (systemic)

Pregnancy Category B (prednisone), C (betamethasone, budesonide, dexamethasone, hydrocortisone, methylprednisolone, prednisolone, triamcinolone), D (cortisone)

Indications

Cortisone, hydrocortisone: Management of adrenocortical insufficiency. **Betamethasone, dexamethasone, hydrocortisone, prednisolone, prednisone, methylprednisolone, triamcinolone:** Used systemically and locally in a wide variety of chronic diseases including: Inflammatory, Allergic, Hematologic, Neoplastic, Autoimmune disorders. **Methylprednisolone, prednisone:** With other immunosuppressants in the prevention of organ rejection in transplantation surgery. Asthma. **Dexamethasone:** Management of cerebral edema: Diagnostic agent in adrenal disorders. **Budesonide:** Treatment of mild to moderate Crohn's disease. **Unlabeled uses:** Short-term administration to high-risk mothers before delivery to prevent respiratory distress syndrome in the newborn (betamethasone, dexamethasone). Adjunctive therapy of hypercalcemia (prednisone, prednisolone, methylprednisolone). Management of acute spinal cord injury (methylprednisolone). Adjunctive management of nausea and vomiting from chemotherapy (dexamethasone, prednisone, prednisolone, methylprednisolone). Management of croup (dexamethasone). Treatment of airway edema prior to extubation (dexamethasone). Facilitation of ventilator weaning in neonates with bronchopulmonary dysplasia (dexamethasone).

C

Action

In pharmacologic doses, all agents suppress inflammation and the normal immune response. All agents have numerous intense metabolic effects (see Adverse Reactions/Side Effects). Suppress adrenal function at chronic doses of *betamethasone*—0.6 mg/day; *cortisone, hydrocortisone*—20 mg/day; *dexamethasone*—0.75 mg/day; *methylprednisolone, triamcinolone*—4 mg/day; *prednisone/prednisolone*—5 mg/day. **Cortisone, hydrocortisone:** Replace endogenous cortisol in deficiency states. **Cortisone, hydrocortisone:** Have potent mineralocorticoid (sodium-retaining) activity. **Prednisolone, prednisone:** Have minimal mineralocorticoid activity. **Betamethasone, dexamethasone, methylprednisolone, triamcinolone:** Have negligible mineralocorticoid activity. **Budesonide:** Local anti-inflammatory activity in the lumen of the GI tract.
Therapeutic Effects: Suppression of inflammation and modification of the normal immune response. Replacement therapy in adrenal insufficiency. **Budesonide:** Improvement in symptoms/sequelae of Crohn's disease.

Pharmacokinetics

Absorption: Well absorbed after oral administration (except budesonide). Sodium phosphate and sodium succinate salts are rapidly absorbed after IM administration. Acetate, acetonide, and diacetate salts are slowly but completely absorbed after IM administration. Absorption from local sites (intra-articular, intralesional) is slow but complete. Bioavailability of budesonide is 9–21%.
Distribution: All are widely distributed, cross the placenta, and probably enter breast milk.
Metabolism and Excretion: All are metabolized mostly by the liver to inactive metabolites. *Cortisone* is converted by the liver to hydrocortisone. *Prednisone* is converted by the liver to prednisolone, which is then metabolized by the liver.
Half-life: *Betamethasone*—3–5 hr (plasma), 36–54 hr (tissue). *Budesonide*—2.0–3.6 hr. *Cortisone*—0.5 hr (plasma), 8–12 hr (tissue). *Dexamethasone*—3–4.5 hr (plasma), 36–54 hr (tissue). *Hydrocortisone*—1.5–2 hr (plasma), 8–12 hr (tissue). *Methylprednisolone*—>3.5 hr (plasma), 18–36 hr (tissue). *Prednisolone*—2.1–3.5 hr (plasma), 18–36 hr (tissue). *Prednisone*—3.4–3.8 hr (plasma), 18–36 hr (tissue). *Triamcinolone*—2–>5 hr (plasma), 18–36 hr (tissue).

TIME/ACTION PROFILE (anti-inflammatory activity)

ROUTE	ONSET	PEAK	DURATION
Betamethasone PO	unknown	1–2 hr	3.25 days
Betamethasone IM (acetate/sodium phosphate)	1–3 hr	unknown	1 wk
Budesonide PO	unknown	unknown	unknown
Cortisone PO	rapid	2 hr	1.25–1.5 days
Dexamethasone PO	unknown	1–3 hr	2.75 days
Dexamethasone IM, IV (sodium phosphate)	rapid	unknown	2.75 days
Hydrocortisone PO	unknown	1–2 hr	1.25–1.5 days
Hydrocortisone IM (sodium succinate)	rapid	1 hr	variable
Hydrocortisone IV (sodium succinate)	rapid	unknown	unknown
Methylprednisolone PO	unknown	1–2 hr	1.25–1.5 days
Methylprednisolone IM (acetate)	6–48 hr	4–8 days	1–4 wk
Methylprednisolone IM, IV (sodium succinate)	rapid	unknown	unknown
Prednisolone PO	unknown	1–2 hr	1.25–1.5 days
Prednisone PO	unknown	unknown	1.25–1.5 days
Triamcinolone PO	unknown	1–2 hr	2.25 days
Triamcinolone IM (acetonide)	24–48 hr	unknown	1–6 wk
Triamcinolone Intralesional (hexacetonide)	slow	unknown	4 days–4 wk

Contraindications/Precautions

Contraindicated in: Active untreated infections (may be used in patients being treated for

♣ = Canadian drug name.
*CAPITALS indicates life-threatening; underlines indicate most frequent.

some forms of meningitis); Lactation (avoid chronic use); Known alcohol, bisulfite, or tartrazine hypersensitivity or intolerance (some products contain these and should be avoided in susceptible patients); Administration of live virus vaccines.
Use Cautiously in: Chronic treatment (will lead to adrenal suppression; use lowest possible dose for shortest period of time); Hypothyroidism; Cirrhosis; Pedi: Children (chronic use will result in decreased growth; use lowest possible dose for shortest period of time); Stress (surgery, infections); supplemental doses may be needed; Potential infections may mask signs (fever, inflammation); OB: Pregnancy (safety not established); Neonates (avoid use of benzyl alcohol containing injectable preparations, use preservative free formulations).

Adverse Reactions/Side Effects

Adverse reactions/side effects are much more common with high-dose/long-term therapy.
CNS: depression, euphoria, headache, increased intracranial pressure (children only), personality changes, psychoses, restlessness. **EENT:** cataracts, increased intraocular pressure. **CV:** hypertension. **GI:** PEPTIC ULCERATION, anorexia, nausea, vomiting. **Derm:** acne, decreased wound healing, ecchymoses, fragility, hirsutism, petechiae. **Endo:** adrenal suppression, hyperglycemia. **F and E:** fluid retention (long-term high doses), hypokalemia, hypokalemic alkalosis. **Hemat:** THROMBOEMBOLISM, thrombophlebitis. **Metab:** weight gain. **MS:** muscle wasting, osteoporosis, aseptic necrosis of joints, muscle pain. **Misc:** cushingoid appearance (moon face, buffalo hump), increased susceptibility to infection.

Interactions

Drug-Drug: ↑ risk of hypokalemia with **thiazide** and **loop diuretics**, or **amphotericin B**. Hypokalemia may ↑ risk of **digoxin** toxicity. May increase requirement for **insulin** or **oral hypoglycemic agents**. **Phenytoin**, **phenobarbital**, and **rifampin** ↑ metabolism; may ↓ effectiveness. **Hormonal contraceptives** may ↓ metabolism. ↑ risk of adverse GI effects with **NSAIDs** (including aspirin). At chronic doses that suppress adrenal function, may ↓ antibody response to and ↑ risk of adverse reactions from **live-virus vaccines**. May increase serum concentrations of **cyclosporine** and **tacrolimus**. May ↑ risk of tendon rupture from **fluoroquinolones**. **Antacids** ↓ absorption of prednisone and dexamethasone. Known inhibitors of the CYP3A4 enzyme ncluding **ketoconazole**, **itraconazole**, **ritonavir**, **indinavir**, **saquinavir**, and **erythromycin** may ↑ blood levels and effects of budesonide (↓ dose may be necessary). May ↓ **isoniazid** levels and effectiveness. May antagonize the effects of **anticholinergic agents** in myastenia gravis.
Drug-Food: Grapefruit juice ↑ serum levels and effects of budesonide (avoid concurrent use).

Route/Dosage

Betamethasone

PO (Adults): 0.6–7.2 mg/day as single daily dose or in divided doses.
PO (Children): *Adrenocortical insufficiency*—17.5 mcg/kg/day (500 mcg/m^2/day) in 3 divided doses. *Other uses*—62.5–250 mcg/kg/day (1.875–7.5 mg/m^2/day) in 3 divided doses.
IM (Adults): 0.5–9 mg as betamethasone sodium phosphate/acetate suspension. *Prevention of respiratory distress syndrome in newborn*—12 mg daily for 2–3 days before delivery (unlabeled).
IM (Children): *Adrenocortical insufficiency*—17.5 mcg/kg/day (500 mcg/m^2/day) in 3 divided doses every 3rd day or 5.8–8.75 mcg/kg (166–250 mcg/m^2)/day as a single dose.

Budesonide

PO (Adults): *Active Crohn's disease*—9 mg once daily in the morning for ≤8 weeks, may repeat 8 wk course for recurring episodes. *Maintenance of remission*—6 mg once daily for up to 3 months, once symptoms are controlled, taper to complete cessation.

Cortisone

PO (Adults): 25–300 mg/day in divided doses q 12–24 hr.
PO (Children): *Adrenocortical insufficiency*—0.7 mg/kg/day (20–25 mg/m^2/day) in divided doses q 8 hr. *Other uses*—2.5–10 mg/kg/day (75–300 mg/m^2/day) in divided doses q 6–8 hr.

Dexamethasone

PO, IM, IV (Adults): *Anti-inflammatory*—0.75–9 mg daily in divided doses q 6–12 hr. *Airway edema or extubation*—0.5–2 mg/kg/day divided q 6 hr; begin 24 hr prior to extubation and continue for 24 hr post-extubation. *Cerebral edema*—10 mg IV, then 4 mg IM or IV q 6 hr until maximal response achieved, then switch to PO regimen and taper over 5–7 days.

PO, IM, IV (Children): *Airway edema or extubation*—0.5–2 mg/kg/day divided q 6 hr; begin 24 hr prior to extubation and continue for 24 hr post-extubation. *Anti-inflammatory*—0.08–0.3 mg/kg/day or 2.5–10 mg/m²/day divided q 6–12 hr. *Physiologic replacement*—0.03–0.15 mg/kg/day or 0.6–0.75 mg/m²/day divided q 6–12 hr.

PO (Adults): *Suppression test*—1 mg at 11 PM or 0.5 mg q 6 hr for 48 hr.

IV (Children): *Chemotherapy induced emesis*—5–20 mg given 15–30 min before treatment. *Cerebral edema*—Loading dose 1–2 mg/kg followed by 1–1.5 mg/kg/day divided q 4–6 hr for 5 days (not to exceed 16 mg/day); then taper over 1–6 wk. *Bacterial meningitis*—0.6 mg/kg/day divided q 6 hr x 4 days (start at time of first antibiotic dose).

IV, PO (Adults): *Chemotherapy induced emesis*—10–20 mg given 15–30 min before each treatment or 10 mg q 12 hr on each treatment day. *Delayed nausea/vomiting*—4–10 mg PO 1–2 times/day for 2–4 days *or* 8 mg PO q 12 hr for 2 days, then 4 mg PO q 12 hr for 2 days *or* 20 mg PO 1 hr before chemotherapy, then 10 mg PO q 12 hr after chemotherapy, then 8 mg PO q 12 hr for 2 days, then 4 mg PO q 12 hr for 2 days.

IS (Adults): 0.4–6 mg/day.

Hydrocortisone

PO (Adults): 20–240 mg/day in 1–4 divided doses.

PO (Children): *Adrenocortical insufficiency*—0.56 mg/kg/day (15–20 mg/m²/day) as a single dose or in divided doses. *Other uses*—2–8 mg/kg/day (60–240 mg/m²/day) as a single dose or in divided doses.

IM, IV (Adults): 100–500 mg q 2–6 hr (range 100–8000 mg/day).

IM, IV (Children): *Adrenocortical insufficiency*—0.186–0.28 mg/kg/day (10–12 mg/m²/day) in 3 divided doses. *Other uses*—0.666–4 mg/kg (20–120 mg/m²) q 12–24 hr.

Methylprednisolone

PO (Adults): *Multiple sclerosis*—160 mg/day for 7 days, then 64 mg every other day for 1 mo. *Other uses*—2–60 mg/day as a single dose or in 2–4 divided doses. *Asthma exacerbations*—120–180 mg/day in divided doses 3–4 times/day for 48 hr, then 60–80 mg/day in 2 divided doses.

PO (Children): *Anti-inflammatory/Immunosuppressive*—0.5–1.7 mg/kg/day (5–25 mg/m²/day) in divided doses q 6–12 hr. *Asthma exacerbations*—1 mg/kg q 6 hr for 48 hr, then 1–2 mg/kg/day (maximum: 60 mg/day) divided twice daily.

IM, IV (Adults): *Most uses: methylprednisolone sodium succinate*—40–250 mg q 4–6 hr. *High-dose "pulse" therapy: methylprednisolone sodium succinate*—30 mg/kg IV q 4–6 hr for up to 72 hr. *Status asthmaticus: methylprednisolone sodium succinate*—2 mg/kg IV, then 0.5–1 mg/kg IV q 6 hr for up to 5 days. *Multiple sclerosis: methylprednisolone sodium succinate*—160 mg/day for 7 days, then 64 mg every other day for 1 mo. *Adjunctive therapy of* Pneumocystis carinii *pneumonia in AIDS patients: methylprednisolone sodium succinate*—30 mg twice daily for 5 days, then 30 mg once daily for 5 days, then 15 mg once daily for 10 days. *Acute spinal cord injury: methylprednisolone sodium succinate*—30 mg/kg IV over 15 min initially, followed in 45 min with a continuous infusion of 5.4 mg/kg/hr for 23 hr (unlabeled).

IM, IV (Children): *Anti-inflammatory/Immunosuppressive*—0.5–1.7 mg/kg/day (5–25 mg/m²/day) in divided doses q 6–12 hr. *Acute spinal cord injury: methylprednisolone sodium succinate*—30 mg/kg IV over 15 min initially, followed in 45 min with a continuous infusion of 5.4 mg/kg/hr for 23 hr (unlabeled). *Status asthmaticus*—2 mg/kg IV, then 0.5–1 mg/kg IV q 6 hr. *Lupus nephritis*—30 mg/kg IV every other day for 6 doses.

IM (Adults): *Methylprednisolone acetate*—40–120 mg daily, weekly, or every 2 wk.

Prednisolone

PO (Adults): *Most uses*—5–60 mg/day as a single dose or in divided doses. *Multiple sclerosis*—200 mg/day for 7 days, then 80 mg every other day for 1 mo. *Asthma exacerbations*—120–180 mg/day in divided doses 3–4 times/day for 48 hrs, then 60–80 mg/day in 2 divided doses.

PO (Children): *Anti-inflammatory/Immunosuppressive*—0.1–2 mg/kg/day in 1–4 divided doses. *Nephrotic syndrome*—2 mg/kg/day (60 mg/m²/day) in 1–3 divided doses daily (maximum dose: 80 mg/day) until urine is protein free for 4–6 weeks, followed by 2 mg/kg/

dose (40 mg/m²/dose) every other day in the morning, gradually taper off over 4–6 weeks. *Asthma exacerbations*—1 mg/kg q 6 hr for 48 hr, then 1–2 mg/kg/day (maximum: 60 mg/day) divided twice daily.

Prednisone

PO (Adults): *Most uses*—5–60 mg/day as a single dose or in divided doses. *Multiple sclerosis*—200 mg/day for 1 wk, then 80 mg every other day for 1 mo. *Adjunctive therapy of* Pneumocystis carinii *pneumonia in AIDS patients*—40 mg twice daily for 5 days, then 40 mg once daily for 5 days, then 20 mg once daily for 10 days.
PO (Children): *Nephrotic syndrome*—2 mg/kg/day initially given in 1–3 divided doses (maximum 80 mg/day) until urine is protein free for 4–6 weeks. Maintenance dose of 2 mg/kg/day every other day in the morning, gradually taper off after 4–6 weeks. *Asthma exacerbation*—1 mg/kg q 6 hr for 48 hr, then 1–2 mg/kg/day (maximum 60 mg/day) in divided doses twice daily.

Triamcinolone

IM (Adults): *Triamcinolone acetonide*—40–80 mg q 4 wk.
IM (Children): *Triamcinolone acetonide*—40 mg q 4 wk or 30–200 mcg/kg (1–6.25 mg/m²) q 1–7 days.

Availability

Betamethasone

Tablets: ✤0.5 mg. **Oral solution (cherry-orange flavor):** 0.6 mg/5 ml. **Effervescent tablets:** ✤0.5 mg. **Extended-release tablets:** ✤1 mg. **Suspension for injection (sodium phosphate and acetate):** 6 mg (total)/ml.

Budesonide

Capsules (enteric-coated): 3 mg.

Cortisone

Tablets: 25 mg.

Dexamethasone

Tablets: 0.5 mg, 0.75 mg, 1 mg, 1.5 mg, 2 mg, 4 mg, 6 mg. **Elixir (raspberry flavor):** 0.5 mg/5 ml. **Oral solution (cherry flavor):** 0.5 mg/5 ml, 1 mg/ml. **Solution for injection (sodium phosphate):** 4 mg/ml, 10 mg/ml.

Hydrocortisone

Tablets: 5 mg, 10 mg, 20 mg. **Powder for injection (sodium succinate):** 100 mg, 250 mg, 500 mg, 1 g.

Methylprednisolone

Tablets: 2 mg, 4 mg, 8 mg, 16 mg, 32 mg. **Powder for injection (sodium succinate):** 40 mg, 125 mg, 500 mg, 1 g, 2 g. **Suspension for injection (acetate):** 20 mg/ml, 40 mg/ml, 80 mg/ml.

Prednisolone

Tablets: 5 mg. **Orally disintegrating tablets (grape flavor):** 10 mg, 15 mg, 30 mg. **Syrup:** 5 mg/5 ml, 15 mg/5 ml. **Oral solution:** 5 mg/5 ml, 15 mg/5 ml.

Prednisone

Tablets: 1 mg, 2.5 mg, 5 mg, 10 mg, 20 mg, 50 mg. **Oral solution:** 5 mg/5 ml, 5 mg/ml.

Triamcinolone

Suspension for injection (acetonide): 10 mg/ml, 40 mg/ml . **Suspension for injection (hexacetonide):** 5 mg/ml, 20 mg/ml.

NURSING IMPLICATIONS

Assessment

- These drugs are indicated for many conditions. Assess involved systems before and periodically during therapy.
- Assess patient for signs of adrenal insufficiency (hypotension, weight loss, weakness, nausea, vomiting, anorexia, lethargy, confusion, restlessness) before and periodically during therapy.
- Monitor intake and output ratios and daily weights. Observe patient for peripheral edema, steady weight gain, rales/crackles, or dyspnea. Notify health care professional if these occur.
- Children should have periodic evaluations of growth.
- **Cerebral Edema:** Assess patient for changes in level of consciousness and headache during therapy.
- **Budesonide:** Assess signs of Crohn's disease (diarrhea, crampy abdominal pain, fever, bleeding from rectum) during therapy.
- ***Lab Test Considerations:*** Monitor serum electrolytes and glucose. May cause hyperglycemia, especially in persons with diabetes. May cause hypokalemia. Patients on prolonged therapy should routinely have CBC, serum electrolytes, and serum and urine glucose evaluated. May ↓ WBCs. May cause hyperglycemia, especially in persons with diabetes. May ↓ serum potassium and calcium and ↑ serum sodium concentrations.

- Guaiac-test stools. Promptly report presence of guaiac-positive stools.
- May ↑ serum cholesterol and lipid values. May ↓ uptake of thyroid ^{123}I or ^{131}I.
- Suppress reactions to allergy skin tests.
- Periodic adrenal function tests may be ordered to assess degree of hypothalamic-pituitary-adrenal axis suppression in systemic and chronic topical therapy. Dexamethasone Suppression Test To diagnose Cushing's syndrome: Obtain baseline cortisol level; administer dexamethasone at 11 PM and obtain cortisol levels at 8 AM the next day. Normal response is a ↓ cortisol level.
- Alternative method: Obtain baseline 24-hr urine for 17-hydroxycorticosteroid (OHCS) concentrations, then begin 48-hr administration of dexamethasone. Second 24-hr urine for 17-OHCS is obtained after 24 hr of dexamethasone.

Potential Nursing Diagnoses

Risk for infection (Side Effects)
Disturbed body image (Side Effects)

Implementation

- Do not confuse prednisone with methylprednisolone or primidone. Do not confuse hydrocortisone with hydrocodone.
- If dose is ordered daily or every other day, administer in the morning to coincide with the body's normal secretion of cortisol.
- Periods of stress, such as surgery, may require supplemental systemic corticosteroids.
- Patients with mild to moderate Crohn's disease may be switched from oral prednisolone without adrenal insufficiency by gradually decreasing prednisolone doses and adding budesonide.
- **PO:** Administer with meals to minimize GI irritation.
- Tablets may be crushed and administered with food or fluids for patients with difficulty swallowing. Capsules should be swallowed whole; do not crush, break, or chew.
- Use calibrated measuring device to ensure accurate dose of liquid forms.
- Avoid consumption of grapefruit juice during therapy with budesonide or methylprednisolone.
- **IM, Subcut:** Shake suspension well before drawing up. IM doses should not be administered when rapid effect is desirable. Do not dilute with other solution or admix. Do not administer suspensions IV.

Dexamethasone Sodium Phosphate

IV Administration

- **Direct IV:** ***Diluent:*** May be given undiluted. ***Concentration:*** 4–10 mg/ml. ***Rate:*** Administer over 1–4 min if dose is <10 mg.
- **Intermittent Infusion:** ***Diluent:*** High-dose therapy should be added to D5W or 0.9% NaCl solution. Solution should be clear and colorless to light yellow; use diluted solution within 24 hr. ***Concentration:*** Up to 10 mg/ml. ***Rate:*** Administer infusions over 15–30 min.
- **Syringe Compatibility:** granisetron, metoclopramide, palonosetron, ranitidine, sufentanil.
- **Syringe Incompatibility:** doxapram, glycopyrrolate, pantoprazole.
- **Y-Site Compatibility:** acyclovir, allopurinol, amifostine, amikacin, amphotericin B cholesteryl, amsacrine, aztreonam, bivalirudin, cefepime, cisatracurium, cisplatin, cladribine, cyclophosphamide, cytarabine, dexmedetomidine, docetaxel, doxorubicin, doxorubicin liposome, etoposide phosphate, famotidine, fentanyl, filgrastim, fluconazole, fludarabine, foscarnet, gallium nitrate, gatifloxacin, gemcitabine, granisetron, heparin, hydromorphone, lansoprazole, levofloxacin, linezolid, lorazepam, melphalan, meperidine, meropenem, methadone, milrinone, morphine, ondansetron, oxaliplatin, paclitaxel, pemetrexed, piperacillin/tazobactam, potassium, propofol, remifentanil, sargramostim, sodium bicarbonate, sufentanil, tacrolimus, teniposide, theophylline, thiotepa, vinorelbine, vitamin B complex with C, zidovudine.
- **Y-Site Incompatibility:** ciprofloxacin, fenoldopam, idarubicin, midazolam, topotecan.
- **Additive Compatibility:** aminophylline, bleomycin, cimetidine, floxacillin, furosemide, granisetron, lidocaine, meropenem, nafcillin, palonosetron, ranitidine.
- **Additive Incompatibility:** daunorubicin, metaraminol, vancomycin.

Hydrocortisone Sodium Succinate

IV Administration

- **Direct IV:** ***Diluent:*** Reconstitute with provided solution (i.e., Act-O-Vials) or 2 ml of bacteriostatic water or saline for injection. ***Concentration:*** 50 mg/ml. ***Rate:*** Administer each 100 mg over at least 30 sec. Doses 500 mg and larger should be infused over at least 10 min.

- **Intermittent/Continuous Infusion:** ***Diluent:*** May be added to 50–1000 ml of D5W, 0.9% NaCl, or D5/0.9% NaCl. Diluted solutions should be used within 24 hr. ***Concentration:*** 1–5 mg/ml. Concentrations of up to 60 mg/ml have been used in fluid restricted adults. ***Rate:*** Administer over 20–30 min or at prescribed rate.
- **Syringe Compatibility:** thiopental.
- **Syringe Incompatibility:** pantoprazole.
- **Y-Site Compatibility:** acyclovir, allopurinol, amifostine, aminophylline, amphotericin B cholesteryl sulfate, ampicillin, amsacrine, argatroban, atracurium, atropine, aztreonam, bivalirudin, calcium gluconate, cefepime, chlordiazepoxide, chlorpromazine, cisatracurium, cladribine, cyanocobalamin, cytarabine, digoxin, diphenhydramine, docetaxel, dopamine, doxorubicin liposome, droperidol, edrophonium, enalaprilat, epinephrine, esmolol, conjugated estrogens, ethacrynate, etoposide, famotidine, fenoldopam, fentanyl, filgrastim, fludarabine, fluorouracil, foscarnet, furosemide, gallium nitrate, gatifloxacin, gemcitabine, granisetron, heparin, hydralazine, inamrinone, insulin, isoproterenol, kanamycin, lidocaine, linezolid, lorazepam, magnesium sulfate, melphalan, meperidine, methoxamine, methylergonovine, morphine, neostigmine, nicardipine, norepinephrine, ondansetron, oxacillin, oxaliplatin, oxytocin, paclitaxel, pancuronium, penicillin G potassium, pentazocine, phytonadione, piperacillin/tazobactam, procainamide, prochlorperazine edisylate, propofol, propranolol, pyridostigmine, remifentanil, scopolamine, sodium bicarbonate, succinylcholine, tacrolimus, teniposide, theophylline, thiotepa, trimethobenzamide, vecuronium, vinorelbine.
- **Y-Site Incompatibility:** ciprofloxacin, diazepam, idarubicin, lansoprazole, midazolam, phenytoin, sargramostim.
- **Additive Compatibility:** amikacin, aminophylline, amphotericin B, calcium chloride, calcium gluconate, daunorubicin, diphenhydramine, lidocaine, magnesium sulfate, mitomycin, mitoxantrone, potassium chloride, vitamin B complex with C.
- **Additive Incompatibility:** bleomycin.

Methylprednisolone Sodium Succinate

IV Administration

- **Direct IV:** ***Diluent:*** Reconstitute with provided solution (Act-O-Vials, Univials, ADD-Vantage vials) or 2 ml of bacteriostatic water (with benzyl alcohol) for injection. Use preservative-free diluent for use in neonates. Acetate injection is not for IV use. ***Concentration:*** Maximum concentration 125 mg/ml. ***Rate:*** Low dose (<1.8 mg/kg or <125 mg/dose): May be administered direct IV push over 1 to several minutes. Moderate dose (>2 mg/kg or 250 mg/dose): give over 15–30 min. High dose (15 mg/kg or >500 mg/dose): give over 30 min. Doses >15 mg/kg or >1 g give over 1 hour.
- **Intermittent/Continuous Infusion:** ***Diluent:*** May be diluted further in D5W, 0.9% NaCl, or D5/0.9% NaCl and administered as intermittent or continuous infusion at the prescribed rate. ***Concentration:*** Maximum concentration 2.5 mg/ml. Solution may form a haze upon dilution.
- **Syringe Compatibility:** granisetron, metoclopramide.
- **Syringe Incompatibility:** pantoprazole.
- **Y-Site Compatibility:** acyclovir, amifostine, amiodarone, amphotericin B cholesteryl sulfate, aztreonam, bivalirudin, cefepime, ceftazidime, cisplatin, cladribine, cyclophosphamide, cytarabine, dexmedetomidine, dopamine, doxorubicin, doxorubicin liposome, enalaprilat, famotidine, fludarabine, gatifloxacin, granisetron, heparin, inamrinone, linezolid, melphalan, meperidine, methotrexate, metronidazole, midazolam, milrinone, morphine, nicardipine, oxaliplatin, pemetrexed, piperacillin/tazobactam, remifentanil, sodium bicarbonate, tacrolimus, teniposide, theophylline, thiotepa, topotecan.
- **Y-Site Incompatibility:** allopurinol, amsacrine, ciprofloxacin, docetaxel, etoposide, fenoldopam, filgrastim, gemcitabine, lansoprazole, ondansetron, paclitaxel, propofol, sargramostim, vinorelbine.
- **Additive Compatibility:** cimetidine, granisetron, heparin, ranitidine, theophylline.

Patient/Family Teaching

- Instruct patient on correct technique of medication administration. Advise patient to take medication as directed. Take missed doses as soon as remembered unless almost time for next dose. Do not double doses. Stopping the medication suddenly may result in adrenal insufficiency (anorexia, nausea, weakness, fatigue, dyspnea, hypotension, hypoglycemia). If these signs appear, notify health care professional immediately. This can be life threatening.

- Corticosteroids cause immunosuppression and may mask symptoms of infection. Instruct patient to avoid people with known contagious illnesses and to report possible infections immediately.
- *Prelone* syrup should not be refrigerated, *Pediapred* solution may be refrigerated, *Orapred* solution should be refrigerated.
- Caution patient to avoid vaccinations without first consulting health care professional.
- Review side effects with patient. Instruct patient to inform health care professional promptly if severe abdominal pain or tarry stools occur. Patient also should report unusual swelling, weight gain, tiredness, bone pain, bruising, nonhealing sores, visual disturbances, or behavior changes.
- Advise patient to notify health care professional of medication regimen before treatment or surgery.
- Discuss possible effects on body image. Explore coping mechanisms.
- Instruct patient to inform health care professional if symptoms of underlying disease return or worsen.
- Advise patient to carry identification describing disease process and medication regimen in the event of emergency in which patient cannot relate medical history.
- Explain need for continued medical follow-up to assess effectiveness and possible side effects of medication. Periodic lab tests and eye exams may be needed.
- **Long-term Therapy:** Encourage patient to eat a diet high in protein, calcium, and potassium, and low in sodium and carbohydrates (see Appendix L). Alcohol should be avoided during therapy.

Evaluation/Desired Outcomes

- Decrease in presenting symptoms with minimal systemic side effects.
- Suppression of the inflammatory and immune responses in autoimmune disorders, allergic reactions, and neoplasms.
- Management of symptoms in adrenal insufficiency.
- Improvement of symptoms/sequelae of Crohn's disease (decreased frequency of liquid stools, decreased abdominal complaints, improved sense of well being).

CORTICOSTEROIDS (TOPICAL/LOCAL)

alclometasone
(al-kloe-**met**-a-sone)
Aclovate

amcinonide (am-**sin**-oh-nide)
Cyclocort

betamethasone
(bay-ta-**meth**-a-sone)
✤Betacort, ✤Betaderm, Beta-Val, ✤Betnovate, ✤Celestoderm, Dermabet, Diprolene, ✤Ectosone, Luxiq, ✤Metaderm, ✤Novobetamet, ✤Prevex, ✤Topilene, ✤Topisone, Valnac

clobetasol (kloe-**bay**-ta-sol)
Clobex, Cormax, ✤Dermovate, Embeline, Embeline E, Olux, Olux-E, Temovate, Temovate E

clocortolone (kloe-**kor**-toe-lone)
Cloderm

desonide (**des**-oh-nide)
Desonate, DesOwen, Verdeso

desoximetasone
(dess-ox-i-**met**-a-sone)
Topicort, Topicort-LP

diflorasone (dye-**flor**-a-sone)
Psorcon

fluocinolone
(floo-oh-**sin**-oh-lone)
Derma-Smoothe/FS, ✤Fluoderm, ✤Fluolar, ✤Fluonide, FS Shampoo, Synalar, ✤Synamol

fluocinonide
(floo-oh-**sin**-oh-nide)
✤Lidemol, Lidex, Lidex-E, ✤Lyderm, ✤Topsyn, Vanos

flurandrenolide
(flure-an-**dren**-oh-lide)
Cordran, Cordran-SP, ✤Drenison

fluticasone (floo-**tik**-a-sone)
Cutivate

halcinonide (hal-**sin**-oh-nide)
Halog

halobetasol (hal-oh-**bay**-ta-sol)
Ultravate

hydrocortisone
(hye-droe-**kor**-ti-sone)
Acticort, Aeroseb-HC, Ala-Cort, Ala-Scalp, Alphaderm, Anusol HC, Bactine, ✤Barriere-HC, Calde-CORT Anti-Itch, Carmol HC, Cetacort, ✤Cortacet, Cortaid, ✤Cortate, Cort-Dome, ✤Cortef Feminine Itch, Corticaine, ✤Corticreme, Cortifair, Cortifoam, Cortizone, Dermacort, DermiCort, Dermtex HC, ✤Emo-Cort, Foille-Cort, Gynecort, Hemril-HC, Hi-Cor, Hycort, ✤Hyderm, Hydro-Tex, Hytone, LactiCare-HC, Lanacort 9-1-1, Lemoderm, Locoid, ✤Novohydrocort, Nutracort, Orabase-HCA, Pandel, Penecort, Pharma-Cort, Prevex HC, Proctocort, Rhulicort, Synacort, Texacort, ✤Unicort, Westcort

mometasone (moe-**met**-a-sone)
✤Elocom, Elocon

prednicarbate (pred-ni-**kar**-bate)
Dermatop

triamcinolone
(trye-am-**sin**-oh-lone)
Kenalog, ✤Triaderm, ✤Trianide, Triderm

Classification
Therapeutic: corticosteroids
Pharmacologic: corticosteroids (topical)

Pregnancy Category C

Indications
Management of inflammation and pruritis associated with various allergic/immunologic skin problems.

Action
Suppress normal immune response and inflammation. **Therapeutic Effects:** Suppression of dermatologic inflammation and immune processes.

Pharmacokinetics
Absorption: Minimal. Prolonged use on large surface areas, application of large amounts, or use of occlusive dressings may ↑ systemic absorption.
Distribution: Remain primarily at site of action.
Metabolism and Excretion: Usually metabolized in skin; some have been modified to resist local metabolism and have a prolonged local effect.
Half-life: *Betamethasone*—3–5 hr (plasma), 36–54 hr (tissue). *Dexamethasone*—3–4.5 hr (plasma), 36–54 hr (tissue). *Hydrocortisone*—1.5–2 hr (plasma), 8–12 hr (tissue). *Triamcinolone*—2–>5 hr (plasma), 18–36 hr (tissue).

TIME/ACTION PROFILE (response depends on condition being treated)

ROUTE	ONSET	PEAK	DURATION
Topical	min–hrs	hrs–days	hrs–days

Contraindications/Precautions
Contraindicated in: Hypersensitivity or known intolerance to corticosteroids or components of vehicles (ointment or cream base, preservative, alcohol); Untreated bacterial or viral infections.
Use Cautiously in: Hepatic dysfunction; Diabetes mellitus, cataracts, glaucoma, or tuberculosis (use of large amounts of high-potency agents may worsen condition); Patients with pre-existing skin atrophy; OB, Lactation: Chronic use at high dosages may result in adrenal suppression in mother and growth suppression in children; Pedi: Children may be more susceptible to adrenal and growth suppression. Clobetasol not recommended for children <12 yr; desoximetasone not recommended for children <10 yr.

Adverse Reactions/Side Effects
Derm: allergic contact dermatitis, atrophy, burning, dryness, edema, folliculitis, hypersen-

sitivity reactions, hypertrichosis, hypopigmentation, irritation, maceration, miliaria, perioral dermatitis, secondary infection, striae. **Misc:** adrenal suppression (increased dose, long-term therapy).

Interactions

Drug-Drug: None significant.

Route/Dosage

Topical (Adults and Children): 1–4 times daily (depends on product, preparation, and condition being treated).

Rect (Adults): hydrocortisone *Retention enema*—100 mg nightly for 21 days or until remission occurs; *aerosol foam*—90 mg 1–2 times/day for 2–3 wk; then adjusted.

Availability

Alclometasone

Cream: 0.05%. **Ointment:** 0.05%.

Amcinonide

Cream: 0.1%. **Lotion:** 0.1%. **Ointment:** 0.1%.

Betamethasone

Cream: 0.05%, 0.1%. **Gel:** 0.05%. **Lotion:** 0.05%, 0.1%. **Ointment:** 0.05%, 0.1%. **Aerosol Foam:** 0.12%. ***In combination with:*** clotrimazole (Lotrisone), calcipotriene (Taclonex); see Appendix B.

Clobetasol

Cream: 0.05%. **Emollient cream:** 0.05%. **Gel:** 0.05%. **Ointment:** 0.05%. **Foam:** 0.05%. **Lotion:** 0.05%. **Scalp solution:** 0.05%. **Shampoo:** 0.05%. **Spray:** 0.05%.

Clocortolone

Cream: 0.1%.

Desonide

Cream: 0.05%. **Foam:** 0.05%. **Gel:** 0.05%. **Ointment:** 0.05%. **Lotion:** 0.05%.

Desoximetasone

Cream: 0.05%, 0.25%. **Gel:** 0.05%. **Ointment:** 0.25%.

Diflorasone

Cream: 0.05%. **Ointment:** 0.05%.

Fluocinolone

Cream: 0.01%, 0.025%. **Ointment:** 0.025%. **Solution:** 0.01%. **Shampoo:** 0.01%. **Oil:** 0.01%.

Fluocinonide

Cream: 0.05%, 0.1%. **Gel:** 0.05%. **Ointment:** 0.05%. **Solution:** 0.05%.

Flurandrenolide

Cream: 0.025%, 0.05%. **Ointment:** 0.025%, 0.05%. **Lotion:** 0.05%. **Tape:** $4\ mcg/m^2$.

Fluticasone

Cream: 0.05%. **Lotion:** 0.05%. **Ointment:** 0.005%.

Halcinonide

Cream: 0.1%. **Ointment:** 0.1%. **Solution:** 0.1%.

Halobetasol

Cream: 0.05%. **Ointment:** 0.05%.

Hydrocortisone

Cream: 0.1%, 0.2%, 0.5%[Rx, OTC], 1%[Rx, OTC], 2.5%. **Gel:** 1%[Rx, OTC]. **Ointment:** 0.1%, 0.2%, 0.5%[Rx, OTC], 1%[Rx, OTC], 2.5%. **Lotion:** 1%[Rx, OTC], 2.5%. **Solution:** 1%, 2.5%. **Spray:** 0.5%[Rx, OTC], 1%[Rx, OTC]. **Rectal suspension:** 100 mg/60 ml. **Rectal cream:** 1%. **Rectal aerosol:** 10%.

Mometasone

Cream: 0.1%. **Ointment:** 0.1%. **Lotion:** 0.1%.

Prednicarbate

Cream: 0.1%.

Triamcinolone

Cream: 0.025%, 0.1%, 0.5%. **Ointment:** 0.025%, 0.1%, 0.5%. **Lotion:** 0.025%, 0.1%. **Spray:** 0.2 mg/2-sec spray. ***In combination with:*** acetic acid, antifungals, anti-infectives, antihistamines, urea, and benzoyl peroxide in various otic and topical preparations. See Appendix B.

NURSING IMPLICATIONS

Assessment

- Assess affected skin before and daily during therapy. Note degree of inflammation and pruritus. Notify physician or other health care professional if symptoms of infection (increased pain, erythema, purulent exudate) develop.
- ***Lab Test Considerations:*** Adrenal function tests may be ordered to assess degree of hypothalamic-pituitary-adrenal (HPA) axis suppression in long-term topical therapy. Children and patients with dose applied to a large area, using an occlusive dressing, or using high-potency products, are at highest risk for HPA suppression.
- May cause ↑ serum and urine glucose concentrations if significant absorption occurs.

Potential Nursing Diagnoses
Risk for impaired skin integrity (Indications)
Risk for infection (Side Effects)

Implementation
- Choice of vehicle depends on site and type of lesion. Ointments are more occlusive and preferred for dry, scaly lesions. Creams should be used on oozing or intertriginous areas, where the occlusive action of ointments might cause folliculitis or maceration. Creams may be preferred for esthetic reasons even though they may dry skin more than ointments. Gels, aerosols, lotions, and solutions are useful in hairy areas.
- **Topical:** Apply *ointments, creams,* or *gels* sparingly as a thin film to clean, slightly moist skin. Wear gloves. Apply occlusive dressing only if specified by physician or other health care professional.
- Apply *lotion, solution,* or *gel* to hair by parting hair and applying a small amount to affected area. Rub in gently. Protect area from washing, clothing, or rubbing until medication has dried. Hair may be washed as usual but not right after applying medication.
- Use *aerosols* by shaking well and spraying on affected area, holding container 3–6 in. away. Spray for about 2 seconds to cover an area the size of a hand. Do not inhale. If spraying near face, cover eyes.

Patient/Family Teaching
- Instruct patient on correct technique of medication administration. Emphasize importance of avoiding the eyes. If a dose is missed, it should be applied as soon as remembered unless almost time for the next dose.
- Caution patient to use only as directed. Avoid using cosmetics, bandages, dressings, or other skin products over the treated area unless directed by health care professional.
- Advise parents of pediatric patients not to apply tight-fitting diapers or plastic pants on a child treated in the diaper area; these garments work as an occlusive dressing and may cause more of the drug to be absorbed.
- Caution women that medication should not be used extensively, in large amounts, or for protracted periods if they are pregnant or planning to become pregnant.
- Advise patient to consult health care professional before using medicine for condition other than indicated.
- Instruct patient to inform health care professional if symptoms of underlying disease return or worsen or if symptoms of infection develop.

Evaluation/Desired Outcomes
- Resolution of skin inflammation, pruritus, or other dermatologic conditions.

cromolyn, **See MAST CELL STABILIZERS.**

cyclobenzaprine
(sye-kloe-**ben**-za-preen)
Amrix, Flexeril

Classification
Therapeutic: skeletal muscle relaxants (centrally acting)

Pregnancy Category B

Indications
Management of acute painful musculoskeletal conditions associated with muscle spasm. **Unlabeled uses:** Management of fibromyalgia.

Action
Reduces tonic somatic muscle activity at the level of the brainstem. Structurally similar to tricyclic antidepressants. **Therapeutic Effects:** Reduction in muscle spasm and hyperactivity without loss of function.

Pharmacokinetics
Absorption: Well absorbed from the GI tract.
Distribution: Unknown.
Protein Binding: 93%.
Metabolism and Excretion: Mostly metabolized by the liver.
Half-life: 1–3 days.

TIME/ACTION PROFILE (skeletal muscle relaxation)

ROUTE	ONSET	PEAK†	DURATION
PO	within 1 hr	3–8 hr	12–24 hr
Extended release	unk	unk	24 hr

†Full effects may not occur for 1–2 wk

Contraindications/Precautions
Contraindicated in: Hypersensitivity; Should not be used within 14 days of MAO inhibitor therapy; Immediate period after MI; Severe or symptomatic cardiovascular disease; Cardiac conduction disturbances; Hyperthyroidism.

Use Cautiously in: Cardiovascular disease; Geri: Appears on Beers list. Poorly tolerated due to anticholinergic effects. Pregnancy, lactation, and children <15 yr (safety not established).

Adverse Reactions/Side Effects

CNS: dizziness, drowsiness, confusion, fatigue, headache, nervousness. **EENT:** dry mouth, blurred vision. **CV:** arrhythmias. **GI:** constipation, dyspepsia, nausea, unpleasant taste. **GU:** urinary retention.

Interactions

Drug-Drug: Additive CNS depression with other **CNS depressants**, including **alcohol**, **antihistamines**, **opioid analgesics**, and **sedative/hypnotics**. Additive anticholinergic effects with **drugs possessing anticholinergic properties**, including **antihistamines**, **antidepressants**, **atropine**, **disopyramide**, **haloperidol**, and **phenothiazines**. Avoid use within 14 days of **MAO inhibitors** (hyperpyretic crisis, seizures, and death may occur). May blunt the response to **guanadrel**.
Drug-Natural Products: Concomitant use of **kava kava**, **valerian**, **chamomile**, or **hops** can ↑ CNS depression.

Route/Dosage

PO (Adults): *Acute painful musculoskeletal conditions*—10 mg 3 times daily (range 20–40 mg/day in 2–4 divided doses; not to exceed 60 mg/day) *or* extended-release—15–30 mg once daily. *Fibromyalgia*—5–40 mg at bedtime (unlabeled).

Availability (generic available)

Tablets: 5 mg, 10 mg. **Cost:** *Generic*—5 mg $18.85/100, 10 mg $18.86/100. **Extended-release capsules:** 15 mg, 30 mg. **Cost:** 15 mg $773.97/90.

NURSING IMPLICATIONS

Assessment

- Assess patient for pain, muscle stiffness, and range of motion before and periodically throughout therapy.
- Geri: Assess geriatric patients for anticholinergic effects (sedation and weakness).

Potential Nursing Diagnoses

Acute pain (Indications)
Impaired physical mobility (Indications)
Risk for injury (Side Effects)

Implementation

- Do not confuse cyclobenzaprine with cyproheptadine.
- **PO:** May be administered with meals to minimize gastric irritation.

Patient/Family Teaching

- Instruct patient to take medication as directed; do not take more than the prescribed amount. Taken missed doses within 1 hr of time ordered; otherwise, return to normal dose schedule. Do not double doses.
- Medication may cause drowsiness, dizziness, and blurred vision. Caution patient to avoid driving or other activities requiring alertness until response to drug is known.
- Advise patient to avoid concurrent use of alcohol or other CNS depressants with this medication.
- If constipation becomes a problem, advise patient that increasing fluid intake and bulk in diet and stool softeners may alleviate this condition.
- Advise patient to notify health care professional if symptoms of urinary retention (distended abdomen, feeling of fullness, overflow incontinence, voiding small amounts) occur.
- Inform patient that good oral hygiene, frequent mouth rinses, and sugarless gum or candy may help relieve dry mouth.

Evaluation/Desired Outcomes

- Relief of muscular spasm in acute skeletal muscle conditions. Maximum effects may not be evident for 1–2 wk. Use is usually limited to 2–3 wk; however, has been effective for at least 12 wk in the management of fibromyalgia.

HIGH ALERT

cyclophosphamide

(sye-kloe-**fos**-fa-mide)
Cytoxan, Neosar, ✤Procytox

Classification
Therapeutic: antineoplastics, immunosuppressants
Pharmacologic: alkylating agents

Pregnancy Category D

Indications

Alone or with other modalities in the management of: Hodgkin's disease, Malignant lymphomas, Multiple myeloma, Leukemias, Mycosis fungoides, Neuroblastoma, Ovarian carcinoma, Breast carcinoma and a variety of other tumors. Minimal change nephrotic syndrome in children. **Unlabeled uses:** Severe active rheumatoid arthritis or Wegener's granulomatosis.

Action

Interferes with DNA replication and RNA transcription, ultimately disrupting protein synthesis (cell-cycle phase–nonspecific). **Therapeutic Effects:** Death of rapidly replicating cells, particularly malignant ones. Also has immunosuppressant action in smaller doses.

Pharmacokinetics

Absorption: Inactive parent drug is well absorbed from the GI tract. Converted to active drug by the liver.
Distribution: Widely distributed. Limited penetration of the blood-brain barrier. Crosses the placenta; enters breast milk.
Metabolism and Excretion: Converted to active drug by the liver; 30% eliminated unchanged by the kidneys.
Half-life: 4–6.5 hr.

TIME/ACTION PROFILE (effects on blood counts)

ROUTE	ONSET	PEAK	DURATION
PO, IV	7 days	7–15 days	21 days

Contraindications/Precautions

Contraindicated in: Hypersensitivity; Pregnancy or lactation.
Use Cautiously in: Active infections; Bone marrow depression; Other chronic debilitating illnesses; Patients with childbearing potential.

Adverse Reactions/Side Effects

Resp: PULMONARY FIBROSIS. **CV:** MYOCARDIAL FIBROSIS, hypotension. **GI:** anorexia, nausea, vomiting. **GU:** HEMORRHAGIC CYSTITIS, hematuria. **Derm:** alopecia. **Endo:** gonadal suppression, syndrome of inappropriate antidiuretic hormone (SIADH). **Hemat:** LEUKOPENIA, thrombocytopenia, anemia. **Metab:** hyperuricemia. **Misc:** secondary neoplasms.

Interactions

Drug-Drug: Phenobarbital or **rifampin** may ↑ toxicity of cyclophosphamide. Concurrent **allopurinol** or **thiazide diuretics** may exaggerate bone marrow depression. May prolong neuromuscular blockade from **succinylcholine**. Cardiotoxicity may be additive with other **cardiotoxic agents (cytarabine, daunorubicin, doxorubicin)**. May ↓ serum **digoxin** levels. Additive bone marrow depression with other **antineoplastics** or **radiation therapy**. May potentiate the effects of **warfarin**. May ↓ antibody response to **live-virus vaccines** and ↑ risk of adverse reactions. Prolongs the effects of **cocaine**.

Route/Dosage

Many regimens are used.
PO (Adults): 1–5 mg/kg/day.
PO (Children): *Induction*—2–8 mg/kg/day (60–250 mg/m^2/day) in divided doses for 6 days or longer. *Maintenance*—2–5 mg/kg (50–150 mg/m^2/day) twice weekly.
IV (Adults): 40–50 mg/kg in divided doses over 2–5 days *or* 10–15 mg/kg q 7–10 days *or* 3–5 mg/kg twice weekly *or* 1.5–3 mg/kg/day. Other regimens may use larger doses.
IV (Children): *Induction*—2–8 mg/kg/day (60–250 mg/m^2/day) in divided doses for 6 days or longer. Total dose for 7 days may be given as a single weekly dose. *Maintenance*—10–15 mg/kg every 7–10 days or 30 mg/kg q 3–4 wk.

Availability (generic available)

Tablets: 25 mg, 50 mg. **Injection:** 100 mg, 200 mg, 500 mg, ✤750 mg, 1 g, 2 g.

NURSING IMPLICATIONS

Assessment

- Monitor blood pressure, pulse, respiratory rate, and temperature frequently during administration. Report significant changes.
- Monitor urinary output frequently during therapy. To reduce the risk of hemorrhagic cystitis, fluid intake should be at least 3000 ml/day for adults and 1000–2000 ml/day for children. May be administered with mesna.
- Monitor for bone marrow depression. Assess for bleeding (bleeding gums, bruising, petechiae, guaiac stools, urine, and emesis) and avoid IM injections and taking rectal temperatures if platelet count is low. Apply pressure to venipuncture sites for 10 min. Assess for signs of infection during neutropenia. Anemia may occur. Monitor for increased fatigue, dyspnea, and orthostatic hypotension.
- Assess nausea, vomiting, and appetite. Weigh weekly. Antiemetics may be given 30 min before administration of medication to minimize GI effects. Anorexia and weight loss can be minimized by feeding frequent light meals.

- Encourage patient to drink 2000–3000 ml/day to promote excretion of uric acid. Alkalinization of the urine may be used to help prevent uric acid nephropathy.
- Assess cardiac and respiratory status for dyspnea, rales/crackles, weight gain, edema. Pulmonary toxicity may occur after prolonged therapy. Cardiotoxicity may occur early in therapy and is characterized by symptoms of CHF.
- ***Lab Test Considerations:*** Monitor CBC with differential and platelet count before and periodically during therapy. The nadir of leukopenia occurs in 7–12 days (recovery in 17–21 days). Leukocytes should be maintained at 2500–4000/mm^3. May also cause thrombocytopenia (nadir 10–15 days), and rarely causes anemia.
- Monitor BUN, creatinine, and uric acid before and frequently during therapy to detect nephrotoxicity.
- Monitor ALT, AST, LDH, and serum bilirubin before and frequently during therapy to detect hepatotoxicity.
- Urinalysis should be evaluated before initiating therapy and frequently during therapy to detect hematuria or change in specific gravity indicative of SIADH.
- May suppress positive reactions to skin tests for *Candida*, mumps, *Trichophyton*, and tuberculin purified-protein derivative (PPD). May also produce false-positive results in Papanicolaou smears.

Potential Nursing Diagnoses

Risk for infection (Side Effects)
Disturbed body image (Side Effects)

Implementation

- ***High Alert:*** Fatalities have occurred with chemotherapeutic agents. Before administering, clarify all ambiguous orders; double-check single, daily, and course-of-therapy dose limits; have second practitioner independently double-check original order, calculations, and infusion pump settings. Do not confuse cyclophosphamide with cyclosporine. Do not confuse Cytoxan (cyclophosphamide) with Cytozar (cytarabine) or Cytotec (misoprostol).
- **PO:** Administer medication on an empty stomach. If severe gastric irritation develops, medication may be given with food.
- Oral solution can be formed by diluting powder for injection in aromatic elixir to a concentration of 1–5 mg of cyclophosphamide/ml. Reconstituted preparations should be refrigerated and used within 2 wk.
- **IV:** Solution for IV administration should be prepared in a biologic cabinet. Wear gloves, gown, and mask while handling IV medication. Discard IV equipment in specially designated containers.
- Prepare IV solution by diluting each 100 mg with 5 ml of sterile water or bacteriostatic water for injection containing parabens. Shake solution gently and allow to stand until clear. Use solution without bacteriostatic water within 6 hr. Solution prepared with bacteriostatic water is stable for 24 hr at room temperature, 6 days if refrigerated.

IV Administration

- **Direct IV:** ***Diluent:*** Administer reconstituted solution undiluted. ***Concentration:*** 20 mg/ml. ***Rate:*** Administer at a rate of 100 mg/min.
- **Intermittent Infusion:** ***Diluent:*** May be further diluted in up to 250 ml of D5W, 0.9% NaCl, 0.45% NaCl, dextrose/saline combinations, LR or dextrose/Ringer's solution. ***Concentration:*** 20–25 mg/ml. ***Rate:*** Administer over 30–60 min.
- **Syringe Compatibility:** bleomycin, cisplatin, doxapram, doxorubicin, droperidol, fluorouracil, furosemide, heparin, leucovorin calcium, methotrexate, metoclopramide, mitomycin, vinblastine, vincristine.
- **Y-Site Compatibility:** allopurinol, amifostine, amikacin, ampicillin, aztreonam, bleomycin, cefazolin, cefepime, cefoperazone, cefotaxime, cefoxitin, cefuroxime, chloramphenicol, chlorpromazine, cimetidine, cisplatin, cladribine, clindamycin, dexamethasone, diphenhydramine, doxorubicin, doxorubicin liposome, doxycycline, droperidol, erythromycin lactobionate, etoposide phosphate, famotidine, filgrastim, fludarabine, fluorouracil, furosemide, ganciclovir, gemcitabine, gentamicin, granisetron, heparin, hydromorphone, idarubicin, kanamycin, leucovorin calcium, linezolid, lorazepam, melphalan, methotrexate, methylprednisolone, metoclopramide, metronidazole, minocycline, mitomycin, morphine, nafcillin, ondansetron, oxacillin,

oxaliplatin, paclitaxel, pemetrexed, penicillin G potassium, piperacillin, piperacillin/tazobactam, prochlorperazine, promethazine, propofol, ranitidine, sargramostim, sodium bicarbonate, teniposide, thiotepa, ticarcillin/clavulanate, tobramycin, topotecan, trimethoprim/sulfamethoxazole, vancomycin, vinblastine, vincristine, vinorelbine.
- **Y-Site Incompatibility:** amphotericin B cholesteryl sulfate, lansoprazole.
- **Additive Compatibility:** fluorouracil, methotrexate, mitoxantrone, ondansetron.

Patient/Family Teaching
- Instruct patient to take dose in early morning. Emphasize need for adequate fluid intake for 72 hr after therapy. Patient should void frequently to decrease bladder irritation from metabolites excreted by the kidneys. Report hematuria immediately. If a dose is missed, contact health care professional.
- Instruct patient to notify health care professional promptly if fever; sore throat; signs of infection; lower back or side pain; difficult or painful urination; sores in the mouth or on the lips; yellow discoloration of skin or eyes; bleeding gums; bruising; petechiae; blood in urine, stool, or emesis; unusual swelling; joint pain; shortness of breath; or confusion occurs. Caution patient to avoid crowds and persons with known infections. Instruct patient to use soft toothbrush and electric razor and to avoid falls. Patient should also be cautioned not to drink alcoholic beverages or to take products containing aspirin or NSAIDs; may precipitate GI hemorrhage.
- Advise patient that this medication may cause sterility and menstrual irregularities or cessation of menses. This drug is also teratogenic, and contraceptive measures should continue for at least 4 mo after completion of therapy.
- Discuss with patient the possibility of hair loss. Explore methods of coping. May also cause darkening of skin and fingernails.
- Instruct patient not to receive any vaccinations without advice of health care professional.

Evaluation/Desired Outcomes
- Decrease in size or spread of malignant tumors.
- Improvement of hematologic status in patients with leukemia. Maintenance therapy is instituted if leukocyte count remains between 2500 and 4000/mm³ and if patient does not demonstrate serious side effects.
- Management of minimal change nephrotic syndrome in children.

cycloSPORINE†
(**sye**-kloe-spor-een)
Neoral, Sandimmune, Gengraf

Classification
Therapeutic: immunosuppressants, antirheumatics (DMARD)
Pharmacologic: polypeptides (cyclic)

Pregnancy Category C

†See Appendix C for ophthalmic use

Indications
PO, IV: Prevention and treatment of rejection in renal, cardiac, and hepatic transplantation (with corticosteroids). **PO:** Treatment of severe active rheumatoid arthritis (Neoral only). Treatment of severe recalcitrant psoriasis in adult nonimmunocompromised patients (Neoral only). **Unlabeled uses:** Management of recalcitrant ulcerative colitis. Treatment of steroid resistant nephrotic syndrome. Treatment of severe steroid resistant autoimmune disease. Prevention and treatment of graft vs. host disease in bone marrow transplant patients.

Action
Inhibits normal immune responses (cellular and humoral) by inhibiting interleukin-2, a factor necessary for initiation of T-cell activity. **Therapeutic Effects:** Prevention of rejection reactions. Slowed progression of rheumatoid arthritis or psoriasis.

Pharmacokinetics
Absorption: Erratically absorbed (range 10–60%) after oral administration, with significant first-pass metabolism by the liver. Microemulsion (Neoral) has better bioavailability.
Distribution: Widely distributed, mainly into extracellular fluid and blood cells. Crosses the placenta; enters breast milk.
Protein Binding: 90–98%.
Metabolism and Excretion: Extensively metabolized by the liver (first pass); excreted in bile, small amounts excreted unchanged in urine.
Half-life: Children—7 hr; adults—19 hr.

TIME/ACTION PROFILE (blood levels)

ROUTE	ONSET	PEAK	DURATION
PO	unknown†	2–6 hr	unknown
IV	unknown	end of infusion	unknown

†Onset of action in rheumatoid arthritis is 4–8 wk and may last 4 wk after discontinuation; for psoriasis, onset is 2–6 wk and lasts 6 wk following discontinuation

Contraindications/Precautions

Contraindicated in: Hypersensitivity to cyclosporine or polyoxyethylated castor oil (vehicle for IV form); Should not be given to pregnant or lactating women unless benefits outweigh risks; Disulfiram therapy or known alcohol intolerance (IV and oral liquid dosage forms contain alcohol); Psoriasis patients receiving immunosuppressants or radiation; Uncontrolled hypertension.

Use Cautiously in: Severe hepatic impairment (dose reduction recommended); Renal impairment (frequent dose changes may be necessary); Active infection; Children (larger or more frequent doses may be required).

Adverse Reactions/Side Effects

CNS: SEIZURES, tremor, confusion, flushing, headache, psychiatric problems. **CV:** hypertension. **GI:** diarrhea, hepatotoxicity, nausea, vomiting, abdominal discomfort, anorexia, pancreatitis. **GU:** nephrotoxicity. **Derm:** hirsutism, acne. **F and E:** hyperkalemia, hypomagnesemia. **Hemat:** anemia, leukopenia, thrombocytopenia. **Metab:** hyperlipidemia, hyperuricemia. **Neuro:** hyperesthesia, paresthesia. **Misc:** gingival hyperplasia, hypersensitivity reactions, infections.

Interactions

Drug-Drug: ↑ blood levels and/or risk of toxicity with **azithromycin, clarithromycin**, **amphotericin B, aminoglycosides, amiodarone, anabolic steroids**, some **calcium channel blockers, cimetidine, colchicine, danazol, erythromycin, fluconazole, fluoroquinolones, ketoconazole, itraconazole, metoclopramide, methotrexate, miconazole, NSAIDs, melphalan**, or **hormonal contraceptives**. ↑ nephrotoxicity with **acyclovir, amphotericin B, aminoglycosides, NSAIDs, trimethoprim, ciprofloxacin**, and **vancomycin**. ↑ immunosuppression with other **immunosuppressants** (cyclophosphamide, azathioprine, corticosteroids). **Quinupristin/dalfopristin** ↑ cyclosporine levels. **Barbiturates, phenytoin, rifampin, rifabutin, carbamazepine**, or **sulfonamides** may ↓ effect of cyclosporine. ↑ risk of hyperkalemia with **potassium-sparing diuretics, potassium supplements**, or **ACE inhibitors**. ↑ serum levels/risk of toxicity from **digoxin** (↓ digoxin dose by 50%). Prolongs the action of **neuromuscular blocking agents**. ↑ risk of seizures with **imipenem/cilastatin**. May ↓ antibody response to **live-virus vaccines** and ↑ risk of adverse reactions. ↑ risk of rhabdomyolysis with **HMG-CoA reductase inhibitors**. Concurrent use with **tacrolimus** should be avoided. **Orlistat** ↓ absorption; avoid concurrent use.

Drug-Natural Products: Concomitant use with **echinacea** and **melatonin** may interfere with immunosuppression. Use with **St. John's wort** may cause ↓ serum levels and organ rejection for transplant patients. Some **HIV protease inhibitors** may ↑ blood levels and the risk of toxicity.

Drug-Food: Concurrent ingestion of **grapefruit or grapefruit juice** ↑ absorption and should be avoided. **Food** ↓ absorption of microemulsion products (Neoral).

Route/Dosage

Doses are adjusted on the basis of serum level monitoring.

Prevention of Transplant Rejection (Sandimmune)

PO (Adults and Children): 14–18 mg/kg/dose 4–12 hr before transplant then 5–15 mg/kg/day divided q 12–24 hr postoperatively, taper by 5% weekly to maintenance dose of 3–10 mg/kg/day.

IV (Adults and Children): 5–6 mg/kg/dose 4–12 hr before transplant, then 2–10 mg/kg/day in divided doses q 8–24 hr; change to PO as soon as possible.

Prevention of Transplant Rejection (Neoral)

PO (Adults and Children): 4–12 mg/kg/day divided q 12 hr (dose varies depending on organ transplanted).

Rheumatoid Arthritis (Neoral only)

PO (Adults and Children): 2.5 mg/kg/day given in 2 divided doses; may increase by 0.5–

0.75 mg/kg/day after 8 and 12 weeks, up to 4 mg/kg/day. Decrease dose by 25–50% if adverse reactions occur.

Severe Psoriasis (Neoral only)
PO (Adults): 2.5 mg/kg/day given in 2 divided doses, for at least 4 wk; then may increase by 0.5 mg/kg/day q 2 wk, up to 4 mg/kg/day. Decrease dose by 25–50% if adverse reactions occur.

Autoimmune Diseases (Neoral only)
PO (Adults and Children): 1–3 mg/kg/day.

Availability (generic available)

Microemulsion soft gelatin capsules (Gengraf, Neoral): 25 mg, 100 mg. **Cost:** *Gengraf*—25 mg $227.97/180, 100 mg $949.52/180; *Neoral*—25 mg $239.96/180, 100 mg $956.36/180. **Microemulsion oral solution (Gengraf, Neoral):** 100 mg/ml. **Cost:** *Neoral*—$301.71/50 ml. **Soft gelatin capsules (Sandimmune):** 25 mg, 100 mg. **Cost:** 25 mg $337.25/180, 100 mg $1,280.00/180. **Oral solution (Sandimmune):** 100 mg/ml. **Cost:** *Neoral*—$363.18/50 ml. **Injection (Sandimmune):** 50 mg/ml in 5-ml ampules.

NURSING IMPLICATIONS

Assessment

- Monitor serum creatinine level, intake and output ratios, daily weight, and blood pressure during therapy. Report significant changes.
- **Prevention of Transplant Rejection:** Assess for symptoms of organ rejection throughout therapy.
- **IV:** Monitor patient for signs and symptoms of hypersensitivity (wheezing, dyspnea, flushing of face or neck) continuously during at least the first 30 min of each treatment and frequently thereafter. Oxygen, epinephrine, and equipment for treatment of anaphylaxis should be available with each IV dose.
- **Arthritis:** Assess pain and limitation of movement prior to and during administration.
- Prior to initiating therapy, perform a physical exam including blood pressure on 2 occasions to determine baseline. Monitor blood pressure every 2 wk during initial 3 mo, then monthly if stable. If hypertension occurs, dose should be reduced.
- **Psoriasis:** Assess skin lesions prior to and during therapy.
- ***Lab Test Considerations:*** Measure serum creatinine, BUN, CBC, magnesium, potassium, uric acid, and lipids at baseline, every 2 wk during initial therapy, and then monthly if stable. Nephrotoxicity may occur; report significant increases.
- May cause hepatotoxicity; monitor for ↑ AST, ALT, alkaline phosphatase, amylase, and bilirubin.
- May cause ↑ serum potassium and uric acid levels and ↓ serum magnesium levels.
- Serum lipid levels may be ↑.
- ***Toxicity and Overdose:*** Evaluate serum cyclosporine levels periodically during therapy. Dose may be adjusted daily, in response to levels, during initiation of therapy. Guidelines for desired serum levels will vary among institutions.

Potential Nursing Diagnoses

Risk for infection (Side Effects)
Acute pain (Indications)

Implementation

- Do not confuse cyclosporine with cyclophosphamide or cycloserine.
- Given with other immunosuppressive agents. Protect transplant patients from staff and visitors who may carry infection. Maintain protective isolation as indicated.
- Microemulsion products (Neoral) and other products (Sandimmune) are not interchangeable.
- **PO:** Draw up oral solution in the pipette provided with the medication. Mix oral solution with milk, chocolate milk, apple juice, or orange juice, preferably at room temperature. Stir well and drink at once. Use a glass container and rinse with more diluent to ensure that total dose is taken. Administer oral doses with meals. Wipe pipette dry; do not wash after use.

IV Administration

- **Intermittent Infusion:** ***Diluent:*** Dilute each 1 ml (50 mg) of IV concentrate immediately before use with 20–100 ml of D5W or 0.9% NaCl for injection. Solution is stable for 24 hr in D5W. In 0.9% NaCl, it is stable for 6 hr in a polyvinylchloride container and 12 hr in a glass container at room temperature. ***Concentration:*** 2.5 mg/ml. ***Rate:*** Infuse slowly over 2–6 hr via infusion pump.
- **Continuous Infusion:** May be administered over 24 hr.
- **Y-Site Compatibility:** lansoprazole, linezolid, propofol, sargramostim.

- **Y-Site Incompatibility:** amphotericin B cholesteryl sulfate, drotrecogin.
- **Additive Incompatibility:** magnesium sulfate.

Patient/Family Teaching

- Instruct patient to take medication at the same time each day and with regard to food, as directed. Do not skip doses or double up on missed doses. Take missed doses as soon as remembered within 12 hr. Do not discontinue medication without advice of health care professional.
- Reinforce the need for lifelong therapy to prevent transplant rejection. Review symptoms of rejection for transplanted organ, and stress need to notify health care professional immediately if they occur.
- Pedi: Review side effects carefully with parents and teach them how to monitor for hypertension, infection, and kidney disease. Instruct parents to notify health care provider if child develops diarrhea, which decreases absorption of cyclosporine and can result in rejection.
- Instruct patient to avoid grapefruit and grapefruit juice to prevent interaction with cyclosporine.
- Advise patient of common side effects (nephrotoxicity, increased blood pressure, hand tremors, increased facial and body hair, gingival hyperplasia). Pedi: Advise parents that if hair growth is excessive and upsetting to the child, depilatories, or hair removal waxing, can be used.
- Teach patient the correct method for monitoring blood pressure. Instruct patient to notify health care professional of significant changes in blood pressure or if hematuria, increased frequency, cloudy urine, decreased urine output, fever, sore throat, tiredness, or unusual bruising occurs.
- Instruct patient on proper oral hygiene. Meticulous oral hygiene and dental examinations for teeth cleaning and plaque control every 3 mo will help decrease gingival inflammation and hyperplasia.
- Instruct patient to consult health care professional before taking any OTC medications or receiving any vaccinations while taking this medication.
- Advise patient to notify health care professional if pregnancy is planned or suspected.
- Emphasize the importance of follow-up exams and lab tests.

Evaluation/Desired Outcomes

- Prevention of rejection of transplanted tissues.
- Decrease in severity of pain.
- Increased ease of joint movement.
- Decrease in progression of psoriasis.

cyproheptadine

(si-proe-**hep**-ta-deen)
Periactin, PMS-Cyproheptadine

Classification
Therapeutic: allergy, cold, and cough remedies, antihistamines

Pregnancy Category B

Indications

Relief of allergic symptoms caused by histamine release including: Seasonal and perennial allergic rhinitis, Chronic urticaria, Cold urticaria. **Unlabeled uses:** Stimulation of appetite.

Action

Antagonizes the effects of histamine at H-receptor sites; does not bind to or inactivate histamine. Also blocks the effects of serotonin, which may result in increased appetite. **Therapeutic Effects:** Decreased symptoms of histamine excess (sneezing, rhinorrhea, nasal and ocular pruritus, ocular tearing and redness). Decreased cold urticaria.

Pharmacokinetics

Absorption: Apparently well absorbed after oral dosing.
Distribution: Unknown.
Metabolism and Excretion: Mostly metabolized by the liver.
Half-life: Unknown.

TIME/ACTION PROFILE (antihistaminic effects)

ROUTE	ONSET	PEAK	DURATION
PO	15–60 min	1–2 hr	8 hr

Contraindications/Precautions

Contraindicated in: Hypersensitivity; Acute attacks of asthma; Lactation; Known alcohol intolerance (syrup only).

Use Cautiously in: Geri: Appears on Beers list. Geriatric patients are sensitive to anticholinergic effects and have increased risk for side effects; Angle-closure glaucoma; Liver disease; Pregnancy (safety not established).

Adverse Reactions/Side Effects

CNS: drowsiness, excitation (increased in children). **EENT:** blurred vision. **CV:** arrhythmias, hypotension, palpitations. **GI:** dry mouth, constipation. **GU:** hesitancy, retention. **Derm:** photosensitivity, rashes. **Misc:** weight gain.

Interactions

Drug-Drug: Additive CNS depression with other **CNS depressants**, including **alcohol**, **opioid analgesics**, and **sedative/hypnotics**. **MAO inhibitors** may intensify and prolong the anticholinergic effects of **antihistamines**.

Route/Dosage

PO (Adults): 4 mg q 8 hr (range 4–20 mg/day in 3 divided doses; up to 0.5 mg/kg/day).
PO (Children 6–14 yr): 2–4 mg q 8–12 hr (not to exceed 16 mg/day).
PO (Children 2–6 yr): 2 mg q 8–12 hr (not to exceed 12 mg/day).

Availability (generic available)

Tablets: 4 mg, ♣4 mg[OTC]. **Syrup:** 2 mg/5 ml, ♣2 mg/5 ml[OTC].

NURSING IMPLICATIONS

Assessment

- Geri: Assess for adverse anticholinergic effects (delirium, acute confusion, dizziness, dry mouth, blurred vision, urinary retention, constipation, tachycardia).
- **Allergy:** Assess symptoms (rhinitis, conjunctivitis, hives) prior to and periodically throughout therapy.
- Assess lung sounds and respiratory function prior to and periodically throughout therapy. May cause thickening of bronchial secretions. Maintain fluid intake of 1500–2000 ml/day to decrease viscosity of secretions.
- **Appetite Stimulant:** Monitor food intake and weight routinely.
- ***Lab Test Considerations:*** May cause false-negative reactions on allergy skin tests; discontinue 72 hr prior to testing.
- Increased serum amylase and prolactin concentrations may occur when cyproheptadine is administered with a thyrotropin-releasing hormone.

Potential Nursing Diagnoses

Ineffective airway clearance (Indications)
Risk for injury (Side Effects)

Implementation

- Do not confuse cyproheptadine with cyclobenzaprine.
- **PO:** Administer with food, water, or milk to minimize gastric irritation.

Patient/Family Teaching

- Instruct patient to take cyproheptadine exactly as directed. Missed dose should be taken as soon as remembered. Do not double doses. Syrup should be accurately measured using calibrated medication cup or measuring device.
- Medication may cause drowsiness. Advise patient to avoid driving or other activities requiring alertness until response to the drug is known.
- Advise patient to use sunscreen and protective clothing to prevent a photosensitivity reaction.
- Caution patient to avoid concurrent use of alcohol and other CNS depressants.
- Advise patient that frequent mouth rinses, good oral hygiene, and sugarless gum or candy may decrease dry mouth. Patient should notify dentist if dry mouth persists for >2 wk.
- Geri: Teach patient and family about anticholinergic effects and to contact a health care provider if such effects persist.

Evaluation/Desired Outcomes

- Alleviation of allergic symptoms.
- Alleviation of cold urticaria.
- Improvement of appetite.

HIGH ALERT

cytarabine (sye-**tare**-a-been)

Ara-C, cytosine arabinoside, ♣Cytosar, Cytosar-U, DepoCyt

Classification
Therapeutic: antineoplastics
Pharmacologic: antimetabolites

Pregnancy Category D

Indications

IV: Used mainly in combination chemotherapeutic regimens for the treatment of leukemias and non-Hodgkin's lymphomas. **IT:** Treatment of lymphomatous meningitis.

C

Action
Inhibits DNA synthesis by inhibiting DNA polymerase (cell-cycle S-phase–specific). **Therapeutic Effects:** Death of rapidly replicating cells, particularly malignant ones.

Pharmacokinetics
Absorption: Absorption occurs from subcut sites, but blood levels are lower than with IV administration; IT administration results in negligible systemic exposure.
Distribution: Widely distributed; IV- and subcut-administered cytarabine crosses the blood-brain barrier but not in sufficient quantities. Crosses the placenta.
Metabolism and Excretion: Metabolized mostly by the liver; <10% excreted unchanged by the kidneys. Metabolism to inactive drug in the CSF is negligible because the enzyme that metabolizes it is present in very low concentrations in the CSF.
Half-life: *IV, subcut*—1–3 hr; *IT*—100–236 hr.

TIME/ACTION PROFILE (IV, subcut—effects on WBCs; IT—levels in CSF)

ROUTE	ONSET	PEAK	DURATION
Subcut, IV (1st phase)	24 hr	7–9 days	12 days
Subcut, IV (2nd phase)	15–24 days	15–24 days	25–34 days
IT	rapid	5 hr	14–28 days

Contraindications/Precautions
Contraindicated in: Hypersensitivity; OB: Pregnancy or lactation; Active meningeal infection (IT only).
Use Cautiously in: Active infections; Decreased bone marrow reserve; Renal/hepatic disease; Other chronic debilitating illnesses; OB: Patients with childbearing potential.

Adverse Reactions/Side Effects
CNS: CNS dysfunction (high dose), confusion, drowsiness, headache. **EENT:** corneal toxicity (high dose), hemorrhagic conjunctivitis (high dose). **Resp:** PULMONARY EDEMA (high dose). **CV:** edema. **GI:** nausea, vomiting, hepatitis, hepatotoxicity, severe GI ulceration (high dose), stomatitis. **GU:** urinary incontinence. **Derm:** alopecia, rash. **Endo:** sterility. **Hemat:** *(less with IT use)*— anemia, leukopenia, thrombocytopenia. **Metab:** hyperuricemia. **Neuro:** *Intrathecal only*— CHEMICAL ARACHNOIDITIS, abnormal gait. **Misc:** cytarabine syndrome, fever.

Interactions
Drug-Drug: ↑ bone marrow depression with other **antineoplastics** or **radiation therapy**. ↑ risk of cardiomyopathy when used in high-dose regimens with **cyclophosphamide**. May ↓ antibody response to **live-virus vaccines** and ↑ risk of adverse reactions. May ↓ absorption of **digoxin** tablets. May ↓ the efficacy of **gentamicin** when used to treat *Klebsiella pneumoniae* infections. Recent treatment with **asparaginase** may ↑ risk of pancreatitis. ↑ neurotoxicity with concurrently administered **IT antineoplastics** (IT only).

Route/Dosage
Dose regimens vary widely.
IV (Adults): *Induction dose*—200 mg/m²/day for 5 days q 2 wk as a single agent *or* 2–6 mg/kg/day (100–200 mg/m²/day) as a single daily dose *or* in 2–3 divided doses for 5–10 days or until remission occurs as part of combination chemotherapy. *Maintenance*—70–200 mg/m²/day for 2–5 days monthly. *Refractory leukemias/lymphomas*—3 g/m² q 12 hr for up to 12 doses.
Subcut, IM (Adults): *Maintenance*—1–1.5 mg/kg q 1–4 wk.
IT (Adults): *Depo Cyt Induction*—50 mg (intraventricular or lumbar puncture) every 14 days for 2 doses (weeks 1 and 3); *consolidation*—50 mg (intraventricular or lumbar puncture) every 14 days for 3 doses (weeks 5, 7, and 9), followed by one additional dose at week 13; *maintenance*—50 mg (intraventricular or lumbar puncture) every 28 days for 4 doses (weeks 17, 21, 25, and 29). If drug-related neurotoxicity occurs, dose should be reduced to 25 mg or discontinued (dexamethasone 4 mg PO/IV twice daily for 5 days should be started concurrently with IT cytarabine).

Availability (generic available)
Powder for injection: 100 mg, 500 mg, 1 g, 2 g. **Sustained-release liposome injection for IT use:** 50 ml/5-ml vial.

NURSING IMPLICATIONS

Assessment
- Monitor for bone marrow depression. Assess for bleeding (bleeding gums, bruising, petec-

hiae, guaiac stools, urine, and emesis) and avoid IM injections and taking rectal temperatures if platelet count is low. Apply pressure to venipuncture sites for 10 min. Assess for signs of infection during neutropenia. Anemia may occur. Monitor for increased fatigue, dyspnea, and orthostatic hypotension.

- Monitor intake and output ratios and daily weights. Report significant changes in totals.
- Monitor for symptoms of gout (increased uric acid, joint pain, edema). Encourage patient to drink at least 2 L of fluid each day. Allopurinol may decrease uric acid levels. Alkalinization of urine may increase excretion of uric acid.
- Assess nutritional status. Nausea and vomiting may occur within 1 hr of administration, especially if IV dose is administered rapidly, less severe if medication is infused slowly. Administering an antiemetic prior to and periodically throughout therapy and adjusting diet as tolerated may help maintain fluid and electrolyte balance and nutritional status.
- Monitor patient for development of *cytarabine* or *ara-C syndrome* (fever, myalgia, bone pain, chest pain, maculopapular rash, conjunctivitis, malaise), which usually occurs 6–12 hr following administration. Corticosteroids may be used for treatment or prevention. If patient responds to corticosteroids, continue cytarabine and corticosteroids.
- Assess patient for respiratory distress and pulmonary edema. Occurs with high doses rarely; may be fatal.
- Monitor patient for signs of anaphylaxis (rash, dyspnea, swelling). Epinephrine, corticosteroids, and resuscitation equipment should be readily available.

IT: Chemical arachnoiditis (nausea, vomiting, headache, fever, back pain, CSF pleocytosis and neck rigidity, neck pain, or meningism) is an expected side effect of IT cytarabine. Incidence and severity of symptoms may be decreased with coadministration of dexamethasone.

- Monitor patients receiving IT therapy continuously for the development of neurotoxicity (myelopathy, personality changes, dysarthria, ataxia, confusion, somnolence, coma). If neurotoxicity develops, decrease amount of subsequent doses and discontinue if neurotoxicity persists. Risk may be increased if cytarabine is administered intrathecally and IV within a few days.
- ***Lab Test Considerations:*** Monitor CBC with differential and platelet count prior to and frequently during therapy. Leukocyte counts begin to drop within 24 hr of administration. The initial nadir occurs in 7–9 days. After a small ↑ in the count, the second, deeper nadir occurs 15–24 days after administration. Platelet counts begin to ↓ 5 days after a dose, with a nadir at 12–15 days. Leukocyte and thrombocyte counts usually begin to ↑ 10 days after the nadirs. Therapy is usually withdrawn if leukocyte count is <1000/mm^3 or platelet count is <50,000/mm^3. Bone marrow aspirations are recommended every 2 wk until remission occurs.
- Monitor renal (BUN and creatinine) and hepatic function (AST, ALT, bilirubin, alkaline phosphatase, and LDH) prior to and routinely during therapy.
- May cause ↑ uric acid concentrations.

Potential Nursing Diagnoses

Risk for infection (Adverse Reactions)
Risk for injury (Side Effects)

Implementation

- ***High Alert:*** Fatalities have occurred with chemotherapeutic agents. Before administering, clarify all ambiguous orders; double-check single, daily, and course-of-therapy dose limits; have second practitioner independently double-check original order, calculations, and infusion pump settings.
- ***High Alert:*** Do not confuse cytarabine with Cytoxan (cyclophosphamide). Do not confuse Cytosar (cytarabine) with Cytovene (ganciclovir) or Cytoxan. Do not confuse high-dose and regular therapy. Fatalities have occurred with high-dose therapy.
- Solution should be prepared in a biologic cabinet. Wear gloves, gown, and mask while handling IV medication. Discard IV equipment in specially designated containers (see Appendix K).
- May be given subcut, direct IV, intermittent IV, continuous IV, or IT.
- **IV, Subcut:** Reconstitute 100-mg vials with 5 ml of bacteriostatic water for injection with benzyl alcohol 0.9% for a concentration of 20 mg/ml. Reconstitute 500-mg vials with 10 ml for a concentration of 50 mg/ml, 1-g vials with 10 ml, and 2-g vials with 20 ml for a concentration of 100 mg/ml. Reconstituted solution is stable for 48 hr. Do not administer a cloudy or hazy solution.

IV Administration

- **Direct IV:** ***Diluent:*** Administer undiluted. ***Concentration:*** 100 mg/ml. ***Rate:*** Administer each 100 mg over 1–3 min.
- **Intermittent Infusion:** ***Diluent:*** May be further diluted in 0.9% NaCl, D5W, D10W, D5/0.9% NaCl, Ringer's solution, LR, or D5/LR. ***Concentration:*** Dilute doses in 100 ml of diluent. ***Rate:*** Infuse over 15–30 min.
- **Continuous Infusion:** Rate and concentration for IV infusion are ordered individually.
- **Syringe Compatibility:** metoclopramide.
- **Y-Site Compatibility:** amifostine, amsacrine, aztreonam, cefepime, chlorpromazine, cimetidine, cladribine, dexamethasone phosphate, diphenhydramine, doxorubicin liposome, droperidol, etoposide phosphate, famotidine, filgrastim, fludarabine, furosemide, gemcitabine, gentamicin, granisetron, heparin, hydrocortisone, hydromorphone, idarubicin, linezolid, lorazepam, melphalan, methotrexate, methylprednisolone, metoclopramide, morphine, ondansetron, paclitaxel, pemetrexed, piperacillin/tazobactam, prochlorperazine, promethazine, propofol, ranitidine, sargramostim, sodium bicarbonate, teniposide, thiotepa, vinorelbine.
- **Y-Site Incompatibility:** allopurinol, amphotericin B cholesteryl sulfate complex, ganciclovir, lansoprazole.
- **Additive Compatibility:** methotrexate, mitoxantrone, ondansetron, potassium chloride, sodium bicarbonate, vincristine.
- **Additive Incompatibility:** fluorouracil, heparin, regular insulin, nafcillin, oxacillin, penicillin G sodium. **IT:** Patients receiving *liposomal cytarabine* should be started on dexamethasone 4 mg twice daily PO or IV for 5 days beginning on the day of liposomal cytarabine injection.
- Allow vial to warm to room temperature. Gently agitate or invert vial to resuspend particles immediately before withdrawal from vial. No further reconstitution or dilution is required with *liposomal cytarabine*. Reconstitute *conventional cytarabine* with preservative-free 0.9% NaCl or autologous spinal fluid. Use immediately to prevent bacterial contamination.
- Liposomal cytarabine must be used within 4 hr of withdrawal from the vial. Discard unused portions. Inject directly into CSF via intraventricular reservoir or by direct injection into lumbar sac. Do not use in-line filters.
- Instruct patient to lie flat for 1 hr following IT injection. Monitor for immediate toxic reactions.

Patient/Family Teaching

- Caution patient to avoid crowds and persons with known infections. Report symptoms of infection (fever, chills, cough, hoarseness, sore throat, lower back or side pain, painful or difficult urination) immediately.
- Instruct patient to report unusual bleeding. Advise patient of thrombocytopenia precautions (use soft toothbrush and electric razor, avoid falls, do not drink alcoholic beverages or take medication containing aspirin or NSAIDs; may precipitate gastric bleeding).
- Instruct patient to inspect oral mucosa for redness and ulceration. If mouth sores occur, advise patient to use sponge brush and rinse mouth with water after eating and drinking. Stomatitis may require treatment with opioid analgesics.
- Advise patient that this medication may have teratogenic effects. Contraception should be used during therapy and for at least 4 mo after therapy is concluded.
- Instruct patient not to receive any vaccinations without advice of health care professional.
- Emphasize the need for periodic lab tests to monitor for side effects.
- **IT:** Inform patient about the expected side effects (headache, nausea, vomiting, fever) and about early signs of neurotoxicity. Instruct patient to notify health care professional if these signs occur.
- Emphasize the importance of taking dexamethasone with lyposomal cytarabine.

Evaluation/Desired Outcomes

- Improvement of hematopoietic values in leukemias.
- Decrease in size and spread of the tumor in non-Hodgkin's lymphomas. Therapy is continued every 2 wk until patient is in complete remission or thrombocyte count or leukocyte count falls below acceptable levels.
- Treatment of lymphomatous meningitis.

daclizumab (da-**kliz**-yoo-mab)
Zenapax

Classification
Therapeutic: immunosuppressants
Pharmacologic: monoclonal antibodies

Pregnancy Category C

Indications
Prevention of acute organ rejection during renal transplantation (with cyclosporine and corticosteroids).

Action
Binds specifically to interleukin-2 (IL-2) receptor sites on activated lymphocytes, acting as an IL-2 receptor antagonist. This prevents further activation of lymphocytes and allograft rejection. **Therapeutic Effects:** Prevention of renal allograft rejection.

Pharmacokinetics
Absorption: IV administration results in complete bioavailability.
Distribution: Crosses the placenta.
Metabolism and Excretion: Binds to lymphocytes.
Half-life: 20 days.

TIME/ACTION PROFILE (saturation of IL-2 receptors)

ROUTE	ONSET	PEAK	DURATION
IV	rapid	after 5th dose	120 days†

†Post-transplantation

Contraindications/Precautions
Contraindicated in: Hypersensitivity.
Use Cautiously in: Geriatric patients; Pregnancy, lactation, or children (has been used in children; increased risk of hypertension and dehydration).

Adverse Reactions/Side Effects
CNS: dizziness, fatigue, headache, insomnia. **Resp:** PULMONARY EDEMA, coughing, dyspnea. **CV:** chest pain, edema, hypertension (↑ in children), hypotension, tachycardia. **GI:** abdominal discomfort, constipation, diarrhea (↑ in children), dyspepsia, epigastric pain, nausea, pyrosis, vomiting (↑ in children). **GU:** dysuria, oliguria, renal tubular necrosis. **Derm:** acne, impaired wound healing, pruritus (↑ in children). **Hemat:** thrombosis. **MS:** arthralgia, back pain, musculoskeletal pain. **Neuro:** tremor. **Misc:** Allergic reactions including ANAPHYLAXIS, fever (↑ in children), post-operative pain (↑ in children), urinary and respiratory tract infection (↑ in children).

Interactions
Drug-Drug: None known.
Drug-Natural Products: Concomitant use with **astragalus**, **echinacea**, and **melatonin** may interfere with immunosuppression.

Route/Dosage
IV (Adults and Children): 1 mg/kg, with 1st dose given no more than 24 hr before transplantation, then q 2 wk for a total of 5 doses.

Availability
Concentrate for injection (must be diluted): 25 mg/5 ml in 5-ml vials.

NURSING IMPLICATIONS

Assessment
- Assess for fluid overload (monitor weight and intake and output, assess for edema and rales/crackles). Notify health care professional if patient has experienced 3% or more weight gain in the previous week. Obtain chest x-ray within 24 hr before beginning therapy. Fluid-overloaded patients are at high risk of developing pulmonary edema. Monitor vital signs and breath sounds closely.
- Monitor for signs of anaphylactic or hypersensitivity reactions (hypotension, bronchospasm, wheezing, laryngeal edema, pulmonary edema, cyanosis, hypoxia, respiratory arrest, cardiac arrhythmia, cardiac arrest, peripheral edema, loss of consciousness, fever, rash, urticaria, diaphoresis, pruritus, and/or injection site reactions) at each dose. Resuscitation equipment should be readily available. If a severe hypersensitivity reaction occurs, therapy with daclizumab should be permanently discontinued.
- Monitor for infection (fever, chills, rash, sore throat, purulent discharge, dysuria). Notify health care professional immediately if these symptoms occur; may necessitate discontinuation of therapy.

Potential Nursing Diagnoses
Risk for infection (Side Effects)
Excess fluid volume (Side Effects)

Implementation

- Daclizumab is usually administered concurrently with cyclosporine and corticosteroids.
- Daclizumab should be used only by physicians experienced in the management of organ transplantation.

IV Administration

- **Intermittent Infusion:** ***Diluent:*** Dilute daclizumab with 50 ml of 0.9% NaCl. Gently invert bag to mix; do not shake to avoid foaming. Solution is clear and colorless; do not administer solutions that are discolored or contain particulate matter. Discard unused portion. Administer within 4 hr or may be refrigerated for up to 24 hr. Discard after 24 hr. ***Rate:*** Administer over 15 min via peripheral or central line.
- **Compatibility:** Do not admix; do not administer in IV line containing other medications. If line must be used for other medications, flush with 0.9% NaCl before and after daclizumab.

Patient/Family Teaching

- Explain that patient will need to resume lifelong therapy with other immunosuppressive drugs after completion of daclizumab course.
- May cause dizziness. Caution patient to avoid driving or other activities requiring alertness until response is known.
- Instruct patient to continue to avoid crowds and persons with known infections; this drug also suppresses the immune system.
- Instruct patient not to receive any vaccinations and to avoid contact with persons receiving oral polio vaccine without advice of health care professional.

Evaluation/Desired Outcomes

- Prevention of acute organ rejection.

---

dalteparin, See HEPARINS (LOW MOLECULAR WEIGHT).

---

dantrolene (dan-troe-leen)

Dantrium

Classification

Therapeutic: skeletal muscle relaxants (direct acting)

Pregnancy Category C

Indications

PO: Treatment of spasticity associated with: Spinal cord injury, Stroke, Cerebral palsy, Multiple sclerosis. Prophylaxis of malignant hyperthermia. **IV:** Emergency treatment of malignant hyperthermia. **Unlabeled uses:** Management of neuroleptic malignant syndrome.

Action

Acts directly on skeletal muscle, causing relaxation by decreasing calcium release from sarcoplasmic reticulum in muscle cells. Prevents intense catabolic process associated with malignant hyperthermia. **Therapeutic Effects:** Reduction of muscle spasticity. Prevention of malignant hyperthermia.

Pharmacokinetics

Absorption: 35% absorbed after oral administration.
Distribution: Unknown.
Metabolism and Excretion: Almost entirely metabolized by the liver.
Half-life: 8.7 hr.

TIME/ACTION PROFILE (effects on spasticity)

ROUTE	ONSET	PEAK	DURATION
PO	1 wk	unknown	6–12 hr
IV	rapid	rapid	unknown

Contraindications/Precautions

Contraindicated in: No contraindications to IV form in treatment of hyperthermia; Pregnancy and lactation; Situations in which spasticity is used to maintain posture or balance.
Use Cautiously in: Cardiac, pulmonary, or previous liver disease; Women, patients >35 yr (increased risk of hepatotoxicity).

Adverse Reactions/Side Effects

CNS: drowsiness, muscle weakness, confusion, dizziness, headache, insomnia, malaise, nervousness. **EENT:** excessive lacrimation, visual disturbances. **Resp:** pleural effusions. **CV:** changes in BP, tachycardia. **GI:** HEPATOTOXICITY, diarrhea, anorexia, cramps, dysphagia, GI bleeding, vomiting. **GU:** crystalluria, dysuria, frequency, erectile dysfunction, incontinence, nocturia. **Derm:** pruritus, sweating, urticaria. **Hemat:** eosinophilia. **Local:** irritation at IV site, phlebitis. **MS:** myalgia. **Misc:** chills, drooling, fever.

Interactions

Drug-Drug: Additive CNS depression with **CNS depressants**, including **alcohol**, **antihista-**

mines, **opioid analgesics**, **sedative/hypnotics**, and parenteral **magnesium sulfate**. ↑ risk of hepatotoxicity with other **hepatotoxic agents** or **estrogens**. ↑ risk of arrhythmias with **verapamil**.
Drug-Natural Products: Concomitant use of **kava kava, valerian, chamomile, or hops can increase CNS depression.**

Route/Dosage

PO (Adults): *Spasticity*—25 mg/day initially; increase by 25 mg/day q 4–7 days until desired response or total of 100 mg 4 times daily is reached. *Prevention of malignant hyperthermia*—4–8 mg/kg/day in 3–4 divided doses for 1–2 days before procedure, last dose 3–4 hr preop. *Post-hyperthermic crisis follow-up*—4–8 mg/kg/day in 3–4 divided doses for 1–3 days after IV treatment.
PO (Children >5 yr): *Spasticity*—0.5 mg/kg twice daily; increase by 0.5 mg/kg/day q 4–7 days until desired response is obtained or dosage of 3 mg/kg 4 times daily is reached (not to exceed 400 mg/day). *Prevention of malignant hyperthermia*—4–8 mg/kg/day in 3–4 divided doses for 1–2 days before procedure, last dose 3–4 hr preop. *Post-hyperthermic crisis follow-up*—4–8 mg/kg/day in 3–4 divided doses for 1–3 days after IV treatment.
IV (Adults and Children): *Treatment of malignant hyperthermia*—at least 1 mg/kg (up to 3 mg/kg), continued until symptoms decrease or a cumulative dose of 10 mg/kg has been given. If symptoms reappear, dose may be repeated. *Prevention of malignant hyperthermia*—2.5 mg/kg before anesthesia.

Availability (generic available)

Capsules: 25 mg, 50 mg, 100 mg. **Powder for injection:** 20 mg/vial.

NURSING IMPLICATIONS

Assessment

- Assess bowel function periodically. Persistent diarrhea may warrant discontinuation of therapy.
- **Muscle Spasticity:** Assess neuromuscular status and muscle spasticity before initiating therapy and periodically during its course to determine response to therapy.
- **Malignant Hyperthermia:** Assess previous anesthesia history of all surgical patients. Also assess for family history of reactions to anesthesia (malignant hyperthermia or perioperative death).
- Monitor ECG, vital signs, electrolytes, and urine output continuously when administering IV for malignant hyperthermia
- Monitor patient for difficulty swallowing and choking during meals on the day of administration.
- ***Lab Test Considerations:*** Monitor liver function frequently during therapy. Liver function abnormalities (↑ AST, ALT, alkaline phosphatase, bilirubin, GGTP) may require discontinuation of therapy.
- Evaluate renal function and CBC before and periodically during therapy in patients receiving prolonged therapy.

Potential Nursing Diagnoses

Impaired physical mobility (Indications)
Acute pain (Indications)
Risk for injury (Side Effects)

Implementation

- Do not confuse Dantrium (dantrolene) with danazol.
- **PO:** If gastric irritation becomes a problem, may be administered with food. Oral suspensions may be made by opening capsules and adding them to fruit juices or other liquid. Drink immediately after mixing.
- Oral dose for spasticity should be divided into 4 doses/day.

IV Administration

- **Direct IV:** ***Diluent:*** Reconstitute each 20 mg with 60 ml of sterile water for injection (without a bacteriostatic agent). Shake until solution is clear. Solution must be used within 6 hr. Administer without further dilution. Protect diluted solution from direct light. ***Concentration:*** 0.333 mg/ml. ***Rate:*** Administer each single dose by rapid continuous IV push through Y-tubing or 3-way stopcock. Follow immediately with subsequent doses as indicated. Medication is very irritating to tissues; observe infusion site frequently to avoid extravasation.
- **Intermittent Infusion:** Prophylactic dose has been administered as an infusion. ***Rate:*** Administer over 1 hr before anesthesia.

Patient/Family Teaching

- Advise patient not to take more medication than the amount prescribed to minimize risk of hepatotoxicity and other side effects. If a dose is missed, do not take unless remembered within 1 hr. Do not double doses.

- May cause dizziness, drowsiness, visual disturbances, and muscle weakness. Advise patient to avoid driving and other activities requiring alertness until response to drug is known. After IV dose for surgery, patients may experience decreased grip strength, leg weakness, light-headedness, and difficulty swallowing for up to 48 hr. Caution patients to avoid activities requiring alertness and to use caution when walking down stairs and eating during this period.
- Advise patient to avoid taking alcohol or other CNS depressants concurrently with this medication.
- Instruct patient to notify health care professional if rash; itching; yellow eyes or skin; dark urine; or clay-colored, bloody, or black, tarry stools occur or if nausea, weakness, malaise, fatigue, or diarrhea persists. May require discontinuation of therapy.
- Advise patient to wear sunscreen and protective clothing to prevent photosensitivity reactions.
- Emphasize the importance of follow-up exams to check progress in long-term therapy and blood tests to monitor for side effects.
- **Malignant Hyperthermia:** Patients with malignant hyperthemia should carry identification describing disease process at all times.

Evaluation/Desired Outcomes

- Relief of muscle spasm in musculoskeletal conditions. One wk or more may be required to see improvement; if there is no observed improvement in 45 days, the medication is usually discontinued.
- Prevention of, or decrease in, temperature and skeletal rigidity in malignant hyperthermia.

daptomycin (dap-to-**mye**-sin)

Cubicin

Classification

Therapeutic: anti-infectives

Pharmacologic: cyclic lipopeptide antibacterial agents

Pregnancy Category B

Indications

Complicated skin and skin structure infections caused by aerobic Gram-positive bacteria.

Action

Causes rapid depolarization of membrane potential following binding to bacterial membrane; this results in inhibition of protein, DNA, and RNA synthesis. **Therapeutic Effects:** Death of bacteria with resolution of infection. **Spectrum:** Active against *Stapylococcus aureus* (including methicillin-resistant strains), *Streptococcus pyogenes*, *Streptococcus agalactiae*, some *Streptococcus dysgalactiae*, and *Enterococcus faecalis* (vancomycin-susceptible strains).

Pharmacokinetics

Absorption: IV administration results in complete bioavailability.

Distribution: Unknown.

Protein Binding: 92%.

Metabolism and Excretion: Metabolism not known; mostly excreted by kidneys.

Half-life: 8.1 hr.

TIME/ACTION PROFILE

ROUTE	ONSET	PEAK	DURATION
IV	rapid	end of infusion	24 hr

Contraindications/Precautions

Contraindicated in: Hypersensitivity.

Use Cautiously in: CCr <30 ml/min (dose reduction required); Geriatric patients (may have ↓ clinical response with ↑ risk of adverse reactions); Pregnancy (use only if clearly needed; Lactation; Children <18 yr (safety not established).

Adverse Reactions/Side Effects

CNS: dizziness. **Resp:** dyspnea. **CV:** hypertension, hypotension. **GI:** PSEUDOMEMBRANOUS COLITIS, constipation, diarrhea, nausea, vomiting, ↑ liver function tests. **GU:** renal failure. **Derm:** pruritus, rash. **Hemat:** anemia. **Local:** injection site reactions. **MS:** ↑ CPK. **Misc:** fever.

Interactions

Drug-Drug: Tobramycin ↑ blood levels. Concurrent **HMG-CoA reductase inhibitors** may ↑ the risk of myopathy.

Route/Dosage

IV (Adults): 4 mg/kg every 24 hr.

Renal Impairment

IV (Adults): *CCr <30 ml/min*—4 mg/kg every 48 hr.

Availability

Powder for injection: 500 mg/vial.

NURSING IMPLICATIONS

Assessment

- Assess patient for infection (vital signs; appearance of wound, sputum, urine, and stool; WBC) at beginning of and throughout therapy.
- Assess for signs of pseudomembranous colitis (diarrhea, abdominal cramping, fever, and bloody stools) during therapy.
- ***Lab Test Considerations:*** Monitor CPK weekly, more frequently in patients with unexplained ↑. Discontinue daptomycin if CPK >1000 units/L and signs and symptoms of myopathy occur.

Potential Nursing Diagnoses

Risk for infection (Indications, Side Effects)

Implementation

IV Administration

- **Intermittent Infusion:** ***Diluent:*** Reconstitute 500-mg vial with 10 ml of 0.9% NaCl. Reconstituted vials are stable for 12 hr at room temperature or 48 hrs if refrigerated. Dilute further in 50 ml of 0.9% NaCl. Solution is stable for 12 hr at room temperature or 48 hr if refrigerated. Do not administer solutions that are cloudy or contain a precipitate. ***Rate:*** Infuse over 30 min.
- **Y-Site Compatibility:** amikacin, aminophylline, amiodarone, ampicillin, ampicillin/sulbactam, argatroban, azithromycin, aztreonam, bumetanide, calcium chloride, calcium gluconate, caspofungin, cefazolin, cefepime, cefotaxime, cefoxitin, ceftazidime, ceftizoxime, ceftriaxone, cefuroxime, chloramphenicol, cimetidine, ciprofloxacin, cisatracurium, clindamycin, cyclosporine, dexamethasone sodium phosphate, diazepam, digoxin, diltiazem, diphenhydramine, dobutamine, dolasetron, dopamine, doxycycline, droperidol, enalaprilat, epinephrine, eptifibatide, ertapenem, erythromycin, esmolol, famotidine, fenoldopam, fentanyl, fluconazole, furosemide, ganciclovir, gentamicin, granisetron, haloperidol, heparin, hydralazine, hydrocortisone sodium succinate, hydromorphone, hydroxyzine, insulin, isoproterenol, ketorolac, labetalol, levofloxacin, lidocaine, linezolid, lorazepam, magnesium sulfate, meperidine, meropenem, methylprednisolone sodium succinate, metoclopramide, metoprolol, midazolam, milrinone, morphine, moxifloxacin, mycophenolate mofetil, nafcillin, nicardipine, nitroprusside, norepinephrine, ondansetron, palonosetron, pamidronate, pancuronium, phenylephrine, piperacillin/tazobactam, potassium chloride, potassium phosphate, procainamide, prochlorperazine, promethazine, propranolol, quinupristin/dalfopristin, ranitidine, sodium bicarbonate, tacrolimus, ticarcillin/clavulanate, tirofiban, tobramycin, trimethoprim/sulfamethoxazole, vasopressin, vecuronium, verapamil, voriconazole, zoledronic acid.
- **Y-Site Incompatibility:** acyclovir, imipenem/cilastatin, metronidazole, nesiritide, nitroglycerin, pantoprazole, phenytoin.
- **Solution Incompatibility:** D5W.

Patient/Family Teaching

- Inform patient of purpose of medication.
- Instruct patient to notify health care professional immediately if diarrhea, abdominal cramping, fever, or bloody stools occur and not to treat with antidiarrheals without consulting health care professionals.
- May cause dizziness. Caution patient to avoid driving or other activities requiring alertness until response to medication is known.

Evaluation/Desired Outcomes

- Resolution of the signs and symptoms of infection. Length of time for complete resolution depends on the organism and site of infection.

darbepoetin (dar-be-**poh**-e-tin)

Aranesp

Classification
Therapeutic: antianemics
Pharmacologic: hormones (rDNA)

Pregnancy Category C

Indications

Anemia associated with chronic renal failure. Chemotherapy-induced anemia in patients with non-myeloid malignancies.

Action

Stimulates erythropoiesis (production of red blood cells). **Therapeutic Effects:** Maintains and may elevate red blood cell counts, decreasing the need for transfusions.

D

♣ = Canadian drug name.
*CAPITALS indicates life-threatening; underlines indicate most frequent.

Pharmacokinetics

Absorption: 30–50% following subcut administration; IV administration results in complete bioavailability.
Distribution: Confined to the intravascular space.
Metabolism and Excretion: Unknown.
Half-life: *Subcut*—49 hr; *IV*—21 hr.

TIME/ACTION PROFILE (increase in RBCs)

ROUTE	ONSET	PEAK	DURATION
IV, subcut	2–6 wks	unknown	unknown

Contraindications/Precautions

Contraindicated in: Hypersensitivity; Uncontrolled hypertension.
Use Cautiously in: History of hypertension; Underlying hematologic diseases, including hemolytic anemia, sickle-cell anemia, thalassemia and porphyria (safety not established); OB, Pedi, Pregnancy, lactation, or children (safety not established).

Adverse Reactions/Side Effects

CNS: SEIZURES, dizziness, fatigue, headache, weakness. **Resp:** cough, dyspnea, bronchitis. **CV:** ARRHYTHMIAS, CHF, MI, STROKE, THROMBOTIC EVENTS (especially with hemoglobin >12 g/dL), edema, hypertension, hypotension, chest pain, transient ischemic attack, thrombotic events. **GI:** abdominal pain, nausea, diarrhea, vomiting, constipation. **Derm:** pruritus. **Hemat:** pure red cell aplasia. **MS:** myalgia, arthralgia, back pain, limb pain. **Misc:** fever, allergic reactions, flu-like syndrome, sepsis, ↑ mortality and ↑ tumor growth (with hemoglobin ≥12 g/dL).

Interactions

Drug-Drug: None reported.

Route/Dosage

Anemia due to Chronic Renal Failure

(Use lowest dose that will gradually increase hemoglobin level and avoid RBC transfusion).
IV, Subcut (Adults): *Starting treatment with darbepoetin (no previous epoetin)*—0.45 mcg/kg once weekly; adjust dose to attain target hemoglobin of 12 g/dl. Dosage adjustments should be made monthly in increments or decrements of 25% of current dose. Some patients may be dosed every 2 weeks. *Conversion from epoetin to darbepoetin*—weekly epoetin dose <2500 units = 6.25 mcg/week darbepoetin, weekly epoetin dose 2500–4999 units = 12.5 mcg/week darbepoetin, weekly epoetin dose 5000–10,999 units = 25 mcg/week darbepoetin, weekly epoetin dose 11,000–17,999 units = 40 mcg/week darbepoetin, weekly epoetin dose 18,000–33,999 units = 60 mcg/week darbepoetin, weekly epoetin dose 34,000–89,999 units = 100 mcg/week darbepoetin, weekly epoetin dose >90,000 units = 200 mcg/week darbepoetin.

Anemia due to Chemotherapy

(Use only for chemotherapy-related anemia and discontinue when chemotherapy course is completed)
Subcut (Adults): 2.25 mcg/kg initially. Adjust dose to attain target hemoglobin. If hemoglobin increases by <1.0 g/dL after 6 weeks of therapy, dose should be increased up to 4.5 mcg/kg. If hemoglobin increases by >1.0 g/dL in 2 weeks or if the hemoglobin >12 g/dL, risk of tumor growth and death increases; decrease dose by approximately 25%. If hemoglobin is >13 g/dL, temporarily withhold until hemoglobin falls to 12 g/dL. Restart at a dose approximately 25%<the previous dose.

Availability

Albumin solution for injection: 25 mcg/ml 1-ml vial, 40 mcg/ml 1-ml vial, 60 mcg/ml 1-ml vial, 100 mcg/ml 1-ml vial, 150 mcg/ml 0.75-ml vial, 200 mcg/ml 1-ml vial, 300 mcg/ml 1-ml vial, 500 mcg/ml 1-ml vial. **Pre-filled syringes:** 60 mcg/0.3 ml, 100 mcg/0.5 ml, 200 mcg/0.4 ml.

NURSING IMPLICATIONS

Assessment

- Monitor blood pressure before and during therapy. Inform physician or other health care professional if severe hypertension is present or if blood pressure begins to increase. Additional antihypertensive therapy may be required during initiation of therapy.
- Monitor response for symptoms of anemia (fatigue, dyspnea, pallor).
- Monitor dialysis shunts (thrill and bruit) and status of artificial kidney during hemodialysis. May need to increase heparin dose to prevent clotting. Monitor patients with underlying vascular disease for impaired circulation.
- Monitor for allergic reactions (rash, utricaria). Discontinue darbepoetin if signs of anaphylaxis (dyspnea, laryngeal swelling) occur.
- ***Lab Test Considerations:*** May cause ↑ in WBCs and platelets. May ↓ bleeding times.

- Monitor serum ferritin, transferrin, and iron levels prior to and during therapy to assess need for concurrent iron therapy. Transferrin saturation should be at least 20% and ferritin should be at least 100 ng/ml.
- Monitor hemoglobin before and weekly during initial therapy, for 4 wk after a change in dose, and regularly after target range has been reached and maintenance dose is determined. Monitor other hematopoietic parameters (CBC with differential and platelet count) before and periodically during therapy. Hemoglobin increases of more than 1.0 g/dl in any 2-week period or hemoglobin >12 g/dL increases the likelihood of life—threatening cardiovascular complications, cardiac arrest, neurologic events (seizures, stroke), hypertensive reactions, CHF, vascular thrombosis/ischemia/infarction, acute MI, and fluid overload/edema. Decrease dose by 25% and monitor hemoglobin weekly for 4 wk. If hemoglobin continues to increase, temporarily withhold until hemoglobin begins to decrease; then re-initiate at a dose 25% lower than previous dose.
- If increase in hemoglobin is less than 1 g/dl over 4 wks and iron stores are adequate, dose may be increased by 25% of previous dose.
- Monitor renal function studies and electrolytes closely; resulting increased sense of well-being may lead to decreased compliance with other therapies for renal failure.

Potential Nursing Diagnoses

Activity intolerance (Indications)

Implementation

- Transfusions are still required for severe symptomatic anemia. Supplemental iron should be initiated with darbepoetin and continued during therapy. Correct deficiencies of folic acid or vitamin B_{12} prior to therapy.
- Institute seizure precautions in patients who experience greater than a 1.0 g/dl increase in hemoglobin in a 2-wk period or exhibit any change in neurologic status.
- *For conversion from epoetin alfa to darbepoetin,* if epoetin was administered 2-3 times/wk administer darbepoetin once a week. If patient was receiving epoetin once/wk, darbepoetin may be administered once every 2 wks. Route of administration should remain consistent.
- Dose adjustments should not be more frequent than once/month.
- Do not shake vial; inactivation of medication may occur. Do not administer vials containing solution that is discolored or contains particulate matter. Discard vial immediately after withdrawing dose. Do not pool unused portions.
- **Subcut:** This route is often used for patients not requiring dialysis.

IV Administration

- **Direct IV:** Administer undiluted. ***Rate:*** May be administered as direct injection or bolus over 1–3 min into IV tubing or via venous line at end of dialysis session.
- **Y-Site Incompatibility:** Do not administer in conjunction with other drugs or solutions.

Patient/Family Teaching

- Explain rationale for concurrent iron therapy (increased red blood cell production requires iron).
- Discuss possible return of menses and fertility in women of childbearing age. Patient should discuss contraceptive options with health care professional.
- Discuss ways of preventing self-injury in patients at risk for seizures. Driving and activities requiring continuous alertness should be avoided.
- Stress importance of compliance with dietary restrictions, medications, and dialysis. Foods high in iron and low in potassium include liver, pork, veal, beef, mustard and turnip greens, peas, eggs, broccoli, kale, blackberries, strawberries, apple juice, watermelon, oatmeal, and enriched bread. Darbepoetin will result in increased sense of well-being, but it does not cure underlying disease.
- **Home Care Issues:** Home dialysis patients determined to be able to safely and effectively administer darbepoetin should be taught proper dosage, administration technique, and disposal of equipment. *Information for Patients and Caregivers* should be provided to patient along with medication.

Evaluation/Desired Outcomes

- Increase in hemoglobin not to exceed 12 g/dl with improvement in symptoms of anemia in patients with chronic renal failure.

darifenacin (dar-i-**fen**-a-sin)
Enablex

Classification
Therapeutic: urinary tract antispasmodics
Pharmacologic: anticholinergics

Pregnancy Category C

Indications
Overactive bladder with symptoms (urge incontinence, urgency, frequency).

Action
Acts as a muscarinic (cholinergic) receptor antagonist; antagonizes bladder smooth muscle contraction. **Therapeutic Effects:** Decreased symptoms of overactive bladder.

Pharmacokinetics
Absorption: 15–19% absorbed.
Distribution: Unknown.
Protein Binding: 98%.
Metabolism and Excretion: Extensively metabolized by the CYP2D6 enzyme system in most individuals; poor metabolizers (7% of Caucasians, 2% of African Americans) have less CYP2D6 activity with less metabolism occurring. Some metabolism via CYP3A4 enzyme system. 60% excreted renally as metabolites, 40% in feces as metabolites.
Half-life: 13–19 hr.

TIME/ACTION PROFILE

ROUTE	ONSET	PEAK	DURATION
Oral	Unk	7 hr	24 hr

Contraindications/Precautions
Contraindicated in: Hypersensitivity; Urinary retention; Gastric retention; Uncontrolled angle-closure glaucoma; Severe hepatic impairment.
Use Cautiously in: Concurrent use of CYP3A4 inhibitors (use lower dose/clinical monitoring may be necessary); Moderate hepatic impairment (lower dose recommended); Bladder outflow obstruction; GI obstructive disorders, decreased GI motility, severe constipation, or ulcerative colitis; Myasthenia gravis; Angle-closure glaucoma; Lactation or children (safety not established); Pregnancy (use only if maternal benefit outweighs fetal risk).

Adverse Reactions/Side Effects
CNS: dizziness. **EENT:** blurred vision. **GI:** constipation, dry mouth, dyspepsia, nausea. **Metab:** heat intolerance.

Interactions
Drug-Drug: Blood levels and risk of toxicity are ↑ by concurrent use of strong CYP3A4 inhibitors including **ketoconazole**, **itraconazole**, **ritonavir**, **nelfinavir**, **clarithromycin**, and **nefazodone**; daily dose should not exceed 7.5 mg. Concurrent use of moderate inhibitors of CYP3A4 especially those with narrow therapeutic indices, including **flecainide**, **thioridazine**, and **tricyclic antidepressants** should be undertaken with caution.

Route/Dosage
PO (Adults): 7.5 mg once daily, may be increased after 2 wk to 15 mg once daily.

Availability
Extended-release tablets: 7.5 mg, 15 mg.

NURSING IMPLICATIONS

Assessment
- Monitor voiding pattern and assess symptoms of overactive bladder (urinary urgency, urinary incontinence, urinary frequency) to and periodically during therapy.

Potential Nursing Diagnoses
Impaired urinary elimination (Indications)

Implementation
- **PO:** Administer once daily without regard to food. Extended-release tablets must be swallowed whole; do not break, crush, or chew.

Patient/Family Teaching
- Instruct patient to take darifenacin as directed. Advise patient to read the *Patient Information* before starting therapy and with each prescription refill. If a dose is missed, skip dose and take next day; do not take 2 doses in same day.
- Do not share darifenacin with others; may be dangerous.
- Inform patient of potential anticholinergic side effects (constipation, urinary retention, blurred vision, heat prostration in a hot environment).
- May cause dizziness and blurred vision. Caution patient to avoid driving and other activities that require alertness until response to medication is known.
- Advise patient to consult health care professional prior to taking Rx, OTC, or herbal products with darifenacin.

Evaluation/Desired Outcomes
- Decrease in symptoms of overactive bladder (urge urinary incontinence, urgency, frequency).

darunavir (da-runa-veer)

Prezista

Classification

Therapeutic: antiretrovirals

Pharmacologic: protease inhibitors

Pregnancy Category B

Indications

HIV infection (with other antiretrovirals) in adults who have already received and progressed on other antiretroviral combinations.

Action

Inhibits HIV-1 protease, selectively inhibiting the cleavage of HIV encoded specific polyproteins in infected cells. This prevents the formation of mature virus particles. **Therapeutic Effects:** Increased CD4 cell counts and decreased viral load with subsequent slowed progression of HIV infection and its sequelae.

Pharmacokinetics

Absorption: *Without ritonavir*—37% absorbed following oral administration; *with ritonavir*—82%. Food increases absorption by 30%.

Distribution: Unknown.

Protein Binding: 95% bound to plasma proteins.

Metabolism and Excretion: Extensively metabolized by CYP3A enzyme system. 41% eliminated unchanged in feces, 8% in urine.

Half-life: 15 hr.

TIME/ACTION PROFILE

ROUTE	ONSET	PEAK	DURATION
PO	unknown	2.5–4 hr	12 hr

Contraindications/Precautions

Contraindicated in: Concurrent dihydroergotamine, ergonovine, ergotamine, methylergonovine, midazolam, pimozide, or triazolam; OB: Lactation; HIV may be transmitted in human milk; Pedi: Safe use in children not established.

Use Cautiously in: Hepatic impairment; Geri: Consider age-related impairment in hepatic function, concurrent chronic disease states and drug therapy; OB: Use in pregnancy only if maternal benefit outweighs fetal risk.

Adverse Reactions/Side Effects

Based on concurrent use with ritonavir. **GI:** constipation, diarrhea, nausea, vomiting. **Endo:** hyperglycemia. **Metab:** body fat redistribution.

Interactions

Drug-Drug: Darunavir and ritonavir are both inhibitors of CYP3A and are metabolized by CYP3A. Multiple drug-drug interactions can be expected with drugs that share, inhibit, or induce these pathways. Consult product information for more specific details. **Carbamazepine**, **phenobarbital**, **rifampin**, and **phenytoin** ↑ metabolism and may ↓ antiretroviral effectiveness, concurrent use is contraindicated. ↓ Metabolism of and may ↑ risk of ergot toxicity with **dihydroergotamine**, **ergonovine**, **ergotamine**, **methylergonovine**; concurrent use is contraindicated. ↓ Metabolism of and may ↑ risk of serious myopathy **lovastatin** and simvastatin **ergonovine**, **ergotamine**; concurrent use is contraindicated. **Atorvastatin** and **pravastatin** may be used in modified doses. ↑ levels and risk of cardiotoxicity with **pimozide**; concurrent use is contraindicated. ↑ levels and risk of excess CNS depression with **midazolam** or **triazolam**; concurrent use is contraindicated. Concurrent use with **efavirenz** results in ↓ darunavir levels and ↑ efavirenz levels; use combination cautiously. Concurrent use with **lopivavir/ritonavir** ↓ darunavir levels and may ↓ antiretroviral effectiveness; although concurrent use is not recommended, additional ritonavir may be required. Concurrent use with **saquinavir** ↓ darunavir levels and may ↓ antiretroviral effectiveness; concurrent use is not recommended. ↑ levels and risk of toxicity with **lidocaine**, **quinidine**, and **amiodarone**; use cautiously and with available blood level monitoring. ↓ levels and may ↓ anticoagulant effect of **warfarin**; monitor INR. ↑ levels and risk of adverse reactions to **trazodone**; use cautiously and decrease dose if necessary. ↑ levels of **clarithromycin**, especially in patients with renal impairment (CCr <60 ml/min); ↓ dose of clarithromycin required. **Ketoconazole** and **itraconazole** may ↑ darunavir levels. Darunavir ↑ levels of **ketoconazole** and **itraconazole**; daily dose of itraconazole or ketoconazole should not be >200 mg. ↓ blood levels and may ↓ antifungal effectiveness of **voriconazole**; avoid concurrent use if possible. Concurrent use with **rifabutin** ↑ rifabutin levels and ↓ darunavir levels (may be due to ritonavir); rifabutin dose should be decreased to 150 mg every other day. ↑ levels and may ↑ risk of adverse cardiovascular side effects of **felodipione**, **nifedipine**, or **nicardipine**; monitor clinical response carefully. **Dexamethasone** ↓ levels and may ↓ antiretroviral effectiveness. May ↑ systemic levels of **inhaled fluticasone**; choose alternative inhaled corticosteroid. ↑ levels of; and may ↑ risk of toxicity with; **cyclosporine**, **tacrolimus**, **sirolimus**; blood level monitoring recommended. ↓ levels and may precipitate opiate abstinence syndrome from **methadone**. ↑ levels of, and ↑ risk of serious toxicity from, **sildenafil**, **tardalafil**, or **vardenafil**; dose reduction required. ↓ levels and may ↓ antidepressant effectiveness of **sertraline** and **paroxetine**; adjust dose by clinical response.

Drug-Natural Products: St. John's wort ↑ metabolism and may ↓ antiretroviral effectiveness.

Route/Dosage

PO (Adults): 600 mg with ritonavir 100 mg twice daily.

Availability

Tablets: 300 mg.

NURSING IMPLICATIONS

Assessment

- Assess patient for change in severity of HIV symptoms and for symptoms of opportunistic infections during therapy.
- Assess for allergy to sulfonamides.
- Monitor patient for development of rash; usually maculopapular and self-limited. Discontinue therapy if severe.
- ***Lab Test Considerations:*** Monitor viral load and CD4 counts regularly during therapy.
- May cause ↑ serum AST, ALT, GGT, total bilirubin, alkaline phosphatase, pancreatic amylase, pancreatic lipase, triglycerides, total cholesterol, and uric acid concentrations.

Potential Nursing Diagnoses

Risk for infection (Indications)
Noncompliance (Patient/Family Teaching)

Implementation

- **PO:** Must be administered with a meal or light snack along with ritonavir 100 mg to be effective. The type of food is not important. Tablets should be swallowed whole with water or milk; do not chew.

Patient/Family Teaching

- Emphasize the importance of taking darunavir with ritonavir exactly as directed, at evenly spaced times throughout day. Do not take more than prescribed amount and do not stop taking without consulting health care professional. If a dose of darunavir or ritonavir is missed by more than 6 hrs, wait and take next dose at regularly scheduled time. If missed by less than 6 hrs, take darunavir and ritonavir immediately and then take next dose at regularly scheduled time. If a dose is skipped, do not double doses. Advise patient to read Patient Information sheet before starting therapy and with each prescription renewal in case changes have been made.
- Instruct patient that darunavir should not be shared with others.
- Advise patient to avoid taking other Rx, OTC, or herbal products without consulting health care professional. These medications interact with many other drugs.
- Inform patient that darunavir does not cure AIDS or prevent associated or opportunistic infections. Darunavir does not reduce the risk of transmission of HIV to others through sexual contact or blood contamination. Caution patient to use a condom during sexual contact and to avoid sharing needles or donating blood to prevent spreading the AIDS virus to others. Advise patient that the long-term effects of darunavir are unknown at this time.
- Inform patient that darunavir may cause hyperglycemia. Advise patient to notify health care professional if increased thirst or hunger; unexplained weight loss; increased urination; fatigue; or dry, itchy skin occurs.
- Advise patients taking oral contraceptives to use a nonhormonal method of birth control during darunavir therapy. Advise female patients to avoid breastfeeding during therapy with darunavir.
- Inform patient that redistribution and accumulation of body fat may occur, causing central obesity, dorsocervical fat enlargement (buffalo hump), peripheral wasting, breast enlargement, and cushingoid appearance. The cause and long-term effects are not known.

- Emphasize the importance of regular follow-up exams and blood counts to determine progress and monitor for side effects.

Evaluation/Desired Outcomes
- Delayed progression of AIDS and decreased opportunistic infections in patients with HIV.
- Decrease in viral load and improvement in CD4 cell counts.

HIGH ALERT

DAUNOrubicin citrate liposome
(daw-noe-**roo**-bi-sin **sy**-trate **lye**-poe-sohm)
DaunoXome

Classification
Therapeutic: antineoplastics
Pharmacologic: anthracyclines

Pregnancy Category D

Indications
Management of advanced Kaposi's sarcoma in HIV-infected patients.

Action
Forms a complex with DNA, which subsequently inhibits DNA and RNA synthesis (cell-cycle phase–nonspecific). Encapsulation in a liposome increases uptake by tumor and decreases systemic toxicity. **Therapeutic Effects:** Death of rapidly replicating cells, particularly malignant ones. Also has immunosuppressive properties.

Pharmacokinetics
Absorption: Administered IV only, resulting in complete bioavailability. DaunoXome is released from the liposome after uptake by tumor.
Distribution: Widely distributed. Crosses the placenta.
Metabolism and Excretion: Extensively metabolized by the liver. Converted partially to a compound that also has antineoplastic activity (daunorubicinol); 40% eliminated by biliary excretion.
Half-life: *Daunorubicin citrate liposome*—55.4 hr. *Daunorubicinol*—26.7 hr.

TIME/ACTION PROFILE (effects on blood counts)

ROUTE	ONSET	PEAK	DURATION
IV	unknown	unknown	unknown

Contraindications/Precautions
Contraindicated in: Hypersensitivity to daunorubucin citrate liposome or any other components in the formulation; Pregnant or lactating women.
Use Cautiously in: Active infections or decreased bone marrow reserve; Geriatric patients or patients with other chronic debilitating illnesses; May reactivate skin lesions produced by previous radiation therapy; Hepatic or renal impairment (dosage reduction recommended if serum creatinine >3 mg/dl or serum bilirubin >1.2 mg/dl); Patients who have received previous anthracycline therapy or who have underlying cardiovascular disease (increased risk of cardiotoxicity); Patients with childbearing potential; Children (safety not established for DaunoXome).

Adverse Reactions/Side Effects
CNS: fatigue, headache, depression, dizziness, insomnia, malaise. **EENT:** rhinitis, abnormal vision, sinusitis. **CV:** CARDIOTOXICITY, chest pain, edema. **GI:** abdominal pain, anorexia, constipation, diarrhea, nausea, stomatitis, tenesmus, vomiting. **GU:** red urine, gonadal suppression. **Derm:** alopecia, increased sweating, pruritus. **Hemat:** anemia, leukopenia, thrombocytopenia. **Local:** phlebitis at IV site. **Metab:** hyperuricemia. **MS:** back pain, arthralgia, myalgia. **Neuro:** neuropathy. **Misc:** *DaunoXome*— allergic reactions, chills, fever, back pain, flushing, chest tightness, influenza-like symptoms.

Interactions
Drug-Drug: Additive myelosuppression with other **antineoplastics**. May decrease antibody response to **live-virus vaccines** and increase risk of adverse reactions. **Cyclophosphamide** increases the risk of cardiotoxicity.

Route/Dosage
Other dose regimens are used. In adults, cumulative dose should not exceed 550 mg/m² (450 mg/m² if previous chest radiation).
IV (Adults): 40 mg/m² q 2 wk.

Renal Impairment

IV (Adults): *Serum creatinine >3 mg/dl*—reduce dose by 50%.

Hepatic Impairment

IV (Adults): *Serum bilirubin 1.2–3 mg/dl*—reduce dose by 25%; *serum bilirubin >3 mg/dl*—reduce dose by 50%.

Availability (generic available)

Liposomal dispersion for injection: 2 mg/ml in 25-ml vial.

NURSING IMPLICATIONS

Assessment

- Monitor vital signs before and frequently during therapy.
- Assess patient for back pain, flushing, and chest tightness. Usually occurs during first 5 min of infusion and subsides with interruption of therapy. Symptoms do not usually recur when infusion is restarted at a slower rate.
- Monitor for bone marrow depression. Assess for bleeding (bleeding gums; bruising; petechiae; guaiac stools, urine, and emesis) and avoid IM injections and taking rectal temperatures if platelet count is low. Apply pressure to venipuncture sites for 10 min. Assess for signs of infection during neutropenia. Anemia may occur. Monitor for increased fatigue, dyspnea, and orthostatic hypotension.
- Assess IV site frequently for inflammation or infiltration. Instruct patient to notify nurse immediately if pain or irritation at injection site occurs. If extravasation occurs, infusion must be stopped and restarted in another vein to avoid damage to subcut tissue. Notify health care professional immediately.
- Monitor intake and output, appetite, and nutritional intake. Assess for nausea and vomiting, which, although mild, may persist for 24–48 hr. Administration of an antiemetic before and periodically during therapy and adjusting diet as tolerated may help maintain fluid and electrolyte balance and nutritional status. Encourage fluid intake of 2000–3000 ml/day. Allopurinol and alkalinization of the urine may be used to help prevent urate stone formation.
- Assess patient for evidence of cardiotoxicity, which manifests as CHF (peripheral edema, dyspnea, rales/crackles, weight gain, jugular venous distention) and usually occurs 1–6 mo after initiation of therapy. Chest x-ray, echocardiography, ECGs, and radionuclide angiography determination of ejection fraction may be ordered before and periodically throughout therapy. A 30% decrease in QRS voltage and decrease in systolic ejection fraction are early signs of cardiotoxicity. Patients who receive total cumulative doses >550/mm^2, who have a history of cardiac disease, or who have received mediastinal radiation are at greater risk of developing cardiotoxicity. May be irreversible and fatal, but usually responds to early treatment.
- ***Lab Test Considerations:*** Monitor uric acid levels.
- Monitor CBC and differential before each course of therapy. May cause severe bone marrow depression, especially granulocytopenia. Repeat blood counts before each dose and do not administer if absolute granulocyte count is <750 cells/mm^3.
- Monitor hepatic and renal function before each dose.

Potential Nursing Diagnoses

Risk for infection (Adverse Reactions)
Decreased cardiac output (Side Effects)

Implementation

- ***High Alert:*** Fatalities have occurred with chemotherapeutic agents. Before administering, clarify all ambiguous orders; double-check single, daily, and course-of-therapy dose limits; have second practitioner independently double-check original order, calculations, and infusion pump settings. Do not confuse daunorubicin citrate liposome (DaunoXome) with daunorubicin hydrochloride (Cerubidine) or with doxorubicin (Adriamycin, Rubex) or doxorubicin hydorchloride liposome (Doxil). To prevent confusion, orders should include generic and brand name.
- Solution should be prepared in a biologic cabinet. Wear gloves, gown, and mask while handling IV medication. Discard IV equipment in specially designated containers.

IV Administration

- **Intermittent Infusion: *Diluent:*** Dilute with D5W. Do not use an in-line filter for infusion. Reconstituted infusion may be stored for up to 6 hr in refrigerator. ***Concentration:*** 1 mg/ml. ***Rate:*** Administer dose over 1 hr.
- **Additive Incompatibility:** Information unavailable. Do not admix with other solutions or medications.

Patient/Family Teaching

- Instruct patient to notify health care professional if fever; chills; sore throat; signs of infection; bleeding gums; bruising; petechiae; or blood in urine, stool, or emesis occurs. Caution patient to avoid crowds and persons with known infections. Instruct patient to use soft toothbrush and electric razor. Patient should be cautioned not to drink alcoholic beverages or take products containing aspirin or NSAIDs.
- Instruct patient to inspect oral mucosa for erythema and ulceration. If ulceration occurs, advise patient to use sponge brush and rinse mouth with water after eating and drinking. Stomatitis pain may require management with opioid analgesics. Period of highest risk is 3–7 days after administration of dose.
- Instruct patient to notify health care professional immediately if irregular heartbeat, shortness of breath, or swelling of lower extremities occurs.
- Discuss with patient possibility of hair loss. Explore methods of coping. Regrowth of hair usually begins within 5 wk after discontinuing therapy.
- Inform patient that medication may turn urine reddish color for 1–2 days after administration.
- Inform patient that this medication may cause irreversible gonadal suppression. Advise patient that this medication may have teratogenic effects. Contraception should be used during therapy and for at least 4 mo after therapy is concluded.
- Instruct patient not to receive any vaccinations without advice of health care professional.
- Emphasize the need for periodic lab tests to monitor for side effects.

Evaluation/Desired Outcomes

- Arrested progression of Kaposi's sarcoma in patients with HIV infection. Therapy is continued until there is evidence of progression (new visceral sites of involvement, progression of visceral disease, development of 10 or more new cutaneous lesions or 25% increase in the number of lesions at baseline, change in character of >25% of lesions from flat to raised, increase in surface area of lesions) or until complications of HIV disease preclude continuation of therapy.

HIGH ALERT

DAUNOrubicin hydrochloride

(daw-noe-**roo**-bi-sin **hye**-dro-**klor**-ide)
Cerubidine

Classification
Therapeutic: antineoplastics
Pharmacologic: anthracyclines

Pregnancy Category D

Indications

In combination with other antineoplastics in the treatment of leukemias.

Action

Forms a complex with DNA, which subsequently inhibits DNA and RNA synthesis (cell-cycle phase-nonspecific). **Therapeutic Effects:** Death of rapidly replicating cells, particularly malignant ones. Also has immunosuppressive properties.

Pharmacokinetics

Absorption: Administered IV only, resulting in complete bioavailability.
Distribution: Widely distributed. Crosses the placenta.
Metabolism and Excretion: Extensively metabolized by the liver. Converted partially to a compound that also has antineoplastic activity (daunorubicinol); 40% eliminated by biliary excretion.
Half-life: *Daunorubicin hydrochloride*—18.5 hr. *Daunorubicinol*—26.7 hr.

TIME/ACTION PROFILE (effects on blood counts)

ROUTE	ONSET	PEAK	DURATION
IV	7–10 days	10–14 days	21 days

Contraindications/Precautions

Contraindicated in: Hypersensitivity to daunorubucin hydrochloride or any other components in the formulation; Symptomatic CHF/arrhythmias; Pregnant or lactating women.
Use Cautiously in: Active infections or decreased bone marrow reserve; Geriatric patients or patients with other chronic debilitating illnesses (dosage reduction recommended for patients ≥60 yr); May reactivate skin lesions produced by previous radiation therapy; Hepat-

ic or renal impairment (dosage reduction recommended if serum creatinine >3 mg/dl or serum bilirubin >1.2 mg/dl); Patients who have received previous anthracycline therapy or who have underlying cardiovascular disease (increased risk of cardiotoxicity); Patients with childbearing potential.

Adverse Reactions/Side Effects

EENT: rhinitis, abnormal vision, sinusitis. **CV:** CARDIOTOXICITY, arrhythmias. **GI:** nausea, vomiting, esophagitis, hepatoxicity, stomatitis. **GU:** red urine, gonadal suppression. **Derm:** alopecia. **Hemat:** anemia, leukopenia, thrombocytopenia. **Local:** phlebitis at IV site. **Metab:** hyperuricemia. **Misc:** chills, fever.

Interactions

Drug-Drug: Additive myelosuppression with other **antineoplastics**. May decrease antibody response to **live-virus vaccines** and increase risk of adverse reactions. **Cyclophosphamide** increases the risk of cardiotoxicity. Increased risk of hepatic toxicity with other **hepatotoxic agents**.

Route/Dosage

Other dose regimens are used. In adults, cumulative dose should not exceed 550 mg/m² (450 mg/m² if previous chest radiation).

IV (Adults <60 yr): 45 mg/m²/day for 3 days in first course, then for 2 days of second course (as part of combination regimen).

IV (Adults ≥60 yr): 30 mg/m²/day for 3 days in first course, then for 2 days of second course (as part of combination regimen).

IV (Children >2 yr): 25 mg/m² once weekly (as part of combination regimen). In children <2 yr or BSA <0.5 m², dosage should be determined on a mg/kg basis.

Availability (generic available)

Powder for injection: 20 mg/vial. **Solution for injection:** 5 mg/ml in 4-ml vials (20 mg).

NURSING IMPLICATIONS

Assessment

- Monitor vital signs before and frequently during therapy.
- Monitor for bone marrow depression. Assess for bleeding (bleeding gums; bruising; petechiae; guaiac stools, urine, and emesis) and avoid IM injections and taking rectal temperatures if platelet count is low. Apply pressure to venipuncture sites for 10 min. Assess for signs of infection during neutropenia. Anemia may occur. Monitor for increased fatigue, dyspnea, and orthostatic hypotension.
- Assess IV site frequently for inflammation or infiltration. Instruct patient to notify nurse immediately if pain or irritation at injection site occurs. If extravasation occurs, infusion must be stopped and restarted in another vein to avoid damage to subcut tissue. Notify physician immediately. Daunorubicin hydrochloride is a vesicant. Standard treatments include local injections of steroids and application of ice compresses.
- Monitor intake and output, appetite, and nutritional intake. Assess for nausea and vomiting, which, although mild, may persist for 24–48 hr. Administration of an antiemetic before and periodically during therapy and adjusting diet as tolerated may help maintain fluid and electrolyte balance and nutritional status. Encourage fluid intake of 2000–3000 ml/day. Allopurinol and alkalinization of the urine may be used to help prevent urate stone formation.
- Assess patient for evidence of cardiotoxicity, which manifests as CHF (peripheral edema, dyspnea, rales/crackles, weight gain, jugular venous distention) and usually occurs 1–6 mo after initiation of therapy. Chest x-ray, echocardiography, ECGs, and radionuclide angiography determination of ejection fraction may be ordered before and periodically throughout therapy. A 30% decrease in QRS voltage and decrease in systolic ejection fraction are early signs of cardiotoxicity. Patients who receive total cumulative doses >550/mm², who have a history of cardiac disease, or who have received mediastinal radiation are at greater risk of developing cardiotoxicity. May be irreversible and fatal, but usually responds to early treatment.
- ***Lab Test Considerations:*** Monitor uric acid levels.
- *Daunorubicin hydrochloride:* Monitor CBC and differential before and periodically throughout therapy. The leukocyte count nadir occurs 10–14 days after administration. Recovery usually occurs within 21 days after administration of daunorubicin hydrochloride.
- Monitor AST, ALT, LDH, and serum bilirubin. May cause transiently ↑ serum alkaline phosphatase, bilirubin, and AST concentrations.

Potential Nursing Diagnoses
Risk for infection (Adverse Reactions)
Decreased cardiac output (Side Effects)

Implementation
- ***High Alert:*** Fatalities have occurred with chemotherapeutic agents. Before administering, clarify all ambiguous orders; double-check single, daily, and course-of-therapy dose limits; have second practitioner independently double-check original order, calculations, and infusion pump settings. Do not confuse daunorubicin hydrochloride (Cerubidine) with daunorubicin citrate liposome (DaunoXome) or with doxorubicin (Adriamycin, Rubex) or doxorubicin hydrochloride liposome (Doxil). To prevent confusion, orders should include generic and brand name.
- Solution should be prepared in a biologic cabinet. Wear gloves, gown, and mask while handling IV medication. Discard IV equipment in specially designated containers.
- **IV:** Reconstitute each 20 mg with 4 ml of sterile water for injection for a concentration of 5 mg/ml. Shake gently to dissolve. Reconstituted medication is stable for 24 hr at room temperature, 48 hr if refrigerated. Protect from sunlight.
- Do not use aluminum needles when reconstituting or injecting daunorubicin hydrochloride, as aluminum darkens the solution.

IV Administration
- **Direct IV:** ***Diluent:*** Dilute further in 10–15 ml of 0.9% NaCl. Administer direct IV push through Y-site into free-flowing infusion of 0.9% NaCl or D5W. ***Rate:*** Administer over at least 2–3 min. Rapid administration rate may cause facial flushing or erythema along the vein.
- **Intermittent Infusion:** ***Diluent:*** May also be diluted in 50–100 mL of 0.9% NaCl. ***Rate:*** Administer 50 ml over 10–15 min or 100 ml over 30–45 min.
- **Y-Site Compatibility:** amifostine, etoposide, filgrastim, gemcitabine, granisetron, melphalan, methotrexate, ondansetron, sodium bicarbonate, teniposide, thiotepa, vinorelbine.
- **Y-Site Incompatibility:** allopurinol, aztreonam, cefepime, fludarabine, lansoprazole, piperacillin/tazobactam.
- **Additive Incompatibility:** Manufacturer does not recommend admixing daunorubicin hydrochloride.

Patient/Family Teaching
- Instruct patient to notify health care professional if fever; chills; sore throat; signs of infection; bleeding gums; bruising; petechiae; or blood in urine, stool, or emesis occurs. Caution patient to avoid crowds and persons with known infections. Instruct patient to use soft toothbrush and electric razor. Patient should be cautioned not to drink alcoholic beverages or take products containing aspirin or NSAIDs.
- Instruct patient to inspect oral mucosa for erythema and ulceration. If ulceration occurs, advise patient to use sponge brush and rinse mouth with water after eating and drinking. Stomatitis pain may require management with opioid analgesics. Period of highest risk is 3–7 days after administration of dose.
- Instruct patient to notify health care professional immediately if irregular heartbeat, shortness of breath, or swelling of lower extremities occurs.
- Discuss with patient possibility of hair loss. Explore methods of coping. Regrowth of hair usually begins within 5 wk after discontinuing therapy.
- Inform patient that medication may turn urine reddish color for 1–2 days after administration.
- Inform patient that this medication may cause irreversible gonadal suppression. Advise patient that this medication may have teratogenic effects. Contraception should be used during therapy and for at least 4 mo after therapy is concluded.
- Instruct patient not to receive any vaccinations without advice of health care professional.
- Emphasize the need for periodic lab tests to monitor for side effects.

Evaluation/Desired Outcomes
- Improvement of hematologic status in patients with leukemia.

HIGH ALERT

decitabine (de-sit-a-been)

Dacogen

Classification
Therapeutic: antineoplastics

Pregnancy Category D

Indications
Treatment of various myelodysplastic syndromes (MDS).

Action
Inhibits DNA methyltransferase, causing apoptosis. Has more effect on rapidly replicating cells. **Therapeutic Effects:** Improved hematologic and clinical manifestations of MDS.

Pharmacokinetics
Absorption: IV administration results in complete bioavailability.
Distribution: Unknown.
Metabolism and Excretion: Mostly metabolized by the liver.
Half-life: 0.5 hr.

TIME/ACTION PROFILE (blood levels)

ROUTE	ONSET	PEAK	DURATION
IV	rapid	end of infusion	unknown

Contraindications/Precautions
Contraindicated in: Hypersensitivity; OB: Pregnancy or lactation.
Use Cautiously in: Patients with child-bearing potential (males and females); Impaired hepatic/renal function; Geri: Elderly patients may be more sensitive to effects; Pedi: Safety in children not established.

Adverse Reactions/Side Effects
CNS: confusion, fatigue, insomnia, depression, lethargy. **EENT:** blurred vision. **Resp:** cough. **CV:** atrial fibrillation, pulmonary edema, tachycardia. **GI:** abdominal pain, constipation, diarrhea, stomatitis, vomiting, abnormal liver function tests. **Derm:** petechiae, rash. **F and E:** edema, hypokalemia, hypomagnesemia, ascites. **Hemat:** BLEEDING, anemia, neutropenia, thrombocytopenia. **Local:** injection site irritation. **Metab:** hyperglycemia. **MS:** arthralgia, myalgia. **Misc:** INFECTION, fever, lymphadenopathy.

Interactions
Drug-Drug: ↑ risk of myelosuppression with other **antineoplastics**, **immunosuppressants**, or **radiation therapy**. May ↓ antibody response to and ↑ risk of adverse reactions from **live virus vaccines**.

Route/Dosage
IV (Adults): *First treatment cycle*—15 mg/m² as a continuous infusion over 3 hours repeated every 8 hours for 3 days. *Subsequent cycles*—cycle should be repeated every 6 wks for a minimum of 4 cycles; treatment may be continued as long as the patient continues to benefit. Dose adjustment/delay may be required for hematologic toxicity, renal or hepatic impairment, or infection.

Availability
Lyophilized powder for injection (requires reconstitution): 50 mg/vial.

NURSING IMPLICATIONS

Assessment
- Monitor for bone marrow depression. Assess for bleeding (bleeding gums, bruising, petechiae, guaiac stools, urine, and emesis) and avoid IM injections and taking rectal temperatures if platelet count is low. Apply pressure to venipuncture sites for 10 min. Assess for signs of infection during neutropenia. Anemia may occur. Monitor for increased fatigue, dyspnea, and orthostatic hypotension.
- ***Lab Test Considerations:*** Monitor CBC prior to each dosing cycle and periodically as needed. May cause neutropenia, thrombocytopenia, and anemia; occur more frequently in 1st or 2nd cycle. Use early institution of growth factors and antimicrobial agents to prevent infections.
- Obtain liver chemistries and serum creatinine prior to initiation of treatment. May cause hyperbilirubinemia and hypoalbuminemia.
- May cause hyperglycemia, hypomagnesemia, hyponatremia, hypokalemia, and hyperkalemia.

Potential Nursing Diagnoses
Risk for infection (Adverse Reactions)

Implementation
- ***High Alert:*** Fatalities have occurred with chemotherapeutic agents. Before administering, clarify all ambiguous orders; double-check single, daily, and course-of-therapy dose limits; have second practitioner independently double-check original order, calculations, and infusion pump settings.

- Solution should be prepared in a biologic cabinet. Wear gloves, gown, and mask while handling IV medication. Discard IV equipment in specially designated containers (see Appendix K).
- Pre-medicate patient with standard antiemetic therapy.
- If hematologic recovery (ANC ≥1,000 cells/mm³ and platelets ≥50,000 cells/mm³) from previous treatment cycle requires more than 6, but less than 8 wks—delay dosing for up to 2 wks and temporarily reduce dose to 11 mg/m² (33 mg/m²/day, 99 mg/m²/cycle) upon restarting therapy.
- If hematologic recovery requires more than 8, but less than 10 wks—Patient should be assessed for disease progression (by bone marrow aspirates); in the absence of progression, delay dose for up to 2 more wks and reduce dose as above upon restarting, then maintain or increase in subsequent cycles as clinically indicated.
- **Intermittent Infusion:** Reconstitute with 10 mL of Sterile Water for injection for a concentration of 5 mg/mL. Immediately after reconstitution, dilute further with 0.9% NaCl, D5W, or LR for a final concentration of 0.1–1.0 mg/mL. Unless used within 15 min of reconstitution, dilute solution must be prepared using cold infusion fluids and refrigerated until administration (maximum of 7 hr). ***Rate:*** Administer over 3 hr.

Patient/Family Teaching

- Caution patient to avoid crowds and persons with known infections. Report symptoms of infection (fever, chills, cough, hoarseness, sore throat, lower back or side pain, painful or difficult urination) immediately.
- Instruct patient to report unusual bleeding. Advise patient of thrombocytopenia precautions (use soft toothbrush and electric razor, avoid falls, do not drink alcoholic beverages or take medication containing aspirin or NSAIDs; may precipitate gastric bleeding).
- Inform patient that this medication may have teratogenic effects. Advise women to avoid becoming pregnant during treatment and advise men not to father a child during or for 2 months after treatment.

Evaluation/Desired Outcomes

- Improved hematologic and clinical manifestations of MDS.

deferoxamine
(de-fer-**ox**-a-meen)
Desferal

Classification
Therapeutic: antidotes
Pharmacologic: heavy metal antagonists

Pregnancy Category C

Indications

Acute toxic iron ingestion. Secondary iron overload syndromes associated with multiple transfusion therapy.

Action

Chelates unbound iron, forming a water-soluble complex (ferrioxamine) in plasma that is easily excreted by the kidneys. **Therapeutic Effects:** Removal of excess iron. Also chelates aluminum.

Pharmacokinetics

Absorption: Poorly absorbed after oral administration. Well absorbed after IM administration and subcut administration.
Distribution: Appears to be widely distributed.
Metabolism and Excretion: Metabolized by tissues and plasma enzymes. Unchanged drug and chelated form excreted by the kidneys; 33% of iron removed is eliminated in the feces via biliary excretion.
Half-life: 1 hr.

TIME/ACTION PROFILE (effects on hematologic parameters)

ROUTE	ONSET	PEAK	DURATION
IV	rapid	unknown	unknown
IM	unknown	unknown	unknown
Subcut	unknown	unknown	unknown

Contraindications/Precautions

Contraindicated in: Severe renal disease; Anuria; OB: Early pregnancy or childbearing potential (however, may be used safely in pregnant patients with moderate-to-severe acute iron intoxication).
Use Cautiously in: Pedi: Children <3 yr (safety not established).

Adverse Reactions/Side Effects

EENT: blurred vision, cataracts, ototoxicity. **CV:** hypotension, tachycardia. **GI:** abdominal pain, diarrhea. **GU:** red urine. **Derm:** erythema, flushing, urticaria. **Local:** induration at injection site, pain at injection site. **MS:** leg cramps. **Misc:** allergic reactions, fever, shock after rapid IV administration.

Interactions

Drug-Drug: Ascorbic acid may ↑ effectiveness of deferoxamine but may also ↑ cardiac iron toxicity.

Route/Dosage

Acute Iron Ingestion

IM, IV (Adults and Children ≥3 yr): 1 g (20 mg/kg or 600 mg/m^2), then 500 mg (10 mg/kg or 300 mg/m^2) q 4 hr for 2 doses. Additional doses of 500 mg (10 mg/kg or 300 mg/m^2) q 4–12 hr may be needed (not to exceed 6 g/24 hr).

Chronic Iron Overload

IM, IV (Adults and Children ≥3 yr): 500 mg–1 g daily; additional doses of 2 g should be given IV for each unit of blood transfused.
Subcut (Adults and Children ≥3 yr): 1–2 g/day (20–40 mg/kg/day) infused over 8–24 hr.

Availability (generic available)

Injection: 500 mg/vial.

NURSING IMPLICATIONS

Assessment

- In acute poisoning, assess time, amount, and type of iron preparation ingested.
- Monitor signs of iron toxicity: early acute (abdominal pain, bloody diarrhea, emesis), late acute (decreased level of consciousness, shock, metabolic acidosis).
- Monitor vital signs closely, especially during IV administration. Report hypotension, erythema, urticaria, or signs of allergic reaction. Keep epinephrine, an antihistamine, and resuscitation equipment close by in the event of an anaphylactic reaction.
- May cause oculotoxicity or ototoxicity. Report decreased visual acuity or hearing loss. Audiovisual exams should be performed every 3 mo in patients with chronic iron overload.
- Monitor intake and output and urine color. Inform physician or other health care professional if patient is anuric. Chelated iron is excreted primarily by the kidneys; urine may turn red.
- ***Lab Test Considerations:*** Monitor serum iron, total iron binding capacity (TIBC), ferritin levels, and urinary iron excretion before and periodically during therapy.
- Monitor liver function studies to assess damage from iron poisoning.

Potential Nursing Diagnoses

Risk for injury poisoning (Indications)

Implementation

- IM route is preferred unless patient is in shock.
- Reconstitute 500-mg vial with 2 ml of sterile water for injection. Dissolve powder completely before administration. Solution is stable for 1 wk after reconstitution if protected from light.
- Used in conjunction with induction of emesis or gastric aspiration and lavage with sodium bicarbonate, and supportive measures for shock and metabolic acidosis in acute poisoning.
- **Trial Dose:** May be administered between 2 and 4 hr after ingestion of iron and after GI tract has been cleaned out. Monitor urine for color change (orange-rose color indicates significant iron ingestion) until serum iron and total iron binding capacity results are available.
- May be administered IM or by IV infusion over 4 hr.
- **IM:** Administer deep IM and massage well. Rotate sites. IM administration may cause transient severe pain.
- **Subcut:** Subcut route used to treat chronically elevated iron therapy is administered into abdominal subcut tissue via infusion pump for 8–24 hr per treatment.
- **IV:** Reconstitute, then further dilute in D5W, 0.9% NaCl, or LR. ***Rate:*** Maximum infusion rate is 15 mg/kg/hr. Rapid infusion rate may cause hypotension, erythema, urticaria, wheezing, convulsions, tachycardia, or shock.
- May be administered at the same time as blood transfusion in persons with chronically elevated serum iron levels. Use separate site for administration.

Patient/Family Teaching

- Reinforce need to keep iron preparations, all medications, and hazardous substances out of the reach of children.

- Reassure patient that red coloration of urine is expected and reflects excretion of excess iron.
- Advise patient not to take vitamin C preparations without consulting health care professional, because tissue toxicity may increase.
- Encourage patients requiring chronic therapy to keep follow-up appointments for lab tests. Eye and hearing exams may be monitored every 3 mo.

Evaluation/Desired Outcomes

- Return of serum iron concentrations to a normal level (50–150 mcg/100 ml).

desipramine

(dess-**ip**-ra-meen)
Norpramin, ✤Pertofrane

Classification
Therapeutic: antidepressants
Pharmacologic: tricyclic antidepressants

Pregnancy Category C

Indications

Depression. **Unlabeled uses:** Chronic pain syndromes. Anxiety. Insomnia.

Action

Potentiates the effect of serotonin and norepinephrine in the CNS. Has significant anticholinergic properties. **Therapeutic Effects:** Antidepressant action (may develop only over several weeks).

Pharmacokinetics

Absorption: Well absorbed from the GI tract.
Distribution: Widely distributed.
Protein Binding: 90–92%.
Metabolism and Excretion: Extensively metabolized by the liver. One metabolite is pharmacologically active (2-hydroxydesipramine). Undergoes enterohepatic recirculation and secretion into gastric juices. Small amounts enter breast milk.
Half-life: 12–27 hr.

TIME/ACTION PROFILE (antidepressant effect)

ROUTE	ONSET	PEAK	DURATION
PO	2–3 wk	2–6 wk	days–wks

Contraindications/Precautions

Contraindicated in: Angle-closure glaucoma; Recent MI, heart failure, known history of QTc prolongation.
Use Cautiously in: Patients with pre-existing cardiovascular disease; Prostatic hyperplasia (↑ susceptibility to urinary retention); History of seizures (threshold may be ↓); May ↑ risk of suicide attempt/ideation especially during early treatment or dose adjustment; risk may be greater in children or adolescents; OB: Use during pregnancy only if potential maternal benefit outweighs risks to fetus; use during lactation may result in neonatal sedation; Pedi: Safety not established in children <12 yr; Geri: ↑ sensitivity to effects.

Adverse Reactions/Side Effects

CNS: drowsiness, fatigue. **EENT:** blurred vision, dry eyes, dry mouth. **CV:** ARRHYTHMIAS, hypotension, ECG changes. **GI:** constipation, drug-induced hepatitis, paralytic ileus, increased appetite, weight gain. **GU:** urinary retention, decreased libido. **Derm:** photosensitivity.
Endo: changes in blood glucose, gynecomastia.
Hemat: blood dyscrasias.

Interactions

Drug-Drug: Desipramine is metabolized in the liver by the cytochrome P450 2D6 enzyme and its action may be affected by drugs which compete for metabolism by or alter the activity of this enzyme including other **antidepressants**, **phenothiazines**, **carbamazepine**, **class 1C antiarrhythmics** (**propafenone**, **flecainide**, **encainide**); when used concurrently dose reduction of one or the other or both may be necessary. Concurrent use of other drugs that inhibit the activity of the enzyme, including **cimetidine**, **quinidine**, **amiodarone**, and **ritonavir** may result in ↑ effects. May cause hypotension, tachycardia, and potentially fatal reactions when used with **MAO inhibitors** (avoid concurrent use—discontinue 2 wk prior to). Concurrent use with **SSRI antidepressants** may result in ↑ toxicity and should be avoided (fluoxetine should be

✤ = Canadian drug name.
*CAPITALS indicates life-threatening; underlines indicate most frequent.

stopped 5 wk before). Concurrent use with **clonidine** may result in hypertensive crisis and should be avoided. **Phenytoin** may ↓ levels and effectiveness; ↑ doses of desipramine may be required to treat depression. Concurrent use with **levodopa** may result in delayed / ↓ absorption of levodopa or hypertension. Blood levels and effects may be ↓ by **rifamycins**, **carbamazepine**, and **barbiturates**. Concurrent use with **moxifloxacin** ↑ risk of adverse cardiovascular reactions. ↑ CNS depression with other **CNS depressants** including **alcohol**, **antihistamines**, **clonidine**, **opioid analgesics**, and **sedative/hypnotics**. **Barbiturates** may alter blood levels and effects. **Adrenergic** and **anticholinergic** side effects may be ↑ with other **agents having these properties**. **Hormonal contraceptives** ↑ levels and may cause toxicity. **Cigarette smoking** may ↑ metabolism and alter effects.
Drug-Natural Products: Concomitant use of **kava kava**, **valerian**, or **chamomile** can ↑ CNS depression. ↑ anticholinergic effects with **jimson weed** and **scopolia**.

Route/Dosage

PO (Adults): 100–200 mg/day as a single dose or in divided doses (up to 300 mg/day).
PO (Geriatric Patients): 25–50 mg/day in divided doses (up to 150 mg/day).
PO (Children >12 yr): 25–50 mg/day in divided doses, increased as needed up to 100 mg/day.
PO (Children 6–12 yr): 10–30 mg/day (1–5 mg/kg/day) in divided doses.

Availability (generic available)

Tablets: 10 mg, 25 mg, 50 mg, 75 mg, 100 mg, 150 mg.

NURSING IMPLICATIONS

Assessment

- Obtain weight and BMI initially and periodically throughout therapy.
- Assess FBS and cholesterol levels for overweight/obese individuals.
- Refer as appropriate for nutrition/weight management and medical management.
- Monitor blood pressure and pulse prior to and during initial therapy. Notify physician or other health care professional of decreases in blood pressure (10–20 mm Hg) or sudden increase in pulse rate. Patients taking high doses or with a history of cardiovascular disease should have ECG monitored prior to and periodically during therapy.
- **Depression:** Monitor mental status (orientation, mood, behavior) frequently. Assess for suicidal tendencies, especially during early therapy. Restrict amount of drug available to patient.
- **Pain:** Assess intensity, quality, and location of pain periodically throughout therapy. Use pain scale to monitor effectiveness of medication.
- ***Lab Test Considerations:*** Assess leukocyte and differential blood counts, liver function, and serum glucose periodically. May cause an ↑ serum bilirubin and alkaline phosphatase. May cause bone marrow depression. Serum glucose may be ↑ or ↓.
- ***Lab Test Considerations:*** Serum levels may be monitored in patients who fail to respond to usual therapeutic dose.

Potential Nursing Diagnoses

Ineffective coping (Indications)
Risk for injury (Side Effects)
Impaired oral mucous membrane (Side Effects)
Impaired urinary elimination (Side Effects)
Chronic pain (Indications)
Risk for constipation (Side Effects)
Sexual dysfunction (Side Effects)

Implementation

- Do not confuse despiramine with clomipramine, imipramine, or nortriptyline.
- Dose increases should be made at bedtime because of sedation. Dose titration is a slow process; may take weeks to months. May give entire dose at bedtime.
- Taper to avoid withdrawal effects. Reduce dose by half for 3 days then reduce again by half for 3 days, then discontinue.
- **PO:** Administer medication with or immediately after a meal to minimize gastric upset. Tablet may be crushed and given with food or fluids.

Patient/Family Teaching

- Instruct patient to take medication as directed. Take missed doses as soon as possible unless almost time for next dose; if regimen is a single dose at bedtime, do not take in the morning because of side effects. Advise patient that drug effects may not be noticed for at least 2 wk. Abrupt discontinuation may cause nausea; vomiting; diarrhea; headache; trouble sleeping, with vivid dreams; and irritability.

- May cause drowsiness and blurred vision. Caution patient to avoid driving and other activities requiring alertness until response to drug is known.
- Orthostatic hypotension, sedation, and confusion are common during early therapy, especially in the elderly. Protect patient from falls. Institute fall precautions. Advise patient to make position changes slowly.
- Advise patient to avoid alcohol or other CNS depressant drugs during and for 3–7 days after therapy has been discontinued.
- Instruct patient to notify health care professional if urinary retention, dry mouth, or constipation persists. Sugarless candy or gum may diminish dry mouth, and an increase in fluids or bulk may prevent constipation. If symptoms persist, dose reduction or discontinuation may be necessary. Consult health care professional if dry mouth persists for more than 2 wk.
- Caution patient to use sunscreen and protective clothing to prevent photosensitivity reactions.
- Inform patient of need to monitor dietary intake. Increase in appetite may lead to undesired weight gain.
- Alert patient that medication may turn urine blue-green in color.
- Advise patient to notify health care professional of medication regimen prior to treatment or surgery.
- Therapy for depression is usually prolonged. Emphasize the importance of follow-up exams to monitor effectiveness and side effects and to improve coping skills.
- Refer to local support group.

Evaluation/Desired Outcomes

- Increased sense of well-being.
- Renewed interest in surroundings.
- Increased appetite.
- Improved energy level.
- Improved sleep.
- Decrease in chronic pain symptoms.
- Full therapeutic effects may be seen 2–6 wk after initiating therapy.

desirudin (des-i-**rude**-in)

Iprivask

Classification

Therapeutic: anticoagulants

Pharmacologic: thrombin inhibitors

Pregnancy Category C

Indications

Prevention of deep-vein thrombosis (DVT) after hip-replacement surgery.

Action

Selectively inhibits free and clot-bound thrombin. Inhibition of thrombin prevents activation of factors V, VIII, and XII; conversion of fibrinogen to fibrin; platelet adhesion and aggregation. **Therapeutic Effects:** Decreased incidence of DVT and subsequent pulmonary embolism after hip-replacement surgery.

Pharmacokinetics

Absorption: Completely absorbed following subcutaneous administration.

Distribution: Binds specifically and directly to thrombin.

Metabolism and Excretion: 40–50% excreted unchanged by kidneys; some metabolism in kidneys and pancreas.

Half-life: 2 hr.

TIME/ACTION PROFILE (effect on aPTT)

ROUTE	ONSET	PEAK	DURATION
Subcut	rapid	1–3 hr	12 hr

Contraindications/Precautions

Contraindicated in: Hypersensitivity to natural or recombinant hirudins; Active bleeding; Coagulation disorders.

Use Cautiously in: Renal impairment (dosage change recommended if CCr ≤60 ml/min); Geriatric patients (due to age-related renal impairment); Hepatic impairment; Pregnancy (use only if benefits to mother outweigh fetal risk); Lactation, children (safety not established).

Exercise Extreme Caution in: Spinal/epidural anesthesia (increased risk of spinal/epidural hematomas and their sequelae, especially when used with NSAIDs, platelet inhibitors, or other anticoagulants).

Adverse Reactions/Side Effects

GI: nausea. **Hemat:** BLEEDING, anemia. **Local:** injection site reactions, wound secretion.

Interactions

Drug-Drug: Dextran 40, systemic corticosteroids, thrombolytics, and other **anticoagulants** ↑ risk of bleeding (discontinue if possible; if not, monitor laboratory and clinical status closely). Agents altering platelet function including **salicylates, NSAIDs, clopidogrel, ticlopidine, dipyridamole**, and **glycoprotein IIb/IIIa antagonists** also ↑ risk of bleeding.

Route/Dosage

Subcut (Adults): 15 mg every 12 hr, start 5–15 min prior to surgery, but after regional block (if used), for up to 12 days.

Renal Impairment

Subcut (Adults): *CCr 31–60 ml/min*—start with 5 mg every 12 hr; further doses determined by daily aPTT; *CCr <31 ml/min*—start with 1.7 mg every 12 hr; further doses determined by daily aPTT.

Availability

Lyophilized powder for injection (requires reconstitution with specific diluent): 15.75 mg/vial with 0.6 ml ampule of diluent (contains mannitol, delivers 15 mg dose).

NURSING IMPLICATIONS

Assessment

- Assess for signs of bleeding (bleeding gums, nosebleed, unusual bruising; black, tarry stools; hematuria; fall in hematocrit or blood pressure; guaiac-positive stools; bleeding from surgical site). Notify physician if these occur.
- Assess patient for evidence of thrombosis. Symptoms depend on area of involvement. Notify physician immediately; may require urgent treatment.
- Monitor patients with epidural catheters frequently for signs of neurological impairment (midline back pain, numbness or weakness in lower limbs, bowel and/or bladder dysfunction). Notify physician immediately if these occur.
- Observe injection sites for hematomas, ecchymosis, or inflammation.
- ***Lab Test Considerations:*** Monitor activated partial thromboplastin time (aPTT) daily in patients with increased risk of bleeding and/or renal impairment. Monitor serum creatinine daily in patients with renal impairment. Peak aPTT should not exceed two times control. Reduce dose or discontinue desirudin until aPTT is <2 times control; resume at a lower dose.
- If a patient is switched from oral anticoagulants to desirudin or from desirudin to oral anticoagulants, measure anticoagulant activity closely.
- Thrombin time is not suitable for monitoring desirudin.
- Monitor CBC. If hematocrit ↓ unexpectedly, assess patient for potential bleeding sites.

Potential Nursing Diagnoses

Ineffective tissue perfusion (Indications)
Risk for injury (Adverse Reactions)

Implementation

- Reconstitute each vial with 0.5 ml of diluent provided for a concentration of 15.75 mg of desirudin/0.5 ml. Shake vial gently until fully reconstituted to a clear colorless solution. Do not administer solutions that are discolored, cloudy, or contain particulate matter. Reconstituted solution should be used immediately, but is stable for 24 hr at room temperature and protected from light. Discard unused solution.
- **Subcut:** Withdraw all reconstituted solution into syringe with a 26- or 27-gauge, 1/2 inch length needle. Inject entire contents subcutaneously which will deliver 15 mg. Patient should be sitting or lying down during administration. Rotate sites between left and right anterolateral and left and right posterolateral thigh or abdominal wall. Inject entire length of needle while pinching skin between thumb and forefinger; continue to pinch skin throughout injection. Do not rub injection site following injection to prevent bruising.
- **Syringe Incompatibility:** Do not mix with other diluents or medications.

Patient/Family Teaching

- Advise patient to report symptoms of unusual bleeding or bruising to health care professional immediately.
- Instruct patient not to take aspirin, NSAIDs, or herbal products during therapy without consulting health care professional.

Evaluation/Desired Outcomes

- Decreased incidence of DVT and subsequent pulmonary embolism after hip-replacement surgery.

desloratadine
(dess-lor-**a**-ta-deen)
Clarinex

Classification
Therapeutic: allergy, cold, and cough remedies, antihistamines
Pharmacologic: piperidines

Pregnancy Category C

Indications
Symptoms of allergic rhinitis (seasonal and perennial). Chronic idiopathic urticaria.

Action
Blocks peripheral effects of histamine released during allergic reactions. **Therapeutic Effects:** Decreased symptoms of allergic reactions (nasal stuffiness, red swollen eyes). Decreased pruritus, reduction in number and size of hives in chronic idiopathic urticaria.

Pharmacokinetics
Absorption: Well absorbed; absorption for orally-disintegrating tablets and oral tablets is identical.
Distribution: Enters breast milk.
Metabolism and Excretion: Extensively metabolized to 3-hydroxydesloratadine, an active metabolite; small percentage of patients may be slow metabolizers.
Half-life: 27 hr.

TIME/ACTION PROFILE (antihistaminic effects)

ROUTE	ONSET	PEAK	DURATION
PO	unknown	3 hr	24 hr

Contraindications/Precautions
Contraindicated in: Hypersensitivity; OB: Lactation.
Use Cautiously in: Patients with hepatic or renal impairment (↓ dose to 5 mg every other day); Geri: Dosing for the elderly should consider ↓ hepatic, renal, or cardiac function, concomitant diseases, other drug therapy and ↑ risk of adverse reactions; Pedi: Children <6 mo (safety not established).

Adverse Reactions/Side Effects
CNS: drowsiness (rare). **EENT:** pharyngitis. **GI:** dry mouth. **Misc:** allergic reactions including ANAPHYLAXIS.

Interactions
Drug-Drug: The following interactions may occur, but are less likely to occur with desloratidine than with more sedating antihistamines. **MAO inhibitors** may ↑ and prolong effects of antihistamines. ↑ CNS depression may occur with other **CNS depressants** including **alcohol**, **antidepressants**, **opioids**, and **sedative/hypnotics**.

Route/Dosage
PO (Adults and Children ≥12 yr): 5 mg once daily.

Hepatic Impairment
Renal Impairment
PO (Adults and Children ≥12 yr): 5 mg every other day.
PO (Children 6–11 yr): 2.5 mg once daily.
PO (Children 12 mo–5 yr): 1.25 mg once daily.
PO (Children 6–12 mo): 1 mg once daily.

Availability
Tablets: 5 mg. **Cost:** $292.91/90. **Orally-disintegrating tablets (RediTabs) (tutti-frutti):** 2.5 mg, 5 mg. **Cost:** 2.5 mg $319.29/90, 5 mg $307.89/90. **Syrup (bubblegum):** 0.5 mg/mL. **Cost:** $168.58/473 ml. ***In combination with:*** pseudoephedrine (Clarinex-D 12 Hour, Clarinex-D 24 Hour; see Appendix B).

NURSING IMPLICATIONS

Assessment
- Assess allergy symptoms (rhinitis, conjunctivitis, hives) before and periodically during therapy.
- Assess lung sounds and character of bronchial secretions. Maintain fluid intake of 1500–2000 ml/day to decrease viscosity of secretions.
- ***Lab Test Considerations:*** May cause false-negative result on allergy skin testing.

Potential Nursing Diagnoses
Ineffective airway clearance (Indications)
Risk for injury (Adverse Reactions)

Implementation
- **PO:** May be administered without regard to meals.
- Pedi: Use calibrated measuring device to ensure accurate dose of syrup for children.
- *For rapidly disintegrating tablets (Reditabs):* Place on tongue. Tablet disintegrates

rapidly. May be taken with or without water. Administer immediately after opening the blister.

Patient/Family Teaching

- Instruct patients to take desloratidine as directed. Do not increase dose or frequency; does not increase effectiveness and may increase side effects.
- May rarely cause drowsiness. Caution patient to avoid driving or other activities requiring alertness until response to medication is known.
- Advise patient to avoid taking alcohol or other CNS depressants concurrently with this drug.
- Advise patient that good oral hygiene, frequent rinsing of mouth with water, and sugarless gum or candy may minimize dry mouth. Patient should notify dentist if dry mouth persists >2 wk.

Evaluation/Desired Outcomes

- Decrease in allergic symptoms.

desmopressin

(des-moe-**press**-in)
DDAVP, DDAVP Rhinal Tube, DDAVP Rhinyle Drops, Octostim, Stimate

Classification
Therapeutic: hormones
Pharmacologic: antidiuretic hormones

Pregnancy Category B

Indications

Intranasal: Management of primary nocturnal enuresis unresponsive to other treatment modalities. **PO, Subcut, IV, Intranasal:** Treatment of diabetes insipidus caused by a deficiency of vasopressin. **Intranasal:** Controls bleeding in certain types of hemophilia and von Willebrand's disease.

Action

An analogue of naturally occurring vasopressin (antidiuretic hormone). Primary action is enhanced reabsorption of water in the kidneys. **Therapeutic Effects:** Prevention of nocturnal enuresis. Maintenance of appropriate body water content in diabetes insipidus. Control of bleeding in certain types of hemophilia or von Willebrand's disease.

Pharmacokinetics

Absorption: 5% absorbed following oral administration; some 10–20% absorbed from nasal mucosa.
Distribution: Distribution not fully known. Enters breast milk.
Metabolism and Excretion: Unknown.
Half-life: 75 min.

TIME/ACTION PROFILE (PO, intranasal = antidiuretic effect; IV = effect on factor VIII activity)

ROUTE	ONSET	PEAK	DURATION
PO	1 hr	4–7 hr	unknown
Intranasal	1 hr	1–5 hr	8–20 hr
IV	within min	15–30 min	3 hr†

†4–24 hr in mild hemophilia A

Contraindications/Precautions

Contraindicated in: Hypersensitivity; Hypersensitivity to chlorobutanol; Patients with type IIB or platelet-type (pseudo) von Willebrand's disease.
Use Cautiously in: Angina pectoris; Hypertension; Pregnancy or lactation (safety not established).

Adverse Reactions/Side Effects

CNS: drowsiness, headache, listlessness. **EENT:** *intranasal*— nasal congestion, rhinitis. **Resp:** dyspnea. **CV:** hypertension, hypotension, tachycardia (large IV doses only). **GI:** mild abdominal cramps, nausea. **GU:** vulval pain. **Derm:** flushing. **F and E:** water intoxication/hyponatremia. **Local:** phlebitis at IV site.

Interactions

Drug-Drug: Chlorpropamide, **clofibrate**, or **carbamazepine** may enhance the antidiuretic response to desmopressin. **Demeclocycline**, **lithium**, or **norepinephrine** may diminish the antidiuretic response to desmopressin. Large doses may enhance the effects of **vasopressors**.

Route/Dosage

Primary Nocturnal Enuresis

Intranasal (Adults and Children ≥6 yr): 20 mcg (10 mcg in each nostril) at bedtime (range 10–40 mcg).

Diabetes Insipidus

PO (Adults): 0.05 mg twice daily; adjusted as needed (usual range 0.1–1.2 mg/day in 2–3 divided doses).
PO (Children): 0.05 mg daily initially; adjusted as needed.

Intranasal (Adults): *Using nasal tube delivery system or spray pump (0.1 mg/ml)*—0.1–0.4 ml/day as a single dose or 2–3 divided doses.
Intranasal (Children 3 mo–12 yr): *Using nasal tube delivery system or spray pump (0.1 mg/ml)*—0.05–0.3 ml/day as a single dose or 2 divided doses.
Subcut, IV (Adults): 2–4 mcg/day in 2 divided doses.

Antihemorrhagic

IV (Adults and Children >3 mo): 0.3 mcg/kg repeated as needed.
Intranasal (Adults and Children ≥50 kg): 1 spray (150 mcg) in each nostril.
Intranasal (Adults and Children <50 kg): 1 spray in one nostril (150 mcg).

Availability

Tablets: 0.1 mg, 0.2 mg. **Nasal spray pump:** 10 mcg/spray—5-ml bottle (0.1 mg/ml) contains 50 doses (DDAVP). **Rhinal tube delivery system-nasal solution:** 2.5-ml vials with applicator tubes (0.1 mg/ml). **Nasal solution:** 1.5 mg/ml (150 mcg/dose) in 2.5-ml bottle (contains 25 doses). **Injection:** 4 mcg/ml.

NURSING IMPLICATIONS

Assessment

- Chronic intranasal use may cause tolerance or if administered more frequently than every 24–48 hr IV tachyphylaxis (short-term tolerance) may develop.
- **Nocturnal Enuresis:** Monitor frequency of enuresis throughout therapy.
- **Diabetes Insipidus:** Monitor urine and plasma osmolality and urine volume frequently. Assess patient for symptoms of dehydration (excessive thirst, dry skin and mucous membranes, tachycardia, poor skin turgor). Weigh patient daily and assess for edema.
- **Hemophilia:** Monitor plasma factor VIII coagulant, factor VIII antigen, and ristocetin cofactor. May also assess activated partial thromboplastin time (aPTT) for hemophilia A and skin bleeding time for von Willebrand's disease. Assess patient for signs of bleeding.
- Monitor blood pressure and pulse during IV infusion.
- Monitor intake and output and adjust fluid intake (especially in children and elderly) to avoid overhydration in patients receiving desmopressin for hemophilia.
- ***Toxicity and Overdose:*** Signs and symptoms of water intoxication include confusion, drowsiness, headache, weight gain, difficulty urinating, seizures, and coma. Treatment of overdose includes decreasing dose and, if symptoms are severe, administration of furosemide.

Potential Nursing Diagnoses

Deficient fluid volume (Indications)
Excess fluid volume (Adverse Reactions)

Implementation

- IV desmopressin has 10 times the antidiuretic effect of intranasal desmopressin.
- **PO:** Begin oral doses 12 hr after last intranasal dose. Monitor response closely.
- **Diabetes Insipidus:** Parenteral dose for antidiuretic effect is administered through direct IV or subcut.
- **Hemophilia:** Parenteral dose for control of bleeding is administered via IV infusion. If used preoperatively, administer 30 min prior to procedure.

IV Administration

- **Direct IV:** (for diabetes insipidus) ***Diluent:*** Administer undiluted. ***Concentration:*** 4 mcg/ml. ***Rate:*** Administer over 1 min.
- **Intermittent Infusion:** (for hemophilia and von Willebrand's disease) ***Diluent:*** Dilute each dose in 50 ml of 0.9% NaCl for adults and children >10 kg and in 10 ml in children weighing <10 kg. ***Rate:*** Infuse slowly over 15–30 min.
- **Y-Site Compatibility:** No information available. **Intranasal:** If intranasal dose is used preoperatively, administer 2 hr before procedure.

Patient/Family Teaching

- Advise patient to notify health care professional if bleeding is not controlled or if headache, dyspnea, heartburn, nausea, abdominal cramps, vulval pain, or severe nasal congestion or irritation occurs.
- Caution patient to avoid concurrent use of alcohol with this medication.
- **Diabetes Insipidus:** Instruct patient on intranasal administration. Medication is supplied with a flexible calibrated catheter (rhinyle). Draw solution into rhinyle. Insert one

end of tube into nostril; blow on the other end to deposit solution deep into nasal cavity. An air-filled syringe may be attached to the plastic catheter for children, infants, or obtunded patients. Tube should be rinsed under water after each use.

- If nasal spray is used, prime pump prior to first use by pressing down 4 times. Caution patient that nasal spray should not be used beyond the labeled number of sprays; subsequent sprays may not deliver accurate dose. Do not attempt to transfer remaining solution to another bottle.
- Instruct patient to take missed doses as soon as remembered but not if it is almost time for the next dose. Do not double doses.
- Advise patient that rhinitis or upper respiratory infection may decrease effectiveness of this therapy. If increased urine output occurs, patient should contact health care professional for dosage adjustment.
- Patients with diabetes insipidus should carry identification at all times describing disease process and medication regimen.

Evaluation/Desired Outcomes

- Decreased frequency of nocturnal enuresis.
- Decrease in urine volume.
- Relief of polydipsia.
- Increased urine osmolality.
- Control of bleeding in hemophilia.

desonide, See CORTICOSTEROIDS (TOPICAL/LOCAL).

desoximetasone, See CORTICOSTEROIDS (TOPICAL/LOCAL).

dexamethasone, See CORTICOSTEROIDS (SYSTEMIC).

dexmethylphenidate

(dex-meth-ill-**fen**-i-date)
Focalin, Focalin XR

Classification
Therapeutic: central nervous system stimulants

Schedule II

Pregnancy Category C

Indications

Adjunctive treatment of ADHD.

Action

Produces CNS and respiratory stimulation with weak sympathomimetic activity. **Therapeutic Effects:** Increased attention span in ADHD.

Pharmacokinetics

Absorption: Readily absorbed following oral administration.
Distribution: Unknown.
Metabolism and Excretion: Mostly metabolized by the liver; inactive metabolites are renally excreted.
Half-life: 2.2 hr.

TIME/ACTION PROFILE (improvement in symptoms)

ROUTE	ONSET	PEAK	DURATION
PO	7 days	1 mo	unknown

Contraindications/Precautions

Contraindicated in: Hypersensitivity; Hyperexcitable states (marked anxiety, agitation, or tension); Hyperthyroidism; Psychotic personalities, suicidal or homicidal tendencies; Glaucoma; Motor tics, family history or diagnosis of Tourette's syndrome; Concurrent use of MAO inhibitors; Should not be used to treat depression or prevent/treat normal fatigue; Psychoses (may exacerbate symptoms).
Use Cautiously in: History of cardiovascular disease; Hyperthyroidism; Hypertension; Diabetes mellitus; Geri: Geriatric/debilitated patients; Continual use (may result in psychological or physical dependence); Seizure disorders (may lower seizure threshold); OB: Pregnancy, lactation, or children <6 yr (safety not established; use in pregnancy only if clearly needed).

Adverse Reactions/Side Effects

CNS: insomnia, nervousness. **EENT:** visual disturbances. **CV:** tachycardia. **GI:** abdominal pain, anorexia, nausea. **Metab:** growth suppression, weight loss (may occur with prolonged use). **Neuro:** twitching. **Misc:** fever.

Interactions

Drug-Drug: Concurrent use with or use within 14 days following discontinuation of **MAO inhibitors** may result in hypertensive crisis and is contraindicated. May ↓ effects of **antihypertensives**. May ↑ effects of **vasopressors**. May cause serious adverse reactions with **clonidine**. May ↑ effects of **warfarin, phe-**

nobarbital, **phenytoin**, some **antidepressants**; dose adjustments may be necessary.

Route/Dosage

Tablets

PO (Adults and Children ≥6 yr): *Patients not previously taking methylphenidate*—2.5 mg twice daily, may be increased weekly as needed up to 10 mg twice daily; *Patients currently taking methylphenidate*—starting dose is 1/2 of the methylphenidate dose, up to 10 mg twice daily.

Extended-release Capsules

PO (Adults): *Patients not previously taking methylphenidate*—10 mg once daily, may be increased by 10 mg after 1 wk to 20 mg/day; *Patients currently taking methylphenidate*—starting dose is 1/2 of the methylphenidate dose, up to 20 mg/day given as a single daily dose; *Patients currently taking dexmethylphenidate*—give same daily dose as a single dose.

PO (Children ≥6 yr): *Patients not previously taking methylphenidate*—5 mg once daily, may be increased by 5 mg weekly up to 20 mg/day; *Patients currently taking methylphenidate*—starting dose is 1/2 of the methylphenidate dose, up to 20 mg/day, given as a single daily dose; *Patients currently taking dexmethylphenidate*—give same daily dose as a single dose.

Availability (generic available)

Tablets: 2.5 mg, 5 mg, 10 mg. **Cost:** *Generic*—2.5 mg $69.90/100, 5 mg $89.90/100, 10 mg $129.90/100. **Extended-release capsules:** 5 mg, 10 mg, 15 mg, 20 mg.

NURSING IMPLICATIONS

Assessment

- Assess child's attention span, impulse control, and interactions with others. Therapy may be interrupted at intervals to determine whether symptoms are sufficient to continue therapy.
- Monitor blood pressure, pulse, and respiration before administering and periodically during therapy.
- Monitor growth, both height and weight, in children on long-term therapy.
- Dexmethylphenidate has the potential for dependence and abuse. Prolonged use may result in tolerance.
- ***Lab Test Considerations:*** Monitor CBC, differential, and platelet count periodically in patients receiving prolonged therapy.

Potential Nursing Diagnoses

Disturbed thought process (Side Effects)

Implementation

- **PO:** Administer twice daily at least 4 hr apart without regard to meals.
- Administer Focalin XR tablets once daily in the morning. Capsules should be swallowed whole. For patients with difficulty swallowing, capsules can be opened and sprinkled on a spoonful of applesauce. Mixture should be consumed immediately; do not store for future use.

Patient/Family Teaching

- Instruct patient to take medication exactly as directed. If more than prescribed amount is taken notify health care professional immediately. If a dose is missed, take the remaining doses for that day at regularly spaced intervals; do not double doses. Take the last dose before 6 PM to minimize the risk of insomnia. Instruct patient not to alter dose without consulting health care professional. Abrupt cessation with high doses may cause extreme fatigue and mental depression.
- Inform patient that sharing this medication may be dangerous.
- Advise patient to check weight 2–3 times weekly and report weight loss to health care professional.
- Advise patient to consult with health care professional prior to taking other prescription, OTC, or herbal products concurrently with dexmethylphenidate.
- May rarely cause dizziness or drowsiness. Caution patient to avoid driving or activities requiring alertness until response to medication is known.
- Inform patient that health care professional may order periodic holidays from the drug to assess progress and to decrease dependence.
- Advise patient to notify health care professional if pregnancy is planned or suspected, or if breastfeeding.
- Caution patients to inform health care professional if they have ever abused or been dependent on alcohol or drugs, or if they are now abusing or dependent on alcohol or drugs.

- Emphasize the importance of routine follow-up exams to monitor progress.
- Advise parents to notify school nurse of medication regimen.

Evaluation/Desired Outcomes

- Improved attention span, decreased impulsiveness, and hyperactivity in ADHD. If improvement is not seen within 1 month, discontinue dexmethylphenidate.

dexrazoxane (dex-ra-zox-ane)

Totect, Zinecard

Classification

Therapeutic: cardioprotective agents

Pregnancy Category C

Indications

Reducing incidence and severity of cardiomyopathy from doxorubicin in women with metastatic breast cancer who have already received a cumulative dose of doxorubicin >300 mg/m^2. Treatment of extravasation resulting from IV anthracycline chemotherapy.

Action

Acts as an intracellular chelating agent. **Therapeutic Effects:** Diminishes the cardiotoxic effects of doxorubicin. Decreased damage from extravasation of anthracyclines.

Pharmacokinetics

Absorption: IV administration results in complete bioavailability.

Distribution: Unknown.

Metabolism and Excretion: Some metabolism occurs; 42% eliminated in urine.

Half-life: 2.1–2.5 hr.

TIME/ACTION PROFILE (cardioprotective effect)

ROUTE	ONSET	PEAK	DURATION
IV	rapid	unknown	unknown

Contraindications/Precautions

Contraindicated in: Any other type of chemotherapy except other anthracyclines (doxorubicin-like agents).

Use Cautiously in: CCr <40 mL/min (dose reduction required); OB: Pregnancy, lactation, or children (safety not established).

Adverse Reactions/Side Effects

Hemat: myelosuppression. **Local:** pain at injection site.

Interactions

Drug-Drug: Myelosuppression may be ↑ by **antineoplastics** or **radiation therapy**. Antitumor effects of concurrent combination chemotherapy with **fluorouracil** and **cyclophosphamide** may be ↓ by dexrazoxane.

Route/Dosage

Cardioprotective

IV (Adults): 10 mg of dexrazoxane/1 mg doxorubicin.

Renal Impairment

IV (Adults): decrease dose by 50%.

Extravasation protection

IV (Adults): 1000 mg/m^2 (maximum 2000 mg) given on days 1 and 2, and followed by a dose of 500 mg/m^2 (maximum 1000 mg) on day 3.

Renal Impairment

IV (Adults CCr <40 mL/min): decrease dose by 50%.

Availability (generic available)

Injection (Zinecard): 250-mg vial, 500-mg vial. **Injection (Totect):** 500-mg vial.

NURSING IMPLICATIONS

Assessment

- **Cardioprotective:** Assess extent of cardiomyopathy (cardiomegaly on x-ray, basilar rales, S gallop, dyspnea, decline in left ventricular ejection fraction) prior to and periodically during therapy.
- **Extravasation protection:** Assess site of extravasation for pain, burning, swelling, and redness.
- ***Lab Test Considerations:*** Monitor CBC and platelet count frequently during therapy. Thrombocytopenia, leukopenia, neutropenia, and granulocytopenia from chemotherapy may be more severe at nadir with dexrazoxane therapy.
- Monitor liver function tests periodically during therapy. May cause reversible ↑ of liver enzymes.

Potential Nursing Diagnoses

Decreased cardiac output (Indications)
Risk for impaired skin integrity (Indications)

Implementation

- Solution should be prepared in a biologic cabinet. Wear gloves, gown, and mask while handling IV medication. Discard IV equipment in specially designated containers (see Appendix K).

- Do not administer solutions that are discolored or contain particulate matter. Reconstituted solution and diluted solution are stable in an IV bag for 6 hr at room temperature or if refrigerated. Discard unused solutions.

IV Administration

- **Cardioprotective:** Doxorubicin should be administered within 30 min following dexrazoxane administration.
- **Direct IV:** ***Diluent:*** Reconstitute dexrazoxane with 0.167 molar (M/6) sodium lactate injection. ***Concentration:*** 10 mg/ml. ***Rate:*** Administer via slow IV push.
- **Intermittent Infusion:** ***Diluent:*** Reconstituted solution may also be diluted with 0.9% NaCl or D5W. Solution is stable for 6 hr at room temperature or refrigerated. ***Concentration:*** 1.3–5 mg/ml. ***Rate:*** May also be administered via rapid IV infusion over 15–30 min.
- **Additive Incompatibility:** Do not mix with other medications. Extravasation Protection. Administer as soon as possible within 6 hr of extravasation. Remove cooling procedures, such as ice packs, at least 15 min before administration to allow sufficient blood flow to area of extravasation.
- **Intermittent Infusion:** ***Diluent:*** Dilute each vial in 50 mL of diluent provided by manufacturer. Add contents of all vials into 1000 mL of 0.9% NaCl for further dilution. Solution is slightly yellow. Use diluted solutions within 2 hrs of dilution. Store at room temperature. ***Rate:*** Administer over 1–2 hrs.

Patient/Family Teaching

- Explain the purpose of the medication to the patient.
- Emphasize the need for continued monitoring of cardiac function.
- Advise patient to notify health care professional if pregnancy is suspected or planned. Dexrazoxane may be teratogenic.

Evaluation/Desired Outcomes

- Reduction of incidence and severity of cardiomyopathy associated with doxorubicin administration in women with metastatic breast cancer.
- Decrease in late sequalae (site pain, fibrosis, atrophy, and local sensory disturbance) following extravasation of anthracycline chemotherapeutic agents.

dextroamphetamine

(dex-troe-am-**fet**-a-meen)
Dexedrine, Dextrostat

Classification
Therapeutic: central nervous system stimulants
Pharmacologic: amphetamines

Schedule II

Pregnancy Category C

Indications

Narcolepsy. Adjunct management of ADHD. **Unlabeled uses:** Exogenous obesity.

Action

Produces CNS stimulation by releasing norepinephrine from nerve endings. Pharmacologic effects: CNS and respiratory stimulation, Vasoconstriction, Mydriasis (pupillary dilation), Contraction of the urinary bladder sphincter. **Therapeutic Effects:** Increased motor activity and mental alertness and decreased fatigue in narcoleptic patients. Increased attention span in ADHD.

Pharmacokinetics

Absorption: Well absorbed.
Distribution: Widely distributed; high concentrations in brain and CSF. Crosses the placenta; enters breast milk; potentially embryotoxic.
Metabolism and Excretion: Some metabolism by the liver. Urinary excretion is pH-dependent. Alkaline urine promotes reabsorption and prolongs action.
Half-life: 10–12 hr (6.8 hr in children).

TIME/ACTION PROFILE (CNS stimulation)

ROUTE	ONSET	PEAK	DURATION
PO	1–2 hr	3 hr	2–10 hr
PO-ER	unknown	unknown	up to 24 hr

Contraindications/Precautions

Contraindicated in: Pregnancy or lactation; Hyperexcitable states, including hyperthyroidism; Psychotic personalities; Suicidal or homicidal tendencies; Glaucoma; Some products con-

tain tartrazine; avoid in patients with known hypersensitivity.
Use Cautiously in: Cardiovascular disease (sudden death has occurred in children with structural cardiac abnormalities or other serious heart problems); Hypertension; Diabetes mellitus; History of substance abuse; Debilitated patients; Continual use (may produce psychological dependence or physical addiction); Geri: Appears on Beers list. Elderly are at increased risk for cardiovascular side effects.

Adverse Reactions/Side Effects

CNS: hyperactivity, insomnia, restlessness, tremor, depression, dizziness, headache, irritability. **CV:** palpitations, tachycardia, arrhythmias, hypertension. **GI:** anorexia, constipation, cramps, diarrhea, dry mouth, metallic taste, nausea, vomiting. **GU:** erectile dysfunction, increased libido. **Derm:** urticaria. **Misc:** physical dependence, psychological dependence.

Interactions

Drug-Drug: ↑ adrenergic effects with other **adrenergics**. Use with **MAO inhibitors** can result in hypertensive crisis. Alkalinizing the urine (**sodium bicarbonate**, **acetazolamide**) prolongs effect. Acidification of urine (**ammonium chloride**, large doses of **ascorbic acid**) ↓ effect. **Phenothiazines** may decrease the effect of dextroamphetamine. May antagonize the response to **antihypertensives**. ↑ risk of cardiovascular side effects with **beta blockers** or **tricyclic antidepressants**.
Drug-Natural Products: St. John's wort may increase serious side effects, concurrent use is not recommended. Use with caffeine-containing herbs (**guarana**, **tea**, **coffee**) ↑ stimulant effect. **St. John's wort** may increase serious side effects, concurrent use is not recommended.

Route/Dosage

Attention-Deficit Hyperactivity Disorder

PO (Adults): 5–40 mg/day in divided doses. Sustained-release capsules should not be used as initial therapy.
PO (Children ≥6 yr): 5 mg 1–2 times daily, increase by 5 mg daily at weekly intervals (maximum: 40 mg/day). Sustained-release capsules should not be used as initial therapy.
PO (Children 3–5 yr): 2.5 mg/day, increase by 2.5 mg daily at weekly intervals (maximum: 40 mg/day).

Narcolepsy

PO (Adults): 5–60 mg/day single dose or in divided doses. Sustained-release capsules should not be used as initial therapy.
PO (Children ≥12 yr): 10 mg/day, increase by 10 mg/day at weekly intervals until response is obtained or 60 mg is reached.
PO (Children 6–12 yr): 5 mg/day, increase by 5 mg/day at weekly intervals until response is obtained or 60 mg is reached.

Exogenous Obesity

PO (Adults and Children >12 yr): 5–30 mg/day in divided doses of 5–10 mg given 30–60 min before meals.

Availability (generic available)

Tablets: 5 mg. **Sustained-release capsules:** 5 mg, 10 mg, 15 mg.

NURSING IMPLICATIONS

Assessment

- Monitor blood pressure, pulse, and respiration before administering and periodically during therapy.
- Geri: Not recommended for use in elderly secondary to risk for hypertension, angina, and MI.
- **ADHD:** Monitor weight biweekly and inform physician of significant loss. Pedi: Monitor height periodically in children; report growth inhibition.
- Assess attention span, impulse control, motor and vocal tics, and interactions with others.
- **Narcolepsy:** Observe and document frequency of narcoleptic episodes.
- May produce a false sense of euphoria and well-being. Provide frequent rest periods and observe patient for rebound depression after the effects of the medication have worn off.
- Has high dependence and abuse potential. Tolerance to medication occurs rapidly; do not increase dose.
- ***Lab Test Considerations:*** May interfere with urinary steroid determinations.
- May cause ↑ plasma corticosteroid concentrations; greatest in evening.

Potential Nursing Diagnoses

Disturbed thought process (Side Effects)

Implementation

- Do not confuse Adderall (dextroamphetamine/amphetamine) with Inderal (propranolol).

D

- Therapy should utilize the lowest effective dose.
- **PO:** Sustained-release capsules should be swallowed whole; do not break, crush, or chew.
- **ADHD:** Pedi: When symptoms are controlled, dose reduction or interruption of therapy may be possible during summer months or may be given on each of the 5 school days with medication-free weekends and holidays.

Patient/Family Teaching

- Instruct patient to take medication at least 6 hr before bedtime to avoid sleep disturbances. Take missed doses as soon as remembered up to 6 hr before bedtime. Do not double doses. Instruct patient not to alter dose without consulting health care professional. Abrupt cessation of high doses may cause extreme fatigue and mental depression.
- Inform patient that the effects of drug-induced dry mouth can be minimized by rinsing frequently with water or chewing sugarless gum or candies.
- Advise patient to avoid the intake of large amounts of caffeine.
- Medication may impair judgment. Advise patients to use caution when driving or during other activities requiring alertness.
- Advise patient to notify health care professional if nervousness, restlessness, insomnia, dizziness, anorexia, or dry mouth becomes severe.
- Inform patient that periodic holiday from the drug may be ordered to assess progress and decrease dependence.

Evaluation/Desired Outcomes

- Improved attention span. Therapy should be interrupted and needs reassessed periodically.
- Decrease in narcoleptic symptoms.

dextromethorphan

(dex-troe-meth-**or**-fan)

✤Balminil DM, Benylin Adult, Benylin Pediatric, ✤Broncho-Grippol-DM, ✤Calmylin #1, Children's Hold, Creo-Terpin, Delsym, Dex-Alone, ✤DM Syrup, Drixoral Liquid Cough Caps, ElixSure Children's Cough Syrup, Hold, ✤Koffex, Little Colds Cough Formula Drops, Mediquell, ✤Neo-DM, ✤Ornex•DM, PediCare Infant's Long Acting Cough Drops, Pertussin Cough Suppressant, Pertussin CS, Pertussin ES, ✤Robidex, Robitussin Cough Calmers, Robitussin CoughGels, Robitussin Maximum Strength Cough Suppressant, Robitussin Pediatric, ✤Sedatuss, Simply Cough, Sucrets Cough Control Formula, TheraFlu Thin Strips Long Acting Cough, Triaminic Thin Strips Long Acting Cough, Vicks 44 Cough Relief, Vicks Formula 44 Pediatric Formula

Classification

Therapeutic: allergy, cold, and cough remedies, antitussives

Pregnancy Category C

Indications

Symptomatic relief of coughs caused by minor viral upper respiratory tract infections or inhaled irritants. Most effective for chronic nonproductive cough. A common ingredient in nonprescription cough and cold preparations.

Action

Suppresses the cough reflex by a direct effect on the cough center in the medulla. Related to opioids structurally but has no analgesic properties. **Therapeutic Effects:** Relief of irritating nonproductive cough.

Pharmacokinetics

Absorption: Rapidly absorbed from the GI tract. Extended-release product is slowly absorbed.
Distribution: Unknown. Probably crosses the placenta and enters breast milk.
Metabolism and Excretion: Metabolized to dextrorphan, an active metabolite. Dextromethorphan and dextrorphan are renally excreted.
Half-life: Unknown.

TIME/ACTION PROFILE (cough suppression)

ROUTE	ONSET	PEAK	DURATION
PO	15–30 min	unknown	3–6 hr†
PO-ER	unknown	unknown	9–12 hr

†Up to 8 hr for gelcaps

Contraindications/Precautions

Contraindicated in: Hypersensitivity; Patients taking MAO inhibitors or SSRIs; Should not be used for chronic productive coughs; Some products contain alcohol and should be avoided in patients with known intolerance.

Use Cautiously in: Cough that lasts more than 1 wk or is accompanied by fever, rash, or headache—health care professional should be consulted; History of drug abuse or drug-seeking behavior (capsules have been abused resulting in deaths); Diabetes (some products contain sucrose); OB: Pregnancy (has been used safely); Pedi: Lactation or children <2 yr (safety not established).

Adverse Reactions/Side Effects

CNS: *high dose*—dizziness, sedation. **GI:** nausea.

Interactions

Drug-Drug: Use with **MAO inhibitors** may result in serotonin syndrome (nausea, confusion, changes in blood pressure); concurrent use should be avoided. ↑ CNS depression with **antihistamines**, **alcohol**, **antidepressants**, **sedative/hypnotics**, or **opioids**. **Amiodarone**, **fluoxetine**, or **quinidine** may ↑ blood levels and adverse reactions from dextromethorphan.

Route/Dosage

PO (Adults and Children >12 yr): 10–20 mg q 4 hr *or* 30 mg q 6–8 hr *or* 60 mg of extended-release preparation bid (not to exceed 120 mg/day).

PO (Children 6–12 yr): 5–10 mg q 4 hr *or* 15 mg q 6–8 hr *or* 30 mg of extended-release preparation q 12 hr (not to exceed 60 mg/day).

PO (Children 2–6 yr): 2.5–5 mg q 4 hr *or* 7.5 mg q 6–8 hr *or* 15 mg of extended-release preparation q 12 hr (not to exceed 30 mg/day).

Availability

Gelcaps: 30 mg^{OTC}. **Lozenges (cherry):** 2.5 mg^{OTC}, 5 mg^{OTC}. **Liquid (cherry, grape):** 3.5 mg/5 ml^{OTC}, 5 mg/5 mL, 7.5 mg/5 ml^{OTC}, 15 mg/5 ml^{OTC}, 30 mg/5 mL^{OTC}. **Syrup (cherry, cherry bubblegum):** 7.5 mg/5 mL^{OTC}, 15 mg/15 ml^{OTC}, 10 mg/5 ml^{OTC}. **Extended-release suspension (orange):** 30 mg/5 ml^{OTC}. **Drops (Grape):** 7.5 mg/0.8 mL^{OTC}, 7.5 mg/1 mL^{OTC}. **Orally-disintegrating strips (cherry, grape):** 7.5 mg^{OTC}, 15 mg^{OTC}. ***In combination with:*** antihistamines, decongestants, and expectorants in cough and cold preparations^{OTC}. See Appendix B.

NURSING IMPLICATIONS

Assessment

- Assess frequency and nature of cough, lung sounds, and amount and type of sputum produced. Unless contraindicated, maintain fluid intake of 1500–2000 ml to decrease viscosity of bronchial secretions.

Potential Nursing Diagnoses

Ineffective airway clearance (Indications)

Implementation

- Do not confuse Benylin (dextromethorphan) with Benadryl (diphenhydramine).
- Dextromethorphan 15–30 mg is equivalent in cough suppression to codeine 8–15 mg.
- **PO:** Do not give fluids immediately after administering to prevent dilution of vehicle. Shake oral suspension well before administration.

Patient/Family Teaching

- Instruct patient to cough effectively: Sit upright and take several deep breaths before attempting to cough.
- Advise patient to minimize cough by avoiding irritants, such as cigarette smoke, fumes, and dust. Humidification of environmental air, frequent sips of water, and sugarless hard candy may also decrease the frequency of dry, irritating cough.
- Caution patient to avoid taking more than the recommended dose or taking alcohol or other CNS depressants concurrently with this medication; fatalities have occurred.
- May occasionally cause dizziness. Caution patient to avoid driving or other activities requiring alertness until response to the medication is known.
- Advise patient that any cough lasting over 1 wk or accompanied by fever, chest pain, persistent headache, or skin rash warrants medical attention.

Evaluation/Desired Outcomes

- Decrease in frequency and intensity of cough without eliminating patient's cough reflex.

diazepam (dye-**az**-e-pam)

✤ Apo-Diazepam, Diastat, ✤ Diazemuls, ✤ Novodipam, ✤ PMS-Diazepam, Valium, ✤ Vivol

Classification
Therapeutic: antianxiety agents, anticonvulsants, sedative/hypnotics, skeletal muscle relaxants (centrally acting)
Pharmacologic: benzodiazepines

Schedule IV

Pregnancy Category D

Indications
Adjunct in the management of: Anxiety Disorder, Athetosis, Anxiety relief prior to cardioversion (injection), Stiffman Syndrome, Preoperative sedation, Conscious sedation (provides light anesthesia and anterograde amnesia). Treatment of status epilepticus/uncontrolled seizures (injection). Skeletal muscle relaxant. Management of the symptoms of alcohol withdrawal. **Unlabeled uses:** Anxiety associated with acute myocardial infarction, insomnia.

Action
Depresses the CNS, probably by potentiating GABA, an inhibitory neurotransmitter. Produces skeletal muscle relaxation by inhibiting spinal polysynaptic afferent pathways. Has anticonvulsant properties due to enhanced presynaptic inhibition. **Therapeutic Effects:** Relief of anxiety. Sedation. Amnesia. Skeletal muscle relaxation. Decreased seizure activity.

Pharmacokinetics
Absorption: Rapidly absorbed from the GI tract. Absorption from IM sites may be slow and unpredictable. Well absorbed (90%) from rectal mucosa.
Distribution: Widely distributed. Crosses the blood-brain barrier. Crosses the placenta; enters breast milk.
Metabolism and Excretion: Highly metabolized by the liver. Some products of metabolism are active as CNS depressants.
Half-life: Neonates: 50–95 hr; Infants 1 month–2 yr: 40–50 hr; Children 2–12 yr: 15–21 hr; Children 12–16 yr: 18–20 hr; Adults: 20–50 hr (up to 100 hr for metabolites).

TIME/ACTION PROFILE (sedation)

ROUTE	ONSET	PEAK	DURATION
PO	30–60 min	1–2 hr	up to 24 hr
IM	within 20 min	0.5–1.5 hr	unknown
IV	1–5 min	15–30 min	15–60 min†
Rectal	2–10 min	1–2 hr	4–12 hr

†In status epilepticus, anticonvulsant duration is 15–20 min

Contraindications/Precautions
Contraindicated in: Hypersensitivity; Cross-sensitivity with other benzodiazepines may occur; Comatose patients; Pre-existing CNS depression; Uncontrolled severe pain; Angle-closure glaucoma; Pregnancy or lactation; Some products contain alcohol, propylene glycol, or tartrazine and should be avoided in patients with known hypersensitivity or intolerance; OB: Increased risk of congenital malformations; Lactation: Recommend to discontinue drug or bottle-feed.
Use Cautiously in: Hepatic dysfunction; Severe renal impairment; Severe pulmonary impairment; History of suicide attempt or drug dependence; Debilitated patients (dose reduction required); Patients with low albumin; Pedi: Metabolites can accumulate in neonates. Injection contains benzyl alcohol which can cause potentially fatal gasping syndrome in neonates; Geri: Long-acting benzodiazepines cause prolonged sedation in the elderly. Appears on Beers list and is associated with increased risk of falls (↓ dose required or consider short-acting benzodiazepine).

Adverse Reactions/Side Effects
CNS: dizziness, drowsiness, lethargy, depression, hangover, ataxia, slurred speech, headache, paradoxical excitation. **EENT:** blurred vision. **Resp:** respiratory depression. **CV:** hypotension (IV only). **GI:** constipation, diarrhea (may be caused by propylene glycol content in oral solution), nausea, vomiting, weight gain. **Derm:** rashes. **Local:** pain (IM), phlebitis (IV), venous thrombosis. **Misc:** physical dependence, psychological dependence, tolerance.

Interactions
Drug-Drug: Alcohol, **antidepressants**, **antihistamines**, and **opioid analgesics**—concurrent use results in additive CNS depression. **Cimetidine**, **hormonal contraceptives**, **disulfiram**, **fluoxetine**, **isoniazid**, **ketoconazole**, **metoprolol**, **propoxyphene**, **propranolol**, or **valproic acid** may decrease the metabolism of diazepam, enhancing its actions. May decrease the efficacy of **levodopa**. **Rifampin** or **barbiturates** may increase the metabolism and decrease effectiveness of diazepam.

Sedative effects may be decreased by **theophylline**. Concurrent use of **ritonavir** is not recommended.

Drug-Natural Products: Concomitant use of **kava kava, valerian**, or **chamomile** can increase CNS depression.

Route/Dosage

Antianxiety

PO (Adults): 2–10 mg 2–4 times daily.

IM, IV (Adults): 2–10 mg, may repeat in 3–4 hrs as needed.

PO (Children >1 mo): 0.12–0.8 mg/kg/day 3–4 times daily.

IM, IV (Children >1 mo): 0.04–0.3 mg/kg/dose q 2–4 hr to a maximum of 0.6 mg/kg within an 8 hr period if necessary.

Precardioversion

IV (Adults): 5–15 mg 5–10 min precardioversion.

Pre-endoscopy

IV (Adults): 2.5–20 mg.

IM (Adults): 5–10 mg 30 min pre-endoscopy.

Pediatric Conscious Sedation for Procedures

PO (Children >1 mo): 0.2–0.3 mg/kg (not to exceed 10 mg/dose) 45–60 min prior to procedure.

Status Epilepticus/Acute Seizure Activity

IV (Adults): 5–10 mg, may repeat q 10–15 min to a total of 30 mg, may repeat regimen again in 2–4 hr (IM route may be used if IV route unavailable); larger doses may be required.

IM, IV (Children ≥5 yr): 0.05–0.3 mg/kg/dose given over 3–5 min q 15–30 min to a total dose of 10 mg, repeat q 2–4 hr.

IM, IV (Children 1 mo–5 yr): 0.05–0.3 mg/kg/dose given over 3–5 min q 15–30 min to maximum dose of 5 mg, repeat in 2–4 hr if needed.

IV (Neonates): 0.1–0.3 mg/kg/dose given over 3–5 min q 15–30 min to maximum dose of 2 mg.

Rect (Adults and Children >12 yr): 0.2 mg/kg; may repeat 4–12 hr later.

Rect (Children 6–11 yr): 0.3 mg/kg; may repeat 4–12 hr later.

Rect (Children 2–5 yr): 0.5 mg/kg; may repeat 4–12 hr later.

Febrile Seizure Prophylaxis

PO (Children >1 mo): 1 mg/kg/day divided q 8 hr at first sign of fever and continue for 24 hr after fever is gone.

Skeletal Muscle Relaxation

PO (Adults): 2–10 mg 3–4 times daily.

PO (Geriatric Patients or Debilitated Patients): 2–2.5 mg 1–2 times daily initially.

PO (Children): 0.12–0.8 mg/kg/day 3–4 times daily.

IM, IV (Adults): 5–10 mg; may repeat in 2–4 hr (larger doses may be required for tetanus).

IM, IV (Geriatric Patients or Debilitated Patients): 2–5 mg; may repeat in 2–4 hr (larger doses may be required for tetanus).

IM, IV (Children ≥5 yr): *Tetanus*—5–10 mg q 3–4 hr.

IM, IV (Children >1 mo): *Tetanus*—1–2 mg q 3–4 hr.

Alcohol Withdrawal

PO (Adults): 10 mg 3–4 times in first 24 hr, decrease to 5 mg 3–4 times daily.

IM, IV (Adults): 10 mg initially, then 5–10 mg in 3–4 hr as needed; larger or more frequent doses have been used.

Psychoneurotic Reactions

IM, IV (Adults): 2–10 mg, may be repeated in 3–4 hr.

Availability (generic available)

Tablets: 2 mg, 5 mg, 10 mg. **Cost:** *Generic*—2 mg $7.99/30, 5 mg $7.99/30, 10 mg $7.99/30. **Oral solution:** 5 mg/ml (Intensol), 1 mg/ml. **Solution for injection:** 5 mg/ml (contains 10% alcohol and 40% propylene glycol). **Rectal gel delivery system:** 2.5 mg, 10 mg, 20 mg.

NURSING IMPLICATIONS

Assessment

- Monitor blood pressure, pulse, and respiratory rate prior to and periodically throughout therapy and frequently during IV therapy.
- Assess IV site frequently during administration; diazepam may cause phlebitis and venous thrombosis.
- Prolonged high-dose therapy may lead to psychological or physical dependence. Restrict amount of drug available to patient. Observe depressed patients closely for suicidal tendencies.
- Conduct regular assessment of continued need for treatment.

- Geri: Assess risk of falls and institute fall prevention strategies.
- **Anxiety:** Assess mental status (orientation, mood, behavior) and degree of anxiety.
- Assess level of sedation (ataxia, dizziness, slurred speech prior to and periodically throughout therapy.
- **Seizures:** Observe and record intensity, duration, and location of seizure activity. The initial dose of diazepam offers seizure control for 15–20 min after administration. Institute seizure precautions.
- **Muscle Spasms:** Assess muscle spasm, associated pain, and limitation of movement prior to and during therapy.
- **Alcohol Withdrawal:** Assess patient experiencing alcohol withdrawal for tremors, agitation, delirium, and hallucinations. Protect patient from injury.
- ***Lab Test Considerations:*** Evaluate hepatic and renal function and CBC periodically during prolonged therapy.
- ***Toxicity and Overdose:*** Flumazenil is an adjunct in the management of toxicity or overdose. (Flumazenil may induce seizures in patients with a history of seizures disorder or who are on tricyclic antidepressants.)

Potential Nursing Diagnoses

Anxiety (Indications)
Impaired physical mobility (Indications)
Risk for injury (Side Effects)
Ineffective coping

Implementation

- Do not confuse diazepam with lorazepam or ditropan.
- Patient should be kept on bedrest and observed for at least 3 hr following parenteral administration.
- If opioid analgesics are used concurrently with parenteral diazepam, decrease opioid dose by $^1/_3$ and titrate dose to effect.
- Use lowest effective dose. Taper by 2 mg every 3 days to decrease withdrawal symptoms. Some patients may require longer taper periods (mos).
- **PO:** Tablets may be crushed and taken with food or water if patient has difficulty swallowing.
- Mix Intensol preparation with liquid or semisolid food such as water, juices, soda, applesauce, or pudding. Administer entire amount immediately. Do not store.
- **IM:** IM injections are painful and erratically absorbed. If IM route is used, inject deeply into deltoid muscle for maximum absorption.

IV Administration

- **IV:** Resuscitation equipment should be available when diazepam is administered IV.
- **Direct IV:** ***Diluent:*** For IV administration do not dilute or mix with any other drug. If direct IV push is not feasible, administer IV push into tubing as close to insertion site as possible. Continuous infusion is not recommended due to precipitation in IV fluids and absorption of diazepam into infusion bags and tubing. Injection may cause burning and venous irritation; avoid small veins. ***Concentration:*** 5 mg/ml. ***Rate:*** Administer slowly at a rate of 5 mg/min in adults. Infants and children should receive 1–2 mg/min. Rapid injection may cause apnea, hypotension, bradycardia, or cardiac arrest.
- **Syringe Compatibility:** cimetidine.
- **Syringe Incompatibility:** doxapram, glycopyrrolate, heparin, hydromorphone, nalbuphine, pantoprazole, sufentanil.
- **Y-Site Compatibility:** dobutamine, fentanyl, methadone, morphine, nafcillin, sufentanil.
- **Y-Site Incompatibility:** amphotericin B cholesteryl sulfate, atracurium, cefepime, dexmedetomidine, diltiazem, fenoldopam, fluconazole, foscarnet, heparin, lansoprazole, linezolid, meropenem, oxaliplatin, pancuronium, potassium chloride, propofol, tirofiban, vecuronium, vitamin B complex with C.
- **Rect:** Do not repeat *Diastat* rectal dose more than 5 times/mo or 1 episode every 5 days. Round dose up to next available dose unit.
- Diazepam injection has been used for rectal administration. Instill via catheter or cannula fitted to the syringe or directly from a 1-ml syringe inserted 4–5 cm into the rectum. A dilution of diazepam injection with propylene glycol containing 1 mg/ml has also been used.
- Do not dilute with other solutions, IV fluids, or medications.

Patient/Family Teaching

- Instruct patient to take medication exactly as directed and not to take more than pre-

scribed or increase dose if less effective after a few weeks without checking with health care professional. Abrupt withdrawal of diazepam may cause insomnia, unusual irritability or nervousness, and seizures. Advise patient that sharing of this medication may be dangerous.
- Medication may cause drowsiness, clumsiness, or unsteadiness. Advise patient to avoid driving or other activities requiring alertness until response to medication is known. ***Geri:*** Advise geriatric patients of increased risk for CNS effects and potential for falls.
- Caution patient to avoid taking alcohol or other CNS depressants concurrently with this medication.
- Advise patient to notify health care professional if pregnancy is suspected or planned.
- Emphasize the importance of follow-up examinations to determine effectiveness of the medication.
- Inform patient that psychotherapy is beneficial in addressing source of anxiety and improving coping skills.
- Teach other methods to decrease anxiety, such as exercise, support groups, relaxation techniques.
- **Seizures:** Patients on anticonvulsant therapy should carry identification describing disease process and medication regimen at all times.
- Carefully review package insert for Diastat rectal gel with patient/caregiver prior to administration.

Evaluation/Desired Outcomes
- Decrease in anxiety level. Full therapeutic antianxiety effects occur after 1–2 wk of therapy.
- Decreased recall of surgical or diagnostic procedures.
- Control of seizures.
- Decrease in muscle spasms.
- Decreased tremulousness and more rational ideation when used for alcohol withdrawal.

DICLOFENAC†
(dye-**kloe**-fen-ak)

diclofenac potassium
Cataflam, ✤Apo–Diclo Rapide

diclofenac sodium
✤Apo-Diclo, Voltaren

diclofenac topical
Solaraze

Classification
Therapeutic: nonopioid analgesics, nonsteroidal anti-inflammatory agents

Pregnancy Category B (topical), C (oral)

†For ophthalmic use see Appendix C

Indications
PO: Management of inflammatory disorders including: Rheumatoid arthritis, Osteoarthritis, Ankylosing spondylitis. Primary dysmenorrhea. Relief of mild to moderate pain. **Topical:** Treatment of actinic keratoses.

Action
Inhibits prostaglandin synthesis. **Therapeutic Effects:** Suppression of pain and inflammation. **Topical:** Clearance of actinic keratosis lesions.

Pharmacokinetics
Absorption: Undergoes first-pass metabolism by liver which results in 50% bioavailability. Oral diclofenac sodium is a delayed-release dosage form. Diclofenac potassium is an immediate-release dosage form. 10% of topically applied diclofenac is systemically absorbed.
Distribution: Crosses the placenta.
Protein Binding: >99%.
Metabolism and Excretion: Metabolized by the liver to several metabolites; 65% excreted in urine, 35% in bile.
Half-life: 2 hr.

TIME/ACTION PROFILE

ROUTE	ONSET	PEAK	DURATION
PO (inflammation)	few days–1 wk	2 wk or more	unknown
PO (pain)	30 min	unknown	up to 8 hr
Topical	unknown	30 days*	unknown

*Complete healing of lesions following cessation of therapy

Contraindications/Precautions
Contraindicated in: Hypersensitivity to diclofenac or other components of formulation; Cross-sensitivity may occur with other NSAIDs including aspirin; Active GI bleeding/ulcer disease; Patients undergoing coronary artery bypass graft surgery.
Use Cautiously in: Severe renal/hepatic disease; Cardiovascular disease or risk factors for cardiovascular disease (may ↑ risk of serious cardiovascular thrombotic events, myocardial

infarction, and stroke, especially with prolonged use); History of porphyria; History of peptic ulcer disease and/or GI bleeding; Geri: Geriatric patients (dosage reduction recommended; more susceptible to adverse reactions, including GI bleeding); Bleeding tendency or concurrent anticoagulant therapy; OB, Lactation: Pregnancy and lactation (not recommended for use during second half of pregnancy); Pedi: Pregnancy, lactation, and children (safety not established).

Adverse Reactions/Side Effects

For oral diclofenac unless noted.

CNS: dizziness, headache. **CV:** hypertension. **EENT:** tinnitus. **GI:** GI BLEEDING, abdominal pain, constipation, diarrhea, dyspepsia, flatulence, heartburn, liver enzyme elevation, nausea, vomiting. **GU:** acute renal failure, hematuria. **Derm:** EXFOLIATIVE DERMATITIS, STEVENS-JOHNSON SYNDROME, TOXIC EPIDERMAL NECROLYSIS, pruritis, rashes, eczema, photosensitivity. **F and E:** edema. **Hemat:** anemia, prolonged bleeding time. **Local:** *Topical only*— contact dermatitis, dry skin, exfoliation. **Misc:** allergic reactions including ANAPHYLAXIS.

Interactions

Primarily noted for oral administration

Drug-Drug: ↑ adverse GI effects with **aspirin**, other **NSAIDs**, or **corticosteroids**. May ↓ effectiveness of **diuretics**, or **antihypertensives**. May ↑ levels/risk of toxicity from **cyclosporine**, **lithium**, or **methotrexate**. ↑ risk of bleeding with some **cephalosporins**, **thrombolytic agents**, **antiplatelet agents**, or **warfarin**. Concurrent use of oral **NSAIDs** during topical diclofenac therapy should be minimized.

Drug-Natural Products: ↑ bleeding risk with **arnica, chamomile, clove, dong quai, feverfew, garlic, ginger, ginkgo, Panax ginseng, and others.**

Route/Dosage

Different formulations of oral diclofenac (diclofenac sodium enteric-coated tablets, diclofenac sodium extended-release tablets, and diclofenac potassium immediate-release tablets are not bioequivalent and should not be substituted on a mg-to-mg basis.

Diclofenac Potassium

PO (Adults): *Analgesic/antidysmenorrheal*—100 mg initially, then 50 mg 3 times daily as needed; *Rheumatoid arthritis*—50 mg 3–4 times daily, after initial response reduced to lowest dose that controls symptoms; *Osteoarthritis*—50 mg 2–3 times daily, after initial response reduced to lowest dose that controls symptoms.

Diclofenac Sodium

PO (Adults): *Rheumatoid arthritis (delayed-release [enteric-coated] tablets)*—50 mg 3–4 times daily *or* 75 mg twice daily; after initial response reduce to lowest dose that controls symptoms (usual maintenance dose 25 mg 3 times daily). *Rheumatoid arthritis (extended-release tablets)*—100 mg once daily, if unsatisfactory response, dose may be ↑ to 100 mg twice daily. *Osteoarthritis (delayed-release [enteric-coated] tablets)*—50 mg 2–3 times daily *or* 75 mg twice daily; after initial response, ↓ to lowest dose that controls symptoms. *Osteoarthritis (extended-release tablets)*—100 mg once daily. *Ankylosing spondylitis (delayed-release [enteric-coated] tablets)*—25 mg 4 times daily, with an additional 25 mg given at bedtime, if necessary.

Topical (Adults): Apply to lesions twice daily for 60–90 days.

Availability (generic available)

Diclofenac potassium immediate-release tablets: 50 mg. **Cost:** *Generic*—$59.98/100. **Diclofenac sodium delayed-release (enteric-coated) tablets:** 25 mg, 50 mg, 75 mg. **Cost:** *Generic*—25 mg $42.80/100, 50 mg $37.08/100, 75 mg $44.98/100. **Diclofenac sodium extended-release tablets:** ✤75 mg, 100 mg. **Cost:** *Generic*—100 mg $208.78/90. **Gel:** 3% in 50- and 100-g tubes. **Cost:** $193.36/50 g, $275.68/100 g. ***In combination with:*** 200 mcg misoprostol (Arthrotec). See Appendix B.

NURSING IMPLICATIONS

Assessment

- Patients who have asthma, aspirin-induced allergy, and nasal polyps are at ↑ risk for developing hypersensitivity reactions.
- **Pain:** Assess pain and limitation of movement; note type, location, and intensity before and 30–60 min after administration.
- **Arthritis:** Assess arthritic pain (note type, location, intensity) and limitation of movement before and periodically during therapy.

- **Actinic Keratosis:** Assess lesions prior to and periodically during therapy.
- ***Lab Test Considerations:*** Diclofenac has minimal effect on bleeding time and platelet aggregation.
- May cause ↓ in hemoglobin and hematocrit.
- Monitor liver function tests within 8 wk of initiating diclofenac therapy and periodically during therapy. May cause ↑ serum alkaline phosphatase, LDH, AST, and ALT concentrations.
- Monitor BUN and serum creatinine periodically during therapy. May cause ↑ BUN and serum creatinine.

Potential Nursing Diagnoses

Acute pain (Indications)
Impaired physical mobility (Indications)

Implementation

- Do not confuse Cataflam (diclofenac) with Catapres (clonidine).
- Administration in higher than recommended doses does not provide increased effectiveness but may cause increased side effects. Use lowest effective dose for shortest period of time.
- **PO:** Take with food or milk to minimize gastric irritation. May take first 1–2 doses on an empty stomach for more rapid onset. Do not crush or chew enteric-coated or extended-release tablets.
- **Dysmenorrhea:** Administer as soon as possible after the onset of menses. Prophylactic treatment has not been shown to be effective.
- **Topical:** Gel should be applied to intact skin; do not use on open wounds. An adequate amount of gel should be applied to cover the entire lesion.

Patient/Family Teaching

- **PO:** Instruct patient to take diclofenac with a full glass of water and to remain in an upright position for 15–30 min after administration. Take missed doses as soon as possible within 1–2 hr if taking once or twice a day or unless almost time for next dose if taking more than twice a day. Do not double doses.
- Caution patient to avoid concurrent use of alcohol, aspirin, acetaminophen, other NSAIDs, or other OTC medications without consulting health care professional.
- May cause drowsiness or dizziness. Caution patient to avoid driving or other activities requiring alertness until response to medication is known.
- Instruct patient to notify health care professional of medication regimen before treatment or surgery.
- Caution patient to wear sunscreen and protective clothing to prevent photosensitivity reactions.
- Instruct female patients to inform health care professional if they plan or suspect pregnancy.
- Advise patient to consult health care professional if rash, itching, visual disturbances, tinnitus, weight gain, edema, black stools, persistent headache, or influenza-like syndrome (chills, fever, muscle aches, pain) occurs.
- **Topical:** Advise patient to minimize use of concurrent NSAIDs during topical therapy.
- Instruct patient to avoid covering lesion with occlusive dressing and to avoid applying sunscreen or cosmetics to the affected area.
- Advise patient that it may take up to 1 mo for complete healing of the lesion to occur.

Evaluation/Desired Outcomes

- Decrease in severity of mild-to-moderate pain.
- Increased ease of joint movement. Patients who do not respond to one NSAID may respond to another. May require 2 wk or more for maximum effects.
- Decrease in or healing of lesions in actinic keratosis. Optimal effect may not be seen until 30 days after discontinuation of therapy. Lesions that do not heal should be re-evaluated.

dicloxacillin, See PENICILLINS, PENICILLINASE RESISTANT.

dicyclomine

(dye-**sye**-kloe-meen)
Bentyl, ✤Bentylol, ✤Formulex, ✤Spasmoban

Classification
Therapeutic: antispasmodics
Pharmacologic: anticholinergics

Pregnancy Category UK

Indications

Management of irritable bowel syndrome in patients who do not respond to usual interventions (sedation/change in diet).

Action
May have a direct and local effect on GI smooth muscle, reducing motility and tone. **Therapeutic Effects:** Decreased GI motility.

Pharmacokinetics
Absorption: Well absorbed after oral and IM administration.
Distribution: Unknown.
Metabolism and Excretion: 80% eliminated in urine, 10% in feces.
Half-life: 1.8 hr (initial phase), 9–10 hr (terminal phase).

TIME/ACTION PROFILE (antispasmodic effect)

ROUTE	ONSET	PEAK	DURATION
PO, IM	unknown	unknown	unknown

Contraindications/Precautions
Contraindicated in: Hypersensitivity; Obstruction of the GI or GU tract; Reflux esophagitis; Severe ulcerative colitis (risk of paralytic ileus); Unstable cardiovascular status; Glaucoma; Myasthenia gravis; Infants <6 mo; Lactation.
Use Cautiously in: High environmental temperatures (risk of heat prostration); Hepatic/renal impairment; Autonomic neuropathy; Cardiovascular disease; Prostatic hyperplasia; Geri: Appears on Beers list. Geriatric patients have increased sensitivity to anticholinergics; Pregnancy (safety not established).

Adverse Reactions/Side Effects
CNS: confusion (increased in geriatric patients), drowsiness, light-headedness (IM only). **EENT:** blurred vision, increased intraocular pressure. **CV:** palpitations, tachycardia. **GI:** PARALYTIC ILEUS, <u>constipation</u>, <u>heartburn</u>, decreased salivation, dry mouth, nausea, vomiting. **GU:** erectile dysfunction, urinary hesitancy, urinary retention. **Derm:** decreased sweating. **Endo:** decreased lactation. **Local:** pain/redness at IM site. **Misc:** allergic reactions including <u>ANAPHYLAXIS</u>.

Interactions
Drug-Drug: Additive anticholinergic effects with other **anticholinergics**, including **antihistamines**, **quinidine**, and **disopyramide**. May alter the absorption of **other orally administered drugs** by slowing motility of the GI tract. **Antacids** or **adsorbent antidiarrheals** decrease the absorption of anticholinergics. May increase GI mucosal lesions in patients taking oral **potassium chloride** tablets. Increased risk of adverse cardiovascular reactions with **cyclopropane** anesthesia.

Route/Dosage
PO (Adults): 10–20 mg 3–4 times daily (up to 160 mg/day).
PO (Children ≥2 yr): 10 mg 3–4 times daily, adjusted as tolerated.
PO (Children 6 mo–2 yr): 5–10 mg 3–4 times daily, adjusted as tolerated.
IM (Adults): 20 mg q 4–6 hr, adjusted as tolerated.

Availability
Tablets: ✣10 mg, 20 mg. **Capsules:** 10 mg, 20 mg. **Syrup:** 10 mg/5 ml. **Solution for injection:** 10 mg/ml.

NURSING IMPLICATIONS

Assessment
- Assess patient for symptoms of irritable bowel syndrome (abdominal cramping, alternating constipation and diarrhea, mucus in stools) before and periodically during therapy.
- Assess patient routinely for abdominal distention and auscultate for bowel sounds. If constipation becomes a problem, increasing fluids and adding bulk to the diet may help alleviate the constipating effects of the drug.
- Monitor intake and output ratios; may cause urinary retention.
- ***Lab Test Considerations:*** Antagonizes effects of pentagastrin and histamine during the gastric acid secretion test. Avoid administration for 24 hr preceding the test.
- ***Toxicity and Overdose:*** Severe anticholinergic symptoms may be reversed with physostigmine or neostigmine.

Potential Nursing Diagnoses
Acute pain (Indications)
Diarrhea (Indications)

Implementation
- **PO:** Administer dicyclomine 30 min–1 hr before meals.
- **IM:** Monitor patient after administration; may cause light-headedness and irritation at injection site.

Patient/Family Teaching
- Instruct patient to take dicyclomine exactly as directed and not to take more than the pre-

✣ = Canadian drug name.
* CAPITALS indicates life-threatening; <u>underlines</u> indicate most frequent.

scribed amount. Missed doses should be taken as soon as remembered if not just before next dose.

- Medication may cause drowsiness and blurred vision. Caution patient to avoid driving or other activities requiring alertness until response to the medication is known.
- Inform patient that frequent oral rinses, sugarless gum or candy, and good oral hygiene may help relieve dry mouth. Consult health care professional regarding use of saliva substitute if dry mouth persists for more than 2 wk.
- Advise patient receiving dicyclomine to make position changes slowly to minimize the effects of drug-induced orthostatic hypotension.
- Caution patient to avoid extremes of temperature. This medication decreases the ability to sweat and may increase the risk of heat stroke.
- Advise patient to consult health care professional before taking any OTC medications concurrently with this therapy.
- Advise patient to notify health care professional immediately if eye pain or increased sensitivity to light occurs. Emphasize the importance of routine eye exams throughout therapy.

Evaluation/Desired Outcomes

- A decrease in the symptoms of irritable bowel syndrome.

diflorasone, See CORTICOSTEROIDS (TOPICAL/LOCAL).

HIGH ALERT

digoxin (di-**jox**-in)

Digitek, Lanoxicaps, Lanoxin

Classification

Therapeutic: antiarrhythmics, inotropics

Pharmacologic: digitalis glycosides

Pregnancy Category C

Indications

Treatment of CHF. Tachyarrhythmias: Atrial fibrillation and atrial flutter (slows ventricular rate), Paroxysmal atrial tachycardia.

Action

Increases the force of myocardial contraction. Prolongs refractory period of the AV node. Decreases conduction through the SA and AV nodes. **Therapeutic Effects:** Increased cardiac output (positive inotropic effect) and slowing of the heart rate (negative chronotropic effect).

Pharmacokinetics

Absorption: 60–80% absorbed after oral administration of tablets; 70-85% absorbed after administration of elixir. Absorption from liquid-filled capsules is 90–100%; 80% absorbed from IM sites (IM route not recommended due to pain/irritation).

Distribution: Widely distributed; crosses placenta and enters breast milk.

Metabolism and Excretion: Excreted almost entirely unchanged by the kidneys.

Half-life: 36–48 hr (increased in renal impairment).

TIME/ACTION PROFILE (antiarrhythmic or inotropic effects, provided that a loading dose has been given)

ROUTE	ONSET	PEAK	DURATION
Digoxin–PO	30–120 min	2–8 hr	2–4 days†
Digoxin–IM	30 min	4–6 hr	2–4 days†
Digoxin–IV	5–30 min	1–4 hr	2–4 days†

†Duration listed is that for normal renal function; in impaired renal function, duration will be longer

Contraindications/Precautions

Contraindicated in: Hypersensitivity; Uncontrolled ventricular arrhythmias; AV block; Idiopathic hypertrophic subaortic stenosis; Constrictive pericarditis; Known alcohol intolerance (elixir only).

Use Cautiously in: Hypokalemia (greatly increases risk of digoxin toxicity); Hypercalcemia (increases risk of toxicity, especially with mild hypokalemia); Hypomagnesemia (may potentiate digoxin toxicity); Diuretic use (may cause electrolyte abnormalities including hypokalemia and hypomagnesemia); Hypothyroidism; Geri: Geriatric patients (very sensitive to toxic effects, dose adjustments required for age-related decrease in renal function and body weight); MI; Renal impairment (dose reduction required); Obesity (dose should be based on ideal body weight); OB: Pregnancy (although safety has not been established, has been used during pregnancy without adverse effects on the fetus); Lactation: Similar concentrations in serum and breast milk result in subtherapeutic levels in infants, use with caution).

Adverse Reactions/Side Effects

CNS: fatigue, headache, weakness. **EENT:** blurred vision, yellow or green vision. **CV:** ARRHYTHMIAS, bradycardia, ECG changes, A-V block, S-A block. **GI:** anorexia, nausea, vomiting, diarrhea. **Endo:** gynecomastia. **Hemat:** thrombocytopenia. **Metab:** electrolyte imbalances with acute digoxin toxicity.

Interactions

Drug-Drug: Thiazide and **loop diuretics**, **piperacillin**, **ticarcillin**, **amphotericin B**, and **corticosteroids**, and excessive use of **laxatives** may cause hypokalemia which may ↑ risk of toxicity. **Amiodarone**, some **benzodiazepines**, **cyclosporine**, **diphenoxylate**, **indomethacin**, **itraconazole**, **propafenone**, **propantheline**, **quinidine**, **quinine**, **spironolactone**, and **verapamil** may ↑ serum levels and may lead to toxicity (serum level monitoring/dose reduction may be required). Blood levels may be ↓ by oral **aminoglycosides**, some **antineoplastics** (**bleomycin**, **carmustine**, **cyclophosphamide**, **cytarabine**, **doxorubicin**, **methotrexate**, **procarbazine**, **vincristine**), **activated charcoal**, **cholestyramine**, **colestipol**, **kaolin/pectin**, **metoclopramide**, **penicillamine**, **rifampin**, or **sulfasalazine**. In a small percentage (10%) of patients gut bacteria metabolize digoxin to inactive compounds; **macrolide anti-infectives** (**erythromycin**, **azithromycin**, **clarithromycin**), **tetracyclines**, by killing these bacteria, will cause ↑ digoxin levels and toxicity; dose may need to be ↓ for up to 9 weeks. Additive bradycardia may occur with **beta blockers** and other **antiarrhythmics** (**quinidine**, **disopyramide**). Concurrent use of **sympathomimetics** may ↑ risk of arrthythmias. **Thyroid hormones** may ↓ therapeutic effects.
Drug-Natural Products: Licorice and stimulant natural products (**aloe**) may ↑ risk of potassium depletion. **St. John's wort** may ↓ digoxin levels and effect.
Drug-Food: Concurrent ingestion of a **high-fiber meal** may ↓ absorption. Administer digoxin 1 hour before or 2 hours after such a meal.

Route/Dosage

For rapid effect, a larger initial loading/digitalizing dose should be given in several divided doses over 12–24 hr. Maintenance doses are determined for digoxin by renal function. All dosing must be evaluated by individual response. In general, doses required for atrial arrhythmias are higher than those for inotropic effect. When determining dose, consider that bioavailability of gelatin capsules (Lanoxicaps) is greater than that of tablets.
IV (Adults): *Digitalizing dose*—0.5–1 mg given as 50% of the dose initially and one quarter of the initial dose in each of 2 subsequent doses at 6-12 hr intervals.
IV (Children >10 yr): *Digitalizing dose*—8–12 mcg/kg given as 50% of the dose initially and one quarter of the initial dose in each of 2 subsequent doses at 6-12 hr intervals.
IV (Children 5–10 yr): *Digitalizing dose*—15–30 mcg/kg given as 50% of the dose initially and one quarter of the initial dose in each of 2 subsequent doses at 6-12 hr intervals.
IV (Children 2–5 yr): *Digitalizing dose*—25–35 mcg/kg given as 50% of the dose initially and one quarter of the initial dose in each of 2 subsequent doses at 6-12 hr intervals.
IV (Children 1–24 mo): *Digitalizing dose*—30–50 mcg/kg given as 50% of the dose initially and one quarter of the initial dose in each of 2 subsequent doses at 6-12 hr intervals.
IV (Infants—full term): 20–30 mcg/kg given as 50% of the dose initially and one quarter of the initial dose in each of 2 subsequent doses at 6-12 hr intervals.
IV (Infants—premature): *Digitalizing dose*—15–25 mcg/kg given as 50% of the dose initially and one quarter of the initial dose in each of 2 subsequent doses at 6-12 hr intervals.
PO (Adults): *Digitalizing dose*—0.75–1.5 mg given as 50% of the dose initially and one quarter of the initial dose in each of 2 subsequent doses at 6–12 hr intervals. *Maintenance dose*—0.125–0.5 mg/day as tablets or 0.350–0.5 mg/day as gelatin capsules, depending on patient's lean body weight, renal function, and serum level.
PO (Geriatric Patients): Daily dosage should not exceed 0.125 mg except when treating atrial fibrillation.
PO (Children >10 yr): *Digitalizing dose*—10–15 mcg/kg given as 50% of the dose initially and one quarter of the initial dose in each of 2 subsequent doses at 6-12 hr intervals. *Maintenance dose*—2.5–5 mcg/kg given daily as a single dose.

D

PO (Children 5–10 yr): *Digitalizing dose*—20–35 mcg/kg given as 50% of the dose initially and one quarter of the initial dose in each of 2 subsequent doses at 6-12 hr intervals. *Maintenance dose*—5–10 mcg/kg given daily in 2 divided doses.
PO (Children 2–5 yr): *Digitalizing dose*—30–40 mcg/kg given as 50% of the dose initially and one quarter of the initial dose in each of 2 subsequent doses at 6-12 hr intervals. *Maintenance dose*—7.5–10 mcg/kg given daily in 2 divided doses.
PO (Children 1–24 mo): *Digitalizing dose*—35–60 mcg/kg given as 50% of the dose initially and one quarter of the initial dose in each of 2 subsequent doses at 6-12 hr intervals. *Maintenance dose*—10–15 mcg/kg given daily in 2 divided doses.
PO (Infants—full term): *Digitalizing dose*—25–35 mcg/kg given as 50% of the dose initially and one quarter of the initial dose in each of 2 subsequent doses at 6-12 hr intervals. *Maintenance dose*—6–10 mcg/kg given daily in 2 divided doses.
PO (Infants—premature): *Digitalizing dose*—20–30 mcg/kg given as 50% of the dose initially and one quarter of the initial dose in each of 2 subsequent doses at 6-12 hr intervals. *Maintenance dose*—5–7.5 mcg/kg given daily in 2 divided doses.

Availability (generic available)

Tablets: 0.125 mg, 0.25 mg. **Cost:** *Lanoxin*—0.125 mg $24.97/90, 0.25 mg $29.97/90; *Generic*—0.125 mg $21.97/90, 0.25 mg $21.97/90. **Capsules:** 0.05 mg, 0.1 mg, 0.2 mg. **Cost:** 0.05 mg $25.99/100, 0.1 mg $33.56/100, 0.2 mg $39.57/100. **Pediatric elixir (lime flavor):** 0.05 mg/ml. **Injection:** 0.25 mg/ml. **Pediatric injection:** 0.1 mg/ml.

NURSING IMPLICATIONS

Assessment

- Monitor apical pulse for 1 full min before administering. Withhold dose and notify physician if pulse rate is <60 bpm in an adult, <70 bpm in a child, or <90 bpm in an infant. Also notify health care professional promptly of any significant changes in rate, rhythm, or quality of pulse.
- Pedi: Heart rate varies in children depending on age, ask physician to specify at what heart rates digoxin should be withheld.
- Monitor blood pressure periodically in patients receiving IV digoxin.
- Monitor ECG throughout IV administration and 6 hours after each dose. Notify health care professional if bradycardia or new arrhythmias occur.
- Observe IV site for redness or infiltration; extravasation can lead to tissue irritation and sloughing.
- Monitor intake and output ratios and daily weights. Assess for peripheral edema, and auscultate lungs for rales/crackles throughout therapy.
- Before administering initial loading dose, determine whether patient has taken any digitalis preparations in the preceding 2–3 wk.
- Geri: Digoxin has been associated with an increased risk of falls in the elderly. Assess for falls risk and implement prevention strategies per facility protocol.
- ***Lab Test Considerations:*** Evaluate serum electrolyte levels (especially potassium, magnesium, and calcium) and renal and hepatic functions periodically during therapy. Notify health care professional before giving dose if patient is hypokalemic. Hypokalemia, hypomagnesemia, or hypercalcemia may make the patient more susceptible to digitalis toxicity. Pedi: Neonates may have falsely elevated serum digoxin concentrations due to a naturally occurring substance chemically similar to digoxin. Geri: Older adults may be toxic even when serum concentrations are within normal range; assess for clinical symptoms of toxicity even when serum levels are normal.
- ***Toxicity and Overdose:*** Therapeutic serum digoxin levels range from 0.5–2 mg/ml. Serum levels may be drawn 6–8 hr after a dose is administered, although they are usually drawn immediately before the next dose. Bacteria in the GI tract can metabolize a substantial amount of digoxin before it is absorbed. Patients receiving erythromycin or tetracycline, which kill gut bacteria, can develop toxicity on their usual doses of digoxin. Geri: Older adults are at increased risk for toxic effects of digoxin (appears on Beers list) due to age-related decreased renal clearance, which can exist even when serum creatinine levels are normal. Digoxin requirements in the older adult may change and a formerly therapeutic dose can become toxic: Observe for signs and symptoms of toxicity. In adults and older children, the first signs of toxicity usually include abdominal pain, anorexia, nausea, vomiting, visual disturbances,

bradycardia, and other arrhythmias. In infants and small children, the first symptoms of overdose are usually cardiac arrhythmias. If these appear, withhold drug and notify physician or health care professional immediately. If signs of toxicity occur and are not severe, discontinuation of digitalis glycoside may be all that is required. If hypokalemia is present and renal function is adequate, potassium salts may be administered. Do not administer if hyperkalemia or heart block exists. **Correct any other electrolyte abnormalities**. Correction of arrhythmias resulting from digitalis toxicity may be attempted with lidocaine, procainamide, quinidine, propranolol, or phenytoin. Temporary ventricular pacing may be useful in advanced heart block. Treatment of life-threatening arrhythmias may include administration of digoxin immune Fab (Digibind), which binds to the digitalis glycoside molecule in the blood and is excreted by the kidneys.

Potential Nursing Diagnoses

Decreased cardiac output (Indications)

Implementation

- ***High Alert:*** Digoxin has a narrow therapeutic range. Medication errors associated with digoxin include miscalculation of pediatric doses and insufficient monitoring of digoxin levels. Have second practitioner independently check original order and dose calculations. Monitor therapeutic drug levels.
- For rapid digitalization, the initial dose is higher than the maintenance dose; 50% of the total digitalizing dose is given initially. The remainder of the dose will be administered in 25% increments at 4-8 hr intervals.
- When changing from parenteral to oral dose forms, dose adjustments may be necessary because of pharmacokinetic variations in percentage of digoxin absorbed: 100 mcg (0.1 mg) digoxin injection or 100 mcg (0.1 mg) liquid-filled capsule = 125 mcg (0.125 mg) tablet or 125 mcg (0.125 mg) of elixir.
- **PO:** Administer oral preparations consistently with regard to meals. Tablets can be crushed and administered with food or fluids if patient has difficulty swallowing. Use calibrated measuring device for liquid preparations; calibrated dropper is not accurate for doses of less than 0.2 mL or 10 mcg. Do not alternate between dose forms; bioavailability of capsules is greater than that of tablets or elixir.
- **IM:** Administer deep into gluteal muscle and massage well to reduce painful local reactions. Do not administer more than 2 ml of digoxin in each IM site. IM administration is not generally recommended.

IV Administration

- **Direct IV:** ***Diluent:*** May be administered undiluted. May also dilute 1 ml of digoxin in 4 ml of sterile water for injection, D5W, or 0.9% NaCl. Less diluent will cause precipitation. Use diluted solution immediately. ***Rate:*** Administer over at least 5 min.
- **Y-Site Compatibility:** acyclovir, amikacin, aminophylline, anidulafungin, atropine, aztreonam, bivalirudin, bumetanide, calcium chloride, calcium gluconate, cefazolin, cefotaxime, cefoxitin, ceftazidime, ceftizoxime, ceftriaxone, cefuroxime, chloramphenicol, cimetidine, ciprofloxacin, cisatracurium, clindamycin, cyclosporine, daptomycin, dexamethasone sodium phosphate, dexmedetomidine, diltiazem, diphenhydramine, dobutamine, dopamine, doxycycline, enalaprilat, epinephrine, ertapenem, erythromycin, esmolol, famotidine, fenoldopam, fentanyl, furosemide, ganciclovir, gentamicin, granisetron, heparin, hydrocortisone sodium succinate, hydromorphone, imipenem/cilastatin, inamrinone, isoproterenol, ketorolac, labetalol, levofloxacin, lidocaine, linezolid, lorazepam, magnesium sulfate, meperidine, meropenem, methylprednisolone sodium succinate, metoclopramide, metoprolol, metronidazole, midazolam, milrinone, morphine, nafcillin, nesiritide, nitroglycerin, nitroprusside, norepinephrine, ondansetron, palonosetron, pantoprazole, penicillin G potassium, phenylephrine, phytonadione, piperacillin/tazobactam, potassium chloride, procainamide, prochlorperazine, promethazine, propranolol, protamine, ranitidine, remifentanil, sodium bicarbonate, tacrolimus, ticarcillin/clavulanate, tirofiban, tobramycin, vancomycin, vasopressin, verapamil, vitamin B complex with C, voriconazole.
- **Y-Site Incompatibility:** amiodarone, amphotericin B cholesteryl sulfate complex, caspofungin, diazepam, fluconazole, foscarnet, lansoprazole, phenytoin, propofol, quinu-

pristin/dalfopristin, trimethoprim/sulfamethoxazole.

Patient/Family Teaching

- Instruct patient to take medication as directed, at the same time each day. Teach parents or caregivers of infants and children how to accurately measure medication. Take missed doses within 12 hr of scheduled dose or not taken at all. Do not double doses. Consult health care professional if doses for 2 or more days are missed. Do not discontinue medication without consulting health care professional.
- Teach patient to take pulse and to contact health care professional before taking medication if pulse rate is <60 or >100.
- Pedi: Teach parents or caregivers that changes in heart rate, especially bradycardia, are among the first signs of digoxin toxicity in infants and children. Instruct parents or caregivers in apical heart rate assessment and ask them to notify a health care professional if heart rate is outside of range set by health care professional before administering the next scheduled dose.
- Review signs and symptoms of digitalis toxicity with patient and family. Advise patient to notify health care professional immediately if these or symptoms of CHF occur. Inform patient that these symptoms may be mistaken for those of colds or flu.
- Instruct patient to keep digoxin tablets in their original container and not to mix in pill boxes with other medications; they may look similar to, and may be mistaken for, other medications.
- Advise patient that sharing of this medication can be dangerous.
- Caution patient to avoid concurrent use of OTC and herbal products without consulting health care professional. Advise patient to avoid taking antacids or antidiarrheals within 2 hr of digoxin.
- Advise patient to notify health care professional of this medication regimen before treatment.
- Patients taking digoxin should carry identification describing disease process and medication regimen at all times.
- Geri: Review fall prevention strategies with older adults and their families.
- ***High Alert:*** Emphasize the importance of routine follow-up exams to determine effectiveness and to monitor for toxicity.

Evaluation/Desired Outcomes

- Decrease in severity of CHF.
- Increase in cardiac output.
- Decrease in ventricular response in atrial tachyarrhythmias.
- Termination of paroxysmal atrial tachycardia.

digoxin immune Fab

(di-**jox**-in im-**myoon** fab)
Digibind, DigiFab

Classification
Therapeutic: antidotes
Pharmacologic: antibody fragments

Pregnancy Category C

Indications

Serious life-threatening overdosage with digoxin.

Action

An antibody produced in sheep that binds antigenically to unbound digoxin in serum. **Therapeutic Effects:** Binding and subsequent removal of digoxin, preventing toxic effects in overdose.

Pharmacokinetics

Absorption: Administered IV only, resulting in complete bioavailability.
Distribution: Widely distributed throughout extracellular space.
Metabolism and Excretion: Excreted by the kidneys as the bound complex (digoxin immune Fab plus digoxin).
Half-life: 14–20 hr.

TIME/ACTION PROFILE (reversal of arrhythmias and hyperkalemia; reversal of inotropic effect may take several hr)

ROUTE	ONSET	PEAK	DURATION
IV	30 min (variable)	unknown	2–6 hr

Contraindications/Precautions

Contraindicated in: No known contraindications.
Use Cautiously in: Known hypersensitivity to sheep proteins or products; Children, pregnancy, or lactation (safety not established).

Adverse Reactions/Side Effects

CV: re-emergence of atrial fibrillation, re-emergence of CHF. **F and E:** HYPOKALEMIA.

Interactions

Drug-Drug: Prevents therapeutic response to **digoxin**.

Route/Dosage

Digibind—38 mg of digoxin immune Fab will bind 0.5 mg of digoxin. Each vial contains 38 mg of digoxin immune Fab; *DigiFab*—40 mg of digoxin immune Fab will bind 0.5 mg of digoxin. Each vial contains 40 mg of digoxin immune Fab.

Known Amount of Digoxin Ingested (Administered)

IV (Adults and Children): *For digitalis glycoside toxicity due to digoxin tablets, oral solution, or IM digoxin*—dose of digoxin ingested (mg) × 0.8/1000 × 38. *For digitalis glycoside toxicity due to digoxin capsules, IV digoxin*—dose of digoxin ingested (mg)/0.5 × 38.

Known Serum Digoxin Concentrations (SDCs)

IV (Adults and Children): *Digibind*—Dose (mg) = SDC (nanograms/ml) × body weight (kg)/100 × 38; *DigiFab*—SDC (nanograms/ml) × body weight (kg)/100 × 40.

Unknown Amount Ingested/SDCs Unavailable

IV (Adults and Children): *Digibind*—760 mg (20 vials); *DigiFab*—800 mg (20 vials).

Toxicity during chronic digoxin therapy

IV (Adults and Children): *Digibind*—228 mg (6 vials); *DigiFab*—240 mg (6 vials).

Availability

Powder for injection, lyophilized (Digibind): 38 mg/vial. **Powder for injection, lyophilized (DigiFab):** 40 mg/vial.

NURSING IMPLICATIONS

Assessment

- Monitor ECG, pulse, blood pressure, and body temperature before and during treatment. Patients with atrial fibrillation may develop a rapid ventricular response as a result of decreased digoxin levels.
- Assess patient for increase in signs of CHF (peripheral edema, dyspnea, rales/crackles, weight gain).
- ***Lab Test Considerations:*** Monitor serum digoxin levels before administration.
- Monitor serum potassium levels frequently during treatment. Before treatment, hyperkalemia usually coexists with toxicity. Levels may decrease rapidly; hypokalemia should be treated promptly.
- Free serum digoxin levels fall rapidly after administration. Total serum concentrations rise suddenly after administration but are bound to the Fab molecule and are inactive. Total serum concentrations will decrease to undetectable levels within several days. Serum digoxin levels are not valid for 5–7 days after administration.

Potential Nursing Diagnoses

Deficient knowledge, related to medication regimen (Patient/Family Teaching)

Implementation

- Cardiopulmonary resuscitation equipment and medications should be available during administration.
- Delay redigitalization for several days until the elimination of digoxin immune Fab from the body is complete.

IV Administration

- **Intermittent Infusion:** ***Diluent:*** Reconstitute each vial in 4 ml of sterile water for injection and mix gently. Solution will contain a concentration of 9.5 mg/ml (*Digibind*) or 10 mg/ml (*DigiFab*). May be further diluted with 0.9% NaCl to achieve the concentration below. Reconstituted solution should be used immediately but is stable for 4 hr if refrigerated. For small doses in infants and children, a reconstituted 38-mg vial can be diluted with 34 ml of 0.9% NaCl (*Digibind*) or 36 ml of 0.9% NaCl (*DigiFab*) for a concentration of 1 mg/ml. ***Concentration:*** 1 mg/ml. ***Rate:*** Infuse over 30 min through a 0.22-micron membrane filter. If cardiac arrest is imminent, rapid direct IV injection may be used. Do not use rapid direct injection in other patients because of increased risk of adverse reactions. Small doses in infants and children may be administered with a tuberculin syringe.
- **Incompatibility:** Information unavailable. Do not mix with other drugs or solutions.

Patient/Family Teaching

- Explain the procedure and purpose of the treatment to the patient.

- Instruct patient notify health care provider immediately if signs of delayed allergic reaction (rash, pruritus, urticaria) occur after hospital discharge.

Evaluation/Desired Outcomes

- Resolution of signs and symptoms of digoxin toxicity.
- Decreased digoxin or level without major side effects.

diltiazem (dil-**tye**-a-zem)

✤Apo-Diltiaz, Cardizem, Cardiazem CD, Cardizem LA, Cardizem SR, Cartia XT, Dilacor XR, Diltia XT, ✤Novo-Diltazem, Nu-Diltiaz, ✤Ratio-Diltiazem CD, ✤Syn-Diltiazem, Taztia XT, Tiazac

Classification

Therapeutic: antianginals, antiarrhythmics (class IV), antihypertensives

Pharmacologic: calcium channel blockers

Pregnancy Category C

Indications

Hypertension. Angina pectoris and vasospastic (Prinzmetal's) angina. Supraventricular tachyarrhythmias and rapid ventricular rates in atrial flutter or fibrillation. **Unlabeled uses:** Management of Raynaud's syndrome.

Action

Inhibits transport of calcium into myocardial and vascular smooth muscle cells, resulting in inhibition of excitation-contraction coupling and subsequent contraction. **Therapeutic Effects:** Systemic vasodilation resulting in decreased blood pressure. Coronary vasodilation resulting in decreased frequency and severity of attacks of angina. Suppression of arrhythmias.

Pharmacokinetics

Absorption: Well absorbed, but rapidly metabolized after oral administration.

Distribution: Unknown.

Protein Binding: 70–80%.

Metabolism and Excretion: Mostly metabolized by the liver (CYP3A4 enzyme system).

Half-life: 3.5–9 hr.

TIME/ACTION PROFILE

ROUTE	ONSET	PEAK	DURATION
PO	30 min	2–3 hr	6–8 hr
PO–SR	unknown	unknown	12 hr
PO–CD, XR, LA	unknown	14 days†	up to 24 hr
IV	2–5 min	2–4 hr	unknown

†Maximum antihypertensive effect with chronic therapy

Contraindications/Precautions

Contraindicated in: Hypersensitivity; Sick sinus syndrome; 2nd- or 3rd-degree AV block (unless an artificial pacemaker is in place); Blood pressure <90 mm Hg; Recent MI or pulmonary congestion; Concurrent use of rifampin.

Use Cautiously in: Severe hepatic impairment (↓ dose recommended); Geri: Geriatric patients (↓ dose/slower IV infusion rate recommended; ↑ risk of hypotension; consider age-related decrease in body mass, decreased hepatic/renal/cardiac function, concurrent drug therapy and other disease states); Severe renal impairment; Serious ventricular arrhythmias or CHF; OB, Lactation, Pedi: Pregnancy, lactation, or children (safety not established).

Adverse Reactions/Side Effects

CNS: abnormal dreams, anxiety, confusion, dizziness, drowsiness, headache, nervousness, psychiatric disturbances, weakness. **EENT:** blurred vision, disturbed equilibrium, epistaxis, tinnitus. **Resp:** cough, dyspnea. **CV:** ARRHYTHMIAS, CHF, peripheral edema, bradycardia, chest pain, hypotension, palpitations, syncope, tachycardia. **GI:** abnormal liver function studies, anorexia, constipation, diarrhea, dry mouth, dysgeusia, dyspepsia, nausea, vomiting. **GU:** dysuria, nocturia, polyuria, sexual dysfunction, urinary frequency. **Derm:** dermatitis, erythema multiforme, flushing, increased sweating, photosensitivity, pruritus/urticaria, rash. **Endo:** gynecomastia, hyperglycemia. **Hemat:** anemia, leukopenia, thrombocytopenia. **Metab:** weight gain. **MS:** joint stiffness, muscle cramps. **Neuro:** paresthesia, tremor. **Misc:** STEVENS-JOHNSON SYNDROME, gingival hyperplasia.

Interactions

Drug-Drug: ↑ hypotension may occur when used with **fentanyl**, other **antihypertensives**, **nitrates**, acute ingestion of **alcohol**, or **quinidine**. Antihypertensive effects may be ↓ by **NSAIDs**. Serum **digoxin** levels may be increased. Concurrent use with **beta blockers**, **digoxin**, **disopyramide**, or **phenytoin** may result in bradycardia, conduction defects, or CHF. **Phenobarbital** and **phenytoin** may ↑ metabolism and ↓ effectiveness. May ↓ metabolism of and ↑ risk of toxicity from **cyclosporine**, **quinidine**, or **carbamazepine**.

Cimetidine and **ranitidine** ↑ blood levels and effects. May increase or decrease the effects of **lithium** or **theophylline**.
Drug-Food: Grapefruit juice ↑ serum levels and effect.

Route/Dosage

PO (Adults): 30–120 mg 3–4 times daily or 60–120 mg twice daily as SR capsules or 180–240 mg once daily as CD or XR capsules or LA tablets (up to 360 mg/day).
IV (Adults): 0.25 mg/kg; may repeat in 15 min with a dose of 0.35 mg/kg. May follow with continuous infusion at 10 mg/hr (range 5–15 mg/hr) for up to 24 hr.

Availability (generic available)

Tablets: 30 mg, 60 mg, 90 mg, 120 mg. **Cost:** *Generic*—30 mg $12.99/90, 60 mg $14.99/90, 90 mg $15.99/90, 120 mg $19.99/90. **Sustained-release capsules:** 60 mg, 90 mg, 120 mg. **Cost:** *Generic*—60 mg $80.30/180, 90 mg $124.76/180, 120 mg $199.13/180. **Extended-release capsules (Cardizem CD, Dilacor XR, Tiazac, Cartia XT, Taztia XT):** 120 mg, 180 mg, 240 mg, 300 mg, 360 mg, 420 mg. **Cost:** *Generic*—120 mg $69.98/90, 180 mg $79.97/90, 240 mg $106.97/90, 300 mg $126.97/90, 360 mg $128.97/90, 420 mg $120.99/90. **Extended-release tablets (Cardizem LA):** 120 mg, 180 mg, 240 mg, 300 mg, 360 mg, 420 mg. **Cost:** 120 mg $183.90/90, 180 mg $189.97/90, 240 mg $225.98/90, 300 mg $330.86/90, 360 mg $339.98/90, 420 mg $363.18/90. **Injection:** 5 mg/ml in 5-, 10-, and 25-ml vials.

NURSING IMPLICATIONS

Assessment

- Monitor blood pressure and pulse prior to therapy, during dose titration, and periodically during therapy. Monitor ECG periodically during prolonged therapy. May cause prolonged PR interval.
- Monitor intake and output ratios and daily weight. Assess for signs of CHF (peripheral edema, rales/crackles, dyspnea, weight gain, jugular venous distention).
- Monitor frequency of prescription refills to determine adherence.
- Patients receiving digoxin concurrently with calcium channel blockers should have routine serum digoxin levels checked and be monitored for signs and symptoms of digoxin toxicity.
- **Angina:** Assess location, duration, intensity, and precipitating factors of patient's anginal pain.
- **Arrhythmias:** Monitor ECG continuously during administration. Report bradycardia or prolonged hypotension promptly. Emergency equipment and medication should be available. Monitor blood pressure and pulse before and frequently during administration.
- ***Lab Test Considerations:*** Total serum calcium concentrations are not affected by calcium channel blockers.
- Monitor serum potassium periodically. Hypokalemia ↑ the risk of arrhythmias and should be corrected.
- Monitor renal and hepatic functions periodically during long-term therapy. May cause ↑ in hepatic enzymes after several days of therapy, which return to normal on discontinuation of therapy.

Potential Nursing Diagnoses

Acute pain (Indications)
Decreased cardiac output (Adverse Reactions)

Implementation

- Do not confuse Cardizem (diltiazem) with Cardene (nicardipine). Do not confuse Cardizem LA with Cardene SR. Do not confuse Tiazac (diltiazem) with Ziac (bisprolol/hydrochlorothiazide).
- **PO:** May be administered without regard to meals. May be administered with meals if GI irritation becomes a problem.
- Do not open, crush, break, or chew sustained-release capsules or tablets. Empty tablets that appear in stool are not significant. Crush and mix diltiazem with food or fluids for patients having difficulty swallowing.

IV Administration

- **Direct IV:** ***Diluent:*** Administer bolus dose undiluted. ***Concentration:*** 5 mg/ml. ***Rate:*** Administer over 2 min.
- **Continuous Infusion:** ***Diluent:*** Dilute 125 mg in 100 ml, 250 mg in 250 ml, or 250 mg in 500 ml of 0.9% NaCl, D5W, or D5/0.45% NaCl. Infusion is stable for 24 hr at room temperature or if refrigerated. ***Concentration:*** 125 mg/125 ml (1 mg/ml), 250 mg/300 ml (0.83 mg/ml), 250 mg/550 ml (0.45 mg/ml). ***Rate:*** See Route/Dosage section. Titrate

to patient's heart rate and blood pressure response.

- **Y-Site Compatibility:** albumin, amikacin, amiodarone, amphotericin B, argatroban, aztreonam, bivalirudin, bumetanide, cefazolin, cefotaxime, cefoxitin, ceftazidime, ceftizoxime, ceftriaxone, cefuroxime, cimetidine, ciprofloxacin, clindamycin, dexamethasone, digoxin, dobutamine, dopamine, doxycycline, epinephrine, erythromycin lactobionate, esmolol, famotidine, fenoldopam, fentanyl, fluconazole, gentamicin, hydromorphone, imipenem/cilastatin, labetalol, levofloxacin, lidocaine, lorazepam, meperidine, metoclopramide, metronidazole, midazolam, milrinone, morphine, multivitamins, nicardipine, nitroglycerin, nitroprusside, norepinephrine, oxacillin, penicillin G potassium, pentamidine, potassium chloride, potassium phosphate, ranitidine, tacrolimus, theophylline, ticarcillin/clavulanate, tirofiban, tobramycin, trimethoprim/sulfamethoxazole, vancomycin, vasopressin, vecuronium.
- **Y-Site Incompatibility:** diazepam, furosemide, lansoprazole, phenytoin, rifampin.

Patient/Family Teaching

- Advise patient to take medication as directed at the same time each day, even if feeling well. Take missed doses as soon as possible unless almost time for next dose; do not double doses. May need to be discontinued gradually.
- Advise patient to avoid large amounts (6–8 glasses of grapefruit juice/day) during therapy.
- Instruct patient on correct technique for monitoring pulse. Instruct patient to contact health care professional if heart rate is <50 bpm.
- Caution patient to change positions slowly to minimize orthostatic hypotension.
- May cause drowsiness or dizziness. Advise patient to avoid driving or other activities requiring alertness until response to the medication is known.
- Instruct patient on importance of maintaining good dental hygiene and seeing dentist frequently for teeth cleaning to prevent tenderness, bleeding, and gingival hyperplasia (gum enlargement).
- Instruct patient to avoid concurrent use of alcohol or OTC medications, especially cough and cold preparations, without consulting health care professional.
- Advise patient to notify health care professional if irregular heartbeats, dyspnea, swelling of hands and feet, pronounced dizziness, nausea, constipation, or hypotension occurs or if headache is severe or persistent.
- Caution patient to wear protective clothing and use sunscreen to prevent photosensitivity reactions.
- **Angina:** Instruct patient on concurrent nitrate or beta-blocker therapy to continue taking both medications as directed and to use SL nitroglycerin as needed for anginal attacks.
- Advise patient to contact health care professional if chest pain does not improve, worsens after therapy, or occurs with diaphoresis; if shortness of breath occurs; or if severe, persistent headache occurs.
- Caution patient to discuss exercise restrictions with health care professional before exertion.
- **Hypertension:** Encourage patient to comply with other interventions for hypertension (weight reduction, low-sodium diet, smoking cessation, moderation of alcohol consumption, regular exercise, and stress management). Medication controls but does not cure hypertension.
- Instruct patient and family in proper technique for monitoring blood pressure. Advise patient to take blood pressure weekly and to report significant changes to health care professional.

Evaluation/Desired Outcomes

- Decrease in blood pressure.
- Decrease in frequency and severity of anginal attacks.
- Decrease in need for nitrate therapy.
- Increase in activity tolerance and sense of well-being.
- Suppression and prevention of tachyarrhythmias.

dimenhyDRINATE

(dye-men-**hye**-dri-nate)
✤Apo-Dimenhydrinate, Calm X, Dimetabs, Dinate, Dramamine, Dramanate, ✤Gravol, Hydrate, ✤PMS-Dimenhydrinate, ✤Traveltabs, Triptone Caplets

D

Classification
Therapeutic: antiemetics, antihistamines

Pregnancy Category B

Indications
Nausea, vomiting, dizziness, and vertigo accompanying motion sickness.

Action
Inhibits vestibular stimulation. Has significant CNS depressant, anticholinergic, antihistaminic, and antiemetic properties. **Therapeutic Effects:** Decreased vestibular stimulation, which may prevent motion sickness.

Pharmacokinetics
Absorption: Well absorbed after oral or IM administration.
Distribution: Probably crosses the placenta and enters breast milk.
Metabolism and Excretion: Metabolized by the liver.
Half-life: Unknown.

TIME/ACTION PROFILE (anti-motion sickness, antiemetic activity)

ROUTE	ONSET	PEAK	DURATION
PO	15–60 min	1–2 hr	3–6 hr
Rect	30–45 min	unknown	6–12 hr
IM	20–30 min	1–2 hr	3–6 hr
IV	rapid	unknown	3–6 hr

Contraindications/Precautions
Contraindicated in: Hypersensitivity; Some products contain alcohol or tartrazine; in patients with known intolerance.
Use Cautiously in: Angle-closure glaucoma; Seizure disorders; Prostatic hyperplasia.

Adverse Reactions/Side Effects
CNS: drowsiness, dizziness, headache, paradoxical excitation (children). **EENT:** blurred vision, tinnitus. **CV:** hypotension, palpitations. **GI:** anorexia, constipation, diarrhea, dry mouth. **GU:** dysuria, frequency. **Derm:** photosensitivity. **Local:** pain at IM site.

Interactions
Drug-Drug: ↑ CNS depression with other **antihistamines**, **alcohol**, **opioid analgesics**, and **sedative/hypnotics**. May mask signs or symptoms of ototoxicity in patients receiving **ototoxic drugs (aminoglycosides, ethacrynic acid)**. ↑ anticholinergic properties with **tricyclic antidepressants**, **quinidine**, or **disopyramide**. **MAO inhibitors** intensify and prolong the anticholinergic effects of antihistamines.

Route/Dosage
PO (Adults): 50–100 mg q 4 hr (not to exceed 400 mg/day).
PO (Children 6–12 yr): 25–50 mg q 6–8 hr (not to exceed 300 mg/day).
Rect (Adults): 50–100 mg q 6–8 hr.
Rect (Children 8–12 yr): 25–50 mg q 8–12 hr.
Rect (Children 6–8 yr): 12.5–25 mg q 8–12 hr.
IM, IV (Adults): 50 mg q 4 hr as needed.
IM, IV (Children): 1.25 mg/kg (37.5 mg/m²) q 6 hr as needed (not to exceed 300 mg/day).

Availability (generic available)
Tablets: 50 mg^OTC. **Chewable tablets (orange flavor):** 50 mg^OTC. **Capsules:** ✤50 mg^OTC. **Extended-release capsules:** ✤25 mg^OTC. **Elixir (cherry flavor):** 12.5 mg/5 ml^OTC, ✤15 mg/5 ml^OTC. **Liquid:** 12.5 mg/4 ml^OTC. **Suppositories:** ✤50 mg^OTC, ✤100 mg^OTC. **Injection:** 50 mg/ml.

NURSING IMPLICATIONS

Assessment
- Assess nausea, vomiting, bowel sounds, and abdominal pain before and after administration of this drug. Dimenhydrinate may mask the signs of an acute abdomen.
- Monitor intake and output, including emesis. Assess for signs of dehydration (excessive thirst, dry skin and mucous membranes, tachycardia, increased urine specific gravity, poor skin turgor).
- ***Lab Test Considerations:*** Will cause false-negative allergy skin test results; discontinue 72 hr before testing.

Potential Nursing Diagnoses
Risk for deficient fluid volume (Indications)
Imbalanced nutrition: less than body requirements (Indications)
Risk for injury (Side Effects)

Implementation
- When used for prophylaxis of motion sickness, administer at least 30 min and preferably 1–2 hr before exposure to conditions that may precipitate motion sickness.

- **PO:** Use calibrated measuring device when administering liquid dose.
- **IM:** Administer into well-developed muscle; massage well.

IV Administration

- **Direct IV:** ***Diluent:*** Dilute 50 mg in 0.9% NaCl for injection. ***Concentration:*** 5 mg/ml. ***Rate:*** Inject over 2 min.
- **Syringe Compatibility:** atropine, codeine, droperidol, fentanyl, heparin, hydromorphone, meperidine, metoclopromide, morphine, pentazocine, perphenazine, ranitidine, scopolamine.
- **Syringe Incompatibility:** butorphanol, chlorpromazine, glycopyrrolate, hydroxyzine, midazolam, nalbuphine, pentobarbital, prochlorperazine, promethazine, thiopental.
- **Y-Site Compatibility:** acyclovir, pantoprazole.
- **Y-Site Incompatibility:** aminophylline, heparin, hydrocortisone sodium succinate, phenobarbital, phenytoin, prednisolone, prochlorperazine, promethazine.
- **Solution Compatibility:** D5W, 0.45% NaCl, 0.9% NaCl, Ringer's solution, lactated Ringer's solution, dextrose/saline combinations, or dextrose/Ringer's combinations.

Patient/Family Teaching

- May cause drowsiness. Caution patient to avoid driving or other activities requiring alertness until response to the drug is known.
- Inform patient that this medication may cause dry mouth. Frequent oral rinses, good oral hygiene, and sugarless gum or candy may minimize this effect.
- Caution patient to avoid alcohol and other CNS depressants concurrently with this medication.
- Advise patient to use sunscreen and protective clothing to prevent photosensitivity reactions.

Evaluation/Desired Outcomes

- Prevention or decreased severity of nausea and vomiting, vertigo, or motion sickness.

dinoprostone

(dye-noe-**prost**-one)
Cervidil Vaginal Insert, Prepidil Endocervical Gel, Prostin E Vaginal Suppository

Classification
Therapeutic: cervical ripening agents
Pharmacologic: oxytocics, prostaglandins

Pregnancy Category C

Indications

Endocervical Gel, Vaginal Insert: Used to "ripen" the cervix in pregnancy at or near term when induction of labor is indicated. Vaginal Suppository: Induction of midtrimester abortion, Management of missed abortion up to 28 wk, Management of nonmetastatic gestational trophoblastic disease (benign hydatidiform mole).

Action

Produces contractions similar to those occurring during labor at term by stimulating the myometrium (oxytocic effect). Initiates softening, effacement, and dilation of the cervix (ripening). Also stimulates GI smooth muscle. **Therapeutic Effects:** Initiation of labor. Expulsion of fetus.

Pharmacokinetics

Absorption: Rapidly absorbed.
Distribution: Unknown. Action is mostly local.
Metabolism and Excretion: Metabolized by enzymes in lung, kidneys, spleen, and liver tissue.
Half-life: Unknown.

TIME/ACTION PROFILE

ROUTE	ONSET	PEAK	DURATION
Cervical ripening (gel)	rapid	30–45 min	unknown
Cervical ripening (insert)	rapid	unknown	12 hr
Abortion time (suppository)	10 min	12–24 hr	2–3 hr

Contraindications/Precautions

Contraindicated in: Hypersensitivity to prostaglandins or additives in the gel or suppository; The gel/insert should be avoided in situations in which prolonged uterine contractions should be avoided, including: Previous cesarean section or uterine surgery, Cephalopelvic disproportion, Traumatic delivery or difficult labor, Multiparity (≥6 term pregnancies), Hyperactive or hypertonic uterus, Fetal distress (if delivery is not imminent), Unexplained vaginal bleeding, Placenta previa, Vasa previa, Active herpes geni-

talis, Obstetric emergency requiring surgical intervention, Situations in which vaginal delivery is contraindicated. Presence of acute pelvic inflammatory disease or ruptured membranes; Concurrent oxytocic therapy (wait for 30 min after removing insert before using oxytocin).
Use Cautiously in: Uterine scarring; Asthma; Hypotension; Cardiac disease; Adrenal disorders; Anemia; Jaundice; Diabetes mellitus; Epilepsy; Glaucoma; Pulmonary, renal, or hepatic disease; Multiparity (up to 5 previous term pregnancies).

Adverse Reactions/Side Effects

Endocervical Gel, Vaginal Insert. **GU:** uterine contractile abnormalities, warm feeling in vagina. **MS:** back pain. **Misc:** fever.
Suppository **CNS:** headache, drowsiness, syncope. **Resp:** coughing, dyspnea, wheezing. **CV:** hypotension, hypertension. **GI:** diarrhea, nausea, vomiting. **GU:** UTERINE RUPTURE, urinary tract infection, uterine hyperstimulation, vaginal/uterine pain. **Misc:** allergic reactions including ANAPHYLAXIS, chills, fever.

Interactions

Drug-Drug: Augments the effects of other **oxytocics**.

Route/Dosage

Cervical Ripening

Vag (Adults, Cervical): *Endocervical gel*—0.5 mg; if response is unfavorable, may repeat in 6 hr (not to exceed 1.5 mg/24 hr). *Vaginal insert*—one 10-mg insert.

Abortifacient

Vag (Adults): One 20-mg suppository, repeat q 3–5 hr (not to exceed 240 mg total or longer than 48 hr).

Availability

Endocervical gel (Prepidil): 0.5 mg dinoprostone in 3 g of gel vehicle in a prefilled syringe with catheters. **Vaginal insert (Cervidil):** 10 mg. **Vaginal suppository (Prostin E Vaginal):** 20 mg.

NURSING IMPLICATIONS

Assessment

- **Abortifacient:** Monitor frequency, duration, and force of contractions and uterine resting tone. Opioid analgesics may be administered for uterine pain.
- Monitor temperature, pulse, and blood pressure periodically throughout therapy. Dinoprostone-induced fever (elevation >1.1°C or 2°F) usually occurs within 15–45 min after insertion of suppository. This returns to normal 2–6 hr after discontinuation or removal of suppository from vagina.
- Auscultate breath sounds. Wheezing and sensation of chest tightness may indicate hypersensitivity reaction.
- Assess for nausea, vomiting, and diarrhea in patients receiving suppository. Vomiting and diarrhea occur frequently. Patient should be premedicated with antiemetic and antidiarrheal.
- Monitor amount and type of vaginal discharge. Notify physician or other health care professional immediately if symptoms of hemorrhage (increased bleeding, hypotension, pallor, tachycardia) occur.
- **Cervical Ripening:** Monitor uterine activity, fetal status, and dilation and effacement of cervix continuously throughout therapy. Assess for hypertonus, sustained uterine contractility, and fetal distress. Insert should be removed at the onset of active labor.

Potential Nursing Diagnoses

Deficient knowledge, related to medication regimen (Patient/Family Teaching)

Implementation

- **Abortifacient:** Warm the suppository to room temperature just before use.
- Wear gloves when handling unwrapped suppository to prevent absorption through skin.
- Patient should remain supine for 10 min after insertion of suppository; then she may be ambulatory.
- **Vaginal Insert:** Place vaginal insert transversely in the posterior vaginal fornix immediately after removing from foil package. Warming of insert and sterile conditions are not required. Use vaginal insert only with a retrieval system. Use minimal amount of water-soluble lubricant during insertion; avoid excess because it may hamper release of dinoprostone from insert. Patient should remain supine for 2 hr after insertion, then may ambulate.
- Vaginal insert delivers dinoprostone 0.3 mg/hr over 12 hr. Remove insert at the onset of

active labor, before amniotomy, or after 12 hr.

- Oxytocin should not be used during or less than 30 min after removal of insert.
- **Endocervical Gel:** Determine degree of effacement before insertion of the endocervical catheter. Do not administer above the level of the internal os. Use a 20-mm endocervical catheter if no effacement is present and a 10-mm catheter if the cervix is 50% effaced.
- Use caution to prevent contact of dinoprostone gel with skin. Wash hands thoroughly with soap and water after administration.
- Bring gel to room temperature just before administration. Do not force warming with external sources (water bath, microwave). Remove peel-off seal from end of syringe; then remove the protective end cap and insert end cap into plunger stopper assembly in barrel of syringe. Aseptically remove catheter from package. Firmly attach catheter hub to syringe tip; click is evidence of attachment. Fill catheter with sterile gel by pushing plunger to expel air from catheter before administration to patient. Gel is stable for 24 mo if refrigerated.
- Patient should be in dorsal position with cervix visualized using a speculum. Introduce gel with catheter into cervical canal using sterile technique. Administer gel by gentle expulsion from syringe and then remove catheter. Do not attempt to administer small amount of gel remaining in syringe. Use syringe for only 1 patient; discard syringe, catheter, and unused package contents after using.
- Patient should remain supine for 15–30 min after administration to minimize leakage from cervical canal.
- Oxytocin may be administered 6–12 hr after desired response from dinoprostone gel. If no cervical/uterine response to initial dose of dinoprostone is obtained, repeat dose may be administered in 6 hr.

Patient/Family Teaching

- Explain purpose of medication and vaginal exams.
- **Abortifacient:** Instruct patient to notify health care professional immediately if fever and chills, foul-smelling vaginal discharge, lower abdominal pain, or increased bleeding occurs.
- Provide emotional support throughout therapy.
- **Cervical Ripening:** Inform patient that she may experience a warm feeling in her vagina during administration.
- Advise patient to notify health care professional if contractions become prolonged.

Evaluation/Desired Outcomes

- Complete abortion. Continuous administration for more than 2 days is not usually recommended.
- Cervical ripening and induction of labor.

diphenhydrAMINE (oral, parenteral)

(dye-fen-**hye**-dra-meen)

✤Allerdryl, Allergy Medication, AllerMax, Banophen, Benadryl Dye-Free Alergy, Benadryl Allergy, Benadryl, Compoz, Compoz Nighttime Sleep Aid, Diphen AF, Diphen Cough, Diphenhist, Dormin, Genahist, 40 Winks, Hyrexin-50, ✤Insomnal, Maximum Strength Nytol, Maximum Strength Sleepinal, Midol PM, Miles Nervine, Nighttime Sleep Aid, Nytol, Scot-Tussin Allergy DM, Siladril, Silphen, Sleep-Eze 3, Sleepwell 2-night, Sominex, Snooze Fast, Sominex, Tusstat, Twilite, Unisom Nighttime Sleep-Aid

Classification

Therapeutic: allergy, cold, and cough remedies, antihistamines, antitussives

Pregnancy Category B

Indications

Relief of allergic symptoms caused by histamine release including: Anaphylaxis, Seasonal and perennial allergic rhinitis, Allergic dermatoses. Parkinson's disease and dystonic reactions from medications. Mild nighttime sedation. Prevention of motion sickness. Antitussive (syrup only).

Action

Antagonizes the effects of histamine at H_1-receptor sites; does not bind to or inactivate histamine. Significant CNS depressant and anticholinergic properties. **Therapeutic Effects:** Decreased symptoms of histamine excess (sneezing, rhinorrhea, nasal and ocular pruritus, ocular tearing and redness, urticaria). Relief of acute dystonic reactions. Prevention of motion sickness. Suppression of cough.

Pharmacokinetics

Absorption: Well absorbed after oral or IM administration but 40–60% of an oral dose reaches systemic circulation due to first-pass metabolism.
Distribution: Widely distributed. Crosses the placenta; enters breast milk.
Metabolism and Excretion: 95% metabolized by the liver.
Half-life: 2.4–7 hr.

TIME/ACTION PROFILE (antihistaminic effects)

ROUTE	ONSET	PEAK	DURATION
PO	15–60 min	2–4 hr	4–8 hr
IM	20–30 min	2–4 hr	4–8 hr
IV	rapid	unknown	4–8 hr

Contraindications/Precautions

Contraindicated in: Hypersensitivity; Acute attacks of asthma; Lactation; Known alcohol intolerance (some liquid products).
Use Cautiously in: Severe liver disease; Angle-closure glaucoma; Seizure disorders; Prostatic hyperplasia; Peptic ulcer; May cause paradoxical excitation in young children; Hyperthyroidism; OB: Safety not established. Lactation: Discontinue drug or bottle-feed; Geri: Appears on Beers list. Geriatric patients are more susceptible to adverse drug reactions and anticholinergic effects (delirium, acute confusion, dizziness, dry mouth, blurred vision, urinary retention, constipation, tachycardia); dosage reduction or non-anticholinergic antihistamine recommended.

Adverse Reactions/Side Effects

CNS: drowsiness, dizziness, headache, paradoxical excitation (increased in children). **EENT:** blurred vision, tinnitus. **CV:** hypotension, palpitations. **GI:** anorexia, dry mouth, constipation, nausea. **GU:** dysuria, frequency, urinary retention. **Derm:** photosensitivity. **Resp:** chest tightness, thickened bronchial secretions, wheezing. **Local:** pain at IM site.

Interactions

Drug-Drug: ↑ risk of CNS depression with other **antihistamines**, **alcohol**, **opioid analgesics**, and **sedative/hypnotics**. ↑ anticholinergic effects with **tricyclic antidepressants**, **quinidine**, or **disopyramide**. **MAO inhibitors** intensify and prolong the anticholinergic effects of antihistamines.
Drug-Natural Products: Concomitant use of **kava kava, valerian, or chamomile, can ↑ CNS depression.**

Route/Dosage

PO (Adults and Children >12 yr): *Antihistaminic/antiemetic/antivertiginic*—25–50 mg q 4–6 hr, not to exceed 300 mg/day. *Antitussive*—25 mg q 4 hr as needed, not to exceed 150 mg/day. *Antidyskinetic*—25–50 mg q 4 hr (not to exceed 400 mg/day). *Sedative/hypnotic*—50 mg 20–30 min before bedtime.
PO (Children 6–12 yr): *Antihistaminic/antiemetic/antivertiginic*—12.5–25 mg q 4–6 hr (not to exceed 150 mg/day). *Antidyskinetic*—1–1.5 mg/kg q 6–8 hr as needed (not to exceed 300 mg/day). *Antitussive*—12.5 mg q 4 hr (not to exceed 75 mg/day). *Sedative/hypnotic*—1 mg/kg/dose 20–30 min before bedtime (not to exceed 50 mg).
PO (Children 2–6 yr): *Antihistaminic/antiemetic/antivertiginic*—6.25–12.5 mg q 4–6 hr (not to exceed 37.5 mg/day). *Antidyskinetic*—1–1.5 mg/kg q 4–6 hr as needed (not to exceed 300 mg/day). *Antitussive*—6.25 mg q 4 hr (not to exceed 37.5 mg/24 hr). *Sedative/hypnotic*—1 mg/kg/dose 20–30 min before bedtime (not to exceed 50 mg).
IM, IV (Adults): 25–50 mg q 4 hr as needed (may need up to 100-mg dose, not to exceed 400 mg/day).
IM, IV (Children): 1.25 mg/kg (37.5 mg/m^2) 4 times daily (not to exceed 300 mg/day).

Availability (generic available)

Capsules: 25 mg[Rx, OTC], 50 mg[Rx, OTC]. **Tablets:** 25 mg[Rx, OTC], 50 mg[Rx, OTC]. **Chewable tablets (grape flavor):** 25 mg[Rx, OTC]. **Elixir (cherry and other flavors):** 12.5 mg/5 ml[Rx, OTC]. **Syrup (cherry and raspberry flavor):** 12.5 mg/5 ml[Rx, OTC]. **Injection:** 10 mg/ml, 50 mg/ml. ***In combination with:*** analgesics, decongestants, and expectorants, in OTC pain, sleep, cough, and cold preparations. See Appendix B.

NURSING IMPLICATIONS

Assessment

- Diphenhydramine has multiple uses. Determine why the medication was ordered and

🍁 = Canadian drug name.
*CAPITALS indicates life-threatening; underlines indicate most frequent.

assess symptoms that apply to the individual patient. Geri: Appears in the Beers list. May cause sedation and confusion due to increased sensitivity to anticholinergic effects. Monitor carefully, assess for confusion, delirium, other anticholinergic side effects and fall risk. Institute measures to prevent falls.

- **Prevention and Treatment of Anaphylaxis:** Assess for urticaria and for patency of airway.
- **Allergic Rhinitis:** Assess degree of nasal stuffiness, rhinorrhea, and sneezing.
- **Parkinsonism and Extrapyramidal Reactions:** Assess movement disorder before and after administration.
- **Insomnia:** Assess sleep patterns.
- **Motion Sickness:** Assess nausea, vomiting, bowel sounds, and abdominal pain.
- **Cough Suppressant:** Assess frequency and nature of cough, lung sounds, and amount and type of sputum produced. Unless contraindicated, maintain fluid intake of 1500–2000 ml daily to decrease viscosity of bronchial secretions.
- **Pruritus:** Assess degree of itching, skin rash, and inflammation.
- ***Lab Test Considerations:*** Diphenhydramine may decrease skin response to allergy tests. Discontinue 4 days before skin testing.

Potential Nursing Diagnoses

Insomnia (Indications)
Risk for deficient fluid volume (Indications)
Risk for injury (Side Effects)

Implementation

- Do not confuse Benadryl (diphenhydramine) with Benylin (dextromethorphan), desipramine (Norpramin) or with dimenhydrinate (Dramamine).
- When used for insomnia, administer 20 min before bedtime and schedule activities to minimize interruption of sleep.
- When used for prophylaxis of motion sickness, administer at least 30 min and preferably 1–2 hr before exposure to conditions that may precipitate motion sickness.
- **PO:** Administer with meals or milk to minimize GI irritation. Capsule may be emptied and contents taken with water or food.
- **IM:** Administer 50 mg/ml into well-developed muscle. Avoid subcut injections.

IV Administration

- **Direct IV:** ***Diluent:*** May be further diluted in 0.9% NaCl, 0.45% NaCl, D5W, D10W, dextrose/saline combinations, Ringer's solution, LR, and dextrose/Ringer's combinations. ***Concentration:*** 25 mg/ml. ***Rate:*** Infuse over 10–15 min at a rate not to exceed 25 mg/min.
- **Syringe Compatibility:** atropine, butorphanol, chlorpromazine, cimetidine, dimenhydrinate, droperidol, fentanyl, fluphenazine, glycopyrrolate, hydromorphone, hydroxyzine, meperidine, metoclopramide, midazolam, morphine, nalbuphine, pentazocine, perphenazine, prochlorperazine, promethazine, ranitidine, scopolamine, sufentanil.
- **Syringe Incompatibility:** haloperidol, pentobarbital, thiopental.
- **Y-Site Compatibility:** abciximab, acyclovir, aldesleukin, amifostine, amsacrine, argatroban, azithromycin, aztreonam, bivalirudin, ciprofloxacin, cisatracurium, cisplatin, cladribine, cyclophosphamide, cytarabine, dexmedetomidine, docetaxel, doxorubicin, doxorubicin liposome, etoposide phosphate, famotidine, fenoldopam, fentanyl, filgrastim, fluconazole, fludarabine, gemcitabine, granisetron, heparin, hydrocortisone, hydromorphone, idarubicin, linezolid, melphalan, meperidine, meropenem, methadone, methotrexate, morphine, ondansetron, oxaliplatin, paclitaxel, pemetrexed, piperacillin/tazobactam, potassium chloride, propofol, remifentanil, sargramostim, sufentanil, tacrolimus, teniposide, thiotepa, vinorelbine, vitamin B complex with C.
- **Y-Site Incompatibility:** allopurinol, amphotericin B cholesteryl sulfate, cefepime, foscarnet, lansoprazole.

Patient/Family Teaching

- Instruct patient to take medication as directed; do not exceed recommended amount. Caution patient not to use oral OTC diphenhydramine products with any other product containing diphenhydramine, including products used topically.
- May cause drowsiness. Caution patient to avoid driving or other activities requiring alertness until response to drug is known.
- Inform patient that this drug may cause dry mouth. Frequent oral rinses, good oral hygiene, and sugarless gum or candy may minimize this effect. Notify health care professional if dry mouth persists for more than 2 wks.
- Teach sleep hygiene techniques (dark room, quiet, bedtime ritual, limit daytime napping,

avoidance of nicotine and caffeine) to patients taking diphenhydramine to aid sleep.

- Advise patient to use sunscreen and protective clothing to prevent photosensitivity reactions.
- Caution patient to avoid use of alcohol and other CNS depressants concurrently with this medication.
- Pedi: Can cause excitation in children. Caution parents or caregivers about proper dose calculation; overdosage, especially in infants and children, can cause hallucinations, seizures, or death.
- Geri: Instruct older adults to avoid OTC products that contain diphenhydramine due to increased sensitivity to anticholinergic effects and potential for adverse reactions related to these effects.
- Advise patients taking diphenhydramine in OTC preparations to notify health care professional if symptoms worsen or persist for more than 7 days.

Evaluation/Desired Outcomes

- Prevention of, or decreased urticaria in, anaphylaxis or other allergic reactions.
- Decreased dyskinesia in parkinsonism and extrapyramidal reactions.
- Sedation when used as a sedative/hypnotic.
- Prevention of, or decrease in, nausea and vomiting caused by motion sickness.
- Decrease in frequency and intensity of cough without eliminating cough reflex.

diphenoxylate/atropine

(dye-fen-**ox**-i-late/**a**-troe-peen)
Logen, Lomanate, Lomotil, Lonox

difenoxin/atropine

(dye-fen-**ox**-in/**a**-troe-peen)
Motofen

Classification
Therapeutic: antidiarrheals
Pharmacologic: anticholinergics

Schedule V (diphenoxylate/atropine), IV (difenoxin/atropine)

Pregnancy Category C

Indications

Adjunctive therapy in the treatment of diarrhea.

Action

Inhibits excess GI motility. Structurally related to opioid analgesics but has no analgesic properties. Atropine added to discourage abuse.
Therapeutic Effects: Decreased GI motility with subsequent decrease in diarrhea.

Pharmacokinetics

Absorption: Well absorbed from the GI tract.
Distribution: Enters breast milk.
Metabolism and Excretion: *Diphenoxylate*—mostly metabolized by the liver with some conversion to an active antidiarrheal compound (difenoxin). *Difenoxin*—metabolized by the liver. Minimal excretion in urine.
Half-life: *Diphenoxylate*—2.5 hr; *difenoxin*—4.5 hr.

TIME/ACTION PROFILE (antidiarrheal action)

ROUTE	ONSET	PEAK	DURATION
Difenoxin–PO	45–60 min	2 hr	3–4 hr
Diphenoxylate–PO	45–60 min	2 hr	3–4 hr

Contraindications/Precautions

Contraindicated in: Hypersensitivity; Severe liver disease; Infectious diarrhea (due to *Escherichia coli*, *Salmonella*, or *Shigella*); Diarrhea associated with pseudomembranous colitis; Dehydrated patients; Angle-closure glaucoma; Children <2 yr; Known alcohol intolerance (some liquid diphenoxylate/atropine products only).
Use Cautiously in: Patients physically dependent on opioids; Inflammatory bowel disease; Geriatric patients (more sensitive to effects); Children (more sensitive to effects, espcially Down's syndrome patients); Prostatic hyperplasia; Pregnancy, lactation, or children <12 yr (safety not established for difenoxin/atropine in children <12 yr; diphenoxylate/atropine should not be used in children <2 yr).

Adverse Reactions/Side Effects

CNS: dizziness, confusion, drowsiness, headache, insomnia, nervousness. **EENT:** blurred vision, dry eyes. **CV:** tachycardia. **GI:** constipation, dry mouth, epigastric distress, ileus, nausea, vomiting. **GU:** urinary retention. **Derm:** flushing.

Interactions

Drug-Drug: Additive CNS depression with other **CNS depressants** including **alcohol**, **antihistamines**, **opioid analgesics**, and **sedative/hypnotics**. Additive anticholinergic properties with other **drugs having anticholinergic properties**, including **tricyclic antidepressants** and **disopyramide**. Use with **MAO inhibitors** may result in hypertensive crisis.

Drug-Natural Products: Increased anticholinergic effects with **angel's trumpet, jimson weed, and scopolia.**

Route/Dosage

Difenoxin/Atropine

Doses given are in terms of difenoxin—each tablet contains 1 mg difenoxin with 0.025 mg of atropine.

PO (Adults): 2 tablets initially, then 1 tablet after each loose stool or every 3–4 hr as needed (not to exceed 8 tablets/day).

Diphenoxylate/Atropine

Adult doses given are in terms of diphenoxylate—each tablet contains 2.5 mg diphenoxylate with 0.025 mg of atropine; pediatric doses are given in mg of diphenoxylate and in ml of diphenoxylate/atropine liquid; each 5 ml of liquid contains 2.5 mg diphenoxylate with 0.025 mg of atropine.

PO (Adults): 5 mg 3–4 times daily initially, then 5 mg once daily as needed (not to exceed 20 mg/day).

PO (Children): *use liquid only*—0.3–0.4 mg/kg/day in 4 divided doses.

Availability

Difenoxin/Atropine

Tablets: 1 mg difenoxin/0.025 mg atropine.

Diphenoxylate/Atropine

Tablets: 2.5 mg diphenoxylate/0.025 mg atropine. **Liquid (cherry flavor):** 2.5 mg diphenoxylate/0.025 mg atropine per 5 ml.

NURSING IMPLICATIONS

Assessment

- Assess the frequency and consistency of stools and bowel sounds prior to and throughout therapy.
- Assess patient's fluid and electrolyte balance and skin turgor for dehydration.
- ***Lab Test Considerations:*** Liver function tests should be evaluated periodically during prolonged therapy.
- Diphenoxylate/atropine may cause increased serum amylase concentrations.

Potential Nursing Diagnosis

Diarrhea (Indications)
Constipation (Side Effects)

Implementation

- Do not confuse Lomotil with Lamictal (lamontrigine) or Lamisil (terbinafine).
- Risk of dependence increases with high-dose, long-term use. Atropine has been added to discourage abuse.
- **PO:** Diphenoxylate/atropine tablets may be administered with food if GI irritation occurs. Tablets may be crushed and administered with patient's fluid of choice. Use calibrated measuring device for liquid preparations.

Patient/Family Teaching

- Instruct patient to take medication exactly as directed. Do not take more than the prescribed amount because of the habit-forming potential and risk of overdose in children. If on a scheduled dosing regimen, missed doses should be taken as soon as possible unless almost time for next dose. Do not double doses.
- Medication may cause drowsiness. Advise patient to avoid driving or other activities requiring alertness until response to drug is known.
- Advise patient that frequent mouth rinses, good oral hygiene, and sugarless gum or candy may relieve dry mouth.
- Caution patient to avoid alcohol and other CNS depressants concurrently with this medication.
- Advise patient to inform health care professional of medication regimen prior to treatment or surgery.
- Instruct patient to notify health care professional if diarrhea persists or if fever, abdominal pain, or palpitations occur.

Evaluation/Desired Outcomes

- Decrease in diarrhea. Treatment of acute diarrhea should be continued for 24–36 hr before it is considered ineffective.

dipyridamole

(dye-peer-**id**-a-mole)
✤Apo-Dipyridamole, Dipridacot, ✤Novodipiradol, Persantine, Persantine IV

Classification
Therapeutic: antiplatelet agents, diagnostic agents (coronary vasodilators)
Pharmacologic: platelet adhesion inhibitors

Pregnancy Category B

Indications
PO: Prevention of thromboembolism in patients with prosthetic heart valves (with warfarin). Maintains patency after surgical grafting procedures, including coronary artery bypass (with aspirin). **IV:** As an alternative to exercise in myocardial perfusion scintigraphy (cardiac stress testing with radiotracer imaging).

Action
PO: Decreases platelet aggregation by inhibiting the enzyme phosphodiesterase. **IV:** Produces coronary vasodilation by inhibiting adenosine uptake. **Therapeutic Effects: PO:** Inhibition of platelet aggregation and subsequent thromboembolic events. **IV:** In diagnostic thallium imaging, dipyridamole dilates normal coronary arteries, reducing flow to vessels that are narrowed and causing abnormal thallium distribution.

Pharmacokinetics
Absorption: Moderately absorbed (30–60%) after oral administration.
Distribution: Widely distributed. Crosses the placenta; enters breast milk.
Metabolism and Excretion: Metabolized by the liver; excreted in the bile.
Half-life: 10 hr.

TIME/ACTION PROFILE (PO = antiplatelet activity, IV = coronary vasodilation)

ROUTE	ONSET	PEAK	DURATION
PO	unknown	unknown	unknown
IV	unknown	6.5 min†	30 min

†From start of infusion

Contraindications/Precautions
Contraindicated in: Hypersensitivity.
Use Cautiously in: Hypotensive patients; Geri: Appears on Beers list. Geriatric patients may be more susceptible to orthostatic hypotension. Patients with platelet defects; Pregnancy (although safety not established, has been used without harm during pregnancy); Lactation or children <12 yr (safety not established).

Adverse Reactions/Side Effects
CNS: dizziness, headache, syncope; *IV only*— transient cerebral ischemia, weakness. **Resp:** *IV only*— bronchospasm. **CV:** *IV only*— MI, hypotension, arrhythmias, flushing. **GI:** nausea, diarrhea, GI upset, vomiting. **Derm:** rash.

Interactions
Drug-Drug: Additive effects with **aspirin** on platelet aggregation. Risk of bleeding may be ↑ when used with **anticoagulants**, **thrombolytic agents**, **NSAIDs**, **cefoperazone**, **cefotetan**, **valproic acid**, or **sulfinpyrazone**. ↑ risk of hypotension with **alcohol**. **Theophylline** may negate the effects of dipyridamole during diagnostic thallium imaging.

Route/Dosage
PO (Adults): 225–400 mg/day in 3–4 divided doses.
IV (Adults): 570 mcg/kg; maximum dose 60 mg.

Availability (generic available)
Tablets: 25 mg, 50 mg, 75 mg, ✤100 mg. **Injection:** 5 mg/ml in 2-ml and 10-ml vials. ***In combination with:*** aspirin (Aggrenox). See Appendix B.

NURSING IMPLICATIONS

Assessment
- **PO:** Monitor blood pressure and pulse before instituting therapy and regularly during period of dosage adjustment. Geri: Assess geriatric patients for orthostatic hypotension.
- **IV:** Monitor vital signs during and for 10–15 min after infusion. Obtain ECG in at least 1 lead. If severe chest pain or bronchospasm occurs, administer IV aminophylline 50–250 mg at a rate of 50–100 mg over 30–60 sec. If hypotension is severe, place patient in a supine position with head tilting down. If chest pain is unrelieved with aminophylline 250 mg, administer nitroglycerin SL. If chest pain is still unrelieved, treat as myocardial infarction.
- ***Lab Test Considerations:*** Bleeding time should be monitored periodically throughout therapy.

Potential Nursing Diagnoses
Decreased cardiac output (Indications)
Acute pain (Indications)

Implementation

- **PO:** Administer with a full glass of water at least 1 hr before or 2 hr after meals for faster absorption. If GI irritation occurs, may be administered with or immediately after meals. Tablets may be crushed and mixed with food if patient has difficulty swallowing. Pharmacist may make a suspension.

IV Administration

- **Intermittent Infusion:** ***Diluent:*** Dilute in at least a 1:2 ratio of 0.45% NaCl, 0.9% NaCl, or D5W for a total volume of 20–50 ml. Undiluted dipyridamole may cause venous irritation. ***Rate:*** Infuse over 4 min.
- **Y-Site Compatibility:** No information available.

Patient/Family Teaching

- **PO:** Instruct patient to take medication at evenly spaced intervals as directed. Take missed doses as soon as remembered unless the next scheduled dose is within 4 hr. Do not double doses. Benefit of medication may not be apparent to patient; encourage patient to continue taking medication as directed.
- Caution patient to change positions slowly to minimize orthostatic hypotension.
- Advise patient to avoid the use of alcohol, as it may potentiate the hypotensive effects. Tobacco products should also be avoided because nicotine causes vasoconstriction.
- Advise patient to consult health care professional before taking OTC medications concurrently with this medication. Aspirin should be taken only if directed and only in dose prescribed. Advise patient to discuss alternatives for pain relief or fever.
- Instruct patient to notify health care professional if unusual bleeding or bruising occurs. Concurrent use of aspirin or warfarin may increase risk of bleeding but is commonly used with specific indications.
- Advise patient to notify health care professional of medication regimen and whether using concurrent aspirin or warfarin therapy.
- **IV:** Instruct patient to notify health care professional immediately if dyspnea or chest pain occurs.

Evaluation/Desired Outcomes

- Prevention of postoperative thromboembolic complications associated with prosthetic heart valves.
- Maintenance of patency after surgical graft procedures.
- Coronary vasodilation in thallium myocardial perfusion imaging.

disopyramide

(dye-soe-**peer**-a-mide)
Norpace, Norpace CR, ✤Rythmodan, ✤Rythmodan-LA

Classification
Therapeutic: antiarrhythmics (class I)

Pregnancy Category C

Indications

Suppression/prevention of unifocal and multifocal PVCs, paired PVCs, and ventricular tachycardia. **Unlabeled uses:** Treatment/prevention of supraventricular tachyarrhythmias.

Action

Decreases myocardial excitability and conduction velocity. Has anticholinergic properties. Little effect on heart rate but has a direct negative inotropic effect. **Therapeutic Effects:** Suppression of ventricular arrhythmias.

Pharmacokinetics

Absorption: Well absorbed from the GI tract.
Distribution: Widely distributed; enters breast milk.
Metabolism and Excretion: Metabolized by the liver; 10% excreted unchanged in the feces, 50% excreted unchanged by the kidneys.
Half-life: 8–18 hr (increased in hepatic or renal impairment).

TIME/ACTION PROFILE (antiarrhythmic effects)

ROUTE	ONSET	PEAK	DURATION
PO	0.5–3.5 hr	2.5 hr	1.5–8.5 hr
PO-CR	0.5–3.5 hr	4.9 hr	12 hr

Contraindications/Precautions

Contraindicated in: Hypersensitivity; Cardiogenic shock; 2nd-degree and 3rd-degree heart block; Sick sinus syndrome (without a pacemaker).
Use Cautiously in: CHF or left ventricular dysfunction (dosage reduction recommended); Hepatic or renal insufficiency (dosage reduction recommended if CCr ≤40 ml/min); Prostatic enlargement; Myasthenia gravis; Glaucoma; Geri: Appears on Beers list. May induce heart failure in elderly patients; Children, pregnancy, or lactation (safety not established).

D

Adverse Reactions/Side Effects

CNS: dizziness, fatigue, headache. **EENT:** blurred vision, dry eyes, dry throat. **CV:** CHF, arrhythmias, AV block, dyspnea, edema, hypotension. **GI:** constipation, dry mouth, abdominal pain, flatulence, nausea. **GU:** urinary hesitancy, urinary retention. **Endo:** hypoglycemia. **Misc:** impaired temperature regulation.

Interactions

Drug-Drug: May potentiate anticoagulant effect of **warfarin**. **Rifampin**, **phenobarbital**, and **phenytoin** may decrease blood levels and effectiveness. **Cimetidine** or **erythromycin** may decrease metabolism and increase blood levels. May have additive toxic cardiac effects when used with other **antiarrhythmics** (prolonged conduction and decreased cardiac output), especially **verapamil**—avoid using disopyramide for 48 hr before or 24 hr after. Anticholinergic side effects may be additive with other **drugs having anticholinergic properties**, including **antihistamines** and **tricyclic antidepressants**. Increased risk of arrhythmias with **pimozide**.
Drug-Natural Products: Increased anticholinergic effects with **angel's trumpet**, **jimson weed**, and **scopolia**.

Route/Dosage

PO (Adults >50 kg): 150 mg q 6 hr (as immediate-release capsules) or 300 mg q 12 hr (as CR or LA dosage form; not to exceed 800 mg/day).
PO (Adults <50 kg or Patients with Poor Left Ventricular Function): 100 mg q 6–8 hr (as immediate-release capsules) or 200 mg q 12 hr (as CR or LA dosage form).
PO (Children 12–18 yr): 6–15 mg/kg daily, in divided doses q 6 hr.
PO (Children 4–12 yr): 10–15 mg/kg daily in divided doses q 6 hr.
PO (Children 1–4 yr): 10–20 mg/kg daily in divided doses q 6 hr.
PO (Children <1 yr): 10–30 mg/kg daily in divided doses q 6 hr.

Renal Impairment

PO (Adults): *CCr >40 ml/min or patients with hepatic impairment*—100 mg q 6 hr; *CCr 30–40 ml/min*—100 mg q 8 hr; *CCr 15–30 ml/min*—100 mg q 12 hr; *CCr <15 ml/min*—100 mg q 24 hr as immediate-release dosage form.

Availability (generic available)

Capsules: 100 mg, 150 mg. **Extended-release capsules:** 100 mg, 150 mg. **Extended-release tablets:** ✤150 mg. **Injection:** ✤10 mg/ml.

NURSING IMPLICATIONS

Assessment

- Monitor blood pressure, pulse, and ECG before and routinely throughout therapy. Check pulse before administering medication; withhold and notify physician or other health care professional if <60 or >120 bpm or if changes in rhythm.
- Monitor intake and output ratios and daily weight; assess for edema and urinary retention daily.
- Assess patient for signs of congestive heart failure (peripheral edema, rales/crackles, dyspnea, weight gain, jugular venous distention). Notify physician or other health care professional if these occur.
- ***Lab Test Considerations:*** Renal and hepatic functions and serum potassium levels should be evaluated periodically throughout therapy.
- May cause elevated serum BUN, cholesterol, and triglyceride levels.
- May cause decreased blood glucose concentrations.

Potential Nursing Diagnoses

Decreased cardiac output (Indications)
Impaired oral mucous membrane (Side Effects)

Implementation

- When changing from quinidine sulfate or procainamide to disopyramide, regular maintenance dose of disopyramide may be given 6–12 hr after last dose of quinidine sulfate or 3–6 hr after last dose of procainamide.
- Extended-release form (CR or LA formulations) is indicated for maintenance therapy only. When changing from regular form to extended-release forms, give the first dose of extended-release form 6 hr after the last regular dose.
- **PO:** Administer medication on an empty stomach, 1 hr before or 2 hr after meals. CR and LA forms must be swallowed whole; do not break open, crush, or chew.

- Pharmacist may prepare a suspension with 100-mg capsules and cherry syrup.

Patient/Family Teaching

- Advise patient to take medication around the clock, exactly as directed. Do not discontinue medication without consulting health care professional. If a dose is missed, take as soon as remembered unless within 4 hr of next dose. Do not double doses.
- Medication may cause dizziness. Caution patients to avoid driving or other activities requiring alertness until response to medication is known.
- Instruct patient to change positions slowly to minimize orthostatic hypotension.
- Advise patient that frequent mouth rinses, good oral hygiene, and sugarless gum or candy may help relieve dry mouth.
- Caution patient to avoid extremes of temperature, because this medication may cause impairment of body temperature regulation. Patient should use sunscreen and protective clothing to prevent photosensitivity reactions.
- Advise patient to consult health care professional before taking OTC medications or alcohol concurrently with this medication.
- If constipation becomes a problem, advise patient that increasing bulk and fluids in the diet and exercising may minimize constipation.
- Instruct patient to notify health care professional if dry mouth, difficult urination, constipation, or blurred vision persists.

Evaluation/Desired Outcomes

- Suppression of PVCs and ventricular tachycardia.
- Prevention of further arrhythmias.

DIURETICS (POTASSIUM-SPARING)

amiloride (a-**mill**-oh-ride)
✤Apo-Amiloride, ✤Midamor

spironolactone
(speer-oh-no-**lak**-tone)
Aldactone, ✤Novospiroton

triamterene (trye-**am**-ter-een)
Dyrenium

Classification
Therapeutic: diuretics
Pharmacologic: potassium-sparing diuretics

Pregnancy Category B (amiloride), C (spironolactone, triamterene)

Indications

Counteract potassium loss caused by other diuretics. Used with other agents (thiazides) to treat edema or hypertension. Primary hyperaldosteronism (spironolactone only). **Unlabeled uses: Spironolactone:** Management of CHF (low doses).

Action

Inhibition of sodium reabsorption in the kidney while saving potassium and hydrogen ions (spironolactone achieves this effect by antagonizing aldosterone receptors). **Therapeutic Effects:** Weak diuretic and antihypertensive response when compared with other diuretics. Conservation of potassium.

Pharmacokinetics

Absorption: *Amiloride*—30–90% absorbed; *spironolactone*—>90% absorbed; *triamterene*—30–70% absorbed.
Distribution: *Amiloride* and *triamterene*—widely distributed; all crosses the placenta and enter breast milk.
Protein Binding: *spironolactone* >90%.
Metabolism and Excretion: *Amiloride*—50% eliminated unchanged in urine, 40% excreted in the feces; *spironolactone*—converted by the liver to its active diuretic compound (canrenone); *triamterene*—80% metabolized by the liver, some excretion of unchanged drug.
Half-life: *Amiloride*—6–9 hr; *spironolactone*—78–84 min (spironolactone); 13–24 hr (canrenone); *triamterene*—1.7–2.5 hr.

TIME/ACTION PROFILE (diuretic effect)

ROUTE	ONSET	PEAK	DURATION
Amiloride	2 hr†	6–10 hr†	24 hr†
Spironolactone	unknown	2–3 days‡	2–3 days‡
Triamterene	2–4 hr†	1–several days‡	7–9 hr†

†Single dose
‡Multiple doses

Contraindications/Precautions

Contraindicated in: Hypersensitivity; Hyperkalemia; Anuria; Acute renal insufficiency; Significant renal dysfunction (CCr ≤30 ml/min or SCr >2.5 mg/dl).

Use Cautiously in: Hepatic dysfunction; Geri: Elderly (presence of age-related renal dysfunction may lead to ↑ risk of hyperkalemia); Diabetes (↑ risk of hyperkalemia); History of gout or kidney stones (triamterene only); Concurrent use of potassium supplements or potassium-containing salt substitutes; OB, Lactation, Pedi, Pregnancy, lactation, or children (safety not established).

Adverse Reactions/Side Effects

CNS: dizziness; *spironolactone only*— clumsiness, headache. **CV:** arrhythmias. **GI:** *amiloride*— constipation, nausea, vomiting. **GU:** *spironolactone*— erectile dysfunction; *triamterene*— nephrolithiasis. **Derm:** *triamterene*— photosensitivity. **Endo:** *spironolactone*— breast tenderness, gynecomastia, irregular menses, voice deepening. **F and E:** hyperkalemia, hyponatremia. **Hemat:** *spironolactone*— agranulocytosis; *triamterene*— hemolytic anemia, thrombocytopenia. **MS:** muscle cramps. **Misc:** allergic reactions.

Interactions

Drug-Drug: ↑ hypotension with acute ingestion of **alcohol**, other **antihypertensives**, or **nitrates**. Use with **ACE inhibitors**, **angiotensin II receptor antagonists**, **NSAIDS**, **potassium supplements**, **cyclosporine**, or **tacrolimus** ↑ risk of hyperkalemia. May ↑ levels/risk of toxicity from **lithium**. Effectiveness may be ↓ by **NSAIDs**. Spironolactone may ↑ effects of **digoxin**.

Route/Dosage

Amiloride

PO (Adults): *HTN*—5–10 mg/day (up to 20 mg).

PO (Children 1–17 yr): 0.4–0.625 mg/kg/day (maximum = 20 mg/day) (unlabeled use).

Spironolactone

PO (Adults): *Edema*—25–200 mg/day in 1–2 divided doses. *HTN*—50–100 mg/day in 1–2 divided doses. *Diuretic-induced hypokalemia*—25–100 mg/day in 1–2 divided doses. *Diagnosis of primary hyperaldosteronism*—100–400 mg/day in 1–2 divided doses. *CHF*—12.5–25 mg/day (unlabeled use).

PO (Children 1–17 yr): *Diuretic, HTN* 1 mg/kg/day in 1–2 divided doses (should not exceed 3.3 mg/kg/day or 100 mg/day) (unlabeled use). *Diagnosis of primary hyperaldosteronism*—125–375 mg/m²/day in 1–2 divided doses (unlabeled use).

PO (Neonates): 1–3 mg/kg/day in 1–2 divided doses.

Triamterene

PO (Adults): *HTN*—100 mg twice daily (not to exceed 300 mg/day; lower doses in combination products).

PO (Children): *HTN*—1–2 mg/kg/day in 2 divided doses; should not exceed 4 mg/kg/day or 300 mg/day.

Availability

Amiloride

Tablets: 5 mg. ***In combination with:*** hydrochlorothiazide (✤Moduret, ✤Novamilor). See Appendix B.

Spironolactone

Tablets: 25 mg, 50 mg, 100 mg. ***In combination with:*** hydrochlorothiazide (Aldactazide, ✤Apo-Spirozide, Spirazide). See Appendix B.

Triamterene

Capsules: 50 mg, 100 mg. ***In combination with:*** hydrochlorothiazide (Apo-Triazide, Dyazide, Maxzide, ✤Novo-Triamzide, ✤Nu-Triazide, ✤ro-Triazide, ✤Riva-Zide). See Appendix B.

NURSING IMPLICATIONS

Assessment

- Monitor intake and output ratios and daily weight during therapy.
- If medication is given as an adjunct to antihypertensive therapy, monitor blood pressure before administering.
- Monitor response of signs and symptoms of hypokalemia (weakness, fatigue, U wave on ECG, arrhythmias, polyuria, polydipsia). Assess patient frequently for development of hyperkalemia (fatigue, muscle weakness, paresthesia, confusion, dyspnea, ECG changes, cardiac arrhythmias). Patients who have diabetes mellitus or kidney disease and geriatric patients are at increased risk of developing these symptoms.
- Periodic ECGs are recommended in patients receiving prolonged therapy.
- ***Lab Test Considerations:*** Serum potassium levels should be evaluated before and

✤ = Canadian drug name.

*CAPITALS indicates life-threatening; underlines indicate most frequent.

routinely during therapy. Withhold drug and notify physician or other health care professional if patient becomes hyperkalemic.

- Monitor BUN, serum creatinine, and electrolytes before and periodically during therapy. May cause ↑ serum magnesium, BUN, creatinine, potassium, and urinary calcium excretion levels. May also cause ↓ sodium levels.
- Discontinue potassium-sparing diuretics 3 days before a glucose tolerance test because of risk of severe hyperkalemia.
- *Spironolactone* may cause false ↑ of plasma cortisol concentrations. Spironolactone should be withdrawn 4–7 days before test.
- Monitor platelet count and total and differential leukocyte count periodically during therapy in patients taking *triamterene*.

Potential Nursing Diagnoses

Excess fluid volume (Indications)

Implementation

- **PO:** Administer in AM to avoid interrupting sleep pattern.
- Administer with food or milk to minimize gastric irritation and to increase bioavailability.
- *Triamterene* capsules may be opened and contents mixed with food or fluids for patients with difficulty swallowing.

Patient/Family Teaching

- Emphasize the importance of continuing to take this medication, even if feeling well. Instruct patient to take medication at the same time each day. Take missed doses as soon as remembered unless almost time for next dose. Do not double doses.
- Caution patient to avoid salt substitutes and foods that contain high levels of potassium or sodium unless prescribed by health care professional.
- May cause dizziness. Caution patient to avoid driving or other activities requiring alertness until response to medication is known.
- Advise patient to consult with health care professional before taking any OTC decongestants, cough or cold preparations, or appetite suppressants concurrently with this medication because of potential for increased blood pressure.
- Advise patients taking *triamterene* to use sunscreen and protective clothing to prevent photosensitivity reactions.
- Instruct patient to notify health care professional of medication regimen before treatment or surgery.
- Advise patient to notify health care professional if muscle weakness or cramps; fatigue; or severe nausea, vomiting, or diarrhea occurs.
- Emphasize the need for follow-up exams to monitor progress.
- **Hypertension:** Reinforce need to continue additional therapies for hypertension (weight loss, restricted sodium intake, stress reduction, moderation of alcohol intake, regular exercise, and cessation of smoking). Medication helps control, but does not cure, hypertension.
- Teach patient and family the correct technique for checking blood pressure weekly.

Evaluation/Desired Outcomes

- Increase in diuresis and decrease in edema while maintaining serum potassium level in an acceptable range.
- Decrease in blood pressure.
- Prevention of hypokalemia in patients taking diuretics.
- Treatment of hyperaldosteronism.

DIURETICS (THIAZIDE)

chlorothiazide
(klor-oh-**thye**-a-zide)
Diuril, Sodium Diuril

chlorthalidone (thiazide–like)
(klor-**thal**-i-doan)
✤Apo-Chlorthalidone, Thalitone

hydrochlorothiazide
(hye-droe-klor-oh-**thye**-a-zide)
✤Apo-Hydro, ✤Bio-Hydrochlorothiazide, ✤DOM-Hydrochlorothiazide, Esedrix, Microzide, ✤Novo-Hydrazide, ✤Nu-Hydro, Oretic, ✤PHL-Hydrochlorothiazide, ✤PMS-Hydrochlorothiazide, ✤U-rozide

Classification
Therapeutic: antihypertensives, diuretics
Pharmacologic: thiazide diuretics

Pregnancy Category B (chlorthalidone, hydrochlorothiazide), C (chlorothiazide)

Indications

Management of mild to moderate hypertension. Treatment of edema associated with: CHF, Renal dysfunction, Cirrhosis, Glucocorticoid therapy, Estrogen therapy.

Action

Increases excretion of sodium and water by inhibiting sodium reabsorption in the distal tubule. Promotes excretion of chloride, potassium, magnesium, and bicarbonate. May produce arteriolar dilation. **Therapeutic Effects:** Lowering of blood pressure in hypertensive patients and diuresis with mobilization of edema.

Pharmacokinetics

Absorption: All are rapidly absorbed after oral administration.
Distribution: All cross the placenta and enter breast milk.
Metabolism and Excretion: All are excreted mainly unchanged by the kidneys.
Half-life: *Chlorothiazide*—1–2 hr; *chlorthalidone*—35–50 hr; *hydrochlorothiazide*—6–15 hr.

TIME/ACTION PROFILE (diuretic effect)

ROUTE	ONSET	PEAK	DURATION
Chlorothiazide PO	2 hr	4 hr	6–12 hr
Chlorothiazide IV	15 min	30 min	2 hr
Chlorthalidone	2 hr	2 hr	48–72 hr
Hydrochlorothiazide†	2 hr	3–6 hr	6–12 hr

†Onset of antihypertensive effect is 3–4 days and does not become maximal for 7–14 days of dosing

Contraindications/Precautions

Contraindicated in: Hypersensitivity (cross-sensitivity with other thiazides or sulfonamides may exist); Some products contain tartrazine and should be avoided in patients with known intolerance; Anuria; Lactation.
Use Cautiously in: Renal or hepatic impairment; OB: Pregnancy (jaundice or thrombocytopenia may be seen in the newborn); Pedi: Avoid use of hydrochlorothiazide oral solution in neonates (contains sodium benzoate, a metabolite of benzyl alcohol, which causes fetal gasping syndrome).

Adverse Reactions/Side Effects

CNS: dizziness, drowsiness, lethargy, weakness. **CV:** hypotension. **GI:** anorexia, cramping, hepatitis, nausea, pancreatitis, vomiting. **Derm:** photosensitivity, rashes. **Endo:** hyperglycemia. **F and E:** hypokalemia, dehydration, hypercalcemia, hypochloremic alkalosis, hypomagnesemia, hyponatremia, hypophosphatemia, hypovolemia. **Hemat:** thrombocytopenia. **Metab:** hypercholesterolemia, hyperuricemia. **MS:** muscle cramps.

Interactions

Drug-Drug: Additive hypotension with other **antihypertensives**, acute ingestion of **alcohol**, or **nitrates**. Additive hypokalemia with **corticosteroids**, **amphotericin B**, **piperacillin**, or **ticarcillin**. ↓ excretion of **lithium**. **Cholestyramine** or **colestipol** ↓ absorption. Hypokalemia ↑ risk of **digoxin** toxicity. **NSAIDs** may ↓ effectiveness.

Route/Dosage

When used as a diuretic in adults, generally given daily, but may be given every other day or 2–3 days/week.

Chlorothiazide

PO (Adults): 125 mg–2 g/day in 1–2 divided doses.
PO (Children >6 mos): 20 mg/kg/day in 1–2 divided doses (maximum dose = 1 g/day).
PO (Neonates ≤6 mo): 10–20 mg/kg q 12 hr (maximum dose = 375 mg/day).
IV (Adults): 500 mg–1 g/day in 1–2 divided doses.
IV (Children >6 mos): 4 mg/kg/day in 1–2 divided doses (maximum dose = 20 mg/kg/day) (unlabeled use).
IV (Neonates ≤6 mo): 1–4 mg/kg q 12 hr (maximum dose = 20 mg/kg/day) (unlabeled use).

Chlorthalidone

PO (Adults): 12.5–100 mg once daily (daily doses above 25 mg are associated with greater likelihood of electrolyte abnormalities).

Hydrochlorothiazide

PO (Adults): 12.5–100 mg/day in 1–2 divided doses (up to 200 mg/day); not to exceed 50 mg/day for hypertension; daily doses above 25 mg are associated with greater likelihood of electrolyte abnormalities.
PO (Children >6 mo): 1–3 mg/kg/day in 2 divided doses (not to exceed 37.5 mg/day).
PO (Children <6 mo): 1–3 mg/kg/day in 2 divided doses.

Availability

Chlorothiazide

Tablets: 250 mg, 500 mg. **Oral suspension:** 250 mg/5 ml. **Powder for injection:** 500 mg.

Chlorthalidone

Tablets: 25 mg, 50 mg, 100 mg. ***In combination with:*** atenolol (Tenoretic), clonidine (Clorpres). See Appendix B.

Hydrochlorothiazide

Tablets: 25 mg, 50 mg. **Capsules:** 12.5 mg. **Oral solution:** 10 mg/ml, 100 mg/ml. ***In combination with:*** numerous antihypertensive agents. See Appendix B.

NURSING IMPLICATIONS

Assessment

- Monitor blood pressure, intake, output, and daily weight and assess feet, legs, and sacral area for edema daily.
- Assess patient, especially if taking digoxin, for anorexia, nausea, vomiting, muscle cramps, paresthesia, and confusion. Notify health care professional if these signs of electrolyte imbalance occur. Patients taking digoxin are at risk of digoxin toxicity because of the potassium-depleting effect of the diuretic.
- If hypokalemia occurs, consideration may be given to potassium supplements or ↓ dose of diuretic.
- Assess patient for allergy to sulfonamides.
- **Hypertension:** Monitor blood pressure before and periodically during therapy.
- Monitor frequency of prescription refills to determine compliance.
- ***Lab Test Considerations:*** Monitor electrolytes (especially potassium), blood glucose, BUN, serum creatinine, and uric acid levels before and periodically throughout therapy.
- May cause ↑ in serum and urine glucose in diabetic patients.
- May cause ↑ in serum bilirubin, calcium, creatinine, and uric acid, and ↓ in serum magnesium, potassium, sodium, and urinary calcium concentrations.
- May cause ↑ serum cholesterol, low-density lipoprotein, and triglyceride concentrations.

Potential Nursing Diagnoses

Excess fluid volume (Indications)
Risk for deficient fluid volume (Side Effects)
Deficient knowledge, related to medication regimen (Patient/Family Teaching)

Implementation

- Administer in the morning to prevent disruption of sleep cycle.
- Intermittent dose schedule may be used for continued control of edema.
- **PO:** May give with food or milk to minimize GI irritation. Tablets may be crushed and mixed with fluid to facilitate swallowing.

IV Administration

- **Intermittent Infusion:** ***Diluent:*** Reconstitute chlorothiazide with at least 18 ml of sterile water for injection. Shake to dissolve. Stable for 24 hr at room temperature. May be given undiluted or may be diluted further with D5W or 0.9% NaCl. ***Concentration:*** Up to 28 mg/ml. ***Rate:*** If administered undiluted may give by direct IV over 3–5 min. If diluted, may run over 30 min.

Patient/Family Teaching

- Instruct patient to take this medication at the same time each day. If a dose is missed, take as soon as remembered but not just before next dose is due. Do not double doses.
- Instruct patient on use of calibrated dropper for measuring hydrochlorothiazide concentrated oral solution.
- Instruct patient to monitor weight biweekly and notify health care professional of significant changes.
- Caution patient to change positions slowly to minimize orthostatic hypotension. This may be potentiated by alcohol.
- Advise patient to use sunscreen and protective clothing to prevent photosensitivity reactions.
- Instruct patient to discuss dietary potassium requirements with health care professional (see Appendix L).
- Instruct patient to notify health care professional of medication regimen before treatment or surgery.
- Advise patient to report muscle weakness, cramps, nausea, vomiting, diarrhea, or dizziness to health care professional.
- Emphasize the importance of routine follow-up exams.
- **Hypertension:** Advise patients to continue taking the medication even if feeling better. Medication controls, but does not cure, hypertension.
- Encourage patient to comply with additional interventions for hypertension (weight reduction, low-sodium diet, regular exercise,

smoking cessation, moderation of alcohol consumption, and stress management).
- Instruct patient and family in correct technique for monitoring weekly blood pressure.
- Advise patient to consult health care professional before taking OTC medication, especially cough or cold preparations, concurrently with this therapy.

Evaluation/Desired Outcomes
- Decrease in blood pressure.
- Increase in urine output.
- Decrease in edema.

divalproex sodium, See **VALPROATES.**

HIGH ALERT

DOBUTamine
(doe-**byoo**-ta-meen)
Dobutrex

Classification
Therapeutic: inotropics
Pharmacologic: adrenergics

Pregnancy Category B

Indications
Short-term (<48 hr) management of heart failure caused by depressed contractility from organic heart disease or surgical procedures.

Action
Stimulates $beta_1$ (myocardial)-adrenergic receptors with relatively minor effect on heart rate or peripheral blood vessels. **Therapeutic Effects:** Increased cardiac output without significantly increased heart rate.

Pharmacokinetics
Absorption: Administered by IV infusion only, resulting in complete bioavailability.
Distribution: Unknown.
Metabolism and Excretion: Metabolized by the liver and other tissues.
Half-life: 2 min.

TIME/ACTION PROFILE (inotropic effects)

ROUTE	ONSET	PEAK	DURATION
IV	1–2 min	10 min	brief (min)

Contraindications/Precautions
Contraindicated in: Hypersensitivity to dobutamine or bisulfites; Idiopathic hypertrophic subaortic stenosis.
Use Cautiously in: History of hypertension (increased risk of exaggerated pressor response); MI; Atrial fibrillation (pretreatment with digitalis glycosides recommended); History of ventricular atopic activity (may be exacerbated); Hypovolemia (correct before administration); Pregnancy or lactation (safety not established); Children (has been used safely in children, although risk of tachycardia is increased).

Adverse Reactions/Side Effects
CNS: headache. **Resp:** shortness of breath. **CV:** hypertension, increased heart rate, premature ventricular contractions, angina pectoris, arrhythmias, hypotension, palpitations. **GI:** nausea, vomiting. **Local:** phlebitis. **Misc:** hypersensitivity reactions including skin rash, fever, bronchospasm or eosinophilia, nonanginal chest pain.

Interactions
Drug-Drug: Use with **nitroprusside** may have a synergistic effect on ↑ cardiac output. **Beta blockers** may negate the effect of dobutamine. ↑ risk of arrhythmias or hypertension with some **anesthetics (cyclopropane, halothane), MAO inhibitors, oxytocics,** or **tricyclic antidepressants.**

Route/Dosage
IV (Adults and Children): Start with low infusion rates (0.5–1 mcg/kg/min), titrated at intervals of a few minutes, guided by the patient's response (range 2–20 mcg/kg/min, up to 40 mcg/kg/min).

Availability
Injection: 12.5 mg/ml in 20-, 40-, and 100-ml vials. **Premixed infusion:** 250 mg/250 ml, 500 mg/500 ml, 500 mg/250 ml, 1000 mg/250 ml.

NURSING IMPLICATIONS

Assessment
- Monitor blood pressure, heart rate, ECG, pulmonary capillary wedge pressure (PCWP),

cardiac output, CVP, and urinary output continuously during the administration. Report significant changes in vital signs or arrhythmias. Consult physician for parameters for pulse, blood pressure, or ECG changes for adjusting dose or discontinuing medication.

- Palpate peripheral pulses and assess appearance of extremities routinely throughout dobutamine administration. Notify physician if quality of pulse deteriorates or if extremities become cold or mottled.
- ***Lab Test Considerations:*** Monitor potassium concentrations during therapy; may cause hypokalemia.
- Monitor electrolytes, BUN, creatinine, and prothrombin time weekly during prolonged therapy.
- ***Toxicity and Overdose:*** If overdose occurs, reduction or discontinuation of therapy is the only treatment necessary because of the short duration of dobutamine.

Potential Nursing Diagnoses

Decreased cardiac output (Indications)
Ineffective tissue perfusion (Indications)

Implementation

- ***High Alert:*** IV vasoactive medications are potentially dangerous. Have second practitioner independently check original order, dosage calculations, and infusion pump settings. Do not confuse dobutamine with dopamine. If available as floor stock, store in separate areas.
- Correct hypovolemia with volume expanders before initiating dobutamine therapy.
- Administer into a large vein and assess administration site frequently. Extravasation may cause pain and inflammation.

IV Administration

- **Continuous Infusion:** ***Diluent:*** Vials must be diluted before use. Dilute 250–1000 mg in 250–500 ml of D5W, 0.9% NaCl, 0.45% NaCl, D5/0.45% NaCl, D5/0.9% NaCl, or LR. Admixed infusions stable for 48 hr at room temperature and 7 days if refrigerated. Premixed infusions are already diluted and ready to use. ***Concentration:*** 0.25–5 mg/ml. ***Rate:*** Based on patient's weight (see Route/Dosage section). Administer via infusion pump to ensure precise amount delivered. Titrate to patient response (heart rate, presence of ectopic activity, blood pressure, urine output, CVP, PCWP, cardiac index). Dose should be titrated so heart rate does not increase by >10% of baseline.
- **Y-Site Compatibility:** amifostine, amikacin, amiodarone, anidulafungin, argatroban, atracurium, atropine, aztreonam, bivalirudin, bumetanide, calcium chloride, calcium gluconate, caspofungin, cimetidine, ciprofloxacin, cisatracurium, cyclosporine, digoxin, cladribine, dexmeditomidine, diazepam, diltiazem, diphenhydramine, docetaxel, dopamine, doxorubicin liposome, doxycycline, enalaprilat, epinephrine, eptifibatide, erythromycin, esmolol, etoposide phosphate, famotidine, fenoldopam, fentanyl, fluconazole, gemcitabine, gentamicin, granisetron, haloperidol, hydromorphone, inamrinone, insulin, isoproterenol, labetalol, levofloxacin, lidocaine, linezolid, lorazepam, magnesium sulfate, meperidine, methylprednisolone sodium succinate, metoclopramide, metoprolol, milrinone, morphine, nafcillin, nicardipine, nitroglycerin, norepinephrine, ondansetron, oxaliplatin, palonosetron, pancuronium, phenylephrine, potassium chloride, procainamide, prochlorperazine, promethazine, propofol, propranolol, protamine, ranitidine, remifentanil, streptokinase, tacrolimus, theophylline, thiotepa, tigecycline, tirofiban, tobramycin, tolazoline, vancomycin, vasopressin, vecuronium, verapamil, voriconazole, zidovudine.
- **Y-Site Incompatibility:** acyclovir, alteplase, aminophylline, amphotericin B cholesteryl sulfate, ampicillin, ampicillin/sulbactam, amphotericin B, cefazolin, cefoxitin, ceftriaxone, cefuroxime, chloramphenicol, ertapenem, foscarnet, ganciclovir, hydrocortisone sodium succinate, indomethacin, ketorolac, lansoprazole, micafungin, pantoprazole, pemetrexed, penicillin G potassium, phenytoin, phytonadione, piperacillin/tazobactam, sodium bicarbonate, thiopental, ticarcillin/clavulanate, trimethoprim/sulfamethoxazole, warfarin.

Patient/Family Teaching

- Explain to patient the rationale for instituting this medication and the need for frequent monitoring.
- Advise patient to inform nurse immediately if chest pain; dyspnea; or numbness, tingling, or burning of extremities occurs.
- Instruct patient to notify nurse immediately of pain or discomfort at the site of administration.

- **Home Care Issues:** Instruct caregiver on proper care of IV equipment.
- Instruct caregiver to report signs of worsening CHF (shortness of breath, orthopnea, decreased exercise tolerance), abdominal pain, and nausea or vomiting to health care professional promptly.

Evaluation/Desired Outcomes

- Increase in cardiac output.
- Improved hemodynamic parameters.
- Increased urine output.

HIGH ALERT

docetaxel (doe-se-**tax**-el)

Taxotere

Classification

Therapeutic: antineoplastics

Pharmacologic: taxoids

Pregnancy Category D

Indications

Breast cancer (locally advanced/metastatic breast cancer or with doxorubicin and cyclophosphamide as adjuvant treatment of node-positive disease). Non–small-cell lung cancer (locally advanced/metastatic) after failure on platinum regimen or with platinum as initial therapy). Advanced metastatic hormone-refractory prostate cancer (with prednisone). Squamous cell carcinoma of the head and neck (inoperable, locally advanced) with cisplatin and fluorouracil.

Action

Interferes with normal cellular microtubule function required for interphase and mitosis. **Therapeutic Effects:** Death of rapidly replicating cells, particularly malignant ones.

Pharmacokinetics

Absorption: IV administration results in complete bioavailability.
Distribution: Unknown.
Metabolism and Excretion: Extensively metabolized by the liver; metabolites undergo fecal elimination.
Half-life: 11.1 hr.

TIME/ACTION PROFILE (effect on blood counts)

ROUTE	ONSET	PEAK	DURATION
IV	rapid	5–9 days	7 days

Contraindications/Precautions

Contraindicated in: Hypersensitivity; Hypersensitivity to polysorbate 80; Known alcohol intolerance; Neutrophil count <1500/mm³; Liver impairment (serum bilirubin >upper limit of normal, ALT and/or AST >1.5 times upper limit of normal, with alkaline phosphatase >2.5 times upper limit of normal); OB: Pregnancy or lactation.
Use Cautiously in: OB: Patients with child-bearing potential.

Adverse Reactions/Side Effects

CNS: fatigue, weakness. **Resp:** bronchospasm. **CV:** ASCITES, CARDIAC TAMPONADE, PERICARDIAL EFFUSION, PULMONARY EDEMA, peripheral edema. **GI:** diarrhea, nausea, stomatitis, vomiting. **Derm:** alopecia, rashes, dermatitis, desquamation, edema, erythema, nail disorders. **Hemat:** anemia, thrombocytopenia, leukopenia. **Local:** injection site reactions. **MS:** myalgia, arthralgia. **Neuro:** neurosensory deficits, peripheral neuropathy. **Misc:** hypersensitivity reactions, including ANAPHYLAXIS.

Interactions

Drug-Drug: ↑ bone marrow depression may occur with other **antineoplastics** or **radiation therapy**. **Cyclosporine**, **ketoconazole**, **erythromycin**, or **troleandomycin** may significantly alter the effects of docetaxel.

Route/Dosage

IV (Adults): *Breast cancer*—60–100 mg/m² every 3 wk; *Breast cancer adjuvant therapy*—75 mg/m² every 3 wk for 6 cycles (with doxorubicin and cyclophosphamide); *Non–small-cell lung cancer*—75 mg/m² every 3 wk (alone or with platinum); *Prostate cancer*—75 mg/m² every 3 wk (with oral prednisone); *Squamous cell cancer*—75 mg/m² every 3 wks for 4 cycles (with cisplatin and fluorouracil).

Availability

Injection concentrate: 20 mg/0.5 ml polysorbate 80 with diluent (13% ethanol), 80 mg/2 ml polysorbate 80 with diluent (13% ethanol).

NURSING IMPLICATIONS

Assessment

- Monitor vital signs before and after administration.
- Assess infusion site for patency. Docetaxel is not a vesicant. If extravasation occurs, discontinue docetaxel immediately and aspirate the IV needle. Apply cold compresses to the site for 24 hr.
- Monitor for hypersensitivity reactions continuously during infusion. These are most common after the first and second doses of docetaxel. Reactions may consist of bronchospasm, hypotension, and/or erythema. Mild to moderate reactions may be treated symptomatically and infusion slowed or stopped until reaction subsides. Severe reactions require discontinuation of therapy and symptomatic treatment. Do not readminister docetaxel to patients with previous severe reactions. Severe edema may also occur. Weigh patients before each treatment. Fluid accumulation may result in edema, ascites, and pleural or pericardial effusions. Pretreatment with corticosteroids (such as dexamethasone 8 mg PO twice daily for 5 days, starting 1 day before docetaxel) is recommended to minimize edema and hypersensitivity reactions. PO furosemide may be used to treat edema.
- Monitor for bone marrow depression. Assess for bleeding (bleeding gums, bruising, petechiae; guaiac stools, urine, and emesis) and avoid IM injections and taking rectal temperatures if platelet count is low. Apply pressure to venipuncture sites for 10 min. Assess for signs of infection during neutropenia. Anemia may occur. Monitor for increased fatigue, dyspnea, and orthostatic hypotension.
- Assess patient for rash. May occur on feet or hands but may also occur on arms, face, or thorax, usually with pruritus. Rash usually occurs within 1 wk after infusion and resolves before next infusion.
- Assess for development of neurosensory deficit (paresthesia, dysesthesia, pain, burning). May also cause weakness. Pyridoxine may be used to minimize symptoms. Severe symptoms may require dose reduction or discontinuation.
- Assess patient for arthralgia and myalgia, which are usually relieved by nonopioid analgesics but may be severe enough to require treatment with opioid analgesics.
- ***Lab Test Considerations:*** Monitor CBC and differential before each treatment. Frequently causes neutropenia (<2000 neutrophils/mm^3); may require dose adjustment. If the neutrophil count is less than 1500/mm^3, dose should be held. Neutropenia is reversible and not cumulative. The nadir is 8 days, with a duration of 7 days. May also cause thrombocytopenia and anemia.
- Monitor liver function studies (AST, ALT, alkaline phosphatase, bilirubin) before each cycle. Doses are usually held if levels are elevated.

Potential Nursing Diagnoses

Risk for infection (Adverse Reactions)
Risk for injury (Adverse Reactions)

Implementation

- ***High Alert:*** Fatalities have occurred with chemotherapeutic agents. Before administering, clarify all ambiguous orders; double-check single, daily, and course-of-therapy dose limits; have second practitioner independently double-check original order, calculations, and infusion pump settings. Do not confuse Taxotere (docetaxel) with Taxol (paclitaxel).
- Solution should be prepared in a biologic cabinet. Wear gloves, gown, and mask while handling medication. Discard IV equipment in specially designated containers.

IV Administration

- **Continuous Infusion: *Diluent:*** Before dilution, allow vials to stand at room temperature for 5 min. Withdraw entire contents of diluent vial and transfer to vial of docetaxel. Rotate vial gently for 15 sec to mix. Do not shake. Solution should be clear but may contain foam at top. Allow to stand for a few minutes to allow foam to dissipate. All foam need not dissipate before continuing preparation. ***Concentration:*** To prepare the solution for infusion, withdraw the required amount of 10 mg/ml solution into syringe and inject into 250 ml of 0.9% NaCl or D5W for a concentration of 0.3–0.9 mg/ml. Rotate infusion container to mix infusion thoroughly. Do not administer solutions that are cloudy or contain a precipitate. Solution does not require an in-line filter. Dilute solutions are stable for 8 hr if refrigerated or at room temperature. ***Rate:*** Administer over 1 hr.
- **Y-Site Compatibility:** acyclovir, amifostine, amikacin, aminophylline, ampicillin, ampi-

cillin/sulbactam, aztreonam, bumetanide, buprenorphine, butorphanol, calcium gluconate, cefazolin, cefepime, cefotaxime, cefotetan, cefoxitin, ceftazidime, ceftizoxime, ceftriaxone, cefuroxime, chlorpromazine, cimetidine, ciprofloxacin, clindamycin, dexamethasone sodium phosphate, diphenhydramine, dobutamine, dopamine, doxycycline, droperidol, enalaprilat, famotidine, fluconazole, furosemide, ganciclovir, gemcitabine, gentamicin, granisetron, haloperidol, heparin, hydrocortisone, hydromorphone, imipenem/cilastatin, leucovorin, lorazepam, LR, magnesium sulfate, mannitol, meperidine, meropenem, mesna, metoclopramide, metronidazole, minocycline, morphine, ondansetron, oxaliplatin, palonosetron, pemetrexed, piperacillin, piperacillin/tazobactam, potassium chloride, prochlorperazine, promethazine, ranitidine, sodium bicarbonate, ticarcillin/clavulanate, tobramycin, trimethoprim/sulfamethoxazole, vancomycin, zidovudine.

- **Y-Site Incompatibility:** amphotericin B, doxorubicin liposome, methylprednisolone, nalbuphine.
- **Additive Incompatibility:** Information unavailable. Do not admix with other drugs or solutions.

Patient/Family Teaching

- Advise patient to notify health care professional if fever >101°F; chills; sore throat; signs of infection; bleeding gums; bruising; petechiae; or blood in urine, stool, or emesis occurs. Caution patient to avoid crowds and persons with known infections. Instruct patient to use soft toothbrush and electric razor.
- Patient should be cautioned not to drink alcoholic beverages or take products containing aspirin or NSAIDs.
- Fatigue is a frequent side effect of docetaxel. Advise patient that frequent rest periods and pacing of activities may minimize fatigue.
- Instruct patient to notify health care professional if abdominal pain, yellow skin, weakness, paresthesia, gait disturbances, swelling of the feet, or joint or muscle aches occur.
- Instruct patient to inspect oral mucosa for redness and ulceration. If mouth sores occur, advise patient to use sponge brush and rinse mouth with water after eating and drinking.
- Discuss with patient the possibility of hair loss. Complete hair loss usually begins after 1 or 2 treatments and is reversible after discontinuation of therapy. Explore coping strategies.
- Instruct patient not to receive any vaccinations without advice of health care professional.
- Emphasize the need for periodic lab tests to monitor for side effects.

Evaluation/Desired Outcomes

- Decrease in size or spread of malignancy in women with advanced breast cancer.
- Decrease in size or spread of malignancy in locally advanced or metastatic non–small-cell lung cancer.
- Decreased size or spread of advanced metastatic hormone-refractory prostate cancer.

docosanol (doe-**koe**-sa-nole)

Abreva

Classification

Therapeutic: antivirals (topical)

Pregnancy Category B

Indications

Treatment of recurrent oral-facial herpes simplex (cold sores, fever blisters).

Action

Prevents herpes simplex virus from entering cells by preventing viral particles from fusing with cell membranes. **Therapeutic Effects:** Reduced healing time. Decreased duration of symptoms (pain, burning, itching, tingling).

Pharmacokinetics

Absorption: Unknown.
Distribution: Unknown.
Metabolism and Excretion: Unknown.
Half-life: Unknown.

TIME/ACTION PROFILE

ROUTE	ONSET	PEAK	DURATION
Topical	unknown	unknown	unknown

Contraindications/Precautions

Contraindicated in: Hypersensitivity to docosanol or any other components of the formula-

♣ = Canadian drug name.

* CAPITALS indicates life-threatening; underlines indicate most frequent.

tion (benzyl alcohol, mineral oil, propylene glycol, or sucrose).

Use Cautiously in: Children <12 yr (safety not established); Pregnancy (use only if clearly needed).

Adverse Reactions/Side Effects

All local reactions occured at site of application

Local: acne, skin, itching, rash.

Interactions

Drug-Drug: None significant.

Route/Dosage

Topical (Adults and Children ≥12 yr): Apply small amount 5 times daily to sores on lips or face until healed.

Availability

Cream: 10% cream in 2 g tubes[OTC].

NURSING IMPLICATIONS

Assessment

- Assess skin lesions prior to and periodically throughout therapy.

Potential Nursing Diagnoses

Impaired skin integrity, impaired (Indications)
Risk for infection, high risk for (Indications)
Deficient knowledge, related to disease processes and medication regimen (Patient/Family Teaching)

Implementation

- **Topical:** Cream should be applied to lesions 5 times daily starting at the first sign of a sore or blister.

Patient/Family Teaching

- Instruct patient on correct technique for application of docosanol. Cream should only be applied to lips and face. Avoid application in or near eyes. Emphasize handwashing following application, or touching lesions to prevent spread to others or to other areas of the body.
- Advise patient to begin application of docosanol at the first sign of a sore or blister, even during prodromal stage (feeling of burning, itching, tingling, or numbness).
- Inform patient that docosanol reduces duration of herpes simplex virus episodes but does not cure virus. Viral reactivation may be triggered by ultraviolet radiation or sun exposure, stress, fatigue, chilling, and windburn. Other possible triggers include fever, injury, menstruation, dental work, and infectious diseases (cold, flu).
- Advise patient to notify health care professional if lesions do not heal in 14 days or if fever, rash, or swollen lymph nodes occur.

Evaluation/Desired Outcomes

- Reduction in duration of symptoms (pain, burning, itching, tingling) of herpes simplex virus episodes.

DOCUSATE (dok-yoo-sate)

docusate calcium
DC Softgels, Dioctocal, Pro-Cal-Sof, Sulfolax, Surfak

docusate sodium
Colace, Correctol Stool Softener, Soft Gels, Diocto, Docu, Docusoft S, DOK, DOS Softgels, DOS, DOSS, DSS, Dulcolax Stool Softener, Ex-Lax Stool Softener, Fleet Sof-Lax, Modane Soft, Phillips Liqui-Gels, Regulax-SS, ✤Regulex, Silace, Soflax, Stool Softener, Therevac SB

Classification
Therapeutic: laxatives
Pharmacologic: stool softeners

Pregnancy Category C

Indications

PO: Prevention of constipation (in patients who should avoid straining, such as after MI or rectal surgery). **Rect:** Used as enema to soften fecal impaction.

Action

Promotes incorporation of water into stool, resulting in softer fecal mass. May also promote electrolyte and water secretion into the colon. **Therapeutic Effects:** Softening and passage of stool.

Pharmacokinetics

Absorption: Small amounts may be absorbed from the small intestine after oral administration. Absorption from the rectum is not known.

Distribution: Unknown.

Metabolism and Excretion: Amounts absorbed after oral administration are eliminated in bile.

Half-life: Unknown.

TIME/ACTION PROFILE (softening of stool)

ROUTE	ONSET	PEAK	DURATION
PO	24–48 hr (up to 3–5 days)	unknown	unknown
Rectal	2–15 min	unknown	unknown

Contraindications/Precautions

Contraindicated in: Hypersensitivity; Abdominal pain, nausea, or vomiting, especially when associated with fever or other signs of an acute abdomen.

Use Cautiously in: Excessive or prolonged use may lead to dependence; Should not be used if prompt results are desired; OB, Lactation: Has been used safely.

Adverse Reactions/Side Effects

EENT: throat irritation. **GI:** mild cramps. **Derm:** rashes.

Interactions

Drug-Drug: None significant.

Route/Dosage

Docusate Calcium

PO (Adults): 240 mg once daily.

Docusate Sodium

PO (Adults and Children >12 yr): 50–400 mg in 1–4 divided doses.

PO (Children 6–12 yr): 40–150 mg in 1–4 divided doses.

PO (Children 3–6 yr): 20–60 mg in 1–4 divided doses.

PO (Children <3 yr): 10–40 mg in 1–4 divided doses.

Rect (Adults): 50–100 mg or 1 unit containing 283 mg docusate sodium, soft soap, and glycerin.

Availability (generic available)

Docusate Calcium

Capsules: 240 mg^{OTC}.

Docusate Sodium

Tablets: 100 mg^{OTC}. **Capsules:** 50 mg^{OTC}, 100 mg^{OTC}, 120 mg^{OTC}, 240 mg^{OTC}, 250 mg^{OTC}. **Syrup:** 20 mg/5 ml^{OTC}. **Liquid:** 150 mg/15 ml^{OTC}. **Enema:** 283 mg/5 ml^{OTC}. ***In combination with:*** stimulant laxatives^{OTC}. See Appendix B.

NURSING IMPLICATIONS

Assessment

- Assess for abdominal distention, presence of bowel sounds, and usual pattern of bowel function.
- Assess color, consistency, and amount of stool produced.

Potential Nursing Diagnoses

Constipation (Indications)

Implementation

- This medication does not stimulate intestinal peristalsis.
- **PO:** Administer with a full glass of water or juice. May be administered on an empty stomach for more rapid results.
- Oral solution may be diluted in milk or fruit juice to decrease bitter taste.
- Do not administer within 2 hr of other laxatives, especially mineral oil. May cause increased absorption.

Patient/Family Teaching

- Advise patients that laxatives should be used only for short-term therapy. Long-term therapy may cause electrolyte imbalance and dependence.
- Encourage patients to use other forms of bowel regulation, such as increasing bulk in the diet, increasing fluid intake (6–8 full glasses/day), and increasing mobility. Normal bowel habits are variable and may vary from 3 times/day to 3 times/wk.
- Instruct patients with cardiac disease to avoid straining during bowel movements (Valsalva maneuver).
- Advise patient not to use laxatives when abdominal pain, nausea, vomiting, or fever is present.
- Advise patient not to take docusate within 2 hr of other laxatives.

Evaluation/Desired Outcomes

- A soft, formed bowel movement, usually within 24–48 hr. Therapy may take 3–5 days for results. Rectal dose forms produce results within 2–15 min.

dofetilide (doe-**fet**il-ide)

Tikosyn

Classification

Therapeutic: antiarrhythmics (class III)

Pregnancy Category C

Indications

Maintenance of normal sinus rhythm (delay in time to recurrence of atrial fibrillation/atrial flutter [AF/AFl]) in patients with AF/AFl lasting more than one week, and who have been converted to normal sinus rhythm. For the conversion of atrial fibrillation and atrial flutter to normal sinus rhythm.

Action

Blocks cardiac ion channels responsible for transport of potassium. Increases monophasic action potential duration. Increases effective refractory period. **Therapeutic Effects:** Prevention of recurrent AF/AFl. Conversion of AF/AFl to normal sinus rhythm.

Pharmacokinetics

Absorption: Well absorbed (>90%) following oral administration.
Distribution: Unknown.
Metabolism and Excretion: 80% excreted by kidneys via cationic renal secretion, mostly as unchanged drug; 20% excreted as inactive metabolites; some metabolism in the liver via cytochrome P450 system (CYP3A4 isoenzyme).
Half-life: 10 hr.

TIME/ACTION PROFILE (blood levels)

ROUTE	ONSET	PEAK	DURATION
PO	within hours	2-3 hr†	12-24 hr

†Steady state levels are achieved after 2–3 days

Contraindications/Precautions

Contraindicated in: Hypersensitivity; Congenital or acquired prolonged QT syndromes; Baseline QT interval or QTc of >440 msec (500 msec in patients with ventricular conduction abnormalities); Creatinine clearance (CCr) <20 ml/min; Concurrent use of verapamil or agents which inhibit the renal cation transport system including cimetidine, ketoconazole, trimethoprim, megestrol or prochlorperazine; Concurrent use of hydrochlorothiazide; OB: Lactation (use should be avoided).
Use Cautiously in: Underlying electrolyte abnormalities (increased risk of serious arrhythmias; correct prior to administration); CCr 20–60 ml/min (dosage reduction recommended); Severe hepatic impairment; OB: Pregnancy (use only when benefit to patient outweighs potential risk to fetus); Pedi: Children <18 yr (safety not established).

Adverse Reactions/Side Effects

CNS: dizziness, headache. **CV:** VENTRICULAR ARRHYTHMIAS, chest pain, QT interval prolongation.

Interactions

Drug-Drug: Hydrochlorothiazide ↑ dofetilide levels and the risk of QT prolongation with arrhythmias; concurrent use is contraindicated. Concurrent use of renal cation transport inhibitors including **cimetidine**, **trimethoprim**, and **ketoconazole** increases blood levels and the risk of serious arrhythmias and is contraindicated. **Amiloride**, **metformin**, **megestrol**, **prochlorperazine**, and **triamterene** may have similar effects. **Phenothiazines**, **tricyclic antidepressants**, some **macrolides** (including **erythromycin** and **telithromycin**, and **fluoroquinolones** may prolong QT interval and ↑ risk of arrhythmias; concurrent use is not recommended. Blood levels and risk of arrhythmias are also ↑ by **verapamil**; concurrent use is contraindicated and a 2-day washout period is recommended). Inhibitors of the cytochrome P450 system (CYP450 3A4 isoenzyme) including **macrolide anti-infectives**, **azole antifungals**, **protease inhibitor antiretrovirals**, **SSRI antidepressants**, **amiodarone**, **cannabinoids**, **diltiazem**, **nefazodone**, **quinine**, and **zafirlukast** may also ↑ blood levels and the risk of arrhythmias and concurrent use should be undertaken with caution. Should not be used concurrently with other **class I or III antiarrhythmics** due to increased risk of arrhythmias. **Phenothiazines** and **tricyclic antidepressants** also prolong QT interval and should not be used concurrently with dofetilide. Hypokalemia or hypomagnesemia from **potassium-depleting diuretics** increases the risk of arrhythmias; correct abnormalities prior to administration. Concurrent use of **digoxin** may also increase the risk of arrhythmias.
Drug-Food: Grapefruit juice may ↑ levels; avoid concurrent use.

Route/Dosage

Dosing should be adjusted according to renal function and assessment of QT interval.
PO (Adults): *Starting dose*—500 mcg twice daily; *maintenance dose*—250 mcg twice daily (not to exceed 500 mcg twice daily).

Renal Impairment

PO (Adults): CCr 40–60 ml/min *Starting dose*—250 mcg twice daily; *maintenance dose*—125 mcg twice daily; CCr 20–40 ml/min *Starting dose*—125 mcg twice daily; *maintenance dose*—125 mcg once daily.

Availability

Capsules: 125 mcg, 250 mcg, 500 mcg.

NURSING IMPLICATIONS

Assessment

- Monitor ECG, pulse, and blood pressure continuously during initiation of therapy and for at least 3 days, then periodically during therapy. Evaluate QTc prior to initiation of therapy and every 3 months during therapy. If QTc exceeds 440 msec (500 msec in patients with ventricular conduction abnormalities), discontinue dofetilide and monitor patient until QTc returns to baseline.
- Assess the patient's medication history including OTC, Rx, and natural/herbal products, with emphasis on those that interact with dofetilide (see Interactions).
- ***Lab Test Considerations:*** Creatinine clearance must be calculated for all patients prior to administration and every 3 months during therapy.

Potential Nursing Diagnoses

Decreased cardiac output (Indications)

Implementation

- Dolfetilide must be initiated or reinitiated in a setting that provides continuous ECG monitoring and has personnel trained in the management of serious ventricular arrhythmias. Due to the potential for life-threatening ventricular arrhythmias, dofetilide is usually used for patients with highly symptomatic AF/AFl.
- Patients with AF should be anticoagulated according to usual protocol prior to electrical or pharmacological cardioversion.
- Make sure patient has an adequate supply of dofetilide prior to discharge to prevent interruption of therapy.
- Patients should not be discharged from the hospital within 12 hrs of electrical or pharmacological conversion to normal sinus rhythm.
- **PO:** Administer at the same time each day without regard to food.

Patient/Family Teaching

- Instruct patient to take medication as directed, even if feeling well. If a dose is missed, do not double next dose. Take next dose at usual time.
- Patient should read the patient package insert prior to initiation of therapy and reread it each time therapy is renewed. Emphasize the need for compliance with therapy, the potential for drug interactions, and the need for periodic monitoring to minimize the risk of serious arrhythmias.
- Instruct patient or family member on how to take pulse. Advise patient to report changes in pulse rate or rhythm to health care professional.
- May cause dizziness. Caution patient to avoid driving or other activities requiring alertness until response to medication is known.
- Advise patient to inform health care professional of medication regimen prior to treatment or surgery.
- Instruct patient not to take OTC medications with dofetilide without consulting health care professional.
- Advise patient to consult health care professional immediately if they faint, become dizzy, or have fast heartbeats. If health care professional is unavailable instruct patient to go to nearest hospital emergency department, take remaining dofetilide capsules, and show them to the doctor or nurse. If symptoms associated with altered electrolyte balance such as excessive or prolonged diarrhea, sweating, or vomiting or loss of appetite or thirst occur health care professional should also be notified immediately.
- Emphasize the importance of routine follow-up exams to monitor progress.

Evaluation/Desired Outcomes

- Prevention of recurrent AF/AFl.
- Conversion of AF/AFl to normal sinus rhythm.
- If patients do not convert to normal sinus rhythm within 24 hr of initiation of therapy, electrical conversion should be considered.

dolasetron (dol-a-se-tron)

Anzemet

Classification

Therapeutic: antiemetics

Pharmacologic: 5-HT_3 antagonists

Pregnancy Category B

Indications

Prevention of nausea and vomiting associated with emetogenic chemotherapy. Prevention and treatment of postoperative nausea/vomiting.

Action

Blocks the effects of serotonin at receptor sites (selective antagonist) located in vagal nerve terminals and in the chemoreceptor trigger zone in the CNS. **Therapeutic Effects:** Decreased incidence and severity of nausea/vomiting associated with emetogenic chemotherapy or surgery.

Pharmacokinetics

Absorption: Well absorbed but rapidly metabolized to hydrodolasetron, the active metabolite.
Distribution: Unknown.
Metabolism and Excretion: 61% of hydrodolasetron is excreted unchanged by the kidneys.
Half-life: *Hydrodolasetron*—8.1 hr (shorter in children).

TIME/ACTION PROFILE (antiemetic effect)

ROUTE	ONSET	PEAK	DURATION
PO	unknown	1–2 hr	up to 24 hr
IV	unknown	15–30 min	up to 24 hr

Contraindications/Precautions

Contraindicated in: Hypersensitivity.
Use Cautiously in: Patients with risk factors for prolongation of cardiac conduction intervals (hypokalemia, hypomagnesemia, concurrent diuretic or antiarrhythmic therapy, congenital QT syndrome, cumulative high-dose anthracycline therapy); Pregnancy or lactation (safety not established).

Adverse Reactions/Side Effects

CNS: headache (increased in cancer patients), dizziness, fatigue, syncope. **CV:** bradycardia, ECG changes, hypertension, hypotension, tachycardia. **GI:** diarrhea, dyspepsia. **GU:** oliguria. **Derm:** pruritus. **Misc:** chills, fever, pain.

Interactions

Drug-Drug: Concurrent **diuretic** or **antiarrhythmic** therapy or cumulative **high-dose anthracycline therapy** may ↑ risk of conduction abnormalities. Blood levels and effects of hydrodolasetron are ↑ by **atenolol** and **cimetidine**. Blood levels and effects of hydrodolasetron are ↓ by **rifampin**.

Route/Dosage

Prevention of Chemotherapy-Induced Nausea/Vomiting

PO (Adults): 100 mg given within 1 hr before chemotherapy.
PO (Children 2–16 yr): 1.8 mg/kg given within 1 hr before chemotherapy (not to exceed 100 mg).
IV (Adults and Children ≥2 yr): 1.8 mg/kg given 30 min before chemotherapy (usual dose in adults is 100 mg; not to exceed 100 mg in children).

Prevention/Treatment of Postoperative Nausea/Vomiting

PO (Adults): 100 mg given within 2 hr before surgery.
PO (Children 2–16 yr): 1.2 mg/kg (up to 100 mg/dose) given within 2 hr before surgery.
IV (Adults): 12.5 mg given 15 min before cessation of anesthesia (prevention) or as soon as nausea or vomiting begins (treatment).
IV (Children 2–16 yr): 0.35 mg/kg (up to 12.5 mg) given 15 min before cessation of anesthesia (prevention) or as soon as nausea or vomiting begins (treatment).

Availability

Tablets: 50 mg, 100 mg. **Injection:** 12.5 mg/0.625 ml ampules, 20 mg/ml in 5-ml vials.

NURSING IMPLICATIONS

Assessment

- Assess patient for nausea, vomiting, abdominal distention, and bowel sounds before and after administration.
- Monitor vital signs after administration. IV administration may be followed by severe hypotension, bradycardia, and syncope.

Potential Nursing Diagnoses

Imbalanced nutrition: less than body requirements (Indications)

Implementation

- **PO:** Administer within 1 hr before chemotherapy or 2 hr before surgery.
- Injectable dolasetron may be mixed in apple or apple-grape juice for oral dosing for pediatric patients. May be stored at room temperature for 2 hr before use.

IV Administration

- **IV:** Administer 30 min before chemotherapy, 15 min before cessation of anesthesia, or postoperatively if nausea and vomiting occur shortly after surgery.
- **Direct IV:** ***Diluent:*** May be administered undiluted. ***Concentration:*** 20 mg/ml. ***Rate:*** Administer over at least 30 sec.
- **Intermittent Infusion:** ***Diluent:*** May be diluted in 0.9% NaCl, D5W, dextrose/saline combinations, D5/LR, LR, or 10% mannitol solution. Solution is clear and colorless. Stable for 24 hr at room temperature or 48 hr if

refrigerated after dilution. ***Concentration:*** Dilute doses in 50 ml diluent. ***Rate:*** Administer each dose as an IV infusion over up to 15 min.
- **Y-Site Compatibility:** azithromycin, dexmeditomidine, fenoldopam, oxaliplatin.
- **Y-Site Incompatibility:** Manufacturer recommends not admixing with other medications.

Patient/Family Teaching
- Advise patient to notify health care professional if nausea or vomiting occurs.

Evaluation/Desired Outcomes
- Prevention of nausea and vomiting associated with emetogenic cancer chemotherapy.
- Prevention and treatment of postoperative nausea and vomiting.

donepezil (doe-nep-i-zill)
Aricept, Aricept ODT

Classification
Therapeutic: anti-Alzheimer's agents
Pharmacologic: cholinergics (cholinesterase inhibitors)

Pregnancy Category C

Indications
Mild to moderate dementia associated with Alzheimer's disease.

Action
Inhibits acetylcholinesterase thus improving cholinergic function by making more acetylcholine available. **Therapeutic Effects:** May temporarily lessen some of the dementia associated with Alzheimer's disease. Enhances cognition. Does not cure the disease.

Pharmacokinetics
Absorption: Well absorbed after oral administration.
Distribution: Unknown.
Protein Binding: 96%.
Metabolism and Excretion: Partially metabolized by the liver (CYP2D6 and CYP3A4 enyzmes) and partially excreted by kidneys (17% unchanged). Two metabolites are pharmacologically active.
Half-life: 70 hr.

TIME/ACTION PROFILE (improvement in symptoms)

ROUTE	ONSET	PEAK	DURATION
PO	unknown	several wk	6 wk†

†Return to baseline after discontinuation

Contraindications/Precautions
Contraindicated in: Hypersensitivity to donepezil or piperidine derivatives.
Use Cautiously in: Patients with underlying cardiac disease, especially sick sinus syndrome or supraventricular conduction defects; Patients with a history of ulcer disease or those currently taking NSAIDs; Patients with a history of seizures; Patients with a history of asthma or obstructive pulmonary disease; OB, Lactation, Pedi: Safety not established; assumed to be secreted in breast milk. Discontinue drug or bottle-feed.

Adverse Reactions/Side Effects
CNS: headache, abnormal dreams, depression, dizziness, drowsiness, fatigue, insomnia, syncope, sedation (unusual). **CV:** atrial fibrillation, hypertension, hypotension, vasodilation. **GI:** diarrhea, nausea, anorexia, vomiting, weight gain (unusual). **GU:** frequent urination. **Derm:** ecchymoses. **Metab:** hot flashes, weight loss. **MS:** arthritis, muscle cramps.

Interactions
Drug-Drug: Exaggerates muscle relaxation from **succinylcholine**. Interferes with the action of **anticholinergics**. ↑ cholinergic effects of **bethanechol**. May ↑ risk of GI bleeding from **NSAIDs**. **Quinidine** and **ketoconazole** ↓ metabolism of donepezil. **Rifampin**, **carbamazepine**, **dexamethasone**, **phenobarbital**, and **phenytoin** induce the enzymes that metabolize donepezil and may ↓ its effects.
Drug-Natural Products: Jimson weed and scopolia may antagonize cholinergic effects.

Route/Dosage

Mild to Moderate Alzheiner's Disease
PO (Adults): 5 mg once daily; after 4–6 wk may increase to 10 mg once daily (dose should not exceed 5 mg/day in frail, elderly females).

Severe Alzheimer's Disease

PO (Adults): 10 mg once daily (dose should not exceed 10 mg/day).

Availability

Tablets: 5 mg, 10 mg. **Cost:** 5 mg $464.97/90, 10 mg $455.97/90. **Orally-disintegrating tablets:** 5 mg, 10 mg. **Cost:** 5 mg $174.65/30, 10 mg $166.85/30.

NURSING IMPLICATIONS

Assessment

- Assess cognitive function (memory, attention, reasoning, language, ability to perform simple tasks) periodically during therapy.
- Administer Mini-Mental Status Exam (MMSE) initially and periodically as a screening tool to rate cognitive functioning.
- Administer Clock Drawing Test initially and periodically as a screening tool to measure severity of dementia.
- Monitor heart rate periodically during therapy. May cause bradycardia.

Potential Nursing Diagnoses

Disturbed thought process (Indications)
Impaired environmental interpretation syndrome (Indications)
Risk for injury (Indications)

Implementation

- **PO:** Administer in the evening just before going to bed. May be taken without regard to food.
- *Oral disintegrating tablets* should be allowed to dissolve on tongue; follow with water.

Patient/Family Teaching

- Emphasize the importance of taking donepezil daily, as directed. Missed doses should be skipped and regular schedule returned to the following day. Do not take more than prescribed; higher doses do not increase effects but may increase side effects.
- Inform patient/family that it may take weeks before improvement in baseline behavior is observed.
- Caution patient and caregiver that donepezil may cause dizziness.
- Advise patient and caregiver to notify health care professional if nausea, vomiting, diarrhea, or changes in color of stool occur or if new symptoms occur or previously noted symptoms increase in severity.
- Advise patient and caregiver to notify health care professional of medication regimen before treatment or surgery.
- Emphasize the importance of follow-up exams to monitor progress; atypical antipsychotics may be used as an adjunct to improve behavior.

Evaluation/Desired Outcomes

- Improvement in cognitive function (memory, attention, reasoning, language, ability to perform simple tasks) in patients with Alzheimer's disease.

HIGH ALERT

DOPamine (dope-a-meen)

Intropin, ✤Revimine

Classification
Therapeutic: inotropics, vasopressors
Pharmacologic: adrenergics

Pregnancy Category C

Indications

Adjunct to standard measures to improve: Blood pressure, Cardiac output, Urine output in treatment of shock unresponsive to fluid replacement.

Action

Small doses (0.5–3 mcg/kg/min) stimulate dopaminergic receptors, producing renal vasodilation. Larger doses (2–10 mcg/kg/min) stimulate dopaminergic and $beta_1$-adrenergic receptors, producing cardiac stimulation and renal vasodilation. Doses greater than 10 mcg/kg/min stimulate alpha-adrenergic receptors and may cause renal vasoconstriction. **Therapeutic Effects:** Increased cardiac output, increased blood pressure, and improved renal blood flow.

Pharmacokinetics

Absorption: Administered IV only, resulting in complete bioavailability.
Distribution: Widely distributed but does not cross the blood-brain barrier.
Metabolism and Excretion: Metabolized in liver, kidneys, and plasma.
Half-life: 2 min.

TIME/ACTION PROFILE (hemodynamic effects)

ROUTE	ONSET	PEAK	DURATION
IV	1–2 min	up to 10 min	<10 min

Contraindications/Precautions

Contraindicated in: Tachyarrhythmias; Pheochromocytoma; Hypersensitivity to bisulfites (some products).
Use Cautiously in: Hypovolemia; Myocardial infarction; Occlusive vascular diseases; Geri: Older patients may be more susceptible to adverse effects; OB, Pedi: Pregnancy, lactation, and children (safety not established).

Adverse Reactions/Side Effects

CNS: headache. **EENT:** mydriasis (high dose). **Resp:** dyspnea. **CV:** arrhythmias, hypotension, angina, ECG change, palpitations, vasoconstriction. **GI:** nausea, vomiting. **Derm:** piloerection. **Local:** irritation at IV site.

Interactions

Drug-Drug: Use with **MAO inhibitors**, **ergot alkaloids** (**ergotamine**), **doxapram**, **guanadrel**, or some **antidepressants** results in severe hypertension. Use with IV **phenytoin** may cause hypotension and bradycardia. Use with **general anesthetics** may result in arrhythmias. **Beta blockers** may antagonize cardiac effects.

Route/Dosage

IV (Adults): *Dopaminergic (renal vasodilation) effects*—0.5–3 mcg/kg/min. *Beta-adrenergic (cardiac stimulation) effects*—2–10 mcg/kg/min. *Alpha-adrenergic (increased peripheral vascular resistance) effects*—10 mcg/kg/min; infusion rate may be increased as needed.
IV (Children): 5–20 mcg/kg/min, depending on desired response (0.5–3 mcg/kg/min has been used to improve renal blood flow).

Availability (generic available)

Injection for dilution: 40 mg/ml, 80 mg/ml, 160 mg/ml. **Premixed injection:** 200 mg/250 ml, 400 mg/250 ml, 800 mg/250 ml, 800 mg/500 ml.

NURSING IMPLICATIONS

Assessment

- Monitor blood pressure, heart rate, pulse pressure, ECG, pulmonary capillary wedge pressure (PCWP), cardiac output, CVP, and urinary output continuously during administration. Report significant changes in vital signs or arrhythmias. Consult physician for parameters for pulse, blood pressure, or ECG changes for adjusting dose or discontinuing medication.
- Monitor urine output frequently throughout administration. Report decreases in urine output promptly.
- Palpate peripheral pulses and assess appearance of extremities routinely during dopamine administration. Notify physician if quality of pulse deteriorates or if extremities become cold or mottled.
- If hypotension occurs, administration rate should be increased. If hypotension continues, more potent vasoconstrictors (norepinephrine) may be administered.
- ***Toxicity and Overdose:*** If excessive hypertension occurs, rate of infusion should be decreased or temporarily discontinued until blood pressure is decreased. Although additional measures are usually not necessary because of short duration of dopamine, phentolamine may be administered if hypertension continues.

Potential Nursing Diagnoses

Decreased cardiac output (Indications)
Ineffective tissue perfusion (Indications)

Implementation

- ***High Alert:*** IV vasoactive medications are potentially dangerous. Have second practitioner independently check original order, dose calculations, and infusion pump settings. Do not confuse dopamine with dobutamine. If both are available as floor stock, store in separate areas.
- Correct hypovolemia with volume expanders before initiating dopamine therapy.
- Extravasation may cause severe irritation, necrosis, and sloughing of tissue. Administer into a large vein and assess administration site frequently. If extravasation occurs, affected area should be infiltrated liberally with 10–15 ml of 0.9% NaCl containing 5–10 mg of phentolamine. Reduce proportionally for pediatric patients. Infiltration within 12 hr of extravasation produces immediate hyperemic changes.

IV Administration

- **Continuous Infusion:** ***Diluent:*** Dopamine vials must be diluted before use. Dilute 200–800 mg of dopamine in 250–500 ml of 0.9% NaCl, D5W, D5/LR, D5/0.45% NaCl, D5/0.9% NaCl, or LR. Admixed solution is stable for 24 hr. Discard solutions that are cloudy, discolored, or contain a precipitate. Premixed infusions are already diluted and ready to use. ***Concentration:*** 0.8–3.2 mg/ml. ***Rate:*** Based on patient's weight (see Route/Dosage section). Infusion must be administered via infusion pump to ensure precise amount delivered. Titrate to response (blood pressure, heart rate, urine output, peripheral perfusion, presence of ectopic activity, cardiac index). Decrease rate gradually when discontinuing to prevent marked decreases in blood pressure.
- **Y-Site Compatibility:** amifostine, amikacin, aminophylline, amiodarone, anidulafungin, argatroban, atracurium, atropine, aztreonam, bivalirudin, bumetanide, calcium chloride, calcium gluconate, caspofungin, cefotaxime, cefoxitin, ceftazidime, ceftizoxime, ceftriaxone, cefuroxime, cimetidine, ciprofloxacin, cisatracurium, cladribine, clindamycin, cyclosporine, daptomycin, dexamethasone sodium phosphate, dexmedetomidine, digoxin, diltiazem, diphenhydramine, dobutamine, docetaxel, doxorubicin liposome, doxycycline, droperidol, enalaprilat, epinephrine, ertapenem, erythromycin, esmolol, etoposide phosphate, famotidine, fenoldopam, fentanyl, fluconazole, foscarnet, gemcitabine, gentamicin, granisetron, haloperidol, heparin, hydrocortisone sodium succinate, hydromorphone, imipenem/cilastatin, inamrinone, isoproterenol, ketorolac, labetalol, levofloxacin, lidocaine, linezolid, lorazepam, magnesium sulfate, meperidine, methylprednisolone sodium succinate, metoclopramide, metoprolol, metronidazole, micafungin, midazolam, milrinone, morphine, nafcillin, nicardipine, nitroglycerin, nitroprusside, norepinephrine, ondansetron, oxaliplatin, palonosetron, pancuronium, pantoprazole, pemetrexed, penicillin G potassium, phenylephrine, phytonadione, piperacillin/tazobactam, potassium chloride, procainamide, prochlorperazine, promethazine, propofol, propranolol, protamine, ranitidine, remifentanil, sargramostim, streptokinase, tacrolimus, theophylline, thiotepa, ticarcillin/clavulanate, tigecycline, tirofiban, tobramycin, tolazoline, vancomycin, vasopressin, vecuronium, verapamil, vitamin B complex with C, voriconazole, warfarin, zidovudine.
- **Y-Site Incompatibility:** acyclovir, alteplase, amphotericin B cholesteryl sulfate, ampicillin, cefazolin, chloramphenicol, diazepam, ganciclovir, indomethacin, insulin, lansoprazole, phenytoin, thiopental, trimethoprim/sulfamethoxazole.

Patient/Family Teaching

- Explain to patient the rationale for instituting this medication and the need for frequent monitoring.
- Advise patient to inform nurse immediately if chest pain; dyspnea; numbness, tingling, or burning of extremities occurs.
- Instruct patient to inform nurse immediately of pain or discomfort at the site of administration.

Evaluation/Desired Outcomes

- Increase in blood pressure.
- Increase in peripheral circulation.
- Increase in urine output.

doxazosin (dox-**ay**-zoe-sin)

Cardura

Classification

Therapeutic: antihypertensives

Pharmacologic: peripherally acting antiadrenergics

Pregnancy Category C

Indications

Hypertension (alone or with other agents). Symptomatic benign prostatic hyperplasia (BPH).

Action

Dilates both arteries and veins by blocking postsynaptic alpha$_1$-adrenergic receptors. **Therapeutic Effects:** Lowering of blood pressure.

Pharmacokinetics

Absorption: Well absorbed following oral administration.

Distribution: Probably enters breast milk; rest of distribution unknown.

Protein Binding: 98–99%.

Metabolism and Excretion: Extensively metabolized by the liver.

Half-life: 22 hr.

TIME/ACTION PROFILE (antihypertensive effect)

ROUTE	ONSET	PEAK	DURATION
PO	1–2 hr	2–6 hr	24 hr

Contraindications/Precautions

Contraindicated in: Hypersensitivity.
Use Cautiously in: Hepatic dysfunction and impaired renal function; Geri: Appears on Beers list. Geriatric patients are at increased risk for hypotension and renal impairment; Pregnancy, lactation, or children (safety not established).

Adverse Reactions/Side Effects

CNS: dizziness, headache, depression, drowsiness, fatigue, nervousness, weakness. **EENT:** abnormal vision, blurred vision, conjunctivitis, epistaxis. **Resp:** dyspnea. **CV:** first-dose orthostatic hypotension, arrhythmias, chest pain, edema, palpitations. **GI:** abdominal discomfort, constipation, diarrhea, dry mouth, flatulence, nausea, vomiting. **GU:** decreased libido, sexual dysfunction. **Derm:** flushing, rash, urticaria. **MS:** arthralgia, arthritis, gout, myalgia.

Interactions

Drug-Drug: ↑ risk of hypotension with acute ingestion of **alcohol**, **sildenafil**, **vardenafil**, other **antihypertensives**, or **nitrates**. May ↓ antihypertensive effect of **clonidine**.

Route/Dosage

PO (Adults): *Hypertension*—1 mg once daily, may be gradually increased at 2-wk intervals to 2–16 mg/day; incidence of postural hypotension greatly increased at doses >4 mg/day. *BPH*—1 mg once daily, may be gradually increased to 8 mg/day.

Availability (generic available)

Tablets: 1 mg, 2 mg, 4 mg, 8 mg. **Cost:** *Generic*—1 mg $49.97/90, 2 mg $43.97/90, 4 mg $59.97/90, 8 mg $62.99/90.

NURSING IMPLICATIONS

Assessment

- Monitor blood pressure and pulse 2–6 hr after first dose, with each increase in dose, and periodically during therapy. Report significant changes.
- Assess patient for first-dose orthostatic hypotension and syncope. Incidence may be dose related. Observe patient closely during this period and take precautions to prevent injury.
- Monitor intake and output ratios and daily weight, and assess for edema daily, especially at beginning of therapy. Report weight gain or edema.
- **BPH:** Assess patient for symptoms of prostatic hyperplasia (urinary hesitancy, feeling of incomplete bladder emptying, interruption of urinary stream, impairment of size and force of urinary stream, terminal urinary dribbling, straining to start flow, dysuria, urgency) prior to and periodically during therapy.

Potential Nursing Diagnoses

Impaired urinary elimination (Indications)
Risk for injury (Side Effects)

Implementation

- Do not confuse Cardura (doxazosin) with Cardene (nicardipine) or Ridaura (auranofin).
- Administer daily dose at bedtime.
- **Hypertension:** May be administered concurrently with a diuretic or other antihypertensive.

Patient/Family Teaching

- Emphasize the importance of continuing to take this medication, even if feeling well. Instruct patient to take medication at the same time each day. Take missed doses as soon as remembered unless almost time for next dose. Do not double doses.
- Doxazosin may cause drowsiness or dizziness. Advise patient to avoid driving or other activities requiring alertness until response to medication is known.
- Caution patient to change positions slowly to decrease orthostatic hypotension.
- Advise patient to consult health care professional before taking any cough, cold, or allergy remedies or herbal products.
- Emphasize the importance of follow-up visits to determine effectiveness of therapy.
- **Hypertension:** Instruct patient and family on proper technique for blood pressure monitoring. Advise them to check blood pressure at least weekly and report significant changes.
- Encourage patient to comply with additional interventions for hypertension (weight reduction, low-sodium diet, smoking cessation,

moderation of alcohol consumption, regular exercise, and stress management).

Evaluation/Desired Outcomes

- Decrease in blood pressure without appearance of side effects.
- Decrease in urinary symptoms of BPH.

doxepin (dox-e-pin)

Sinequan, ✤Triadapin, Zonalon

Classification

Therapeutic: antianxiety agents, antidepressants, antihistamines (topical)

Pharmacologic: tricyclic antidepressants

Pregnancy Category C

Indications

PO: Depression. **Topical:** Short-term control of pruritus associated with: Eczematous dermatitis, Lichen simplex chronicus. **Unlabeled uses:** POChronic pain syndromes: Pruritus, Dermatitis, Anxiety, Insomnia.

Action

PO Prevents the reuptake of norepinephrine and serotonin by presynaptic neurons; resultant accumulation of neurotransmitters potentiates their activity. Also possesses significant anticholinergic properties. **Topical:** Antipruritic action due to antihistaminic properties. **Therapeutic Effects:** PORelief of depression. Decreased anxiety. **Topical:** Decreased pruritus.

Pharmacokinetics

Absorption: Well absorbed from the GI tract, although much is metabolized on first pass through the liver. Some systemic absorption follows topical application.

Distribution: Widely distributed. Enters breast milk; probably crosses the placenta.

Metabolism and Excretion: Metabolized by the liver. Some conversion to active antidepressant compound. May re-enter gastric juice via secretion from enterohepatic circulation, where more absorption may occur.

Half-life: 8–25 hr.

TIME/ACTION PROFILE (antidepressant activity)

ROUTE	ONSET	PEAK	DURATION
PO	2–3 wk	up to 6 wk	days–weeks

Contraindications/Precautions

Contraindicated in: Hypersensitivity; Some products contain bisulfites and should be avoided in patients with known intolerance; Untreated angle-closure glaucoma; Period immediately after myocardial infarction; history of QTc prolongation, heart failure, cardiac arrhythmia.

Use Cautiously in: Geri: Pre-existing cardiovascular disease (increased risk of adverse reactions); Prostatic enlargement (more susceptible to urinary retention); Seizures; OB: Use during pregnancy only if potential maternal benefit outweighs risks to fetus; use during lactation may result in neonatal sedation. Recommend discontinuing drug or bottle-feed; Pedi: May ↑ risk of suicide attempt/ideation especially during dose early treatment or dose adjustment; risk may be greater in children or adolescents; Pedi: Safety not established in children <12 yr; Geri: Appears on Beers list and is associated with increased falls risk secondary to anticholinergic and sedative effects. Geriatric patients should have initial dosage reduction.

Adverse Reactions/Side Effects

CNS: fatigue, sedation, agitation, confusion, hallucinations. **EENT:** blurred vision, increased intraocular pressure. **CV:** hypotension, arrhythmias, ECG abnormalities. **GI:** constipation, dry mouth, hepatitis, increased appetite, weight gain, nausea, paralytic ileus. **GU:** urinary retention, decreased libido. **Derm:** photosensitivity, rashes. **Hemat:** blood dyscrasias. **Misc:** hypersensitivity reactions.

Interactions

Apply to both topical and oral use

Drug-Drug: Doxepin is metabolized in the liver by the cytochrome P450 2D6 enzyme and its action may be affected by drugs that compete for metabolism by this enzyme including other **antidepressants**, **phenothiazines**, **carbamazepine**, **class 1C antiarrhythmics** (**propafenone**, **flecainide**); when used concurrently, dosage ↓ of one or the other or both may be necessary. Concurrent use of other drugs that inhibit the activity of the enzyme, including **cimetidine**, **quinidine**, **amiodarone**, and **ritonavir**, may result in ↑ effects of doxepin. May cause hypotension, tachycardia, and potentially fatal reactions when used with **MAO inhibitors** (avoid concurrent use—discontinue 2 wk prior to doxepin). Concurrent use with **SSRI antidepressants** may result in ↑ toxicity and should be avoided (fluoxetine should be stopped 5 wk before). Concurrent use with **clonidine** may result in hypertensive crisis and should be avoided. Concurrent use with **levodopa** may result in delayed / ↓ absorption of levodopa or

hypertension. Blood levels and effects may be ↓ by **rifamycins**. ↑ CNS depression with other **CNS depressants** including **alcohol**, **antihistamines**, **clonidine**, **opioid analgesics**, and **sedative/hypnotics**. **Barbiturates** may alter blood levels and effects. **Adrenergic** and **anticholinergic** side effects may be ↑ with other **agents having these properties**. **Phenothiazines** or **hormonal contraceptives** ↑ levels and may cause toxicity. **Smoking** may increase metabolism and alter effects.
Drug-Natural Products: Concomitant use of **kava kava, valerian, or chamomile can increase CNS depression. Increased anticholinergic effects with jimson weed and scopolia.**

Route/Dosage

PO (Adults): *Antidepressant/anti-anxiety*—25 mg 3 times daily, may be increased as needed (up to 150 mg/day in outpatients or 300 mg/day in inpatients; some patients may require only 25–50 mg/day). Once stabilized, entire daily dose may be given at bedtime. *Antipruritic*—10 mg at bedtime initially, may be increased up to 25 mg.
PO (Geriatric Patients): *Antidepressant*—25–50 mg/day initially, may be increased as needed.
Topical (Adults): Apply 4 times daily (wait 3–4 hr between applications) for up to 8 days.

Availability (generic available)

Capsules: 10 mg, 25 mg, 50 mg, 75 mg, 100 mg, 150 mg. **Oral concentrate:** 10 mg/ml. **Topical cream:** 5%.

NURSING IMPLICATIONS

Assessment

- Monitor blood pressure and pulse rate prior to and during initial therapy. Patients taking high doses or with a history of cardiovascular disease should have ECG monitored prior to and periodically during therapy.
- Assess for sexual dysfunction (decreased libido; erectile dysfunction).
- Assess weight and BMI initially and throughout treatment. Obtain FBS and cholesterol levels in overweight/obese individuals.
- Geri: Assess falls risk and institute fall prevention strategies. Assess for anticholinergic effects.
- **Depression:** Assess mental status (orientation, mood, behavior) frequently. Confusion, agitation, and hallucinations may occur during initiation of therapy and may require dosage reduction. Assess for suicidal tendencies, especially during early therapy. Restrict amount of drug available to patient.
- **Anxiety:** Assess degree and manifestations of anxiety prior to and during therapy.
- **Pain:** Assess the type, location, and severity of pain prior to and periodically during therapy. Use pain scale to assess effectiveness of therapy.
- **Topical:** Assess pruritic area prior to and periodically during therapy.
- ***Lab Test Considerations:*** Monitor WBC and differential blood counts, hepatic function, and serum glucose periodically. May cause ↑ serum bilirubin and alkaline phosphatase levels. May cause bone marrow depression. Serum glucose may be ↑ or ↓.

Potential Nursing Diagnoses

Ineffective coping (Indications)
Risk for injury (Side Effects)
Sexual dysfunction (Side Effects)

Implementation

- Do not confuse doxepin with doxycycline.
- May be given as a single dose at bedtime to minimize sedation during the day. Dose increases should be made at bedtime because of sedation. Dose titration is a slow process; may take weeks to months.
- To avoid withdrawal, taper by 50% for 3 days, then 50% again for 3 days, then discontinue.
- **PO:** Administer medication with or immediately following a meal to minimize gastric irritation. Capsules may be opened and mixed with foods or fluids if patient has difficulty swallowing.
- Oral concentrate must be diluted in at least 120 ml of water, milk, or fruit juice. Do not mix with carbonated beverages or grape juice. Use calibrated measuring device to ensure accurate amount.
- **Topical:** Apply thin film of doxepin cream only to affected areas, and rub in gently. Apply only to affected skin; not for ophthalmic, oral, or intravaginal use.

Patient/Family Teaching

- Inform patient that systemic side effects may occur with oral or topical use.

- May cause drowsiness and blurred vision. Caution patient to avoid driving and other activities requiring alertness until response to the medication is known.
- Orthostatic hypotension, sedation, and confusion are common during early therapy, especially in geriatric patients. Protect patient from falls. Institute fall precautions. Advise patient to change positions slowly.
- Advise patient to avoid alcohol or other CNS depressant drugs during and for at least 3–7 days after therapy has been discontinued.
- Instruct patient to notify health care professional if urinary retention occurs or if dry mouth or constipation persists. Sugarless candy or gum may diminish dry mouth, and an increase in fluid intake or bulk may prevent constipation. If symptoms persist, dose reduction or discontinuation may be necessary. Consult health care professional if dry mouth persists for more than 2 wk.
- Advise patient to notify health care professional of medication regimen prior to treatment or surgery.
- **PO:** Instruct patient to take medication as directed. Take missed doses as soon as possible unless almost time for next dose; if regimen is a single dose at bedtime, do not take in the morning because of side effects. Advise patient that drug effects may not be noticed for at least 2 wk. Abrupt discontinuation may cause nausea, vomiting, diarrhea, headache, trouble sleeping with vivid dreams, and irritability.
- Refer appropriate individuals for weight management.
- Caution patient to use sunscreen and protective clothing to prevent photosensitivity reactions.
- Inform patient that urine may turn blue-green in color.
- Inform patient of need to monitor dietary intake. Increase in appetite is possible and may lead to undesired weight gain.
- Therapy for depression is usually prolonged. Emphasize the importance of follow-up exams to monitor effectiveness and side effects.
- Refer patient to psychotherapy to improve coping skills and to local support group.
- **Topical:** Instruct patient to apply a thin film of medication exactly as directed; do not use more medication than directed, apply to a larger area than directed, use more often than directed, or use longer than 8 days.
- Inform patient that topical preparation may cause burning, stinging, swelling, increased itching, or worsening of eczema. Notify health care professional if these symptoms become bothersome.
- Caution patient not to use occlusive dressings; may increase systemic absorption.
- Advise patient to notify health care professional if excessive drowsiness occurs with topical application. Number of applications per day, amount of cream applied, or area of application may be reduced. May require discontinuation of therapy.

Evaluation/Desired Outcomes

- Increased sense of well-being.
- Renewed interest in surroundings.
- Increased appetite.
- Improved energy level.
- Improved sleep.
- Decrease in anxiety.
- Decrease in chronic pain. Patients may require 2–6 wk of oral therapy before full therapeutic effects of medication are evident.
- Decrease in pruritus associated with eczema.

---

doxercalciferol, See VITAMIN D COMPOUNDS.

HIGH ALERT

DOXOrubicin hydrochloride

(dox-oh-**roo**-bi-sin hye-droe-**klor**-ide)

Adriamycin PFS, Adriamycin RDF, Rubex

Classification

Therapeutic: antineoplastics

Pharmacologic: anthracyclines

Pregnancy Category D

Indications

Alone or with other modalities in the treatment of various solid tumors including: Breast, Ovarian, Bladder, Bronchogenic carcinoma, Malignant lymphomas, and leukemias.

Action

Inhibits DNA and RNA synthesis by forming a complex with DNA; action is cell-cycle S-phase–specific. Also has immunosuppressive properties. **Therapeutic Effects:** Death of rapidly replicating cells, particularly malignant ones.

Pharmacokinetics

Absorption: Administered IV only, resulting in complete bioavailability.
Distribution: Widely distributed; does not cross the blood-brain barrier; extensively bound to tissues.
Metabolism and Excretion: Mostly metabolized by the liver. Converted by liver to an active compound. Excreted predominantly in the bile, 50% as unchanged drug. Less than 5% eliminated unchanged in the urine.
Half-life: 16.7 hr.

TIME/ACTION PROFILE (effect on blood counts)

ROUTE	ONSET	PEAK	DURATION
IV	10 days	14 days	21–24 days

Contraindications/Precautions

Contraindicated in: Hypersensitivity; Pregnancy or lactation.
Use Cautiously in: History of cardiac disease or high cumulative doses of anthracyclines; Depressed bone marrow reserve; Liver impairment (reduce dose if serum bilirubin >1.2 mg/dl); Children, geriatric patients, mediastinal radiation, concurrent cyclophosphamide (risk of cardiotoxicity); Patients with childbearing potential.

Adverse Reactions/Side Effects

Resp: recall pneumonitis. **CV:** CARDIOMYOPATHY, ECG changes. **GI:** diarrhea, esophagitis, nausea, stomatitis, vomiting. **GU:** red urine. **Derm:** alopecia, photosensitivity. **Endo:** sterility, prepubertal growth failure with temporary gonadal impairment (children only). **Hemat:** anemia, leukopenia, thrombocytopenia. **Local:** phlebitis at IV site, tissue necrosis. **Metab:** hyperuricemia. **Misc:** hypersensitivity reactions.

Interactions

Drug-Drug: ↑ bone marrow depression with other **antineoplastics** or **radiation therapy**. Pediatric patients who have received concurrent doxorubicin and **dactinomycin** have an ↑ risk of recall pneumonitis at variable times following local radiation therapy. May ↑ skin reactions at previous **radiation therapy** sites. If **paclitaxel** is administered first, clearance of doxorubicin is ↓ and the incidence and severity of neutropenia and stomatitis are ↑ (problem is diminished if doxorubicin is administered first). Hematologic toxicity is ↑ and prolonged by concurrent use of **cyclosporine**; risk of coma and seizures is also ↑. Incidence and severity of neutropenia and thrombocytopenia are ↑ by concurrent **progesterone**. **Phenobarbital** may ↑ clearance and decrease effects of doxorubicin. Doxorubicin may ↓ metabolism and ↑ effects of **phenytoin**. **Streptozocin** may ↑ the half-life of doxorubicin (dosage ↓ of doxorubicin recommended). May ↑ risk of hemorrhagic cystitis from **cyclophosphamide** or hepatitis from **mercaptopurine**. Cardiac toxicity may be ↑ by **radiation therapy** or **cyclophosphamide**. May ↓ antibody response to **live-virus vaccines** and ↑ risk of adverse reactions.

Route/Dosage

Other regimens are used.
IV (Adults): 60–75 mg/m² daily, repeat q 21 days; or 25–30 mg/m² daily for 2–3 days, repeat q 3–4 wk or 20 mg/m²/wk. Total cumulative dose should not exceed 550 mg/m² without monitoring of cardiac function or 400 mg/m² in patients with previous chest radiation or other cardiotoxic chemotherapy.
IV (Children): 30 mg/m²/day for 3 days every 4 wk.

Hepatic Impairment

IV (Adults): Serum bilirubin 1.2–3mg/dl—50% of usual dose; serum bilirubin 3.1–5 mg/dl—25% of usual dose.

Availability (generic available)

Powder for injection: 10-mg, 20-mg, 50-mg, 100-mg, 150-mg vials. **Injection:** 2 mg/ml.

NURSING IMPLICATIONS

Assessment

- Monitor blood pressure, pulse, respiratory rate, and temperature frequently during administration. Report significant changes.
- Monitor for bone marrow depression. Assess for bleeding (bleeding gums, bruising, petechiae, guaiac stools, urine, and emesis) and avoid IM injections and taking rectal temperatures if platelet count is low. Apply pressure to venipuncture sites for 10 min. Assess for signs of infection during neutropenia. Anemia

may occur. Monitor for increased fatigue, dyspnea, and orthostatic hypotension.

- Monitor intake and output ratios, and report occurrence of significant discrepancies. Encourage fluid intake of 2000–3000 ml/day. Allopurinol and alkalinization of the urine may be used to decrease serum uric acid levels and to help prevent urate stone formation.
- Severe and protracted nausea and vomiting may occur as early as 1 hr after therapy and may last 24 hr. Administer parenteral antiemetics 30–45 min prior to therapy and routinely around the clock for the next 24 hr as indicated. Monitor amount of emesis and notify physician or other health care professional if emesis exceeds guidelines to prevent dehydration.
- Monitor for development of signs of cardiac toxicity, which may be either acute and transient (ST segment depression, flattened T wave, sinus tachycardia, and extrasystoles) or late onset (usually occurs 1–6 mo after initiation of therapy) and characterized by intractable CHF (peripheral edema, dyspnea, rales/crackles, weight gain). Chest x-ray, echocardiography, ECGs, and radionuclide angiography may be ordered prior to and periodically during therapy. Cardiotoxicity is more prevalent in children younger than 2 yr and geriatric patients. Dexrazoxane may be used to prevent cardiotoxicity in patients receiving cumulative doses of >300 mg/m^2.
- Assess injection site frequently for redness, irritation, or inflammation. Doxorubicin is a vesicant but may infiltrate painlessly even if blood returns on aspiration of infusion needle. Severe tissue damage may occur if doxorubicin extravasates. If extravasation occurs, stop infusion immediately, restart, and complete dose in another vein. Local infiltration of antidote is not recommended. Apply ice packs and elevate and rest extremity for 24–48 hr to reduce swelling, then resume normal activity as tolerated. If swelling, redness, and/or pain persists beyond 48 hr, immediate consultation for possible débridement is indicated.
- Assess oral mucosa frequently for development of stomatitis. Increased dosing interval and/or decreased dosing is recommended if lesions are painful or interfere with nutrition.
- ***Lab Test Considerations:*** Monitor CBC and differential prior to, and periodically during, therapy. The WBC nadir occurs 10–14 days after administration, and recovery usually occurs by the 21st day. Thrombocytopenia and anemia may also occur. Increased dosing interval and/or decreased dose is recommended if ANC is <1000 cells/mm^3 and/or platelet count is <50,000 cells/mm^3.
- Monitor renal (BUN and creatinine) and hepatic (AST, ALT, LDH, and serum bilirubin) function prior to, and periodically during, therapy. Dose reduction is required for bilirubin >1.2 mg/dl or serum creatinine >3 mg/dl.
- May cause ↑ serum and urine uric acid concentrations.

Potential Nursing Diagnoses

Risk for infection (Adverse Reactions)
Decreased cardiac output (Adverse Reactions)

Implementation

- ***High Alert:*** Fatalities have occurred with incorrect administration of chemotherapeutic agents. Before administering, clarify all ambiguous orders; double-check single, daily, and course-of-therapy dose limits; have second practitioner independently double-check original order, calculations, and infusion pump settings. Do not confuse doxorubicin hydrochloride (Adriamycin, Rubex) with doxorubicin hydrochloride liposome (Doxil) or with daunorubicin hydrochloride (Cerubidine) or daunorubicin citrate liposome (DaunoXome) or with idarubicin. Do not confuse adriamycin with idamycin. Clarify orders that do not include generic and brand names.
- Solution should be prepared in a biologic cabinet. Wear gloves, gown, and mask while handling medication. Discard IV equipment in specially designated containers (see Appendix K).
- Aluminum needles may be used to administer doxorubicin but should not be used during storage, because prolonged contact results in discoloration of solution and formation of a dark precipitate. Solution is red.

IV Administration

- **Direct IV:** ***Diluent:*** Dilute each 10 mg with 5 ml of 0.9% NaCl (nonbacteriostatic) for injection. Shake to dissolve completely. Do not add to IV solution. Reconstituted medication is stable for 24 hr at room temperature and 48 hr if refrigerated. Protect from sunlight. ***Concentration:*** 2 mg/ml. ***Rate:*** Administer each dose over 3–5 minutes through Y-site of a free-flowing infusion of 0.9% NaCl or D5W. Facial flushing and erythema along involved vein frequently occur when administration is too rapid.

- **Syringe Compatibility:** bleomycin, cisplatin, cyclophosphamide, droperidol, leucovorin calcium, methotrexate, metoclopramide, mitomycin, vincristine.
- **Syringe Incompatibility:** furosemide, heparin.
- **Y-Site Compatibility:** amifostine, aztreonam, bleomycin, chlorpromazine, cimetidine, cisplatin, cladribine, cyclophosphamide, dexamethasone, diphenhydramine, droperidol, etoposide phosphate, famotidine, filgrastim, fludarabine, fluorouracil, gemcitabine, granisetron, hydromorphone, leucovorin calcium, linezolid, lorazepam, melphalan, methotrexate, methylprednisolone, metoclopramide, mitomycin, morphine, ondansetron, oxaliplatin, paclitaxel, prochlorperazine edisylate, promethazine, ranitidine, sargramostim, sodium bicarbonate, teniposide, thiotepa, topotecan, vinblastine, vincristine, vinorelbine.
- **Y-Site Incompatibility:** allopurinol, amphotericin B cholesteryl sulfate, cefepime, ganciclovir, lansoprazole, pemetrexed, piperacillin/tazobactam, propofol.

Patient/Family Teaching

- Instruct patient to notify health care professional promptly if fever; sore throat; signs of infection; bleeding gums; bruising; petechiae; blood in stools, urine, or emesis; increased fatigue; dyspnea; or orthostatic hypotension occurs. Caution patient to avoid crowds and persons with known infections. Instruct patient to use soft toothbrush and electric razor and to avoid falls. Caution patient not to drink alcoholic beverages or take medication containing aspirin or NSAIDs, because these may precipitate gastric bleeding.
- Instruct patient to report pain at injection site immediately.
- Instruct patient to inspect oral mucosa for erythema and ulceration. If ulceration occurs, advise patient to use sponge brush, rinse mouth with water after eating and drinking, and confer with health care professional if mouth pain interferes with eating. Pain may require treatment with opioid analgesics. The risk of developing stomatitis is greatest 5–10 days after a dose; the usual duration is 3–7 days.
- Advise patient that this medication may have teratogenic effects. Contraception should be used during and for at least 4 mo after therapy is concluded. Inform patient before initiating therapy that this medication may cause irreversible gonadal suppression.
- Instruct patient to notify health care professional immediately if irregular heartbeat, shortness of breath, swelling of lower extremities, or skin irritation (swelling, pain, or redness of feet or hands) occurs.
- Discuss the possibility of hair loss with patient. Explore methods of coping. Regrowth usually occurs 2–3 mo after discontinuation of therapy.
- Instruct patient not to receive any vaccinations without advice of health care professional.
- Inform patient that medication may cause urine to appear red for 1–2 days.
- Instruct patient to notify health care professional if skin irritation occurs at site of previous radiation therapy.
- Advise family and/or caregivers to take precautions (i.e., latex gloves) in handling body fluids for at least 5 days posttreatment.
- Emphasize the need for periodic lab tests to monitor for side effects.

Evaluation/Desired Outcomes

- Decrease in size or spread of malignancies in solid tumors.
- Improvement of hematologic status in leukemias.

HIGH ALERT

DOXOrubicin hydrochloride liposome

(dox-oh-**roo**-bi-sin hye-droe-**klor**-ide **lye**-poe-sohm)

Doxil

Classification

Therapeutic: antineoplastics

Pharmacologic: anthracyclines

Pregnancy Category D

Indications
AIDS-related Kaposi's sarcoma (KS) in patients who cannot tolerate conventional therapy. Ovarian carcinoma. Multiple myeloma with bortezomib in patients who have not previously received bortezomib and have received at least one prior therapy.

Action
Inhibits DNA and RNA synthesis by forming a complex with DNA; action is cell-cycle S-phase–specific. Also has immunosuppressive properties. Encapsulation in a liposome increases uptake by tumors, prolongs action, and may decrease some toxicity. **Therapeutic Effects:** Death of rapidly replicating cells, particularly malignant ones.

Pharmacokinetics
Absorption: Administered IV only, resulting in complete bioavailability.
Distribution: Widely distributed; does not cross the blood-brain barrier; extensively bound to tissues (↑ concentrations delivered to KS lesions due to liposomal carrier).
Metabolism and Excretion: Mostly metabolized by the liver with conversion to an active compound. Excreted mostly in bile, 50% as unchanged drug. <5% eliminated unchanged in the urine.
Half-life: 55 hr.

TIME/ACTION PROFILE (effect on blood counts)

ROUTE	ONSET	PEAK	DURATION
IV	10 days	14 days	21–24 days

Contraindications/Precautions
Contraindicated in: Hypersensitivity; OB: Pregnancy or lactation.
Use Cautiously in: Pre-existing cardiac disease or ↑ cumulative doses of anthracyclines; Depressed bone marrow reserve; Liver impairment (dose reduction required if serum bilirubin >1.2 mg/dl); Geri, Pedi: Children, geriatric patients, prior mediastinal radiation, concurrent cyclophosphamide (increased risk of cardiotoxicity); OB: Patients with childbearing potential.

Adverse Reactions/Side Effects
CNS: weakness. **CV:** CARDIOMYOPATHY. **GI:** nausea, diarrhea, increased alkaline phosphatase, moniliasis, stomatitis, vomiting. **Derm:** alopecia, palmar-plantar erythrodysesthesia. **Hemat:** anemia, leukopenia, thrombocytopenia. **Local:** injection site reactions. **Misc:** ANAPHYLACTOID ALLERGIC REACTIONS, acute infusion-related reactions, fever.

Interactions
Drug-Drug: ↑ bone marrow depression with other **antineoplastics** or **radiation therapy**. Pediatric patients who have received concurrent doxorubicin and **dactinomycin** have ↑ risk of recall pneumonitis following local radiation therapy. May ↑ skin reactions at previous **radiation therapy** sites. If **paclitaxel** is administered first, clearance of doxorubicin is ↓ and incidence and severity of neutropenia and stomatitis are ↑ (problem is less if doxorubicin is administered first). Hematologic toxicity is ↑ by concurrent use of **cyclosporine**; risk of coma and seizures is also ↑. Incidence and severity of neutropenia and thrombocytopenia are ↑ by concurrent **progesterone**. **Phenobarbital** may ↑ clearance and ↓ effects of doxorubicin. Doxorubicin may ↓ metabolism and ↑ effects of **phenytoin**. **Streptozocin** may ↑ the half-life of doxorubicin (dose reduction of doxorubicin recommended). May ↑ risk of hemorrhagic cystitis from **cyclophosphamide** or hepatitis from **mercaptopurine**. Cardiac toxicity may be ↑ by **radiation therapy** or **cyclophosphamide**. May ↓ antibody response to **live-virus vaccines** and ↑ risk of adverse reactions.

Route/Dosage
Other regimens are used.
IV (Adults): *AIDS-related KS*—20 mg/m² every 3 wk; *metastatic ovarian cancer*–40–50 mg/m² every 4 wk; *Multiple myeloma*—30 mg/m² on day 4 after following borezomib for up to 8 cycles.

Availability
Liposomal dispersion for injection: 20 mg/10 ml in 10-ml and 25 ml vials.

NURSING IMPLICATIONS

Assessment
- Monitor blood pressure, pulse, respiratory rate, and temperature frequently during administration. Report significant changes.
- Monitor for acute infusion-related reactions consisting of flushing, shortness of breath, facial swelling, headache, chills, chest pain, back pain, chest or throat tightness, fever, tachycardia, pruritus, rash, cyanosis, syncope, bronchospasm, asthma, apnea, which may be accompanied by hypotension. Reac-

tions usually resolve over 1 day and are usually limited to first dose. Slowing infusion rate may minimize this reaction. Reaction is thought to be due to liposome.

- Observe for signs and symptoms of anaphylaxis (rash, pruritus, laryngeal edema, wheezing). Discontinue doxorubicin and notify health care professional immediately if these problems occur. Keep epinephrine, an antihistamine, and resuscitation equipment close by in case of an anaphylactic reaction.
- Monitor for bone marrow depression. Assess for bleeding (bleeding gums, bruising, petechiae, guaiac stools, urine, and emesis) and avoid IM injections and taking rectal temperatures if platelet count is low. Apply pressure to venipuncture sites for 10 min. Assess for signs of infection during neutropenia. Anemia may occur. Monitor for increased fatigue, dyspnea, and orthostatic hypotension.
- Monitor intake and output ratios, and report occurrence of significant discrepancies. Encourage fluid intake of 2000–3000 ml/day. Allopurinol and alkalinization of the urine may be used to decrease serum uric acid levels and to help prevent urate stone formation.
- Severe and protracted nausea and vomiting may occur as early as 1 hr after therapy and may last 24 hr. Administer parenteral antiemetics 30–45 min prior to therapy and routinely around the clock for the next 24 hr as indicated. Monitor amount of emesis and notify health care professional if emesis exceeds guidelines to prevent dehydration.
- Monitor for development of signs of cardiac toxicity, which may be either acute and transient (ST segment depression, flattened T wave, sinus tachycardia, and extrasystoles) or late onset (usually occurs 1–6 mo after initiation of therapy) and characterized by intractable CHF (peripheral edema, dyspnea, rales/crackles, weight gain); occurs more frequently in patients receiving a cumulative dose of ≥550 mg/m². Chest x-ray, echocardiography, ECGs, and radionuclide angiography may be ordered prior to, and periodically during, therapy. Cardiotoxicity is more prevalent in children younger than 2 yr and geriatric patients. Dexrazoxane may be used to prevent cardiotoxicity in patients receiving cumulative doses of >300 mg/m².
- Assess injection site frequently for redness, irritation, or inflammation. Doxorubicin is a vesicant but may infiltrate painlessly even if blood returns on aspiration of infusion needle. Severe tissue damage may occur if doxorubicin extravasates. If extravasation occurs, stop infusion immediately, restart, and complete dose in another vein. Local infiltration of antidote is not recommended. Apply ice packs and elevate and rest extremity for 24–48 hr to reduce swelling, then resume normal activity as tolerated. If swelling, redness, and/or pain persists beyond 48 hr, immediate consultation for possible débridement is indicated.
- Assess oral mucosa frequently for development of stomatitis. Increased dosing interval and/or decreased dose is recommended if lesions are painful or interfere with nutrition.
- Monitor for skin toxicity with prolonged use; palmar-plantar erythrodysesthesia usually occurs after 6 wk of treatment and consists of swelling, pain, and erythema of the hands and feet. This may progress to desquamation but usually regresses after 2 wk. In severe cases, modification and delay of future doses of doxorubicin liposome may be necessary.
- ***Lab Test Considerations:*** Monitor CBC and differential prior to, and periodically during, therapy. The WBC nadir occurs 10–14 days after administration, and recovery usually occurs by the 21st day. Thrombocytopenia and anemia may also occur. ↑ dosing interval and/or ↓ dose is recommended if ANC is <1000 cells/mm³ and/or platelet count is <50,000 cells/mm³.
- Monitor renal (BUN and creatinine) and hepatic (AST, ALT, LDH, and serum bilirubin) function prior to and periodically during therapy. Dose reduction is required for bilirubin >1.2 mg/dl or serum creatinine >3 mg/dl.
- May cause ↑ serum and urine uric acid concentrations.

Potential Nursing Diagnoses

Risk for infection (Adverse Reactions)
Decreased cardiac output (Adverse Reactions)

Implementation

- ***High Alert:*** Fatalities have occurred with incorrect administration of chemotherapeutic agents. Before administering, clarify all ambiguous orders; double-check single, daily, and course-of-therapy dose limits; have second practitioner independently double-check original order, calculations, and infusion pump settings. Do not confuse doxorubicin hydrochloride liposome (Doxil) with doxorubicin hydrochloride (Adriamycin, Rubex) or with daunorubicin hydrochloride (Cerubidine) or daunorubicin citrate liposome (DaunoXome). Clarify orders that do not include generic and brand names.

- Prepare solution in a biologic cabinet. Wear gloves, gown, and mask while handling medication. Discard IV equipment in specially designated containers.
- Aluminum needles may be used to administer doxorubicin but should not be used during storage, because prolonged contact results in discoloration of solution and formation of a dark precipitate. Solution is red.

IV Administration

- **Intermittent Infusion:** ***Diluent:*** Dilute dose, up to 90 mg, in 250 ml of D5W. Do not dilute with other diluents or diluents containing a bacteriostatic agent. Solution is not clear, but a translucent red liposomal dispersion. Do not use in-line filters. Refrigerate diluted solutions and administer within 24 hr of dilution. ***Concentration:*** 0.36 mg/ml. ***Rate:*** Initial rate of infusion should be 1 mg/min to minimize risk of infusion reactions. If no reactions occur, increase rate to complete administration within 1 hr. Do not administer as a bolus or undiluted solution. Rapid infusion may increase infusion-related reactions.
- **Y-Site Compatibility:** acyclovir, allopurinol, aminophylline, ampicillin, aztreonam, bleomycin, butorphanol, calcium gluconate, carboplatin, cefazolin, cefepime, cefoxitin, ceftizoxime, ceftriaxone, chlorpromazine, cimetidine, ciprofloxacin, cisplatin, clindamycin, cyclophosphamide, cytarabine, dacarbazine, dexamethasone sodium phosphate, diphenhydramine, dobutamine, dopamine, droperidol, enalaprilat, etoposide, famotidine, fluconazole, fluorouracil, furosemide, ganciclovir, gentamicin, granisetron, haloperidol, heparin, hydrocortisone sodium succinate, hydromorphone, ifosfamide, leucovorin, lorazepam, magnesium sulfate, mesna, methotrexate, methylprednisolone sodium succinate, metronidazole, ondansetron, piperacillin, potassium chloride, prochlorperazine, ranitidine, ticarcillin/clavulanate, tobramycin, trimethoprim/sulfamethoxazole, vancomycin, vinblastine, vincristine, vinorelbine, zidovudine.
- **Y-Site Incompatibility:** amphotericin B, amphotericin B cholesteryl sulfate complex, buprenorphine, cefoperazone, ceftazidime, docetaxel, mannitol, meperidine, metoclopramide, mitoxantrone, morphine, ofloxacin, paclitaxel, piperacillin/tazobactam, promethazine, sodium bicarbonate.
- **Additive Incompatibility:** Do not admix with other solutions or medications.

Patient/Family Teaching

- Instruct patient to notify health care professional promptly if fever; sore throat; signs of infection; bleeding gums; bruising; petechiae; blood in stools, urine, or emesis; increased fatigue; dyspnea; or orthostatic hypotension occurs. Caution patient to avoid crowds and persons with known infections. Instruct patient to use soft toothbrush and electric razor and to avoid falls. Caution patient not to drink alcoholic beverages or take medication containing aspirin or NSAIDs; may precipitate gastric bleeding.
- Instruct patient to report pain at injection site immediately.
- Instruct patient to inspect oral mucosa for erythema and ulceration. If ulceration occurs, advise patient to use sponge brush, rinse mouth with water after eating and drinking, and confer with health care professional if mouth pain interferes with eating. Pain may require treatment with opioid analgesics. The risk of developing stomatitis is greatest 5–10 days after a dose; the usual duration is 3–7 days.
- Advise patient that this medication may have teratogenic effects. Contraception should be used during and for at least 4 mo after therapy is concluded. Inform patient before initiating therapy that this medication may cause irreversible gonadal suppression.
- Instruct patient to notify health care professional immediately if irregular heartbeat, shortness of breath, swelling of lower extremities, or skin irritation (swelling, pain, or redness of feet or hands) occurs.
- Discuss the possibility of hair loss with patient. Explore methods of coping. Regrowth usually occurs 2–3 mo after discontinuation of therapy.

- Instruct patient not to receive any vaccinations without advice of health care professional.
- Inform patient that medication may cause urine to appear red for 1–2 days.
- Instruct patient to notify health care professional if skin irritation occurs at site of previous radiation therapy.
- Advise family and/or caregivers to take precautions (i.e., latex gloves) in handling body fluids for at least 5 days posttreatment.
- Emphasize the need for periodic lab tests to monitor for side effects.

Evaluation/Desired Outcomes

- Decrease in size or spread of malignancies.
- Arrested progression of KS in patients with HIV infection.

doxycycline, See TETRACYCLINES.

droperidol (droe-per-i-dole)

Inapsine

Classification

Therapeutic: sedative/hypnotics

Pharmacologic: butyrophenones

Pregnancy Category C

Indications

Used to produce tranquilization and as an adjunct to general and regional anesthesia. **Unlabeled uses:** Useful in decreasing postoperative or postprocedure nausea and vomiting.

Action

Similar to haloperidol—alters the action of dopamine in the CNS. **Therapeutic Effects:** Tranquilization. Suppression of nausea and vomiting in selected situations.

Pharmacokinetics

Absorption: Well absorbed following IM administration.

Distribution: Appears to cross the blood-brain barrier and placenta.

Metabolism and Excretion: Mainly metabolized by the liver. Only 10% excreted unchanged by the kidneys.

Half-life: 2.2 hr.

TIME/ACTION PROFILE (sedation)

ROUTE	ONSET	PEAK	DURATION*
IM, IV	3–10 min	30 min	2–4 hr

*Listed as duration of tranquilization; alterations in consciousness may last up to 12 hr

Contraindications/Precautions

Contraindicated in: Hypersensitivity; Known intolerance; Angle-closure glaucoma; Bone marrow depression; CNS depression; Severe liver or cardiac disease; Known or suspected QT prolongation.

Use Cautiously in: Geriatric, debilitated, or severely ill patients (smaller doses should be used); Diabetic patients; Respiratory insufficiency; Prostatic hyperplasia; CNS tumors; Intestinal obstruction; Seizures (may lower seizure threshold); Severe liver disease; Pregnancy, lactation, and children <2 yr (although safety not established, droperidol has been used during cesarean section without respiratory depression in the newborn); Age >65 yr, concurrent benzodiazepines, volatile anesthetics, IV opioids (may increase risk of serious arrhythmias); use lower initial doses.

Exercise Extreme Caution in: Patients with risk factors for prolonged QT syndrome (CHF, bradycardia, diuretic use, cardiac hypertrophy, hypokalemia, hypomagnesema) or other drugs known to prolong QT interval.

Adverse Reactions/Side Effects

CNS: SEIZURES, extrapyramidal reactions, abnormal EEG, anxiety, confusion, dizziness, excessive sedation, hallucinations, hyperactivity, mental depression, nightmares, restlessness, tardive dyskinesia. **CV:** ARRHYTHMIAS (including torsades de pointes), QT prolongation. **EENT:** blurred vision, dry eyes. **Resp:** bronchospasm, laryngospasm. **CV:** hypotension, tachycardia. **GI:** constipation, dry mouth. **Misc:** chills, facial sweating, shivering.

Interactions

Drug-Drug: Additive hypotension with **antihypertensives** or **nitrates**. Additive CNS depression with other **CNS depressants**, including **alcohol**, **antihistamines**, **antidepressants**, **opioid analgesics**, and other **sedatives**. Concurrent use of **drugs known to prolong QT interval** (↑ risk of potentially life-threatening arrhythmias).

Drug-Natural Products: Concomitant use of **kava kava**, **valerian**, **chamomile**, or **hops** can ↑ CNS depression.

Route/Dosage

Premedication/Use Without Premedication in Diagnostic Procedures

IV, IM (Adults): 2.5–initially, 30–60 min prior to induction of anesthesia; additional doses of 1.25 mg IV may be needed, but should be undertaken with caution.
IM, IV (Children 2–12 yr): 0.1 mg/kg maximum initial dose.

Adjunct to General Anesthesia

IV (Adults): 2.5 mg, additional doses of 1.25 mg IV may be needed, but should be undertaken with caution.
IM, IV (Children 2–12 yr): 0.1 mg/kg maximum initial dose.

Adjunct in Regional Anesthesia

IM, IV (Adults): 2.5 mg.

Antiemetic

IV (Adults): 0.5–1.25 mg q 4 hr as needed (unlabeled).

Availability (generic available)

Injection: 2.5 mg/ml.

NURSING IMPLICATIONS

Assessment

- Monitor blood pressure and heart rate frequently during therapy. Report significant changes immediately. Hypotension may be treated with parenteral fluids if hypovolemia is a causal factor. Vasopressors (norepinephrine, phenylephrine) may be needed. Avoid use of epinephrine, because droperidol reverses its pressor effects and may cause paradoxical hypotension.
- Assess 12-lead ECG in all patients prior to administration to determine if prolonged QT interval is present. Do not administer to patients with a prolonged QT interval. Monitor ECG prior to, during, and for 2–3 hr after treatment to monitor for arrhythmias.
- Assess patient for level of sedation following administration.
- Observe patient for extrapyramidal symptoms (dystonia, oculogyric crisis, extended neck, flexed arms, tremor, restlessness, hyperactivity, anxiety) throughout therapy. Notify physician or other health care professional should these occur. An anticholinergic antiparkinsonian agent may be used to treat these symptoms.
- **Nausea and Vomiting:** Assess nausea, vomiting, hydration status, bowel sounds, and abdominal pain prior to and following administration.

Potential Nursing Diagnoses

Risk for injury (Side Effects)

Implementation

IV Administration

- **Direct IV:** ***Diluent:*** Administer undiluted. ***Concentration:*** 2.5 mg/ml. ***Rate:*** Administer each dose slowly over 30–60 sec.
- **Intermittent Infusion:** ***Diluent:*** May be added to D5W, 0.9% NaCl, or LR. ***Rate:*** Administer by slow IV infusion. Titrate according to patient response.
- **Syringe Compatibility:** atropine, bleomycin, butorphanol, chlorpromazine, cimetidine, cisplatin, cyclophosphamide, dimenhydrinate, diphenhydramine, doxorubicin, fentanyl, glycopyrrolate, hydroxyzine, meperidine, metoclopramide, midazolam, mitomycin, morphine, nalbuphine, pentazocine, perphenazine, prochlorperazine, promethazine, scopolamine, vinblastine, vincristine.
- **Syringe Incompatibility:** fluorouracil, furosemide, heparin, leucovorin calcium, methotrexate, ondansetron, pentobarbital.
- **Y-Site Compatibility:** amifostine, azithromycin, aztreonam, bivalirudin, bleomycin, buprenorphine, cisatracurium, cladribine, cisplatin, cyclophosphamide, cytarabine, dexmedetomidine, docetaxel, doxorubicin, doxorubicin liposome, etoposide, famotidine, fenoldopam, filgrastim, fluconazole, fludarabine, gemcitabine, granisetron, hydrocortisone sodium succinate, idarubicin, linezolid, melphalan, meperidine, metoclopramide, mitomycin, ondansetron, oxaliplatin, paclitaxel, potassium chloride, propofol, remifentanil, sargramostim, teniposide, thiotepa, vinblastine, vincristine, vinorelbine, vitamin B complex with C.
- **Y-Site Incompatibility:** allopurinol sodium, amphotericin B cholesteryl sulfate complex, cefepime, fluorouracil, foscarnet, furosemide, lansoprazole, leucovorin calcium, nafcillin, pemetrexed, piperacillin/tazobactam.
- **Additive Incompatibility:** barbiturates.

D

Patient/Family Teaching

- Caution patient to change positions slowly to minimize orthostatic hypotension.
- Medication causes drowsiness. Advise patient to call for assistance during ambulation and transfer.

Evaluation/Desired Outcomes

- General quiescence and reduced motor activity.
- Decreased nausea and vomiting.

drotrecogin (dro-tre-**coe**-gin)

Xigris

Classification
Therapeutic: anti-infectives
Pharmacologic: activated protein C, human

Pregnancy Category C

Indications

To reduce mortality in adult patients with sepsis.

Action

Probably acts by suppressing widespread inflammation associated with sepsis. **Therapeutic Effects:** Decrease mortality due to sepsis.

Pharmacokinetics

Absorption: IV administration results in complete bioavailability.
Distribution: Unknown.
Metabolism and Excretion: Unknown.
Half-life: Unknown.

TIME/ACTION PROFILE (activity)

ROUTE	ONSET	PEAK	DURATION
IV	unknown	end of infusion	unknown

Contraindications/Precautions

Contraindicated in: Hypersensitivity; Patients with a high risk of bleeding, including those with: active internal bleeding, recent (within 3 months) stroke, recent (within 2 months) intracranial or intraspinal injury or severe head trauma, any trauma associated with an increased risk of life-threatening bleeding, presence of an epidural catheter, intracranial neoplasm/mass lesion/cerebral herniation. Patients not expected to survive due to pre-existing medical condition(s); HIV-positive patients with CD-4 cell counts ≤50/mm³; Chronic dialysis patients; Patients who have undergone bone marrow, lung, liver, pancreas, or small bowel transplantation; OB: Lactation.

Use Cautiously in: Concurrent therapeutic heparin therapy (≥15 units/kg/hr), recent (within 3 days) thrombolytic therapy, recent (within 7 days) oral anticoagulants or glycoprotein IIb/IIIa inhibitors, recent (within 7 days) aspirin therapy >650 mg/day or other platelet inhibitors; Platelet count <30,000 x 10^6 /L; Prothrombin time—INR >3.0; Recent (within 6 wk) GI bleeding; Recent (within 3 mos) ischemic stroke; Intracranial arteriovenous malformation or aneurysm; Known bleeding diathesis; Chronic severe hepatic disease; Any other serious bleeding risk; Surgical procedures (discontinue 2 hr before; resume 12 hr after if hemostasis is achieved); OB: Pregnancy (use only if clearly needed); Pedi: Children (safety not established).

Adverse Reactions/Side Effects

Hemat: BLEEDING.

Interactions

Drug-Drug: Risk of serious bleeding may be ↑ by **antiplatelet agents**, **anticoagulants**, **thrombolytic agents**, or **other agents that may affect coagulation**.
Drug-Natural Products: Risk of bleeding may be ↑ by **arnica**, **chamomile**, **clove**, **dong quai**, **feverfew**, **garlic**, **ginger**, **gingko**, **Panax ginseng**, and others.

Route/Dosage

IV (Adults): 24 mcg/kg/hr for 96 hr.

Availability

Powder for intravenous infusion (requires reconstitution): 5-mg vial, 20-mg vial.

NURSING IMPLICATIONS

Assessment

- Assess for signs of bleeding and hemorrhage (bleeding gums; nosebleed; unusual bruising; tarry, black stools; hematuria; fall in hematocrit or blood pressure; guaiac-positive stools, urine, or nasogastric aspirate) throughout therapy. If clinically important bleeding occurs, stop drotrecogin infusion immediately. Assess other agents used that may affect coagulation. Once hemostasis is achieved, reinstitution of drotrecogin may be reconsidered.

- Assess patient for infection (vital signs; appearance of wound, sputum, urine, and stool; WBC) at beginning of and during therapy.
- ***Lab Test Considerations:*** Most patients with severe sepsis have coagulopathy prolonging activated partial thromboplastin time (aPTT) and prothrombin time (PT). Drotrecogin may also affect aPTT, but has minimal effect on PT. Use PT to monitor coagulation status of patients receiving drotrecogin.

Potential Nursing Diagnoses

Ineffective tissue perfusion, impaired (Indications)

Implementation

- Drotrecogin should be discontinued 2 hr prior to invasive surgical procedures or procedures with a risk of bleeding. Once hemostasis is achieved, drotrecogin may be started 12 hr after the procedure.

IV Administration

- **Intermittent Infusion:** Calculate dose and number of 5-mg or 20-mg vials needed (vials contain excess to facilitate delivery). Reconstitute 5-mg vials with 2.5 ml and 20-mg vials with 10 ml sterile water for injection for a concentration of 2 mg/ml. Add sterile water slowly to vial; avoid inverting or shaking. Gently swirl until powder is completely dissolved. ***Diluent:*** Reconstituted solution must be diluted further with 0.9% NaCl. Withdraw amount of reconstituted solution needed from vial and add to infusion bag of 0.9% NaCl; direct stream to side of the bag to avoid agitating solution. Gently invert bag to mix. Reconstituted solution must be used within 3 hr and IV administration must be completed within 14 hr of preparation of IV solution. Do not administer if discolored or contains particulate matter. If infusion is interrupted, restart at initial infusion rate and continue to complete recommended infusion. ***Concentration:*** 100–1000 mcg/ml. When using low concentrations (<200 mcg/ml) at low flow rates (<5 ml/hr), prime infusion set for approximately 15 min at a flow rate of 5 ml/hr. ***Rate:*** Administer at a rate of 24 mcg/kg/hr for 96 hr. Do not use bolus dosing or dose escalation.
- **Y-Site Incompatibility:** Administer via a dedicated IV line or a dedicated lumen of a multilumen central venous catheter
- **Solution Compatibility:** May be administered only with 0.9% NaCl, LR, dextrose, or dextrose/saline combinations.

Patient/Family Teaching

- Explain purpose of medication to patient.

Evaluation/Desired Outcomes

- Reduction of mortality in adult patients with severe sepsis.

duloxetine (do-**lox**-e-teen)

Cymbalta

Classification

Therapeutic: antidepressants

Pharmacologic: selective serotonin and norepinephrine reuptake inhibitors—SSNRIs

Pregnancy Category C

Indications

Major depressive disorder. Management of diabetic peripheral neuropathic pain. Generalized anxiety disorder (DPNP). **Unlabeled uses:** Stress urinary incontinence. Neuropathic pain/chronic pain. Fibromyalgia. Generalized Anxiety Disorder (GAD).

Action

Inhibits serotonin and norepinephrine reuptake in the CNS. Both antidepressant and pain inhibition are centrally mediated. **Therapeutic Effects:** Decreased depressive symptomatology. Decreased neuropathic pain. Decreased symptoms of anxiety.

Pharmacokinetics

Absorption: Well absorbed following oral administration.

Distribution: Unknown.

Protein Binding: Highly (>90%) protein-bound.

Metabolism and Excretion: Mostly metabolized, primarily by the CYP2D6 and CYP1A2 enzyme pathways.

Half-life: 12 hr.

TIME/ACTION PROFILE (blood levels)

ROUTE	ONSET	PEAK	DURATION
PO	unknown	6 hr	12 hr

Contraindications/Precautions

Contraindicated in: Hypersensitivity; Concurrent MAO inhibitor therapy; Uncontrolled angle-closure glaucoma; End stage renal disease;

Chronic hepatic impairment or substantial alcohol use (increased risk of hepatitis); Lactation: May enter breast milk; discontinue or bottle-feed.
Use Cautiously in: History of suicide attempt or ideation; History of mania (may activate mania/hypomania); Concurrent use of other centrally-acting drugs (↑ risk of adverse reactions); History of seizure disorder; Controlled angle-closure glaucoma; Diabetic patients and those with renal impairment (consider lower initial dose with gradual increase); OB: Use during third trimester may result in neonatal serotonin syndrome requiring prolonged hospitalization, respiratory and nutritional support; Pedi: May ↑ risk of suicide attempt/ideation especially during dose early treatment or dose adjustment; risk may be greater in children or adolescents (safe use in children/adolescents not established).

Adverse Reactions/Side Effects

CNS: SEIZURES, fatigue, drowsiness, insomnia, activation of mania, dizziness, nightmares. **EENT:** blurred vision, ↑ intraocular pressure. **CV:** ↑ blood pressure. **GI:** ↓ appetite, constipation, dry mouth, nausea, diarrhea, ↑ liver enzymes, gastritis, hepatitis, vomiting. **GU:** dysuria, abnormal orgasm, erectile dysfunction, ↓ libido, urinary hesitation. **Derm:** ↑ sweating, pruritus, rash. **Neuro:** tremor.

Interactions

Drug-Drug: Concurrent use with **MAO inhibitors** may result in serious potentially fatal reactions (do not use within 14 days of discontinuing MAOI. Wait at least 5 days after stopping duloxetine to start MAOI). ↑ risk of hepatotoxicity with chronic **alcohol** abuse. Drugs that affect serotonergic neurotransmitter systems, including **linezolid**, **tramadol**, and **triptans** ↑ risk of serotonin syndrome. **Drugs that inhibit CYP1A2**, including **fluvoxamine** and some **fluoroquinolones** ↑ levels of duloxetine and should be avoided. **Drugs that inhibit CYP2D6**, including **paroxetine**, **fluoxetine**, and **quinidine**, ↑ levels of duloxetine and may increase the risk of adverse reactions. Duloxetine also inhibits CYP2D6 and may ↑ levels of drugs metabolized by CYP2D6, including **tricyclic antidepressants**, **phenothiazines**, and **class 1C antiarrhythmics (propafenone** and **flecainide)**; concurrent use should be undertaken with caution. ↑ risk of serious arrhythmias with **thioridazine**; avoid concurrent use.
Drug-Natural Products: Use with **St. John's wort ↑ of serotonin syndrome.**

Route/Dosage

PO (Adults): *Antidepressant*—20–30 mg twice daily; *for neuropathic pain or generalized anxiety disorder*—60 mg once daily.

Renal Impairment

PO (Adults): start with lower dose and increase gradually.

Availability

Capsules: 20 mg, 30 mg, 60 mg. **Cost:** 20 mg $320.96/90, 30 mg $345.99/90, 60 mg $347.98/90.

NURSING IMPLICATIONS

Assessment

- Assess for sexual dysfunction (erectile dysfunction; decreased libido).
- Monitor blood pressure before and periodically during therapy. Sustained hypertension may be dose related; decrease dose or discontinue therapy if this occurs.
- Monitor appetite and nutritional intake. Weigh weekly. Report continued weight loss. Adjust diet as tolerated to support nutritional status.
- **Depression:** Assess mental status (orientation, mood, and behavior). Inform health care professional if patient demonstrates significant increase in anxiety, nervousness, or insomnia.
- Assess suicidal tendencies in both adults and children, especially in early therapy or during dose changes. Restrict amount of drug available to patient.
- **Pain:** Assess intensity, quality, and location of pain periodically during therapy. Use pain scale. May require several weeks for effects to be seen.
- ***Lab Test Considerations:*** May cause ↑ ALT, AST, bilirubin, CPK, and alkaline phosphatase.

Potential Nursing Diagnoses

Ineffective coping (Indications)
Risk for suicide (Adverse Reactions)
Chronic pain (Indications)

Implementation

- **PO:** May be administered without regard to meals. Capsules should be swallowed whole. Do not crush, chew, or open and sprinkle contents on food or liquids; may affect enteric coating.

Patient/Family Teaching

- Instruct patient to take duloxetine as directed at the same time each day. Take missed doses as soon as possible unless time for next dose. Do not stop abruptly; must be decreased gradually.
- Encourage patient and family to be alert for emergence of anxiety, agitation, panic attacks, insomnia, irritability, hostility, impulsivity, akathisia, hypomania, mania, worsening of depression and suicidal ideation, especially during early antidepressant therapy. If these symptoms occur, notify health care professional.
- May cause drowsiness. Caution patient to avoid driving or other activities requiring alertness until response to medication is known.
- Advise patient to consult health care professional prior to taking any Rx, OTC, or herbal products.
- Instruct patient to notify health care professional if signs of liver damage (pruritus, dark urine, jaundice, right upper quadrant tenderness, unexplained "flu-like" symptoms) occur.
- Advise patient to avoid taking alcohol during duloxetine therapy.
- Instruct patient to notify health care professional if pregnancy is planned or suspected or if breastfeeding.
- Refer patient/family to local support group.

Evaluation/Desired Outcomes

- Increased sense of well-being.
- Renewed interest in surroundings. Need for therapy should be periodically reassessed. Patients may notice improvement within 1–4 wks, but should be advised to continue therapy as directed. Therapy is usually continued for several months.
- Decrease in neuropathic pain associated with diabetic peripheral neuropathy.

dutasteride (doo-**tas**-te-ride)

Avodart

Classification

Therapeutic: benign prostatic hyperplasia (BPH) agents

Pharmacologic: androgen inhibitors

Pregnancy Category X

Indications

Management of the symptoms of benign prostatic hyperplasia (BPH) in men with an enlarged prostate gland.

Action

Inhibits the enzyme 5-alpha-reductase, which is responsible for converting testosterone to its potent metabolite 5-alpha-dihydrotestosterone in the prostate gland and other tissues. 5-Alpha-dihydrotestosterone is partly responsible for prostatic hyperplasia. **Therapeutic Effects:** Reduced prostate size with associated decrease in urinary symptoms.

Pharmacokinetics

Absorption: Well absorbed (60%) following oral administration; also absorbed through skin.

Distribution: 11.5% of serum concentration partitions into semen.

Protein Binding: 99% bound to albumin; 96.6 % bound to alpha-1 glycoprotein.

Metabolism and Excretion: Mostly metabolized by the liver via the CYP3A4 metabolic pathway; metabolites are excreted in feces.

Half-life: 5 wk.

TIME/ACTION PROFILE (reduction in dihydrotestosterone levels†)

ROUTE	ONSET	PEAK	DURATION
PO	unknown	1-2 wk	unknown

†Symptoms may only improve over 3–12 mo

Contraindications/Precautions

Contraindicated in: Hypersensitivity; Cross-sensitivity with other 5-alpha-reductase inhibitors may occur; Women; Children.

Use Cautiously in: Hepatic impairment.

Adverse Reactions/Side Effects

GU: decreased libido, ejaculation disorders, erectile dysfunction. **Endo:** gynecomastia.

Interactions

Drug-Drug: Blood levels and effects may be increased by **ritonavir**, **ketoconazole**, **vera-**

pamil, **diltiazem**, **cimetidine**, **ciprofloxacin**, or other **CYP3A4 enzyme inhibitors**.

Route/Dosage

PO (Adults): 0.5 mg once daily.

Availability

Soft gelatin capsules: 0.5 mg. **Cost:** $269.97/90.

NURSING IMPLICATIONS

Assessment

- Assess patient for symptoms of prostatic hyperplasia (urinary hesitancy, feeling of incomplete bladder emptying, interruption of urinary stream, impairment of size and force of urinary stream, terminal urinary dribbling, straining to start flow, dysuria, urgency) before, and periodically throughout, therapy.
- Digital rectal examinations should be performed before and periodically throughout therapy for BPH.
- ***Lab Test Considerations:*** Serum prostate-specific antigen (PSA) concentrations, which are used to screen for prostate cancer, decrease by about 20% within the 1st mo of therapy and stabilize at about 50% of the pretreatment level within 6 mo. New baseline PSA concentrations should be established at 3 and 6 mo of therapy and evaluated periodically throughout therapy.

Potential Nursing Diagnoses

Impaired urinary elimination (Indications)

Implementation

- **PO:** Administer once daily with or without meals. Do not crush, break, or chew capsule.

Patient/Family Teaching

- Instruct patient to take dutasteride at the same time each day as directed, even if symptoms improve or are unchanged. If a dose is missed, take as soon as remembered later in the day or omit dose. Do not make up by taking double doses the next day.
- Caution patient that sharing of dutasteride may be dangerous.
- Inform patient that the volume of ejaculate may be decreased during therapy but that this will not interfere with normal sexual function.
- Caution patient that dutasteride poses a potential risk to a male fetus. Women who are pregnant or may become pregnant should avoid exposure to semen of a partner taking dutasteride and should not handle dutasteride because of the potential for absorption.
- Advise patient to avoid donating blood for at least 6 mo after last dose of dutasteride to prevent a pregnant female from receiving dutasteride through a blood transfusion.
- Emphasize the importance of periodic follow-up exams to determine whether a clinical response has occurred.

Evaluation/Desired Outcomes

- Decrease in urinary symptoms of BPH.

econazole, See ANTIFUNGALS (TOPICAL).

efavirenz (e-fav-i-renz)
Sustiva

Classification
Therapeutic: antiretrovirals
Pharmacologic: non-nucleoside reverse transcriptase inhibitors

Pregnancy Category D

Indications
HIV infection (in combination with one or more other antiretroviral agents).

Action
Inhibits HIV reverse transcriptase, which results in disruption of DNA synthesis. **Therapeutic Effects:** Slowed progression of HIV infection and decreased occurrence of sequelae. Increases CD4 cell counts and decreases viral load.

Pharmacokinetics
Absorption: 50% absorbed when ingested following a high-fat meal.
Distribution: 99.5–99.75% bound to plasma proteins; enters CSF.
Metabolism and Excretion: Mostly metabolized by the liver.
Half-life: *Following single dose*—52–76 hr. *Following multiple doses*—40–55 hr.

TIME/ACTION PROFILE (blood levels)

ROUTE	ONSET	PEAK	DURATION
PO	rapid	3–5 hr	24 hr

Contraindications/Precautions
Contraindicated in: Hypersensitivity; Concurrent midazolam, triazolam, ergot derivatives, or voriconazole.
Use Cautiously in: History of mental illness or substance abuse (↑ risk of psychiatric symptomatology); History of hepatic impairment (including hepatitis B or C infection or concurrent therapy with hepatotoxic agents); Pedi: Children (increased incidence of rash); OB: Pregnancy or lactation (use in pregnancy only if other options have been exhausted; breastfeeding not recommended in HIV-infected patients).

Adverse Reactions/Side Effects
CNS: abnormal dreams, depression, dizziness, drowsiness, fatigue, headache, impaired concentration, insomnia, nervousness, psychiatric symptomatology. **GI:** nausea, abdominal pain, anorexia, diarrhea, dyspepsia, flatulence. **GU:** hematuria, renal calculi. **Derm:** RASH, increased sweating, pruritus. **Neuro:** hypoesthesia.

Interactions
Drug-Drug: ↑ levels of **midazolam, triazolam,** or **ergot alkaloids** when used concurrently; may result in potentially serious adverse reactions including arrhythmias, CNS, and respiratory depression. Induces (stimulates) the hepatic cytochrome P450 3A4 enzyme system and would be expected to influence the effects of other drugs that are metabolized by this system; efavirenz itself is also metabolized by this system. ↑ risk of CNS depression with other **CNS depressants**, including **alcohol, antidepressants, antihistamines**, and **opioid analgesics**. Concurrent use with **ritonavir** ↑ levels of both agents and the likelihood of adverse reactions, especially hepatotoxicity. May alter the effectiveness of **hormonal contraceptives**. Significantly ↓ **voriconazole** levels; concurrent use is contraindicated. ↓ **indinavir** blood levels (indinavir dosage ↑ recommended). ↓ **saquinavir** blood levels (avoid using saquinavir as the only protease inhibitor with efavirenz). May alter the effects of **warfarin**.
Drug-Natural Products: Use with **St. John's wort** may cause ↓ levels and effectiveness, including development of drug resistance.
Drug-Food: Ingestion following a high-fat meal increases absorption by 50%.

Route/Dosage
PO (Adults and Children >40 kg): 600 mg once daily.
PO (Children 32.5–40 kg): 400 mg once daily.
PO (Children 25–32.5 kg): 350 mg once daily.
PO (Children 20–25 kg): 300 mg once daily.
PO (Children 15–20 kg): 250 mg once daily.
PO (Children 10–15 kg): 200 mg once daily.

Availability
Capsules: 50 mg, 100 mg, 200 mg. **Tablets:** 600 mg. ***In combination with:*** emtricitabine and tenofovir (Atripla) (See Appendix B).

NURSING IMPLICATIONS

Assessment

- Assess for change in severity of HIV symptoms and for symptoms of opportunistic infections during therapy.
- Assess for rash, especially during 1st month of therapy. Onset is usually within 2 wk and resolves with continued therapy within 1 mo. May range from mild maculopapular with erythema and pruritus to exfoliative dermatitis and Stevens-Johnson syndrome. Occurs more often and may be more severe in children. If rash is severe or accompanied by blistering, desquamation, mucosal involvement, or fever, therapy must be discontinued immediately. Efavirenz may be reinstated concurrently with antihistamines or corticosteroids in patients discontinuing due to rash.
- Assess patient for CNS and psychiatric symptoms (dizziness, impaired concentration, somnolence, abnormal dreams, insomnia) during therapy. Symptoms usually begin during 1st or 2nd day of therapy and resolve after 2–4 wk. Administration at bedtime may minimize symptoms. Concurrent use with alcohol or psychoactive agents may cause additive CNS symptoms.
- ***Lab Test Considerations:*** Monitor viral load and CD4 cell count regularly during therapy.
- Monitor liver function tests in patients with a history of hepatitis B or C. May cause ↑ serum AST, ALT, and GGT concentrations. If moderate to severe liver function test abnormalities occur, efavirenz doses should be held until levels return to normal. Discontinue if liver function abnormalities recur when therapy is resumed.
- May cause ↑ in total cholesterol and serum triglyceride levels.
- May cause false-positive urine cannabinoid results.

Potential Nursing Diagnoses

Risk for infection (Indications)
Noncompliance (Patient/Family Teaching)

Implementation

- **PO:** May be administered with or without food. Avoid taking with a high-fat meal.

Patient/Family Teaching

- Emphasize the importance of taking efavirenz as directed. It must always be used in combination with other antiretroviral drugs. Do not take more than prescribed amount and do not stop taking without consulting health care professional. Take missed doses as soon as remembered; do not double doses.
- Instruct patient that efavirenz should not be shared with others.
- May cause dizziness, impaired concentration, or drowsiness. Caution patient to avoid driving or other activities requiring alertness until response to medication is known.
- Advise patient to avoid taking other medications, prescription or OTC, or herbal products without consulting health care professional.
- Inform patient that efavirenz does not cure AIDS or prevent associated or opportunistic infections. Efavirenz does not reduce the risk of transmission of HIV to others through sexual contact or blood contamination. Caution patient to use a condom and to avoid sharing needles or donating blood to prevent spreading the AIDS virus to others. Advise patient that the long-term effects of efavirenz are unknown at this time.
- Advise patients taking oral contraceptives to use a nonhormonal method of birth control during efavirenz therapy and to notify health care professional if they become pregnant while taking efavirenz.
- Instruct patient to notify health care professional immediately if rash occurs.
- Emphasize the importance of regular follow-up exams and blood counts to determine progress and monitor for side effects.

Evaluation/Desired Outcomes

- Delayed progression of AIDS and decreased opportunistic infections in patients with HIV.
- Decrease in viral load and increase in CD4 cell counts.

eletriptan (e-le-**trip**-tan)
Relpax

Classification
Therapeutic: vascular headache suppressants
Pharmacologic: 5-HT_1 agonists

Pregnancy Category C

Indications

Acute treatment of migraine headache.

Action

Acts as an agonist at specific 5-hydroxy-tryptamine receptor sites in intracranial blood vessels and sensory trigeminal nerves. **Therapeutic Effects:** Cranial vessel vasoconstriction with resultant decrease in migraine headache.

Pharmacokinetics

Absorption: 50% absorbed after oral administration.
Distribution: Enters breast milk.
Metabolism and Excretion: Mostly metabolized by the liver via the CYP3A4 enzyme system.
Half-life: 4 hr.

TIME/ACTION PROFILE (decreased migraine pain)

ROUTE	ONSET	PEAK	DURATION
PO	within 2 hr	2 hr	up to 24 hr

Contraindications/Precautions

Contraindicated in: Hypersensitivity; Hemiplegic or basilar migraine; Ischemic cardiovascular, cerebrovascular, or peripheral vascular syndromes (including ischemic bowel disease); History of significant cardiovascular disease; Uncontrolled hypertension; Severe hepatic impairment; Should not be used within 24 hr of other 5-HT_1 agonists or ergot-type compounds (dihydroergotamine); Should not be used within 72 hr of potent CYP3A4 inhibitors including ketoconazole, itraconazole, nefazodone, clarithromycin, ritonavir, and nelfinavir.
Use Cautiously in: Geriatric patients; Pregnancy, lactation, or children <18 yr (safety not established; use during pregnancy only if potential benefits justify potential risk to fetus).
Exercise Extreme Caution in: Cardiovascular risk factors (hypertension, hypercholesterolemia, cigarette smoking, obesity, diabetes, strong family history, menopausal women, or men >40 yr); use only if cardiovascular status has been evaluated and determined to be safe and 1st dose is administered under supervision.

Adverse Reactions/Side Effects

CNS: dizziness, drowsiness, weakness. **CV:** chest tightness/pressure. **GI:** abdominal pain, dry mouth, dysphagia, nausea. **Neuro:** paresthesia.

Interactions

Drug-Drug: Blood levels and risk of adverse reactions are increased by potent **CYP3A4 inhibitors** (including **ketoconazole**, **itraconazole**, **nefazodone**, **clarithromycin**, **ritonavir**, and **nelfinavir**); use within 72 hr is contraindicated. Concurrent use (within 24 hr of each other) with ergot-containing drugs (**dihydroergotamine**) may result in prolonged vasospastic reactions and should be avoided.

Route/Dosage

PO (Adults): 20 or 40 mg; may be repeated in 2 hr if initial response is inadequate (not to exceed 80 mg/24 hr or treatment of 3 headaches/mo).

Availability

Tablets: 20 mg, 40 mg. **Cost:** 20 mg $113.61/6, 40 mg $113.99/6.

NURSING IMPLICATIONS

Assessment

- Assess pain location, intensity, character, duration, and associated symptoms (photophonia, phonophobia, nausea, vomiting) during migraine attack.

Potential Nursing Diagnoses

Acute pain (Indications)

Implementation

- **PO:** Administer at the first sign of a headache. If after the initial dose, headache improves but then returns, dose may be repeated at least 2 hr after initial dose. If initial dose is ineffective, second dose is unlikely to be effective.

Patient/Family Teaching

- Instruct patient that eletriptan should only be used during a migraine attack. Eletriptan is used for treatment of a migraine attack, not for prevention.
- Instruct patient to take eletriptan at the first sign of a migraine, but may be administered at any time during attack. Allow at least 2 hr between doses and do not use more than 80 mg/day or 3 attacks/mo.
- Caution patient not to take eletriptan within 24 hr of other vascular headache suppressants.
- Advise patient that lying down in a darkened room after eletriptan administration may further help relieve headache.
- Advise patient to notify health care professional if she plans or suspects pregnancy, or if breastfeeding.
- Advise patient to notify health care professional before next dose of eletriptan if pain or

tightness in the chest occurs. If chest pain is severe or does not subside, notify health care professional immediately. If feelings of tingling, heat, flushing, heaviness, pressure, drowsiness, dizziness, tiredness, or sickness develop, discuss with health care provider at next visit.
- May cause drowsiness or dizziness. Caution patient to avoid driving or other activities requiring alertness until response to medication is known.
- Advise patient to avoid alcohol, which aggravates headaches, during therapy.

Evaluation/Desired Outcomes
- Relief of migraine attack.

emtricitabine
(em-tri-**si**-ti-been)
Emtriva

Classification
Therapeutic: antiretrovirals
Pharmacologic: nucleoside reverse transcriptase inhibitors

Pregnancy Category B

Indications
HIV infection (with other antiretrovirals).

Action
Phosphorylated intracellularly where it inhibits HIV reverse transcriptase, resulting in viral DNA chain termination. **Therapeutic Effects:** Slowed progression of HIV infection and decreased occurrence of sequelae. Increases CD4 cell counts and decreases viral load.

Pharmacokinetics
Absorption: Rapidly and extensively absorbed; 93% bioavailable.
Distribution: Unknown.
Metabolism and Excretion: Some metabolism, 86% renally excreted, 14% fecal excretion.
Half-life: 10 hr.

TIME/ACTION PROFILE (blood levels*)

ROUTE	ONSET	PEAK	DURATION
PO	rapid	1–2 hr	24 hr

*Normal renal function

Contraindications/Precautions
Contraindicated in: Hypersensitivity; Lactation: Lactation (breast-feeding is not recommended in HIV-infected patients); Pedi: Children <18 yr (safety not established).
Use Cautiously in: Geri: Elderly (may be at ↑ risk for adverse effects); Hepatitis B infection (may exacerbate following discontinuation); Renal impairment; OB: Pregnancy (use only if clearly needed).

Adverse Reactions/Side Effects
CNS: dizziness, headache, insomnia, weakness, depression, nightmares. **GI:** abdominal pain, diarrhea, nausea, SEVERE HEPATOMEGALY WITH STEATOSIS, dyspepsia, vomiting. **Derm:** rash, skin discoloration. **F and E:** LACTIC ACIDOSIS. **MS:** arthralgia, myalgia. **Neuro:** neuropathy, paresthesia. **Resp:** cough, rhinitis. **Misc:** fat redistribution.

Interactions
Drug-Drug: None noted.

Route/Dosage
PO (Adults ≥18 yr): 200 mg once daily.

Renal Impairment
PO (Adults ≥18 yr): *CCr 30–49 ml/min*—200 mg every 48 hr; *CCr 15–29 ml/min*—200 mg every 72 hr; *CCr <15 ml/min*—200 mg every 96 hr.

Availability
Capsules: 200 mg. **Oral solution (cotton candy flavor):** 10 mg/mL in 270-ml bottles. ***In combination with:*** efavirenz and emtricitabine (Atripla); tenofovir (Truvada). See Appendix B.

NURSING IMPLICATIONS

Assessment
- Assess patient for change in severity of HIV symptoms and for symptoms of opportunistic infections during therapy.
- May cause lactic acidosis and severe hepatomegaly with steatosis. These events are more likely to occur if patients are female, obese, or receiving nucleoside analogue medications for extended periods of time. Monitor patient for signs (increased serum lactate levels, elevated liver enzymes, liver enlargement on palpation). Therapy should be suspended if clinical or laboratory signs occur.
- Test patients for chronic hepatitis B virus (HBV) before initiating therapy. Emtricitabine is not indicated for treatment of HBV. Exacerbations of HBV have occurred upon discontinuation of emtricitabine.

- ***Lab Test Considerations:*** Monitor viral load and CD4 cell count regularly during therapy.
- May cause ↑ AST, ALT, bilirubin, creatine kinase, serum amylase, serum lipase, and triglycerides. May cause ↑ or ↓ serum glucose. May cause ↓ neutrophil count.

Potential Nursing Diagnoses

Risk for infection (Indications)
Noncompliance (Patient/Family Teaching)

Implementation

- **PO:** May be administered with or without food.

Patient/Family Teaching

- Emphasize the importance of taking emtricitabine exactly as directed. It must always be used in combination with other antiretroviral drugs. Do not take more than prescribed amount and do not stop taking without consulting health care professional. Take missed doses as soon as remembered, but not if almost time for next dose; do not double doses.
- Instruct patient that emtricitabine should not be shared with others.
- Inform patient that emtricitabine does not cure AIDS or prevent associated or opportunistic infections. Emtricitabine does not reduce the risk of transmission of HIV to others through sexual contact or blood contamination. Caution patient to use a condom and to avoid sharing needles or donating blood to prevent spreading the AIDS virus to others. Advise patient that the long-term effects of emtricitabine are unknown at this time.
- Instruct patient to notify health care professional immediately if symptoms of lactic acidosis (tiredness or weakness, unusual muscle pain, trouble breathing, stomach pain with nausea and vomiting, cold especially in arms or legs, dizziness, fast or irregular heartbeat) or if signs of hepatotoxicity (yellow skin or whites of eyes, dark urine, light colored stools, lack of appetite for several days or longer, nausea, abdominal pain) occur. These symptoms may occur more frequently in patients that are female, obese, or have been taking medications like emtricitabine for a long time.
- Inform patient that redistribution of body fat (central obesity, dorsocervical fat enlargement or buffalo hump, peripheral and facial wasting, breast enlargement, cushingoid appearance) and skin discoloration (hyperpigmentation on palms and soles) may occur.
- Emphasize the importance of regular follow-up exams and blood counts to determine progress and monitor for side effects.
- Advise patient to notify health care professional if she plans or suspects pregnancy or is breastfeeding.

Evaluation/Desired Outcomes

- Delayed progression of AIDS and decreased opportunistic infections in patients with HIV.
- Decrease in viral load and increase in CD4 cell counts.

enalapril/enalaprilat, See ANGIOTENSIN-CONVERTING ENZYME (ACE) INHIBITORS.

enfuvirtide (en-**foo**-veer-tide)

Fuzeon

Classification
Therapeutic: antiretrovirals
Pharmacologic: fusion inhibitors

Pregnancy Category B

Indications

Management of HIV infection in combination with other antiretrovirals in patients with evidence of progressive HIV-1 replication despite ongoing treatment.

Action

Prevents entry of HIV-1 into cells by interfering with the fusion of the virus with cellular membranes. **Therapeutic Effects:** Decreased replication of the HIV virus. Slowed progression of HIV infection with decreased occurrence of sequelae. Improved CD4 cell count.

Pharmacokinetics

Absorption: 84% absorbed following subcutaneous administration.
Distribution: 5.5 L.
Protein Binding: 92% bound to plasma proteins.
Metabolism and Excretion: Broken down into component amino acids and then recycled in body pool.
Half-life: 3.8 hr.

TIME/ACTION PROFILE (blood levels)

ROUTE	ONSET	PEAK	DURATION
Subcut	Unknown	8 hr	12 hr

Contraindications/Precautions

Contraindicated in: Hypersensitivity; Lactation (breast feeding not recommended in HIV-infected patients).

Use Cautiously in: Pregnancy (use only if clearly indicated); Children <6 yr (safety not established).

Adverse Reactions/Side Effects

CNS: fatigue. **EENT:** conjunctivitis. **Resp:** cough, pneumonia, sinusitis. **GI:** diarrhea, nausea, abdominal pain, anorexia, dry mouth, pancreatitis, weight loss. **Local:** injection site reactions. **MS:** myalgia, limb pain. **Misc:** hypersensitivity reactions, herpes simplex.

Interactions

Drug-Drug: None noted.

Route/Dosage

Subcut (Adults): 90 mg twice daily.

Subcut (Children 6–16 yr): 2 mg/kg twice daily (not to exceed 90 mg/dose).

Availability

Lyophilized powder for subcut administration: 108 mg/vial (to deliver a 90 mg/1 ml concentration).

NURSING IMPLICATIONS

Assessment

- Assess patient for change in severity of HIV symptoms and for symptoms of opportunistic infections throughout therapy.
- Assess patient for injection site reactions (pain, discomfort, induration, erythema, nodules and cysts, pruritus, ecchymosis). These are common, may require analgesics and limitation of physical activities.
- Assess patient for signs and symptoms of pneumonia (cough with fever, rapid breathing, dyspnea) during therapy. Notify health care professional immediately if these appear. Patients at higher risk for pneumonia include patients with low initial CD4 cell count, high initial viral load, IV drug use, smoking, and prior history of lung disease.
- Monitor patient for signs of hypersensitivity reactions (rash, fever, nausea and vomiting, chills, rigors, hypotension, elevated serum liver transaminases). If these occur, discontinue and do not restart enfuvirtide.
- ***Lab Test Considerations:*** Monitor viral load and CD4 cell count regularly during therapy.
- May cause eosinophilia, ↑ serum amylase, lipase, triglycerides, ALT, AST, creatine phosphokinase, and GGT.

Potential Nursing Diagnoses

Risk for infection (Indications)
Noncompliance (Patient/Family Teaching)

Implementation

- Reconstitute vial with 1.1 ml of sterile water for injection and gently tap vial for 10 sec and roll between hands to avoid foaming and ensure all particles come in contact with the liquid and no drug remains on vial wall. Allow vial to stand until powder goes completely into solution; may take up to 45 min or roll vial gently between hands until completely dissolved. Solutions should be clear and colorless; do not administer solutions that are discolored or contain bubbles or particulate matter. Inject immediately or refrigerate for up to 24 hr after reconstitution. Bring to room temperature and inspect solution before administering. Discard any unused drug.
- **Subcut:** Administer in the upper arm, abdomen, or anterior thigh. Rotate sites; do not inject into sites with previous injection site reactions, moles, scars, bruises, or within 2 inches of the navel.
- **Syringe Incompatibility:** Do not mix other medications in the same syringe.

Patient/Family Teaching

- Instruct patient on the correct technique for administering enfuvirtide. Review patient information sheet, preparation of dose, administration sites and technique, and disposal of equipment into a puncture-resistant container. First injection should be administered under supervision of a health care professional and technique should be re-evaluated periodically. Instruct patient to contact www.FUZEON.com or 1-877-4-FUZEON (1-877-438-9366) for more information.
- Emphasize the importance of administering enfuvirtide exactly as directed. It must always be used in combination with other antiretrovirals. Do not take more than prescribed amount and do not stop taking without consulting health care professional. If a dose is missed, take as soon as remembered then return to regular schedule. If close to time for the next dose, wait and administer next dose

as regularly scheduled; do not administer two doses at same time. If too much is administered, notify health care professional promptly.

- Instruct patient that enfuvirtide should not be shared with others.
- Inform patient that enfuvirtide does not cure AIDS or prevent opportunistic infections. Enfuvirtide does not reduce the risk of transmission of HIV to others through sexual contact or blood contamination. Caution patient to use a condom and to avoid sharing needles or donating blood. Advise patient that the long-term effects of enfuvirtide are unknown at this time.
- May cause dizziness. Caution patient to avoid driving or other activities requiring alertness until response to medication is known.
- Advise patient to notify health care professional if she plans or suspects pregnancy or if breastfeeding.
- Instruct patient to notify health care professional if signs of injection site infection (oozing, increasing heat, swelling, redness, or pain), pneumonia, or hypersensitivity occur.
- Emphasize the importance of regular follow-up exams and blood counts to determine progress and monitor for side effects.

Evaluation/Desired Outcomes

- Decreased replication of the HIV virus.
- Slowed progression of HIV infection with decreased occurrence of sequelae.
- Improved CD4 count.

enoxaparin, See HEPARINS (LOW MOLECULAR WEIGHT).

entacapone (en-**tak**-a-pone)

Comtan

Classification

Therapeutic: antiparkinson agents

Pharmacologic: catechol-O-methyltransferase inhibitors

Pregnancy Category C

Indications

With levodopa/carbidopa to treat idiopathic Parkinson's disease when signs and symptoms of end-of-dose "wearing-off" (so-called fluctuating patients) occur.

Action

Acts as a selective and reversible inhibitor of the enzyme catechol *O*-methyltransferase (COMT). Inhibition of this enzyme prevents the breakdown of levodopa, increasing availability to the CNS. **Therapeutic Effects:** Prolongs duration of response to levodopa with end-of-dose motorfluctuations. Decreased signs and symptoms of Parkinson's disease.

Pharmacokinetics

Absorption: 35% absorbed following oral administration; absorption is rapid.

Distribution: Unknown.

Protein Binding: 98%.

Metabolism and Excretion: Minimal amounts excreted unchanged; highly metabolized followed by biliary excretion.

Half-life: *Initial phase*—0.4–0.7 hr; *second phase*—2.4 hr.

TIME/ACTION PROFILE (inhibition of COMT)

ROUTE	ONSET	PEAK	DURATION
PO	unknown	unknown	up to 8 hr

Contraindications/Precautions

Contraindicated in: Hypersensitivity; Concurrent nonselective MAO inhibitor therapy.

Use Cautiously in: Hepatic impairment; Concurrent use of drugs that are metabolized by COMT; Pregnancy, lactation, or children (safety not established).

Adverse Reactions/Side Effects

CNS: NEUROLEPTIC MALIGNANT SYNDROME, dizziness, hallucinations, syncope. **Resp:** pulmonary infiltrates, pleural effusion, pleural thickening. **CV:** hypotension. **GI:** abdominal pain, diarrhea, nausea (during initiation), retroperitoneal fibrosis. **GU:** brownish-orange discoloration of urine. **MS:** RHABDOMYOLYSIS. **Neuro:** dyskinesia.

Interactions

Drug-Drug: Concurrent use with selective **MAO inhibitors** is not recommended; both agents inhibit the metabolic pathways of catecholamines. Concurrent use of drugs that are metabolized by COMT such as **isoproterenol**, **epinephrine**, **norepinephrine**, **dopamine**, **dobutamine**, and **methyldopa** may ↑ risk of tachycardia, increased blood pressure, and arrhythmias. **Probenecid**, **cholestyramine**, **erythromycin**, **rifampin**, **ampicillin**, and **chloramphenicol** may interfere with biliary elimination of entacapone; concurrent use should be undertaken with caution.

Route/Dosage

PO (Adults): 200 mg with each dose of levodopa/carbidopa up to a maximum of 8 times daily.

Availability

Tablets: 200 mg. ***In combination with:*** levodopa/carbidopa (Stalevo), see Appendix B.

NURSING IMPLICATIONS

Assessment

- Assess parkinsonian and extrapyramidal symptoms (restlessness or desire to keep moving, rigidity, tremors, pill rolling, mask-like face, shuffling gait, muscle spasms, twisting motions, difficulty speaking or swallowing, loss of balance control) prior to and during therapy. Dyskinesia may increase with therapy.
- Monitor patient for development of diarrhea. Usually occurs within 4 to 12 wk of start of therapy, but may occur as early as the first week and as late as months after initiation of therapy.
- Monitor patient for signs similar to neuroleptic malignant syndrome (elevated temperature, muscular rigidity, altered consciousness, elevated CPK). Symptoms have been associated with rapid dose reduction or withdrawal of other dopaminergic drugs. Withdrawal should be gradual.

Potential Nursing Diagnoses

Impaired physical mobility (Indications)
Risk for injury (Indications)

Implementation

- **PO:** Always administer entacapone with levodopa/carbidopa. Entacapone has no antiparkinsonism effects of its own.

Patient/Family Teaching

- Encourage patient to take entacapone as directed. Missed doses should be taken as soon as possible, up to 2 hr before the next dose. Taper gradually when discontinuing or a withdrawal reaction may occur.
- May cause dizziness or hallucinations. Advise patient to avoid driving or other activities that require alertness until response to the drug is known.
- Inform patient that nausea may occur, especially at initiation of therapy. Therapy may cause change in urine color to brownish orange.
- Caution patient to change positions slowly to minimize orthostatic hypotension.
- Instruct patient to notify health care professional if pregnancy is planned or suspected.
- Emphasize the importance of routine follow-up exams.

Evaluation/Desired Outcomes

- Decreased signs and symptoms of Parkinson's disease.

entecavir (en-tek-aveer)

Baraclude

Classification
Therapeutic: antivirals
Pharmacologic: nucleoside analogues

Pregnancy Category C

Indications

Chronic hepatitis B infection with evidence of active disease.

Action

Phosphorylated intracellularly to active form which acts as an analogue of guanosine, interfering with viral DNA synthesis. **Therapeutic Effects:** Decreased hepatic damage due to chronic hepatitis B infection.

Pharmacokinetics

Absorption: Well absorbed following oral administration.
Distribution: Extensive tissue distribution.
Metabolism and Excretion: 62–73% excreted unchanged by kidneys.
Half-life: Plasma—128–149 hr; intracellular—15 hr.

TIME/ACTION PROFILE (blood levels)

ROUTE	ONSET	PEAK	DURATION
PO	rapid	0.5–1 hr	24 hr

Contraindications/Precautions

Contraindicated in: Hypersensitivity; Lactation.
Use Cautiously in: Renal impairment (dose reduction recommended if CCr <50 mL/min; Liver transplant recipients (careful monitoring of renal function recommended); Elderly patients (may have age-related decrease in renal

function); Children <16 yr (safety not established); Pregnancy (use only if clearly needed, considering benefits and risks).

Adverse Reactions/Side Effects

CNS: dizziness, fatigue, headache. **GI:** dyspepsia, nausea. **F and E:** LACTIC ACIDOSIS.

Interactions

Drug-Drug: Concurrent use of drugs which may impair renal function may ↑ blood levels and risk of toxicity.

Route/Dosage

PO (Adults and Children >16 yr): 0.5 mg once daily; *history of lamivudine resistance*—1 mg once daily

Renal Impairment

PO (Adults and Children >16 yr): *CCr 30–50 mL/min*—0.25 mg once daily, *history of lamivudine resistance*—0.5 mg once daily; *CCr 10– <30 mL/min*—0.15 mg once daily, *history of lamivudine resistance*—0.3 mg once daily; *CCr <10 mL/min*—0.05 mg once daily, *history of lamivudine resistance*—0.1 mg once daily.

Availability

Tablets: 0.5 mg, 1 mg. **Oral solution (orange):** 0.05 mg/mL.

NURSING IMPLICATIONS

Assessment

- Monitor signs of hepatitis (jaundice, fatigue, anorexia, pruritus) during and for several months following discontinuation of therapy. Exacerbations may occur when therapy is discontinued.
- ***Lab Test Considerations:*** Monitor liver function closely during and for several months following discontinuation of therapy. May cause ↑ AST, ALT, bilirubin, amylase, lipase, creatinine and serum glucose. May cause ↓ serum albumin.

Potential Nursing Diagnoses

Risk for infection (Indications)
Noncompliance (Patient/Family Teaching)

Implementation

- **PO:** Administer on an empty stomach at least 2 hr before or after a meal. Oral solution is ready to use and should not be diluted or mixed with water or any other liquid. Hold spoon in a vertical position and fill gradually to mark corresponding to the prescribed dose. Rinse dosing spoon with water after each daily dose. Store in outer carton at room temperature. After opening, solution can be used until expiration date on bottle.

Patient/Family Teaching

- Instruct patient to read the *Patient Information* with each refill and to take entecavir as directed. Take missed doses as soon as possible unless almost time for next dose. Do not run out of entecavir, get more when supply runs low. Do not double doses. Emphasize the importance of compliance with full course of therapy, not taking more than the prescribed amount, and not discontinuing without consulting health care professional. Inform patient that hepatitis exacerbation may occur upon discontinuation of therapy. Caution patient not to share medication with others.
- Inform patient that entecavir does not cure HBV disease, but may lower the amount of HBV in the body, lower the ability of HBV to multiply and infect new liver cells, and may improve the condition of the liver. Entecavir does not reduce the risk of transmission of HBV to others through sexual contact or blood contamination. Caution patient to use a condom during sexual contact and avoid sharing needles or donating blood to prevent spreading HBV to others.
- Advise patient to notify health care professional promptly if signs of lactic acidosis (weakness or tiredness; unusual muscle pain; trouble breathing; stomach pain with nausea and vomiting; feeling cold, especially in arms or legs; dizziness, fast or irregular heartbeat) or hepatotoxicity (jaundice, dark urine, light-colored bowel movements, anorexia, nausea, lower stomach pain) occur.
- May cause dizziness. Caution patient to avoid driving or other activities requiring alertness until response to medication is known.
- Advise patient to consult health care professional before taking other Rx, OTC, or herbal products with entecavir.
- Advise patient to notify health care professional if pregnancy is planned or suspected or if breastfeeding.

- Emphasize the importance of regular follow-up exams and blood tests to determine progress and monitor for side effects.

Evaluation/Desired Outcomes

- Decreased hepatic damage due to chronic hepatitis B infection.

EPIDURAL LOCAL ANESTHETICS

bupivacaine (byoo-**pi**-vi-kane)
Marcaine, Sensorcaine

ropivacaine (**roe**-pi-vi-kane)
Naropin

Classification
Therapeutic: epidural local anesthetics, anesthetics—topical/local

Pregnancy Category B (ropivacaine), C (bupivacaine)

Indications

Local or regional anesthesia or analgesia for surgical, obstetric, or diagnostic procedures.

Action

Local anesthetics inhibit initiation and conduction of sensory nerve impulses by altering the influx of sodium and efflux of potassium in neurons, slowing or stopping pain transmission. Epidural administration allows action to take place at the level of the spinal nerve roots immediately adjacent to the site of administration. The catheter is placed as close as possible to the dermatomes (skin surface areas innervated by a single spinal nerve or group of spinal nerves) that, when blocked, will produce the most effective spread of analgesia for the site of injury.
Therapeutic Effects: Decreased pain or induction of anesthesia; low doses have minimal effect on sensory or motor function; higher doses may produce complete motor blockade.

Pharmacokinetics

Absorption: Systemic absorption follows epidural administration, but amount absorbed depends on dose.
Distribution: Agents are lipid soluble, which selectively keeps them in the epidural space and limits systemic absorption. If systemic absorption occurs, these agents are widely distributed and cross the placenta.
Metabolism and Excretion: Small amounts that may reach systemic circulation are mostly metabolized by the liver. Very little excreted unchanged in the urine.
Half-life: *Bupivacaine*—1.5–5 hr (after epidural use); *ropivacaine*—4.2 hr (after epidural use).

TIME/ACTION PROFILE (analgesia)

ROUTE	ONSET	PEAK	DURATION
Epidural	10–30 min	unknown	2-8 hr†

†Duration of anesthetic block

Contraindications/Precautions

Contraindicated in: Hypersensitivity; cross-sensitivity with other amide local anesthetics may occur (lidocaine, mepivacaine, prilocaine); Bupivacaine contains bisulfites and should be avoided in patients with known intolerance; OB: Obstetrical paracervical block anesthesia (bupivacaine only).
Use Cautiously in: Concurrent use of other local anesthetics; Liver disease; Concurrent use of anticoagulants (including low-dose heparin and low-molecular-weight heparins/heparinoids); ↑ the risk of spinal/epidural hematomas; Pedi: Children (safety not established).

Adverse Reactions/Side Effects

CNS: SEIZURES, anxiety, dizziness, headache, irritability. **EENT:** blurred vision, tinnitus. **CV:** CARDIOVASCULAR COLLAPSE, arrhythmias, bradycardia, hypotension, tachycardia. **GI:** nausea, vomiting. **GU:** urinary retention. **Derm:** pruritus. **F and E:** metabolic acidosis. **Neuro:** circumoral tingling/numbness, tremor. **Misc:** allergic reactions, fever.

Interactions

Drug-Drug: Additive toxicity may occur with concurrent use of other **amide local anesthetics** (including **lidocaine**, **mepivacaine**, and **prilocaine**). Use of bupivacaine solution containing epinephrine with **MAO inhibitors** may cause hypertension. **Fluvoxamine**, **amiodarone**, **ciprofloxacin**, and **propofol** may ↑ effects of ropivacaine.

Route/Dosage

Solutions containing preservatives should not be used for caudal or epidural blocks.

Bupivacaine

Epidural: (Adults and Children >12 yr): 10–20 ml of 0.25% (partial to moderate block), 0.5% (moderate to complete block), or 0.75% (complete block) solution. Administer in increments of 3–5 ml allowing sufficient time to detect toxic signs/symptoms of inadvertent IV or IT administration. A test dose of 2–3 ml of 0.5% with epinephrine solution is recommended prior to epidural blocks.

Ropivacaine

Surgical Anesthesia

Epidural: (Adults): *Lumbar epidural*—15–30 ml of 0.5% solution or 15–25 ml of 0.75% solution or 15–20 ml of 1% solution; *Lumbar epidural for cesarean section*—20–30 ml of 0.5% solution or 15–20 ml of 0.75% solution; *Thoracic epidural*—5–15 ml of 0.5–0.75% solution.

Labor Pain

Epidural: (Adults): *Lumbar epidural*—10–20 ml of 0.2% solution initially, then continuous infusion of 6–14 ml/hr of 0.2% solution with incremental injection of 10–15 ml/hr of 0.2% solution.

Postoperative Pain

Epidural: (Adults): *Lumbar or thoracic epidural*—Continuous infusion of 6–14 ml/hr of 0.2% solution.

Availability

Bupivacaine

Solution for injection (preservative-free): 0.25%, 0.5%, 0.75%. ***In combination with:*** epinephrine 1:200,000

Ropivacaine

Solution for injection (preservative-free): 0.2%, 0.5%, 0.75%, 1%.

NURSING IMPLICATIONS

Assessment

- **Systemic Toxicity:** Assess for systemic toxicity (circumoral tingling and numbness, ringing in ears, metallic taste, dizziness, blurred vision, tremors, slow speech, irritability, twitching, seizures, cardiac dysrhythmias) each shift. Report to physician or other health care professional.
- **Orthostatic Hypotension:** Monitor blood pressure, heart rate, and respiratory rate continuously while patient is receiving this medication. Mild hypotension is common because of the effect of local anesthetic block of nerve fibers on the sympathetic nervous system, causing vasodilation. Significant hypotension and bradycardia may occur, especially when rising from a prone position or following large dose increases or boluses. Treatment of unresolved hypotension may include hydration, decreasing the epidural infusion rate, and/or removal of local anesthetic from analgesic solution.
- **Unwanted Motor and Sensory Deficit:** The goal of adding low-dose local anesthetics to epidural opioids for pain management is to provide analgesia, not to produce anesthesia. Patients should be able to ambulate if their condition allows, and epidural analgesic should not hamper this important recovery activity. However, many factors, including location of the epidural catheter, local anesthetic dose, and variability in patient response, can result in patients experiencing unwanted motor and sensory deficits. Pain is the first sensation lost, followed by temperature, touch, proprioception, and skeletal muscle tone.
- Assess for sensory deficit every shift. Ask patient to point to numb and tingling skin areas (numbness and tingling at the incision site is common and usually normal). Notify physician or other health care professional of unwanted motor and sensory deficits
- Unwanted motor and sensory deficits often can be corrected with simple treatment. For example, a change in position may relieve temporary sensory loss in an extremity. Minor extremity muscle weakness is often treated by decreasing the epidural infusion rate and keeping the patient in bed until the weakness resolves. Sometimes removing the local anesthetic from the analgesic solution is necessary, such as when signs of local anesthetic toxicity are detected or when simple treatment of motor and sensory deficits has been unsuccessful.

Potential Nursing Diagnoses

Acute pain, acute (Indications)
Impaired physical mobility (Side Effects)

Implementation

- See Route and Dosage section.

Patient/Family Teaching

- Instruct patient to notify nurse if signs or symptoms of systemic toxicity occur.
- Advise patient to request assistance during ambulation until orthostatic hypotension and motor deficits are ruled out.

Evaluation/Desired Outcomes

- Decrease in postoperative pain without unwanted sensory or motor deficits.

HIGH ALERT

epinephrine (e-pi-**nef**-rin)
Adrenalin, Ana-Guard, Asthma-Haler Mist, AsthmaNefrin (racepinephrine), EpiPen, microNefrin, Nephron, Primatene, Sus-Phrine, S-2

Classification
Therapeutic: antiasthmatics, bronchodilators, vasopressors
Pharmacologic: adrenergics

Pregnancy Category C

See Appendix C for ophthalmic use

Indications

Subcut, IV, Inhaln: Management of reversible airway disease due to asthma or COPD. **Subcut, IV:** Management of severe allergic reactions. **IV, Intracardiac, Intratracheal, Intraosseous (part of advanced cardiac life support [ACLS] and pediatric advanced life support [PALS] guidelines):** Management of cardiac arrest (unlabeled). **Inhaln:** Management of upper airway obstruction and croup (racemic epinephrine). **Local/Spinal:** Adjunct in the localization/prolongation of anesthesia.

Action

Results in the accumulation of cyclic adenosine monophosphate (cAMP) at beta-adrenergic receptors. Affects both $beta_1$ (cardiac)-adrenergic receptors and $beta_2$ (pulmonary)-adrenergic receptor sites. Produces bronchodilation. Also has alpha-adrenergic agonist properties, which result in vasoconstriction. Inhibits the release of mediators of immediate hypersensitivity reactions from mast cells. **Therapeutic Effects:** Bronchodilation. Maintenance of heart rate and blood pressure. Localization/prolongation of local/spinal anesthetic.

Pharmacokinetics

Absorption: Well absorbed following subcut administration; some absorption may occur following repeated inhalation of large doses.
Distribution: Does not cross the blood-brain barrier; crosses the placenta and enters breast milk.
Metabolism and Excretion: Action is rapidly terminated by metabolism and uptake by nerve endings.
Half-life: Unknown.

TIME/ACTION PROFILE (bronchodilation)

ROUTE	ONSET	PEAK	DURATION
Inhaln	1 min	unknown	1–3 hr
Subcut	5–10 min	20 min	<1–4 hr
IM	6–12 min	unknown	<1–4 hr
IV	rapid	20 min	20–30 min

Contraindications/Precautions

Contraindicated in: Hypersensitivity to adrenergic amines; Cardiac arrhythmias; Some products may contain bisulfites or fluorocarbons (in some inhalers) and should be avoided in patients with known hypersensitivity or intolerance.
Use Cautiously in: Cardiac disease (angina, tachycardia, MI); Hypertension; Hyperthyroidism; Diabetes; Cerebral arteriosclerosis; Glaucoma (except for ophthalmic use); Elderly patients (more susceptible to adverse reactions; may require dosage reduction); Pregnancy (near term) and lactation; Excessive use may lead to tolerance and paradoxical bronchospasm (inhaler).

Adverse Reactions/Side Effects

CNS: nervousness, restlessness, tremor, headache, insomnia. **Resp:** paradoxical bronchospasm (excessive use of inhalers). **CV:** angina, arrhythmias, hypertension, tachycardia. **GI:** nausea, vomiting. **Endo:** hyperglycemia.

Interactions

Drug-Drug: Concurrent use with other **adrenergic agents** will have additive adrenergic side effects. Use with **MAO inhibitors** may lead to hypertensive crisis. **Beta blockers** may negate therapeutic effect. **Tricyclic antidepressants** enhance pressor response to epinephrine.
Drug-Natural Products: Use with caffeine-containing herbs (**cola nut**, **guarana**, **mate**, **tea**, **coffee**) ↑ stimulant effect.

Route/Dosage

Subcut, IM (Adults): *Anaphylactic reactions/asthma*—0.1–0.5 mg (single dose not to exceed 1 mg); may repeat q 10–15 min for anaphylactic shock or q 20 min–4 hr for asthma.
Subcut (Children >1 month): *Anaphylactic reactions/asthma*—0.01 mg/kg (not to exceed 0.5 mg/dose) q 15 min for 2 doses, then q 4 hr.
IV (Adults): *Severe anaphylaxis*—0.1–0.25 mg q 5–15 min; may be followed by 1–4 mcg/

min continuous infusion; *cardiopulmonary resuscitation (ACLS guidelines)*—1 mg q 3–5 min; *bradycardia (ACLS guidelines)*—2–10 mcg/min).

IV (Children): *Severe anaphylaxis*—0.1 mg (less in younger children); may be followed by 0.1 mcg/kg/min continuous infusion (may be increased up to 1.5 mcg/kg/min); *symptomatic bradycardia/pulseless arrest (PALS guidelines)*—0.01 mg/kg, may be repeated q 3–5 min higher doses (up to 0.1–0.2 mg/kg) may be considered; may also be given by the intraosseous route. May also be given by the endotracheal route in doses of 0.1–0.2 mg/kg diluted to a volume of 3–5 ml with normal saline followed by several positive pressure ventilations.

Inhaln (Adults): *Metered-dose inhaler*—1 inhalation (160–250 mcg), may be repeated after 1–2 min; additional doses may be repeated q 3 hr; *inhalation solution*—1 inhalation of 1% solution; may be repeated after 1–2 min; additional doses may be given q 3 hr; *racepinephrine*—Via hand nebulizer, 2–3 inhalations of 2.25% solution; may repeat in 5 min with 2–3 more inhalations, up to 4–6 times daily.

Inhaln (Children >1 month): 0.25–0.5 mL of 2.25% racemic epinephrine solution diluted in 3 ml normal saline.

IV, Intratracheal (Neonates): 0.01–0.03 mg/kg q 3–5 min as needed.

IM (Children >1 month <30 kg): 0.15 mg (EpiPen Jr); >30 kg: 0.3 mg (EpiPen).

Intracardiac (Adults): 0.3–0.5 mg.

Endotracheal (Adults): *Cardiopulmonary resuscitation (ACLS guidelines)*—2–2.5 mg.

Topical (Adults and Children ≥6 yr): *Nasal decongestant*—Apply 1% solution as drops, spray, or with a swab.

Intraspinal (Adults and Children): 0.2–0.4 ml of 1:1000 solution.

With Local Anesthetics (Adults and Children): Use 1:200,000 solution with local anesthetic.

Availability (generic available)

Inhalation aerosol: 0.125% (≥300 inhalations/15 ml)OTC, 0.5% (≥300 inhalations/15 ml)OTC, 300 mcg/spray (≥300 inhalations/15 ml)OTC. **Inhalation solution:** 1%OTC. **Injection:** 0.1 mg/ml (1:10,000), 1 mg/ml (1:1000). **Auto-injector (EpiPen):** 0.15 mg/0.3 ml (1:2000), 0.3 mg/0.3 ml (1:1000). **Cost:** 0.15 mg $56.48/syringe, 0.3 mg $58.99/syringe. **Topical solution:** 0.1%.

NURSING IMPLICATIONS

Assessment

- **Bronchodilator:** Assess lung sounds, respiratory pattern, pulse, and blood pressure before administration and during peak of medication. Note amount, color, and character of sputum produced, and notify health care professional of abnormal findings.
- Monitor pulmonary function tests before and periodically throughout therapy to determine effectiveness of medication.
- Observe for paradoxical bronchospasm (wheezing). If condition occurs, withhold medication and notify health care professional immediately.
- Observe patient for drug tolerance and rebound bronchospasm. Patients requiring more than 3 inhalation treatments in 24 hr should be under close supervision. If minimal or no relief is seen after 3–5 inhalation treatments within 6–12 hr, further treatment with aerosol alone is not recommended
- Assess for hypersensitivity reaction (rash; urticaria; swelling of the face, lips, or eyelids). If condition occurs, withhold medication and notify health care professional immediately.
- **Vasopressor:** Monitor blood pressure, pulse, ECG, and respiratory rate frequently during IV administration. Continuous ECG monitoring, hemodynamic parameters, and urine output should be monitored continuously during IV administration.
- Monitor for chest pain, arrhythmias, heart rate >110 bpm, and hypertension. Consult physician for parameters of pulse, blood pressure, and ECG changes for adjusting dosage or discontinuing medication.
- **Shock:** Assess volume status. Hypovolemia should be corrected prior to administering epinephrine IV.
- **Nasal Decongestant:** Assess patient for nasal and sinus congestion prior to and periodically during therapy.
- ***Lab Test Considerations:*** May cause transient ↓ in serum potassium concentrations with nebulization or at higher than recommended doses.

- May cause an ↑ in blood glucose and serum lactic acid concentrations.
- ***Toxicity and Overdose:*** Symptoms of overdose include persistent agitation, chest pain or discomfort, decreased blood pressure, dizziness, hyperglycemia, hypokalemia, seizures, tachyarrhythmias, persistent trembling, and vomiting, Treatment includes discontinuing adrenergic bronchodilator and other beta-adrenergic agonists and symptomatic, supportive therapy. Cardioselective beta blockers are used cautiously, because they may induce bronchospasm.

Potential Nursing Diagnoses

Ineffective airway clearance (Indications)
Ineffective tissue perfusion (Indications)

Implementation

- ***High Alert:*** Patient harm or fatalities have occurred from medication errors with epinephrine. Epinephrine is available in various concentrations, strengths, and percentages and is used for different purposes. Packaging labels may be easily confused or the products incorrectly diluted. Dilutions should be prepared by a pharmacist. IV doses should be expressed in milligrams not ampules, concentration, or volume. Prior to administration, have second practitioner independently check original order, dose calculations, concentration, route of administration, and infusion pump settings.
- Medication should be administered promptly at the onset of bronchospasm.
- Use a tuberculin syringe with a 26-gauge ½-in. needle for subcut injection to ensure that correct amount of medication is administered.
- Tolerance may develop with prolonged or excessive use. Effectiveness may be restored by discontinuing for a few days and then readministering.
- Do not use solutions that are pinkish or brownish or that contain a precipitate.
- For anaphylactic shock, volume replacement should be administered concurrently with epinephrine. Antihistamines and corticosteroids may be used in conjunction with epinephrine.
- **IM, Subcut:** Medication can cause irritation of tissue. Rotate injection sites to prevent tissue necrosis. Massage injection sites well after administration to enhance absorption and to decrease local vasoconstriction. Avoid IM administration in gluteal muscle.

IV Administration

- **Direct IV:** ***Diluent:*** The 1:10,000 solution can be administered undiluted. Dilute 1 mg (1 ml) of a 1:1000 solution in 9 ml of 0.9% NaCl to prepare a 1:10,000 solution. ***Concentration:*** 0.1 mg/ml (1:10,000). ***Rate:*** Administer each 1 mg (10 ml) of a 1:10,000 solution over at least 1 min; more rapid administration may be used during cardiac resuscitation. Follow each dose with 20 ml IV saline flush.
- **Continuous Infusion:** ***Diluent:*** Dilute 1 mg (1 ml) of a 1:1000 solution in 250 ml of D5W or 0.9% NaCl. Protect from light. Infusion stable for 24 hr. ***Concentration:*** 4 mcg/ml. ***Rate:*** See Route/Dosage section. Titrate to response (blood pressure, heart rate, respiratory rate).
- **Y-Site Compatibility:** amikacin, amiodarone, anidulafungin, atracurium, atropine, aztreonam, bivalirudin, bumetanide, calcium chloride, calcium gluconate, caspofungin, cefazolin, cefotaxime, cefoxitin, ceftazidime, ceftizoxime, ceftriaxone, cefuroxime, chloramphenicol, cimetidine, cisatracurium, clindamycin, cyclosporine, daptomycin, dexamethasone sodium phosphate, dexmedetomidine, digoxin, diltiazem, diphenhydramine, dobutamine, dopamine, doxycycline, enalaprilat, ertapenem, erythromycin, esmolol, famotidine, fenoldopam, fentanyl, fluconazole, furosemide, gentamicin, granisetron, heparin, hydrocortisone sodium succinate, hydromorphone, imipenem/cilastatin, inamrinone, isoproterenol, ketorolac, labetalol, levofloxacin, lidocaine, linezolid, lorazepam, magnesium sulfate, meperidine, methylprednisolone sodium succinate, metoclopramide, metoprolol, metronidazole, midazolam, milrinone, morphine, nafcillin, nicardipine, nitroglycerin, nitroprusside, norepinephrine, ondansetron, palonosetron, pancuronium, pantoprazole, penicillin G potassium, phenylephrine, phytonadione, piperacillin/tazobactam, potassium chloride, procainamide, prochlorperazine, promethazine, propofol, propranolol, protamine, quinupristin/dalfopristin, ranitidine, remifentanil, tacrolimus, ticarcillin/clavulanate, tigecycline, tirofiban, tobramycin, vancomycin, vasopressin, vecuronium, verapamil, vitamin B complex with C, voriconazole, warfarin.
- **Y-Site Incompatibility:** acyclovir, aminophylline, ampicillin, diazepam, ganciclovir,

micafungin, phenytoin, sodium bicarbonate, thiopental, trimethoprim/sulfamethoxazole.

- **Inhaln:** When using epinephrine inhalation solution, 10 drops of 1% base solution should be placed in the reservoir of the nebulizer.
- The 2.25% inhalation solution of racepinephrine must be diluted for use in the combination nebulizer/respirator.
- Allow 1–2 min to elapse between inhalations of epinephrine inhalation solution, epinephrine inhalation aerosol, or epinephrine bitartrate inhalation aerosol to make certain the second inhalation is necessary.
- When epinephrine is used concurrently with corticosteroid or ipratropium inhalations, administer bronchodilator first and other medications 5 min apart to prevent toxicity from inhaled fluorocarbon propellants.
- **Endotracheal:** Epinephrine can be injected directly into the bronchial tree via the endotracheal tube if the patient has been intubated. Perform 5 rapid insufflations; forcefully administer 10 ml containing 2–2.5 mg epinephrine (1 mg/ml) directly into tube; follow with 5 quick insufflations.

Patient/Family Teaching

- Instruct patient to take medication exactly as directed. If on a scheduled dosing regimen, take a missed dose as soon as possible; space remaining doses at regular intervals. Do not double doses. Caution patient not to exceed recommended dose; may cause adverse effects, paradoxical bronchospasm, or loss of effectiveness of medication.
- Instruct patient to contact health care professional immediately if shortness of breath is not relieved by medication or is accompanied by diaphoresis, dizziness, palpitations, or chest pain.
- Advise patient to consult health care professional before taking any OTC medications or alcoholic beverages concurrently with this therapy. Caution patient also to avoid smoking and other respiratory irritants.
- **Inhaln:** Review correct administration technique (aerosolization, IPPB, metered-dose inhaler) with patient. See Appendix D for administration with metered-dose inhaler. Wait 1–5 min before administering next dose. Mouthpiece should be washed after each use.
- Do not spray inhaler near eyes.
- Instruct patient to save inhaler; refill canisters may be available.
- Advise patients to use bronchodilator first if using other inhalation medications, and allow 5 min to elapse before administering other inhalant medications, unless otherwise directed.
- Advise patient to rinse mouth with water after each inhalation dose to minimize dry mouth.
- Advise patient to maintain adequate fluid intake (2000–3000 ml/day) to help liquefy tenacious secretions.
- Advise patient to consult health care professional if respiratory symptoms are not relieved or worsen after treatment or if chest pain, headache, severe dizziness, palpitations, nervousness, or weakness occurs.
- Instruct patient to notify health care professional if contents of one canister are used up in less than 2 wk.
- **Auto-injector:** Instruct patients using auto-injector for anaphylactic reactions to remove gray safety cap, placing black tip on thigh at right angle to leg. Press hard into thigh until auto-injector functions, hold in place several seconds, remove, and discard properly. Massage injected area for 10 sec. Pedi: Teach parents or caregivers signs and symptoms of anaphlyaxis, how to use auto-injector safely, and to get the child to a hospital as soon as possible. Instruct parents or caregivers to teach child how to manage his or her allergy, how to self inject, and what to do in an emergency. For children too young to self-inject and who will be separated from parent, tell parents to always discuss allergy and use of auto-injector with responsible adult.

Evaluation/Desired Outcomes

- Prevention or relief of bronchospasm.
- Increase in ease of breathing.
- Prevention of bronchospasm or reduction of frequency of acute asthma attacks in patients with chronic asthma.
- Prevention of exercise-induced asthma.
- Reversal of signs and symptoms of anaphylaxis.
- Increase in cardiac rate and output, when used in cardiac resuscitation.
- Increase in blood pressure, when used as a vasopressor.

E

- Localization of local anesthetic.
- Decrease in sinus and nasal congestion.

HIGH ALERT

epirubicin (ep-i-**roo**-bi-sin)
Ellence

Classification
Therapeutic: antineoplastics
Pharmacologic: anthracyclines

Pregnancy Category D

Indications
A component of adjuvant therapy for evidence of axillary tumor involvement following resection of primary breast cancer.

Action
Inhibits DNA and RNA synthesis by forming a complex with DNA. **Therapeutic Effects:** Death of rapidly replicating cells, particularly malignant ones.

Pharmacokinetics
Absorption: IV administration results in complete bioavailability.
Distribution: Rapidly and widely distributed; concentrates in RBCs.
Metabolism and Excretion: Extensively and rapidly metabolized by the liver and other tissues.
Half-life: 35 hr.

TIME/ACTION PROFILE (effect on WBCs)

ROUTE	ONSET	PEAK	DURATION
IV	unknown	10–14 days	21 days

Contraindications/Precautions
Contraindicated in: Hypersensitivity to epirubicin, other anthracyclines, or related compounds; Baseline neutrophil count <1500 cells/mm^3; Severe myocardial insufficiency or recent MI; Previous anthracyclines up to the maximum cumulative dose; Severe hepatic dysfunction; OB: Pregnancy or lactation; Concurrent cimetidine therapy.
Use Cautiously in: Severe renal impairment (serum creatinine >5 mg/dl); lower doses should be considered; Hepatic impairment (dose reduction recommended for bilirubin >1.2 mg/dl or AST >2–4 times upper limit of normal); Female patients ≥70 yr (increased risk of toxicity); Depressed bone marrow reserve; OB: Patients with childbearing potential; Pedi: Pediatric patients (safety not established; increased risk of acute cardiotoxicity and chronic CHF).

Adverse Reactions/Side Effects
CNS: lethargy. **CV:** CARDIOTOXICITY (dose-related). **GI:** nausea, vomiting, anorexia, diarrhea, mucositis. **Derm:** alopecia, flushing, itching, photosensitivity, radiation-recall reaction, rash, skin/nail hyperpigmentation. **Endo:** gonadal suppression. **Hemat:** LEUKOPENIA, anemia, thrombocytopenia, treatment-related leukemia/myelodysplastic syndromes. **Local:** injection site reactions, phlebitis at IV site, tissue necrosis. **Metab:** hot flashes, hyperuricemia. **Misc:** ANAPHYLAXIS, INFECTION.

Interactions
Drug-Drug: Cimetidine increases blood levels and the risk of serious toxicity; concurrent use should be avoided. Additive hematologic and gastrointestinal toxicity with other **antineoplastics** or **radiation therapy**. May decrease the antibody response to **live-virus vaccines** and increase the risk of adverse reactions.

Route/Dosage
IV (Adults): 100–120 mg/m^2 repeated in 3–4 wk cycles (total dose may be given on day 1 or split and given in equally divided doses on day 1 and day 8 of each cycle (combination regimens may employ concurrent 5-fluorouracil and cyclophosphamide).

Hepatic Impairment
IV (Adults): *Bilirubin 1.2—3 mg/dl or AST 2–4 times upper limit of normal*—use 50% of recommended starting dose; *bilirubin >3 mg/dl or AST >4 times upper limit of normal*—use 25% of recommended starting dose.

Availability
Solution for injection (red): 50-mg/25-ml single-use vial, 200-mg/100-ml single-use vial.

NURSING IMPLICATIONS

Assessment
- Monitor for bone marrow depression. Assess for bleeding (bleeding gums, bruising, petechiae, guaiac stools, urine, and emesis) and avoid IM injections and taking rectal temperatures if platelet count is low. Apply pressure to venipuncture sites for 10 min. Assess for signs of infection during neutropenia. Anemia may occur. Monitor for increased fatigue, dyspnea, and orthostatic hypotension.

- Severe nausea and vomiting may occur. Parenteral antiemetic agents should be administered 30–45 min prior to therapy and routinely around the clock for the next 24 hr as indicated. Monitor amount of emesis and notify physician or other health care professional if emesis exceeds guidelines to prevent dehydration.
- Cardiac function, measured by ECG and a multigated radionuclide angiography (MUGA) scan or an ECHO, should be measured prior to therapy. Repeated evaluations of left ventricular ejection fraction should be performed during therapy. Monitor for development of signs of cardiac toxicity, which may occur early (ST-T wave changes, sinus tachycardia, and extrasystoles) or late (may occur months to years after termination of therapy). Delayed cardiac toxicity is characterized by cardiomyopathy, tachycardia, peripheral edema, dyspnea, rales/crackles, weight gain, hepatomegaly, ascites, pleural effusion. Toxicity is usually dependent on cumulative dose.
- Assess injection site frequently for redness, irritation, or inflammation. Burning or stinging during infusion may indicate infiltration and infusion should be discontinued and restarted in another vein. Epirubicin is a vesicant but may infiltrate painlessly even if blood returns on aspiration of infusion needle. Severe tissue damage may occur if epirubicin extravasates. If extravasation occurs, stop infusion immediately, restart, and complete dose in another vein.
- Assess oral mucosa frequently for development of stomatitis (pain, burning, erythema, ulcerations, bleeding, infection). Increased dosing interval and/or decreased dosing is recommended if lesions are painful or interfere with nutrition.
- ***Lab Test Considerations:*** Monitor CBC and differential before and during each cycle of therapy. Epirubicin should not be administered to patients with a baseline neutrophil count <1500 cells/mm^3. The WBC nadir occurs 10–14 days after administration, and recovery usually occurs by the 21st day. Severe thrombocytopenia and anemia may also occur.
- Monitor renal (BUN and creatinine) and hepatic (AST, ALT, LDH, and serum bilirubin) function prior to and periodically during therapy. Dose reduction is required for bilirubin >1.2 mg/dl, AST 2–4 times the upper limit of normal, or serum creatinine >5 mg/dl.

Potential Nursing Diagnoses

Risk for infection (Adverse Reactions)
Decreased cardiac output (Adverse Reactions)

Implementation

- ***High Alert:*** Fatalities have occurred with incorrect administration of chemotherapeutic agents. Before administering, clarify all ambiguous orders; double-check single, daily, and course-of-therapy dose limits; have second practitioner independently double-check original order, calculations and infusion pump settings. Epirubicin should be administered only under the supervision of a physician experienced in the use of cancer chemotherapeutic agents.
- Solution should be prepared in a biologic cabinet. Wear gloves, gown, and mask while handling medication. Discard IV equipment in specially designated containers.
- Prophylactic anti-infective therapy with trimethoprim/sulfamethoxazole or a fluoroquinolone and antiemetic therapy should be administered prior to administration of epirubicin.
- Do not administer subcut or IM.

IV Administration

- **Intermittent Infusion:** ***Diluent:*** Administer undiluted. Solution is clear red. Use epirubicin within 24 hr of penetration of rubber stopper. Discard unused solution. ***Concentration:*** 2 mg/ml. ***Rate:*** Administer initial dose of 100–120 mg/m^2 over 15–20 min through Y-site of a free-flowing infusion of 0.9% NaCl or D5W. Lower doses may be infused for shorter periods, but not less than over 3 min. Do not administer via direct IV push. Facial flushing and erythema along involved vein frequently occur when administration is too rapid. Venous sclerosis may result from injection into a small vein or repeated injections into the same vein. Avoid veins over joints or in extremities with compromised venous or lymphatic drainage.
- **Syringe Incompatibility:** Do not mix in syringe with other drugs or with alkaline solutions, fluorouracil, heparin, ifosfamide.

- **Y-Site Compatibility:** oxaliplatin.

Patient/Family Teaching

- Instruct patient to notify health care professional promptly if fever; sore throat; signs of infection; bleeding gums; bruising; petechiae; blood in stools, urine, or emesis; increased fatigue; dyspnea; or orthostatic hypotension occurs. Caution patient to avoid crowds and persons with known infections. Instruct patient to use soft toothbrush and electric razor and to avoid falls. Patient should be cautioned not to drink alcoholic beverages or take medication containing aspirin or NSAIDs, because these may precipitate gastric bleeding.
- Instruct patient to report pain at injection site immediately.
- Instruct patient to inspect oral mucosa for erythema and ulceration. If ulceration occurs, advise patient to use sponge brush, rinse mouth with water after eating and drinking, and confer with health care professional if mouth pain interferes with eating. Pain may require treatment with opioid analgesics. Patients usually recover by the third week of therapy.
- Advise patient that this medication may have teratogenic effects. Contraception should be used during and for at least 4 mo after therapy is concluded. Inform patient before initiating therapy that this medication may cause irreversible gonadal suppression.
- Instruct patient to avoid taking cimetidine, OTC or Rx, during therapy, and to consult health care professional prior to taking other Rx, OTC, or herbal products.
- Instruct patient to notify health care professional immediately if vomiting, dehydration, fever, evidence of infection, symptoms of CHF, or pain at injection site occurs. Patients should be informed of the risk of irreversible cardiac damage and treatment-related leukemia.
- Discuss the possibility of hair loss with patient. Explore methods of coping. Regrowth usually occurs 2–3 month after discontinuation of therapy.
- Instruct patient not to receive any vaccinations without advice of health care professional.
- Inform patient that medication may cause urine to appear red for 1–2 days.
- Instruct patient to notify health care professional if skin irritation occurs at site of previous radiation therapy. May cause hyperpigmentation of the skin and nails. Advise patient to use sunscreen and protective clothing to prevent photosensitivity reactions.
- Emphasize the need for periodic lab tests to monitor for side effects.

Evaluation/Desired Outcomes

- Decrease in size or spread of malignancies in patients with axillary node tumor involvement following resection of primary breast cancer.

eplerenone (e-**ple**-re-none)

Inspra

Classification

Therapeutic: antihypertensives

Pharmacologic: aldosterone antagonists

Pregnancy Category B

Indications

Hypertension (alone, or with other agents).

Action

Blocks the effects of aldosterone by attaching to mineralocorticoid receptors. **Therapeutic Effects:** Lowering of blood pressure.

Pharmacokinetics

Absorption: Well absorbed following oral administration.

Distribution: Unknown.

Metabolism and Excretion: Mostly metabolized by the liver (CYP3A4 enzyme system); <5% excreted unchanged by the kidneys.

Half-life: 4–6 hr.

TIME/ACTION PROFILE (antihypertensive effect)

ROUTE	ONSET	PEAK	DURATION
PO	Unknown	4 wk	Unknown

Contraindications/Precautions

Contraindicated in: Serum potassium >5.5 mEq/L; Type 2 diabetes with microalbuminuria (increased risk of hyperkalemia); Serum creatinine >2.0 mg/dL in males or >1.8 mg/dL in females; CCr <50 ml/min; Concurrent use of potassium-sparing diuretics; Concurrent use of strong inhibitors of the CYP3A4 enzyme system (ketoconazole, itraconazole); Lactation.

Use Cautiously in: Severe hepatic impairment; Concurrent use of ACE inhibitors or angiotensin II receptor antagonists (increased risk of hyperkalemia); Pregnancy (use only if clearly needed); Children (safety not established).

Adverse Reactions/Side Effects

CNS: dizziness, fatigue. **GI:** abnormal liver function tests, abdominal pain, diarrhea. **GU:** albuminuria. **Endo:** abnormal vaginal bleeding, gynecomastia. **F and E:** HYPERKALEMIA. **Metab:** hypercholesterolemia, hypertriglyceridemia. **Misc:** flu-like symptoms.

Interactions

Drug-Drug: Concurrent use of strong inhibitors of the CYP3A4 enzyme system (**ketoconazole**, **itraconazole**) significantly ↑ effects of eplenerone and should be avoided. Concurrent use of weak inhibitors of the CYP3A4 enzyme system (**erythromycin**, **saquinavir**, **fluconazole**, **verapamil**) may ↑ effects of eplerenone; initial dose of eplerenone should be ↓ by 50%. **NSAIDs** may ↓ antihypertensive effects. Concurrent use of **ACE inhibitors** or **Angiotensin II receptor blockers** may ↑ risk of hyperkalemia.

Route/Dosage

PO (Adults): 50 mg once daily initially; may be increased to 50 mg twice daily; *patients receiving concurrent weak CYP3A4 inhibitors (erythromycin, saquinavir, verapamil, fluconazole)*—25 mg once daily initially.

Availability

Tablets: 25 mg, 50 mg, 100 mg.

NURSING IMPLICATIONS

Assessment

- Monitor blood pressure periodically during therapy.
- Monitor prescription refills to determine adherence.
- ***Lab Test Considerations:*** May cause hyperkalemia. Monitor serum potassium levels every 2 wk for the first 1–2 mo, then monthly thereafter.
- May cause ↓ serum sodium and ↑ serum triglyceride, cholesterol, ALT, GGT, creatinine, and uric acid levels.

Potential Nursing Diagnoses

Decreased cardiac output (Indications)
Noncompliance (Patient/Family Teaching)

Implementation

- **PO:** Administer once daily. May be increased to twice daily if response is inadequate.

Patient/Family Teaching

- Instruct patient to take medication as directed at the same time each day, even if feeling well.
- Encourage patient to comply with additional interventions for hypertension (weight reduction, discontinuation of smoking, moderation of alochol consumption, regular exercise, stress management). Medication controls, but does not cure, hypertension.
- Instruct patient and family on correct technique for monitoring blood pressure. Advise them to monitor blood pressure at least weekly, and notify health care professional of significant changes.
- Inform patient not to use potassium supplements, salt substitutes containing potassium, or other Rx or OTC medications without consulting health care professional.
- May cause dizziness. Caution patient to avoid driving or other activities requiring alertness until response to medication is known.
- Advise patient to inform health care professional of treatment regimen prior to treatment or surgery.

Evaluation/Desired Outcomes

- Decrease in blood pressure without appearance of side effects.

epoetin (e-**poe**-e-tin)

Epogen, EPO, ✦Eprex, erythropoietin, Procrit

Classification
Therapeutic: antianemics
Pharmacologic: hormones

Pregnancy Category C

Indications

Anemia associated with chronic renal failure. Anemia secondary to zidovudine (AZT) therapy in HIV-infected patients. Anemia from chemotherapy in patients with nonmyeloid malignancies. Reduction of need for transfusions after surgery.

Action

Stimulates erythropoiesis (production of red blood cells). **Therapeutic Effects:** Maintains and may elevate RBCs, decreasing the need for transfusions.

Pharmacokinetics
Absorption: Well absorbed after subcut administration.
Distribution: Unknown.
Metabolism and Excretion: Unknown.
Half-life: 4–13 hr.

TIME/ACTION PROFILE (increase in RBCs)

ROUTE	ONSET†	PEAK	DURATION
IV, subcut	7–10 days	within 2 mos	2 wk‡

†Increase in reticulocytes
‡After discontinuation

Contraindications/Precautions
Contraindicated in: Hypersensitivity to albumin or mammalian cell-derived products; Uncontrolled hypertension; Patients with erythropoietin levels >200 mU/ml.
Use Cautiously in: History of seizures; History of porphyria; Pregnancy or lactation.

Adverse Reactions/Side Effects
CNS: SEIZURES, headache. **CV:** hypertension, thrombotic events such as myocardial infarction or stroke (↑ in hemodialysis patients or hemoglobin ≥12 g/dL). **Derm:** transient rashes. **Endo:** restored fertility, resumption of menses. **Misc:** ↑ mortality and ↑ tumor growth (with hemoglobin ≥12 g/dL).

Interactions
Drug-Drug: May increase the requirement for **heparin** anticoagulation during hemodialysis.

Route/Dosage
(Use lowest dose that will gradually increase hemoglobin level and avoid RBC transfusion).

Anemia of Chronic Renal Failure
Subcut, IV (Adults): 50–100 units/kg 3 times weekly initially, then adjust dose based on hematocrit.
Subcut, IV (Children): 50 units/kg 3 times weekly initially, then adjust dose based on hematocrit.

Anemia Secondary to AZT Therapy
Subcut, IV (Adults): 100 units/kg 3 times weekly for 8 wk; if inadequate response, may increase by 50–100 units/kg every 4–8 wk, up to 300 units/kg 3 times weekly.

Anemia from Chemotherapy
(Use only for chemotherapy-related anemia and discontinue when chemotherapy course is completed)
Subcut (Adults): 150 units/kg 3 times weekly; may increase after 8 wk up to 300 units/kg 3 times weekly.

Surgery
Subcut (Adults): 300 units/kg/day for 10 days before surgery, day of surgery, and 4 days after *or* 600 units/kg 21, 14, and 7 days before surgery and on day of surgery.

Availability
Injection: 2000 units/ml, 3000 units/ml, 4000 units/ml, 10,000 units/ml, 20,000 units/ml.

NURSING IMPLICATIONS
Assessment
- Monitor blood pressure before and during therapy. Inform physician or other health care professional if severe hypertension is present or if blood pressure begins to increase. Additional antihypertensive therapy may be required during initiation of therapy.
- Monitor for symptoms of anemia (fatigue, dyspnea, pallor).
- Monitor dialysis shunts (thrill and bruit) and status of artificial kidney during hemodialysis. Heparin dose may need to be increased to prevent clotting. Patients with underlying vascular disease should be monitored for impaired circulation.
- ***Lab Test Considerations:*** May cause ↑ in WBCs and platelets. May ↓ bleeding times.
- Serum ferritin, transferrin, and iron levels should also be monitored to assess need for concurrent iron therapy. Transferrin saturation should be at least 20% and ferritin should be at least 100 mg/ml.
- **Anemia of Chronic Renal Failure:** Monitor hematocrit before and twice weekly during initial therapy, for 2–6 wk after a change in dose, and regularly after target range (30–36%) has been reached and maintenance dose is determined. Monitor other hematopoietic parameters (CBC with differential and platelet count) before and periodically during therapy. If hemoglobin exceeds 12 g/dL or increases more than 1 g/dL in a 2-wk period, risk of life—threatening cardiovascular complications and seizures increases. Decrease dose by 25% and monitor hemoglobin twice weekly for 2–6 wk. If increase in hemoglobin continues and exceeds 12 g/dL, dose should be withheld until hemoglobin begins to decrease; epoetin is then re-initiated at a

lower dose. If hemoglobin increase of 1 g/dL is not achieved after a 4-wk period and iron stores are adequate, dose may be incrementally increased at 4–wk intervals until desired response is attained.

- Monitor renal function studies and electrolytes closely; resulting increased sense of well-being may lead to decreased compliance with other therapies for renal failure. Increases in BUN, creatinine, uric acid, phosphorus, and potassium may occur.
- **Anemia Secondary to Zidovudine Therapy:** Before initiating therapy, determine serum erythropoietin level before transfusion. Patients receiving zidovudine with endogenous serum erythropoietin levels >500 mU/ml may not respond to therapy. Monitor hematocrit weekly during dosage adjustment. If response does not reduce transfusion requirements or increase hematocrit effectively after 8 wk of therapy, dose may be increased by 50–100 units/kg 3 times weekly. Evaluate response and adjust dose by 50–100 units/kg every 4–8 wk thereafter. If a satisfactory response is not obtained with a dose of 300 units/kg 3 times weekly, it is unlikely that a higher dose will produce a response. Once the desired response is attained, maintenance dose is titrated based on variations of zidovudine dose and intercurrent infections. If hemoglobin exceeds 13 g/dL, discontinue dose until hemoglobin drops to 12 g/dL, then decrease dose by 25%.
- **Anemia from Chemotherapy:** Monitor hemoglobin weekly until stable. Patients with lower baseline serum erythropoietin levels may respond more rapidly; not recommended if levels >200 mU/ml. If response is not adequate after 8 wk of therapy, dose may be increased up to 300 units/kg 3 times weekly. If no response is obtained to this dose, it is unlikely that higher doses will produce a response. If hemoglobin exceeds 12 g/dL or increases >1 g/dL in any 2–wk period, risk of life—threatening cardiovascular complications, tumor growth and death increases; decrease dose by 25%. If hemoglobin exceeds 13 g/dL, hold dose until it falls to 12 g/dL, then decrease dose by 25%.
- **Surgery:** Determine that hematocrit is >10 to ≤13 g/dL before therapy.

Potential Nursing Diagnoses

Activity intolerance (Indications)
Noncompliance (Patient/Family Teaching)

Implementation

IV Administration

- Transfusions are still required for severe symptomatic anemia. Supplemental iron should be initiated with epoetin and continued throughout therapy
- Institute seizure precautions in patients who experience greater than a 4-point increase in hematocrit in a 2-wk period or exhibit any change in neurologic status. Risk of seizures is greatest during the first 90 days of therapy.
- Do not shake vial; inactivation of medication may occur. Discard vial immediately after withdrawing dose from single-use 1-ml vial. Refrigerate multidose 2-ml vial; stable for 21 days after initial entry.
- **Subcut:** This route is often used for patients not requiring dialysis
- May be admixed in syringe immediately before administration with 0.9% NaCl with benzyl alcohol 0.9% in a 1:1 ratio to prevent injection site discomfort.
- **Direct IV:** ***Diluent:*** Administer undiluted or dilute with an equal amount of 0.9% NaCl. ***Concentration:*** 1,000–40,000 units/ml. ***Rate:*** May be administered as direct injection or bolus over 1–3 minutes into IV tubing or via venous line at end of dialysis session.

Patient/Family Teaching

- Explain rationale for concurrent iron therapy (increased red blood cell production requires iron).
- Discuss possible return of menses and fertility in women of childbearing age. Patient should discuss contraceptive options with health care professional.
- Discuss ways of preventing self-injury in patients at risk for seizures. Driving and activities requiring continuous alertness should be avoided.
- **Anemia of Chronic Renal Failure:** Stress importance of compliance with dietary restrictions, medications, and dialysis. Foods high in iron and low in potassium include liver, pork, veal, beef, mustard and turnip greens, peas, eggs, broccoli, kale, blackberries, strawberries, apple juice, watermelon, oatmeal, and enriched bread. Epoetin will re-

sult in increased sense of well-being, but it does not cure underlying disease.

- **Home Care Issues:** Home dialysis patients determined to be able to safely and effectively administer epoetin should be taught proper dosage, administration technique, and disposal of equipment. *Information for Home Dialysis Patients* should be provided to patient along with medication.

Evaluation/Desired Outcomes

- Increase in hematocrit to 30–36% with improvement in symptoms of anemia in patients with chronic renal failure.
- Increase in hematocrit in anemia secondary to zidovudine therapy.
- Increase in hematocrit in patients with anemia resulting from chemotherapy.
- Reduction of need for transfusions after surgery.

eprosartan, See ANGIOTENSIN II RECEPTOR ANTAGONISTS.

HIGH ALERT

eptifibatide (ep-ti-**fib**-a-tide)

Integrilin

Classification

Therapeutic: antiplatelet agents

Pharmacologic: glycoprotein IIb/IIIa inhibitors

Pregnancy Category B

Indications

Acute coronary syndrome (unstable angina/non–Q-wave MI), including patients who will be managed medically and those who will undergo percutaneous coronary intervention (PCI) that may consist of percutaneous transluminal angioplasty (PCTA) or atherectomy. Treatment of patients undergoing PCI. Usually used concurrently with aspirin and heparin.

Action

Decreases platelet aggregation by reversibly antagonizing the binding of fibrinogen to the glycoprotein IIb/IIIa binding site on platelet surfaces. **Therapeutic Effects:** Inhibition of platelet aggregation resulting in decreased incidence of new MI, death, or refractory ischemia, reducing the need for repeat urgent cardiac intervention.

Pharmacokinetics

Absorption: IV administration results in complete bioavailability.
Distribution: Unknown.
Metabolism and Excretion: 50% excreted by the kidneys.
Half-life: 2.5 hr.

TIME/ACTION PROFILE (effects on platelet function)

ROUTE	ONSET	PEAK	DURATION
IV	immediate	following bolus	brief†

†Inhibition is reversible following cessation of infusion

Contraindications/Precautions

Contraindicated in: Hypersensitivity; Active internal bleeding or history of bleeding within previous 30 days; Severe uncontrolled hypertension (systolic BP >200 mm Hg and/or diastolic BP >110 mm Hg); Major surgical procedure within 6 wk; History of hemorrhagic stroke or other stroke within 30 days; Concurrent use of other glycoprotein IIb/IIIa receptor antagonists; Platelet count <100,000/mm^3; Severe renal insufficiency (serum creatinine ≥4 mg/dl) or dependency on renal dialysis.
Use Cautiously in: Geri: ↑ risk of bleeding; Renal insufficiency (↓ infusion rate if CCr <50 ml/min); OB, Pedi: Pregnancy, lactation, or children (safety not established; use in pregnancy only if clearly needed).

Adverse Reactions/Side Effects

Noted for patients receiving heparin and aspirin in addition to eptifibatide. **CV:** hypotension. **Hemat:** BLEEDING (including GI and intracranial bleeding, hematuria, and hematomas).

Interactions

Drug-Drug: ↑ risk of bleeding with other drugs that affect hemostasis (**heparins**, **warfarin**, **NSAIDs**, **thrombolytic agents**, **abciximab**, **dipyridamole**, **ticlopidine**, **clopidogrel**, some **cephalosporins**, **valproates**).
Drug-Natural Products: ↑ bleeding risk with **arnica, chamomile, clove, dong quai, feverfew, garlic, ginger, ginkgo,** and **Panax ginseng.**

Route/Dosage

Acute Coronary Syndrome

IV (Adults ≤121 kg): 180 mcg/kg as a bolus dose, followed by 2 mcg/kg/min until hospital discharge or surgical intervention (up to 72 hr).

Percutaneous Coronary Intervention
IV (Adults): 180 mcg/kg as a bolus dose, immediately before PCI, followed by 2 mcg/kg/min infusion; a second bolus of 180 mcg/kg is given 10 min after first bolus; infusion should continue for 18–24 or hospital discharge (minimum of 12 hr)

Renal Impairment
IV (Adults CCr <50 mL/min): 180 mcg/kg bolus followed by 1 mcg/kg/min infusion; second bolus of 180 mcg/kg is given 10 min after first bolus for patients undergoing PCI.

Availability
Solution for injection: 20 mg/10 ml, 75 mg/100 ml, 200 mg/100 ml.

NURSING IMPLICATIONS

Assessment

- Assess for bleeding. Most common sites are arterial access site for cardiac catheterization or GI or GU tract. Arterial and venous punctures, IM injections, and use of urinary catheters, nasotracheal intubation, and NG tubes should be minimized. Noncompressible sites for IV access should be avoided. If bleeding cannot be controlled with pressure, discontinue eptifibatide and heparin immediately.
- ***Lab Test Considerations:*** Prior to eptifibatide therapy, assess hemoglobin or hematocrit, platelet count, serum creatinine, and PT/aPTT. Activated clotting time (ACT) should also be measured in patients undergoing PCI.
- Maintain the aPTT between 50 and 70 sec unless PCI is to be performed. Maintain ACT between 300 and 350 sec during PCI.
- Arterial sheath should not be removed unless aPTT <45 sec.
- If platelet count decreases to <100,000 and is confirmed, eptifibatide and heparin should be discontinued and condition monitored and treated.

Potential Nursing Diagnoses

Ineffective tissue perfusion (Indications)

Implementation

- ***High Alert:*** Accidental overdose of antiplatelet medications has resulted in patient harm or death from internal hemorrhage or intracranial bleeding. Have second practitioner independently check original order, dose calculations, and infusion pump settings.
- Most patients receive heparin and aspirin concurrently with eptifibatide.
- After PCI, femoral artery sheath may be removed during eptifibatide treatment only after heparin has been discontinued and its effects mostly reversed.
- Do not administer solutions that are discolored or contain particulate matter. Discard unused portion.

IV Administration

- **Direct IV:** ***High Alert: Diluent:*** Withdraw appropriate loading dose from bolus vial (20 mg/10ml vial) into a syringe. Administer undiluted. ***Concentration:*** 2 mg/ml. ***Rate:*** Administer over 1–2 min.
- **Continuous Infusion:** ***Diluent:*** Administer undiluted directly from the 100-ml vial via an infusion pump. ***Concentration:*** 0.75 mg/ml or 2 mg/ml (depends on vial used). ***Rate:*** Based on patient's weight (see Route/Dosage section).
- **Y-Site Compatibility:** alteplase, amiodarone, argatroban, atropine, bivalirudin, daptomycin, dobutamine, ertapenem, heparin, lidocaine, meperidine, metoprolol, micafungin, midazolam, morphine, nitroglycerin, palonosetron, potassium chloride, verapamil.
- **Y-Site Incompatibility:** furosemide.
- **Solution Compatibility:** 0.9% NaCl, D5/0.9% NaCl.

Patient/Family Teaching

- Inform patient of the purpose of eptifibatide.
- Instruct patient to notify health care professional immediately if any bleeding is noted.

Evaluation/Desired Outcomes

- Inhibition of platelet aggregation, resulting in decreased incidence of new MI, death, or refractory ischemia with the need for repeat urgent cardiac intervention.

---

ergocalciferol, **See VITAMIN D COMPOUNDS.**

---

ergonovine (er-goe-**noe**-veen)
ergometrine, Ergotrate

Classification
Therapeutic: none assigned
Pharmacologic: oxytocics

Pregnancy Category UK

Indications
Prevention and treatment of postpartum or postabortion hemorrhage caused by uterine atony or involution. **Unlabeled uses:** As a diagnostic agent to provoke coronary artery spasm.

Action
Directly stimulates uterine and vascular smooth muscle. **Therapeutic Effects:** Uterine contraction.

Pharmacokinetics
Absorption: Well absorbed after oral or IM administration.
Distribution: Unknown.
Metabolism and Excretion: Unknown. Probably metabolized by the liver.
Half-life: Unknown.

TIME/ACTION PROFILE (uterine contractions)

ROUTE	ONSET	PEAK	DURATION
PO	5–15 min	unknown	≥3 hr
IM	2–5 min	unknown	≥3 hr
IV	immediate	unknown	45 min

Contraindications/Precautions
Contraindicated in: Hypersensitivity; Avoid chronic use; Should not be used to induce labor.
Use Cautiously in: Hypertensive or eclamptic patients (increased susceptibility to hypertensive and arrhythmogenic side effects); Severe hepatic or renal disease; Sepsis; Third stage of labor.

Adverse Reactions/Side Effects
CNS: dizziness, headache. **EENT:** tinnitus. **Resp:** dyspnea. **CV:** arrhythmias, chest pain, hypertension, palpitations. **GI:** nausea, vomiting. **Derm:** sweating. **Misc:** allergic reactions.

Interactions
Drug-Drug: Excessive vasoconstriction may result when used with other **vasopressors**, such as **dopamine** or **nicotine**. May ↑ the risk of adverse reactions with **bromocriptine**.

Route/Dosage
Oxytocic
PO, SL (Adults): 0.2–0.4 mg q 6–12 hr (usual course is 48 hr).
IM, IV (Adults): 200 mcg (0.2 mg) q 2–4 hr for up to 5 doses.

Provocative Agent for Coronary Artery Spasm
IV (Adults): 50 mcg (0.05 mg) q 5 min until chest pain occurs or a total dose of 400 mcg (0.4 mg) has been given (unlabeled).

Availability
Tablets: 0.2 mg. **Injection:** 0.2 mg/ml, ✤0.25 mg/ml.

NURSING IMPLICATIONS

Assessment
- Monitor blood pressure, pulse, and respirations every 15–30 min until transfer to the postpartum unit, then every 1–2 hr. Report hypertension, chest pain, arrhythmias, headache, or change in neurologic status.
- Monitor amount and type of vaginal discharge. Report symptoms of hemorrhage (increased bleeding, hypotension, pallor, tachycardia) immediately.
- Palpate uterine fundus; note position and consistency. Notify physician or other health care professional if fundus fails to contract in response to ergonovine. Assess patient for severe cramping; dose may be decreased.
- Assess for signs of ergotism (cold, numb fingers and toes; nausea; vomiting; diarrhea; headache; muscle pain; weakness).
- If patient fails to respond to ergonovine, check serum calcium level. Correction of hypocalcemia may restore responsiveness.
- ***Lab Test Considerations:*** May cause ↓ serum prolactin level, which inhibits synthesis of breast milk.
- ***Toxicity and Overdose:*** Toxicity, initially manifested as ergotism, may cause seizures and gangrene. Seizures are treated with anticonvulsants. Vasodilators and heparin may be ordered to improve circulation to extremities.

Potential Nursing Diagnoses
Ineffective tissue perfusion (Indications)
Risk for injury (Side Effects)

Implementation
- Do not administer solution that is discolored or contains a precipitate.
- **PO:** Administration is usually limited to 48 hr postpartum, by which time the danger of hemorrhage from uterine atony has passed.
- Tablets may be administered SL.

- **IM:** The preferred route is IM. Firm uterine contractions are produced within a few minutes. Dose may need to be repeated every 2–4 hr for full therapeutic effect.

IV Administration

- **Direct IV:** The IV route is reserved for severe uterine bleeding. ***Diluent:*** Dilute with 5 mL of 0.9% NaCl. ***Rate:*** Administer slow IV push over at least 1 min through Y-site injection of an IV of D5W or 0.9% NaCl.

Patient/Family Teaching

- Review symptoms of toxicity with patient. Instruct the patient to report occurrence of these immediately.
- Inform patient that uterine cramping demonstrates effectiveness of therapy.
- Explain need for pad count to determine degree of bleeding. Instruct patient to report immediately an increase in degree of bleeding or passage of clots.
- Instruct patient to report breastfeeding difficulties.
- Caution patient not to smoke while receiving ergonovine; nicotine is also a vasoconstrictor.

Evaluation/Desired Outcomes

- Uterine contraction and cramping in the prevention or cessation of uterine hemorrhage after delivery or abortion.
- Vasoconstriction of the coronary arteries when used as a diagnostic agent.

ergotamine (er-**got**-a-meen)
Ergomar

dihydroergotamine
(dye-hye-droe-er-**got**-a-meen)
D.H.E. 45, Migranal

Classification
Therapeutic: vascular headache suppressants
Pharmacologic: ergot alkaloids

Pregnancy Category X

Indications

Treatment of vascular headaches including: Migraine with or without aura, Cluster headaches.

Action

Vasoconstriction of dilated blood vessels by stimulating alpha-adrenergic and serotonergic (5-HT) receptors. Larger doses may produce alpha-adrenergic blockade and vasodilation. **Therapeutic Effects:** Constriction of dilated carotid artery bed with resolution of vascular headache.

Pharmacokinetics

Absorption: *Ergotamine*—Unpredictably absorbed (60%) from the GI tract (may be enhanced by caffeine). Sublingual absorption is very poor. *Dihydroergotamine*—Rapidly absorbed after IM and subcut administration, 32% absorbed from nasal mucosa.
Distribution: Ergotamine crosses the blood-brain barrier and enters breast milk.
Protein Binding: *Dihydroergotamine*—90%; *ergotamine*—93–98%.
Metabolism and Excretion: Both ergotamine and dihydroergotamine are 90% metabolized by the liver (CYP3A4 enzyme system). Some metabolites are active.
Half-life: *Ergotamine*—1.5–2.5 hr. *Dihydroergotamine*—9–10 hr.

TIME/ACTION PROFILE (relief of headache)

ROUTE	ONSET	PEAK	DURATION
PO	1–2 hr (variable)	1–5 hr	unknown
Nasal	within 30 min	unknown	unknown
SL	unknown	unknown	unknown
IM, subcut	15–30 min	15 min–2 hr	8 hr
IV	<5 min	15 min–2 hr	8 hr

Contraindications/Precautions

Contraindicated in: Peripheral vascular disease; Ischemic heart disease; Uncontrolled hypertension; Severe renal or liver disease; Malnutrition; Known alcohol intolerance (dihydroergotamine injection only); OB, Lactation: Pregnancy and lacation; Concurrent use of CYP3A4 inhibitors (protease inhibitors and macrolide anti-infectives).
Use Cautiously in: Illnesses associated with peripheral vascular pathology such as diabetes mellitus; Concurrent administration of other vasconstrictor agents; Pedi: Children (safety not established).

Adverse Reactions/Side Effects

CNS: dizziness. **EENT:** rhinitis (nasal). **CV:** MI, hypertension, angina pectoris, arterial spasm, intermittent claudication. **GI:** abdominal pain, nausea, vomiting, altered taste *(nasal)*, diarrhea, polydipsia. **MS:** extremity stiffness, muscle pain, stiff neck, stiff shoulders. **Neuro:** leg weakness, numbness or tingling in fingers or toes. **Misc:** fatigue.

Interactions

Drug-Drug: Concurrent use of potent inhibitors of the CYP3A4 enzyme system, including protease inhibitors (**ritonavir**, **nelfinavir**, and **indinavir**) some macrolide anti-infectives (**erythromycin**, **clarithromycin**, and **troleandomycin**) and some azole antifungals (**ketoconazole**, **itraconazole**) may produce serious life-threatening peripheral ischemia and is contraindicated. Concurrent use with **beta blockers**, **hormonal contraceptives**, or **nicotine** (heavy smoking) may ↑ risk of peripheral vasoconstriction. Dihydroergotamine antagonizes the antianginal effects of **nitrates**. Concurrent use with **vasoconstrictors** may have ↑ effects (avoid concurrent use). Concurrent use with **almotriptan**, **frovatriptan**, **naratriptan**, **rizatriptan**, **sumatriptan**, and **zolmitriptan** may result in prolonged vasoconstriction (allow 24 hr between use).

Route/Dosage

Ergotamine

PO, SL (Adults): 1–2 mg initially, then 1–2 mg q 30 min until attack subsides or a total of 6 mg has been given. Should not be used more than twice weekly, with at least 5 days between courses; 1–2 mg PO at bedtime daily for 10–14 days have been used to terminate series of cluster headaches.

Dihydroergotamine

IM, Subcut (Adults): 1 mg; may repeat in 1 hr to a total of 3 mg (not to exceed 3 mg/day or 6 mg/wk).
IV (Adults): 0.5 mg; may repeat in 1 hr (not to exceed 2 mg/day or 6 mg/wk). For chronic intractable headache, 0.5–1 mg q 8 hr may be given until relief is obtained (not to exceed 6 mg/wk).
Intranasal (Adults): 1 spray (0.5 mg) in each nostril, repeat after 15 min (2 mg total dose); not to exceed 3 mg/24 hr or 4 mg/wk.

Availability

Ergotamine

Sublingual tablets: 2 mg. ***In combination with:*** caffeine, barbiturates, and belladonna alkaloids in preparations for vascular headaches. See Appendix B.

Dihydroergotamine

Injection: 1 mg/ml (contains alcohol). **Nasal spray:** 4 mg/1 ml in 1-ml ampules with nasal spray applicator. ***In combination with:*** *Ergotamine*—caffeine, barbiturates, and belladonna alkaloids in preparations for vascular headaches. See Appendix B.

NURSING IMPLICATIONS

Assessment

- Assess frequency, location, duration, and characteristics (pain, nausea, vomiting, visual disturbances) of chronic headaches. During acute attack, assess type, location, and intensity of pain before and 60 min after administration.
- Monitor blood pressure and peripheral pulses periodically during therapy. Report any increases in blood pressure.
- Assess for signs of ergotism (cold, numb fingers and toes; nausea; vomiting; headache; muscle pain; weakness).
- Assess for nausea and vomiting. Ergotamine stimulates the chemoreceptor trigger zone. Metoclopramide or a phenothiazine antiemetic may be given orally as prophylaxis 1 hr before administration of dihydroergotamine IV. Oral administration may decrease risk of extrapyramidal reactions and other side effects encountered with IV administration.
- ***Toxicity and Overdose:*** Toxicity is manifested by severe ergotism (chest pain, abdominal pain, persistent paresthesia in the extremities) and gangrene. Vasodilators, dextran, or heparin may be ordered to improve circulation.

Potential Nursing Diagnoses

Acute pain (Indications)
Risk for injury (Side Effects)
Deficient knowledge, related to medication regimen (Patient/Family Teaching)

Implementation

- Do not confuse Cafergot (ergotamine/caffeine) with Carafate (sucralfate).
- Administer as soon as patient reports prodromal symptoms or headache. **SL:** Allow tablet to dissolve under tongue. Do not allow patient to eat, drink, or smoke while tablet is dissolving.

IV Administration

- **Direct IV:** ***Diluent:*** Dihydroergotamine may be administered undiluted. ***Concentration:*** 1 mg/ml. ***Rate:*** Administer over 1 min.

Patient/Family Teaching

- Instruct patient to take ergotamine at the first sign of an impending headache and not to exceed the maximum dose prescribed.
- Encourage patient to rest in a quiet, dark room after taking ergotamine.
- Review symptoms of toxicity. Instruct patient to report these promptly.
- Caution patient not to smoke and to avoid exposure to cold; these vasoconstrictors may further impair peripheral circulation.
- May cause dizziness. Caution patient to avoid driving and other activities requiring alertness until response to the drug is known.
- Advise patient to avoid alcohol, which may precipitate vascular headaches.
- Instruct female patients to inform health care professional if they plan or suspect pregnancy. Ergotamine should not be taken during pregnancy.
- **Subcut, IM:** Inject at the first sign of a headache and repeat at 1-hr intervals up to 3 doses. Once minimal effective dose is determined, adjust dose for subsequent attacks.
- **Intranasal:** Instruct patient in proper use of nasal spray. Prime nasal sprayer 4 times before dose. Administer 1 spray to each nostril followed in 15 min by an additional spray in each nostril for a total of 4 sprays. Do not tilt head or sniff after spray. Do not use more than amount instructed. Discard ampule within 8 hr of opening. Do not refrigerate. Assembly may be used for 4 treatments; then discard.
- Advise patient not to use *Migranal* to prevent a headache if there are no symptoms or if headache is different from typical migraine.
- Instruct patient to notify health care professional if numbness or tingling in fingers or toes; pain, tightness, or discomfort in chest; muscle pain or cramps in arms or legs; weakness in legs; temporary speeding or slowing of heart rate; or swelling or itching occurs.

Evaluation/Desired Outcomes

- Relief of pain from vascular headaches.

erlotinib (er-**lo**-ti-nib)
Tarceva

Classification
Therapeutic: antineoplastics
Pharmacologic: enzyme inhibitors

Pregnancy Category D

E

Indications

Locally advanced/metastatic non-small cell lung cancer which has not responded to previous chemotherapy.

Action

Inhibits the enzyme tyrosine kinase which is associated with human epidermal growth factor receptor (EGFR); blocks growth stimulation signals in cancer cells. **Therapeutic Effects:** Decreased spread of lung cancer with increased survival.

Pharmacokinetics

Absorption: 60% absorbed; bioavailability increased to 100% with food.
Distribution: Unknown.
Protein Binding: 93% protein bound.
Metabolism and Excretion: Mostly metabolized by the liver (CYP3A4 enzyme system).
Half-life: 36 hr.

TIME/ACTION PROFILE (blood levels)

ROUTE	ONSET	PEAK	DURATION
Oral	unknown	4 hr	24 hr

Contraindications/Precautions

Contraindicated in: Pregnancy or lactation.
Use Cautiously in: Hepatic impairment; Previous chemotherapy/radiation, pre-existing lung disease, metastatic lung disease (may ↑ risk of interstitial lung disease); Patients with child-bearing potential; Children (safety not established).

Adverse Reactions/Side Effects

CNS: fatigue. **EENT:** conjunctivitis, corneal ulceration. **Resp:** INTERSTITIAL LUNG DISEASE, dyspnea, cough. **GI:** diarrhea, abdominal pain, anorexia, nausea, stomatitis, vomiting, ↑ liver transaminases. **Derm:** rash, dry skin, pruritus.

Interactions

Drug-Drug: Strong inhibitors of CYP3A4, including **atazanavir, clarithromycin, indinavir, itraconazole, ketoconazole, nefazodone, nelfinavir, ritonavir, saquinavir, telithromycin,** or **voriconazole** ↑ erlotinib levels and the risk of toxicity; dosage reduction should be considered. Strong inducers of CYP3A4, including **rifampin** ↓ levels of erlotinib and may ↓ response; alternative therapy or ↑ dose should be considered. May ↑ risk of bleeding with **warfarin**.

Route/Dosage

PO (Adults): 150 mg daily taken at least 1 hr before or 2 hr after food.

Availability

Tablets: 25 mg, 100 mg, 150 mg.

NURSING IMPLICATIONS

Assessment

- Assess respiratory status prior to and periodically during therapy. If dyspnea, cough or fever occur, discontinue erlotinib, assess for interstitial lung disease, and institute treatment as needed.
- Assess for diarrhea. Usually responds to loperamide but may require dose reduction or discontinuation of therapy.
- ***Lab Test Considerations:*** Monitor liver function tests (AST, ALT, bilirubin, alkaline phosphatase) periodically during therapy. Dose reduction or discontinuation of therapy should be considered if severe changes in liver function occur.
- Monitor INR regularly in patients taking warfarin. May cause ↑ INR.

Potential Nursing Diagnoses

Ineffective breathing pattern (Side Effects)

Implementation

- **PO:** Administer at least 1 hr before or 2 hrs after food.

Patient/Family Teaching

- Instruct patient to take erlotinib as directed.
- Caution patient to use contraceptive during and for at least 2 wks after completion of therapy.
- Advise patient to notify health care professional if severe or persistent diarrhea, nausea, anorexia, vomiting, onset or worsening of unexplained dyspnea or cough, or eye irritation occur.

Evaluation/Desired Outcomes

- Decrease in spread of non-small cell lung cancer with increased survival.

ertapenem (er-ta-**pen**-em)

Invanz

Classification
Therapeutic: anti-infectives
Pharmacologic: carbapenems

Pregnancy Category B

Indications

Moderate to severe: complicated intra-abdominal infections, complicated skin and skin structure infections, community acquired pneumonia, complicated urinary tract infections (including pyelonephritis), acute pelvic infections including postpartum endomyometritis, septic abortion, and post surgical gynecologic infections. Prophylaxis of surgical site infection following elective colorectal surgery.

Action

Therapeutic Effects: Bactericidal action against susceptible bacteria. **Spectrum:** Active against the following aerobic gram-positive organisms *Staphylococcus aureus* (methicillin-susceptible strains only), *Staphylococcus epidermidis, Streptococcus agalactiae, S. pneumoniae* (penicillin-susceptible strains only), and *S. pyogenes*. Also active against the following gram-negative aerobic organisms *Escherichia coli, Haemophilus influenzae* (beta-lactamase negative strains), *Klebsiella pneumonia, Moraxella catarrhalis,* and *Providencia rettgeri*. Addition anaerobic spectrum includes *Bacteroides fragilis, B. distasonis, B. ovatus, B. thetaiotamicron, B. uniformis, B. vulgatis, Clostridium clostrioforme, Eubacterium lentum, Peptostreptococcus, Porphyromonas asaccharolytica,* and *Prevotella bivia*.

Pharmacokinetics

Absorption: 90% after IM administration; IV administration results in complete bioavailability.
Distribution: Enters breast milk.
Metabolism and Excretion: Mostly excreted by the kidneys.
Half-life: 1.8 hr (increased in renal impairment).

TIME/ACTION PROFILE (blood levels)

ROUTE	ONSET	PEAK	DURATION
IM	rapid	2 hr	24 hr
IV	rapid	end of infusion	24 hr

Contraindications/Precautions

Contraindicated in: Hypersensitivity; Cross-sensitivity may occur with penicillins, cephalosporins and other carbapenems; Hypersensitivity to lidocaine (may be used as a diluent for IM administration).

Use Cautiously in: History of multiple hypersensitivity reactions; Seizure disorders; Geri: Geriatric patients (↑ sensitivity and age-related ↓ in renal function); Renal impairment; OB, Pedi: Pregnancy, lactation, or children <18 yr (safety not established, use during lactation only when benefits outweigh risks, use in pregnancy only if clearly needed).

Adverse Reactions/Side Effects

CNS: SEIZURES, headache. **GI:** PSEUDOMEMBRANOUS COLITIS, diarrhea, nausea, vomiting. **GU:** vaginitis. **Local:** phlebitis at IV site, pain at IM site. **Misc:** hypersensitivity reaction including ANAPHYLAXIS.

Interactions

Drug-Drug: Probenecid decreases excretion and increases blood levels.

Route/Dosage

IV, IM (Adults and Children 13 yrs or older): 1 g once daily for up to 14 days (IV) or 7 days (IM).

IV, IM (Children 3 months-12 yrs): 15 mg/kg twice daily (not to exceed 1 g/day) for up to 14 days (IV) or 7 days (IM).

Renal Impairment

IM, IV (Adults): *CCr ≤30 ml/min/1.73m²*—500 mg once daily.

Availability

Powder for injection: 1 g/vial.

NURSING IMPLICATIONS

Assessment

- Assess for infection (vital signs; appearance of wound, sputum, urine, and stool; WBC) at beginning of and during therapy.
- Obtain a history before initiating therapy to determine previous use of and reactions to penicillins, cephalosporins or carbapenems. Persons with a negative history of penicillin sensitivity may still have an allergic response.
- Obtain specimens for culture and sensitivity before initiating therapy. First dose may be given before receiving results.
- Observe patient for signs and symptoms of anaphylaxis (rash, pruritus, laryngeal edema, wheezing). Discontinue the drug and notify the physician immediately if these occur. Have epinephrine, an antihistamine, and resuscitative equipment close by in the event of an anaphylactic reaction.
- ***Lab Test Considerations:*** May cause ↑ AST, ALT, serum alkaline phosphatase levels.
- May cause ↑ platelet and eosinophil counts.

Potential Nursing Diagnoses

Risk for infection (Indications, Side Effects)

Implementation

- **IM:** Reconstitute 1-g vial with 3.2 ml of 1% lidocaine without epinephrine. Shake well to form solution. Immediately withdraw contents and inject deep into large muscle mass. Use reconstituted solution within 1 hr.

IV Administration

- **Intermittent Infusion:** ***Diluent:*** Reconstitute 1-g vial with 10 ml of sterile water for injection or 0.9% NaCl and shake well. Further dilute in 50 ml of 0.9% NaCl. Administer within 6 hr of reconstitution. ***Rate:*** Infuse over 30 min.
- **Y-Site Compatibility:** acyclovir, amikacin, aminophylline, amphotericin B liposome, argatroban, azithromycin, aztreonam, bumetanide, calcium chloride, calcium gluconate, chloramphenicol, cimetidine, ciprofloxacin, cisatracurium, cyclosporine, daptomycin, dexamethasone sodium phosphate, digoxin, diltiazem, diphenhydramine, dolasetron, dopamine, doxycycline, enalaprilat, epinephrine, eptifibatide, erythromycin, esmolol, famotidine, fenoldopam, fluconazole, furosemide, ganciclovir, gentamicin, granisetron, haloperidol, heparin, hydromorphone, insulin, isoproterenol, ketorolac, labetalol, levofloxacin, lidocaine, linezolid, lorazepam, magnesium sulfate, meperidine, methylprednisolone sodium succinate, metoclopramide, metronidazole, milrinone, morphine, nesiritide, nitroglycerin, nitroprusside, norepinephrine, pancuronium, pantoprazole, phenylephrine, potassium chloride, potassium phosphate, procainamide, propranolol, ranitidine, sodium bicarbonate, tacrolimus, tigecycline, tirofiban, tobramycin, trimethoprim/sulfamethoxazole, vancomycin, vasopressin, vecuronium, voriconazole, zoledronic acid.
- **Y-Site Incompatibility:** amiodarone, anidulafungin, caspofungin, diazepam, dobutamine, droperidol, hydralazine, hydroxyzine, midazolam, nicardipine, ondansetron, phe-

nytoin, prochlorperazine, promethazine, quinupristin/dalfopristin, verapamil.

Patient/Family Teaching

- Advise patient to report the signs of superinfection (black, furry overgrowth on the tongue; vaginal itching or discharge; loose or foul-smelling stools) and allergy. Consult health care professional before treating with antidiarrheals.
- Caution patient to notify health care professional if fever and diarrhea occur, especially if stool contains blood, pus, or mucus. Advise patient not to treat diarrhea without consulting health care professional. May occur up to several weeks after discontinuation of medication.

Evaluation/Desired Outcomes

- Resolution of the signs and symptoms of infection. Length of time for complete resolution depends on the organism and site of infection.

ERYTHROMYCIN†

(eh-rith-roe-**mye**-sin)

erythromycin base
✤Apo-Erythro-EC, E-Base, E-Mycin, ✤Erybid, Eryc, Ery-Tab, ✤Erythromid, ✤Novo-rythro, PCE

erythromycin estolate
Ilosone, ✤Novo-rythro

erythromycin ethylsuccinate
✤Apo-Erythro-ES, E.E.S, EryPed

erythromycin gluceptate

erythromycin lactobionate
Erythrocin

erythromycin stearate
Erythrocin, ✤Novo-rythro

erythromycin (topical)
Akne-Mycin, Del-Mycin, A/T/S, E/Gel, Emgel, Erycette, Erygel, Ery-Max, Erysol, ETS, ✤Sans-Acne, Staticin, Theramycin Z, T-Stat

Classification
Therapeutic: anti-infectives
Pharmacologic: macrolides

Pregnancy Category B

†See Appendix C for ophthalmic use

Indications

IV, PO: Infections caused by susceptible organisms including: Upper and lower respiratory tract infections, Otitis media (with sulfonamides), Skin and skin structure infections, Pertussis, Diphtheria, Erythrasma, Intestinal amebiasis, Pelvic inflammatory disease, Nongonococcal urethritis, Syphilis, Legionnaires' disease, Rheumatic fever. Useful when penicillin is the most appropriate drug but cannot be used because of hypersensitivity, including: Streptococcal infections, Treatment of syphilis or gonorrhea. **Topical:** Treatment of acne.

Action

Suppresses protein synthesis at the level of the 50S bacterial ribosome. **Therapeutic Effects:** Bacteriostatic action against susceptible bacteria. **Spectrum:** Active against many gram-positive cocci, including: Streptococci, Staphylococci. Gram-positive bacilli, including: *Clostridium*, *Corynebacterium*. Several gram-negative pathogens, notably: *Neisseria*, *Legionella pneumophila*. *Mycoplasma* and *Chlamydia* are also usually susceptible.

Pharmacokinetics

Absorption: Variable absorption from the duodenum after oral administration (dependent on salt form). Absorption of enteric-coated products is delayed. Minimal absorption may follow topical or ophthalmic use.
Distribution: Widely distributed. Minimal CNS penetration. Crosses placenta; enters breast milk.
Protein Binding: 70–80%; 96% for estolate.
Metabolism and Excretion: Partially metabolized by the liver, excreted mainly unchanged in the bile; small amounts excreted unchanged in the urine.
Half-life: Neonates: 2.1 hr; Adults: 1.4–2 hr.

TIME/ACTION PROFILE (blood levels)

ROUTE	ONSET	PEAK	DURATION
PO	1 hr	1–4 hr	6–12 hr
IV	rapid	end of infusion	6–12 hr

Contraindications/Precautions

Contraindicated in: Hypersensitivity; Hepatic dysfunction (estolate salt); Concurrent pimozide; Known alcohol intolerance (most topicals); Tartrazine sensitivity (some products contain tartrazine—FDC yellow dye #5); OB: Estolate salt is contraindicated in pregnancy due to potential for hepatic dysfunction; Products

containing benzyl alcohol should be avoided in neonates.
Use Cautiously in: Liver/renal disease; OB: Salts other than the estolate may be used in pregnancy to treat chlamydial infections or syphilis; Geri: ↑ risk of ototoxicity if parenteral dose >4 g/day, ↑ risk of QTc prolongation.

Adverse Reactions/Side Effects

CNS: seizures (rare). **EENT:** ototoxicity. **CV:** QTC PROLONGATION (may result in Torsades de Pointes), VENTRICULAR ARRHYTHMIAS,. **GI:** nausea, vomiting, abdominal pain, cramping, diarrhea, drug-induced hepatitis, infantile hypertrophic pyloric stenosis, drug-induced pancreatitis (rare). **Derm:** rashes. **Local:** phlebitis at IV site. **Misc:** allergic reactions, superinfection.

Interactions

Drug-Drug: Concurrent use with **pimozide** ↑ risk of serious arrhythmias (concurrent use contraindicated); similar effects may occur with **diltiazem**, **verapamil**, **ketoconazole**, **itraconazole**, **nefazodone**, and **protease inhibitors**; avoid concurrent use. ↑ blood levels and effects of **silfenafil**, **tadalafil** and **vardenafil**; use lower doses. Concurrent **rifabutin** or **rifampin** may ↓ effect of erythromycin and ↑ risk of adverse GI reactions. ↑ levels and risk of toxicity from **alfentanil**, **alprazolam**, **buspirone**, **clozapine**, **bromocriptine**, **theophylline**, **carbamazepine**, **cyclosporine**, **cylostazol diazepam**, **disopyramide**, **ergot alkaloids**, **felodipine**, **warfarin**, **methylprednisolone**, **midazolam**, **quinidine**, **rifabutin**, **tacrolimus**, **triazolam**, or **vinblastine**. Concurrent **HMG-CoA reductase inhibitors** ↑ risk of myopathy/rhabdomyolysis. May ↑ serum **digoxin** levels in a few patients. **Theophylline** may ↓ blood levels. Beneficial effects may be ↓ by **clindamycin** or **lincomycin**.

Route/Dosage

250 mg of erythromycin base, estolate, or stearate = 400 mg of erythromycin ethylsuccinate.

Most Infections

PO (Adults): *Base, estolate, stearate*—250 mg q 6 hr, *or* 333 mg q 8 hr, *or* 500 mg q 12 hr. *Ethylsuccinate*—400 mg q 6 hr *or* 800 mg q 12 hr.
PO (Children >1 mo): *Base and ethylsuccinate*—30–50 mg/kg/day divided q 6–8 hr (maximum 2 g/day as base or 3.2 g/day as ethylsuccinate) *Estolate.*—30–50 mg/kg/day divided q 6–12 hr (maximum 2 g/day). *Stearate*—30–50 mg/kg/day divided q 6 hr (maximum 2 g/day).
PO (Neonates): *Ethylsuccinate*—20–50 mg/kg/day divided q 6–12 hrs.
IV (Adults): *Gluceptate and lactobionate only*—250–500 mg (up to 1 g) q 6 hr.
IV (Children >1 mo): *Gluceptate and lactobionate only*—15–50 mg/kg/day divided q 6 hr, maximum 4 g/day.

Acne

Topical (Adults and Children >12 yr): 2% ointment, gel, or solution bid.

Availability (generic available)

Erythromycin Base

Enteric-coated tablets: 250 mg, 333 mg. **Tablets with polymer-coated particles:** 333 mg, 500 mg. **Film-coated tablets:** 500 mg. **Delayed-release capsules:** 250 mg.

Erythromycin Estolate

Tablets: 500 mg. **Capsules:** 250 mg. **Oral suspension (orange flavor):** 125 mg/5 ml. **Oral suspension (cherry flavor):** 250 mg/5 ml.

Erythromycin Ethylsuccinate

Chewable tablets (fruit flavor): 200 mg. **Tablets:** 400 mg. **Oral suspension (fruit flavor, cherry):** 200 mg/5 ml. **Oral suspension (orange, banana flavors):** 400 mg/5 ml. **Drops (fruit flavor):** 100 mg/2.5 ml.

Erythromycin Gluceptate

Powder for injection: 500 mg, 1 g.

Erythromycin Lactobionate

Powder for injection: 500 mg, 1 g.

Erythromycin Stearate

Film-coated tablets: 250 mg.

Topical Preparations

Topical ointment: 2%. **Topical gel:** 2%. **Topical solution:** 2%. ***In combination with:*** sulfisoxazole (Eryzole, Pediazole) and benzoyl peroxide (Benzamycin). See Appendix B.

NURSING IMPLICATIONS

Assessment

- Assess patient for infection (vital signs; appearance of wound, sputum, urine, and stool; WBC) at beginning of and during therapy.

E

- Obtain specimens for culture and sensitivity before initiating therapy. First dose may be given before receiving results.
- ***Lab Test Considerations:*** Monitor liver function tests periodically on patients receiving high-dose, long-term therapy.
- May cause ↑ serum bilirubin, AST, ALT, and alkaline phosphatase concentrations.
- May cause false ↑ of urinary catecholamines.

Potential Nursing Diagnoses

Risk for infection (Indications, Side Effects)
Noncompliance (Patient/Family Teaching)

Implementation

- Do not confuse erythromycin with azithromycin. Do not confuse Erythrocin (erythromycin) with Ethmozine (morizocine).
- **PO:** Administer around the clock. *Erythromycin film-coated tablets (base and stearate)* are absorbed better on an empty stomach, at least 1 hr before or 2 hr after meals; may be taken with food if GI irritation occurs. *Enteric-coated erythromycin (base and estolate)* may be taken without regard to meals. *Erythromycin ethylsuccinate* is best absorbed when taken with meals. Take each dose with a full glass of water.
- Use calibrated measuring device for liquid preparations. Shake well before using.
- Chewable tablets should be crushed or chewed and not swallowed whole.
- Do not crush or chew delayed-release capsules or tablets; swallow whole. *Erythromycin base delayed-release capsules* may be opened and sprinkled on applesauce, jelly, or ice cream immediately before ingestion. Entire contents of the capsule should be taken.

IV Administration

- **IV:** ***Diluent:*** Add 10 ml of sterile water for injection without preservatives to 250- or 500-mg vials and 20 ml to 1-g vial. Solution is stable for 7 days after reconstitution if refrigerated
- **Intermittent Infusion:** ***Concentration:*** Dilute to a final concentration of 1–5 mg/ml in 0.9% NaCl or D5W. ***Rate:*** Administer slowly over 20–60 min to avoid phlebitis. Assess for pain along vein; slow rate if pain occurs; apply ice and notify physician or other health care professional if unable to relieve pain.
- **Continuous Infusion:** May also be administered as an infusion in a dilution of 1 g/liter of 0.9% NaCl, D5W, or LR over 4 hr.

Erythromycin Gluceptate

- **Syringe Incompatibility:** heparin.
- **Additive Compatibility:** calcium gluconate, heparin, hydrocortisone sodium succinate, potassium chloride, sodium bicarbonate.
- **Additive Incompatibility:** pentobarbital, secobarbital.

Erythromycin Lactobionate

- **Syringe Incompatibility:** heparin.
- **Y-Site Compatibility:** acyclovir, amiodarone, bivalirudin, cyclophosphamide, dexmedetomidine, diltiazem, enalaprilat, esmolol, famotidine, fenoldopam, foscarnet, heparin, hydromorphone, idarubicin, labetalol, lorazepam, magnesium sulfate, meperidine, midazolam, morphine, multivitamins, nicardipine, perphenazine, tacrolimus, theophylline, vitamin B complex with C, zidovudine.
- **Y-Site Incompatibility:** cefepime, ceftazidime.
- **Additive Compatibility:** cimetidine, hydrocortisone sodium succinate, pentobarbital, potassium chloride, ranitidine, sodium bicarbonate.
- **Additive Incompatibility:** heparin, metoclopramide, vitamin B complex with C.
- **Topical:** Cleanse area before application. Wear gloves during application.

Patient/Family Teaching

- Instruct patient to take medication around the clock and to finish the drug completely as directed, even if feeling better. Take missed doses as soon as remembered, with remaining doses evenly spaced throughout day. Advise patient that sharing of this medication may be dangerous.
- May cause nausea, vomiting, diarrhea, or stomach cramps; notify health care professional if these effects persist or if severe abdominal pain, yellow discoloration of the skin or eyes, darkened urine, pale stools, or unusual tiredness develops. May cause infantile hypertrophic pyloric stenosis in infants; notify health care professional if vomiting and irritability occur.
- Advise patient to report signs of superinfection (black, furry overgrowth on the tongue; vaginal itching or discharge; loose or foul-smelling stools).
- Instruct patient to notify health care professional if symptoms do not improve.

Evaluation/Desired Outcomes
- Resolution of the signs and symptoms of infection. Length of time for complete resolution depends on the organism and site of infection.
- Improvement of acne lesions.

escitalopram
(ess-sit-**al**-o-pram)
Lexapro

Classification
Therapeutic: antidepressants
Pharmacologic: selective serotonin reuptake inhibitors (SSRIs)

Pregnancy Category C

Indications
Major depressive disorder. Generalized anxiety disorder (GAD). **Unlabeled uses:** Panic disorder. Obsessive-compulsive disorder (OCD). Post-traumatic stress disorder (PTSD). Social anxiety discorder (social phobia). Premenstrual dysphoric disorder (PMDD).

Action
Selectively inhibits the reuptake of serotonin in the CNS. **Therapeutic Effects:** Antidepressant action.

Pharmacokinetics
Absorption: 80% absorbed following oral administration.
Distribution: Enters breast milk.
Metabolism and Excretion: Mostly metabolized by the liver (primarily CYP3A4 and CYP2C19 isoenzymes); 7% excreted unchanged by kidneys.
Half-life: Increased in geriatric patients and patients with hepatic impairment.

TIME/ACTION PROFILE (antidepressant effect)

ROUTE	ONSET	PEAK	DURATION
PO	within 1–4 wk	Unknown	Unknown

Contraindications/Precautions
Contraindicated in: Hypersensitivity; Concurrent MAO inhibitors; Concurrent use of citalopram.
Use Cautiously in: History of mania (may activate mania/hypomania); History of seizures; Patients at risk for suicide; Hepatic impairment (dose reduction recommended); Geri: Hepatic impairment or geriatric patients (↓ doses recommended); Severe renal impairment; OB: Neonates exposed to SSRI in 3rd trimester may develop drug discontinuation syndrome including respiratory distress, feeding difficulty, and irritability. Weigh risks and benefits; Lactation: May cause adverse effects in infant; risk/benefit should be considered; Pedi: May ↑ risk of suicide attempt/ideation especially during early treatment or dose adjustment in children/adolescents (unlabeled for pediatric use).

E

Adverse Reactions/Side Effects
CNS: insomnia, dizziness, drowsiness, fatigue. **GI:** diarrhea, nausea, abdominal pain, constipation, dry mouth, indigestion. **GU:** anorgasmia, decreased libido, ejaculatory delay, erectile dysfunction. **Derm:** increased sweating. **Endo:** syndrome on inappropriate secretion of antidiuretic hormone (SIADH). **F and E:** hyponatremia. **Metab:** increased appetite.

Interactions
Drug-Drug: May cause serious, potentially fatal reactions when used with **MAO inhibitors**; allow at least 14 days between escitalopram and **MAO inhibitors**. Use cautiously with other **centrally acting drugs** (including **alcohol**, **antihistamines**, **opioid analgesics**, and **sedative/hypnotics**; concurrent use with **alcohol** is not recommended). Concurrent use with **sumatriptan** or other **5-HT$_3$ agonist vascular headache suppressants** may result in weakness, hyperreflexia, and incoordination. **Cimetidine** ↑ blood levels of escitalopram. Serotonergic effects may be ↑ by **lithium** (concurrent use should be carefully monitored). **Carbamazepine** may ↓ blood levels. May ↑ blood levels of **metoprolol**. Concurrent use with **tricyclic antidepressants** should be undertaken with caution because of altered pharmacokinetics.
Drug-Natural Products: ↑ risk of serotonin syndrome with **St. John's wort** and **SAMe**.

Route/Dosage
PO (Adults): 10 mg once daily, may be increased to 20 mg once daily after one week.

Hepatic Impairment
PO (Adults): 10 mg once daily.

PO (Geriatric Patients): 10 mg once daily.

Availability

Tablets: 5 mg, 10 mg, 20 mg. **Cost:** 5 mg $214.97/90, 10 mg $228.97/90, 20 mg $239.97/90. **Oral solution (peppermint):** 1 mg/ml in 240-ml bottles. **Cost:** $131.64/240 ml.

NURSING IMPLICATIONS

Assessment

- Monitor mood changes and level of anxiety during therapy.
- Assess for suicidal tendencies, especially during early therapy. Restrict amount of drug available to patient. Risk may be increased for children or adolescents. After starting therapy, children and adolescents should be seen by health care professional at least weekly for 4 wks, every 2 wks for next 4 wks, and on advice of health care professional thereafter.
- Assess for sexual dysfunction (erectile dysfunction; decreased libido).

Potential Nursing Diagnoses

Ineffective coping (Indications)
Post-trauma syndrome (Indications)
Risk for injury (Side Effects)
Sexual dysfunction (Side Effects)

Implementation

- Do not administer escitalopram and citalopram concomitantly. Taper to avoid potential withdrawal reactions. Reduce dose by 50% for 3 days, then again by 50% for 3 days, then discontinue.
- **PO:** Administer as a single dose in the morning or evening without regard to meals.

Patient/Family Teaching

- Instruct patient to take escitalopram as directed. Take missed doses on the same day as soon as remembered and consult health care professional. Resume regular dosing schedule next day. Do not double doses. Do not stop abruptly, should be discontinued gradually.
- May cause dizziness. Caution patient to avoid driving or other activities requiring alertness until response to medication is known.
- Advise patient to avoid alcohol and other CNS-depressant drugs during therapy and to consult a health care professional before taking other Rx or OTC medications or herbal products.
- Instruct female patients to notify health care professional if pregnancy is planned or suspected or if they plan to breastfeed an infant.
- Caution patients that escitalopram should not be used for at least 14 days after discontinuing MAO inhibitors, and at least 14 days should be allowed after stopping escitalopram before starting an MAO inhibitor.
- Emphasize importance of follow-up exams to monitor progress.
- Encourage patient participation in psychotherapy to improve coping skills.
- Refer patient/family to local support groups.

Evaluation/Desired Outcomes

- Increased sense of well-being.
- Renewed interest in surroundings. May require 1–4 wk of therapy to obtain antidepressant effects. Full antidepressant effects occur in 4–6 wks.
- Decrease in anxiety.

HIGH ALERT

esmolol (es-moe-lole)

Brevibloc

Classification

Therapeutic: antiarrhythmics (class II)
Pharmacologic: beta blockers

Pregnancy Category C

Indications

Management of sinus tachycardia and supraventricular arrhythmias.

Action

Blocks stimulation of $beta_1$ (myocardial)-adrenergic receptors. Does not usually affect $beta_2$ (pulmonary, vascular, or uterine)-receptor sites. **Therapeutic Effects:** Decreased heart rate. Decreased AV conduction.

Pharmacokinetics

Absorption: IV administration results in complete bioavailability.

Distribution: Rapidly and widely distributed.

Metabolism and Excretion: Metabolized by enzymes in RBCs and liver.

Half-life: 9 min.

TIME/ACTION PROFILE (antiarrhythmic effect)

ROUTE	ONSET	PEAK	DURATION
IV	within minutes	unknown	1–20 min

Contraindications/Precautions

Contraindicated in: Uncompensated CHF; Pulmonary edema; Cardiogenic shock; Bradycardia or heart block; Known alcohol intolerance.

Use Cautiously in: Geri: Geriatric patients (increased sensitivity to the effects of beta blockers); Thyrotoxicosis (may mask symptoms); Diabetes mellitus (may mask symptoms of hypoglycemia); Patients with a history of severe allergic reactions (intensity of reactions may be increased); OB, Pedi: Pregnancy, lactation, or children (safety not established; neonatal bradycardia, hypotension, hypoglycemia, and respiratory depression may occur rarely).

Adverse Reactions/Side Effects

CNS: fatigue, agitation, confusion, dizziness, drowsiness, weakness. **CV:** hypotension, peripheral ischemia. **GI:** nausea, vomiting. **Derm:** sweating. **Local:** injection site reactions.

Interactions

Drug-Drug: General anesthesia, IV **phenytoin**, and **verapamil** may cause additive myocardial depression. Additive bradycardia may occur with **digoxin**. Additive hypotension may occur with other **antihypertensives**, acute ingestion of **alcohol**, or **nitrates**. Concurrent use with **amphetamine**, **cocaine**, **ephedrine**, **epinephrine**, **norepinephrine**, **phenylephrine**, or **pseudoephedrine** may result in unopposed alpha-adrenergic stimulation (excessive hypertension, bradycardia). Concurrent **thyroid** administration may decrease effectiveness. May alter the effectiveness of **insulins** or **oral hypoglycemic agents** (dosage adjustments may be necessary). May ↓ effectiveness of **theophylline**. May ↓ beneficial beta cardiovascular effects of **dopamine** or **dobutamine**. Use cautiously within 14 days of **MAO inhibitor** therapy (may result in hypertension).

Route/Dosage

IV (Adults): *Antiarrhythmic*—500-mcg/kg loading dose over 1 min initially, followed by 50-mcg/kg/min infusion for 4 min; if no response within 5 min, give 2nd loading dose of 500 mcg/kg over 1 min, then increase infusion to 100 mcg/kg/min for 4 min. If no response, repeat loading dose of 500 mcg/kg over 1 min and increase infusion rate by 50-mcg/kg/min increments (not to exceed 200 mcg/kg/min for 48 hr). As therapeutic end point is achieved, eliminate loading doses and decrease dose increments to 25 mg/kg/min. *Intraoperative antihypertensive/antiarrhythmic*—250–500-mcg/kg loading dose over 1 min initially, followed by 50-mcg/kg/min infusion for 4 min; if no response within 5 min, give 2nd loading dose of 250–500 mcg/kg over 1 min, then increase infusion to 100 mcg/kg/min for 4 min. If no response, repeat loading dose of 250–500 mcg/kg over 1 min and increase infusion rate by 50-mcg/kg/min increments (not to exceed 200 mcg/kg/min for 48 hr).

IV (Children): *Antiarrhythmic*—50 mcg/kg/min, may be increased q 10 min up to 300 mcg/kg/min.

Availability

Solution for injection (prediluted for use as loading dose): 10 mg/ml in 10-ml vials, 20 mg/ml in 5-ml vials. **Solution for injection (must be diluted to prepare continuous infusion):** 250 mg/ml in 10-ml ampules. **Premixed infusion:** 2000 mg/100 ml, 2500 mg/250 ml.

NURSING IMPLICATIONS

Assessment

- Monitor blood pressure, ECG, and pulse frequently during dose adjustment period and periodically during therapy. The risk of hypotension is greatest within the first 30 min of initiating esmolol infusion.
- Monitor intake and output ratios and daily weights. Assess routinely for signs and symptoms of CHF (dyspnea, rales/crackles, weight gain, peripheral edema, jugular venous distention).
- Assess infusion site frequently throughout therapy. Concentrations >10 mg/ml may cause redness, swelling, skin discoloration, and burning at the injection site. Do not use butterfly needles for administration. If venous irritation occurs, stop the infusion and resume at another site.
- ***Toxicity and Overdose:*** Monitor patients receiving esmolol for signs of overdose

(bradycardia, severe dizziness or fainting, severe drowsiness, dyspnea, bluish fingernails or palms, seizures). Notify physician immediately if these signs occur: IV glucagon and symptomatic care are used in the treatment of esmolol overdose. Because of the short action of esmolol, discontinuation of therapy may relieve acute toxicity.

Potential Nursing Diagnoses

Decreased cardiac output (Side Effects)

Implementation

- ***High Alert:*** IV vasoactive medications are inherently dangerous. Esmolol is available in different concentrations; fatalities have occurred when loading dose vial is confused with concentrated solution for injection, which contains 2,500 mg in 10 ml (250 mg/ml) and must be diluted. Before administering, have second practitioner independently check original order, dose calculations, and infusion pump settings.
- ***High Alert:*** Do not confuse Brevibloc (esmolol) with Brevital (methohexital). If both are available as floor stock, store in separate areas.
- To convert to other antiarrhythmics following esmolol administration, administer the 1st dose of the antiarrhythmic agent and decrease the esmolol dose by 50% after 30 min. If an adequate response is maintained for 1 hr following the 2nd dose of the antiarrhythmic agent, discontinue esmolol.

IV Administration

- **Direct IV:** ***Diluent:*** The 10 mg/ml and 20 mg/ml vials should be used for the loading dose. These vials are already diluted. No further dilution is needed. *The 250 mg/ml ampule should not be used for the loading dose.* ***Concentration:*** 10 mg/ml or 20 mg/ml (depends upon the vial used). ***Rate:*** Administer over 1 min.
- **Continuous Infusion:** ***Diluent:*** Remove 10 ml from a 250 ml bag of D5W, D5/0.45% NaCl, D5/0.9% NaCl, 0.45% NaCl, 0.9% NaCl, or LR and add 2500 mg (10 ml) from the 250 mg/ml ampule. Alternatively, remove 20 ml from a 500 ml bag of an appropriate diluent and add 5000 mg (20 ml) from two 250 mg/ml ampules. Admixed solution is stable for 24 hr at room temperature. Premixed infusions are already diluted and ready to use. Solution is clear, colorless to light yellow. ***Concentration:*** 10 mg/ml. ***Rate:*** Based on patient's weight (see Route/Dosage section). Titration of dose is based on desired heart rate or undesired decrease in blood pressure. Esmolol infusions should not be abruptly discontinued; the infusion rate should be tapered.
- **Y-Site Compatibility:** amikacin, aminophylline, amiodarone, atropine, atracurium, aztreonam, bivalirudin, bumetanide, butorphanol, calcium chloride, calcium gluconate, caspofungin, cefazolin, cefotaxime, cefoxitin, ceftazidime, ceftizoxime, ceftriaxone, cefuroxime, cimetidine, cisatracurium, clindamycin, cyclosporine, daptomycin, dexmedetomidine, digoxin, diltiazem, diphenhydramine, dobutamine, dopamine, doxycycline, enalaprilat, epinephrine, ertapenem, erythromycin lactobionate, famotidine, fenoldopam, fentanyl, fluconazole, gentamicin, granisetron, heparin, hydrocotrisone sodium succinate, hydromorphone, hydroxyzine, imipenem/cilastatin, insulin, isoproterenol, labetalol, levofloxacin, lidocaine, linezolid, lorazepam, magnesium sulfate, methyldopate, meperidine, metoclopramide, metoprolol, metronidazole, micafungin, midazolam, morphine, nicardipine, nitroglycerin, nitroprusside, norepinephrine, ondansetron, palonosetron, pancuronium, penicillin G potassium, phenylephrine, phytonadione, piperacillin/tazobactam, potassium chloride, potassium phosphate, procainamide, prochlorperazine, promethazine, propofol, propranolol, protamine, quinupristin/dalfopristin, ranitidine, remifentanil, sodium bicarbonate, tacrolimus, ticarcillin/clavulanate, tirofiban, tobramycin, trimethoprim/sulfamethoxazole, vancomycin, vasopressin, vecuronium, verapamil, voriconazole.
- **Y-Site Incompatibility:** acyclovir, amphotericin B cholesteryl sulfate, dexamethoasone sodium phosphate, diazepam, furosemide, ganciclovir, ketorolac, lansoprazole, pantoprazole, warfarin.

Patient/Family Teaching

- May cause drowsiness. Caution patients receiving esmolol to call for assistance during ambulation or transfer.
- Advise patients to change positions slowly to minimize orthostatic hypotension.
- Patients with diabetes should closely monitor blood glucose, especially if weakness, malaise, irritability, or fatigue occurs. Medication does not block dizziness or sweating as signs of hypoglycemia.

Evaluation/Desired Outcomes

- Control of arrhythmias without appearance of detrimental side effects.

esomeprazole

(es-o-**mep**-ra-zole)
Nexium

Classification
Therapeutic: antiulcer agents
Pharmacologic: proton-pump inhibitors

Pregnancy Category B

Indications

GERD including: erosive esophagitis. Hypersecretory conditions, including Zollinger-Ellison syndrome. With amoxicillin and clarithromycin to eradicate *Helicobacter pylori* in duodenal ulcer disease or history of duodenal ulcer disease. Decrease risk of gastric ulcer during continuous NSAID therapy.

Action

Binds to an enzyme on gastric parietal cells in the presence of acidic gastric pH, preventing the final transport of hydrogen ions into the gastric lumen. **Therapeutic Effects:** Diminished accumulation of acid in the gastric lumen with lessened gastroesophageal reflux. Healing of duodenal ulcers. Decreased incidence of gastric ulcer during continuous NSAID therapy.

Pharmacokinetics

Absorption: 90% absorbed following oral administration; food decreases absorption.
Distribution: Unknown.
Protein Binding: 97%.
Metabolism and Excretion: Extensively metabolized by the liver (cytochrome P450 [CY P450] system, primarily CY P2 C19 isoenzyme); <1% excreted unchanged in urine.
Half-life: 1.0–1.5 hr.

TIME/ACTION PROFILE (blood levels*)

ROUTE	ONSET	PEAK	DURATION
PO	rapid	1.6 hr	24 hr
IV	rapid	end of infusion	24 hr

*Resolution of symptoms takes 5–8 days

Contraindications/Precautions

Contraindicated in: Hypersensitivity; OB: Lactation (not recommended).

Use Cautiously in: Severe hepatic impairment (daily dose should not exceed 20 mg); Geri: Increased risk of hip fractures in patients using high-doses for >1 year; OB: Pregnancy (use only if clearly needed); Pedi: Children <18 yr (safety not established).

E

Adverse Reactions/Side Effects

CNS: headache. **GI:** abdominal pain, constipation, diarrhea, dry mouth, flatulence, nausea.

Interactions

Drug-Drug: May ↓ absorption and effects of drugs where gastric pH is a determinant of bioavailability, including **digoxin**, **ketoconazole**, and **iron salts**. May ↑ risk of bleeding with **warfarin** (monitor INR and PT).

Route/Dosage

Gastroesophageal Reflux Disease

PO (Adults): *Healing of erosive esophagitis*—20 mg or 40 mg once daily for 4–8 wks; *maintenance of healing of erosive esophagitis*—20 mg once daily; *symptomatic GERD*—20 mg once daily for 4 wks (additional 4 wks may be considered for nonresponders).
PO (Children 12–17 yrs): *Short-term treatment of GERD*—20 mg or 20 mg once daily up to 8 wks.
IV (Adults): 20 or 40 mg once daily.

H. pylori Eradication to Reduce the Risk of Duodenal Ulcer Recurrence (Triple Therapy)

PO (Adults): 40 mg once daily for 10 days with amoxicillin 1000 mg twice daily for 10 days and clarithromycin 500 mg twice daily for 10 days.

Decrease Gastric Ulcer During Continuous NSAID Therapy

PO (Adults): 20 or 40 mg once daily for up to 6 mo.

Pathological Hypersecretory Conditions Including Zollinger-Ellison Syndrome

PO (Adults): 40 mg twice daily.

Severe Hepatic Impairment

PO, IV (Adults): Daily dose should not exceed 20 mg.

Availability

Delayed-release capsules: 20 mg, 40 mg. **Cost:** 20 mg $430.97/90, 40 mg $425.97/90. **Delayed-release oral suspension packets:** 20 mg, 40 mg. **Powder for injection (re-**

quires reconstitution): 20 mg/vial, 40 mg/vial.

NURSING IMPLICATIONS

Assessment

- Assess patient routinely for epigastric or abdominal pain and frank or occult blood in the stool, emesis, or gastric aspirate.
- ***Lab Test Considerations:*** May cause ↑ serum creatinine, uric acid, total bilirubin, alkaline phosphatase, AST, and ALT.
- May alter hemoglobin, WBC, platelets, serum sodium, potassium, and thyroxine levels.

Potential Nursing Diagnoses

Acute pain (Indications)

Implementation

- Antacids may be used while taking esomeprazole.
- **PO:** Administer at least 1 hr before meals. Capsules should be swallowed whole.
- **Delayed-release capsules:** For patients with difficulty swallowing, place 1 tbsp of applesauce in an empty bowl. Open capsule and carefully empty the pellets inside onto applesauce. Mix pellets with applesauce and swallow immediately. Applesauce should not be hot and should be soft enough to swallow without chewing. Do not store applesauce mixture for future use. Tap water, orange juice, apple juice, and yogurt have also been used. Do not crush or chew pellets.
- **For patients with an NG tube,** delayed-release capsules can be opened and intact granules emptied into a 60-ml syringe and mixed with 50 ml of water. Replace plunger and shake syringe vigorously for 15 sec. Hold syringe with tip up and check for granules in tip. Attach syringe to NG tube and administer solution. After administering, flush syringe with additional water. Do not administer if granules have dissolved or disintegrated. Administer immediately after mixing.
- **Delayed-release oral suspension:** Mix contents of packet with 1 tablespoon (15 ml) of water, leave 2-3 min to thicken, stir and drink within 30 minutes.
- **For delayed-release oral suspension nasogastric or gastric tube:** Add 15 ml of water to a syringe and then add contents of packet. Shake the syringe, leave 2–3 min to thicken. Shake the syringe and inject through the nasogastric or gastric tube within 30 min.
- **Direct IV:** Reconstitute each vial with 5 mL of 0.9% NaCl, LR, or D5W. Do not administer solutions that are discolored or contain a precipitate. Stable at room temperature for up to 12 hr. ***Rate:*** Administer over at least 3 min.
- **Intermittent Infusion:** Dilute reconstituted solution to a volume of 50 ml. Solutions diluted with 0.9% NaCl or LR are stable for 12 hr and those diluted with D5W are stable for 6 hr at room temperature. ***Rate:*** Administer over 10–30 min.
- **Y-Site Incompatibility:** Do not administer with other medications or solutions. Flush line with 0.9% NaCl, LR, or D5W before and after administration.

Patient/Family Teaching

- Instruct patient to take medication as directed for the full course of therapy, even if feeling better. Take missed doses as soon as remembered but not if almost time for next dose. Do not double doses.
- Advise patient to avoid alcohol, products containing aspirin or NSAIDs, and foods that may cause an increase in GI irritation.
- Advise patient to report onset of black, tarry stools; diarrhea; abdominal pain; or persistent headache to health care professional promptly.

Evaluation/Desired Outcomes

- Decrease in abdominal pain or prevention of gastric irritation and bleeding. Healing of duodenal ulcers can be seen on X-ray examination or endoscopy.
- Decrease in symptoms of GERD. Sustained resolution of symptoms usually occurs in 5–8 days. Therapy is continued for 4–8 wk after initial episode.
- Decreased incidence of gastric ulcer during continuous NSAID therapy.
- Eradication of *H. Pylori* in duodenal ulcer disease.
- Decrease in symptoms of hypersecretory conditions, including Zollinger-Ellison.

ESTRADIOL (es-tra-**dye**-ole)

Estrace, Gynodiol

estradiol acetate
Femtrace

estradiol cypionate
depGynogen, Depo-Estradiol, Depogen, Dura-Estrin, E-Cypionate,

Estragyn LA 5, Estro-Cyp, Estrofem, Estroject-LA, Estro-L.A

estradiol valerate
Clinagen LA, Delestrogen, Dioval, Duragen, Estra-L, Estro-Span, ✤Femogex, Gynogen L.A, Menaval, Valergen

estradiol topical emulsion
Estrasorb

estradiol topical gel
Divigel, Elestrin, EstroGel

estradiol transdermal spray
EvaMist

estradiol transdermal system
Alora, Climara, Esclim, Estraderm, FemPatch, Menostar, Vivelle

estradiol vaginal tablet
Vagifem

estradiol vaginal ring
Femring, Estring

Classification
Therapeutic: hormones
Pharmacologic: estrogens

Pregnancy Category X

Indications

PO, IM, Topical, Transdermal: Replacement of estrogen (HRT) to diminish moderate to severe vasomotor symptoms of menopause and of various estrogen deficiency states including: Female hypogonadism, Ovariectomy, Primary ovarian failure. Treatment and prevention of postmenopausal osteoporosis (not vaginal dose forms). **PO:** Inoperable metastatic postmenopausal breast or prostate carcinoma. **Vag:** Management of atrophic vaginitis that may occur with menopause (low dose), bothersome systemic symptoms of menopause (higher dose). Concurrent use of progestin is recommended during cyclical therapy to decrease the risk of endometrial carcinoma in patients with an intact uterus.

Action

Estrogens promote growth and development of female sex organs and the maintenance of secondary sex characteristics in women. Metabolic effects include reduced blood cholesterol, protein synthesis, and sodium and water retention. **Therapeutic Effects:** Restoration of hormonal balance in various deficiency states, including menopause. Treatment of hormone-sensitive tumors.

Pharmacokinetics

Absorption: Well absorbed after oral administration. Readily absorbed through skin and mucous membranes.
Distribution: Widely distributed. Crosses the placenta and enters breast milk.
Metabolism and Excretion: Mostly metabolized by the liver and other tissues. Enterohepatic recirculation occurs, and more absorption may occur from the GI tract.
Half-life: Gel: 36 hr.

TIME/ACTION PROFILE (estrogenic effects)

ROUTE	ONSET	PEAK	DURATION
PO	unknown	unknown	unknown
IM	unknown	unknown	unknown
TD	unknown	unknown	3–4 days (Estraderm), 7 days (Climara)
Topical	unknown	unknown	uknown
Vaginal ring	unknown	unknown	90 days
Vaginal tablet	unknown	unknown	3–4 days

Contraindications/Precautions

Contraindicated in: Thromboembolic disease; Undiagnosed vaginal bleeding; OB: Pregnancy (may result in harm to the fetus); Lactation.
Use Cautiously in: Underlying cardiovascular disease; Severe hepatic or renal disease; May increase the risk of endometrial carcinoma; History of porphyria.

Adverse Reactions/Side Effects

CNS: headache, dizziness, lethargy. **EENT:** intolerance to contact lenses, worsening of myopia or astigmatism. **CV:** MI, THROMBOEMBOLISM, edema, hypertension. **GI:** nausea, weight changes, anorexia, increased appetite, jaundice, vomiting. **GU:** *women*— amenorrhea, dysmenorrhea, breakthrough bleeding, cervical erosions, loss of libido, vaginal candidiasis; *men*— impotence, testicular atrophy. **Derm:** oily skin, acne, pigmentation, urticaria. **Endo:** gynecomastia (men), hyperglycemia. **F and E:** hypercal-

✤ = Canadian drug name.
* CAPITALS indicates life-threatening; underlines indicate most frequent.

cemia, sodium and water retention. **MS:** leg cramps. **Misc:** breast tenderness.

Interactions

Drug-Drug: May alter requirement for **warfarin**, **oral hypoglycemic agents**, or **insulins**. **Barbiturates** or **rifampin** may ↓ effectiveness. **Smoking** ↑ risk of adverse CV reactions.

Route/Dosage

Estrogens should be used in the lowest doses for the shortest period of time consistent with desired therapeutic outcome.

Symptoms of Menopause, Atrophic Vaginitis, Female Hypogonadism, Ovarian Failure/Osteoporosis

PO (Adults): 0.45–2 mg daily or in a cycle.
IM (Adults): 1–5 mg monthly (estradiol cypionate) *or* 10–20 mg (estradiol valerate) monthly.
Topical: Emulsion *(Estrasorb)* **(Adults):** Apply two 1.74 g pouches (4.35 mg estradiol) daily.
Gel **(Adults):** Apply contents of one packet *(Divigel)* or one actuation from pump *(EstroGel, Elestrin)* daily.
Spray *EvaMist* **(Adults):** 1 spray daily, may be increased to 2–3 sprays daily.
Transdermal (Adults): *Alora, Estraderm*—50- or 100-mcg/24-hr transdermal patch applied twice weekly. *Climara*—50–100-mcg/24-hr patch applied weekly. *FemPatch*—25-mcg/24-hr patch applied q 7 days. *Vivelle*—37.5–100-mcg/24 hr transdermal patch applied twice weekly. *Menostar*—14-mcg/24-hr patch applied q 7 days. Progestin may be administered for 10–14 days of each month.
Vag (Adults): *Cream*—2–4 g (0.2–0.4 mg estradiol) daily for 1–2 wk, then decrease to 1–2 g/day for 1–2 wk; then maintenance dose of 1 g 1–3 times weekly for 3 wk, then off for 1 wk; then repeat cycle once vaginal mucosa has been restored; *Vaginal ring (Estring)*—2-mg (releases 7.5 mcg estradiol/24 hr) q 3 mo; *Vaginal ring (Femring)*—12.4 mg (releases 50 mcg estradiol/24 hr) q 3 mo or 24.8 mg (releases 100 mcg estradiol/24 hr) q 3 mo (*Femring* requires concurrent progesterone) *Vaginal tablet*—25-mcg once daily for 2 wk, then twice weekly.

Postmenopausal Breast Carcinoma

PO (Adults): 10 mg 3 times daily.

Prostate Carcinoma

PO (Adults): 1–2 mg 3 times daily.
IM (Adults): 30 mg q 1–2 wk (estradiol valerate).

Availability

Tablets: 0.45 mg, 0.5 mg, 0.9 mg, 1 mg, 1.8 mg, 2 mg. **Cost:** *Generic*—0.5 mg $22.17/100, 1 mg $15.52/100, 2 mg $33.30/100. **Injection (valerate in oil):** 10 mg/ml, 20 mg/ml, 40 mg/ml. **Injection (cypionate in oil):** 5 mg/ml. **Topical emulsion:** 4.35 mg/1.74 g pouch in boxes of 14 pouches in a one-month supply carton of 56 pouches. **Topical gel packet:** 0.25 g packet, 0.5 g packet, 1 g packet. **Topical gel pump (0.06%):** 0.87 g/actuation, 1.25 g/actuation. **Transdermal Spray:** metered dose pump contains 8.1 mL, delivers 56 sprays of 1.53 mg each. **Transdermal system:** 14 mcg/24-hr release rate, 25 mcg/24-hr release rate, 37.5 mcg/24-hr release rate, 50 mcg/24-hr release rate, 60 mcg/24–hr release rate, 75 mcg/24-hr release rate, 100 mcg/24-hr release rate. **Cost:** *Generic*—25 mcg/24–hr release rate $36.99/4 patches, 37.5 mcg/24–hr release rate $39.35/4 patches, 50 mcg/24–hr release rate $29.97/4 patches, 60 mcg/24–hr release rate $39.99/4 patches, 75 mcg/24–hr release rate $35.99/4 patches, 100 mcg/24–hr release rate $31.46/4 patches. **Vaginal cream:** 100 mcg/g. **Vaginal ring (Estring):** 2 mg (releases 7.5 mcg/day over 90 days). **Vaginal ring (Femring):** 12.4 mg (releases 50 mcg/day over 90 days), 24.8 mg (releases 100 mcg/day over 90 days). **Vaginal tablet:** 25 mcg. **Cost:** $75.81/18 tablets.

NURSING IMPLICATIONS

Assessment

- Assess blood pressure before and periodically during therapy.
- Monitor intake and output ratios and weekly weight. Report significant discrepancies or steady weight gain.
- **Menopause:** Assess frequency and severity of vasomotor symptoms.
- ***Lab Test Considerations:*** May cause ↑ HDL, phospholipids, and triglycerides and ↓ serum LDL and total cholesterol concentrations.
- May cause ↑ serum glucose, sodium, cortisol, prolactin, prothrombin, and factor VII, VIII, IX, and X levels. May ↓ serum folate, pyridoxine, antithrombin III, and urine pregnanediol concentrations.
- Monitor hepatic function before and periodically during therapy.

- May cause false interpretations of thyroid function tests, false ↑ in norepinephrine platelet-induced aggregability, and false ↓ in metyrapone tests.
- May cause hypercalcemia in patients with metastatic bone lesions.

Potential Nursing Diagnoses

Sexual dysfunction (Indications)

Implementation

- Do not confuse Estraderm (estradiol) with Testaderm (testosterone).
- **PO:** Administer with or immediately after food to reduce nausea.
- **Vag:** Manufacturer provides applicator with cream. Dose is marked on the applicator. Wash applicator with mild soap and warm water after each use.
- **Transdermal:** When switching from PO form, begin transdermal therapy 1 wk after the last dose or when symptoms reappear.
- **Topical:** In a comfortable position, apply *Estrasorb* to clean, dry skin of thighs each morning. Open each foil pouch individually. Cut or tear the first pouch at the notches near the top of the pouch. Apply the contents of the pouch to the top of the left thigh; push entire contents from bottom through neck of pouch. Using one or both hands rub the emulsion into the thigh and calf for 3 min until completely absorbed. Rub any excess remaining on hands into buttocks. Repeat procedure with second pouch on right leg. Allow application sites to dry completely before covering with clothing to prevent transfer. Wash hands with soap and water to remove residual estradiol.
- Apply *Divigel* individual-use once-daily packets of quick drying gel to an area measuring 5 inches by 7 inches (size of 2 palm prints) on the thigh. Do not wash area for at least 1 hr after gel has dried.
- Spray *EvaMist* on inside of forearm at the same time each day. Do not massage or rub the spray into the skin. Allow to dry for 2 min before dressing and 30 min before washing. Never spray *EvaMist* around breast or vagina Do not use more than 56 doses, even if fluid remains in pump.
- **IM:** Injection has oil base. Roll syringe to ensure even dispersion. Administer deep IM. Avoid IV administration.

Patient/Family Teaching

- Instruct patient on correct method of administration. Instruct patient to take medication as directed. Take missed doses as soon as remembered as long as it is not just before next dose. If a dose of *EvaMist* is missed, apply if more than 12 hr before next dose; if less than 12 hrs, omit dose and return to regular schedule. Do not double doses.
- Explain dose schedule and maintenance routine. Discontinuing medication suddenly may cause withdrawal bleeding.
- If nausea becomes a problem, advise patient that eating solid food often provides relief.
- Advise patient to report signs and symptoms of fluid retention (swelling of ankles and feet, weight gain), thromboembolic disorders (pain, swelling, tenderness in extremities, headache, chest pain, blurred vision), mental depression, or hepatic dysfunction (yellowed skin or eyes, pruritus, dark urine, light-colored stools) to health care professional.
- Instruct patient to stop taking medication and notify health care professional if pregnancy is suspected.
- Advise patient to notify health care professional of medication regimen before treatment or surgery.
- Caution patient that cigarette smoking during estrogen therapy may cause increased risk of serious side effects, especially for women over age 35.
- Caution patient to use sunscreen and protective clothing to prevent increased pigmentation.
- Advise patient treated for osteoporosis that exercise has been found to arrest and reverse bone loss. The patient should discuss any exercise limitations with health care professional before beginning program.
- Inform patient that estrogens should not be used to decrease risk of cardiovascular disease. Estrogens may increase risk of cardiovascular disease and breast cancer.
- Emphasize the importance of routine follow-up physical exams, including blood pressure; breast, abdomen, and pelvic examinations; Papanicolaou smears every 6–12 mo; and mammogram every 12 mo or as directed. Health care professional will evaluate possibility of discontinuing medication every 3–6 mo. If on continuous (not cyclical) therapy

or without concurrent progestins, endometrial biopsy may be recommended, if uterus is intact.

- **Vag:** Instruct patient in the correct use of applicator. Patient should remain recumbent for at least 30 min after administration. May use sanitary napkin to protect clothing, but do not use tampon. If a dose is missed, do not use the missed dose, but return to regular dosing schedule.
- Instruct patient to use applicator provided with vaginal tablet. Insert as high up in the vagina as comfortable, without using force.
- **Vaginal Ring:** Instruct patient to press ring into an oval and insert into the upper third of the vaginal vault. Exact position is not critical. Once ring is inserted, patient should not feel anything. If discomfort is felt, ring is probably not in far enough; gently push farther into vagina. Leave in place continuously for 90 days. Ring does not interfere with sexual intercourse. If straining at defecation makes ring move to lower vagina, push up with finger. If expelled totally, rinse ring with lukewarm water and reinsert. To remove, hook a finger through the ring and pull it out.
- **Transdermal:** Instruct patient to wash and dry hands first. Apply disc to intact skin on hairless portion of abdomen (do not apply to breasts or waistline). Press disc for 10 sec to ensure contact with skin (especially around edges). Avoid areas where clothing may rub disc loose. Change site with each administration to prevent skin irritation. Do not reuse site for 1 wk; disc may be reapplied if it falls off.

Evaluation/Desired Outcomes

- Resolution of menopausal vasomotor symptoms.
- Decreased vaginal and vulvar itching, inflammation, or dryness associated with menopause.
- Normalization of estrogen levels in patients with ovariectomy or hypogonadism.
- Control of the spread of advanced metastatic breast or prostate cancer.
- Prevention of osteoporosis.

estrogens, conjugated (equine) (ess-troe-jenz)

✤C.E.S, ✤Congest, Premarin

estrogens,conjugated(synthetic,A)

Cenestin

estrogens,conjugated(synthetic,B)

Enjuvia

Classification

Therapeutic: hormones

Pharmacologic: estrogens

Pregnancy Category X

Indications

PO: Treatment of moderate to severe vasomotor symptoms of menopause. Estrogen deficiency states, including: Female hypogonadism, Ovariectomy, Primary ovarian failure. Prevention of postmenopausal osteoporosis. Advanced inoperable metastatic breast and prostatic carcinoma. **IM, IV:** Uterine bleeding resulting from hormonal imbalance. **Vag:** Management of atrophic vaginitis. Concurrent use of progestin is recommended during cyclical therapy to decrease the risk of endometrial carcinoma in patients with an intact uterus.

Action

Estrogens promote the growth and development of female sex organs and the maintenance of secondary sex characteristics in women. **Therapeutic Effects:** Restoration of hormonal balance in various deficiency states and treatment of hormone-sensitive tumors.

Pharmacokinetics

Absorption: Well absorbed after oral administration. Readily absorbed through skin and mucous membranes.

Distribution: Widely distributed. Crosses placenta and enters breast milk.

Metabolism and Excretion: Mostly metabolized by liver and other tissues. Enterohepatic recirculation occurs, with more absorption from GI tract.

Half-life: Unknown.

TIME/ACTION PROFILE (estrogenic effects†)

ROUTE	ONSET	PEAK	DURATION
PO	rapid	unknown	24 hr
IM	delayed	unknown	6–12 hr
IV	rapid	unknown	6–12 hr

†Tumor response may take several weeks

Contraindications/Precautions

Contraindicated in: Thromboembolic disease (e.g. DVT, PE, MI, stroke); Undiagnosed vaginal bleeding; History of breast cancer; History of estrogen-dependent cancer; Liver dysfunction; OB: Pregnancy (may result in harm to the fetus); OB: Lactation.

Use Cautiously in: Long-term use (more than 4–5 yr); may increase risk of myocardial infarction, stroke, invasive breast cancer, pulmonary emboli, deep vein thrombosis and dementia in postmenopausal women; Underlying cardiovascular disease; Hypertriglyceridemia; May increase the risk of endometrial carcinoma.

Adverse Reactions/Side Effects

(systemic use) **CNS:** headache, dizziness, insomnia, lethargy, mental depression. **CV:** MI, THROMBOEMBOLISM, edema, hypertension. **GI:** nausea, weight changes, anorexia, increased appetite, jaundice, vomiting. **GU:** *women*— amenorrhea, breakthrough bleeding, dysmenorrhea, cervical erosion, loss of libido, vaginal candidiasis; *men*— impotence, testicular atrophy. **Derm:** acne, oily skin, pigmentation, urticaria. **Endo:** gynecomastia (men), hyperglycemia. **F and E:** hypercalcemia, sodium and water retention. **MS:** leg cramps. **Misc:** breast tenderness.

Interactions

Drug-Drug: May alter requirement for **warfarin**, **oral hypoglycemic agents**, or **insulins**. **Barbiturates**, **carbamazepine**, or **rifampin** may ↓ effectiveness. **Smoking** ↑ risk of adverse CV reactions. **Erythromycin**, **clarithromycin**, **itraconazole**, **ketoconazole**, and **ritonavir** may ↑ risk of adverse effects.

Drug-Natural Products: Grapefruit juice may ↑ risk of adverse effects.

Route/Dosage

Estrogens should be used in the lowest doses for the shortest period of time consistent with desired therapeutic outcome.

Ovariectomy, Primary Ovarian Failure

PO (Adults): 1.25 mg daily administered cyclically (3 wk on, 1 wk off).

Osteoporosis/Menopausal Symptoms

PO (Adults): 0.3–1.25 mg daily or in a cycle.

Female Hypogonadism

PO (Adults): 0.3–0.625 mg daily administered cyclically (3 wk on, 1 wk off).

Inoperable Breast Carcinoma—Men and Postmenopausal Women

PO (Adults): 10 mg 3 times daily.

Inoperable Prostate Carcinoma

PO (Adults): 1.25–2.5 mg 3 times daily.

Uterine Bleeding

IM, IV (Adults): 25 mg, may repeat in 6–12 hr if necessary.

Atrophic Vaginitis

PO (Adults): 0.3–1.25 mg daily.

Vag (Adults): 1.25–2.5 mg (2–4 g cream) daily for 3 wk, off for 1 wk, then repeat.

Availability (generic available)

Tablets: 0.3 mg, 0.45 mg, 0.625 mg, 0.9 mg, 1.25 mg. **Cost:** *Premarin*—0.3 mg $166.63/100, 0.45 mg $139.97/100, 0.625 mg $136.95/100, 0.9 mg $139.97/100, 1.25 mg $126.46/100. **Powder for injection:** 25 mg/vial. **Vaginal cream:** 0.625 mg/g. **Cost:** $85.99/42.5-g tube. ***In combination with:*** medroxyprogesterone (Prempro and Premphase [compliance package]). See Appendix B.

NURSING IMPLICATIONS

Assessment

- Assess blood pressure before and periodically during therapy.
- Monitor intake and output ratios and weekly weight. Report significant discrepancies or steady weight gain.
- **Menopause:** Assess frequency and severity of vasomotor symptoms.
- ***Lab Test Considerations:*** May cause ↑ HDL and triglycerides, and ↓ serum LDL and total cholesterol concentrations.
- May cause ↑ serum glucose, sodium, cortisol, prolactin, prothrombin, and factor VII, VIII, IX, and X levels. May ↓ serum folate, pyridoxine, antithrombin III, and urine pregnanediol concentrations.
- Monitor hepatic function before and periodically during therapy.
- May cause false interpretations of thyroid function tests.
- May cause hypercalcemia in patients with metastatic bone lesions.

Potential Nursing Diagnoses

Sexual dysfunction (Indications)

Implementation

- Estrogens should be used in the lowest doses for the shortest period of time consistent with desired therapeutic outcome.

- **PO:** Administer with or immediately after food to reduce nausea.
- **Vag:** Manufacturer provides applicator with cream. Dose is marked on the applicator. Wash applicator with mild soap and warm water after each use.
- **IM:** To reconstitute, withdraw at least 5 ml of air from dry container and then slowly introduce the sterile diluent (bacteriostatic water for injection) against the container side. Gently agitate container to dissolve; do not shake vigorously. Solution is stable for 60 days if refrigerated. Do not use if precipitate is present or if solution is darkened.
- IV is preferred parenteral route because of rapid response.

IV Administration

- **Direct IV:** ***Diluent:*** Reconstitute as for IM. Inject into distal port tubing of free-flowing IV of 0.9% NaCl, D5W, or lactated Ringer's solution. ***Concentration:*** 5 mg/ml. ***Rate:*** Administer slowly (no faster than 5 mg/min) to prevent flushing.
- **Y-Site Compatibility:** heparin, potassium chloride, vitamin B complex with C.
- **Additive Incompatibility:** ascorbic acid or acidic solutions.

Patient/Family Teaching

- Instruct patient to take oral medication as directed. Take missed doses as soon as remembered, but not just before next dose. Do not double doses.
- Explain dosage schedule and maintenance routine. Discontinuing medication suddenly may cause withdrawal bleeding. Bleeding is anticipated during the week when conjugated estrogens are withheld.
- If nausea becomes a problem, advise patient that eating solid food often provides relief.
- Advise patient to report signs and symptoms of fluid retention (swelling of ankles and feet, weight gain), thromboembolic disorders (pain, swelling, tenderness in extremities; headache; chest pain; blurred vision), depression, hepatic dysfunction (yellowed skin or eyes, pruritus, dark urine, light-colored stools), or abnormal vaginal bleeding to health care professional.
- Instruct patient to stop taking medication and notify health care professional if pregnancy is suspected.
- Caution patient that cigarette smoking during estrogen therapy may increase risk of serious side effects, especially for women over age 35.
- Caution patient to use sunscreen and protective clothing to prevent increased pigmentation.
- Advise patient to notify health care professional of medication regimen before treatment or surgery.
- Advise patient treated for osteoporosis that exercise has been found to arrest and reverse bone loss. The patient should discuss any exercise limitations with health care professional before beginning program.
- Emphasize the importance of routine follow-up physical exams, including blood pressure; breast, abdomen, and pelvic examinations; Papanicolaou smears every 6–12 mo; and mammogram every 12 mo or as directed. Health care professional will evaluate possibility of discontinuing medication every 3–6 mo. If on continuous (not cyclical) therapy or without concurrent progestins, endometrial biopsy may be recommended if uterus is intact.
- Inform patient that estrogens should not be used to decrease risk of cardiovascular disease. Estrogens may increase risk of cardiovascular disease and breast cancer.
- **Vag:** Instruct patient in the correct use of applicator. Patient should remain recumbent for at least 30 min after administration. May use sanitary napkin to protect clothing, but do not use tampon. If a dose is missed, do not use the missed dose, but return to regular dosing schedule.

Evaluation/Desired Outcomes

- Resolution of menopausal vasomotor symptoms.
- Decreased vaginal and vulvar itching, inflammation, or dryness associated with menopause.
- Normalization of estrogen levels in patients with ovariectomy or hypogonadism.
- Control of the spread of advanced metastatic breast or prostate cancer.
- Prevention of osteoporosis.

estropipate (ess-troe-**pi**-pate)

Ogen, Ortho-Est, piperazine estrone sulfate

Classification
Therapeutic: hormones
Pharmacologic: estrogens

Pregnancy Category X

Indications
PO: As part of HRT in the treatment of vasomotor symptoms of menopause. Treatment of various estrogen deficiency states, including: Female hypogonadism, Ovariectomy, Primary ovarian failure. Adjunctive therapy of postmenopausal osteoporosis. **Vag:** Management of atrophic vaginitis. Concurrent use of progestin is recommended during cyclical therapy to decrease the risk of endometrial carcinoma in patients with an intact uterus.

Action
Estrogens promote the growth and development of female sex organs and the maintenance of secondary sex characteristics in women. Metabolic effects include reduced blood cholesterol, protein synthesis, and sodium and water retention. **Therapeutic Effects:** Restoration of hormonal balance in various deficiency states.

Pharmacokinetics
Absorption: Well absorbed after oral administration. Readily absorbed through skin and mucous membranes.
Distribution: Widely distributed. Crosses the placenta and enters breast milk.
Metabolism and Excretion: Mostly metabolized by the liver and other tissues. Enterohepatic recirculation occurs, and more absorption may occur from the GI tract.
Half-life: Unknown.

TIME/ACTION PROFILE (estrogenic effects)

ROUTE	ONSET	PEAK	DURATION
PO	unknown	unknown	24 hr

Contraindications/Precautions
Contraindicated in: Thromboembolic disease; Undiagnosed vaginal bleeding; Pregnancy (may result in harm to the fetus); Lactation.
Use Cautiously in: Underlying cardiovascular disease; Severe hepatic or renal disease; May increase the risk of endometrial carcinoma.

Adverse Reactions/Side Effects
(systemic use) **CNS:** headache, dizziness, lethargy, mental depression. **EENT:** intolerance to contact lenses, worsening of myopia or astigmatism. **CV:** MI, THROMBOEMBOLISM, edema, hypertension. **GI:** nausea, weight changes, anorexia, increased appetite, jaundice, vomiting. **GU:** *women*— amenorrhea, breakthrough bleeding, dysmenorrhea, cervical erosion, loss of libido, vaginal candidiasis; *men*— erectile dysfunction, testicular atrophy. **Derm:** acne, oily skin, pigmentation, urticaria. **Endo:** gynecomastia (men), hyperglycemia. **F and E:** hypercalcemia, sodium and water retention. **MS:** leg cramps. **Misc:** breast tenderness.

Interactions
Drug-Drug: May alter requirement for **warfarin**, **oral hypoglycemic agents**, or **insulins**. **Barbiturates** or **rifampin** may ↓ effectiveness. **Smoking** ↑ the risk of adverse cardiovascular reactions.

Route/Dosage
Vasomotor Symptoms of Menopause/ Atrophic Vaginitis/Osteoporosis
PO (Adults): 0.75–6 mg daily or in a cycle.
Vag (Adults): 3–6 mg (2–4 g of 0.15% cream) daily for 3 wk, then off for 1 wk, then repeat cycle.

Female Hypogonadism/Ovarian Failure
PO (Adults): 1.5–9 mg daily or in a cycle.

Availability (generic available)
Tablets: 0.75 mg, 1.5 mg, 3 mg, 6 mg estropipate. **Vaginal cream:** 1.5 mg/g.

NURSING IMPLICATIONS
Assessment
- Assess blood pressure before and periodically throughout therapy.
- Monitor intake and output ratios and weekly weight. Report significant discrepancies or steady weight gain.
- **Menopause:** Assess frequency and severity of vasomotor symptoms.
- ***Lab Test Considerations:*** May cause increased HDL, phospholipids, and triglycerides, and decreased serum LDL and total cholesterol concentrations.
- May cause increased serum glucose, sodium, cortisol, prolactin, prothrombin, and factor VII, VIII, IX, and X levels. May decrease serum folate, pyridoxine, antithrombin III, and urine pregnanediol concentrations.

- Monitor hepatic function before and periodically throughout therapy.
- May cause false interpretations of thyroid function tests, false increases in norepinephrine platelet-induced aggregability, and false decreases in metyrapone tests.

Potential Nursing Diagnoses
Sexual dysfunction (Indications)

Implementation
- **PO:** Administer PO doses with or immediately after food to reduce nausea.
- **Vag:** Manufacturer provides applicator with cream. Dose is marked on the applicator. Wash applicator with mild soap and warm water after each use.

Patient/Family Teaching
- Instruct patient to take oral medication as directed. If a dose is missed, take as soon as remembered as long as it is not just before next dose. Do not double doses.
- Explain medication schedule to women on 21-day cycle followed by 7 days of not taking medication. Encourage patient to take medication at the same time each day.
- If nausea becomes a problem, advise patient that eating solid food often provides relief.
- Advise patient to report signs and symptoms of fluid retention (swelling of ankles and feet, weight gain), thromboembolic disorders (pain, swelling, or tenderness in extremities; headache; chest pain; blurred vision), mental depression, hepatic dysfunction (yellowed skin or eyes, pruritus, dark urine, light-colored stools), or abnormal vaginal bleeding to health care professional.
- Instruct patient to stop taking medication and notify health care professional if pregnancy is suspected.
- Caution patient that cigarette smoking during estrogen therapy may increase risk of serious side effects, especially for women over age 35.
- Caution patient to use sunscreen and protective clothing to prevent increased pigmentation.
- Advise patient to notify health care professional of medication regimen before treatment or surgery.
- Advise patient treated for osteoporosis that exercise has been found to arrest and reverse bone loss. The patient should discuss any exercise limitations with health care professional before beginning program.
- Emphasize the importance of routine follow-up physical exams, including blood pressure; breast, abdomen, and pelvic examinations; Papanicolaou smears every 6–12 mo; and mammogram every 12 mo or as directed. Health care professional will evaluate possibility of discontinuing medication every 3–6 mo. If on continuous (not cyclical) therapy or without concurrent progestins, endometrial biopsy may be recommended, if uterus is intact.
- **Vag:** Instruct patient in the correct use of applicator. Patient should remain recumbent for at least 30 min after administration. May use sanitary napkin to protect clothing, but do not use tampon. If a dose is missed, do not use the missed dose, but return to regular dosing schedule.

Evaluation/Desired Outcomes
- Resolution of menopausal vasomotor symptoms.
- Decreased vaginal and vulvar itching, inflammation, or dryness associated with menopause.
- Normalization of estrogen levels in patients with ovariectomy or hypogonadism.
- Prevention of osteoporosis.

eszopiclone (es-zop-i-klone)
Lunesta

Classification
Therapeutic: sedative/hypnotics
Pharmacologic: cyclopyrrolones

Schedule IV

Pregnancy Category C

Indications
Insomnia.

Action
Interacts with GABA-receptor complexes; not a benzodiazepine. **Therapeutic Effects:** Improved sleep with decreased latency and increased maintenance of sleep.

Pharmacokinetics
Absorption: Rapidly absorbed after oral administration.
Distribution: Unknown.
Metabolism and Excretion: Extensively metabolized by the liver (CYP3A4 and CYP2E1 enzyme systems); metabolites are renally excreted, <10% excreted unchanged in urine.

Half-life: 6 hr.

TIME/ACTION PROFILE (blood levels)

ROUTE	ONSET	PEAK	DURATION
PO	rapid	1 hr	6 hr

Contraindications/Precautions

Contraindicated in: No known contraindications.

Use Cautiously in: Geri: Geriatric/debilitated patients (may have ↓ metabolism or increased sensitivity; use lower initial dose); Conditions that may alter metabolic or hemodynamic function; Severe hepatic impairment (use lower initial dose); OB, Pedi: Lactation and children <18 yr (safety not established); Pregnancy (safety not established; use only if maternal benefit justifies fetal risk).

Adverse Reactions/Side Effects

CNS: abnormal thinking, behavior changes, depression, hallucinations, headache, sleep-driving. **CV:** chest pain, peripheral edema. **GI:** dry mouth, unpleasant taste. **Derm:** rash.

Interactions

Drug-Drug: ↑ risk of CNS depression with other **CNS depressants** including **antihistamines**, **antidepressants**, **opioids**, **sedative/hypnotics** and **antipsychotics**. ↑ levels and risk of CNS depression with **drugs that inhibit the CYP3A4 enzyme system**, including **ketoconazole**, **itraconazole**, **clarithromycin**, **nefazodone**, **ritonavir** and **nelfinavir**. Levels and effectiveness may be ↓ by **drugs that induce the CYP3A4 enzyme system**, including **rifampicin**.

Route/Dosage

PO (Adults): 2 mg immediately before bedtime, may be raised to 3 mg if needed (3 mg dose is more effective for sleep maintenance); *geriatric patients*—1 mg immediately before bedtime for patients with difficulty falling asleep, 2 mg for patients who difficulty staying asleep.

Hepatic Impairment

PO (Adults): *Severe hepatic impairment*—1 mg immediately before bedtime.

PO (Adults receiving concurrent CYP3A4 inhibitors): 1 mg immediately before bedtime, may be raised to 2 mg if needed.

Availability

Tablets: 1 mg, 2 mg, 3 mg. **Cost:** 1 mg $136.69/30, 2 mg $139.97/30, 3 mg $139.98/30.

NURSING IMPLICATIONS

Assessment

- Assess sleep patterns prior to and during administration. Continued insomnia after 7–10 days of therapy may indicate primary psychiatric or mental illness.
- Assess mental status and potential for abuse prior to administration. Prolonged use (>7–10 days) may lead to physical and psychological dependence. Limit amount of drug available to the patient.

Potential Nursing Diagnoses

Insomnia (Indications)

Implementation

- **PO:** Onset is rapid. Administer immediately before going to bed or after patient has gone to bed and has experienced difficulty falling asleep, only on nights when patient is able to get 8 or more hours of sleep before being active again.
- Swallow tablet whole; do not break, crush, or chew.
- Eszopiclone is more effective if not taken with or before a high-fat, heavy meal.

Patient/Family Teaching

- Instruct patient to take eszopiclone immediately before going to bed, as directed. Taking prior to going to bed may result in short-term memory impairment, hallucinations, impaired coordination, and dizziness. Do not increase dose or discontinue without notifying health care professional. Dose may need to be decreased gradually to minimize withdrawal symptoms. Rebound insomnia may occur upon discontinuation and usually resolves within 1–2 nights.
- May cause daytime drowsiness. Caution patient to avoid driving or other activities requiring alertness until response to medication is known.
- Advise patient to notify health care professional before taking any Rx, OTC, or herbal products with eszopiclone.
- Caution patient to avoid concurrent use of alcohol or other CNS depressants.

- Advise patient to notify health care professional if pregnancy is planned or suspected.

Evaluation/Desired Outcomes

- Decreased sleep latency and improved sleep maintenance.

etanercept (e-tan-er-sept)

Enbrel

Classification

Therapeutic: antirheumatics (DMARDs)

Pharmacologic: anti-TNF agents

Pregnancy Category B

Indications

To decrease progression, signs and symptoms of rheumatoid arthritis, juvenile arthritis, ankylosing spondylitis, psoriatic arthritis or plaque psoriasis when response has been inadequate to other disease-modifying agents. May be used with other agents.

Action

Binds to tumor necrosis factor (TNF), making it inactive. TNF is a mediator of inflammatory response. **Therapeutic Effects:** Decreased inflammation and slowed progression of arthritis, sponlylitis or psoriasis.

Pharmacokinetics

Absorption: 60% absorbed after subcut administration.
Distribution: Unknown.
Metabolism and Excretion: Unknown.
Half-life: 115 hr (range 98–300 hr).

TIME/ACTION PROFILE (symptom reduction)

ROUTE	ONSET	PEAK	DURATION
Subcut	2–4 wk	unknown	unknown

Contraindications/Precautions

Contraindicated in: Hypersensitivity; Sepsis; OB: Lactation; Untreated infections; Wegener's granulomatosis (receiving immunosuppressive agents); Concurrent cyclophosphamide or anakinra.
Use Cautiously in: Pre-existing or recent demyelinating disorders (multiple sclerosis, myelitis, optic neuritis); History of tuberculosis (increased risk of reactivation); Underlying chronic diseases which may predispose to infections (advanced or poorly-controlled diabetes mellitus); Latex allergy (needle cover of diluent syringe contains latex); Geri: May have ↑ risk of infection; Pedi: Children with significant exposure to varicella virus (temporarily discontinue etanercept; consider varicella zoster immune globulin); OB: Pregnancy (use only if needed).

Adverse Reactions/Side Effects

CNS: headache, dizziness, weakness. **EENT:** rhinitis, pharyngitis, sinusitis. **Resp:** upper respiratory tract infection, cough, respiratory disorder. **GI:** abdominal pain, dyspepsia. **Derm:** rash. **Hemat:** pancytopenia. **Local:** injection site reactions. **Misc:** INFECTIONS, ↑ risk of malignancies.

Interactions

Drug-Drug: Concurrent use with **anakinra** ↑ risk of serious infections (not recommended). Concurrent use of **cyclophosphamide** may ↑ risk of malignancies. May decrease the antibody response to **live-virus vaccine** and increase the risk of adverse reactions (do not administer concurrently).

Route/Dosage

Subcut (Adults): *Adult rheumatoid arthritis, ankylosing spondylitis, psoriatic arthritis*—50 mg once weekly; *adult plaque psoriasis*—50 mg twice weekly for 3 mos, then 50 mg once weekly, may also be given as 25–50 mg once weekly as an initial dose.
Subcut (Children 4–17 yr): *>63 kg*—0.8 mg/kg/wk (up to 50 mg) as a single injection; *31–62 kg*—0.8 mg/kg/wk either as two injections on the same day or divided and given on two separate days 3–4 days apart; *<31 kg*—0.8 mg/kg/wk as a single injection.

Availability

Pre-filled syringes: 50 mg/ml. **Powder for injection:** 25 mg/vial.

NURSING IMPLICATIONS

Assessment

- Assess range of motion, degree of swelling, and pain in affected joints before and periodically during therapy.
- Assess patient for injection site reaction (erythema, pain, itching, swelling). Reactions are usually mild to moderate and last 3–5 days after injection.
- Monitor patients who develop a new infection while taking etanercept closely. Discontinue therapy in patients who develop a serious infection or sepsis. Do not initiate therapy in patients with active infections.

Potential Nursing Diagnoses

Impaired physical mobility (Indications)
Acute pain (Indications)

Implementation

- Needle cover of the pre-filled syringe contains latex and should not be handled by people with latex allergies.
- **Subcut:** Prepare injection with single dose pre-filled syringe or multi-dose vial for reconstitution.
- Solution in pre-filled syringe may be allowed to reach room temperature (15–30 min); do not remove needle cap during this time.
- For multi-dose vial, reconstitute with 1 ml of the bacteriostatic sterile water supplied by manufacturer for a concentration of 25 mg/mL. If the vial is used for multiple doses, use a 25-gauge needle for reconstituting and withdrawing solution and apply "Mixing Date" sticker with date of reconstitution entered. Inject diluent slowly into vial to avoid foaming. Some foaming will occur. Swirl gently for dissolution; do not shake or vigorously agitate to prevent excess foaming. Solution should be clear and colorless; do not administer solution that is discolored or contains particulate matter. Dissolution usually takes <10 min. Withdraw solution into syringe. Some foam may remain in vial. Amount in syringe should approximate 1 ml. Do not filter reconstituted solution during preparation or administration. Attach a 27-gauge needle to inject. Administer as soon as possible after reconstitution; stable up to 6 hr if refrigerated. Solution and pre-filled syringes are stable if refrigerated and used within 14 days.
- May be injected into abdomen, thigh, or upper arm. Rotate sites. Do not administer within 1 inch of an old site or into area that is tender, red, hard, or bruised.
- **Syringe Incompatibility:** Do not mix with other solutions or dilute with other diluents.

Patient/Family Teaching

- Instruct patient on self-administration technique, storage, and disposal of equipment. First injection should be administered under the supervision of health care professional. Provide patient with a puncture-proof container for used equipment.
- Advise patient not to receive live vaccines during therapy. Parents should be advised that children should complete immunizations to date before initiation of etanercept. Patients with significant exposure to varicella virus (chickenpox) should temporarily discontinue therapy and varicella immune globulin should be considered.
- Advise patient that methotrexate, analgesics, NSAIDs, corticosteroids, and salicylates may be continued during therapy.
- Instruct patient to notify health care professional if upper respiratory or other infections occur. Therapy may need to be discontinued if serious infection occurs.

Evaluation/Desired Outcomes

- Reduction in symptoms of rheumatoid arthritis. Symptoms may return within 1 mo of discontinuation of therapy.

ethambutol

(e-**tham**-byoo-tole)
♣Etibi, Myambutol

Classification
Therapeutic: antituberculars

Pregnancy Category C

Indications

Active tuberculosis or other mycobacterial diseases (with at least one other drug).

Action

Inhibits the growth of mycobacteria. **Therapeutic Effects:** Tuberculostatic effect against susceptible organisms.

Pharmacokinetics

Absorption: Rapidly and well absorbed (80%) from the GI tract.
Distribution: Widely distributed; crosses blood-brain barrier in small amounts; crosses placenta and enters breast milk.
Metabolism and Excretion: 50% metabolized by the liver, 50% eliminated unchanged by the kidneys.
Half-life: 3.3 hr (increased in renal or hepatic impairment).

TIME/ACTION PROFILE (blood levels)

ROUTE	ONSET	PEAK	DURATION
PO	rapid	2–4 hr	24 hr

Contraindications/Precautions

Contraindicated in: Hypersensitivity; Optic neuritis.

Use Cautiously in: Renal and severe hepatic impairment (dosage reduction required); Children <13 yr (safety not established); Pregnancy (although safety not established, ethambutol has been used with isoniazid in pregnant women without adverse effects on the fetus); Lactation.

Adverse Reactions/Side Effects

CNS: confusion, dizziness, hallucinations, headache, malaise. **EENT:** optic neuritis. **GI:** HEPATITIS, abdominal pain, anorexia, nausea, vomiting. **Metab:** hyperuricemia. **MS:** joint pain. **Neuro:** peripheral neuritis. **Misc:** anaphylactoid reactions, fever.

Interactions

Drug-Drug: Neurotoxicity may be ↑ with other **neurotoxic agents**.

Route/Dosage

PO (Adults and Children >13 yr): 15–25 mg/kg/day (maximum 2.5 g/day) *or* 50 mg/kg (up to 2.5 g) twice weekly *or* 25–30 mg/kg (up to 2.5 g) 3 times weekly.

Availability (generic available)

Tablets: 100 mg, 400 mg.

NURSING IMPLICATIONS

Assessment

- Mycobacterial studies and susceptibility tests should be performed before and periodically during therapy to detect possible resistance.
- Assess lung sounds and character and amount of sputum periodically during therapy.
- Assessments of visual function should be made frequently during therapy. Advise patient to report blurring of vision, constriction of visual fields, or changes in color perception immediately. Visual impairment, if not identified early, may lead to permanent sight impairment.
- ***Lab Test Considerations:*** Monitor renal and hepatic functions, CBC, and uric acid levels routinely therapy. Frequently causes elevated uric acid concentrations, which may precipitate an attack of gout.

Potential Nursing Diagnoses

Risk for infection (Indications)
Disturbed sensory perception (Side Effects)

Implementation

- Ethambutol is given as a single daily dose and should be taken at the same time each day. Some regimens require dosing 2–3 times/week. Usually administered concurrently with other antitubercular medications to prevent development of bacterial resistance.
- **PO:** Administer with food or milk to minimize GI irritation.

Patient/Family Teaching

- Instruct patient to take medication as directed. Take missed doses as soon as possible unless almost time for next dose; do not double up on missed doses. A full course of therapy may take months to years. Do not discontinue without consulting health care professional, even though symptoms may disappear.
- Advise patient to notify health care professional if pregnancy is suspected.
- Instruct patient to notify health care professional if no improvement is seen in 2–3 wk. Health care professional should also be notified if unexpected weight gain or decreased urine output occurs.
- Emphasize the importance of routine exams to evaluate progress and ophthalmic examinations if signs of optic neuritis occur.

Evaluation/Desired Outcomes

- Resolution of clinical symptoms of tuberculosis.
- Decrease in acid-fast bacteria in sputum samples.
- Improvement seen in chest x-rays. Therapy for tuberculosis is usually continued for at least 1–2 yr.

---

ethinyl estradiol/desogestrel, See CONTRACEPTIVES, HORMONAL.

---

ethinyl estradiol/drospirenone, See CONTRACEPTIVES, HORMONAL.

---

ethinyl estradiol/ethynodiol, See CONTRACEPTIVES, HORMONAL.

ethinyl estradiol/etonogestrel, See CONTRACEPTIVES, HORMONAL.

ethinyl estradiol/levonorgestrel, See CONTRACEPTIVES, HORMONAL.

ethinyl estradiol/norgestimate, See CONTRACEPTIVES, HORMONAL.

ethinyl estradiol/norgestrel, See CONTRACEPTIVES, HORMONAL.

ethinyl estradiol/norethindrone, See CONTRACEPTIVES, HORMONAL.

ethinyl estradiol/norelgestromin, See CONTRACEPTIVES, HORMONAL.

etidronate (eh-tih-**droe**-nate)

✤Didrocal, Didronel

Classification

Therapeutic: bone resorption inhibitors, hypocalcemics

Pharmacologic: biphosphonates

Pregnancy Category B (oral), C (intravenous)

Indications

Treatment of Paget's disease of bone. Treatment and prophylaxis of heterotopic calcification associated with total hip replacement or spinal cord injury. Used with other agents (saline diuresis) in the management of hypercalcemia associated with malignancies.

Action

Blocks the growth of calcium hydroxyapatite crystals by binding to calcium phosphate. **Therapeutic Effects:** Decreased bone resorption and turnover.

Pharmacokinetics

Absorption: Absorption is generally poor (1–6%) after oral administration.

Distribution: Half of the absorbed dose is bound to hydroxyapatite crystals in areas of increased osteogenesis.

Metabolism and Excretion: Unabsorbed drug is eliminated in the feces; 50% of the absorbed dose is excreted unchanged by the kidneys.

Half-life: 5–7 hr.

TIME/ACTION PROFILE

ROUTE	ONSET	PEAK	DURATION
PO (Paget's disease)	1 mo†	unknown	1 yr
PO (heterotopic calcification)	unknown	unknown	several months
IV‡ (hypercalcemia)	24 hr	3 days	11 days

†As measured by decreased urinary hydroxyproline

‡As measured by decreased urinary calcium excretion

Contraindications/Precautions

Contraindicated in: Hypersensitivity; Severe renal impairment (serum creatinine >5 mg/dl); Hypercalcemia due to hyperparathyroidism.

Use Cautiously in: Long bone fractures; CHF; Hypocalcemia; Hypovitaminosis D; Moderate renal impairment (dosage reduction recommended if serum creatinine 2.5–4.9 mg/dl); OB, Lactation, Pedi: Pregnancy, lactation, or children (safety not established).

Adverse Reactions/Side Effects

GI: diarrhea, nausea; *IV*— loss of taste, metallic taste. **GU:** nephrotoxicity. **Derm:** rash. **MS:** bone pain, bone tenderness, microfractures.

Interactions

Drug-Drug: Antacids, **mineral supplements**, or **buffers** (as in **didanosine**) containing **calcium**, **aluminum**, **iron**, or **magnesium** may ↓ absorption of etidronate. Hypocalcemic effect may be additive with **calcitonin**.

Drug-Food: Foods containing large amounts of **calcium**, **aluminum**, **iron**, or **magnesium** may ↓ absorption of etidronate.

Route/Dosage

Paget's Disease

PO (Adults): 5–10 mg/kg/day single dose for up to 6 mo *or* 11–20 mg/kg/day for not more than 3 mo.

Heterotopic Ossification (Hip Replacement)

PO (Adults): 20 mg/kg/day for 1 mo before and 3 mo after surgery.

Heterotopic Ossification (Spinal Cord Injury)

PO (Adults): 20 mg/kg/day for 2 wk, then decreased to 10 mg/kg/day for 10 wk.

Hypercalcemia

PO (Adults): 20 mg/kg/day for 30–90 days.
IV (Adults): 7.5 mg/kg/day for 3 days; has also been given as a single dose of 25–30 mg/kg over 24 hr. May be followed by oral therapy.

Availability

Tablets: 200 mg, 400 mg. **Injection:** 50 mg/ml in 6-ml ampules.

NURSING IMPLICATIONS

Assessment

- Assess patient for bone pain, weakness, or loss of function before and throughout therapy. Bone pain may persist or increase in patients with Paget's disease; it usually subsides days to months after therapy is discontinued. Confer with physician or other health care professional regarding analgesic to control pain.
- **Heterotopic Ossification:** Monitor for inflammation and pain at the site and loss of function if ossification occurs near a joint.
- **Hypercalcemia:** Monitor symptoms of hypercalcemia (nausea, vomiting, anorexia, weakness, constipation, thirst, and cardiac arrhythmias).
- Observe patient carefully for evidence of hypocalcemia (paresthesia, muscle twitching, laryngospasm, colic, cardiac arrhythmias, and Chvostek's or Trousseau's sign). Protect symptomatic patients by elevating and padding side rails; keep bed in low position. Risk of hypocalcemia is greatest after 3 days of continuous IV therapy.
- ***Lab Test Considerations:*** Etidronate interferes with bone uptake of technetium 99 in diagnostic scans.
- *Paget's disease:* Decreased urinary excretions of hydroxyproline and serum alkaline phosphatase are often the first clinical signs of effectiveness. These values are monitored every 3 mo. Treatment is restarted when levels return to 75% of pretreatment values. Serum phosphate levels are also monitored before and 4 wk after beginning therapy. Dosage may be reduced if serum phosphate is elevated without corresponding decrease in urinary excretion of hydroxyproline or serum alkaline phosphatase.
- *Hypercalcemia:* Monitor serum calcium and albumin levels to determine effectiveness of therapy.
- Monitor BUN and creatine before and periodically throughout course of therapy. Stable or reversible increases in BUN and creatinine may occur in patients with hypercalcemia.

Potential Nursing Diagnoses

Acute pain (Indications, Side Effects)
Risk for injury (Indications)

Implementation

- Do not confuse etidronate with etomidate.
- **Hypercalcemia:** Used as adjunctive treatment after IV hydration and loop diuretics have restored urine output.
- Oral doses may be started on the day after the last IV infusion.
- **PO:** Administer on empty stomach, because food decreases absorption.

IV Administration

- **Intermittent Infusion:** ***Diluent:*** Dilute in at least 250 mL of 0.9% NaCl or D5W. Solution is stable for 48 hr. Oral etidronate may be started on the day after last infusion. ***Rate:*** Infuse doses of 7.5 mg/kg over at least 2 hr.
- **Continuous Infusion:** ***Diluent:*** May also dilute 25–30 mg/kg single dose in 1000 mL of 0.9% NaCl. ***Rate:*** Administer over 24 hr.

Patient/Family Teaching

- Advise patient to take as directed. If dose is missed, take as soon as remembered unless almost time for next dose. Do not double up on doses. Dose should not be taken within 2 hr of eating (especially products high in calcium) or taking vitamins or antacids, because absorption will be impaired.
- Instruct patient to notify health care professional if diarrhea occurs. Health care professional may divide the dose throughout the day to control diarrhea.
- Encourage patients to comply with diet recommendations. Diet should contain adequate amounts of calcium and vitamin D (see Appendix L).
- Advise patient to notify health care professional if pain appears or worsens during therapy.

- Explain to patient receiving IV dose that metallic taste is not uncommon and usually disappears in a few hours.
- Advise patient to report signs of hypercalcemic relapse (bone pain, anorexia, nausea, vomiting, thirst, lethargy) to health care professional promptly.
- Emphasize need for keeping follow-up appointments to monitor progress, even after medication is discontinued, to detect relapse.

Evaluation/Desired Outcomes

- Lowered serum calcium levels.
- Decreased bone pain and fractures in Paget's disease.
- Prevention or treatment of heterotopic ossification. Normal serum calcium levels are usually attained in 2–8 days in hypercalcemia associated with bony metastasis. Therapy may be repeated once after 1 wk.

etodolac (ee-**toe**-doe-lak)

Lodine, Lodine XL

Classification

Therapeutic: antirheumatics, nonopioid analgesics

Pharmacologic: pyranocarboxylic acid

Pregnancy Category C

Indications

Osteoarthritis. Rheumatoid arthritis. Mild to moderate pain (not XL tablets).

Action

Inhibits prostaglandin synthesis. Also has uricosuric action. **Therapeutic Effects:** Suppression of inflammation. Decreased severity of pain.

Pharmacokinetics

Absorption: Well absorbed after oral administration.

Distribution: Widely distributed,.

Protein Binding: >99%.

Metabolism and Excretion: Mostly metabolized by the liver; <1% excreted unchanged in urine.

Half-life: 6–7 hr (single dose); 7.3 hr (chronic dosing).

TIME/ACTION PROFILE (analgesic effect)

ROUTE	ONSET	PEAK	DURATION
PO (analgesic)	0.5 hr	1–2 hr	4–12 hr
PO (anti-inflammatory)	days–wks	unknown	6–12 hr†

†Up to 24 hr as XL (extended-release) tablet

Contraindications/Precautions

Contraindicated in: Hypersensitivity; Active GI bleeding or ulcer disease; Cross-sensitivity may exist with other NSAIDs, including aspirin.

Use Cautiously in: Cardiovascular disease or risk factors for cardiovascular disease (may ↑ risk of serious cardiovascular thrombotic events, myocardial infarction, and stroke, especially with prolonged use) Renal, or hepatic disease; Geri: Geriatric patients (increased risk of GI bleeding); History of ulcer disease; OB: Pregnancy (not recommended for use during second half of pregnancy); OB, Pedi: Lactation or children (safety not established).

Adverse Reactions/Side Effects

CNS: depression, dizziness, drowsiness, insomnia, malaise, nervousness, syncope, weakness. **EENT:** blurred vision, photophobia, tinnitus. **Resp:** asthma. **CV:** CHF, edema, hypertension, palpitations. **GI:** GI BLEEDING, <u>dyspepsia</u>, abdominal pain, constipation, diarrhea, drug-induced hepatitis, dry mouth, flatulence, gastritis, nausea, stomatitis, thirst, vomiting. **GU:** dysuria, renal failure, urinary frequency. **Derm:** EXFOLIATIVE DERMATITIS, STEVENS-JOHNSON SYNDROME, TOXIC EPIDERMAL NECROLYSIS, ecchymoses, flushing, hyperpigmentation, pruritus, rashes, sweating. **Hemat:** anemia, prolonged bleeding time, thrombocytopenia. **Misc:** allergic reactions including ANAPHYLAXIS, ANGIOEDEMA, chills, fever.

Interactions

Drug-Drug: Concurrent use with **aspirin** may ↓ effectiveness. ↑ adverse GI effects with **aspirin**, other **NSAIDs**, **potassium supplements**, **corticosteroids**, **antiplatelet agents**, or **alcohol**. Chronic use with **acetaminophen** may ↑ risk of adverse renal reactions. May ↓ effectiveness of **diuretic** or **antihypertensive** therapy. May ↑ serum **lithium** levels and ↑ risk of toxicity. ↑ risk of toxicity from **methotrexate**. ↑ risk of bleeding with **cefotetan**, **cefoperazone**, **valproic acid**, **thrombolytics**, **antiplatelet agents**, or **anticoagu-**

lants. Increased risk of adverse hematologic reactions with **antineoplastics** or **radiation therapy**. May increase the risk of nephrotoxicity from **cyclosporine**.
Drug-Natural Products: ↑ risk of bleeding with **arnica**, **chamomile**, **clove**, **dong quai**, **fever few**, **garlic**, **ginkgo**, and **Panax ginseng**.

Route/Dosage

PO (Adults): *Analgesia*—200–400 mg q 6–8 hr (not to exceed 1200 mg/day). *Osteoarthritis/rheumatoid arthritis*—300 mg 2–3 times daily, 400 mg twice daily, or 500 mg twice daily; may also be given as 400–1200 mg once daily as XL tablets.

Availability (generic available)

Capsules: 200 mg, 300 mg. **Tablets:** 400 mg, 500 mg. **Extended-release tablets (XL):** 400 mg, 600 mg.

NURSING IMPLICATIONS

Assessment

- Patients who have asthma, aspirin-induced allergy, and nasal polyps are at increased risk for developing hypersensitivity reactions. Monitor for rhinitis, asthma, and urticaria.
- **Osteoarthritis/Rheumatoid Arthritis:** Assess pain and range of movement before and 1–2 hr after administration.
- **Pain:** Assess location, duration, and intensity of the pain before and 60 min after administration.
- ***Lab Test Considerations:*** May cause ↓ hemoglobin, hematocrit, leukocyte, and platelet counts.
- Monitor liver function tests within 8 wk of initiating etodolac therapy and periodically during therapy. May cause ↑ serum alkaline phosphatase, LDH, AST, and ALT concentrations.
- Monitor BUN, serum creatinine, and electrolytes periodically during therapy. May cause ↑ BUN, serum creatinine, and electrolyte concentrations and ↓ urine electrolyte concentrations.
- May cause ↓ serum and ↑ urine uric acid concentrations.

Potential Nursing Diagnoses

Acute pain (Indications)
Impaired physical mobility (Indications)

Implementation

- Do not confuse Lodine (etodolac) with codeine or iodine.
- Administration in higher-than-recommended doses does not provide increased effectiveness but may cause increased side effects.
- Use lowest effective dose for shortest period of time.
- **PO:** For rapid initial effect, administer 30 min before or 2 hr after meals. May be administered with food, milk, or antacids containing aluminum or magnesium to decrease GI irritation.
- Do not crush, break, or chew extended-release tablets.

Patient/Family Teaching

- Advise patients to take etodolac with a full glass of water and to remain in an upright position for 15–30 min after administration.
- Instruct patient to take medication as directed. Take missed doses as soon as possible within 1–2 hr if taking twice/day, or unless almost time for next dose if taking more than twice/day. Do not double doses.
- Etodolac may occasionally cause drowsiness or dizziness. Advise patient to avoid driving or other activities requiring alertness until response to the medication is known.
- Caution patient to avoid the concurrent use of alcohol, aspirin, acetaminophen, NSAIDs, or other OTC medications without consultation with health care professional.
- Advise patient to inform health care professional of medication regimen before treatment or surgery.
- Advise patient to consult health care professional if rash, itching, visual disturbances, tinnitus, weight gain, edema, black stools, persistent headache, or influenza-like syndrome (chills, fever, muscle aches, pain) occurs.

Evaluation/Desired Outcomes

- Decreased severity of pain.
- Improved joint mobility. Patients who do not respond to one NSAID may respond to another. May require 2 wk or more for maximum anti-inflammatory effects.

---

etonorgestrel, See CONTRACEPTIVES, HORMONAL.

HIGH ALERT

ETOPOSIDES (e-toe-poe-sides)

etoposide
VePesid, VP-16

etoposide phosphate
Etopophos

Classification
Therapeutic: antineoplastics
Pharmacologic: podophyllotoxin derivatives

Pregnancy Category D

Indications
Refractory testicular neoplasms (used in combination with other chemotherapeutic agents in patients who have already received chemotherapy, surgery, or radiation) (IV only). Small cell lung carcinoma (first-line therapy, used in combination with other chemotherapeutic agents) (oral and IV). **Unlabeled uses:** Lymphomas and some leukemias. Uterine cancer. Brain tumors.

Action
Damages DNA before mitosis (cycle-dependent and phase-specific). **Therapeutic Effects:** Death of rapidly replicating cells, particularly malignant ones.

Pharmacokinetics
Absorption: Variably absorbed after oral administration. After IV administration, etoposide phosphate is rapidly converted to etoposide.
Distribution: Rapidly distributed, poorly enters the CSF; probably crosses placenta; enters breast milk.
Protein Binding: 97%.
Metabolism and Excretion: Some metabolism by the liver with biliary excretion, 44% excreted in feces; 45% excreted unchanged by the kidneys.
Half-life: 4–11 hr.

TIME/ACTION PROFILE (noted as effects on blood counts)

ROUTE	ONSET	PEAK	DURATION
Etoposide PO	unknown	7–14 days (granulocytes); 9–16 days (platelets)	20 days
Etoposide IV	7–14 days	7–14 days granulocytes; 9–16 days (platelets)	20 days
Etoposide phosphate IV	Unknown	12–19 days (granulocytes); 10–15 days (platelets)	21 days

Contraindications/Precautions
Contraindicated in: Hypersensitivity; OB, Lactation: Pregnancy and lactation; Known intolerance to benzyl alcohol, polysorbate 80, polyethylene glycol (IV etoposide only), or dextran (IV etoposide phosphate only).
Use Cautiously in: Patients with childbearing potential; Active infections; Decreased bone marrow reserve; Hypoalbuminemia; Renal/hepatic impairment (dosage modification may be necessary); Other chronic debilitating illnesses; Geri: Elderly (may be at ↑ risk for adverse effects); Pedi: Children (safety and effectiveness not established).

Adverse Reactions/Side Effects
CNS: dizziness, drowsiness, fatigue. **CV:** <u>hypotension</u> (IV). **GI:** <u>anorexia</u>, <u>diarrhea</u>, <u>nausea</u>, <u>vomiting</u>, abdominal pain, stomatitis, taste alteration. **Derm:** <u>alopecia</u>, pruritis, rashes, urticaria. **Endo:** sterility. **Hemat:** <u>anemia</u>, <u>leukopenia</u>, <u>thrombocytopenia</u>. **Local:** phlebitis at IV site. **Neuro:** peripheral neuropathy. **Misc:** allergic reactions including <u>ANAPHYLAXIS</u>, fever.

Interactions
Drug-Drug: ↑ bone marrow depression with other **antineoplastics** or **radiation therapy**. May alter immune response to **live-virus vaccines** and ↑ risk of adverse reactions.

Route/Dosage
Other regimens are used. Dosages below are expressed as the desired etoposide dosage.

Testicular Neoplasms
IV (Adults): Dosage ranges from 50–100 mg/m^2 daily for 5 days to 100 mg/m^2 on days 1, 3, and 5; repeat at 3–4 wk intervals.

Small-Cell Carcinoma of the Lung
PO (Adults): Dosage ranges from 70 mg/m^2 (rounded to the nearest 50 mg) daily for 4 days to 100 mg/m^2 (rounded to the nearest 50 mg) daily for 5 days; repeat at 3–4 wk intervals.
IV (Adults): Dosages range from 35 mg/m^2 daily for 4 days to 50 mg/m^2 daily for 5 days; repeat at 3–4 wk intervals.

Availability

Etoposide

Capsules: 50 mg. **Injection:** 20 mg/ml.

Etoposide Phosphate

Powder for injection: 100 mg/vial (with dextran).

NURSING IMPLICATIONS

Assessment

- Monitor blood pressure before and every 15 min during infusion. If hypotension occurs, stop infusion and notify physician or other health care professional. After stabilizing blood pressure with IV fluids and supportive measures, infusion may be resumed at slower rate.
- Monitor for hypersensitivity reaction (fever, chills, dyspnea, pruritus, urticaria, bronchospasm, tachycardia, hypotension). If these occur, stop infusion and notify physician. Keep epinephrine, an antihistamine, corticosteroids, volume expanders, and resuscitative equipment close by in the event of an anaphylactic reaction.
- Assess for signs of infection (fever, chills, cough, hoarseness, lower back or side pain, sore throat, difficult or painful urination). Notify physician if these symptoms occur.
- Assess for bleeding (bleeding gums, bruising, petechiae, guaiac test stools, urine, and emesis). Avoid IM injections and taking rectal temperatures. Apply pressure to venipuncture sites for 10 min.
- Monitor intake and output, appetite, and nutritional intake. Etoposide causes mild-to-moderate nausea and vomiting. Prophylactic antiemetics may ↓ frequency and duration of nausea and vomiting.
- Adjust diet as tolerated to help maintain fluid and electrolyte balance and nutritional status.
- ***Lab Test Considerations:*** Monitor CBC and differential before and periodically during therapy. The nadir of leukopenia occurs in 7–14 days (etoposide) or 12–19 days (etoposide phosphate). Notify physician if leukocyte count is $<1000/mm^3$. The nadir of thrombocytopenia occurs in 9–16 days. Notify physician if the platelet count is $<75,000/mm^3$. Recovery of leukopenia and thrombocytopenia occurs in 20 days.
- Monitor liver function studies (AST, ALT, LDH, bilirubin) and renal function studies (BUN, creatinine) before and periodically during therapy to detect hepatotoxicity and nephrotoxicity.

Potential Nursing Diagnoses

Risk for injury (Side Effects)
Risk for infection (Side Effects)

Implementation

- ***High Alert:*** Fatalities have occurred with incorrect administration of chemotherapeutic agents. Before administering, clarify all ambiguous orders; double-check single, daily, and course-of-therapy dose limits; have second practitioner independently double-check original order, calculations and infusion pump settings. Do not confuse VePesid (etoposide) with Versed (midazolam). Do not confuse etoposide (VePesid) with etoposide phosphate (Etopophos).
- Solution should be prepared in a biologic cabinet. Wear gloves, gown, and mask while handling medication. Discard equipment in designated containers.
- Avoid contact with skin. Use Luer-Lok tubing to prevent accidental leakage. If contact with skin occurs, immediately wash skin with soap and water.
- **PO:** Capsules should be refrigerated. Capsules are stable for 24 mo when refrigerated.

Etoposide (VePesid)

IV Administration

- **Intermittent Infusion:** ***Diluent:*** Dilute 5-ml vial with D5W or 0.9% NaCl. ***Concentration:*** 200–400 mcg/ml. The 200-mcg/ml solution is stable for 96 hr. The 400-mcg/ml solution is stable for 48 hr. Concentrations >400 mcg/ml are not recommended, because crystallization is likely. Discard solution if crystals are present. ***Rate:*** Infuse slowly over 30–60 min. Temporary hypotension may occur with infusion rates shorter than 30 min.
- **Y-Site Compatibility:** allopurinol, amifostine, aztreonam, cladribine, doxorubicin liposome, fludarabine, gemcitabine, granisetron, melphalan, methotrexate, mitoxandrone, ondansetron, paclitaxel, piperacillin/tazobactam, sargramostim, sodium bicarbonate, teniposide, thiotepa, topotecan, vinorelbine.
- **Y-Site Incompatibility:** cefepime, filgrastim, idarubicin.
- **Additive Compatibility:** carboplatin, cisplatin, cytarabine, floxuridine, fluorouracil, ifosfamide, mitoxantrone, ondansetron.

Etoposide phosphate (Etopophos)

IV Administration

- **Intermittent Infusion:** Reconstitute each vial with 5 or 10 ml of sterile water, D5W, or 0.9% NaCl for a concentration of 20 or 10 mg/ml, respectively. ***Diluent:*** May be administered undiluted or diluted with D5W or 0.9% NaCl. ***Concentration:*** Undiluted: 10–20 mg/ml; Diluted: as low as 0.1 mg/ml. Reconstituted solutions are stable for 24 hr at room temperature or if refrigerated. ***Rate:*** Administer over 5–210 min.
- **Y-Site Compatibility:** acyclovir, amikacin, aminophylline, ampcillin, ampicillin/sulbactam, aztreonam, bleomycin, bumetanide, buprenorphine, butorphanol, calcium gluconate, carboplatin, carmustine, cefazolin, cefotaxime, cefotetan, cefoxitin, ceftazidime, ceftizoxime, ceftriaxone, cefuroxime, cimetidine, ciprofloxacin, cisplatin, clindamycin, cyclophosphamide, cytarabine, dacarbazine, dactinomycin, daunorubicin, dexamethasone sodium phosphate, diphenhydramine, dobutamine, dopamine, doxorubicin, doxycycline, droperidol, enalaprilat, famotidine, floxuridine, fluconazole, fludarabine, fluorouracil, furosemide, ganciclovir, gemcitabine, gentamicin, granisetron, haloperidol, heparin, hydrocortisone, hydromorphone, idarubicin, ifosfamide, leucovorin calcium, linezolid, lorazepam, magnesium sulfate, mannitol, meperidine, mesna, methotrexate, metoclopramide, metronidazole, mitoxantrone, morphine, nalbuphine, ofloxacin, ondansetron, oxaliplatin, paclitaxel, piperacillin, piperacillin/tazobactam, potassium chloride, promethazine, ranitidine, sodium bicarbonate, streptozocin, teniposide, thiotepa, ticarcillin/clavulanate, tobramycin, trimethoprim/sulfamethoxazole, vancomycin, vinblastine, vincristine, zidovudine.
- **Y-Site Incompatibility:** amphotericin B, cefepime, chlorpromazine, imipenem/cilastatin, lansoprazole, methylprednisolone, mitomycin, prochlorperazine.

Patient/Family Teaching

- Instruct patient to take etoposide exactly as directed, even if nausea or vomiting occurs. If vomiting occurs shortly after dose is taken, consult physician. If a dose is missed, do not take at all.
- Advise patient to notify health care professional if fever; chills; sore throat or other signs of infection; bleeding gums; bruising; petechiae; or blood in urine, stool, or emesis occurs. Caution patient to avoid crowds and persons with known infections. Instruct patient to use soft toothbrush and electric razor. Caution patient not to drink alcoholic beverages or take products containing aspirin or NSAIDs.
- Instruct patient to notify health care professional if rapid heartbeat, difficulty breathing, abdominal pain, yellow skin, weakness, paresthesia, or gait disturbances occur.
- Instruct patient to inspect oral mucosa for redness and ulceration. If mouth sores occur, advise patient to use sponge brush and rinse mouth with water after eating and drinking. Viscous lidocaine swishes may be used if pain interferes with eating. Stomatitis pain may require treatment with opioid analgesics.
- Discuss with patient the possibility of hair loss. Explore coping strategies.
- Advise patient to use contraception.
- Instruct patient not to receive any vaccinations without advice of physician.
- Emphasize the need for periodic lab tests to monitor for side effects.

Evaluation/Desired Outcomes

- Decrease in size or spread of testicular or small cell lung cancer.

exenatide (ex-**en**-a-tide)

Byetta

Classification
Therapeutic: antidiabetics
Pharmacologic: incretrin mimetic agents

Pregnancy Category C

Indications

Type 2 diabetes uncontrolled by metformin, a sulfonylurea, or a thiazolidinedione (or a combination of these agents)

Action

Mimics the action of incretin which promotes endogenous insulin secretion and promotes other mechanisms of glucose-lowering. **Therapeutic Effects:** Improved control of blood glucose.

Pharmacokinetics

Absorption: Well absorbed following subcutaneous administration.
Distribution: Unknown.
Metabolism and Excretion: Excreted mostly by glomerular filtration followed by degradation.
Half-life: 2.4 hr.

TIME/ACTION PROFILE (effects on postprandial blood glucose)

ROUTE	ONSET	PEAK	DURATION
subcut	within 30 min	2.1 hr	8 hr

Contraindications/Precautions

Contraindicated in: Hypersensitivity; Type 1 diabetes or diabetic ketoacidosis; End-stage renal disease (CCr <30 mL/min); Severe gastrointestinal disease; OB: Lactation.
Use Cautiously in: (dose adjustment may be necessary); OB: Use in pregnancy only if potential maternal benefit outweighs fetal risk); Pedi: Safety not established.

Adverse Reactions/Side Effects

CV: dizziness, headache, jitteryness, weakness. **GI:** diarrhea, nausea, vomiting, dyspepsia, gastroinestinal reflux. **Derm:** hyperhydrosis. **Metab:** ↓ appetite, weight loss.

Interactions

Drug-Drug: Concurrent use with **sulfonlyureas** may ↑ risk of hypoglycemia (↓ dose of sulfonylurea if hypoglycemia occurs). Due to slowed gastric emptying, may decrease absorption of **orally administered medications**, especially those requiring rapid GI absorption or require a specific level for efficacy (**anti-infectives, oral contraceptives**).

Route/Dosage

Subcut (Adults): 5 mcg within 60 min before morning and evening meal; after one month, dose may be increased to 10 mcg depending on response.

Availability

Solution for subcutaneous injection: 250 mcg/ml in prefilled pen-injector that delivers either 5 mcg/dose (1.2-ml pen) or 10 mcg/dose (2.4-ml pen) for 60 doses (30 days of twice daily dosing). **Cost:** $200.98/1.2-ml pen, $225.99/2.4-ml pen.

NURSING IMPLICATIONS

Assessment

- Observe for signs and symptoms of hypoglycemic reactions (abdominal pain, sweating, hunger, weakness, dizziness, headache, drowsiness, tremor, tachycardia, anxiety, confusion, irritability, jitteryness), especially when combined with oral sulfonylureas.
- ***Lab Test Considerations:*** Monitor serum glucose and glycolysated hemoglobin periodically during therapy to evaluate effectiveness of therapy.

Potential Nursing Diagnoses

Imbalanced nutrition: more than body requirements (Indications)
Noncompliance (Patient/Family Teaching)

Implementation

- Some medications may need to be taken 1 hr before exenatide.
- Patients stabilized on a diabetic regimen who are exposed to stress, fever, trauma, infection, or surgery may require administration of insulin.
- **Subcut:** Follow directions for *New Pen Setup* in *Information for Patient* prior to use of each new pen. Administer exenatide in thigh, abdomen, or upper arm at any time within the 60–min period **before** the morning and evening meals. Do not administer after a meal. Solution should be clear and colorless; do not administer solutions that are discolored or contain particulate matter. Refrigerate; discard pen 30 days after 1st use, even if some drug remains in pen. Do not freeze. Do not store pen with needle attached; medication may leak from pen or air bubbles may form in the cartridge.

Patient/Family Teaching

- Instruct patient to take exenatide as directed within 60 min before a meal. Do not take after a meal. If a dose is missed, skip the dose and take the next dose at the prescribed time. Do not take an extra dose or increase the amount of the next dose to make up for missed dose.
- Instruct patient in proper technique for administration, timing of dose and concurrent oral medications, storage of medication and disposal of used needles. Patients should read the "Information for Patient" insert prior to initiation of therapy and with each Rx refill. Advise patient that New Pen Setup should be done only with each new pen, not with each dose.
- Inform patient that pen needles are not included with pen and must be purchased separately. Advise patient which needle length and

gauge should be used. Caution patient not to share pen and needles.

- Explain to patient that exenatide helps control hyperglycemia but does not cure diabetes. Therapy is usually long term.
- Encourage patient to follow prescribed diet, medication, and exercise regimen to prevent hyperglycemic or hypoglycemic episodes.
- Review signs of hypoglycemia and hyperglycemia with patient. If hypoglycemia occurs, advise patient to take a glass of orange juice or 2–3 tsp of sugar, honey, or corn syrup dissolved in water, and notify health care professional. Risk of hypoglycemia is increased if sulfonureas are taken concurrently with exenatide.
- Inform patient that therapy may result in reduction of appetite, food intake, and/or body weight. Dose modification is not necessary. Nausea is more common at initiation of therapy and usually decreases over time.
- Advise patient to notify health care professional before taking any Rx, OTC, and herbal products. Exenatide delays stomach emptying. Some medications (such as anti-infectives and oral contraceptives) may need to be taken 1 hr before exenatide injection.
- Instruct patient in proper testing of blood glucose and urine ketones. These tests should be monitored closely during periods of stress or illness and health care professional notified if significant changes occur.
- Advise patient to notify health care professional if pregnancy is suspected or planned.
- Advise patient to inform health care professional of medication regimen before treatment or surgery.
- Advise patient to carry a form of sugar (sugar packets, candy) and identification describing disease process and medication regimen at all times.
- Emphasize the importance of routine follow-up exams and regular testing of blood glucose and glycosylated hemoglobin.

Evaluation/Desired Outcomes

- Control of blood glucose levels without the appearance of hypoglycemic or hyperglycemic episodes.

ezetimibe (e-zet-i-mibe)

✤Ezetrol, Zetia

Classification
Therapeutic: lipid-lowering agents
Pharmacologic: cholesterol absorption inhibitors

Pregnancy Category C

Indications

Alone or with other agents (HMG-CoA reductase inhibitors) in the management of dyslipidemias including primary hypercholesterolemia, homozygous familial hypercholesterolemia and homozygous sitosterolemia.

Action

Inhibits absorption of cholesterol in the small intestine. **Therapeutic Effects:** Lowering of cholesterol, a known risk factor for atherosclerosis.

Pharmacokinetics

Absorption: Following absorption, rapidly converted to ezetimibe-glucaronide, which is active. Bioavailability is variable.
Distribution: Unknown.
Metabolism and Excretion: Undergoes enterhepatic recycling, mostly eliminated in feces, minimal renal excretion.
Half-life: 22 hr.

TIME/ACTION PROFILE

ROUTE	ONSET	PEAK	DURATION
PO	unknown	unknown	unknown

Contraindications/Precautions

Contraindicated in: Hypersensitivity; Acute liver disease or unexplained laboratory evidence of liver disease (when used with HMG-CoA reductase inhibitor); Moderate or severe hepatic insufficiency; Concurrent use of fibrates.
Use Cautiously in: OB: Lactation (use only if benefit to mother outweighs possible risks to infant); OB, Pedi: Pregnancy or children <10 yr (safety not established).

Adverse Reactions/Side Effects

GI: cholecystitis, cholelithiasis, ↑ hepatic transaminases (with HMG-CoA reductase inhibitors), nausea, pancreatitis. **Derm:** rash. **Misc:** ANGIOEDEMA.

Interactions

Drug-Drug: Effects may be ↓ by **cholestyramine** or other **bile acid sequestrants**. Con-

✤ = Canadian drug name.
* CAPITALS indicates life-threatening; underlines indicate most frequent.

current use of **fibrates** may ↑ blood levels of ezetimibe and also ↑ the risk of cholelithiasis. **Cyclosporine** may ↑ ezetimibe levels. May ↑ risk of rhabdomyolysis when used with **HMG CoA-reductase inhibitors**.

Route/Dosage

PO (Adults): 10 mg once daily.

Availability

Tablets: 10 mg. **Cost:** $265.98/90. ***In combination with:*** simvastatin (Vytorin); see Appendix B.

NURSING IMPLICATIONS

Assessment

- Obtain a diet history, especially with regard to fat consumption.
- ***Lab Test Considerations:*** Evaluate serum cholesterol and triglyceride levels before initiating, after 2–4 wk of therapy, and periodically thereafter.
- May cause ↑ liver transaminases when administered with HMG-CoA reductase inhibitors. Monitor liver enzymes prior to initiation and during therapy according to recommendations of HMG-CoA reductase inhibitor. Elevations are usually asymptomatic and return to baseline with continued therapy.

Potential Nursing Diagnoses

Noncompliance, related to diet and medication regimen (Patient/Family Teaching)

Implementation

- **PO:** Administer without regard to meals. May be taken at the same time as HMG-CoA reductase inhibitors.

Patient/Family Teaching

- Instruct patient to take medication as directed, at the same time each day, even if feeling well. Take missed doses as soon as remembered, but do not take more than 1 dose/day. Medication helps control but does not cure elevated serum cholesterol levels.
- Advise patient that this medication should be used in conjunction with diet restrictions (fat, cholesterol, carbohydrates, alcohol), exercise, and cessation of smoking. Ezetimibe does not assist with weight loss.
- Instruct female patients to notify health care professional promptly if pregnancy is planned or suspected or if breast feeding. If regimen includes HMG-CoA reductase inhibitors, they are contraindicated in pregnancy.
- Instruct patient to notify health care professional if unexplained muscle pain, tenderness, or weakness occur. Risk may increase when used with HMG CoA reductase inhibitors.
- Advise patient to avoid taking OTC medications or natural/herbal products without consulting health care professional.
- Advise patient to notify health care professional of medication regimen prior to treatment or surgery.
- Emphasize the importance of follow-up exams to determine effectiveness and to monitor for side effects.

Evaluation/Desired Outcomes

- Decrease in serum LDL and total cholesterol levels.
- Increase in HDL cholesterol levels.

famciclovir
(fam-**sye**-kloe-veer)
Famvir

Classification
Therapeutic: antivirals

Pregnancy Category B

Indications
Acute herpes zoster infections (shingles). Treatment/suppression of recurrent herpes genitalis in immunocompetent patients. Treatment of recurrent mucocutaneous herpes simplex virus (HSV) infection in HIV-infected patients.

Action
Inhibits viral DNA synthesis in herpes-infected cells only. **Therapeutic Effects:** Decreased duration of herpes zoster infection with decreased duration of viral shedding. Decreased lesion formation and improved healing in recurrent HSV infection.

Pharmacokinetics
Absorption: Following absorption, famciclovir is rapidly converted in the intestinal wall to penciclovir, the active compound.
Distribution: Unknown.
Metabolism and Excretion: Penciclovir is mostly excreted by the kidneys.
Half-life: *Penciclovir*—2.1–3 hr (increased in renal impairment).

TIME/ACTION PROFILE (penciclovir blood levels)

ROUTE	ONSET	PEAK	DURATION
PO	rapid	0.9 hr	8–12 hr

Contraindications/Precautions
Contraindicated in: Hypersensitivity.
Use Cautiously in: Patients with impaired renal function (increased dosage interval/decreased dose recommended if CCr <40–60 ml/min); Geri: Geriatric patients (because of age-related decrease in renal function); OB, Pedi: Pregnancy, lactation, or children <18 yr (safety not established).

Adverse Reactions/Side Effects
CNS: headache, dizziness, fatigue. **GI:** diarrhea, nausea, vomiting.

Interactions
Drug-Drug: Probenecid increases plasma concentration of penciclovir.

Route/Dosage
Herpes Zoster
PO (Adults): 500 mg q 8 hr for 7 days.

Renal Impairment
PO (Adults): *CCr 40–59 ml/min*—500 mg q 12 hr; *CCr 20–39ml/min*—500 mg q 24 hr; *CCr <20 ml/min*—250 mg q 24 hr; *Hemodialysis*—250 mg after each dialysis.

Recurrent Genital Herpes Simplex Infections
PO (Adults): 1000 mg twice daily for one day.

Renal Impairment
PO (Adults): *CCr 40–59 mL/min*– 500 mg twice daily for one day; *CCr 20–39 mL/min*– 500 mg as a single dose; *CCr <20 ml/min*—250 mg as a single dose; *Hemodialysis*—250 mg as a single dose after dialysis.

Suppression of Recurrent Herpes Simplex Infections
PO (Adults): 250 mg q 12 hr for up to 1 yr.

Renal Impairment
PO (Adults): *CCr 20–39 ml/min*—125 mg q 12 hr for 5 days; *CCr <20 ml/min*—125 mg q 24 hr for 5 days; *Hemodialysis*—125 mg after each dialysis.

Recurrent Herpes Labialis Infections (cold sores)
PO (Adults): 1500 mg as a single dose.

Renal Impairment
PO (Adults): *CCr 40–59 mL/min*—750 mg as a single dose; *CCr 20–39 mL/min*—500 mg as a single dose; *CCr <20 ml/min*—250 mg as a single dose; *Hemodialysis*—250 mg as a single dose after dialysis.

Herpes Simplex in HIV-Infected Patients
PO (Adults): 500 mg q 12 hr for 7 days.

Renal Impairment
PO (Adults): *CCr 20–39 ml/min*—500 mg q 24 hr for 7 days; *CCr <20 ml/min*—250 mg q 24 hr for 7 days; *Hemodialysis*—250 mg after each dialysis.

Availability
Tablets: 125 mg, 250 mg, 500 mg.

NURSING IMPLICATIONS

Assessment

- Assess lesions prior to and daily during therapy.
- Assess patient for postherpetic neuralgia periodically during and following therapy.

Potential Nursing Diagnoses

Risk for impaired skin integrity (Indications)
Risk for infection (Indications, Patient/Family Teaching)

Implementation

- Famciclovir therapy should be started as soon as herpes zoster is diagnosed, at least within 72 hr, preferably within 48 hr.
- **PO:** Famciclovir may be administered without regard to meals.

Patient/Family Teaching

- Instruct patient to take famciclovir as directed for the full course of therapy. If a dose is missed, take as soon as remembered if not just before next dose.
- Inform patient that famciclovir does not prevent the spread of infection to others. Until all lesions have crusted, precautions should be taken around others who have not had chickenpox or varicella vaccine or people who are immunosuppressed.
- Advise patient that condoms should be used during sexual contact and that no sexual contact should be made while lesions are present.
- Instruct women with genital herpes to have yearly Papanicolaou smears because these women may be more likely to develop cervical cancer.

Evaluation/Desired Outcomes

- Decrease in time to full crusting, loss of vesicles, loss of ulcers, and loss of crusts in patients with acute herpes zoster (shingles).
- Crusting over and healing of lesions in herpes labialis, genital herpes and in recurrent mucocutaneous HSV infection in HIV-infected patients.
- Prevention of recurrence of herpes genitalis.

famotidine, See HISTAMINE H_2 ANTAGONISTS.

felodipine (fe-loe-di-peen)

Plendil, ✤Renedil

Classification
Therapeutic: antianginals, antihypertensives
Pharmacologic: calcium channel blockers

Pregnancy Category C

Indications

Management of hypertension, angina pectoris, and vasospastic (Prinzmetal's) angina.

Action

Inhibits the transport of calcium into myocardial and vascular smooth muscle cells, resulting in inhibition of excitation-contraction coupling and subsequent contraction. **Therapeutic Effects:** Systemic vasodilation resulting in decreased blood pressure. Coronary vasodilation resulting in decreased frequency and severity of attacks of angina.

Pharmacokinetics

Absorption: Well absorbed after oral administration, but extensively metabolized, resulting in decreased bioavailability.
Distribution: Unknown.
Protein Binding: >99%.
Metabolism and Excretion: Mostly metabolized; minimal amounts excreted unchanged by kidneys.
Half-life: 11–16 hr.

TIME/ACTION PROFILE (antihypertensive effect)

ROUTE	ONSET	PEAK	DURATION
PO	1 hr	2–4 hr	up to 24 hr

Contraindications/Precautions

Contraindicated in: Hypersensitivity (cross-sensitivity may occur); Sick sinus syndrome; 2nd- or 3rd-degree AV block (unless an artificial pacemaker is in place); Blood pressure <90 mm Hg.
Use Cautiously in: Severe hepatic impairment (dose reduction recommended); Geri: Geriatric patients (dose reduction recommended; increased risk of hypotension); Severe renal impairment; History of serious ventricular arrhythmias or CHF; OB, Lactation, Pedi: Pregnancy, lactation, or children (safety not established).

Adverse Reactions/Side Effects

CNS: headache, abnormal dreams, anxiety, confusion, dizziness, drowsiness, nervousness, psychiatric disturbances, weakness. **EENT:** blurred vision, disturbed equilibrium, epistaxis, tinnitus. **Resp:** cough, dyspnea. **CV:** ARRHYTHMIAS, CHF, peripheral edema, bradycardia, chest pain, hypotension, palpitations, syncope, tachycardia. **GI:** abnormal liver function studies, anorexia, constipation, diarrhea, dry mouth, dysgeusia, dyspepsia, nausea, vomiting. **GU:** dysuria, nocturia, polyuria, sexual dysfunction, urinary frequency. **Derm:** dermatitis, erythema multiforme, flushing, increased sweating, photosensitivity, pruritus/urticaria, rash. **Endo:** gynecomastia, hyperglycemia. **Hemat:** anemia, leukopenia, thrombocytopenia. **Metab:** weight gain. **MS:** joint stiffness, muscle cramps. **Neuro:** paresthesia, tremor. **Misc:** STEVENS-JOHNSON SYNDROME, gingival hyperplasia.

Interactions

Drug-Drug: Additive hypotension may occur when used concurrently with **fentanyl**, other **antihypertensives**, **nitrates**, acute ingestion of **alcohol**, or **quinidine**. Antihypertensive effects may be ↓ by concurrent use of **NSAIDs**. Concurrent use with **beta blockers**, **digoxin**, **disopyramide**, or **phenytoin** may result in bradycardia, conduction defects, or CHF. **Ketoconazole**, **itraconazole**, **propranolol** and **erythromycin** ↓ metabolism, increase blood levels and the risk of toxicity (dose reduction may be necessary).
Drug-Food: Grapefruit and **grapefruit juice** ↑ serum levels and effect.

Route/Dosage

PO (Adults): 5 mg/day (2.5 mg/day in geriatric patients); may increase q 2 wk (range 5–10 mg/day; not to exceed 10 mg/day).

Availability (generic available)

Extended-release tablets: 2.5 mg, 5 mg, 10 mg. **Cost:** *Generic*—2.5 mg $89.96/90, 5 mg $85.97/90, 10 mg $139.97/90. ***In combination with:*** enalapril (Lexxel). See Appendix B.

NURSING IMPLICATIONS

Assessment

- Monitor blood pressure and pulse before therapy, during dosage titration, and periodically throughout therapy. Monitor ECG periodically during prolonged therapy.
- Monitor intake and output ratios and daily weight. Assess for signs of CHF (peripheral edema, rales/crackles, dyspnea, weight gain, jugular venous distention).
- **Angina:** Assess location, duration, intensity, and precipitating factors of patient's anginal pain.
- **Hypertension:** Check frequency of refills to monitor adherence.
- ***Lab Test Considerations:*** Total serum calcium concentrations are not affected by calcium channel blockers.
- Monitor serum potassium periodically. Hypokalemia ↑ risk of arrhythmias and should be corrected.
- Monitor renal and hepatic functions periodically during long-term therapy. May cause ↑ in hepatic enzymes after several days of therapy, which return to normal upon discontinuation of therapy.

Potential Nursing Diagnoses

Ineffective tissue perfusion (Indications)
Acute pain (Indications)

Implementation

- Do not confuse Plendil (felodipine) with pindolol.
- **PO:** May be administered without regard to meals. May be administered with meals if GI irritation becomes a problem.
- Do not crush, break, or chew sustained-release tablets. Empty tablets that appear in stool are not significant.

Patient/Family Teaching

- Advise patient to take medication as directed, even if feeling well. If a dose is missed, take as soon as possible unless almost time for next dose; do not double doses. May need to be discontinued gradually.
- Instruct patient on correct technique for monitoring pulse. Instruct patient to contact health care professional if heart rate is <50 bpm.
- Advise patient to avoid grapefruit or grapefruit juice during therapy.
- Caution patient to change positions slowly to minimize orthostatic hypotension.
- May cause drowsiness or dizziness. Advise patient to avoid driving or other activities requiring alertness until response to the medication is known.
- Instruct patient on importance of maintaining good dental hygiene and seeing dentist frequently for teeth cleaning to prevent tenderness, bleeding, and gingival hyperplasia (gum enlargement).

- Instruct patient to avoid concurrent use of alcohol or OTC medications, especially cold preparations, without consulting health care professional.
- Advise patient to notify health care professional if irregular heartbeat, dyspnea, swelling of hands and feet, pronounced dizziness, nausea, constipation, or hypotension occurs or if headache is severe or persistent.
- Caution patient to wear protective clothing and to use sunscreen to prevent photosensitivity reactions.
- Advise patient to inform health care professional of medication regimen before treatment or surgery.
- **Angina:** Instruct patient on concurrent nitrate or beta-blocker therapy to continue taking both medications as directed and to use SL nitroglycerin as needed for anginal attacks.
- Advise patient to contact health care professional if chest pain does not improve or worsens after therapy, occurs with diaphoresis or shortness of breath, or if severe, persistent headache occurs.
- Caution patient to discuss exercise restrictions with health care professional before exertion.
- **Hypertension:** Encourage patient to comply with other interventions for hypertension (weight reduction, low-sodium diet, smoking cessation, moderation of alcohol consumption, regular exercise, and stress management). Medication controls but does not cure hypertension.
- Instruct patient and family in proper technique for monitoring blood pressure. Advise patient to take blood pressure weekly and to report significant changes.

Evaluation/Desired Outcomes

- Decrease in blood pressure.
- Decrease in frequency and severity of anginal attacks.
- Decrease in need for nitrate therapy.
- Increase in activity tolerance and sense of well-being.

fenofibrate (fen-o-fi-brate)

Antara, Lipofen, ✤Lipidil Micro, ✤Lipidil Supra, Lofibra, Tricor, Triglide

Classification
Therapeutic: lipid-lowering agents
Pharmacologic: fibric acid derivatives

Pregnancy Category C

Indications

With dietary therapy to decrease LDL cholesterol, total cholesterol, triglycerides, and apolipoprotein B in adult patients with hypercholesterolemia or mixed dyslipidemia. With dietary management in the treatment of hypertriglyceridemia (types IV and V hyperlipidemia) in patients who are at risk for pancreatitis and do not respond to nondrug therapy.

Action

Fenofibric acid primarily inhibits triglyceride synthesis. **Therapeutic Effects:** Lowering of cholesterol and triglycerides with subsequent decreased risk of pancreatitis.

Pharmacokinetics

Absorption: Well absorbed (60%) after oral administration; absorption is increased by food.
Distribution: Unknown.
Protein Binding: 99%.
Metabolism and Excretion: Rapidly converted to fenofibric acid, which is the active metabolite; fenofibric acid is metabolized by the liver. Fenofibric acid and its metabolites are primarily excreted in urine (60%).
Half-life: 20 hr.

TIME/ACTION PROFILE (lowering of triglycerides)

ROUTE	ONSET	PEAK	DURATION
PO	unknown	2 wk	unknown

Contraindications/Precautions

Contraindicated in: Hypersensitivity; Hepatic impairment (including primary biliary cirrhosis); Pre-existing gallbladder disease; Severe renal impairment; Concurrent use of HMG-CoA reductase inhibitors; OB: Lactation.
Use Cautiously in: Concurrent warfarin therapy; OB, Pedi: Pregnancy or children (use in pregnancy only if benefits outweigh risks to the fetus; safety not established).

Adverse Reactions/Side Effects

CNS: fatigue/weakness, headache. **CV:** arrhythmias. **GI:** cholelithiasis, pancreatitis. **Derm:** rash, urticaria. **MS:** rhabdomyolysis. **Misc:** hypersensitivity reactions.

Interactions

Drug-Drug: ↑ anticoagulant effects of **warfarin**. Concurrent use with **HMG-CoA reductase inhibitors** ↑ risk of rhabdomyolysis (combined use should be avoided). Absorption is ↓ by **bile acid sequestrants** (fenofibrate should be given 1 hr before or 4–6 hr after). ↑ risk of nephrotoxicity with **cyclosporine**.

Route/Dosage

Primary Hypercholesterolemia/Mixed Dyslipidemia

PO (Adults): *Antara*—130 mg/day initially; *Lofibra*—200 mg/day initially; *Tricor*—145 mg/day initially; *Triglide*—160 mg/day initially; *Lipofen*—50 mg daily; *Lipidil Supra*—160 mg daily.

Hypertriglyceridemia

PO (Adults): *Antara*—43–130 mg/day; *Lofibra*—67–200 mg/day initially; *Tricor*—48–145 mg/day initially; *Triglide*—50–160 mg/day initially; *Lipofen*—50 mg daily; *Lipidil Supra*—160 mg daily.

Renal impairment/Geriatric patients

PO (Adults): *Antara*—43 mg/day; *Lofibra*—67 mg/day; *Tricor*—48 mg/day.

Availability

Tablets (Tricor): 48 mg, 145 mg. **Cost:** 48 mg $109.97/90, 145 mg $299.96/90. **Tablets (Triglide):** 50 mg, 160 mg. **Micronized tablets (Lofibra):** 54 mg, 160 mg. **Cost:** 160 mg $189.97/90. **Microcoated tablets (Lipidil Supra):** 100 mg, 160 mg. **Micronized capsules (Antara):** 43 mg, 130 mg. **Cost:** 43 mg $116.96/90, 130 mg $318.93/90. **Capsules (Lipofen):** 50 mg, 100 mg, 150 mg. **Micronized capsules (Lofibra):** 67 mg, 134 mg, 200 mg. **Cost:** *Generic*—67 mg $76.39/90, 134 mg $147.00/90, 200 mg $226.87/90. **Micronized capsules (Lipidil Micro):** 67 mg, 200 mg.

NURSING IMPLICATIONS

Assessment

- Obtain a diet history, especially with regard to fat consumption. Every attempt should be made to obtain normal serum triglyceride levels with diet, exercise, and weight loss in obese patients before fenofibrate therapy is instituted.
- Assess patient for cholelithiasis. If symptoms occur, gallbladder studies are indicated. Therapy should be discontinued if gallstones are found.
- ***Lab Test Considerations:*** Monitor serum lipids before therapy to determine consistent elevations, then monitor periodically during therapy.
- Monitor serum AST and ALT periodically during therapy. May cause ↑ levels. Therapy should be discontinued if levels rise >3 times the normal limit.
- If patient develops muscle tenderness during therapy, CPK levels should be monitored. If CPK levels are markedly ↑ or myopathy occurs, therapy should be discontinued.
- May cause mild to moderate ↓ in hemoglobin, hematocrit, and WBCs. Monitor periodically during first 12 mo of therapy. Levels usually stabilize during long-term therapy.
- Patients taking anticoagulants concurrently should have prothrombin levels monitored frequently until levels stabilize.

Potential Nursing Diagnoses

Noncompliance (Patient/Family Teaching)

Implementation

- Patients should be placed on a triglyceride-lowering diet before therapy and remain on this diet throughout therapy.
- Dose may be increased after repeated serum triglyceride levels every 4–8 wk.
- Brands are not interchangeable.
- **PO:** Administer *Antara, Lipofen, Lipidil Micro, Lipidil Supra, Lofibra,* and *Tricor* products with meals. *Triglide* formulation may be taken without regard to meals.

Patient/Family Teaching

- Instruct patient to take medication as directed, not to skip doses or double up on missed doses. Medication helps control but does not cure elevated serum triglyceride levels.
- Advise patient that this medication should be used in conjunction with diet restrictions (fat, cholesterol, carbohydrates, alcohol), exercise, and cessation of smoking.
- Instruct patient to notify health care professional if unexplained muscle pain, tenderness, or weakness occurs, especially if accompanied by fever or malaise.

- Instruct female patients to notify health care professional promptly if pregnancy is planned or suspected.
- Advise patient to notify health care professional of medication regimen before treatment or surgery.
- Emphasize the importance of follow-up exams to determine effectiveness and to monitor for side effects.

Evaluation/Desired Outcomes

- Decrease in serum triglycerides and cholesterol to normal levels. Therapy should be discontinued in patients who do not have an adequate response in 2 months of therapy.

fenoldopam

(fen-**ole**-doe-pam)
Corlopam

Classification
Therapeutic: antihypertensives
Pharmacologic: vasodilators

Pregnancy Category B

Indications

Short-term (<48 hr), in-hospital management of hypertensive emergencies, including malignant hypertension with end-organ deterioration.

Action

Acts as an agonist at dopamine d_1-like receptors. Also binds to alpha-adrenergic receptors. Acts as a vasodilator. **Therapeutic Effects:** Rapid lowering of blood pressure.

Pharmacokinetics

Absorption: IV administration results in complete bioavailability.
Distribution: Unknown.
Metabolism and Excretion: Mostly metabolized by the liver; 90% of metabolites are excreted in urine, 10% in feces.
Half-life: 5–10 min.

TIME/ACTION PROFILE (effect on blood pressure)

ROUTE	ONSET	PEAK	DURATION
IV	rapid	15 min	1–4 hr

Contraindications/Precautions

Contraindicated in: Hypersensitivity to fenoldopam or sulfites; Concurrent beta blocker therapy (will prevent reflex tachycardia).
Use Cautiously in: Glaucoma or intraocular hypertension; Pregnancy, lactation, or children (safety not established).

Adverse Reactions/Side Effects

CNS: headache, nervousness/anxiety, dizziness. **CV:** hypotension, tachycardia, ECG changes, peripheral edema. **GI:** nausea, abdominal pain, constipation, diarrhea, vomiting. **Derm:** flushing, sweating. **F and E:** hypokalemia. **Local:** injection site reactions. **MS:** back pain.

Interactions

Drug-Drug: Concurrent use with **beta blockers** may result in excessive hypotension (concurrent use should be avoided).

Route/Dosage

IV (Adults): 0.01–1.6 mcg/kg/min.

Availability

Concentrate for injection: 10 mg/ml in 1- and 2-ml single-use ampules (with sodium meta-bisulfite).

NURSING IMPLICATIONS

Assessment

- Monitor blood pressure, heart rate, and ECG frequently throughout therapy; continuous monitoring is preferred. Consult physician for parameters.
- ***Lab Test Considerations:*** Monitor serum potassium concentrations every 6 hr during therapy. May cause hypokalemia. Treat with oral or IV potassium supplementation.

Potential Nursing Diagnoses

Ineffective tissue perfusion (Indications)

Implementation

IV Administration

- Administer via continuous infusion; do not use bolus doses. Avoid hypotension and rapid decreases in blood pressure. Initial dose titration should occur no more frequently than every 15 min and less frequently as desired blood pressure is reached. Increments of 0.05 to 0.1 mcg/kg/min are recommended for titration. Lower initial doses (0.03 to 0.1 mcg/kg/min) titrated slowly have been associated with less reflex tachycardia than higher initial doses
- Infusion can be abruptly discontinued or gradually tapered before discontinuation. Oral therapy with other antihypertensives can begin anytime after the blood pressure is sta-

ble. Do not administer beta blockers concurrently with fenoldopam.

- **Continuous Infusion:** ***Diluent:*** Dilute 4 ml (40 mg of drug) with 1000 ml, 2 ml (20 mg of drug) with 500 ml, or 1 ml (10 mg of drug) with 250 ml of 0.9% NaCl or D5W. Infusion is stable for 24 hrs at room temperature. ***Concentration:*** 40 mcg/ml. ***Rate:*** Based on patient's weight (see Route/Dosage section). Titrate to desired effect. Administer via infusion pump to ensure accurate dosage rate.
- **Y-Site Compatibility:** alfentanil, amikancin, aminocaproic acid, amiodarone, ampicillin/sulbactam, argatroban, atracurium, atropine, azithromycin, aztreonam, butorphanol, calcium chloride, calcium gluconate, caspofungin, cefazolin, cefepime, cefotaxime, ceftazidime, ceftizoxime, ceftriaxone, cefuroxime, chloramphenicol, cimetidine, ciprofloxacin, cisatracurium, clindamycin, cyclosporine, daptomycin, dexmedetomidine, digoxin, diltiazem, diphenhydramine, dobutamine, dolasetron, dopamine, doxycycline, droperidol, enalaprilat, epinephrine, ertapenem, erythromycin, esmolol, famotidine, fentanyl, fluconazole, gentamicin, granisetron, haloperidol, heparin, hydralazine, hydrocortisone sodium succinate, hydromorphone, imipenem/cilastatin, inamrinone, insulin, isoproterenol, labetalol, levofloxacin, lidocaine, linezolid, lorazepam, magnesium sulfate, mannitol, meperidine, metoclopramide, metoprolol, metronidazole, micafungin, midazolam, milrinone, morphine, nafcillin, nalbuphine, naloxone, nicardipine, nitroglycerin, nitroprusside, norepinephrine, ondansetron, palonosetron, pancuronium, phenylephrine, piperacillin/tazobactam, potassium chloride, potassium phosphate, procainamide, promethazine, propofol, propranolol, quinupristin/dalfopristin, ranitidine, remifentanil, rocuronium, sufentanil, tacrolimus, theophylline, ticarcillin/clavulanate, tirofiban, tobramycin, trimethoprim/sulfamethoxazole, vancomycin, vasopressin, vecuronium, verapamil, voriconazole.
- **Y-Site Incompatibility:** acyclovir, aminophylline, amphotericin B, ampicillin, bumetanide, cefoxitin, dexamethasone sodium phosphate, diazepam, fosphenytoin, furosemide, ganciclovir, ketorolac, meropenem, methohexital, methylprednisolone sodium succinate, pantoprazole, pentobarbital, phenytoin, prochlorperazine, sodium bicarbonate, thiopental.

Patient/Family Teaching

- Explain purpose of medication to patient.
- Advise patient to report headache or pain at the injection site.

Evaluation/Desired Outcomes

- Decrease in blood pressure without the appearance of side effects.

fentanyl buccal (fen-ta-nil)

Fentora

Classification

Therapeutic: opioid analgesics

Pharmacologic: opioid agonists

Schedule II

Pregnancy Category C

Indications

Management of breakthrough pain in cancer patients already receiving and tolerant to opioid therapy for pain (60 mg/day of oral morphine or equivalent).

Action

Binds to opiate receptors in the CNS, altering the response to and perception of pain. **Therapeutic Effects:** Decrease in severity of breakthrough pain.

Pharmacokinetics

Absorption: 65% absorbed from the buccal mucosa; 50% is absorbed transmucosally, remainder is swallowed and is absorbed slowly from the GI tract. Buccal absorption is enhanced by an effervescent reaction in the dose form. Bioavailability is greater than transmucosal fentanyl (Actiq).

Distribution: Readily crosses the placenta and enters breast milk.

Protein Binding: 80–85%.

Metabolism and Excretion: >90% metabolized by the liver and intestinal mucosa (CYP3A4 enzyme system; 7% excreted unchanged in urine.

Half-life: *100 mcg tablet*—2.6 hr; *200 mcg tablet*—4.4 hr; *100 mcg tablet*—2.6 hr; *400* *mcg tablet*—11.0 hr; *800 mcg tablet*—11.7 hr.

TIME/ACTION PROFILE (decreased pain)

ROUTE	ONSET	PEAK	DURATION
Buccal	15 min	40–60 min	60 min

Contraindications/Precautions

Contraindicated in: Known intolerance or hypersensitivity; Acute/postoperative pain; Opioid non-tolerant patients; OB: Labor and delivery; OB: Lactation.

Use Cautiously in: Chronic obstructive pulmonary disease; History of substance abuse; Severe renal/hepatic impairment, CYP3A4 inhibitors (use lowest effective starting dose); Bradyarrhythmias; Geri: Patients >65 yr may be more sensitive to effects and may have an ↑ risk of adverse reactions; titrate dosage carefully; Pedi: Children <18 yr (safety not established).

Exercise Extreme Caution in: Head injuries/increased intracranial pressure.

Adverse Reactions/Side Effects

Opioid side effects increase with increased dosage.

CNS: <u>dizziness</u>, <u>drowsiness</u>, <u>headache</u>, confusion, depression, fatigue, insomnia, weakness. **Resp:** RESPIRATORY DEPRESSION, cough, dyspnea. **GI:** <u>application site reactions</u>, <u>constipation</u>, <u>nausea</u>, <u>vomiting</u>, abdominal pain, anorexia, diarrhea. **F and E:** dehydration, edema. **Misc:** physical dependence, psychological dependence.

Interactions

Drug-Drug: CNS depressants, including other **opioids**, **sedative/hypnotics**, **general anesthetics**, **phenothiazines**, **skeletal muscle relaxants**, **sedating antihistamines**, and **alcohol** may ↑ CNS depression, hypoventilation and hypotension. Concurrent use of **agents that induce CYP3A4 enzyme activity** may ↓ analgesia. Concurrent use with **CYP3A4 inhibitors** including **ritonavir**, **ketoconazole**, **itraconazole**, **clarithromycin**, **nelfinavir**, **nefazodone**, **diltiazem**, **erythromycin**, **amprenavir**, **aprepitant**, **fluconazole**, **fosamprenavir**, and **verapamil** may significantly ↑ blood levels and ↑ risk of respiratory and CNS depression; careful monitoring and dose adjustment is recommended. Should not be used within 14 days of **MAO inhibitors** (may result in severe and unpredictable reactions).

Drug-Food: Grapefruit juice is a moderate inhibitor of the CYP3A4 enzyme system; concurrent use may ↑ blood levels and the risk of respiratory and CNS depression. Careful monitoring and dose adjustment is recommended.

Route/Dosage

Buccal (Adults): 100 mcg, then titrated to dose that provides adequate analgesia with tolerable side effects.

Availability

Buccal tablets: 100 mcg, 200 mcg, 400 mcg, 600 mcg, 800 mcg.

NURSING IMPLICATIONS

Assessment

- Monitor type, location, and intensity of pain before and 15 min after administration of buccal fentanyl.
- Assess blood pressure, pulse, and respirations before and periodically during administration. If respiratory rate is <10 min, assess level of sedation. Physical stimulation may be sufficient to prevent hypoventilation. Subsequent doses may need to be decreased. Patients tolerant to opioid analgesics are usually tolerant to the respiratory depressant effects also.
- Monitor for application site reactions (paresthesia, ulceration, bleeding, pain, ulcer, irritation). Reactions are usually self-limited and rarely require discontinuation.
- ***Lab Test Considerations:*** May cause anemia, neutropenia, thrombocytopenia, and leukopenia.
- May cause hypokalemia, hypoalbuminemia, hypercalcemia, hypomagnesemia, and hyponatremia.
- ***Toxicity and Overdose:*** If an opioid antagonist is required to reverse respiratory depression or coma, naloxone (Narcan) is the antidote. Dilute the 0.4-mg ampule of naloxone in 10 ml of 0.9% NaCl and administer 0.5 ml (0.02 mg) by direct IV push every 2 min. For patients weighing <40 kg, dilute 0.1 mg of naloxone in 10 ml of 0.9% NaCl for a concentration of 10 mcg/ml and administer 0.5 mcg every 2 min. Use extreme caution when titrating dose in patients physically dependent on opioid analgesics to avoid withdrawal, seizures, and severe pain. Duration of respiratory depression may be longer than duration of opioid antagonist, requiring repeated doses.

Potential Nursing Diagnoses

Acute pain (Indications)
Risk for injury (Adverse Reactions)

Implementation

- ***High Alert:*** Accidental overdosage of opioid analgesics has resulted in fatalities. Before administering, clarify all ambiguous orders; have second practitioner independently check original order and dose calculations.
- Patients considered opioid-tolerant are those who are taking ≥60 mg of oral morphine/day, at least 25 mcg transdermal fentanyl/hr, 30 mg of oxycodone/day, 8 mg of hydromorphone/day or an equianalgesic dose of another opioid for ≥1 wk.
- ***High Alert:*** Dose may be lethal to a child; keep out of reach of children.
- Do not substitute fentanyl buccal for fentanyl oral transmucosal; doses are not equivalent.
- **Buccal:** For patients not previously using transmucosal fentanyl, initial dose should be 100 mcg. Titrate to provide adequate relief while minimizing side effects. For patients switching from oral transmucosal fentanyl to fentanyl buccal, if transmucosal dose is 200–400 mcg, switch to 100 mcg buccal; if transmucosal dose is 600–800 mcg, switch to 200 mcg buccal; if transmucosal dose is 1200–1600 mcg, switch to 400 mcg buccal fentanyl.
- Dose may be repeated once during a single episode of breakthrough pain if not adequately relieved. Re-dose may occur 30 min after start of administration of fentanyl buccal and the same dose should be used.
- If more than one dose is required per breakthrough pain episode for several consecutive episodes, dose of maintenance opioid and fentanyl buccal should be adjusted. To increase dose, use multiples of 100 mcg tablet, use two 100 mcg tablets (one on each side of mouth in buccal cavity). If unsuccessful in controlling breakthrough pain episode, two 100 mcg tablets may be placed on each side of mouth in buccal cavity (four 100 mcg tablets). Titrate above 400 mcg by 200 mcg increments. To reduce risk of overdose, patients should have only one strength available at any one time.
- Once a successful dose has been established, if more than 4 breakthrough pain episodes/day occur, re-evaluate opioid dose for persistent pain.

Patient/Family Teaching

- Instruct patient to take fentanyl buccal exactly as directed. Do not take more often than prescribed, keep out of reach of children, protect it from being stolen, and do not share with others, even if they have the same symptoms. Open blister pouch only when ready to administer. Do not attempt to push tablet through blister, may cause damage to tablet. Open by tearing along perforations to separate from blister card. Then bend blister unit on line where indicated. Blister backing should then be peeled to expose tablets. Use immediately; do not store, may damage integrity of tablet. Tablets are not to be sucked, chewed or swallowed whole; this will reduce medication effectiveness. Place between cheek and gum above a molar and allow medication to dissolve, usually 14–25 min. May cause bubbling sensation between teeth and gum while tablet dissolves. Do not attempt to split tablet. After 30 min, if remnants of tablet remain, swallow with glass of water. Advise patient to review *Medication Guide* each time fentanyl buccal is dispensed; new information may be available. Advise patient to notify health care professional if breakthrough pain is not alleviated or worsens.
- Caution patient to make position changes slowly to minimize orthostatic hypotension.
- Medication causes dizziness and drowsiness. Advise patient to call for assistance during ambulation and transfer, and to avoid driving or other activities requiring alertness until response to medication is known.
- Instruct patient to avoid concurrent use of alcohol or other CNS depressants, such as sleep aids.
- Advise patient to notify health care professional if sores on gums or inside cheek become a problem.
- Instruct patient to notify health care professional before taking Rx, OTC, or herbal products.
- Advise patient to notify health care professional if pregnancy is planned or suspected or if breastfeeding.
- Inform patient if medication is no longer needed they should contact Cephalon at

1-800-896-5855 or remove from blister pack and flush any remaining product down toilet.

Evaluation/Desired Outcomes

- Decrease in severity of pain during episodes of breakthrough pain in patients receiving long-acting opioids.

HIGH ALERT

fentanyl (oral transmucosal) (fen-ta-nil)

Actiq

Classification

Therapeutic: opioid analgesics
Pharmacologic: opioid agonists

Schedule II

Pregnancy Category C

Indications

Management of breakthrough cancer pain in patients with malignancies who are already receiving and are tolerant to opioid therapy for their underlying cancer pain.

Action

Binds to opiate receptors in the CNS, altering response to and perception of pain. **Therapeutic Effects:** Decreased pain.

Pharmacokinetics

Absorption: Initial rapid absorption (25%) from buccal mucosa is followed by more prolonged absorption (25%) from GI tract (combined bioavailability 50%).
Distribution: Highly lipid soluble; rapidly distributes to brain, heart, lungs, kidneys, and spleen, followed by slower distribution to muscle and fat.
Metabolism and Excretion: Mostly metabolized by liver and intestinal mucosa; <7% excreted unchanged in urine.
Half-life: 7 hr.

TIME/ACTION PROFILE (analgesia)

ROUTE	ONSET	PEAK	DURATION
Oral/transmucosal	rapid	15–30 min	several hrs

Contraindications/Precautions

Contraindicated in: Hypersensitivity; Management of acute or postoperative pain; Opioid-naive (nontolerant) patients; Lactation.
Use Cautiously in: Bradyarrhythmias; Concurrent use of CNS active drugs; Chronic pulmonary disease or predisposition to hypoventilation; Hepatic or renal impairment; Geri: Elderly patients may be more sensitive to effects; OB, Pedi: Pregnancy or children <16 yr (safety not established).
Exercise Extreme Caution in: Increased intracranial pressure or altered consciousness.

Adverse Reactions/Side Effects

Includes effects seen with concurrent use of longer-acting opioids.
CNS: dizziness, drowsiness, abnormal thinking, confusion, hallucinations, headache, insomnia, nervousness, weakness. **EENT:** abnormal vision. **Resp:** RESPIRATORY DEPRESSION, dyspnea. **CV:** hypotension. **GI:** nausea, constipation, dry mouth, vomiting. **Derm:** pruritus, rash, sweating. **Neuro:** abnormal gait.

Interactions

Drug-Drug: Should not be used within 14 days of **MAO inhibitors** because of possible severe and unpredictable reactions. Concurrent use of other **CNS depressants**, including **sedative/hypnotics**, **antidepressants**, other **opioid analgesics**, **skeletal muscle relaxants**, **sedating antihistamines**, or **alcohol** may produce ↑ sedation, hypoventilation, and hypotension. Concomitant use of **CYP3A4 inhibitors** including **ritonavir**, **ketoconazole**, **itraconazole**, **clarithromycin**, **nelfinavir**, **nefazodone**, **diltiazem**, **apretitant**, **fluconazole**, **fosamprenavir**, **verapamil**, and **erythromycin** may result in ↑ plasma levels and ↑ risk of CNS and respiratory depression. Administration of **partial-antagonist opioid analgesics** or **opioid antagonists** will precipitate withdrawal in physically dependent patients. **Buprenorphine**, **nalbuphine**, or **pentazocine** may ↓ analgesia.
Drug-Food: Grapefruit juice is a moderate inhibitor of the CYP3A4 enzyme system; concurrent use may ↑ blood levels and the risk of respiratory and CNS depression. Careful monitoring and dose adjustment is recommended.

Route/Dosage

Transmucosal (Adults): *Dose titration*—One 200 mcg *Actiq* unit dissolved in mouth (see Implementation section) over 15 min; additional unit may be used 15 min after first unit is completed. If more than one unit is required per episode (as evaluated over several episodes), dose may be increased as required to control pain. Optimal usage/titration should result in using no more than 4 units/day.

Availability

Lozenge on a stick (berry flavor-sugar free): 200 mcg, 400 mcg, 600 mcg, 800 mcg, 1200 mcg, 1600 mcg.

NURSING IMPLICATIONS

Assessment

- Monitor type, location, and intensity of pain before and 15 min after administration of transmucosal fentanyl.
- Assess blood pressure, pulse, and respirations before and periodically during administration. If respiratory rate is <10 min, assess level of sedation. Physical stimulation may be sufficient to prevent hypoventilation. Subsequent doses may need to be decreased by 25–50%. Patients tolerant to opioid analgesics are usually tolerant to the respiratory depressant effects also.
- ***Toxicity and Overdose:*** If an opioid antagonist is required to reverse respiratory depression or coma, naloxone (Narcan) is the antidote. Dilute the 0.4-mg ampule of naloxone in 10 ml of 0.9% NaCl and administer 0.5 ml (0.02 mg) by direct IV push every 2 min. For patients weighing <40 kg, dilute 0.1 mg of naloxone in 10 ml of 0.9% NaCl for a concentration of 10 mcg/ml and administer 0.5 mcg every 2 min. Use extreme caution when titrating dose in patients physically dependent on opioid analgesics to avoid withdrawal, seizures, and severe pain.

Potential Nursing Diagnoses

Acute pain (Indications)
Risk for injury (Adverse Reactions)

Implementation

- ***High Alert:*** Accidental overdosage of opioid analgesics has resulted in fatalities. Before administering, clarify all ambiguous orders; have second practitioner independently check original order and dose calculations.
- Patients considered opioid-tolerant are those who are taking ≥60 mg of oral morphine/day, 50 mcg transdermal fentanyl/hr, or an equianalgesic dose of another opioid for ≥1 wk.
- ***High Alert:*** Supplied in individually sealed child-resistant foil pouches. Dose may be lethal to a child; keep out of reach of children.
- **Transmucosal:** Open the foil package immediately before use. Instruct patient to place unit in the mouth between the cheek and lower gum, moving it from one side to the other using the handle. Patient should suck, not chew, the lozenge. If it is chewed and swallowed, lower peak concentrations and lower bioavailability may occur. Instruct patient to consume lozenge over 15-min period; longer or shorter periods may be less efficacious. If signs of excessive opioid effects occur, remove from patient's mouth immediately and decrease future doses.
- Initial dose for breakthrough pain should be 200 mcg. Six 200-mcg units should be prescribed and should be used before increasing to a higher dose. If one unit is ineffective, a second unit may be started 15 min after the completion of the first unit. Do not use more than 2 units during a single episode of breakthrough pain during titration phase. With each new dose during titration, 6 units should be prescribed, allowing treatment of several episodes of breakthrough pain. Adequate dose is determined based on effective analgesia with acceptable side effects. Side effects during titration period are usually greater than after effective dose is determined.
- Once an effective dose is determined, instruct patient to limit dose to 4 units/day. If >4 units/day are required, consider increasing the dose of the long-acting opioid.
- Discontinue with a gradual decrease in dose to prevent signs and symptoms of abrupt withdrawal.
- To dispose of remaining unit, remove drug matrix from handle by grasping with tissue paper and separating with a twisting motion. Flush remaining drug matrix down toilet. Drug remaining on handle may be removed by placing under running warm water until dissolved. Dispose of drug-free handle according to institutional protocol.
- ***High Alert:*** Partially consumed units are no longer protected by child-resistant pouch; dose may still be fatal. A temporary child-resistant storage bottle is provided for partially consumed units that cannot be disposed of properly.

Patient/Family Teaching

- Instruct patient in proper use, storage, and disposal of unit. Review *Patient Leaflet* describing use of this medication with patient. Advise patient to notify health care professional if excessive opioid effects occur or if >4 units/day are required to control pain.
- Caution patient to make position changes slowly to minimize orthostatic hypotension.
- Medication causes dizziness and drowsiness. Advise patient to call for assistance during ambulation and transfer, and to avoid driving or other activities requiring alertness until response to medication is known.
- Instruct patient to avoid concurrent use of alcohol or other CNS depressants.
- Inform patient that this drug may contain sugar and may cause dry mouth. Advise patient to maintain good oral hygiene and have regular dental exams.

Evaluation/Desired Outcomes

- Decrease in severity of pain during episodes of breakthrough pain in patients receiving long-acting opioids.

HIGH ALERT

fentanyl (parenteral)

(**fen**-ta-nil)
Sublimaze

Classification
Therapeutic: opioid analgesics
Pharmacologic: opioid agonists

Schedule II

Pregnancy Category C

Indications

Analgesic supplement to general anesthesia; usually with other agents (ultra–short-acting barbiturates, neuromuscular blocking agents, and inhalation anesthetics) to produce balanced anesthesia. Induction/maintenance of anesthesia (with oxygen or oxygen/nitrous oxide and a neuromuscular blocking agents). Neuroleptanalgesia/neuroleptanesthesia (with or without nitrous oxide). Supplement to regional/local anesthesia. Preoperative and postoperative analgesia. **Unlabeled uses:** Continuous IV infusion as part of PCA.

Action

Binds to opiate receptors in the CNS, altering the response to and perception of pain. Produces CNS depression. **Therapeutic Effects:** Supplement in anesthesia. Decreased pain.

Pharmacokinetics

Absorption: Well absorbed after IM administration.
Distribution: Unknown.
Metabolism and Excretion: Mostly metabolized by the liver, 10–25% excreted unchanged by the kidneys.
Half-life: Children: Bolus dose—2.4 hr, long-term continuous infusion—11–36 hr; Adults: 2–4 hr (increased after cardiopulmonary bypass and in geriatric patients).

TIME/ACTION PROFILE (analgesia*)

ROUTE	ONSET	PEAK	DURATION
IM	7–15 min	20–30 min	1–2 hr
IV	1–2 min	3–5 min	0.5–1 hr

*Respiratory depression may last longer than analgesia

Contraindications/Precautions

Contraindicated in: Hypersensitivity; Cross-sensitivity among agents may occur; Known intolerance.
Use Cautiously in: Geriatric, debilitated, or critically ill patients; Diabetes; Severe renal, pulmonary or hepatic disease; CNS tumors; Increased intracranial pressure; Head trauma; Adrenal insufficiency; Undiagnosed abdominal pain; Hypothyroidism; Alcoholism; Cardiac disease (arrhythmias); Pregnancy and lactation.

Adverse Reactions/Side Effects

CNS: confusion, paradoxical excitation/delirium, postoperative depression, postoperative drowsiness. **EENT:** blurred/double vision. **Resp:** APNEA, LARYNGOSPASM, allergic bronchospasm, respiratory depression. **CV:** arrhythmias, bradycardia, circulatory depression, hypotension. **GI:** biliary spasm, nausea/vomiting. **Derm:** facial itching. **MS:** skeletal and thoracic muscle rigidity (with rapid IV infusion).

Interactions

Drug-Drug: Avoid use in patients who have received **MAO inhibitors** within the previous 14 days (may produce unpredictable, potentially fatal reactions). Concomitant use of **CYP3A4 inhibitors** including **ritonavir**, **ketoconazole**, **itraconazole**, **clarithromycin**, **nelfinavir**, **nefazodone**, **diltiazem**, **aprepitant**, **fluconazole**, **fosamprenavir**, **verapamil**, and **erythromycin** may result in ↑ plasma levels and ↑ risk of CNS and respiratory depres-

sion. Additive CNS and respiratory depression with other **CNS depressants**, including **alcohol**, **antihistamines**, **antidepressants**, other **sedative/hypnotics**, and other **opioid analgesics**. ↑ risk of hypotension with **benzodiazepines**. **Nalbuphine**, **buprenorphine**, or **pentazocine** may ↓ analgesia.
Drug-Food: Grapefruit juice is a moderate inhibitor of the CYP3A4 enzyme system; concurrent use may ↑ blood levels and the risk of respiratory and CNS depression. Careful monitoring and dose adjustment is recommended.

Route/Dosage

Preoperative Use

IM, IV (Adults and Children >12 yr): 50–100 mcg 30–60 min before surgery.

Adjunct to General Anesthesia

IM, IV (Adults and Children >12 yr): *Low dose–minor surgery*—2 mcg/kg. *Moderate dose–major surgery*—2–20 mcg/kg. *High dose–major surgery*—20–50 mcg/kg.

Adjunct to Regional Anesthesia

IM, IV (Adults and Children >12 yr): 50–100 mcg.

Postoperative Use (Recovery Room)

IM, IV (Adults and Children >12 yr): 50–100 mcg; may repeat in 1–2 hr.

General Anesthesia

IV (Adults and Children >12 yr): 50–100 mcg/kg (up to 150 mcg/kg).
IV (Children 1–12 yr): 2–3 mcg/kg.

Sedation/Analgesia

IV (Adults and Children >12 yr): 0.5–1 mcg/kg/dose, may repeat after 30–60 min.
IV (Children 1–12 yr): *Bolus*—1–2 mcg/kg/dose, may repeat at 30–60 min intervals. *Continuous infusion*—1–5 mcg/kg/hr following bolus dose.
IV (Neonates): *Bolus*—0.5–3 mcg/kg/dose. *Continuous infusion*—0.5–2 mcg/kg/hr following bolus dose. *Continuous infusion during ECMO*—5–10 mcg/kg bolus followed by 1–5 mcg/kg/hr, may require up to 20 mcg/kg/hr after 5 days of therapy.

Availability (generic available)

Injection: 0.05 mg/ml. ***In combination with:*** droperidol (Innovar). See Appendix B.

NURSING IMPLICATIONS

Assessment

- Monitor respiratory rate and blood pressure frequently throughout therapy. Report significant changes immediately. The respiratory depressant effects of fentanyl may last longer than the analgesic effects. Initial doses of other opioids should be reduced by 25–33% of the usually recommended dose. Monitor closely.
- Geri: Opioids have been associated with increased risk of falls in geriatric patients. Assess risk and implement fall prevention strategies.
- **IV, IM:** Assess type, location, and intensity of pain before and 30 min after IM administration or 3–5 min after IV administration when fentanyl is used to treat pain.
- ***Lab Test Considerations:*** May cause ↑ serum amylase and lipase concentrations.
- ***Toxicity and Overdose:*** Symptoms of toxicity include respiratory depression, hypotension, arrhythmias, bradycardia, and asystole. Atropine may be used to treat bradycardia. If respiratory depression persists after surgery, prolonged mechanical ventilation may be required. If an opioid antagonist is required to reverse respiratory depression or coma, naloxone (Narcan) is the antidote. Dilute the 0.4-mg ampule of naloxone in 10 ml of 0.9% NaCl and administer 0.5 ml (0.02 mg) by direct IV push every 2 min. Pedi: For children and patients weighing <40 kg, dilute 0.1 mg of naloxone in 10 ml of 0.9% NaCl for a concentration of 10 mcg/ml and administer 0.5 mcg/kg every 2 min. Titrate dose to avoid withdrawal, seizures, and severe pain. Administration of naloxone in these circumstances, especially in cardiac patients, has resulted in hypertension and tachycardia, occasionally causing left ventricular failure and pulmonary edema.

Potential Nursing Diagnoses

Acute pain (Indications)
Ineffective breathing pattern (Adverse Reactions)
Risk for injury (Side Effects)

Implementation

- ***High Alert:*** Accidental overdosage of opioid analgesics has resulted in fatalities. Before administering, clarify all ambiguous orders;

have second practitioner independently check original order, dose calculations, route of administration, and infusion pump programming. Do not confuse fentanyl with alfentanil or sufentanil.

- Benzodiazepines may be administered before or after administration of fentanyl to reduce the induction dose requirements, decrease the time to loss of consciousness, and produce amnesia. This combination may also increase the risk of hypotension.
- ***High Alert:*** Opioid antagonists, oxygen, and resuscitative equipment should be readily available during the administration of fentanyl. Fentanyl derivatives should be administered IV only in monitored anesthesia care settings (operating room, emergency department, ICU) with immediate access to life-support equipment and should be administered only by personnel trained in resuscitation and emergency airway management.

IV Administration

- **Direct IV:** ***Diluent:*** Administer undiluted. ***Concentration:*** 50 mcg/ml. ***Rate:*** Injections should be administered slowly over 1–3 min. Administer doses >5 mcg/kg over 5–10 min. Slow IV administration may reduce the incidence and severity of muscle rigidity, bradycardia, or hypotension. Neuromuscular blocking agents may be administered concurrently to decrease chest wall muscle rigidity.
- **Intermittent Infusion:** ***Diluent:*** May be diluted in D5W or 0.9% NaCl. ***Concentration:*** Up to 50 mcg/ml. ***Rate:*** see Direct IV.
- **Syringe Compatibility:** atracurium, atropine, chlorpromazine, cimetidine, dimenhydrinate, diphenhydramine, droperidol, heparin, hydromorphone, hydroxyzine, meperidine, metoclopramide, midazolam, morphine, perphenazine, prochlorperazine edisylate, promethazine, ranitidine, scopolamine.
- **Syringe Incompatibility:** pantoprazole, pentobarbital.
- **Y-Site Compatibility:** abciximab, amiodarone, amphotericin cholesteryl sulfate, argatroban, atracurium, atropine, bivalirudin, cisatracurium, dexamethasone sodium phosophate, diazepam, diltiazem, diphenhydramine, dobutamine, dopamine, doxapram, enalaprilat, epinephrine, esmolol, etomidate, fenoldopam, furosemide, haloperidol, heparin, hydrocortisone sodium succinate, hydromorphone, ketorolac, labetalol, lansoprazole, levofloxacin, linezolid, lorazepam, metoclopramide, midazolam, milrinone, morphine, nafcillin, nicardipine, nitroglycerin, norepinephrine, oxaliplatin, pancuronium, phenobarbital, potassium chloride, propofol, ranitidine, remifentanil, sargramostim, scopolamine, vecuronium, vitamin B complex with C.
- **Additive Compatibility:** bupivacaine, ropivacaine.
- **Additive Incompatibility:** methohexital, pentobarbital, thiopental.

Patient/Family Teaching

- Discuss the use of anesthetic agents and the sensations to expect with the patient before surgery.
- Explain pain assessment scale to patient.
- Caution patient to change positions slowly to minimize orthostatic hypotension. Geri: Geriatric patients may be a greater risk for orthostatic hypotension and, consequently, falls. Teach patient to take precautions until drug effects have completely resolved.
- Medication causes dizziness and drowsiness. Advise patient to call for assistance during ambulation and transfer and to avoid driving or other activities requiring alertness for 24 hr after administration during outpatient surgery.
- Instruct patient to avoid alcohol or other CNS depressants for 24 hr after administration for outpatient surgery.

Evaluation/Desired Outcomes

- General quiescence.
- Reduced motor activity.
- Pronounced analgesia.

HIGH ALERT

fentanyl (transdermal)

(**fen**-ta-nil)

Duragesic

Classification

Therapeutic: opioid analgesics, anesthetic adjuncts

Pharmacologic: opioid agonists

Schedule II

Pregnancy Category C

Indications

Moderate to severe chronic pain requiring continuous opioid analgesic therapy for an extended time at a dosage of 25 mcg/hr or more of the transdermal system. Transdermal fentanyl is not recommended for the control of postoperative, mild, or intermittent pain, nor should it be used for short term-pain relief.

Action

Binds to opiate receptors in the CNS, altering the response to and perception of pain. **Therapeutic Effects:** Decrease in severity of chronic pain.

Pharmacokinetics

Absorption: Well absorbed (92% of dose) through skin surface under transdermal patch, creating a depot in the upper skin layers. Release from transdermal system into systemic circulation increases gradually to a constant rate, providing continuous delivery for 72 hr.
Distribution: Crosses the placenta; enters breast milk.
Metabolism and Excretion: Mostly metabolized by the liver (CYP3A4 enzyme system); 10–25% excreted unchanged by the kidneys.
Half-life: 17 hr after removal of a single application patch, increases to 21 hr after removal of multiple patches (because of continued release from deposition of drug in skin layers).

TIME/ACTION PROFILE (decreased pain)

ROUTE	ONSET	PEAK	DURATION
Transdermal	6 hr†	12–24 hr	72 hr‡

†Achievement of blood levels associated with analgesia. Maximal response and dose titration may take up to 6 days
‡While patch is worn

Contraindications/Precautions

Contraindicated in: Hypersensitivity to fentanyl or adhesives; Known intolerance; Acute pain (onset not rapid enough); Alcohol intolerance (small amounts of alcohol released into skin); OB: Not recommeded during labor and delivery, avoid during lactation.
Use Cautiously in: Geri: Patients >60 yr, cachectic or debilitated patients (dose reduction suggested because of altered drug disposition); Diabetes; Patients with severe pulmonary or hepatic disease; CNS tumors; Increased intracranial pressure; Head trauma; Adrenal insufficiency; Undiagnosed abdominal pain; Hypothyroidism; Alcoholism; Cardiac disease (particularly bradyarrhythmias); Fever or situations that increase body temperature (increases release of fentanyl from delivery system); Titration period (additional analgesics may be required); Pedi: Children (safety not established for children <2 yr; pediatric patients initiating therapy at 25 mcg/hr should be opioid tolerant and receiving at least 60 mg oral morphine equivalents per day.

Adverse Reactions/Side Effects

CNS: confusion, sedation, weakness, dizziness, restlessness. **Resp:** APNEA, bronchoconstriction, laryngospasm, respiratory depression. **CV:** bradycardia. **GI:** anorexia, constipation, dry mouth, nausea, vomiting. **Derm:** sweating, erythema. **Local:** application site reactions. **MS:** skeletal and thoracic muscle rigidity. **Misc:** physical dependence, psychological dependence.

Interactions

Drug-Drug: Avoid use in patients who have received **MAO inhibitors** within the previous 14 days (may produce unpredictable, potentially fatal reactions). Concomitant use of **CYP3A4 inhibitors** including **ritonavir**, **ketoconazole**, **itraconazole**, **clarithromycin**, **nelfinavir**, **nefazodone**, **diltiazem**, **aprepitant**, **fluconazole**, **fosamprenavir**, **verapamil**, and **erythromycin** may result in ↑ plasma levels and ↑ risk of CNS and respiratory depression. Levels and effectiveness may be ↓ by **drugs that induce the CYP3A4 enzyme**. ↑ CNS and respiratory depression with other **CNS depressants**, including **alcohol**, **antihistamines**, **antidepressants**, **sedative/hypnotics**, and other **opioids**.
Drug-Natural Products: Concomitant use of **kava kava**, **valerian**, or **chamomile** can ↑ CNS depression.
Drug-Food: Grapefruit juice is a moderate inhibitor of the CYP3A4 enzyme system; concurrent use may ↑ blood levels and the risk of respiratory and CNS depression. Careful monitoring and dose adjustment is recommended.

Route/Dosage

Transdermal (Adults): 25 mcg/hr is the initial dose; patients who have not been receiving opioids should receive not more that 25 mcg/hr. To calculate the dosage of transdermal fentanyl required in patients who are already receiving opioid analgesics, assess the 24-hr requirement of currently used opioid. Using the equianalgesic table in Appendix J, convert this to an equivalent amount of morphine/24 hr. Conversion to fentanyl transdermal may be accomplished by using the fentanyl conversion table (Appendix J). During dosage titration, additional short-acting opioids should be available for any breakthrough pain that may occur. Morphine 10 mg IM or 60 mg PO q 4 hr (60 mg/24 hr IM or 360 mg/24 hr PO) is considered to be approximately equivalent to transdermal fentanyl 100 mcg/hr. Transdermal patch lasts 72 hr in most patients. Some patients require a new patch every 48 hr.

Transdermal (Adults >60 yr, Debilitated, or Cachectic Patients): Initial dose should be 25 mcg/hr unless previous opioid use was >135 mg morphine PO/day (or other opioid equivalent).

Availability (generic available)

Transdermal systems: 12.5 mcg/hr, 25 mcg/hr, 50 mcg/hr, 75 mcg/hr, 100 mcg/hr.

NURSING IMPLICATIONS

Assessment

- Assess type, location, and intensity of pain before and 24 hr after application and periodically during therapy. Monitor pain frequently during initiation of therapy and dose changes to assess need for supplementary analgesics for breakthrough pain.
- Assess blood pressure, pulse, and respirations before and periodically during administration. If respiratory rate is <10/min, assess level of sedation. Physical stimulation may be sufficient to prevent significant hypoventilation. Dose may need to be decreased by 25–50%. Initial drowsiness will diminish with continued use.
- Prolonged use may lead to physical and psychological dependence and tolerance. This should not prevent patient from receiving adequate analgesia. Most patients who receive opioid analgesics for pain do not develop psychological dependence.
- Progressively higher doses may be required to relieve pain with long-term therapy. It may take up to 6 days after increasing doses to reach equilibrium, so patients should wear higher dose through 2 applications before increasing dose again.
- Assess bowel function routinely. Prevent constipation with increased intake of fluids and bulk, and laxatives to minimize constipating effects. Administer stimulant laxatives routinely if opioid use exceeds 2–3 days, unless contraindicated.
- ***Lab Test Considerations:*** May ↑ plasma amylase and lipase levels.
- ***Toxicity and Overdose:*** If an opioid antagonist is required to reverse respiratory depression or coma, naloxone (Narcan) is the antidote. Dilute the 0.4-mg ampule of naloxone in 10 ml of 0.9% NaCl and administer 0.5 ml (0.02 mg) by direct IV push every 2 min. For patients weighing <40 kg, dilute 0.1 mg of naloxone in 10 ml of 0.9% NaCl for a concentration of 10 mcg/ml and administer 0.5 mcg/kg every 2 min. Titrate dose to avoid withdrawal, seizures, and severe pain. Monitor patient closely; dose may need to be repeated or may need to be administered as an infusion because of long duration of action despite removal of patch.

Potential Nursing Diagnoses

Acute pain (Indications)
Risk for injury (Side Effects)

Implementation

- ***High Alert:*** Accidental overdose of opioid analgesics has resulted in fatalities. Before administering, clarify ambiguous orders; have second practitioner independently check original order and dose calculations.
- Duragesic-12 delivers 12.5 mcg/hr of fentanyl. Use supplemental doses of short-acting opioid analgesics to manage pain until relief is obtained with the transdermal system. Patients may continue to require supplemental opioids for breakthrough pain. If >100 mcg/hr is required, use multiple transdermal systems.
- Dose is titrated based on the patient's report of pain until adequate analgesia (50% reduction in patient's pain rating on numerical or visual analogue scale or patient reports satisfactory relief) is attained. Dose is determined by calculating the previous 24-hr analgesic requirement and converting to the equianalgesic morphine dose using Appendix J. The conversion ratio from morphine to transdermal fentanyl is conservative; 50% of patients may require a dose increase after initial application. Increase after 3 days based on required daily doses of supplemental analgesics. Increases should be based on ratio of 45 mg/24 hr of oral morphine to 12.5 mcg/hr increase in transdermal fentanyl dose.

- Coadministration with nonopioid analgesics may have additive analgesic effects and permit lower opioid doses.
- To convert to another opioid analgesic, remove transdermal fentanyl system and begin treatment with half the equianalgesic dose of the new analgesic in 12–18 hr.
- Medication should be discontinued gradually after long-term use to prevent withdrawal symptoms.
- **Transdermal:** Apply system to flat, nonirritated, and nonirradiated site such as chest, back, flank, or upper arm. If skin preparation is necessary, use clear water and clip, do not shave, hair. Allow skin to dry completely before application. Apply immediately after removing from package. Do not alter the system (i.e., cut) in any way before application. Remove liner from adhesive layer and press firmly in place with palm of hand for 30 sec, especially around the edges, to make sure contact is complete. For continued use, remove used system and fold so that adhesive edges are together. Flush system down toilet immediately on removal. Apply new system to a different site. Discard unused systems by removing from pouch and flushing down toilet.

Patient/Family Teaching

- Instruct patient in how and when to ask for pain medication.
- Instruct patient in correct method for application and disposal of transdermal system. Fatalities have occurred from children having access to improperly discarded patches. May be worn while bathing, showering, or swimming.
- May cause drowsiness or dizziness. Caution patient to call for assistance when ambulating or smoking and to avoid driving or other activities requiring alertness until response to medication is known.
- Advise patient to change positions slowly to minimize dizziness.
- Caution patient to avoid concurrent use of alcohol or other CNS depressants with this medication.
- Advise patient that fever, electric blankets, heating pads, saunas, hot tubs, and heated water beds increase the release of fentanyl from the patch.
- Advise patient that good oral hygiene, frequent mouth rinses, and sugarless gum or candy may decrease dry mouth.

Evaluation/Desired Outcomes

- Decrease in severity of pain without a significant alteration in level of consciousness, respiratory status, or blood pressure.

F

ferrous fumarate, See IRON SUPPLEMENTS.

ferrous gluconate, See IRON SUPPLEMENTS.

ferrous sulfate, See IRON SUPPLEMENTS.

fexofenadine

(fex-oh-**fen**-a-deen)
Allegra

Classification
Therapeutic: allergy, cold, and cough remedies, antihistamines

Pregnancy Category C

Indications

Relief of symptoms of seasonal allergic rhinitis. Management of chronic idiopathic urticaria.

Action

Antagonizes the effects of histamine at peripheral histamine–1 (H_1) receptors, including pruritus and urticaria. Also has a drying effect on the nasal mucosa. **Therapeutic Effects:** Decreased sneezing, rhinorrhea, itchy eyes, nose, and throat associated with seasonal allergies. Decreased urticaria.

Pharmacokinetics

Absorption: Rapidly absorbed after oral administration.
Distribution: Unknown.
Metabolism and Excretion: 80% excreted in urine, 11% excreted in feces.
Half-life: 14.4 hr (increased in renal impairment).

TIME/ACTION PROFILE (antihistaminic effect)

ROUTE	ONSET	PEAK	DURATION
PO	within 1 hr	2–3 hr	12–24 hr

Contraindications/Precautions

Contraindicated in: Hypersensitivity.

Use Cautiously in: Impaired renal function (increased dosing interval recommended); OB, Pedi: Pregnancy or lactation (safety not established).

Adverse Reactions/Side Effects

CNS: drowsiness, fatigue. **GI:** dyspepsia. **Endo:** dysmenorrhea.

Interactions

Drug-Drug: Magnesium- and **aluminum-containing antacids** ↓ absorption and may decrease effectiveness.

Drug-Food: Apple, **orange**, and **grapefruit juice** ↓ absorption and may decrease effectiveness.

Route/Dosage

PO (Adults and Children ≥12 yr): 60 mg twice daily, or 180 mg once daily.

PO (Children 2–11 yr): 30 mg twice daily.

PO (Children 6 months-2 yr): 15 mg twice daily.

Renal Impairment

PO (Adults): 60 mg once daily as a starting dose.

PO (Children 6–11 yr): 30 mg once daily as a starting dose.

Availability (generic available)

Tablets: 30 mg, 60 mg, 180 mg. **Cost:** *Generic*—30 mg $49.97/90, 60 mg $99.97/90, 180 mg $161.97/90. **Suspension (raspberry–cream):** 30 mg/5 mL in 30-ml and 300-ml bottles. **Cost:** $59.07/300 ml. ***In combination with:*** pseudoephedrine (Allegra-D). See Appendix B.

NURSING IMPLICATIONS

Assessment

- Assess allergy symptoms (rhinitis, conjunctivitis, hives) before and periodically during therapy.
- Assess lung sounds and character of bronchial secretions. Maintain fluid intake of 1500–2000 ml/day to decrease viscosity of secretions.
- ***Lab Test Considerations:*** Will cause false-negative reactions on allergy skin tests; discontinue 3 days before testing.

Potential Nursing Diagnoses

Ineffective airway clearance (Indications)
Risk for injury (Adverse Reactions)

Implementation

- **PO:** Administer with food or milk to decrease GI irritation. Capsules and tablets should be taken with water or milk, not juice.

Patient/Family Teaching

- Instruct patient to take medication as directed. Take missed doses as soon as remembered unless almost time for next dose.
- Inform patient that drug may cause drowsiness, although it is less likely to occur than with other antihistamines. Avoid driving or other activities requiring alertness until response to drug is known.
- Instruct patient to contact health care professional if symptoms persist.

Evaluation/Desired Outcomes

- Decrease in allergic symptoms.
- Decrease in urticaria.

filgrastim (fil-**gra**-stim)

Neupogen, G-CSF, granulocyte colony stimulating factor

Classification

Therapeutic: colony-stimulating factors

Pregnancy Category C

Indications

Prevention of febrile neutropenia and associated infection in patients who have received bone marrow–depressing antineoplastics for the treatment of nonmyeloid malignancies. Reduction of time for neutrophil recovery and duration of fever in patients undergoing induction and consolidation chemotherapy for acute myelogenous leukemia. Reduction of time to neutrophil recovery and sequelae of neutropenia in patients with nonmyeloid malignancies undergoing myeloablative chemotherapy followed by bone marrow transplantation. Mobilization of hematopoietic progenitor cells into peripheral blood for collection by leukapheresis. Management of severe chronic neutropenia. **Unlabeled uses:** Neutropenia associated with HIV infection.

Action

A glycoprotein, filgrastim binds to and stimulates immature neutrophils to divide and differentiate. Also activates mature neutrophils.
Therapeutic Effects: Decreased incidence of infection in patients who are neutropenic from chemotherapy or other causes. Improved harvest of progenitor cells for bone marrow transplantation.

Pharmacokinetics

Absorption: Well absorbed after subcut administration.
Distribution: Unknown.
Metabolism and Excretion: Unknown.
Half-life: 3.5 hr.

TIME/ACTION PROFILE

ROUTE	ONSET	PEAK	DURATION
IV, subcut	unknown	unknown	4 days†

†Return of neutrophil count to baseline

Contraindications/Precautions

Contraindicated in: Hypersensitivity to filgrastim or *Escherichia coli*–derived proteins.
Use Cautiously in: Malignancy with myeloid characteristics; Pre-existing cardiac disease; Pregnancy, lactation, or children (safety not established).

Adverse Reactions/Side Effects

Hemat: excessive leukocytosis. **Local:** pain, redness at subcut site. **MS:** medullary bone pain.

Interactions

Drug-Drug: Simultaneous use with **antineoplastics** may have adverse effects on rapidly proliferating neutrophils—avoid use for 24 hr before and 24 hr after chemotherapy. **Lithium** may potentiate the release of neutrophils; concurrent use should be undertaken cautiously.

Route/Dosage

After Myelosuppressive Chemotherapy

IV, Subcut (Adults): 5 mcg/kg/day as a single injection daily for up to 2 wk. Dosage may be increased by 5 mcg/kg during each cycle of chemotherapy, depending on blood counts.

After Bone Marrow Transplantation

IV, Subcut (Adults): 10 mcg/kg/day as a 4- or 24-hr IV infusion or as a continuous subcut infusion; initiate at least 24 hr after chemotherapy and at least 24 hr after bone marrow transplantation. Subsequent dosage is adjusted according to blood counts.

Peripheral Blood Progenitor Cell Collection and Therapy

Subcut (Adults): 10 mcg/kg/day as a bolus or continuous infusion for at least 4 days before first leukapheresis and continued until last leukapheresis; dosage modification suggested if WBC >100,000 cells/mm³.

Severe Chronic Neutropenia

Subcut (Adults): *Congenital neutropenia*—6 mcg/kg twice daily. *Idiopathic/cyclical neutropenia*—5 mcg/kg daily (decrease if ANC remains >10,000/mm³).

Availability

Injection: 300 mcg/ml in 1- and 1.6-ml vials.

NURSING IMPLICATIONS

Assessment

- Monitor heart rate, blood pressure, and respiratory status before and periodically during therapy.
- Assess bone pain throughout therapy. Pain is usually mild to moderate and controllable with nonopioid analgesics, but may require treatment with opioid analgesics, especially in patients receiving high-dose IV therapy.
- ***Lab Test Considerations:*** *After chemotherapy,* obtain a CBC with differential, including examination for the presence of blast cells, and platelet count before chemotherapy and twice weekly during therapy to avoid leukocytosis. Monitor ANC. A transient rise is seen 1–2 days after initiation of therapy, but therapy should not be discontinued until ANC >10,000/mm³.
- *After bone marrow transplant,* the daily dose is titrated by the neutrophil response. When the ANC is >1000/mm³ for 3 consecutive days, the dose should be reduced by 5 mcg/kg/day. If the ANC remains >1000/mm³ for 3 or more consecutive days, filgrastim is discontinued. If the ANC decreases to <1000/mm³, filgrastim should be resumed at 5 mcg/kg/day.
- *For chronic severe neutropenia,* monitor CBC with differential and platelet count twice weekly during initial 4 wk of therapy and during 2 wk after any dose adjustment.

- May cause ↓ platelet count and transient increases in uric acid, LDH, and alkaline phosphatase concentrations.

Potential Nursing Diagnoses
Risk for infection (Indications)
Acute pain (Side Effects)

Implementation
- Administer no earlier than 24 hr after cytotoxic chemotherapy, at least 24 hr after bone marrow infusion, and not during the 24 hr before administration of chemotherapy.
- Refrigerate; do not freeze. Do not shake. May warm to room temperature for up to 6 hr before injection. Discard if left at room temperature for >6 hr. Vial is for 1-time use only.
- **Subcut:** If dose requires >1 ml of solution, may be divided into 2 injection sites.
- May also be administered as a continuous subcut infusion over 24 hr after bone marrow transplantation.

IV Administration
- **Continuous Infusion:** ***Diluent:*** Dilute in D5W. Refrigerate; do not freeze. Do not shake. May warm to room temperature for up to 6 hr before injection. Vial is for 1-time use only. ***Concentration:*** Dilute to a final concentration of at least 15 mcg/ml. If the final concentration is <15 mcg/ml, human albumin in a concentration of 2 mg/ml must be added to D5W before filgrastim to prevent adsorption of the components of the drug delivery system. ***Rate:*** *After chemotherapy* dose is administered via infusion over 15–60 min.
- *After chemotherapy* dose may also be administered as a continuous infusion.
- *After bone marrow transplant,* dose should be administered as an infusion over 4 or 24 hr.
- **Y-Site Compatibility:** acyclovir, allopurinol, amikacin, aminophylline, ampicillin, ampicillin/sulbactam, aztreonam, bleomycin, bumetanide, buprenorphine, butorphanol, calcium gluconate, carboplatin, carmustine, cefazolin, cefotetan, ceftazidime, chlorpromazine, cimetidine, cisplatin, cyclophosphamide, cytarabine, dacarbazine, daunorubicin, dexamethasone, diphenhydramine, doxorubicin, doxycycline, droperidol, enalaprilat, famotidine, floxuridine, fluconazole, fludarabine, ganciclovir, granisetron, haloperidol, hydrocortisone, hydromorphone, idarubicin, ifosfamide, leucovorin calcium, lorazepam, mechlorethamine, melphalan, meperidine, mesna, methotrexate, metoclopramide, mitoxantrone, morphine, nalbuphine, ondansetron, potassium chloride, promethazine, ranitidine, sodium bicarbonate, streptozocin, ticarcillin/clavulanate, tobramycin, trimethoprim/sulfamethoxazole, vancomycin, vinblastine, vincristine, vinorelbine, zidovudine.
- **Y-Site Incompatibility:** amphotericin B, cefepime, cefotaxime, cefoxitin, ceftizoxime, ceftriaxone, cefuroxime, clindamycin, dactinomycin, etoposide, fluorouracil, furosemide, heparin, mannitol, methylprednisolone sodium succinate, metronidazole, mitomycin, piperacillin, prochlorperazine, thiotepa.

Patient/Family Teaching
- **Home Care Issues:** Instruct patient on correct technique and proper disposal for home administration. Caution patient not to reuse needle, vial, or syringe. Provide patient with a puncture-proof container for needle and syringe disposal.

Evaluation/Desired Outcomes
- Decreased incidence of infection in patients who receive bone marrow–depressing antineoplastics.
- Reduction of duration and sequelae of neutropenia after bone marrow transplantation.
- Reduction of the incidence and duration of sequelae of neutropenia in patients with severe chronic neutropenia.
- Improved harvest of progenitor cells for bone marrow transplantation.

finasteride (fi-nas-teer-ide)
Propecia, Proscar

Classification
Therapeutic: hair regrowth stimulants
Pharmacologic: androgen inhibitors

Pregnancy Category X

Indications
Benign prostatic hyperplasia (BPH); can be used with doxazosin. Androgenetic alopecia (male pattern baldness) in men only.

Action
Inhibits the enzyme 5-alpha-reductase, which is responsible for converting testosterone to its potent metabolite 5-alpha-dihydrotestosterone in prostate, liver, and skin; 5-alpha-dihydrotestosterone is partially responsible for prostatic

hyperplasia and hair loss. **Therapeutic Effects:** Reduced prostate size with associated decrease in urinary symptoms. Decreases hair loss; promotes hair regrowth.

Pharmacokinetics

Absorption: Well absorbed after oral administration (63%).
Distribution: Enters prostatic tissue and crosses the blood-brain barrier. Remainder of distribution not known.
Protein Binding: 90%.
Metabolism and Excretion: Mostly metabolized; 39% excreted in urine as metabolites; 57% excreted in feces.
Half-life: 6 hr (range 6–15 hr; slightly increased in patients >70 yr).

TIME/ACTION PROFILE (reduction in dihydrotestosterone levels†)

ROUTE	ONSET	PEAK	DURATION
PO	rapid	8 hr	2 wk

†Clinical effects as noted by urinary tract symptoms and hair regrowth may not be evident for several months and remain for 4 mo after discontinuation

Contraindications/Precautions

Contraindicated in: Hypersensitivity; Women.
Use Cautiously in: Patients with hepatic impairment or obstructive uropathy.

Adverse Reactions/Side Effects

GU: decreased libido, decreased volume of ejaculate, erectile dysfunction.

Interactions

Drug-Drug: None noted.

Route/Dosage

PO (Adults): *BPH*—5 mg once daily (Proscar); *androgenetic alopecia*—1 mg/day (Propecia).

Availability (generic available)

Tablets: 1 mg (Propecia), 5 mg (Proscar). **Cost:** *Propecia*—1 mg $177.97/90; *Generic*—5 mg $199.98/90.

NURSING IMPLICATIONS

Assessment

- Assess for symptoms of prostatic hyperplasia (urinary hesitancy, feeling of incomplete bladder emptying, interruption of urinary stream, impairment of size and force of urinary stream, terminal urinary dribbling, straining to start flow, dysuria, urgency) before and periodically during therapy.
- Digital rectal examinations should be performed before and periodically during therapy for BPH.
- ***Lab Test Considerations:*** Serum prostate-specific antigen (PSA) concentrations, which are used to screen for prostate cancer, may be evaluated before and periodically during therapy. Finasteride may cause a ↓ in serum PSA levels.

Potential Nursing Diagnoses

Impaired urinary elimination (Indications)

Implementation

- **PO:** Administer once daily with or without meals.

Patient/Family Teaching

- Instruct patient to take finasteride as directed, even if symptoms improve or are unchanged. At least 6–12 mo of therapy may be necessary to determine whether or not an individual will respond to finasteride.
- Inform patient that the volume of ejaculate may be decreased during therapy but that this will not interfere with normal sexual function. Sexual dysfunction side effects will diminish over time.
- Caution patient that finasteride poses a potential risk to a male fetus. Women who are pregnant or may become pregnant should avoid exposure to semen of a partner taking finasteride and should not handle crushed finasteride because of the potential for absorption.
- Emphasize the importance of periodic follow-up exams to determine whether a clinical response has occurred.

Evaluation/Desired Outcomes

- Decrease in urinary symptoms of benign prostatic hyperplasia.
- Hair regrowth in androgenetic alopecia. Evidence of hair growth usually requires 3 mo or longer. Continued use is recommended to sustain benefit. Withdrawal leads to reversal of effect within 12 mo.

flavocoxid (fla-vo-**cox**-id)
Limbrel

Classification
Therapeutic: nonopioid analgesics
Pharmacologic: flavanoids

Pregnancy Category UK

Indications
Dietary management of osteoarthritis; considered to be a medical food product.

Action
Anti-inflammatory and analgesic properties related to inhibition of prostaglandin synthesis by inhibiting cyclo-oxygenase (not COX-2 selective) and other mediators of inflammation. **Therapeutic Effects:** Decreased pain/inflammation associated with osteoarthritis, with improved mobility.

Pharmacokinetics
Absorption: Some intestinal conversion prior to absorption, remainder unknown.
Distribution: Unknown.
Metabolism and Excretion: Mostly metabolized by the liver.
Half-life: Unknown.

TIME/ACTION PROFILE (analgesic effect)

ROUTE	ONSET	PEAK	DURATION
PO	within 1–2 hr	unknown	12 hr

Contraindications/Precautions
Contraindicated in: Hypersensitivity; Pregnancy, lactation or children <18 yr.
Use Cautiously in: History of GI bleeding.

Adverse Reactions/Side Effects
CV: ↑ blood pressure, ↑ in varicose veins. **GI:** GI upset. **Derm:** psoriasis.

Interactions
Drug-Drug: None noted.

Route/Dosage
PO (Adults): 250 mg every 12 hr (up to 250 mg three times daily has been used).

Availability
Capsules: 250 mg.

NURSING IMPLICATIONS

Assessment
- Assess pain (note type, location, and intensity), range of motion, degree of swelling, and stiffness in affected joints before and periodically during therapy.

Potential Nursing Diagnoses
Chronic pain (Indications)

Implementation
- **PO:** Administer flavocoxid twice daily.

Patient/Family Teaching
- Instruct patient to take flavocoxid as directed. Do not increase does without consulting health care professional.

Evaluation/Desired Outcomes
- Decrease in pain and stiffness, and improved mobility in patients with osteoarthritis.

flecainide (**flek**-a-nide)
Tambocor

Classification
Therapeutic: antiarrhythmics (class IC)

Pregnancy Category C

Indications
Life-threatening ventricular arrhythmias, including ventricular tachycardia. Supraventricular tachyarrhythmias including: Paroxysmal supraventricular tachycardia (PSVT), Paroxysmal atrial fibrillation/flutter (PAF). **Unlabeled uses:** Single dose treatment of atrial fibrillation.

Action
Slows conduction in cardiac tissue by altering transport of ions across cell membranes. **Therapeutic Effects:** Suppression of arrhythmias.

Pharmacokinetics
Absorption: Well absorbed from the GI tract following oral administration.
Distribution: Widely distributed.
Metabolism and Excretion: Mostly metabolized by liver; 30% excreted unchanged by kidneys.
Half-life: 11–14 hr.

TIME/ACTION PROFILE (antiarrhythmic effects)

ROUTE	ONSET	PEAK	DURATION
PO	days	days–weeks	12 hr

Contraindications/Precautions
Contraindicated in: Hypersensitivity; Cardiogenic shock.
Use Cautiously in: CHF (dosage reduction may be required); Pre-existing sinus node dys-

function or 2nd- or 3rd-degree heart block (without a pacemaker); Renal impairment (dosage reduction required if CCr <35 ml/min); Pregnancy, lactation, or children (safety not established).

Adverse Reactions/Side Effects

CNS: dizziness, anxiety, fatigue, headache, mental depression. **EENT:** blurred vision, visual disturbances. **CV:** ARRHYTHMIAS, CHEST PAIN, CHF. **GI:** anorexia, constipation, drug-induced hepatitis, nausea, stomach pain, vomiting. **Derm:** rashes. **Neuro:** tremor.

Interactions

Drug-Drug: ↑ risk of arrhythmias with other **antiarrhythmics**, including **calcium channel blockers**. **Disopyramide**, **beta blockers**, or **verapamil** may have ↑ myocardial depressant effects; combination use should be undertaken cautiously. **Amiodarone** doubles serum flecainide levels (↓ flecainide dose by 50%). Increases serum **digoxin** levels by a small amount (15–25%). Concurrent **beta blocker** therapy may cause ↑ levels of beta blocker and flecainide. **Alkalinizing agents** promote reabsorption, ↑ blood levels, and may cause toxicity. **Acidifying agents** ↑ renal elimination and may ↓ effectiveness of flecainide (if urine pH <5).
Drug-Food: Foods that ↑ urine pH to >7 result in ↑ levels (strict **vegetarian diet**). **Foods or beverages that ↓ urine pH** to <5 ↑ renal elimination and may ↓ effectiveness of flecainide **(acidic juices)**.

Route/Dosage

Ventricular Tachycardia

PO (Adults): 100 mg q 12 hr initially, increased by 50 mg bid until response is obtained or maximum total daily dose of 400 mg is reached. Some patients may require q 8 hr dosing.

Renal Impairment

PO (Adults): *CCr <35 ml/min*—100 mg once a day or 50 mg q 12 hr initially; further dosing on the basis of frequent blood level monitoring.

PSVT/PAF

PO (Adults): 50 mg q 12 hr initially, increased by 50 mg bid until response is obtained or maximum total daily dose of 300 mg is reached. Some patients may require q 8 hr dosing.

Atrial Fibrillation (unlabeled)

PO (Adults): 200 mg or 300 mg single dose.

Availability (generic available)

Tablets: 50 mg, 100 mg, 150 mg.

NURSING IMPLICATIONS

Assessment

- Monitor ECG or Holter monitor prior to and periodically during therapy. May cause QRS widening, PR prolongation, and QT prolongation.
- Monitor blood pressure and pulse periodically during therapy.
- Monitor intake and output ratios and daily weight. Assess patient for signs of CHF (peripheral edema, rales/crackles, dyspnea, weight gain, jugular venous distention).
- ***Lab Test Considerations:*** Evaluate renal, pulmonary, and hepatic functions and CBC periodically on patients receiving long-term therapy. Flecainide should be discontinued if bone marrow depression occurs.
- May cause ↑ in serum alkaline phosphatase during prolonged therapy.
- ***Toxicity and Overdose:*** Therapeutic blood levels range from 0.2 to 1.0 mcg/ml. Monitor plasma trough levels frequently during dose adjustment in patients with severe renal or hepatic disease or in patients with CHF and moderate renal impairment.

Potential Nursing Diagnoses

Decreased cardiac output (Adverse Reactions)

Implementation

- Previous antiarrhythmic therapy (except lidocaine) should be withdrawn 2–4 half-lives before starting flecainide.
- Therapy should be initiated in a hospital setting to monitor for increase in arrhythmias.
- Dose adjustments should be at least 4 days apart because of the long half-life of flecainide.
- **PO:** May be administered with meals if GI irritation becomes a problem.

Patient/Family Teaching

- Instruct patient to take medication around the clock as directed at evenly spaced intervals, even if feeling better. Take missed doses as soon as remembered if within 6 hr; omit if remembered later. Gradual dosage reduction may be necessary.

- May cause dizziness or visual disturbances. Caution patient to avoid driving and other activities requiring alertness until response to medication is known.
- Advise patient to notify health care professional of medication regimen prior to treatment or surgery.
- Instruct patient to notify health care professional if chest pain, shortness of breath, or diaphoresis occurs.
- Advise patient to carry identification describing disease process and medication regimen at all times.
- Emphasize the importance of follow-up exams to monitor progress.

Evaluation/Desired Outcomes

- Decrease in frequency of life-threatening ventricular arrhythmias.
- Decrease in supraventricular tachyarrhythmias.

fluconazole (floo-**kon**-a-zole)

Diflucan

Classification

Therapeutic: antifungals (systemic)

Pregnancy Category C

Indications

PO, IV: Fungal infections caused by susceptible organisms, including: Oropharyngeal or esophageal candidiasis, Serious systemic candidal infections, Urinary tract infections, Peritonitis, Cryptococcal meningitis. Prevention of candidiasis in patients who have undergone bone marrow transplantation. **PO:** Single-dose oral treatment of vaginal candidiasis. **Unlabeled uses:** Prevention of recurrent vaginal yeast infections.

Action

Inhibits synthesis of fungal sterols, a necessary component of the cell membrane. **Therapeutic Effects:** Fungistatic action against susceptible organisms. May be fungicidal in higher concentrations. **Spectrum:** *Cryptococcus neoformans*, *Candida*, spp.

Pharmacokinetics

Absorption: Well absorbed after oral administration.

Distribution: Widely distributed, good penetration into CSF, saliva, sputum, vaginal fluid, skin, eye, and peritoneum. Excreted in breast milk.

Metabolism and Excretion: >80% excreted unchanged by the kidneys; <10% metabolized by the liver.

Half-life: Premature neonates: 46–74 hr; Children: 19–25 hr (PO) and 15–17 hr (IV); Adults: 30 hr (increased in renal impairment).

TIME/ACTION PROFILE (blood levels)

ROUTE	ONSET	PEAK	DURATION
PO	unknown	2–4 hr	24 hr
IV	rapid	end of infusion	24 hr

Contraindications/Precautions

Contraindicated in: Hypersensitivity to fluconazole or other azole antifungals; Concurrent use with pimozide.

Use Cautiously in: Renal impairment (dose reduction required if CCr <50 ml/min); Geri: Increased risk of adverse reactions (rash, vomiting, diarrhea, seizures); consider age-related decrease in renal function in determining dose; Underlying liver disease; OB, Pedi: Pregnancy, lactation, or children (safety not established).

Adverse Reactions/Side Effects

Incidence of adverse reactions is increased in HIV patients.

CNS: headache, dizziness, seizures. **GI:** HEPATOTOXICITY, abdominal discomfort, diarrhea, nausea, vomiting. **Derm:** exfoliative skin disorders including STEVENS-JOHNSON SYNDROME. **Endo:** hypokalemia, hypertriglyceridemia. **Misc:** allergic reactions, including ANAPHYLAXIS.

Interactions

Drug-Drug: ↑ activity of **warfarin**. **Rifampin**, **rifabutin**, and **isoniazid** ↓ levels. Fluconazole at doses >200 mg/day may inhibit the CYP3A4 enzyme system and effect the activity of drugs metabolized by this system. ↑ hypoglycemic effects of **tolbutamide**, **glyburide**, or **glipizide**. ↑ levels and risk of toxicity from **cyclosporine**, **rifabutin**, **tacrolimus**, **theophylline**, **zidovudine**, **alfentanil**, and **phenytoin**. ↑ levels and effects of **benzodiazepines**, **zolpidem**, **bispirone**, **nisoldipine**, **tricyclic antidepressants**, and **losartan**. May ↑ risk of bleeding with **warfarin**. May antagonize effects of **amphotericin B**.

Route/Dosage

Oropharyngeal Candidiasis

PO, IV (Adults): 200 mg initially, then 100 mg daily for at least 2 wk.

PO, IV (Children >14 days): 6 mg/kg initially, then 3 mg/kg/day for at least 2 wk.
PO, IV (Neonates <14 days, 30–36 weeks gestation): same dose as older children except frequency is q 48 hr; Premature neonates <29 weeks gestation: 5–6 mg/kg/dose q 48–72 hr.

Esophageal Candidiasis

PO, IV (Adults): 200 mg initially, then 100 mg once daily for at least 3 wk (up to 400 mg/day).
PO, IV (Children >14 days): 6 mg/kg initially, then 3–12 mg/kg/day for at least 3 wk.
PO, IV (Neonates <14 days, 30–36 weeks gestation): same dose as older children except frequency is q 48 hr; Premature neonates <29 weeks gestation: 5–6 mg/kg/dose q 48–72 hr.

Vaginal Candidiasis

PO (Adults): 150-mg single dose; prevention of recurrence (unlabeled)—150 mg daily for 3 days then weekly for 6 mo.

Systemic Candidiasis

PO, IV (Adults): 400 mg/day initially, then 200–800 mg/day for 28 days.
PO, IV (Children >14 days): 6–12 mg/kg/day for 28 days.
PO, IV (Neonates <14 days, 30–36 weeks gestation): same dose as older children except frequency is q 48 hr; Premature neonates <29 weeks gestation: 5–6 mg/kg/dose q 48–72 hr.

Cryptococcal Meningitis

PO, IV (Adults): *Treatment*—400 mg once daily until favorable clinical response, then 200–800 mg once daily for at least 10–12 wk after clearing of CSF; change to oral therapy as soon as possible. *Suppressive therapy*—200 mg once daily.
PO, IV (Children >14 days): 12 mg/kg/day initially, then 6–12 mg/kg/day for at least 10–12 wk after clearing of CSF; change to oral therapy as soon as possible. *Suppressive therapy*—6 mg/kg/day.
PO, IV (Neonates <14 days, 30–36 weeks gestation): same dose as older children except frequency is q 48 hr; Premature neonates <29 weeks gestation: 5–6 mg/kg/dose q 48–72 hr.

Prevention of Candidiasis after Bone Marrow Transplant

PO, IV (Adults): 400 mg once daily; begin several days before procedure if severe neutropenia is expected, and continue for 7 days after ANC >1000/mm^3.

PO, IV (Children >14 days): 10–12 mg/kg/day, not to exceed 600 mg/day.

Renal Impairment

PO, IV (Adults): *CCr 11–50 ml/min*—50% of the usual dose.

Availability (generic available)

Tablets: 50 mg, 100 mg, 150 mg, 200 mg. **Cost:** *Generic*—100 mg $109.99/30, 150 mg $167.19/12, 200 mg $247.57/30. **Oral suspension (orange flavor):** 10 mg/ml in 35-ml bottle, 40 mg/ml in 35-ml bottle. **Cost:** $25.99/35 ml. **Premixed infusion:** 2 mg/ml in 100- or 200-ml bottles/containers.

NURSING IMPLICATIONS

Assessment

- Assess infected area and monitor CSF cultures before and periodically during therapy.
- Specimens for culture should be taken before instituting therapy. Therapy may be started before results are obtained.
- ***Lab Test Considerations:*** Monitor BUN and serum creatinine before and periodically during therapy; patients with renal dysfunction will require dose adjustment.
- Monitor liver function tests before and periodically during therapy. May cause ↑ AST, ALT, serum alkaline phosphate, and bilirubin concentrations.

Potential Nursing Diagnoses

Risk for infection (Indications)

Implementation

- Do not confuse Diflucan (fluconazole) with Diprivan (propofol).
- **PO:** Shake oral suspension well before administration.

IV Administration

- **Intermittent Infusion:** ***Diluent:*** Premixed infusions are pre-diluted and ready to use. Do not unwrap until ready to use. Do not administer solution that is cloudy or has a precipitate. Check for leaks by squeezing inner bag. If leaks are found, discard container as unsterile. ***Concentration:*** 2 mg/ml. ***Rate:*** Infuse over 1–2 hr. Do not exceed a rate of 200 mg/hr. Pedi: For children receiving doses >6 mg/kg/day, give over 2 hours.
- **Y-Site Compatibility:** acyclovir, aldesleukin, amifostine, amikacin, aminophylline, amiodarone, anidulafungin, ampicillin/sul-

bactam, atropine, aztreonam, benztropine, bivalirudin, bumetanide, calcium chloride, caspofungin, cefazolin, cefepime, cefoxitin, ceftizoxime, cimetidine, cisatracurium, cyclosporine, daptomycin, dexamethasone sodium phosphate, dexmedetomidine, diltiazem, diphenhydramine, dobutamine, docetaxel, dopamine, doxorubicin liposome, doxycycline, droperidol, drotrecogin, enalaprilat, epinephrine, ertapenem, esmolol, etoposide phosphate, famotidine, fenoldopam, fentanyl, filgrastim, fludarabine, foscarnet, ganciclovir, gemcitabine, gentamicin, granisetron, heparin, hydrocortisone, hydromorphone, insulin, isoproterenol, immune glogulin, ketorolac, labetalol, lansoprazole, leucovorin, levofloxacin, lidocaine, linezolid, lorazepam, melphanan, magnesium sulfate, meperidine, meropenem, methylprednisolone sodium succinate, metoclopramide, metoprolol, metronidazole, midazolam, morphine, nafcillin, nitroglycerin, nitroprusside, norepinephrine, ondansetron, paclitaxel, palonosetron, pancuronium, pemetrexed, penicillin G potassium, phenytoin, phytonadione, piperacillin/tazobactam, potassium chloride, procainamide, prochlorperazine, promethazine, propofol, propranolol, quinapristin-dalfopristin, ranitidine, remifentanil, sargramostim, sodium bicarbonate, tacrolimus, teniposide, theophylline, thiotepa, ticarcillin/clavulanate, tigecycline, tirofiban, tobramycin, vancomycin, vasopressin, vecuronium, verapamil, vinorelbine, voriconazole, zidovudine.

- **Y-Site Incompatibility:** amphotericin B, amphotericin B cholesteryl sulfate, ampicillin, calcium gluconate, cefotaxime, ceftriaxone, cefuroxime, chloramphenicol, clindamycin, diazepam, digoxin, furosemide, haloperidol, hydroxyzine, imipenem/cilastatin, pantoprazole, pentamidine, trimethoprim/sulfamethoxazole.

Patient/Family Teaching

- Instruct patient to take medication as directed, even if feeling better. Doses should be taken at the same time each day. Take missed doses as soon as remembered, but not if almost time for next dose. Do not double doses.
- Instruct patient to notify health care professional if skin rash, abdominal pain, fever, or diarrhea becomes pronounced, if signs and symptoms of liver dysfunction (unusual fatigue, anorexia, nausea, vomiting, jaundice, dark urine, or pale stools) occur, if unusual bruising or bleeding occur, or if no improvement is seen within a few days of therapy.

Evaluation/Desired Outcomes

- Resolution of clinical and laboratory indications of fungal infections. Full course of therapy may require weeks or months of treatment after resolution of symptoms.
- Prevention of candidiasis in patients who have undergone bone marrow transplantation.
- Decrease in skin irritation and vaginal discomfort in patients with vaginal candidiasis. Diagnosis should be reconfirmed with smears or cultures before a second course of therapy to rule out other pathogens associated with vulvovaginitis. Recurrent vaginal infections may be a sign of systemic illness.

fludrocortisone

(floo-droe-**kor**-ti-sone)
Florinef

Classification
Therapeutic: hormones
Pharmacologic: corticosteroids (mineralocorticoid)

Pregnancy Category C

Indications

Sodium loss and hypotension associated with adrenocortical insufficiency (given with hydrocortisone or cortisone). Management of sodium loss due to congenital adrenogenital syndrome (congenital adrenal hyperplasia). **Unlabeled uses:** Idiopathic orthostatic hypotension (with increased sodium intake). Type IV renal tubular acidosis.

Action

Causes sodium reabsorption, hydrogen and potassium excretion, and water retention by its effects on the distal renal tubule. **Therapeutic Effects:** Maintenance of sodium balance and blood pressure in patients with adrenocortical insufficiency.

Pharmacokinetics

Absorption: Well absorbed following oral administration.
Distribution: Widely distributed; probably enters breast milk.
Protein Binding: High.

Metabolism and Excretion: Mostly metabolized by the liver.
Half-life: 3.5 hr.

TIME/ACTION PROFILE (mineralocorticoid activity)

ROUTE	ONSET	PEAK	DURATION
PO	unknown	unknown	1–2 days

Contraindications/Precautions

Contraindicated in: Hypersensitivity.
Use Cautiously in: CHF; Addison's disease (patients may have exaggerated response); Pregnancy, lactation, or children (safety not established).

Adverse Reactions/Side Effects

CNS: dizziness, headache. **CV:** CHF, arrhythmias, edema, hypertension. **GI:** anorexia, nausea. **Endo:** adrenal suppression, weight gain. **F and E:** hypokalemia, hypokalemic alkalosis. **MS:** arthralgia, muscular weakness, tendon contractures. **Neuro:** ascending paralysis. **Misc:** hypersensitivity reactions.

Interactions

Drug-Drug: Use with **thiazide** or **loop diuretics**, **piperacillin**, or **amphotericin B** may result in ↑ risk of hypokalemia. Hypokalemia may ↑ risk of **digoxin** toxicity. May produce prolonged neuromuscular blockade following the use of **nondepolarizing neuromuscular blocking agents**. **Phenobarbital** or **rifampin** may ↑ metabolism and ↓ effectiveness of fludrocortisone.
Drug-Food: Large amounts of **salt** or **sodium-containing foods** may cause excessive sodium retention and potassium loss.

Route/Dosage

PO (Adults): *Adrenocortical insufficiency*—100 mcg/day (range 100 mcg 3 times weekly—200 mcg daily). Doses as small as 50 mcg daily may be required by some patients. Use with 10–37.5 mg cortisone daily or 10–30 mg hydrocortisone daily. *Adrenogenital syndrome*—100–200 mcg/day. *Idiopathic hypotension*—50–200 mcg/day (unlabeled).
PO (Children): 50–100 mcg/day.

Availability (generic available)

Tablets: 100 mcg (0.1 mg).

NURSING IMPLICATIONS

Assessment

- Monitor blood pressure periodically during therapy. Report significant changes. Hypotension may indicate insufficient dose.
- Monitor for fluid retention (weigh daily, assess for edema, and auscultate lungs for rales/crackles).
- Monitor patients with Addison's disease closely and stop treatment if a significant increase in weight or blood pressure, edema, or cardiac enlargement occurs. Patients with Addison's disease are more sensitive to the action of fludrocortisone and may have an exaggerated response.
- ***Lab Test Considerations:*** Monitor serum electrolytes periodically during therapy. Fludrocortisone causes ↓ serum potassium levels.

Potential Nursing Diagnoses

Deficient fluid volume (Indications)
Excess fluid volume (Side Effects)

Implementation

- **PO:** Tablets are scored and may be broken if dose adjustment is necessary.

Patient/Family Teaching

- Instruct patient to take medication as directed. Take missed doses as soon as remembered but not just before next dose is due. Explain that lifelong therapy may be necessary and that abrupt discontinuation may lead to addisonian crisis. Patient should keep an adequate supply available at all times.
- Advise patient to follow dietary modification prescribed by health care professional. Instruct patient to follow a diet high in potassium (see Appendix L). Amount of sodium allowed in diet varies with pathophysiology.
- Instruct patient to inform health care professional if weight gain or edema, muscle weakness, cramps, nausea, anorexia, or dizziness occurs.
- Advise patient to carry identification at all times describing disease process and medication regimen.

Evaluation/Desired Outcomes

- Normalization of fluid and electrolyte balance without the development of hypokalemia or hypertension.

flumazenil (flu-maz-e-nil)

Anexate, Romazicon

Classification
Therapeutic: antidotes
Pharmacologic: benzodiazepines

Pregnancy Category C

Indications

Complete/partial reversal of effects of benzodiazepines used as general anesthetics, or during diagnostic or therapeutic procedures. Management of intentional or accidental overdose of benzodiazepines.

Action

Flumazenil is a benzodiazepine derivative that antagonizes the CNS depressant effects of benzodiazepine compounds. It has no effect on CNS depression from other causes, including opioids, alcohol, barbiturates, or general anesthetics. **Therapeutic Effects:** Reversal of benzodiazepine effects.

Pharmacokinetics

Absorption: IV administration results in complete bioavailability.
Distribution: Unknown.
Protein Binding: 50% primarily to albumin.
Metabolism and Excretion: Metabolism of flumazenil occurs primarily in the liver.
Half-life: Children: 20–75 min; Adults: 41–79 min.

TIME/ACTION PROFILE (reversal of benzodiazepine effects)

ROUTE	ONSET	PEAK	DURATION
IV	1–2 min	6–10 min	1–2 hr†

†Depends on dose/concentration of benzodiazepine and dose of flumazenil

Contraindications/Precautions

Contraindicated in: Hypersensitivity to flumazenil or benzodiazepines; Patients receiving benzodiazepines for life-threatening medical problems, including status epilepticus or increased intracranial pressure, should not be given flumazenil; Serious cyclic antidepressant overdosage.
Use Cautiously in: Mixed CNS depressant overdose (effects of other agents may emerge when benzodiazepine effect is removed); History of seizures (seizures are more likely to occur in patients who are experiencing sedative/hypnotic withdrawal, who have recently received repeated doses of benzodiazepines, or who have a previous history of seizure activity); Head injury (may increase intracranial pressure and risk of seizures); Severe hepatic impairment; Pregnancy, lactation (safety not established); Pedi: children <2 yr (safety not established).

Adverse Reactions/Side Effects

CNS: SEIZURES, dizziness, agitation, confusion, drowsiness, emotional lability, fatigue, headache, sleep disorders. **EENT:** abnormal hearing, abnormal vision, blurred vision. **CV:** arrhythmias, chest pain, hypertension. **GI:** nausea, vomiting, hiccups. **Derm:** flushing, sweating. **Local:** pain/injection-site reactions, phlebitis. **Neuro:** paresthesia. **Misc:** rigors, shivering.

Interactions

Drug-Drug: None significant.

Route/Dosage

Reversal of Conscious Sedation or General Anesthesia

IV (Adults): 0.2 mg. Additional doses may be given at 1-min intervals until desired results are obtained, up to a total dose of 1 mg. If resedation occurs, regimen may be repeated at 20-min intervals, not to exceed 3 mg/hr.
IV (Children): 0.01 mg/kg (up to 0.2 mg); if the desired level of consciousness is not obtained after waiting an additional 45 sec, further injections of 0.01 mg/kg (up to 0.2 mg) can be administered and repeated at 60-sec intervals when necessary (up to a maximum of 4 additional times) to a maximum total dose of 0.05 mg/kg or 1 mg, whichever is lower. The dose should be individualized based on the patient's response.

Suspected Benzodiazepine Overdose

IV (Adults): 0.2 mg. Additional 0.3 mg may be given 30 sec later. Further doses of 0.5 mg may be given at 1-min intervals, if necessary, to a total dose of 3 mg. Usual dose required is 1–3 mg. If resedation occurs, additional doses of 0.5 mg/min for 2 min may be given at 20-min intervals (given no more than 1 mg at a time, not to exceed 3 mg per hour).
IV (Children): *Unlabeled*—0.01 mg/kg (maximum dose 0.2 mg) with repeat doses every minute up to a cumulative dose of 1 mg. As an alternative to repeat doses, continuous infusions of 0.005–0.01 mg/kg/hr have been used.

Availability (generic available)

Injection: 0.1 mg/ml in 5- and 10-ml vials.

NURSING IMPLICATIONS

Assessment

- Assess level of consciousness and respiratory status before and during therapy. Observe patient for at least 2 hr after administration for the appearance of resedation. Hypoventilation may occur.
- **Overdose:** Attempt to determine time of ingestion and amount and type of benzodiazepine taken. Knowledge of agent ingested allows an estimate of duration of CNS depression.

Potential Nursing Diagnoses

Risk for injury (Indications)
Risk for poisoning (Indications)

Implementation

- Ensure that patient has a patent airway before administration of flumazenil.
- Observe IV site frequently for redness or irritation. Administer through a free-flowing IV infusion into a large vein to minimize pain at the injection site.
- Optimal emergence should be undertaken slowly to decrease undesirable effects including confusion, agitation, emotional lability, and perceptual distortion.
- Institute seizure precautions. Seizures are more likely to occur in patients who are experiencing sedative/hypnotic withdrawal, patients who have recently received repeated doses of benzodiazepines, or those who have a previous history of seizure activity. Seizures may be treated with benzodiazepines, barbiturates, or phenytoin. Larger than normal doses of benzodiazepines may be required.
- **Suspected Benzodiazepine Overdose:** If no effects are seen after administration of flumazenil, consider other causes of decreased level of consciousness (alcohol, barbiturates, opioid analgesics).

IV Administration

- **Direct IV:** ***Diluent:*** May be administered undiluted or diluted in syringe with D5W, 0.9% NaCl, or LR. Diluted solution should be discarded after 24 hr. ***Concentration:*** Up to 0.1 mg/ml. ***Rate:*** Administer each dose over 15–30 sec into free-flowing IV in a large vein. Do not exceed 0.2 mg/min in children or 0.5 mg/min in adults.

Patient/Family Teaching

- Flumazenil does not consistently reverse the amnestic effects of benzodiazepines. Provide patient and family with written instructions for postprocedure care. Inform family that patient may appear alert at the time of discharge but the sedative effects of the benzodiazepine may recur. Instruct patient to avoid driving or other activities requiring alertness for at least 24 hr after discharge.
- Instruct patient not to take any alcohol or nonprescription drugs for at least 18–24 hr after discharge.
- Resumption of usual activities should occur only when no residual effects of the benzodiazepine remain.

Evaluation/Desired Outcomes

- Improved level of consciousness.
- Decrease in respiratory depression caused by benzodiazepines.

flunisolide, See CORTICOSTEROIDS (INHALATION), CORTICOSTEROIDS (NASAL).

fluocinolone, See CORTICOSTEROIDS (TOPICAL/LOCAL).

fluocinonide, See CORTICOSTEROIDS (TOPICAL/LOCAL).

FLUOROQUINOLONES
(floor-oh-**kwin**-oh-lones)

ciprofloxacin†
(sip-roe-**flox**-a-sin)
✤Apo-Ciproflox, Cipro, Cipro XR, Proquin XR

gemifloxacin (gem-i-**flox**-a-sin)
Factive

levofloxacin (le-voe-**flox**-a-sin)
Levaquin, ✤Novo-Levofloxacin

moxifloxacin† (mox-i-**flox**-a-sin)
Avelox

norfloxacin† (nor-**flox**-a-sin)
✤Apo-Norfloxacin, ✤Co-Norfloxacin, Noroxin, ✤Novo-Norfloxacin,

✤PMS-Norfloxacin, ✤Riva-Norfloxacin

ofloxacin† (oh-**flox**-a-sin)
✤Apo-Ofloxacin, Floxin

Classification
Therapeutic: anti-infectives
Pharmacologic: fluoroquinolones

Pregnancy Category C

†See Appendix C for ophthalmic use

Indications

PO, IV: Treatment of the following bacterial infections: Urinary tract infections including cystitis and prostatitis (ciprofloxacin, levofloxacin, norfloxacin, ofloxacin), Gonorrhea (may not be considered first-line agents due to increasing resistance), Gynecologic infections (ciprofloxacin, norfloxacin, ofloxacin), Respiratory tract infections including acute sinusitis, acute exacerbations of chronic bronchitis, and pneumonia (not norfloxacin), Skin and skin structure infections (levofloxacin, moxifloxacin, ciprofloxacin, ofloxacin), Bone and joint infections (ciprofloxacin), Infectious diarrhea (ciprofloxacin), Intra-abdominal infections (ciprofloxacin, moxifloxacin). Febrile neutropenia (ciprofloxacin). Post-exposure treatment of inhalational anthrax (ciprofloxacin, levofloxacin).

Action

Inhibit bacterial DNA synthesis by inhibiting DNA gyrase. **Therapeutic Effects:** Death of susceptible bacteria. **Spectrum:** Broad activity includes many gram-positive pathogens: Staphylococci including methicillin-resistant *Staphylococcus aureus*, *Staphylococcus epidermidis*, *S. saprophyticus*, *Streptococcus pneumoniae*, *S. pyogenes*, and *Bacillus anthracis*. Gram-negative spectrum notable for activity against: *Escherichia coli*, *Klebsiella*, *Enterobacter*, *Salmonella*, *Shigella*, *Proteus*, *Providencia*, *Morganella morganii*, *Pseudomonas aeruginosa*, *Serratia*, *Haemophilus*, *Acinetobacter*, *Neisseria gonorrhoeae*, *Moraxella catarrhalis*, *Campylobacter*. Additional spectrum includes: *Chlamydia pneumoniae*, *Legionella pneumoniae*, and *Mycoplasma pneumoniae*.

Pharmacokinetics

Absorption: Well absorbed after oral administration (*ciprofloxacin*—70%; *moxifloxacin*—90%; *gemifloxacin*—71%; *levofloxacin*—99%; *norfloxacin*—30–40%; *ofloxacin*—98%.
Distribution: Widely distributed. High tissue and urinary levels are achieved. All agents appear to cross the placenta. *Ciprofloxacin,* and *ofloxacin* enter breast milk.
Metabolism and Excretion: *Ciprofloxacin*—15% metabolized by the liver, 40–50% excreted unchanged by the kidneys; *gemifloxacin*—Minimal metabolism, 61% excreted unchanged in feces, 36% excreted unchanged in urine; *levofloxacin*—87% excreted unchanged in urine, small amounts metabolized; *moxifloxacin*—mostly metabolized by the liver, 20% excreted unchanged in urine, 25% excreted unchanged in feces; *norfloxacin*—10% metabolized by the liver, 30% excreted unchanged by the kidneys, 30% excreted unchanged in feces; *ofloxacin*—70–80% excreted unchanged by the kidneys.
Half-life: *Ciprofloxacin*—4 hr; *gemifloxacin*—7 hr; *levofloxacin*—8 hr; *moxifloxacin*—12 hr; *norfloxacin*—6.5 hr; *ofloxacin*—5–7 hr (all are increased in renal impairment).

TIME/ACTION PROFILE (blood levels)

ROUTE	ONSET	PEAK	DURATION
Ciprofloxacin—PO	rapid	1–2 hr	12 hr
Ciprofloxacin—PO-ER	rapid	1–4 hr	24 hr
Ciprofloxacin—IV	rapid	end of infusion	12 hr
Gemifloxacin—PO	rapid	0.5—2 hr	24 hr
Levofloxacin—PO	rapid	1–2 hr	24 hr
Levofloxacin—IV	rapid	end of infusion	24 hr
Moxifloxacin—PO	within 1 hr	1–3 hr	24 hr
Moxifloxacin—IV	rapid	end of infusion	24 hr
Norfloxacin—PO	rapid	2–3 hr	12 hr
Ofloxacin—PO	rapid	1–2 hr	12 hr
Ofloxacin—IV	rapid	end of infusion	12 hr

Contraindications/Precautions

Contraindicated in: Hypersensitivity. Cross-sensitivity among agents within class may occur; **Gemifloxacin and moxifloxacin:** Concurrent use of amiodarone, disopyramide, erythromycin, pentamidine, phenothiazines, procainamide, quinidine, sotalol, or tricyclic antidepressants; Known QT prolongation or concurrent use of agents causing prolongation; OB: Pregnancy (do not use unless potential benefit outweighs potential fetal risk); Pedi: Use only for treatment of anthrax and complicated UTIs in children 1–17 yrs due to possible arthropathy.

Use Cautiously in: Known or suspected CNS disorder; Renal impairment (dosage reduction if CCr ≤50 ml/min for ciprofloxacin, levofloxacin, ofloxacin; ≤30 ml/min for norfloxacin; <40 ml/min for gemifloxacin); Cirrhosis (levofloxacin or norfloxacin); Geri: Geriatric patients (↑ risk of adverse reactions); Lactation: safety not established except for treatment of anthrax.

Adverse Reactions/Side Effects

CNS: SEIZURES, dizziness, headache, insomnia, acute psychoses, agitation, confusion, drowsiness. **CV:** *gemifloxacin, levofloxacin, moxifloxacin*—ARRHYTHMIAS, QT prolongation, vasodilation. **GI:** PSEUDOMEMBRANOUS COLITIS, diarrhea, nausea, abdominal pain, increased liver function tests (ciprofloxacin, moxifloxacin), vomiting. **GU:** vaginitis. **Derm:** photosensitivity, rash. **Endo:** hyperglycemia, hypoglycemia. **Local:** phlebitis at IV site. **MS:** tendinitis, tendon rupture. **Misc:** hypersensitivity reactions including ANAPHYLAXIS, STEVENS-JOHNSON SYNDROME.

Interactions

Drug-Drug: ↑ risk of QTc prolongation and life-threatening arrhythmias with concurrent use of gemifloxacin and moxifloxacin and **amiodarone**, **disopyramide**, **erythromycin**, **pentamidine**, **phenothiazines, procainamide**, **quinidine**, **sotalol**, and **tricyclic antidepressants** (concurrent use should be avoided). ↑ serum **theophylline** levels and may lead to toxicity. Administration with **magnesium and aluminum-containing antacids**, **iron salts**, **bismuth subsalicylate**, **sucralfate**, **didanosine**, and **zinc salts** ↓ absorption of fluoroquinolones. May ↑ the effects of **warfarin**. Ciprofloxacin may ↓ blood levels and effectiveness of **phenytoin**. Serum levels of fluoroquinolones may be ↓ by **antineoplastics**. **Cimetidine** may interfere with elimination of fluoroquinolones. Beneficial effects of ciprofloxacin may be antagonized by **nitrofurantoin**. **Probenecid** ↓ renal elimination of fluoroquinolones. May ↑ risk of nephrotoxicity from **cyclosporine**. Concurrent use of ciprofloxacin with **foscarnet** may ↑ risk of seizures. Concurrent therapy with **corticosteroids** may ↑ the risk of tendon rupture. May ↑ risk of hypoglycemia when used with **antidiabetic agents**.

Drug-Natural Products: Fennel ↓ the absorption of ciprofloxacin.

Drug-Food: Absorption is impaired by **concurrent tube feeding** (because of metal cations). Absorption is ↓ if taken with **dairy products** or **calcium-fortified juices.**

Route/Dosage

Ciprofloxacin

PO (Adults): *Most infections*—500–750 mg q 12 hr. *Complicated urinary tract infections*—500 mg q 12 hr for 7–14 days (immediate-release); *or* 1000 mg q 24 hr for 7–14 days (extended-release). *Uncomplicated urinary tract infections*—250 mg every 12 hr for 3 days (immediate-release) *or* 500 mg every 24 hr for 3 days (extended-release). *Gonorrhea*—250-mg single dose. *Inhalational anthrax (post exposure) or cutaneous anthrax*—500 mg every 12 hr for 60 days.

PO (Children 1–17 yr): *Complicated urinary tract infections*—10–15 mg/kg q 12 hr (not to exceed 750 mg/dose) for 10–21 days. *Inhalational anthrax (post-exposure) or cutaneous anthrax*—10–15 mg/kg q 12 hr (not to exceed 500 mg/dose) for 60 days.

IV (Adults): *Most infections*—400 mg q 12 hr. *Complicated urinary tract infections*—400 mg q 12 hr for 7–14 days. *Uncomplicated urinary tract infections*—200 mg q 12 hr for 7–14 days. *Inhalational anthrax (post exposure)*—400 mg q 12 hr for 60 days.

IV (Children 1–17 yr): *Inhalational anthrax (post exposure)*—10 mg/kg q 12 hr (not to exceed 400 mg/dose) for 60 days; *Complicated urinary tract infections*—6–10 mg/kg q 8 hr (not to exceed 400 mg/dose) for 10–21 days.

Renal Impairment

PO (Adults): *CCr 30–50 ml/min*—250–500 mg q 12 hr; *CCr 5–29 ml/min*—250–500 mg q 18 hr (immediate-release) *or* 500 mg q 24 hr (extended-release).

IV (Adults): *CCr 5–29 ml/min*—200–400 mg q 18–24 hr.

Gemifloxacin

PO (Adults): *Acute bacterial exacerbation of chronic bronchitis*—320 mg once daily for 5 days; *Community-acquired-pneumonia (CAP) caused by Klebsiella pneumoniae, Mo-*

F

raxella catarrhalis, and multidrug resistant strains of S. pneumonia—320 mg once daily for 7 days. *Community-acquired-pneumonia (CAP) caused by S. pneumonia, Haemophilus influenzae, Mycoplasma pneumoniae, or Chlamydia pneumonia, and multidrug resistant strains of S. pneumonia*—320 mg once daily for 5 days.

Renal Impairment

PO (Adults): *CCr ≤40 ml/min* 160 mg once daily for 5 days.

Levofloxacin

PO, IV (Adults): *Most infections*—250–750 mg q 24 hr; *inhalational anthrax (post-exposure)*—500 mg once daily for 60 days.

Renal Impairment

PO, IV (Adults): *Normal renal function dosing of 750 mg/day:—CCr 20–49 ml/min*—750 mg q 48 hr; *CCr 10–19 ml/min*—750 mg initially, then 500 mg q 48 hr; *Normal renal function dosing of 500 mg/day:—CCr 20–49 ml/min*—500 mg initially then 250 mg q 24 hr; *CCr 10–19 ml/min*—500 mg initially then 250 mg q 48 hr. *Normal renal function dosing of 250 mg/day:—CCr 10–19 ml/min*—250 mg q 48 hr.

Moxifloxacin

PO, IV (Adults): *Bacterial sinusitis*—400 mg once daily for 10 days. *Community-acquired pneumonia*—400 mg once daily for 7–14 days. *Acute bacterial exacerbation of chronic bronchitis*—400 mg once daily for 5 days. *Complicated intraabdominal infection*—400 mg once daily for 5–14 days. *Urethritis/cervicitis*—300 mg q 12 hr for 7 days. *Skin/skin structure infections*—400 mg/day for 7–21 days.

Norfloxacin

PO (Adults): *Uncomplicated urinary tract infections*—400 mg q 12 hr for 3–14 days. *Complicated urinary tract infections*—400 mg q 12 hr for 10–21 days. *Gonorrhea*—800-mg single dose. *Prostatitis*—400 mg q 12 hr for 4–6 wk.

Renal Impairment

PO (Adults): *CCr ≤30 ml/min*—400 mg once daily.

Ofloxacin

PO (Adults): *Most infections*—400 mg q 12 hr. *Prostatitis*—300 mg q 12 hr for 6 wk. *Uncomplicated urinary tract infections*—200 mg q 12 hr for 3–7 days. *Complicated urinary tract infections*—200 mg q 12 hr for 10 days. *Gonorrhea*—400-mg single dose.

Otic (Adults and Children ≥6 mo): *Otitis Externa 6 months to 13 yr*—5 drops instilled into affected ear once daily for 7 days; *Otitis Externa ≥13 yr*—10 drops instilled into affected ear once daily for 7 days. *Acute Otitis Media in pediatric patients 1–12 yr old with tympanostomy tubes*—5 drops instilled into the affected ear twice daily for 10 days. *Chronic Suppurative Otitis Media with perforated tympanic membranes in patients ≥12 yr*—10 drops instilled into the affected ear twice daily for 14 days.

Renal Impairment

PO, IV (Adults): *CCr 20–50 ml/min*—100% of the usual dose q 24 hr; *CCr <20 ml/min*—50% of the usual dose q 24 hr.

Availability

Ciprofloxacin

Tablets: 100 mg, 250 mg, 500 mg, 750 mg. **Extended-release tablets:** 500 mg, 1000 mg. **Oral suspension (strawberry flavor):** 250 mg/5 ml, 500 mg/5 ml. **Solution for injection:** 10 mg/ml. **Premixed infusion:** 200 mg/100 ml D5W, 400 mg/200 ml D5W. ***In combination with:*** hydrocortisone (Cipro HC) (see Appendix B).

Gemifloxacin

Tablets: 320 mg.

Levofloxacin

Tablets: 250 mg, 500 mg, 750 mg. **Cost:** 250 mg $199.98/20, 500 mg $231.98/20, 750 mg $429.99/20. **Oral solution:** 25 mg/ml. **Solution for injection:** 25 mg/ml. **Premixed infusion:** 250 mg/50 ml D5W, 500 mg/100 ml D5W, 750 mg/150 ml D5W.

Moxifloxacin

Tablets: 400 mg. **Cost:** $160.21/14. **Premixed infusion:** 400 mg/250 ml 0.8% NaCl.

Norfloxacin

Tablets: 400 mg.

Ofloxacin

Tablets: 200 mg, 300 mg, 400 mg. **Cost:** *Generic*—200 mg $77.13/20, 300 mg $91.42/20, 400 mg $83.33/20. **Otic solution:** 0.3% in 5- and 10-ml dropper bottles and 0.25 ml single-dispensing containers. **Cost:** *Generic*—$55.99/5 ml, $92.99/10 ml.

NURSING IMPLICATIONS

Assessment

- Assess for infection (vital signs; appearance of wound, sputum, urine, and stool; WBC; urinalysis; frequency and urgency of urination; cloudy or foul-smelling urine) prior to and during therapy.
- Obtain specimens for culture and sensitivity before initiating therapy. First dose may be given before receiving results.
- Observe for signs and symptoms of anaphylaxis (rash, pruritus, laryngeal edema, wheezing). Discontinue drug and notify physician or other health care professional immediately if these problems occur. Keep epinephrine, an antihistamine, and resuscitation equipment close by in case of an anaphylactic reaction. Patients taking *gemifloxacin* who are at greater risk for rash are those receiving gemifloxacin for >7 days, <40 yrs of age, females, and postmenopausal females receiving hormone replacement therapy.
- ***Lab Test Considerations:*** May cause ↑ serum AST, ALT, LDH, bilirubin, and alkaline phosphatase.
- May also cause ↑ or ↓ serum glucose.
- Moxifloxacin may cause hyperglycemia, hyperlipidemia, and altered prothrombin time. It may also cause ↑ WBC; ↑ serum calcium, chloride, albumin, and globulin; and ↓ glucose, hemoglobin, RBCs, neutrophils, eosinophils, and basophils.
- Monitor prothrombin time closely in patients receiving fluoroquinolones and warfarin; may enhance the anticoagulant effects of warfarin.

Potential Nursing Diagnoses

Risk for infection (Patient/Family Teaching)

Implementation

- Do confuse norfloxacin with Norflex (orphenadrine).
- **PO:** Administer *norfloxacin* and *ofloxacin* on an empty stomach 1 hr before or 2 hr after meals, with a full glass of water. *Moxifloxacin, levofloxacin,* and *gemifloxacin* may be administered without regard to meals. Should be taken at least 2 hr (3 hr for gemifloxacin, 4 hr for moxifloxacin) before or 2 hr (8 hr for moxifloxacin) after antacids or other products containing calcium, iron, zinc, magnesium, or aluminum.
- If gastric irritation occurs, ciprofloxacin may be administered with meals.
- Ciprofloxacin 5% and 10% oral suspension should not be administered through a feeding tube (may ↓ absorption). Shake solution for 15 seconds prior to administration. Do not chew microcapsules in solution.
- *Gemifloxacin* and *ciprofloxacin extended-release tablets* should be swallowed whole; do not crush, break, or chew.

Ciprofloxacin

IV Administration

- **Intermittent Infusion: *Diluent:*** Dilute with 0.9% NaCl or D5W. Stable for 14 days at refrigerated or room temperature. ***Concentration:*** 1–2 mg/ml. ***Rate:*** Administer over 60 min into a large vein to minimize venous irritation.
- **Y-Site Compatibility:** amifostine, amiodarone, anidulafungin, aztreonam, bivalirudin, calcium gluconate, ceftazidime, cisatracurium, dexmedetomidine, digoxin, diltiazem, diphenhydramine, dobutamine, docetaxel, dopamine, doxorubicin liposome, etoposide, fenoldopam, gemcitabine, gentamicin, granisetron, lidocaine, linezolid, lorazepam, LR, metoclopramide, midazolam, midodrine, milrinone, piperacillin, potassium acetate, potassium chloride, promethazine, quinupristin-dalfopristin, ranitidine, remifentanil, 0.9% NaCL, tacrolimus, teniposide, thiotepa, tobramycin, verapamil.
- **Y-Site Incompatibility:** Manufacturer recommends temporarily discontinuing other solutions when administering ciprofloxacin, aminophylline, ampicillin/sulbactam, azithromycin, cefepime, dexamethasone, drotrecogin, furosemide, heparin, hydrocortisone, lansoprazole, methylprednisolone, pemetrexed, phenytoin, potassium phosphates, propofol, sodium phosphates, warfarin.

Levofloxacin

IV Administration

- **Intermittent Infusion: *Diluent:*** Dilute with 0.9% NaCl, D5W, dextrose/saline combinations, 5% sodium bicarbonate, Plasmalyte 56, or sodium lactate. Also available in premixed bottles and flexible containers with D5W, which need no further dilution. Discard unused solution. Diluted solution is stable for 72 hr at room temperature and 14 days if refrigerated. ***Concentration:*** 5 mg/ml. ***Rate:*** Administer by infusion over at least 60 min for 250 mg or 500 mg doses and over 90 min for 750 mg dose. Avoid rapid bolus injection to prevent hypotension.

- **Y-Site Compatibility:** amikacin, aminophylline, ampicillin, bivalirudin, caffeine citrate, cefotaxime, cimetidine, clindamycin, dexamethasone, dexmedetomidine, dobutamine, dopamine, epinephrine, fenoldopam, fentanyl, gentamicin, isoproterenol, lidocaine, linezolid, lorazepam, metoclopramide, morphine, oxacillin, pancuronium, penicillin G, phenobarbital, phenylephrine, sodium bicarbonate, vancomycin.
- **Y-Site Incompatibility:** acyclovir, alprostadil, azithromycin, drotrecogin, furosemide, heparin, indomethacin, lansoprazole, nitroglycerin, nitroprusside, propofol.
- **Additive Compatibility:** linezolid.

Moxifloxacin

IV Administration

- **Intermittent Infusion:** ***Diluent:*** Premixed bags are diluted in sodium chloride 0.8% and should not be further diluted. Use transfer set whose piercing pin does not require excessive force; insert with a gentle twisting motion until pin is firmly seated. ***Concentration:*** 1.6 mg/ml. ***Rate:*** Administer over 60 min. Avoid rapid or bolus infusion.
- **Solution Compatibility:** 0.9% NaCl, D5W, D10W, LR.
- **Y-Site Incompatibility:** Temporarily discontinue administration of other solutions during moxifloxacin.

Patient/Family Teaching

- Instruct patient to take medication as directed at evenly spaced times and to finish drug completely, even if feeling better. Take missed doses as soon as possible, unless almost time for next dose. Do not double doses. Advise patient that sharing of this medication may be dangerous.
- Advise patients to notify health care professional immediately if they are taking theophylline.
- Encourage patient to maintain a fluid intake of at least 1500–2000 ml/day to prevent crystalluria.
- Advise patient that antacids or medications containing iron or zinc will decrease absorption. *Ciprofloxacin, levofloxacin, norfloxacin,* and *ofloxacin* should be taken at least 2 hr before (3 hr for *gemifloxacin*, 4 hr for *moxifloxacin*) or 2 hr after (8 hr for *moxifloxacin*) these products.
- May cause dizziness and drowsiness. Caution patient to avoid driving or other activities requiring alertness until response to medication is known.
- Advise patient to notify health care professional of any personal or family history of QTc prolongation or proarrhythmic conditions such as recent hypokalemia, significant bradycardia, or recent myocardial ischemia. Patients with this history should not receive fluoroquinolones.
- Caution patient to use sunscreen and protective clothing to prevent phototoxicity reactions during and for 5 days after therapy. Notify health care professional if a sunburn-like reaction or skin eruption occurs.
- Instruct patients being treated for gonorrhea that partners also must be treated.
- Instruct patient to consult health care professional before taking any other Rx, OTC, or herbal products.
- Advise patient to report signs of superinfection (furry overgrowth on the tongue, vaginal itching or discharge, loose or foul-smelling stools).
- Instruct patient to notify health care professional if fever and diarrhea develop, especially if stool contains blood, pus, or mucus. Advise patient not to treat diarrhea without consulting health care professional.
- Instruct patient to notify health care professional immediately if rash, jaundice, signs of hypersensitivity, or tendon (shoulder, hand, Achilles, and other) pain or inflammation occur. Increased risk in >65 yrs old, taking corticosteroids concurrently, and taking ciprofloxacin, ofloxacin, and levofloxacin. Therapy should be discontinued.

Evaluation/Desired Outcomes

- Resolution of the signs and symptoms of infection. Time for complete resolution depends on organism and site of infection.
- Post exposure treatment of inhalational anthrax or cutaneous anthrax (ciprofloxacin and levofloxacin).

HIGH ALERT

fluorouracil

(flure-oh-**yoor**-a-sill)
Adrucil, Efudex, Fluoroplex, 5-FU

Classification
Therapeutic: antineoplastics
Pharmacologic: antimetabolites

Pregnancy Category D

Indications

IV: Used alone and in combination with other modalities (surgery, radiation therapy, other antineoplastics) in the treatment of: Colon cancer, Breast cancer, Rectal cancer, Gastric cancer, Pancreatic carcinoma. **Topical:** Management of multiple actinic (solar) keratoses and superficial basal cell carcinomas.

Action

Inhibits DNA and RNA synthesis by preventing thymidine production (cell-cycle S-phase–specific). **Therapeutic Effects:** Death of rapidly replicating cells, particularly malignant ones.

Pharmacokinetics

Absorption: Minimal absorption (5–10%) after topical application.
Distribution: Widely distributed; concentrates and persists in tumors.
Metabolism and Excretion: Converted to an active metabolite; undergoes hepatic metabolism with small amounts excreted unchanged in urine.
Half-life: 20 hr.

TIME/ACTION PROFILE (IV = effects on blood counts, Top = dermatologic effects)

ROUTE	ONSET	PEAK	DURATION
IV	1–9 days	9–21 days (nadir)	30 days
Top	2–3 days	2–6 wk	1–2 mo

Contraindications/Precautions

Contraindicated in: Hypersensitivity; Pregnancy or lactation.
Use Cautiously in: Infections; Depressed bone marrow reserve; Other chronic debilitating illnesses; Obese patients, patients with edema or ascites (dose should be based on ideal body weight).

Adverse Reactions/Side Effects

More likely to occur with systemic use than with topical use.
CNS: acute cerebellar dysfunction. **GI:** diarrhea, nausea, stomatitis, vomiting. **Derm:** alopecia, maculopapular rash, local inflammatory reactions (topical only), melanosis of nails, nail loss, palmar-plantar erythrodysesthesia, phototoxicity. **Endo:** sterility. **Hemat:** anemia, leukopenia, thrombocytopenia. **Local:** thrombophlebitis. **Misc:** fever.

Interactions

Drug-Drug: Combination chemotherapy with **irinotecan** may produce unacceptable toxicity (dehydration, neutropenia, sepsis). Additive bone marrow depression with other **bone marrow depressants**, including other **antineoplastics** and **radiation therapy**. May decrease antibody response to **live-virus vaccines** and increase risk of adverse reactions.

Route/Dosage

Doses may vary greatly, depending on tumor, patient condition, and protocol used.

Advanced Colorectal Cancer

IV (Adults): 370 mg/m² preceded by leucovorin *or* 425 mg/m² preceded by leucovorin daily for 5 days. May be repeated q 4–5 wk.

Other Tumors

IV (Adults): *Initial dose*—12 mg/kg/day for 4 days, then 1 day of rest, then 6 mg/kg every other day for 4–5 doses *or* 7–12 mg/kg/day for 4 days followed by 3-day rest, then 7–10 mg/kg q 3–4 days for 3 doses. *Maintenance*—7–12 mg/kg q 7–10 days *or* 300–500 mg/m²/day for 4–5 days, repeated monthly (no single daily dose should exceed 800 mg). **Poor-Risk Patients:** 3–6 mg/kg/day on days 1–3, 3 mg/kg/day on days 5, 7, 9 (not to exceed 400 mg/dose). Doses of 370–425 mg/m²/day for 5 days have been used in combination with leucovorin.

Actinic (Solar) Keratoses/Superficial Basal Cell Carcinomas

Topical (Adults): *Actinic/solar keratoses*—1% solution or cream 1–2 times daily to lesions on head, neck, or chest; 2–5% solution or cream may be needed for hands. *Superficial basal cell carcinomas*—5% solution or cream twice daily for 3–6 wk (up to 12 wk).

Availability

Injection: 50 mg/ml in 10-ml ampules or 10-, 20-, and 100-ml vials. **Cream:** 1%, 5%. **Solution:** 1%, 2%, 5%.

NURSING IMPLICATIONS

Assessment

- Monitor vital signs before and frequently during therapy.
- Assess mucous membranes, number and consistency of stools, and frequency of vomiting. Assess for signs of infection (fever, chills, sore throat, cough, hoarseness, pain in lower back or side, difficult or painful urination). Assess for bleeding (bleeding gums; bruising; petechiae; and guaiac test stools, urine, and emesis). Avoid IM injections and taking rectal temperatures. Apply pressure to venipuncture sites for 10 min. Notify physician if symptoms of toxicity (stomatitis or esophagopharyngitis, uncontrollable vomiting, diarrhea, GI bleeding, myocardial ischemia, leukocyte count <3500/mm^3, platelet count <100,000/mm^3, or hemorrhage from any site) occur; drug will need to be discontinued. May be reinitiated at a lower dose when side effects have subsided
- Assess IV site frequently for inflammation or infiltration. Patient should notify nurse if pain or irritation at injection site occurs. May cause thrombophlebitis. If extravasation occurs, infusion must be stopped and restarted in another vein to avoid damage to subcut tissue. Report immediately. Standard treatment includes application of ice compresses.
- Assess skin for palmar-plantar erythrodysesthesia (tingling of hands and feet followed by pain, erythema, and swelling) throughout therapy.
- Monitor intake and output, appetite, and nutritional intake. GI effects usually occur on 4th day of therapy. Adjusting diet as tolerated may help maintain fluid and electrolyte balance and nutritional status
- Monitor patient for cerebellar dysfunction (weakness, ataxia, dizziness). This may persist after discontinuation of therapy.
- **Topical:** Inspect involved skin before and throughout therapy.
- ***Lab Test Considerations:*** May cause ↓ in plasma albumin.
- Monitor hepatic (AST, ALT, LDH, and serum bilirubin), renal, and hematologic (hematocrit, hemoglobin, leukocyte, platelet count) functions before and periodically throughout therapy. Monitor CBC daily during IV therapy. Report WBC of <3500/mm^3 or platelets <100,000/mm^3 immediately; they are criteria for discontinuation. Nadir of leukopenia usually occurs in 9–14 days, with recovery by day 30. May also cause thrombocytopenia.
- May cause ↑ in urine excretion of 5-hydroxyindoleacetic acid (5-HIAA).

Potential Nursing Diagnoses

Risk for infection (Side Effects)
Imbalanced nutrition: less than body requirements (Side Effects)

Implementation

- ***High Alert:*** Fatalities have occurred with incorrect administration of chemotherapeutic agents. Before administering, clarify all ambiguous orders; double-check single, daily, and course-of-therapy dose limits; have second practitioner independently double-check original order, calculations and infusion pump settings. The number 5 in 5-fluorouracil is part of the drug name and does not refer to the dosage.
- Solution should be prepared in a biologic cabinet. Wear gloves, gown, and mask while handling IV medication. Discard IV equipment in specially designated containers.

IV Administration

- **Direct IV:** ***Diluent:*** May be administered undiluted. ***Concentration:*** 50 mg/ml. ***Rate:*** Rapid IV push administration (over 1–2 min) is most effective, but there is a more rapid onset of toxicity.
- **Intermittent Infusion:** ***Diluent:*** May be diluted with D5W or 0.9% NaCl. Use plastic IV tubing and IV bags to maintain greater stability of medication. Solution is stable for 24 hr at room temperature; do not refrigerate. Solution is colorless to faint yellow. Discard highly discolored or cloudy solution. If crystals form, dissolve by warming solution to 140°F, shaking vigorously, and cooling to body temperature. ***Concentration:*** Up to 50 mg/ml. ***Rate:*** Onset of toxicity is greatly delayed by administering an infusion over 2–8 hr.
- **Syringe Compatibility:** bleomycin, cisplatin, cyclophosphamide, furosemide, heparin, leucovorin, methotrexate, metoclopramide, mitomycin, vinblastine, vincristine.
- **Syringe Incompatibility:** droperidol, epirubicin.

- **Y-Site Compatibility:** allopurinol, amifostine, aztreonam, bleomycin, cefepime, cisplatin, cyclophosphamide, doxorubicin, doxorubicin liposome, etoposide, fludarabine, furosemide, gemcitabine, granisetron, heparin, hydrocortisone, leucovorin, linezolid, mannitol, melphalan, methotrexate, metoclopramide, mitomycin, paclitaxel, pemetrexed, piperacillin/tazobactam, potassium chloride, propofol, sargramostim, teniposide, thiotepa, vinblastine, vincristine, vitamin B complex with C.
- **Y-Site Incompatibility:** aldesleukin, amphotericin B cholesteryl sulfate complex, droperidol, filgrastim, lansoprazole, topotecan, vinorelbine.
- **Additive Compatibility:** bleomycin, cyclophosphamide, D5/LR, etoposide, floxuridine, ifosfamide, methotrexate, mitoxantrone, vincristine.
- **Additive Incompatibility:** carboplatin, cisplatin, cytarabine, diazepam, doxorubicin, epirubicin, fentanyl, leucovorin, metoclopramide, morphine.
- **Topical:** Consult health care professional before administering topical preparations to determine which skin preparation regimen should be followed. Tight occlusive dressings are not advised because of irritation to surrounding healthy tissue. A loose gauze dressing for cosmetic purposes is usually preferred. Wear gloves when applying medication. Do not use metallic applicator.

Patient/Family Teaching

- Instruct patient to notify health care professional if fever; chills; sore throat; signs of infection; yellowing of skin or eyes; abdominal pain; joint or flank pain; swelling of feet or legs; bleeding gums; bruising; petechiae; or blood in urine, stool, or emesis occurs. Caution patient to avoid crowds and persons with known infections. Instruct patient to use soft toothbrush and electric razor. Patients should be cautioned not to drink alcoholic beverages or take products containing aspirin or NSAIDs.
- Advise patient to rinse mouth with clear water after eating and drinking and to avoid flossing to minimize stomatitis. Viscous lidocaine may be used if mouth pain interferes with eating. Stomatitis pain may require treatment with opioid analgesics.
- Discuss with patient the possibility of hair loss. Explore methods of coping.
- Review with patient the need for contraception during therapy.
- Caution patient to use sunscreen and protective clothing to prevent phototoxicity reactions.
- Instruct patient not to receive any vaccinations without advice of health care professional.
- Emphasize the importance of routine follow-up lab tests to monitor progress and to check for side effects.
- **Topical:** Instruct patient in correct application of solution or cream. Emphasize importance of avoiding the eyes; caution should also be used when applying medication near mouth and nose. If patient uses clean finger to self-administer, emphasize importance of washing hands thoroughly after application. Explain that erythema, scaling, and blistering with pruritus and burning sensation are expected. Therapy is discontinued when erosion, ulceration, and necrosis occur in 2–6 wk (10–12 wk for basal cell carcinomas). Skin heals 4–8 wk later.

Evaluation/Desired Outcomes

- Tumor regression.
- Removal of solar keratoses or superficial basal cell skin cancers.

fluoxetine (floo-ox-uh-teen)
Prozac, Prozac Weekly, Sarafem

Classification
Therapeutic: antidepressants
Pharmacologic: selective serotonin reuptake inhibitors (SSRIs)

Pregnancy Category B

Indications

Various forms of depression. OCD. Bulimia nervosa. Panic disorder. **Sarafem:** Management of premenstrual dysphoric disorder (PMDD). **Unlabeled uses:** Anorexia nervosa: ADHD, Diabetic neuropathy, Fibromyalgia, Obesity, Raynaud's phenomenon, Social anxiety disorder (social phobia), Post-traumatic stress disorder (PTSD).

F

Action
Selectively inhibits the reuptake of serotonin in the CNS. **Therapeutic Effects:** Antidepressant action. Decreased behaviors associated with: panic disorder, bulimia. Decreased mood alterations associated with PMDD.

Pharmacokinetics
Absorption: Well absorbed after oral administration.
Distribution: Crosses the blood-brain barrier.
Protein Binding: 94.5%.
Metabolism and Excretion: Converted by the liver to norfluoxetine, another antidepressant compound; fluoxetine and norfluoxetine are mostly metabolized by the liver; 12% excreted by kidneys as unchanged fluoxetine, 7% as unchanged norfluoxetine.
Half-life: 1–3 days (norfluoxetine 5–7 days).

TIME/ACTION PROFILE (antidepressant effect)

ROUTE	ONSET	PEAK	DURATION
PO	1–4 wk	unknown	2 wk

Contraindications/Precautions
Contraindicated in: Hypersensitivity; Concurrent use or use within 14 days of discontinuing MAO inhibitors (fluoxetine should be discontinued 5 weeks before MAO therapy is initiated).
Use Cautiously in: Severe hepatic or renal impairment (lower/less frequent dose may be necessary); History of seizures; Debilitated patients (↑ risk of seizures); Diabetes mellitus; Patients with concurrent chronic illness, or multiple drug therapy (dose adjustments may be necessary); Patients with impaired hepatic function (lower doses/increased dosing interval may be necessary); May ↑ risk of suicide attempt/ideation especially during early treatment or dose adjustment; OB: Use during third trimester may result in neonatal serotonin syndrome requiring prolonged hospitalization, respiratory and nutritional support. May cause sedation in infant; Lactation: May cause sedation in infant; discontinue drug or bottle-feed; Pedi: Risk of suicide ideation or attempt may be greater in children or adolescents (safe use in children <8 yr not established); Geri: Appears on Beers list. Geriatric patients are at increased risk for excessive CNS stimulation, sleep disturbances, and agitation.

Adverse Reactions/Side Effects
CNS: SEIZURES, anxiety, drowsiness, headache, insomnia, nervousness, abnormal dreams, dizziness, fatigue, hypomania, mania, weakness. **EENT:** stuffy nose, visual disturbances. **Resp:** cough. **CV:** chest pain, palpitations. **GI:** diarrhea, abdominal pain, abnormal taste, anorexia, constipation, dry mouth, dyspepsia, nausea, vomiting, weight loss. **GU:** sexual dysfunction, urinary frequency. **Derm:** excessive sweating, pruritus, erythema nodusum, flushing, rashes. **Endo:** dysmenorrhea. **MS:** arthralgia, back pain, myalgia. **Neuro:** tremor. **Misc:** allergic reactions, fever, flu-like syndrome, hot flashes, sensitivity reaction.

Interactions
Drug-Drug: Discontinue use of **MAO inhibitors** for 14 days before fluoxetine therapy; combined therapy may result in confusion, agitation, seizures, hypertension, and hyperpyrexia (serotonin syndrome). Fluoxetine should be discontinued for at least 5 wk before MAO inhibitor therapy is initiated. Inhibits the activity of cytochrome P450 2D6 enzyme in the liver and ↑ effects of drugs metabolized by this enzyme system. **Medications that inhibit the P450 enzyme system** (including **ritonavir**, **saquinavir**, and **efavirenz**) may ↑ risk of developing the serotonin syndrome). For concurrent use with **ritonavir** ↓ fluoxetine dose by 70%; if initiating fluoxetine, start with 10 mg/day dose. ↓ metabolism and ↑ effects of **alprazolam** (decrease alprazolam dose by 50%). ↑ CNS depression with **alcohol**, **antihistamines**, other **antidepressants**, **opioid analgesics**, or **sedative/hypnotics**. ↑ risk of side effects and adverse reactions with other **antidepressants**, **tryptophan**, **risperidone**, or **phenothiazines**. May ↑ effectiveness/risk of toxicity from **carbamazepine**, **clozapine**, **digoxin**, **haloperidol**, **phenytoin**, **lithium**, or **warfarin**. May ↓ the effects of **buspirone**. **Cyproheptadine** may decrease or reverse effects of fluoxetine. May ↑ sensitivity to **adrenergics** and increase the risk of serotonin syndrome. May alter the activity of other **drugs that are highly bound to plasma proteins**.
Drug-Natural Products: ↑ risk of serotonin syndrome with **St. John's wort** and **SAMe.**

Route/Dosage
PO (Adults): *Depression, OCD*—20 mg/day in the morning. After several weeks, may increase by 20 mg/day at weekly intervals. Doses greater than 20 mg/day should be given in 2 di-

vided doses, in the morning and at noon (not to exceed 80 mg/day). Patients who have been stabilized on the 20 mg/day dose may be switched over to delayed-release capsules (Prozac Weekly) at dose of 90 mg weekly, initiated 7 days after the last 20 mg dose. *Panic disorder*—10 mg/day initially, may increase after one week to 20 mg/day (usual dose is 20 mg, but may be increased as needed/tolerated up to 60 mg/day). *Bulimia nervosa*—60 mg/day (may need to titrate up to dosage over several days). *PMDD*—20 mg/day (not to exceed 80 mg/day) *or* 20 mg/day starting 14 days prior to expected onset on menses, continued through first full day of menstruation, repeated with each cycle.

PO (Geriatric Patients): *Depression*—10 mg/day in the morning initially, may be increased (not to exceed 60 mg/day).

PO (Children 7–17 yr): *adolescents and higher weight children*— 10 mg/day may be increased after 2 wk to 20 mg/day; additional increases may be made after several more weeks (range 20–60 mg/day); *lower-weight children*—10 mg/day initially, may be increased after several more weeks (range 20–30 mg/day).

Availability (generic available)

Tablets: 10 mg, 20 mg. **Cost:** *Generic*—10 mg $47.98/90, 20 mg $62.97/90. **Capsules:** 10 mg, 20 mg, 40 mg. **Cost:** *Generic*—10 mg $48.97/90, 20 mg $26.99/90, 40 mg $119.97/90. **Delayed-release capsules (Prozac Weekly):** 90 mg. **Cost:** $110.99/4. **Oral solution (mint flavor):** 20 mg/5 ml. **Cost:** *Generic*—$72.98/120 ml. ***In combination with:*** olanzapine (Symbyax; see Appendix B).

NURSING IMPLICATIONS

Assessment

- Monitor mood changes. Inform health care professional if patient demonstrates significant increase in anxiety, nervousness, or insomnia.
- Assess for suicidal tendencies, especially during early therapy. Restrict amount of drug available to patient
- Monitor appetite and nutritional intake. Weigh weekly. Notify health care professional of continued weight loss. Adjust diet as tolerated to support nutritional status
- Assess patient for sensitivity reaction (urticaria, fever, arthralgia, edema, carpal tunnel syndrome, rash, hives, lymphadenopathy, respiratory distress) and notify health care professional if present; symptoms usually resolve by stopping fluoxetine but may require administration of antihistamines or corticosteroids.
- Assess for sexual side effects (erectile dysfunction; decreased libido).
- **OCD:** Assess patient for frequency of obsessive-compulsive behaviors. Note degree to which these thoughts and behaviors interfere with daily functioning.
- **Bulimia Nervosa:** Assess frequency of binge eating and vomiting during therapy.
- **PMDD:** Monitor patient's mood prior to and periodically during therapy.
- ***Lab Test Considerations:*** Monitor CBC and differential periodically during therapy. Notify physician or other health care professional if leukopenia, anemia, thrombocytopenia, or increased bleeding time occurs.
- Proteinuria and mild ↑ in AST may occur during sensitivity reactions.
- May cause ↑ in serum alkaline phosphatase, ALT, BUN, creatine phosphokinase; hypouricemia, hypocalcemia, hypoglycemia or hyperglycemia, and hyponatremia.

Potential Nursing Diagnoses

Ineffective coping (Indications)
Risk for injury (Side Effects)
Sexual dysfunction (Side Effects)

Implementation

- Do not confuse Sarafem (fluoxetine) with Serophene (clomiphene).
- **PO:** Administer as a single dose in the morning. Some patients may require increased amounts, in divided doses, with a 2nd dose at noon.
- May be administered with food to minimize GI irritation.

Patient/Family Teaching

- Instruct patient to take fluoxetine as directed. If a dose is missed, omit and return to regular schedule. Do not double doses or discontinue without consulting health care professional; discontinuation may cause anxiety, insomnia, nervousness.
- May cause drowsiness, dizziness, impaired judgment, and blurred vision. Caution patient

to avoid driving and other activities requiring alertness until response to the drug is known.
- Advise patient to avoid alcohol or other CNS depressant drugs during therapy and to consult health care professional before taking other medications or natural/herbal products with fluoxetine.
- Caution patient to change positions slowly to minimize dizziness.
- Inform patient that frequent mouth rinses, good oral hygiene, and sugarless gum or candy may minimize dry mouth. If dry mouth persists for more than 2 wk, consult health care professional regarding use of saliva substitute.
- Instruct female patients to inform health care professional if pregnancy is planned or suspected.
- Caution patient to wear protective clothing and use sunscreen to prevent photosensitivity reactions.
- Inform patient that medication may cause decreased libido.
- Advise patient to notify health care professional if symptoms of sensitivity reaction occur or if headache, nausea, anorexia, anxiety, or insomnia persists.
- Emphasize the importance of follow-up exams to monitor progress. Encourage patient participation in psychotherapy to improve coping skills.
- May be augmented with benzodiazepine to treat jitteriness or anxiety.
- Refer patient/family to local support group.

Evaluation/Desired Outcomes
- Increased sense of well-being.
- Renewed interest in surroundings. May require 1–4 wk of therapy to obtain antidepressant effects.
- Decrease in obsessive-compulsive behaviors.
- Decrease in binge eating and vomiting in patients with bulimia nervosa.
- Decreased incidence frequency of panic attacks.
- Decreased mood alterations associated with PMDD.

fluphenazine (floo-**fen**-a-zeen)
✤Apo-Fluphenazine, ✤Modecate Concentrate, ✤PMS-Fluphenazine, Prolixin, Prolixin Decanoate

Classification
Therapeutic: antipsychotics
Pharmacologic: phenothiazines

Pregnancy Category C

Indications
Acute and chronic psychoses.

Action
Alters the effects of dopamine in the CNS. Has anticholinergic and alpha-adrenergic blocking activity. **Therapeutic Effects:** Diminished signs and symptoms of psychoses.

Pharmacokinetics
Absorption: Well absorbed after PO/IM administration. Decanoate salt in sesame oil has delayed onset and prolonged action because of delayed release from oil vehicle and subsequent delayed release from fatty tissues.
Distribution: Widely distributed. Crosses the blood-brain barrier. Crosses the placenta; enters breast milk.
Protein Binding: ≥90%.
Metabolism and Excretion: Highly metabolized by the liver; undergo enterohepatic recirculation.
Half-life: *Fluphenazine hydrochloride*—33 hr; *fluphenazine decanoate*—6.8–9.6 days.

TIME/ACTION PROFILE (antipsychotic activity)

ROUTE	ONSET	PEAK	DURATION
PO hydrochloride	1 hr	unknown	6–8 hr
IM decanoate	24–72 hr	48–96 hr	≥4 wk

Contraindications/Precautions
Contraindicated in: Hypersensitivity; Cross-sensitivity with other phenothiazines may exist; Subcortical brain damage; Severe CNS depression; Coma; Bone marrow depression; Liver disease; Hypersensitivity to sesame oil (decanoate salt); Some products contain alcohol or tartrazine and should be avoided in patients with known intolerance; Concurrent use of drugs that prolong the QT interval; Pedi: Safety not established in children <6 months.
Use Cautiously in: Cardiovascular disease; Parkinson's disease; Angle-closure glaucoma; Myasthenia gravis; Prostatic hypertrophy; Seizure disorders; OB, Lactation: Enters breast milk, not recommended; Geri: Initial dosage re-

duction may be necessary in geriatric or debilitated patients.

Adverse Reactions/Side Effects

CNS: NEUROLEPTIC MALIGNANT SYNDROME, extrapyramidal reactions, sedation, tardive dyskinesia. **EENT:** blurred vision, dry eyes. **CV:** hypertension, hypotension, tachycardia. **GI:** anorexia, constipation, drug-induced hepatitis, dry mouth, ileus, nausea, weight gain. **GU:** urinary retention. **Derm:** photosensitivity, pigment changes, rashes. **Endo:** galactorrhea. **Hemat:** AGRANULOCYTOSIS, leukopenia, thrombocytopenia. **Misc:** allergic reactions.

Interactions

Drug-Drug: Concurrent use with drugs that prolong the QT interval, including **antiarrhythmics**, **pimozide**, **erythromycin**, **clarithromycin**, **fluoroquinolones**, **methadone**, and **tricyclic antidepressants** may ↑ the risk for arrhythmias; concurrent use should be avoided. Additive hypotension with **antihypertensives**. Additive CNS depression with other **CNS depressants**, including **alcohol**, **antidepressants**, **antihistamines**, **opioids**, **sedative/hypnotics**, or **general anesthetics**. **Phenobarbital** may increase metabolism and decrease effectiveness of fluphenazine. May ↑ the risk of **lithium** toxicity. **Aluminum-containing antacids** may decrease oral absorption of fluphenazine. May decrease anti-Parkinson activity of **levodopa** and **bromocriptine**. May decrease the vasopressor response to **epinephrine** and **norepinephrine**. **Beta-blockers**, **chlorpromazine**, **chloroquine**, **delavirdine**, **fluoxetine**, **paroxetine**, **quinidine**, **quinine**, **ritonavir**, and **ropinirole** may ↑ the effects of fluphenazine. Increased risk of anticholinergic effects with other **agents having anticholinergic properties**, including **antihistamines**, **tricyclic antidepressants**, **disopyramide**, or **quinidine**. **Metoclopramide** may ↑ the risk of extrapyramidal reactions.

Route/Dosage

Fluphenazine Decanoate

IM (Adults): 12.5–25 mg initially; may be repeated q 3 wk. Dosage may be slowly increased as needed (not to exceed 100 mg/dose).

Fluphenazine Hydrochloride

PO (Adults): 0.5–10 mg/day in divided doses q 6–8 hr (maximum dose = 40 mg/day).

PO (Geriatric Patients or Debilitated Patients): 1–2.5 mg/day initially; increase dose every 4–7 days by 1–2.5 mg/day as needed (max dose = 20 mg/day).

IM (Adults): 1.25–2.5 mg q 6–8 hr.

Availability (generic available)

Fluphenazine decanoate injection: 25 mg/ml, ✤100 mg/ml. **Fluphenazine hydrochloride tablets:** 1 mg, 2.5 mg, 5 mg[Rx], 10 mg. **Fluphenazine hydrochloride elixir (orange flavor):** 2.5 mg/5 ml. **Fluphenazine hydrochloride concentrate:** 5 mg/ml. **Fluphenazine hydrochloride injection:** 2.5 mg/ml.

NURSING IMPLICATIONS

Assessment

- Assess patient's mental status (orientation, mood, behavior) before and periodically during therapy.
- Monitor blood pressure (sitting, standing, lying), ECG, pulse, and respiratory rate before and frequently during the period of dose adjustment. May cause Q-wave and T-wave changes in ECG.
- Observe patient carefully when administering oral medication to ensure that medication is actually taken and not hoarded.
- Assess fluid intake and bowel function. Increased bulk and fluids in the diet help minimize constipation.
- Monitor patient for onset of akathisia (restlessness or desire to keep moving) and extrapyramidal side effects (*parkinsonian*—difficulty speaking or swallowing, loss of balance control, pill rolling, mask-like face, shuffling gait, rigidity, tremors; *dystonic*—muscle spasms, twisting motions, twitching, inability to move eyes, weakness of arms or legs) every 2 mo during therapy and 8–12 wk after therapy has been discontinued. Reduction in dose or discontinuation of medication may be necessary. Benztropine or diphenhydramine may be used to control these symptoms.
- Monitor for tardive dyskinesia (uncontrolled rhythmic movement of mouth, face, and extremities; lip smacking or puckering; puffing of cheeks; uncontrolled chewing; rapid or

worm-like movements of tongue). Report immediately; may be irreversible.
- Monitor for development of neuroleptic malignant syndrome (fever, respiratory distress, tachycardia, seizures, diaphoresis, arrhythmias, hypertension or hypotension, pallor, tiredness, severe muscle stiffness, loss of bladder control). Report immediately.
- ***Lab Test Considerations:*** Evaluate CBC, liver function tests, and ocular examinations periodically during therapy. May cause ↓ hematocrit, hemoglobin, leukocytes, granulocytes, and platelets. May cause ↑ bilirubin, AST, ALT, and alkaline phosphatase. Agranulocytosis may occur after 4–10 wk of therapy with recovery 1–2 wk after discontinuation. May recur if medication is restarted. Liver function abnormalities may require discontinuation of therapy.

Potential Nursing Diagnoses
Disturbed thought process (Indications)
Noncompliance (Patient/Family Teaching)

Implementation
- Slight yellow to amber color does not alter potency.
- To prevent contact dermatitis, avoid getting liquid preparations on hands and wash hands thoroughly if spillage occurs.
- Injectable forms must be drawn up with a dry syringe and dry 21-gauge needle to prevent clouding of the solution.
- **PO:** Dilute concentrate just before administration in 120–240 ml of water, milk, carbonated beverage, soup, or tomato or fruit juice. Do not mix with beverages containing caffeine (cola, coffee), tannics (tea), or pectinates (apple juice).
- **Subcut:** Fluphenazine decanoate is dissolved in sesame oil for long duration of action. It may be administered subcut or IM. 12.5 mg of fluphenazine decanoate given every 3 wk is approximately equivalent to 10 mg/day orally of fluphenazine hydrochloride.
- **IM:** IM dose of fluphenazine hydrochloride is usually 30–50% of oral dose. Because fluphenazine hydrochloride has a shorter duration of action, it is used initially to determine the patient's response to the drug and to treat the acutely agitated patient.
- Administer deep IM, using a dry syringe and 21-gauge needle, into dorsal gluteal site. Instruct patient to remain recumbent for 30 min to prevent hypotension.
- **Syringe Compatibility:** Fluphenazine hydrocholride is compatible in syringe with benztropine, diphenhydramine, hydroxyzine.

Patient/Family Teaching
- Advise patient to take medication exactly as directed and not to skip doses or double up on missed doses. If a dose is missed, take within 1 hr or skip dose and return to regular schedule if taking more than 1 dose/day; take as soon as possible unless almost time for next dose if taking 1 dose/day. Abrupt withdrawal may lead to gastritis, nausea, vomiting, dizziness, headache, tachycardia, and insomnia.
- Inform patient of possibility of extrapyramidal symptoms and tardive dyskinesia. Caution patient to report these symptoms immediately to health care professional.
- Advise patient to change positions slowly to minimize orthostatic hypotension.
- Medication may cause drowsiness. Caution patient to avoid driving or other activities requiring alertness until response to medication is known.
- Caution patient to avoid taking alcohol or other CNS depressants concurrently with this medication.
- Advise patient to use sunscreen and protective clothing when exposed to the sun. Exposed surfaces may develop a blue-gray pigmentation, which may fade after discontinuation of the medication. Extremes of temperature should also be avoided because this drug impairs body temperature regulation.
- Advise patient that good oral hygiene, frequent rinsing of mouth with water, and sugarless gum or candy may help relieve dry mouth. Health care professional should be notified if dry mouth persists beyond 2 wk.
- Instruct patient to notify health care professional promptly if sore throat, fever, unusual bleeding or bruising, rash, weakness, tremors, visual disturbances, dark-colored urine, or clay-colored stools occur.
- Advise patient to notify health care professional of medication regimen before treatment or surgery.
- Emphasize the importance of routine follow-up exams, including ocular exams, with long-term therapy and continued participation in psychotherapy.

Evaluation/Desired Outcomes
- Decrease in excitable, paranoic, or withdrawn behavior.

flurandrenolide, See CORTICOSTEROIDS (TOPICAL/LOCAL).

flurazepam (flur-az-e-pam)

♣Apo-Flurazepam, Dalmane, ♣Novoflupam, ♣Somnol

Classification
Therapeutic: sedative/hypnotics
Pharmacologic: benzodiazepines

Schedule IV

Pregnancy Category UK

Indications
Short-term management of insomnia (<4 wk).

Action
Depresses the CNS, probably by potentiating GABA, an inhibitory neurotransmitter. **Therapeutic Effects:** Relief of insomnia.

Pharmacokinetics
Absorption: Well absorbed after oral administration.
Distribution: Widely distributed; crosses blood-brain barrier. Probably crosses the placenta and enters breast milk. Accumulation of drug occurs with chronic dosing.
Protein Binding: 97% (one of the active metabolites).
Metabolism and Excretion: Metabolized by the liver; some metabolites have hypnotic activity.
Half-life: 2.3 hr (half-life of active metabolite may be 30–200 hr).

TIME/ACTION PROFILE (hypnotic activity)

ROUTE	ONSET	PEAK	DURATION
PO	15–45 min	0.5–1 hr	7–8 hr

Contraindications/Precautions
Contraindicated in: Impaired repiratory function; Impaired repiratory function; Sleep apnea; Hypersensitivity; Cross-sensitivity with other benzodiazepines may exist; Pre-existing CNS depression; Severe uncontrolled pain; Angle-closure glaucoma; OB: Infants may experience withdrawal effects; Lactation: Enters breast milk; discontinue or bottle-feed.
Use Cautiously in: Hepatic dysfunction (dosage reduction may be necessary); History of suicide attempt or drug dependence; Geri: Appears on Beers list and is associated with increased falls risk in geriatric patients; Debilitated patients (initial dose reduction may be necessary); Pedi: Safety not established in children <15 yr.

Adverse Reactions/Side Effects
CNS: abnormal thinking, behavior changes, confusion, daytime drowsiness, decreased concentration, dizziness, hallucinations, headache, lethargy, mental depression, paradoxical excitation, sleep—driving. **EENT:** blurred vision. **GI:** constipation, diarrhea, nausea, vomiting. **Derm:** rashes. **Neuro:** ataxia. **Misc:** physical dependence, psychological dependence, tolerance.

Interactions
Drug-Drug: Concurrent use with **alcohol**, **antidepressants**, **antihistamines**, and **opioids** may result in additive CNS depression. **Cimetidine**, **hormonal contraceptives**, **disulfiram**, **fluoxetine**, **isoniazid**, **ketoconazole**, **metoprolol**, **propoxyphene**, **propranolol**, or **valproic acid** may ↓ metabolism of flurazepam, enhancing its actions. May ↓ efficacy of **levodopa**. **Rifampin** or **barbiturates** may ↑ metabolism and decrease ↓ effectiveness of flurazepam. Sedative effects may be ↓ by **theophylline**.
Drug-Natural Products: Concomitant use of **kava kava**, **valerian**, **chamomile**, or **hops** can ↑ CNS depression.

Route/Dosage
PO (Adults): 15–30 mg at bedtime.
PO (Geriatric Patients or Debilitated Patients): 15 mg initially, may be increased.

Availability (generic available)
Capsules: 15 mg, 30 mg. **Tablets:** 15 mg, 30 mg.

NURSING IMPLICATIONS

Assessment
- Assess sleep patterns before and periodically throughout therapy.
- Assess mental status (orientation, mood, behavior) and potential for abuse prior to administering medication.
- Prolonged use may lead to psychological or physical dependence. Restrict amount of

♣ = Canadian drug name.
*CAPITALS indicates life-threatening; underlines indicate most frequent.

drug available to patient, especially if patient is depressed, suicidal, or has a history of addiction.
- Geri: Assess fall risk and institute prevention strategies.

Potential Nursing Diagnoses
Insomnia (Indications)
Ineffective coping (Indications)
Sleep deprivation (Indications)
Risk for falls (Side Effects)
Acute confusion (Side Effects)
Risk for injury (Side Effects)

Implementation
- Do not confuse flurazepam with temazepam.
- Supervise ambulation and transfer of patients after administration. Remove cigarettes. Two side rails should be raised and call bell within reach at all times.
- When discontinuing, taper to decrease chance of withdrawal effects (may take months in some patients).
- **PO:** Capsules may be opened and mixed with food or fluids for patients having difficulty swallowing.

Patient/Family Teaching
- Advise patient to take medication exactly as directed.
- Teach sleep hygiene techniques (dark room, quiet, bedtime ritual, limit daytime napping, avoidance of nictotine and caffeine).
- Maximum hypnotic properties are apparent 2–3 nights after initiating therapy and may last 1–2 nights after therapy is discontinued.
- Medication may cause daytime drowsiness. Caution patient to avoid driving and other activities requiring alertness until response to medication is known.
- Caution patient to avoid taking alcohol or other CNS depressants concurrently with this medication.
- Refer for psychotherapy if ineffective coping is basis for sleep pattern disturbance.
- OB: Instruct patient to contact health care professional immediately if pregnancy is planned or suspected.
- Geri: Caution patient or family to institute fall prevention strategies at home.
- Instruct patient to contact health care professional immediately if pregnancy is planned or suspected.

Evaluation/Desired Outcomes
- Improvement in sleep patterns (decreased number of night time awakenings, improved sleep onset, and increased total sleep time).

fluticasone, See CORTICOSTEROIDS (INHALATION), CORTICOSTEROIDS (NASAL), CORTICOSTEROIDS (TOPICAL/LOCAL).

fluvastatin, See HMG-CoA REDUCTASE INHIBITORS (statins).

fluvoxamine
(floo-**voks**-a-meen)
Luvox

Classification
Therapeutic: antidepressants, antiobsessive agents
Pharmacologic: selective serotonin reuptake inhibitors (SSRIs)

Pregnancy Category C

Indications
Obsessive-compulsive disorder (OCD). **Unlabeled uses:** Depression. Generalized anxiety disorder (GAD). Post-traumatic stress disorder (PSTD).

Action
Inhibits the reuptake of serotonin in the CNS. **Therapeutic Effects:** Decrease in obsessive-compulsive behaviors.

Pharmacokinetics
Absorption: 53% absorbed after oral administration.
Distribution: Excreted in breast milk; enters the CNS. Remainder of distribution not known.
Metabolism and Excretion: Eliminated mostly by the kidneys.
Half-life: 13.6–15.6 hr.

TIME/ACTION PROFILE (improvement on obsessive-compulsive behaviors)

ROUTE	ONSET	PEAK	DURATION
PO	within 2–3 wk	several mo	unknown

Contraindications/Precautions
Contraindicated in: Hypersensitivity to fluvoxamine or other SSRIs; Concurrent use or use within 14 days of discontinuing MAOI, alosetron, pimozide, thioridazine, or tizanidine.
Use Cautiously in: Impaired hepatic function; OB: Neonates exposed to SSRI in third trimester

may develop drug discontinuation syndrome including respiratory distress, feeding difficulty, and irritability; Lactation: Discontinue drug or bottle-feed; Pedi: Safety not established in children <8 yr; Geri: Geriatric patients may have increased sensitivity; recommend lower initial dose and slower dosage titration.

Adverse Reactions/Side Effects

CNS: sedation, dizziness, drowsiness, headache, insomnia, nervousness, weakness, agitation, anxiety, apathy, emotional lability, manic reactions, mental depression, psychotic reactions, syncope. **EENT:** sinusitis. **Resp:** cough, dyspnea. **CV:** edema, hypertension, palpitations, postural hypotension, tachycardia, vasodilation. **GI:** constipation, diarrhea, dry mouth, dyspepsia, nausea, anorexia, dysphagia, elevated liver enzymes, flatulence, weight gain (unusual), vomiting. **GU:** decreased libido/sexual dysfunction. **Derm:** excessive sweating. **Metab:** weight gain, weight loss. **MS:** hypertonia, myoclonus/twitching. **Neuro:** hypokinesia/hyperkinesia, tremor. **Misc:** allergic reactions, chills, flu-like symptoms, tooth disorder/caries, yawning.

Interactions

Drug-Drug: Serious, potentially fatal reactions (serotonin syndrome) may occur with **MAO inhibitors**. **Smoking** may ↓ effectiveness of fluvoxamine. Concurrent use with **tricyclic antidepressants** may ↑ plasma levels of fluvoxamine. ↓ metabolism and may ↑ effects of some **beta blockers (propranolol)**, **alosetron** (avoid concurrent use), some **benzodiazepines** (avoid concurrent **diazepam**), **carbamazepine**, **methadone**, **lithium**, **theophylline** (↓ dose to 33% of usual dose), **tolbutamide**, **warfarin**, and **L-tryptophan**. ↑ blood levels and risk of toxicity from **clozapine** (dosage adjustments may be necessary).

Route/Dosage

PO (Adults): *Initial dose*—50 mg daily at bedtime; increase by 50 mg q 4–7 days until desired effect is achieved. If daily dose >100 mg, give in two equally divided doses or give a larger dose at bedtime (not to exceed 300 mg/day). *Maintenance dose*—Make periodic adjustments to maintain lowest possible dose to control symptoms.

PO (Children 8–17 yr): 25 mg at bedtime, may increase by 25 mg/day q 4–7 days (not to exceed 200 mg/day; daily doses >50 mg should be given in divided doses with a larger dose at bedtime).

Hepatic Impairment

PO (Adults): 25 mg daily at bedtime initially, slower titration and longer dosing intervals should be used.

Availability

Tablets: 25 mg, 50 mg, 100 mg.

NURSING IMPLICATIONS

Assessment

- Monitor mood changes. Assess patient for frequency of obsessive-compulsive behaviors. Note degree to which these thoughts and behaviors interfere with daily functioning. Inform health care professional if patient demonstrates significant increase in anxiety, nervousness, or insomnia.
- Assess for suicidal tendencies, especially during early therapy. Restrict amount of drug available to patient.
- Monitor appetite and nutritional intake. Weigh weekly. Report significant changes in weight. Adjust diet as tolerated to support nutritional status.
- ***Toxicity and Overdose:*** Common symptoms of toxicity include drowsiness, vomiting, diarrhea, and dizziness. Coma, tachycardia, bradycardia, hypotension, ECG abnormalities, liver function abnormalities, and convulsions may also occur. Treatment is symptomatic and supportive.

Potential Nursing Diagnoses

Ineffective coping (Indications)
Risk for injury (Side Effects)

Implementation

- Taper to avoid withdrawal effects. Reduce dose by 50% for 3 days, then reduce by 50% for 3 days, then discontinue.
- **PO:** Initial therapy is administered as a single bedtime dose. May be increased every 4–7 days as tolerated.
- Fluvoxamine may be given without regard to meals.

Patient/Family Teaching

- Instruct patient to take fluvoxamine exactly as directed. Do not skip or double up on missed doses. Improvement in symptoms may be no-

F

ticed in 2–3 wk, but medication should be continued as directed.

- May cause drowsiness and dizziness. Caution patient to avoid driving and other activities requiring alertness until response to medication is known.
- Advise patient to avoid alcohol or other CNS depressants during therapy and to consult health care professional before taking other medications with fluvoxamine.
- Instruct female patients to notify health care professional if breastfeeding or if pregnancy is planned or suspected.
- Advise patient to notify health care professional if rash or hives occur or if headache, nausea, anorexia, anxiety, or insomnia persists.
- Emphasize the importance of follow-up exams to monitor progress.
- Advise patient to avoid use of caffeine (chocolate, tea, cola).
- Refer patient to psychotherapy to improve coping skills and/or to an OCD support group.

Evaluation/Desired Outcomes

- Decrease in symptoms of obsessive-compulsive disorder.

folic acid (foe-lik a-sid)

✤Apo-Folic, folate, Folvite, ✤Novofolacid, vitamin B

Classification

Therapeutic: antianemics, vitamins

Pharmacologic: water soluble vitamins

Pregnancy Category A

Indications

Prevention and treatment of megaloblastic and macrocytic anemias. Given during pregnancy to promote normal fetal development.

Action

Required for protein synthesis and red blood cell function. Stimulates the production of red blood cells, white blood cells, and platelets. Necessary for normal fetal development. **Therapeutic Effects:** Restoration and maintenance of normal hematopoiesis.

Pharmacokinetics

Absorption: Well absorbed from the GI tract and IM and subcut sites.

Distribution: Half of all stores are in the liver. Enters breast milk. Crosses the placenta.

Protein Binding: Extensive.

Metabolism and Excretion: Converted by the liver to its active metabolite, dihydrofolate reductase. Excess amounts are excreted unchanged by the kidneys.

Half-life: Unknown.

TIME/ACTION PROFILE (increase in reticulocyte count)

ROUTE	ONSET	PEAK	DURATION
PO, IM, subcut, IV	30–60 min	1 hr	unknown

Contraindications/Precautions

Contraindicated in: Uncorrected pernicious, aplastic, or normocytic anemias (neurologic damage will progress despite correction of hematologic abnormalities); Preparations containing benzyl alcohol should not be used in newborns.

Use Cautiously in: Undiagnosed anemias.

Adverse Reactions/Side Effects

Derm: rashes.

CNS: irritability, difficulty sleeping, malaise, confusion. **Misc:** fever.

Interactions

Drug-Drug: Pyrimethamine, **methotrexate**, **trimethoprim**, and **triamterene** prevent the activation of folic acid (leucovorin should be used instead to treat overdoses of these drugs). Absorption of folic acid is ↓ by **sulfonamides** (including **sulfasalazine**), **anatacids**, and **cholestyramine**. Folic acid requirements are ↑ by **estrogens**, **phenytoin**, **phenobarbital**, **primidone**, **carbamazepine**, or **corticosteroids**. May ↓ **phenytoin** serum concentration.

Route/Dosage

Therapeutic Dose (Folic acid deficiency)

PO, IM, IV, Subcut (Adults and Children >11 yr): 1 mg/day initial dosage then 0.5 mg/day maintenance dose.

PO, IM, IV, Subcut (Children >1 yr): 1 mg/day initial dosage then 0.1–0.4 mg/day maintenance dose.

PO, IM, IV, Subcut (Infants): 15 mcg/kg/dose daily or 50 mcg/day.

Recommended Daily Allowance

PO (Adults and Children >15 yr): 0.2 mg/day.

PO (Adults, Pregnant or Lactating): 0.4 mg/day.
PO (Children 11–14 yr): 0.15 mg/day.
PO (Children 7–10 yr): 0.1 mg/day.
PO (Children 4–6 yr): 0.075 mg/day.
PO (Infants 6 months–3 yr): 0.05 mg/day.

Availability (generic available)

Tablets: 0.4 mg, 0.8 mg, 1 mg, ✤5 mg. **Injection:** 5 mg/ml. ***In combination with:*** other vitamins and minerals as multiple vitamins Rx, OTC.

NURSING IMPLICATIONS

Assessment

- Assess patient for signs of megaloblastic anemia (fatigue, weakness, dyspnea) before and periodically throughout therapy.
- ***Lab Test Considerations:*** Monitor plasma folic acid levels, hemoglobin, hematocrit, and reticulocyte count before and periodically during therapy.
- May cause ↓ serum concentrations of other B complex vitamins when given in high continuous doses.

Potential Nursing Diagnoses

Imbalanced nutrition: less than body requirements (Indications)
Activity intolerance (Indications)

Implementation

- Do not confuse folic acid with folinic acid (leucovorin calcium).
- Because of infrequency of solitary vitamin deficiencies, combinations are commonly administered (see Appendix B).
- May be given subcut, deep IM, or IV when PO route is not feasible.
- **PO:** Antacids should be given at least 2 hr after folic acid; folic acid should be given 2 hr before or 4–6 hr after cholestyramine. A 50-mcg/ml oral solution may be extemporaneously prepared by pharmacy for use in neonates and infants.
- **IV:** Solution ranges from yellow to orange-yellow in color.

IV Administration

- **Direct IV:** ***Diluent:*** Dilute with dextrose or 0.9%NaCl. ***Concentration:*** 0.1 mg/ml. ***Rate:*** 5 mg/min.
- **Continuous Infusion:** May be added to hyperalimentation solution.
- **Y-Site Compatibility:** famotidine.
- **Additive Compatibility:** D20W.
- **Additive Incompatibility:** D50W, calcium gluconate.

Patient/Family Teaching

- Encourage patient to comply with diet recommendations of health care professional. Explain that the best source of vitamins is a well-balanced diet with foods from the four basic food groups. A diet low in vitamin B and folate will be used to diagnose folic acid deficiency without concealing pernicious anemia.
- Foods high in folic acid include vegetables, fruits, and organ meats; heat destroys folic acid in foods.
- Patients self-medicating with vitamin supplements should be cautioned not to exceed RDA. The effectiveness of megadoses for treatment of various medical conditions is unproven and may cause side effects.
- Explain that folic acid may make urine more intensely yellow.
- Instruct patient to notify health care professional if rash occurs, which may indicate hypersensitivity.
- Emphasize the importance of follow-up exams to evaluate progress.

Evaluation/Desired Outcomes

- Reticulocytosis 2–5 days after beginning therapy.
- Resolution of symptoms of megaloblastic anemia.

HIGH ALERT

fondaparinux

(fon-da-**par**-i-nux)
Arixtra

Classification
Therapeutic: anticoagulants
Pharmacologic: active factor X inhibitors

Pregnancy Category B

Indications

Prevention and treatment of deep vein thrombosis and pulmonary embolism. **Unlabeled uses:** Systemic anticoagulation for other diagnoses.

Action

Binds selectively to antithrombin III (AT III). This binding potentiates the neutralization (inactivation) of active factor X (Xa). **Therapeutic Effects:** Interruption of the coagulation cascade resulting in inhibition of thrombus formation. Prevention of thrombus formation decreases the risk of pulmonary emboli.

Pharmacokinetics

Absorption: 100% absorbed following subcutaneous administration.
Distribution: Distributes mainly throughout the intravascular space.
Metabolism and Excretion: Eliminated mainly unchanged in urine.
Half-life: 17–21 hr.

TIME/ACTION PROFILE (anticoagulant effect)

ROUTE	ONSET	PEAK	DURATION
Subcut	rapid	3 hr	24 hr

Contraindications/Precautions

Contraindicated in: Hypersensitivity; Severe renal impairment (CCr <30 ml/min; increased risk of bleeding); Body weight <50 kg in patients undergoing hip replacement (markedly increased risk of bleeding); Active major bleeding; Bacterial endocarditis; Thrombocytopenia due to fonaparinux antibodies.
Use Cautiously in: Mild-to-moderate renal impairment; Retinopathy (hypertensive or diabetic); Untreated hypertension; Recent history of ulcer disease; History of congenital or acquired bleeding disorder; Geri: Patients >65 yr (increased risk of bleeding); Malignancy; History of heparin-induced thrombocytopenia; OB, Pedi: Pregnancy, lactation, or children (safety not established; use during pregnancy only if clearly needed)
Exercise Extreme Caution in: Severe uncontrolled hypertension; Bleeding disorders; GI bleeding/ulceration/pathology; Hemorrhagic stroke; Recent CNS or ophthalmologic surgery; Active GI bleeding/ulceration; Spinal/epidural anesthesia or spinal puncture (increased risk of spinal/epidural hematoma that may lead to long-term or permanent paralysis).

Adverse Reactions/Side Effects

CNS: confusion, dizziness, headache, insomnia. **CV:** edema, hypotension. **GI:** constipation, diarrhea, dyspepsia, increased serum aminotransferases, nausea, vomiting. **GU:** urinary retention. **Derm:** bullous eruption, hematoma, purpura, rash. **Hemat:** bleeding, thrombocytopenia. **F and E:** hypokalemia. **Misc:** fever, increased wound drainage.

Interactions

Drug-Drug: Risk of bleeding may be ↑ by concurrent use of **warfarin** or **drugs that affect platelet function**, including **aspirin**, **NSAIDs**, **dipyridamole**, some **cephalosporins**, **valproates**, **clopidogrel**, **ticlopidine**, **abciximab**, **eftifibatide**, **tirofiban**, and **dextran**.
Drug-Natural Products: ↑ risk of bleeding with **arnica**, **chamomile**, **clove**, **dong quai**, **feverfew**, **garlic**, **ginger**, **gingko**, **Panax ginseng**, and others.

Route/Dosage

Treatment of DVT/PE

Subcut (Adults): *<50 kg* 5—mg once daily for at least 5 days until therapeutic anticoagulation with warfarin is achieved (INR >2 for two consecutive days); warfarin may be started within 72 hr of fondaparinux (has been used for up to 26 days). *50–100 kg*—7.5 mg once daily for at least 5 days until therapeutic anticoagulation with warfarin is achieved (INR >2 for two consecutive days). *>100 kg*—10 mg once daily for at least 5 days until therapeutic anticoagulation-with warfarin is achieved (INR >2 for for two consecutive days); warfarin may be started within 72 hr of fondaparinux.

Prevention of DVT/PE

Subcut (Adults): 2.5 mg once daily, starting 6–8 hr after surgery, continuing for 5–9 days (up to 11 days) following abdominal surgery or knee/hip replacement or continuing for 24 days following hip fracture surgery (up to 32 days).

Availability

Solution for subcut injection: 2.5 mg/0.5 ml in prefilled syringes, 5 mg/0.4 ml in prefilled syringes, 7.5 mg/0.6 ml in prefilled syringes, 10 mg/0.8 ml in prefilled syringes.

NURSING IMPLICATIONS

Assessment

- Assess for signs of bleeding and hemorrhage (bleeding gums; nosebleed; unusual bruising; black, tarry stools; hematuria; fall in hematocrit; sudden drop in blood pressure; guaiac positive stools); bleeding from surgical site. Notify physician if these occur.
- Assess for evidence of additional or increased thrombosis. Symptoms will depend on area of involvement. Monitor neurological status fre-

quently for signs of impairment. May require urgent treatment.

- ***Lab Test Considerations:*** Monitor platelet count closely; may cause thrombocytopenia. If platelet count is <100,000/mm^3, discontinue fondaparinux.
- Fondaparinux is not accurately measured by prothrombin time (PT), activated thromboplastin time (aPTT), or international standards of heparin or low-molecular-weight heparins. If unexpected changes in coagulation parameters or major bleeding occurs, discontinue fondaparinux.
- Monitor CBC, serum creatinine levels, and stool occult blood tests routinely during therapy.
- May cause asymptomatic ↑ in AST and ALT. Elevations are fully reversible and not associated with ↑ in bilirubin.

Potential Nursing Diagnoses

Ineffective tissue perfusion (Indications)
Risk for injury (Side Effects)

Implementation

- Fondaparinux cannot be used interchangeably with heparin, low-molecular-weight heparins, or heparinoids as they differ in manufacturing process, anti-Xa and anti-IIa activity, units, and dosage. Each of these medications has its own instructions for use.
- Initial dose should be administered 6-8 hr after surgery. Administration before 6 hr after surgery has been associated with risk of major bleeding.
- **Subcut:** Administer subcut only into fatty tissue, alternating sites between right and left anterolateral or posterolateral abdominal wall. Inject entire length of needle at a 45° or 90° angle into a skin fold held between thumb and forefinger; hold skin fold throughout injection. Do not aspirate or massage. Rotate sites frequently. Do not administer IM because of danger of hematoma formation. Solution should be clear; do not inject solution containing particulate matter. Do not mix with other injections.
- Fondaparinux is provided in a single-dose prefilled syringe with an automatic needle protection system. Do not expel air bubble from prefilled syringe before injection to prevent loss of drug.

Patient/Family Teaching

- Advise patient to report any symptoms of unusual bleeding or bruising, dizziness, itching, rash, fever, swelling, or difficulty breathing to health care professional immediately.
- Instruct patient not to take aspirin or NSAIDs without consulting health care professional during therapy.

Evaluation/Desired Outcomes

- Prevention and treatment of deep vein thrombosis and pulmonary embolism.

formoterol (for-**mo**-te-role)

Foradil, Perforomist

Classification
Therapeutic: bronchodilators
Pharmacologic: adrenergics

Pregnancy Category C

Indications

Long-term maintenance treatment of asthma. Prevention of bronchospasm in reversible obstructive airways disease, including. Long-term management of bronchoconstriction associated with COPD including chronic bronchitis and emphysema. Acute prevention of exercise-induced bronchospasm, when used on an occasional, as needed, basis. Maintenance treatment of emphysema and chronic bronchitis.

Action

Produces accumulation of cyclic adenosine monophosphate (cAMP) at beta-adrenergic receptors, resulting in relaxation of airway smooth muscle. Relatively specific for beta$_2$ (pulmonary) receptors. **Therapeutic Effects:** Bronchodilation.

Pharmacokinetics

Absorption: Following inhalation, majority of inhaled drug is swallowed and absorbed.
Distribution: Unknown.
Metabolism and Excretion: Mostly metabolized by the liver; 10–18% excreted unchanged in urine.
Half-life: 10 hr.

TIME/ACTION PROFILE (bronchodilation)

ROUTE	ONSET	PEAK	DURATION
inhalation	15 min	1–3 hr	12 hr

Contraindications/Precautions

Contraindicated in: Hypersensitivity; Acute attack of asthma (onset of action is delayed).
Use Cautiously in: Cardiovascular disease (including angina and hypertension); Diabetes; Glaucoma; Hyperthyroidism; Pheochromocytoma; Excessive use (may lead to tolerance and paradoxical bronchospasm); OB, Pedi: Pregnancy, lactation, or children <5 yr (may inhibit contractions during labor; use only if potential benefits outweigh risks).

Adverse Reactions/Side Effects

CNS: dizziness, fatigue, headache, insomnia, malaise, nervousness. **Resp:** PARADOXICAL BRONCHOSPASM. **CV:** angina, arrhythmias, hypertension, hypotension, palpitations, tachycardia. **GI:** dry mouth, nausea. **F and E:** hypokalemia. **Metab:** hyperglycemia, metabolic acidosis. **MS:** muscle cramps. **Neuro:** tremor. **Misc:** allergic reactions including ANAPHYLAXIS.

Interactions

Drug-Drug: Concurrent use with **MAO inhibitors, tricyclic antidepressants** or other **agents that may prolong the QTc interval** may result in serious arrhythmias and should be undertaken with extreme caution. ↑ risk of hypokalemia with **theophylline**, **corticosteroids**, **potassium-losing diuretics**. **Beta blockers** may ↓ therapeutic effects of formoterol. ↑ adrenergic effects may occur with concurrent use of **adrenergics**.

Route/Dosage

Maintenance Treatment of Asthma

Inhaln (Adults and Children ≥5 yr): 1 capsule (12 mcg) every 12 hr using the Aerolizer Inhaler.

Prevention of Exercise-Induced Bronchospasm

Inhaln (Adults and Children ≥12 yr): 1 capsule (12 mcg) at least 15 min before exercise on an occasional as-needed basis.

Maintenance Treatment of Emphysema and Chronic Bronchitis

Inhaln (Adults): 20 mcg/2 mL-unit-dose vial twice daily via jet nebulizer.

Availability

Capsule for Aerolizer use: 12 mcg. **Vials for nebulization:** 20 mcg/2 mL. ***In combination with:*** budesonide (Symbicort; see Appendix B).

NURSING IMPLICATIONS

Assessment

- Assess lung sounds, pulse, and blood pressure before administration and during peak of medication. Note amount, color, and character of sputum produced. Closely monitor patients on higher dose for adverse effects.
- Monitor pulmonary function tests before initiating and periodically therapy to determine effectiveness of medication.
- Observe for paradoxical bronchospasm (wheezing). If condition occurs, withhold medication and notify physician or other health care provider immediately.
- Monitor ECG periodically during therapy. May cause prolonged QTc interval.
- Monitor patient for signs of anaphylaxis (dyspnea, rash, laryngeal edema) throughout therapy.
- ***Lab Test Considerations:*** May cause ↑ serum glucose and decreased serum potassium.

Potential Nursing Diagnoses

Ineffective airway clearance (Indications)

Implementation

- **Inhaln:** *For use with inhaler:* Place capsule in the well of the Aerolizer Inhaler with dry hands; do not expose to moisture. The capsule is pierced by pressing and releasing the buttons on the side of the device. Medication is dispersed into the air stream when patient inhales rapidly and deeply through mouthpiece. Capsules are only to be used with Aerolizer Inhaler and should not be taken orally. Store capsules in the blister and only remove immediately before use. Store inhaler in a level, horizontal position. Aerolizer Inhaler should never be washed and should be kept dry.
- Do not use a spacer with fomoterol.
- To use, pull off the Aerolizer cover. Hold the base of the inhaler firmly, and twist mouthpiece in the direction of the arrow to open. Push the buttons in to make sure four pins are visible in the capsule well on each side. Remove capsule from blister pack immediately before use. Separate one blistered cap-

sule by tearing at perforations. With foil-side up, fold back along perforation and flatten. Starting at slit, tear off corner; separate and peel foil from paper backing and remove capsule. Place capsule in the capsule chamber in the base of the Aerolizer Inhaler. Never place a capsule directly into the mouthpiece. Twist the mouthpiece back to the closed position. With the mouthpiece upright, simultaneously press both buttons only once. A click should be heard as the capsule is being pierced. Release buttons; if buttons stick in depressed position grasp wings on buttons and retract before inhalation. With patient sitting or standing in a comfortable upright position, exhale fully. Do not exhale into the device. Tilt head back slightly and breathe in rapidly but steadily. A sweet taste will be experienced and a whirring noise heard. If no whirring is heard, the capsule may be stuck. Open inhaler and loosen capsule allowing it to spin freely. Do not repeatedly press buttons to loosen capsule. Hold breath for as long as comfortably possible after removing inhaler from mouth. Open inhaler to see if any powder is still in capsule. If powder is found, repeat inhalation steps. After use, open, remove and discard empty capsule.

- **Inhaln:** *For use with nebulizer:* Administer via standard jet nebulizer via mouthpiece or face mask. Remove vial from foil immediately prior to use and discard via after use. May be stored in refrigerator for up to 3 months.

Patient/Family Teaching

- Instruct patient to take fomoterol as directed. Do not discontinue therapy without discussing with health care professional, even if feeling better. If on a scheduled dosing regimen, take a missed dose as soon as remembered, spacing remaining doses at regular intervals. Do not double doses. Use a rapid-acting bronchodilator if symptoms occur before next dose is due. Caution patient not to use more than 2 times a day or less than 12 hr apart; may cause adverse effects, paradoxical bronchospasm, or loss of effectiveness of medication Instruct patient to review medication guide with each Rx refill.
- Advise patient to have a rapid-acting bronchodilator available for use at all times for symptomatic relief of acute asthma attacks.
- Instruct patient to contact health care professional immediately if shortness of breath is not relieved by medication or nausea, vomiting, shakiness, headache, fast or irregular heartbeat, or sleeplessness occur.
- Instruct patient to notify health care professional if there is no response to the usual dose of fomoterol. Asthma and treatment regimen should be re-evaluated and corticosteroids should be considered. Need for increased use to treat symptoms indicates decrease in asthma control and need to reevaluate therapy.
- Advise patient to consult health care professional before taking any Rx, OTC, or herbal products or alcohol concurrently with this therapy. Caution patient also to avoid smoking and other respiratory irritants.
- Advise patient to notify health care professional if pregnancy is planned or suspected, or if nursing.
- **Inhaler:** Instruct patient on correct technique for use of Aerolizer Inhaler. Advise patient always to use new Aerolizer Inhaler that comes with each refill. Take sticker with "use by" date written by pharmacist from the outside of the box and place it on the Aerolizer Inhaler cover. If the date is blank, count 4 months from the date of purchase and write date on sticker. Use new inhaler and blister pack following the "use by" date.
- Inform patient that in rare cases capsule might break into small pieces. These pieces should be retained by the screen in the inhaler, however in rare instances tiny pieces may reach mouth or throat after inhalation. Shattering of capsule is less likely to happen if storage conditions are strictly followed, capsules removed from blister immediately before use, and capsules are only pierced once.

Evaluation/Desired Outcomes

- Prevention of bronchospasm.

fosamprenavir calcium
(fos-am-**pren**-a-veer)
Lexiva

Classification
Therapeutic: antiretrovirals
Pharmacologic: protease inhibitors

Pregnancy Category C

Indications
With other antiretrovirals in the management of HIV infection.

Action
Inhibits the action of HIV protease and prevents the cleavage of viral polyproteins. **Therapeutic Effects:** Increased CD4 cell counts and decreased viral load with subsequent slowed progression of HIV and its sequelae.

Pharmacokinetics
Absorption: Fosamprenavir is a prodrug. Following oral administration, it is rapidly converted to amprenavir by the gut lining during absorption.
Distribution: Penetration into RBCs is concentration dependent.
Metabolism and Excretion: Mostly metabolized the liver (CYP3A4 enzyme system). Minimal renal excretion.
Half-life: 7.7 hr.

TIME/ACTION PROFILE (blood levels)

ROUTE	ONSET	PEAK	DURATION
PO	rapid	1.5–4 hr	12–24 hr

Contraindications/Precautions
Contraindicated in: Hypersensitivity, sulfonamide/sulfa hypersensitivity; Severe hepatic impairment; Concurrent use of flecainide, propafenone, rifampin, ergot derivatives, St. John's wort, lovastatin, simvastatin, pimozide, delavirdine, midazolam or triazolam.
Use Cautiously in: Geri: Geriatric patients (consider age-related decrease in body mass, cardiac/hepatic/renal impairment, concurrent illness and medications); Mild to moderate hepatic impairment; Concurrent use of medications handled by or affecting the CYP3A4 enzyme system (may require serum level monitoring, dose or dosing interval alterations); OB, Pedi: Pregnancy, lactation, children (safety not established; breast feeding not recommended in HIV-infected patients).

Adverse Reactions/Side Effects
Reflects use with other antiretrovirals.
CNS: headache, fatigue, mood disorders. **GI:** diarrhea, nausea, vomiting, abdominal pain, ↑ liver enzymes. **Derm:** rash. **Endo:** glucose intolerance. **Hemat:** neutropenia. **Metab:** fat redistribution, ↑ triglycerides. **Misc:** allergic reactions including STEVENS-JOHNSON SYNDROME, inflammatory response to opportunistic infection.

Interactions
Drug-Drug: Amprenavir, the active moiety of fosamprenavir is metabolized by CYP3A4; it also inhibits and induces this enzyme system. The action of any other medication that is also handled by or affects this system may be altered by concurrent use. Concurrent use of **flecainide**, **propafenone**, **rifampin**, **ergot derivatives** (**dihydroergotamine**, **ergotamine**, **ergonovine**, **methylergonovine**), **fluticasone lovastatin**, **simvastatin**, **pimozide**, **delavirdine**, **midazolam** or **triazolam** may result in serious, potentially life-threatening adverse reactions including arrhythmias, excessive sedation, myopathy or loss of virologic response and is contraindicated. Blood levels are ↓ by **efavirenz** (additional ritonavir may be required when used together), **nevirapine**, **lopinavir/ritonavir**, **saquinavir**, **carbamazepine**, **phenobarbital**, **phenytoin**, **dexamethasone**, **histamine H_2-receptor antagonists**, and **proton-pump inhibitors**; monitor for ↓ antiretroviral activity. Levels are ↑ by **indinavir** and **nelfinavir**. May ↓ **methadone** and **paroxetine** levels. ↑ levels and risk of toxicity from **amiodarone**, **lidocaine**, **quinidine** (monitor blood levels), **ketoconazole**, and **itraconazole** (dose of itraconazole or ketoconazole should not exceed 200 mg/day when fosamprenavir is used with ritonavir or 400 mg/day when used without), **rifabutin** (monitor for neutropenia, ↓ rifabutin dose by 50% when used with fosamprenavir or by 75% when used with fosamprenavir with ritonavir), **atorvastatin** and **rosuvastatin** (dose not to exceed 20 mg/day or consider other HMG-CoA reductase inhibitors), **cyclsosporine** or **tacrolimus** (monitor blood levels of immunosuppressants), **calcium channel blockers** (clinical monitoring recommended), some **benzodiazepines** (**alprazolam**, **clorazepate**, **diazepam**, **flurazepam** (dose reduction of benzodiazepine may be needed), **sildenafil**, **tadalafil**, and **vardenafil** (use

cautiously; ↓ dose of sildenafil to 25 mg every 48 hr, for tadalafil single dose should not exceed 10 mg in any 72 hr period, dose of vardenafil should not exceed 2.5 mg every 24 hr if used without ritonavir or 2.5 mg every 72 hr with ritonavir with monitoring for toxicity) and **tricyclic antidepressants** (blood level monitoring recommended). May alter the effects of **warfarin** (monitor INR) or **hormonal contraceptives** (use alternative method of contraception).
Drug-Natural Products: Concurrent use of **St. John's wort** is contraindicated; ↓ blood levels and may lead to ↓ virologic response.

Route/Dosage

PO (Adults): *Treatment-naive patients without ritonavir*—1400 mg twice daily; *treatment-naive patients with ritonavir*—1400 mg once daily with ritonavir 100 or 200 mg once daily, or 700 mg twice daily with ritonavir 100 mg twice daily. *Protease inhibitor–experienced patients*—700 mg twice daily with ritonavir 100 mg twice daily. If efavirenz is added to a once daily regimen using both fosamprenavir and ritonavir, an additional 100 mg of ritonavir (total of 300 mg) should be given.

Hepatic Impairment

PO (Adults mild-moderate hepatic impairment): 700 mg twice daily without ritonavir.

Availability

Tablets: 700 mg.

NURSING IMPLICATIONS

Assessment

- Assess patient for change in severity of HIV symptoms and for symptoms of opportunistic infections throughout therapy.
- Assess patient for allergy to sulfonamides. May exhibit cross-sensitivity.
- Assess patient for skin reactions throughout therapy. Reactions may be severe and life threatening. Discontinue therapy if severe reactions or moderate rashes with systemic symptoms occur.
- ***Lab Test Considerations:*** Monitor viral load and CD4 cell count regularly during therapy.
- May cause ↑ serum glucose, and triglyceride levels.
- May cause ↑ AST and ALT levels.
- May cause neutropenia.

Potential Nursing Diagnoses

Risk for infection (Indications)
Noncompliance (Patient/Family Teaching)

Implementation

- **PO:** May be administered with or without food.

Patient/Family Teaching

- Emphasize the importance of taking fosamprenavir exactly as directed. Advise patient to read the Patient Information that comes with the prescription prior to initiation of therapy and with each prescription refill. Fosamprenavir must always be used in combination with other antiretroviral drugs. Do not take more than prescribed amount and do not stop taking without consulting health care professional. Take missed doses as soon as remembered, then return to regular schedule. If a dose is skipped, do not double the next doses.
- Instruct patient that fosamprenavir should not be shared with others.
- Inform patient that fosamprenavir does not cure AIDS or prevent associated or opportunistic infections. Fosamprenavir does not reduce the risk of transmission of HIV to others through sexual contact or blood contamination. Caution patient to use a condom and to avoid sharing needles or donating blood to prevent spreading the AIDS virus to others. Advise patient that the long-term effects of fosamprenavir are unknown at this time.
- Emphasize the importance of providing health care professional with accurate current drug history and notifying health care professional before taking any prescription or OTC medications or herbal products because of potentially serious drug interactions.
- May decrease effectiveness of hormonal contraceptives; advise patient to use a nonhormonal form of contraception during therapy.
- Instruct patient to notify health care professional if nausea, vomiting, diarrhea, or rash occurs.
- Emphasize the importance of regular follow-up exams and blood counts to determine progress and monitor for side effects.

Evaluation/Desired Outcomes

- Delayed progression of AIDS and decreased opportunistic infections in patients with HIV.

- Decrease in viral load and increase in CD4 cell counts.

foscarnet (foss-**kar**-net)
Foscavir

Classification
Therapeutic: antivirals

Pregnancy Category C

Indications
Treatment of cytomegalovirus (CMV) retinitis in HIV-infected patients (alone or with ganciclovir). Treatment of acyclovir-resistant mucocutaneous herpes simplex virus (HSV) infections in immunocompromised patients.

Action
Prevents viral replication by inhibiting viral DNA-polymerase and reverse transcriptase. **Therapeutic Effects:** Virustatic action against susceptible viruses including CMV.

Pharmacokinetics
Absorption: IV administration results in complete bioavailability.
Distribution: Variable penetration into CSF. May concentrate in and be slowly released from bone.
Metabolism and Excretion: 80–90% excreted unchanged in urine.
Half-life: 3 hr (in patients with normal renal function); longer half-life of 90 hr may reflect release of drug from bone.

TIME/ACTION PROFILE

ROUTE	ONSET	PEAK	DURATION
IV	rapid	end of infusion	8–24 hr

Contraindications/Precautions
Contraindicated in: Hypersensitivity.
Use Cautiously in: Renal impairment (dose reduction required if CCr ≤1.4–1.6 ml/min/kg; see product information); History of seizures; OB, Pedi: Pregnancy, lactation, or children (safety not established).

Adverse Reactions/Side Effects
CNS: SEIZURES, headache, anxiety, confusion, dizziness, fatigue, malaise, mental depression, weakness. **EENT:** conjunctivitis, eye pain, vision abnormalities. **Resp:** coughing, dyspnea. **CV:** chest pain, ECG abnormalities, edema, palpitations. **GI:** diarrhea, nausea, vomiting, abdominal pain, abnormal taste sensation, anorexia, constipation, dyspepsia. **GU:** renal failure, albuminuria, dysuria, nocturia, polyuria, urinary retention. **Derm:** increased sweating, pruritus, rash, skin ulceration. **F and E:** hypocalcemia, hypokalemia, hypomagnesemia, hyperphosphatemia, hypophosphatemia. **Hemat:** anemia, granulocytopenia, leukopenia. **Local:** pain/inflammation at injection site. **MS:** arthralgia, myalgia, back pain, involuntary muscle contraction. **Neuro:** ataxia, hypoesthesia, neuropathy, paresthesia, tremor. **Misc:** fever, chills, flu-like syndrome, lymphoma, sarcoma.

Interactions
Drug-Drug: Concurrent use with parenteral **pentamidine** may result in severe, life-threatening hypocalcemia. Risk of nephrotoxicity may be ↑ by concurrent use of other **nephrotoxic agents (amphotericin B, aminoglycosides)**.

Route/Dosage
IV (Adults): *CMV retinitis*—60 mg/kg q 8 hr or 90 mg/kg q 12 hr for 2–3 wk, then 90–120 mg/kg/day as a single dose. Dosage reduction required for any degree of renal impairment; *HSV*—40 mg/kg q 8–12 hr for 2–3 wk or until healing occurs.

Availability (generic available)
Injection: 6000 mg/250 ml, 12,000 mg/500 ml.

NURSING IMPLICATIONS

Assessment
- **CMV Retinitis:** Diagnosis of CMV retinitis should be determined by ophthalmoscopy before treatment with foscarnet. Ophthalmologic examinations should also be performed at the conclusion of induction and every 4 wk during maintenance therapy.
- Culture for CMV (urine, blood, throat) may be taken before administration. However, a negative CMV culture does not rule out CMV retinitis.
- **HSV Infections:** Assess lesions before and daily during therapy.
- ***Lab Test Considerations:*** Monitor serum creatinine before and 2–3 times weekly during induction therapy and at least once every 1–2 wk during maintenance therapy. Monitor 24-hr CCr before and periodically throughout therapy. If CCr drops below 0.4 ml/min/kg, foscarnet should be discontinued.

- Monitor serum calcium, magnesium, potassium, and phosphorus before and 2–3 times weekly during induction therapy and at least weekly during maintenance therapy. May cause concentrations.
- May cause anemia, granulocytopenia, leukopenia, and thrombocytopenia. May cause ↑ AST and ALT levels and abnormal A-G ratios.

Potential Nursing Diagnoses

Risk for infection (Indications)

Implementation

- Patient should be adequately hydrated with 750–1000 ml of 0.9% NaCl or D5W before first infusion to establish diuresis, then 750–1000 ml with 120 mg/kg of foscarnet or 500 ml with 40–60 mg/kg of foscarnet should be administered with each dose to prevent renal toxicity.

IV Administration

- **Intermittent Infusion:** ***Diluent:*** May be administered via central line undiluted. If administered via peripheral line, *must* be diluted with D5W or 0.9% NaCl to prevent vein irritation. Do not administer solution that is discolored or contains particulate matter. Use diluted solution within 24 hr. ***Concentration:*** Undiluted: 24 mg/ml; Diluted: 12 mg/ml.
- Dose is based on patient weight; excess solution may be discarded from bottle before administration to prevent overdosage.
- Patients who experience progression of CMV retinitis during maintenance therapy may be re-treated with induction therapy followed by maintenance therapy. ***Rate:*** Administer at a rate not to exceed 1 mg/kg/min.
- Infuse solution via infusion pump to ensure accurate infusion rate.
- **Y-Site Compatibility:** aldesleukin, amikacin, aminophylline, ampicillin, aztreonam, cefazolin, cefoxitin, ceftazidime, ceftizoxime, ceftriaxone, cefuroxime, chloramphenicol, cimetidine, clindamycin, dexamethasone sodium phosphate, dopamine, erythromycin lactobionate, fluconazole, flucytosine, furosemide, gentamicin, heparin, hydrocortisone, hydromorphone, imipenen-cilastatin, metoclopramide, metronidazole, morphine, nafcillin, oxacillin, penicillin G potassium, phenytoin, piperacillin, ranitidine, ticarcillin/clavulanate, tobramycin.
- **Y-Site Incompatibility:** Manufacturer recommends that foscarnet not be administered concurrently with other drugs or solutions in the same IV catheter except D5W or 0.9% NaCl, acyclovir, amphotericin B, diazepam, digoxin, diphenhydramine, dobutamine, droperidol, ganciclovir, haloperidol, leucovorin, midazolam, pentamidine, prochlorperazine, promethazine, trimetrexate.

Patient/Family Teaching

- Inform patient that foscarnet is not a cure for CMV retinitis. Progression of retinitis may continue in immunocompromised patients during and after therapy. Advise patients to have regular ophthalmologic exams.
- Advise patient to notify health care professional immediately if perioral tingling or numbness in the extremities or paresthesia occurs during or after infusion. If these signs of electrolyte imbalance occur during administration, infusion should be stopped and lab samples for serum electrolyte concentrations obtained immediately.
- Emphasize the importance of frequent follow-up exams to monitor renal function and electrolytes.

Evaluation/Desired Outcomes

- Management of the symptoms of CMV retinitis in patients with AIDS.
- Crusting over and healing of skin lesions in HSV infections.

fosinopril, See ANGIOTENSIN-CONVERTING ENZYME (ACE) INHIBITORS.

fosphenytoin (foss-**fen**-i-toyn)

Cerebyx

Classification

Therapeutic: anticonvulsants

Pregnancy Category D

Indications

Short-term (<5 day) parenteral management of generalized, convulsive status epilepticus when use of phenytoin is not feasible. Treatment and prevention of seizures during neurosurgery when use of phenytoin is not feasible.

Action
Limits seizure propagation by altering ion transport. May also decrease synaptic transmission. Fosphenytoin is rapidly converted to phenytoin, which is responsible for its pharmacologic effects. **Therapeutic Effects:** Diminished seizure activity.

Pharmacokinetics
Absorption: Rapidly converted to phenytoin after IV administration and completely absorbed after IM administration.
Distribution: Distributes into CSF and other body tissues and fluids. Enters breast milk; crosses the placenta, achieving similar maternal/fetal levels. Preferentially distributes into fatty tissue.
Protein Binding: *Fosphenytoin*—95–99%; *phenytoin*—90–95%.
Metabolism and Excretion: Mostly metabolized by the liver; minimal amounts excreted in the urine.
Half-life: *Fosphenytoin*—15 min; *phenytoin*—22 hr (range 7–42 hr).

TIME/ACTION PROFILE (anticonvulsant effect)

ROUTE	ONSET	PEAK	DURATION
IM	unknown	30 min	up to 24 hr
IV	15–45 min	15–60 min	up to 24 hr

Contraindications/Precautions
Contraindicated in: Hypersensitivity; Sinus bradycardia, sinoatrial block, 2nd- or 3rd-degree AV heart block or Adams-Stokes syndrome.
Use Cautiously in: Hepatic or renal disease (increased risk of adverse reactions; dose reduction recommended for hepatic impairment); OB: Safety not established; may result in fetal hydantoin syndrome if used chronically or hemorrhage in the newborn if used at term; Lactation: Safety not established.

Adverse Reactions/Side Effects
CNS: dizziness, drowsiness, nystagmus, agitation, brain edema, headache, stupor, vertigo. **EENT:** amblyopia, deafness, diplopia, tinnitus. **CV:** hypotension (with rapid IV administration), tachycardia. **GI:** dry mouth, nausea, taste perversion, tongue disorder, vomiting. **Derm:** pruritus, rash, STEVENS-JOHNSON SYNDROME. **MS:** back pain. **Neuro:** ataxia, dysarthria, extrapyramidal syndrome, hypesthesia, incoordination, paresthesia, tremor. **Misc:** pelvic pain.

Interactions
Drug-Drug: Disulfiram, acute ingestion of **alcohol**, **amiodarone**, **ethosuximide**, **isoniazid**, **chloramphenicol**, **sulfonamides**, **fluoxetine**, **gabapentin**, **H2 antagonists**, **benzodiazepines**, **omeprazole**, **ketoconazole**, **fluconazole**, **estrogens**, **succinamides**, **halothane**, **methylphenidate**, **phenothiazines**, **salicylates**, **ticlopidine**, **tolbutamide**, **topiramate**, **trazodone**, **felbamate**, and **cimetidine** may ↑ phenytoin blood levels . **Barbiturates**, **carbamazepine**, **reserpine**, and chronic ingestion of **alcohol** may ↓ phenytoin blood levels. Phenytoin may decrease the effects of **amiodarone**, **benzodiazepines**, **carbamazepine**, **chloramphenicol**, **corticosteroids**, **disopyramide**, **warfarin**, **felbamate**, **doxycycline**, **lamotrigine**, **oral contraceptives**, **paroxetine**, **propafenone**, **rifampin**, **ritonavir**, **quinidine**, **tacrolimus**, **theophylline**, **topiramate**, **tricyclic antidepressants**, **zonisamide**, **methadone**, **cyclosporine**, and **estrogens**. IV phenytoin and **dopamine** may cause additive hypotension. Additive CNS depression with other **CNS depressants**, including **alcohol**, **antihistamines**, **antidepressants**, **opioids**, and **sedative/hypnotics**. **Antacids** may ↓ absorption of orally administered phenytoin. ↑ systemic clearance of antileukemic drugs **teniposide** and **methotrexate** which has been associated with a worse event free survival. **Phenytoin** use is not recommended in children undergoing chemotherapy for acute lymphocytic leukemia. **Calcium** and **sucralfate** ↓ phenytoin absorption.

Route/Dosage
Note: Doses of fosphenytoin are expressed as phenytoin sodium equivalents [PE].

Status Epilepticus
IV (Adults): 15–20 mg PE/kg.

Nonemergent and Maintenance Dosing
IV, IM (Adults and Children >16 yr): *Loading dose*—10–20 mg PE/kg. *Maintenance dose*—4–6 mg PE/kg/day.
IV, IM (Children 10–16 yr): 6–7 mg PE/kg/day.
IV, IM (Children 7–9 yr): 7–8 mg PE/kg/day.
IV, IM (Children 4–6 yr): 7.5–9 mg PE/kg/day.
IV, IM (Children 0.5–3 yr): 8–10 mg PE kg/day.
IV, IM (Infants): 5 mg PE kg/day.
IV, IM (Neonates): 5–8 mg PE/kg/day.

Availability
Injection: 50 mgPE/ml.

NURSING IMPLICATIONS

Assessment

- **Seizures:** Assess location, duration, frequency, and characteristics of seizure activity. EEG may be monitored periodically during therapy.
- Monitor blood pressure, ECG, and respiratory function continuously during administration of fosphenytoin and during period when peak serum phenytoin levels occur (15–30 min after administration).
- Observe patient for development of rash. Discontinue fosphenytoin at the first sign of skin reactions. Serious adverse reactions such as exfoliative, purpuric, or bullous rashes or the development of lupus erythematosus, Stevens-Johnson syndrome, or toxic epidermal necrolysis preclude further use of phenytoin or fosphenytoin. If less serious skin eruptions (measles-like or scarlatiniform) occur, fosphenytoin may be resumed after complete clearing of the rash. If rash reappears, further use of fosphenytoin or phenytoin should be avoided.
- ***Lab Test Considerations:*** Fosphenytoin contains 0.0037 mmol phosphate per mg PE. Monitor serum phosphate concentrations in patients with renal insufficiency; may cause ↑ phosphate concentrations.
- May cause ↑ serum alkaline phosphatase, GTT, and glucose levels.
- Fosphenytoin therapy may be monitored using phenytoin levels. Optimal total plasma phenytoin concentrations are typically 10–20 mcg/ml (unbound plasma phenytoin concentrations of 1–2 mcg/ml).
- ***Toxicity and Overdose:*** Serum phenytoin levels should not be monitored until complete conversion from fosphenytoin to phenytoin has occurred (2 hr after IV or 4 hr after IM administration): Initial signs and symptoms of phenytoin toxicity include nystagmus, ataxia, confusion, nausea, slurred speech, and dizziness.

Potential Nursing Diagnoses

Risk for injury (Indications)

Deficient knowledge, related to medication regimen (Patient/Family Teaching)

Implementation

- Do not confuse fosphenytoin (Cerebyx) with celocoxib (Celebrex) or citalopram (Celexa).
- Implement seizure precautions.
- When substituting *fosphenytoin* for oral *phenytoin* therapy, the same total daily dose may be given as a single dose. Unlike parenteral phenytoin, fosphenytoin may be given safely by the IM route.
- The anticonvulsant effect of fosphenytoin is not immediate. Additional measures (including parenteral benzodiazepines) are usually required in the immediate management of status epilepticus. Loading dosage of *fosphenytoin* should be followed with the institution of maintenance anticonvulsant therapy.

IV Administration

- **Direct IV:** *Diluent:* D5W or 0.9% NaCl. *Concentration:* 1.5–25 mg PE/ml. May be refrigerated for up to 48 hr. ***Rate:*** Administer at a rate of <150 mg PE/min in adults and <3 mg/kg/min in children to minimize risk of hypotension.
- **Y-Site Compatibility:** lorazepam, phenobarbital.
- **Y-Site Incompatibility:** fenoldopam, midazolam.
- **Additive Incompatibility:** Information unavailable. Do not admix with other solutions or medications.

Patient/Family Teaching

- May cause drowsiness or dizziness. Caution patient to avoid driving or other activities requiring alertness until response to medication is known. Do not resume driving until physician gives clearance based on control of seizure disorder.
- Advise patient to carry identification describing disease process and medication regimen at all times.
- Advise patient to notify health care professional if skin rash, severe nausea or vomiting, drowsiness, slurred speech, unsteady gait, swollen glands, bleeding or tender gums, yellow skin or eyes, joint pain, fever, sore throat, unusual bleeding or bruising, or persistent headache occurs.
- Advise female patients to use an additional nonhormonal method of contraception during therapy and until next menstrual period. Instruct patient to notify health care professional if pregnancy is planned or suspected.
- Emphasize the importance of routine exams to monitor progress. Patient should have rou-

tine physical exams, especially monitoring skin and lymph nodes, and EEG testing.

Evaluation/Desired Outcomes

- Decrease or cessation of seizures without excessive sedation.

frovatriptan (froe-va-**trip**-tan)
Frova

Classification
Therapeutic: vascular headache suppressants
Pharmacologic: 5-HT_1 agonists

Pregnancy Category C

Indications

Acute treatment of migraine headache.

Action

Acts as an agonist at specific 5-HT receptor sites in intracranial blood vessels and sensory trigeminal nerves. **Therapeutic Effects:** Cranial vessel vasoconstriction with associated decrease in release of neuropeptides and resultant decrease in migraine headache.

Pharmacokinetics

Absorption: 20–30% following oral administration.
Distribution: Unknown.
Metabolism and Excretion: Mostly metabolized by the liver (P450 1A2 enzyme system); some metabolites eliminated in urine, <10% excreted unchanged.
Half-life: 26 hr.

TIME/ACTION PROFILE (blood levels)

ROUTE	ONSET	PEAK	DURATION
PO	unknown	2–4 hr	unknown

Contraindications/Precautions

Contraindicated in: Hypersensitivity; History, symptoms or findings consistent with;: ischemic heart disease, coronary artery vasospasm, other significant underlying cardiovascular disease Cerebrovascular syndromes including;: strokes of any type, transient ischemic attacks Uncontrolled hypertension; Hemiplegic or basilar migraine; Peripheral vascular disease, including ischemic bowel disease; Should not be used within 24 hr of any other 5-HT agonist or ergot-type compounds (dihydroergotamine); Children <18 yr.
Use Cautiously in: Elderly patients (may be more susceptible to adverse cardiovascular effects); Pregnancy or lactation (safety not established).
Exercise Extreme Caution in: Cardiovascular risk factors (hypertension, hypercholesterolemia, cigarette smoking, obesity, diabetes, strong family history, menopausal women or men >40 yr); use only if cardiovascular status has been evaluated and determined to be safe and first dose is administered under supervision.

Adverse Reactions/Side Effects

CNS: dizziness, drowsiness, fatigue. **CV:** CORONARY ARTERY VASOSPASM, MI, VENTRICULAR FIBRILLATION, VENTRICULAR TACHYCARDIA, chest pain, myocardial ischemia. **GI:** dry mouth, dyspepsia, nausea. **Derm:** flushing. **MS:** skeletal pain. **Neuro:** paresthesia. **Misc:** pain.

Interactions

Drug-Drug: Blood levels may be increased by **hormonal contraceptives** or **propranolol**. Blood levels may be decreased by **ergotamine**. Increased risk of serious vasospastic reactions with **dihydroergotamine** (concurrent use contraindicated).

Route/Dosage

PO (Adults): 2.5 mg; if there has been initial relief, a second tablet may be taken after at least 2 hr (daily dose should not exceed 3 tablets and should not be used to treat more than 4 attacks/30-day period).

Availability

Tablets: 2.5 mg.

NURSING IMPLICATIONS

Assessment

- Assess pain location, intensity, duration, and associated symptoms (photophobia, phonophobia, nausea, vomiting) during migraine attack.

Potential Nursing Diagnoses

Acute pain (Indications)

Implementation

- **PO:** Tablets may be administered at any time after the headache starts.

Patient/Family Teaching

- Inform patient that frovatriptan should be used only during a migraine attack. It is meant to be used to relieve migraine attack but not to prevent or reduce the number of attacks.

- Instruct patient to administer frovatriptan as soon as symptoms appear, but it may be administered any time during an attack. If migraine symptoms return, a second dose may be used. Allow at least 2 hr between doses, and do not use more than 3 tablets in any 24-hr period.
- If dose does not relieve headache, additional frovatriptan doses are not likely to be effective; notify health care professional.
- Advise patient that lying down in a darkened room following frovatriptan administration may further help relieve headache.
- Caution patient not to use frovatriptan if she is pregnant, suspects she is pregnant, plans to become pregnant, or is breastfeeding. Adequate contraception should be used during therapy.
- May cause dizziness or drowsiness. Caution patient to avoid driving or other activities requiring alertness until response to medication is known.
- Advise patient to notify health care professional prior to next dose of frovatriptan if pain or tightness in the chest occurs during use. If pain is severe or does not subside, notify health care professional immediately. If wheezing; heart throbbing; swelling of eyelids, face, or lips; skin rash; skin lumps; or hives occur, notify health care professional immediately and do not take more frovatriptan without approval of health care professional. If feelings of tingling, heat, flushing, heaviness, pressure, drowsiness, dizziness, tiredness, or sickness develop, discuss with health care professional at next visit.
- Advise patient to avoid alcohol, which aggravates headaches, during frovatriptan use.

Evaluation/Desired Outcomes

- Relief of migraine attack.

furosemide (fur-**oh**-se-mide)

✤Apo-Furosemide, Lasix, ✤Lasix Special, ✤Novosemide, ✤Nu-Furosemide, ✤PMS-Furosemide

Classification
Therapeutic: diuretics
Pharmacologic: loop diuretics

Pregnancy Category C

Indications

Edema due to heart failure, hepatic impairment or renal disease. Hypertension.

Action

Inhibits the reabsorption of sodium and chloride from the loop of Henle and distal renal tubule. Increases renal excretion of water, sodium, chloride, magnesium, potassium, and calcium. Effectiveness persists in impaired renal function. **Therapeutic Effects:** Diuresis and subsequent mobilization of excess fluid (edema, pleural effusions). Decreased blood pressure.

Pharmacokinetics

Absorption: 60–67% absorbed after oral administration (↓ in acute CHF and in renal failure); also absorbed from IM sites.
Distribution: Crosses placenta, enters breast milk.
Protein Binding: 91–99%.
Metabolism and Excretion: Minimally metabolized by liver, some nonhepatic metabolism, some renal excretion as unchanged drug.
Half-life: 30–60 min (↑ in renal impairment).

TIME/ACTION PROFILE (diuretic effect)

ROUTE	ONSET	PEAK	DURATION
PO	30–60 min	1–2 hr	6–8 hr
IM	10–30 min	unknown	4–8 hr
IV	5 min	30 min	2 hr

Contraindications/Precautions

Contraindicated in: Hypersensitivity; Cross-sensitivity with thiazides and sulfonamides may occur; Hepatic coma or anuria; Some liquid products may contain alcohol, avoid in patients with alcohol intolerance.
Use Cautiously in: Severe liver disease (may precipitate hepatic coma; concurrent use with potassium-sparing diuretics may be necessary); Electrolyte depletion; Geri: Geriatric patients may have increased risk of side effects, especially hypotension and electrolyte imbalance, at usual doses; Diabetes mellitus; Increasing azo-

temia; Pregnancy and lactation; Pedi: Increased risk of renal calculi and patent ductus arteriosis in premature neonates.

Adverse Reactions/Side Effects

CNS: blurred vision, dizziness, headache, vertigo. **EENT:** hearing loss, tinnitus. **CV:** hypotension. **GI:** anorexia, constipation, diarrhea, dry mouth, dyspepsia, nausea, pancreatitis, vomiting. **GU:** excessive urination. **Derm:** photosensitivity, pruritis, rash. **Endo:** hyperglycemia, hyperuricemia. **F and E:** dehydration, hypocalcemia, hypochloremia, hypokalemia, hypomagnesemia, hyponatremia, hypovolemia, metabolic alkalosis. **Hemat:** APLASTIC ANEMIA, AGRANULOCYTOSIS, hemolytic anemia, leukopenia, thrombocytopenia. **MS:** muscle cramps. **Neuro:** paresthesia. **Misc:** fever, increased BUN, nephrocalcinosis.

Interactions

Drug-Drug: ↑ hypotension with **antihypertensives**, **nitrates**, or acute ingestion of **alcohol**. ↑ risk of hypokalemia with other **diuretics**, **amphotericin B**, **stimulant laxatives**, and **corticosteroids**. Hypokalemia may ↑ risk of **digoxin** toxicity and ↑ risk of arrhythmia in patients taking drugs that prolong the QT interval. ↓ **lithium** excretion, may cause **lithium** toxicity. ↑ risk of ototoxicity with **aminoglycosides**. **NSAIDS** ↓ effects of furosemide. ↓ effects of furosemide when given at same time as **sucralfate**, **cholestyramine**, or **colestipol**. ↑ risk of **salicylate** toxicity (with use of high-dose **salicylate** therapy).

Route/Dosage

Edema

PO (Adults): 20–80 mg/day as a single dose initially, may repeat in 6–8 hr; may increase dose by 20–40 mg q 6–8 hr until desired response. Maintenance doses may be given once or twice daily (doses up to 2.5 g/day have been used in patients with congestive heart failure or renal disease). *Hypertension*—40 twice daily initially (when added to regimen, decrease dose of other antihypertensives by 50%); adjust further dosing based on response; *Hypercalcemia*—120 mg/day in 1–3 doses.

PO (Children >1 month): 2 mg/kg as a single dose; may be increased by 1–2 mg/kg q 6–8 hr (maximum dose = 6 mg/kg).

PO (Neonates): 1–4 mg/kg/dose 1–2 times/day.

IM, IV (Adults): 20–40 mg, may repeat in 1–2 hr and increase by 20 mg every 1–2 hr until response is obtained, maintenance dose may be given q 6–12 hr; *Continuous infusion*—Bolus 0.1 mg/kg followed by 0.1 mg/kg/hr, double q 2 hr to a maximum of 0.4 mg/kg/hr.

IM, IV (Children): 1–2 mg/kg/dose q 6–12 hr *Continuous infusion*—0.05 mg/kg/hr, titrate to clinical effect.

IM, IV (Neonates): 1–2 mg/kg/dose q 12–24 hr.

Hypertension

PO (Adults): 40 twice daily initially (when added to regimen, decrease dose of other antihypertensives by 50%); adjust further dosing based on response.

Availability (generic available)

Tablets: 20 mg, 40 mg, 80 mg, ✱500 mg. **Cost:** *Generic*—20 mg $10.99/100, 40 mg $8.99/100, 80 mg $16.99/100. **Oral solution (10 mg/ml-orange flavor, 8 mg/ml-pineapple-peach flavor):** 8 mg/ml, 10 mg/ml. **Cost:** *Generic*—10 mg/ml $13.99/60 ml. **Solution for injection:** 10 mg/ml.

NURSING IMPLICATIONS

Assessment

- Assess fluid status. Monitor daily weight, intake and output ratios, amount and location of edema, lung sounds, skin turgor, and mucous membranes. Notify physician or other health care professional if thirst, dry mouth, lethargy, weakness, hypotension, or oliguria occurs.
- Monitor blood pressure and pulse before and during administration. Monitor frequency of prescription refills to determine compliance in patients treated for hypertension.
- Geri: Diuretic use is associated with increased risk for falls in older adults. Assess falls risk and implement fall prevention strategies.
- Assess patients receiving digoxin for anorexia, nausea, vomiting, muscle cramps, paresthesia, and confusion. Patients taking digoxin are at increased risk of digoxin toxicity because of the potassium-depleting effect of the diuretic. Potassium supplements or potassium-sparing diuretics may be used concurrently to prevent hypokalemia.
- Assess patient for tinnitus and hearing loss. Audiometry is recommended for patients receiving prolonged high-dose IV therapy. Hearing loss is most common after rapid or high-dose IV administration in patients with

decreased renal function or those taking other ototoxic drugs.

- Assess for allergy to sulfonamides.
- ***Lab Test Considerations:*** Monitor electrolytes, renal and hepatic function, serum glucose, and uric acid levels before and periodically throughout therapy. Commonly ↓ serum potassium. May cause ↓ serum sodium, calcium, and magnesium concentrations. May also cause ↑ BUN, serum glucose, creatinine, and uric acid levels.

Potential Nursing Diagnoses

Excess fluid volume (Indications)
Deficient fluid volume (Side Effects)

Implementation

- Do not confuse furosemide with torsemide.
- If administering twice daily, give last dose no later than 5pm to minimize disruption of sleep cycle.
- IV route is preferred over IM route for parenteral administration.
- **PO:** May be taken with food or milk to minimize gastric irritation. Tablets may be crushed if patient has difficulty swallowing.
- Do not administer discolored solution or tablets.

IV Administration

- **Direct IV:** ***Diluent:*** Administer undiluted (larger doses may be diluted and administered as intermittent infusion [see below]). ***Concentration:*** 10 mg/ml. ***Rate:*** Administer at a rate of 20 mg/min. Pedi: Administer at a maximum rate of 0.5 mg/kg/min (for doses <120 mg) or 4 mg/min (for doses >120 mg).
- **Intermittent Infusion:** ***Diluent:*** Dilute larger doses in 50 ml of D5W or 0.9% NaCl. Infusion stable for 24 hr at room temperature. Do not refrigerate. Protect from light. ***Concentration:*** Final concentration should not exceed 10 mg/ml. ***Rate:*** Administer at a rate not to exceed 4 mg/min (for doses >120 mg) in adults to prevent ototoxicity. Use an infusion pump to ensure accurate dosage.
- **Continuous Infusion:** ***Diluent:*** May dilute in D5W or 0.9% NaCl. May also administer as undiluted drug. Protect from light. ***Concentration:*** Final concentration should not exceed 10 mg/ml. ***Rate:*** See Route/Dosage section.
- **Y-Site Compatibility:** acyclovir, amikacin, aminophylline, amphotericin B cholesteryl sulfate, anidulafungin, argatroban, atropine, aztreonam, bivalirudin, calcium chloride, calcium gluconate, cefazolin, cefepime, cefotaxime, cefoxitin, ceftazidime, ceftizoxime, ceftriaxone, cefuroxime, chloramphenicol, clindamycin, cyclosporine, daptomycin, dexamethasone, digoxin, enalaprilat, epinephrine, ertapenem, fentanyl, ganciclovir, granisetron, heparin, hydrocortisone sodium succinate, hydromorphone, imipenem, insulin, ketorolac, lidocaine, linezolid, lorazepam, meropenem, methylprednisolone, metoprolol, metronidazole, micafungin, nafcillin, nitroglycerin, nitroprusside, palonosetron, pantoprazole, penicillin G potassium, phytonadione, piperacillin/tazobactam, potassium chloride, procainamide, propofol, propranolol, ranitidine, sodium bicarbonate, tacrolimus, thiopental, ticarcillin/clavulanate, tirofiban, tobramycin, vitamin B complex with C, voriconazole.
- **Y-Site Incompatibility:** azithromycin, caspofungin, cimetidine, ciprofloxacin, diazepam, diltiazem, diphenhydramine, doxycycline, droperidol, eptifibatide, erythromycin, esmolol, fenoldopam, filgrastim, hydroxyzine, labetalol, lansoprazole, levofloxacin, midazolam, milrinone, nesiritide, nicardipine, ondansetron, phenytoin, prochlorperazine, promethazine, protamine, quinupristin/dalfopristin, sulfamethoxazole/trimethoprim, vecuronium, vinblastine, vincristine, vinorelbine.

Patient/Family Teaching

- Instruct patient to take furosemide as directed. Take missed doses as soon as possible; do not double doses.
- Caution patient to change positions slowly to minimize orthostatic hypotension. Caution patient that the use of alcohol, exercise during hot weather, or standing for long periods during therapy may enhance orthostatic hypotension.
- Instruct patient to consult health care professional regarding a diet high in potassium (see Appendix L).
- Advise patient to notify health care professional of weight gain more than 3 lbs in one day.

- Advise patient to consult health care professional before taking OTC medication or herbal products concurrently with this therapy.
- Instruct patient to notify health care professional of medication regimen before treatment or surgery.
- Caution patient to use sunscreen and protective clothing to prevent photosensitivity reactions.
- Advise patient to contact health care professional immediately if muscle weakness, cramps, nausea, dizziness, numbness, or tingling of extremities occurs.
- Advise diabetic patients to monitor blood glucose closely; may cause increased blood glucose levels.
- Emphasize the importance of routine follow-up examinations.
- Geri: Caution older patients or their caregivers about increased risk for falls. Suggest strategies for fall prevention.
- **Hypertension:** Advise patients on antihypertensive regimen to continue taking medication even if feeling better. Furosemide controls but does not cure hypertension.
- Reinforce the need to continue additional therapies for hypertension (weight loss, exercise, restricted sodium intake, stress reduction, regular exercise, moderation of alcohol consumption, cessation of smoking).

Evaluation/Desired Outcomes

- Decrease in edema.
- Decrease in abdominal girth and weight.
- Increase in urinary output.
- Decrease in blood pressure.

gabapentin (ga-ba-**pen**-tin)
Neurontin

Classification
Therapeutic: analgesic adjuncts, anticonvulsants, mood stabilizers

Pregnancy Category C

Indications
Partial seizures (adjunct treatment). Post-herpetic neuralgia. **Unlabeled uses:** Chronic pain. Prevention of migraine headache. Bipolar disorder. Anxiety.

Action
Mechanism of action is not known. May affect transport of amino acids across and stabilize neuronal membranes. **Therapeutic Effects:** Decreased incidence of seizures. Decreased post-herpetic pain.

Pharmacokinetics
Absorption: Well absorbed after oral administration by active transport. At larger doses, transport becomes saturated and absorption decreases (bioavailability ranges from 60% for a 300-mg dose to 35% for a 1600-mg dose).
Distribution: Crosses blood-brain barrier; enters breast milk.
Metabolism and Excretion: Eliminated mostly by renal excretion of unchanged drug.
Half-life: 5–7 hr (normal renal function); up to 132 hr in anuria.

TIME/ACTION PROFILE (blood levels)

ROUTE	ONSET	PEAK	DURATION
PO	rapid	2–4 hr	8 hr

Contraindications/Precautions
Contraindicated in: Hypersensitivity.
Use Cautiously in: Renal insufficiency (↓ dose and/or ↑ dosing interval if CCr ≤60 ml/min); Geri: Geriatric patients (because of age-related ↓ in renal function); OB, Pedi: Safety not established for children <3 yr and pregnant women; Lactation: Discontinue drug or bottle-feed.

Adverse Reactions/Side Effects
CNS: confusion,, depression, drowsiness, sedation, anxiety, concentration difficulties (children), dizziness, emotional lability (children), hostility, hyperkinesia (children), malaise, vertigo, weakness. **EENT:** abnormal vision, nystagmus. **CV:** hypertension. **GI:** weight gain, anorexia, flatulence, gingivitis. **MS:** arthralgia. **Neuro:** ataxia, altered reflexes, hyperkinesia, paresthesia. **Misc:** facial edema.

Interactions
Drug-Drug: Antacids may ↓ absorption of gabapentin. ↑ risk of CNS depression with other **CNS depressants**, including **alcohol**, **antihistamines**, **opioids**, and **sedative/hypnotics**. **Morphine** ↑ gabapentin levels and may ↑ risk of toxicity, dosage adjustments may be required.
Drug-Natural Products: Kava kava, **valerian**, or **chamomile** can ↑ CNS depression.

Route/Dosage

Epilepsy
PO (Adults and Children >12 yr): 300 mg 3 times daily initially. Titration may be continued until desired (range is 900–1800 mg/day in 3 divided doses; doses should not be more than 12 hr apart). Doses up to 2400–3600 mg/day have been well tolerated.
PO (Children ≥5–12 yr): 10–15 mg/kg/day in 3 divided doses initially titrated upward over 3 days to 25–35 mg/kg/day in 3 divided doses; dosage interval should not exceed 12 hr (doses up to 50 mg/kg/day have been used).
PO (Children 3–4 yrs): 10–15 mg/kg/day in 3 divided doses initially titrated upward over 3 days to 40 mg/kg/day in 3 divided doses; dosage interval should not exceed 12 hr (doses up to 50 mg/kg/day have been used).

Renal Impairment
PO (Adults and Children >12 yr): *CCr 30–60 ml/min*—300 mg twice daily; *CCr 15–30 ml/min*—300 mg once daily; *CCr <15 ml/min*—300 mg once every other day; further adjustments are based on clinical response.

Post-Herpetic Neuralgia
PO (Adults): 300 mg once daily on first day, 300 mg twice daily on second day, then 300 mg three times/day on day 3, may then be titrated upward as needed up to 600 mg three times/day.

Availability (generic available)
Capsules: 100 mg, 300 mg, 400 mg. **Cost:** *Generic*—100 mg $64.96/270, 300 mg $169.97/270, 400 mg $209.98/270. **Tablets:** 100 mg, 300 mg, 400 mg, 600 mg, 800 mg.

Cost: *Generic*—600 mg $229.96/270, 800 mg $199.96/270. **Oral solution (cool strawberry anise flavor):** 250 mg/5 ml. **Cost:** $130.10/470 ml.

NURSING IMPLICATIONS

Assessment

- **Seizures:** Assess location, duration, and characteristics of seizure activity.
- **Postherpetic Neuralgia & Chronic Pain:** Assess location, characteristics, and intensity of pain periodically during therapy.
- **Migraine Prophylaxis:** Monitor frequecy and intensity of pain on pain scale.
- ***Lab Test Considerations:*** May cause false-positive readings when testing for urinary protein with *Ames N-Multistix SG* dipstick test; use sulfosalicylic acid precipitation procedure.
- May cause leukopenia.

Potential Nursing Diagnoses

Risk for injury (Side Effects)
Chronic pain (Indications)
Risk for aspiration (Adverse Reactions)
Ineffective coping (Indications)

Implementation

- **PO:** May be administered without regard to meals.
- 600 mg and 800 mg tablets are scored and can be broken to administer a half-tablet. If half-tablet is used, administer other half at the next dose. Discard half-tablets not used within several days.
- Gabapentin should be discontinued gradually over at least 1 wk. Abrupt discontinuation may cause increase in seizure frequency.

Patient/Family Teaching

- Instruct patient to take medication exactly as directed. Patients on tid dosing should not exceed 12 hr between doses. Take missed doses as soon as possible; if less than 2 hr until next dose, take dose immediately and take next dose 1–2 hr later, then resume regular dosing schedule. Do not double doses. Do not discontinue abruptly; may cause increase in frequency of seizures.
- Advise patient not to take gabapentin within 2 hr of an antacid.
- Gabapentin may cause dizziness and drowsiness. Caution patient to avoid driving or activities requiring alertness until response to medication is known. Seizure patients should not resume driving until physician gives clearance based on control of seizure disorder.
- Advise female patient to notify health care professional if pregnancy is planned or suspected or if she intends to breastfeed or is breastfeeding an infant.
- Instruct patient to notify health care professional of medication regimen before treatment or surgery.
- Advise patient to carry identification describing disease process and medication regimen at all times.
- Refer patients with bipolar disorder to Manic-Depressive and Depressive Association for support.

Evaluation/Desired Outcomes

- Decreased frequency of or cessation of seizures.
- Decreased post-herpetic neuralgia pain.
- Decreased intensity of chronic pain.
- Decreased frequency of migraine headaches.
- Increased mood stability.

galantamine (ga-lant-a-meen)
Razadyne, Razadyne ER

Classification
Therapeutic: anti-Alzheimer's agents
Pharmacologic: cholinergics (cholinesterase inhibitors)

Pregnancy Category B

Indications

Mild to moderate dementia of the Alzheimer's type.

Action

Enhances cholinergic function by reversible inhibition of cholinesterase. **Therapeutic Effects:** Decreased dementia (temporary) associated with Alzheimer's disease. Cognitive enhancer.

Pharmacokinetics

Absorption: Well absorbed (90%) following oral administration.
Distribution: Unknown.
Metabolism and Excretion: Mostly metabolized by the liver; 20% excreted unchanged in urine.
Half-life: 7 hr.

TIME/ACTION PROFILE (antihcholinesterase activity)

ROUTE	ONSET	PEAK	DURATION
PO	unknown	1 hr	12 hr
PO-ER	unknown	1 hr	24 hr

Contraindications/Precautions

Contraindicated in: Hypersensitivity; Severe hepatic or renal impairment; Children or lactation.

Use Cautiously in: Patients with supraventricular cardiac conduction defects or concurrent use of drugs that may slow heart rate (increased risk of bradycardia); History of ulcer disease/GI bleeding/concurrent NSAID use; Severe asthma or obstructive pulmonary disease; Mild to moderate renal impairment (avoid use if CCr <9 ml/min); Mild to moderate hepatic impairment (cautious dose titration recommended); May increase risk of cardiovascular mortality; OB: Use only if potential benefit outweighs potential risk to fetus.

Adverse Reactions/Side Effects

CNS: fatigue, dizziness, headache, syncope. **CV:** bradycardia, chest pain. **GI:** anorexia, diarrhea, dyspepsia, flatulence, nausea, vomiting. **GU:** bladder outflow obstruction, incontinence. **Neuro:** tremor. **Misc:** weight loss.

Interactions

Drug-Drug: Will ↑ neuromuscular blockade from **succinylcholine-type neuromuscular blocking agents**. May ↑ effects of other **cholinesterase inhibitors** or other **cholinergic agonists**, including **bethanechol**. May ↓ effectiveness of **anticholinergic medications**. Blood levels and effects may be ↑ by **ketoconazole**, **paroxetine**, **amitriptyline**, **fluvoxamine**, or **quinidine**.

Route/Dosage

PO (Adults): *Immediate-release tablets*—4 mg twice daily initially, dose increments of 4 mg should be made at 4 wk intervals, up to 12 mg twice daily. Doses up to 16 mg twice daily have been used (range 16–32 mg/day; *Extended-release capsules*—8mg/day as a single dose in the morning, may be increased to 16 mg/day after 4 wk, then up to 24 mg/day after 4 wk, increments based on benefit/tolerability.

Renal Impairment

PO (Adults): *Moderate renal impairment*—Daily dose should not exceed 16 mg.

Hepatic Impairment

PO (Adults): *Moderate hepatic impairment*—Daily dose should not exceed 16 mg.

Availability

Immediate-release tablets: 4 mg, 8 mg, 12 mg. **Extended-release capsules:** 8 mg, 16 mg, 24 mg. **Oral solution:** 4 mg/ml in 100 ml bottles.

G

NURSING IMPLICATIONS

Assessment

- Assess cognitive function (memory, attention, reasoning, language, ability to perform simple tasks) periodically during therapy.
- Monitor heart rate periodically during therapy. May cause bradycardia.

Potential Nursing Diagnoses

Disturbed thought process (Indications)
Risk for injury (Indications)
Impaired environmental interpretation syndrome (Indications)

Implementation

- Patient should be maintained on a stable dose for a minimum of 4 weeks prior to increasing dose.
- If dose has been interrupted for several days or longer, restart at the lowest dose and escalate to the current dose.
- **PO:** Administer twice daily, preferably with morning and evening meal. Administration with food, the use of antiemetic medications, and ensuring adequate fluid intake may decrease nausea and vomiting.
- Administer extended-release capsules in the morning, preferably with food. *Razadyne XR* can be opened and sprinkled on applesauce or yogurt; should be consumed within 10 min.
- Use pipette provided with oral solution to administer accurate amount.

Patient/Family Teaching

- Emphasize the importance of taking galantamine daily, as directed. Instruct patient and/or caregiver in correct use of pipette if using oral solution. Skip missed doses and return to regular schedule the following day; do not double doses. Do not discontinue abruptly;

although no increase in frequency of adverse events may occur, beneficial affects of galantamine are lost when the drug is discontinued.

- Caution patient and caregiver that galantamine may cause dizziness.
- Advise patient and caregiver to notify health care professional if nausea or vomiting persists beyond 7 days or if new symptoms occur or previously noted symptoms increase in severity.
- Advise patient and caregiver to notify health care professional of medication regimen prior to treatment or surgery.
- Emphasize the importance of follow-up exams to monitor progress.
- Teach patient and caregivers that improvements in cognitive functioning may take weeks to months to stabilize.
- Caution that disease is not cured and degenerative process is not reversed.

Evaluation/Desired Outcomes

- Improvement in cognitive function (memory, attention, reasoning, language, ability to perform simple tasks) in patients with Alzheimer's disease.

ganciclovir (gan-**sye**-kloe-vir)

Cytovene, Vitrasert

Classification

Therapeutic: antivirals

Pregnancy Category C

Indications

IV: Treatment of cytomegalovirus (CMV) retinitis in immunocompromised patients, including HIV-infected patients (may be used with foscarnet). Prevention of CMV infection in transplant patients at risk. **PO:** Maintenance treatment of stable CMV retinitis in immunocompromised patients after initial IV treatment and prevention of CMV retinitis in patients with advanced HIV infection.

Action

CMV converts ganciclovir to its active form (ganciclovir phosphate) inside the host cell, where it inhibits viral DNA polymerase. **Therapeutic Effects:** Antiviral effect directed preferentially against CMV-infected cells.

Pharmacokinetics

Absorption: 5–9% absorbed after oral administration. IV administration results in complete bioavailability. Action of intravitreal implant is local.

Distribution: Widely distributed; enters CSF.

Metabolism and Excretion: 90% excreted unchanged by the kidneys.

Half-life: 2.9 hr (increased in renal impairment).

TIME/ACTION PROFILE (antiviral levels)

ROUTE	ONSET	PEAK	DURATION
PO	rapid	1.8–3 hr	3–8 hr
IV	rapid	end of infusion	12–24 hr
Intravitreal	rapid	unknown	5–8 mo

Contraindications/Precautions

Contraindicated in: Hypersensitivity to ganciclovir or acyclovir.

Use Cautiously in: Renal impairment (dose reduction required if CCr <80 ml/min); Geriatric patients (dose reduction recommended); Bone marrow depression or immunosuppression; Pregnancy, lactation, or children (safety not established).

Adverse Reactions/Side Effects

CNS: SEIZURES, abnormal dreams, coma, confusion, dizziness, drowsiness, headache, malaise, nervousness. **EENT:** retinal detachment; *intravitreal only*—decreased visual acuity, vitreous hemorrhage, hyphema, intraocular pressure spikes, lens opacities, macular abnormalities, optic nerve changes, uveitis. **Resp:** dyspnea. **CV:** arrhythmias, edema, hypertension, hypotension. **GI:** GI BLEEDING, abdominal pain, increased liver enzymes, nausea, vomiting. **GU:** gonadal suppression, hematuria, renal toxicity. **Derm:** alopecia, photosensitivity, pruritus, rash, urticaria. **Endo:** hypoglycemia. **Hemat:** neutropenia, thrombocytopenia, anemia, eosinophilia. **Local:** pain/phlebitis at IV site. **Neuro:** ataxia, tremor. **Misc:** fever.

Interactions

Drug-Drug: ↑ risk of bone marrow depression with **antineoplastics**, **radiation therapy**, or **zidovudine**. Toxicity may be ↑ by **probenecid**. ↑ risk of seizures with **imipenem/cilastatin**. Concurrent use of other **nephrotoxic drugs**, **cyclosporine**, or **amphotericin B** ↑ risk of nephrotoxicity.

Route/Dosage

IV (Adults): *Induction*—5 mg/kg q 12 hr for 14–21 days. *Maintenance regimen*—5 mg/kg/day or 6 mg/kg for 5 days of each week. If progression occurs, increase to q 12 hr regimen.

Prevention—5 mg/kg q 12 hr for 7–14 days, then 5 mg/kg/day or 6 mg/kg for 5 days of each week.
PO (Adults): *Maintenance regimen*—1000 mg 3 times daily (with food) or 500 mg 6 times daily; *Prevention of CMV retinitis in advanced HIV infection*—1000 mg 3 times daily.
Intravitreal (Adults): 4.5 mg implant.

Availability (generic available)

Capsules: 250 mg, 500 mg. **Powder for injection:** 500 mg/vial. **Intravitreal insert:** 4.5 mg.

NURSING IMPLICATIONS

Assessment

- Diagnosis of CMV retinitis should be determined by ophthalmoscopy before treatment with ganciclovir.
- Culture for CMV (urine, blood, throat) may be taken before administration. However, a negative CMV culture does not rule out CMV retinitis. If symptoms do not respond after several weeks, resistance to ganciclovir may have occurred. Ophthalmologic exams should be performed weekly during induction and every 2 wk during maintenance or more frequently if the macula or optic nerve is threatened. Progression of CMV retinitis may occur during or after ganciclovir treatment.
- Assess for signs of infection (fever, chills, cough, hoarseness, lower back or side pain, sore throat, difficult or painful urination). Notify physician or other health care professional if these symptoms occur.
- Assess for bleeding (bleeding gums, bruising, petechiae; guaiac stools, urine, and emesis). Avoid IM injections and taking rectal temperatures. Apply pressure to venipuncture sites for 10 min.
- ***Lab Test Considerations:*** Monitor neutrophil and platelet count at least every 2 days during bid therapy and weekly thereafter. Granulocytopenia usually occurs during the first 2 wk of treatment but may occur anytime during therapy. Do not administer if neutrophil count $<500/mm^3$ or platelet count $<25,000/mm^3$. Recovery begins within 3–7 days of discontinuation of therapy.
- Monitor BUN and serum creatinine at least once every 2 wk throughout therapy.
- Monitor liver function tests (AST, ALT, serum bilirubin, alkaline phosphatase) periodically during therapy. May cause ↑ levels.
- May cause ↓ blood glucose.

Potential Nursing Diagnoses

Risk for infection (Indications, Patient/Family Teaching)

Implementation

- Do not confuse Cytovene (ganciclovir) with Cytosar (cytarabine).
- Solution should be prepared in a biologic cabinet. Wear gloves, gown, and mask while handling medication. Discard IV equipment in specially designated containers.
- Do not administer subcut or IM; severe tissue irritation may result.
- **PO:** Administer capsules with food.
- **IV:** Observe infusion site for phlebitis. Rotate infusion site to prevent phlebitis.
- Maintain adequate hydration throughout therapy.

IV Administration

- **Intermittent Infusion:** Reconstitute 500 mg with 10 ml of sterile water for injection for a concentration of 50 mg/ml. Do not reconstitute with bacteriostatic water with parabens; precipitation will occur. Shake well to dissolve completely. Discard vial if particulate matter or discoloration occurs. Reconstituted solution is stable for 12 hr at room temperature; do not refrigerate.
- ***Diluent:*** Dilute in 100 ml of D5W, 0.9% NaCl, Ringer's or LR. Once diluted for infusion, solution should be used within 24 hr. Refrigerate but do not freeze. ***Concentration:*** 10 mg/ml. ***Rate:*** Administer slowly, via infusion pump, over 1 hr using an in-line filter. Rapid administration may increase toxicity.
- **Y-Site Compatibility:** allopurinol, amphotericin B cholesteryl sulfate, cisplatin, cyclophosphamide, docetaxel, doxorubicin liposome, enalaprilat, etoposide phosphate, filgrastim, fluconazole, granisetron, lansoprazole, linezolid, melphalan, methotrexate, paclitaxel, pemetrexed, propofol, remifentanil, teniposide, thiotepa.
- **Y-Site Incompatibility:** aldesleukin, amifostine, amsacrine, aztreonam, cefepime, cytarabine, doxorubicin, fludarabine, foscarnet, gemcitabine, ondansetron, piperacillin/

tazobactam, sargramostim, tacrolimus, vinorelbine.

Patient/Family Teaching

- Instruct patient to take ganciclovir with food, exactly as directed.
- Inform patient that ganciclovir is not a cure for CMV retinitis. Progression of retinitis may continue in immunocompromised patients during and after therapy. Advise patients to have regular ophthalmic exams at least every 6 wk. Duration of therapy for CMV prevention is based on the duration and degree of immunosuppression.
- Advise patient to notify health care professional if fever; chills; sore throat; other signs of infection; bleeding gums; bruising; petechiae; or blood in urine, stool, or emesis occurs. Caution patient to avoid crowds and persons with known infections. Instruct patient to use soft toothbrush and electric razor. Patient should be cautioned not to drink alcoholic beverages or take products containing aspirin or NSAIDs.
- Advise patient that ganciclovir may have teratogenic effects. A nonhormonal method of contraception should be used during and for at least 90 days after therapy.
- Caution patient to use sunscreen and protective clothing to prevent photosensitivity reactions.
- Emphasize the importance of frequent follow-up exams to monitor blood counts.

Evaluation/Desired Outcomes

- Management of the symptoms of CMV retinitis in immunocompromised patients.
- Prevention of CMV retinitis in transplant patients at risk.

gefitinib (je-fit-in-ib)

Iressa

Classification
Therapeutic: antineoplastics
Pharmacologic: enzyme inhibitors

Pregnancy Category D

Indications

Patients who are currently benefiting from or have benefited from gefitinib in the past for treatment of non-small cell lung cancer.

Action

Inhibits activation of kinases found in transmembrane cell surface receptors, including epidermal growth factor receptor (EGFR-TK). **Therapeutic Effects:** Death of rapidly replicating cells, particularly malignant ones.

Pharmacokinetics

Absorption: 60% absorbed following oral administration.
Distribution: Extensively distributed.
Metabolism and Excretion: Mostly metabolized by the liver (CYP3A4 enzyme system); excreted in feces, <4% excreted in urine.
Half-life: 48 hr.

TIME/ACTION PROFILE

ROUTE	ONSET	PEAK	DURATION
PO	unknown	unknown	unknown

Contraindications/Precautions

Contraindicated in: Hypersensitivity; OB: Pregnancy, lactation, children.
Use Cautiously in: Idiopathic pulmonary fibrosis (↑ risk of pulmonary toxicity); Concurrent use of strong inhibitors of the CYP3A4 enzyme system (may increase risk of toxicity).

Adverse Reactions/Side Effects

CNS: weakness. **EENT:** aberrant eyelash, conjunctivitis, corneal erosion/ulcer, eye pain, ↓ vision. **CV:** peripheral edema. **Resp:** PULMONARY TOXICITY, dyspnea. **GI:** diarrhea, nausea, vomiting, anorexia, hepatotoxicity, mouth ulceration. **Derm:** acne, dry skin, rash, pruritus. **Metab:** weight loss. **Misc:** allergic reactions including ANGIOEDEMA.

Interactions

Drug-Drug: Strong inducers of the CYP3A4 enzyme system, including **rifampin** and **phenytoin** ↓ blood levels and effects (consider ↑ dose of gefitinib to 500 mg/day). Strong inhibitors of the CYP3A4 enzyme system, including **ketoconazole** and **itraconazole** ↑ blood levels and effects (use with caution). Absorption and efficacy may be ↓ by **drugs that ↑ gastric pH** including **cimetidine** and **ranitidine**. May ↑ the risk of bleeding with **warfarin**. Concurrent use with **vinorelbine** may ↑ risk/severity of neutropenia.

Route/Dosage

PO (Adults): 250 mg once daily.

Availability

Tablets: 250 mg.

NURSING IMPLICATIONS

Assessment

- Assess for signs of pulmonary toxicity (dyspnea, cough, fever). If interstitial lung disease is confirmed, discontinue gefitinib and treat appropriately.

- Assess patient for eye symptoms such as pain during therapy. May require interruption of therapy and removal of aberrant eyelash. After symptoms and eye changes have resolved, may reinstate therapy.
- ***Lab Test Considerations:*** Monitor liver function tests periodically. May cause ↑ transaminases, bilirubin, and alkaline phosphatase. Discontinue gefitinib if elevations are severe.
- Monitor for changes in prothrombin time and INR in patients taking warfarin. May cause ↑ levels.

Potential Nursing Diagnoses

Diarrhea (Adverse Reactions)
Impaired skin integrity (Side Effects)
Ineffective breathing pattern (Adverse Reactions)

Implementation

- **PO:** Administer one tablet daily without regard to food.
- May interrupt therapy briefly (14 days) for patients with poorly tolerated diarrhea with dehydration or skin adverse reactions. Follow by restarting 250 mg dose.

Patient/Family Teaching

- Instruct patient to take gefitinib as directed.
- Advise patient to notify health care professional promptly if severe persistent diarrhea, nausea, vomiting, or anorexia occur; if shortness of breath or cough occur or worsen; or if eye irritation or other new symptoms develop.
- Instruct patient to notify health care professional if pregnancy is planned or suspected or if breastfeeding.

Evaluation/Desired Outcomes

- Decrease in size and spread of tumors in non-small cell lung cancer.

HIGH ALERT

gemcitabine (jem-**site**-a-been)

Gemzar

Classification
Therapeutic: antineoplastics
Pharmacologic: antimetabolites, nucleoside analogues

Pregnancy Category D

Indications

Pancreatic cancer (locally advanced or metastatic). Inoperable locally advanced/metastatic non-small cell lung cancer (with cisplatin). Metastatic breast cancer (with paclitaxel). Advanced ovarian cancer that has relapsed 6 months after completion of platinum-based therapy (with carboplatin).

Action

Interferes with DNA synthesis (cell-cycle phase–specific). **Therapeutic Effects:** Death of rapidly replicating cells, particularly malignant ones.

Pharmacokinetics

Absorption: IV administration results in complete bioavailability.
Distribution: Unknown.
Metabolism and Excretion: Converted in cells to active diphosphate and triphosphate metabolites; these are excreted primarily by the kidneys.
Half-life: 32–94 min.

TIME/ACTION PROFILE (effect on blood counts)

ROUTE	ONSET	PEAK	DURATION
IV	unknown	unknown	unknown

Contraindications/Precautions

Contraindicated in: Hypersensitivity; OB: Pregnancy or lactation.
Use Cautiously in: History of cardiovascular disease; Impaired hepatic or renal function (increased risk of toxicity); OB: Patients with child-bearing potential; Other chronic debilitating illness.

Adverse Reactions/Side Effects

Resp: PULMONARY TOXICITY, dyspnea, bronchospasm. **CV:** ARRHYTHMIAS, CEREBROVASCULAR ACCIDENT, MI, edema, hypertension. **GI:** HEPATOTOXICITY, diarrhea, nausea, stomatitis, transient elevation of hepatic transaminases, vomiting. **GU:** HEMOLYTIC UREMIC SYNDROME, hematuria, proteinuria. **Derm:** alopecia, rash. **Hemat:** anemia, leukopenia, thrombocytopenia. **Local:** injection site reactions. **Neuro:** paresthesias. **Misc:** flu-like symptoms, fever, anaphylactoid reactions.

Interactions

Drug-Drug: ↑ bone marrow depression with other **antineoplastics** or **radiation therapy**. May ↓ antibody response to **live virus vaccines** and ↑ risk of adverse reactions.

Route/Dosage

Other regimens are used.

Pancreatic Cancer

IV (Adults): 1000 mg/m² once weekly for 7 wk, followed by a week of rest. May be followed by cycles of once-weekly administration for 3 wk followed by a week of rest.

Non-Small Cell Lung Cancer (with Cisplatin)

IV (Adults): 1000 mg/m² on days 1, 8, and 15 of each 28-day cycle (cisplatin is also given on day 1) *or* 1250 mg/m² on days 1 and 8 of each 21-day cycle (cisplatin is also given on day 1).

Breast Cancer

IV (Adults): 1250 mg/m² on days 1 and 8 of each 21-day cycle (paclitaxel is also given on day 1).

Ovarian Cancer

IV (Adults): 1000 mg/m² on days 1 and 8 of each 21–day cycle.

Availability

Powder for injection: 200 mg in 10-ml vial, 1 g in 50-ml vial. **Cost:** 200 mg $117.95/10-ml vial, 1 g $589.90/50-ml vial.

NURSING IMPLICATIONS

Assessment

- Monitor vital signs before and frequently during therapy.
- Assess injection site during administration. Although gemcitabine is not considered a vesicant, local reactions may occur.
- Monitor for bone marrow depression. Assess for bleeding (bleeding gums, bruising, petechiae; guaiac stools, urine, and emesis) and avoid IM injections and taking rectal temperatures if platelet count is low. Apply pressure to venipuncture sites for 10 min. Assess for signs of infection during neutropenia. Anemia may occur. Monitor for increased fatigue, dyspnea, and orthostatic hypotension.
- Monitor intake and output, appetite, and nutritional intake. Mild to moderate nausea and vomiting occur frequently. Antiemetics may be used prophylactically.
- ***Lab Test Considerations:*** Monitor CBC, including differential and platelet count, before each dose. Dose guidelines are based on the CBC. *For single-agent use:* If the absolute granulocyte count is >1000 and platelet count is >100,000, the full dose may be administered. If the absolute granulocyte count is 500–999 or platelet count is 50,000–99,000, 75% of the dose may be given. If the absolute granulocyte count is <500 or the platelet count is <50,000, withhold further doses. *For gemcitabine with paclitaxel (breast cancer):* If the absolute granulocyte count is >1200 and platelet count is >75,000, the full dose may be administered. If the absolute granulocyte count is 1000–1199 or platelet count is 50,000–75,000, 75% of the dose may be given. If the absolute granulocyte count is 700–999 or platelet count is ≥50,000, 50% of the dose may be given. If the absolute granulocyte count is <700 or the platelet count is <50,000, withhold further doses.
- Monitor serum creatinine, potassium, calcium, and magnesium in patients taking cisplatin with gemcitabine. *For gemcitabine with carboplatin (ovarian cancer):* If the absolute granulocyte count is >1500 and platelet count is >100,000, the full dose may be administered. If the absolute granulocyte count is 1000–1499 or platelet count is 75,000–99,000, 75% of the dose may be given. If the absolute granulocyte count is <1000 or the platelet count is <75,000, withhold further doses.
- Monitor hepatic and renal function before and periodically during therapy. May cause transient ↑ in serum AST, ALT, alkaline phosphatase, and bilirubin concentrations.
- May also cause ↑ BUN and serum creatinine concentrations, proteinuria, and hematuria.

Potential Nursing Diagnoses

Risk for infection (Adverse Reactions)

Implementation

- ***High Alert:*** Fatalities have occurred with incorrect administration of chemotherapeutic agents. Before administering, clarify all ambiguous orders; double-check single, daily, and course-of-therapy dose limits; have second practitioner independently double-check original order, calculations and infusion pump settings.

- Solution should be prepared in a biologic cabinet. Wear gloves, gown, and mask while handling IV medication. Discard IV equipment in specially designated containers.

IV Administration

- **Intermittent Infusion:** To reconstitute, add 5 ml of 0.9% NaCl without preservatives to 200-mg vial or 25 ml of 0.9% NaCl to the 1-g vial of gemcitabine for a concentration of 40 mg/ml. Incomplete dissolution may result in concentrations greater than 40 mg/ml. ***Diluent:*** May be further diluted with 0.9% NaCl. Solution is colorless to light straw color. Do not administer solutions that are discolored or contain particulate matter. Solution is stable for 24 hr at room temperature. Discard unused portions. Do not refrigerate; crystallization may occur. ***Concentration:*** 0.1–38 mg/ml. ***Rate:*** Administer dose over 30 min. Infusions longer than 60 min have a greater incidence of toxicity.
- **Y-Site Compatibility:** amifostine, amikacin, aminophylline, ampicillin, ampicillin/sulbactam, aztreonam, bleomycin, bumetanide, buprenorphine, butorphanol, calcium gluconate, carboplatin, carmustine, cefazolin, cefotetan, cefoxitin, ceftazidime, ceftizoxime, ceftriaxone, cefuroxime, chlorpromizine, cimetidine, ciprofloxacin, cisplatin, clindamycin, cyclophosphamide, cytarabine, dactinomycin, daunorubicin, dexrazoxane, diphenhydramine, dobutamine, docetaxel, dopamine, doxorubicin, doxycycline, droperidol, enalaprilat, etoposide, etoposide phosphate, famotidine, floxuridine, fluconazole, fludarabine, fluorouracil, gentamicin, granisetron, haloperidol, heparin, hydrocortisone, hydromorphone, idarubicin, ifosfamide, leucoverin, linezolid, lorazepam, mannitol, meperidine, mesna, metoclopramide, metronidazole, mitoxantrone, morphine, nalbuphine, ofloxacin, ondansetron, oxaliplatin, paclitaxel, potassium chloride, promethazine, ranitidine, sodium bicarbonate, streptozocin, teniposide, thiotepa, ticarcillin/clavulanate, tobramycin, topotecan, trimethoprim/sulfamethoxazole, vancomycin, vinblastine, vincristine, vinorelbine, zidovudine.
- **Y-Site Incompatibility:** acyclovir, amphotericin B, cefotaxime, furosemide, ganciclovir, imipenem-cilastatin, irinotecan, lansoprazole, methotrexate, methoprednisolone, mitomycin, pemetrexed, piperacillin, piperacillin/tazobactam, prochlorperazine.

Patient/Family Teaching

- Instruct patient to notify health care professional if fever; chills; sore throat; signs of infection; bleeding gums; bruising; petechiae; or blood in urine, stool, or emesis occurs. Caution patient to avoid crowds and persons with known infections. Instruct patient to use soft toothbrush and electric razor. Patient should be cautioned not to drink alcoholic beverages or take products containing aspirin or NSAIDs.
- Instruct patient to inspect oral mucosa for erythema and ulceration. If ulceration occurs, advise patient to use sponge brush and rinse mouth with water after eating and drinking. Stomatitis pain may require management with opioid analgesics.
- Instruct patient to notify health care professional if flu-like symptoms (fever, anorexia, headache, cough, chills, myalgia), swelling of the feet or legs, or shortness of breath occurs.
- Discuss with patient the possibility of hair loss. Explore methods of coping.
- Advise patient that this medication may have teratogenic effects. Contraception should be used during therapy.
- Instruct patient not to receive any vaccinations without advice of health care professional.
- Emphasize the need for periodic lab tests to monitor for side effects.

Evaluation/Desired Outcomes

- Palliative, symptomatic improvement in patients with pancreatic cancer.
- Decrease in size and spread of malignancy in lung, ovarian, and breast cancer.

gemfibrozil (gem-**fye**-broe-zil)

Lopid

Classification

Therapeutic: lipid-lowering agents

Pharmacologic: fibric acid derivatives

Pregnancy Category C

Indications

Management of type II-b hyperlipidemia (decreased HDLs, increased LDLs, increased triglycerides) in patients who do not yet have clinical coronary artery disease and have failed therapy with diet, exercise, weight loss, or other agents (niacin, bile acid sequestrants).

Action
Inhibits peripheral lipolysis. Decreases triglyceride production by the liver. Decreases production of the triglyceride carrier protein. Increases HDL. **Therapeutic Effects:** Decreased plasma triglycerides and increased HDL.

Pharmacokinetics
Absorption: Well absorbed after oral administration.
Distribution: Unknown.
Metabolism and Excretion: Some metabolism by the liver, 70% excreted by the kidneys (mostly unchanged), 6% excreted in feces.
Half-life: 1.3–1.5 hr.

TIME/ACTION PROFILE (triglyceride-VLDL–lowering effect)

ROUTE	ONSET	PEAK	DURATION
PO	2–5 days	4 wk	several mo

Contraindications/Precautions
Contraindicated in: Hypersensitivity; Primary biliary cirrhosis; Concurrent use of HMG-CoA reductase inhibitors.
Use Cautiously in: Gallbladder disease; Liver disease; Severe renal impairment; Pregnancy, lactation, or children (safety not established).

Adverse Reactions/Side Effects
CNS: dizziness, headache. **EENT:** blurred vision. **GI:** abdominal pain, diarrhea, epigastric pain, flatulence, gallstones, heartburn, nausea, vomiting. **Derm:** alopecia, rashes, urticaria. **Hemat:** anemia, leukopenia. **MS:** myositis.

Interactions
Drug-Drug: May ↑ the effects of **warfarin** or **sulfonylurea oral hypoglycemic agents**. Concurrent use with **HMG-CoA reductase inhibitors** may ↑ the risk of rhabdomyolysis (avoid concurrent use). May ↓ the effect of **cyclosporine**.

Route/Dosage
PO (Adults): 600 mg twice daily 30 min before breakfast and dinner.

Availability (generic available)
Tablets: 600 mg. **Cost:** *Generic*—$45.97/180. **Capsules:** ✤300 mg.

NURSING IMPLICATIONS

Assessment
- Obtain patient's diet history, especially regarding fat and alcohol consumption.
- ***Lab Test Considerations:*** Serum triglyceride and cholesterol levels should be monitored before and periodically throughout therapy. LDL and VLDL levels should be assessed before and periodically throughout therapy. Medication should be discontinued if paradoxical increase in lipid levels occurs.
- Liver function tests should be assessed before and periodically throughout therapy. May cause an increase in serum bilirubin, alkaline phosphatase, CK, LDH, AST, and ALT. If hepatic function tests rise significantly, therapy should be discontinued and not resumed.
- CBC and electrolytes should be evaluated every 3–6 mo and then yearly throughout course of therapy. May cause mild decrease in hemoglobin, hematocrit, and leukocyte counts. May cause a decrease in serum potassium concentrations.
- May cause slight increase in serum glucose.

Potential Nursing Diagnoses
Noncompliance (Patient/Family Teaching)

Implementation
- Do not confuse Lopid (gemfibrozil) with Levbid (hyoscyamine).
- **PO:** Administer 30 min before breakfast or dinner.

Patient/Family Teaching
- Instruct patient to take medication exactly as directed, not to skip doses or double up on missed doses. If a dose is missed, take as soon as remembered unless almost time for next dose.
- Advise patient that this medication should be used in conjunction with dietary restrictions (fat, cholesterol, carbohydrates, alcohol), exercise, and cessation of smoking.
- Instruct patient to notify health care professional promptly if any of the following symptoms occur: severe stomach pains with nausea and vomiting, fever, chills, sore throat, rash, diarrhea, muscle cramping, general abdominal discomfort, or persistent flatulence.

Evaluation/Desired Outcomes
- Decrease in serum triglyceride and cholesterol levels and improved HDL to total cholester-

ol ratios. If response is not seen within 3 mo, medication is usually discontinued.

gemifloxacin, See FLUOROQUINOLONES.

gentamicin, See AMINOGLYCOSIDES.

glimepiride, See HYPOGLYCEMIC AGENTS, ORAL.

glipiZIDE, See HYPOGLYCEMIC AGENTS, ORAL.

glucagon (gloo-ka-gon)

GlucaGen

Classification

Therapeutic: hormones

Pharmacologic: pancreatics

Pregnancy Category B

Indications

Acute management of severe hypoglycemia when administration of glucose is not feasible. Facilitation of radiographic examination of the GI tract. **Unlabeled uses:** Antidote to: Beta blockers, Calcium channel blockers.

Action

Stimulates hepatic production of glucose from glycogen stores (glycogenolysis). Relaxes the musculature of the GI tract (stomach, duodenum, small bowel, and colon), temporarily inhibiting movement. Has positive inotropic and chronotropic effects. **Therapeutic Effects:** Increase in blood glucose. Relaxation of GI musculature, facilitating radiographic examination.

Pharmacokinetics

Absorption: Well absorbed following IM and subcut administration.

Distribution: Unknown.

Metabolism and Excretion: Extensively metabolized by the liver, plasma, and kidneys.

Half-life: 8–18 min.

TIME/ACTION PROFILE

ROUTE	ONSET	PEAK	DURATION
IM (hyperglycemic action)	within 10 min	30 min	12–27 min
IV (hyperglycemic action)	1 min	5 min	9–17 min
Subcut (hyperglycemic action)	within 10 min	30–45 min	60–90 min
IV (effect on GI musculature)	45 sec (for 0.25–2-mg dose)	unknown	9–17 min (0.25–0.5-mg dose); 22–25 min (2-mg dose)
IM (effect on GI musculature)	8–10 min (1-mg dose); 4–7 min (2-mg dose)	unknown	9–27 min (1-mg dose); 21–32 min (2-mg dose)

Contraindications/Precautions

Contraindicated in: Hypersensitivity; Pheochromocytoma; Some products contain glycerin and phenol—avoid use in patients with hypersensitivities to these ingredients.

Use Cautiously in: History suggestive of insulinoma or pheochromocytoma; Prolonged fasting, starvation, adrenal insufficiency or chronic hypoglycemia (low levels of releasable glucose); When used to inhibit GI motility, use cautiously in geriatric patient with cardiac disease or diabetics; OB: Should be used during pregnancy only if clearly needed; Lactation: Safety not established.

Adverse Reactions/Side Effects

CV: hypotension. **GI:** <u>nausea</u>, <u>vomiting</u>. **Misc:** hypersensitivity reactions including ANAPHYLAXIS.

Interactions

Drug-Drug: Large doses may enhance the effect of **warfarin**. Negates the response to **insulin** or **oral hypoglycemic agents**. **Phenytoin** inhibits the stimulant effect of glucagon on insulin release. Hyperglycemic effect is intensified and prolonged by **epinephrine**. Patients on concurrent **beta blocker** therapy may have a greater increase in heart rate and blood pressure.

Route/Dosage

Hypoglycemia

IV, IM, Subcut (Adults and Children ≥20 kg): 1 mg; may be repeated in 15 min if necessary.

IV, IM, Subcut (Children <20 kg): 0.5 mg or 0.02–0.03 mg/kg; may be repeated in 15 min if necessary.

Radiographic Examination of the GI Tract

IM, IV (Adults): 0.25–2 mg; depending on location and duration of examination (0.5 mg IV or 2 mg IM for relaxation of stomach, for examination of the colon 2 mg IM 10 min before procedure).

Antidote (unlabeled)

IV (Adults): *To beta blockers*—50–150 mcg (0.05–0.15 mg)/kg, followed by 1–5 mg/hr infusion. *To calcium channel blockers*—2 mg; additional doses determined by response.

Availability

Powder for injection: 1-mg (equivalent to 1 unit) vials as an emergency kit for low blood glucose and a diagnostic kit.

NURSING IMPLICATIONS

Assessment

- Assess for signs of hypoglycemia (sweating, hunger, weakness, headache, dizziness, tremor, irritability, tachycardia, anxiety) prior to and periodically during therapy.
- Assess neurologic status throughout therapy. Institute safety precautions to protect patient from injury caused by seizures, falling, or aspiration. For insulin shock therapy, 0.5–1 mg is administered after 1 hr of coma; patient usually awakens in 10–25 min. If no response occurs, repeat the dose. Feed patient supplemental carbohydrates orally to replenish liver glycogen and prevent secondary hypoglycemia as soon as possible after awakening, especially pediatric patients.
- Assess nutritional status. Patients who lack liver glycogen stores (starvation, chronic hypoglycemia, adrenal insufficiency) will require glucose instead of glucagon.
- Assess for nausea and vomiting after administration of dose. Protect patients with depressed level of consciousness from aspiration by positioning on side; ensure that a suction unit is available. Notify health care professional if vomiting occurs; patient will require parenteral glucose to prevent recurrent hypoglycemia.
- ***Lab Test Considerations:*** Monitor serum glucose levels throughout episode, during treatment, and for 3–4 hr after patient regains consciousness. Use of bedside fingerstick blood glucose determination methods is recommended for rapid results. Follow-up lab results may be ordered to validate fingerstick values, but do not delay treatment while awaiting lab results, as this could result in neurologic injury or death.
- Large doses of glucagon may cause a ↓ in serum potassium concentrations.

Potential Nursing Diagnoses

Risk for injury (Indications)
Noncompliance (Patient/Family Teaching)

Implementation

- May be given subcut, IM, or IV. Reconstitute with diluent supplied in kit by manufacturer. Inspect solution prior to use; use only clear, water-like solution. Solution is stable for 48 hr if refrigerated, 24 hr at room temperature. Unmixed medication should be stored at room temperature.
- Administer supplemental carbohydrates IV or orally to facilitate increase of serum glucose levels.

IV Administration

- **Direct IV:** ***Diluent:*** Reconstitute each vial with 1 ml of an appropriate diluent. For doses ≤2 mg, use diluent provided by manufacturer. For doses >2 mg, use sterile water for injection instead of diluent supplied by manufacturer to minimize risk of thrombophlebitis, CNS toxicity, and myocardial depression from phenol preservative in diluent supplied by manufacturer. Reconstituted vials should be used immediately. ***Concentration:*** Not exceed 1 mg/ml. ***Rate:*** Administer at a rate not exceeding 1 mg/min. May be administered through IV line containing D5W.
- **Continuous Infusion:** ***Diluent:*** Reconstitute vials as per directions above (use sterile water for injection). Further dilute 10 mg of glucagon in 100 ml of D5W. ***Concentration:*** 0.1 mg/ml. ***Rate:*** See Route/Dosage section.
- **Y-Site Compatibility:** No information available.

Patient/Family Teaching

- Teach patient and family signs and symptoms of hypoglycemia. Instruct patient to take oral glucose as soon as symptoms of hypoglycemia occur—glucagon is reserved for episodes when patient is unable to swallow because of decreased level of consciousness.
- **Home Care Issues:** Instruct family on correct technique to prepare, draw up, and

administer injection. Health care professional must be contacted immediately after each dose for orders regarding further therapy or adjustment of insulin dose or diet.

- Advise family that patient should receive oral glucose when alertness returns.
- Instruct family to position patient on side until fully alert. Explain that glucagon may cause nausea and vomiting. Aspiration may occur if patient vomits while lying on back.
- Instruct patient to check expiration date monthly and to replace outdated medication immediately.
- Review hypoglycemic medication regimen, diet, and exercise programs.
- Patients with diabetes mellitus should carry a source of sugar (such as a packet of sugar or candy) and identification describing disease process and treatment regimen at all times.

Evaluation/Desired Outcomes

- Increase of serum glucose to normal levels with improved level of consciousness.
- Smooth muscle relaxation of the stomach, duodenum, and small and large intestine in patients undergoing radiologic examination of the GI tract.

glyBURIDE, See HYPOGLYCEMIC AGENTS, ORAL.

glycopyrrolate

(glye-koe-**pye**-roe-late)

Robinul, Robinul-Forte

Classification

Therapeutic: antispasmodics

Pharmacologic: anticholinergics

Pregnancy Category B

Indications

Inhibits salivation and excessive respiratory secretions when given preoperatively. Reverses some of the secretory and vagal actions of cholinesterase inhibitors used to treat nondepolarizing neuromuscular blockade (cholinergic adjunct). Adjunctive management of peptic ulcer disease.

Action

Inhibits the action of acetylcholine at postganglionic sites located in smooth muscle, secretory glands, and the CNS (antimuscarinic activity). Low doses decrease sweating, salivation, and respiratory secretions. Intermediate doses result in increased heart rate. Larger doses decrease GI and GU tract motility. **Therapeutic Effects:** Decreased GI and respiratory secretions.

Pharmacokinetics

Absorption: Incompletely absorbed (10%) after oral administration. Well absorbed after IM administration.

Distribution: Distribution not fully known. Does not significantly cross the blood-brain barrier or eye. Crosses the placenta.

Metabolism and Excretion: Eliminated primarily unchanged in the feces, via biliary excretion.

Half-life: 1.7 hr (0.6–4.6 hr).

TIME/ACTION PROFILE (anticholinergic effects)

ROUTE	ONSET	PEAK	DURATION
PO	1 hr	unknown	8–12 hr
IM	15–30 min	30–45 min	2–7 hr*
IV	1–10 min	unknown	2–7 hr*

*Antisecretory effect lasts up to 7 hr; vagal blockade lasts 2–3 hr

Contraindications/Precautions

Contraindicated in: Hypersensitivity; Angle-closure glaucoma; Acute hemorrhage; Tachycardia secondary to cardiac insufficiency or thyrotoxicosis; Pedi: Injection contains benzyl alcohol and should not be given to neonates; Myasthenia gravis; Obstructive uropathy; Paralytic ileus.

Use Cautiously in: Geri: Geriatric have increased sensitivity to anticholinergic drugs and are more susceptible to adverse reactions. Pedi: Young children and infants have increased sensitivity to anticholinergic drugs and are more susceptible to adverse reactions; Patients who may have intra-abdominal infections; Prostatic hyperplasia; Chronic renal, hepatic, pulmonary, or cardiac disease; Down syndrome and children with spastic paralysis or brain damage (may be hypersensitive to antimuscarinic effects); Pregnancy and lactation (safety not established).

Adverse Reactions/Side Effects

CNS: confusion, drowsiness. **EENT:** blurred vision, cycloplegia, dry eyes, mydriasis. **CV:** tachycardia, orthostatic hypotension, palpitations. **GI:** dry mouth, constipation. **GU:** urinary hesitancy, retention.

Interactions

Drug-Drug: Additive anticholinergic effects with other **anticholinergics**, including **antihistamines**, **phenothiazines, meperidine, amantadine, tricyclic antidepressants**, **quinidine**, and **disopyramide**. May alter the absorption of other **orally administered drugs** by slowing motility of the GI tract. **Antacids** or **adsorbent antidiarrheal agents** ↓ absorption of anticholinergics. May ↑ GI mucosal lesions in patients taking oral **potassium chloride** tablets. ↑ risk of adverse cardiovascular reactions with **cyclopropane** anesthesia. Concurrent use may ↓ absorption of **ketoconazole** (administer 2 hr after ketoconazole).

Route/Dosage

Control of Secretions during Surgery

IM (Adults): 4.4 mcg/kg 30–60 min preop (not to exceed 0.1 mg).
IM (Children >2 yr): 4.4 mcg/kg 30–60 min preop.
IM (Children <2 yr): 4.4–8.8 mcg/kg 30–60 min preop.

Control of Secretions (chronic)

IM, IV (Children): 4–10 mcg/kg/dose q 3–4 hr.
PO (Children): 40–100 mcg/kg/dose 3–4 times/day.

Cholinergic Adjunct

IV (Adults and Children): 200 mcg for each 1 mg of neostigmine or 5 mg of pyridostigmine given at the same time.

Antiarrhythmic

IV (Adults): 100 mcg, may be repeated q 2–3 min.
IV (Children): 4.4 mcg/kg (up to 100 mcg); may be repeated q 2–3 min.

Peptic Ulcer

PO (Adults): 1–2 mg 2–3 times daily. An additional 2 mg may be given at bedtime; may be decreased to 1 mg twice daily (not to exceed 8 mg/day).
IM, IV (Adults): 100–200 mcg q 4 hr up to 4 times daily.

Availability (generic available)

Tablets: 1 mg, 2 mg. **Injection:** 200 mcg (0.2 mg)/ml.

NURSING IMPLICATIONS

Assessment

- Assess heart rate, blood pressure, and respiratory rate before and periodically during parenteral therapy.
- Pedi: Assess for hyperexcitability, a paradoxical response that may occur in children.
- Monitor intake and output ratios in geriatric or surgical patients; glycopyrrolate may cause urinary retention. Instruct patient to void before parenteral administration.
- Assess patient routinely for abdominal distention and auscultate for bowel sounds. If constipation becomes a problem, increasing fluids and adding bulk to the diet may help alleviate the constipating effects of the drug.
- Periodic intraocular pressure determinations should be made for patients receiving long-term therapy.
- ***Lab Test Considerations:*** Antagonizes effects of pentagastrin and histamine during the gastric acid secretion test. Avoid administration for 24 hr preceding the test.
- May cause ↓ uric acid levels in patients with gout or hyperuricemia.
- ***Toxicity and Overdose:*** If overdosage occurs, neostigmine is the antidote.

Potential Nursing Diagnoses

Impaired oral mucous membrane (Side Effects)
Constipation (Side Effects)

Implementation

- Do not administer cloudy or discolored solution.
- **PO:** Administer 30–60 min before meals to maximize absorption.
- Do not administer within 1 hr of antacids or antidiarrheal medications.
- Oral dose is 10 times the parenteral dose.
- **IM:** May be administered undiluted (200 mcg/ml).

IV Administration

- **Direct IV:** ***Diluent:*** May be given undiluted through Y-site. ***Concentration:*** 200 mcg/ml. ***Rate:*** Administer at a maximum rate of 20 mcg over 1 min.
- **Syringe Compatibility:** chlorpromazine, cimetidine, codeine, diphenhydramine, droperidol, hydromorphone, hydroxyzine, levorphanol, lidocaine, meperidine, midazolam,

morphine, nalbuphine, neostigmine, ondansetron, oxymorphone, prochlorperazine, promethazine, pyridostigmine, ranitidine, triflupromazine.
- **Syringe Incompatibility:** chloramphenicol, dexamethasone, diazepam, dimenhydrinate, methohexital, pentazocine, pentobarbital, secobarbital, sodium bicarbonate, thiopental.
- **Y-Site Compatibility:** propofol.
- **Solution Compatibility:** D5/0.45% NaCl, D5W, 0.9% NaCl, Ringer's solution. Administer immediately after admixing.
- **Additive Incompatibility:** methylprednisolone sodium succinate.

Patient/Family Teaching

- Instruct patient to take glycopyrrolate exactly as directed and not to take more than the prescribed amount. Take missed doses as soon as remembered if not just before next dose.
- Medication may cause drowsiness and blurred vision. Caution patient to avoid driving or other activities requiring alertness until response to the medication is known.
- Inform patient that frequent oral rinses, sugarless gum or candy, and good oral hygiene may help relieve dry mouth. Consult health care professional regarding use of saliva substitute if dry mouth persists for more than 2 wk.
- Advise patient to change positions slowly to minimize the effects of drug-induced orthostatic hypotension.
- Caution patient to avoid extremes of temperature. This medication decreases the ability to sweat and may increase the risk of heat stroke.
- Advise patient to notify health care professional immediately if eye pain or increased sensitivity to light occurs. Emphasize the importance of routine eye exams throughout therapy.
- Advise patient to consult health care professional before taking any OTC medications concurrently with this therapy.
- Geri: Advise geriatric patients about increased susceptibility to side effects and to call health care professional immediately if they occur.

Evaluation/Desired Outcomes

- Mouth dryness preoperatively.
- Reversal of cholinergic medications.
- Decrease in GI motility and pain in patients with peptic ulcer disease.

granisetron (gra-**nees**-e-tron)
Kytril

Classification
Therapeutic: antiemetics
Pharmacologic: $5\text{-}HT_3$ antagonists

Pregnancy Category B

Indications

Prevention of nausea and vomiting due to: emetogenic chemotherapy, radiation therapy. Prevention and treatment of postoperative nausea and vomiting.

Action

Blocks the effects of serotonin at receptor sites (selective antagonist) located in vagal nerve terminals and in the chemoreceptor trigger zone in the CNS. **Therapeutic Effects:** Decreased incidence and severity of nausea and vomiting following emetogenic chemotherapy, radiation therapy or surgery.

Pharmacokinetics

Absorption: 50% absorbed following oral administration.
Distribution: Distributes into erythrocytes; remainder of distribution is unknown.
Metabolism and Excretion: Mostly metabolized by the liver; 12% excreted unchanged in urine.
Half-life: *Patients with cancer*—8–9 hr (range 0.9–31.1 hr); *healthy volunteers*—4.9 hr (range 0.9–15.2 hr); *geriatric patients*—7.7 hr (range 2.6–17.7 hr).

TIME/ACTION PROFILE

ROUTE	ONSET	PEAK	DURATION
PO	rapid	60 min	24 hr
IV	rapid	30 min	up to 24 hr

Contraindications/Precautions

Contraindicated in: Hypersensitivity; Some products contain benzyl alcohol; avoid use in neonates.
Use Cautiously in: OB: Pregnancy or lactation (safety not established); Pedi: Children <2 yr (safe use of IV route not established); Pedi: Chil-

dren <18 yr (safe use of PO route not established).

Adverse Reactions/Side Effects

CNS: headache, agitation, anxiety, CNS stimulation, drowsiness, weakness. **CV:** hypertension. **GI:** constipation, diarrhea, elevated liver enzymes, taste disorder. **Misc:** anaphylactoid reactions, fever.

Interactions

Drug-Drug: ↑ risk of extrapyramidal reactions with other **agents causing extrapyramidal reactions**.

Route/Dosage

Prevention of Nausea and Vomiting Due to Emetogenic Chemotherapy

PO (Adults): 1 mg twice daily; 1st dose given at least 60 min prior to chemotherapy and 2nd dose 12 hr later only on days when chemotherapy is administered; may also be given as 2 mg once daily at least 60 min prior to chemotherapy.
IV (Adults and Children 2–16 yr): 10 mcg/kg within 30 min prior to chemotherapy.

Prevention of Nausea and Vomiting Associated with Radiation Therapy

PO (Adults): 2 mg taken once daily within 1 h of radiation therapy.

Prevention and Treatment of Postoperative Nausea and Vomiting

IV (Adults): *Prevention*—1 mg prior to induction or anesthesia or just prior to reversal of anesthesia; *Treatment*—1 mg.

Availability

Tablets: 1 mg. **Cost:** $131.99/2. **Oral solution (orange flavor):** 2 mg/10 ml in 30 ml bottles. **Solution for injection:** 1 mg/ml.

NURSING IMPLICATIONS

Assessment

- Assess patient for nausea, vomiting, abdominal distention, and bowel sounds prior to and following administration.
- Assess for extrapyramidal symptoms (involuntary movements, facial grimacing, rigidity, shuffling walk, trembling of hands) during therapy. This occurs rarely and is usually associated with concurrent use of other drugs known to cause this effect.
- ***Lab Test Considerations:*** May cause ↑ AST and ALT levels.

Potential Nursing Diagnoses

Imbalanced nutrition: less than body requirements (Indications)

Implementation

- For chemotherapy or radiation, granisetron is administered only on the day(s) chemotherapy or radiation is given. Continued treatment when not on chemotherapy or radiation therapy has not been found to be useful.
- **PO:** Administer 1st dose up to 1 hr before chemotherapy or radiation therapy and 2nd dose 12 hr after the first.
- 2 tsp oral solution are equal to 2 mg granisetron.

IV Administration

- **Direct IV:** ***Diluent:*** May be administered undiluted or diluted in 20–50 ml of 0.9% NaCl or D5W. Solution should be prepared at time of administration but is stable for 24 hr at room temperature. ***Concentration:*** Up to 1 mg/ml. ***Rate:*** Administer undiluted granisetron over 30 sec or as a diluted solution over 30 min–1 hr.
- **Syringe Compatibility:** dexamethasone, methylprednisolone.
- **Y-Site Compatibility:** acyclovir, allopurinol, amifostine, amikacin, aminophylline, amphotericin B cholesteryl sulfate, ampicillin, ampicillin-sulbactam, amsacrine, aztreonam, bleomycin, bumetanide, buprenorphine, butorphanol, calcium gluconate, carboplatin, carmustine, cefazolin, cefepime, cefotaxime, cefotetan, cefoxitin, ceftazidime, ceftizoxime, ceftriaxone, cefuroxime, chlorpromazine, cimetidine, ciprofloxacin, cisplatin, cladribine, clindamycin, cyclophosphamide, cytarabine, dacarbazine, dactinomycin, daunorubicin, dexamethasone, dexmedetomidine, diphenhydramine, dobutamine, docetaxel, dopamine, doxorubicin, doxorubicin liposome, doxycycline, droperidol, enalaprilat, etoposide, etoposide phosphate, famotidine, fenoldopam, filgrastim, floxuridine, fluconazole, fludarabine, fluorouracil, furosemide, ganciclovir, gemcitabine, gentamicin, haloperidol, heparin, hydrocortisone, hydromorphone, idarubicin, ifosfamide, imipenem/cilastatin, leucovorin, linezolid, lorazepam, magnesium sulfate, mechlorethamine, melphalan, meperidine, mesna, methotrexate, methylprednisolone, metoclopramide, metronidazole, mitomycin, mitoxantrone, morphine, nalbuphine, ofloxacin, oxaliplatin, paclitaxel, pemetrexed, piperacil-

lin, piperacillin-tazobactam, potassium chloride, prochlorperazine, promethazine, propofol, ranitidine, sargramostim, sodium bicarbonate, streptozocin, teniposide, thiotepa, ticarcillin/clavulanate, tobramycin, topotecan, trimethoprim/sulfamethoxazole, vancomycin, vinblastine, vincristine, vinorelbine, zidovudine.

- **Y-Site Incompatibility:** amphotericin B, lansoprazole.
- **Additive Incompatibility:** Granisetron should not be admixed with other medications.

Patient/Family Teaching

- Advise patient to notify health care professional immediately if involuntary movement of eyes, face, or limbs occurs.

Evaluation/Desired Outcomes

- Prevention of nausea and vomiting associated with emetogenic cancer chemotherapy or radiation therapy.
- Prevention and treatment of postoperative nausea and vomiting.

GROWTH HORMONES

somatropin (recombinant)

(soe-ma-**troe**-pin)

Genotropin, Humatrope, Norditropin, Nutropin, Nutropin AQ, Saizen, Serostim, Serostim LQ, Tev-Tropin, Zorbtive

Classification

Therapeutic: hormones

Pharmacologic: growth hormones

Pregnancy Category B (Serostim and Zorbtive), C (all others)

Indications

Growth failure in children due to chronic renal insufficiency. Growth failure in children due to deficiency of growth hormone. Short stature associated with Turner's syndrome. Short stature associated with or Noonan's syndrome (Norditropin only). Growth hormone deficiency in adults (Humatrope, Nutropin, Norditropin). Short stature (Humatrope). AIDS wasting or cachexia (Serostim only). Increases spinal bone density in childhood–onset growth hormone–deficient patients (somatropin). As part of a comprehensive treatment program for Short Bowel Syndrome (Zorbtive).

Action

Produce growth (skeletal and cellular). Metabolic actions include: Increased protein synthesis, Increased carbohydrate metabolism, Lipid mobilization, Retention of sodium, phosphorus, and potassium. Somatropin has the same amino acid sequence as naturally occurring growth hormone; somatrem has 1 additional amino acid. Both are produced by recombinant DNA techniques. Growth hormone enhances GI tract mucosal transport of water, electrolytes and nutrients. **Therapeutic Effects:** Increased skeletal growth in children with growth hormone deficiency. Replacement of somatropin in deficient adults. Decreased wasting in patients with AIDS. Increased bone density in adult growth hormone–deficient patients. Enhanced GI absorption of water, electrolytes and nutrients in short bowel syndrome.

Pharmacokinetics

Absorption: Well absorbed.
Distribution: Localize to highly perfused organs (liver, kidneys).
Metabolism and Excretion: Broken down in renal cells to amino acids that are recirculated; some liver metabolism.
Half-life: *Subcut*—3.8 hr; *IM*—4.9 hr.

TIME/ACTION PROFILE (growth)

ROUTE	ONSET	PEAK	DURATION
IM, subcut	within 3 mo	unknown	12–48 hr

Contraindications/Precautions

Contraindicated in: Closure of epiphyses; Active neoplasia; Hypersensitivity to growth hormone, *m*-cresol or glycerin (somatropin) or benzyl alcohol (Zorbtive); Acute critical illness (therapy should not be initiated) or respiratory failure; Diabetic retinopathy; Prader-Willi syndrome with obesity and respiratory impairment (risk of fatal complications; can be used only if growth hormone deficiency is documented); OB: Use only if clearly needed.
Use Cautiously in: Growth hormone deficiency due to intracranial lesion; Coexisting adrenocorticotropic hormone (ACTH) deficiency; Diabetes (may cause insulin resistance); Thyroid dysfunction; Lactation: Safety not established;

G

Geri: ↑ sensitivity, ↑ risk of adverse reactions; use lower starting dose and smaller dose increments.

Adverse Reactions/Side Effects

CV: edema of the hands and feet. **Endo:** hyperglycemia, hypothyroidism, insulin resistance. **Local:** pain at injection site. **MS:** arthralgia; *Serostim only*—carpal tunnel syndrome, musculoskeletal pain.

Interactions

Drug-Drug: Excessive **corticosteroid** use (equivalent to 10–15 mg/m^2 /day) may ↓ response to somatropin.

Route/Dosage

Somatrem (Protropin)

IM, Subcut (Children): up to 0.3 mg (0.9 unit)/kg weekly; subcut route is preferred.

Somatropin (Genotropin)

Subcut (Children): 0.16–0.24 mg/kg/wk divided in 6–7 daily doses.
Subcut (Adults): 0.04–0.8 mg/kg/wk divided in 6–7 daily doses.

Somatropin (Humatrope)

Subcut (Adults): 0.018 unit/kg/day (up to 0.0375 unit/kg/day).
IM, Subcut (Children): 0.18 mg/kg (0.54 unit/kg)/wk given in divided doses on 3 alternating days or 6 times weekly (up to 0.3 mg/kg or 0.9 unit/kg/wk).

Somatropin (Nutropin/Nutropin AQ)

Subcut (Children): *Growth hormone inadequacy*—0.3 mg/kg. *Chronic renal insufficiency*—0.35 mg/kg (1.05 units/kg)/wk given as daily injections. *Turner's syndrome*—≤0.375 mg/kg (1.125 units/kg)/wk in 3–7 divided doses.
Subcut (Adults): <0.006 mg/kg daily; may be increased to 0.025 mg/kg/day in patients <35 yrs or 0.0125 mg/kg in patients >35 yrs.

Somatropin (Norditropin)

Subcut (Adults): 0.005 mg/kg/day, may be increased to 0.01 mg/kg/day after 4 wk.
Subcut (Children): 0.024–0.034 mg/kg 6–7 times weekly (up to 0.066 mg/kg/day in Noonan's syndrome).

Somatropin (Saizen)

Subcut, IM (Children): 0.06 mg (0.18 unit/kg) 3 times weekly.

Somatropin (Serostim)

Subcut (Adults): *>55 kg*—6 mg once daily; *45–55 kg*—5 mg once daily; *35–45 kg*—4 mg once daily; *<35 kg*—0.1 mg/kg once daily.

Somatropin (Tev-Tropin)

Subcut (Children): up to 0.1 mg/kg three times weekly.

Somatropin (Zorbtive)

Subcut (Adults): 0.1 mg/kg/day for 4 wk (not to exceed 8 mg/dose), dose may be stopped for 5 days and resumed at half dose for fluid retention or arthalgias.

Availability

Somatropin/Genotropin

Powder for injection: 1.5-mg intra-mix cartridge (delivers 1.3 mg), 5.8-mg intra-mix cartridge (delivers 5 mg), 5.8-mg intra-mix cartridge (delivers 5 mg) as Pen 5 system, 13.8-mg intra-mix cartridge (delivers 12 mg), 13.8-mg intra-mix cartridge (delivers 12 mg) as Pen 12 system, MiniQuick system 0.2 mg, MiniQuick system 0.4 mg, MiniQuick system 0.6 mg, MiniQuick system 0.8 mg, MiniQuick system 1 mg, MiniQuick system 1.4 mg, MiniQuick system 1.6 mg, MiniQuick system 1.8 mg, MiniQuick system 2 mg.

Humatrope

Powder for injection: 5 mg/vial.

Norditropin

Powder for injection: 4 mg (12 units)/vial, 5 mg (13 units)/vial, 8 mg (24 units)/vial, 10 mg (26 units)/vial. **Cartridges for injection (using Nordipen):** 5 mg/1.5 ml, 10 mg/1.5 ml, 15 mg/1.5 ml.

Nutropin

Powder for injection: 5 mg (13 units)/vial, 10 mg (26 units)/vial.

Nutropin AQ

Solution for injection (AQ): 5 mg (15 units)/ml in 2-ml vial.

Saizen

Powder for injection: 5 mg (15 units)/vial, 6 mg (18 units)/vial.

Serostim

Powder for injection: 6 mg (15 units)/vial.
Liquid for injection: 6 mg/0.5 mL cartridge.

Tev-Tropin

Powder for injection: 5 mg (15 units)/vial.

Zorbtive

Powder for injection: 4-, 5- or 6-mg vials, 8.8 mg multidose vials.

NURSING IMPLICATIONS

Assessment

- **Growth Failure:** Monitor bone age annually and growth rate determinations, height, and weight every 3–6 mo during therapy.
- **AIDS Wasting/Cachexia:** Re-evaluate treatment in patients who continue to lose weight in first 2 wk of treatment.
- ***Lab Test Considerations:*** Monitor thyroid function prior to and during therapy. May decrease T^4, radioactive iodine uptake, and thyroxine-binding capacity. Hypothyroidism necessitates concurrent thyroid replacement for growth hormone to be effective. Serum inorganic phosphorus, alkaline phosphatase, and parathyroid hormone may ↑ with somatropin therapy.
- Monitor blood glucose periodically during therapy. Diabetic patients may require ↑ insulin dose.
- Monitor for development of neutralizing antibodies if growth rate does not exceed 2.5 cm/6 mo.
- Monitor alkaline phosphatase closely in patients with adult growth hormone deficiency.

Potential Nursing Diagnoses

Disturbed body image (Indications)

Implementation

- Rotate injection sites with each injection.
- **Somatropin:** Reconstitute 5-mg vial with 1.5–5 ml of sterile water for injection provided by manufacturer (contains preservative *m*-cresol), aiming the liquid against glass vial wall. Do not shake; swirl gently to dissolve. Solution is clear; do not use solutions that are cloudy or contain a precipitate. Stable for 14 days when refrigerated; do not freeze.
- **Genotropin intra-mix:** Dissolve powder with solution provided with 2-chamber cartridge as directed. Gently tip cartridge upside down a few times until contents are completely dissolved. The 1.5-mg cartridge is stable following dilution for 24 hr if refrigerated. The 5.8-mg and 13.8-mg cartridges contain preservatives and are stable for 14 days if refrigerated.
- **Genotropin Pen:** Prepare and administer as directed in patient instruction insert. Store in the refrigerator.
- **Genotropin MiniQuick:** For single use only. Inject immediately after reconstitution; may be refrigerated for 24 hr after reconstitution. Follow directions on patient package insert for reconstitution and administration.
- **Humatrope:** Reconstitute each 5-mg vial with 1.5–5 ml of diluent provided. Stable for 14 days if refrigerated.
- **Norditropin:** Reconstitute each 4-mg or 8-mg vial with 2 ml of diluent. Use reconstituted vials within 14 days. If using cartridges for the Nordipen, each cartridge has a corresponding color-coded pen which is graduated to deliver the appropriate dose based on the concentration of norditropin in the cartridge. Color coding of cartridge and pen must match.
- **Nutropin/Nutropin AQ:** Reconstitute 5-mg vial with 1–5 ml and 10-mg vial with 1–10 ml of bacteriostatic water for injection. Reconstituted vials are stable for 14 days (Nutropin) or 28 days (Nutropin AQ) if refrigerated.
- **Saizen:** Reconstitute each 5-mg vial with 1–3 ml of bacteriostatic water for injection. Reconstituted vials are stable for 14 days if refrigerated. To use cool.click needle-free injector, wind the device to energize the spring, and draw medication into the Crystal Check nozzle. Using firm pressure at the injection site, hold the injector at a 90° angle and press the blue actuator button.
- **Serostim:** Reconstitute each vial with 1 ml of sterile water for injection. Use within 24 hr of reconstitution.
- **Tev-tropin:** Reconstitute with 1–5 mL or 0.9% NaCl. May be cloudy if refrigerated. Allow to warm to room temperature. If remains solution cloudy or contains particulate matter, do not use.
- **Zorbtive:** Reconstitute each 4-, 5-, or 6-mg vial with 0.5–1 mL of sterile water for injection and each 8.8 mg vial with 1 or 2 mL bacteriostatic water for injection. Solution should be clear upon reconstitution. Do not administer if cloudy upon reconstitution (4-, 5-, or 6-mg vials) or after refrigeration (8.8-mg vial). After refrigeration may contain small particles which should disappear when allowed to warm to room temperature. Solution reconstituted with bacteriostatic water is stable for 14 days if refrigerated.
- **Subcut:** Injection volume for *somatropin* should not exceed 1 ml.

Patient/Family Teaching

- Instruct patient and parents on correct procedure for reconstituting medication, site selection, technique for IM or subcut injection, and disposal of needles and syringes. Review dosage schedule. Parents should report persistent pain or edema at injection site.
- Explain rationale for prohibition of use for increasing athletic performance. Administration to persons without growth hormone deficiency or after epiphyseal closure may result in acromegaly (coarsening of facial features; enlarged hands, feet, and internal organs; increased blood glucose; hypertension).
- Emphasize need for regular follow-up with endocrinologist to ensure appropriate growth rate, to evaluate lab work, and to determine bone age by x-ray exam.
- Assure parents and child that these dose forms are synthetic and therefore not capable of transmitting Creutzfeldt-Jakob disease, as was the original somatropin, which was extracted from human cadavers.

Evaluation/Desired Outcomes

- Child's attainment of adult height in growth failure secondary to pituitary growth hormone deficiency. Therapy is limited to period before closure of epiphyseal plates (approximately up to 14–15 yr in girls, 15–16 yr in boys).
- Replacement of somatropin in deficient adults.
- Decreased wasting in patients with AIDS.
- Enhanced GI absorption of water, electrolytes and nutrients in short bowel syndrome.

guaifenesin (gwye-**fen**-e-sin)

Alfen Jr, Altarussin, ✤Benylin-E, Breonesin, ✤Calmylin Expectorant, Diabetic Tussin, Ganidin NR, Guiatuss, Hytuss, Hytuss-2X, Mucinex, Naldecon Senior EX, Organidin NR, ✤Resyl, Robitussin, Scottussin Expectorant, Siltussin SA, Siltussin DAS

Classification

Therapeutic: allergy, cold, and cough remedies, expectorants

Pregnancy Category C

Indications

Coughs associated with viral upper respiratory tract infections.

Action

Reduces viscosity of tenacious secretions by increasing respiratory tract fluid. **Therapeutic Effects:** Mobilization and subsequent expectoration of mucus.

Pharmacokinetics

Absorption: Well absorbed after oral administration.

Distribution: Unknown.

Metabolism and Excretion: Renally excreted as metabolites.

Half-life: Unknown.

TIME/ACTION PROFILE (expectorant action)

ROUTE	ONSET	PEAK	DURATION
PO	30 min	unknown	4–6 hr
PO-ER	unknown	unknown	12 hr

Contraindications/Precautions

Contraindicated in: Hypersensitivity; Some products contain alcohol and should be avoided in patients with known intolerance; Some products contain aspartame and should be avoided in patients with phenylketonuria.

Use Cautiously in: Cough lasting >1 wk or accompanied by fever, rash, or headache; Pregnancy (although safety has not been established, guaifenesin has been used without adverse effects); Patients receiving disulfiram (liquid products may contain alcohol); Diabetic patients (some products may contain sugar); Children (check age limitations on specific dose forms).

Adverse Reactions/Side Effects

CNS: dizziness, headache. **GI:** nausea, diarrhea, stomach pain, vomiting. **Derm:** rashes, urticaria.

Interactions

Drug-Drug: None significant.

Route/Dosage

PO (Adults): 200–400 mg q 4 hr or 600–1200 mg q 12 hr as extended-release product (not to exceed 2400 mg/day).

PO (Children 6–12 yr): 100–200 mg q 4 hr or 600 mg q 12 hr as extended-release product (not to exceed 1200 mg/day).

PO (Children 2–6 yr): 50–100 mg q 4 hr (not to exceed 600 mg/day).

Availability (generic available)

Syrup: 100 mg/5 ml^{OTC}. **Oral solution:** 100 mg/5 ml$^{Rx, OTC}$, 200 mg/5 ml^{OTC}. **Capsules:** 200 mg^{OTC}. **Tablets:** 100 mg^{OTC}, 200 mg$^{Rx, OTC}$, 1200 mg. **Extended-release tablets (Mucinex):**

600 mg, 1200 mg. ***In combination with:*** analgesics/antipyretics, antihistamines, decongestants, and cough suppressants[Rx, OTC].

NURSING IMPLICATIONS

Assessment

- Assess lung sounds, frequency and type of cough, and character of bronchial secretions periodically during therapy. Maintain fluid intake of 1500–2000 ml/day to decrease viscosity of secretions.

Potential Nursing Diagnoses

Ineffective airway clearance (Indications)

Implementation

- **PO:** Administer each dose of guaifenesin followed by a full glass of water to decrease viscosity of secretions.
- Extended-release tablets should be swallowed whole; do not open, crush, break, or chew.

Patient/Family Teaching

- Instruct patient to cough effectively. Patient should sit upright and take several deep breaths before attempting to cough.
- Inform patient that drug may occasionally cause dizziness. Avoid driving or other activities requiring alertness until response to drug is known.
- Advise patient to limit talking, stop smoking, maintain moisture in environmental air, and take some sugarless gum or hard candy to help alleviate the discomfort caused by a chronic nonproductive cough.
- Instruct patient to contact health care professional if cough persists longer than 1 wk or is accompanied by fever, rash, or persistent headache or sore throat.

Evaluation/Desired Outcomes

- Easier mobilization and expectoration of mucus from cough associated with upper respiratory infection.

G

halcinonide, See CORTICOSTEROIDS (TOPICAL/LOCAL).

halobetasol, See CORTICOSTEROIDS (TOPICAL/LOCAL).

haloperidol (ha-loe-**per**-i-dole)

♣Apo-Haloperidol, Haldol, Haldol Decanoate, ♣Haldol LA, ♣Novo-Peridol, ♣Peridol, ♣PMS Haloperidol

Classification
Therapeutic: antipsychotics
Pharmacologic: butyrophenones

Pregnancy Category C

Indications

Acute and chronic psychotic disorders including: schizophrenia, manic states, drug-induced psychoses. Schizophrenic patients who require long-term parenteral (IM) antipsychotic therapy. Also useful in managing aggressive or agitated patients. Tourette's syndrome. Severe behavioral problems in children which may be accompanied by: unprovoked, combative, explosive hyperexcitability, hyperactivity accompanied by conduct disorders (short-term use when other modalities have failed). Considered second-line treatment after failure with atypical antipsychotic. **Unlabeled uses:** Nausea and vomiting from surgery or chemotherapy.

Action

Alters the effects of dopamine in the CNS. Also has anticholinergic and alpha-adrenergic blocking activity. **Therapeutic Effects:** Diminished signs and symptoms of psychoses. Improved behavior in children with Tourette's syndrome or other behavioral problems.

Pharmacokinetics

Absorption: Well absorbed following PO/IM administration. Decanoate salt is slowly absorbed and has a long duration of action.
Distribution: Concentrates in liver. Crosses placenta; enters breast milk.
Protein Binding: 90%.
Metabolism and Excretion: Mostly metabolized by the liver.
Half-life: 21–24 hr.

TIME/ACTION PROFILE (antipsychotic activity)

ROUTE	ONSET	PEAK	DURATION
PO	2 hr	2–6 hr	8–12 hr
IM	20–30 min	30–45 min	4–8 hr†
IM (decanoate)	3–9 days	unknown	1 mo

†Effect may persist for several days

Contraindications/Precautions

Contraindicated in: Hypersensitivity; Angle-closure glaucoma; Bone marrow depression; CNS depression; Severe liver or cardiovascular disease (Q-T interval prolonging conditions); Some products contain tartrazine, sesame oil, or benzyl alcohol and should be avoided in patients with known intolerance or hypersensitivity.
Use Cautiously in: Debilitated patients (dose reduction required); Cardiac disease; Diabetes; Respiratory insufficiency; Prostatic hyperplasia; CNS tumors; Intestinal obstruction; Seizures; OB: Safety not established; Lactation: Discontinue drug or bottle-feed; Geri: Dosage reduction required due to increased sensitivity.

Adverse Reactions/Side Effects

CNS: SEIZURES, extrapyramidal reactions, confusion, drowsiness, restlessness, tardive dyskinesia. **EENT:** blurred vision, dry eyes. **Resp:** respiratory depression. **CV:** hypotension, tachycardia. **GI:** constipation, dry mouth, anorexia, drug-induced hepatitis, ileus, weight gain. **GU:** urinary retention. **Derm:** diaphoresis, photosensitivity, rashes. **Endo:** galactorrhea, amenorrhea. **Hemat:** anemia, leukopenia. **Metab:** hyperpyrexia. **Misc:** NEUROLEPTIC MALIGNANT SYNDROME, hypersensitivity reactions.

Interactions

Drug-Drug: ↑ hypotension with **antihypertensives**, **nitrates**, or acute ingestion of **alcohol**. ↑ anticholinergic effects with **drugs having anticholinergic properties**, including **antihistamines**, **antidepressants**, **atropine**, **phenothiazines**, **quinidine**, and **disopyramide**. ↑ CNS depression with other **CNS depressants**, including **alcohol**, **antihistamines**, **opioid analgesics**, and **sedative/**

hypnotics. Concurrent use with **epinephrine** may result in severe hypotension and tachycardia. May ↓ therapeutic effects of **levodopa**. Acute encephalopathic syndrome may occur when used with **lithium**. Dementia may occur with **methyldopa**.
Drug-Natural Products: Kava kava, **valerian**, or **chamomile** can ↑ CNS depression.

Route/Dosage

Haloperidol

PO (Adults): 0.5–5 mg 2–3 times daily. Patients with severe symptoms may require up to 100 mg/day.
PO (Geriatric Patients or Debilitated Patients): 0.5–2 mg twice daily initially; may be gradually increased as needed.
PO (Children 3–12 yr or 15–40 kg): 50 mcg/kg/day in 2–3 divided doses; may increase by 500 mcg (0.5 mg)/day q 5–7 days as needed (up to 75 mcg/kg/day for nonpsychotic disorders or Tourette's syndrome or 150 mcg/kg/day for psychoses).
IM (Adults): 2–5 mg q 1–8 hr (not to exceed 100 mg/day).
IV (Adults): 0.5–5 mg, may be repeated q 30 min (unlabeled).

Haloperidol Decanoate

IM (Adults): 10–15 times the previous daily PO dose but not to exceed 100 mg initially, given monthly (not to exceed 300 mg/mo).

Availability (generic available)

Tablets: 0.5 mg, 1 mg, 2 mg, 5 mg, 10 mg, 20 mg. **Oral concentrate:** 2 mg/ml. **Haloperidol injection:** 5 mg/ml. **Haloperidol decanoate injection:** 50 mg/ml, 100 mg/ml.

NURSING IMPLICATIONS

Assessment

- Assess mental status (orientation, mood, behavior) prior to and periodically during therapy.
- Assess positive (hallucination, delusions) and negative (social isolation) symptoms of schizophrenia.
- Monitor blood pressure (sitting, standing, lying) and pulse prior to and frequently during the period of dose adjustment. May cause QT interval changes on ECG.
- Observe patient carefully when administering medication, to ensure that medication is actually taken and not hoarded.
- Monitor intake and output ratios and daily weight. Assess patient for signs and symptoms of dehydration (decreased thirst, lethargy, hemoconcentration), especially in geriatric patients.
- Assess fluid intake and bowel function. Increased bulk and fluids in the diet help minimize constipating effects.
- Monitor patient for onset of akathisia (restlessness or desire to keep moving), which may appear within 6 hr of 1st dose and may be difficult to distinguish from psychotic agitation. Benztropine may be used to differentiate agitation from akathisia. Observe closely for extrapyramidal side effects (*parkinsonian*—difficulty speaking or swallowing, loss of balance control, pill rolling of hands, mask-like face, shuffling gait, rigidity, tremors; and *dystonic*—muscle spasms, twisting motions, twitching, inability to move eyes, weakness of arms or legs). Trihexyphenidyl or benztropine may be used to control these symptoms. Benzodiazepines may alleviate akathisia.
- Monitor for tardive dyskinesia (uncontrolled rhythmic movement of mouth, face, and extremities; lip smacking or puckering; puffing of cheeks; uncontrolled chewing; rapid or worm-like movements of tongue, excessive eye blinking). Report immediately; may be irreversible.
- Monitor for development of neuroleptic malignant syndrome (fever, respiratory distress, tachycardia, seizures, diaphoresis, hypertension or hypotension, pallor, tiredness, severe muscle stiffness, loss of bladder control). Report symptoms immediately. May also cause leukocytosis, elevated liver function tests, elevated CPK.
- ***Lab Test Considerations:*** Monitor CBC with differential and liver function tests periodically during therapy.

Potential Nursing Diagnoses

Disturbed thought process (Indications)
Disturbed sensory perception (specify: visual, auditory, kinesthetic, gustatory, tactile, olfactory) (Indications)

Implementation

- Avoid skin contact with oral solution; may cause contact dermatitis.
- **PO:** Administer with food or full glass of water or milk to minimize GI irritation.
- Use calibrated measuring device for accurate dosage. Do not dilute concentrate with coffee

or tea; may cause precipitation. Should be given undiluted, but if necessary may dilute in at least 60 ml of liquid.

- **IM:** Inject slowly, using 2-in., 21-gauge needle into well-developed muscle via Z-track technique. Do not exceed 3 ml per injection site. Slight yellow color does not indicate altered potency. Keep patient recumbent for at least 30 min following injection to minimize hypotensive effects.

IV Administration

- **IV:** Haloperidol decanoate should not be administered IV.
- **Direct IV:** ***Diluent:*** May be administered undiluted for rapid control of acute psychosis or delirium. ***Concentration:*** 5 mg/ml. ***Rate:*** Administer at a rate of 5 mg/min.
- **Intermittent Infusion:** ***Diluent:*** May be diluted in 30–50 ml of D5W. ***Rate:*** Infuse over 30 min.
- **Y-Site Compatibility:** amifostine, amphotericin B liposome, amsacrine, aztreonam, bivalirudin, caspofungin, cimetidine, cisatracurium, cladribine, daptomycin, dexmedetomidine, diltiazem, dobutamine, docetaxel, dopamine, doxorubicin liposome, ertapenem, etoposide phosphate, famotidine, fenoldopam, fentanyl, filgrastim, gemcitabine, granisetron, hydromorphone, lidocaine, levofloxacin, linezolid, lorazepam, melphalan, methadone, midazolam, morphine, nitroglycerin, norepinephrine, ondansetron, oxaliplatin, paclitaxel, palonosetron, pemetrexed, phenylephrine, propofol, quinupristin/dalfopristin, remifentanil, sufentanil, tacrolimus, teniposide, theophylline, thiotepa, tigecycline, tirofiban, voriconazole, vinorelbine.
- **Y-Site Incompatibility:** acyclovir, allopurinol, aminophylline, amphotericin B cholesteryl sulfate, ampicillin, ampicillin/sulbactam, bumetanide, calcium chloride, cefazolin, cefepime, cefotaxime, cefoxitin, ceftazidime, ceftizoxime, ceftriaxone, cefuroxime, chloramphenicol, clindamycin, dexamethasone sodium phosphate, diazepam, fluconazole, foscarnet, furosemide, ganciclovir, heparin, hydralazine, imipenem/cilastatin, ketorolac, lansoprazole, magnesium sulfate, methylprednisolone sodium succinate, metronidazole, nafcillin, pantoprazole, penicillin G potassium, phenytoin, piperacillin/tazobactam, potassium chloride, sargramostim, sodium bicarbonate, ticarcillin/clavulanate, trimethoprim/sulfamethoxazole.

Patient/Family Teaching

- Advise patient to take medication as directed. Take missed doses as soon as remembered, with remaining doses evenly spaced throughout the day. May require several weeks to obtain desired effects. Do not increase dose or discontinue medication without consulting health care professional. Abrupt withdrawal may cause dizziness; nausea; vomiting; GI upset; trembling; or uncontrolled movements of mouth, tongue, or jaw.
- Inform patient of possibility of extrapyramidal symptoms and tardive dyskinesia. Caution patient to report symptoms immediately.
- Advise patient to change positions slowly to minimize orthostatic hypotension.
- May cause drowsiness. Caution patient to avoid driving or other activities requiring alertness until response to medication is known.
- Caution patient to avoid taking alcohol or other CNS depressants concurrently with this medication.
- Advise patient to use sunscreen and protective clothing when exposed to the sun to prevent photosensitivity reactions. Extremes of temperature should also be avoided, because this drug impairs body temperature regulation.
- Instruct patient to use frequent mouth rinses, good oral hygiene, and sugarless gum or candy to minimize dry mouth.
- Advise patient to notify health care professional of medication regimen prior to treatment or surgery.
- Instruct patient to notify health care professional promptly if weakness, tremors, visual disturbances, dark-colored urine or clay-colored stools, sore throat, or fever is noted.
- Encourage continued participation in psychotherapy.
- Provide positive reinforcement for medication compliance.
- Refer to local support group.
- Emphasize the importance of routine follow-up exams to monitor response to medication and detect side effects.

H

Evaluation/Desired Outcomes

- Decrease in hallucinations, insomnia, agitation, hostility, and delusions.
- Decreased tics and vocalization in Tourette's syndrome.
- Improved behavior in children with severe behavioral problems. If no therapeutic effects are seen in 2–4 wk, dosage may be increased.

HIGH ALERT

heparin (hep-a-rin)

Calcilean, Calciparine, Hepalean, Heparin Leo, Hep-Lock, Hep-Lock U/P

Classification
Therapeutic: anticoagulants
Pharmacologic: antithrombotics

Pregnancy Category C

Indications

Prophylaxis and treatment of various thromboembolic disorders including: Venous thromboembolism, Pulmonary emboli, Atrial fibrillation with embolization, Acute and chronic consumptive coagulopathies, Peripheral arterial thromboembolism. Used in very low doses (10–100 units) to maintain patency of IV catheters (heparin flush).

Action

Potentiates the inhibitory effect of antithrombin on factor Xa and thrombin. In low doses, prevents the conversion of prothrombin to thrombin by its effects on factor Xa. Higher doses neutralize thrombin, preventing the conversion of fibrinogen to fibrin. **Therapeutic Effects:** Prevention of thrombus formation. Prevention of extension of existing thrombi (full dose).

Pharmacokinetics

Absorption: Erratically absorbed following subcut or IM administration.
Distribution: Does not cross the placenta or enter breast milk.
Protein Binding: Very high (to low-density lipoproteins, globulins, and fibrinogen).
Metabolism and Excretion: Probably removed by the reticuloendothelial system (lymph nodes, spleen).
Half-life: 1–2 hr (increases with increasing dose); affected by obesity, renal and hepatic function, malignancy, presence of of pulmonary embolism, and infections.

TIME/ACTION PROFILE (anticoagulant effect)

ROUTE	ONSET	PEAK	DURATION
Heparin subcut	20–60 min	2 hr	8–12 hr
Heparin IV	immediate	5–10 min	2–6 hr

Contraindications/Precautions

Contraindicated in: Hypersensitivity; Uncontrolled bleeding; Severe thrombocytopenia; Open wounds (full dose); Products containing benzyl alcohol should not be used in premature infants.
Use Cautiously in: Severe liver or kidney disease; Retinopathy (hypertensive or diabetic); Untreated hypertension; Ulcer disease; Spinal cord or brain injury; History of congenital or acquired bleeding disorder; Malignancy; OB: May be used during pregnancy, but use with caution during the last trimester and in the immediate postpartum period; Geri: Women >60 yr have increased risk of bleeding.
Exercise Extreme Caution in: Severe uncontrolled hypertension; Bleeding disorders; GI bleeding/ulceration etc; Bacterial endocarditis, bleeding disorders; GI bleeding/ulceration/pathology; Hemorrhagic stroke; Recent CNS or ophthalmologic surgery; Active GI bleeding/ulceration; History of thrombocytopenia related to heparin.

Adverse Reactions/Side Effects

GI: drug-induced hepatitis. **Derm:** alopecia (long-term use), rashes, urticaria. **Hemat:** BLEEDING, anemia, thrombocytopenia (can occur up to several weeks after discontinuation of therapy). **Local:** pain at injection site. **MS:** osteoporosis (long-term use). **Misc:** fever, hypersensitivity.

Interactions

Heparin is frequently used concurrently or sequentially with other agents affecting coagulation. The risk of potentially serious interactions is greatest with full anticoagulation.
Drug-Drug: Risk of bleeding may be ↑ by concurrent use of **drugs that affect platelet function**, including **aspirin**, **NSAIDs**, **clopi-**

dogrel, **dipyridamole**, some **penicillins**, **ticlopidine**, **abciximab**, **eptifibitide**, **tirofiban**, and **dextran**. Risk of bleeding may be ↑ by concurrent use of **drugs that cause hypoprothrombinemia**, including **quinidine**, **cefoperazone**, **cefotetan**, and **valproic acid**. Concurrent use of **thrombolytics** ↑ risk of bleeding. Heparins affect the prothrombin time used in assessing the response to **warfarin**. **Digoxin**, **tetracyclines**, **nicotine**, and **antihistamines** may ↓ anticoagulant effect of heparin. **Streptokinase** may be followed by relative resistance to heparin.
Drug-Natural Products: ↑ risk of bleeding with **arnica, anise, chamomile, clove, dong quai, fever few, garlic, ginger,** and **Panax ginseng.**

Route/Dosage

Therapeutic Anticoagulation

IV (Adults): *Intermittent bolus*—10,000 units, followed by 5000–10,000 units q 4–6 hr. *Continuous infusion*—5000 units (35–70 units/kg), followed by 20,000–40,000 units infused over 24 hr (approx. 1000 units/hr or 15–18 units/kg/hr).
IV (Children >1 yr): *Intermittent bolus*—50–100 units/kg, followed by 50–100 units/kg q 4 hr. *Continuous infusion*—Loading dose 75 units/kg, followed by 20 units/kg/hr, adjust to maintain aPTT of 60–85 seconds.
IV (Neonates and Infants <1yr): *Continuous infusion*—Loading dose 75 units/kg, followed by 28 units/kg/hr, adjust to maintain aPTT of 60–85 seconds.
Subcut (Adults): 5000 units IV, followed by initial subcut dose of 10,000–20,000 units, then 8000–10,000 units q 8 hr or 15,000–20,000 units q 12 hr.

Prophylaxis of Thromboembolism

Subcut (Adults): 5000 units q 8–12 hr (may be started 2 hr prior to surgery).

Cardiovascular Surgery

IV (Adults): At least 150 units/kg (300 units/kg if procedure <60 min; 400 units/kg if >60 min).
IA (Neonates, Infants and Children): 100–150 units/kg via an artery prior to cardiac catheterization.

Line Flushing

IV (Adults and Children): 10–100 units/ml (10 units/ml for infants <10 kg, 100 units/ml for all others) solution to fill heparin lock set to needle hub; replace after each use.

Total Parenteral Nutrition

IV (Adults and Children): 05–1 units/ml (final solution concentration) to maintain line patency.

Arterial Line Patency

IA (Neonates): 0.5–2 units/ml.

Availability (generic available)

Heparin Sodium

Solution for injection: 10 units/ml, 100 units/ml, 1000 units/ml, 5000 units/ml, 7500 units/ml, 10,000 units/ml, 20,000 units/ml, 40,000 units/ml. **Premixed solution:** 1000 units/500 ml, 2000 units/1000 ml, 12,500 units/250 ml, 25,000 units in 250 and 500 ml.

NURSING IMPLICATIONS

Assessment

- Assess for signs of bleeding and hemorrhage (bleeding gums; nosebleed; unusual bruising; black, tarry stools; hematuria; fall in hematocrit or blood pressure; guaiac-positive stools). Notify physician if these occur.
- Assess patient for evidence of additional or increased thrombosis. Symptoms will depend on area of involvement.
- Monitor patient for hypersensitivity reactions (chills, fever, urticaria). Report signs to physician.
- **Subcut:** Observe injection sites for hematomas, ecchymosis, or inflammation.
- ***Lab Test Considerations:*** Monitor activated partial thromboplastin time (aPTT) and hematocrit prior to and periodically throughout therapy. When *intermittent IV* therapy is used, draw aPTT levels 30 min before each dose during initial therapy and then periodically. During *continuous* administration, monitor aPTT levels every 4 hr during early therapy. For *Subcut* therapy, draw blood 4–6 hr after injection.
- Monitor platelet count every 2–3 days throughout therapy. May cause mild thrombocytopenia, which appears on 4th day and resolves despite continued heparin therapy. Heparin-induced thrombocytopenia (HIT), a

more severe form which necessitates discontinuing medication, may develop on 8th day of therapy; may reduce platelet count to as low as 5000/mm^3 and lead to increased resistance to heparin therapy. HIT may progress to development of venous and arterial thrombosis (HITT) and may occur up to several wks after discontinuation. Patients who have received a previous course of heparin may be at higher risk for severe thrombocytopenia for several months after the initial course.

- May cause prolonged prothrompintine (PT) levels, ↑ serum thyroxine, T_3 resin and false-negative ^{125}I fibrinogen uptake tests.
- May cause ↓ serum triglyceride and cholesterol levels and ↑ plasma free fatty acid concentrations.
- May also cause hyperkalemia and ↑ AST and ALT levels.
- ***Toxicity and Overdose:*** Protamine sulfate is the antidote. Due to short half-life, overdose can often be treated by withdrawing the drug.

Potential Nursing Diagnoses

Ineffective tissue perfusion (Indications)
Risk for injury (Side Effects)

Implementation

- ***High Alert:*** Unintended concomitant use of two heparin products (unfractionated heparin and LMW heparins) has resulted in serious harm or death. Review patients' recent (emergency department, operating room) and current medication administration records before administering any heparin or LMW heparin product. Dose calculation and infusion pump programming errors have also occurred. Have second practitioner independently check original order, dose calculation and infusion pump settings. Do not confuse heparin with Hespan (hetastarch in sodium chloride). Do not confuse vials of heparin with vials of insulin.
- Inform all personnel caring for patient of anticoagulant therapy. Venipunctures and injection sites require application of pressure to prevent bleeding or hematoma formation. IM injections of other medications should be avoided, because hematomas may develop.
- In patients requiring long-term anticoagulation, oral anticoagulant therapy should be instituted 4–5 days prior to discontinuing heparin therapy.
- Solution is colorless to slightly yellow.

IV Administration

- **Subcut:** Administer deep into subcut tissue. Alternate injection sites between the left and right abdominal wall above the iliac crest. Inject entire length of needle at a 45° or 90° angle into a skin fold held between thumb and forefinger; hold skin fold throughout injection. Do not aspirate or massage. Rotate sites frequently. Do not administer IM because of danger of hematoma formation. Solution should be clear; do not inject solution containing particulate matter
- **Direct IV:** ***Diluent:*** Loading dose administered undiluted. ***Concentration:*** Varies depending upon vial used. ***Rate:*** Administer over at least 1 min. Loading dose given before continuous infusion.
- **Continuous Infusion:** ***Diluent:*** Heparin vials must be diluted. Dilute 25,000 units of heparin in 250–500 ml of 0.9% NaCl or D5W. Premixed infusions are already diluted and ready to use. Admixed solutions stable for 24 hr at room temperature or if refrigerated. Premixed infusion stable for 30 days once overwrap removed. ***Concentration:*** 50–100 units/ml. ***Rate:*** See Route/Dosage section. Adjust to maintain therapeutic aPTT. Use an infusion pump to ensure accuracy. Flush to prevent clot formation in intermittent infusion (heparin lock) sets, inject dilute heparin solution of 10–100 units/0.5–1 ml after each medication injection or every 8–12 hr. To prevent incompatibility of heparin with medication, flush lock set with sterile water or 0.9% NaCl for injection before and after medication is administered.
- **Y-Site Compatibility:** acyclovir, aminophylline, amphotericin B liposome, anidulafungin, atropine, aztreonam, betamethasone, bivalirudin, bumetanide, calcium chloride, calcium gluconate, cefazolin, cefotaxime, cefoxitin, ceftazidime, ceftizoxime, ceftriaxone, cefuroxime, chloramphenicol, chlordiazepoxide, cimetidine, clindamycin, conjugated estrogens, cyclosporine, daptomycin, dexamethasone, digoxin, dopamine, enalaprilat, epinephrine, eptifibatide, ertapenem, ethacrynate, famotidine, fenoldopam, fentanyl, fluconazole, flumazenil, furosemide, ganciclovir, gemcitabine, granisetron, hydralazine, hydrocortisone, hydromorphone, imipenem/cilastatin, insulin, isoproterenol, ketorolac, lansoprazole, linezolid, lorazepam, magnesium sulfate, meropenem, metoclopramide,

metoprolol, metronidazole, micafungin, midazolam, milrinone, morphine, nafcillin, nitroglycerin, nitroprusside, norepinephrine, ondansetron, palonosetron, pancuronium, pantoprazole, penicillin G potassium, phenylephrine, phytonadione, piperacillin/tazobactam, potassium chloride, procainamide, propofol, propranolol, ranitidine, scopolamine, sodium bicarbonate, sulfamethoxazole/trimethoprim, tacrolimus, ticarcillin/clavulanate, tigecycline, tirofiban, vasopressin, vecuronium, verapamil, voriconazole, warfarin.

- **Y-Site Incompatibility:** alteplase, amikacin, amiodarone, amphotericin B cholesteryl sulfate, caspofungin, ciprofloxacin, diazepam, doxycycline, filgrastim, gentamicin, haloperidol, hydroxyzine, levofloxacin, nesiritidne, phenytoin, quinupristin/dalfopristin, reteplase, tobramycin, vancomycin.
- **Additive Compatibility:** It is recommended that heparin not be mixed in solution with other medications when given for anticoagulation, even those that are compatible, because changes in rate of heparin infusion may be required that would also affect admixtures. If heparin is added to an admixture, the following drugs are compatible:, aminophylline, amphotericin, calcium gluconate, cefepime, chloramphenicol, clindamycin, colistimethate, dopamine, enalaprilat, esmolol, fluconazole, flumazenil, furosemide, lidocaine, magnesium sulfate, meropenem, methyldopate, methylprednisolone, nafcillin, octreotide, potassium chloride, ranitidine, sodium bicarbonate, verapamil, vitamin B complex, vitamin B complex with C. Also compatible with TPN solutions or fat emulsion.
- **Additive Incompatibility:** alteplase, amikacin, ciprofloxacin, cytarabine, daunorubicin, erythromycin lactobionate, gentamicin, hyaluronidase, kanamycin, meperidine, morphine, streptomycin.

Patient/Family Teaching

- Advise patient to report any symptoms of unusual bleeding or bruising to health care professional immediately.
- Instruct patient not to take medications containing aspirin or NSAIDs while on heparin therapy.
- Caution patient to avoid IM injections and activities leading to injury and to use a soft toothbrush and electric razor during heparin therapy.
- Advise patient to inform health care professional of medication regimen prior to treatment or surgery.
- Patients on anticoagulant therapy should carry an identification card with this information at all times.

Evaluation/Desired Outcomes

- Prolonged partial thromboplastin time (PTT) of 1.5–2.5 times the control, without signs of hemorrhage.
- Prevention of deep vein thrombosis and pulmonary emboli.
- Patency of IV catheters.

H

HIGH ALERT

HEPARINS (LOW MOLECULAR WEIGHT)

dalteparin (dal-**te**-pa-rin)
Fragmin

enoxaparin (e-nox-a-**pa**-rin)
Lovenox

tinzaparin (tin-za-**pa**-rin)
Innohep

Classification
Therapeutic: anticoagulants
Pharmacologic: antithrombotics

Pregnancy Category B

Indications

Enoxaparin and dalteparin: Prevention of venous thromboembolism (VTE) (deep vein thrombosis (DVT) and/or pulmonary embolism (PE)) in surgical or medical patients. **Dalteparin only:** Extended treatment of symptomatic DVT and/or PE in patients with cancer. **Enoxaparin and tinzaparin:** Treatment of DVT with or without PE (with warfarin). **Enoxaparin and dalteparin only:** Prevention of ischemic complications (with aspirin) from unstable angina and non-ST-segment-elevation MI. **Enoxaparin only:** Treatment of acute ST-segment-elevation MI (with thrombolytics or percutaneous coronary intervention).

Action

Potentiate the inhibitory effect of antithrombin on factor Xa and thrombin. **Therapeutic Effects:** Prevention of thrombus formation.

Pharmacokinetics

Absorption: Well absorbed after subcut administration (87% for dalteparin and tinzaparin, 92% for enoxaparin).
Distribution: Unknown.
Metabolism and Excretion: *Dalteparin*—unknown; *enoxaparin*—primarily eliminated renally; *tinzaparin*—partially metabolized, elimination is primarily renal.
Half-life: *Dalteparin*—2.1–2.3 hr; *enoxaparin*—3–6 hr; *tinzaparin*—3.9 hr (all are ↑ in renal insufficiency).

TIME/ACTION PROFILE (anticoagulant effect)

ROUTE	ONSET	PEAK	DURATION
Dalteparin subcut	rapid	4 hr	up to 24 hr
Enoxaparin subcut	unknown	3–5 hr	12 hr
Tinzaparin subcut	rapid	4–6 hr	24 hr

Contraindications/Precautions

Contraindicated in: Hypersensitivity to specific agents or pork products; cross-sensitivity may occur; Some products contain sulfites or benzyl alcohol and should be avoided in patients with known hypersensitivity or intolerance; Active major bleeding; History of heparin-induced thrombocytopenia; *Dalteparin*—regional anesthesia during treatment for unstable angina/non–Q-wave MI.
Use Cautiously in: Severe liver or kidney disease (adjust dose of enoxaparin if CCr <30 ml/min); Women <45 kg or men <57 kg; Retinopathy (hypertensive or diabetic); Untreated hypertension; Geri: Geriatric patients (may have ↑ risk of bleeding due to age-related decrease in renal function); Recent history of ulcer disease; History of congenital or acquired bleeding disorder; OB, Lactation, Pedi: Pregnancy, lactation, or children (safety not established; should not be used in pregnant patients with prosthetic heart valves without careful monitoring).
Exercise Extreme Caution in: Spinal/epidural anesthesia (increased risk of spinal/epidural hematomas, especially with concurrent NSAIDs, repeated or traumatic epidural puncture, or indwelling epidural catheter); Severe uncontrolled hypertension; Bacterial endocarditis, bleeding disorders.

Adverse Reactions/Side Effects

CNS: dizziness, headache, insomnia. **CV:** edema. **GI:** constipation, nausea, reversible increase in liver enzymes, vomiting. **GU:** urinary retention. **Derm:** ecchymoses, pruritus, rash, urticaria. **Hemat:** BLEEDING, anemia, thrombocytopenia. **Local:** erythema at injection site, hematoma, irritation, pain. **Misc:** fever.

Interactions

Drug-Drug: Risk of bleeding may be ↑ by concurrent use of **drugs that affect platelet function and coagulation**, including **warfarin**, **aspirin**, **NSAIDs**, **dipyridamole**, some **penicillins**, **clopidogrel**, **ticlopidine**, **abciximab**, **eptifibatide**, **tirofiban**, **thrombolytics** and **dextran**.
Drug-Natural Products: ↑ bleeding risk with, **arnica, chamomile, clove, feverfew, garlic, ginger, ginkgo, Panax ginseng,** and **others.**

Route/Dosage

Dalteparin

Subcut (Adults): *Prophylaxis of DVT following abdominal surgery*—2500 IU 1–2 hr before surgery, then once daily for 5–10 days; *Prophylaxis of VTE in high-risk patients undergoing abdominal surgery*—5000 IU evening before surgery, then once daily for 5–10 days *or* in patients with malignancy, 2500 IU 1–2 hr before surgery, another 2500 IU 12 hr later, then 5000 IU once daily for 5–10 days; *Prophylaxis of VTE in patients undergoing hip replacement surgery*—2500 IU within 2 hr before surgery, then 2500 IU 4–8 hr after surgery, then 5000 IU once daily (start at least 6 hr after postsurgical dose) for 5–10 days *or* 5000 IU evening before surgery (10–14 hr before surgery), then 5000 IU 4–8 hr after surgery, then 5000 IU once daily for 5–10 days *or* 2500 IU 4–8 hr after surgery, then 5000 IU once daily (start at least 6 hr after postsurgical dose); *Prophylaxis of VTE in medical patients with severely restricted mobility during acute illness*—5000 IU once daily for 12 to 14 days. *Unstable angina/non–ST—segment—elevation MI*—120 IU/kg (not to exceed 10,000 IU) q 12 hr for 5–8 days with concurrent aspirin; *Extended treatment of symptomatic VTE in cancer patients*—200 IU/kg (not to exceed 18,000 IU) once daily for first 30 days, followed by 150 IU/kg (not to exceed 18,000 IU) once daily through 6th month.

Renal Impairment

Subcut (Adults): *Cancer patients receiving extended treatment of symptomatic VTE with CCr ≤30 ml/min*- Monitor anti-Xa levels (target 0.5–1.5 IU/ml).

Enoxaparin

Subcut (Adults): *VTE prophylaxis in patients undergoing knee replacement surgery*—30 mg q 12 hr starting 12–24 hr postop for 7–10 days; *VTE prophylaxis in patients undergoing hip replacement surgery*—30 mg q 12 hr starting 12–24 hr postop *or* 40 mg once daily starting 12 hr before surgery (either dose may be continued for 7–14 days; continued prophylaxis with 40 mg once daily may be continued for up to 3 wk); *VTE prophylaxis following abdominal surgery*—40 mg once daily starting 2 hr before surgery and then continued for 7–12 days or until ambulatory (up to 14 days); *VTE prophylaxis in medical patients with acute illness*—40 mg once daily for 6–14 days; *Treatment of DVT/PE (outpatient)*—1 mg/kg q 12 hr. Warfarin should be started within 72 hr; enoxaparin may be continued for a minimum of 5 days and until therapeutic anticoagulation with warfarin is achieved (INR >2 for two consecutive days); *Treatment of DVT/PE (inpatient)*—1 mg/kg q 12 hr *or* 1.5 mg/kg once daily. Warfarin should be started within 72 hr; enoxaparin may be continued for a minimum of 5 days and until therapeutic anticoagulation with warfarin is achieved (INR >2 for two consecutive days); *Unstable angina/non—ST—segment—elevation MI* –1 mg/kg q 12 hr for 2–8 days (with aspirin).

IV, Subcut (Adults <75 yr): *Acute ST—segment—elevation MI*—Administer single IV bolus of 30 mg plus 1 mg/kg subcut dose (maximum of 100 mg for first 2 doses only), followed by 1 mg/kg subcut q 12 hrs. The usual duration of treatment is 2–8 days. In patients undergoing percutaneous coronary intervention, if last subcut dose was <8 hr before balloon inflation, no additional dosing needed; if last subcut dose was ≥8 hr before balloon inflation, administer single IV bolus of 0.3 mg/kg.

Subcut (Adults ≥75 yr): *Acute ST—segment—elevation MI*—0.75 mg/kg every 12 hrs (no IV bolus needed) (maximum of 75 mg for first 2 doses only; no initial bolus). The usual duration of treatment is 2–8 days.

Renal Impairment

Subcut (Adults CCr <30 ml/min): *VTE prophylaxis for abdominal or knee/hip replacement surgery*—30 mg once daily. *Treatment of DVT/PE*—1 mg/kg once daily. *Unstable angina/non-ST-segment-elevation MI*—1 mg/kg once daily. *Acute ST-segment-elevation MI (patients <75 yr)*—Single IV bolus of 30 mg plus 1 mg/kg subcut dose, followed by 1 mg/kg subcut once daily. *Acute ST-segment-elevation MI (patients ≥75 yr)*—1 mg/kg once daily (no initial bolus).

Tinzaparin

Subcut (Adults): *Treatment of deep vein thrombosis*—175 anti-Xa IU/kg once daily for at least 6 days and until adequate anticoagulation is achieved with warfarin (INR >2 for two consecutive days).

Availability

Dalteparin

Solution for injection (prefilled syringes): 2500 IU/0.2 ml, 5000 IU/0.2 ml, 7500 IU/0.3 ml, 10,000 IU/0.4 ml, 10,000 IU/1 ml, 12,500 IU/0.5 ml, 15,000 IU/0.6 ml, 18,000 IU/0.72 ml. **Solution for injection (multidose vials):** 10,000 IU/ml in 9.5-ml vials, 25,000 IU/ml in 3.8-ml vials.

Enoxaparin

Solution for injection (prefilled syringes): 30 mg/0.3 ml, 40 mg/0.4 ml, 60 mg/0.6 ml, 80 mg/0.8 ml, 100 mg/1 ml, 120 mg/0.8 ml, 150 mg/ml. **Solution for injection (multidose vials):** 300 mg/3 ml.

Tinzaparin

Solution for injection: 20,000 anti-Xa units/ml in 2-ml vials.

NURSING IMPLICATIONS

Assessment

- Assess for signs of bleeding and hemorrhage (bleeding gums; nosebleed; unusual bruising; black, tarry stools; hematuria; fall in hematocrit or blood pressure; guaiac-positive stools); bleeding from surgical site. Notify physician or other health care professional if these occur.
- Assess for evidence of additional or increased thrombosis. Symptoms depend on area of in-

volvement. Monitor neurological status frequently for signs of neurological impairment. May require urgent treatment.

- Monitor for hypersensitivity reactions (chills, fever, urticaria). Report signs to physician or other health care professional.
- Monitor patients with epidural catheters frequently for signs and symptoms of neurologic impairment.
- **Subcut:** Observe injection sites for hematomas, ecchymosis, or inflammation.
- ***Lab Test Considerations:*** Monitor CBC, platelet count, and stools for occult blood periodically during therapy. If thrombocytopenia occurs (platelet count <100,000/mm^3), discontinue therapy. If hematocrit ↓ unexpectedly, assess patient for potential bleeding sites. For *dalteparin* use for extended treatment of symptomatic VTE in cancer patients, if platelets ↓ to 50,000–100,000/mm^3, reduce dose to 2500 IU once daily until recovery to ≥100,000/mm^3; if platelets <50,000/mm^3, discontinue until count returns to ≥50,000/mm^3.
- Special monitoring of aPTT is not necessary. Monitoring of anti-Xa levels may be considered in patients who are obese or have renal dysfunction (for *enoxaparin*, obtain 4 hr after injection).
- May cause ↑ in AST and ALT levels.
- ***Toxicity and Overdose:*** For *enoxaparin* overdose, protamine sulfate 1 mg for each mg of *enoxaparin* should be administered by slow IV injection. For *dalteparin* overdose, protamine sulfate 1 mg for each 100 anti-factor Xa IU of *dalteparin* should be administered by slow IV injection. If the aPTT measured 2–4 hr after protamine administration remains prolonged, a 2nd infusion of protamine 0.5 mg/100 anti-factor Xa IU of *dalteparin* may be administered.

Potential Nursing Diagnoses

Ineffective tissue perfusion (Indications)
Risk for injury (Side Effects)

Implementation

- ***High Alert:*** Unintended concomitant use of two heparin products (unfractionated heparin and LMW heparins) has resulted in serious harm and death. Review patients' recent and current medication administration records before administering any heparin or low-molecular-weight heparin product.
- Cannot be used interchangeably (unit for unit) with unfractionated heparin or other low-molecular-weight heparins.
- **Subcut:** Administer deep into subcut tissue. Alternate injection sites daily between the left and right anterolateral and left and right posterolateral abdominal wall, the upper thigh, or buttocks. Inject entire length of needle at a 45° or 90° angle into a skin fold held between thumb and forefinger; hold skin fold throughout injection. Do not aspirate or massage. Rotate sites frequently. Do not administer IM because of danger of hematoma formation. Solution should be clear; do not inject solution containing particulate matter.
- If excessive bruising occurs, ice cube massage of site before injection may lessen bruising.
- **Enoxaparin:** To avoid the loss of drug, do not expel the air bubble from the syringe before the injection.
- **Subcut:** Per manufacturer's recommendations, to enhance absorption, inject enoxaparin into left or right anterolateral or posterolateral abdominal wall only.
- To minimize risk of bleeding after vascular instrumentation for unstable angina, recommended intervals between doses should be followed closely. Leave vascular access sheath in place for 6–8 hr after enoxaparin dose. Give next enoxaparin dose ≥6–8 hr after sheath removal. Observe site for bleeding or hematoma formation.
- **Direct IV:** Use multidose vial for bolus injections. Administer through a pre-exsting IV line. Flush line with 0.9% NaCl or D5W before and after administration.
- **Tinzaparin:** Tinzaparin should be administered daily for at least 6 days and until patient is adequately anticoagulated with warfarin (INR at least 2.0 for 2 consecutive days). Warfarin therapy should be started within 1–3 days of tinzaparin initiation.

Patient/Family Teaching

- Advise patient to report any symptoms of unusual bleeding or bruising, dizziness, itching, rash, fever, swelling, or difficulty breathing to health care professional immediately.
- Instruct patient not to take aspirin or NSAIDs without consulting health care professional while on therapy.

Evaluation/Desired Outcomes

- Prevention of DVT and pulmonary emboli (enoxaparin and dalteparin only).

- Resolution of DVT and pulmonary embolism (enoxaparin and tinzaparin only).
- Prevention of ischemic complications (with aspirin) in patients with unstable angina or non–ST—segment—elevation MI (enoxaparin and dalteparin only).
- Prevention of recurrent MI or death in patients with acute ST-segment-elevation MI (enoxaparin only).

HISTAMINE H_2 ANTAGONISTS

cimetidine (sye-**me**-ti-deen)
✤Apo-Cimetidine, ✤Dom-Cimetidine, ✤Gen-Cimetidine, ✤Novo-Cimetine, ✤Nu-Cimet, ✤PMS-Cimetidine, Tagamet, Tagamet HB

famotidine (fa-**moe**-ti-deen)
✤Acid Control, ✤Apo-Famotidine, ✤Gen-Famotidine, Maximum Strength Pepcid, Mylanta AR, ✤Novo-Famotidine, ✤Nu-Famotidine, Pepcid, Pepcid AC, Pepcid AC Acid Controller, Pepcid RPD, ✤Ulcidine

nizatidine (ni-**za**-ti-deen)
✤Apo-Nizatidine, Axid, Axid AR, ✤Dom-Nizatidine, ✤Gen-Nizatidine, ✤Novo-Nizatidine, ✤PHL-Nizatidine, ✤PMS-Nizatidine

ranitidine (ra-**ni**-ti-deen)
Apo-Ranitidine, ✤Dom-Ranitidine, ✤Gen-Ranitidine, ✤Novo-Ranitidine, ✤Nu-Ranitidine, ✤PHL-Ranitidine, ✤PMS-Ranitidine, ✤Ratio-Ranitidine, ✤Riva-Ranitidine, Zantac, Zantac 75

Classification
Therapeutic: antiulcer agents
Pharmacologic: histamine H2 antagonists

Pregnancy Category B

Indications

Short-term treatment of active duodenal ulcers and benign gastric ulcers. Maintenance therapy for duodenal and gastric ulcers after healing of active ulcers. Management of GERD. Treatment of heartburn, acid indigestion, and sour stomach (OTC use). **Cimetidine, famotidine, ranitidine:** Management of gastric hypersecretory states (Zollinger-Ellison syndrome). **Cimetidine, famotidine, ranitidine IV:** Prevention and treatment of stress-induced upper GI bleeding in critically ill patients. **Ranitidine:** Treatment of and maintenance therapy for erosive esophagitis. **Unlabeled uses:** Management of GI symptoms associated with the use of NSAIDs. Prevention of acid inactivation of supplemental pancreatic enzymes in patients with pancreatic insufficiency. Management of urticaria.

H

Action

Inhibits the action of histamine at the H_2-receptor site located primarily in gastric parietal cells, resulting in inhibition of gastric acid secretion. **Therapeutic Effects:** Healing and prevention of ulcers. Decreased symptoms of gastroesophageal reflux. Decreased secretion of gastric acid.

Pharmacokinetics

Absorption: *Cimetidine*—well absorbed after oral and IM administration. *Famotidine*—40–45% absorbed after oral administration. *Nizatidine*—70–95% absorbed after oral administration. *Ranitidine*—50% absorbed after PO and IM administration.
Distribution: All agents enter breast milk and cerebrospinal fluid.
Metabolism and Excretion: *Cimetidine*—30% metabolized by the liver; remainder is eliminated unchanged by the kidneys. *Famotidine*—up to 70% excreted unchanged by the kidneys, 30–35% metabolized by the liver. *Nizatidine*—60% excreted unchanged by the kidneys; some hepatic metabolism; at least 1 metabolite has histamine-blocking activity. *Ranitidine*—metabolized by the liver, mostly on first pass; 30% excreted unchanged by the kidneys after PO administration, 70% after parenteral administration.
Half-life: *Cimetidine*—2 hr; *famotidine*—2.5–3.5 hr; *nizatidine*—1.6 hr; *ranitidine*—2–2.5 hr (all are ↑ in renal impairment).

TIME/ACTION PROFILE

ROUTE	ONSET	PEAK	DURATION
Cimetidine PO	30 min	45–90 min	4–5 hr
Cimetidine IM, IV	10 min	30 min	4–5 hr

Famotidine PO	within 60 min	1–4 hr	6–12 hr
Famotidine IV	within 60 min	0.5–3 hr	8–15 hr
Nizatidine PO	unknown	unknown	8–12 hr
Ranitidine PO	unknown	1–3 hr	8–12 hr
Ranitidine IM	unknown	15 min	8–12 hr
Ranitidine IV	unknown	15 min	8–12 hr

Contraindications/Precautions

Contraindicated in: Hypersensitivity; Some products contain alcohol and should be avoided in patients with known intolerance; Some products contain aspartame and should be avoided in patients with phenylketonuria.
Use Cautiously in: Renal impairment (more susceptible to adverse CNS reactions; increased dosage interval recommended for *cimetidine* and *nizatidine* if CCr ≤50 ml/min, and for *famotidine* and *ranitidine* if CCr <50 ml/min; Hepatic impairment (for *ranitidine*); Acute porphyria (for *ranitidine*); Geri: Geriatric patients (more susceptible to adverse CNS reactions; dosage reduction recommended); OB, Lactation: Pregnancy or lactation.

Adverse Reactions/Side Effects

CNS: confusion, dizziness, drowsiness, hallucinations, headache. **CV:** ARRHYTHMIAS. **GI:** constipation, diarrhea, drug-induced hepatitis (nizatidine, cimetidine), nausea. **GU:** decreased sperm count, erectile dysfunction (cimetidine). **Endo:** gynecomastia. **Hemat:** AGRANULOCYTOSIS, APLASTIC ANEMIA, anemia, neutropenia, thrombocytopenia. **Local:** pain at IM site. **Misc:** hypersensitivity reactions, vasculitis.

Interactions

Drug-Drug: Cimetidine is a moderate inhibitor of the CYP1A2, CYP2C9, CYP2D6, and CYP3A4 isoenzymes in the liver; may lead to ↑ levels and toxicity with **benzodiazepines** (especially **chlordiazepoxide**, **diazepam**, and **midazolam**), some **beta blockers** (**labetalol**, **metoprolol**, **propranolol**), **caffeine**, **calcium channel blockers**, **carbamazepine**, **cyclosporine**, **dofetilide**, **lidocaine**, **metronidazole**, **mexiletine**, **nefazodone**, **pentoxifylline**, **phenytoin**, **procainamide**, **propafenone**, **quinidine**, **metformin**, **risperidone**, **ritonavir**, **ropinirole**, **selective serotonin reuptake inhibitors**, **sildenafil**, **sulfonylureas**, **tacrolimus**, **theophylline**, **tricyclic antidepressants**, **venlafaxine** and **warfarin**. Famotidine, nizatidine, and ranitidine have a much smaller and less significant effect on the metabolism of other drugs. Cimetidine may ↑ myelosuppressive effects of **carmustine** (avoid concurrent use). All agents ↓ absorption of **atazanavir**, **delavirdine**, **ketoconazole**, and **itraconazole**.

Route/Dosage

Cimetidine

PO (Adults): *Short-term treatment of active ulcers*—300 mg 4 times daily *or* 800 mg at bedtime *or* 400–600 mg twice daily (not to exceed 2.4 g/day) for up to 8 wk. *Duodenal ulcer prophylaxis*—300 mg twice daily *or* 400 mg at bedtime. *GERD*—400 mg q 6 hr *or* 800 mg twice daily for 12 wk. *Gastric hypersecretory conditions*—300–600 mg q 6 hr (up to 2400 mg/day). *OTC use*—up to 200 mg may be taken twice daily (for not more than 2 wk).
PO (Children): *Short-term treatment of active ulcers*—5–10 mg/kg q 6 hr.
IM, IV (Adults): *Short-term treatment of active ulcers*—300 mg q 6 hr (not to exceed 2.4 g/day). *Continuous IV infusion*—900 mg infused over 24 hr (37.5 mg/hr); may be preceded by a 150-mg bolus dose. *Gastric hypersecretory conditions*—300–600 mg q 6 hr (not to exceed 2.4 g/day). *Prevention of upper GI bleeding in critically ill patients*—50 mg/hr.
IM, IV (Children): *Short-term treatment of active ulcers*—5–10 mg/kg q 6 hr.

Renal Impairment

IV, PO (Adults): *CCr 10–50 ml/min*—Administer 50% of normal dose; *CCr <10 ml/min*—Administer 25% of normal dose; *prevention of upper GI bleeding in critically ill patients if CCr <30 ml/min*—25 mg/hr.

Renal Impairment

PO (Children): 10–15 mg/kg/day.

Famotidine

PO (Adults): *Short-term treatment of active duodenal ulcers*—40 mg/day at bedtime or 20 mg twice daily for up to 8 wk. *Treatment of benign gastric ulcers*—40 mg/day at bedtime. *Maintenance treatment of duodenal ulcers*—20 mg once daily at bedtime. *GERD*—20 mg twice daily for up to 6 wk; up to 40 mg twice daily for up to 12 wk for esophagitis with erosions, ulcerations, and continuing symptoms. *Gastric hypersecretory conditions*—20 mg q 6 hr initially, up to 160 mg q 6 hr. *OTC use*—10 mg for relief of symptoms; for prevention—10 mg 60 min before eating or take 10 mg as chewable tablet 15 minutes before heartburn-inducing

foods or beverages (not to exceed 20 mg/24 hr for up to 2 wk).
PO, IV (Children 1–16 yr): *Peptic ulcer*—0.5 mg/kg/day as a single bedtime dose or in 2 divided doses (up to 40 mg daily); *GERD*—1 mg/kg/day in 2 divided doses (up to 80 mg twice daily).
PO (Infants >3 mo—1 yr): *GERD*—0.5 mg/kg/dose twice daily.
PO (Infants and neonates <3 mo): *GERD*—0.5 mg/kg/dose once daily.
IV (Adults): 20 mg q 12 hr.

Renal Impairment

PO (Adults): *CCr <50 ml/min*—administer normal dose q 36–48 hr *or* 50% of normal dose at normal dosing interval. *CCr <10 ml/min*—dosing interval may need to be ↑ to q 36–48 hr.

Nizatidine

PO (Adults): *Short-term treatment of active duodenal or benign gastric ulcers*—300 mg once daily at bedtime. *Maintenance treatment of duodenal ulcers*—150 mg once daily at bedtime. *GERD*—150 mg twice daily. *OTC use*—75 mg twice daily given 30–60 min before foods or beverages expected to cause symptoms.

Renal Impairment

PO (Adults): *Short-term treatment of active ulcers—CCr 20–50 ml/min*—150 mg once daily; *CCr <20 ml/min*—150 mg every other day. *Maintenance treatment of duodenal ulcers—CCr 20–50 ml/min*—150 mg every other day; *CCr <20 ml/min*—150 mg every 3 days.

Ranitidine

PO (Adults): *Short-term treatment of active duodenal of benign gastric ulcers*—150 mg twice daily *or* 300 mg once daily at bedtime. *Maintenance treatment of duodenal or gastric ulcers*—150 mg once daily at bedtime. *GERD*—150 mg twice daily. *Erosive esophagitis*—150 mg 4 times daily initially, then 150 mg twice daily as maintenance. *Gastric hypersecretory conditions*—150 mg twice daily initially; up to 6 g/day have been used. *OTC use*—75 mg 30–60 min before foods or beverages expected to cause symptoms (up to twice daily) (not to be used for more than 2 wk).
PO (Children 1 mo-16 yr): *Treatment of gastric/duodenal ulcers* 2–4 mg/kg/day in 2 divided doses (up to 300 mg/day) *Maintenance treatment of ulcers*—2–4 mg/kg once daily (up to 150 mg/day); *GERD/erosive esophagitis*—5–10 mg/kg/day in 2 divided doses (up to 300 mg/day for GERD or 600 mg/day for erosive esophagitis).
PO (Neonates): 2 mg/kg/day in 2 divided doses.
IV, IM (Adults): 50 mg q 6–8 hr. *Continuous IV infusion*—6.25 mg/hr. *Gastric hypersecretory conditions*—1 mg/kg/hr; may be ↑ by 0.5 mg/kg/hr (not to exceed 2.5 mg/kg/hr).
IV, IM (Children 1 mo-16 yr): *Treatment of gastric/duodenal ulcers*—2–4 mg/kg/day divided q 6–8 hr (up to 200 mg/day). *Continuous infusion*—1 mg/kg/dose followed by 0.08–0.17 mg/kg/hr.
IV (Neonates): 1.5 mg/kg/dose load, then in 12 hr start maintenance of 1.5–2 mg/kg/day divided q 12 hr. *Continuous IV infusion*—1.5 mg/kg/dose load followed by 0.04–0.08 mg/kg/hr infusion.

Renal Impairment

PO (Adults): *CCr<50 ml/min*—150 mg q 24 hr.

Renal Impairment

IV (Adults): *CCr<50 ml/min*—50 mg q 24 hr.

Availability

Cimetidine

Tablets: 200 mg[Rx, OTC], 300 mg, 400 mg, ✤600 mg, 800 mg. **Oral liquid (mint-peach flavor):** 200 mg/5 ml[OTC], 300 mg/5 ml. **Premixed infusion:** 300 mg/50 ml 0.9% NaCl. **Solution for injection:** 150 mg/ml.

Famotidine

Tablets: 10 mg[OTC], 20 mg[Rx, OTC], 40 mg. **Gelcaps:** 10 mg[OTC]. **Oral suspension (cherry-banana-mint flavor):** 40 mg/5 ml. **Premixed infusion:** 20 mg/50 ml 0.9% NaCl. **Solution for injection:** 10 mg/ml. ***In combination with:*** calcium carbonate and magnesium hydroxide[OTC] (Pepcid Complete, see Appendix B).

Nizatidine

Tablets: 75 mg[OTC]. **Capsules:** 150 mg, 300 mg. **Oral solution (bubble gum flavor):** 15 mg/mL.

Ranitidine

Tablets: 75 mg[OTC], 150 mg, 300 mg. **Cost:** *Generic*—150 mg $23.99/180, 300 mg $24.84/90. **Capsules:** 150 mg, 300 mg. **Cost:** *Generic*—150 mg $89.95/180, 300 mg $79.99/90. **Effer-**

vescent tablets (EFFERdose): 25 mg. **Syrup (peppermint flavor):** 15 mg/ml. **Cost:** $330.01/473 ml. **Premixed infusion:** 50 mg/ 50 ml 0.45% NaCl. **Solution for injection:** 25 mg/ml.

NURSING IMPLICATIONS

Assessment

- Assess for epigastric or abdominal pain and frank or occult blood in the stool, emesis, or gastric aspirate.
- Geri: Assess geriatric and debilitated patients routinely for confusion. Report promptly.
- ***Lab Test Considerations:*** Monitor CBC with differential periodically during therapy.
- Antagonize effects of pentagastrin and histamine during gastric acid secretion testing. Avoid administration for 24 hr before the test.
- May cause false-negative results in skin tests using allergenic extracts. Histamine H_2 antagonists should be discontinued 24 hr before the test.
- May cause ↑ in serum transaminases and serum creatinine.
- Serum prolactin concentration may be ↑ after IV bolus of *cimetidine*. May also cause ↓ parathyroid concentrations.
- *Nizatidine* may cause ↑ alkaline phosphatase concentrations.
- *Ranitidine* and *famotidine* may cause false-positive results for urine protein; test with sulfosalicylic acid.

Potential Nursing Diagnoses

Acute pain (Indications)

Implementation

- **PO:** Administer with meals or immediately afterward and at bedtime to prolong effect.
- If antacids or sucralfate are used concurrently for relief of pain, avoid administration of antacids within 30 min-1 hr of the H_2 antagonist and take sucralfate 2 hr after H_2 antagonist; may ↓ absorption of H_2 antagonist.
- Doses administered once daily should be administered at bedtime to prolong effect.
- Shake oral suspension before administration. Discard unused suspension after 30 days.
- Remove foil from *ranitidine effervescent tablets* and dissolve in 6–8 oz water before drinking.

Cimetidine

IV Administration

- **Direct IV:** ***Diluent:*** 0.9% NaCl, D5W, D10W, D5/LR, D5/0.9% NaCl, D5/0.45% NaCl, D5/0.25% NaCl, Ringer's or LR, or sodium bicarbonate. ***Concentration:*** 15 mg/ ml. ***Rate:*** Administer over at least 5 min (minimum 5 min). Rapid administration may cause hypotension and arrhythmias.
- **Intermittent Infusion:** ***Diluent:*** See Direct IV. Diluted solution is stable for 48 hr at room temperature. Refrigeration may cause cloudiness but will not affect potency. Do not use solution that is discolored or contains precipitate. ***Concentration:*** 6 mg/ml. ***Rate:*** Administer over 15–30 min.
- **Continuous Infusion:** Dilute cimetidine 900 mg in 100–1000 ml of compatible solution (see Direct IV). ***Rate:*** Usually infused at a rate of 37.5 mg/hr or greater but should be individualized.
- **Continuous Infusion:** ***Diluent:*** Dilute 4 ml (40 mg of drug) with 1000 ml, 2 ml (20 mg of drug) with 500 ml, or 1 ml (10 mg of drug) with 250 ml of 0.9% NaCl or D5W. Infusion is stable for 24 hrs at room temperature. ***Concentration:*** 40 mcg/ml. ***Rate:*** Based on patient's weight (see Route/Dosage section). Titrate to desired effect. Administer via infusion pump to ensure accurate dosage rate.
- **Syringe Compatibility:** atropine, butorphanol, diazepam, diphenhydramine, doxapram, droperidol, fentanyl, glycopyrrolate, hydromorphone, hydroxyzine, lorazepam, meperidine, midazolam, morphine, nafcillin, nalbuphine, penicillin G sodium, pentazocine, perphenazine, prochlorperazine, promethazine, scopolamine, sodium acetate, sodium chloride, sodium lactate, sterile water.
- **Y-Site Compatibility:** alfentanil, amikacin, aminocaproic acid, amiodarone, ampicillin/ sulbactam, argatroban, atracurium, atropine, azithromycin, aztreonam, butorphanol, calcium chloride, calcium gluconate, caspofungin, cefazolin, cefepime, cefotaxime, ceftazidime, ceftizoxime, ceftriaxone, cefuroxime, chloramphenicol, cimetidine, ciprofloxacin, cisatracurium, clindamycin, cyclosporine, daptomycin, dexmedetomidine, digoxin, diltiazem, diphenhydramine, dobutamine, dolasetron, dopamine, doxycycline, droperidol, enalaprilat, epinephrine, ertapenem, erythromycin, esmolol, famotidine, fentanyl, fluconazole, gentamicin, granisetron, haloperidol, heparin, hydralazine, hydrocortisone sodium succinate, hydromorphone, imipenem/cilastatin, inamrinone,

insulin, isoproterenol, labetalol, levofloxacin, lidocaine, linezolid, lorazepam, magnesium sulfate, mannitol, meperidine, metoclopramide, metoprolol, metronidazole, micafungin, midazolam, milrinone, morphine, nafcillin, nalbuphine, naloxone, nicardipine, nitroglycerin, nitroprusside, norepinephrine, ondansetron, palonosetron, pancuronium, phenylephrine, piperacillin/tazobactam, potassium chloride, potassium phosphate, procainamide, promethazine, propofol, propranolol, quinupristin/dalfopristin, ranitidine, remifentanil, rocuronium, sufentanil, tacrolimus, theophylline, ticarcillin/clavulanate, tirofiban, tobramycin, trimethoprim/sulfamethoxazole, vancomycin, vasopressin, vecuronium, verapamil, voriconazole.

- **Y-Site Incompatibility:** acyclovir, aminophylline, amphotericin B, ampicillin, bumetanide, cefoxitin, dexamethasone sodium phosphate, diazepam, fosphenytoin, furosemide, ganciclovir, ketorolac, meropenem, methohexital, methylprednisolone sodium succinate, pantoprazole, pentobarbital, phenytoin, prochlorperazine, sodium bicarbonate, thiopental, promazine.
- **Syringe Incompatibility:** chlorpromazine, pentobarbital, secobarbital.
- **Y-Site Compatibility:** acyclovir, amifostine, aminophylline, atracurium, anakinra, anidulafungin, aztreonam, bivalirudin, cisatracurium, cisplatin, cladribine, cyclophosphamide, cytarabine, dexmedetomidine, diltiazem, docetaxel, doxorubicin, doxorubicin liposome, enalaprilat, esmolol, etoposide phosphate, fenoldopam, filgrastim, fluconazole, fludarabine, foscarnet, gemcitabine, granisetron, haloperidol, heparin, idarubicin, inamrinone, labetalol, levofloxacin, linezolid, melphalan, meropenem, methotrexate, midazolam, milrinone, nicardipine, ondansetron, oxaliplatin, paclitaxel, pancuronium, pemetrexed, piperacillin/tazobactam, propofol, remifentanil, sargramostim, tacrolimus, teniposide, theophylline, thiotepa, tolazoline, topotecan, vecuronium, vinorelbine, zidovudine.
- **Y-Site Incompatibility:** allopurinol, amphotericin B cholesteryl sulfate, amsacrine, cefepime, indomethacin, lansoprazole, warfarin.

Famotidine

IV Administration

- **Direct IV:** ***Diluent:*** 0.9% NaCl, D5W, D10W, or LR. ***Concentration:*** 4 mg/ml. ***Rate:*** Administer at a rate of 10 mg/min. Rapid administration may cause hypotension.
- **Intermittent Infusion:** ***Diluent:*** Dilute each 20 mg in 100 ml of 0.9% NaCl, D5W, D10W, or LR. Diluted solution is stable for 48 hr at room temperature. Do not use solution that is discolored or contains a precipitate. ***Concentration:*** 0.2 mg/ml. ***Rate:*** Administer over 15–30 min.
- **Y-Site Compatibility:** acyclovir, allopurinol, amifostine, aminophylline, amiodarone, ampicillin, ampicillin/sulbactam, amsacrine, anakinra, atropine, aztreonam, bivalirudin, calcium gluconate, cefazolin, cefotaxime, cefoxitin, ceftazidime, ceftizoxime, ceftriaxone, cefuroxime, chlorpromazine, cisatracurium, cisplatin, cladribine, cyclophosphamide, cytarabine, dexamethasone, dexmedetomidine, dextran 40, digoxin, diphenhydramine, dobutamine, docetaxel, dopamine, doxorubicin, doxorubicin liposome, droperidol, enalaprilat, epinephrine, erythromycin lactobionate, esmolol, etoposide phosphate, fenoldopam, filgrastim, fluconazole, fludarabine, folic acid, gatifloxin, gemcitabine, gentamicin, granisetron, haloperidol, heparin, hydrocortisone, hydrocortisone sodium succinate, hydromorphone, imipenem/cilastatin, inamrinone, insulin, isoproterenol, labetalol, lidocaine, linezolid, lorazepam, magnesium sulfate, melphalan, meperidine, methotrexate, methylprednisolone, metoclopramide, midazolam, morphine, nafcillin, nicardipine, nitroglycerin, nitroprusside, norepinephrine, ondansetron, oxaliplatin, oxacillin, paclitaxel, pemetrexed, perphenazine, phenylephrine, phenytoin, phytonadione, potassium chloride, potassium phosphate, procainamide, propofol, remifentanil, sargramostim, sodium bicarbonate, teniposide, theophylline, thiamine, thiotepa, ticarcillin, ticarcillin/clavulanate, tirofiban, verapamil, vinorelbine.
- **Y-Site Incompatibility:** amphotericin B cholesteryl sulfate, azithromycin, cefepime, lansoprazole, piperacillin/tazobactam.

H

Ranitidine

IV Administration

- **Direct IV:** ***Diluent:*** 0.9% NaCl or D5W for injection. ***Concentration:*** 2.5 mg/ml. ***Rate:*** Administer over at least 5 min not to exceed 10 mg/min. Rapid administration may cause hypotension and arrhythmias.
- **Intermittent Infusion:** ***Diluent:*** See Direct IV. Diluted solution is stable for 48 hr at room temperature. Do not use solution that is discolored or that contains precipitate. ***Concentration:*** 0.5 mg/ml. ***Rate:*** Administer over 15–30 min.
- **Continuous Infusion:** Add ranitidine to D5W for a concentration of 150 mg/250 ml (no greater than 2.5 mg/ml for Zollinger-Ellison patients). ***Rate:*** Administer at a rate of 6.25 mg/hr. In patients with Zollinger-Ellison syndrome, start infusion at 1 mg/kg/hr. If gastric acid output is >10 mEq/hr or patient becomes symptomatic after 4 hr, adjust dose by 0.5 mg/kg/hr increments and remeasure gastric output.
- **Syringe Compatibility:** atropine, cyclizine, dexamethasone, dimenhydrinate, diphenhydramine, fentanyl, glycopyrrolate, heparin, hydromorphone, meperidine, metoclopramide, morphine, nalbuphine, pentazocine, perphenazine, prochlorperazine, promethazine, scopolamine, thiethylperazine.
- **Syringe Incompatibility:** hydroxyzine, midazolam, pantoprazole, pentobarbital, phenobarbital.
- **Y-Site Compatibility:** acyclovir, aldesleukin, allopurinol, amifostine, aminophylline, amsacrine, atracurium, aztreonam, bivalirudin, cefazolin, cefepime, cefoxitin, ceftazidime, ceftizoxime, ciprofloxacin, cisatracurium, cisplatin, cladribine, cyclophosphamide, cytarabine, dexmedetomidine, diltiazem, dobutamine, docetaxel, dopamine, doxorubicin, doxorubicin liposome, enalaprilat, epinephrine, esmolol, etoposide phosphate, fenoldopam, fentanyl, filgrastim, fluconazole, fludarabine, foscarnet, furosemide, gemcitabine, granisetron, heparin, hydromorphone, idarubicin, labetalol, linezolid, lorazepam, melphalan, meperidine, methotrexate, midazolam, milrinone, morphine, nicardipine, nitroglycerin, norepinephrine, ondansetron, oxaliplatin, paclitaxel, pancuronium, pemetrexed, piperacillin/tazobactam, procainamide, propofol, remifentanil, sargramostim, tacrolimus, teniposide, theophylline, thiopental, thiotepa, vecuronium, vinorelbine, warfarin, zidovudine.
- **Y-Site Incompatibility:** amphotericin B cholesteryl sulfate, insulin, lansoprazole.
- **Additive Compatibility:** amikacin, aminophylline, chloramphenicol, ciprofloxacin, dexamethasone, dobutamine, dopamine, doxycycline, furosemide, gentamicin, heparin, insulin, regular, lidocaine, methylprednisolone, penicillin G potassium, penicillin G sodium, potassium chloride, tobramycin, vancomycin.
- **Additive Incompatibility:** amphotericin B, phytonadione.

Patient/Family Teaching

- Instruct patient to take medication as directed for the full course of therapy, even if feeling better. Take missed doses as soon as remembered but not if almost time for next dose. Do not double doses.
- Advise patients taking OTC preparations not to take the maximum dose continuously for more than 2 wk without consulting health care professional. Notify health care professional if difficulty swallowing occurs or abdominal pain persists.
- Inform patient that smoking interferes with the action of histamine antagonists. Encourage patient to quit smoking or at least not to smoke after last dose of the day.
- May cause drowsiness or dizziness. Caution patient to avoid driving or other activities requiring alertness until response to the drug is known.
- Advise patient to avoid alcohol, products containing aspirin or NSAIDs, and foods that may cause an increase in GI irritation.
- Inform patient that increased fluid and fiber intake and exercise may minimize constipation.
- Advise patient to report onset of black, tarry stools; fever; sore throat; diarrhea; dizziness; rash; confusion; or hallucinations to health care professional promptly.

Evaluation/Desired Outcomes

- Decrease in abdominal pain.
- Treatment and prevention of gastric or duodenal irritation and bleeding. Healing of duodenal ulcers can be seen by x-rays or endoscopy. Therapy is continued for at least 6 wk in treatment of ulcers but not usually longer than 8 wk.
- Decreased symptoms of esophageal reflux.

- Treatment of heartburn, acid indigestion, and sour stomach (OTC use).

HMG-CoA REDUCTASE INHIBITORS (statins)

atorvastatin (a-**tore**-va-stat-in)
Lipitor

fluvastatin (**floo**-va-sta-tin)
Lescol, Lescol XL

lovastatin (**loe**-va-sta-tin)
Altoprev, Mevacor

pravastatin (**pra**-va-sta-tin)
Pravachol

rosuvastatin (roe-**soo**-va-sta-tin)
Crestor

simvastatin (**sim**-va-sta-tin)
Zocor

Classification
Therapeutic: lipid-lowering agents
Pharmacologic: HMG-CoA reductase inhibitors

Pregnancy Category X

Indications

Adjunctive management of primary hypercholesterolemia and mixed dyslipidemias. **Atorvastatin:** Primary prevention of cardiovascular disease (↓ risk of MI or stroke) in patients with multiple risk factors for coronary heart disease CHD or type 2 diabetes mellitus (also ↓ risk of angina or revascsularization procedures in patients with multiple risk factors for CHD). **Atorvastatin and Pravastatin:** Secondary prevention of cardiovascular disease (↓ risk of MI, stroke, revascularization procedures, angina, and hospitalizations for CHF) in patients with clinically evident CHD. **Fluvastatin:** Secondary prevention of coronary revascularizations procedures in patients with clinically evident CHD. **Fluvastatin, lovastatin, and rosuvastatin:** Slow progression of coronary atherosclerosis in patients with CHD. **Lovastatin:** Primary prevention of CHD (↓ risk of MI, unstable angina, and coronary revascularization) in patients without symptomatic cardiovascular disease with ↑ total and low-density lipoprotein (LDL) cholesterol and ↓ high-density lipoprotein (HDL) cholesterol. **Pravastatin:** Primary prevention of CHD (↓ risk of MI, coronary revascularization, and cardiovascular mortality) in patients without clinically evident CHD. **Simvastatin:** Secondary prevention of cardiovascular events (↓ risk of MI, coronary revascularization, stroke, and cardiovascular mortality) in patients with clinically evident CHD or those at high-risk for CHD (history of diabetes, peripheral arterial disease, or stroke).

Action

Inhibit an enzyme, 3-hydroxy-3-methylglutaryl-coenzyme A (HMG-CoA) reductase, which is responsible for catalyzing an early step in the synthesis of cholesterol. **Therapeutic Effects:** Lowers total and LDL cholesterol and triglycerides. Slightly increase HDL. Slows of the progression of coronary atherosclerosis with resultant decrease in CHD-related events (all agents except rosuvastatin have indication for ↓ events).

Pharmacokinetics

Absorption: *Atorvastatin*—rapidly absorbed but undergoes extensive GI and hepatic metabolism, resulting in 14% bioavailability; *fluvastatin*—98% absorbed after oral administration, but undergoes extensive first-pass metabolism resulting in 24% bioavailability; *lovastatin, pravastatin*—poorly and variably absorbed after oral administration; *rosuvastatin*—20% absorbed following oral administration; *simvastatin*—85% absorbed but rapidly metabolized.
Distribution: *Atorvastatin*—probably enters breast milk. *Fluvastatin*—enters breast milk. *Lovastatin*—crosses the blood-brain barrier and placenta. *Pravastatin*—small amounts enter breast milk. *Rosuvastatin and simvastatin*—unknown.
Protein Binding: *Atorvastatin, fluvastatin, and simvastatin*—>98%.
Metabolism and Excretion: All agents are extensively metabolized by the liver *atorvastatin*—<2%, *lovastatin*—10%, *fluvastatin*—5%, *pravastatin*—20% and *simvastatin*—13%.
Half-life: *Atorvastatin*—14 hr; *fluvastatin*—1.2 hr; *lovastatin*—3 hr; *pravastatin*—1.3–2.7 hr; *rosuvastatin*—19 hr; *simvastatin*—unknown.

TIME/ACTION PROFILE (cholesterol-lowering effect)

ROUTE	ONSET	PEAK	DURATION*
Atorvastatin	unknown	unknown	20–30 hr
Fluvastatin	1–2 wk	4–6 wk	unknown
Lovastatin	2 wk	4–6 wk	6 wk
Pravastatin	several days	2–4 wk	unknown
Rosuvastatin	unknown	2–4 wk	unknown
Simvastatin	several days	2–4 wk	unknown

*After discontinuation

Contraindications/Precautions

Contraindicated in: Hypersensitivity; Active liver disease or unexplained persistent ↑ in AST or ALT; OB, Lactation: Pregnancy or lactation (potential for fetal anomalies); Concurrent use of gemfibrozil or azole antifungals; Concurrent use of nelfinavir or ritonavir (with lovastatin or simvastatin).

Use Cautiously in: History of liver disease; Alcoholism; *Rosuvastatin only*—patients with Asian ancestry (may have ↑ blood levels and ↑ risk of rhabdomyolysis); *Atorvastatin, lovastatin, rosuvastatin, and simvastatin only*—concurrent use of gemfibrozil, azole antifungals, macrolides, protease inhibitors, niacin, cyclosporine, amiodarone or verapamil (↑ risk of myopathy/rhabdomyolysis); Renal impairment; OB: Women of childbearing age; Pedi: Children <8 yr (safety not established; some products approved for use in older children only).

Adverse Reactions/Side Effects

CNS: dizziness, headache, insomnia, weakness. **CV:** chest pain, peripheral edema. **EENT:** rhinitis; *lovastatin*— blurred vision. **Resp:** bronchitis. **GI:** abdominal cramps, constipation, diarrhea, flatus, heartburn, altered taste, drug-induced hepatitis, dyspepsia, elevated liver enzymes, nausea, pancreatitis. **GU:** erectile dysfunction. **Derm:** rashes, pruritus. **MS:** RHABDOMYOLYSIS, arthralgia, arthritis, myalgia, myositis. **Misc:** hypersensitivity reactions.

Interactions

Atorvastatin, lovastatin, simvastatin, and rosuvastatin are metabolized by the CYP3A4 metabolic pathway. Fluvastatin is metabolized by CYP2C9. Pravastatin is not metabolized by the CYPP450 system.

Drug-Drug: Atorvastatin, lovastatin and simvastatin may interact with **CYP3A4 inhibitors**. Bioavailability and effectiveness may be ↓ by **cholestyramine** and **colestipol**. Risk of myopathy with atorvastatin, lovastatin, and simvastatin is ↑ with **amiodarone**, **cyclosporine**, **gemfibrozil**, **clofibrate**, **diltiazem**, **verapamil**, **erythromycin**, **clarithromycin**, **telithromycin**, **nefazodone**, large doses of **niacin**, **azole antifungals**, **nelfinavir**, **saquinavir**, and **ritonavir**. Atorvastatin, fluvastatin, and simvastatin may slightly ↑ serum **digoxin** levels. Atorvastatin and rosuvastatin may ↑ levels of **hormonal contraceptives**. Atorvastatin, fluvastatin, lovastatin, rosuvastatin, and simvastatin may ↑ risk of bleeding with **warfarin**. **Isradipine** may ↓ the effectiveness of lovastatin. **Alcohol**, **cimetidine**, **ranitidine**, and **omeprazole** may ↑ fluvastatin levels. **Rifampin** may ↓ fluvastatin levels. **Antacids** ↓ absorption of rosuvastatin (administer 2 hr after rosuvastatin. **Lopinavir/ritonavir** may ↑ rosuvastatin levels. **Cyclosporine** ↑ levels and risk of toxicity of rosuvastatin (dosage adjustment required). Fluvastatin ↑ levels of **glyburide**; **glyburide** ↑ fluvastatin levels (monitoring of both agents recommended). Fluvastatin ↑ levels of **phenytoin**; **phenytoin** ↑ fluvastatin levels (monitoring of both agents recommended).

Drug-Natural Products: St. John's wort may ↓ levels and effectiveness (lovastatin and simvastatin).

Drug-Food: Large quantities of **grapefruit juice** ↑ blood levels and ↑ risk of rhabdomyolysis. **Food** enhances blood levels of lovastatin.

Route/Dosage

Atorvastatin

PO (Adults): 10—20 mg once daily initially (may start with 40 mg/day if LDL should be lowered by >45%); may be increased q 2–4 wk up to 80 mg/day.

PO (Children 10–17 yr): 10 mg/day initially, may be ↑ q 4 wk up to 20 mg/day.

Fluvastatin

PO (Adults): 20 mg (capsule) once daily at bedtime (may start with 40 mg once daily at bedtime if LDL needs to be lowered by ≥25%). May be ↑ to 80 mg once daily (as extended-release tablet) or 40 mg twice daily (capsule).

Lovastatin

PO (Adults): 20 mg once daily with evening meal. May be ↑ at 4-wk intervals to a maximum of 80 mg/day (immediate-release) or 60 mg/day (extended-release); initiate at 10 mg/day in patients receiving cyclosporine or other immunosuppressants and do not exceed 20 mg/day;

should not exceed 40 mg/day (immediate-release) or 20 mg/day (extended-release) if receiving verapamil or amiodarone; should not exceed 20 mg/day if receiving danazol or niacin (>1 g/day).

Renal Impairment

PO (Adults): *CCr <30 ml/min*—dosage should not exceed 20 mg/day unless carefully titrated.

PO (Children/Adolescents 10-17 yr): *Familial heterozygous hypercholesterolemia*—10-40 mg/day adjusted at 4 wk intervals.

Pravastatin

PO (Adults): 40 mg once daily at bedtime; may be ↑ at 4–wk intervals up to maximum of 80 mg/day. *Concurrent cyclosporine therapy*—initial dose is 10 mg/day and should not exceed 20 mg/day.

PO (Children 14-18 yrs): 40 mg once daily.

PO (Children 8-13 yrs): 20 mg once daily.

Hepatic/Renal Impairment

PO (Adults): 10–20 mg once daily at bedtime; ↑ at 4–wk intervals as needed (usual range = 10–20 mg/day).

Rosuvastatin

PO (Adults): 10 mg once daily initially (range 5–20 mg initially); dose may be adjusted at 2–4 wk intervals, some patients may require up to 40 mg/day (associated with ↑ risk of rhabdomyolysis); *Patients with Asian ancestry*—initial dose should not exceed 5 mg/day *Concurrent cyclosporine therapy*—dose should not exceed 5 mg/day; *Concurrent gemfibrozil or lopinavir/ritonavir therapy*—dose should not exceed 10 mg/day (avoid if possible)

Renal Impairment

PO (Adults): *CCr <30 ml/min*—5 mg once daily intially; dose may be ↑ but should not exceed 10 mg/day.

Simvastatin

PO (Adults): 5–80 mg once daily in the evening. *Concurrent cyclosporine or danazol therapy*—Initiate at 5 mg once daily; dose should not exceed 10 mg/day. *Concurrent fibrate or niacin therapy* -Dose should not exceed 10 mg/day. *Concurrent amiodarone or verapamil therapy* -Dose should not exceed 20 mg/day.

PO (Children and adolescents 10–17 yr): 10 mg once daily initially, may be ↑ at 4–wk intervals up to 40 mg/day (not to exceed 10 mg/day in patients receiving cyclosporine, danazol, fibrates, or niacin or 20 mg/day in patients receiving amiodarone or verapamil)

Renal Impairment

PO (Adults): *CCr <10 ml/min* –5 mg/day initially, titrate carefully.

Availability

Atorvastatin

Tablets: 10 mg, 20 mg, 40 mg, 80 mg. **Cost:** 10 mg $237.99/90, 20 mg $321.97/90, 40 mg $325.97/90, 80 mg $329.97/90. ***In combination with:*** amlodipine (Caduet); see Appendix B.

Fluvastatin

Capsules: 20 mg, 40 mg. **Cost:** 20 mg $205.97/90, 40 mg $205.97/90. **Extended-release tablets:** 80 mg. **Cost:** 80 mg $265.99/90.

Lovastatin

Immediate-release tablets: 10 mg, 20 mg, 40 mg. **Cost:** 10 mg $89.70/60, 20 mg $158.19/60, 40 mg $284.76/60. **Extended-release tablets:** 10 mg, 20 mg, 40 mg, 60 mg. ***In combination with:*** Niacin (Advicor). See Appendix B.

Pravastatin

Tablets: 10 mg, 20 mg, 40 mg, 80 mg. **Cost:** 10 mg $169.97/90, 20 mg $44.67/90, 40 mg $49.97/90, 80 mg $379.72/90.

Rosuvastatin

Tablets: 5 mg, 10 mg, 20 mg, 40 mg. **Cost:** 5 mg $275.96/90, 10 mg $275.96/90, 20 mg $275.96/90, 40 mg $278.96/90.

Simvastatin

Tablets: 5 mg, 10 mg, 20 mg, 40 mg, 80 mg. **Cost:** *Generic*—5 mg $45.97/90, 10 mg $49.97/90, 20 mg $73.97/90, 40 mg $75.97/90, 80 mg $89.97/90. ***In combination with:*** Ezetimibe (Vytorin). See Appendix B.

NURSING IMPLICATIONS

Assessment

- Obtain a dietary history, especially with regard to fat consumption.
- ***Lab Test Considerations:*** Evaluate serum cholesterol and triglyceride levels before initiating, after 4–6 wk of therapy, and periodically thereafter.

- Monitor liver function tests, including AST, before, at 12 wk after initiation of therapy or after dose elevation, and then q 6 mo. If AST levels ↑ to 3 times normal, HMG-CoA reductase inhibitor therapy should be reduced or discontinued. May also cause ↑ alkaline phosphatase and bilirubin levels.
- If patient develops muscle tenderness during therapy, monitor CK levels. If CK levels are >10 times the upper limit of normal or myopathy occurs, therapy should be discontinued.

Potential Nursing Diagnoses

Noncompliance (Patient/Family Teaching)

Implementation

- Do not confuse Pravachol (pravastatin) with Prevacid (lansoprazole).
- **PO:** Administer *lovastatin* with food. Administration on an empty stomach decreases absorption by approximately 30%. Initial once-daily dose is administered with the evening meal.
- Administer extended-release tablets at bedtime. Extended-release tablets should be swallowed whole, do not crush, break, or chew.
- Administer *fluvastatin, pravastatin,* and *simvastatin* once daily in the evening. *Atorvastatin* and *rosuvastatin* can be taken any time of day. May be administered without regard to food.
- Avoid large amounts of grapefruit juice during therapy; may ↑ risk of toxicity.
- If *fluvastatin* or *pravastatin* is administered in conjunction with bile acid sequestrants (cholestyramine, colestipol), administer at least 4 hr after bile acid sequestrant.
- If *rosuvastatin* is administered in conjunction with magnesium or aluminum-containing antacids, administer antacid at least 2 hr after *rosuvastatin*.

Patient/Family Teaching

- Instruct patient to take medication as directed and not to skip doses or double up on missed doses. Advise patient to avoid drinking more that 200 mL/day of grapefruit juice during therapy. Medication helps control but does not cure elevated serum cholesterol levels.
- Advise patient that this medication should be used in conjunction with diet restrictions (fat, cholesterol, carbohydrates, alcohol), exercise, and cessation of smoking.
- Instruct patient to notify health care professional if unexplained muscle pain, tenderness, or weakness occurs, especially if accompanied by fever or malaise.
- Advise patient to avoid taking Rx, OTC, or herbal products without consulting with a health care professional.
- OB: Instruct female patients to notify health care professional promptly if pregnancy is planned or suspected.
- Advise patient to notify health care professional of medication regimen before treatment or surgery.
- Emphasize the importance of follow-up exams to determine effectiveness and to monitor for side effects.

Evaluation/Desired Outcomes

- Decrease in sLDL and total cholesterol levels.
- Increase in HDL cholesterol levels.
- Decrease in triglyceride levels.
- Slowing of the progression of coronary artery disease.

human papillomavirus quadravalent (types 6, 11, 16, 18) recombinant vaccine

(**hyoo**-man pa-pil-**lo**-ma)
Gardasil

Classification
Therapeutic: vaccines/immunizing agents

Indications

Prevention of squamous cell cervical cancer, other cervical and vaginal neoplasias and genital warts.

Action

Vaccination results in antibodies to HPV viruses that are causative agents for squamous cell cervical cancer and genital warts. **Therapeutic Effects:** Prevention of squamous cell cervical cancer and genital warts.

Pharmacokinetics

Absorption: Well absorbed following IM administration.
Distribution: Unk.
Metabolism and Excretion: Unk.
Half-life: Unk.

TIME/ACTION PROFILE (antibody response)

ROUTE	ONSET	PEAK	DURATION
IM	unknown	1 mo*	unknown

*After third vaccination

Contraindications/Precautions

Contraindicated in: Hypersensitivity; Thrombocytopenia/bleeding disorder; OB: Pregnancy. **Use Cautiously in:** Current/recent febrile illness; Immunosuppression may ↓ antibody response; OB: Use cautiously during lactation; Pedi: Safety in children <9 yr not established.

Adverse Reactions/Side Effects

Local: injection site reactions. **Misc:** ANAPHYLAXIS (RARE).

Interactions

Drug-Drug: Immunosuppressants or **antineoplastics** may ↓ antibody response.

Route/Dosage

IM (Adults and Children—females 9–26 yr): Three 0.5 ml doses at 0, 2 and 6 months.

Availability

Sterile preparation for intramuscular administration: 20 mcg of HPV 6 L1 protein, 40 mcg of HPV 11 L1 protein, 40 mcg of HPV 16 L1 protein, and 20 mcg of HPV 18 L1 protein/0.5-mL dose.

NURSING IMPLICATIONS

Assessment

- Assess vital signs prior to administration. Do not administer to patient with a current or recent febrile illness; low grade fever (<100°F) and mild upper respiratory infection and usually not contraindicated.

Potential Nursing Diagnoses

Risk for infection (Indications)

Implementation

- **General:** Vaccine is not intended for treatment of active genital warts or cervical cancer and will not protect from diseases not caused by HPV.
- **IM:** Prefilled syringe is for single use; do not use for more than one person. Administer as supplied; do not dilute; administer full dose. Shake well prior to administration to maintain suspension of vaccine. Solution is cloudy and white; do not administer solution that is discolored or contains particulate matter. If using single-dose vial, withdraw 0.5 mL dose and administer entire contents of syringe. Administer intramuscularly in the deltoid or in the high anterolateral area of the thigh.

Patient/Family Teaching

- Provide information about vaccine and the importance of completing immunization series unless contraindicated to patient and guardian.
- Inform patient that vaccine does not replace routine cervical cancer screening or prevent other sexually transmitted diseases; such screening should be continued as usual.
- Advise patient to consult health care professional prior to taking Rx, OTC, or herbal products.
- Advise patient to notify health care professional if pregnancy is planned or suspected. Women exposed to vaccine during pregnancy are encouraged to call manufacturer pregnancy registry at 800-986-8999.
- Instruct patient to report any adverse reactions to health care professional.

Evaluation/Desired Outcomes

- Prevention of cervical cancer, genital warts, cervical adenocarcinoma in situ, cervical, vulvar, and vaginal intraepithelial neoplasia caused by HPV.

hydrALAZINE

(hye-**dral**-a-zeen)

Apresoline, ✤Novo-Hylazin

Classification

Therapeutic: antihypertensives

Pharmacologic: vasodilators

Pregnancy Category C

Indications

Moderate to severe hypertension (with a diuretic). **Unlabeled uses:** CHF unresponsive to conventional therapy with digoxin and diuretics.

Action

Direct-acting peripheral arteriolar vasodilator. **Therapeutic Effects:** Lowering of blood pressure in hypertensive patients and decreased afterload in patients with CHF.

Pharmacokinetics

Absorption: Rapidly absorbed following oral administration; well absorbed from IM sites. **Distribution:** Widely distributed. Crosses the placenta; enters breast milk in minimal concentrations.

Metabolism and Excretion: Mostly metabolized by the GI mucosa and liver.
Half-life: 2–8 hr.

TIME/ACTION PROFILE (antihypertensive effect)

ROUTE	ONSET	PEAK	DURATION
PO	45 min	2 hr	2–4 hr
IM	10–30 min	1 hr	3–8 hr
IV	5–20 min	15–30 min	2–6hr

Contraindications/Precautions

Contraindicated in: Hypersensitivity; Some products contain tartrazine and should be avoided in patients with known intolerance.
Use Cautiously in: Cardiovascular or cerebrovascular disease; Severe renal and hepatic disease (dose modification may be necessary); Pregnancy and lactation (has been used safely during pregnancy).

Adverse Reactions/Side Effects

CNS: dizziness, drowsiness, headache. **CV:** tachycardia, angina, arrhythmias, edema, orthostatic hypotension. **GI:** diarrhea, nausea, vomiting. **Derm:** rashes. **F and E:** sodium retention. **MS:** arthralgias, arthritis. **Neuro:** peripheral neuropathy. **Misc:** drug-induced lupus syndrome.

Interactions

Drug-Drug: ↑ hypotension with acute ingestion of **alcohol**, other **antihypertensives**, or **nitrates**. **MAO inhibitors** may exaggerate hypotension. May ↓ pressor response to **epinephrine**. **NSAIDs** may ↓ antihypertensive response. **Beta blockers** ↓ tachycardia from hydralazine (therapy may be combined for this reason). **Metoprolol** and **propranolol** ↑ hydralazine levels. ↑ blood levels of **metoprolol** and **propranolol**.

Route/Dosage

PO (Adults): *Hypertension*—10 mg 4 times daily initially. After 2–4 days may increase to 25 mg 4 times daily for the rest of the 1st week; may then increase to 50 mg 4 times daily (up to 300 mg/day). Once maintenance dose is established, twice-daily dosing may be used. *CHF*—25–37.5 mg 4 times daily; may be increased up to 300 mg/day in 3–4 divided doses.
PO (Children >1 month): Initial—0.75–1 mg/kg/day in 2–4 divided doses, not to exceed 25 mg/dose; may increase gradually to 5 mg/kg/day in infants and 7.5 mg/kg/day in children (not to exceed 200 mg/day) in 2–4 divided doses.
IM, IV (Adults): *Hypertension*—5–40 mg repeated as needed. *Eclampsia*—5 mg q 15–20 min; if no response after a total of 20 mg, consider an alternative agent.
IM, IV (Children >1 month): Initial—0.1–0.2 mg/kg/dose (not to exceed 20 mg) q 4–6 hr as needed, up 1.7–3.5 mg/kg/day in 4–6 divided doses.

Availability (generic available)

Tablets: 10 mg, 25 mg, 50 mg, 100 mg. **Cost:** *Generic*—10 mg $23.30/100, 25 mg $22.90/100, 50 mg $23.30/100, 100 mg $66.65/100. **Injection:** 20 mg/ml. ***In combination with:*** isosorbide dinitrate (BiDil). See Appendix B.

NURSING IMPLICATIONS

Assessment

- Monitor blood pressure and pulse frequently during initial dose adjustment and periodically during therapy. Report significant changes.
- Monitor frequency of prescription refills to determine adherence.
- ***Lab Test Considerations:*** Monitor CBC, electrolytes, LE cell prep, and ANA titer prior to and periodically during prolonged therapy.
- May cause a positive direct Coombs' test result.

Potential Nursing Diagnoses

Ineffective tissue perfusion (Indications)
Noncompliance (Patient/Family Teaching)

Implementation

- Do not confuse hydralazine with hydroxyzine.
- IM or IV route should be used only when drug cannot be given orally.
- May be administered concurrently with diuretics or beta blockers to permit lower doses and minimize side effects.
- **PO:** Administer with meals consistently to enhance absorption.
- Pharmacist may prepare oral solution from hydralazine injection for patients with difficulty swallowing.

IV Administration

- **Direct IV:** ***Diluent:*** Administer undiluted. Use solution as quickly as possible after drawing through needle into syringe. ***Concentration:*** 20 mg/ml. ***Rate:*** Administer over at least 1 min. Pedi: Administer at a rate of 0.2 mg/kg/min in children. Monitor blood pressure and pulse in all patients frequently after injection.

- **Y-Site Compatibility:** daptomycin, diltiazem, fenoldopam, granisetron, heparin, hydrocortisone, hydromorphone, linezolid, palonosetron, potassium chloride, tacrolimus, tirofiban, verapamil, vitamin B complex with C, voriconazole.
- **Y-Site Incompatibility:** acyclovir, aminophylline, ampicillin, caspofungin, cefazolin, cefotaxime, cefoxitin, ceftazidime, ceftizoxime, ceftriaxone, cefuroxime, chloramphenicol, diazepam, ertapenem, furosemide, ganciclovir, haloperidol, lorazepam, methylprednisolone sodium succinate, nafcillin, nesiritide, nitroprusside, pantoprazole, phenytoin, procainamide, trimethoprim/sulfamethoxazole.
- **Solution Compatibility:** 0.45% NaCl, 0.9% NaCl, LR.
- **Solution Incompatibility:** D5W.

Patient/Family Teaching

- Emphasize the importance of continuing to take this medication, even if feeling well. Instruct patient to take medication at the same time each day; last dose of the day should be taken at bedtime. Take missed doses as soon as remembered; do not double doses. If more than 2 doses in a row are missed, consult health care professional. Must be discontinued gradually to avoid sudden increase in blood pressure. Hydralazine controls but does not cure hypertension.
- Encourage patient to comply with additional interventions for hypertension (weight reduction, low-sodium diet, smoking cessation, moderation of alcohol intake, regular exercise, and stress management). Instruct patient and family on proper technique for blood pressure monitoring. Advise them to check blood pressure at least weekly and report significant changes.
- Patients should weigh themselves twice weekly and assess feet and ankles for fluid retention.
- May occasionally cause drowsiness. Advise patient to avoid driving or other activities requiring alertness until response to medication is known.
- Caution patient to avoid sudden changes in position to minimize orthostatic hypotension.
- Advise patient to consult health care professional before taking any Rx, OTC, or herbal cough, cold, or allergy remedies.
- Instruct patient to notify health care professional of medication prior to treatment or surgery.
- Advise patient to notify health care professional immediately if general tiredness; fever; muscle or joint aching; chest pain; skin rash; sore throat; or numbness, tingling, pain, or weakness of hands and feet occurs. Vitamin B_6 (pyridoxine) may be used to treat peripheral neuritis.
- Emphasize the importance of follow-up exams to evaluate effectiveness of medication.

Evaluation/Desired Outcomes

- Decrease in blood pressure without appearance of side effects.
- Decreased afterload in patients with CHF.

hydralazine/isosorbide dinitrate

(hye-**dral**-a-zeen eye-so-**sor**-bide di-**ni**-trate)

BiDil

Classification

Therapeutic: vasodilators

Pharmacologic: vasodilators, nitrates

Pregnancy Category C

Indications

Management of heart failure in black patients.

Action

BiDil is a fixed-dose combination of **isosorbide dinitrate**, a vasodilator with effects on both arteries and veins, and **hydralazine**, a predominantly arterial vasodilator. **Therapeutic Effects:** Improved survival, increased time to hospitalization and decreased symptoms of heart failure in black patients.

Pharmacokinetics

See pharmacokinetic sections in hydralazine and isosorbide dinitrate monographs of Davis's Drug Guide for Nurses for more information.

Absorption: *Hydralazine*—10–26% absorbed in CHF patients, absorption can be saturated leading to large increases in absorption with higher doses; *isosorbide dinitrate*—vari-

H

able absorbed (10–90%) reflecting first-pass hepatic metabolism.
Distribution: *Hydralazine*—widely distributed, crosses the placenta, minimal amounts in breast milk; *isosorbide dinitrate*—accumulates in muscle and venous wall.
Metabolism and Excretion: *Hydralazine*—mostly metabolized by GI mucosa and liver; *isosorbide dinitrate*—undergoes extensive first-pass metabolism in the liver mostly metabolized by the liver, some metabolites are vasodilators.
Half-life: *Hydralazine*—4 hr; *isosorbide dinitrate*—2 hr.

TIME/ACTION PROFILE (effect on blood pressure)

ROUTE	ONSET	PEAK	DURATION
hydralazine	45 min	2 hr	2–4 hr
isosorbide	15–40 min	unknown	4 hr

Contraindications/Precautions

Contraindicated in: Hypersensitivity to either component.
Use Cautiously in: Pedi: Children <18 yr or lactation (safety not established); Hydralazine-Cardiovascular or cerebrovascular disease; Severe renal/hepatic disease (dose modification may be necessary); Pregnancy and lactation (has been used safely during pregnancy); isosorbide dinitrate. Head trauma or cerebral hemorrhage; Geriatric patients (start with lower doses); OB: Pregnancy (may compromise maternal/fetal circulation) or lactation (safety not established).

Adverse Reactions/Side Effects

Hydralazine **CNS:** dizziness, drowsiness, headache. **CV:** tachycardia, angina, arrhythmias, edema, orthostatic hypotension. **GI:** diarrhea, nausea, vomiting. **Derm:** rashes. **F and E:** sodium retention. **MS:** arthralgias, arthritis. **Neuro:** peripheral neuropathy. **Misc:** drug-induced lupus syndrome.
isosorbide dinitrate **CNS:** dizziness, headache, apprehension, weakness. **CV:** hypotension, tachycardia, paradoxic bradycardia, syncope. **GI:** abdominal pain, nausea, vomiting. **Misc:** cross-tolerance, flushing, tolerance.

Interactions

Drug-Drug: ↑ risk of hypotension with **phosphodiesterase inhibitors** (**sildenafil**, **vardenafil**, or **tadalafil**) other **antihypertensives**, acute ingestion of **alcohol**, **beta blockers**, **calcium channel blockers**, and **phenothiazines**. **MAO inhibitors** may exaggerate hypotension. May reduce the pressor response to **epinephrine**. **Beta blockers** ↓ tachycardia from hydralazine (therapy may be combined for this reason). **Metoprolol** and **propranolol** increase hydralazine levels. Hydralazine ↑ blood levels of **metoprolol** and **propranolol**.

Route/Dosage

PO (Adults): 1 tablet three times daily, may be increased to 2 tablets three times daily.

Availability

Tablets: hydralazine 37.5 mg/isosorbide dinitrate 20 mg.

NURSING IMPLICATIONS

Assessment

- Monitor blood pressure and pulse routinely during period of dosage adjustment. Symptomatic hypotension may occur even with small doses. Use caution with patients who are volume depleted or hypotensive.
- ***Lab Test Considerations:*** If symptoms of systemic lupus erythematosus (SLE) occur obtain a CBC and ANA titer. If positive for SLE, carefully weigh risks/benefits of continued therapy.

Potential Nursing Diagnoses

Ineffective tissue perfusion (Indications)
Activity intolerance (Indications)

Implementation

- Dose may be titrated rapidly over 3–5 days, but may need to decrease if side effects occur. May decrease to one-half tablet three time daily if intolerable side effects occur. Titrate up as soon as side effects subside.

Patient/Family Teaching

- Instruct patient to take medication as directed on a regular schedule.
- Caution patient to make position changes slowly to minimize orthostatic hypotension.
- May cause dizziness. Caution patient to avoid driving or other activities requiring alertness until response to medication is known.
- Advise patient to avoid concurrent use of alcohol or medications for erectile dysfunction with this medication. Patient should also consult health care professional before taking Rx, OTC, or herbal products while taking this medication.
- Caution patient that inadequate fluid intake or excessive fluid loss from perspiration, diarrhea or vomiting may lead to a fall in blood

pressure, dizziness or syncope. If syncope occurs, discontinue medication and notify health care professional promptly.

- Inform patient that headache is a common side effect that should decrease with continuing therapy. Aspirin or acetaminophen may be ordered to treat headache. Notify health care professional if headache is persistent or severe. Do not alter dose to avoid headache.
- Advise patient to notify health care professional if symptoms of systemic lupus erythematosus occur (arthralgia, fever, chest pain, prolonged malaise or other unexplained symptoms).

Evaluation/Desired Outcomes

- Improved survival, increased time to hospitalization and decreased symptoms of heart failure in black patients.

HIGH ALERT

hydrocodone

(hye-droe-**koe**-done)
Hycodan, Tussigon (U.S. antitussive formulations contain homatropine)

hydrocodone/acetaminophen
Anexsia, Co-Gesic, Lorcet-HD, Lortab, Norco, Vicodin, Zydone

hydrocodone/aspirin
Azdone

hydrocodone/ibuprofen
Vicoprofen

Classification
Therapeutic: allergy, cold, and cough remedies (antitussive), opioid analgesics
Pharmacologic: opioid agonists/nonopioid analgesic combinations

Schedule III (in combination)

Pregnancy Category C (with acetaminophen, or ibuprofen), D (with aspirin)

For information on the acetaminophen, aspirin, and ibuprofen components of these formulations, see the acetaminophen, aspirin, and ibuprofen monographs

Indications

Used mainly in combination with nonopioid analgesics (acetaminophen/aspirin/ibuprofen) in the management of moderate to severe pain. Antitussive (usually in combination products with decongestants).

Action

Bind to opiate receptors in the CNS. Alter the perception of and response to painful stimuli while producing generalized CNS depression: Suppress the cough reflex via a direct central action. **Therapeutic Effects:** Decrease in severity of moderate pain. Suppression of the cough reflex.

Pharmacokinetics

Absorption: Well absorbed following oral administration.
Distribution: Unknown.
Metabolism and Excretion: Mostly metabolized by the liver; eliminated in the urine (50–60% as metabolites, 15% as unchanged drug).
Half-life: 2.2 hr.

TIME/ACTION PROFILE (analgesic effect)

ROUTE	ONSET	PEAK	DURATION
PO	10–30 min	30–60 min	4–6 hr

Contraindications/Precautions

Contraindicated in: Hypersensitivity to hydrocodone (cross-sensitivity may exist to other opioids); Hypersensitivity to acetaminophen/aspirin/ibuprofen (for combination products); Aspirin- and ibuprofen-containing products should be avoided in patients with bleeding disorders or thrombocytopenia; Acetaminophen should be avoided in patients with severe hepatic or renal disease; Ibuprofen-containing products should be avoided in patients undergoing coronary artery bypass graft surgery; OB, Lactation: Pregnancy or lactation (avoid chronic use); Products containing alcohol, aspartame, saccharin, sugar, or tartrazine (FDC yellow dye #5) should be avoided in patients who have hypersensitivity or intolerance to these compounds.
Use Cautiously in: Head trauma; Increased intracranial pressure; Severe renal, hepatic, or pulmonary disease; Cardiovascular disease (ibuprofen-containing products only); History of peptic ulcer disease (ibuprofen-containing products only); Alcoholism; Geriatric or debilitated patients (initial dosage reduction required; more prone to CNS depression, constipation); Patients with undiagnosed abdominal

H

pain; Prostatic hyperplasia; Pedi: Children (safety not established).

Adverse Reactions/Side Effects

Noted for hydrocodone only; see acetaminophen/aspirin/ibuprofen monographs for specific information on individual components.

CNS: confusion, dizziness, sedation, euphoria, hallucinations, headache, unusual dreams. **EENT:** blurred vision, diplopia, miosis. **Resp:** respiratory depression. **CV:** hypotension, bradycardia. **GI:** constipation, dyspepsia, nausea, vomiting. **GU:** urinary retention. **Derm:** sweating. **Misc:** physical dependence, psychological dependence, tolerance.

Interactions

Drug-Drug: Use with extreme caution in patients receiving **MAO inhibitors** (may produce severe, unpredictable reactions—do not use within 14 days of each other). Additive CNS depression with **alcohol**, **antihistamines**, and **sedative/hypnotics**. Administration of partial antagonist opioids (**buprenorphine**, **butorphanol**, **nalbuphine**, or **pentazocine**) may ↓ analgesia or precipitate opioid withdrawal in physically dependent patients.

Drug-Natural Products: Concomitant use of **kava kava**, **valerian**, **skullcap**, **chamomile**, or **hops** can increase CNS depression.

Route/Dosage

PO (Adults): *Analgesic*—2.5–10 mg q 3–6 hr as needed; if using combination products, acetaminophen or aspirin dosage should not exceed 4 g/day and should not exceed 5 tablets/day of ibuprofen-containing products; *Antitussive*—5 mg q 4–6 hr as needed.

PO (Children): *Analgesic (2–13 yr)*—0.14 mg/kg q 4–6 hr. *Antitussive (6–12 yr)*—2.5 mg q 4–6 hr.

Availability

Hydrocodone

Hydrocodone tablets: 🍁5 mg (Hycodan). **Hydrocodone syrup:** 🍁5 mg/ml (Hycodan, Robidone).

Hydrocodone/Acetaminophen

Tablets: 2.5 mg hydrocodone/500 mg acetaminophen, 5 mg hydrocodone/400 mg acetaminophen (Zydone), 5 mg hydrocodone/325 mg acetaminophen (Anexsia 5/325, Norco), 5 mg hydrocodone/500 mg acetaminophen (Anexsia 5/500, Co-Gesic, Lorcet, Lortab 5/500, Vicodin), 7.5 mg hydrocodone/325 mg acetaminophen (Anexsia 7.5/325, Norco), 7.5 mg hydrocodone/400 mg acetaminophen (Zydone), 7.5 mg hydrocodone/500 mg acetaminophen, 7.5 mg hydrocodone/650 mg acetaminophen (Anexsia 7.5/650), 7.5 mg hydrocodone/750 mg acetaminophen (Vicodin ES), 10 mg hydrocodone/325 mg acetaminophen (Norco), 10 mg hydrocodone/400 mg acetaminophen (Zydone), 10 mg hydrocodone/500 mg acetaminophen (Lortab 10/500), 10 mg hydrocodone/650 mg acetaminophen, 10 mg hydrocodone/660 mg acetaminophen (Vicodin HP), 10 mg hydrocodone/750 mg acetaminophen (Anexsia 10/750). **Capsules:** 5 mg hydrocodone/500 mg acetaminophen (Lorcet-HD). **Elixir/oral solution:** 2.5 mg hydrocodone plus 167 mg acetaminophen/5 ml.

Hydrocodone/Aspirin

Tablets: 5 mg hydrocodone/500 mg aspirin (Azdone).

Hydrocodone/Ibuprofen

Tablets: 7.5 mg hydrocodone/200 mg ibuprofen.

NURSING IMPLICATIONS

Assessment

- Assess blood pressure, pulse, and respirations before and periodically during administration. If respiratory rate is <10/min, assess level of sedation. Physical stimulation may be sufficient to prevent significant hypoventilation. Dose may need to be decreased by 25–50%. Initial drowsiness will diminish with continued use.
- Assess bowel function routinely. Prevention of constipation should be instituted with increased intake of fluids and bulk, and laxatives to minimize constipating effects. Stimulant laxatives should be administered routinely if opioid use exceeds 2–3 days, unless contraindicated.
- **Pain:** Assess type, location, and intensity of pain prior to and 1 hr (peak) following administration. When titrating opioid doses, increases of 25–50% should be administered until there is either a 50% reduction in the patient's pain rating on a numerical or visual analogue scale or the patient reports satisfactory pain relief. A repeat dose can be safely administered at the time of the peak if previous dose is ineffective and side effects are minimal.
- An equianalgesic chart (see Appendix J) should be used when changing routes or when changing from one opioid to another

- Prolonged use may lead to physical and psychological dependence and tolerance. This should not prevent patient from receiving adequate analgesia. Most patients who receive opioids for pain do not develop psychological dependence. If progressively higher doses are required, consider conversion to a stronger opioid.
- **Cough:** Assess cough and lung sounds during antitussive use.
- ***Lab Test Considerations:*** May cause ↑ plasma amylase and lipase concentrations.
- ***Toxicity and Overdose:*** If an opioid antagonist is required to reverse respiratory depression or coma, naloxone (Narcan) is the antidote. Dilute the 0.4-mg ampule of naloxone in 10 ml of 0.9% NaCl and administer 0.5 ml (0.02 mg) by direct IV push every 2 min. For children and patients weighing <40 kg, dilute 0.1 mg of naloxone in 10 ml of 0.9% NaCl for a concentration of 10 mcg/ml and administer 0.5 mcg/kg every 2 min. Titrate dose to avoid withdrawal, seizures, and severe pain.

Potential Nursing Diagnoses

Acute pain (Indications)
Disturbed sensory perception (visual, auditory) (Side Effects)
Risk for injury (Side Effects)

Implementation

- ***High Alert:*** Accidental overdosage of opioid analgesics has resulted in fatalities. Before administering, clarify all ambiguous orders; have second practitioner independently check original order and dose calculations. Do not confuse hydrocodone with hydrocortisone.
- Explain therapeutic value of medication prior to administration to enhance the analgesic effect.
- Regularly administered doses may be more effective than prn administration. Analgesic is more effective if given before pain becomes severe.
- Combination with nonopioid analgesics may have additive analgesic effects and permit lower doses. Maximum doses of nonopioid agents limit the titration of hydrocodone doses.
- Medication should be discontinued gradually after long-term use to prevent withdrawal symptoms.
- **PO:** May be administered with food or milk to minimize GI irritation.

Patient/Family Teaching

- Advise patient to take medication exactly as directed and not to take more than the recommended amount. Severe and permanent liver damage may result from prolonged use or high doses of acetaminophen. Renal damage may occur with prolonged use of acetaminophen, aspirin, or ibuprofen. Doses of nonopioid agents should not exceed the maximum recommended daily dose.
- Instruct patient on how and when to ask for pain medication.
- May cause drowsiness or dizziness. Advise patient to call for assistance when ambulating or smoking. Caution patient to avoid driving or other activities requiring alertness until response to the medication is known.
- Advise patient to change positions slowly to minimize orthostatic hypotension.
- Caution patient to avoid concurrent use of alcohol or other CNS depressants with this medication.
- Encourage patient to turn, cough, and breathe deeply every 2 hr to prevent atelectasis.
- Advise patient that good oral hygiene, frequent mouth rinses, and sugarless gum or candy may decrease dry mouth.

Evaluation/Desired Outcomes

- Decrease in severity of pain without a significant alteration in level of consciousness or respiratory status.
- Suppression of nonproductive cough.

hydrochlorothiazide, See DIURETICS (THIAZIDE).

hydrocortisone, See CORTICOSTEROIDS (SYSTEMIC), CORTICOSTEROIDS (TOPICAL/LOCAL).

H

HIGH ALERT

hydromorphone

(hye-droe-**mor**-fone)

Dilaudid, Dilaudid-HP, Hydrostat IR, PMS Hydromorphone

Classification

Therapeutic: allergy, cold, and cough remedies (antitussives), opioid analgesics

Pharmacologic: opioid agonists

Schedule II

Pregnancy Category C

Indications

Moderate to severe pain (alone and in combination with nonopioid analgesics); extended release product for opioid-tolerant patients requiring around-the-clock management of persistent pain. Antitussive (lower doses).

Action

Binds to opiate receptors in the CNS. Alters the perception of and response to painful stimuli while producing generalized CNS depression. Suppresses the cough reflex via a direct central action. **Therapeutic Effects:** Decrease in moderate to severe pain. Suppression of cough.

Pharmacokinetics

Absorption: Well absorbed following oral, rectal, subcut, and IM administration. Extended-release product results in an initial release of drug, followed by a second sustained phase of absorption.

Distribution: Widely distributed. Crosses the placenta; enters breast milk.

Metabolism and Excretion: Mostly metabolized by the liver.

Half-life: *Oral, immediate release, or injection*—2–4 hr.

TIME/ACTION PROFILE (analgesic effect)

ROUTE	ONSET	PEAK	DURATION
PO	30 min	30–90 min	4–5 hr
Subcut	15 min	30–90 min	4–5 hr
IM	15 min	30–60 min	4–5 hr
IV	10–15 min	15–30 min	2–3 hr
Rect	15–30 min	30–90 min	4–5 hr

Contraindications/Precautions

Contraindicated in: Hypersensitivity; Some products contain bisulfites and should be avoided in patients with known hypersensitivity; OB, Lactation: Avoid chronic use during pregnancy or lactation.

Use Cautiously in: Head trauma; Increased intracranial pressure; Severe renal, hepatic, or pulmonary disease; Hypothyroidism; Adrenal insufficiency; Alcoholism; Geri: Geriatric or debilitated patients (dose reduction recommended); Undiagnosed abdominal pain; Prostatic hypertrophy.

Adverse Reactions/Side Effects

CNS: confusion, sedation, dizziness, dysphoria, euphoria, floating feeling, hallucinations, headache, unusual dreams. **EENT:** blurred vision, diplopia, miosis. **Resp:** respiratory depression. **CV:** hypotension, bradycardia. **GI:** constipation, dry mouth, nausea, vomiting. **GU:** urinary retention. **Derm:** flushing, sweating. **Misc:** physical dependence, psychological dependence, tolerance.

Interactions

Drug-Drug: Exercise extreme caution with **MAO inhibitors** (may produce severe, unpredictable reactions—reduce initial dose of hydromorphone to 25% of usual dose, discontinue MAO inhibitors 2 wk prior to hydromorphone). ↑ risk of CNS depression with **alcohol**, **antidepressants**, **antihistamines**, and **sedative/hypnotics** including **benzodazepines** and **phenothiazines**. Administration of partial antagonists (**buprenorphine**, **butorphanol**, **nalbuphine**, or **pentazocine**) may precipitate opioid withdrawal in physically dependent patients. **Nalbuphine** or **pentazocine** may ↓ analgesia.

Drug-Natural Products: Concomitant use of **kava kava**, **valerian**, **chamomile**, or **hops** can ↑ CNS depression.

Route/Dosage

Doses depend on level of pain and tolerance.

Analgesic

PO (Adults ≥50 kg): 4–8 mg q 3–4 hr initially (some patients may respond to doses as small as 2 mg initially).

PO (Adults and Children <50 kg): 0.06 mg/kg q 3–4 hr initially, younger children may require smaller initial doses of 0.03 mg/kg. Maximum dose 5 mg.

IV, IM, Subcut (Adults ≥50 kg): 1.5 mg q 3–4 hr as needed initially; may be increased.

IV, IM, Subcut (Adults and Children <50 kg): 0.015 mg/kg mg q 3–4 hr as needed initially; may be increased.

IV (Adults): *Continuous infusion (unlabeled)*—0.2–30 mg/hr depending on previous opioid use. An initial bolus of twice the hourly rate in mg may be given with subsequent breakthrough boluses of 50–100% of the hourly rate in mg.
Rect (Adults): 3 mg q 6–8 hr initially as needed.

Antitussive
PO (Adults and Children >12 yr): 1 mg q 3–4 hr.
PO (Children 6–12 yr): 0.5 mg q 3–4 hr.

Availability (generic available)
Tablets: 2 mg, 3 mg, 4 mg, 8 mg. **Oral solution:** 5 mg/5 ml. **Injection:** 1 mg/ml, 2 mg/ml, 4 mg/ml, 10 mg/ml. **Suppositories:** 3 mg. ***In combination with:*** guaifenesin and alcohol (Dilaudid Cough Syrup). See Appendix B.

NURSING IMPLICATIONS

Assessment

- Assess blood pressure, pulse, and respirations before and periodically during administration. If respiratory rate is <10/min, assess level of sedation. Dose may need to be decreased by 25–50%. Initial drowsiness will diminish with continued use. Geri, Pedi: Assess geriatric and pediatric patients frequently; more sensitive to the effects of opioid analgesics and may experience side effects and respiratory complications more frequently.
- Assess bowel function routinely. Institute prevention of constipation with increased intake of fluids and bulk, and laxatives to minimize constipating effects. Administer stimulant laxatives routinely if opioid use exceeds 2–3 days, unless contraindicated.
- **Pain:** Assess type, location, and intensity of pain prior to and 1 hr following IM and 5 min (peak) following IV administration. When titrating opioid doses, increases of 25–50% should be administered until there is either a 50% reduction in the patient's pain rating on a numerical or visual analogue scale or the patient reports satisfactory pain relief. When titrating doses of short-acting hydromorphone, a repeat dose can be safely administered at the time of the peak if previous dose is ineffective and side effects are minimal.
- Patients on a continuous infusion should have additional bolus doses provided every 15–30 min, as needed, for breakthrough pain. The bolus dose is usually set to the amount of drug infused each hour by continuous infusion
- An equianalgesic chart (see Appendix J) should be used when changing routes or when changing from one opioid to another
- Prolonged use may lead to physical and psychological dependence and tolerance. This should not prevent patient from receiving adequate analgesia. Most patients who receive hydromorphone for pain do not develop psychological dependence. Progressively higher doses may be required to relieve pain with long-term therapy.
- **Cough:** Assess cough and lung sounds during antitussive use.
- ***Lab Test Considerations:*** May ↑ plasma amylase and lipase concentrations.
- ***Toxicity and Overdose:*** If an opioid antagonist is required to reverse respiratory depression or coma, naloxone (Narcan) is the antidote. Dilute the 0.4-mg ampule of naloxone in 10 ml of 0.9% NaCl and administer 0.5 ml (0.02 mg) by direct IV push every 2 min. For children and patients weighing <40 kg, dilute 0.1 mg of naloxone in 10 ml of 0.9% NaCl for a concentration of 10 mcg/ml and administer 0.5 mcg every 2 min. Titrate dose to avoid withdrawal, seizures, and severe pain.

Potential Nursing Diagnoses

Acute pain (Indications)
Disturbed sensory perception (visual, auditory) (Side Effects)
Risk for injury (Side Effects)

Implementation

- ***High Alert:*** Accidental overdosage of opioid analgesics has resulted in fatalities. Before administering, clarify all ambiguous orders; have second practitioner independently check original order, dose calculations, and infusion pump settings. Do not confuse with meperidine or morphine; fatalities have occurred. Do not confuse high-potency (HP) dose forms with regular dose forms. Pedi: Medication errors with opioid analgesics are common in pediatric patients; do not misinterpret or miscalculate doses. Use appropriate measuring devices.

- Explain therapeutic value of medication prior to administration to enhance the analgesic effect.
- Regularly administered doses may be more effective than prn administration. Analgesic is more effective if given before pain becomes severe.
- Coadministration with nonopioid analgesics may have additive analgesic effects and permit lower opioid doses.
- Medication should be discontinued gradually after long-term use to prevent withdrawal symptoms.
- **PO:** May be administered with food or milk to minimize GI irritation.

IV Administration

- **Direct IV:** ***Diluent:*** Dilute with at least 5 ml of sterile water or 0.9% NaCl for injection. Inspect solution for particulate matter. Slight yellow color does not alter potency. Store at room temperature. ***Rate:*** Administer slowly, at a rate not to exceed 2 mg over 3–5 min.
- ***High Alert:*** Rapid administration may lead to increased respiratory depression, hypotension, and circulatory collapse.
- **Syringe Compatibility:** atropine, bupivacaine, ceftazidime, chlorpromazine, cimetidine, diphenhydramine, fentanyl, glycopyrrolate, hydroxyzine, lorazepam, metoclopramide, midazolam, pentobarbital, potassium chloride, prochlorperazine, promethazine, ranitidine, scopolamine, thiethylperazine.
- **Syringe Incompatibility:** ampicillin, diazepam, heparin, hyaluronidase, pantoprazole, phenobarbital, phenytoin.
- **Y-Site Compatibility:** acyclovir, allopurinol, amifostine, amikacin, amsacrine, atropine, aztreonam, bivalirudin, cefepime, cefoperazone, cefotaxime, cefoxitin, ceftazidime, ceftizoxime, cefuroxime, chloramphenicol, cisatracurium, cisplatin, cladribine, clindamycin, cyclophosphamide, cytarabine, dexamethasone, dexmedetomidine, diltiazem, diphenhydramine, dobutamine, docetaxel, dopamine, doxorubicin, doxorubicin liposome, doxycycline, epinephrine, erythromycin lactobionate, etoposide, famotidine, fenoldopam, fentanyl, filgrastim, fludarabine, foscarnet, furosemide, gemcitabine, gentamicin, granisetron, haloperidol, heparin, kanamycin, ketorolac, labetalol, linezolid, lorazepam, magnesium sulfate, melphalan, methotrexate, methotrimeprizine, metoclopramide, metronidazole, midazolam, milrinone, morphine, nafcillin, nitroglycerin, norepinephrine, ondansetron, oxaliplatin, paclitaxel, pemetrexed, penicillin G potassium, piperacillin/tazobactam, propofol, ranitidine, remifentanil, scopolamine, tacrolimus, teniposide, thiotepa, tobramycin, trimethoprim/sulfamethoxazole, vancomycin, vecuronium, vinorelbine.
- **Y-Site Incompatibility:** amphotericin B cholesteryl sulfate complex, lansoprazole, phenytoin, sargramostim, thiopental.
- **Additive Compatibility:** bupivicaine, clonidine, heparin, midazolam, ondansetron, potassium chloride.
- **Additive Incompatibility:** sodium bicarbonate, thiopental.
- **Solution Compatibility:** D5W, D5/0.45% NaCl, D5/0.9% NaCl, D5/LR, D5/Ringer's solution, 0.45% NaCl, 0.9% NaCl, Ringer's and LR.

Patient/Family Teaching

- Instruct patient on how and when to ask for pain medication.
- May cause drowsiness or dizziness. Advise patient to call for assistance when ambulating or smoking. Caution patient to avoid driving or other activities requiring alertness until response to medication is known.
- Advise patient to change positions slowly to minimize orthostatic hypotension.
- Instruct patient to avoid concurrent use of alcohol or other CNS depressants.
- Encourage patient to turn, cough, and breathe deeply every 2 hr to prevent atelectasis.
- **Home Care Issues:** Explain to patient and family how and when to administer hydromorphone and how to care for infusion equipment properly. Pedi: Teach parents or caregivers how to accurately measure liquid medication and to use only the measuring device dispensed with the medication.
- Emphasize the importance of aggressive prevention of constipation with the use of hydromorphone.

Evaluation/Desired Outcomes

- Decrease in severity of pain without a significant alteration in level of consciousness or respiratory status.
- Suppression of cough.

hydroxychloroquine

(hye-drox-ee-**klor**-oh-kwin)

Plaquenil

Classification
Therapeutic: antimalarials, antirheumatics (DMARDs)

Pregnancy Category C

Indications
Suppression/chemoprophylaxis of malaria. Treatment of severe rheumatoid arthritis/systemic lupus erythematosus.

Action
Inhibits protein synthesis in susceptible organisms by inhibiting DNA and RNA polymerase. **Therapeutic Effects:** Death of plasmodia responsible for causing malaria. Also has anti-inflammatory properties.

Pharmacokinetics
Absorption: Highly variable (31–100%) following oral administation.
Distribution: Widely distributed; high concentrations in RBCs; crosses the placenta; excreted into breast milk.
Metabolism and Excretion: Partially metabolized by the liver to active metabolites; partially excreted unchanged by the kidneys.
Half-life: 72–120 hr.

TIME/ACTION PROFILE (blood levels)

ROUTE	ONSET	PEAK	DURATION
PO	rapid†	1–2 hr	days–weeks

†Onset of antirheumatic action may take 6 wk

Contraindications/Precautions
Contraindicated in: Hypersensitivity to hydroxychloroquine or chloroquine; Previous visual damage from hydroxychloroquine or chloroquine.
Use Cautiously in: Concurrent use of hepatotoxic drugs; History of liver disease or alcoholism or renal impairment; Severe neurological disorders; Severe blood disorders; Retinal or visual field changes; G6PD deficiency; Psoriasis; Bone marrow depression; Obesity (determine dose by ideal body weight); Pregnancy or lactation (avoid use unless treating/preventing malaria or treating amebic abscess); Children (long-term use increased sensitivity to effects).

Adverse Reactions/Side Effects
CNS: SEIZURES, aggressiveness, anxiety, apathy, confusion, fatigue, headache, irritability, personality changes, psychoses. **EENT:** keratopathy, ototoxicity, retinopathy, tinnitus, visual disturbances. **CV:** ECG changes, hypotension. **GI:** abdominal cramps, anorexia, diarrhea, epigastric discomfort, nausea, vomiting, hepatic failure. **Derm:** bleaching of hair, alopecia, hyperpigmentation, photosensitivity, Stevens-Johnson syndrome. **Hemat:** AGRANULOCYTOSIS, APLASTIC ANEMIA, leukopenia, thrombocytopenia. **Neuro:** neuromyopathy, peripheral neuritis.

Interactions
Drug-Drug: May ↑ the risk of hepatotoxicity when administered with **hepatotoxic drugs**. May ↑ the risk of hematologic toxicity when administered with **penicillamine**. May ↑ risk of dermatitis when administered with other **agents having dermatologic toxicity**. May ↓ serum titers of rabies antibody when given concurrently with **human diploid cell rabies vaccine**. **Urinary acidifiers** may ↑ renal excretion. May ↑ serum levels of **digoxin**.

Route/Dosage
Antimalarial doses expressed as mg of base; antirheumatic and lupus doses expressed as mg of hydroxychloroquine sulfate (200 mg hydroxychloroquine sulfate = 155 mg of hydroxychloroquine base).

Malaria
PO (Adults): *Suppression or chemoprophylaxis*—310 mg once weekly; start 1–2 wk prior to entering malarious area; continue for 4 wk after leaving area. *Treatment*—620 mg, then 310 mg at 6 hr, 24 hr, and 48 hr after initial dose.
PO (Children): *Suppression or chemoprophylaxis*—5 mg/kg once weekly; start 1–2 wk prior to entering malarious area; continue for 4 wk after leaving area. *Treatment*—10 mg/kg initially, then 5 mg/kg at 6–8 hr, 24 hr, and 48 hr after initial dose.

Rheumatoid Arthritis
PO (Adults): 400–600 mg once daily initially, maintenance 200–400 mg/day divided 1–2 times/day.
PO (Children): 3–5 mg/kg/day divided 1–2 times/day to a maximum of 400 mg/day; not to exceed 7 mg/kg/day.

Systemic Lupus Erythematosus
PO (Adults): 400 mg once or twice daily, maintenance 200–400 mg/day.

PO (Children): 3–5 mg/kg/day divided 1–2 times/day to a maximum of 400 mg/day; not to exceed 7 mg/kg/day.

Availability
Tablets: 200 mg (155-mg base).

NURSING IMPLICATIONS

Assessment
- Assess deep tendon reflexes periodically to determine muscle weakness. Therapy may be discontinued should this occur.
- Patients on prolonged high-dose therapy should have eye exams prior to and every 3–6 mo during therapy to detect retinal damage.
- **Malaria or Lupus Erythematosus:** Assess patient for improvement in signs and symptoms of condition daily throughout course of therapy.
- **Rheumatoid Arthritis:** Assess patient monthly for pain, swelling, and range of motion.
- ***Lab Test Considerations:*** Monitor CBC and platelet count periodically throughout therapy. May cause decreased RBC, WBC, and platelet counts. If severe decreases occur that are not related to the disease process, hydroxychloroquine should be discontinued.

Potential Nursing Diagnoses
Risk for infection (Indications)
Chronic pain (Indications)

Implementation
- **PO:** Administer with milk or meals to minimize GI distress.
- Tablets may be crushed and placed inside empty capsules for patients with difficulty swallowing. Contents of capsules may also be mixed with a teaspoonful of jam, jelly, or Jell-O prior to administration.
- **Malaria Prophylaxis:** Hydroxychloroquine therapy should be started 2 wk prior to potential exposure and continued for 4–6 wk after leaving the malarious area.

Patient/Family Teaching
- Instruct patient to take medication exactly as directed and continue full course of therapy even if feeling better. Missed doses should be taken as soon as remembered unless it is almost time for next dose. Do not double doses.
- Advise patients to avoid use of alcohol while taking hydroxychloroquine.
- Caution patient to keep hydroxychloroquine out of reach of children; fatalities have occurred with ingestion of 3 or 4 tablets.
- Explain need for periodic ophthalmic exams for patients on prolonged high-dose therapy. Advise patient that the risk of ocular damage may be decreased by the use of dark glasses in bright light. Protective clothing and sunscreen should also be used to reduce risk of dermatoses.
- Advise patient to notify health care professional promptly if sore throat, fever, unusual bleeding or bruising, blurred vision, visual changes, ringing in the ears, difficulty hearing, or muscle weakness occurs.
- **Malaria Prophylaxis:** Review methods of minimizing exposure to mosquitoes with patients receiving hydroxychloroquine prophylactically (use repellent, wear long-sleeved shirt and long trousers, use screen or netting).
- Advise patient to notify health care professional if fever develops while traveling or within 2 mo of leaving an endemic area.
- **Rheumatoid Arthritis:** Instruct patient to contact health care professional if no improvement is noticed within a few days. Treatment for rheumatoid arthritis may require up to 6 mo for full benefit.

Evaluation/Desired Outcomes
- Prevention or resolution of malaria.
- Improvement in signs and symptoms of rheumatoid arthritis.
- Improvement in symptoms of lupus erythematosus.

hydrOXYzine (hye-**drox**-i-zeen)
✤Apo-Hydroxyzine, Atarax, Hyzine-50, ✤Multipax, ✤Novohydroxyzin, Vistaril

Classification
Therapeutic: antianxiety agents, antihistamines, sedative/hypnotics

Pregnancy Category C

Indications
Treatment of anxiety. Preoperative sedation. Antiemetic. Antipruritic. May be combined with opioid analgesics.

Action
Acts as a CNS depressant at the subcortical level of the CNS. Has anticholinergic, antihistaminic,

and antiemetic properties. Blocks histamine 1 receptors. **Therapeutic Effects:** Sedation. Relief of anxiety. Decreased nausea and vomiting. Decreased allergic symptoms associated with release of histamine, including pruritus.

Pharmacokinetics

Absorption: Well absorbed following PO/IM administration.
Distribution: Unknown.
Metabolism and Excretion: Completely metabolized by the liver; eliminated in the feces via biliary excretion.
Half-life: 3 hr.

TIME/ACTION PROFILE (sedative, antiemetic, antipruritic effects)

ROUTE	ONSET	PEAK	DURATION
PO	15–30 min	2–4 hr	4–6 hr
IM	15–30 min	2–4 hr	4–6 hr

Contraindications/Precautions

Contraindicated in: Hypersensitivity; OB: Potential for congenital defects (oral clefts and hypoplasia of cerebral hemisphere; Lactation: Safety not established.
Use Cautiously in: Severe hepatic dysfunction; OB: Has been used safely during labor; Pedi: Injection contains benzyl alcohol, which can cause potentially fatal gasping syndrome in neonates; Geri: Appears on *Beers list*. Geriatric patients are more susceptible to adverse reactions due to anticholinergic effects; dosage reduction recommended.

Adverse Reactions/Side Effects

CNS: drowsiness, agitation, ataxia, dizziness, headache, weakness. **Resp:** wheezing. **GI:** dry mouth, bitter taste, constipation, nausea. **GU:** urinary retention. **Derm:** flushing. **Local:** pain at IM site, abscesses at IM sites. **Misc:** chest tightness.

Interactions

Drug-Drug: Additive CNS depression with other **CNS depressants**, including **alcohol**, **antidepressants**, **antihistamines**, **opioid analgesics**, and **sedative/hypnotics**. Additive anticholinergic effects with other **drugs possessing anticholinergic properties**, including **antihistamines**, **antidepressants**, **atropine**, **haloperidol**, **phenothiazines**, **quinidine**, and **disopyramide**. Can antagonize the vasopressor effects of **epinephrine**.
Drug-Natural Products: Concomitant use of **kava kava**, **valerian**, or **chamomile** can ↑ CNS depression. ↑ anticholinergic effects with **angel's trumpet**, **jimson weed**, and **scopolia.**

Route/Dosage

PO (Adults): *Antianxiety*—25–100 mg 4 times/day, not to exceed 600 mg/day. *Preoperative sedation*—50–100 mg single dose. *Antipruritic*—25 mg 3–4 times daily.
PO (Children):—2 mg/kg/day divided q 6–8 hr.
IM (Adults): *Preoperative sedation*—25–100 mg single dose. *Antiemetic, adjunct to opioid analgesics*—25–100 mg q 4–6 hr as needed.
IM (Children): 0.5–1 mg/kg q 4–6 hr as needed.

Availability (generic available)

Tablets: 10 mg, 25 mg, 50 mg, 100 mg. **Capsules:** ✤ 10 mg, 25 mg, 50 mg, 100 mg. **Syrup:** 10 mg/5 ml. **Oral suspension:** 25 mg/5 ml. **Injection:** 25 mg/ml, 50 mg/ml.

NURSING IMPLICATIONS

Assessment

- Assess patient for profound sedation and provide safety precautions as indicated (side rails up, bed in low position, call bell within reach, supervision of ambulation and transfer). Geri: Older adults are more sensitive to CNS and anticholinergic effects (delirium, acute confusion, dizziness, dry mouth, blurred vision, urinary retention, constipation, tachycardia). Monitor for drowsiness, agitation, over sedation, and other systemic side effects. Assess falls risk and implement prevention strategies.
- **Anxiety:** Assess mental status (orientation, mood, and behavior).
- **Nausea and Vomiting:** Assess degree of nausea and frequency and amount of emesis.
- **Pruritus:** Assess degree of itching and character of involved skin.
- ***Lab Test Considerations:*** May cause false-negative skin test results using allergen extracts. Discontinue hydroxyzine at least 72 hr before test.

Potential Nursing Diagnoses

Anxiety (Indications)

Impaired skin integrity (Indications)
Risk for injury (Side Effects)
Ineffective coping (Side Effects)

Implementation

- Do not confuse hydroxyzine with hydralazine or Atarax (hydroxyzine) with Ativan (lorazepam).
- **PO:** Tablets may be crushed and capsules opened and administered with food or fluids for patients having difficulty swallowing.
- Shake suspension well before administration.
- **IM:** Administer *only* IM deep into well-developed muscle, preferably with Z-track technique. Injection is extremely painful. Do not use deltoid site. If must be administered to children, midlateral muscles of the thigh are preferred. Significant tissue damage, necrosis, and sloughing may result from subcut or intra-arterial injections. Hemolysis may result from IV injections. Rotate injection sites frequently.
- **Syringe Compatibility:** atropine, butorphanol, chlorpromazine, cimetidine, codeine, diphenhydramine, doxapram, droperidol, fentanyl, fluphenazine, glycopyrrolate, hydromorphone, lidocaine, meperidine, metoclopramide, midazolam, morphine, nalbuphine, oxymorphone, pentazocine, perphenazine, procaine, prochlorperazine, promethazine, scopolamine, sufentanil.
- **Syringe Incompatibility:** dimenhydrinate, haloperidol, heparin, ketorolac, pentobarbital, ranitidine.

Patient/Family Teaching

- Instruct patient to take medication exactly as directed. Missed doses should be taken as soon as remembered unless it is almost time for next dose; do not double doses.
- May cause drowsiness or dizziness. Caution patient to avoid driving and other activities requiring alertness until response to medication is known. Geri: Warn patients or caregivers that older adults are at increased risk for CNS effects and falls.
- Advise patient to avoid concurrent use of alcohol or other CNS depressants with this medication.
- Inform patient that frequent mouth rinses, good oral hygiene, and sugarless gum or candy may help decrease dry mouth. If dry mouth persists for more than 2 wk, consult dentist about saliva substitute.
- If used for anxiety, advise patient that psychotherapy is beneficial in addressing sources of anxiety and improving coping skills.
- Teach other methods to decrease anxiety, such as increased exercise, support groups, and relaxation techniques.

Evaluation/Desired Outcomes

- Decrease in anxiety.
- Relief of nausea and vomiting.
- Relief of pruritus.
- Sedation when used as a sedative/hypnotic.

hyoscyamine

(hi-oh-**si**-a-meen)
Anaspaz, A-Spas S/L, Cystospaz, Cystospaz-M, Donnamar, ED-SPAZ, Gastrosed, Levsinex, Levsin, Levbid, L-hyoscyamine, NuLev

Classification
Therapeutic: antispasmodics
Pharmacologic: anticholinergics

Pregnancy Category C

Indications

Control of gastric secretion, visceral spasm, hypermotility in spastic colitis, spastic bladder, pylorospasm, and related abdominal cramps. Decreases symptoms of various functional intestinal disorders including mild dysenteries, diverticulitis, infant colic, biliary and renal colic. Adjunctive therapy in peptic ulcer disease, irritable bowel syndrome, neurogenic bowel disturbances. Decreases pain and hypersecretion associated with pancreatitis. Relief of symptoms of acute rhinitis. Decreases rigidity and tremors associated with parkinsonism and controls related sialorrhea and hyperhidrosis. May also be used to manage anticholinesterase poisoning. Management of cystitis or renal colic. Management of some forms of heart block due to vagal activity. **IM, IV, Subcut** Facilitation of diagnostic hypotonic duodenography; may also increase radiologic visibility of the kidneys. Preoperative administration decreases secretions and blocks bradycardia associated with some forms of anesthesia and related surgical agents.

Action

Inhibits the muscarinic effect of acetylcholine in smooth muscle, secretory glands and the CNS. Small doses decrease salivary and bronchial secretions and decrease sweating; intermediate doses dilate the pupil, inhibit accommodation, increase heart rate (vagolytic action); large doses decrease GI and GU motility, further increase in dose decreases gastric acid secretion. **Therapeutic Effects:** Decreased secretions with decreased GI and GU symptomatology. Increased heart rate.

Pharmacokinetics

Absorption: Well absorbed; food does not affect absorption.
Distribution: Crosses the placenta and blood-brain barrier; enters breast milk.
Metabolism and Excretion: Excreted mostly unchanged by the kidneys.
Half-life: 3.5 hr.

TIME/ACTION PROFILE (GI effects)

ROUTE	ONSET	PEAK	DURATION
PO	20–30 min	unknown	4–6 hr
IM, IV, subcut	2–3 min	unknown	4–6 hr

Contraindications/Precautions

Contraindicated in: Hypersensitivity; Angle-closure glaucoma; synechiae; Tachycardia or unstable cardiovascular status; GI obstructive disease, paralytic ileus, intestinal atony, severe ulcerative colitis; Obstructive uropathy; Myasthenia gravis; Lactation; Products containing benzyl alcohol should not be used in newborn or immature infants; Some products contain alcohol, sulfites, or tartrazine and should be avoided in patients with known intolerance/hypersensitivity; Phenylketonuria (NuLev contains aspartame).
Use Cautiously in: History of cardiovascular disease including CHF, arrhythmias, hypertension, tachycardia, or coronary artery disease; Renal disease or prostatic hyperplasia; Hepatic disease, early ileus, or reflux esophagitis; Autonomic neuropathy; Hyperthyroidism; Geri: Appears on Beers list. Geriatric patients have increased sensitivity to anticholinergics.; Infants, small children, blondes, Down's syndrome, brain damage, or spastic paralysis (increased sensitivity); Pregnancy (may cause fetal tachycardia; safety not established).

Adverse Reactions/Side Effects

CNS: confusion/excitement (especially in geriatric patients), dizziness, flushing, headache, insomnia, lightheadedness (IM, IV, subcut), nervousness. **EENT:** blurred vision, cycloplegia, increased intraocular pressure, mydriasis, photophobia. **CV:** palpitations, tachycardia. **GI:** dry mouth, altered taste perception, bloated feeling, constipation, nausea, paralytic ileus, vomiting. **GU:** erectile dysfunction, urinary hesitancy/retention. **Derm:** decreased sweating, urticaria. **Local:** local irritation (IM, IV, subcut). **Misc:** allergic reactions including ANAPHYLAXIS, fever (especially in children), suppression of lactation.

Interactions

Drug-Drug: Concurrent administration with **amantadine** ↑ anticholinergic side effects (may require dose reduction). ↑ effects of **atenolol**. Concurrent use with **phenothiazines** may result in ↓ effect of phenothiazine and ↑ anticholinergic side effects (dose reduction may be necessary). ↑ anticholinergic side effects with **tricyclic antidepressants**.

Route/Dosage

PO, SL (Adults): 0.125–0.25 mg 3–4 times daily or 0.375–0.75 mg as sustained release form every 12 hr.
PO (Children 2–<12 yr): *orally disintegrating tablets (NuLev)*—0.0625–0.125 mg (1/2–1 tablet) every 4 hr, up to 6 times/day.
PO (Children 34–36 kg): 125–187 mcg every 4 hr as needed.
PO (Children 22.7–33 kg): 94–125 mcg every 4 hr as needed.
PO (Children 13.6–22.6 kg): 63 mcg every 4 hr as needed.
PO (Children 9.1–13.5 kg): 31.3 mcg every 4 hr as needed.
PO (Children 6.8–9 kg): 25 mcg every 4 hr as needed.
PO (Children 4.5–6.7 kg): 18.8 mcg every 4 hr as needed.
PO (Children 3.4–4.4 kg): 15.6 mcg every 4 hr as needed.
PO (Children 2.3–3.3 kg): 12.5 mcg every 4 hr as needed.
IM, IV, Subcut (Adults): *Gastrointestinal anticholinergic*—0.25–0.5 mg 3–4 times daily as needed; *preoperative prophylaxis of secretions*—0.5 mg or 0.005 mg/kg 30–60 min before anesthesia; *antiarrhythmic*—0.125 mg IV repeated as needed; *cholinergic adjunct (cu-*

H

rariform block)—0.2 mg for each 1 mg of neostigmine.
IM, IV, Subcut (Children ≥2 yr): *preoperative prophylaxis of secretions*—0.005 mg/kg 30–60 min before anesthesia.

Availability (generic available)
Tablets: 0.125 mg, 0.15 mg. **Sublingual tablets:** 0.125 mg, 0.375 mg. **Orally-disintegrating tablets (contains aspartame) (mint):** 0.125 mg. **Extended-release tablets:** 0.375 mg. **Timed-release capsules:** 0.375 mg. **Solution (drops) (orange):** 0.125 mg/ml. **Elixir (orange):** 0.125 mg/5 ml. **Injection:** 0.5 mg/ml.

NURSING IMPLICATIONS

Assessment
- Assess vital signs and ECG tracings frequently during IV drug therapy. Report any significant changes in heart rate or blood pressure, or increased ventricular ectopy or angina to physician promptly.
- Monitor intake and output ratios in elderly or surgical patients because hyoscyamine may cause urinary retention
- Assess patients routinely for abdominal distention and auscultate for bowel sounds. If constipation becomes a problem, increasing fluids and adding bulk to the diet may help alleviate constipation.
- ***Toxicity and Overdose:*** If overdose occurs, physostigmine is the antidote.

Potential Nursing Diagnoses
Decreased cardiac output (Indications)
Impaired oral mucous membrane (Side Effects)
Constipation (Side Effects)

Implementation
- Do not confuse Levbid (hyoscyamine) with Lithobid (lithium) Lopid (gemfibrozil) or Lorabid (loracarbef).
- **PO:** Oral doses are usually given 30 min before meals.

IV Administration
- **Direct IV:** ***Diluent:*** May give IV undiluted or dilute in 10 mL of sterile water. ***Rate:*** No rate information available, give slowly.

Patient/Family Teaching
- Instruct patient to take exactly as directed. Take missed doses as soon as remembered unless almost time for next dose. Do not double doses.
- May cause drowsiness. Caution patients to avoid driving or other activities requiring alertness until response to medication is known.
- Instruct patient that oral rinses, sugarless gum or candy, and frequent oral hygiene may help relieve dry mouth.
- Caution patients that hyoscyamine impairs heat regulation. Strenuous activity in a hot environment may cause heat stroke.
- Instruct patient to consult health care professional before taking any Rx, OTC, or herbal products concurrently with hyoscyamine.
- Inform male patients with benign prostatic hyperplasia that hyoscyamine may cause urinary hesitancy and retention. Changes in urinary stream should be reported to health care professional.

Evaluation/Desired Outcomes
- Increase in heart rate.
- Dryness of mouth.
- Reversal of muscarinic effects.

HIGH ALERT

HYPOGLYCEMIC AGENTS, ORAL

glimepiride (glye-**me**-pye-ride)
Amaryl, ✤Apo-Glimepiride, ✤Co-Glimepiride

glipiZIDE (**glip**-i-zide)
Glucotrol, Glucotrol XL

glyBURIDE (**glye**-byoo-ride)
✤Apo-Glyburide, DiaBeta, ✤Dom-Glyburide, ✤Euglucon, ✤Gen-Glybe, Glynase PresTab, Micronase

Classification
Therapeutic: antidiabetics
Pharmacologic: sulfonylureas

Pregnancy Category B (glyburide [Micronase, Glynase PresTab]), C (glimepiride, glipizide, and glyburide [Diabeta])

Indications
Control of blood glucose in type 2 diabetes mellitus when diet therapy fails. Require some pancreatic function.

Action
Lower blood glucose by stimulating the release of insulin from the pancreas and increasing the

sensitivity to insulin at receptor sites. May also decrease hepatic glucose production. **Therapeutic Effects:** Lowering of blood glucose in diabetic patients.

Pharmacokinetics

Absorption: All agents are well absorbed after oral administration.
Distribution: *Glyburide*—reaches high concentrations in bile and crosses the placenta.
Protein Binding: *Glimepiride* –99.5%, *glipizide* 99%, *glyburide* 99%,.
Metabolism and Excretion: All agents are mostly metabolized by the liver. *Glimepiride*—converted to a metabolite with some hypoglycemic activity.
Half-life: *Glimepiride*—5–9.2; *glipizide*—2.1–2.6 hr; *glyburide*—10 hr.

TIME/ACTION PROFILE (hypoglycemic activity)

ROUTE	ONSET	PEAK	DURATION
Glimepiride	unknown	2–3 hr	24 hr
Glipizide	15–30 min	1–2 hr	up to 24 hr
Glyburide	45–60 min	1.5–3 hr	24 hr

Contraindications/Precautions

Contraindicated in: Hypersensitivity; Hypersensitivity with sulfonamides (cross-sensitivity may occur); Type 1 diabetes; Diabetic coma or ketoacidosis.
Use Cautiously in: Geri: Elderly (↑ sensitivity; dosage reduction may be required); Renal or hepatic dysfunction (↑ risk of hypoglycemia); Infection, trauma, or surgery (may alter requirements for control of blood glucose); Impaired pituitary, or adrenal function; Prolonged nausea or vomiting; Debilitated or malnourished patients (↑ risk of hypoglycemia); OB, Lactation: Pregnancy or lactation (safety not established; insulin recommended during pregnancy); Pedi: Children (safety and effectiveness not established).

Adverse Reactions/Side Effects

CNS: dizziness, drowsiness, headache, weakness. **GI:** constipation, cramps, diarrhea, drug-induced hepatitis, heartburn, increased appetite, nausea, vomiting. **Derm:** photosensitivity, rashes. **Endo:** hypoglycemia. **F and E:** hyponatremia. **Hemat:** APLASTIC ANEMIA, agranulocytosis, leukopenia, pancytopenia, thrombocytopenia.

Interactions

Drug-Drug: Effectiveness may be ↓ by concurrent use of **diuretics**, **corticosteroids**, **phenothiazines**, **oral contraceptives**, **estrogens**, **thyroid preparations**, **phenytoin**, **niacin**, **sympathomimetics**, and **isoniazid**. **Alcohol**, **androgens (testosterone)**, **chloramphenicol**, **MAO inhibitors**, **NSAIDs**, **salicylates**, **sulfonamides**, and **warfarin** may ↑ risk of hypoglycemia. **Fluoroquinolones** may ↑ effects of glyburide. Concurrent use with **warfarin** may alter the response to both agents (↑ effects of both initially, then ↓ activity); close monitoring recommended during any changes in dosage. **Beta blockers** may mask the signs and symptoms of hypoglycemia.

Route/Dosage

Glimepiride

PO (Adults): 1–2 mg once daily initially; may ↑ q 1–2 wk up to 8 mg/day (usual range 1–4 mg/day).
PO (Geriatric Patients): 1 mg/day initially.

Glipizide

PO (Adults): 5 mg/day initially, may be ↑ by 2.5–5 mg/day at weekly intervals as needed; maximum dose = 40 mg/day (immediate-release), 20 mg/day (XL); XL dosage form is given once daily. Doses >15 mg/day should be given as 2 divided doses of immediate-release tablets (not XL).
PO (Geriatric Patients): 2.5 mg/day initially.

Glyburide

The nonmicronized formulation (Diabeta or Micronase) cannot be used interchangeably with the micronized formulation (Glynase PresTab)

PO (Adults): *DiaBeta/Micronase (nonmicronized)*—2.5–5 mg once daily initially; may be ↑ by 2.5–5 mg/day at weekly intervals (range 1.25–20 mg/day). *Glynase PresTab (micronized)*—1.5–3 mg/day initially; may be ↑ by 1.5 mg/day at weekly intervals (range 0.75–12 mg/day; doses >6 mg/day should be given as divided doses).
PO (Geriatric Patients): *DiaBeta/Micronase (nonmicronized)*—1.25 mg/day initially; may be ↑ by 2.5 mg/day at weekly intervals. *Glynase PresTab (micronized)*—0.75 mg/day; may be ↑ by 1.5 mg/day at weekly intervals.

Availability

Glimepiride

Tablets: 1 mg, 2 mg, 4 mg. ***In combination with:*** pioglitazone (Duetact); rosiglitazone (Avandaryl) See Appendix B.

Glipizide

Tablets: 5 mg, 10 mg. **Cost:** *Generic*—5 mg $16.65/100, 10 mg $12.22/100. **Extended-release tablets:** 2.5 mg, 5 mg, 10 mg. **Cost:** *Generic*—2.5 mg $32.97/90, 5 mg $32.97/90, 10 mg $59.97/90. ***In combination with:*** metformin (Metaglip); see Appendix B.

Glyburide

Tablets: 1.25 mg, 2.5 mg, 5 mg. **Micronized tablets:** 1.5 mg, 3 mg, 6 mg. ***In combination with:*** metformin (Glucovance). See Appendix B.

NURSING IMPLICATIONS

Assessment

- Observe for signs and symptoms of hypoglycemic reactions (sweating, hunger, weakness, dizziness, tremor, tachycardia, anxiety).
- Assess patient for allergy to sulfonamides.
- Patients on concurrent beta-blocker therapy may have very subtle signs of hypoglycemia.
- ***Lab Test Considerations:*** Monitor serum glucose and glycosylated hemoglobin periodically during therapy to evaluate effectiveness of treatment.
- Monitor CBC periodically during therapy. Report ↓ in blood counts promptly.
- May cause an ↑ in AST, LDH, BUN, and serum creatinine.
- ***Toxicity and Overdose:*** Overdose is manifested by symptoms of hypoglycemia. Mild hypoglycemia may be treated with administration of oral glucose. Severe hypoglycemia should be treated with IV D50W followed by continuous IV infusion of more dilute dextrose solution at a rate sufficient to keep serum glucose at approximately 100 mg/dl.

Potential Nursing Diagnoses

Imbalanced nutrition: more than body requirements (Indications)
Noncompliance (Patient/Family Teaching)

Implementation

- ***High Alert:*** Accidental administration of oral hypoglycemic agents to non-diabetic adults and children has resulted in serious harm or death. Before administering, confirm that patient has type 2 diabetes.
- ***High Alert:*** Several oral hypoglycemic agents are subject to sound-alike or look-alike confusion: Do not confuse glipizide with glyburide. Do not confuse Glucotrol with Glucotrol XL. Do not confuse micronase (glyburide) with Micro-K (potassium).
- Patients stabilized on a diabetic regimen who are exposed to stress, fever, trauma, infection, or surgery may require administration of insulin.
- To convert from other oral hypoglycemic agents, gradual conversion is not required. For insulin dosage of less than 20 units/day, change to oral hypoglycemic agents can be made without gradual dose adjustment. Patients taking 20 or more units/day should convert gradually by receiving oral agent and a 25–30% reduction in insulin dose every day or every 2nd day with gradual insulin dose reduction as tolerated. Monitor serum or urine glucose and ketones at least 3 times/day during conversion.
- **PO:** May be administered once in the morning with breakfast or divided into 2 doses.
- Administer *glipizide* 30 min before a meal.
- Do not administer *nonmicronized glyburide* with a meal high in fat. *Micronized glyburide* cannot be substituted for *nonmicronized glyburide*. These preparations are not equivalent.

Patient/Family Teaching

- Instruct patient to take medication at same time each day. Take missed doses as soon as remembered unless almost time for next dose. Do not take if unable to eat.
- Explain to patient that this medication controls hyperglycemia but does not cure diabetes. Therapy is long term.
- Review signs of hypoglycemia and hyperglycemia with patient. If hypoglycemia occurs, advise patient to take a glass of orange juice or 2–3 tsp of sugar, honey, or corn syrup dissolved in water or an appropriate number of glucose tablets and notify health care professional.
- Encourage patient to follow prescribed diet, medication, and exercise regimen to prevent hypoglycemic or hyperglycemic episodes.
- Instruct patient in proper testing of serum glucose and ketones. These tests should be closely monitored during periods of stress or illness and health care professional notified if significant changes occur.

- May occasionally cause dizziness or drowsiness. Caution patient to avoid driving or other activities requiring alertness until response to medication is known.
- Caution patient to avoid other medications, especially alcohol, while on this therapy without consulting health care professional.
- Concurrent use of alcohol may cause a disulfiram-like reaction (abdominal cramps, nausea, flushing, headaches, and hypoglycemia).
- Insulin is the recommended method of controlling blood glucose during pregnancy. Counsel female patients to use a form of contraception other than oral contraceptives and to notify health care professional promptly if pregnancy is planned or suspected.
- Caution patient to use sunscreen and protective clothing to prevent photosensitivity reactions.
- Advise patient to inform health care professional of medication regimen before treatment or surgery.
- Advise patient to carry a form of sugar (sugar packets, candy) and identification describing disease process and medication regimen at all times.
- Advise patient to notify health care professional promptly if unusual weight gain, swelling of ankles, drowsiness, shortness of breath, muscle cramps, weakness, sore throat, rash, or unusual bleeding or bruising occurs.
- Emphasize the importance of routine follow-up exams.

Evaluation/Desired Outcomes

- Control of blood glucose levels without the appearance of hypoglycemic or hyperglycemic episodes.

H

ibandronate (i-ban-dro-nate)
Boniva

Classification
Therapeutic: bone resorption inhibitors
Pharmacologic: biphosphonates

Pregnancy Category C

Indications
Treatment/prevention of postmenopausal osteoporosis.

Action
Inhibits resorption of bone by inhibiting ostoclast activity. **Therapeutic Effects:** Reversal/prevention of progression of osteoporosis with decreased fractures.

Pharmacokinetics
Absorption: 0.6% absorbed following oral administration (significantly decreased by food).
Distribution: Rapidly binds to bone.
Protein Binding: 90.9–99.5%.
Metabolism and Excretion: 50–60% excreted in urine; unabsorbed drug is eliminated in feces.
Half-life: *PO*—10–60 hr; *IV*—4.6–25.5 hrs.

TIME/ACTION PROFILE

ROUTE	ONSET	PEAK	DURATION
PO	unknown	0.5–2 hr	up to 1 mo
IV	unknown	3 hr	up to 3 mo

Contraindications/Precautions
Contraindicated in: Hypersensitivity; Uncorrected hypocalcemia; Inability to stand/sit upright for at least 60 min; CCr <30 ml/min.
Use Cautiously in: Geri: Consider age-related decreases in body mass, renal and hepatic function, concurrent disease states and drug therapy; Concurrent use of NSAIDs or aspirin; OB: Pregnancy (use only if potential benefit outweighs risks to mother and fetus); OB: Lactation; Pedi: Children <18 yr (safety not established).

Adverse Reactions/Side Effects
GI: diarrhea, dyspepsia, esophagitis, esophageal/gastric ulcer. **MS:** injection site reactions, pain in arms/legs.

Interactions
Drug-Drug: Calcium, aluminum, magnesium, and **iron**-containing products, including **antacids** ↓ absorption (ibandronate should be taken 60 min before). Concurrent use of **NSAIDs** including **aspirin**, may ↑ risk of gastric irritation.
Drug-Food: Milk and other foods ↓ absorption.

Route/Dosage
PO (Adults): 2.5 mg once daily or 150 mg once monthly.
IV (Adults): 3 mg every 3 months.

Availability
Tablets: 2.5 mg, 150 mg. **Cost:** 150 mg $254.00/3. **Injection:** 3 mg/3 mL in prefilled single-use syringe.

NURSING IMPLICATIONS

Assessment
- **Osteoporosis:** Assess patients for low bone mass before and periodically during therapy.
- ***Lab Test Considerations:*** Assess serum calcium before and periodically during therapy. Hypocalcemia and vitamin D deficiency should be treated before initiating ibandronate therapy.
- May cause ↓ total alkaline phosphatase levels.
- May cause hypercholesterolemia.

Potential Nursing Diagnoses
Risk for injury (Indications)

Implementation
- **PO:** Administer first thing in the morning with 6–8 oz plain water 30 min before other medications, beverages, or food.
- *Once-monthly tablet* should be administered on the same date each month.

IV Administration
- **IV:** Administer using prefilled syringe. Do not administer solution that is discolored or contain particulate matter. Administer IV only; other routes may cause tissue damage. ***Rate:*** Administer as a 15–30 second bolus.
- **Y-Site Incompatibility:** Do not administer with calcium-containing solutions or other IV drugs.

Patient/Family Teaching
- Advise patient to eat a balanced diet and consult health care professional about the need for supplemental calcium and vitamin D. Wait at least 60 min after administration before taking supplemental calcium and vitamin D.

♣ = Canadian drug name.
*CAPITALS indicates life-threatening; underlines indicate most frequent.

I

- Encourage patient to participate in regular exercise and to modify behaviors that increase the risk of osteoporosis (stop smoking, reduce alcohol consumption).
- Advise female patient to notify health care professional if pregnancy is planned or suspected or if she is breastfeeding.
- **PO:** Instruct patient on the importance of taking as directed, first thing in the morning, 60 min before other medications, beverages, or food. Ibandronate should be taken with 6–8 oz plain water (mineral water, orange juice, coffee, and other beverages decrease absorption). Do not chew or suck on tablet. If a dose is missed, skip dose and resume the next morning; do not double doses or take later in the day. If a once-monthly dose is missed and the next scheduled dose is >7 days away, take in the morning following the date it is remembered. Resume original schedule the following month. If the next dose is <7 days away, omit dose and take next scheduled dose. Do not discontinue without consulting health care professional.
- Caution patient to remain upright for 60 min following dose to facilitate passage to stomach and minimize risk of esophageal irritation.
- **IV:** Advice patient that IV doses should not be administered sooner that every 3 months. If a dose is missed, have health care professional administer as soon as possible; next injection should be scheduled 3 months from last injection.

Evaluation/Desired Outcomes

- Prevention of or decrease in the progression of osteoporosis in postmenopausal women.

ibuprofen, oral

(eye-byoo-**proe**-fen)

✤Actiprofen, Advil, Advil Migraine Liqui-Gels, ✤Apo-Ibuprofen, Children's Advil, Children's Motrin, Excedrin IB, Genpril, Haltran, Junior Strength Advil, Menadol, Medipren, Midol Maximum Strength Cramp Formula, Motrin, Motrin Drops, Motrin IB, Motrin Junior Strength, Motrin Migraine Pain, ✤Novo-Profen, Nu-Ibuprofen, Nuprin, PediaCare Children's Fever

Classification
Therapeutic: antipyretics, antirheumatics, nonopioid analgesics, nonsteroidal anti-inflammatory agents
Pharmacologic: nonopioid analgesics

Pregnancy Category B (first trimester)

Indications

Mild to moderate pain or dysmenorrhea. Inflammatory disorders including: Rheumatoid arthritis (including juvenile), Osteoarthritis. Lowering of fever. **Unlabeled uses:** Slows progression of lung disease in cystic fibrosis patients >5 yrs of age (high doses).

Action

Inhibits prostaglandin synthesis. **Therapeutic Effects:** Decreased pain and inflammation. Reduction of fever.

Pharmacokinetics

Absorption: Well absorbed (80%) from the GI tract.
Distribution: Does not enter breast milk in significant amounts.
Protein Binding: 99%.
Metabolism and Excretion: Mostly metabolized by the liver; small amounts (1%) excreted unchanged by the kidneys.
Half-life: Children: 1–2 hr; Adults: 2–4 hr.

TIME/ACTION PROFILE

ROUTE	ONSET	PEAK	DURATION
PO (antipyretic)	0.5–2.5 hr	2–4 hr	6–8 hr
PO (analgesic)	30 min	1–2 hr	4–6 hr
PO (anti-inflammatory)	7 days	1–2 wk	unknown

Contraindications/Precautions

Contraindicated in: Hypersensitivity; Cross-sensitivity may exist with other NSAIDs, including aspirin; Active GI bleeding or ulcer disease; Chewable tablets contain aspartame and should not be used in patients with phenylketonuria; Peri-operative pain from coronary artery bypass graft (CABG) surgery.
Use Cautiously in: Cardiovascular disease (may ↑ risk of cardiovascular events); Renal or hepatic disease, dehydration, or patients on nephrotoxic drugs (may ↑ risk of renal toxicity); Aspirin triad patients (asthma, nasal polyps, and aspirin intolerance); can cause fatal anaphylactoid reactions; Geri: Increased risk of adverse reactions secondary to age-related de-

crease in renal and hepatic function, concurrent illnesses, and medications; Chronic alcohol use/abuse; History of ulcer disease (may ↑ risk of GI bleeding); OB: Not recommended for pregnant patients; has been associated with persistent pulmonary hypertension in infants; Lactation: Has been used safely; Pedi: Safety not established for infants <6 mo.

Adverse Reactions/Side Effects

CNS: headache, dizziness, drowsiness, psychic disturbances. **EENT:** amblyopia, blurred vision, tinnitus. **CV:** arrhythmias, edema. **GI:** GI BLEEDING, HEPATITIS, constipation, dyspepsia, nausea, vomiting, abdominal discomfort. **GU:** cystitis, hematuria, renal failure. **Derm:** EXFOLIATIVE DERMATITIS, STEVENS-JOHNSON SYNDROME, TOXIC EPIDERMAL NECROLYSIS, rashes. **Hemat:** blood dyscrasias, prolonged bleeding time. **Misc:** allergic reactions including ANAPHYLAXIS.

Interactions

Drug-Drug: May limit the cardioprotective effects of low-dose **aspirin**. Concurrent use with **aspirin** may ↓ effectiveness of ibuprofen. Additive adverse GI side effects with **aspirin**, **oral potassium** and other **NSAIDs**, **corticosteroids**, or **alcohol**. Chronic use with **acetaminophen** may ↑ risk of adverse renal reactions. May ↓ effectiveness of **diuretics** or **antihypertensives**. May ↑ hypoglycemic effects of **insulin** or **oral hypoglycemic agents**. May slightly ↑ serum **digoxin** levels. May ↑ serum **lithium** levels and risk of toxicity. ↑ risk of toxicity from **methotrexate**. **Probenecid** ↑ risk of toxicity from ibuprofen. ↑ risk of bleeding with **cefotetan**, **cefoperazone**, **valproic acid**, **thrombolytics**, **warfarin**, and **drugs affecting platelet function** including **clopidogrel**, **ticlopidine**, **abciximab**, **eptifibatide**, or **tirofiban**. ↑ risk of adverse hematologic reactions with **antineoplastics** or **radiation therapy**. ↑ risk of nephrotoxicity with **cyclosporine**.
Drug-Natural Products: ↑ bleeding risk with, **arnica**, **chamomile**, **feverfew**, **garlic**, **ginger**, **ginkgo**, **Panax ginseng**, and others.

Route/Dosage

Analgesia

PO (Adults): *Anti-inflammatory*—400–800 mg 3–4 times daily (not to exceed 3600 mg/day). *Analgesic/antidysmenorrheal/antipyretic*—200–400 mg q 4–6 hr (not to exceed 1200 mg/day).
PO (Children 6 mo–12 yr): *Anti-inflammatory*—30–50 mg/kg/day in 3–4 divided doses (maximum dose: 2.4 g/day). *Antipyretic*—5 mg/kg for temperature <102.5°F (39.17°C) or 10 mg/kg for higher temperatures (not to exceed 40 mg/kg/day); may be repeated q 4–6 hr. *Cystic fibrosis (unlabeled)*—20–30 mg/kg/day divided twice daily.
PO (Infants and Children): *Analgesic*—4–10 mg/kg/dose q 6–8 hr.

Pediatric OTC Dosing

PO (Children 11 yr—72–95 lb): 300 mg q 6–8 hr.
PO (Children 9–10 yr—60–71 lb): 250 mg q 6–8 hr.
PO (Children 6–8 yr—48–59 lb): 200 mg q 6–8 hr.
PO (Children 4–5 yr—36–47 lb): 150 mg q 6–8 hr.
PO (Children 2–3 yr—24–35 lb): 100 mg q 6–8 hr.
PO (Children 12–23 mo—-18–23 lb): 75 mg q 6–8 hr.
PO (Infants 6–11 mo—12–17 lb): 50 mg q 6–8 hr.

Availability (generic available)

Tablets: 100 mg[OTC], 200 mg[OTC], 300 mg, 400 mg, 600 mg, 800 mg. **Capsules (liqui-gels):** 200 mg[OTC]. **Chewable tablets (fruit, grape, orange, and citrus flavor):** 50 mg[OTC], 100 mg[OTC]. **Liquid (berry flavor):** 100 mg/5 ml[OTC]. **Oral suspension (fruit, berry, grape flavor):** 100 mg/5 ml[OTC], 100 mg/2.5 ml[OTC]. **Pediatric drops (berry flavor):** 50 mg/1.25 ml[OTC]. ***In combination with:*** decongestants, [OTC], hydrocodone (Vicoprofen), oxycodone (Combunox). See Appendix B.

NURSING IMPLICATIONS

Assessment

- Patients who have asthma, aspirin-induced allergy, and nasal polyps are at increased risk for developing hypersensitivity reactions. Assess for rhinitis, asthma, and urticaria.
- Geri: Higher risk for poor outcomes or death from GI bleeding. Age-related renal impairment increases risk of hepatic and renal toxicity. Assess for signs and symptoms of GI bleeding (tarry stools, lightheadedness, hy-

potension), renal dysfunction (elevated BUN and creatinine levels, decreased urine output), and hepatic impairment (elevated liver enzymes, jaundice).
- **Pain:** Assess pain (note type, location, and intensity) prior to and 1–2 hr following administration.
- **Arthritis:** Assess pain and range of motion prior to and 1–2 hr following administration.
- **Fever:** Monitor temperature; note signs associated with fever (diaphoresis, tachycardia, malaise).
- ***Lab Test Considerations:*** BUN, serum creatinine, CBC, and liver function tests should be evaluated periodically in patients receiving prolonged therapy.
- Serum potassium, BUN, serum creatinine, alkaline phosphatase, LDH, AST, and ALT may show ↑ levels. Blood glucose, hemoglobin, and hematocrit concentrations, leukocyte and platelet counts, and CCr may be ↓.
- May cause prolonged bleeding time; may persist for <1 day following discontinuation.

Potential Nursing Diagnoses

Acute pain (Indications)
Impaired physical mobility (Indications)

Implementation

- Administration of higher than recommended doses does not provide increased pain relief but may increase incidence of side effects.
- Geri: Use lowest effective dose for shortest period of time.
- Coadministration with opioid analgesics may have additive analgesic effects and may permit lower opioid doses.
- **PO:** For rapid initial effect, administer 30 min before or 2 hr after meals. May be administered with food, milk, or antacids to decrease GI irritation. Tablets may be crushed and mixed with fluids or food; 800-mg tablet can be dissolved in water.
- **Dysmenorrhea:** Administer as soon as possible after the onset of menses. Prophylactic treatment has not been shown to be effective.

Patient/Family Teaching

- Advise patients to take ibuprofen with a full glass of water and to remain in an upright position for 15–30 min after administration.
- Instruct patient to take medication as directed. Take missed doses as soon as remembered but not if almost time for next dose. Do not double doses. Pedi: Teach parents or caregivers to calculate and measure doses accurately and to use measuring device supplied with product.
- May cause drowsiness or dizziness. Advise patient to avoid driving or other activities requiring alertness until response to medication is known.
- Caution patient to avoid the concurrent use of alcohol, aspirin, acetaminophen, or other OTC or herbal products without consulting health care professional.
- Advise patient to inform health care professional of medication regimen prior to treatment or surgery.
- Caution patient to wear sunscreen and protective clothing to prevent photosensitivity reactions.
- Instruct patients not to take OTC ibuprofen preparations for more than 10 days for pain or more than 3 days for fever, and to consult health care professional if symptoms persist or worsen. Many OTC products contain ibuprofen; avoid duplication.
- Pedi: Teach parents or caregivers to check labels of all OTC products to prevent administration of more than one ibuprofen product.
- Caution patient that use of ibuprofen with 3 or more glasses of alcohol per day may increase the risk of GI bleeding.
- Advise patient to consult health care professional if rash, itching, visual disturbances, tinnitus, weight gain, edema, black stools, persistent headache, or influenza-like syndrome (chills, fever, muscle aches, pain) occurs.
- Pedi: Advise parents or caregivers not to administer ibuprofen to children who may be dehydrated (can occur with vomiting, diarrhea, or poor fluid intake); dehydration increases risk of renal dysfuntion.

Evaluation/Desired Outcomes

- Decrease in severity of pain.
- Improved joint mobility. Partial arthritic relief is usually seen within 7 days, but maximum effectiveness may require 1–2 wk of continuous therapy. Patients who do not respond to one NSAID may respond to another.
- Reduction in fever.

ibutilide (eye-**byoo**-ti-lide)
Corvert

Classification
Therapeutic: antiarrhythmics (class III)

Pregnancy Category C

Indications
Rapid conversion of recent-onset atrial flutter or fibrillation to normal sinus rhythm, including management of atrial flutter or fibrillation occurring within 1 wk of coronary artery bypass or cardiac valve surgery.

Action
Activates slow inward current of sodium in cardiac tissue, resulting in delayed repolarization, prolonged action potential duration, and increased refractoriness. Mildly slows sinus rate and AV conduction. **Therapeutic Effects:** Conversion to normal sinus rhythm.

Pharmacokinetics
Absorption: IV administration results in complete bioavailability.
Distribution: Unknown.
Metabolism and Excretion: Highly metabolized by the liver, 1 metabolite is active; metabolites excreted by kidneys.
Half-life: 6 hr (2–12 hr).

TIME/ACTION PROFILE (antiarrhythmic effect)

ROUTE	ONSET	PEAK	DURATION
IV	within 30–90 min	unknown	up to 24 hr

Contraindications/Precautions
Contraindicated in: Hypersensitivity.
Use Cautiously in: CHF or left ventricular dysfunction (↑ risk of more serious arrhythmias during infusion); Pregnancy, lactation, or children <18 yr (safety not established).

Adverse Reactions/Side Effects
CNS: headache. **CV:** arrhythmias. **GI:** nausea.

Interactions
Drug-Drug: Amiodarone, **disopyramide**, **procainamide**, **quinidine**, and **sotalol** should not be given concurrently or within 4 hr because of additive effects on refractoriness. Proarrhythmic effects may be ↑ by **phenothiazines**, **tricyclic** and **tetracyclic antidepressants**, some **antihistamines**, and **histamine H_2-receptor blocking agents**; concurrent use should be avoided.

Route/Dosage
Atrial Fibrillation/Flutter
IV (Adults ≥60 kg): 1 mg infusion; may be repeated 10 min after end of first infusion.
IV (Adults <60 kg): 0.01 mg/kg infusion; may be repeated 10 min after end of first infusion.

Atrial Fibrillation/Flutter After Cardiac Surgery
IV (Adults ≥60 kg): 0.5 mg infusion, may be repeated once.
IV (Adults <60 kg): 0.005 mg/kg infusion, may be repeated once.

Availability
Solution for injection: 0.1 mg/ml in 10-ml vial.

NURSING IMPLICATIONS

Assessment
- Monitor ECG continuously throughout and for 4 hr after infusion or until QT interval normalizes. Discontinue if arrhythmia terminates or if sustained ventricular tachycardia, prolonged QT, or QT develops. Ibutilide may have proarrhythmic effects. These arrhythmias may be serious and potentially life threatening. Clinicians trained to treat ventricular arrhythmias, medications, and equipment (defibrillator/cardioverter) should be available during therapy and monitoring of patient.

Potential Nursing Diagnoses
Decreased cardiac output (Indications)

Implementation
- Oral antiarrhythmic therapy may be instituted 4 hr after ibutilide infusion.

IV Administration
- **Intermittent Infusion:** ***Diluent:*** May be administered undiluted or diluted in 50 ml of 0.9% NaCl or D5W. Diluted solution is stable for 24 hr at room temperature or 48 hr if refrigerated. ***Concentration:*** Undiluted: 0.1 mg/ml; Diluted: 0.017 mg/ml. ***Rate:*** Administer over 10 min.
- **Additive Incompatibility:** Information unavailable; do not admix with other solutions or medications.

Patient/Family Teaching

- Inform patient of the purpose of ibutilide.

Evaluation/Desired Outcomes

- Conversion of recent-onset atrial flutter or fibrillation to normal sinus rhythm.

idarubicin (eye-da-**roo**-bi-sin)

Idamycin

Classification

Therapeutic: antineoplastics

Pharmacologic: anthracyclines

Pregnancy Category D

Indications

Acute myelogenous leukemia in adults (with other agents).

Action

Inhibits nucleic acid synthesis. **Therapeutic Effects:** Death of rapidly replicating cells, particularly malignant ones.

Pharmacokinetics

Absorption: IV administration results in complete bioavailability.

Distribution: Rapidly distributed with extensive tissue binding. High degree of cellular uptake.

Metabolism and Excretion: Extensive hepatic and extrahepatic metabolism. One metabolite is active (idarubicinol). Primarily eliminated via biliary excretion.

Half-life: 22 hr (range 4–46 hr).

TIME/ACTION PROFILE (effects on blood counts)

ROUTE	ONSET	PEAK	DURATION
IV	Unknown	10–14 days	21 days

Contraindications/Precautions

Contraindicated in: Pregnancy or lactation.

Use Cautiously in: Children (safety not established); Patients with childbearing potential; Active infection; Decreased bone marrow reserve; Geriatric patients; Other chronic debilitating illnesses; Hepatic impairment (dose reduction may be required; avoid if bilirubin ≥5 mg/dl); Renal impairment; Pre-existing cardiac disease; Previous daunorubicin or doxorubicin therapy.

Adverse Reactions/Side Effects

CNS: headache, mental status changes. **Resp:** pulmonary toxicity, pulmonary allergic reactions. **CV:** ARRHYTHMIAS, CARDIOTOXICITY, CHF. **GI:** abdominal cramps, diarrhea, mucositis, nausea, vomiting. **Derm:** alopecia, photosensitivity, rashes. **Endo:** gonadal suppression. **Hemat:** BLEEDING, anemia, leukopenia, thrombocytopenia. **Local:** phlebitis at IV site. **Metab:** hyperuricemia. **Neuro:** peripheral neuropathy. **Misc:** fever.

Interactions

Drug-Drug: ↑ myelosuppression with other **antineoplastics** or **radiation therapy**. May ↓ antibody response to and ↑ risk of adverse reactions from **live-virus vaccines**.

Route/Dosage

IV (Adults): 12 mg/m² daily for 3 days in combination with cytarabine.

Availability (generic available)

Powder for injection: 5-mg vials, 10-mg vials.

NURSING IMPLICATIONS

Assessment

- Monitor blood pressure, pulse, respiratory rate, and temperature frequently during administration. Report significant changes.
- Monitor for bone marrow depression. Assess for bleeding (bleeding gums, bruising, petechiae, guaiac stools, urine, and emesis) and avoid IM injections and taking rectal temperatures if platelet count is low. Apply pressure to venipuncture sites for 10 min. Assess for signs of infection during neutropenia. Anemia may occur. Monitor for increased fatigue, dyspnea, and orthostatic hypotension.
- Monitor intake and output ratios. Report significant discrepancies. Encourage fluid intake of 2000–3000 ml/day. Allopurinol and alkalinization of the urine may be used to decrease serum uric acid levels and to help prevent urate stone formation.
- Severe and protracted nausea and vomiting may occur as early as 1 hr after therapy and may last 24 hr. Parenteral antiemetics should be administered 30–45 min prior to therapy and routinely around the clock for the next 24 hr as indicated. Monitor amount of emesis; report emesis exceeding guidelines to prevent dehydration.
- Monitor for development of signs of myocardial toxicity manifested by life-threatening arrhythmias, cardiomyopathy, and CHF (peripheral edema, dyspnea, rales/crackles, weight gain). Chest x-ray, ECG, echocardiography, and radionuclide angiography determinations of ejection fraction should be mon-

itored prior to and periodically during therapy.

- Assess injection site frequently for redness, irritation, or inflammation. May infiltrate painlessly. If extravasation occurs, infusion must be stopped and restarted elsewhere to avoid damage to subcut tissue. Treatment of extravasation includes rest and elevation of the extremity and application of intermittent ice packs (apply for 30 min immediately and 30 min qid for 3 days). If pain, erythema, or vesication persists longer than 48 hr, immediate plastic surgery may be warranted.
- ***Lab Test Considerations:*** Monitor CBC, differential, and platelet count prior to and frequently during therapy. Nadirs of leukopenia and thrombocytopenia are 10–14 days, with recovery occurring 21 days after a dose.
- Monitor renal and hepatic function prior to and periodically during therapy. Idarubicin may cause hyperuricemia. May also cause transient ↑ in AST, ALT, LDH, serum alkaline phosphatase, and bilirubin.

Potential Nursing Diagnoses

Risk for infection (Adverse Reactions)
Imbalanced nutrition: less than body requirements (Adverse Reactions)

Implementation

- Do not confuse Adriamycin (doxorubicin hydrochloride) with Idamycin (idarubicin).
- Solution should be prepared in a biologic cabinet. Wear gloves, gown, and mask while handling medication. Discard IV equipment in specially designated containers.
- See cytarabine monograph for specific information on administration of cytarabine with idarubicin.
- Do not administer subcut or IM and avoid extravasation; may cause severe tissue necrosis.

IV Administration

- **Direct IV:** ***Diluent:*** 0.9% NaCl (nonbacteriostatic) for injection. Reconstitute 5-mg and 10-mg vials with 5 ml and 10 ml, respectively. ***Concentration:*** 1 mg/ml. Vial contents are under pressure; use care when inserting needle
- Reconstituted medication is stable for 72 hr at room temperature and 7 days if refrigerated. ***Rate:*** Administer each dose slowly over 10–30 min through Y-site of a free-flowing infusion of 0.9% NaCl or D5W. Tubing may be attached to a butterfly needle and injected into a large vein.
- **Y-Site Compatibility:** amifostine, amikacin, aztreonam, cimetidine, cladribine, cyclophosphamide, cytarabine, diphenhydramine, droperidol, erythromycin lactobionate, etoposide phosphate, filgrastim, gemcitabine, granisetron, imipenem/cilastatin, magnesium sulfate, mannitol, melphalan, metoclopramide, potassium chloride, ranitidine, sargramostim, thiotepa, vinorelbine.
- **Y-Site Incompatibility:** acyclovir, allopurinol, ampicillin/sulbactam, cefazolin, cefepime, ceftazidime, clindamycin, dexamethasone, etoposide, furosemide, gentamicin, heparin, hydrocortisone sodium succinate, lorazepam, meperidine, methotrexate, piperacillin/tazobactam, sodium bicarbonate, teniposide, vancomycin, vincristine.

Patient/Family Teaching

- Instruct patient to notify health care professional promptly if fever; sore throat; signs of infection; bleeding gums; bruising; petechiae; blood in stools, urine, or emesis; increased fatigue; dyspnea; or orthostatic hypotension occurs. Caution patient to avoid crowds and persons with known infections. Instruct patient to use soft toothbrush and electric razor and to avoid falls. Caution patient not to drink alcoholic beverages or take medication containing aspirin or NSAIDs, as these may precipitate gastric bleeding.
- Instruct patient to report pain at injection site immediately.
- Instruct patient to inspect oral mucosa for erythema and ulceration. If ulceration occurs, advise patient to use sponge brush, rinse mouth with water after eating and drinking, and confer with health care professional if mouth pain interferes with eating. Further courses of idarubicin should be withheld until recovery from mucositis, and subsequent doses should be decreased by 25%. Stomatitis pain may require treatment with opioid analgesics.
- Advise patient that this medication may have teratogenic effects. Contraception should be practiced during and for at least 4 mo after therapy is concluded.
- Instruct patient to notify health care professional immediately if irregular heartbeat,

I

shortness of breath, or swelling of lower extremities occurs.
- Advise patient to wear sunscreen and protective clothing to prevent photosensitivity reactions.
- Discuss with patient the possibility of hair loss. Explore methods of coping.
- Instruct patient not to receive any vaccinations without advice of health care professional.
- Inform patient that urine may turn a reddish color.
- Emphasize the need for periodic lab tests to monitor for side effects.

Evaluation/Desired Outcomes
- Improvement of hematologic status in leukemias.

ifosfamide (eye-foss-fam-ide)
Ifex

Classification
Therapeutic: antineoplastics
Pharmacologic: alkylating agents

Pregnancy Category D

Indications
Germ cell testicular carcinoma (with other agents). Used with mesna, which prevents ifosfamide-induced hemorrhagic cystitis.

Action
Following conversion to active compounds, interferes with DNA replication and RNA transcription, ultimately disrupting protein synthesis (cell-cycle phase–nonspecific).
Therapeutic Effects: Death of rapidly replicating cells, particularly malignant ones.

Pharmacokinetics
Absorption: Administered IV only; inactive prior to conversion to metabolites.
Distribution: Excreted in breast milk.
Metabolism and Excretion: Metabolized by the liver to active antineoplastic compounds.
Half-life: 15 hr.

TIME/ACTION PROFILE (effects on blood counts)

ROUTE	ONSET	PEAK	DURATION
IV	unknown	7–14 days	21 days

Contraindications/Precautions
Contraindicated in: Hypersensitivity; Pregnancy or lactation.
Use Cautiously in: Patients with childbearing potential; Active infections; Decreased bone marrow reserve; Geriatric patients; Other chronic debilitating illness; Impaired renal function; Children.

Adverse Reactions/Side Effects
CNS: CNS toxicity (somnolence, confusion, hallucinations, coma), cranial nerve dysfunction, disorientation, dizziness. **CV:** cardiotoxicity. **GI:** nausea, vomiting, anorexia, constipation, diarrhea, hepatotoxicity. **GU:** hemorrhagic cystitis, dysuria, sterility, renal toxicity. **Derm:** alopecia. **Hemat:** anemia, leukopenia, thrombocytopenia. **Local:** phlebitis. **Misc:** allergic reactions.

Interactions
Drug-Drug: ↑ myelosuppression with other **antineoplastics** or **radiation therapy**. Toxicity may be ↑ by **allopurinol** or **phenobarbital**. May ↓ antibody response to and ↑ risk of adverse reactions from **live-virus vaccines**.

Route/Dosage
Other Regimens are Used
IV (Adults): 1.2 g/m^2/day for 5 days; coadminister with mesna. May repeat cycle q 3 wk.

Availability
Injection: 1- and 3-g vials. ***In combination with:*** mesna (in a kit).

NURSING IMPLICATIONS

Assessment
- Monitor blood pressure, pulse, respiratory rate, and temperature frequently during administration. Report significant changes.
- Monitor urinary output frequently during therapy. Notify physician if hematuria occurs. To reduce the risk of hemorrhagic cystitis, fluid intake should be at least 3000 ml/day for adults and 1000–2000 ml/day for children. Mesna is given concurrently to prevent hemorrhagic cystitis.
- Monitor neurologic status. Ifosfamide should be discontinued if severe CNS symptoms (agitation, confusion, hallucinations, unusual tiredness) occur. Symptoms usually abate within 3 days of discontinuation of ifosfamide but may persist for longer; fatalities have been reported.
- Assess nausea, vomiting, and appetite. Weigh weekly. Premedication with an antiemetic may be used to minimize GI effects. Adjust diet as tolerated.
- Monitor for bone marrow depression. Assess for bleeding (bleeding gums, bruising, petec-

hiae, guaiac stools, urine, and emesis) and avoid IM injections and taking rectal temperatures if platelet count is low. Apply pressure to venipuncture sites for 10 min. Assess for signs of infection during neutropenia. Anemia may occur. Monitor for increased fatigue, dyspnea, and orthostatic hypotension.

- ***Lab Test Considerations:*** Monitor CBC, differential, and platelet count prior to and periodically during therapy. Withhold dose and notify physician if WBC <2000/mm³ or platelet count is <50,000/mm³. Nadir of leukopenia and thrombocytopenia occurs within 7–14 days and usually recovers within 21 days of therapy.
- Urinalysis should be evaluated before each dose. Withhold dose and notify physician if urinalysis shows >10 RBCs per high-power field.
- May cause ↑ in liver enzymes and serum bilirubin.
- Monitor AST, ALT, serum alkaline phosphatase, bilirubin, and LDH prior to and periodically during therapy. Ifosfamide may cause ↑ in liver enzymes and serum bilirubin.
- Monitor BUN, serum creatinine, phosphate, and potassium periodically during therapy.

Potential Nursing Diagnoses

Risk for infection (Side Effects)
Disturbed body image (Side Effects)

Implementation

- Solution should be prepared in a biologic cabinet. Wear gloves, gown, and mask while handling IV medication. Discard IV equipment in specially designated containers.

IV Administration

- **IV: *Diluent:*** Sterile water or bacteriostatic water for injection containing parabens. Prepare solution by diluting each 1-g vial with 20 ml of diluent. Use solution prepared without bacteriostatic water within 6 hr. Solution prepared with bacteriostatic water is stable for 1 wk at 30°C or 6 wk at 5°C
- **Intermittent Infusion: *Concentration:*** May be further diluted to a concentration of 0.6 to 20 mg/ml (maximum 40 mg/ml) in D5W, 0.9% NaCl, LR, or sterile water for injection. ***Rate:*** Administer over at least 30 min.
- **Continuous Infusion:** Has also been administered as a continuous infusion over 72 hr.
- **Syringe Compatibility:** epirubicin, mesna.
- **Y-Site Compatibility:** allopurinol, amifostine, amphotericin B cholesteryl sulfate, aztreonam, doxorubicin liposome, etoposide phosphate, filgrastim, fludarabine, gemcitabine, granisetron, lansoprazole, linezolid, melphalan, ondansetron, oxaliplatin, paclitaxel, pemetrexed, piperacillin/tazobactam, propofol, sargramostim, sodium bicarbonate, teniposide, thiotepa, topotecan, vinorelbine.
- **Y-Site Incompatibility:** cefepime, methotrexate.
- **Additive Compatibility:** carboplatin, cisplatin, epirubicin, etoposide, fluorouracil, mesna.

Patient/Family Teaching

- Emphasize need for adequate fluid intake throughout therapy. Patient should void frequently to decrease bladder irritation from metabolites excreted by the kidneys. Notify health care professional immediately if hematuria is noted.
- Instruct patient to notify health care professional promptly if fever; chills; cough; hoarseness; sore throat; signs of infection; lower back or side pain; painful or difficult urination; bleeding gums; bruising; petechiae; blood in urine, stool, or emesis; or confusion occurs.
- Caution patient to avoid crowds and persons with known infections. Instruct patient to use soft toothbrush and electric razor and to avoid falls. Patients should also be cautioned not to drink alcoholic beverages or to take products containing aspirin or NSAIDs, as these may precipitate GI hemorrhage.
- Review with patient the need for contraception during therapy.
- Discuss with patient the possibility of hair loss. Explore methods of coping.
- Instruct patient not to receive any vaccinations without advice of health care professional; ifosfamide may decrease antibody response to and increase risk of adverse reactions from live-virus vaccines.

Evaluation/Desired Outcomes

- Decrease in size or spread of malignant germ cell testicular carcinoma.

HIGH ALERT

imatinib (i-mat-i-nib)
Gleevec

Classification
Therapeutic: antineoplastics
Pharmacologic: enzyme inhibitors

Pregnancy Category D

Indications
Newly diagnosed Philadelphia positive (Ph+) chronic myeloid leukemia (CML). CML in blast crisis, accelerated phase, or in chronic phase after failure of interferon-alpha treatment. Kit (CD117) positive. Metastatic/unresectable malignant gastrointestinal stomal tumors (GIST). Pediatric patients with Ph+ CML after failure of bone marrow transplant or resistance to interferon-alpha. Adult patients with relapsed or refractory Ph+ acute lymphoblastic leukemia (ALL). Myelodysplastic/myelyproliferative disease (MDS/MPD). Aggressive systemic mastocytosis (ASM). Hypereosinophilic syndrome and/or chronic eosinophilic leukemia (HES/CEL). Unresectable, recurrent, or metastatic dermatofibrosarcoma protuberans (DFSP).

Action
Inhibits kinases which may be produced by malignant cell lines. **Therapeutic Effects:** Inhibits production of malignant cell lines with decreased proliferation of leukemic cells in CML, HES/CEL, and ALL and malignant cells in GIST, MDS/MPD, ASM, and DFSP.

Pharmacokinetics
Absorption: Well absorbed (98%) following oral administration.
Distribution: Unknown.
Protein Binding: 95%.
Metabolism and Excretion: Mostly metabolized by the CYP3A4 enzyme system to N-demethyl imatinib, which is as active as imatinib. Excreted mostly in feces as metabolites. 5% excreted unchanged in urine.
Half-life: *Imatinib*—18 hr; *N-desmethyl imatinib*—40 hr.

TIME/ACTION PROFILE (blood levels of imatinib)

ROUTE	ONSET	PEAK	DURATION
PO	unknown	2–4 hr	24 hr

Contraindications/Precautions
Contraindicated in: Hypersensitivity; OB: Potential for fetal harm; Lactation: Potential for serious adverse reactions in nursing infants; breast-feeding should be avoided.
Use Cautiously in: Hepatic impairment (dose reduction recommended if bilirubin >3 times normal or liver transaminases >5 times normal); Cardiac disease (severe congestive heart failure and left ventricular dysfunction may occur); Pedi: Safety not established for children <3 yr; Geri: Increased risk of edema.

Adverse Reactions/Side Effects
CNS: fatigue, headache, weakness. **Resp:** cough, dyspnea, epistaxis, nasopharyngitis, pneumonia. **GI:** HEPATOTOXICITY, abdominal pain, anorexia, constipation, diarrhea, dyspepsia, nausea, vomiting. **Derm:** petechiae, pruritus, skin rash. **F and E:** edema (including pleural effusion, pericardial infusion, anasarca, superficial edema and fluid retention), hypokalemia. **Hemat:** BLEEDING, NEUTROPENIA, THROMBOCYTOPENIA. **Metab:** weight gain. **MS:** arthralgia, muscle cramps, musculoskeletal pain, myalgia. **Misc:** fever, night sweats.

Interactions
Drug-Drug: Blood levels and effects are ↑ by concurrent **ketoconazole**. Blood levels and effects may be ↓ by **phenytoin**. ↑ blood levels of **simvastatin**. Imatinib inhibits the following enzyme systems: CYP2C9, CYP2D6, CYP3A4/5 and may be expected to alter the effects of other drugs metabolized by these systems.

Route/Dosage

Chronic Myeloid Leukemia
PO (Adults): *Chronic phase*—400 mg once daily, may be increased to 600 mg once daily; *accelerated phase or blast crisis*—600 mg once daily; may be increased to 800 mg/day given as 400 mg twice daily based on response and circumstances.
PO (Children): *Newly diagnosed Ph+ CML*-340 mg/m²/day (not to exceed 600 mg); *CML recurrent after failure of bone marrow transplant or resistance to interferon-alpha*—260 mg/m²/day.

Hepatic Impairment
PO (Adults and Children): Decrease dose by 25% in patients with severe hepatic impairment.

Gastrointestinal Stromal Tumors
PO (Adults): 400 mg/day or 600 mg/day as a single dose.

Ph+ Acute Lymphoblastic Leukemia
PO (Adults): 600 mg/day.

Myelodysplastic/Myeloproliferative Diseases
PO (Adults): 400 mg/day.

Aggressive Systemic Mastocytosis
PO (Adults): 400 mg/day. *For patients with eosinophilia*—100 mg/day; increase to 400 mg if well tolerated and response insufficient.

Hypereosinophilic Syndrome and/or Chronic Eosinophilic Leukemia
PO (Adults): 400 mg/day. *For patients with FIP1L1–PDGFRa fusion kinase* 100 mg/day; increase to 400 mg if well tolerated and response insufficient.

Dermatofibrosarcoma Protuberans
PO (Adults): 800 mg/day.

Availability
Tablets: 100 mg, 400 mg.

NURSING IMPLICATIONS

Assessment
- Monitor for fluid retention. Weigh regularly, and assess for signs of pleural effusion, pericardial effusion, pulmonary edema, ascites (dyspnea, periorbital edema, swelling in feet and ankles, weight gain). Evaluate unexpected weight gain. Edema is usually managed with diuretics. General fluid retention is usually dose related, more common in accelerated phase or blast crisis, and is more common in the elderly. Treatment usually involves diuretics, supportive therapy, and interruption of imatinib.
- Monitor vital signs; may cause fever.
- ***Lab Test Considerations:*** Monitor liver function before and monthly during treatment or when clinically indicated. May cause ↑ transamininases and bilirubin which usually lasts 1 wk and may require dose reduction or interruption. If bilirubin is >3 times the upper limit of normal or transaminases are >5 times the upper limit of normal withhold dose until bilirubin levels return to <1.5 times the upper limit of normal and transaminase levels to <2.5 times the upper limit of normal. Treatment may then be continued at reduced levels (patients on 400 mg/day should receive 300 mg/day and patients receiving 600 mg/day should receive 400 mg/day).
- Monitor CBC weekly for the first month, biweekly for the second month, and periodically during therapy. May cause neutropenia and thrombocytopenia, usually lasting 2–3 wk or 3–4 wk, respectively, and anemia. Usually requires dose reduction, but may require discontinuation. (see Implementation).
- May cause hypokalemia.

Potential Nursing Diagnoses
Risk for injury (Adverse Reactions)

Implementation
- ***High Alert:*** Fatalities have occurred with incorrect administration of chemotherapeutic agents. Before administering, clarify all ambiguous orders; double-check single, daily, and course-of-therapy dose limits; have second practitioner independently double-check original order and dose calculations. Therapy should be initiated by physician experienced in the treatment of patients with chronic myeloid leukemia.
- Patients requiring anticoagulation should receive low-molecular-weight or standard heparin, not warfarin.
- Treatment should be continued as long as patient continues to benefit.
- **PO:** Administer with food and a full glass of water to minimize GI irritation.
- Tablets may be dispersed in water or apple juice (50 ml for the 100 mg and 100 ml for the 400 mg tablet) and stirred with a spoon for patients unable to swallow pills. Administer immediately after suspension.
- Patients receiving *chronic phase, myelodysplastic/myeloproliferative disease, aggressive systemic mastocytosis, and hypereosinophilic syndrome and/or chronic eosinophilic leukemia* treatment who develop an ANC $<1.0 \times 10^9$ /L and/or platelets $<50 \times 10^9$ L should stop imatinib until ANC $\geq 1.5 \times 10^9$ /L and platelets are $\geq 75 \times 10^9$ /L. Then resume imatinib treatment at 400 mg or 600 mg/day.
- *Patients receiving accelerated phase and blast crisis treatment or Ph+ acute lymphoblastic leukemia* who develop an ANC $<0.5 \times 10^9$ /L and/or platelets $<10 \times 10^9$ /L should determine if cytopenia is related to leukemia via marrow aspirate or biopsy. If cytopenia is unrelated to leukemia, reduce dose to 400 mg/day. If cytopenia persists for 2 wks, reduce dose to 300 mg/day. If cytopenia persists for 4 wks and is still unrelated to leukemia, stop imatinib until ANC $\geq 1 \times 10^9$ /L and

platelets are ≥20 × 10^9 /L. Then resume imatinib treatment at 300 mg/day.

- *Patients receiving aggressive systemic mastocytosis with eosinophilia or hypereosinohpilic syndrome and/or chronic eosinophilic leukemia with FIP1L1–PDGFRa fusion kinase* who develop ANC <1.0 x 10^9 /L and platelets <50 x 10^9 /L should stop imatinib until ANC ≥1.5 x 10^9 /L and platelets ≥75 x 10^9 /L. Resume treatment at previous dose.

Patient/Family Teaching

- Explain purpose of imatinib to patient.

Evaluation/Desired Outcomes

- Decrease in production of leukemic cells in patients with CML, HES/CEL, and ALL and malignant cells in GIST, MDS/MPD, ASM, and DFSP.

imipenem/cilastatin

(i-me-**pen**-em/sye-la-**stat**-in)
Primaxin

Classification
Therapeutic: anti-infectives
Pharmacologic: carbapenems

Pregnancy Category C

Indications

Treatment of: Lower respiratory tract infections, Urinary tract infections, Abdominal infections, Gynecologic infections, Skin and skin structure infections, Bone and joint infections, Bacteremia, Endocarditis, Polymicrobic infections.

Action

Imipenem binds to the bacterial cell wall, resulting in cell death. Combination with cilastatin prevents renal inactivation of imipenem, resulting in high urinary concentrations. Imipenem resists the actions of many enzymes that degrade most other penicillins and penicillin-like anti-infectives. **Therapeutic Effects:** Bactericidal action against susceptible bacteria. **Spectrum:** Spectrum is broad. Active against most gram-positive aerobic cocci: *Streptococcus pneumoniae*, Group A beta-hemolytic streptococci, *Enterococcus*, *Staphylococcus aureus*. Active against many gram-negative bacillary organisms: *Escherichia coli*, *Klebsiella*, *Acinetobacter*, *Proteus*, *Serratia*, *Pseudomonas aeruginosa*. Also displays activity against: *Salmonella*, *Shigella*, *Neisseria gonorrhoeae*, Numerous anaerobes.

Pharmacokinetics

Absorption: Well absorbed after IM administration (imipenem 95%, cilastatin 75%). IV administration results in complete bioavailability.
Distribution: Widely distributed. Crosses the placenta; enters breast milk.
Metabolism and Excretion: *Imipenem and cilastatin*—70% excreted unchanged by the kidneys.
Half-life: *Imipenem and cilastatin*—1 hr (prolonged in renal impairment).

TIME/ACTION PROFILE (blood levels)

ROUTE	ONSET	PEAK	DURATION
IM	rapid	1–2 hr	12 hr
IV	rapid	end of infusion	6–8 hr

Contraindications/Precautions

Contraindicated in: Hypersensitivity; Cross-sensitivity may occur with penicillins and cephalosporins.
Use Cautiously in: Previous history of multiple hypersensitivity reactions; Seizure disorders; Geriatric patients; Renal impairment (dose reduction required if CCr ≤70 ml/min/1.73 m^2); Pregnancy, lactation, or children (safety not established).

Adverse Reactions/Side Effects

CNS: SEIZURES, dizziness, somnolence. **CV:** hypotension. **GI:** PSEUDOMEMBRANOUS COLITIS, diarrhea, nausea, vomiting. **Derm:** rash, pruritus, sweating, urticaria. **Hemat:** eosinophilia. **Local:** phlebitis at IV site. **Misc:** allergic reaction including ANAPHYLAXIS, fever, superinfection.

Interactions

Drug-Drug: Do not admix with **aminoglycosides** (inactivation may occur). **Probenecid** ↓ renal excretion and ↑ blood levels. ↑ risk of seizures with **ganciclovir** or **cyclosporine** (avoid concurrent use of ganciclovir).

Route/Dosage

IV (Adults): *Mild infections*—250–500 mg q 6 hr. *Moderate infections*—500 mg q 6–8 hr *or* 1 g q 8 hr. *Serious infections*—500 mg q 6 hr to 1 g q 6–8 hr.
IV (Children ≥3 mo [non-CNS infections]): 15–25 mg/kg q 6 hr; higher doses have been used in older children with cystic fibrosis.
IV (Children 4 wk–3 mo): 25 mg/kg q 6 hr.
IV (Children 1–4 wk): 25 mg/kg q 8 hr.
IV (Children <1 wk): 25 mg/kg q 12 hr.
IM (Adults): 500–750 mg q 12 hr.
IM (Children): 10–15 mg/kg q 6 hr.

Renal Impairment

IV (Adults): If dose for normal renal function is 1 g/day *CCr 41–70 ml/min*—125–250 mg q 6–8 hr, *CCr 21–40 ml/min*—125–250 mg q 8–12 hr, *CCr 6–20 ml/min*—125–250 mg q 12 hr; if dose for normal renal function is 1.5 g/day *CCr 41–70 ml/min*—125–250 mg q 6–8 hr, *CCr 21–40 ml/min*—125–250 mg q 8–12 hr, *CCr 6–20 ml/min*—125–250 mg q 12 hr; if dose for normal renal function is 2 g/day *CCr 41–70 ml/min*—125–500 mg q 6–8 hr, *CCr 21–40 ml/min*—125–250 mg q 8–12 hr, *CCr 6–20 ml/min*—125–250 mg q 12 hr; if dose for normal renal function is 3 g/day *CCr 41–70 ml/min*—250–500 mg q 6–8 hr, *CCr 21–40 ml/min*—250–500 mg q 6–8 hr, *CCr 6–20 ml/min*—250–500 mg q 12 hr; if dose for normal renal function is 4 g/day *CCr 41–70 ml/min*—250–750 mg q 6–8 hr, *CCr 21–40 ml/min*—250–500 mg q 6–8 hr, *CCr 6–20 ml/min*—250 –250 mg q 12 hr.

Availability

Powder for IV injection: 250 mg imipenem/250 mg cilastatin, 500 mg imipenem/500 mg cilastatin. **Powder for IM injection:** 500 mg imipenem/500 mg cilastatin, 750 mg imipenem/750 mg cilastatin.

NURSING IMPLICATIONS

Assessment

- Assess patient for infection (vital signs; appearance of wound, sputum, urine, and stool; WBC) at beginning of and throughout therapy.
- Obtain a history before initiating therapy to determine previous use of and reactions to penicillins. Persons with a negative history of penicillin sensitivity may still have an allergic response.
- Obtain specimens for culture and sensitivity before initiating therapy. First dose may be given before receiving results.
- Observe patient for signs and symptoms of anaphylaxis (rash, pruritus, laryngeal edema, wheezing). Discontinue the drug and notify the physician immediately if these occur. Have epinephrine, an antihistamine, and resuscitative equipment close by in the event of an anaphylactic reaction.
- ***Lab Test Considerations:*** BUN, AST, ALT, LDH, serum alkaline phosphatase, bilirubin, and creatinine may be transiently ↑.
- Hemoglobin and hematocrit concentrations may be ↓.
- May cause positive direct Coombs' test.

Potential Nursing Diagnoses

Risk for infection (Indications, Side Effects)

Implementation

- **IM: Only the IM formulation can be used for IM administration.** Reconstitute 500-mg vial with 2 ml and 750-mg vial with 3 ml of lidocaine without epinephrine. Shake well to form a suspension. Withdraw and inject entire contents of vial IM.

IV Administration

- **Intermittent Infusion: Only the IV formulation can be used for IV administration.** ***Diluent:*** Reconstitute each 250- or 500-mg vial with 10 ml of D5W or 0.9% NaCl and shake well. Further dilute in 100 ml of D5W or 0.9% NaCl. Solution may range from clear to yellow in color. Infusion is stable for 4 hr at room temperature and 24 hr if refrigerated. ***Concentration:*** 2.5 mg/ml (with 250-mg vial); 5 mg/ml (with 500-mg vial). ***Rate:*** Infuse doses ≤500 mg over 20–30 min. Infuse doses ≥750 mg over 40–60 min. Pedi: Infuse doses ≤500 mg over 15–30 min. Infuse doses >500 mg over 40–60 min.
- Rapid infusion may cause nausea and vomiting. If these symptoms develop, slow infusion.
- **Y-Site Compatibility:** acyclovir, amifostine, amikacin, anidulafungin, atropine, aztreonam, bumetanide, caspofungin, cefazolin, cefepime, cefotaxime, cefoxitin, ceftazidime, ceftizoxime, cefuroxime, chloramphenicol, cimetidine, cisatracurium, clindamycin, cyclosporine, dexamethasone sodium phosphate, digoxin, diltiazem, diphenhydramine, docetaxel, dopamine, doxycycline, enalaprilat, epinephrine, erythromycin, esmolol, famotidine, fenoldopam, fentanyl, fludarabine, foscarnet, furosemide, gentamicin, granisetron, heparin, hydrocortisone sodium succinate, hydromorphone, idarubicin, insulin, isoproterenol, ketorolac, labetalol, levofloxacin, lidocaine, linezolid, magnesium sulfate, melphalan, methotrexate, methylprednisolone sodium succinate, metoclopramide, metoprolol, metronidazole, morphine, nafcillin, nitroglycerin, norepinephrine, ondansetron, pantoprazole, penicillin G potassium, phenylephrine, phytonadione, potassium chloride,

propranolol, propofol, protamine, ranitidine, remifentanil, tacrolimus, teniposide, thiotepa, ticarcillin/clavulanate, tigecycline, tirofiban, tobramycin, vancomycin, vasopressin, verapamil, vinorelbine, voriconazole, zidovudine.

- **Y-Site Incompatibility:** alopurinol, amiodarone, amphotericin B cholesteryl sulfate, azithromycin, ceftriaxone, daptomycin, diazepam, drotrecogin, etoposide phosphate, fluconazole, galliun nitrate, ganciclovir, gemcitabine, haloperidol, lansoprazole, lorazepam, meperidine, midazolam, milrinone, phenytoin, prochlorperazine, quinupristin/dalfopristin, sargramostim, sodium bicarbonate, trimethoprim/sulfamethoxazole.
- **Additive Incompatibility:** May be inactivated if administered concurrently with aminoglycosides. If administered concurrently, administer in separate sites, if possible, at least 1 hr apart. If second site is unavailable, flush lines between medications.

Patient/Family Teaching

- Advise patient to report the signs of superinfection (black, furry overgrowth on the tongue; vaginal itching or discharge; loose or foul-smelling stools) and allergy. Consult health care professional before treating with antidiarrheals.
- Caution patient to notify health care professional if fever and diarrhea occur, especially if stool contains blood, pus, or mucus. Advise patient not to treat diarrhea without consulting health care professional. May occur up to several weeks after discontinuation of medication.

Evaluation/Desired Outcomes

- Resolution of the signs and symptoms of infection. Length of time for complete resolution depends on the organism and site of infection.

imipramine (im-ip-ra-meen)

✤Apo-Imipramine, ✤Impril, Norfranil, ✤Novopramine, Tipramine, Tofranil, Tofranil PM

Classification
Therapeutic: antidepressants
Pharmacologic: tricyclic antidepressants

Pregnancy Category C

Indications

Various forms of depression. Enuresis in children. **Unlabeled uses:** Adjunct in the management of chronic pain, incontinence (in adults), vascular headache prophylaxis, cluster headache, insomnia.

Action

Potentiates the effect of serotonin and norepinephrine. Has significant anticholinergic properties. **Therapeutic Effects:** Antidepressant action that develops slowly over several weeks.

Pharmacokinetics

Absorption: Well absorbed from the GI tract.
Distribution: Widely distributed. Probably crosses the placenta and enters breast milk.
Protein Binding: 89–95%.
Metabolism and Excretion: Extensively metabolized by the liver, mostly on first pass; some conversion to active compounds. Undergoes enterohepatic recirculation and secretion into gastric juices.
Half-life: 8–16 hr.

TIME/ACTION PROFILE (antidepressant effect)

ROUTE	ONSET	PEAK	DURATION
PO, IM	hours	2–6 wk	weeks

Contraindications/Precautions

Contraindicated in: Hypersensitivity; Cross-sensitivity with other antidepressants may occur; Angle-closure glaucoma; Hypersensitivity to tartrazine or sulfites (in some preparations); Recent MI, known history of QTc prolongation, heart failure.
Use Cautiously in: Pre-existing cardiovascular disease; Seizures or history of seizure disorder; May ↑ risk of suicide attempt/ideation especially during early treatment or dose adjustment; OB: Drug is present in breast milk; discontinue imipramine or bottle feed; Pedi: Suicide risk may be greater in children or adolescents. Safety not established in children <6 yr; Geri: Geriatric patients (more susceptible to adverse reactions). Geriatric males with prostatic hyperplasia are more susceptible to urinary retention.

Adverse Reactions/Side Effects

CNS: drowsiness, fatigue, agitation, confusion, hallucinations, insomnia. **EENT:** blurred vision, dry eyes. **CV:** ARRHYTHMIAS, hypotension, ECG changes. **GI:** constipation, dry mouth, nausea, paralytic ileus, weight gain. **GU:** urinary retention, decreased libido. **Derm:** photosensitivity. **Endo:** gynecomastia. **Hemat:** blood dyscrasias.

Interactions

Drug-Drug: May cause hypotension, tachycardia, and potentially fatal reactions when used with **MAO inhibitors** (avoid concurrent use—discontinue 2 wk prior to imipramine). Concurrent use with **SSRI antidepressants** may result in increased toxicity and should be avoided (**fluoxetine** should be stopped 5 wk before). Concurrent use with **clonidine** may result in hypertensive crisis and should be avoided. Imipramine is metabolized in the liver by the **cytochrome P450 2D6 enzyme** and its action may be affected by drugs that compete for metabolism by this enzyme including **other antidepressants**, **phenothiazines**, **carbamazepine**, **class 1C antiarrhythmics** (**propafenone**, **flecainide**); when used concurrently, dose reduction of one or the other or both may be necessary. Concurrent use of other drugs that inhibit the activity of the enzyme, including **cimetidine**, **quinidine**, **amiodarone**, and **ritonavir**, may result in ↑ effects of imipramine. Concurrent use with **levodopa** may result in delayed/ ↓ absorption of levodopa or hypertension. Blood levels and effects may be ↓ by **rifamycins**. ↑ CNS depression with other CNS **depressants** including **alcohol**, **antihistamines**, **clonidine**, **opioids**, and **sedative/hypnotics**. **Barbiturates** may alter blood levels and effects. **Adrenergic** and **anticholinergic** side effects may be ↑ with other **agents having these properties**. **Phenothiazines** or **hormonal contraceptives** ↑ levels and may cause toxicity. **Cigarette smoking (nicotine)** may increase metabolism and alter effects.

Drug-Natural Products: Concomitant use of **kava kava, valerian,** or **chamomile can** ↑ **CNS depression.** ↑ **anticholinergic effects** with **jimson weed** and **scopolia.**

Route/Dosage

PO (Adults): 25–50 mg 3–4 times daily (not to exceed 300 mg/day); total daily dose may be given at bedtime.

PO (Geriatric Patients): 25 mg at bedtime initially, up to 100 mg/day in divided doses.

PO (Children >12 yr): *Antidepressant*—25–50 mg/day in divided doses (not to exceed 100 mg/day).

PO (Children 6–12 yr): *Antidepressant*—10–30 mg/day in 2 divided doses.

PO (Children ≥6 yr): *Enuresis*—25 mg once daily 1 hr before bedtime; increase if necessary by 25 mg at weekly intervals to 50 mg in children <12 yr, up to 75 mg in children >12 yr.

IM (Adults): Up to 100 mg/day in divided doses (not to exceed 300 mg/day).

Availability (generic available)

Tablets: 10 mg, 25 mg, 50 mg, ✤75 mg. **Capsules:** 75 mg, 100 mg, 125 mg, 150 mg. **Injection:** 12.5 mg/ml.

NURSING IMPLICATIONS

Assessment

- Monitor blood pressure and pulse rate prior to and during initial therapy.
- Monitor plasma levels in treatment-resisant patients.
- Monitor weight and BMI initially and periodically throughout therapy.
- For overweight/obese individuals, obtain FBS and cholesterol levels Refer as appropriate for nutrition/weight management and medical management.
- Obtain weight and BMI initially and regularly throughout therapy.
- Assess for sexual dysfunction (decreased libido; erectile dysfunction).
- Pedi, Geri: Monitor baseline and periodic ECGs in elderly patients or patients with heart disease and before increasing dose with children treated for enuresis. May cause prolonged PR and QT intervals and may flatten T waves.
- **Depression:** Assess mental status (orientation, mood, behavior) frequently. Confusion, agitation, and hallucinations may occur during initiation of therapy and may require dosage reduction. Assess for suicidal tendencies, especially during early therapy. Restrict amount of drug available to patient.
- **Enuresis:** Assess frequency of bedwetting during therapy. Ask patient or caretaker to maintain diary.
- **Pain:** Assess location, duration, and severity of pain periodically during therapy. Use pain scale to monitor effectiveness of therapy.
- ***Lab Test Considerations:*** Assess leukocyte and differential blood counts and renal and hepatic functions prior to and periodically during prolonged or high-dose therapy.

- Serum levels may be monitored in patients who fail to respond to usual therapeutic dose. Therapeutic plasma concentration range for depression is 150–300 mg/ml.
- May cause alterations in blood glucose levels.
- ***Toxicity and Overdose:*** Symptoms of acute overdose include disturbed concentration, confusion, restlessness, agitation, seizures, drowsiness, mydriasis, arrhythmias, fever, hallucinations, vomiting, and dyspnea: Treatment of overdose includes gastric lavage, activated charcoal, and a stimulant cathartic. Maintain respiratory and cardiac function (monitor ECG for at least 5 days) and temperature. Medications may include digoxin for CHF, antiarrhythmics, and anticonvulsants.

Potential Nursing Diagnoses

Ineffective coping (Indications)
Chronic pain (Indications)
Impaired urinary elimination (Indications, Side Effects)
Sexual dysfunction (Side Effects)

Implementation

- Do not confuse imipramine with desipramine.
- Dose increases should be made at bedtime because of sedation. Dose titration is a slow process; may take weeks to months. May be given as a single dose at bedtime to minimize sedation during the day.
- Taper to avoid withdrawal effects. Reduce by 50% for 3 days, then reduce by 50% for 3 days, then discontinue.
- **PO:** Administer medication with or immediately following a meal to minimize gastric irritation.
- **IM:** May be slightly yellow or red in color. Crystals may develop if solution is cool; place ampule under warm running water for 1 min to dissolve.

Patient/Family Teaching

- Instruct patient to take medication as directed. Take missed doses as soon as possible unless almost time for next dose; if regimen is a single dose at bedtime, do not take in the morning because of side effects. Advise patient that drug effects may not be noticed for at least 2 wk. Abrupt discontinuation may cause nausea, vomiting, diarrhea, headache, trouble sleeping with vivid dreams, and irritability.
- May cause drowsiness and blurred vision. Caution patient to avoid driving and other activities requiring alertness until response to drug is known.
- Instruct patient to notify health care professional if visual changes occur. Inform patient that periodic glaucoma testing may be needed during long-term therapy.
- Caution patient to change positions slowly to minimize orthostatic hypotension.
- Advise patient to avoid alcohol or other CNS depressant drugs during therapy and for at least 3–7 days after therapy has been discontinued.
- Instruct patient to notify health care professional if urinary retention, dry mouth, or constipation persists. Sugarless candy or gum may diminish dry mouth and an increase in fluid intake or bulk may prevent constipation. If symptoms persist, dose reduction or discontinuation may be necessary. Consult health care professional if dry mouth persists for more than 2 wk.
- Caution patient to use sunscreen and protective clothing to prevent photosensitivity reactions.
- Alert patient that urine may turn blue-green in color.
- Inform patient of need to monitor dietary intake, as possible increase in appetite may lead to undesired weight gain. Inform patient that increased amounts of riboflavin in the diet may be required; consult health care professional.
- Advise patient to notify health care professional of medication regimen prior to treatment or surgery.
- Therapy for depression is usually prolonged. Emphasize the importance of follow-up exams to evaluate progress and improve coping skills.
- Pedi: Inform parents that the side effects most likely to occur include nervousness, insomnia, unusual tiredness, and mild nausea and vomiting. Notify health care professional if these symptoms become pronounced.
- Advise parents to keep medication out of reach of children to prevent inadvertent overdose.
- Refer to local support group.

Evaluation/Desired Outcomes

- Increased sense of well-being.
- Renewed interest in surroundings.
- Increased appetite.
- Improved energy level.
- Pain relief.
- Diminished incidence of enuresis.

- Improved sleep in patients treated for depression. Patient may require 2–6 wk of therapy before full therapeutic effects of medication are noticeable.
- Control of bedwetting in children >6 yr.
- Decrease in chronic neurogenic pain.

imiquimod (i-mi-kwi-mod)

Aldara

Classification

Therapeutic: antivirals

Pharmacologic: immune response modifiers

Pregnancy Category B

Indications

External genital or perianal warts/condylomata (condyloma acuminatum). Typical, nonhyperkeratotic, nonhypertrophic actinic keratoses on the face or scalp. Biopsy-confirmed, primary superficial basal cell carcinoma.

Action

May induce the formation of interferons that have antiproliferative and antiviral properties. **Therapeutic Effects:** Regression of external genital or perianal warts/condylomata, actinic keratoses, or basal cell carcinoma lesions.

Pharmacokinetics

Absorption: Minimal absorption.
Distribution: Action is primarily local.
Metabolism and Excretion: <0.9% excreted in urine and feces.
Half-life: Unknown.

TIME/ACTION PROFILE (regression of lesions)

ROUTE	ONSET	PEAK	DURATION
Topical	days–wks	10–16 wk	unknown

Contraindications/Precautions

Contraindicated in: None known.
Use Cautiously in: Previous treatment/surgery in affected area (area should be healed prior to use); Pre-existing inflammatory skin lesions (may be exacerbated); Immunocompromised patients (safety not established); Pregnancy, lactation, or children <12 yr (safety not established).

Adverse Reactions/Side Effects

Local: <u>irritation</u>, <u>pain</u>, <u>pruritis</u>, <u>burning</u>, <u>swelling</u>, fungal infections (women).

Interactions

Drug-Drug: None known.

Route/Dosage

External Genital Warts

Topical (Adults and Children >12 yr): Apply thin layer to warts at bedtime every other day (3 times weekly); leave on for 6–10 hr, then rinse off with mild soap and water. Repeat until lesions are completely cleared or up to 16 wk.

Actinic Keratoses

Topical (Adults): Apply thin layer to clean, dry affected area twice weekly; leave on for 8 hr, then rinse off with mild soap and water. Continue for 16 wk.

Superficial Basal Cell Carcinoma

Topical (Adults): Apply thin layer to clean, dry affected area 5 times per week; leave on for 8 hr, then rinse off with mild soap and water. Continue for 6 wk.

Availability

Cream: 5% in single-use packets in boxes of 12. **Cost:** $185.59/box.

NURSING IMPLICATIONS

Assessment

- Assess affected area(s) prior to and periodically during therapy.

Potential Nursing Diagnoses

Risk for infection (Indications)
Risk for infection (Patient/Family Teaching)

Implementation

- **Topical:** Apply a thin film to clean and dry skin as directed prior to bedtime. Rub in well and leave on skin for time period specified. Remove by washing with mild soap and water. Discard unused cream from single-dose packet. A rest period of several days may be taken if required for patient comfort or severity of skin reaction. Resume therapy when reaction subsides.
- Do not use occlusive dressings. If covering is needed, use cotton gauze or cotton underclothes.

Patient/Family Teaching

- Instruct patient on proper application technique. Emphasize the importance of washing

hands before and after application and avoiding contact with eyes. Advise patient not to use more cream than was prescribed. Missed doses should be applied as soon as possible; then return to regular schedule.
- Advise patient to delay next dose for several days when experiencing discomfort or severe reactions. Notify health care professional if severe reactions occur.
- Advise patient to avoid sharing this medication with others.
- Instruct patient to avoid contact with affected areas while the cream is on the skin. Wash cream off of genital areas before engaging in sexual activities. Inform patient that oils in the cream weaken latex contraceptive devices, such as cervical caps, condoms, and diaphragms.
- Advise patient to avoid use of other topical medications on same treatment area unless recommended by health care professional.

Evaluation/Desired Outcomes
- Healing of genital or perianal warts. Treatment is continued until wart is healed or up to 16 wk.
- Healing of actinic keratosis. Treatment is continued for 16 wk.
- Resolution of superficial basal cell carcinoma lesions. Treatment is continued for 6 wk.

HIGH ALERT

INSULINS (rapid acting)
(**in**-su-lin)

insulin aspart, rDNA origin
Novolog

insulin lispro, rDNA origin
Humalog

insulin glulisine
Apidra

Classification
Therapeutic: antidiabetics, hormones
Pharmacologic: pancreatics

Pregnancy Category B (insulin aspart, insulin lispro), C (insulin glulisine)

See Appendix M for more information concerning insulins

Indications
Control of hyperglycemia in patients with type 1 or type 2 diabetes mellitus.

Action
Lower blood glucose by: stimulating glucose uptake in skeletal muscle and fat, inhibiting hepatic glucose production. Other actions: inhibition of lypolysis and proteolysis, enhanced protein synthesis. These are rapid-acting insulins with a more rapid onset and shorter duration than regular insulin; should be used with an intermediate- or long-acting insulin. **Therapeutic Effects:** Control of hyperglycemia in diabetic patients.

Pharmacokinetics
Absorption: Very rapidly absorbed from subcut administration sites.
Distribution: Widely distributed.
Metabolism and Excretion: Metabolized by liver, spleen, kidney, and muscle.
Half-life: *Insulin aspart*—1–1.5 hr; *insulin lispro* -1 hr; *insulin glulisine*—42 min.

TIME/ACTION PROFILE (hypoglycemic effect)

ROUTE	ONSET	PEAK	DURATION
Insulin aspart	10–20 min	1–3 hr	3–5 hr
Insulin glulisine	within 15 min	1 hr	2–4 hr
Insulin lispro	within 15 min	1–1.5 hr	3–4 hr

Contraindications/Precautions
Contraindicated in: Hypoglycemia; Allergy or hypersensitivity to a particular type of insulin, preservatives, or other additives.
Use Cautiously in: Stress and infection (may temporarily ↑ insulin requirements); Renal/hepatic dysfunction (may ↓ insulin requirements); OB: Pregnancy (may temporarily ↑ insulin requirements); Pedi: Children <3 yr (for insulin lispro), <6 yr (for insulin aspart) (safety not established).

Adverse Reactions/Side Effects
Endo: HYPOGLYCEMIA. **Local:** erythema, lipodystrophy, pruritis, swelling. **Misc:** allergic reactions including ANAPHYLAXIS.

Interactions
Drug-Drug: Beta blockers, clonidine, and **reserpine** may mask some of the signs and symptoms of hypoglycemia. **Corticosteroids, thyroid supplements, estrogens, isoniazid, niacin, phenothiazines**, and **rifampin** may ↑ insulin requirements. **Alcohol, ACE inhibitors, MAO inhibitors, octreotide,**

oral hypoglycemic agents, and **salicylates**, may ↓ insulin requirements.
Drug-Natural Products: Glucosamine may worsen blood glucose control. **Fenugreek**, **chromium**, and **coenzyme Q-10** may produce additive hypoglycemic effects.

Route/Dosage

Dose depends on blood glucose, response, and many other factors. Only insulin aspart and insulin glulisine can be administered IV.
Subcut (Adults and Children): Total insulin dose determined by needs of patient; generally 0.5–1 unit/kg/day; 50–70% of this dose may be given as meal-related boluses of rapid-acting insulin, and the remainder as an intermediate or long-acting insulin. *Subcutaneous infusion pump* —~50% of total dose can be given as meal-related boluses and ~50% of total dose can be given as basal infusion.

Availability

Insulin aspart: 100 units/ml in 10 mL vials and 3 mL disposable delivery devices. **Cost:** $88.99/10-ml vial *NovoLog Pens (3 ml)*—$166.39/5 pens. **Insulin glulisine:** 100 units/mL in 10 mL vials and 3 ml disposable delivery devices. **Cost:** $79.99/10-ml vial. **Insulin lispro:** 100 units/mL in 10-mL vials and 3 mL disposable delivery device. **Cost:** $85.99/10-ml vial *Humalog Pens (3 ml)*—$172.05/5 pens. ***In combination with:*** **Insulin lispro 75/25 mix (Humalog Mix 75/25):** 75% lispro insulin protamine suspension and 25% insulin lispro mix 100 units/mL in 10 mL vials and 3 mL disposable delivery devices. **Cost:** $91.25/10-ml vial *Humalog Mix 75/25 Pens (3 ml)*—$147.50/5 pens. **Insulin lispro 50/50 mix (Humalog Mix 50/50):** 50% lispro insulin protamine suspension and 50% insulin lispro mix 100 units/mL in 10 ml vials and 3 mL disposable delivery devices.

NURSING IMPLICATIONS

Assessment

- Assess for symptoms of hypoglycemia (anxiety; restlessness; tingling in hands, feet, lips, or tongue; chills; cold sweats; confusion; cool, pale skin; difficulty in concentration; drowsiness; nightmares or trouble sleeping; excessive hunger; headache; irritability; nausea; nervousness; tachycardia; tremor; weakness; unsteady gait) and hyperglycemia (confusion, drowsiness; flushed, dry skin; fruit-like breath odor; rapid, deep breathing, polyuria; loss of appetite; nausea; vomiting; unusual thirst) periodically during therapy.
- Monitor body weight periodically. Changes in weight may necessitate changes in insulin dose.
- Assess patient for signs of allergic reactions (rash, shortness of breath, wheezing, rapid pulse, sweating, low blood pressure) during therapy.
- ***Lab Test Considerations:*** May cause ↓ serum inorganic phosphate, magnesium, and potassium levels.
- Monitor blood glucose every 6 hr during therapy, more frequently in ketoacidosis and times of stress. A1C may also be monitored every 3–6 mo to determine effectiveness.
- ***Toxicity and Overdose:*** Overdose is manifested by symptoms of hypoglycemia. Mild hypoglycemia may be treated by ingestion of oral glucose. Severe hypoglycemia is a life-threatening emergency; treatment consists of IV glucose, glucagon, or epinephrine.

Potential Nursing Diagnoses

Noncompliance (Patient/Family Teaching)

Implementation

- ***High Alert:*** Insulin-related medication errors have resulted in patient harm and death. Clarify ambiguous orders; do not accept orders using the abbreviation "u" for units, (can be misread as a zero or the numeral 4; has resulted in tenfold overdoses).
- Insulins are available in different types and strengths. Check type, dose, and expiration date with another licensed nurse. Do not interchange insulins without consulting physician or other health care professional.
- Use *only* insulin syringes to draw up dose. The unit markings on the insulin syringe must match the insulin's units/ml.
- *Insulin aspart, insulin glulisine,* and *insulin lispro* may be mixed with NPH insulin. When mixing insulins, draw insulin aspart, insulin glulisine, or insulin lispro into syringe first to avoid contamination of rapid-acting insulin vial. Mixed insulins should never be used in a pump or for IV infusion.
- Store vials in refrigerator. Vials may also be kept at room temperature for up to 28 days. Do not use if cloudy, discolored, or unusually viscous. Cartridges and pens should be stored

at room temperature and used within 28 days.

- Because of their short duration, *insulin lispro, insulin glulisine* and *insulin aspart*, must be used with a longer-acting insulin or insulin infusion pump. In patients with type 2 diabetes, *insulin lispro* may be used without a longer-acting insulin when used in combination with an oral sulfonylurea agent.
- **Subcut:** Administer into abdominal wall, thigh, or upper arm subcut. Rotate injection sites.
- Administer *insulin aspart* within 5–10 min before a meal.
- When used as meal time insulin, administer *insulin glulisine* 15 min before or within 20 min after starting a meal.
- Administer *insulin lispro* within 15 min before or immediately after a meal.
- May also be administered subcut via external insulin pump. Do not mix with other insulins or solution when used with a pump. The insulin in the reservoir, the infusion set, and the infusion site should be changed q 48 hr. Discard cartridges after 48 hrs (7 days for insulin lispro), even if solution remains.
- **IV:** *Insulin aspart* and *insulin glulisine* may be administered IV in selected situations under appropriate medical supervision. Should be diluted to a concentration of 1 unit/ml in 0.9% NaCl (D5W may also be used with *insulin aspart*). *Insulin lispro* should not be administered IV.

Patient/Family Teaching

- Instruct patient on proper technique for administration. Include type of insulin, equipment (syringe, cartridge pens, external puml, alcohol swabs), storage, and place to discard syringes. Discuss the importance of not changing brands of insulin or syringes, selection and rotation of injection sites, and compliance with therapeutic regimen.
- Demonstrate technique for mixing insulins by drawing up insulin aspart, insulin glulisine, or insulin lispro first. Roll intermediate-acting insulin vial between palms to mix, rather than shaking (may cause inaccurate dose).
- Explain to patient that this medication controls hyperglycemia but does not cure diabetes. Therapy is long term.
- Instruct patient in proper testing of serum glucose and ketones. These tests should be closely monitored during periods of stress or illness and health care professional notified of significant changes.
- Emphasize the importance of compliance with nutritional guidelines and regular exercise as directed by health care professional.
- Advise patient to consult health care professional prior to using alcohol or other Rx, OTC, or herbal products concurrently with insulin.
- Advise patient to notify health care professional of medication regimen prior to treatment or surgery.
- Advise patient to notify health care professional if nausea, vomiting, or fever develops, if unable to eat regular diet, or if blood glucose levels are not controlled.
- Instruct patient on signs and symptoms of hypoglycemia and hyperglycemia and what to do if they occur.
- Advise patient to notify health care professional if pregnancy is planned or suspected or if breastfeeding or planning to breastfeed.
- Patients with diabetes mellitus should carry a source of sugar (candy, glucose gel) and identification describing their disease and treatment regimen at all times.
- Emphasize the importance of regular follow-up, especially during first few weeks of therapy.

Evaluation/Desired Outcomes

- Control of blood glucose levels without the appearance of hypoglycemic or hyperglycemic episodes.

indapamide (in-dap-a-mide)

Lozide, Lozol

Classification

Therapeutic: antihypertensives, diuretics
Pharmacologic: thiazide-like diuretics

Pregnancy Category B

Indications

Mild to moderate hypertension. Edema associated with CHF and other causes.

Action

Increases excretion of sodium and water by inhibiting sodium reabsorption in the distal tubule. Promotes excretion of chloride, potassium, magnesium, and bicarbonate. May produce arteriolar dilation. **Therapeutic Effects:** Lowering of blood pressure in hypertensive patients and diuresis with subsequent mobilization of edema.

Pharmacokinetics

Absorption: Well absorbed from the GI tract after oral administration.
Distribution: Widely distributed.
Metabolism and Excretion: Mostly metabolized by the liver. Small amounts (7%) excreted unchanged by the kidneys.
Half-life: 14–18 hr.

TIME/ACTION PROFILE (antihypertensive effect)

ROUTE	ONSET	PEAK	DURATION
PO (single dose)	unknown	24 hr	unknown
PO (multiple dose)	1–2 wk	8–12 wk	up to 8 wk

Contraindications/Precautions

Contraindicated in: Hypersensitivity; Cross-sensitivity with sulfonamides may occur; Anuria; Lactation.
Use Cautiously in: Renal or severe hepatic impairment; Geriatric patients (increased sensitivity); Pregnancy or children (safety not established).

Adverse Reactions/Side Effects

CNS: dizziness, drowsiness, lethargy. **CV:** arrhythmias, hypotension. **GI:** anorexia, cramping, nausea, vomiting. **Derm:** photosensitivity, rashes. **Endo:** hyperglycemia. **F and E:** hypokalemia, dehydration, hypochloremic alkalosis, hyponatremia, hypovolemia. **Metab:** hyperuricemia. **MS:** muscle cramps.

Interactions

Drug-Drug: Additive hypotension with other **antihypertensives**, **nitrates**, or acute ingestion of **alcohol**. Additive hypokalemia with **corticosteroids**, **amphotericin B**, **piperacillin**, or **ticarcillin**. ↓ the excretion of **lithium**; may cause toxicity. Hypokalemia may ↑ risk of **digoxin** toxicity.
Drug-Natural Products: Licorice and **stimulant laxative herbs (aloe, senna)** may ↑ risk of potassium depletion.

Route/Dosage

PO (Adults): *Hypertension*—1.25–5 mg daily in the morning; may be increased at 4-wk intervals up to 5 mg/day. *Edema secondary to CHF*—2.5 mg daily in the morning; may be increased after 1 wk to 5 mg/day.

Availability (generic available)

Tablets: 1.25 mg, 2.5 mg. **Cost:** *Generic*—1.25 mg $12.60/90, 2.5 mg $12.60/90.

NURSING IMPLICATIONS

Assessment

- Monitor blood pressure, intake and output, and daily weight and assess feet, legs, and sacral area for edema daily.
- Assess patient, especially if taking digoxin, for anorexia, nausea, vomiting, muscle cramps, paresthesia, and confusion; report signs of electrolyte imbalance. Patients taking digoxin have an increased risk of digitalis toxicity due to the potassium-depleting effect of the diuretic.
- Assess patient for allergy to sulfonamides.
- ***Lab Test Considerations:*** Monitor electrolytes (especially potassium), blood glucose, BUN, serum creatinine, and uric acid levels periodically throughout therapy. May cause decreased potassium, sodium, and chloride concentrations. May increase serum glucose; diabetic patients may require increased oral hypoglycemic or insulin dosage. Increases uric acid level an average of 1.0 mg/100 ml; may precipitate an episode of gout.

Potential Nursing Diagnoses

Excess fluid volume (Indications)
Risk for deficient fluid volume (Side Effects)

Implementation

- Administer in the morning to prevent disruption of sleep cycle.
- **PO:** May be given with food or milk to minimize GI irritation.

Patient/Family Teaching

- Instruct patient to take this medication at the same time each day. If a dose is missed, take as soon as remembered but not just before next dose is due. Do not double doses. Advise patients using indapamide for hypertension to continue taking the medication even if feeling well. Indapamide controls but does not cure hypertension.
- Caution patient to change positions slowly to minimize orthostatic hypotension. This may be potentiated by alcohol.
- Advise patient to use sunscreen (avoid those containing PABA) and protective clothing

when in the sun to prevent photosensitivity reactions.

- Instruct patient to follow a diet high in potassium (see Appendix L).
- Advise patient to report muscle weakness, cramps, nausea, or dizziness to health care professional.
- Advise patient to consult health care professional before taking OTC medication concurrently with this therapy.
- Emphasize the importance of routine follow-up exams.
- **Hypertension:** Instruct patient and family on proper technique of blood pressure monitoring. Advise them to check blood pressure at least weekly and to report significant changes.
- Encourage patient to comply with additional interventions for hypertension (weight reduction, low-sodium diet, regular exercise, smoking cessation, moderation of alcohol consumption, and stress management).

Evaluation/Desired Outcomes

- Control of hypertension.
- Decrease in edema secondary to CHF.

indomethacin

(in-doe-**meth**-a-sin)

✤Apo-Indomethacin, ✤Indameth, ✤Indocid, Indocin, Indocin I.V, ✤Indocin PDA, Indocin SR, Indochron E-R, ✤Novo-Methacin, ✤Nu-Indo

Classification

Therapeutic: antirheumatics, ductus arteriosus patency adjuncts (IV only), nonsteroidal anti-inflammatory agents

Pregnancy Category B (first trimester)

Indications

PO: Inflammatory disorders including: Rheumatoid arthritis, Gouty arthritis, Osteoarthritis, Ankylosing spondylitis. Generally reserved for patients who do not respond to less toxic agents. **IV:** Alternative to surgery in the management of patent ductus arteriosus in premature neonates.

Action

Inhibits prostaglandin synthesis. **Therapeutic Effects: PO:** Suppression of pain and inflammation. **IV:** Closure of patent ductus arteriosus.

Pharmacokinetics

Absorption: Well absorbed after oral administration in adults, incomplete oral absorption in neonates.

Distribution: Crosses the blood-brain barrier and the placenta. Enters breast milk.

Protein Binding: 99%.

Metabolism and Excretion: Mostly metabolized by the liver.

Half-life: Neonates <2 weeks: 20 hr; >2 weeks: 11 hr; Adults: 2.6–11 hr.

TIME/ACTION PROFILE

ROUTE	ONSET	PEAK	DURATION
PO (analgesic)	30 min	0.5–2 hr	4–6 hr
PO-ER (analgesic)	30 min	unknown	4–6 hr
PO (anti-inflammatory)	up to 7 days	1–2 wk	4–6 hr
PO-ER (anti-inflammatory)	up to 7 days	1–2 wk	4–6 hr
IV (closure of PDA)	up to 48 hr	unknown	unknown

Contraindications/Precautions

Contraindicated in: Hypersensitivity; Known alcohol intolerance (suspension); Cross-sensitivity may exist with other NSAIDs, including aspirin; Active GI bleeding; Ulcer disease; Proctitis or recent history of rectal bleeding; Necrotizing enterocolitis in neonates; Intraventricular hemorrhage; Thrombocytopenia.

Use Cautiously in: Severe cardiovascular, renal, or hepatic disease; History of ulcer disease; Epilepsy; Hypertension; Geri: Geriatric patients are at increased risk for adverse reactions including dizziness and GI bleeding; Pregnancy or lactation (not recommended during 2nd half of pregnancy); Lactation.

Adverse Reactions/Side Effects

CNS: dizziness, drowsiness, headache, psychic disturbances. **EENT:** blurred vision, tinnitus. **CV:** hypertension, edema. **GI:** *PO*— DRUG-INDUCED HEPATITIS, GI BLEEDING, constipation, dyspepsia, nausea, vomiting, discomfort, necrotizing enterocolitis. **GU:** cystitis, hematuria, renal failure. **Derm:** rashes. **F and E:** hyperkalemia; *IV*— dilutional hyponatremia; *IV*— hypoglycemia. **Hemat:** thrombocytopenia, blood dyscrasias, prolonged bleeding time. **Local:** phlebitis at IV site. **Misc:** allergic reactions including ANAPHYLAXIS.

Interactions

Drug-Drug: Concurrent use with **aspirin** may ↓ effectiveness. Additive adverse GI effects with **aspirin**, other **NSAIDs**, **corticosteroids**, or **alcohol**. Chronic use of **acetaminophen** ↑ risk of adverse renal reactions. May ↓ effectiveness of **diuretics** or **antihypertensives**. May ↑ hypoglycemia from **insulins** or **oral hypoglycemic agents**. May ↑ risk of toxicity from **lithium** or **zidovudine** (avoid concurrent use with zidovudine). ↑ risk of toxicity from **methotrexate**. **Probenecid** ↑ risk of toxicity from indomethacin. ↑ risk of bleeding with **cefotetan**, **cefoperazone**, **valproic acid**, **thrombolytics**, **warfarin**, and **drugs affecting platelet function** including **clopidogrel**, **ticlopidine**, **abciximab**, **eptifibatide**, or **tirofiban**. ↑ risk of adverse hematologic reactions with **antineoplastics** or **radiation therapy**. ↑ risk of nephrotoxicity with **cyclosporine**. Concurrent use with **potassium-sparing diuretics** may result in hyperkalemia. May ↑ levels of **digitalis glycosides methotrexate lithium** and **aminoglycosides** when used IV in neonates.
Drug-Natural Products: ↑ bleeding risk with **anise**, **arnica**, **chamomile**, **clove**, **dong quai**, **feverfew**, **garlic**, **ginger**, **ginkgo**, and **Panax ginseng**.

Route/Dosage

Anti-inflammatory

PO (Adults): *Antiarthritic*—25–50 mg 2–4 times daily *or* 75-mg extended-release capsule once or twice daily (not to exceed 200 mg or 150 mg of SR/day). A single bedtime dose of 100 mg may be used. *Antigout*—100 mg initially, followed by 50 mg 3 times daily for relief of pain, then decreased further.
PO (Children >2 yr): 1–2 mg/kg/day in 2–4 divided doses (not to exceed 4 mg/kg/day or 150–200 mg/day).

Closure of Patent Ductus Arteriosus

IV (Neonates): 0.2 mg/kg initially, then 2 subsequent doses at 12–24 hr intervals of 0.1 mg/kg if age <48 hr at time of initial dose; 0.2 mg/kg if 2–7 days at initial dose; 0.25 mg/kg if age >7 days at initial dose.

Availability (generic available)

Capsules: 25 mg, 50 mg. **Sustained-release capsules:** 75 mg. **Oral suspension (fruit mint, pineapple coconut mint flavors):** 25 mg/5 ml. **Powder for injection:** 1-mg vials.

NURSING IMPLICATIONS

Assessment

- Patients who have asthma, aspirin-induced allergy, and nasal polyps are at increased risk for developing hypersensitivity reactions. Monitor for rhinitis, asthma, and urticaria.
- **Arthritis:** Assess limitation of movement and pain—note type, location, and intensity before and 1–2 hr after administration.
- **Patent Ductus Arteriosus:** Monitor respiratory status, heart rate, blood pressure, echocardiogram, and heart sounds routinely throughout therapy.
- Monitor intake and output. Fluid restriction is usually instituted throughout therapy.
- ***Lab Test Considerations:*** Evaluate BUN, serum creatinine, CBC, serum potassium levels, and liver function tests periodically in patients receiving prolonged therapy.
- Serum potassium, BUN, serum creatinine, AST, and ALT tests may show ↑ levels. Blood glucose concentrations may be altered. Hemoglobin and hematocrit concentrations, leukocyte and platelet counts, and CCr may be ↓.
- Urine glucose and urine protein concentrations may be ↑.
- Leukocyte and platelet count may be ↓. Bleeding time may be prolonged for several days after discontinuation.

Potential Nursing Diagnoses

Acute pain (Indications)
Impaired physical mobility (Indications)

Implementation

- If prolonged therapy is used, dose should be reduced to the lowest level that controls symptoms.
- **PO:** Administer after meals, with food, or with antacids to decrease GI irritation. Do not crush, break, or chew sustained-release capsules.
- Shake suspension before administration. Do not mix with antacid or any other liquid.

IV Administration

- **Direct IV:** ***Diluent:*** Preservative-free 0.9% NaCl or preservative-free sterile water. Reconstitute with 1 or 2 ml of diluent. ***Concentration:*** 0.5–1 mg/ml. Reconstitute immediately before use and discard any unused solution. Do not dilute further or admix. Do not administer via umbilical catheter into vessels near the superior mesenteric artery, as these can cause vasoconstriction and compromise blood flow to the intestines. Do not administer intra-arterially. ***Rate:*** Administer over 20–30 min. Avoid extravasation, as solution is irritating to tissues.

- **Y-Site Compatibility:** furosemide, insulin, nitroprusside, potassium chloride, sodium bicarbonate.
- **Y-Site Incompatibility:** calcium gluconate, cimetidine, dobutamine, dopamine, gentamicin, levofloxacin, tobramycin, tolazoline.

Patient/Family Teaching

- Advise patient to take this medication with a full glass of water and to remain in an upright position for 15–30 min after administration.
- Instruct patient to take medication exactly as directed. Take missed doses as soon as remembered if not almost time for next dose. Do not double doses.
- May cause drowsiness or dizziness. Advise patient to avoid driving or other activities requiring alertness until response to medication is known.
- Caution patient to avoid the concurrent use of alcohol, aspirin, other NSAIDs, acetaminophen, or other OTC medications without consulting health care professional.
- Caution patient to wear sunscreen and protective clothing to prevent photosensitivity reactions.
- Advise patient to inform health care professional of medication regimen before treatment or surgery.
- Instruct patient to notify health care professional if rash, itching, chills, fever, muscle aches, visual disturbances, weight gain, edema, abdominal pain, black stools, or persistent headache occurs.
- **Patent Ductus Arteriosus:** Explain to parents the purpose of medication and the need for frequent monitoring.

Evaluation/Desired Outcomes

- Decrease in severity of moderate pain.
- Improved joint mobility. Partial arthritic relief is usually seen within 2 wk, but maximum effectiveness may require up to 1 mo of continuous therapy. Patients who do not respond to one NSAID may respond to another.
- Successful closure of patent ductus arteriosus.

infliximab (in-**flix**-i-mab)

Remicade

Classification

Therapeutic: antirheumatics (DMARDs), gastrointestinal anti-inflammatories—therapeutic

Pharmacologic: monoclonal antibodies

Pregnancy Category C

Indications

Active rheumatoid arthritis (moderate to severe, with methotrexate). Active Crohn's disease (moderate to severe). Active psoriatic arthritis. Active ankylosing spondylitis. Active ulcerative colitis (moderate to severe) with inadequate response to conventional therapy: reducing signs and symptoms, and inducing and maintaining clinical remission and mucosal healing, and eliminating corticosteroid use. Plaque psoriasis (chronic severe).

Action

Neutralizes and prevents the activity of tumor necrosis factor-alpha (TNF-alpha), resulting in anti-inflammatory and antiproliferative activity. **Therapeutic Effects:** Decreased pain and swelling, decreased rate of joint destruction and improved physical function in ankylosing spondylitis, rheumatoid or psoriatic arthritis. Reduction and maintenance of closure of fistulae in Crohn's disease. Decreased symptoms, maintaining remission and mucosal healing with decreased corticosteroid use in ulcerative colitis. Decrease in induration, scaling and erythema of psoriatic lesions.

Pharmacokinetics

Absorption: IV administration results in complete bioavailability.
Distribution: Predominantly distributed within the vascular compartment.
Metabolism and Excretion: Unknown.
Half-life: 9.5 days.

TIME/ACTION PROFILE (symptoms of Crohn's disease)

ROUTE	ONSET	PEAK	DURATION
IV	1–2 wk	unknown	12–48 wk†

†After infusion

Contraindications/Precautions

Contraindicated in: Hypersensitivity to infliximab, murine (mouse) proteins, or other components in the formulation; OB: Lactation; CHF.

Use Cautiously in: Patients being retreated after 2 yr without treatment (increased risk of adverse reactions); History of tuberculosis or exposure (latent tuberculosis should be treated prior to infliximab therapy); Geri: Geriatric patients; OB: Pregnancy (use only if clearly needed); Pedi: Children (safety not established).

Adverse Reactions/Side Effects

CNS: fatigue, headache, anxiety, depression, dizziness, insomnia. **EENT:** conjunctivitis. **Resp:** upper respiratory tract infection, bronchitis, cough, dyspnea, laryngitis, pharyngitis, respiratory tract allergic reaction, rhinitis, sinusitis. **CV:** chest pain, hypertension, hypotension, pericardial effusion, tachycardia, CHF. **GI:** abdominal pain, nausea, vomiting, constipation, diarrhea, dyspepsia, flatulence, hepatotoxicity, intestinal obstruction, oral pain, tooth pain, ulcerative stomatitis. **GU:** dysuria, urinary frequency, urinary tract infection. **Derm:** acne, alopecia, dry skin, ecchymosis, eczema, erythema, flushing, hematoma, increased sweating, hot flushes, pruritus, urticaria, rash. **Hemat:** neutropenia. **MS:** arthralgia, arthritis, back pain, involuntary muscle contractions, myalgia. **Neuro:** paresthesia. **Misc:** INFECTIONS (including reactivation tuberculosis, pneumonia and invasive fungal infections), fever, infusion reactions, chills, flu-like syndrome, herpes simplex, herpes zoster, hypersensitivity reactions, ↑ risk of lymphoma, lupus-like syndrome, moniliasis, pain, peripheral edema, vasculitis.

Interactions

Drug-Drug: None significant.

Route/Dosage

Rheumatoid arthritis

IV (Adults): 3 mg/kg followed by 3 mg/kg 2 and 6 wk after initial dose and then every 8 wk; dose may be adjusted in partial responders up to 10 mg/kg or treatment as often as every 4 wk (used with methotrexate).

Crohn's Disease

IV (Adults): *Moderate-to-severe Crohn's disease*—5 mg/kg as a single infusion. *Fistulizing Crohn's disease*—5 mg/kg repeated 2 and 6 wk after initial infusion; maintenance dose of 5 mg/kg may be given q 8 wk.

Ankylosing spondylitis

IV (Adults): 5 mg/kg given as an infusion repeated 2 and 6 wk later, then every 6 wk.

Psoriatic Arthritis

IV (Adults): 5 mg/kg given as an infusion repeated 2 and 6 weeks later, then every 8 wk thereafter (with or without methotrexate).

Ulcerative Colitis

IV (Adults): 5 mg/kg given as an infusion regimen at 0, 2 and 6 wk followed by a maintenance regimen of 5 mg/kg every 8 wk thereafter.

Psoriasis

IV (Adults): 5 mg/kg given as an infusion regimen at 0, 2 and 6 wk followed by a maintenance regimen of 5 mg/kg every 8 wk thereafter.

Availability

Powder for injection: 100 mg/vial.

NURSING IMPLICATIONS

Assessment

- Assess for infusion-related reactions (fever, chills, urticaria, pruritus) during and for 2 hr after infusion. Symptoms usually resolve when infusion is discontinued. Reactions are more common after 1st or 2nd infusion. Frequency of reactions may be reduced with immunosuppressant agents.
- Assess for latent tuberculosis with a tuberculin skin test prior to initiation of therapy. Treatment of latent tuberculosis should be initiated prior to therapy with infliximab.
- Observe patient for hypersensitivity reactions (urticaria, dyspnea, hypotension) during infusion. Discontinue infliximab if severe reaction occurs. Have medications (antihistamines, acetaminophen, corticosteroids, epinephrine) and equipment readily available in the event of a severe reaction.
- **Rheumatoid Arthritis:** Assess pain and range of motion prior to and periodically during therapy.
- **Crohn's Disease and Ulcerative Colitis:** Assess for signs and symptoms before, during, and after therapy.
- **Psoriasis:** Assess lesions periodically during therapy.
- ***Lab Test Considerations:*** May cause ↑ in positive ANA. Frequency may be decreased with baseline immunosuppressant therapy.
- Monitor liver function tests periodically during therapy. May cause mild to moderate AST

and ALT ↑ without progressing to liver dysfunction. If patient develops jaundice or liver enzyme elevations ≥5 times the upper limits of normal, discontinue infliximab.
- Monitor CBC with differential periodically during therapy. May cause leukopenia, neutropenia, thrombocytopenia, and pancytopenia. Discontinue infliximab is symptoms of blood dyscrasias (persistent fever) occur.

Potential Nursing Diagnoses
Acute pain, chronic (Indications)
Diarrhea (Indications)

Implementation
IV Administration
- **Intermittent Infusion:** Calculate the total number of vials needed. ***Diluent:*** Reconstitute each vial with 10 ml of sterile water for injection using a syringe with a 21-gauge needle or smaller. Direct stream to sides of vial. Do not use if vacuum is not present in vial. Gently swirl solution by rotating vial to dilute; do not shake. May foam on reconstitution; allow to stand for 5 min. Solution is colorless to light yellow and opalescent; a few translucent particles may develop because infliximab is a protein. Do not use if opaque particles, discoloration, or other particles occur. Withdraw volume of total infliximab dose from infusion container containing 250 ml with 0.9% NaCl. ***Concentration:*** Slowly add total dose of infliximab for a concentration ranging from 0.4 to 4 mg/ml. Mix gently. Infusion should begin within 3 hr of preparation. Solution is incompatible with polyvinyl chloride equipment. Prepare in glass infusion bottle or polypropylene or polyolefin bags. Do not reuse or store any portion of infusion solution. ***Rate:*** Administer over at least 2 hr through polyethylene-lined administration set with an in-line, sterile, nonpyrogenic, low protein-building filter with ≤1.2-micron pore size.
- **Y-Site Incompatibility:** Do not administer concurrently in the same line with any other agents.

Patient/Family Teaching
- Advise patient that adverse reactions (myalgia, rash, fever, polyarthralgia, pruritus) may occur 3–12 days after delayed (>2 yr) retreatment with infliximab. Symptoms usually decrease or resolve within 1–3 days. Instruct patient to notify health care professional if symptoms occur.
- May cause dizziness. Caution patient to avoid driving or other activities requiring alertness until response to medication is known.

Evaluation/Desired Outcomes
- Decreased pain and swelling with decreased rate of joint destruction and improved physical function in patients with ankylosing spondylitis, psoriatic, or rheumatoid arthritis.
- Decrease in the signs and symptoms of Crohn's disease and a decrease in the number of draining enterocutaneous fistulas. Decreased symptoms, maintaining remission and mucosal healing with decreased corticosteroid use in ulcerative colitis.
- Decrease in induration, scaling and erythema of psoriatic lesions.

HIGH ALERT

INSULIN (mixtures)
(**in**-su-lin)

insulin lispro protamine suspension/insulin lispro solution mixtures, rDNA origin
Humalog Mix 75/25, Humalog Mix 50/50

insulin aspart protamine suspension/insulin aspart solution mixtures, rDNA origin
NovoLog Mix 70/30

NPH/regular insulin mixtures
Humulin 50/50, Humulin 70/30, Novolin 70/30

Classification
Therapeutic: antidiabetics, hormones
Pharmacologic: pancreatics

Pregnancy Category B (insulin lispro protamine/insulin lispro solution mixture), C (insulin aspart protamine/insulin aspart solution mixture. NPH/regular insulin mixture)

See Appendix M for more information concerning insulins

Indications
Control of hyperglycemia in patients with type 1 or type 2 diabetes mellitus.

Action
Lower blood glucose by: stimulating glucose uptake in skeletal muscle and fat, inhibiting hepatic glucose production. Other actions: inhibition

of lipolysis and proteolysis, enhanced protein synthesis. **Therapeutic Effects:** Control of hyperglycemia in diabetic patients.

Pharmacokinetics

Absorption: Well absorbed from subcutaneous administration sites. Absorption rate is determined by type of insulin, injection site, volume of injectate, and other factors.
Distribution: Widely distributed.
Metabolism and Excretion: Metabolized by liver, spleen, kidney, and muscle.
Half-life: 5–6 min (prolonged in patients with diabetes; biologic half-life is 1–1.5 hr;).

TIME/ACTION PROFILE (hypoglycemic effect)

ROUTE	ONSET	PEAK	DURATION
insulin lispro protamine suspension/ insulin lispro solution mixture subcut	15–30 min	2.8 hr	24 hr
insulin aspart protamine suspension/ insulin aspart solution mixture subcut	15 min	1–4 hr	18–24 hr
NPH/Regular Insulin mixture subcutaneous	30 min	4–8 hr	24 hr

Contraindications/Precautions

Contraindicated in: Hypoglycemia; Allergy or hypersensitivity to a particular type of insulin, preservatives, or other additives.
Use Cautiously in: Stress and infection (may temporarily ↑ insulin requirements); Renal/ hepatic impairment (may ↓ insulin requirements); OB: Pregnancy (may temporarily ↑ insulin requirements); Pedi: Children <18 yr (safety of Humalog not established).

Adverse Reactions/Side Effects

Endo: HYPOGLYCEMIA. **Local:** erythema, lipodystrophy, pruritis, swelling. **Misc:** allergic reactions including ANAPHYLAXIS.

Interactions

Drug-Drug: Beta blockers, **clonidine**, and **reserpine** may mask some of the signs and symptoms of hypoglycemia. **Corticosteroids**, **thyroid supplements**, **estrogens**, **isoniazid**, **niacin**, **phenothiazines**, and **rifampin** may ↑ insulin requirements. **Alcohol**, **ACE inhibitors**, **MAO inhibitors**, **octreotide**, **oral hypoglycemic agents**, and **salicylates**, may ↓ insulin requirements.
Drug-Natural Products: Glucosamine may worsen blood glucose control. **Fenugreek**, **chromium**, and **coenzyme Q-10** may produce additive hypoglycemic effects.

Route/Dosage

Dose depends on blood glucose, response, and many other factors.
Subcut (Adults and Children): 0.5–1 unit/ kg/day. *Adolescents during rapid growth*—0.8–1.2 units/kg/day.

Availability

NPH insulin/regular insulin suspension mixture: 70 units NPH/30 units regular insulin/ ml—Novolin 70/30, Humulin 70/30 (100 units/ ml total) in 10-ml vials and 3-ml disposable delivery devices[OTC], 50 units NPH/50 units regular insulin/ml—Humulin 50/50 (100 units/ml total) in 10-ml vials[OTC]. **Cost:** *Humulin 70/30 or Novolin 70/30*—$42.99/10-ml vial; *Humulin 50/50*—$36.99/10-ml vial; *Humulin 70/30 pen (3 ml)*—$117.03/5 pens; *Novolin 70/30 Penfill (3 ml)*—$116.72/5 pens. **Insulin lispro protamine suspension/insulin lispro solution mixture:** 75% insulin lispro protamine suspension and 25% insulin lispro solution mix—Humalog Mix 75/25 100 units/mL in 10-mL vials and 3-mL disposable delivery devices, 50% insulin lispro protamine suspension and 50% insulin lispro solution mix—Humalog Mix 50/50 100 units/mL in 10-mL vials and 3-mL disposable delivery devices. **Cost:** $91.25/ 10-ml vial *Humalog Mix 75/25 Pens (3 ml)*—$147.50/5 pens. **Insulin aspart protamine suspension/insulin aspart solution mixture:** 70% insulin aspart protamine suspension and 30% insulin aspart solution mix—NovoLog Mix 70/30 100 units/mL in 10-mL vials and 3-mL disposable delivery devices. **Cost:** *Novolog Mix 70/30 Pens (3 ml)*—$166.38/5 pens.

NURSING IMPLICATIONS

Assessment

- Assess for symptoms of hypoglycemia (anxiety; restlessness; tingling in hands, feet, lips, or tongue; chills; cold sweats; confusion; cool, pale skin; difficulty in concentration; drowsiness; excessive hunger; headache; irritability; nightmares or trouble sleeping; nausea; nervousness; tachycardia; tremor; weakness; unsteady gait) and hyperglycemia (confusion, drowsiness; flushed, dry skin; fruit-like breath odor; rapid, deep breathing, polyuria; loss of appetite; nausea; vomiting; unusual thirst) periodically during therapy.
- Monitor body weight periodically. Changes in weight may necessitate changes in insulin dose.
- ***Lab Test Considerations:*** May cause ↓ serum inorganic phosphate, magnesium, and potassium levels.
- Monitor blood glucose every 6 hr during therapy, more frequently in ketoacidosis and times of stress. A1C may also be monitored every 3–6 mo to determine effectiveness.
- ***Toxicity and Overdose:*** Overdose is manifested by symptoms of hypoglycemia. Mild hypoglycemia may be treated by ingestion of oral glucose. Severe hypoglycemia is a life-threatening emergency; treatment consists of IV glucose, glucagon, or epinephrine.

Potential Nursing Diagnoses

Noncompliance (Patient/Family Teaching)

Implementation

- ***High Alert:*** Insulin-related medication errors have resulted in patient harm and death. Clarify ambiguous orders; do not accept orders using the abbreviation "u" for units, (can be misread as a zero or the numeral 4; has resulted in tenfold overdoses).
- Insulins are available in different types and strengths. Check type, dose, and expiration date with another licensed nurse. Do not interchange insulins without consulting physician or other health care professional.
- Use *only* insulin syringes to draw up dose. The unit markings on the insulin syringe must match the insulin's units/ml.
- Store insulin in refrigerator. May also be kept at room temperature for up to 28 days. Do not use if cloudy, discolored, or unusually viscous. Humalog pens must be discarded after 10 days. NovoLog pens must be discarded after 14 days.
- NPH insulins should not be used in the management of ketoacidosis.
- **Subcut:** Rotate injection sites.
- Administer into abdominal wall, thigh, or upper arm subcutaneously.

Patient/Family Teaching

- Instruct patient on proper technique for administration. Include type of insulin, equipment (syringe, cartridge pens, alcohol swabs), storage, and place to discard syringes. Discuss the importance of not changing brands of insulin or syringes, selection and rotation of injection sites, and compliance with therapeutic regimen.
- Explain to patient that this medication controls hyperglycemia but does not cure diabetes. Therapy is long term.
- Instruct patient in proper testing of serum glucose and ketones. These tests should be closely monitored during periods of stress or illness and health care professional notified of significant changes.
- Emphasize the importance of compliance with nutritional guidelines and regular exercise as directed by health care professional.
- Advise patient to consult health care professional prior to using alcohol or other Rx, OTC, or herbal products concurrently with insulin.
- Advise patient to notify health care professional of medication regimen prior to treatment or surgery.
- Advise patient to notify health care professional if nausea, vomiting, or fever develops, if unable to eat regular diet, or if blood glucose levels are not controlled.
- Instruct patient on signs and symptoms of hypoglycemia and hyperglycemia and what to do if they occur.
- Advise patient to notify health care professional if pregnancy is planned or suspected or if breastfeeding or planning to breastfeed.
- Patients with diabetes mellitus should carry a source of sugar (candy, glucose gel) and identification describing their disease and treatment regimen at all times.
- Emphasize the importance of regular follow-up, especially during first few weeks of therapy.

Evaluation/Desired Outcomes

- Control of blood glucose levels in diabetic patients without the appearance of hypoglycemic or hyperglycemic episodes.

HIGH ALERT

INSULINS (short acting)
(in-su-lin)

insulin, regular (injection, concentrated)
Humulin R, Humulin R U-500 (concentrated), ✤Insulin-Toronto, Novolin R

Classification
Therapeutic: antidiabetics, hormones
Pharmacologic: pancreatics

Pregnancy Category B

See Appendix M for more information concerning insulins

Indications
Control of hyperglycemia in patients with type 1 or type 2 diabetes; can be used to treat diabetic ketoacidosis. *Concentrated insulin U-500*: Only for use in patients with insulin requirements >200 units/day. **Unlabeled uses:** Treatment of hyperkalemia.

Action
Lower blood glucose by: stimulating glucose uptake in skeletal muscle and fat, inhibiting hepatic glucose production. Other actions: inhibition of lipolysis and proteolysis, enhanced protein synthesis. **Therapeutic Effects:** Control of hyperglycemia in diabetic patients.

Pharmacokinetics
Absorption: Rapidly absorbed from subcutaneous administration sites.
Distribution: Widely distributed.
Metabolism and Excretion: Metabolized by liver, spleen, kidney, and muscle.
Half-life: 30–60 min.

TIME/ACTION PROFILE (hypoglycemic effect)

ROUTE	ONSET	PEAK	DURATION
Regular insulin IV	10–30 min	15–30 min	30–60 min
Regular insulin subcut	30–60 min	2–4 hr	5–7 hr

Contraindications/Precautions
Contraindicated in: Hypoglycemia; Allergy or hypersensitivity to a particular type of insulin, preservatives, or other additives.
Use Cautiously in: Stress and infection (may temporarily ↑ insulin requirements); Renal/hepatic impairment (may ↓ insulin requirements); OB: Pregnancy (may temporarily ↑ insulin requirements).

Adverse Reactions/Side Effects
Endo: HYPOGLYCEMIA. **Local:** erythema, lipodystrophy, pruritis, swelling. **Misc:** allergic reactions including ANAPHYLAXIS.

Interactions
Drug-Drug: Beta blockers, **clonidine**, and **reserpine** may mask some of the signs and symptoms of hypoglycemia. **Corticosteroids**, **thyroid supplements**, **estrogens**, **isoniazid**, **niacin**, **phenothiazines**, and **rifampin** may ↑ insulin requirements. **Alcohol**, **ACE inhibitors**, **MAO inhibitors**, **octreotide**, **oral hypoglycemic agents**, and **salicylates**, may ↓ insulin requirements.
Drug-Natural Products: Glucosamine may worsen blood glucose control. **Fenugreek**, **chromium**, and **coenzyme Q-10** may produce additive hypoglycemic effects.

Route/Dosage
Dose depends on blood glucose, response, and many other factors.

Ketoacidosis—Regular Insulin Only (100 units/ml)
IV (Adults): 0.1 unit/kg/hr as a continuous infusion.
IV (Children): Loading dose-0.1 unit/kg, then maintenance continuous infusion 0.05–0.2 unit/kg/hr, titrate to optimal rate of decrease of serum glucose of 80–100 mg/dL/hr.

Maintenance Therapy
Subcut (Adults and Children): 0.5–1 unit/kg/day. *Adolescents during rapid growth*—0.8–1.2 units/kg/day.

Treatment of Hyperkalemia
Subcut, IV (Adults and Children): dextrose 0.5–1 g/kg combined with insulin 1 unit for every 4–5 g dextrose given.

Availability
Insulin injection (regular insulin): 100 units/ml in 10 ml vials and 3 ml disposable delivery devices OTC. **Regular (concentrated) insulin injection:** 500 units/ml in 20-ml vials.

✤ = Canadian drug name.
*CAPITALS indicates life-threatening; underlines indicate most frequent.

NURSING IMPLICATIONS

Assessment

- Assess for symptoms of hypoglycemia (anxiety; restlessness; tingling in hands, feet, lips, or tongue; chills; cold sweats; confusion; cool, pale skin; difficulty in concentration; drowsiness; nightmares or trouble sleeping; excessive hunger; headache; irritability; nausea; nervousness; tachycardia; tremor; weakness; unsteady gait) and hyperglycemia (confusion, drowsiness; flushed, dry skin; fruit-like breath odor; rapid, deep breathing, polyuria; loss of appetite; nausea; vomiting; unusual thirst) periodically during therapy.
- Monitor body weight periodically. Changes in weight may necessitate changes in insulin dose.
- ***Lab Test Considerations:*** May cause ↓ serum inorganic phosphate, magnesium, and potassium levels.
- Monitor blood glucose every 6 hr during therapy, more frequently in ketoacidosis and times of stress. A1C may also be monitored every 3–6 mo to determine effectiveness.
- ***Toxicity and Overdose:*** Overdose is manifested by symptoms of hypoglycemia. Mild hypoglycemia may be treated by ingestion of oral glucose. Severe hypoglycemia is a life-threatening emergency; treatment consists of IV glucose, glucagon, or epinephrine.

Potential Nursing Diagnoses

Noncompliance (Patient/Family Teaching)

Implementation

- ***High Alert:*** Insulin-related medication errors have resulted in patient harm and death. Clarify ambiguous orders; do not accept orders using the abbreviation "u" for units, (can be misread as a zero or the numeral 4; has resulted in tenfold overdoses). Insulins are available in different types and strengths. Check type, dose, and expiration date with another licensed nurse. Do not interchange insulins without consulting physician or other health care professional.
- Do not confuse regular **concentrated (U-500)** insulin with regular insulin.
- Use *only* insulin syringes to draw up dose. The unit markings on the insulin syringe must match the insulin's units/ml. Special syringes for doses <50 units are available. Prior to withdrawing dose, rotate vial between palms to ensure uniform solution; do not shake.
- When mixing insulins, draw regular insulin into syringe first to avoid contamination of regular insulin vial. Mixed insulins should never be used in a pump or for IV infusion.
- Store insulin in refrigerator. May also be kept at room temperature for up to 28 days. Do not use if cloudy, discolored, or unusually viscous.
- **Subcut:** Rotate injection sites.
- Administer into abdominal wall, thigh, or upper arm subcutaneously.
- Administer *regular insulin* within 15–30 min before a meal.

IV Administration

- **IV:** Regular insulin is the *only* insulin that can be administered IV.
- ***High Alert:*** Regular (concentrated) insulin U-500 should not be given IV.
- **Direct IV:** May be administered IV undiluted directly into vein or through Y-site. ***Rate:*** Administer up to 50 units over 1 min.
- **Continuous Infusion:** ***Diluent:*** May be diluted in commonly used IV solutions as an infusion; however, insulin potency may be reduced by at least 20–80% by the plastic or glass container or tubing before reaching the venous system. ***Concentration:*** 0.2–1 unit/ml. ***Rate:*** Rate should be ordered by physician (usually 0.05–0.2 units/kg/hr), and infusion should be placed on an IV pump for accurate administration.
- Rate of administration should be decreased when serum glucose level reaches 250 mg/100 ml.
- **Y-Site Compatibility:** amiodarone, ampicillin, ampicillin-sulbactam, aztreonam, cefazolin, cefepime, ceftazidime, dobutamine, doxapram, esmolol, famotadine, gentamicin, heparin, imipenem-cilastatin, indomethacin, magnesium sulfate, meperidine, meropenem, midazolam, milrinone, morphine, nitroglycerin, nitroprusside, oxytocin, pantoprazole, pentobarbital, potassium chloride, propofol, ritodrine, sodium bicarbonate, tacrolimus, terbutaline, ticarcillin, ticarcillin/clavulanate, tobramycin, vancomycin, vitamin B complex with C.
- **Y-Site Incompatibility:** dopamine, drotrecogin, nafcillin, norepinephrine, ranitidine.
- **Additive Compatibility:** May be added to total parenteral nutrition (TPN) solutions.

Patient/Family Teaching

- Instruct patient on proper technique for administration. Include type of insulin, equipment (syringe, cartridge pens, alcohol swabs), storage, and place to discard sy-

ringes. Discuss the importance of not changing brands of insulin or syringes, selection and rotation of injection sites, and compliance with therapeutic regimen.
- Demonstrate technique for mixing insulins by drawing up regular insulin and rolling intermediate-acting insulin vial between palms to mix, rather than shaking (may cause inaccurate dose).
- Explain to patient that this medication controls hyperglycemia but does not cure diabetes. Therapy is long term.
- Instruct patient in proper testing of serum glucose and ketones. These tests should be closely monitored during periods of stress or illness and health care professional notified of significant changes.
- Emphasize the importance of compliance with nutritional guidelines and regular exercise as directed by health care professional.
- Advise patient to consult health care professional prior to using alcohol or other Rx, OTC, or herbal products concurrently with insulin.
- Advise patient to notify health care professional of medication regimen prior to treatment or surgery.
- Advise patient to notify health care professional if nausea, vomiting, or fever develops, if unable to eat regular diet, or if blood glucose levels are not controlled.
- Instruct patient on signs and symptoms of hypoglycemia and hyperglycemia and what to do if they occur.
- Advise patient to notify health care professional if pregnancy is planned or suspected or if breastfeeding or planning to breastfeed.
- Patients with diabetes mellitus should carry a source of sugar (candy, glucose gel) and identification describing their disease and treatment regimen at all times.
- Emphasize the importance of regular follow-up, especially during first few weeks of therapy.

Evaluation/Desired Outcomes
- Control of blood glucose levels in diabetic patients without the appearance of hypoglycemic or hyperglycemic episodes.

HIGH ALERT

INSULINS (intermediate-acting) (in-su-lin)

NPH insulin (isophane insulin suspension)

Humulin N, ✤Novolin ge NPH, Novolin N

Classification

Therapeutic: antidiabetics, hormones

Pharmacologic: pancreatics

Pregnancy Category B

See Appendix M for more information concerning insulins

Indications
Control of hyperglycemia in patients with type 1 or type 2 diabetes mellitus.

Action
Lower blood glucose by: stimulating glucose uptake in skeletal muscle and fat, inhibiting hepatic glucose production. Other actions: inhibition of lipolysis and proteolysis, enhanced protein synthesis. **Therapeutic Effects:** Control of hyperglycemia in diabetic patients.

Pharmacokinetics
Absorption: Well absorbed from subcutaneous administration sites; rate of absorption may vary by site or volume of injection and other factors.
Distribution: Widely distributed.
Metabolism and Excretion: Metabolized by liver, spleen, kidney, and muscle.
Half-life: 5–6 min (prolonged in patients with diabetes; biologic half-life is 1–1.5 hr).

TIME/ACTION PROFILE (hypoglycemic effect)

ROUTE	ONSET	PEAK	DURATION
NPH	1–2 hr	4–12 hr	18–24 hr

Contraindications/Precautions
Contraindicated in: Hypoglycemia; Allergy or hypersensitivity to a particular type of insulin, preservatives, or other additives.
Use Cautiously in: Stress and infection (may temporarily ↑ insulin requirements); Renal/hepatic impairment (may ↓ insulin requirements; OB: Pregnancy (may temporarily ↑ insulin requirements).

Adverse Reactions/Side Effects

Endo: HYPOGLYCEMIA. **Local:** lipodystrophy, pruritus, erythema, swelling. **Misc:** allergic reactions including ANAPHYLAXIS.

Interactions

Drug-Drug: Beta blockers, **clonidine**, and **reserpine** may mask some of the signs and symptoms of hypoglycemia. **Corticosteroids**, **thyroid supplements**, **estrogens**, **isoniazid**, **niacin**, **phenothiazines**, and **rifampin** may ↑ insulin requirements. **Alcohol**, **ACE inhibitors**, **MAO inhibitors**, **octreotide**, **oral hypoglycemic agents**, and **salicylates**, may ↓ insulin requirements.

Drug-Natural Products: Glucosamine may worsen blood glucose control. **Fenugreek**, **chromium**, and **coenzyme Q-10** may produce additive hypoglycemic effects.

Route/Dosage

Dose depends on blood glucose, response, and many other factors.

Subcut (Adults and Children): 0.5–1 unit/kg/day. *Adolescents during rapid growth*—0.8–1.2 units/kg/day.

Availability

Isophane insulin suspension (NPH insulin): 100 units/ml in 10-ml vials and 3-ml disposable delivery devices. **Cost:** $42.99/10-ml vial *Humulin N pen (3 ml)*—$124.90/5 pens; *Novolin N Penfill (3 ml)*—$107.13/5 pens. ***In combination with:*** regular insulin as 70/30 (NPH/Regular) mixture (Humulin 70/30, Novolin 70/30) and 50/50 mixture (Humulin 50/50).

NURSING IMPLICATIONS

Assessment

- Assess for symptoms of hypoglycemia (anxiety; restlessness; mood changes; tingling in hands, feet, lips, or tongue; chills; cold sweats; confusion; cool, pale skin; difficulty in concentration; drowsiness; excessive hunger; headache; irritability; nightmares or trouble sleeping; nausea; nervousness; tachycardia; tremor; weakness; unsteady gait) and hyperglycemia (confusion, drowsiness; flushed, dry skin; fruit-like breath odor; rapid, deep breathing, polyuria; loss of appetite; nausea; vomiting; unusual thirst) periodically during therapy.
- Monitor body weight periodically. Changes in weight may necessitate changes in insulin dose.
- ***Lab Test Considerations:*** May cause ↓ serum inorganic phosphate, magnesium, and potassium levels.
- Monitor blood glucose every 6 hr during therapy, more frequently in ketoacidosis and times of stress. A1C may also be monitored every 3–6 mo to determine effectiveness.
- ***Toxicity and Overdose:*** Overdose is manifested by symptoms of hypoglycemia. Mild hypoglycemia may be treated by ingestion of oral glucose. Severe hypoglycemia is a life-threatening emergency; treatment consists of IV glucose, glucagon, or epinephrine.

Potential Nursing Diagnoses

Noncompliance (Patient/Family Teaching)

Implementation

- ***High Alert:*** Insulin-related medication errors have resulted in patient harm and death. Clarify ambiguous orders; do not accept orders using the abbreviation "u" for units, (can be misread as a zero or the numeral 4; has resulted in tenfold overdoses).
- Insulins are available in different types and strengths. Check type, dose, and expiration date with another licensed nurse. Do not interchange insulins without consulting physician or other health care professional.
- Use *only* insulin syringes to draw up dose. The unit markings on the insulin syringe must match the insulin's units/ml.
- When mixing insulins, draw regular insulin, insulin aspart, insulin glulisine, or insulin lispro into syringe first to avoid contamination of regular insulin vial. Mix insulin glulisine *only* with NPH insulin. Mixed insulins should never be used in a pump or for IV infusion.
- Store insulin vials in refrigerator. May also be kept at room temperature for up to 28 days. Humulin N pens should be kept at room temperature and should be discarded after 14 days. Do not use if cloudy, discolored, or unusually viscous.
- Because of short duration of *insulin lispro, insulin glulisine,* and *insulin aspart*, supplementation with longer-acting insulin may be necessary to control blood glucose levels.
- When transferring from once-daily NPH human insulin to *insulin glargine*, the dose usually remains unchanged. When transferring from twice-daily NPH human insulin to insulin glargine, the initial dose of insulin glargine is usually reduced by 20%.
- NPH insulin should not be used in the management of ketoacidosis.

- **Subcut:** Rotate injection sites.
- Administer into abdominal wall, thigh, or upper arm subcutaneously.
- Administer *NPH insulin* within 30–60 min before a meal.

Patient/Family Teaching

- Instruct patient on proper technique for administration. Include type of insulin, equipment (syringe, cartridge pens, alcohol swabs), storage, and place to discard syringes. Discuss the importance of not changing brands of insulin or syringes, selection and rotation of injection sites, and compliance with therapeutic regimen.
- Demonstrate technique for mixing insulins by drawing up regular insulin, insulin aspart, or insulin lispro first and rolling intermediate-acting insulin vial between palms to mix, rather than shaking (may cause inaccurate dose).
- Explain to patient that this medication controls hyperglycemia but does not cure diabetes. Therapy is long term.
- Instruct patient in proper testing of serum glucose and ketones. These tests should be closely monitored during periods of stress or illness and health care professional notified of significant changes.
- Emphasize the importance of compliance with nutritional guidelines and regular exercise as directed by health care professional.
- Advise patient to consult health care professional prior to using alcohol or other Rx, OTC, or herbal products concurrently with insulin.
- Advise patient to notify health care professional of medication regimen prior to treatment or surgery.
- Advise patient to notify health care professional if nausea, vomiting, or fever develops, if unable to eat regular diet, or if blood glucose levels are not controlled.
- Instruct patient on signs and symptoms of hypoglycemia and hyperglycemia and what to do if they occur.
- Advise patient to notify health care professional if pregnancy is planned or suspected or if breastfeeding or planning to breastfeed.
- Patients with diabetes mellitus should carry a source of sugar (candy, glucose gel) and identification describing their disease and treatment regimen at all times.
- Emphasize the importance of regular follow-up, especially during first few weeks of therapy.

Evaluation/Desired Outcomes

- Control of blood glucose levels in diabetic patients without the appearance of hypoglycemic or hyperglycemic episodes.

HIGH ALERT

INSULINS (long-acting)

(in-su-lin)

insulin detemir
Levemir

insulin glargine
Lantus

Classification
Therapeutic: antidiabetics, hormones
Pharmacologic: pancreatics

Pregnancy Category C

See Appendix M for more information concerning insulins

Indications

Control of hyperglycemia in patients with type 1 or type 2 diabetes mellitus.

Action

Lower blood glucose by: stimulating glucose uptake in skeletal muscle and fat, inhibiting hepatic glucose production. Other actions: inhibition of lipolysis and proteolysis, enhanced protein synthesis. **Therapeutic Effects:** Control of hyperglycemia in diabetic patients.

Pharmacokinetics

Absorption: Physiochemical characteristics of long-acting insulins result in delayed and prolonged absorption.
Distribution: Widely distributed.
Metabolism and Excretion: Metabolized by liver, spleen, kidney, and muscle.
Half-life: 5–6 min (prolonged in patients with diabetes); biologic half-life is 1–1.5 hr; *insulin detemir* 5–7 hr (dose-dependent).

TIME/ACTION PROFILE (hypoglycemic effect)

ROUTE	ONSET	PEAK	DURATION
Insulin detemir	3–4 hr	3–14 hr†	24 hr
Insulin glargine	3–4 hr	none†	24 hr

†Small amounts of insulin glargine and insulin detemir are slowly released, resulting in a relatively constant effect over time.

Contraindications/Precautions

Contraindicated in: Hypoglycemia; Allergy or hypersensitivity to a particular type of insulin, preservatives, or other additives.
Use Cautiously in: Stress and infection (may temporarily ↑ insulin requirements); Renal/hepatic impairment (may ↓ insulin requirements); OB: Pregnancy (may temporarily ↑ insulin requirements); Pedi: Children <6 yr (safety not established).

Adverse Reactions/Side Effects

Endo: HYPOGLYCEMIA. **Local:** lipodystrophy, pruritis, erythema, swelling. **Misc:** allergic reactions including ANAPHYLAXIS.

Interactions

Drug-Drug: Beta blockers, **clonidine**, and **reserpine** may mask some of the signs and symptoms of hypoglycemia. **Corticosteroids**, **thyroid supplements**, **estrogens**, **isoniazid**, **niacin**, **phenothiazines**, and **rifampin** may ↑ insulin requirements. **Alcohol**, **ACE inhibitors**, **MAO inhibitors**, **octreotide**, **oral hypoglycemic agents**, and **salicylates** may ↓ insulin requirements.
Drug-Natural Products: Glucosamine may worsen blood glucose control. **Fenugreek**, **chromium**, and **coenzyme Q-10** may produce additive hypoglycemic effects.

Route/Dosage

Insulin Detemir

Subcut (Adults and Children ≥6 yr): *Type 2 diabetes patients who are insulin-naive*—0.1–0.2 units/kg once daily in the morning *or* 10 units once or twice daily. *Patients with type 1 or 2 diabetes receiving basal insulin or basal bolus therapy*—May substitute on an equivalent unit-per-unit basis.

Insulin Glargine

Subcut (Adults and Children ≥6 yr): *Type 1 diabetes*—Administer 50–75% of daily insulin requirements once daily. *Initiation in patients with type 2 diabetes already being treated with oral antidiabetic agents*—10 units once daily; then adjust on the basis of the patient's needs (range 2–100 units/day). *Patients already receiving insulin*—When switching from once daily NPH, same dose of insulin glargine can be administered once daily. When switching from twice daily NPH, use 80% of the total daily NPH dose and administer once daily. Dose can then be adjusted on the basis of the patient's needs.

Availability

Insulin detemir: 100 units/ml in 10 ml vials and 3 ml cartidges or prefilled syringes. **Cost:** $84.15/10-ml vial. **Insulin glargine:** 100 units/ml in 10-ml vials and 3-ml cartridges or prefilled disposable pens. **Cost:** $84.99/10-ml vial.

NURSING IMPLICATIONS

Assessment

- Assess patient for signs and symptoms of hypoglycemia (anxiety; restlessness; mood changes; tingling in hands, feet, lips, or tongue; chills; cold sweats; confusion; cool, pale skin; difficulty in concentration; drowsiness; nightmares or trouble sleeping; excessive hunger; headache; irritability; nausea; nervousness; tachycardia; tremor; weakness; unsteady gait) and hyperglycemia (confusion, drowsiness; flushed, dry skin; fruit-like breath odor; rapid, deep breathing, polyuria; loss of appetite; nausea; vomiting; tiredness; unusual thirst) periodically during therapy.
- Monitor body weight periodically. Changes in weight may necessitate changes in insulin dose.
- ***Lab Test Considerations:*** Monitor blood glucose every 6 hr during therapy, more frequently in ketoacidosis and times of stress. A1C may also be monitored every 3–6 mo to determine effectiveness.
- ***Toxicity and Overdose:*** Overdose is manifested by symptoms of hypoglycemia. Mild hypoglycemia may be treated by ingestion of oral glucose. Severe hypoglycemia is a life-threatening emergency; treatment consists of IV glucose, glucagon, or epinephrine. Recovery from hypoglycemia may be delayed due to the prolonged effect of long-acting insulins.

Potential Nursing Diagnoses

Noncompliance (Patient/Family Teaching)

Implementation

- ***High Alert:*** Insulin-related medication errors have resulted in patient harm and death. Clarify ambiguous orders; do not accept orders using the abbreviation "u" for units, (can be misread as a zero or the numeral 4; has resulted in tenfold overdoses).
- Insulins are available in different types and strengths. Check type, dose, and expiration date with another licensed nurse. Do not interchange insulins without consulting physician or other health care professional.
- Use *only* insulin syringes to draw up dose. The unit markings on the insulin syringe must match the insulin's units/ml. Special syringes for doses <50 units are available. Prior to withdrawing dose, rotate vial between palms to ensure uniform solution; do not shake.
- ***High Alert:*** Do not mix *insulin glargine* or *insulin detemir* with any other insulin or solution, or use syringes containing any other medicinal product or residue. If giving with a short-acting insulin, use separate syringes and different injection sites. Solution should be clear and colorless with no particulate matter.
- Do not use if cloudy, discolored, or unusually viscous. Store unopened vials and cartridges of *insulin glargine* and *insulin detemir* in the refrigerator; do not freeze. If unable to refrigerate, the 10-ml vial of *insulin glargine* can be kept in a cool place unrefrigerated for up to 28 days. Once the cartridge is placed in an OptiPen One, do not refrigerate. After initial use, *insulin detemir* vials, cartridges, or a prefilled syringe may be stored in a cool place for 42 days. Do not store in-use cartridges and prefilled syringes in refrigerator or with needle in place. Keep away from direct heat and sunlight.
- When transferring from once-daily NPH human insulin to *insulin glargine*, the dose usually remains unchanged. When transferring from twice-daily NPH human insulin to insulin glargine, the initial dose of insulin glargine is usually reduced by 20%.
- NPH insulins should not be used in the management of ketoacidosis.
- **Subcut:** Rotate injection sites.
- Administer *insulin glargine* once daily at the same time each day.
- Administer *daily insulin detemir* with evening meal or at bedtime. With *twice daily insulin detemir*, administer evening dose with evening meal, at bedtime, or 12 hrs after morning dose.
- Do not administer *insulin detemir* or *insulin glargine* IV or in insulin pumps.

Patient/Family Teaching

- Instruct patient on proper technique for administration. Include type of insulin, equipment (syringe, cartridge pens, alcohol swabs), storage, and place to discard syringes. Discuss the importance of not changing brands of insulin or syringes, selection and rotation of injection sites, and compliance with therapeutic regimen. Patients taking insulin detemir should be given the *Patient Information* circular for this product.
- Explain to patient that this medication controls hyperglycemia but does not cure diabetes. Therapy is long term.
- Instruct patient in proper testing of serum glucose and ketones. These tests should be closely monitored during periods of stress or illness and health care professional notified of significant changes.
- Emphasize the importance of compliance with nutritional guidelines and regular exercise as directed by health care professional.
- Advise patient to consult health care professional prior to using alcohol or other Rx, OTC, or herbal products concurrently with insulin.
- Advise patient to notify health care professional of medication regimen prior to treatment or surgery.
- Advise patient to notify health care professional if nausea, vomiting, or fever develops, if unable to eat regular diet, or if blood glucose levels are not controlled.
- Instruct patient on signs and symptoms of hypoglycemia and hyperglycemia and what to do if they occur.
- Advise patient to notify health care professional if pregnancy is planned or suspected or if breastfeeding or planning to breastfeed.
- Patients with diabetes mellitus should carry a source of sugar (candy, glucose gel) and identification describing their disease and treatment regimen at all times.

- Emphasize the importance of regular follow-up, especially during first few weeks of therapy.

Evaluation/Desired Outcomes

- Control of blood glucose levels in diabetic patients without the appearance of hypoglycemic or hyperglycemic episodes.

INTERFERONS, ALPHA
(in-ter-**feer**-onz)

peginterferon alpha-2a
Pegasys

interferon alpha-2b (recombinant)
Intron A

peginterferon alpha-2b (pegylated)
Pegintron

interferon alpha-n3 (human)
Alferon N

Classification
Therapeutic:
Pharmacologic: interferons

Pregnancy Category C

Indications

Peginterferon alpha–2a: Treatment of: Chronic hepatitis C (alone or with ribavirin), Chronic hepatitis B. **Interferon alpha-2b:** Treatment of: Hairy cell leukemia, Malignant melanoma, AIDS-related Kaposi's sarcoma, Condylomata acuminata (intralesional), Chronic hepatitis B, Chronic hepatitis C (with oral ribavirin) which has relapsed following previous treatment with interferon alone, Follicular non-Hodgkin's lymphoma. **Peginterferon alpha–2b:** Chronic hepatitis C (alone or with ribavirin). **Interferon alpha-n3:** Treatment of condylomata acuminata (intralesional).

Action

Interferons are proteins capable of modifying the immune response and have antiproliferative action against tumor cells. Interferon alpha-2b is produced by recombinant DNA techniques, peginterferon is a 'pegylated' formulation of interferon alpha-2b formulated to have a longer duration of action; interferon alpha-n3 is from pooled human leukocytes. Interferons also have antiviral activity. **Therapeutic Effects:** Antineoplastic, antiviral, and antiproliferative activity. Decreased progression of hepatic damage (for patients with hepatitis).

Pharmacokinetics

Absorption: Not absorbed orally. Well absorbed (>80%) following IM and subcut administration. Minimal systemic absorption follows intralesional administration.
Distribution: Unknown.
Metabolism and Excretion: Filtered by the kidneys and subsequently degraded in the renal tubule; *peginterferon alpha-2b*—30% renally excreted.
Half-life: *Peginterferon alpha-2a*—50–160 hr; *interferon alpha-2b*—2–3 hr; *peginterferon alpha-2b*–40 hr.

TIME/ACTION PROFILE (clinical effects)

ROUTE	ONSET	PEAK	DURATION
Interferon alpha-2b IM, subcut	1–3 mo	unknown	unknown (CR)
Interferon alpha-2b IM, subcut	unknown	3–5 days	3–5 days (BC)
Interferon alpha-2b IM, subcut	2 wk	unknown	unknown (LFT)
Interferon alpha-2b and n3	unknown	4–8 wk	unknown (IL)
peginterferon alpha-2b subcut	unknown	6 mos or more	unknown

BC = effects on platelet counts; CR = clinical response; IL= regression of lesions; LFT = effects on liver function in patients with hepatitis

Contraindications/Precautions

Contraindicated in: Hypersensitivity to alpha interferons or human serum albumin; Autoimmune hepatitis; Hepatic decompensation (Child-Pugh class B and C) before or during therapy; Pedi: Products containing benzyl alcohol should not be used in neonates.
Use Cautiously in: Severe cardiovascular, pulmonary, renal, or hepatic disease; Active infections; Underyling CNS pathology or psychiatric history; Decreased bone marrow reserve or underlying immunosuppression; Current history of chickenpox, herpes zoster, or herpes labialis (may reactivate or disseminate disease); Previous or concurrent radiation therapy; Autoimmune disorders (may ↑ risk of exacerbation); Geri: Increases risk of adverse reactions; OB, Pedi: Childbearing potential, pregnancy, lactation and children <3 yr (safety not established).

Exercise Extreme Caution in: History of depression/suicide attempt.

Adverse Reactions/Side Effects

All are more prominent with subcut, IV, or IM administration.

CNS: NEUROPSYCHIATRIC DISORDERS, confusion, depression, dizziness, fatigue, headache, insomnia, irritability, anxiety. **EENT:** blurred vision, nose bleeds, rhinitis. **CV:** ISCHEMIC DISORDERS, arrhythmias, chest pain, edema. **GI:** COLITIS, PANCREATITIS, anorexia, abdominal pain, diarrhea, dry mouth, nausea, taste disorder, vomiting, weight loss, drug-induced hepatitis, flatulence. **Derm:** alopecia, dry skin, pruritus, rash, sweating. **Endo:** thyroid disorders. **Hemat:** LEUKOPENIA, THROMBOCYTOPENIA, anemia, hemolytic anemia (with ribavirin). **MS:** arthralgia, myalgia, leg cramps. **Neuro:** paresthesia. **Resp:** cough, dyspnea. **Local:** injection site reactions. **Misc:** AUTOIMMUNE DISORDERS, INFECTIOUS DISORDERS, allergic reactions including ANAPHYLAXIS, chills, fever, flu-like syndrome.

Interactions

Drug-Drug: Additive myelosuppression with other **antineoplastic agents** or **radiation therapy**. ↑ CNS depression may occur with **CNS depressants**, including **alcohol**, **antihistamines**, **sedative/hypnotics**, and **opioids**. May ↓ metabolism and ↑ blood levels and toxicity of **theophylline** and **methadone**. ↑ risk of adverse reactions with **zidovudine**. **Ribavirin** ↑ risk of hemolytic anemia, especially if CCr <50 mL/min (avoid if possible). May ↓ effects of **immunosuppressant agents**.

Route/Dosage

Peginterferon Alpha-2a

Subcut (Adults): *Chronic hepatitis C*—180 mcg once weekly for 48 wk for Genotypes 1,4 (24 wk for Genotypes 2,3). *Patients with chronic hepatitis C co-infected with HIV*—180 mcg once weekly for 48 wk.

Interferon Alpha-2b

IV (Adults): *Malignant melanoma (induction)*—20 million units/m² for 5 days of each week for 4 wk initially, followed by subcut maintenance dosing.

IM, Subcut (Adults): *Hairy cell leukemia*—2 million units/m² IM or subcut 3 times weekly for up to 6 mo. *Malignant melanoma (maintenance)*—10 million units/m² subcut 3 times weekly for 48 wk, following initial IV dosing. *AIDS-related Kaposi's sarcoma*—30 million units/m² IM or subcut 3 times weekly until disease progression or maximum response has been achieved after 16 wk. *Chronic hepatitis C*—3 million units Im or subcut 3 times weekly. If normalization of ALT occurs after 16 wk of therapy, continue treatment for total of 18–24 mo. If normalization of ALT does not occur after 16 wk of therapy, may consider discontinuing treatment. *Chronic hepatitis B*—5 million units/day IM or subcut *or* 10 million units IM or subcut 3 times weekly for 16 wk. *Follicular non-Hodgkin's lymphoma*—5 million units subcut 3 times weekly for up to 18 mo (to be used following completion of anthracycline-containing chemotherapy).

Subcut (Children >3 yr): *Chronic hepatitis B*—3 million units/m² 3 times weekly for the first week of therapy then increase to 6 million units/m² 3 times weekly (not to exceed 10 million units/dose) for 16 to 24 weeks.

IL (Adults): *Condylomata acuminata*—1 million units/lesion 3 times weekly for 3 wk; treat only 5 lesions per course. An additional course of treatment may be initiated at 12–16 wk.

Peginterferon Alpha-2b

Monotherapy

Subcut (Adults): *137–160 kg*—150 mcg once weekly for 1 yr. *107–136 kg*—120 mcg once weekly for 1 yr. *89–106 kg*—96 mcg once weekly for 1 yr. *73–88 kg*—80 mcg once weekly for 1 year. *57–72 kg*—64 mcg once weekly for 1 yr. *46–56 kg*—50 mcg once weekly for 1 yr. *37–45 kg*—40 mcg once weekly for 1 yr.

In Combination with Ribavirin (Rebetol)

Subcut (Adults): *>85 kg* –150 mcg once weekly. *76–85 kg*—120 mcg once weekly. *61–75 kg*—96 mcg once weekly. *51–60 kg*—80 mcg once weekly. *40–50 kg*—64 mcg once weekly. *<40 kg*—50 mcg once weekly.

Interferon Alpha-n3

IL (Adults): 250,000 units/lesion twice weekly for up to 8 wk; for large lesions, divide dose and inject at several sites.

Availability

Peginterferon Alpha-2a

Solution for injection: 180 mcg/ml in single use vials. **Prefilled syringes:** 180 mcg/0.5 ml.

Interferon Alpha-2b

Powder for injection: 10-million-unit single-use vial, 18-million-unit single-use vial, 50-million-unit single-use vial. **Solution for injection:** 10-million-unit single-use vial, 18-million-unit single-use vial, 18-million-unit multidose pen, 25-million-unit multidose vial, 30-million-unit multidose pen, 60-million-unit multidose pen. ***In combination with:*** oral ribavarin (Rebetrol) as a combination package (Rebetron). See Appendix B. (in various dosage packages).

Peginterferon alpha-2b

Powder for injection (Redipen system or vials): 50 mcg/0.5 ml, 80 mcg/0.5 ml, 120 mcg/0.5 ml, 150 mcg/0.5 ml.

Interferon Alpha-n3

Solution for injection: 5 million units/ml.

NURSING IMPLICATIONS

Assessment

- Assess for signs of neuropsychiatric disorders (irritability, anxiety, depression, suicidal ideation, aggressive behavior). May require discontinuation of therapy.
- Monitor for signs of infection (vital signs, WBC) during therapy. Discontinue drug therapy in cases of severe infection, and antibiotic therapy instituted
- Assess for cardiovascular disorders (pulse, blood pressure, chest pain). An ECG should be performed before and periodically during the course of therapy in patients with a history of cardiovascular disease
- Assess for signs of colitis (abdominal pain, bloody diarrhea, fever) and pancreatitis (nausea, vomiting, abdominal pain) during therapy. Discontinue therapy if these occur; may be fatal. Colitis usually resolves within 1–3 wks of discontinuation
- Assess for development of flu-like syndrome (fever, chills, myalgia, headache). Symptoms often appear suddenly 3–6 hr after therapy. Symptoms tend to decrease, even with continued therapy. Acetaminophen may be used for control of these symptoms
- Monitor for bone marrow depression. Assess for bleeding (bleeding gums; bruising; petechiae; guaiac stools, urine, and emesis) and avoid IM injections and rectal temperatures if platelet count is low. Apply pressure to venipuncture sites for 10 min. Assess for signs of infection during neutropenia. Anemia may occur. Monitor for increased fatigue, dyspnea, and orthostatic hypotension
- May cause nausea and vomiting. Antiemetics may be used prophylactically. Monitor intake and output, daily weight, and appetite. Adjust diet as tolerated for anorexia. Encourage fluid intake of at least 2 liters/day
- Assess pulmonary status (lung sounds, respirations) periodically during therapy
- Perform a baseline eye exam in all patients prior to initiation of therapy. Eye exams should be performed periodically during therapy in patients with pre-existing diabetic or hypertensive retinopathy. Discontinue therapy if patients develop new or worsening eye disorders
- Assess for signs of thyroid dysfunction, as hypothyroidism or hyperthyroidism may occur. Discontinue therapy if the patient's thyroid function cannot be controlled with medications (e.g. thyroid hormone supplementation, antithyroid medications).
- **Kaposi's Sarcoma:** Monitor number, size, and character of lesions prior to and throughout therapy.
- ***Lab Test Considerations:*** **Systemic:** Monitor for CBC and differential prior to and periodically during therapy. May cause leukopenia, neutropenia, thrombocytopenia, decreased hemoglobin and hematocrit, and hemolytic anemia. The nadirs of leukopenia and thrombocytopenia occur in 3–5 days, with recovery 3–5 days after withdrawal of *interferon alpha-2b*. For malignant melanoma, if granulocyte count $>250/mm^3$ but $<500/mm^3$, discontinue *interferon alpha-2b* until platelet or granulocyte counts return to normal or baseline levels, then reinstitute at 50% of dose. If granulocyte count $<250/mm^3$ with *interferon alpha-2b*, discontinue permanently. For follicular non-Hodgkin's lymphoma, if granulocyte count $<1000/mm^3$ or platelet count $<50,000/mm^3$, discontinue *interferon alpha-2b*. *Peginterferon alpha-2b* should be discontinued if granulocyte count $<1000/mm^3$ or platelet count $<50,000/mm^3$. *Peginterferon alpha-2a* should be discontinued if ANC$<500/mm^3$ or platelet count $<25,000/mm^3$ and then may be restarted at a lower dose if the ANC$>1000/mm^3$.
- Platelet count should be $\geq 90,000$ cells/mm^3 and ANC ≥ 1500 cells/mm^3 prior to initiation of peginterferon therapy. Commonly causes ↓ hemoglobin, hematocrit, WBC, ANC, lym-

phocytes and platelet counts within first 2 wks of therapy.
- Monitor liver function tests (AST, ALT, LDH, bilirubin, alkaline phosphatase), triglycerides, and renal function tests (BUN, creatinine, uric acid, urinalysis) prior to and periodically during therapy. CCr should be >50 ml/min prior to initiation of peginterferon therapy.
- Monitor TSH at baseline and if patients develop symptoms consistent with hypothyroidism or hyperthyroidism.
- **Hairy Cell Leukemia:** Monitor number of peripheral blood hairy cells and bone marrow hairy cells prior to and during therapy.

Potential Nursing Diagnoses

Risk for injury (Side Effects)
Risk for infection (Side Effects)

Implementation

- Solution should be prepared in a biologic cabinet. Wear gloves, gown, and mask while handling medication. Discard equipment in specially designated containers (see Appendix K).

Interferon Alpha-2b

- **IM, Subcut:** Subcut route is preferred for patients with a platelet count <50,000/mm^3.
- Reconstitute 10-, 18-, and 50-million-unit vials with 1 ml of diluent provided by manufacturer (sterile water for injection). Agitate gently. Solution may be colorless to light yellow. Solution should be used immediately; stable for up to 24 hr if refrigerated.
- The solution for injection vials do not require reconstitution prior to use and may be used for IM, subcut, or intralesional administration.
- The solution for injection in multidose pens are for subcut use only. Only the needles provided in the package should be used with the pen. A new needle should be used with each dose. Follow instructions in *Medication Guide* for use of multidose pens.
- **IL:** Reconstitute 10-million-unit vial with 1 ml of diluent provided by manufacturer (sterile water for injection). Use a TB syringe with 25–30-gauge needle to administer. Each 0.1-ml dose is injected into the center of the base of the wart using the intradermal injection approach. As many as 5 lesions can be treated at one time.

IV Administration

- **Intermittent Infusion:** (For malignant melanoma). ***Diluent:*** Add 1 ml of diluent provided by manufacturer (sterile water for injection) to vial. Further dilute appropriate dose in 100 ml of 0.9% NaCl. Solution should be used immediately; stable for 24 hr if refrigerated. The solution for injection vials are not recommended for IV administration. ***Concentration:*** Final concentration of infusion should not be less than 10 million units/100 ml. ***Rate:*** Infuse over 20 min.

Peginterferon Alpha–2a

- Vials and pre-filled syringes should be stored in refrigerator. Do not administer solution that is cloudy or contains a precipitate.
- Follow instructions in *Medication Guide* for use of pre-filled syringes.

Peginterferon Alpha–2b

- Reconstitute vial with 0.7 mL of diluent provided by manufacturer (sterile Water for injection). Administer immediately; stable for 24 hr if refrigerated. Solution should be clear and colorless. Discard unused solution.
- *For PEG Intron Redipen* To reconstitute the drug, hold the Redipen upright (dose button down) and press 2 halves of pen together until a click is heard. Gently invert the pen to mix the solution (do not shake). Solution should be clear and colorless. Follow instructions in *Medication Guide* for *RediPen* use. Dispose of *RediPen* and other materials in puncture-resistant container.

Interferon Alpha-N3

- Vials should be refrigerated.

Patient/Family Teaching

- Advise patient to take medication as directed. If a dose is missed, omit dose and return to the regular schedule. The patient should notify the health care professional if more than 1 dose is missed.
- **Home Care Issues:** Instruct patient and family on preparation and correct technique for administration of injection and care and disposal of equipment. Advise patient to read *Medication Guide* prior to administration and with each prescription refill to check for changes. Explain to patient that brands should not be switched without consulting health care professional; may result in a change of dose.

- Discuss possibility of flu-like reaction 3–6 hr after dose. Acetaminophen may be taken prior to injection and every 3–4 hr afterward as needed to control symptoms.
- Review side effects with patient. Interferon may be temporarily discontinued or dose decreased by 50% if serious side effects occur.
- Instruct patient to notify health care professional promptly if fever; chills; cough; hoarseness; sore throat; signs of infection; lower back or side pain; painful or difficult urination; bleeding gums; bruising; petechiae; blood in stools, urine, or emesis; increased fatigue; dyspnea; or orthostatic hypotension occurs. Caution patient to avoid crowds and persons with known infections. Instruct patient to use soft toothbrush and electric razor and to avoid falls. Caution patient not to drink alcoholic beverages or take medication containing aspirin or NSAIDs; may precipitate gastric bleeding.
- Inform patient of the potential for depression and advise patient to notify health care professional if depression occurs.
- Discuss with patient the possibility of hair loss. Explore coping strategies.
- Explain to patient that fertility may be impaired and that contraception is needed during treatment to prevent potential harm to the fetus.
- Instruct patient not to receive any vaccinations without advice of health care professional.
- Emphasize need for periodic lab tests to monitor for side effects.
- Inform patient that peginterferon alpha-2a may not reduce the risk of transmission of HCV to others or prevent cirrhosis, liver failure, or liver cancer.

Evaluation/Desired Outcomes

- Normalized blood parameters (hemoglobin, neutrophils, platelets, monocytes, and bone marrow and peripheral hairy cells) in hairy cell leukemia. Response may not be seen for 6 mo with *interferon alpha-2b*.
- Decrease in the size and number of lesions in Kaposi's sarcoma. Therapy may be required for 6 months before full response is seen. Therapy is continued until disease progresses or a maximum response has been achieved after 4 mo of therapy.
- Improved hematologic parameters in patients with chronic myelogenous leukemia.
- Increase in time to relapse and overall survival in patients with malignant melanoma.
- Disappearance of or decrease in size and number of genital warts. Condylomata acuminata usually respond in 4–8 wk. A second course of therapy may be required if genital warts persist and laboratory values remain in acceptable limits.
- Decrease in symptoms and improvement in liver function tests and ↓ progression of hepatic damage in patients with hepatitis B or hepatitis C infection.

INTERFERONS, BETA
(in-ter-**feer**-on)

interferon beta-1a
Avonex, Rebif

interferon beta-1b
Betaseron

Classification
Therapeutic: anti–multiple sclerosis agents
Pharmacologic: interferons

Pregnancy Category C

Indications
Relapsing forms of multiple sclerosis.

Action
Antiviral and immunoregulatory properties produced by interacting with specific receptor sites on cell surfaces may explain beneficial effects. Produced by recombinant DNA technology. **Therapeutic Effects:** Reduce incidence of relapse (neurologic dysfunction) and slow physical disability.

Pharmacokinetics
Absorption: *Interferon beta-1b*—50% absorbed following subcut administration.
Distribution: Unknown.
Metabolism and Excretion: Unknown.
Half-life: *Interferon beta-1a*—69 hr (subcut), 10 hr (IM); *interferon beta-1b*—8 min–4.3 hr.

TIME/ACTION PROFILE (serum concentrations)

ROUTE	ONSET	PEAK	DURATION
Interferon beta-1a IM, subcut	unknown	3–15 h	unknow
Interferon beta-1b subcut	rapid	16 h	unknown

Contraindications/Precautions
Contraindicated in: Hypersensitivity to natural or recombinant interferon beta or human albumin.

Use Cautiously in: History of suicide attempt or depression; History of seizures (interferon beta-1a); Cardiovascular disease; Liver disease (interferon beta-1a); History of alcohol abuse (interferon beta-1a); Patients with childbearing potential; Pregnancy, lactation, or children <18 yr (safety not established).

Adverse Reactions/Side Effects

CNS: SEIZURES (↑ WITH INTERFERON BETA-1A), depression, dizziness, fatigue, headache, insomnia, drowsiness, incoordination, rigors, suicidal ideation. **EENT:** sinusitis, vision abnormalities. **Resp:** dyspnea, upper respiratory tract infection. **CV:** chest pain, edema, hypertension. **GI:** constipation, nausea, vomiting, abdominal pain, autoimmune hepatitis, dry mouth, elevated liver function tests. **GU:** cystitis, erectile dysfunction, polyuria, urinary incontinence. **Derm:** rashes, alopecia. **Endo:** menstrual disorders, hyperthyroidism, hypothyroidism, menorrhagia, spontaneous abortion. **Hemat:** neutropenia, anemia, eosinophilia, thrombocytopenia. **Local:** injection-site reactions, injection site necrosis. **MS:** myalgia, arthralgia, muscle spasm. **Misc:** allergic reactions including ANAPHYLAXIS, chills, fever, flu-like symptoms, pain.

Interactions

(All interactions below are for Interferon beta-1b)

Drug-Drug: ↑ myelosuppression may occur with other myelosuppressives including **antineoplastics**. Concurrent use of **hepatotoxic agents** may ↑ the risk of hepatotoxicity (↑ liver enzymes).

Drug-Natural Products: Avoid concommitant use with immmunomodulating natural products such as **astragalus**, **echinacea**, and **melatonin**.

Route/Dosage

Interferon Beta-1a

IM (Adults): *Avonex*—30 mcg once weekly.

Subcut (Adults): *Rebif (target dose of 22 mcg 3 times/wk)*—Start with 4.4 mcg 3 times/wk for 2 wk, then ↑ to 11 mcg 3 times/wk for 2 wk, then ↑ to maintenance dose of 22 mcg 3 times/wk. *Rebif (target dose of 44 mcg 3 times/wk)*—Start with 8.8 mcg 3 times/wk for 2 wk, then ↑ to 22 mcg 3 times/wk for 2 wk, then ↑ to maintenance dose of 44 mcg 3 times/wk.

Interferon Beta-1b

Subcut (Adults): *Betaseron*—Initiate with 0.0625 mg (2 million units) every other day and then ↑ dose by 0.0625 mg q 2 wk over a 6-wk period up to target dose of 0.25 mg (8 million units) every other day.

Availability

Interferon Beta-1a (Avonex)

Powder for injection: 30 mcg/vial. **Prefilled syringes (Avonex):** 30 mcg/0.5 ml. **Prefilled syringes (Rebif):** 22 mcg/0.5 ml, 44 mcg/0.5 ml, titration pack of 6 syringes prefilled with 8.8 mcg/0.2 ml and 6 syringes prefilled with 22 mcg/0.5 ml.

Interferon Beta-1b

Powder for injection (Betaseron): 0.3 mg (9.6 million units)/vial.

NURSING IMPLICATIONS

Assessment

- Assess frequency of exacerbations of symptoms of multiple sclerosis periodically during therapy.
- Monitor patient for signs of depression during therapy. If depression occurs, notify physician or other health care professional immediately.
- ***Lab Test Considerations:*** Monitor hemoglobin, WBC, platelets, and blood chemistries including liver function tests prior to and 1, 3, and 6 mo after initiation of therapy and periodically thereafter. Therapy may be temporarily discontinued if the absolute neutrophil count is <750/mm^3, if AST or ALT exceeds 10 times the upper limit of normal, or if serum bilirubin exceeds 5 times the upper limit of normal. Once the absolute neutrophil count is >750/mm^3 or the hepatic enzymes have returned to normal, therapy can be restarted at 50% of the original dose.
- Thyroid function tests should be monitored every 6 mo, especially in patients with a history of thyroid abnormalities.

Potential Nursing Diagnoses

Deficient knowledge, related to medication regimen (Patient/Family Teaching)

Implementation

- Do not confuse products. Interferon beta-1a and interferon beta-1b are not interchangeable.

- **Interferon Beta-1a:** *Avonex:* Reconstitute with 1.1 ml of diluent and swirl gently to dissolve. Do not shake the vial. Inject into the thigh or upper arm. Keep reconstituted solution in refrigerator; inject within 6 hr of reconstitution.
- *Rebif:* Administer subcut via prefilled, single-use syringe at the same time (afternoon or evening) on the same days (Monday, Wednesday, Friday) at least 48 hr apart each wk. Rotate sites with each injection to minimize risk of injection site reactions. Discard unused portions. Store in refrigerator.
- **Interferon Beta-1b:** To reconstitute, inject 1.2 ml of diluent supplied into interferon beta-1b vial for a concentration of 0.25 mg/ml. Swirl gently to dissolve completely; do not shake. Do not use solutions that are discolored or contain particulate matter. Keep reconstituted solution refrigerated; inject within 3 hr of reconstitution.
- Following reconstitution, withdraw 1 ml into a syringe with a 27-gauge needle and inject subcut into arm, abdomen, hip, or thigh. Rotate sites with each injection to minimize risk of injection site reactions. Discard unused portion; vials are for single dose only.

Patient/Family Teaching

- **Home Care Issues:** Instruct patient in correct technique for injection and care and disposal of equipment. Caution patient not to reuse needles or syringes and provide patient with a puncture-resistant container for disposal.
- Instruct patient to take medication as directed; do not change dose or schedule without consulting health care professional. Patients should receive a medication guide with each product.
- Inform patient that flu-like symptoms (fever, chills, myalgia, sweating, malaise) may occur during therapy. Acetaminophen may be used for relief of fever and myalgias.
- Advise patient to notify health care professional if pregnancy is planned or suspected. May cause spontaneous abortion.

Evaluation/Desired Outcomes

- Decrease in the frequency of relapse (neurologic dysfunction) in patients with relapsing-remitting multiple sclerosis.

IODINE, IODIDE

potassium iodide†
Pima, SSKI, ThyroSafe, ThyroShield

strong iodine solution
Lugol's solution

Classification
Therapeutic: antithyroid agents
Pharmacologic: iodine containing agents

Pregnancy Category D

†For more information on potassium iodide as a radiation protectant see *Potassium Iodide as a Thyroid Blocking Agent in Radiation Emergencies* at www.fda.gov

Indications

Adjunct with other antithyroid drugs in preparation for thyroidectomy. Treatment of thyrotoxic crisis. Radiation protectant following radiation emergencies or administration of radioactive iodine.

Action

Rapidly inhibits the release and synthesis of thyroid hormones. Decreases the vascularity of the thyroid gland. Decreases thyroidal uptake of radioactive iodine following radiation emergencies or administration of radioactive isotopes of iodine. Iodine is a necessary component of thyroid hormone. **Therapeutic Effects:** Control of hyperthyroidism. Decreased bleeding during thyroid surgery. Decreased incidence of thyroid cancer following radiation emergencies.

Pharmacokinetics

Absorption: Converted in the GI tract and enters the circulation as iodine; also absorbed through skin and lungs; may also be obtained via recycling of iodothyronines.
Distribution: Concentrates in the thyroid gland and muscle; also found in skin, skeleton, breasts, and hair. Readily crosses the placenta; enters breast milk.
Metabolism and Excretion: Taken up by the thyroid gland, then eliminated via kidneys, liver, skin, lungs, and intestines.
Half-life: Unknown.

TIME/ACTION PROFILE (effects on thyroid)

ROUTE	ONSET	PEAK	DURATION
PO	24 hr	10–15 days	variable†

†Radiation protection lasts 24 hr

Contraindications/Precautions

Contraindicated in: Hypersensitivity; Hyperkalemia; Pulmonary edema; Impaired renal function.

Use Cautiously in: Tuberculosis; Bronchitis; Cardiovascular disease; OB, Pedi: Pregnancy or lactation (although iodine is required during pregnancy, excess amounts may cause thyroid abnormalities/goiter in the newborn; excess use during lactation may cause skin rash or thyroid suppression in the infant).

Adverse Reactions/Side Effects

CNS: confusion, weakness. **GI:** GI BLEEDING, diarrhea, nausea, vomiting. **Derm:** acneiform eruptions. **Endo:** hypothyroidism, goiter, hyperthyroidism. **F and E:** hyperkalemia. **Neuro:** tingling. **MS:** joint pain. **Misc:** hypersensitivity, iodism.

Interactions

Drug-Drug: Use with **lithium** may cause ↑ hypothyroidism. ↑ antithyroid effect of **methimazole** and **propylthiouracil**. ↑ hyperkalemia may result from combined use with **potassium-sparing diuretics, ACE inhibitors, angiotensin II receptor antagonists** or **potassium supplements**.

Route/Dosage

Preparation for Thyroidectomy

PO (Adults and Children): *Strong iodine solution*—3–5 drops (0.1–0.3 ml) 3 times daily for 10 days prior to surgery. *Potassium iodide saturated solution* (SSKI)— 1–5 drops (50–250 mg) 3 times daily for 10 days prior to surgery.

Hyperthyroidism

PO (Adults and Children): *Strong iodine solution*—1 ml in water 3 times daily. *Potassium iodide saturated solution (SSKI)*—6–10 drops (300–500 mg) 3 times daily.

PO (Infants <1 yr): 3–5 drops (150–250 mg) 3 times daily.

Radiation Protectant to Radioactive Isotopes of Iodine

PO (Adults): *Pima*—195 mg once daily for 10 days (start 24 hr prior to exposure (continue until risk of exposure has passed or other measures have been implemented).

PO (Children >1 yr): 130 mg once daily for 10 days (start 24 hr prior to exposure).

PO (Infants <1 yr): 65 mg once daily for 10 days (start 24 hr prior to exposure).

Reduction of Thyroid Cancer after Nuclear Accident

PO (Adults and Children >68 kg, including pregnant/lactating women): *Iosat, ThyroSafe, ThyroShield*—130 mg once daily (continue until risk of exposure has passed or other measures have been implemented).

PO (Children 3–18 yr): 65 mg once daily.

PO (Children 1 mo-3 yr): 32.5 mg once daily.

PO (Infants <1 mo): 16.25 mg once daily.

Availability

Potassium Iodide

Oral solution: 65 mg/ml (ThyroShield), 1 g potassium iodide/ml (SSKI). **Syrup (Pima) (black-raspberry flavor):** 325 mg potassium iodide/5 ml. **Tablets:** 65 mg^{OTC}, 130 mg^{OTC} (available only through state and federal agencies).

Strong Iodine Solution

Oral solution: Iodine 50 mg/ml plus potassium iodide 100 mg/ml.

NURSING IMPLICATIONS

Assessment

- Assess for signs and symptoms of iodism (metallic taste, stomatitis, skin lesions, cold symptoms, severe GI upset). Report these symptoms promptly to physician.
- Monitor response symptoms of hyperthyroidism (tachycardia, palpitations, nervousness, insomnia, diaphoresis, heat intolerance, tremors, weight loss).
- Monitor for hypersensitivity reaction (rash, pruritus, laryngeal edema, wheezing). Discontinue drug and notify physician immediately if these problems occur.
- ***Lab Test Considerations:*** Monitor thyroid function before and periodically during therapy. May alter results of radionuclide thyroid imaging and may ↓ thyroidal uptake of ^{131}I, ^{123}I, and sodium pertechnetate ^{99m}Tc in thyroid uptake tests.
- Monitor serum potassium levels periodically during therapy.
- ***Lab Test Considerations:*** Monitor thyroid stimulating hormone (TSH) and free T_4 in neonates (within the first month of life) treated with potassium iodide for development of hypothyroidism. Thyroid hormone therapy should be instituted if hypothyroidism develops.

Potential Nursing Diagnoses

Deficient knowledge, related to medication regimen (Patient/Family Teaching)

Implementation

- Do not confuse iodine with Lodine (etodolac).
- For protection against inhaled radioiodines, administer potassium iodide prior to or immediately coincident with passage of the radioactive cloud, though a substantial protective effect lasts 3-4 hr after exposure.
- **PO:** Mix solutions in a full glass of fruit juice, water, broth, formula, or milk. Administer after meals to minimize GI irritation.
- Solution is normally clear and colorless. Darkening upon standing does not affect potency of drug. Solutions that are brownish yellow should be discarded.
- Crystals may form, especially if refrigerated, but redissolve upon warming and shaking.

Patient/Family Teaching

- Instruct patient to take medication as directed. Take missed doses as soon as possible but not just before next dose; do not double doses.
- Instruct patient to report suspected pregnancy to health care professional before therapy is initiated.
- Advise patient to consult health care professional about avoiding foods high in iodine (seafood, iodized salt, cabbage, kale, turnips) or potassium (see Appendix L).
- Advise patient to consult health care professional before using OTC or herbal cold remedies. Some cold remedies use iodide as an expectorant.
- **Hyperthyroidism:** Instruct patient to take medication as ordered. Missing a dose may precipitate hyperthyroidism.

Evaluation/Desired Outcomes

- Resolution of the symptoms of thyroid crisis.
- Decrease in size and vascularity of the gland before thyroid surgery. Use of iodides in the treatment of hyperthyroidism is usually limited to 2 wk.
- Protection of the thyroid gland from the effects of radioactive iodine.

ipratropium

(i-pra-**troe**-pee-um)
Atrovent HFA

Classification
Therapeutic: allergy, cold, and cough remedies, bronchodilators
Pharmacologic: anticholinergics

Pregnancy Category B

Indications

Inhaln: Maintenance therapy of reversible airway obstruction due to COPD, including chronic bronchitis and emphysema. **Intranasal:** Rhinorrhea associated with allergic and nonallergic perennial rhinitis (0.03% solution) or the common cold (0.06% solution). **Unlabeled uses: Inhaln:** Adjunctive management of bronchospasm caused by asthma.

Action

Inhaln: Inhibits cholinergic receptors in bronchial smooth muscle, resulting in decreased concentrations of cyclic guanosine monophosphate (cGMP). Decreased levels of cGMP produce local bronchodilation. **Intranasal:** Local application inhibits secretions from glands lining the nasal mucosa. **Therapeutic Effects: Inhaln:** Bronchodilation without systemic anticholinergic effects. **Intranasal:** Decreased rhinorrhea.

Pharmacokinetics

Absorption: Minimal systemic absorption (2% for inhalation solution; 20% for inhalation aerosol; <20% following nasal use).
Distribution: 15% of dose reaches lower airways after inhalation.
Metabolism and Excretion: Small amounts absorbed are metabolized by the liver.
Half-life: 2 hr.

TIME/ACTION PROFILE (bronchodilation)

ROUTE	ONSET	PEAK	DURATION
Inhalation	1–3 min	1–2 hr	4–6 hr
Intranasal	15 min	unknown	6–12 hr

Contraindications/Precautions

Contraindicated in: Hypersensitivity to ipratropium, atropine, belladonna alkaloids, or bromide. Avoid use during acute bronchospasm; **Note: Atrovent HFA has replaced the discontinued Atrovent CFC (chlorofluorocarbon). Soy and CFC-allergic patients can now safely use the Atrovent HFA formulation. However, Combivent (ipratropium/albuterol combination) MDI does contain soya lecithin and is contraindicated in pa-**

tients with a history of hypersensitivity to soy and peanut.
Use Cautiously in: Patients with bladder neck obstruction, prostatic hyperplasia, glaucoma, or urinary retention; Geri: May be more sensitive to effects.

Adverse Reactions/Side Effects

CNS: dizziness, headache, nervousness. **EENT:** blurred vision, sore throat; *nasal only*— epistaxis, nasal dryness/irritation. **Resp:** bronchospasm, cough. **CV:** hypotension, palpitations. **GI:** GI irritation, nausea. **Derm:** rash. **Misc:** allergic reactions.

Interactions

Drug-Drug: ↑ anticholinergic properties with other **drugs having anticholinergic properties (antihistamines, phenothiazines, disopyramide)**.

Route/Dosage

Inhaln (Adults and Children >12 yr): *Metered-dose inhaler (nonacute)*—2 inhalations 4 times daily (not to exceed 12 inhalations/24 hr or more frequently than q 4 hr). *Acute exacerbations*—4–8 puffs using a spacer device as needed. *Via nebulization (nonacute)*—2504 times daily given q 6 hr. *Acute exacerbations* —500 mcg q 30 min for 3 doses then q 2–4 hr as needed.
Inhaln (Children 5–12 yr): *Metered dose inhaler (nonacute)*—1–2 inhalations q 6 hr as needed (not to exceed 12 inhalations/24 hr). *Acute exacerbations*—4–8 puffs as needed *Via nebulization (nonacute)*—250–500 mcg 4 times daily given q 6 hr. *Acute exacerbations*—250 mcg q 20 min for 3 doses then q 2–4 hr as needed.
Inhaln (Infants): *Nebulization*—125–250 mcg 3 times a day.
Inhaln (Neonates): *Nebulization*—25 mcg/kg/dose 3 times a day.
Intranasal (Adults and Children >6 yr): *0.03 % solution*—2 sprays in each nostril 2–3 times daily (21 mcg/spray).
Inhaln (Adults and Children >5 yr): *0.06% solution* –2 sprays in each nostril 3–4 times daily (42 mcg/spray).

Availability (generic available)

Aerosol inhaler (HFA) (chlorofluorocarbon-free): 17 mcg/spray in 12.9-g canister (200 inhalations). **Inhalation solution:** ✤0.0125%, 0.02% in single-dose vials containing 500 mcg, ✤0.025%. **Nasal spray:** 0.03% solution—21 mcg/spray in 30-ml bottle (345 sprays/bottle), 0.06% solution—42 mcg/spray in 15-ml bottle (165 sprays). ***In combination with:*** albuterol (Combivent, Duoneb). See Appendix B.

NURSING IMPLICATIONS

Assessment

- Assess for allergy to atropine and belladonna alkaloids; patients with these allergies may also be sensitive to ipratropium. Atrovent HFA MDI does not contain CFC or soy and may be used safely in soy or CFC-allergic patients. However, Combivent MDI should be avoided in soy- or peanut-allergic patients.
- **Inhaln:** Assess respiratory status (rate, breath sounds, degree of dyspnea, pulse) before administration and at peak of medication. Consult physician or other health care professional about alternative medication if severe bronchospasm is present; onset of action is too slow for patients in acute distress. If paradoxical bronchospasm (wheezing) occurs, withhold medication and notify physician or other health care professional immediately.
- **Nasal Spray:** Assess patient for rhinorrhea.

Potential Nursing Diagnoses

Ineffective airway clearance (Indications)
Activity intolerance (Indications)

Implementation

- Do not confuse Atrovent with Alupent (metaproterenol).
- **Inhaln:** See Appendix D for administration of inhalation medications.
- When ipratropium is administered concurrently with other inhalation medications, administer adrenergic bronchodilators first, followed by ipratropium, then corticosteroids. Wait 5 min between medications.
- Solution for *nebulization* can be diluted with preservative-free 0.9% NaCl. Diluted solution should be used within 24 hr at room temperature or 48 hr if refrigerated. Solution can be mixed with preservative-free albuterol, cromolyn, or metaproterenol if used within 1 hr of mixing.

Patient/Family Teaching

- Instruct patient in proper use of inhaler, nebulizer, or nasal spray and to take medication as directed. Take missed doses as soon as remembered unless almost time for the next dose; space remaining doses evenly during day. Do not double doses.

- Advise patient that rinsing mouth after using inhaler, good oral hygiene, and sugarless gum or candy may minimize dry mouth. Health care professional should be notified if stomatitis occurs or if dry mouth persists for more than 2 wk.
- **Inhalation:** Caution patient not to exceed 12 doses within 24 hr. Patient should notify health care professional if symptoms do not improve within 30 min after administration of medication or if condition worsens.
- Explain need for pulmonary function tests prior to and periodically during therapy to determine effectiveness of medication.
- Caution patient to avoid spraying medication in eyes; may cause blurring of vision or irritation.
- Advise patient to inform health care professional if cough, nervousness, headache, dizziness, nausea, or GI distress occurs.
- **Nasal Spray:** Instruct patient in proper use of nasal spray. Clear nasal passages gently before administration. Do not inhale during administration, so medication remains in nasal passages. Prime pump initially with 7 actuations. If used regularly, no further priming is needed. If not used in 24 hr, prime with 2 actuations. If not used for >7 days, prime with 7 actuations.
- Advise patient to contact health care professional if symptoms do not improve within 1–2 wk or if condition worsens.

Evaluation/Desired Outcomes
- Decreased dyspnea.
- Improved breath sounds.
- Decrease in rhinorrhea from perennial rhinitis or the common cold.

irbesartan, See ANGIOTENSIN II RECEPTOR ANTAGONISTS.

irinotecan (eye-ri-noe-**tee**-kan)
Camptosar

Classification
Therapeutic: antineoplastics
Pharmacologic: enzyme inhibitors

Pregnancy Category D

Indications
Metastatic colorectal cancer (with 5-fluorouracil and leucovorin).

Action
Interferes with DNA synthesis by inhibiting the enzyme topoisomerase. **Therapeutic Effects:** Death of rapidly replicating cells, particularly malignant ones.

Pharmacokinetics
Absorption: IV administration results in complete bioavailability.
Distribution: Unknown.
Protein Binding: *Irinotecan*—30–68%; *SN-38 (active metabolite)*—95%.
Metabolism and Excretion: Converted by the liver to SN–38, its active metabolite, which is also metabolized by the liver. Small amounts excreted by kidneys.
Half-life: 6 hr.

TIME/ACTION PROFILE (hematologic effects)

ROUTE	ONSET	PEAK	DURATION
IV	unknown	21–29 days	27–34 days

Contraindications/Precautions
Contraindicated in: Hypersensitivity; OB: Pregnancy or lactation.
Use Cautiously in: Previous pelvic or abdominal irradiation or age ≥65 yr (increased risk of myelosuppression); Presence of infection, underlying bone marrow depression, or concurrent chronic illness; History of prior pelvic/abdominal irradiation and serum bilirubin >1–2 mg/dl (initial dosage reduction recommended); Geri: ↑ sensitivity to adverse effects (myelosuppression); initiate at lower dose; Previous severe myelosuppression or diarrhea (reinstitute at lower dose following resolution); Patients with genetically reduced UGT1A1 activity (↑ risk of neutropenia); OB: Patients with childbearing potential; Pedi: Children (safety not established).

Adverse Reactions/Side Effects
CNS: dizziness, headache, insomnia, weakness. **EENT:** rhinitis. **Resp:** coughing, dyspnea. **CV:** edema, vasodilation. **GI:** DIARRHEA, ELEVATED LIVER ENZYMES, abdominal pain/cramping, anorexia, constipation, dyspepsia, flatulence, nausea, stomatitis, vomiting, abdominal enlargement, colonic ulceration. **Derm:** alopecia, rash, sweating. **F and E:** dehydration. **Hemat:** anemia, leukopenia, neutropenia, thrombocytopenia.

Local: injection site reactions. **Metab:** weight loss. **MS:** back pain. **Misc:** chills, fever.

Interactions

Drug-Drug: Combination with **fluorouracil** may result in serious toxicity (dehydration, neutropenia, sepsis). ↑ bone marrow depression may occur with other **antineoplastics** or **radiation therapy**. **Laxatives** should be avoided (diarrhea may be ↑). **Diuretics** ↑ risk of dehydration (may discontinue during therapy). **Dexamethasone** used as an antiemetic ↑ risk of hyperglycemia and lymphocytopenia. **Prochlorperazine** given on the same day as irinotecan ↑ risk of akathisia.
Drug-Natural Products: St. John's wort ↑ increases levels and risk of toxicity.

Route/Dosage

Other regimens are used; careful modification required for all levels of toxicity/tolerance.

Single Agent

IV (Adults): *Weekly dosage schedule*—125 mg/m² once weekly for 4 wk, followed by a 2-wk rest period. Cycle may be repeated using doses which depend on patient tolerance and degree of toxicity encountered. *Once-every-3-wk schedule*—350 mg/m² once every 3 wk.
IV (Geriatric Patients >70 yr): Initiate at 300 mg/m² every 3 wk.

Hepatic Impairment

IV (Adults): *Bilirubin 1–2 mg/dl and history of prior pelvic/abdominal irradiation—Weekly dosage schedule*—Initiate therapy at lower dose (100 mg/m²); once weekly for 4 wk, followed by a 2-wk rest period. Cycle may be repeated with dose adjusted as tolerated. *Once-every-3-wk schedule*—300 mg/m² once every 3 wk, dose adjusted as tolerated as low as 200 mg/m² and further adjusted in 50-mg increments.

As Part of Combination Therapy with Leucovorin and 5-Fluorouracil

IV (Adults): *Regimen 1 (Bolus regimen)*—125 mg/m² once weekly for 4 wk, followed by a 2-wk rest period. Cycle may be repeated using doses that depend on patient tolerance and degree of toxicity encountered; *Regimen 2 (Infusional regimen)*—180 mg/m² every 2 wk for 3 doses, followed by a 3-wk rest period. Cycle may be repeated using doses that depend on patient tolerance and degree of toxicity encountered.

Availability

Solution for injection: 20 mg/ml in 2-ml[Rx] and 5-ml vials.

NURSING IMPLICATIONS

Assessment

- Monitor vital signs frequently during administration.
- Monitor for bone marrow depression. Assess for bleeding (bleeding gums, bruising, petechiae, guaiac stools, urine, and emesis) and avoid IM injections and taking rectal temperatures if platelet count is low. Apply pressure to venipuncture sites for 10 min. Assess for signs of infection during neutropenia. Anemia may occur. Monitor for increased fatigue, dyspnea, and orthostatic hypotension.
- Monitor closely for the development of diarrhea. Two types may occur. The early type occurs within 24 hr of administration and may be preceded by cramps and sweating. Atropine 0.25–1 mg IV may be given to decrease symptoms. Potentially life-threatening diarrhea may occur more than 24 hr after a dose and may be accompanied by severe dehydration and electrolyte imbalance. Loperamide 4 mg initially, followed by 2 mg every 2 hr until diarrhea ceases for at least 12 hr (or 4 mg every 4 hr if given during sleeping hours) should be administered promptly to treat late-occurring diarrhea. Do not administer loperamide at these doses for >48 hr. Careful fluid and electrolyte replacement should be instituted to prevent complications. Subsequent doses should be delayed in patients with active diarrhea until diarrhea is resolved for 24 hr. If diarrhea is grade 2, 3, or 4, decrease subsequent doses of irinotecan.
- Nausea and vomiting are common. Pretreatment with dexamethasone 10 mg along with agents such as ondansetron or granisetron should be started on the same day as irinotecan at least 30 min before administration. Prochlorperazine may be used on subsequent days but may increase risk of akathisia if given on the same day as irinotecan.
- Assess IV site frequently for inflammation. Avoid extravasation. If extravasation occurs, infusion must be stopped and restarted in another vein to avoid damage to subcut tissue. Flushing site with sterile water and applica-

tion of ice over the extravasated site are recommended.

- ***Lab Test Considerations:*** Monitor CBC with differential and platelet count prior to each dose. Temporarily discontinue irinotecan if absolute neutrophil count is <500 cells/mm³ or if neutropenic fever occurs. Administration of a colony-stimulating factor may be considered if clinically significant decreases in WBC (<2000/mm³), neutrophil count (<1000/mm³), hemoglobin (<9 g/dl), or platelet count (<100,000 cells/mm³) occur.
- May cause ↑ serum alkaline phosphatase and AST concentrations.

Potential Nursing Diagnoses

Risk for infection (Adverse Reactions)

Implementation

- Solution should be prepared in a biologic cabinet. Wear gloves, gown, and mask while handling IV medication. Discard IV equipment in specially designated containers.

IV Administration

- **Intermittent Infusion: *Diluent:*** Dilute before infusion with D5W or 0.9% NaCl. ***Concentration:*** 0.12–2.8 mg/ml. Usual diluent is 500 ml of D5W. Solution is pale yellow. Do not administer solutions that are cloudy or contain particulate matter. Solution is stable for 24 hr at room temperature or 48 hr if refrigerated. To prevent microbial contamination, solutions should be used within 24 hr of dilution if refrigerated or 6 hr at room temperature. Do not refrigerate solutions diluted with 0.9% NaCl. ***Rate:*** Administer dose over 90 min.
- **Y-Site Compatibility:** oxaliplatin, palonosetron.
- **Y-Site Incompatibility:** gemcitabine, pemetrexed.
- **Additive Incompatibility:** Information unavailable. Do not admix with other solutions or medications.

Patient/Family Teaching

- Instruct patient to report occurrence of diarrhea to health care professional immediately, especially if it occurs more than 24 hr after dose. Diarrhea may be accompanied by severe dehydration and electrolyte imbalance. It may be life-threatening and should be treated promptly.
- Instruct patient to notify health care professional promptly if fever; chills; sore throat; signs of infection; bleeding gums; bruising; petechiae; blood in urine, stool, or emesis occurs. Caution patient to avoid crowds and persons with known infections. Instruct patient to use soft toothbrush and electric razor. Caution patient not to drink alcoholic beverages or take products containing aspirin or other NSAIDs.
- Instruct patient to notify nurse of pain at injection site immediately.
- Instruct patient to notify health care professional if vomiting, fainting, or dizziness occurs.
- Discuss with patient possibility of hair loss. Explore methods of coping.
- Advise patient that this medication may have teratogenic effects. Contraception should be used during therapy.
- Instruct patient not to receive any vaccinations without consulting health care professional.
- Emphasize the need for periodic lab tests to monitor for side effects.

Evaluation/Desired Outcomes

- Decrease in size and spread of malignancy.

IRON SUPPLEMENTS

carbonyl iron (100%)
(**kar**-bo-nil **eye**-ern)
Feosol, Icar

ferrous fumarate (33% elemental iron) (**fer**-us **fyoo**-ma-rate)
Femiron, Feostat, Fumasorb, Fumerin, Hemocyte, Neo-Fer, ✤Nephro-Fer, ✤Novofumar, ✤Palafer, Span-FF

ferrous gluconate (12% elemental iron) (**fer**-us **gloo**-koe-nate)
✤Apo-Ferrous Gluconate, Fergon, Ferralet, ✤Fertinic, ✤Novoferrogluc, Simron

ferrous sulfate (30% elemental iron) (**fer**-us **sul**-fate)
✤Apo-Ferrous Sulfate, ED-IN-SOL, Fe50, Feosol, Feratab, Fergen-sol, Fer-In-Sol, Fer-Iron, ✤Fero-Grad, ✤Novoferrosulfa, ✤PMS Ferrous Sulfate, Slow FE

iron dextran (**eye**-ern **dex**-tran)
DexFerrum, InFeD

iron polysaccharide
(**eye**-ern poll-ee-**sak**-a-ride)
Hytinic, Niferex, Nu-Iron

iron sucrose (**eye**-ern**su**-krose)
Venofer

sodium ferric gluconate complex
(**so**-dee-yum**ferr**-ic**gloo**-ko-nate)
Ferrlecit

Classification
Therapeutic: antianemics
Pharmacologic: iron supplements

Pregnancy Category A (ferrous gluconate, ferrous sulfate, iron polysaccharide), B (sodium ferric gluconate, iron sucrose), C (iron dextran)

Indications

PO: Prevention/treatment of iron-deficiency anemia. **IM, IV:** *Iron dextran*—Treatment of iron-deficiency anemia in patients who cannot tolerate or receive oral iron. *Sodium ferric gluconate complex*—Treatment of iron deficiency in patients undergoing chronic hemodialysis or peritoneal dialysis who are concurrently receiving erythropoietin. Treatment of iron-deficiency anemia in patients with chronic kidney disease including patients who are not on dialysis (with or without erythropoietin) and patients dependent on dialysis (with erythropoietin).

Action

An essential mineral found in hemoglobin, myoglobin, and many enzymes. Enters the bloodstream and is transported to the organs of the reticuloendothelial system (liver, spleen, bone marrow), where it is separated out and becomes part of iron stores. **Therapeutic Effects:** Prevention/treatment of iron deficiency.

Pharmacokinetics

Absorption: 5–10% of dietary iron is absorbed (up to 30% in deficiency states). Therapeutically administered PO iron may be 60% absorbed via an active and passive transport process. Well absorbed following IM administration.
Distribution: Remains in the body for many months. Crosses the placenta; enters breast milk.
Protein Binding: ≥90%.
Metabolism and Excretion: Mostly recycled; small daily losses occurring via desquamation, sweat, urine, and bile.
Half-life: *Iron dextran, iron sucrose*—6 hr.

TIME/ACTION PROFILE (effects on erythropoiesis)

ROUTE	ONSET	PEAK	DURATION
PO	4 days	7–10 days	2–4 mo
IM, IV	4 days	1–2 wk	wks–mos

Contraindications/Precautions

Contraindicated in: Hemochromatosis, hemosiderosis, or other evidence of iron overload; Anemias not due to iron deficiency; Some products contain alcohol, tartrazine, or sulfites and should be avoided in patients with known intolerance or hypersensitivity.
Use Cautiously in: PO: Peptic ulcer; Ulcerative colitis or regional enteritis (condition may be aggravated); Alcoholism; Severe hepatic impairment; Severe renal impairment (oral products); Pre-existing cardiovascular disease (iron dextran) (may be exacerbated by adverse reactions to this drug); Significant allergies or asthma (iron dextran); Rheumatoid arthritis (iron dextran) (may have exacerbation of joint swelling); OB: Pregnancy or lactation (safety of some parenteral products not established); Pedi: Safety not established for infants <4 mo (iron dextran) or children <6 yr (sodium ferric gluconate complex); safety may not be established for other products in the pediatric population.

Adverse Reactions/Side Effects

CNS: *IM, IV*— SEIZURES, dizziness, headache, syncope. **CV:** *IM, IV*— hypotension, hypertension, tachycardia. **GI:** nausea; *PO*— constipation, dark stools, diarrhea, epigastric pain, GI bleeding; *IM, IV*— taste disorder, vomiting. **Derm:** *IM, IV*— flushing, urticaria. **Resp:** *IV*— cough, dyspnea. **Local:** pain at IM site (iron dextran), phlebitis at IV site, skin staining at IM site (iron dextran). **MS:** *IM, IV*— arthralgia, myalgia. **Misc:** *PO*— staining of teeth (liquid preparations); *IM, IV*— allergic reactions including ANAPHYLAXIS, fever, lymphadenopathy, sweating.

Interactions

Drug-Drug: Oral iron supplements ↓ absorption of **tetracyclines**, **bisphosphonates**, **fluoroquinolones**, **levothyroxine**, **mycophenolate mofetil**, and **penicillamine** (si-

multaneous administration should be avoided). ↓ absorption of and may ↓ effects of **levodopa** and **methyldopa**. Concurrent administration of **H_2 antagonists**, **proton pump inhibitors**, and **cholestyramine** may ↓ absorption of iron. Doses of **ascorbic acid** ≥200 mg may ↑ absorption of iron up to ≥30%. **Chloramphenicol** and **vitamin E** may ↓ hematologic response to iron therapy.
Drug-Food: Iron absorption is ↓ 33–50% by concurrent administration of food.

Route/Dosage

Oral Iron Dosage for Iron Deficiency (expressed as mg elemental iron, note individual salt forms, multiple ones exist—see approximate equivalent doses below for dose conversions).

Approximate Equivalent Doses (mg of iron salt): *Ferrous fumarate*—197; *Ferrous gluconate*—560; *Ferrous sulfate*—324; *Ferrous sulfate, exsiccated*—217.
PO (Adults): *Deficiency*—120–240 mg/day (2–3 mg/kg/day) in 2–4 divided doses. *Prophylaxis* —60–100 mg/day.
PO (Infants and Children): *Severe deficiency*—4–6 mg/kg/day in 3 divided doses. *Mild to moderate deficiency*—3 mg/kg/day in 1–2 divided doses. *Prophylaxis*—1–2 mg/kg/day in 1–2 divided dose (maximum: 15 mg/day).
PO (Neonates, Premature): 2–4 mg/kg/day in 1–2 divided doses, maximum: 15 mg/day.

Iron Dextran

IM, IV (Adults and Children): Test dose of 0.5 ml (25 mg) is given 1 hr prior to therapy.
IM, IV (Infants): Test dose of 0.25 ml (12.5 mg) is given 1 hr prior to therapy.
IM, IV (Adults and Children >15 kg): *Iron deficiency*—Total dose (ml) = 0.0442 × (desired Hgb – actual Hgb) × lean body weight (kg) + [0.26 × lean body weight (kg)]. Divided up and given in small daily doses until total is reached; not to exceed 100 mg/day. *Total dose IV infusion*—Total dose may be diluted and infused over 4–5 hr following a test dose of 10 drops (unlabeled).
IM, IV (Adults): *Blood loss*—Dose (ml) = (Blood loss [ml] × hematocrit) × 0.02.
IM, IV (Children 5–15 kg): *Iron deficiency*—Total dose (ml) = 0.042 (desired Hgb – actual Hgb) × weight (kg) + [0.26 × weight (kg)]. / Divided up and given in small daily doses until total is reached; not to exceed 25 mg/day in children <5 kg; 50 mg/day in children 5–10 kg; or 100 mg/day in children >10 kg.

Iron Polysaccharide Complex

PO (Adults): 50–100 mg twice daily of tablets/elixir or 150–300 mg/day of the capsules.
PO (Children >6yr): 50–100 mg/day (may be given in divided doses).
PO (Infants): 1–2 mg/kg/day.
PO (Adults—Pregnant Women): 30–60 mg/day.

Iron Sucrose

IV (Adults): *Hemodialysis dependent patients*—100 mg (5 ml) during each dialysis session for 10 doses (total of 1000 mg), additional smaller doses may be necessary; *Peritoneal dialysis dependent patients*— 300 mg (15 ml) infusion, followed by another 300 mg (15 ml) infusion 14 days later, followed by 400 mg (20 ml) infusion 14 days later; *Non-dialysis dependent patients*—200 mg (10 ml) on 5 different days within a 14 day period to a total of 1000 mg, may also be given as infusion of 500 mg on day 1 and day 14.

Sodium Ferric Gluconate Complex

IV (Adults): 10 ml (125 mg elemental iron) repeated during 8 sequential dialysis treatments to a total cumulative dose of 1 g.
IV (Children >6 yr): 0.12 ml/kg (not to exceed 125 mg/dose) repeated during 8 sequential dialysis treatments.

Availability

Carbonyl Iron (100% Iron)

Tablets: 50 mg[OTC]. **Oral suspension:** 15 mg/1.25 ml in 118-ml bottles[OTC].

Ferrous Fumarate (33% Elemental Iron)

Tablets: 63 mg[OTC], 195 mg[OTC], 200 mg[OTC], 324 mg[OTC], 325 mg[OTC]. **Chewable tablets:** 100 mg[OTC]. **Controlled-release capsules:** 325 mg[OTC]. **Suspension (butterscotch flavor):** 100 mg/5 ml[OTC], ✤300 mg/5 ml[OTC]. **Drops:** 45 mg/0.6 ml[OTC], ✤60 mg/1 ml[OTC].

Ferrous Gluconate (11.6% Elemental Iron)

Tablets: 300 mg[OTC], 320 mg[OTC], 325 mg[OTC]. **Sustained-release tablets:** 320 mg[OTC]. **Soft gelatin capsules:** 86 mg[OTC]. **Elixir:** 300 mg/5 ml[OTC]. **Syrup:** ✤300 mg/5 ml[OTC].

Ferrous Sulfate (20–30% Elemental Iron)

Tablets: 195 mg[OTC], 300 mg[OTC], 325 mg[OTC]. **Capsules:** 150 mg[OTC], 250 mg[OTC]. **Timed-release tablets:** 525 mg[OTC]. **Syrup:** 90 mg/5 ml[OTC]. **Elixir:** 220 mg/5 ml[OTC]. **Drops:** 75 mg/0.6 ml[OTC], 125 mg/1 ml[OTC].

Iron Dextran
Injection: 50 mg/ml.
Iron Polysaccharide (mg Iron)
Capsules: 150 mg[OTC]. **Elixir:** 100 mg/5 ml[OTC].
Tablets: 50 mg[OTC].
Iron Sucrose
Aqueous complex for injection: 20 mg/ml in 5-ml single-use vial (100 mg).
Sodium Ferric Gluconate Complex
Injection: 62.5 mg/5 ml in 5-ml ampules.

NURSING IMPLICATIONS

Assessment

- Assess nutritional status and dietary history to determine possible cause of anemia and need for patient teaching.
- Assess bowel function for constipation or diarrhea. Notify health care professional and use appropriate nursing measures should these occur.
- **Iron Dextran, Iron Sucrose, and Sodium Ferric Gluconate Complex:** Monitor blood pressure and heart rate frequently following IV administration until stable. Rapid infusion rate may cause hypotension and flushing.
- Assess patient for signs and symptoms of anaphylaxis (rash, pruritus, laryngeal edema, wheezing). Notify physician immediately if these occur. Keep epinephrine and resuscitation equipment close by in the event of an anaphylactic reaction.
- ***Lab Test Considerations:*** Monitor hemoglobin, hematocrit, and reticulocyte values prior to and every 3 wk during the first 2 mo of therapy and periodically thereafter. Serum ferritin and iron levels may also be monitored to assess effectiveness of therapy.
- Occult blood in stools may be obscured by black coloration of iron in stool. Guaiac test results may occasionally be false-positive.
- **Iron Dextran:** Monitor hemoglobin, hematocrit, reticulocyte values, transferrin, ferritin, total iron-binding capacity, and plasma iron concentrations periodically during therapy. Serum ferritin levels peak in 7–9 days and return to normal in 3 wk. Serum iron determinations may be inaccurate for 1–2 wk after therapy with large doses; therefore, hemoglobin and hematocrit are used to gauge initial response.
- May impart a brownish hue to blood drawn within 4 hr of administration. May cause false ↑ in serum bilirubin and false decrease in serum calcium values.
- Prolonged PTT may be calculated when blood sample is anticoagulated with citrate dextrose solution; use sodium citrate instead.
- **Iron Sucrose:** Monitor hemoglobin, hematocrit, serum ferritin, and transferritin saturation prior to and periodically during therapy. Transferrin saturation values increase rapidly after IV administration; therefore, serum iron values may be reliably obtained 48 hr after IV administration. Withhold iron therapy if evidence of iron overload occurs.
- May cause ↑ liver enzymes.
- ***Toxicity and Overdose:*** Early symptoms of overdose include stomach pain, fever, nausea, vomiting (may contain blood), and diarrhea. Late symptoms include bluish lips, fingernails, and palms; drowsiness; weakness; tachycardia; seizures; metabolic acidosis; hepatic injury; and cardiovascular collapse. Patient may appear to recover prior to the onset of late symptoms. Therefore, hospitalization continues for 24 hr after patient becomes asymptomatic to monitor for delayed onset of shock or GI bleeding. Late complications of overdose include intestinal obstruction, pyloric stenosis, and gastric scarring: If patient is comatose or seizing, gastric lavage with sodium bicarbonate is performed. Deferoxamine is the antidote. Additional supportive treatments to maintain fluid and electrolyte balance and correction of metabolic acidosis are also indicated, If signs of overdose occur during IV administration of iron sucrose, treatment includes IV fluids, corticosteroids, and/or antihistamines. Administering at a slower rate usually relieves symptoms.

Potential Nursing Diagnoses

Activity intolerance (Indications)

Implementation

- Discontinue oral iron preparations prior to parenteral administration.
- Sodium ferric gluconate and iron sucrose are for IV use only.
- **PO:** Oral preparations are most effectively absorbed if administered 1 hr before or 2 hr after meals. If gastric irritation occurs, administer with meals. Take tablets and capsules with a full glass of water or juice. Do not crush or chew enteric-coated tablets and do not open capsules.

- Liquid preparations may stain teeth. Dilute in water or fruit juice, full glass (240 ml) for adults and ½ glass (120 ml) for children, and administer with a straw or place drops at back of throat.
- Avoid using antacids, coffee, tea, dairy products, eggs, or whole-grain breads with or within 1 hr after administration of ferrous salts. Iron absorption is decreased by 33% if iron and calcium are given with meals. If calcium supplementation is needed, calcium carbonate does not decrease absorption of iron salts if supplements are administered between meals.
- **Iron Dextran:** The 2-ml ampule may be used for IM or IV administration.
- Prior to initial IM or IV dose, a test dose of 25 mg should be given by the same route as the dose will be given, to determine reaction. The IV test dose should be administered over 5 min. The IM dose should be administered in the same injection site and by same technique as the therapeutic dose. The remaining portion may be administered after 1 hr, if no adverse symptoms have occurred.
- **IM:** Inject deeply via Z-track technique into upper outer quadrant of buttock, never into arm or other exposed areas. Use a 2–3 in, 19- or 20-gauge needle. Change needles between withdrawal from container and injection to minimize staining of subcut tissues. Stains are usually permanent.

IV Administration

- **IV: Iron Dextran:** Following IV administration, patient should remain recumbent for at least 30 min to prevent orthostatic hypotension
- **Direct IV:** ***Diluent:*** May administer undiluted or dilute in 0.9% NaCl or D5W. ***Concentration:*** 50 mg/ml. ***Rate:*** Administer slowly at a rate of 50 mg (1 ml) over at least 1 min.
- **Intermittent Infusion:** May be diluted in 200–1000 ml of 0.9% NaCl or D5W; 0.9% NaCl is the preferred diluent; dilution in D5W increases incidence of pain and phlebitis. ***Rate:*** Administer over 1–6 hr following a test dose of 10 drops/min for 10 min. Flush line with 10 ml of 0.9% NaCl at completion of infusion.
- **Y-Site Incompatibility:** Discontinue other IV solutions during infusion.
- **Additive Incompatibility:** Manufacturers recommend that iron dextran not be mixed with other solutions; however, iron dextran has been added to total parenteral nutrition solutions. **Sodium Ferric Gluconate Complex:** ***Diluent:*** Dilute test dose in 50 ml of 0.9% NaCl and administer IV over 60 min
- To administer therapeutic dose of 10 ml (125 mg of elemental iron) dilute in 100 ml of 0.9% NaCl. Dialysis patients frequently require a cumulative dose of 1 g of elemental iron, administered over 8 sessions of sequential dialysis. ***Concentration:*** 12.5 mg/ml. ***Rate:*** Administer at a maximum rate of 12.5 mg/min. **Iron Sucrose:** Each 5-ml vial contains 100 mg of elemental iron.
- *Hemodialysis*—Most patients require a minimum cumulative dose of 1000 mg of elemental iron, administered over 10 sequential dialysis sessions, to achieve a favorable hemoglobin or hematocrit response.
- Solution is brown. Inspect for particulate matter or discoloration. Do not administer solutions that contain particulate matter or are discolored.
- **Direct IV:** May be administered undiluted by slow injection into dialysis line. ***Rate:*** Administer at a rate of 1 ml undiluted solution per minute, not to exceed one vial per injection. Discard any unused portion.
- **Intermittent Infusion:** May also be administered via infusion, into dialysis line for hemodialysis patients. May reduce risk of hypotensive episodes. ***Diluent:*** Each vial must be diluted in a maximum of 100 ml of 0.9% NaCl immediately prior to infusion. Unused diluted solution should be discarded. ***Concentration:*** 1–2 mg/ml. ***Rate:*** Infuse at a rate of 100 mg of iron over at least 15 min, large doses (500 mg) should be given over 3.5–4 hrs.
- **Intermittent Infusion:** *For peritoneal dialysis patients*—***Diluent:*** Dilute each dose in a maximum of 250 mL of 0.9% NaCl. ***Rate:*** Administer doses of 300 mg over 1.5 hrs and doses of 400 mg over 2.5 hrs.
- **Direct IV:** *For non-dialysis dependent patients*—May be administered as a slow injection of 200 mg undiluted. ***Rate:*** Administer over 2–5 min.
- **Intermittent Infusion:** Dilute 500 mg in 250 ml 0.9% NaCl. ***Rate:*** Infuse over 3.5–4 hr on days 1 and 14. May cause hypotension; monitor closely.
- **Additive Incompatibility:** Do not mix iron sucrose with other medications or add to parenteral nutrition solutions for IV infusion.

Patient/Family Teaching

- Explain purpose of iron therapy to patient.
- Encourage patient to comply with medication regimen. Take missed doses as soon as remembered within 12 hr; otherwise, return to regular dosing schedule. Do not double doses.
- Advise patient that stools may become dark green or black and that this change is harmless.
- Instruct patient to follow a diet high in iron (see Appendix L).
- Discuss with parents the risk of children's overdosing on iron. Medication should be stored in the original childproof container and kept out of reach of children. Do not refer to vitamins as candy. In the event of a suspected overdose, parents or guardians should contact the poison control center (1-800-222-1222) or emergency medical services (911) immediately.
- **Iron Dextran:** Delayed reaction may occur 1–2 days after administration and last 3–4 days if IV route used, 3–7 days with IM route. Instruct patient to contact physician if fever, chills, malaise, muscle and joint aches, nausea, vomiting, dizziness, and backache occur.
- **Iron sucrose and sodium ferric gluconate complex:** Instruct patient to immediately report symptoms of hypersensitivity reaction to health care professional.

Evaluation/Desired Outcomes

- Increase in hemoglobin, which may reach normal parameters after 1–2 mo of therapy. May require 3–6 mo for normalization of body iron stores.
- Improvement in iron deficiency anemia or anemia of chronic renal failure.

---

isocarboxazid, See MONOAMINE OXIDASE (MAO) INHIBITORS.

---

isoniazid (eye-soe-**nye**-a-zid)

INH, ♣Isotamine, Nydrazid, ♣PMS Isoniazid, Laniazid

Classification
Therapeutic: antituberculars

Pregnancy Category C

Indications

First-line therapy of active tuberculosis, in combination with other agents. Prevention of tuberculosis in patients exposed to active disease (alone).

Action

Inhibits mycobacterial cell wall synthesis and interferes with metabolism. **Therapeutic Effects:** Bacteriostatic or bactericidal action against susceptible mycobacteria.

Pharmacokinetics

Absorption: Well absorbed following PO/IM administration.
Distribution: Widely distributed; readily crosses the blood-brain barrier. Crosses the placenta; enters breast milk in concentrations equal to plasma.
Metabolism and Excretion: 50% metabolized by the liver at rates that vary widely among individuals; 50% excreted unchanged by the kidneys.
Half-life: 1–4 hr.

TIME/ACTION PROFILE (blood levels)

ROUTE	ONSET	PEAK	DURATION
PO	rapid	1–2 hr	up to 24 hr
IM	rapid	1–2 hr	up to 24 hr

Contraindications/Precautions

Contraindicated in: Hypersensitivity; Acute liver disease; Previous hepatitis from isoniazid.
Use Cautiously in: History of liver damage or chronic alcohol ingestion; Black and Hispanic women, women in the postpartum period, or patients >50 yr (increased risk of drug-induced hepatitis); Severe renal impairment (dosage reduction may be necessary); Malnourished patients, patients with diabetes, or chronic alcoholics (increased risk of neuropathy); Pregnancy and lactation (although safety is not established, isoniazid has been used with ethambutol to treat tuberculosis in pregnant women without harm to the fetus).

Adverse Reactions/Side Effects

CNS: psychosis, seizures. **EENT:** visual disturbances. **GI:** DRUG-INDUCED HEPATITIS, nausea, vomiting. **Derm:** rashes. **Endo:** gynecomastia. **Hemat:** blood dyscrasias. **Neuro:** peripheral neuropathy. **Misc:** fever.

♣ = Canadian drug name.

* CAPITALS indicates life-threatening; underlines indicate most frequent.

Interactions

Drug-Drug: Additive CNS toxicity with other **antituberculars**. **BCG vaccine** may not be effective during isoniazid therapy. Isoniazid inhibits the metabolism of **phenytoin**. **Aluminum-containing antacids** may decrease absorption. Psychotic reactions and coordination difficulties may result with **disulfiram**. Concurrent administration of **pyridoxine** may prevent neuropathy. Increased risk of hepatotoxicity with other **hepatotoxic agents** including **alcohol** and **rifampin**. Isoniazid may decrease blood levels and effectiveness of **ketoconazole**. Concurrent use with **carbamazepine** increases carbamazepine blood levels and risk of hepatotoxicity.
Drug-Food: Severe reactions may occur with ingestion of foods containing high concentrations of **tyramine** (see Appendix L).

Route/Dosage

PO, IM (Adults): 300 mg/day (5 mg/kg) *or* 15 mg/kg (up to 900 mg) 2–3 times weekly.
PO, IM (Children): 10–20 mg/kg/day (up to 300 mg/day) *or* 20–40 mg/kg (up to 900 mg) 2–3 times weekly.

Availability (generic available)

Tablets: 50 mg, 100 mg, 300 mg. **Syrup (orange, raspberry flavor):** 50 mg/5 ml. **Injection:** 100 mg/ml. ***In combination with:*** rifampin (Rifamate) or with rifampin and pyrazinamide (Rifater). See Appendix B.

NURSING IMPLICATIONS

Assessment

- Mycobacterial studies and susceptibility tests should be performed prior to and periodically throughout therapy to detect possible resistance.
- ***Lab Test Considerations:*** Hepatic function should be evaluated prior to and monthly throughout therapy. Increased AST, ALT, and serum bilirubin may indicate drug-induced hepatitis. Black and Hispanic women, postpartal women, and patients >50 yr are at highest risk. The risk is lower in children; therefore, liver function tests are usually ordered less frequently for children.
- ***Toxicity and Overdose:*** If isoniazid overdosage occurs, treatment with pyridoxine (vitamin B) is instituted.

Potential Nursing Diagnoses

Risk for infection (Indications)
Noncompliance (Patient/Family Teaching)

Implementation

- **PO:** May be administered with food or antacids if GI irritation occurs, although antacids containing aluminum should not be taken within 1 hr of administration.
- **IM:** Medication may cause discomfort at injection site. Massage site after administration and rotate injection sites.
- Solution may form crystals at low temperatures; crystals will redissolve upon warming to room temperature.

Patient/Family Teaching

- Advise patient to take medication exactly as directed. If a dose is missed, take as soon as possible unless almost time for next dose; do not double up on missed doses. Emphasize the importance of continuing therapy even after symptoms have subsided. Therapy may be continued for 6 mo–2 yr.
- Advise patient to notify health care professional promptly if signs and symptoms of hepatitis (yellow eyes and skin, nausea, vomiting, anorexia, dark urine, unusual tiredness, or weakness) or peripheral neuritis (numbness, tingling, paresthesia) occur. Pyridoxine may be used concurrently to prevent neuropathy. Any changes in visual acuity, eye pain, or blurred vision should also be reported immediately.
- Caution patient to avoid the use of alcohol during this therapy, as this may increase the risk of hepatotoxicity. Ingestion of Swiss or Cheshire cheeses, fish (tuna, skipjack, and sardinella), and possibly tyramine-containing foods (see Appendix L) should also be avoided, as they may result in redness or itching of the skin; hot feeling; rapid or pounding heartbeat; sweating; chills; cold, clammy feeling; headache; or light-headedness.
- Emphasize the importance of regular follow-up physical and ophthalmologic exams to monitor progress and to check for side effects.

Evaluation/Desired Outcomes

- Resolution of signs and symptoms of tuberculosis.
- Negative sputum cultures.
- Prevention of activation of tuberculosis in persons known to have been exposed.

ISOSORBIDE

isosorbide dinitrate

(eye-soe-**sor**-bide dye-**nye**-trate)

♣Apo-ISDN, ♣Cedocard-SR, ♣Coronex, Dilatrate-SR, Isordil, ♣Novosorbide, ♣PMS-Isosorbide

isosorbide mononitrate

(eye-soe-**sor**-bide mo-noe-**nye**-trate)

♣Apo-ISMN, IMDUR, ISMO, Monoket

Classification

Therapeutic: antianginals

Pharmacologic: nitrates

Pregnancy Category C

Indications

Acute treatment of anginal attacks (SL only). Prophylactic management of angina pectoris. Treatment of chronic CHF (unlabeled).

Action

Produce vasodilation (venous greater than arterial). Decrease left ventricular end–diastolic pressure and left ventricular end–diastolic volume (preload). Net effect is reduced myocardial oxygen consumption. Increase coronary blood flow by dilating coronary arteries and improving collateral flow to ischemic regions. **Therapeutic Effects:** Relief and prevention of anginal attacks.

Pharmacokinetics

Absorption: Isosorbide dinitrate undergoes extensive first-pass metabolism by the liver, resulting in 25% bioavailability; isosorbide mononitrate has 100% bioavailability (does not undergo first-pass metabolism).

Distribution: Unknown.

Metabolism and Excretion: Isosorbide dinitrate is metabolized by the liver to 2 active metabolites (5–mononitrate and 2–mononitrate). Isosorbide mononitrate is primarily meteabolized by the liver to inactive metabolites; primarily excreted in urine as metabolites.

Half-life: *Isosorbide dinitrate*—1 hr; *isosorbide mononitrate*—5 hr.

TIME/ACTION PROFILE (cardiovascular effects)

ROUTE	ONSET	PEAK	DURATION
ISDN-SL	2–10 min	unknown	1–2 hr
ISDN-PO	45–60 min	unknown	4 hr
ISDN-PO-ER	30 min	unknown	up to 12 hr
ISMN-PO	30–60 min	unknown	7 hr
ISMN-ER	unknown	unknown	12 hr

Contraindications/Precautions

Contraindicated in: Hypersensitivity; Concurrent use of sildenafil, vardenafil or tadalafil.

Use Cautiously in: Volume depleted patients; Right ventricular infarction; Hypertrophic cardiomyopathy; Geri: Older patients may be more sensitive to hypotension (start with lower doses); OB: Pregnancy (may compromise maternal/fetal circulation) or lactation; Pedi: Children (safety not established).

Adverse Reactions/Side Effects

CNS: dizziness, headache. **CV:** hypotension, tachycardia, paradoxic bradycardia, syncope. **GI:** nausea, vomiting. **Misc:** flushing, tolerance.

Interactions

Drug-Drug: Concurrent use of **sildenafil**, **tadalafil**, or **vardenafil** may result in significant and potentially fatal hypotension (do not use these drugs within 24 hr of isosorbide dinitrate or mononitrate). Additive hypotension with **antihypertensives**, acute ingestion of **alcohol**, **beta blockers**, **calcium channel blockers**, and **phenothiazines**.

Route/Dosage

Isosorbide Dinitrate

SL (Adults): *Acute attack of angina pectoris*—2.5–5 mg may be repeated q 5–10 min for 3 doses in 15–30 min. *Prophylaxis of angina pectoris*—2.5–5 mg given 15 mm prior to activities known to provoke angina.

PO (Adults): *Prophylaxis of angina pectoris*—5–20 mg 2–3 times daily; usual maintenance dose is 10–40 mg q 6 hr (immediate-release) or 40–80 mg q 8–12 hr (sustained-release).

Isosorbide Mononitrate

PO (Adults): *ISMO, Monoket*—5–20 mg twice daily with the 2 doses given 7 hr apart. *Imdur*—30–60 mg once daily; may increase to 120 mg once daily (maximum dose = 240 mg/day).

Availability (generic available)

Isosorbide Dinitrate

Sublingual tablets: 2.5 mg, 5 mg. **Cost:** *Generic*—2.5 mg $39.16/100, 5 mg $18.59/100. **Tablets:** 5 mg, 10 mg, 20 mg, 30 mg, 40 mg. **Cost:** *Isordil*—40 mg $91.49/100; *Generic*—5 mg $31.23/100, 10 mg $35.45/100, 20 mg $18.85/100, 30 mg $23.32/100. **Extended-release tablets:** ✤20 mg, 40 mg. **Cost:** *Generic*—40 mg $71.29/100. **Sustained-release capsules:** 40 mg. ***In combination with:*** hydralazine (BiDil). See Appendix B.

Isosorbide Mononitrate

Tablets (ISMO, Monoket): 10 mg, 20 mg. **Cost:** *Generic*—10 mg $45.99/180, 20 mg $48.98/180. **Extended-release tablets (Imdur):** 30 mg, 60 mg, 120 mg. **Cost:** *Generic*—30 mg $35.99/90, 60 mg $34.97/90, 120 mg $46.97/90.

NURSING IMPLICATIONS

Assessment

- Assess location, duration, intensity, and precipitating factors of anginal pain.
- Monitor blood pressure and pulse routinely during period of dosage adjustment.
- ***Lab Test Considerations:*** Excessive doses may ↑ methemoglobin concentrations.

Potential Nursing Diagnoses

Ineffective tissue perfusion (Indications)
Activity intolerance (Indications)

Implementation

Isosorbide Dinitrate

- **PO:** Extended-release capsules should be swallowed whole. Do not crush, break, or chew. **SL:** tablets should be held under tongue until dissolved.
- Avoid eating, drinking, or smoking until tablet is dissolved. Replace tablet if inadvertently swallowed.

Isosorbide Mononitrate

- Do not confuse Imdur with Imuran, Inderal, or K-Dur. Do not confuse Monoket with Monopril (fosinopril).
- **PO:** Extended-release tablets should be swallowed whole. Do not crush, break, or chew.

Patient/Family Teaching

- Instruct patient to take medication as directed, even if feeling better. Take missed doses as soon as remembered; doses of isosorbide dinitrate should be taken at least 2 hr apart (6 hr with extended-release preparations); daily doses of isosorbide mononitrate should be taken 7 hr apart. Do not double doses. Do not discontinue abruptly.
- Caution patient to make position changes slowly to minimize orthostatic hypotension.
- May cause dizziness. Caution patient to avoid driving or other activities requiring alertness until response to medication is known.
- Instruct patient to take last dose of day (when taking 2–4 doses/day) no later than 7 pm to prevent the development of tolerance.
- Advise patient to avoid concurrent use of alcohol with this medication. Patient should also consult health care professional before taking Rx, OTC, or herbal products while taking isosorbide.
- Inform patient that headache is a common side effect that should decrease with continuing therapy. Aspirin or acetaminophen may be ordered to treat headache. Notify health care professional if headache is persistent or severe. Do not alter dose to avoid headache.
- Advise patient to notify health care professional if dry mouth or blurred vision occurs.

Evaluation/Desired Outcomes

- Decrease in frequency and severity of anginal attacks.
- Increase in activity tolerance.

isradipine (is-ra-di-peen)

DynaCirc, DynaCirc CR

Classification

Therapeutic: antianginals, antihypertensives
Pharmacologic: calcium channel blockers

Pregnancy Category C

Indications

Management of hypertension, angina pectoris, and vasospastic (Prinzmetal's) angina.

Action

Inhibits the transport of calcium into myocardial and vascular smooth muscle cells, resulting in inhibition of excitation-contraction coupling and subsequent contraction. **Therapeutic Effects:** Systemic vasodilation resulting in decreased blood pressure. Coronary vasodilation resulting in decreased frequency and severity of attacks of angina.

Pharmacokinetics

Absorption: Well absorbed following oral administration but extensively metabolized, resulting in decreased bioavailability.

Distribution: Unknown.
Protein Binding: 95%.
Metabolism and Excretion: Completely metabolized by the liver.
Half-life: 8 hr.

TIME/ACTION PROFILE (cardiovascular effects†)

ROUTE	ONSET	PEAK	DURATION
PO	<2 hr	2–3 hr	12 hr
PO-CR	2 hr	8–10 hr	24 hr

†For single doses, maximal antihypertensive effect during chronic dosing may take 2–4 wk

Contraindications/Precautions
Contraindicated in: Hypersensitivity; Sick sinus syndrome; 2nd- or 3rd-degree AV block (unless an artificial pacemaker is in place); Blood pressure <90 mm Hg.
Use Cautiously in: Severe hepatic impairment (dose reduction recommended); Geri: Geriatric patients (dose reduction recommended for most agents; increased risk of hypotension); Severe renal impairment; History of serious ventricular arrhythmias or CHF; OB, Lactation, Pedi: Pregnancy, lactation, or children (safety not established).

Adverse Reactions/Side Effects
CNS: abnormal dreams, anxiety, confusion, dizziness, drowsiness, headache, nervousness, psychiatric disturbances, weakness. **EENT:** blurred vision, disturbed equilibrium, epistaxis, tinnitus. **Resp:** cough, dyspnea. **CV:** ARRHYTHMIAS, CHF, peripheral edema, bradycardia, chest pain, hypotension, palpitations, syncope, tachycardia. **GI:** abnormal liver function studies, anorexia, constipation, diarrhea, dry mouth, dysgeusia, dyspepsia, nausea, vomiting. **GU:** dysuria, nocturia, polyuria, sexual dysfunction, urinary frequency. **Derm:** dermatitis, erythema multiforme, flushing, increased sweating, photosensitivity, pruritus/urticaria, rash. **Endo:** gynecomastia, hyperglycemia. **Hemat:** anemia, leukopenia, thrombocytopenia. **Metab:** weight gain. **MS:** joint stiffness, muscle cramps. **Neuro:** paresthesia, tremor. **Misc:** STEVENS-JOHNSON SYNDROME, gingival hyperplasia.

Interactions
Drug-Drug: Additive hypotension may occur when used concurrently with **fentanyl**, other **antihypertensives**, **nitrates**, acute ingestion of **alcohol**, or **quinidine**. Antihypertensive effects may be decreased by concurrent use of **NSAIDs**. Concurrent use with **beta blockers**, **digoxin**, **disopyramide**, or **phenytoin** may result in bradycardia, conduction defects, or CHF.
Drug-Food: Grapefruit and **grapefruit juice** ↑ serum levels and effect.

Route/Dosage
PO (Adults): 2.5 mg twice daily; may be increased q 2–4 wk by 5 mg/day (not to exceed 20 mg/day) *or* 5 mg once daily as CR tablets; may be increased q 2–4 wk by 5 mg/day (not to exceed 20 mg/day).

Availability
Capsules: 2.5 mg, 5 mg. **Controlled-release tablets:** 5 mg, 10 mg.

NURSING IMPLICATIONS

Assessment
- Monitor blood pressure and pulse prior to and periodically throughout therapy. Monitor ECG periodically in patients receiving prolonged therapy.
- Monitor intake and output ratios and daily weight. Assess patient for signs of CHF (peripheral edema, rales/crackles, dyspnea, weight gain, jugular venous distention).
- **Angina:** Assess location, duration, intensity, and precipitating factors of patient's anginal pain.
- ***Lab Test Considerations:*** Total serum calcium concentrations are not affected by calcium channel blockers.
- Monitor serum potassium periodically. Hypokalemia increases risk of arrhythmias; should be corrected.
- Monitor renal and hepatic functions periodically during long-term therapy. Several days of therapy may cause increase in hepatic enzymes, which return to normal upon discontinuation of therapy.

Potential Nursing Diagnoses
Decreased cardiac output (Side Effects)

Implementation
- **PO:** May be administered without regard to meals. May be administered with meals if GI irritation becomes a problem.
- Do not open, crush, break, or chew controlled-release tablets.

Patient/Family Teaching

- Advise patient to take medication exactly as directed, even if feeling well. If a dose is missed, take as soon as possible unless almost time for next dose; do not double doses. May need to be discontinued gradually.
- Advise patient to avoid grapefruit or grapefruit juice during therapy.
- Caution patient to change positions slowly to minimize orthostatic hypotension.
- May cause dizziness. Advise patient to avoid driving or other activities requiring alertness until response to the medication is known.
- Instruct patient to avoid concurrent use of alcohol or OTC medications without consulting health care professional.
- Caution patient to wear protective clothing and use sunscreen to prevent photosensitivity reactions.
- Advise patient to notify health care professional if irregular heartbeats, dyspnea, swelling of hands and feet, rash, pronounced dizziness, nausea, constipation, or hypotension occurs.
- **Angina:** Instruct patient on concurrent nitrate or beta-blocker therapy to continue taking both medications as directed and to use SL nitroglycerin as needed for anginal attacks.
- Inform patient that anginal attacks may occur 30 min after administration because of reflex tachycardia. This is usually temporary and is not an indication for discontinuation.
- Advise patient to contact health care professional if chest pain does not improve, worsens after therapy, or occurs with diaphoresis or if shortness of breath or persistent headache occurs.
- Caution patient to discuss exercise restrictions with health care professional prior to exertion.
- **Hypertension:** Encourage patient to comply with other interventions for hypertension (weight reduction, low-sodium diet, smoking cessation, moderation of alcohol consumption, regular exercise, and stress management). Medication controls but does not cure hypertension.
- Instruct patient and family in proper technique for monitoring BP. Advise patient to take BP weekly and to report significant changes to health care professional.

Evaluation/Desired Outcomes

- Decrease in blood pressure.
- Decrease in frequency and severity of anginal attacks.
- Decrease in need for nitrate therapy.
- Increase in activity tolerance and sense of well-being.

itraconazole (it-tra-**kon**-a-zole)

Sporanox

Classification

Therapeutic: antifungals (systemic)

Pregnancy Category C

Indications

Histoplasmosis. Blastomycosis. Aspergillosis. Onychomycosis of the fingernail or toenail caused by *tinea unguium* in nonimmunocompromised patients (oral capsules only). Oropharyngeal esophageal candidiasis.

Action

Inhibits enzymes necessary for integrity of the fungal cell membrane. **Therapeutic Effects:** Fungistatic effects against susceptible organisms. **Spectrum:** Active against *Histoplasma capsulatum*, *Blastomyces dermatitidis*, *Cryptococcus neoformans*, *Aspergillus fumigatus*, *Trichophyton* spp., *Candida*, and *Tinea unguium*.

Pharmacokinetics

Absorption: Oral absorption is enhanced by food.

Distribution: Tissue concentrations are higher than plasma concentrations. Does not enter CSF; enters breast milk.

Protein Binding: *Itraconazole*—99.8%; *hydroxyitraconazole*—99.5%.

Metabolism and Excretion: Mostly metabolized by the liver and excreted in feces. Hydroxyitraconazole, the major metabolite, has antifungal activity.

Half-life: 21 hr.

TIME/ACTION PROFILE (blood levels)

ROUTE	ONSET	PEAK	DURATION
PO	rapid	4 hr	12–24 hr
IV	unknown	end of infusion	12–24 hr

Contraindications/Precautions

Contraindicated in: Hypersensitivity. Cross-sensitivity with other azole antifungals (**miconazole**, **ketoconazole**) may occur; OB: Lactation; Concurrent **quinidine**, **dofetilide**,

pimozide, oral **midazolam**, **triazolam**, **ergot alkaloids (dihydroergotamine**, **ergonovine**, **ergotamine**, **methylergonovine)**, **simvastatin**, or **lovastatin**; Severe renal impairment (CCr <30 ml/min); CHF or other evidence of ventricular dysfunction.
Use Cautiously in: Patients with hepatic impairment (dosage reduction may be required); Patients with achlorhydria or hypochlorhydria (absorption will be decreased); OB, Pedi: Pregnancy or children (safety not established).

Adverse Reactions/Side Effects

CNS: dizziness, drowsiness, fatigue, headache, malaise. **EENT:** tinnitus. **CV:** CHF, edema, hypertension. **GI:** HEPATOXICITY, nausea, abdominal pain, anorexia, diarrhea, flatulence, vomiting. **GU:** albuminuria, decreased libido, erectile dysfunction. **Derm:** TOXIC EPIDERMAL NECROLYSIS, photosensitivity, pruritus, rash. **Endo:** adrenal insufficiency. **F and E:** hypokalemia. **MS:** rhabdomyolysis. **Misc:** allergic reactions including ANAPHYLAXIS, fever.

Interactions

Drug-Drug: Itraconazole is a potent inhibitor of the P450 3A hepatic enzyme, which can ↑ blood levels and effects of other drugs which are metabolized by this system. ↑ risk of potentially fatal arrhythmias with **quinidine**, **dofetilide**, or **pimozide** (concurrent use is contraindicated and may result in QTc prolongation, torsades de pointes, ventricular arrthythmias, and sudden death). ↑ risk of excessive sedation with **midazolam** or **triazolam**, ↑ risk of adverse CNS reactions with **pimozide**, and ↑ risk of myopathy with **simvastatin** or **lovastatin** (concurrent use contraindicated). Concurrent use with **ergot alkaloids (dihydroergotamine**, **ergonovine**, **ergotamine**, **methylergonovine)** ↑ risk of vasoconstriction and is contraindicated. May also ↑ blood levels and the risk of toxicity from **warfarin**, **ritonavir**, **indinavir**, **saquinavir**, **vinca alkaloids**, **busulfan**, **cilostazol diazepam**, **eletriptan felodipine**, **isradipine**, **nicardipine**, **nifedipine**, **nimodipine**, **cyclosporine vardenafil**, **tacrolimus**, **sildenafil methylprednisolone**, **digoxin**, and **quinidine**. May also ↓ metabolism and ↑ effects of **budesonide**, **dexamethasone**, and **methylprednisolone**. Absorption ↓ by **antacids**, **histamine H_2 blockers**, **sucralfate**, **gastric acid-pump inhibitors**, or other **agents that increase gastric pH**, including the buffer in **didanosine** (take 2 hr after itraconazole). **Phenytoin**, **phenobarbital**, **isoniazid**, **rifampin**, **rifabutin**, and **carbamazepine** ↑ metabolism and ↓ blood levels of itraconazole (↑ dosage may be necessary). Itraconazole ↓ metabolism and may ↑ effects of **phenytoin** and **oral hypoglycemic agents**. If hypokalemia occurs, the risk of **digoxin** toxicity is ↑. Blood levels of itraconazole may be ↑ by **clarithromycin**, **erythromycin ritonavir**, and **indinavir**.
Drug-Food: Food ↑ absorption.

Route/Dosage

Aspergillosis

PO (Adults): 200 mg once or twice daily for a minimum of 3 mo.

Blastomycosis, Histoplasmosis

PO (Adults): 200 mg once daily; may be increased by 100 mg/day up to 200 mg twice daily.

Onychomycosis

PO (Adults): *Toenail fungus with or without fingernail fungus*—200 mg/day for 12 consecutive wk. *Fingernail fungus*—200 mg twice daily for 1 wk, then 3 wk without therapy, then 200 mg twice daily an additional wk–6 mo.

Candidiasis

PO (Adults): *Oropharyngeal candidiasis*—200 mg (20 ml) daily for 1–2 wk. *Oropharyngeal candidiasis unresponsive to fluconazole*—100 mg (10 ml) twice daily for at least 2–4 wk. *Esophageal candidiasis*—100 mg (10 ml) once daily for at least 3 wk.

Availability

Capsules: 100 mg. **Oral solution (cherry caramel):** 10 mg/ml.

NURSING IMPLICATIONS

Assessment

- Assess for signs and symptoms of infection (vital signs, lung sounds, sputum, WBC, oral and pharyngeal mucosa, nail beds) before and periodically during therapy.
- Obtain specimens for culture before instituting therapy. Therapy may be started before results are obtained.
- ***Lab Test Considerations:*** Monitor hepatic function tests before and periodically during therapy, especially in patients with pre-ex-

isting hepatic function abnormalities. Discontinue itraconazole if abnormal values persist or worsen.

- Monitor serum potassium. May cause hypokalemia.

Potential Nursing Diagnoses

Risk for infection (Indications)
Noncompliance (Patient/Family Teaching)

Implementation

- Do not interchange capsules and oral solution. Only oral solution is effective for oropharyngeal candidiasis. Oral solution is not recommended for initial treatment of patients at risk for systemic candidiasis.
- **Capsules:** Administer with a full meal to minimize nausea and vomiting and to increase absorption.
- Do not administer with antacids or other medications that may increase gastric pH; may decrease absorption of itraconazole.
- **Oral Solution:** Administer without food if possible. Swish solution in mouth vigorously, 10 ml at a time, for several seconds, then swallow.

Patient/Family Teaching

- Instruct patient to take medication as directed, even if feeling better. Doses should be taken at the same time each day.
- May occasionally cause drowsiness. Caution patient to avoid driving or other activities requiring alertness until response to medication is known.
- Instruct patient to notify health care professional if signs and symptoms of liver dysfunction (unusual fatigue, anorexia, nausea, vomiting, jaundice, dark urine, or pale stools) or CHF (dyspnea, peripheral edema, weight gain) occur. If signs of CHF occur, discontinue itraconazole and notify health care professional immediately.
- Advise patient to consult health care professional before taking any Rx, OTC, or herbal medications concurrently with itraconazole.
- Advise patient to use sunscreen and wear protective clothing to prevent photosensitivity reactions.

Evaluation/Desired Outcomes

- Resolution of clinical and laboratory indications of fungal infections. Minimal treatment for systemic fungal infections is 3 mo. Inadequate period of treatment may lead to recurrence of active infection.

kanamycin, See AMINOGLYCOSIDES.

ketoconazole (systemic)†

(kee-toe-**koe**-na-zole)
Nizoral

Classification
Therapeutic: antifungals (systemic)

Pregnancy Category C

†For topical use, see Antifungals (topical)

Indications

Treatment of: Candidiasis (disseminated and mucocutaneous), Chromomycosis, Coccidioidomycosis, Histoplasmosis, Paracoccidioidomycosis. **Unlabeled uses:** Treatment of advanced prostate cancer. Treatment of Cushing's syndrome.

Action

Disrupts fungal cell membrane. Interferes with fungal metabolism. Also inhibits the production of adrenal steroids. **Therapeutic Effects:** Fungistatic or fungicidal action against susceptible organisms, depending on organism and site of infection. **Spectrum:** Active against many pathogenic fungi, including: *Blastomyces*, *Candida*, *Coccidioides*, *Cryptococcus*, *Histoplasma*, many dermatophytes.

Pharmacokinetics

Absorption: Absorption from the GI tract is pH dependent; increasing pH decreases absorption.
Distribution: Widely distributed. CNS penetration is unpredictable and minimal. Crosses the placenta; enters breast milk.
Protein Binding: 99%.
Metabolism and Excretion: Partially metabolized by the liver. Excreted in feces via biliary excretion.
Half-life: 8 hr.

TIME/ACTION PROFILE (blood levels)

ROUTE	ONSET	PEAK	DURATION
PO	rapid	1–4 hr	24 hr

Contraindications/Precautions

Contraindicated in: Hypersensitivity; Pregnancy or lactation; Concurrent triazolam.
Use Cautiously in: History of liver disease; Achlorhydria or hypochlorhydria; Alcoholism.

Adverse Reactions/Side Effects

CNS: dizziness, drowsiness. **EENT:** photophobia. **GI:** DRUG-INDUCED HEPATITIS, <u>nausea</u>, <u>vomiting</u>, abdominal pain, constipation, diarrhea, flatulence. **GU:** azoospermia, decreased male libido, menstrual irregularities, oligospermia. **Derm:** rashes. **Endo:** gynecomastia.

Interactions

Drug-Drug: Ketoconazole inhibits the hepatic P450 3A4 enzyme system, which results in ↓ metabolism and possibly ↑ effects and/or toxicity from **cyclosporine**, **tacrolimus**, **corticosteroids** (dosage reduction may be necessary), **calcium channel blockers**, **sulfonylurea**, **oral hypoglycemic agents**, **quinidine**, **buspirone**, **clarithromycin**, **troleandomycin**, **erythromycin**, **cyclophosphamide**, **phenytoin**, **warfarin** (↑ risk of bleeding), **tamoxifen**, **tricyclic antidepressants**, **carbamazepine**, **nisoldipine**, **zolpidem**, **vinca alkaloids**, **ifosfamide**, some **benzodiazepines** (effect may persist for several days; use of **triazolam** is contraindicated), **alfentanil**, **fentanyl**, **sufentanil**, **donepezil**, **atorvastatin**, **lovastatin**, **simvastatin**, **amprenavir**, **indinavir** (dosage ↓ of indinavir recommended), **nelfinavir**, **ritonavir**, **saquinavir**, **quinidine**, **sildenafil** and **vardenafil** (dosage adjustments may be necessary). May alter the effectiveness of **hormonal contraceptives** (alternative method of contraception recommended). Drugs that ↑ gastric pH, including **antacids**, **histamine H_2 antagonists**, **didanosine** (chewable tablets, because of buffer), and **gastric acid–pump inhibitors** ↓ absorption (wait 2 hr before administration of ketoconazole). **Sucralfate** and **isoniazid** also ↓ bioavailability. ↑ hepatotoxicity with other **hepatotoxic agents**, including **alcohol**. Disulfiram-like reaction may occur with **alcohol**. **Rifampin** or **isoniazid** may ↓ levels and effectiveness. May ↓ absorption and effectiveness of **theophylline**.

Route/Dosage

PO (Adults): *Antifungal*—200–400 mg/day, single dose. *Prostate cancer*—400 mg 3 times daily (unlabeled).
PO (Children >2 yr): 3.3–6.6 mg/kg/day, single dose.

Availability (generic available)
Tablets: 200 mg. **Oral suspension:** ✤100 mg/5 ml.

NURSING IMPLICATIONS

Assessment
- Assess patient for symptoms of infection prior to and periodically during therapy.
- Specimens for culture should be taken prior to instituting therapy. Therapy may be started before results are obtained.
- ***Lab Test Considerations:*** Monitor hepatic function tests prior to and monthly for 3–4 mo and then periodically during therapy. May cause ↑ AST, ALT, serum alkaline phosphatase, and bilirubin concentrations. Ketoconazole should be discontinued if even minor abnormalities occur.
- May cause ↓ serum testosterone concentrations.

Potential Nursing Diagnoses
Risk for infection (Indications)
Noncompliance (Patient/Family Teaching)

Implementation
- Do not confuse Nizoral (ketoconazole) with Neoral (cyclosporine).
- **PO:** Administer with meals or snacks to minimize nausea and vomiting.
- Shake suspension well prior to administration.
- Do not administer histamine H_2 antagonists or antacids within 2 hr of ketoconazole.
- For patients with achlorhydria, dissolve each tablet in 4 ml of aqueous solution of 0.2 N hydrochloric acid. Use a glass or plastic straw to avoid contact with teeth and follow with a glass of water, swished in mouth and swallowed.

Patient/Family Teaching
- Instruct patient to take medication as directed, at the same time each day, even if feeling better. Take missed doses as soon as remembered; if almost time for next dose, space missed dose and next dose 10–12 hr apart.
- May cause dizziness or drowsiness. Caution patient to avoid driving or other activities requiring alertness until response to medication is known.
- Advise patient to avoid taking OTC antacids within 2 hr of ketoconazole.
- Caution patient to wear sunglasses and to avoid prolonged exposure to bright light to prevent photophobic reactions.
- Advise patient to use a nonhormonal form of contraception during ketoconazole therapy.
- Advise patient to avoid concurrent use of alcohol while taking ketoconazole; may cause a disulfiram-like reaction (flushing, rash, peripheral edema, nausea, headache) and increase the risk of hepatotoxicity.
- Instruct patient to notify health care professional if abdominal pain, fever, or diarrhea becomes pronounced or if signs and symptoms of liver dysfunction (unusual fatigue, anorexia, nausea, vomiting, jaundice, dark urine, or pale stools) occur.

Evaluation/Desired Outcomes
- Resolution of clinical and laboratory indications of fungal infections.
- Minimal treatment for candidiasis is 1–2 wk and for other systemic mycoses is 6 mo.
- Chronic mucocutaneous candidiasis usually requires maintenance therapy.

ketoconazole, See ANTIFUNGALS (TOPICAL).

ketoprofen (kee-toe-**proe**-fen)
Actron, ✤Apo-Keto, ✤Apo-Keto-E, Orudis, ✤Orudis-E, Orudis KT, ✤Orudis-SR, Oruvail, ✤Rhodis

Classification
Therapeutic: antipyretics, antirheumatics, nonopioid analgesics, nonsteroidal anti-inflammatory agents
Pharmacologic: nonopioid analgesics

Pregnancy Category B (first trimester)

Indications
Inflammatory disorders, including: Rheumatoid arthritis, Osteoarthritis. Mild to moderate pain, including dysmenorrhea and fever.

Action
Inhibits prostaglandin synthesis. **Therapeutic Effects:** Suppression of pain and inflammation. Reduction of fever.

Pharmacokinetics
Absorption: Well absorbed from the GI tract.
Distribution: Unknown.
Protein Binding: 99%.
Metabolism and Excretion: Mostly (60%) metabolized by the liver; some renal excretion.
Half-life: 2–4 hr.

TIME/ACTION PROFILE

ROUTE	ONSET	PEAK	DURATION
PO (analgesic)	within 60 min	1 hr	4–6 hr
PO (anti-inflammatory)	few days–1 wk	unknown	up to 24 hr (SR products)

Contraindications/Precautions

Contraindicated in: Hypersensitivity; Cross-sensitivity may exist with other NSAIDs, including aspirin; Active GI bleeding; Ulcer disease; Some products contain tartrazine and should be avoided in patients with known intolerance; Peri-operative pain from coronary artery bypass graft (CABG) surgery.
Use Cautiously in: Cardiovascular disease or risk factors for cardiovascular disease (may ↑ risk of serious cardiovascular thrombotic events, myocardial infarction, and stroke, especially with prolonged use); Severe renal, or hepatic disease; History of ulcer disease; Renal impairment (dosage reduction suggested); Geri: Extended-release product should not be used in geriatric patients, patients of small stature, or patients with renal impairment; Geriatric patients (increased risk of GI bleeding); Chronic alcohol use/abuse; OB, Pedi: Pregnancy, lactation, or children (safety not established; avoid use during 2nd half of pregnancy).

Adverse Reactions/Side Effects

CNS: drowsiness, headache, dizziness. **EENT:** blurred vision, tinnitus. **CV:** edema. **GI:** DRUG-INDUCED HEPATITIS, GI BLEEDING, constipation, diarrhea, dyspepsia, nausea, vomiting, anorexia, discomfort, flatulence. **GU:** cystitis, hematuria, renal failure. **Derm:** EXFOLIATIVE DERMATITIS, STEVENS-JOHNSON SYNDROME, TOXIC EPIDERMAL NECROLYSIS, photosensitivity, rashes. **Endo:** gynecomastia. **Hemat:** blood dyscrasias, prolonged bleeding time. **MS:** myalgia. **Misc:** allergic reactions including ANAPHYLAXIS, fever.

Interactions

Drug-Drug: Aspirin alters distribution, metabolism, and excretion of ketoprofen (concurrent use not recommended). ↑ adverse GI effects with other **NSAIDs, corticosteroids**, or **alcohol**. Chronic use with **acetaminophen** may ↑ risk of adverse renal reactions. May ↓ effectiveness of **diuretics** or **antihypertensives**. May ↑ hypoglycemic effects of **insulin** or **sulfonylurea oral hypoglycemic agents**. May ↑ serum **lithium** levels and increase the risk of toxicity. ↑ risk of toxicity from **methotrexate**. **Probenecid** ↑ risk of toxicity from ketoprofen (concurrent use not recommended). ↑ risk of bleeding with **cefotetan, cefoperazone, valproic acid, thrombolytic agents, clopidogrel, ticlopidine, eptifibatide, tirofiban**, or **anticoagulants**. ↑ risk of adverse hematologic reactions with **antineoplastics** or **radiation therapy**. ↑ risk of nephrotoxicity with **cyclosporine**.
Drug-Natural Products: ↑ bleeding risk with **arnica, chamomile, clove, dong quai, feverfew, garlic, ginger, ginkgo**, and **Panax ginseng**.

Route/Dosage

PO (Adults): *Anti-inflammatory*—150–300 mg/day in 3–4 divided doses or 150–200 mg once daily as extended-release product. *Analgesic*—25–50 mg q 6–8 hr. *OTC analgesic/antipyretic*—12.5 mg q 4–6 hr; if relief is not obtained 1 hr after first dose, an additional dose may be given. An initial dose of 25 mg may be used (not to exceed 25 mg/4–6 hr or 75 mg/24 hr).

Availability (generic available)

Tablets: 12.5 mg[OTC]. **Capsules:** 25 mg, 50 mg, 75 mg. **Extended-release capsules:** 100 mg, 150 mg, 200 mg.

NURSING IMPLICATIONS

Assessment

- Patients who have asthma, aspirin-induced allergy, and nasal polyps are at increased risk for developing hypersensitivity reactions. Assess for rhinitis, wheezing, and urticaria.
- **Arthritis:** Assess pain and range of motion prior to and 1 hr following administration.
- **Pain:** Assess pain (note type, location, and intensity) prior to and 1 hr following administration.
- **Fever:** Monitor temperature; note signs associated with fever (diaphoresis, tachycardia, malaise).
- ***Lab Test Considerations:*** Evaluate BUN, serum creatinine, CBC, and liver function tests periodically in patients receiving prolonged therapy.
- Serum potassium, BUN, serum creatinine, alkaline phosphatase, LDH, AST, and ALT tests

may show ↑ levels. Blood glucose, hemoglobin and hematocrit concentrations, leukocyte and platelet counts, and CCr may be ↓.
- May prolong bleeding time by 3–4 min.
- May alter results of urine albumin, bilirubin, 17-ketosteroid, and 17-hydroxycorticosteroid determinations.

Potential Nursing Diagnoses

Acute pain (Indications)
Impaired physical mobility (Indications)

Implementation

- Do not confuse Oruvail (ketoprofen) with Elavil (amitriptyline).
- Administration in higher-than-recommended doses does not provide increased effectiveness but may cause increased side effects. Use lowest effective dose for shortest period of time.
- Coadministration with opioid analgesics may have additive analgesic effects and may permit lower opioid doses.
- Analgesic is more effective if given before pain becomes severe.
- **PO:** For rapid initial effect, administer 30 min before or 2 hr after meals. Capsules may be administered with food, milk, or antacids containing aluminum hydroxide and magnesium hydroxide to decrease GI irritation.
- Extended-release capsules should be swallowed whole; do not open or chew.
- **Dysmenorrhea:** Administer as soon as possible after the onset of menses. Prophylactic treatment has not been proved effective.

Patient/Family Teaching

- Advise patient to take this medication with a full glass of water and to remain in an upright position for 15–30 min after administration.
- Instruct patient to take medication exactly as directed. Take missed doses as soon as remembered but not if almost time for the next dose. Do not double doses.
- May cause drowsiness or dizziness. Advise patient to avoid driving or other activities requiring alertness until response to medication is known.
- Caution patient to avoid the concurrent use of alcohol, aspirin, acetaminophen, or other OTC medications without consulting health care professional.
- Advise patient to inform health care professional of medication regimen prior to treatment or surgery.
- Caution patient to wear sunscreen and protective clothing to prevent photosensitivity reactions.
- Instruct patients not to take OTC ketoprofen preparations for more than 10 days for pain or more than 3 days for fever and to consult health care professional if symptoms persist or worsen.
- Caution patient that use of ketoprofen with 3 or more glasses of alcohol may increase risk of GI bleeding.
- Advise patient to consult health care professional if rash, itching, visual disturbances, tinnitus, weight gain, edema, black stools, persistent headache, or influenza-like syndrome (chills, fever, muscle aches, pain) occurs.

Evaluation/Desired Outcomes

- Improved joint mobility.
- Decrease in severity of pain. Improvement in arthritis may be seen in a few days to 1 wk; 1–2 wk may be required for maximum effectiveness. Patients who do not respond to one NSAID may respond to another.
- Reduction of fever.

ketorolac† (kee-**toe**-role-ak)

Toradol

Classification

Therapeutic: nonsteroidal anti-inflammatory agents, nonopioid analgesics
Pharmacologic: pyrroziline carboxylic acid

Pregnancy Category C

†See Appendix C for ophthalmic use

Indications

Short-term management of pain (not to exceed 5 days total for all routes combined).

Action

Inhibits prostaglandin synthesis, producing peripherally mediated analgesia. Also has antipyretic and anti-inflammatory properties. **Therapeutic Effects:** Decreased pain.

Pharmacokinetics

Absorption: Rapidly and completely absorbed following all routes of administration.
Distribution: Enters breast milk in low concentrations.
Metabolism and Excretion: <50% metabolized by the liver. Ketorolac and its metabolites

are excreted primarily by the kidneys (92%); 6% excreted in feces.
Half-life: 4.5 hr (range 3.8–6.3 hr; increased in geriatric patients and patients with impaired renal function).

TIME/ACTION PROFILE (analgesic effects)

ROUTE	ONSET	PEAK	DURATION
PO	unknown	2–3 hr	4–6 hr or longer
IM, IV	10 min	1–2 hr	6 hr or longer

Contraindications/Precautions

Contraindicated in: Hypersensitivity; Cross-sensitivity with other NSAIDs may exist; OB: Labor, delivery or lactation; Pre- or perioperative use; Known alcohol intolerance (injection only); Perioperative pain from coronary artery bypass graft (CABG) surgery.
Use Cautiously in: Cardiovascular disease or risk factors for cardiovascular disease (may ↑ risk of serious cardiovascular thrombotic events, myocardial infarction, and stroke, especially with prolonged use); History of GI bleeding; Renal impairment (dosage reduction may be required); Geri: Appears on Beers list. Geriatric patients have increased risk of GI bleeding; OB, Pedi: Pregnancy and children (use not recommended during 2nd half of pregnancy).

Adverse Reactions/Side Effects

CNS: drowsiness, abnormal thinking, dizziness, euphoria, headache. **Resp:** asthma, dyspnea. **CV:** edema, pallor, vasodilation. **GI:** GI BLEEDING, abnormal taste, diarrhea, dry mouth, dyspepsia, GI pain, nausea. **GU:** oliguria, renal toxicity, urinary frequency. **Derm:** EXFOLIATIVE DERMATITIS, STEVENS-JOHNSON SYNDROME, TOXIC EPIDERMAL NECROLYSIS, pruritus, purpura, sweating, urticaria. **Hemat:** prolonged bleeding time. **Local:** injection site pain. **Neuro:** paresthesia. **Misc:** allergic reactions including, anaphylaxis.

Interactions

Drug-Drug: Concurrent use with **aspirin** may ↓ effectiveness. ↑ adverse GI effects with **aspirin**, other **NSAIDs**, **potassium supplements**, **corticosteroids**, or **alcohol**. Chronic use with **acetaminophen** may ↑ risk of adverse renal reactions. May ↓ effectiveness of **diuretics** or **antihypertensives**. May ↑ serum **lithium** levels and ↑ risk of toxicity. ↑ risk of toxicity from **methotrexate**. ↑ risk of bleeding with **cefotetan**, **cefoperazone**, **valproic acid**, **clopidogrel**, **ticlopidine**, **tirofiban**, **eptifibatide**, **thrombolytic agents**, or **anticoagulants**. ↑ risk of adverse hematologic reactions with **antineoplastics** or **radiation therapy**. May ↑ risk of nephrotoxicity from **cyclosporine**. **Probenecid** ↑ ketorolac blood levels and the risk of adverse reactions (concurrent use should be avoided).
Drug-Natural Products: ↑ bleeding risk with **arnica**, **chamomile**, **clove**, **dong quai**, **feverfew**, **garlic**, **ginger**, **ginkgo**, and **Panax ginseng**.

Route/Dosage

Oral therapy is indicated only as a continuation of parenteral therapy; parenteral therapy should not exceed 20 doses/5 days. Total duration of therapy by all routes should not exceed 5 days.
PO (Adults <65 yr): 20 mg initially, followed by 10 mg q 4–6 hr as needed (not to exceed 40 mg/day).
PO (Adults ≥65 yr, <50 kg, or with renal impairment): 10 mg q 4–6 hr as needed (not to exceed 40 mg/day).
IM (Adults <65 yr): *Single dose*—60 mg. *Multiple dosing*—30 mg q 6 hr (not to exceed 120 mg/day).
IM (Adults ≥65 yr, <50 kg, or with renal impairment): *Single dose*—30 mg. *Multiple dosing*—15 mg q 6 hr (not to exceed 60 mg/day).
IV (Adults <65 yr): *Single dose*—30 mg. *Multiple dosing*—30 mg q 6 hr (not to exceed 120 mg/day).
IV (Adults ≥65 yr, <50 kg, or with renal impairment): *Single dose*—15 mg. *Multiple dosing*—15 mg q 6 hr (not to exceed 60 mg/day).

Availability (generic available)

Tablets: 10 mg. **Cost:** *Generic*—$16.66/20. **Injection:** 15 mg/ml in 1-ml preloaded syringes, 30 mg/ml in 1- and 2-ml preloaded syringes.

NURSING IMPLICATIONS

Assessment

- Patients who have asthma, aspirin-induced allergy, and nasal polyps are at increased risk for developing hypersensitivity reactions. Assess for rhinitis, asthma, and urticaria.

K

- **Pain:** Assess pain (note type, location, and intensity) prior to and 1–2 hr following administration.
- ***Lab Test Considerations:*** Evaluate liver function tests, especially AST and ALT, periodically in patients receiving prolonged therapy. May cause ↑ levels.
- May cause prolonged bleeding time that may persist for 24–48 hr following discontinuation of therapy.
- May cause ↑ BUN, serum creatinine, or potassium concentrations.

Potential Nursing Diagnoses

Acute pain (Indications)

Implementation

- Do not confuse Toradol (ketorolac) with Torecan (thiethylperazine) or tramadol (Ultram).
- Administration in higher-than-recommended doses does not provide increased effectiveness but may cause increased side effects. Duration of ketorolac therapy, by all routes combined, should not exceed 5 days. Use lowest effective dose for shortest period of time.
- Coadministration with opioid analgesics may have additive analgesic effects and may permit lower opioid doses.
- **PO:** Ketorolac therapy should always be given initially by the IM or IV route. Use oral therapy *only* as a continuation of parenteral therapy.

IV Administration

- **Direct IV:** Administer undiluted. ***Concentration:*** 15–30 mg/ml. ***Rate:*** Administer over at least 15 sec.
- **Syringe Compatibility:** sufentanil.
- **Syringe Incompatibility:** haloperidol, hydroxyzine, nalbuphine, prochlorperazine, promethazine, thiethylperazine.
- **Y-Site Compatibility:** cisatracurium, dexmedetomidine, fentanyl, hydromorphone, methadone, morphine, remifentanil, sufentanil.
- **Y-Site Incompatibility:** azithromycin, fenoldopam.
- **Solution Compatibility:** D5/0.9% NaCl, D5W, Ringer's injection, lactated Ringer's injection, 0.9% NaCl.

Patient/Family Teaching

- Instruct patient on how and when to ask for pain medication.
- Instruct patient to take medication exactly as directed. Take missed doses as soon as remembered if not almost time for next dose. Do not double doses. Do not take more than prescribed or for longer than 5 days.
- May cause drowsiness or dizziness. Advise patient to avoid driving or other activities requiring alertness until response to the medication is known.
- Caution patient to avoid the concurrent use of alcohol, aspirin, NSAIDs, acetaminophen, or other OTC medications without consulting health care professional.
- Advise patient to inform health care professional of medication regimen prior to treatment or surgery.
- Advise patient to consult health care professional if rash, itching, visual disturbances, tinnitus, weight gain, edema, black stools, persistent headache, or influenza-like syndrome (chills, fever, muscle aches, pain) occurs.

Evaluation/Desired Outcomes

- Decrease in severity of pain. Patients who do not respond to one NSAID may respond to another.

HIGH ALERT

labetalol (la-**bet**-a-lole)
Trandate

Classification
Therapeutic: antianginals, antihypertensives
Pharmacologic: beta blockers

Pregnancy Category C

Indications
Management of hypertension.

Action
Blocks stimulation of beta$_1$ (myocardial)- and beta$_2$ (pulmonary, vascular, and uterine)-adrenergic receptor sites. Also has alpha$_1$-adrenergic blocking activity, which may result in more orthostatic hypotension. **Therapeutic Effects:** Decreased blood pressure.

Pharmacokinetics
Absorption: Well absorbed but rapidly undergoes extensive first-pass hepatic metabolism, resulting in 25% bioavailability.
Distribution: Some CNS penetration; crosses the placenta.
Metabolism and Excretion: Undergoes extensive hepatic metabolism.
Half-life: 3–8 hr.

TIME/ACTION PROFILE (cardiovascular effects)

ROUTE	ONSET	PEAK	DURATION
PO	20 min–2 hr	1–4 hr	8–12 hr
IV	2–5 min	5 min	16–18 hr

Contraindications/Precautions
Contraindicated in: Uncompensated CHF; Pulmonary edema; Cardiogenic shock; Bradycardia or heart block.
Use Cautiously in: Renal impairment; Hepatic impairment; Geriatric patients (increased sensitivity to beta blockers; initial dosage reduction recommended); Pulmonary disease (including asthma); Diabetes mellitus (may mask signs of hypoglycemia); Thyrotoxicosis (may mask symptoms); Patients with a history of severe allergic reactions (intensity of reactions may be increased); Pregnancy, lactation, or children (safety not established; may cause fetal/neonatal bradycardia, hypotension, hypoglycemia, or respiratory depression).

Adverse Reactions/Side Effects
CNS: fatigue, weakness, anxiety, depression, dizziness, drowsiness, insomnia, memory loss, mental status changes, nightmares. **EENT:** blurred vision, dry eyes, nasal stuffiness. **Resp:** bronchospasm, wheezing. **CV:** ARRHYTHMIAS, BRADYCARDIA, CHF, PULMONARY EDEMA, orthostatic hypotension. **GI:** constipation, diarrhea, nausea. **GU:** erectile dysfunction, decreased libido. **Derm:** itching, rashes. **Endo:** hyperglycemia, hypoglycemia. **MS:** arthralgia, back pain, muscle cramps. **Neuro:** paresthesia. **Misc:** drug-induced lupus syndrome.

Interactions
Drug-Drug: General anesthesia, IV, and **verapamil** may cause additive myocardial depression. Additive bradycardia may occur with **digoxin**. Additive hypotension may occur with other **antihypertensives**, acute ingestion of **alcohol**, or **nitrates**. Concurrent **thyroid** administration may ↓ effectiveness. May alter the effectiveness of **insulin** or **oral hypoglycemic agents** (dose adjustments may be necessary). May ↓ the effectiveness of **adrenergic bronchodilators** and **theophylline**. May ↓ beneficial beta cardiovascular effects of **dopamine** or **dobutamine**. Use cautiously within 14 days of **MAO inhibitor** therapy (may result in hypertension). Effects may be ↑ by **propranolol** or **cimetidine**. Concurrent **NSAIDs** may ↓ antihypertensive action.

Route/Dosage
PO (Adults): 100 mg twice daily initially, may be increased by 100 mg twice daily q 2–3 days as needed (usual range 400–800 mg/day in 2–3 divided doses; doses up to 1.2–2.4 g/day have been used).
IV (Adults): 20 mg (0.25 mg/kg) initially, additional doses of 40–80 mg may be given q 10 min as needed (not to exceed 300 mg total dose) *or* 2 mg/min infusion (range 50–300 mg total dose required).

Availability (generic available)
Tablets: 100 mg, 200 mg, 300 mg. **Cost:** *Generic*—100 mg $54.00/180, 200 mg $76.99/180, 300 mg $101.99/180. **Injection:** 5 mg/ml.

🍁 = Canadian drug name.
* CAPITALS indicates life-threatening; underlines indicate most frequent.

NURSING IMPLICATIONS

Assessment

- Monitor blood pressure and pulse frequently during dose adjustment and periodically during therapy. Assess for orthostatic hypotension when assisting patient up from supine position.
- Check frequency of refills to determine compliance.
- Patients receiving *labetalol IV* must be supine during and for 3 hr after administration. Vital signs should be monitored every 5–15 min during and for several hours after administration.
- Monitor intake and output ratios and daily weight. Assess patient routinely for evidence of fluid overload (peripheral edema, dyspnea, rales/crackles, fatigue, weight gain, jugular venous distention).
- ***Lab Test Considerations:*** May cause ↑ BUN, serum lipoprotein, potassium, triglyceride, and uric acid levels.
- May cause ↑ ANA titers.
- May cause ↑ in blood glucose levels.
- May cause ↑ serum alkaline phosphatase, LDH, AST, and ALT levels. Discontinue if jaundice or laboratory signs of hepatic function impairment occur.
- ***Toxicity and Overdose:*** Monitor patients receiving beta blockers for signs of overdose (bradycardia, severe dizziness or fainting, severe drowsiness, dyspnea, bluish fingernails or palms, seizures). Notify physician or other health care professional immediately if these signs occur: Glucagon has been used to treat bradycardia and hypotension.

Potential Nursing Diagnoses

Decreased cardiac output (Side Effects)
Noncompliance (Patient/Family Teaching)

Implementation

- ***High Alert:*** IV vasoactive medications are inherently dangerous. Before administering intravenously, have second practitioner independently check original order, dosage calculations, and infusion pump settings. Do not confuse labetalol with Lamictil.
- Discontinuation of concurrent clonidine should take place gradually, with beta blocker discontinued first. Then, after several days, discontinue clonidine.
- **PO:** Take apical pulse prior to administering. If <50 bpm or if arrhythmia occurs, withhold medication and notify physician or other health care professional.
- Administer with meals or directly after eating to enhance absorption.

IV Administration

- **Direct IV:** ***Diluent:*** Administer undiluted. ***Concentration:*** 5 mg/ml. ***Rate:*** Administer slowly over 2 min.
- **Continuous Infusion:** ***Diluent:*** Add 200 mg of labetalol to 160 ml of diluent. May also be administered as undiluted drug. Compatible diluents include D5W, 0.9% NaCl, D5/0.9% NaCl, and LR. ***Concentration:*** Diluted: 1 mg/ml; Undiluted: 5 mg/ml. ***Rate:*** Administer at a rate of 2 mg/min. Titrate for desired response. Infuse via infusion pump to ensure accurate dosage.
- **Y-Site Compatibility:** amikacin, aminophylline, amiodarone, atropine, aztreonam, ampicillin, bivalirudin, bumetanide, butorphanol, calcium chloride, calcium gluconate, caspofungin, cefazolin, ceftazidine, ceftizoxime, cimetidine, cyclosporine, daptomycin, digoxin, diltiazem, diphenhydramine, dobutamine, dopamine, doxycycline, enalaprilat, epinephrine, ertapenem, erythromycin lactobionate, esmolol, famotidine, fenoldopam, fentanyl, fluconazole, ganciclovir, gentamicin, granisetron, hydromorphone, imipenem/cilastatin, isoproterenol, levofloxacin, lidocaine, linezolid, lorazepam, magnesium sulfate, meperidine, methylprednisolone sodium succinate, metoclopramide, metronidazole, midazolam, milrinone, morphine, nicardipine, nitroglycerin, nitroprusside, norepinephrine, penicillin G, palonosetron, phenylephrine, phytonadione, potassium chloride, potassium phosphate, procainamide, prochlorperazine, promethazine, propofol, protamine, quinupristin/dalfopristin, ranitidine, sodium bicarbonate, tacrolimus, ticarcillin/clavulanate, tirofiban, tobramycin, trimethoprim/sulfamethoxazole, vancomycin, vasopressin, vecuronium, verapamil, voriconazole.
- **Y-Site Incompatibility:** acyclovir, amphotericin B cholesteryl sulfate complex, cefotaxime, cefoxitin, ceftriaxone, cefuroxime, dexamethasone sodium phosphate, diazepam, furosemide, hydrocortisone sodium succinate, insulin, ketorolac, lansoprazole, micafungin, nafcillin, pantoprazole, phenytoin, piperacillin/tazobactam, warfarin.

Patient/Family Teaching

- Instruct patient to take medication as directed, at the same time each day, even if feeling well; do not skip or double up on missed doses. Take missed doses as soon as possible up to 8 hr before next dose. Abrupt withdrawal may precipitate life-threatening arrhythmias, hypertension, or myocardial ischemia.
- Advise patient to make sure enough medication is available for weekends, holidays, and vacations. A written prescription may be kept in wallet in case of emergency.
- Teach patient and family how to check pulse and blood pressure. Instruct them to check pulse daily and blood pressure biweekly. Advise patient to hold dose and contact health care professional if pulse is <50 bpm or blood pressure changes significantly.
- May cause drowsiness or dizziness. Caution patients to avoid driving or other activities that require alertness until response to the drug is known. Caution patients receiving labetalol IV to call for assistance during ambulation or transfer.
- Advise patients to make position changes slowly to minimize orthostatic hypotension, especially during initiation of therapy or when dose is increased. Patients taking oral labetalol should be especially cautious when drinking alcohol, standing for long periods, or exercising, and during hot weather, because orthostatic hypotension is enhanced.
- Caution patient that this medication may increase sensitivity to cold.
- Instruct patient to consult health care professional before taking any Rx, OTC, or herbal products, especially cold preparations, concurrently with this medication.
- Patients with diabetes should closely monitor blood glucose, especially if weakness, malaise, irritability, or fatigue occurs. Medication may mask tachycardia and increased blood pressure as signs of hypoglycemia, but dizziness and sweating may still occur.
- Advise patient to notify health care professional if slow pulse, difficulty breathing, wheezing, cold hands and feet, dizziness, light-headedness, confusion, depression, rash, fever, sore throat, unusual bleeding, or bruising occurs.
- Instruct patient to inform health care professional of medication regimen prior to treatment or surgery.
- Advise patient to carry identification describing disease process and medication regimen at all times.
- **Hypertension:** Reinforce the need to continue additional therapies for hypertension (weight loss, sodium restriction, stress reduction, regular exercise, moderation of alcohol consumption, and smoking cessation). Medication controls but does not cure hypertension.

Evaluation/Desired Outcomes

- Decrease in blood pressure.

lactulose (lak-tyoo-lose)

Cephulac, Cholac, Chronulac, Constilac, Constulose, Duphalac, Enulose, Evalose, Heptalac, Kristalose, ✤Lactulax, Lactulose PSE, Portalac

Classification
Therapeutic: laxatives
Pharmacologic: osmotics

Pregnancy Category B

Indications

Treatment of chronic constipation in adults and geriatric patients. Adjunct in the management of portal-systemic (hepatic) encephalopathy (PSE).

Action

Increases water content and softens the stool. Lowers the pH of the colon, which inhibits the diffusion of ammonia from the colon into the blood, thereby reducing blood ammonia levels. **Therapeutic Effects:** Relief of constipation. Decreased blood ammonia levels with improved mental status in PSE.

Pharmacokinetics

Absorption: Less than 3% absorbed after oral administration.
Distribution: Unknown.
Metabolism and Excretion: Absorbed lactulose is excreted unchanged in the urine. Unabsorbed lactulose is metabolized by colonic bacteria to lactic, acetic, and formic acids.
Half-life: Unknown.

TIME/ACTION PROFILE (relief of constipation)

ROUTE	ONSET	PEAK	DURATION
PO	24–48 hr	unknown	unknown

Contraindications/Precautions

Contraindicated in: Patients on low-galactose diets.

Use Cautiously in: Diabetes mellitus; Excessive or prolonged use (may lead to dependence); OB, Lactation, Pedi: Pregnancy, lactation, or children (safety not established).

Adverse Reactions/Side Effects

GI: belching, cramps, distention, flatulence, diarrhea. **Endo:** hyperglycemia (diabetic patients).

Interactions

Drug-Drug: Should not be used with other **laxatives** in the treatment of hepatic encephalopathy (leads to inability to determine optimal dose of lactulose). **Anti-infectives** may diminish effectiveness in treatment of hepatic encephalopathy.

Route/Dosage

Constipation

PO (Adults): 15–30 ml/day up to 60 ml/day as liquid or 10–20 g as powder for oral solution (up to 40 g/day has been used).

PO (Children): 7.5 ml daily (unlabeled).

PSE

PO (Adults): 30–45 ml 3–4 times/day; may be given q 1–2 hr initially to induce laxation.

PO (Infants): 2.5–10 ml daily in divided doses (unlabeled).

PO (Children and Adolescents): 40–90 ml daily in divided doses (unlabeled).

Rect (Adults): 300 ml diluted and administered as a retention enema q 4–6 hr.

Availability (generic available)

Syrup (cola flavor): 10 g lactulose/15 ml. **Single-use packets (Kristalose):** 10 g (equal to 15 mL liquid lactulose), 20 g (equal to 30 mL liquid lactulose).

NURSING IMPLICATIONS

Assessment

- Assess patient for abdominal distention, presence of bowel sounds, and normal pattern of bowel function.
- Assess color, consistency, and amount of stool produced.
- **PSE:** Assess mental status (orientation, level of consciousness) before and periodically throughout course of therapy.
- ***Lab Test Considerations:*** Decreases blood ammonia concentrations by 25–50%.
- May cause increased blood glucose levels in diabetic patients.
- Monitor serum electrolytes periodically when used chronically. May cause diarrhea with resulting hypokalemia and hypernatremia.

Potential Nursing Diagnoses

Constipation (Indications)

Implementation

- When used in hepatic encephalopathy, dosage should be adjusted until patient averages 2–3 soft bowel movements per day. During initial therapy, 30–45 ml may be given hourly to induce rapid laxation.
- Darkening of solution does not alter potency.
- **PO:** Mix with fruit juice, water, milk, or carbonated citrus beverage to improve flavor. Administer with a full glass (240 ml) of water or juice. May be administered on an empty stomach for more rapid results.
- Dissolve single dose packets (Kristalose) in 4 oz of water. Solution should be colorless to slightly pale yellow.
- **Rect:** To administer enema, use rectal balloon catheter. Mix 300 ml of lactulose with 700 ml of water or 0.9% NaCl. Enema should be retained for 30–60 min. If inadvertently evacuated, may repeat administration.

Patient/Family Teaching

- Encourage patients to use other forms of bowel regulation, such as increasing bulk in the diet, increasing fluid intake, and increasing mobility. Normal bowel habits are individualized and may vary from 3 times/day to 3 times/wk.
- Caution patients that this medication may cause belching, flatulence, or abdominal cramping. Health care professional should be notified if this becomes bothersome or if diarrhea occurs.

Evaluation/Desired Outcomes

- Passage of a soft, formed bowel movement, usually within 24–48 hr.
- Clearing of confusion, apathy, and irritation and improved mental status in PSE. Improvement may occur within 2 hr after enema and 24–48 hr after oral administration.

lamivudine (la-mi-vyoo-deen)
Epivir, Epivir HBV, 3TC

Classification
Therapeutic: antiretrovirals, antivirals
Pharmacologic: nucleoside reverse transcriptase inhibitors

Pregnancy Category C

Indications
HIV infection (with other antiretrovirals). Chronic hepatitis B infection. **Unlabeled uses:** Part of HIV-postexposure prophylaxis with zidovudine and indinavir.

Action
After intracellular conversion to its active form (lamivudine-5-triphosphate), inhibits viral DNA synthesis by inhibiting the enzyme reverse transcriptase. **Therapeutic Effects:** Slows the progression of HIV infection and decreases the occurrence of its sequelae. Increases CD4 cell counts and decreases viral load. Protection from liver damage caused by chronic hepatitis B infection; decreases viral load.

Pharmacokinetics
Absorption: Well absorbed after oral administration (86% in adults, 66% in infants and children).
Distribution: Distributes into the extravascular space. Some penetration into CSF; remainder of distribution unknown.
Metabolism and Excretion: Mostly excreted unchanged in urine; <5% metabolized by the liver.
Half-life: *Adults*—3.7 hr; *children*—2 hr.

TIME/ACTION PROFILE (blood levels)

ROUTE	ONSET	PEAK	DURATION
PO	unknown	0.9 hr†	12 hr

†On an empty stomach; peak levels occur at 3.2 hr if lamivudine is taken with food. Food does not affect total amount of drug absorbed

Contraindications/Precautions
Contraindicated in: Hypersensitivity; Lactation.
Use Cautiously in: Impaired renal function (increased dosing interval/decreased dose recommended if CCr <50 ml/min); Women, prolonged exposure, obesity, history of liver disease (increased risk of lactic acidosis and severe hepatomegaly with steatosis); Coinfection with hepatitis B (hepatitis may recur after discontinuation of lamivudine); Geriatric patients (dosage reduction may be necessary); Pregnancy or children <3 mo (safety not established).
Exercise Extreme Caution in: Pediatric patients with a history of pancreatitis (use only if no alternative).

Adverse Reactions/Side Effects
Noted for combination of lamivudine plus zidovudine.
CNS: SEIZURES, fatigue, headache, insomnia, malaise, depression, dizziness. **Resp:** cough. **GI:** HEPATOMEGALY WITH STEATOSIS, PANCREATITIS (↑ in pediatric patients), anorexia, diarrhea, nausea, vomiting, abdominal discomfort, abnormal liver function studies, dyspepsia. **Derm:** alopecia, erythema multiforme, rashes, urticaria. **Endo:** hyperglycemia. **F and E:** lactic acidosis. **Hemat:** anemia, neutropenia, pure red cell aplasia. **MS:** musculoskeletal pain, arthralgia, muscle weakness, myalgia, rhabdomyolysis. **Neuro:** neuropathy. **Misc:** hypersensitivity reactions including ANAPHYLAXIS and STEVENS-JOHNSON SYNDROME.

Interactions
Drug-Drug: Trimethoprim/sulfamethoxazole ↑ lamivudine blood levels (dosage alteration may be necessary in renal impairment). ↑ risk of pancreatitis with concurrent use of other **drugs causing pancreatitis**. ↑ risk of neuropathy with concurrent use of other **drugs causing neuropathy**. Combination therapy with **tenofovir** and **abacavir** may lead to virologic nonresponse and should not be used.

Route/Dosage
HIV infection
PO (Adults and Children >12 yr and ≥50 kg): 150 mg twice daily.
PO (Adults <50 kg): 2 mg/kg twice daily.
PO (Children 3 mo–12 yr): 4 mg/kg twice daily (up to 150 mg twice daily).

Renal Impairment
PO (Adults): *CCr 30–49 ml/min*—150 mg once daily; *CCr 15–29 ml/min*—150 mg first dose, then 10 mg once daily; *CCr 5–14 ml/min*—150 mg first dose, then 50 mg once daily; *CCr <5 ml/min*—50 mg first dose, then 25 mg once daily.

Chronic Hepatitis B
PO (Adults): 100 mg once daily.

Renal Impairment

PO (Adults): *CCr 30–49 ml/min*—100 mg first dose, then 50 mg once daily; *CCr 15–29 ml/min*—100 mg first dose, then 25 mg once daily; *CCr 5–14 ml/min*—35 mg first dose, then 15 mg once daily; *CCr <5 ml/min*—35 mg first dose, then 10 mg once daily.
PO (Children 2–17 yr): 3 mg/kg once daily (up to 100 mg/day).

Availability

Epivir

Tablets: 150 mg, 300 mg. **Oral solution (strawberry-banana flavor):** 10 mg/ml in 240-ml bottles.

Epivir HBV

Tablets: 100 mg. **Oral solution (strawberry-banana flavor):** 5 mg/ml in 240 ml bottles. ***In combination with:*** zidovudine (Combivir); zidovudine and abacavir (Trizivir). See Appendix B.

NURSING IMPLICATIONS

Assessment

- **HIV:** Assess patient for change in severity of symptoms of HIV infection and for symptoms of opportunistic infection during therapy.
- Monitor patient for signs and symptoms of peripheral neuropathy (tingling, burning, numbness, or pain in hands or feet); may be difficult to differentiate from peripheral neuropathy of severe HIV disease. May require discontinuation of therapy
- Assess patient, especially pediatric patients, for signs of pancreatitis (nausea, vomiting, abdominal pain) periodically during therapy. May require discontinuation of therapy.
- **Chronic Hepatitis B Infection:** Monitor signs of hepatitis (jaundice, fatigue, anorexia, pruritus) during therapy.
- ***Lab Test Considerations:*** Monitor viral load and CD4 levels before and periodically during therapy.
- Monitor serum amylase, lipase, and triglycerides periodically during therapy. Elevated serum levels may indicate pancreatitis and require discontinuation.
- Monitor liver function. May cause elevated levels of AST, ALT, CPK, bilirubin, and alkaline phosphatase, which usually resolve after interruption of therapy. Lactic acidosis may occur with hepatic toxicity causing hepatic steatosis; may be fatal, especially in women.
- May rarely cause neutropenia and anemia.

Potential Nursing Diagnoses

Risk for infection (Indications)

Implementation

- Do not confuse lamivudine with lamontrigine. Do not confuse Epivir tablets and oral solution with Epivir-HBV tablets and oral solutions. Epivir Tablets and Oral Solution contain a higher dose of the same active ingredient (lamivudine) than in Epivir-HBV Tablets and Oral Solution. Epivir-HBV was developed for patients with hepatitis B and should not be used for patients dually infected with HIV and hepatitis B; use may lead to lamivudine-resistant HIV due to subtherapeutic dose.
- **PO:** May be administered without regard to food.

Patient/Family Teaching

- Instruct patient to take lamivudine as directed, every 12 hr. Explain the difference between Epivir and Epivir-HBV to patients. Emphasize the importance of compliance with full course of therapy, not taking more than the prescribed amount, and not discontinuing without consulting health care professional. Take missed doses as soon as possible unless almost time for next dose. Do not double doses. Caution patient not to share medication with others.
- Inform patient that lamivudine does not cure HIV disease or prevent associated or opportunistic infections. Lamivudine does not reduce the risk of transmission of HIV to others through sexual contact or blood contamination. Caution patient to use a condom during sexual contact and avoid sharing needles or donating blood to prevent spreading HIV to others. Advise patient that the long-term effects of lamivudine are unknown at this time.
- Instruct patient to notify health care professional promptly if signs of peripheral neuropathy or pancreatitis occur.
- Advise patient not to take other OTC or prescription medications or herbal products without consulting health care professional.
- Emphasize the importance of regular follow-up exams and blood tests to determine progress and monitor for side effects.

Evaluation/Desired Outcomes

- Slowing of the progression of HIV infection and its sequelae.

- Decrease in viral load and improvement in CD4 levels in patients with advanced HIV infection.
- Protection from liver damage caused by chronic hepatitis B infection; decreases viral load.

lamotrigine (la-moe-tri-jeen)
Lamictal

Classification
Therapeutic: anticonvulsants

Pregnancy Category C

Indications
Adjunct treatment of partial seizures in adults with epilepsy. Lennox-Gastaut syndrome. Primary generalized tonic-clonic seizures in adults and children ≥2 yrs. Conversion to monotherapy in adults with partial seizures receiving a single enzyme-inducing antiepileptic drug. Maintenance treatment of bipolar disorder.

Action
Stabilizes neuronal membranes by inhibiting sodium transport. **Therapeutic Effects:** Decreased incidence of seizures. Delayed time to recurrence of mood episodes.

Pharmacokinetics
Absorption: 98% absorbed following oral administration.
Distribution: Enters breast milk. Highly bound to melanin-containing tissues (eyes, pigmented skin).
Metabolism and Excretion: Mostly metabolized by the liver to inactive metabolites; 10% excreted unchanged by the kidneys.
Half-life: Children taking enzyme-inducing antiepileptic drugs (AEDs): 7–10 hr; Children taking enzyme inducers and valproic acid (VPA): 15–27 hr; Children taking VPA: 44–94 hr; Adults: 25.4 hr (during chronic therapy of lamotrigine alone).

TIME/ACTION PROFILE (blood levels)

ROUTE	ONSET	PEAK	DURATION
PO	unknown	1.4–4.8 hr	unknown

Contraindications/Precautions
Contraindicated in: Hypersensitivity; Lactation.
Use Cautiously in: Patients with reduced renal function, impaired cardiac function, and impaired hepatic function (lower maintenance doses may be required); Prior history of rash to lamotrigine; OB: Exposure during first trimester (may ↑ risk of cleft lip/palate).

Adverse Reactions/Side Effects
CNS: ataxia, dizziness, headache, behavior changes, depression, drowsiness, insomnia, tremor. **EENT:** blurred vision, double vision, rhinitis. **GI:** nausea, vomiting. **GU:** vaginitis. **Derm:** photosensitivity, rash (higher incidence in children, patients taking VPA, high initial doses, or rapid dose increases). **MS:** arthralgia. **Misc:** allergic or hypersensitivity reactions including Stevens-Johnson syndrome.

Interactions
Drug-Drug: Concurrent use with **carbamazepine** may result in ↓ levels of lamotrigine and ↑ levels of an active metabolite of carbamazepine. Lamotrigine levels are ↓ by concurrent use of **phenobarbital**, **phenytoin**, or **primidone**. Concurrent use with **valproic acid** results in a twofold ↑ in lamotrigine levels, ↑ incidence of rash, and a ↓ in valproic acid level (lamotrigine dose should be ↓ by at least 50%). **Oral contraceptives** may ↓ serum levels of lamotrigine (dose adjustments may be necessary when starting and stopping oral contraceptives).

Route/Dosage

Epilepsy

In Combination with Other Antiepileptic Agents
PO (Adults and Children >12 yr): *Patients taking carbamazepine, phenobarbital, phenytoin, or primidone*—50 mg daily as a single dose for first 2 wk, then 50 mg twice daily for next 2 wk; then increase by 100 mg/day on a weekly basis to maintenance dose of 150–250 mg twice daily (not to exceed 500 mg/day). *Patients taking carbamazepine, phenobarbital, phenytoin, or primidone with valproic acid*—25 mg every other day for first 2 wk, then 25 mg once daily for next 2 wk; then increase by 25–50 mg/day every 1–2 wk to maintenance dose of 50–200 mg twice daily (not to exceed 400 mg/day).
PO (Children 2–12 yr): *Patients taking carbamazepine, phenobarbital, phenytoin, or*

primidone—0.6 mg/kg/day in 2 divided doses (rounded down to nearest whole tablet) for first 2 wk, then 1.2 mg/kg in 2 divided doses (rounded down to nearest whole tablet) for next 2 wk; then increase by 1.2 mg/kg/day (rounded down to nearest whole tablet) q 1–2 wk to maintenance dose of 5–15 mg/kg day (not to exceed 400 mg/day in 2 divided doses). *Patients taking valproic acid*—0.15 mg/kg/day in 1–2 divided doses (rounded down to nearest whole tablet) for first 2 wk; (if initial calculated dose is 2.5–5 mg/day, then initial dose should be 5 mg every other day for 2 wk; if patient weighs between 6.7–14 kg, use 2 mg every other day for 2 wk). Then 0.3 mg/kg in 1–2 divided doses (rounded down to nearest whole tablet) for next 2 wk; then increase by 0.3 mg/kg/day (rounded down to nearest whole tablet) q 1–2 wk to maintenance dose of 1–5 mg/kg day (not to exceed 200 mg/day in 1–2 divided doses). *Patients taking antiepileptic drugs other than carbamazepine, phenobarbital, phenytoin, primidone, or valproate*—0.3 mg/kg/day in 2 divided doses (rounded down to nearest whole tablet) for first 2 wk, then 0.6 mg/kg in 2 divided doses (rounded down to nearest whole tablet) for next 2 wk; then increase by 0.6 mg/kg/day (rounded down to nearest whole tablet) q 1–2 wk to maintenance dose of 5–15 mg/kg day (not to exceed 300 mg/day in 2 divided doses).

Conversion to Monotherapy

PO (Adults ≥16 yr): 50 mg/day for 2 wk, then 50 mg twice daily for 2 wk, then increase by 100 mg/day q 1–2 wk to maintenance dose of 300–500 mg/day in 2 divided doses; when target level is reached, decrease other antiepileptic by 20% weekly over 4 wk.

Bipolar Disorder

Escalation Regimen

PO (Adults): *Patients not taking cabamazepine, valproate or other enzyme-inducing drugs*—25 mg/day for 2 wk, then 50 mg/day for 2 wk, then 100 mg/day for 1 wk, then 200 mg/day; *Patients taking valproate*—25 mg every other day for 2 wk, then 25 mg/day for 2 wk, then 50 mg/day for one wk, then 100 mg/day; *Patients taking cabamazepine (or other enzyme inducers), but not taking valporate* 50 mg/day for 2 wk, then 100 mg/day (in divided doses) for 2 wk, then 200 mg/day (in divided doses) for one wk, then 300 mg/day (in divided doses) for one week, then up to 400 mg/day (in divided doses).

Dosage Adjustment Following Discontinuation of Other Psychotropics

PO (Adults): *Following discontinuation of other psychotropics*—maintain previous dose; *following discontinuation of valproate*—100 mg/day, then increase to 150 mg/day for one wk, then 200 mg/day; *following discontinuation of carbamazepine or other enzyme-inducers*—400 mg/day for one wk, then 300 mg/day for one wk, then 200 mg/day.

Availability (generic available)

Tablets: 25 mg, 100 mg, 150 mg, 200 mg. **Cost:** 25 mg $668.97/180, 100 mg $708.97/180, 150 mg $819.90/180, 200 mg $905.89/180. **Chewable dispersible tablets:** 2 mg, 5 mg, 25 mg. **Cost:** *Generic*—5 mg $453.96/180, 25 mg $489.92/180.

NURSING IMPLICATIONS

Assessment

- Assess patient for skin rash frequently during therapy. Discontinue lamotrigine at first sign of rash; may be life threatening. Stevens-Johnson syndrome or toxic epidermal necrolysis may develop. Rash usually occurs during the initial 2–8 wk of therapy and is more frequent in patients taking multiple antiepileptic agents, especially valproic acid, and much more frequent in patients <16 yr.
- Monitor for hypersensitivity reactions (fever, lymphadenopathy with or without rash) If cause cannot be determined, discontinue lamotrigine immediately.
- **Seizures:** Assess location, duration, and characteristics of seizure activity.
- **Bipolar disorders:** Assess mood, ideation, and behaviors frequently. Initiate suicide precautions if indicated.
- ***Lab Test Considerations:*** Lamotrigine plasma concentrations may be monitored periodically during therapy, especially in patients concurrently taking other anticonvulsants. Therapeutic plasma concentration range has not been established, proposed therapeutic range: 1–5 mcg/ml.

Potential Nursing Diagnoses

Risk for impaired skin integrity (Adverse Reactions)
Risk for injury (Side Effects)

Implementation

- Do not confuse lamotrigine (Lamictal) with terbinafine (Lamisil), diphenoxylate/atropine (Lomotil) or lamivudine (Epivir).

- **PO:** May be administered without regard to meals.
- Lamotrigine should be discontinued gradually over at least 2 wk, unless safety concerns require a more rapid withdrawal. Abrupt discontinuation may cause increase in seizure frequency.
- **Chewable/Dispersible Tablets:** May be swallowed whole, chewed, or dispersed in water or dispersed in fruit juice. If chewed, follow with water or fruit juice to aid in swallowing. Only use whole tablets, do not attempt to administer partial quantities of dispersible tablets.

Patient/Family Teaching

- Instruct patient to take medication exactly as directed. Take missed doses as soon as possible unless almost time for next dose. Do not double doses. Do not discontinue abruptly; may cause increase in frequency of seizures.
- Advise patient to notify health care professional immediately if skin rash, fever, or swollen lymph glands occur or if frequency of seizures increases.
- May cause dizziness, drowsiness, and blurred vision. Caution patient to avoid driving or activities requiring alertness until response to medication is known. Do not resume driving until physician gives clearance based on control of seizure disorder.
- Caution patient to wear sunscreen and protective clothing to prevent photosensitivity reactions.
- Advise patient to notify health care professional if pregnancy is planned or suspected or if patient intends to breastfeed or is breastfeeding.
- Instruct patient to notify health care professional of medication regimen prior to treatment or surgery.
- Advise patient to carry identification at all times describing disease process and medication regimen.

Evaluation/Desired Outcomes

- Decrease in the frequency of or cessation of seizures.
- Decreased incidence of mood swings in bipolar disorders.

lansoprazole

(lan-**soe**-pra-zole)
Prevacid

Classification
Therapeutic: antiulcer agents
Pharmacologic: proton-pump inhibitors

Pregnancy Category B

Indications

Erosive esophagitis. Duodenal ulcers (with or without anti-infectives for *Helicobacter pylori*). Active benign gastric ulcer. Short-term treatment of symptomatic GERD. Healing and risk reduction of NSAID-associated gastric ulcer. Pathologic hypersecretory conditions, including Zollinger-Ellison syndrome.

Action

Binds to an enzyme in the presence of acidic gastric pH, preventing the final transport of hydrogen ions into the gastric lumen. **Therapeutic Effects:** Diminished accumulation of acid in the gastric lumen, with lessened acid reflux. Healing of duodenal ulcers and esophagitis.

Pharmacokinetics

Absorption: 80% absorbed after oral administration.
Distribution: Unknown.
Protein Binding: 97%.
Metabolism and Excretion: Extensively metabolized by the liver to inactive compounds. Converted intracellularly to at least two other antisecretory compounds.
Half-life: Children: 1.2–1.5 hr; Adults: 1.3–1.7 hr (↑ in geriatric patients and patients with impaired hepatic function).

TIME/ACTION PROFILE (acid suppression)

ROUTE	ONSET	PEAK	DURATION
PO	rapid	1.7 hr	more than 24 hr

Contraindications/Precautions

Contraindicated in: Hypersensitivity.
Use Cautiously in: Geri: Geriatric patients (maintenance dose should not exceed 30 mg/day unless additional acid suppression is required); Solutabs contain aspartame; use caution when used in phenylketonurics; Severe hepatic impairment (not to exceed 30 mg/day in

these patients); OB, Lactation, Pedi: Safety not established for pregnant or breastfeeding women or for children <1 yr.

Adverse Reactions/Side Effects

CNS: dizziness, headache. **GI:** diarrhea, abdominal pain, nausea. **Derm:** rash.

Interactions

Drug-Drug: Sucralfate ↓ absorption of lansoprazole (take 30 min before sucralfate). May ↓ absorption of drugs requiring acid pH, including **ketoconazole**, **itraconazole**, **ampicillin esters**, **iron salts**, and **digoxin**. May ↑ risk of bleeding with **warfarin** (monitor INR/PT).

Route/Dosage

PO (Adults and Children ≥12 yr): *Short-term treatment of duodenal ulcer*—15 mg once daily for 4 wk; *H. pylori eradication to reduce the risk of duodenal ulcer recurrence*—30 mg twice daily with clarithromycin 500 mg twice daily and amoxicillin 1000 mg twice daily for 10–14 days (triple therapy) or 30 mg three times daily with 1000 mg amoxicillin three times daily for 14 days (dual therapy); *maintenance of healed duodenal ulcers*—15 mg once daily; *short-term treatment of gastric ulcers/healing of NSAID-associated gastric ulcer*—30 mg once daily for up to 8 wk; *risk reduction of NSAID-associated gastric ulcer*—15 mg once daily for up to 12 wk; *short-term treatment of symptomatic GERD*—15 mg once daily for up to 8 wk; *short-term treatment of erosive esophagitis*—30 mg once daily for up to 8 wk (8 additional weeks may be necessary); *maintenance of healing of erosive esophagitis*—15 mg once daily; *pathologic hypersecretory conditions*—60 mg once daily intially, up to 90 mg twice daily (daily dose >120 mg should be given in divided doses).

PO (Children 1–11 yr and >30 kg): *GERD*—30 mg once to twice daily.

PO (Children 1–11 yr and 10–30 kg): *GERD*—15 mg once or twice daily.

PO (Children 1–11 yr and <10 kg): *GERD*—7.5 mg once daily.

PO (Children 3 mo—14 yrs): *Altenative weight-based dosing*—0.5–1.6 mg/kg once daily.

Availability

Delayed-release capsules: 15 mg, 30 mg. **Cost:** 15 mg $136.28/30, 30 mg $444.38/100. **Delayed-release orally disintegrated tablets (SoluTabs):** 15 mg, 30 mg. **Delayed-release oral suspension packets:** 15 mg, 30 mg. ***In combination with:*** amoxicillin and clarithromycin as part of a compliance package (Prevpac), naproxen as part of a combination package (Prevacid NapraPac). See Appendix B.

NURSING IMPLICATIONS

Assessment

- Assess patient routinely for epigastric or abdominal pain and for frank or occult blood in stool, emesis, or gastric aspirate.
- ***Lab Test Considerations:*** May cause abnormal liver function tests, including increased AST, ALT, alkaline phosphatase, LDH, and bilirubin.
- May cause ↑ serum creatinine and ↑ or ↓ electrolyte levels.
- May alter RBC, WBC, and platelet levels.
- May also cause ↑ gastrin levels, abnormal A/G ratio, hyperlipidemia, and ↑ or ↓ cholesterol.
- Monitor INR and prothrombin time in patients taking warfarin.

Potential Nursing Diagnoses

Acute pain (Indications)

Implementation

- Do not confuse Prevacid (lansoprazole) with Pravachol (pravastatin).
- **PO:** Administer before meals. Capsules may be opened and sprinkled on 1 tbsp of applesauce, pudding, cottage cheese, or yogurt and swallowed immediately for patients with difficulty swallowing. Do not crush or chew capsule contents.
- For patients with an NG tube, capsules may be opened and intact granules may be mixed in 40 ml of apple, cranberry, grape, orange, pineapple, prune, or V8 vegetable juice and injected through the NG tube into stomach. Flush NG tube with additional apple juice to clear tube. If administered via jejunostomy tube, lansoprazole should be prepared as a suspension with 2.5 ml of 4.2% sodium bicarbonate and 2.5 ml water.
- *Orally disintegrating tablets* may be placed on tongue, allowed to disintegrate and swallowed with or without water. For administration via oral syringe or nasogastric tube, *Prevacid SoluTab* can be administered by placing a 15 mg tablet in oral syringe and drawing up 4 mL of water, or a 30 mg tablet in oral syringe and drawing up 10 mL of water. Shake gently to allow for a quick dispersal.

After tablet has dispersed, administer the contents within 15 minutes. Refill syringe with 2 mL (5 mL for the 30 mg tablet) of water, shake gently, and administer any remaining contents and flush nasogastric tube. .
- *Granules for oral suspension* may be prepared by emptying packet into 2 tbsp of water. Do not use other liquids or foods. Do not chew granules. Stir well and drink immediately. If material remains in glass, add water and drink immediately. Do not administer oral suspension through enteral tubes.
- Antacids may be used concurrently.

Patient/Family Teaching
- Instruct patient to take medication as directed for the full course of therapy, even if feeling better.
- Advise patient to avoid alcohol, products containing aspirin or NSAIDs, and foods that may cause an increase in GI irritation.
- May occasionally cause dizziness. Caution patient to avoid driving and other activities that require alertness until response to medication is known.
- Advise patient to report onset of black, tarry stools; diarrhea; or abdominal pain to health care professional promptly.

Evaluation/Desired Outcomes
- Decrease in abdominal pain or prevention of gastric irritation and bleeding. Healing of duodenal ulcers can be seen on x-ray examination or endoscopy. Therapy is continued for at least 2–4 wk. Therapy for pathologic hypersecretory conditions may be long term.
- Healing in patients with erosive esophagitis. Therapy is continued for up to 8 wk, and an additional 8-wk course may be used for patients who do not heal in 8 wk or whose ulcer recurs.

lanthanum carbonate
(**lan**-than-um)
Fosrenol

Classification
Therapeutic: hypophosphatemics
Pharmacologic: phosphate binders

Pregnancy Category C

Indications
Reduction of serum phosphate levels associated with end-stage renal disease.

Action
Dissociates in the upper GI tract forming lanthanate ions, which form an insoluble complex with phosphate. **Therapeutic Effects:** Decreased serum phosphate levels.

Pharmacokinetics
Absorption: Negligible absorption.
Distribution: Stays within the GI tract.
Metabolism and Excretion: Eliminated almost entirely in feces.
Half-life: 53 hr (in plasma).

TIME/ACTION PROFILE (effect on phosphate levels)

ROUTE	ONSET	PEAK	DURATION
PO	unknown	2–3 wk	unknown

Contraindications/Precautions
Contraindicated in: Children; Pregnancy.
Use Cautiously in: Peptic ulcer disease, ulcerative colitis, Crohn's disease, any predisposition to bowel obstruction; Lactation (safety not established).

Adverse Reactions/Side Effects
GI: <u>nausea</u>, <u>vomiting</u>, diarrhea.

Interactions
Drug-Drug: Drugs known to interact with antacids may interact with lanthanum carbonate; separate dosing by 2 hr.

Route/Dosage
PO (Adults): 750–1500 mg/day in divided doses; may be titrated upward every 2–3 wk in increments of 750 mg/day up to 3750 mg/day (usual range 1500–3000 mg/day).

Availability
Chewable tablets: 250 mg, 500 mg.

NURSING IMPLICATIONS

Assessment
- Assess patient for nausea and vomiting during therapy.
- ***Lab Test Considerations:*** Monitor serum phosphate levels prior to and periodically during therapy.

Potential Nursing Diagnoses
Nausea (Side Effects)

Implementation

- Divide total daily dose and administer with meals.
- **PO:** Administer with or immediately after meals. Tablets should be chewed completely before swallowing; intact tablets should not be swallowed.

Patient/Family Teaching

- Instruct patient to take lanthanum as directed.

Evaluation/Desired Outcomes

- Decrease in serum phosphate to below than 6.0 mg/dL in patients with end-stage renal disease.

lapatinib (la-pat-i-nib)

Tykerb

Classification

Therapeutic: antineoplastics

Pharmacologic: enzyme inhibitors, kinase inhibitors

Pregnancy Category D

Indications

Advanced metastatic breast cancer with tumor overexpression of the Human Epidermal Receptor Type 2 (HER2) and past therapy with an anthracycline, a taxane and trastuzumab; used in combination with capecitabine (Xeloda).

Action

Acts as an inhibitor of intracellular tyrosine kinase affecting Epidermal Growth Factor (EGFR, ErbB1) and HER2 (ErbB2). Inhibits the growth of ErbB-driven tumors. Effect is additive with capecitabine. **Therapeutic Effects:** Decreased/slowed spread of metastatic breast cancer.

Pharmacokinetics

Absorption: Incompletely and variably absorbed following oral administration blood levels are increased by food.
Distribution: Unknown.
Protein Binding: >99%.
Metabolism and Excretion: Extensively metabolized by, mostly by CYP3A4 and CYP3A5 enzyme systems; <2% excreted by kidneys.
Half-life: 24 hr.

TIME/ACTION PROFILE (blood levels)

ROUTE	ONSET	PEAK	DURATION
PO	unknown	4 hr	24 hr

Contraindications/Precautions

Contraindicated in: Decreased left ventricular ejection fraction (Grade 2 or greater); OB: Pregnancy or lactation.
Use Cautiously in: Concurrent use of CYP3A4 inhibitors including ketoconazole, itraconazole, clarithromycin, atazanavir, indinavir, nefazodone, nelfinavir, ritoanvir, saquinavir, telithromycin, and voriconazole should be avoided (if necessary, dosage reduction of lapatinib is required); Concurrent use of CYP3A4 inducers including dexamathasone, phenytoin, carbamazepine, rifampin, rifabutin, rifapentin and phenobarbital may decrease levels and effectiveness and should be avoided (if necassary, dosage of lapatinib may be titrated upward to 4500 mg/day as tolerated); Severe hepatic impairment (dosage reduction recommended for Child-Pugh Class C); Known QTc prolongation or co-existing risk factors of QTc prolongation including hypokalemia, hypomagnesemia, concurrent anti-arrhythmics or medications that are known to prolong QTc; Geri: Elderly patients may be more sensitive to effects; Pedi: Safety in children has not been established.

Adverse Reactions/Side Effects

CNS: fatigue, insomnia. **Resp:** dyspnea, interstitial lung disease, pneumonitis. **CV:** ↓ left ventricular ejection fraction. **GI:** diarrhea, nausea, vomiting, dyspepsia, ↑ liver enzymes, stomatitis. **Derm:** palmar-plantar erythrodysesthesia, rash, dry skin. **Hemat:** neutropenia. **MS:** back pain, extremity pain.

Interactions

Drug-Drug: Lapatinib inhibits CYP3A4, CYP28 and P-glycoprotein; concurrent use of drugs which are substrates for these enzyme should be undertaken with caution. Concurrent use of **CYP3A4 inhibitors** including **ketoconazole**, **itraconazole**, **clarithromycin**, **atazanavir**, **indinavir**, **nefazodone**, **nelfinavir**, **ritonavir**, **saquinavir**, **telithromycin**, and **voriconazole** may ↑ blood levels and the risk of toxicity. Concurrent use should be avoided, but if necessary dosage of lapatinib should be decreased. Concurrent use of **CYP3A4 inducers** including **dexamathasone**, **phenytoin**, **carbamazepine**, **rifampin**, **rifabutin**, **rifapentin**, and **phenobarbital** may ↓ blood levels

and effectiveness and should be avoided. If necassary, dosage of lapatinib may be titrated upward to 4500 mg/day as tolerated.
Drug-Food: Concurrent **grapefruit** may ↑ blood levels and the risk of toxicity and should be avoided.

Route/Dosage

PO (Adults): 1250 mg (5 tablets) once daily for 21 days.

Hepatic Impairment

PO (Adults): *Severe hepatic impairment*—750 mg/day.

Availability

Tablets: 250 mg.

NURSING IMPLICATIONS

Assessment

- Evaluate left ventricular ejection fraction (LVEF) prior to therapy to determine if within institution's normal limits. Continue to monitor periodically during therapy to ensure it does not fall below limits. If LVEF decreases to Grade 2 or greater discontinue therapy. If it returns to normal and patient is asymptomatic after 2 wks, may restart therapy at a reduced dose of 1000 mg/day.
- Monitor ECG prior to and periodically during therapy to monitor QT.
- Monitor for respiratory status for symptoms of interstitial lung disease and pneumonitis (dyspnea, cough); may require discontinuation of therapy.
- ***Lab Test Considerations:*** Monitor serum potassium and magnesium prior to and periodically during therapy.

Potential Nursing Diagnoses

Diarrhea (Adverse Reactions)

Implementation

- Administer anti-diarrheals prior to therapy to prevent severe diarrhea.
- Correct hypokalemia and hypomagnesemia prior to therapy.
- **PO:** Administer 5 tablets once daily at least 1 hr before or 1 hr after a meal for 21 days. Capecitabine is taken with food or 30 min after meals twice daily.

Patient/Family Teaching

- Instruct patient to take lapatinib as directed and to review the *Patient Information Sheet* prior to therapy and with each refill for new information If a dose is missed take as soon remembered that day. If a day is missed, skip the dose; do not double doses. Caution patient not to share this medication with others, even with same condition; may be harmful.
- Advise patient to avoid drinking grapefruit juice or eating grapefruit during therapy.
- Advise patient to report signs or decreased LVEF (shortness of breath, palpitations, fatigue) to health care professional promptly.
- Instruct patient to notify health care professional before taking any Rx, OTC, or herbal products during therapy.
- Advise patient that lapatinib may cause diarrhea, which may become severe. Instruct patient in how to prevent and manage diarrhea.
- Advise female patients to notify health care professional if pregnancy is planned or suspected; therapy may be teratogenic.

Evaluation/Desired Outcomes

- Decreased/slowed spread of metastatic breast cancer.

L

leflunomide (le-flu-noe-mide)

Arava

Classification
Therapeutic: antirheumatics (DMARDs)
Pharmacologic: immune response modifiers

Pregnancy Category X

Indications

Rheumatoid arthritis (disease-modifying agent).

Action

Inhibits an enzyme required for pyrimidine synthesis; has antiproliferative and anti-inflammatory effects. **Therapeutic Effects:** Decreased pain and inflammation, slowed structural progression and improved physical function.

Pharmacokinetics

Absorption: Tablets are 80% absorbed following oral administration; rapidly converted to the M1 metabolite, which is responsible for pharmacologic activity.
Distribution: Crosses the placenta.
Protein Binding: 99%.

Metabolism and Excretion: Extensively metabolized with metabolites excreted in urine (43%) and feces (48%). Also undergoes biliary recycling.
Half-life: 14–18 days.

TIME/ACTION PROFILE (antirheumatic effect)

ROUTE	ONSET	PEAK	DURATION
PO	1 mo	3–6 mo	wks–mos†

†Due to persistence of active metabolite

Contraindications/Precautions

Contraindicated in: Hypersensitivity; OB: Women who are or may become pregnant; Compromised immune function, including bone marrow dysplasia or severe uncontrolled infection; Concurrent vaccination with live vaccines; Pedi: Children <18 yr; OB: Lactation.
Use Cautiously in: Renal insufficiency; OB: Women with childbearing potential; OB: Men attempting to father a child.
Exercise Extreme Caution in: Significant hepatic impairment, including positive serology for hepatitis B or C; or concurrent use of other hepatotoxic agents (↑ risk of hepatotoxicity).

Adverse Reactions/Side Effects

CNS: headache, dizziness, weakness. **Resp:** bronchitis, increased cough, pharyngitis, pneumonia, respiratory infection, rhinitis, sinusitis. **CV:** chest pain, hypertension. **GI:** diarrhea, nausea, abdominal pain, abnormal liver enzymes, hepatotoxicity (rare), anorexia, dyspepsia, gastroenteritis, mouth ulcers, vomiting. **GU:** urinary tract infection. **Derm:** alopecia, rash, dry skin, eczema, pruritus. **F and E:** hypokalemia. **Metab:** weight loss. **MS:** arthralgia, back pain, joint disorder, leg cramps, synovitis, tenosynovitis. **Neuro:** paresthesia. **Misc:** allergic reactions, flu syndrome, infections including SEPSIS, pain.

Interactions

Drug-Drug: Cholestyramine and **activated charcoal** cause a rapid and significant ↓ in blood levels of active metabolite. Concurrent use of **methotrexate** and other **hepatotoxic drugs** ↑ risk of hepatotoxicity. Concurrent administration of **rifampin** ↑ blood levels of the active metabolite. May ↑ risk of bleeding with **warfarin**.

Route/Dosage

PO (Adults): *Loading dose*—100 mg daily for 3 days; *maintenance dosing*—20 mg/day (if intolerance occurs, dose may be decreased to 10 mg/day).

Availability

Tablets: 10 mg, 20 mg, 100 mg.

NURSING IMPLICATIONS

Assessment

- Assess range of motion and degree of swelling and pain in affected joints before and periodically during therapy.
- ***Lab Test Considerations:*** Monitor liver function throughout therapy. Assess ALT at baseline, then monthly during initial 6 mo of therapy, then every 6–8 wks. If given concurrently with methotrexate, monitor ALT, AST, and serum albumin monthly. May cause ↑ ALT and AST, which are usually reversible with reduction in dose or discontinuation, but may be fatal. If ALT is 2–3 times the upper limit of normal, reduce dose to 10 mg/day and continue therapy. Monitor closely after dose reduction; plasma levels may not ↓ for several weeks due to long half-life. If ALT ↑ of 2–3 times the upper limit of normal persists despite dose reduction or if ALT >3 times the upper limit of normal occurs, discontinue leflunomide and administer cholestyramine (see Toxicity and Overdose). Monitor closely and readminister cholestyramine as indicated.
- Monitor CBC with platelets monthly for 6 mo following initiation of therapy and every 6–8 wks thereafter. If used with methotrexate or other immunosuppressive therapy continue monitoring monthly. If bone marrow depression occurs, discontinue leflunomide and begin decreasing levels with cholestyramine (see Implementation).
- May rarely cause ↑ of alkaline phosphatase and bilirubin.
- ***Toxicity and Overdose:*** If overdose or significant toxicity occurs, cholestyramine 8 g 3 times a day for 24 hr, or activated charcoal orally or via nasogastric tube, 50 g every 6 hr for 24 hr, is recommended to accelerate elimination.

Potential Nursing Diagnoses

Impaired physical mobility (Indications)
Acute pain (Indications)

Implementation

- **PO:** Initiate therapy with loading dose of 100 mg/day for 3 days, followed by 20 mg/day dose. May decrease to 10 mg/day if not well tolerated.

- **Drug Elimination Procedure:** Recommended to achieve nondectable plasma levels <0.02 mg/L after stopping treatment with leflunomide. Administer cholestyramine 8 g 3 times daily for 11 days. (Days do not need to be consecutive unless rapid lowering of levels is desired.) Verify plasma levels <0.02 mg/L by 2 separate tests at least 14 days apart. If plasma levels >0.02 mg/L, consider additional cholestyramine treatment. Plasma levels may take up to 2 yr to reach nondetectable levels without drug elimination procedure.

Patient/Family Teaching

- Instruct patient to take leflunomide as directed.
- May cause dizziness. Caution patient to avoid driving or other activities requiring alertness until response to medication is known.
- Caution patients of childbearing age that leflunomide has teratogenic effects. Women wishing to become pregnant must undergo the drug elimination procedure (see Implementation) and verify that the M1 metabolite plasma levels are <0.02 mg/L. Men wishing to father a child should also take cholestyramine 8 g 3 times daily for 11 days to minimize any possible risk.
- Advise patient to consult health care professional prior to taking other medications or herbal products concurrently with leflunomide. Aspirin, NSAIDs, or low-dose corticosteroids may be continued during therapy, but other agents for treatment of rheumatoid arthritis may require discontinuation.
- Discuss the possibility of hair loss with patient. Explore methods of coping.
- Instruct patient to avoid vaccinations with live vaccines during and following therapy without consulting health care professional.

Evaluation/Desired Outcomes

- Decrease in signs and symptoms of rheumatoid arthritis and slowing of structural damage as evidenced by x-ray erosions and joint narrowings.
- Improved physical function.

lepirudin (rDNA)

(le-**peer**-yoo-din)
Refludan

Classification
Therapeutic: anticoagulants
Pharmacologic: thrombin inhibitors

Pregnancy Category B

Indications

Management of thromboembolic disease and prevention of its complications in patients who have experienced heparin-induced thrombocytopenia.

Action

Acts as an anticoagulant by inhibiting the action of thrombin. Produced by recombinant DNA technology. **Therapeutic Effects:** Anticoagulation with prevention of thromboembolic complications.

Pharmacokinetics

Absorption: IV administration results in complete bioavailability.
Distribution: Distributes mainly to extracellular fluids.
Metabolism and Excretion: Metabolized by release of amino acids caused by breakdown of drug; 48% excreted unchanged in urine.
Half-life: 1.3 hr.

TIME/ACTION PROFILE (anticoagulant effect)

ROUTE	ONSET	PEAK	DURATION
IV	within 30–90 min	unknown	up to 24 hr

Contraindications/Precautions

Contraindicated in: Hypersensitivity.
Use Cautiously in: Recent puncture of large vessels/organ biopsy; Vessel/organ anomaly; Recent CVA, stroke, intracerebral surgery or other neuroaxial procedure; Severe uncontrolled hypertension; Severe renal impairment (CCr <15 ml/min); Bacterial endocarditis; Hemorrhagic diatheses; Recent major surgery; Recent major bleeding; Severe liver impairment; Moderate renal impairment (reduced bolus and maintenance infusion rate recommended if CCr 15<50 ml/min); Pregnancy, lactation or children (safety not established).

Adverse Reactions/Side Effects

Hemat: BLEEDING. **Misc:** allergic reactions including ANAPHYLAXIS.

L

🍁 = Canadian drug name.
*CAPITALS indicates life-threatening; underlines indicate most frequent.

Interactions

Drug-Drug: ↑ risk of bleeding with **thrombolytic agents**, **NSAIDs**, **valproic acid**, **cefotetan**, **cefoperazone**, **platelet aggregation inhibitors** including **aspirin**, **dipyridamole**, **clopidogrel**, **ticlopidine**, **tirofiban**, and **eptifibatide**.

Route/Dosage

IV (Adults): 0.4 mg/kg (not to exceed 44 mg) as a bolus over 15–20 sec, followed by 0.15 mg/kg/hr (not to exceed 16.5 mg/hr) initially, further adjustments made on the basis of laboratory assessment (aPTT) but should not exceed infusion rate of 0.21 mg/kg/hr without checking for coagulation abnormalities.

Renal Impairment

IV (Adults): 0.2 mg/kg as a bolus over 15–20 sec, then if *CCr 45–60 ml/min*—0.075 mg/kg/hr; if *CCr 30–44 ml/min*—0.045 mg/kg/hr; if *CCr 15–29 ml/min*—0.0225 mg/kg/hr.

Availability

Powder for injection: 50 mg/vial.

NURSING IMPLICATIONS

Assessment

- Assess patient for signs of bleeding and hemorrhage (bleeding gums, nosebleed, unusual bruising, black tarry stools, hematuria, fall in hematocrit or blood pressure, guaiac-positive stools). Notify physician if these occur.
- Monitor patient for hypersensitivity reactions (chills, fever, urticaria). Report signs to physician.
- ***Lab Test Considerations:*** Dose is adjusted according to aPTT ratio (patient aPTT at a given time over aPTT reference value, usually median of laboratory normal range for aPTT). Target range for aPTT ratio during treatment should be 1.5–2.5.
- Determine baseline aPTT prior to therapy; therapy should not be started in patients with an aPTT ratio of >2.5.
- First aPTT should be drawn 4 hr after initiation of therapy, then at least daily during therapy. More frequent monitoring is required in patients with serious liver injury or renal impairment.
- If aPTT ratio is out of target range, confirm ratio before modifying dose, unless clinically necessitated. If the confirmed ratio is above the target range, stop infusion for 2 hr. Restart infusion at 50% of previous dose without bolus and determine aPTT ratio in 4 hr.
- If confirmed ratio is below target range, increase infusion in steps of 20% and determine ratio in 4 hr.
- ***Toxicity and Overdose:*** If life-threatening bleeding occurs and excessive plasma levels of lepirudin are suspected, immediately stop infusion, determine aPTT and other coagulation levels, determine hemoglobin and prepare for blood transfusion. No specific antidote for lepirudin is available.

Potential Nursing Diagnoses

Ineffective tissue perfusion (Indications)
Risk for injury (Side Effects)

Implementation

- Inform all personnel caring for patient of anticoagulant therapy. Venipunctures and injection sites require application of pressure to prevent bleeding or hematoma formation. IM injections of other medications should be avoided, as hematomas may develop.
- In patients scheduled to receive coumadin derivatives for oral anticoagulation, lepirudin dose should be gradually decreased to reach an aPTT ratio just above 1.5 before initiating oral anticoagulant therapy.

IV Administration

- **Direct IV:** ***Diluent:*** Reconstitute each vial with 1 ml of sterile water for injection or 0.9% NaCl. Shake gently. Transfer contents of vial into a 10-ml syringe and dilute to a total volume of 10 ml with sterile water for injection, 0.9% NaCl, or D5W. Clear, colorless solution should be obtained within a few seconds to 3 min. Do not use solutions that are cloudy or contain particulate matter. Solution is stable for 24 hr at room temperature. ***Concentration:*** 5 mg/ml. ***Rate:*** Administer slowly over 15–20 sec.
- **Continuous Infusion:** ***Diluent:*** Reconstitute 2 vials (50 mg each) with 1 ml each of sterile water for injection or 0.9% NaCl. Transfer the contents into an infusion bag containing 500 ml or 250 ml of 0.9% NaCl or D5W. Solution is stable for 24 hr at room temperature. ***Concentration:*** 0.2–0.4 mg/ml. ***Rate:*** Based on patient's weight (see Route/Dosage section). Use an infusion pump to ensure accuracy.
- **Y-Site Compatibility:** amiodarone.

Patient/Family Teaching

- Advise patient to report any symptoms of unusual bleeding or bruising to health care professional immediately.

- Caution patient to avoid IM injections and activities leading to injury and to use a soft toothbrush and electric razor during therapy.

Evaluation/Desired Outcomes

- Range of aPTT ratio from 1.5–2.5, without signs of hemorrhage.
- Treatment and prevention of thromboembolic disease and its sequelae.

letrozole (let-roe-zole)

Femara

Classification

Therapeutic: antineoplastics

Pharmacologic: aromatase inhibitors

Pregnancy Category D

Indications

First-line treatment of post-menopausal women with hormone receptor positive or hormone receptor unknown metastatic or advanced breast cancer. Advanced breast cancer in postmenopausal patients with disease progression despite antiestrogen therapy. Extended adjuvant treatment of post-menopausal early breast cancer already treated with 5 yr of tamoxifen.

Action

Inhibits the enzyme aromatase, which is partially responsible for conversion of precursors to estrogen. **Therapeutic Effects:** Lowers levels of circulating estrogen, which may halt progression of estrogen-sensitive breast cancer. Decreased risk of recurrence/metastatic disease.

Pharmacokinetics

Absorption: Rapidly and completely absorbed.
Distribution: Unknown.
Metabolism and Excretion: Mostly metabolized by the liver.
Half-life: 2 days.

TIME/ACTION PROFILE (effect on lowering of serum estradiol levels)

ROUTE	ONSET	PEAK	DURATION
PO	unknown	2–3 days	unknown

Contraindications/Precautions

Contraindicated in: Hypersensitivity; Premenopausal women; OB: Pregnancy.
Use Cautiously in: Severe hepatic impairment; OB, Pedi: Lactation or children (safety not established).

Adverse Reactions/Side Effects

CNS: anxiety, depression, dizziness, drowsiness, fatigue, headache, vertigo, weakness. **Resp:** coughing, dyspnea, pleural effusion. **CV:** chest pain, edema, hypertension, cerebrovascular events, thromboembolic events. **GI:** nausea, abdominal pain, anorexia, constipation, diarrhea, dyspepsia, vomiting. **Derm:** alopecia, hot flashes, increased sweating, pruritus, rash. **F and E:** hypercalcemia. **Metab:** hypercholesterolemia, weight gain. **MS:** musculoskeletal pain, arthralgia, fractures.

Interactions

Drug-Drug: None significant.

Route/Dosage

PO (Adults): 2.5 mg daily.

Availability

Tablets: 2.5 mg.

NURSING IMPLICATIONS

Assessment

- Assess patient for pain and other side effects periodically throughout therapy.
- ***Lab Test Considerations:*** May cause elevated GTT and cholesterol levels.

Potential Nursing Diagnoses

Acute pain (Side Effects)

Implementation

- **PO:** May be taken without regard to food.

Patient/Family Teaching

- Instruct patient to take medication as directed.
- Inform patient of potential for adverse reactions and advise her to notify health care professional if side effects are problematic.
- Caution women who are perimenopausal or who recently became menopausal to use adequate contraception during therapy; letrozole may cause fetal harm.

Evaluation/Desired Outcomes

- Slowing of disease progression in women with advanced breast cancer.
- Decreased risk of recurrence/metastatic disease.

leucovorin calcium

(loo-koe-**vor**-in)

citrovorum factor, folinic acid, Wellcovorin

Classification

Therapeutic: antidotes (for methotrexate), vitamins

Pharmacologic: folic acid analogues

Pregnancy Category C

Indications

Minimizes hematologic effects of high-dose methotrexate therapy (leucovorin rescue). Advanced colorectal carcinoma (with 5-fluorouracil). Management of overdoses/prevention of toxicity from folic acid antagonists (pyrimethamine, trimethoprim, trimetrexate). Folic acid deficiency (megaloblastic anemia) unresponsive to oral replacement.

Action

The reduced form of folic acid that serves as a cofactor in the synthesis of DNA and RNA. **Therapeutic Effects:** Reversal of toxic effects of folic acid antagonists. Reversal of folic acid deficiency.

Pharmacokinetics

Absorption: Well absorbed (38%) following PO administration. Bioavailability decreases with larger doses. Oral absorption is saturated at doses >25 mg.

Distribution: Widely distributed. Concentrates in the CNS and liver.

Metabolism and Excretion: Extensively converted to tetrahydrofolic derivatives, including 5-methyltetrahydrofolate, a major storage form.

Half-life: 3.5 hr.

TIME/ACTION PROFILE (serum folate levels)

ROUTE	ONSET	PEAK	DURATION
PO	20–30 min	unknown	3–6 hr
IM	10–20 min	unknown	3–6 hr
IV	<5 min	unknown	3–6 hr

Contraindications/Precautions

Contraindicated in: Hypersensitivity; Preparations containing benzyl alcohol should not be used in neonates.

Use Cautiously in: Undiagnosed anemia (may mask the progression of pernicious anemia); Pregnancy and lactation (safety not established but has been used safely to treat megaloblastic anemia in pregnancy); Coadministration with high-dose methotrexate requires crucial timing of dosing and knowledge of methotrexate levels; Ascites; Renal failure; Dehydration; Pleural effusions; Urine pH <7.

Adverse Reactions/Side Effects

Hemat: thrombocytosis (intra-arterial methotrexate only). **Misc:** allergic reactions (rash, urticaria, wheezing).

Interactions

Drug-Drug: May ↓ anticonvulsant effect of **barbiturates**, **phenytoin**, or **primidone**. High doses of the liquid contain significant **alcohol** and may cause ↑ CNS depression when used with **CNS depressants**. Concurrent use with **trimethoprim/sulfamethoxazole** may result in ↓ anti-infective efficacy and poor therapeutic outcome when used to treat *Pneumocystis carinii* pneumonia in HIV patients. May ↑ therapeutic effects and toxicity of **fluorouracil**; therapy may be combined for this purpose.

Route/Dosage

High-Dose Methotrexate—Leucovorin Rescue. Must start within 24 hr of methotrexate.

PO, IM, IV (Adults and Children): *Normal methotrexate elimination*—10 mg/m² q 6 hr (1st dose IV/IM, then change to PO) until methotrexate level is $<5 \times 10^{-8}$ M (0.05 micromolar). Larger doses/longer duration may be required in patients with aciduria, ascites, dehydration, renal impairment, GI obstruction, pleural/peritoneal effusions. Dose of leucovorin should be determined on the basis of plasma methotrexate levels.

Advanced Colorectal Cancer

IV (Adults): 200 mg/m² followed by 5-fluorouracil 370 mg/m² or leucovorin 20 mg/m² is followed by 5-fluorouracil 425 mg/m². Regimen is given daily for 5 days q 4–5 wk.

Prevention of Hematologic Toxicity from Trimetrexate

PO, IV (Adults and Children): 20 mg/m² q 6 hr continued for 72 hr after last trimetrexate dose (oral doses should be rounded up to the next 25 mg); both trimetrexate and leucovorin doses require adjustment for hematologic toxicity.

Prevention of Hematologic Toxicity from Pyrimethamine

PO, IV (Adults and Children): 5–15 mg/day.

Inadvertent Overdose of Folic Acid Antagonists

IM, IV (Adults and Children): *Methotrexate–large doses*—75 mg IV followed by 12 mg IM q 6 hr for 4 doses; *methotrexate–average doses*—6–12 mg IM q 6 hr for 4 doses; *other folic acid antagonists*—amount equal in mg to folic acid antagonist.

Megaloblastic Anemia

PO, IM, IV (Adults and Children): Up to 1 mg/day (up to 6 mg/day for dihydrofolate reductase deficiency).

Availability (generic available)

Tablets: 5 mg, 10 mg, 15 mg, 25 mg. **Solution for injection:** 3 mg/ml in 1-ml ampules, 5 mg/ml. **Powder for injection:** 50-, 100-, and 350-mg vials.

NURSING IMPLICATIONS

Assessment

- Assess patient for nausea and vomiting secondary to methotrexate therapy or folic acid antagonists (pyrimethamine and trimethoprim) overdose. Parenteral route may be necessary to ensure that patient receives dose.
- Monitor for development of allergic reactions (rash, urticaria, wheezing). Notify physician if these occur.
- **Megaloblastic Anemia:** Assess degree of weakness and fatigue.
- **Leucovorin rescue:** Monitor serum methotrexate levels to determine dosage and effectiveness of therapy. Leucovorin calcium levels should be equal to or greater than methotrexate level. Rescue continues until serum methotrexate level is <5 × 10M.
- Monitor CCr and serum creatinine prior to and every 24 hr during therapy to detect methotrexate toxicity. An increase >50% over the pretreatment concentration at 24 hr is associated with severe renal toxicity.
- Monitor urine pH every 6 hr during therapy; pH should be maintained >7 to decrease nephrotoxic effects of high-dose methotrexate. Sodium bicarbonate or acetazolamide may be ordered to alkalinize urine.
- *Megaloblastic anemia*—Monitor plasma folic acid levels, hemoglobin, hematocrit, and reticulocyte count prior to and periodically during therapy.

Potential Nursing Diagnoses

Risk for injury (Indications)
Imbalanced nutrition: less than body requirements (Indications)

Implementation

- Do not confuse folinic acid (leucovorin calcium) with folic acid. Do not confuse leucovorin with leukeran (chlorambucil) or leukine (sargramostim).
- Make sure leucovorin calcium is available before administering high-dose methotrexate. Administration must be initiated within 24 hr of methotrexate therapy.
- Administer as soon as possible after toxic dose of folic acid antagonists (pyrimethamine and trimethoprim). Effectiveness of therapy begins to decrease 1 hr after overdose.
- **PO:** Parenteral therapy should be used in patients with GI toxicity, with nausea and vomiting, or with doses >25 mg.
- **IM:** IM route is preferred for treatment of megaloblastic anemia. Ampules of leucovorin calcium injection for IM use do not require reconstitution.

IV Administration

- **Direct IV:** ***Diluent:*** To reconstitute 50-mg vial of leucovorin calcium for injection, add 5 ml of bacteriostatic water or sterile water for injection for a concentration of 10 mg/ml. Use 10-ml diluent for 100-mg vial. The 350-mg vial should be reconstituted with 17 ml of diluent for a concentration of 20 mg/ml. If dose is >10 mg/m^2, do not use product containing benzyl alcohol. Use immediately if reconstituted with sterile water for injection. Stable for 7 days when reconstituted with bacteriostatic water. ***Concentration:*** 10 mg/ml. ***Rate:*** Rate should not exceed 160 mg/min.
- **Intermittent Infusion:** May be diluted in 100–500 ml of D5W, D10W, 0.9% NaCl, Ringer's or LR. Stable for 24 hr
- **Y-Site Compatibility:** amifostine, aztreonam, bleomycin, cefepime, cisplatin, cladribine, cyclophosphamide, docetaxel, doxorubicin, doxorubicin liposome, etoposide phosphate, filgrastim, fluconazole, fluorouracil, furosemide, gemcitabine, granisetron, heparin, linezolid, methotrexate, metoclopramide, mitomycin, oxaliplatin, piperacil-

lin/tazobactam, tacrolimus, teniposide, thiotepa, vinblastine, vincristine.

- **Y-Site Incompatibility:** amphotericin B cholesteryl sulfate complex, droperidol, foscarnet, lansoprazole, sodium bicarbonate.

Patient/Family Teaching

- Explain purpose of medication to patient. Emphasize need to take exactly as ordered. Advise patient to contact health care professional if a dose is missed.
- **Leucovorin Rescue:** Instruct patient to drink at least 3 liters of fluid each day during leucovorin rescue.
- **Folic Acid Deficiency:** Encourage patient to eat a diet high in folic acid (meat proteins; bran; dried beans; and green, leafy vegetables).

Evaluation/Desired Outcomes

- Reversal of bone marrow and GI toxicity in patients receiving methotrexate or in overdose of folic acid antagonists.
- Increased sense of well-being and increased production of normoblasts in patients with megaloblastic anemia.

leuprolide (loo-proe-lide)

Eligard, Lupron, Lupron Depot, Lupron Depot-PED, Lupron Depot-3 Month, Viadur

Classification

Therapeutic: antineoplastics

Pharmacologic: hormones, gonadotropin-releasing hormones

Pregnancy Category X

Indications

Injection, depot or implant: Advanced prostate cancer in patients who are unable to tolerate orchiectomy or estrogen therapy (may be used in combination with flutamide or bicalutamide): Management of central precocious puberty (CPP). **3.75-mg depot only:** Endometriosis: Uterine fibroids (with iron therapy).

Action

A synthetic analogue of luteinizing hormone–releasing hormone (LHRH). Initially causes a transient increase in testosterone; however, with continuous administration, testosterone levels are decreased. Reduces gonadotropins, testosterone, and estradiol. **Therapeutic Effects:** Decreased testosterone levels and resultant decrease in spread of prostate cancer. Reduction of pain/lesions in endometriosis. Decreased growth of fibroids. Delayed puberty.

Pharmacokinetics

Absorption: Rapidly and almost completely absorbed following subcut administration. More slowly absorbed following IM administration of depot form; consistent levels maintained following implant.

Distribution: Unknown.

Metabolism and Excretion: Unknown.

Half-life: 3 hr.

TIME/ACTION PROFILE (effect on hormone levels)

ROUTE	ONSET†	PEAK‡	DURATION§
Subcut	within 1st week	2–4 wk	4–12 wk
IM	within 1st week	2–4 wk	4–12 wk
IM-depot	within 1st week	2–4 wk	4–12 wk
implant	3 days	2 wk	12 mos

†Initial transient increase in testosterone and estradiol levels

‡Maximum decline in testosterone and estradiol levels

§Restoration of normal pituitary–gonadal function; in amenorrheic patients, normal menses usually returns 60–90 days after treatment is discontinued

Contraindications/Precautions

Contraindicated in: Intolerance to synthetic analogues of LHRH (GnRH); Pregnancy or lactation (depot form).

Use Cautiously in: Hypersensitivity to benzyl alcohol (results in induration and erythema at subcut site).

Adverse Reactions/Side Effects

CNS: dizziness, headache, syncope; *depot*— drowsiness, personality disorder; *Subcut*— anxiety, blurred vision, lethargy, memory disorder, mood swings; *implant*— insomnia. **EENT:** blurred vision; *Subcut*— hearing disorder. **Resp:** hemoptysis; *depot*— epistaxis, throat nodules; *Subcut*— cough, pleural rub, pulmonary fibrosis, pulmonary infiltrate. **CV:** MI, PULMONARY EMBOLI, angina, arrhythmias; *depot*— vasodilation; *Subcut*— transient ischemic attack/stroke; *implant*— edema. **GI:** anorexia, diarrhea, dysphagia, nausea, vomiting; *depot*— gingivitis; *Subcut*— GI BLEEDING, hepatic dysfunction, peptic ulcer, rectal polyps, taste disorders. **GU:** decreased testicular size, dysuria, incontinence, testicular pain; *depot*— cervix disorder; *Subcut*— bladder spasm, penile swelling, prostate pain, urinary obstruction. **Derm:** *depot*— hair growth, rash; *Subcut*— dry skin, hair loss, pigmentation, skin cancer, skin lesions. **Endo:** breast swelling, breast tenderness, diabetes. **F and E:** hypercalcemia, lower extremity edema. **Local:** burning, itching, swelling at injection site; *implant*— pain. **Hemat:** *implant*— anemia. **Metab:** *depot*— hyperuricemia, increased bone density. **MS:** fibromyalgia, transient increase in bone pain (prostate cancer only); *Subcut*— ankylosing spondylitis, joint pain, pelvic fibrosis, temporal bone pain. **Neuro:** *Subcut*— peripheral neuropathy. **Misc:** hot flashes, chills, decreased libido, fever; *depot*— body odor, epistaxis.

Interactions

Drug-Drug: ↑ antineoplastic effects with **antiandrogens (megestrol, flutamide)**.

Route/Dosage

Prostate Cancer

Subcut (Adults): 1 mg/day *or* 7.5 mg once monthly, 22.5 mg every 3 mo, 30 mg every 4 mo or 45 mg every 6 mo as long-acting/depot injection.
IM (Adults): 7.5 mg once monthly, 22.5 mg every 3 mo or 30 mg every 4 mo.
Implant (Adults): one implant (72 mg) every 12 months.

Endometriosis/Fibroids

IM (Adults): 3.75 mg once monthly, or 11.25 every 3 mo, or 30 mg every 4 mo.

Central Precocious Puberty (CPP)

Subcut (Children): 50 mcg/kg/day, may be increased by 10 mcg/kg/day as required.
IM (Children >37.5 kg): 15 mg q 4 wk.
IM (Children 25–37.5 kg): 11.25 mg q 4 wk.
IM (Children ≤25 kg): 7.5 mg q 4 wk.

Availability (generic available)

Solution for injection (Lupron and others): 5 mg/ml in 2.8-ml vial. **Lyophilized microspheres for depot injection (Lupron Depot):** 3.75-mg single-use vial, 7.5-mg single-use vial. **Lyophilized microspheres for pediatric depot injection (Lupron Depot-Ped):** 7.5-mg, 11.25-mg, 15—mg single-use kits. **Lyophilized microspheres for 3-mo depot injection (Lupron Depot—3 month):** 22.5-mg single-use kits. **Lyophilized microspheres for 4-mo depot injection (Lupron Depot—4 month:** 30 mg. **Polymeric matrix injectable formulation for subcut use (Eligard):** 7.5 mg, 22.5 mg, 30 mg, 45 mg. **Implant (Viadur):** 72 mg.

NURSING IMPLICATIONS

Assessment

- **Prostate Cancer:** Assess patient for an increase in bone pain, especially during the first few weeks of therapy. Monitor patients with vertebral metastases for increased back pain and decreased sensory/motor function.
- Monitor intake and output ratios; assess for bladder distention in patients with urinary tract obstruction during initiation of therapy.
- **Fibroids:** Assess patient for severity of symptoms (bloating, pelvic pain, pressure, excessive vaginal bleeding) periodically during therapy.
- **Endometriosis:** Assess patient for endometrial pain prior to and periodically during therapy.
- **CPP:** Prior to therapy, diagnosis of CPP should be confirmed by onset of secondary sex characteristics in girls <8 yr or boys <9 yr; a complete physical and endocrinologic examination, including height, weight, hand and wrist x-ray; total sex steroid level (estradiol or testosterone); adrenal steroid level; beta human chorionic gonadotropin level; GnRH stimulation test; and computerized tomography of the head must be performed. These parameters are monitored after 1–2 mo and every 6–12 mo during therapy.
- Assess patient for signs of precocious puberty (menses, breast development, testicular growth) periodically during therapy. Dose is increased until no progression of the disease is noted either clinically or by lab test parameters, then usually maintained throughout therapy. Discontinuation of therapy should be considered before age 11 in girls and age 12 in boys.
- ***Lab Test Considerations:*** Initially ↑, then ↓ luteinizing hormone (LH) and follicle-stimulating hormone (FSH). This leads to castration levels of testosterone in boys 2–4 wk after initial increase in concentrations.
- Monitor testosterone, prostatic acid phosphate, and prostate-specific antigen (PSA) levels to evaluate response to therapy. Tran-

sient ↑ in levels may occur during the 1st month of therapy for prostate cancer.
- May cause ↑ BUN, serum calcium, uric acid, hypoproteinemia, LDH, alkaline phosphatase, AST, hyperglycemia, hyperlipidemia, hyperphosphatemia, WBC, PT, or PTT. May also cause ↓ platelets and serum potassium.

Potential Nursing Diagnoses
Sexual dysfunction (Side Effects)

Implementation
- **Subcut:** *Eligard subcut formulation:* Bring to room temperature before mixing. Assemble the Eligard kit and reconstitute solution using syringes provided, as directed by manufacturer. Mix in syringes as directed by manufacturer, do not shake. Solution must reach room temperature before administration and must be administered within 30 min of mixing, or be discarded. Solution is light tan to tan in color. Inject into abdomen, upper buttocks, or anywhere that has adequate amounts of subcut tissue without excessive pigment, nodules, lesions, or hair. Vary site with each injection.
- **IM:** Use syringe supplied by manufacturer. Rotate sites.
- Leuprolide depot is *only* for IM injection.
- *Lupron Depot formulation:* To reconstitute a single vial, use a 22-gauge needle; withdraw 1 ml of diluent and inject into vial to mix. To mix 2 or more vials, withdraw 0.5 ml and inject into each vial for a total volume of 1 ml. Do not use vial if clumping or caking of microspheres (powder) is evident. Shake each vial well; suspension will appear milky. Withdraw entire contents of all vials into syringe and inject immediately. Patients may store medication at room temperature.
- Store at room temperature; stable for 24 hr following reconstitution.
- *12-mo implant:* Implant is inserted in the inner aspect of the upper arm and provides continuous release of leuprolide for 12 mo. At the end of 12 mo, implant must be removed; a new implant may be inserted for continuous therapy.

Patient/Family Teaching
- Advise patient that medication may cause hot flashes. Notify health care professional if these become bothersome.
- **Prostate Cancer:** Instruct patient and family on subcut injection technique. Review patient insert provided with leuprolide patient-administration kit.
- Instruct patient to take medication exactly as directed. If a dose is missed, take as soon as remembered unless not remembered until next day.
- Advise patient that bone pain may increase at initiation of therapy. This will resolve with time. Patient should discuss with health care professional use of analgesics to control pain
- Instruct patient to notify health care professional promptly if difficulty urinating, weakness, or numbness occurs.
- **Endometriosis:** Advise patient to use a form of contraception other than oral contraceptives during therapy. Inform patient that amenorrhea is expected but does not guarantee contraception.
- **Central Precocious Puberty:** Instruct patient and family on the proper technique for subcut injection. Emphasize the importance of administering the medication at the same time each day. Rotate injection sites periodically.
- Inform patient and parents that if injections are not given daily, pubertal process may be reactivated.
- Advise patient and parents that during the first 2 mo of therapy patient may experience a light menstrual flow or spotting. Health care professional should be notified if this continues beyond 2nd mo.
- Instruct patient and parents to notify health care professional immediately if irritation at the injection site or unusual signs or symptoms occur.

Evaluation/Desired Outcomes
- Decrease in the spread of prostate cancer.
- Decrease in lesions and pain in endometriosis.
- Resolution of the signs of CCP.
- Improvement in preoperative hematologic parameters in patients with anemia from uterine fibroids.

levalbuterol

(leev-al-**byoo**-ter-ole)
Xopenex

Classification
Therapeutic: bronchodilators
Pharmacologic: adrenergics

Pregnancy Category C

Indications

Bronchospasm due to reversible airway disease (short-term control agent).

Action

R-enantiomer of racemic albuterol. Binds to beta-2 adrenergic receptors in airway smooth muscle leading to activation of adenylcyclase and increased levels of cyclic-3', 5'-adenosine monophosphate (cAMP). Increases in cAMP activate kinases, which inhibit the phosphorylation of myosin and decrease intracellular calcium. Decreased intracellular calcium relaxes bronchial smooth muscle. **Therapeutic Effects:** Relaxation of airway smooth muscle with subsequent bronchodilation. Relatively selective for beta-2 (pulmonary) receptors.

Pharmacokinetics

Absorption: Some absorption occurs following inhalation.
Distribution: Unknown.
Metabolism and Excretion: Metabolized in the liver to an inactive sulfate and 3–6% excreted unchanged in the urine.
Half-life: 3.3–4 hr.

TIME/ACTION PROFILE (bronchodilation)

ROUTE	ONSET	PEAK	DURATION
Inhaln	10–17 min	90 min	5–6 hr

Contraindications/Precautions

Contraindicated in: Hypersensitivity to levalbuterol or albuterol.
Use Cautiously in: Cardiovascular disorders (including coronary insufficiency, hypertension, and arrhythmias); History of seizures; Hypokalemia; Hyperthyroidism; Diabetes mellitus; Unusual sensitivity to adrenergic amines; Pregnancy, lactation, or children <2 yr (safety not established).
Exercise Extreme Caution in: Concurrent use or use within 2 weeks of **tricyclic antidepressants** or **MAO inhibitors** (may increase the risk of adverse cardiovascular reactions).

Adverse Reactions/Side Effects

CNS: anxiety, dizziness, headache, nervousness. **Resp:** increased cough, paradoxical bronchospasm, turbinate edema. **CV:** tachycardia. **GI:** dyspepsia. **Endo:** hyperglycemia. **F and E:** hypokalemia. **Neuro:** tremor.

Interactions

Drug-Drug: Concurrent use or use within 2 weeks of **tricyclic antidepressants** or **MAO inhibitors** may ↑ risk of adverse cardiovascular reactions (use with extreme caution). **Beta blockers** block the beneficial pulmonary effects of adrenergic bronchodilators (choose cardioselective beta blockers if necessary and with caution). May ↑ risk of hypokalemia from **potassium-losing diuretics**. May ↓ serum **digoxin** levels. May ↑ risk of arrhythmias with **hydrocarbon inhalation anesthetics** or **cocaine**.
Drug-Natural Products: Use with caffeine-containing herbs (**guarana**, **tea**, **coffee**) ↑ stimulant effect.

Route/Dosage

Inhaln (Adults and Children >12 yr): 0.63 mg via nebulization three times daily (every 6–8 hr); may be increased to 1.25 mg three times daily (every 6–8 hr).
Inhaln (Children 6–11 yr): 0.31 mg three times daily (not exceed 0.63 mg three times daily).
Inhaln (Children 2–11 yr): 0.16–1.25 mg single doses have been used safely.

Availability

Inhalation solution: 0.31 mg/3 ml in green foil pouch containing 12 vials, 0.63 mg/3 ml in yellow foil pouch containing 12 vials, 1.25 mg/3 ml in red foil pouch containing 12 vials, 1.25 mg/0.5 ml in unit-dose vials. **Cost:** 0.31 mg/3 ml $83.76/24 vials, 0.63 mg/3 ml $84.15/24 vials, 1.25 mg/3 ml $85.00/24 vials.

NURSING IMPLICATIONS

Assessment

- Assess lung sounds, pulse, and blood pressure before administration and during peak of medication. Note amount, color, and character of sputum produced. Closely monitor patients on higher dose for adverse effects.

- Monitor pulmonary function tests before initiating therapy and periodically during course to determine effectiveness of medication.
- Observe for paradoxical bronchospasm (wheezing). If condition occurs, withhold medication and notify physician or other health care provider immediately.
- ***Lab Test Considerations:*** May cause ↑ serum glucose and ↓ serum potassium.

Potential Nursing Diagnoses
Ineffective airway clearance (Indications)

Implementation
Inhaln: Allow at least 1 min between inhalations of aerosol medication.
- For nebulization, levalbuterol solution does not require dilution prior to administration. Once the foil pouch is opened, vials must be used within 2 weeks; open vials may be stored for 1 week. Discard vial if solution is not clear or colorless.

Patient/Family Teaching
- Instruct patient in the proper use of the nebulizer (see Appendix D) and to take levalbuterol exactly as directed. Caution patient not to exceed recommended dose; may cause adverse effects, paradoxical bronchospasm, or loss of effectiveness of medication.
- Advise patient to consult health care professional before taking any OTC medications or alcohol concurrently with this therapy. Caution patient to also avoid smoking and other respiratory irritants.
- Instruct patient to contact health care professional immediately if shortness of breath is not relieved by medication or is accompanied by diaphoresis, dizziness, palpitations, or chest pain.
- Advise patients to use levalbuterol first if using other inhalation medications, and allow 5 min to elapse before administering other inhalant medications unless otherwise directed.
- Advise patient to rinse mouth with water after each inhalation dose to minimize dry mouth.
- Instruct patient to notify health care professional if no response to the usual dose of levalbuterol.

Evaluation/Desired Outcomes
- Prevention or relief of bronchospasm.

levetiracetam
(le-ve-teer-**a**-se-tam)
Keppra

Classification
Therapeutic: anticonvulsants
Pharmacologic: pyrrolidines

Pregnancy Category C

Indications
Partial onset seizures (adjunct). Primary generalized tonic-clonic seizures in patients 6 yrs of age and older. Myoclonic seizures in adults with myoclonic epilepsy (adjunct).

Action
Appears to inhibit burst firing without affecting normal neuronal excitability and may selectively prevent hypersynchronization of epileptiform burst firing and propagation of seizure activity. **Therapeutic Effects:** Decreased incidence and severity of seizures.

Pharmacokinetics
Absorption: Rapidly and completely absorbed following oral administration.
Distribution: Unknown.
Metabolism and Excretion: 66% excreted unchanged by the kidneys; some metabolism by the liver (metabolites inactive).
Half-life: 7.1 hr (increased in renal impairment).

TIME/ACTION PROFILE (blood levels)

ROUTE	ONSET	PEAK	DURATION
PO	rapid	1–1.5 hr†	12 hr

†1 hr in the fasting state, 1.5 hr when taken with food

Contraindications/Precautions
Contraindicated in: Hypersensitivity; OB: Lactation.
Use Cautiously in: Geri: Renal elimination decreased; dose reduction may be necessary; Renal impairment (dose reduction recommended if CCr ≤80 ml/minr.); Pedi: Children <4 yr (safety not established); OB: Use only during pregnancy if potential benefit justifies potential risk to fetus.

Adverse Reactions/Side Effects
CNS: dizziness, fatigue/somnolence, weakness, behavioral abnormalities. **Neuro:** coordination difficulties (adults only).

Interactions
Drug-Drug: None noted.

Route/Dosage
PO, IV (Adults): 500 mg twice daily initially; may be increased by 1000 mg/day at 2 wk intervals up to 3000 mg/day.

PO (Children 6–16 yrs): 10 mg/kg twice daily; may be increased at 2 wk intervals by 20 mg/kg increments up to 60 mg/kg/day.

Renal Impairment

PO (Adults): *CCr 50–80 ml/min*—500–1000 mg q 12 hr initially; *CCr 30–50 ml/min*—250–750 mg q 12 hr initially; *CCr <30 ml/min*—250–500 mg q 12 hr initially.

PO (Children and Adolescents 4–15 yr): 20 mg/kg/day in 2 divided doses initially, may be increased by 20 mg/kg/day every 2 wk up to 60 mg/kg/day in 2 divided doses as tolerated.

Availability

Tablets: 250 mg, 500 mg, 750 mg, 100 mg. **Cost:** 250 mg $385.94/180, 500 mg $519.93/180, 750 mg $699.95/180, 1000 mg $1,021.30/180. **Oral solution (grape-flavored):** 100 mg/ml in 480-ml bottles. **Cost:** $282.43/480 ml. **Injection:** 100 mg/mL in 5 mL vials.

NURSING IMPLICATIONS

Assessment

- Assess location, duration, and characteristics of seizure activity.
- Assess patient for CNS adverse effects throughout therapy. These adverse effects are categorized as somnolence and fatigue (asthenia), coordination difficulties (ataxia, abnormal gait, or incoordination), and behavioral abnormalities (agitation, hostility, anxiety, apathy, emotional lability, depersonalization, depression) and usually occur during the first 4 wk of therapy.
- ***Lab Test Considerations:*** May cause ↓ RBC and WBC and abnormal liver function tests.

Potential Nursing Diagnoses

Risk for injury (Side Effects)

Implementation

- Do not confuse Keppra with Kaletra (lopinavir/ritonavir).
- IV doses should be used temporarily when oral route is not feasible. To convert IV to PO, equivalent dose and frequency may be used.
- **PO:** May be administered without regard to meals.
- Administer tablets whole; do not administer partial tablets.
- Pedi: Patients <20 kg should receive oral solution. Administer with calibrated measuring device for accurate dose.
- Discontinue gradually to minimize the risk of increase in seizure frequency.

IV Administration

- **Intermittent Infusion:** ***Diluent:*** Dilute dose in 100 mL of 0.9% NaCl, D5W, or LR. Do not administer solutions that are cloudy or contain particulate matter. ***Rate:*** Infuse over 15 min.
- **Y-Site Compatibility:** diazepam, lorazepam, valproate.

Patient/Family Teaching

- Instruct patient to take medication as directed. *Pedi:* Explain to parents the importance of using calibrated measuring device for accurate dosing. Take missed doses as soon as possible unless almost time for next dose. Do not double doses. Do not discontinue abruptly; may cause increase in frequency of seizures.
- May cause dizziness and somnolence. Caution patient to avoid driving or activities requiring alertness until response to medication is known. Do not resume driving until physician gives clearance based on control of seizure disorder.
- Advise patient to notify health care professional if pregnancy is planned or suspected.
- Instruct patient to notify health care professional of medication regimen prior to treatment or surgery.
- Advise patient to carry identification describing disease process and medication regimen at all times.

Evaluation/Desired Outcomes

- Decrease in the frequency of or cessation of seizures.

levodopa (lee-voe-doe-pa)

Dopar, Larodopa, L-dopa

carbidopa/levodopa

(kar-bi-doe-pa/lee-voe-doe-pa)
Parcopa, Sinemet, Sinemet CR

Classification
Therapeutic: antiparkinson agents
Pharmacologic: dopamine agonists

Pregnancy Category, UK (levodopa), C (carbidopa/levodopa)

Indications
Parkinson's disease. Not useful for drug-induced extrapyramidal reactions.

Action
Levodopa is converted to dopamine in the CNS, where it serves as a neurotransmitter. Carbidopa, a decarboxylase inhibitor, prevents peripheral destruction of levodopa. **Therapeutic Effects:** Relief of tremor and rigidity in Parkinson's syndrome.

Pharmacokinetics
Absorption: Well absorbed following oral administration.
Distribution: Widely distributed. *Levodopa*—enters the CNS in small concentrations. *Carbidopa*—does not cross the blood-brain barrier but does cross the placenta. Both enter breast milk.
Metabolism and Excretion: *Levodopa*—mostly metabolized by the GI tract and liver. *Carbidopa*—30% excreted unchanged by the kidneys.
Half-life: *Levodopa*—1 hr; *carbidopa*—1–2 hr.

TIME/ACTION PROFILE (antiparkinson effects)

ROUTE	ONSET	PEAK	DURATION
Carbidopa	unknown	unknown	5–24 hr
Levodopa	10–15 min	unknown	5–24 hr or more
Carbidopa/levodopa sustained release	unknown	2 hr	12 hr

Contraindications/Precautions
Contraindicated in: Hypersensitivity; Angle-closure glaucoma; MAO inhibitor therapy; Malignant melanoma; Undiagnosed skin lesions; OB: Lactation; Some products contain tartrazine, phenylalanine or aspartame and should be avoided in patients with known hypersensitivity.
Use Cautiously in: History of cardiac, psychiatric, or ulcer disease; OB, Pedi: Pregnancy or children <18 yr (safety not established).

Adverse Reactions/Side Effects
CNS: <u>involuntary movements</u>, anxiety, dizziness, hallucinations, memory loss, psychiatric problems. **EENT:** blurred vision, mydriasis. **GI:** <u>nausea</u>, <u>vomiting</u>, anorexia, dry mouth, hepatotoxicity. **Derm:** melanoma. **Hemat:** hemolytic anemia, leukopenia. **Misc:** darkening of urine or sweat.

Interactions
Drug-Drug: Use with **MAO inhibitors** may result in hypertensive reactions. ↑ risk of arrhythmias with **inhalation hydrocarbon anesthetics** (especially **halothane**; if possible discontinue 6–8 hr before anesthesia). **Phenothiazines**, **haloperidol**, **papaverine**, **phenytoin**, and **reserpine** may ↓ effect of levodopa. Large doses of **pyridoxine** may ↓ beneficial effects of levodopa. Concurrent use with **methyldopa** may alter the effectiveness of levodopa and ↑ risk of CNS side effects. ↑ hypotension may result with concurrent **antihypertensives**. **Anticholinergics** may ↓ absorption of levodopa. ↑ risk of adverse reactions with **selegilene** or **cocaine**.
Drug-Natural Products: Kava kava may ↓ levodopa effectiveness.
Drug-Food: Ingestion of foods containing large amounts of **pyridoxine** may ↓ effect of levodopa.

Route/Dosage

Levodopa
PO (Adults): 250 mg 2–4 times daily; may increase by 100–750 mg q 3–7 days until desired effect is achieved (not to exceed 8 g/day).

Carbidopa/Levodopa
Tablets contain 10/100, 25/100, 25/250 mg
PO (Adults): *Patients not currently receiving levodopa*—10 mg carbidopa/100 mg levodopa 3–4 times daily or 25 mg carbidopa/100 mg levodopa 3 times daily; may be increased every 1–2 days until desired effect is achieved. *Conversion from levodopa alone (<1.5 g/day)*—25 mg carbidopa/100 mg levodopa 3–4 times daily; may be increased every 1–2 days until desired effect is achieved. *Conversion from levodopa alone (>1.5 g/day)*—25 mg carbidopa/250 mg levodopa 3–4 times daily; may be increased every 1–2 days until desired effect is achieved.

Carbidopa/Levodopa Extended-Release

Extended-release (ER) tablets contain 25/100 or 50/200 of carbidopa and levodopa, respectively

PO (Adults): *Patients not currently receiving levodopa*—50 mg carbidopa/200 mg levodopa twice daily (minimum of 6 hr apart) initially. *Conversion from levodopa alone*—initiate therapy at 25% of the daily dose of levodopa; for moderate disease start with 50 mg carbidopa/200 mg levodopa twice daily. *Conversion from standard carbidopa/levodopa*—initiate therapy with at least 10% more levodopa content/day (may need up to 30% more) given at 4–8 hr intervals while awake. Allow 3 days between dosage changes; some patients may require larger doses and shorter dosing intervals.

Availability

Levodopa

Tablets: 100 mg, 250 mg, 500 mg. **Capsules:** 100 mg, 250 mg, 500 mg.

Carbidopa/Levodopa

Tablets: 10 mg carbidopa/100 mg levodopa, 25 mg carbidopa/100 mg levodopa, 25 mg carbidopa/250 mg levodopa. **Orally-disintegrating tablets (mint):** 10 mg carbidopa/100 mg levodopa, 25 mg carbidopa/100 mg levodopa, 25 mg carbidopa/250 mg levodopa. **Extended-release tablets:** 25 mg carbidopa/100 mg levodopa, 50 mg carbidopa/200 mg levodopa. ***In combination with:*** entacapone (Stalevo[Rx]. See Appendix B).

NURSING IMPLICATIONS

Assessment

- Assess parkinsonian symptoms (akinesia, rigidity, tremors, pill rolling, shuffling gait, mask-like face, twisting motions, and drooling) during therapy. "On-off phenomenon" may cause symptoms to appear or improve suddenly.
- Assess blood pressure and pulse frequently during period of dose adjustment.
- ***Lab Test Considerations:*** May cause false-positive test results in Coombs' test, serum and urine uric acid, serum gonadotropin, urine norepinephrine, and urine protein concentrations.
- Dipstick for urine ketones may reveal false-positive results.
- Monitor hepatic and renal function and CBC periodically in patients on long-term therapy. May cause ↑ BUN, AST, ALT, bilirubin, alkaline phosphatase, LDH, and serum protein-bound iodine concentrations.
- ***Toxicity and Overdose:*** Assess for signs of toxicity (involuntary muscle twitching, facial grimacing, spasmodic eye winking, exaggerated protrusion of tongue, behavioral changes). Consult physician or other health care professional if symptoms occur.

Potential Nursing Diagnosis

Impaired physical mobility (Indications)
Risk for injury (Indications)

Implementation

- Do not confuse levodopa with methyldopa.
- In the carbidopa/levodopa combination, the number following the drug name represents the milligrams of each respective drug.
- Wait 8 hr after last levodopa dose before switching patient to carbidopa/levodopa. Carbidopa reduces the need for levodopa by 75%. Administering carbidopa shortly after a full dose of levodopa may result in toxicity.
- In preoperative patients or patients who are NPO, confer with physician or other health care professional about continuing medication administration.
- **PO:** Administer food shortly after medication to minimize gastric irritation; taking food before or concurrently may retard levodopa's effects but may be necessary to minimize GI irritation. If patient has difficulty swallowing, confer with pharmacist.
- Controlled-release tablets may be administered as whole or half tablets, but they should not be crushed or chewed.
- For *orally disintegrating tablets,* just prior to administration remove tablet from bottle with dry hands. Immediately place tablet on top of tongue. Tablet will dissolve in seconds, then swallow with saliva. Administration with liquid is not necessary.

Patient/Family Teaching

- Instruct patient to take this drug as directed. Take missed doses as soon as remembered, unless next scheduled dose is within 2 hr; do not double doses.
- Explain that gastric irritation may be decreased by eating food shortly after taking medications but that high-protein meals may

impair levodopa's effects. Dividing the daily protein intake among all the meals may help ensure adequate protein intake and drug effectiveness. Do not drastically alter diet during levodopa therapy without consulting health care professional.

- May cause drowsiness or dizziness. Advise patient to avoid driving and other activities that require alertness until response to drug is known.
- Caution patient to change positions slowly to minimize orthostatic hypotension. Health care professional should be notified if orthostatic hypotension occurs.
- Instruct patient that frequent rinsing of mouth, good oral hygiene, and sugarless gum or candy may decrease dry mouth.
- Caution patient to monitor skin lesions for any changes. Health care professional should be notified promptly because carbidopa/levodopa may activate malignant melanoma.
- Advise patient to confer with health care professional before taking OTC medications, especially cold remedies. Patients receiving only levodopa should avoid multivitamins. Large amounts of vitamin B_6 (pyridoxine) may interfere with the action of levodopa.
- Inform patient that harmless darkening of urine or sweat may occur.
- Advise patient to notify health care professional if palpitations, urinary retention, involuntary movements, behavioral changes, severe nausea and vomiting, or new skin lesions occur. Dosage reduction may be required.

Evaluation/Desired Outcomes

- Resolution of parkinsonian signs and symptoms. Therapeutic effects usually become evident after 2–3 wk of therapy but may require up to 6 mo. Patients who take this medication for several years may experience a decrease in the effectiveness of this drug. Effectiveness may sometimes be restored after a "drug holiday."

---

levofloxacin, See FLUOROQUINOLONES.

---

levonorgestrel, See CONTRACEPTIVES, HORMONAL.

---

levothyroxine, See THYROID PREPARATIONS.

HIGH ALERT

LIDOCAINE

lidocaine (parenteral)
(**lye**-doe-kane)
LidoPen, Xylocaine, ✤Xylocard

lidocaine (local anesthetic)
Xylocaine

lidocaine (mucosal)
Anestacon, Xylocaine Viscous

lidocaine patch
Lidoderm

lidocaine (topical)
L-M-X 4, L-M-X 5, Solarcaine Aloe Extra Burn Relief, Xylocaine, Zilactin-L

Classification
Therapeutic: anesthetics—topical/local, antiarrhythmics (class IB)

Pregnancy Category B

Indications

IV: Ventricular arrhythmias. **IM:** Self-injected or when IV unavailable (during transport to hospital facilities). **Local:** Infiltration/mucosal/topical anesthetic. **Patch:** Pain due to post-herpetic neuralgia.

Action

IV, IM: Suppresses automaticity and spontaneous depolarization of the ventricles during diastole by altering the flux of sodium ions across cell membranes with little or no effect on heart rate. **Local:** Produces local anesthesia by inhibiting transport of ions across neuronal membranes, thereby preventing initiation and conduction of normal nerve impulses.
Therapeutic Effects: Control of ventricular arrhythmias. Local anesthesia.

Pharmacokinetics

Absorption: Well absorbed after administration into the deltoid muscle; some absorption follows local use.
Distribution: Widely distributed. Concentrates in adipose tissue. Crosses the blood-brain barrier and placenta; enters breast milk.

Metabolism and Excretion: Mostly metabolized by the liver; <10% excreted in urine as unchanged drug.
Half-life: Biphasic—initial phase, 7–30 min; terminal phase, 90–120 min; increased in CHF and liver impairment.

TIME/ACTION PROFILE (IV, IM = antiarrhythmic effects; local = anesthetic effects)

ROUTE	ONSET	PEAK	DURATION
IV	immediate	immediate	10–20 min (up to several hours after continuous infusion)
IM	5–15 min	20–30 min	60–90 min
Local	rapid	unknown	1–3 hr

Contraindications/Precautions

Applies mainly to systemic use.
Contraindicated in: Hypersensitivity; cross-sensitivity may occur; Third-degree heart block.
Use Cautiously in: Liver disease, CHF, patients weighing <50 kg, and geriatric patients (reduce bolus and/or maintenance dose); Respiratory depression; Shock; Heart block; Pregnancy or lactation (safety not established); Children (safety not established for transdermal patch).

Adverse Reactions/Side Effects

Applies mainly to systemic use.
CNS: SEIZURES, confusion, drowsiness, blurred vision, dizziness, nervousness, slurred speech, tremor. **EENT:** *mucosal use*— decreased or absent gag reflex. **CV:** CARDIAC ARREST, arrhythmias, bradycardia, heart block, hypotension. **GI:** nausea, vomiting. **Resp:** bronchospasm. **Local:** stinging, burning, contact dermatitis, erythema. **Misc:** allergic reactions, including ANAPHYLAXIS.

Interactions

Applies mainly to systemic use.
Drug-Drug: ↑ cardiac depression and toxicity with **phenytoin, amiodarone, quinidine, procainamide**, or **propranolol**. **Cimetidine, azole antifungals, clarithromycin, erythromycin, fluoxetine, nefazodone, paroxetine, protease inhibitors, ritonavir, verapamil**, and **beta blockers** may ↓ metabolism and ↑ risk of toxicity. Lidocaine may ↑ levels of **calcium channel blockers**, certain **benzodiazepines, cyclosporine, fluoxetine, lovastatin, simvastatin, mirtazapine, paroxetine, ritonavir, tacrolimus, theophylline, tricyclic antidepressnts**, and **venlafaxine**. Effects of lidocaine may be ↓ by **carbamazepine, phenobarbital, phenytoin**, and **rifampin**.

Route/Dosage

Ventricular Tachycardia (with a Pulse) or Pulseless Ventricular Tachycardia/ Ventricular Fibrillation

IV (Adults): 1–1.5 mg/kg bolus; may repeat doses of 0.5–0.75 mg/kg q 5–10 min up to a total dose of 3 mg/kg; may then start continuous infusion of 1–4 mg/min.
Endotracheal (Adults): Give 2–2.5 times the IV loading dose down the endotracheal tube, followed by a 10-ml saline flush.
IV (Children): 1 mg/kg bolus (not to exceed 100 mg), followed by 20–50 mcg/kg/min continuous infusion (range 20–50 mcg/kg/min); may administer second bolus of 0.5–1 mg/kg if delay between bolus and continuous infusion.
Endotracheal (Children): Give 2–3 mg/kg down the endotracheal tube followed by a 5-ml saline flush.
IM (Adults and Children ≥50 kg): 300 mg (4.5 mg/kg); may be repeated in 60–90 min.

Local

Infiltration (Adults and Children): Infiltrate affected area as needed (increased amount and frequency of use increases likelihood of systemic absorption and adverse reactions).
Topical (Adults): Apply to affected area 2–3 times daily.
Mucosal (Adults): *For anesthetizing oral surfaces*—20 mg as 2 sprays/quadrant (not to exceed 30 mg/quadrant) may be used. 15 ml of the viscous solution may be used q 3 hr for oral or pharyngeal pain. *For anesthetizing the female urethra*—3–5 ml of the jelly or 20 mg as 2% solution may be used. *For anesthetizing the male urethra*—5–10 ml of the jelly or 5–15 ml of 2% solution may be used before catheterization or 30 ml of jelly before cystoscopy or similar procedures. Topical solutions may be used to anesthetize mucous membranes of the larynx, trachea, or esophagus.
Patch (Adults): Up to 3 patches may be applied once for up to 12 hr in any 24-hr period; consider smaller areas of application in geriatric or debilitated patients.

L

Availability (generic available)

Auto-injector for IM injection: 300 mg/3 ml. **Direct IV injection:** 10 mg/ml (1%), 20 mg/ml (2%). **For IV admixture:** 100 mg/ml (10%). **Premixed solution for IV infusion:** 4 mg/ml (0.4%), 8 mg/ml (0.8%). **Injection for local infiltration/nerve block:** 0.5%, 1%, 2%, 4%. ***In combination with:*** epinephrine for local infiltration. **Cream:** 4%^{OTC}. **Gel:** 0.5%^{OTC}, 2.5%^{OTC}. **Jelly:** 2%. **Liquid:** 5%. **Ointment:** 5%. **Transdermal system:** 5% patch. **Cost:** $189.98/box of 30 patches. **Solution:** 4%. **Spray:** 10%. **Viscous solution:** 2%. ***In combination with:*** prilocaine (as EMLA cream, Oraquix); with tetracaine (Synera); with bupivacaine (Duocaine); with epinephrine (LidoSite).

NURSING IMPLICATIONS

Assessment

- **Antiarrhythmic:** Monitor ECG continuously and blood pressure and respiratory status frequently during administration.
- **Anesthetic:** Assess degree of numbness of affected part.
- ***Lab Test Considerations:*** Serum electrolyte levels should be monitored periodically during prolonged therapy.
- IM administration may cause ↑ CPK levels.
- ***Toxicity and Overdose:*** Serum lidocaine levels should be monitored periodically during prolonged or high-dose IV therapy. Therapeutic serum lidocaine levels range from 1.5 to 5 mcg/ml: Signs and symptoms of toxicity include confusion, excitation, blurred or double vision, nausea, vomiting, ringing in ears, tremors, twitching, seizures, difficulty breathing, severe dizziness or fainting, and unusually slow heart rate, If symptoms of overdose occur, stop infusion and monitor patient closely.

Potential Nursing Diagnoses

Decreased cardiac output (Indications)
Acute pain (Indications)

Implementation

- ***High Alert:*** Lidocaine is readily absorbed through mucous membranes. Inadvertent overdosage of lidocaine jelly and spray has resulted in patient harm or death from neurologic and/or cardiac toxicity. Do not exceed recommended dosages.
- **Throat Spray:** Ensure that gag reflex is intact before allowing patient to drink or eat.
- **IM:** IM injections are recommended only when ECG monitoring is not available and benefits outweigh risks. Administer IM injections only into deltoid muscle while frequently aspirating to prevent IV injection.

IV Administration

- **Direct IV:** Only 1% and 2% solutions are used for direct IV injection. ***Diluent:*** Administer undiluted. ***Rate:*** Administer loading dose over 2–3 min. Follow by IV continuous infusion.
- **Continuous Infusion:** ***Diluent:*** Lidocaine vials need to be further diluted. Dilute 2 g of lidocaine in 250 ml or 500 ml of D5W or 0.9% NaCl. Admixed infusion stable for 24 hr at room temperature. Premixed infusions are already diluted and ready to use. ***Concentration:*** 4–8 mg/ml. ***Rate:*** See Route/Dosage section. Administer via infusion pump for accurate dose.
- **Y-Site Compatibility:** alteplase, amikacin, aminophylline, amiodarone, argatroban, atropine, aztreonam, bivalirudin, bumetanide, calcium chloride, calcium gluconate, cefazolin, cefotaxime, cefoxitin, ceftazidime, ceftizoxime, ceftriaxone, cefuroxime, chloramphenicol, cimetidine, ciprofloxacin, cisatracurium, clindamycin, cyclosporine, daptomycin, dexamethasone sodium phosphate, dexmedetomidine, digoxin, diltiazem, diphenhydramine, dobutamine, dopamine, doxycycline, enalaprilat, epinephrine, eptifibatide, ertapenem, erythromycin, esmolol, etomidate, famotidine, fenoldopam, fentanyl, fluconazole, furosemide, gentamicin, granisetron, haloperidol, heparin, hydrocortisone sodium succinate, imipenem/cilastatin, inamrinone, insulin, isoproterenol, ketorolac, labetalol, levofloxacin, linezolid, lorazepam, magnesium sulfate, meperidine, methylprednisolone sodium succinate, metoclopramide, metoprolol, metronidazole, micafungin, midazolam, morphine, nafcillin, nicardipine, nitroglycerin, nitroprusside, norepinephrine, ondansetron, palonosetron, penicillin G potassium, phenylephrine, phytonadione, piperacillin/tazobactam, potassium chloride, procainamide, prochlorperazine, promethazine, propofol, propranolol, protamine, quinupristin/dalfopristin, ranitidine, remifentanil, sodium bicarbonate, streptokinase, tacrolimus, theophylline, ticarcillin/clavulanate, tigecycline, tirofiban, tobramycin, van-

comycin, vasopressin, verapamil, vitamin B complex with C, voriconazole, warfarin.

- **Y-Site Incompatibility:** acyclovir, amphotericin B cholesteryl sulfate complex, caspofungin, diazepam, ganciclovir, lansoprazole, pantoprazole, phenytoin, thiopental, trimethoprim/sulfamethoxazole.
- **Infiltration:** Lidocaine with epinephrine may be used to minimize systemic absorption and prolong local anesthesia.

Patient/Family Teaching

- May cause drowsiness and dizziness. Advise patient to call for assistance during ambulation and transfer.
- **IM:** Available in LidoPen Auto-Injector for use outside the hospital setting. Advise patient to telephone health care professional immediately if symptoms of a heart attack occur. Do not administer unless instructed by health care professional. To administer, remove safety cap and place back end on thickest part of thigh or deltoid muscle. Press hard until needle prick is felt. Hold in place for 10 sec, then massage area for 10 sec. Do not drive after administration unless absolutely necessary.
- **Topical:** Apply *Lidoderm Patch* to intact skin to cover the most painful area. Patch may be cut to smaller sizes with scissors before removing release liner. Clothing may be worn over patch. If irritation or burning sensation occurs during application, remove patch until irritation subsides. Wash hands after application; avoid contact with eyes. Dispose of used patch to avoid access by children or pets.

Evaluation/Desired Outcomes

- Decrease in ventricular arrhythmias.
- Local anesthesia.

lidocaine/prilocaine

(**lye**-doe-kane/**pri**-loe-kane)
EMLA

Classification
Therapeutic: anesthetics—topical/local

Pregnancy Category B

Indications

Produces local anesthesia prior to minor painful procedures including: Insertion of cannulae or needles, Arterial/venous/lumbar puncture, Intramuscular injections, Subcutaneous injections, Dermal procedures, Laser treatments, Circumcision. When applied to genital mucous membranes in preparation for superficial minor surgery or as preparation for infiltration anesthesia.

Action

Produces local anesthesia by inhibiting transport of ions across neuronal membranes, thereby preventing initiation and conduction of normal nerve impulses. Combination of two anesthetics is applied as a system consisting of a cream under an occlusive dressing. Active drug is released into the dermal and epidermal skin layers, resulting in accumulation of local anesthetic in the regions of dermal pain receptors and nerve endings. **Therapeutic Effects:** Anesthetic action localized to the area of the application.

Pharmacokinetics

Absorption: Small amounts are systemically absorbed during 4-hr placement of EMLA system.
Distribution: Small amounts absorbed are widely distributed and cross the placenta and blood-brain barrier.
Metabolism and Excretion: *Lidocaine*—mostly metabolized by the liver. *Prilocaine*—metabolized by the liver and kidneys.
Half-life: *Lidocaine*—7–30 min first phase, 90–120 min terminal phase; *Prilocaine*—10–50 min.

TIME/ACTION PROFILE (local anesthesia)

ROUTE	ONSET	PEAK	DURATION†
Top	15 min	3 hr	1–2 hr

†Following removal of occlusive dressing

Contraindications/Precautions

Contraindicated in: Hypersensitivity to lidocaine, prilocaine, or any other amide-type local anesthetic; Hypersensitivity to any other product in the formulation; Should not be applied to middle ear; Pedi: Congenital or idiopathic methemoglobinemia; Infants <6 mo who are receiving methemoglobin-inducing agents.
Use Cautiously in: Repeated use or use on large areas of skin (more likely to result in systemic absorption); Geri: Elderly, acutely ill, or debilitated patients (increased risk of absorp-

tion and systemic effects); Severe liver disease; Any conditions associated with methemoglobinemia (including glucose-6-phosphate dehydrogenase deficiency); Pedi: Neonates and children <20 kg or 37 weeks gestation (area/duration of treatment should be limited); Lactation.

Adverse Reactions/Side Effects

Local: blanching, redness, alteration in temperature sensation, edema, itching, rash. **Misc:** allergic reactions including ANAPHYLAXIS.

Interactions

Drug-Drug: Concurrent use with **class I antiarrhythmics** including **tocainide** and **mexiletine** may result in adverse cardiovascular effects. Concurrent use with other **local anesthetics** may result in ↑ toxicity. Concurrent use with **sulfonamides** in children ↑ the risk of methemoglobinemia (avoid concurrent use in children <12 mo).

Route/Dosage

Topical (Adults and Children): *Minor dermal procedures including venipuncture and IV cannulation*—2.5 g (½ of the 5-g tube) applied to 20–25 cm^2 (2 in by 2 in) area of skin, covered with an occlusive dressing applied for at least 1 hr. *Major dermal procedures including split-thickness skin graft harvesting*—2 g/10 cm^2 area of skin, covered with an occlusive dressing for at least 2 hr. *Adult male genital skin*—as an adjunct prior to local anesthetic infiltration, apply a thick layer (1 g/10 cm^2) to skin surface for 15 min; local infiltration anesthesia should be performedimmediately after removal of cream. *Adult female genital mucous membranes*—apply a thick layer (5–log) for 5–10 min.

Topical (Children 7–12 yr and >20 kg): Dose should not exceed 20 g over more than 200 cm^2 for more than 4 hr.

Topical (Children 1–6 yr and >10 kg): Dose should not exceed 10 g over more than 100 cm^2 for more than 4 hr.

Topical (Children 3 mo–12 mo and >5 kg): Dose should not exceed 2 g over more than 20 cm^2 for more than 4 hr.

Topical (Children 0–3 mo or <5 kg): Dose should not exceed 1 g over more than 10 cm^2 for more than 1 hr.

Availability (generic available)

Cream: 2.5% lidocaine with 2.5% prilocaine in 5- and 30-g tubes.

NURSING IMPLICATIONS

Assessment

- Assess application site for open wounds. Apply only to intact skin.
- Assess application site for anesthesia following removal of system and prior to procedure.

Potential Nursing Diagnosis

Acute pain (Indications)

Implementation

- **Topical:** When used for minor dermal procedures (venipuncture, IV cannulation, arterial puncture, lumbar puncture), apply the 2.5-g tube of cream (½ of the 5-g tube) to each 2 in. by 2 in. area of skin in a *thick* layer at the site of the impending procedure. Remove the center cutout piece from an occlusive dressing (supplied with the 5-g tube) and peel the paper liner from the paper-framed dressing. Cover the lidocaine/prilocaine cream so that there is a *thick* layer of cream underneath the occlusive dressing. Do not spread out or rub in the cream. Smooth the dressing edges carefully and ensure it is secure to avoid leakage. Remove the paper frame and mark the time of application on the occlusive dressing. Lidocaine/prilocaine cream must be applied *at least 1 hr* before the start of a minor dermal procedure (venipuncture, IV cannulation). Anesthesia may be more profound with 90 min–2 hr application. Remove the occlusive dressing and wipe off the lidocaine/prilocaine cream. Clean the entire area with antiseptic solution and prepare the patient for the procedure.
- For major dermal procedures (skin graft harvesting), follow the same procedure using larger amounts of lidocaine/prilocaine cream and the appropriate-size occlusive dressing. Lidocaine/prilocaine cream must be applied *at least 2 hr* before major dermal procedures.

Patient/Family Teaching

- Explain the purpose of cream and occlusive dressing to patient and parents. Inform the patient that lidocaine/prilocaine cream may block all sensations in the treated skin. Caution patient to avoid trauma to the area from scratching, rubbing, or exposure to extreme heat or cold temperatures until all sensation has returned.

- **Home Care Issues:** Instruct patient or parent in proper application. Provide a diagram of location for application.

Evaluation/Desired Outcomes

- Anesthesia in the area of application.

lindane (lin-dane)

gamma benzene hexachloride, ✤GBH, G-Well, ✤Hexit, ✤PMS Lindane, Scabene

Classification

Therapeutic: pediculocides, scabicides

Pregnancy Category B

Indications

Second-line treatment of parasitic arthropod infestation (scabies and head, body, and crab lice) for use only in patients who are intolerant to or do not respond to less toxic agents.

Action

Causes seizures and death in parasitic arthropods. **Therapeutic Effects:** Cure of infestation by parasitic arthropods.

Pharmacokinetics

Absorption: Significant systemic absorption (9–13%) greater with topical application to damaged skin.
Distribution: Stored in fat.
Metabolism and Excretion: Metabolized by the liver.
Half-life: 17–22 hr (infants and children).

TIME/ACTION PROFILE (antiparasitic action)

ROUTE	ONSET	PEAK	DURATION
Top	rapid	6 hr	190 min

Contraindications/Precautions

Contraindicated in: Hypersensitivity; Areas of skin rash, abrasion, or inflammation (absorption is increased); History of seizures; Lactation; Premature neonates (increased risk of CNS toxicity).
Use Cautiously in: Pregnancy (do not exceed recommended dose; do not use >2 courses of therapy); Children ≤2 yr, geriatric patients, patients with skin conditions (increased risk of systemic absorption and CNS side effects).

Adverse Reactions/Side Effects

All adverse reactions except dermatologic are signs of systemic absorption and toxicity.
CNS: SEIZURES, headache. **CV:** tachycardia. **GI:** nausea, vomiting. **Derm:** contact dermatitis (repeated application), local irritation.

Interactions

Drug-Drug: Concurrent use of **medications that lower seizure threshold** (may ↑ risk of seizures). Simultaneous topical use of **skin, scalp,** or **hair** products may increase systemic absorption.

Route/Dosage

Scabies

Topical (Adults and Children >1 month): 1% lotion applied to all skin surfaces from neck to toes; wash off 6 hr after application in infants, after 6–8 hr in children or after 8–12 hr in adults; may require a 2nd treatment 1 wk later.

Head Lice or Crab Lice

Topical (Adults and Children): 15–30 ml of shampoo applied and lathered for 4 min; may require a 2nd treatment 1 wk later.

Availability (generic available)

Lotion: 1%. **Shampoo:** 1%.

NURSING IMPLICATIONS

Assessment

- Assess skin and hair for signs of infestation before and after treatment.
- Examine family members and close contacts for infestation. When used in treatment of pediculosis pubis or scabies, sexual partners should receive concurrent prophylactic therapy.

Potential Nursing Diagnoses

Risk for impaired skin integrity (Indications)

Implementation

- Due to serious side effects, no more than 2 oz may be dispensed at a time and no refills are allowed.
- **Topical:** When applying medication to another person, wear gloves to prevent systemic absorption.
- Do not apply to open wounds (scratches, cuts, sores on skin or scalp) to minimize systemic absorption. Avoid contact with the eyes. If eye contact occurs, flush thoroughly with

water and notify physician or other health care professional.
- Institute appropriate isolation techniques.
- **Lotion:** Instruct patient to bathe with soap and water. Dry skin well and allow to cool before application. Apply lotion in amount sufficient to cover entire body surface with a thin film from neck down (60 ml for an adult). Leave medication on for an age-appropriate time frame (see Route/Dosage), then remove by washing. If rash, burning, or itching develops, wash off medication and notify physician or other health care professional.
- **Shampoo:** Use a sufficient amount of shampoo to wet hair and scalp (30 ml for short hair, 45 ml for medium hair, 60 ml for long hair). Rub thoroughly into hair and scalp and leave in place for 4 min. Then use enough water to work up a good lather; follow with thorough rinsing and drying. If applied in shower or bath, do not let shampoo run down on other parts of body or into water in which patient is sitting. When hair is dry, use fine-toothed comb to remove remaining nits or nit shells. Shampoo may also be used on combs and brushes to prevent spread of infestation.

Patient/Family Teaching
- Instruct patient on application technique and provide with a medication guide. Patient should repeat therapy only at the recommendation of health care professional. Discuss hygienic measures to prevent and to control infestation. Discuss potential for infectious contacts with patient. Explain why household members should be examined and sexual partners treated simultaneously.
- Instruct patient to wash all recently worn clothing and used bed linens and towels in very hot water or to dry clean to prevent reinfestation or spreading.
- Instruct patient not to apply other oils or creams during therapy; these increase the absorption of lindane and may lead to toxicity.
- Explain to patient that itching may persist after treatment; consult health care professional about use of topical hydrocortisone or systemic antihistamines.
- Advise patient that eyelashes can be treated by applying petroleum jelly 3 times/day for 1 wk.
- Instruct patient not to reapply sooner than 1 wk if live mites appear.
- **Shampoo:** Advise patient that shampoo should not be used as a regular shampoo in the absence of infestation. Emphasize need to avoid contact with eyes.
- Pedi: Advise parents to monitor young children closely for evidence of CNS toxicity (seizures, dizziness, clumsiness, fast heartbeat, muscle cramps, nervousness, restlessness, irritability, nausea, vomiting) during and immediately after treatment.
- Pedi: Cover hands of young children to prevent accidental ingestion from thumbsucking.

Evaluation/Desired Outcomes
- Resolution of signs of infestation with scabies or lice.

linezolid (li-**nez**-o-lid)
Zyvox

Classification
Therapeutic: anti-infectives
Pharmacologic: oxazolidinones

Pregnancy Category C

Indications
Treatment of: Infections caused by vancomycin-resistant *Enterococcus faecium*, Nosocomial pneumonia caused by *S. aureus* (methicillin-susceptible and -resistant strains), Complicated skin/skin structure infections caused by *S. aureus* (methicillin-susceptible and -resistant strains), *Streptococcus pyogenes* or *S. agalactiae* (including diabetic foot infections), Uncomplicated skin/skin structure infections caused by *Staphylococcus aureus* (methicillin-susceptible and -resistant strains), *Streptococcus pyogenes*, Community-acquired pneumonia caused by *Streptococcus pneumoniae* (including multi-drug resistant strains) or *Staphylococcus aureus* (methicillin-susceptible strains only).

Action
Inhibits bacterial protein synthesis at the level of the 23S ribosome of the 50S subunit. **Therapeutic Effects:** Bactericidal action against streptococci; bacteriostatic action against enterococci and staphylococci.

Pharmacokinetics
Absorption: Rapidly and extensively (100%) absorbed following oral administration.
Distribution: Readily distributes to well-perfused tissues.
Metabolism and Excretion: 65% metabolized, mostly by the liver; 30% excreted unchanged by the kidneys.

Half-life: 6.4 hr.

TIME/ACTION PROFILE

ROUTE	ONSET	PEAK	DURATION
PO	rapid	1–2 hr	12 hr
IV	rapid	end of infusion	12 hr

Contraindications/Precautions

Contraindicated in: Hypersensitivity; Phenylketonuria (suspension contains aspartame).
Use Cautiously in: Thrombocytopenia, concurrent use of antiplatelet agents or bleeding diathesis (platelet counts should be monitored more frequently); OB: Pregnancy or lactation (safety not established).

Adverse Reactions/Side Effects

CV: headache, insomnia. **GI:** PSEUDOMEMBRANOUS COLITIS, diarrhea, increased liver function tests, nausea, taste alteration, vomiting. **F and E:** lactic acidosis. **Hemat:** thrombocytopenia. **Neuro:** optic neuropathy, peripheral neuropathy.

Interactions

Drug-Drug: Linezolid has monoamine oxidase inhibitory properties; response to **indirect-acting sympathomimetics**, **vasopressors**, **SSRIs** or **dopaminergic agents** may be ↑. Initial doses of **adrenergics** such as **dopamine** or **epinephrine** should be ↓ and carefully titrated.
Drug-Food: Because of monoamine oxidase inhibitory properties, consumption of large amounts of foods or beverages containing **tyramine** should be avoided (↑ risk of pressor response. See Appendix L).

Route/Dosage

Vancomycin-Resistant *Enterococcus faecium* Infections

PO, IV (Adults): 600 mg every 12 hr for 14–28 days.
PO, IV (Children birth–11 yr): (in the first week of life, pre-term neonates may initially receive 10 mg/kg every 12 hr).

Pneumonia, Complicated Skin/Skin Structure Infections

PO, IV (Adults): 600 mg every 12 hr for 10–14 days.
PO, IV (Children birth–11 yr): 10 mg/kg every 8 hr for 10–14 days (in the first week of life, pre-term neonates may initially receive 10 mg/kg every 12 hr).

Uncomplicated Skin/Skin Structure Infections

PO (Adults): 400 mg q 12 hr for 10–14 days.
PO, IV (Children 5–11 yr): 10 mg/kg every 12 hr for 10–14 days.
PO, IV (Children <5 yr): 10 mg/kg every 8 hr for 10–14 days (in the first week of life, pre-term neonates may initially receive 10 mg/kg every 12 hr).

Availability

Oral suspension (orange): 20 mg/ml. **Tablets:** 400 mg, 600 mg. **Cost:** 600 mg $2,213.46/30. **Premixed infusion:** 200 mg/100 ml, 400 mg/200 ml, 600 mg/300 ml.

L

NURSING IMPLICATIONS

Assessment

- Assess for infection (vital signs; appearance of wound, sputum, urine, and stool; WBC) at beginning of and during therapy.
- Obtain specimens for culture and sensitivity prior to initiating therapy. First dose may be given before receiving.
- May cause lactic acidosis. Notify health care professional if recurrent nausea and vomiting, unexplained acidosis or low bicarbonate levels occur.
- Monitor visual function in patients receiving linezolid for ≥3 months or who report visual symptoms (changes in acuity or color vision, blurred vision, visual field defect) regardless of length of therapy. If optic neuropathy occurs therapy should be reconsidered.
- **Pseudomembranous Colitis:** Assess bowel status (bowel sounds, frequency and consistency of stools, presence of blood in stools) during therapy.
- ***Lab Test Considerations:*** May cause bone marrow suppression, anemia, leukopenia, pancytopenia. Monitor CBC and platelet count weekly, especially in patients who are at risk for increased bleeding, who have pre-existing bone marrow suppression, who receive concurrent medications that may cause myelosuppression, or who may require >2 weeks of therapy. Discontinue therapy if bone marrow suppression occurs or worsens.
- May cause ↑ AST, ALT, LDH, alkaline phosphatase and BUN.

Potential Nursing Diagnoses
Risk for infection (Indications)

Implementation
- Dose adjustment is not necessary when switching from IV to oral dose.
- **PO:** May be administered with or without food.
- Before using oral solution gently invert 3–5 times to mix; do not shake. Store at room temperature.

IV Administration
- **Intermittent Infusion:** ***Diluent:*** Premixed infusions are already diluted and ready to use. Solution is yellowish in color which may intensify over time without affecting its potency. ***Concentration:*** 2 mg/ml. ***Rate:*** Infuse over 30–120 minutes. Flush line before and after infusion.
- **Y-Site Compatibility:** acyclovir, alfentanil, amikacin, aminophylline, amiodarone, ampicillin, ampicillin/sulbactam, anidulafungin, aztreonam, buprenorphine, butorphanol, bumetanide, calcium chloride, calcium gluconate, carboplatin, caspofungin, cefazolin, cefepime, cefotaxime, cefoxitin, ceftazidime, ceftizoxime, ceftriaxone, cefuroxime, chloramphenicol, cimetidine, ciprofloxacin, cisatracurium, cisplatin, clindamycin, cyclophosphamide, cyclosporine, cytarabine, daptomycin, dexamethasone sodium phosphate, dexmedetomidine, digoxin, diltiazem, diphenhydramine, dobutamine, dolasetron, dopamine, dexmedetomidinedoxorubicin, doxycycline, droperidol, enalaprilat, epinephrine, ertapenem, esmolol, dexmedetomidineetoposide phosphate, famotidine, fenoldopam, fentanyl, fluconazole, fluorouracil, furosemide, ganciclovir, gemcitabine, gentamicin, granisetron, haloperidol, heparin, hydralazine, hydrocortisone, hydromorphone, imipenem/cilastatin, insulin, isoproterenol, ketorolac, labetalol, leucovorin, levofloxacin, lidocaine, lorazepam, magnesium sulfate, mannitol, meperidine, meropenem, methotrexate, methylprednisolone, metoclopramide, metoprolol, metronidazole, midazolam, milrinone, morphine, nafcillin, nalbuphine, naloxone, nicardipine, nitroglycerin, nitroprusside, norepinephrine, ondansetron, paclitaxel, pentobarbital, phenobarbital, palonosetron, pancuronium, phenylephrine, piperacillin/tazobactam, potassium chloride, potassium phosphate, procainamide, prochlorperazine, promethazine, propranolol, quinupristin/dalfopristin, ranitidine, remifentanil, sodium bicarbonate, sufentanil, tacrolimus, theophylline, ticarcillin/clavulanate, tigecycline, tirofiban, tobramycin, trimethoprim/sulfamethoxazole, vancomycin, vasopressin, vecuronium, verapamil, vincristine, voriconazole, zidovudine.
- **Y-Site Incompatibility:** amphotericin B, chlorpromazine, diazepam, pantoprazole, pentamidine, phenytoin.

Patient/Family Teaching
- Advise patients taking oral linezolid to take as directed, for full course of therapy, even if feeling better. Take missed doses as soon as remembered unless almost time for next dose; do not double dose.
- Instruct patient to avoid large quantities of foods or beverages containing tyramine (see Appendix L). May cause hypertensive response.
- Instruct patient to notify health care professional if patient has a history of hypertension and before patient takes other Rx, OTC, or herbal products, especially cold remedies, decongestants, or antidepressants.
- Advise patient to notify health care professional if no improvement is seen in a few days.

Evaluation/Desired Outcomes
- Resolution of signs and symptoms of infection. Length of time for complete resolution depends on organism and site of infection.

---

liothyronine, See **THYROID PREPARATIONS.**

---

liotrix, See **THYROID PREPARATIONS.**

---

lisinopril, See **ANGIOTENSIN-CONVERTING ENZYME (ACE) INHIBITORS.**

---

lithium (lith-ee-um)
✤Carbolith, ✤Duralith, Eskalith, ✤Lithizine, Lithobid

Classification
Therapeutic: mood stabilizers

Pregnancy Category D

Indications
Manic episodes of manic depressive illness (treatment, maintenance, prophylaxis).

Action
Alters cation transport in nerve and muscle. May also influence reuptake of neurotransmitters. **Therapeutic Effects:** Prevents/decreases incidence of acute manic episodes.

Pharmacokinetics
Absorption: Completely absorbed after oral administration.
Distribution: Widely distributed into many tissues and fluids; CSF levels are 50% of plasma levels. Crosses the placenta; enters breast milk.
Metabolism and Excretion: Excreted almost entirely unchanged by the kidneys.
Half-life: 20–27 hr.

TIME/ACTION PROFILE (antimanic effects)

ROUTE	ONSET	PEAK	DURATION
PO, PO–ER	5–7 days	10–21 days	days

Contraindications/Precautions
Contraindicated in: Hypersensitivity; Severe cardiovascular or renal disease; Dehydrated or debilitated patients; Should be used only where therapy, including blood levels, may be closely monitored; Some products contain alcohol or tartrazine and should be avoided in patients with known hypersensitivity or intolerance.
Use Cautiously in: Any degree of cardiac, renal, or thyroid disease; Diabetes mellitus; Pregnancy/Lactation: Safety not established; Geri: Initial dosage reduction recommended.

Adverse Reactions/Side Effects
CNS: SEIZURES, fatigue, headache, impaired memory, ataxia, sedation, confusion, dizziness, drowsiness, psychomotor retardation, restlessness, stupor. **EENT:** aphasia, blurred vision, dysarthria, tinnitus. **CV:** ARRHYTHMIAS, ECG changes, edema, hypotension. **GI:** abdominal pain, anorexia, bloating, diarrhea, nausea, dry mouth, metallic taste. **GU:** polyuria, glycosuria, nephrogenic diabetes insipidus, renal toxicity. **Derm:** acneiform eruption, folliculitis, alopecia, diminished sensation, pruritus. **Endo:** hypothyroidism, goiter, hyperglycemia, hyperthyroidism. **F and E:** hyponatremia. **Hemat:** leukocytosis. **Metab:** weight gain. **MS:** muscle weakness, hyperirritability, rigidity. **Neuro:** tremors.

Interactions
Drug-Drug: May prolong the action of **neuromuscular blocking agents**. ↑ risk of neurologic toxicity with **haloperidol** or **molindone**. **Diuretics**, **methyldopa**, **probenecid**, **fluoxetine**, and **NSAIDs** may ↑ risk of toxicity. Blood levels may be ↑ by **ACE inhibitors**. Lithium may ↓ effects of **chlorpromazine**. **Chlorpromazine** may mask early signs of lithium toxicity. Hypothyroid effects may be additive with **potassium iodide** or **antithyroid agents**. **Aminophylline**, **phenothiazines**, and **drugs containing large amounts of sodium** ↑ renal elimination and ↓ effectiveness. **Psyllium** can ↓ **lithium** levels.
Drug-Natural Products: Caffeine-containing herbs (**cola nut, guarana, mate, tea, coffee**) may ↓ **lithium** serum levels and efficacy.
Drug-Food: Large changes in **sodium** intake may alter the renal elimination of lithium. ↑ sodium intake will ↑ renal excretion.

Route/Dosage
Precise dosing is based on serum lithium levels. 300 mg lithium carbonate contains 8–12 mEq lithium.
PO (Adults and Children ≥12 yr): *Tablets/capsules*—300–600 mg 3 times daily initially; usual maintenance dose is 300 mg 3–4 times daily. *Slow-release capsules*—200–300 mg 3 times daily initially; increased up to 1800 mg/day in divided doses. Usual maintenance dose is 300–400 mg 3 times daily. *Extended-release tablets*—450–900 mg twice daily *or* 300–600 mg 3 times daily initially; usual maintenance dose is 450 mg twice daily *or* 300 mg 3 times daily.
PO (Children <12 yr): 15–20 mg (0.4–0.5 mEq)/kg/day in 2–3 divided doses; dosage may be adjusted weekly.

Availability (generic available)
Capsules: 150 mg, 300 mg, 600 mg. **Cost:** *Generic*—150 mg $18.88/100, 300 mg $17.77/100, 600 mg $42.30/100—$0. **Tablets:** 300 mg. **Controlled-release tablets:** 300 mg, 450 mg. **Cost:** *Generic*—300 mg

= Canadian drug name.
*CAPITALS indicates life-threatening; underlines indicate most frequent.

$39.97/100, 450 mg $48.32/100. **Slow-release tablets:** 300 mg. **Syrup:** 300 mg (8 mEq lithium)/5 ml. **Cost:** $60.00/500 ml.

NURSING IMPLICATIONS

Assessment

- Assess mental status (orientation, mood, behavior) initially and periodically. Assess manic symptoms with Young Mania Rating Scale (YMRS) at baseline and periodically through treatment in patients with mania. Initiate suicide precautions if indicated.
- Monitor intake and output ratios. Report significant changes in totals. Unless contraindicated, fluid intake of at least 2000–3000 ml/day should be maintained. Weight should also be monitored at least every 3 mo.
- ***Lab Test Considerations:*** Evaluate renal and thyroid function, WBC with differential, serum electrolytes, and glucose periodically during therapy.
- ***Lab Test Considerations:*** EKG for patients >50 years old.
- ***Toxicity and Overdose:*** Monitor serum lithium levels twice weekly during initiation of therapy and every 2–3 mo during chronic therapy. Draw blood samples in the morning immediately before next dose. Therapeutic levels range from 0.5 to 1.5 mEq/L: Assess patient for signs and symptoms of lithium toxicity (vomiting, diarrhea, slurred speech, decreased coordination, drowsiness, muscle weakness, or twitching). If these occur, report before administering next dose.

Potential Nursing Diagnoses

Disturbed thought process (Indications)
Ineffective coping (Indications)
Imbalanced nutrition: risk for more than body requirements (Side Effects)

Implementation

- Do not confuse Lithobid (lithium) with Levbid (hyoscyamine).
- **PO:** Administer with food or milk to minimize GI irritation. Extended-release preparations should be swallowed whole; do not break, crush, or chew.

Patient/Family Teaching

- Instruct patient to take medication as directed, even if feeling well. Take missed doses as soon as remembered unless within 2 hr of next dose (6 hr if extended release).
- Lithium may cause dizziness or drowsiness. Caution patient to avoid driving or other activities requiring alertness until response to medication is known.
- Advise patient that psychotherapy is beneficial in improving coping skills.
- Low sodium levels may predispose patient to toxicity. Advise patient to drink 2000–3000 ml fluid each day and eat a diet with consistent and moderate sodium intake. Excessive amounts of coffee, tea, and cola should be avoided because of diuretic effect. Avoid activities that cause excess sodium loss (heavy exertion, exercise in hot weather, saunas). Notify health care professional of fever, vomiting, and diarrhea, which also cause sodium loss.
- Advise patient that weight gain may occur. Review principles of a low-calorie diet.
- Instruct patient to consult health care professional before taking OTC medications or herbal products concurrently with this therapy.
- Advise patient to use contraception and to consult health care professional if pregnancy is suspected.
- Review side effects and symptoms of toxicity with patient. Instruct patient to stop medication and report signs of toxicity to health care professional promptly.
- Explain to patients with cardiovascular disease or over 40 yr of age the need for ECG evaluation before and periodically during therapy. Patient should inform health care professional if fainting, irregular pulse, or difficulty breathing occurs.
- Emphasize the importance of periodic lab tests to monitor for lithium toxicity.

Evaluation/Desired Outcomes

- Resolution of the symptoms of mania (hyperactivity, pressured speech, poor judgment, need for little sleep).
- Decreased incidence of mood swings in bipolar disorders.
- Improved affect in unipolar disorders. Improvement in condition may require 1–3 wk.
- Remission of depressive symptoms.

loperamide (loe-**per**-a-mide)

Diar-aid Caplets, Imodium, Imodium A-D, Kaopectate II Caplets, Maalox Antidiarrheal Caplets, Neo-Diaral, Pepto Diarrhea Control

Classification
Therapeutic: antidiarrheals

Pregnancy Category B

Indications
Adjunctive therapy of acute diarrhea. Chronic diarrhea associated with inflammatory bowel disease. Decreases the volume of ileostomy drainage.

Action
Inhibits peristalsis and prolongs transit time by a direct effect on nerves in the intestinal muscle wall. Reduces fecal volume, increases fecal viscosity and bulk while diminishing loss of fluid and electrolytes. **Therapeutic Effects:** Relief of diarrhea.

Pharmacokinetics
Absorption: Not well absorbed following oral administration.
Distribution: Unknown. Does not cross the blood-brain barrier.
Protein Binding: 97%.
Metabolism and Excretion: Metabolized partially by the liver, undergoes enterohepatic recirculation; 30% eliminated in the feces. Minimal excretion in the urine.
Half-life: 10.8 hr.

TIME/ACTION PROFILE (relief of diarrhea)

ROUTE	ONSET	PEAK	DURATION
PO	1 hr	2.5–5 hr	10 hr

Contraindications/Precautions
Contraindicated in: Hypersensitivity; Patients in whom constipation must be avoided; Abdominal pain of unknown cause, especially if associated with fever; Alcohol intolerance (liquid only).
Use Cautiously in: Hepatic dysfunction; Geri: Increased sensitivity to effects; OB, Pedi: Pregnancy, lactation, or children <2 yr (safety not established).

Adverse Reactions/Side Effects
CNS: drowsiness, dizziness. **GI:** constipation, abdominal pain/distention/discomfort, dry mouth, nausea, vomiting. **Misc:** allergic reactions.

Interactions
Drug-Drug: ↑ CNS depression with other **CNS depressants**, including **alcohol**, **antihistamines**, **opioid analgesics**, and **sedative/hypnotics**. ↑ anticholinergic properties with other **drugs having anticholinergic properties**, including **antidepressants** and **antihistamines**.
Drug-Natural Products: Kava kava, **valerian**, **skullcap**, **chamomile**, or **hops** can ↑ CNS depression.

Route/Dosage
PO (Adults): 4 mg initially, then 2 mg after each loose stool. Maintenance dose usually 4–8 mg/day in divided doses (not to exceed 8 mg/day for OTC use or 16 mg/day for Rx use).
PO (Children 9–11 yr or 30–47 kg): 2 mg initially; then 1 mg after each loose stool (not to exceed 6 mg/24 hr; OTC use should not exceed 2 days).
PO (Children 6–8 yr or 24–30 kg): 1 mg initially, then 1 mg after each loose stool (not to exceed 4 mg/24 hr; OTC use should not exceed 2 days).

Availability (generic available)
Tablets: 2 mg[OTC]. **Capsules:** 2 mg. **Liquid (mint):** 1 mg/5 ml[OTC]. ***In combination with:*** simethicone (Immodium Advanced[OTC], see Appendix B).

NURSING IMPLICATIONS

Assessment
- Assess frequency and consistency of stools and bowel sounds prior to and during therapy.
- Assess fluid and electrolyte balance and skin turgor for dehydration.

Potential Nursing Diagnoses
Diarrhea (Indications)
Risk for injury (Side Effects)

Implementation
- **PO:** Administer with clear fluids to help prevent dehydration, which may accompany diarrhea.

Patient/Family Teaching
- Instruct patient to take medication as directed. Do not take missed doses, and do not double doses. In acute diarrhea, medication may be ordered after each unformed stool.

Advise patient not to exceed the maximum number of doses.

- May cause drowsiness. Advise patient to avoid driving or other activities requiring alertness until response to drug is known.
- Advise patient that frequent mouth rinses, good oral hygiene, and sugarless gum or candy may relieve dry mouth.
- Caution patient to avoid using alcohol and other CNS depressants concurrently with this medication.
- Instruct patient to notify health care professional if diarrhea persists or if fever, abdominal pain, or distention occurs.

Evaluation/Desired Outcomes

- Decrease in diarrhea.
- In acute diarrhea, treatment should be discontinued if no improvement is seen in 48 hr.
- In chronic diarrhea, if no improvement has occurred after at least 10 days of treatment with maximum dose, loperamide is unlikely to be effective.

lopinavir/ritonavir

(loe-**pin**-a-veer/ri-**toe**-na-veer)
Kaletra

Classification
Therapeutic: antiretrovirals
Pharmacologic: protease inhibitors, metabolic inhibitors

Pregnancy Category C

Indications

HIV infection (with other antiretrovirals).

Action

Lopinavir: Inhibits HIV viral protease. **Ritonavir:** Although ritonavir has antiretroviral activity of its own (inhibits the action of HIV protease and prevents the cleavage of viral polyproteins), it is combined with lopinavir to inhibit the metabolism of lopinavir thus increasing its plasma levels. **Therapeutic Effects:** Increased CD4 cell counts and decreased viral load with subsequent slowed progression of HIV infection and its sequelae.

Pharmacokinetics

Absorption: Well absorbed following oral administration; food enhances absorption.
Distribution: *Ritonavir*—poor CNS penetration.
Protein Binding: *Lopinavir*—98–99 % bound to plasma proteins.
Metabolism and Excretion: *Lopinavir*—completely metabolized in the liver by cytochrome P450 P3A (CY P450 P3A); ritonavir is a potent inhibitor of this enzyme. *Ritonavir*—highly metabolized by the liver (by CY P450 P3A and CY P2D6 enzymes); one metabolite has antiretroviral activity; 3.5% excreted unchanged in urine.
Half-life: *Lopinavir*—5–6 hr; *ritonavir*—3–5 hr.

TIME/ACTION PROFILE (blood levels)

ROUTE	ONSET	PEAK	DURATION
Lopinavir PO	rapid	4 hr	12 hr
Ritonavir PO	rapid	4 hr*	12 hr

*Non-fasting

Contraindications/Precautions

Contraindicated in: Hypersensitivity; Concurrent use of dihydroergotamine, ergotamine, ergonovine, flecainide, methylergonovine, midazolam, pimozide, propafenone, amiodaroneand triazolam, which are highly dependent on CY P3A or CY P2D6 for metabolism and for which ↑ blood levels may result in serious and/or life-threatening events; Concurrent use with simastatin, lovastatin, St. John's wort (hypericum perforatum) is not recommended; Hypersensitivity or intolerance to alcohol or castor oil (present in capsules and liquid).
Use Cautiously in: Known alcohol intolerance (oral solution contains alcohol); Concurrent use with atorvastatin (may increase risk of rhabdomyolysis); Concurrent use of antiarrhythmics including lidocaine and quinidine (therapeutic blood level monitoring recommended); Concurrent use of anticonvulsants including carbamazepine, phenobarbital or phenytoin (may decrease effectiveness of lopinavir); Concurrent use of dihydropyridine calcium channel blockers including felodipine, nifedipine and nicardipine (clinical monitoring recommended due to increased levels of calcium channel blocker); Impaired hepatic function, history of hepatitis (for ritonavir content); OB: Pregnancy or lactation (safety not established; breastfeeding not recommended in HIV-infected patients).
Exercise Extreme Caution in: Concurrent use with sildenafil, vardenafil or tadalafil should be undertaken with extreme caution and may result in hypotension, syncope, visual changes and prolonged erection.

Adverse Reactions/Side Effects

CNS: headache, insomnia, weakness. **GI:** diarrhea (↑ in children), abdominal pain, nausea, pancreatitis, taste aversion (in children), vomiting (↑ in children). **Derm:** rash.

Interactions

Drug-Drug: Concurrent use of **flecainide**, **amiodarone**, **propafenone**, **dihydroergotamine**, **ergonovine**, **ergotamine**, **methylergonovine**, **pimozide**, **midazolam**, and **triazolam**, is contraindicated because of the risk of potentially serious, life-threatening drug interactions. Concurrent use with **sildenafil**, **vardenafil** or **tadalafil** should be undertaken with extreme caution and may result in hypotension, syncope, visual changes and prolonged erection (dose reduction of sildenafil to 25 mg every 48 hr with monitoring recommended). Concurrent use with **rifampin** ↓ effectiveness of antiretroviral therapy and should not be undertaken. Should not be used concurrently with **simvastatin** or **lovastatin** due to ↑ risk of rhabdomyolysis; similar risk exists for **atorvastatin** (use lowest possible dose with careful monitoring). Concurrent use with **efavirenz** or **nevirapine** ↓ lopinavir/ritonavir levels and effectiveness; dose increase may be necessary. **Delavirdine** ↑ lopinavir levels. ↑ levels of **lidocaine** and **quinidine** (blood level monitoring recommended). Concurrent use of anticonvulsants including **carbamazepine**, **phenobarbital**, or **phenytoin** may ↓ effectiveness of lopinavir. ↑ levels of **dihydropyridine calcium channel blockers** including **felodipine**, **nifedipine**, and **nicardipine** (clinical monitoring recommended). May alter levels and effectiveness of **warfarin**. ↑ levels of **clarithromycin** (dose reduction recommended for patients with CCr ≤60 ml/min. ↑ blood levels of **itraconazole** and **ketoconazole** (high antifungal doses not recommended). ↑ levels of **rifabutin** (dose reduction recommended). ↓ blood levels of **atovaquone** (may require dosage increase). **Dexamethasone** ↓ blood levels and may ↓ effectiveness of lopinavir. Oral solution contains alcohol may produce intolerance when administered with **disulfiram** or **metronidazole**. May ↑ levels and risk of toxicity with immunosuppressant including **cyclosporine** or **tacrolimus** (blood level monitoring recommended). May ↓ levels and effects of **methadone** (dose of **methadone** may need to be ↑). May ↓ levels and contraceptive efficacy of some estrogen-based **hormonal contraceptives** including **ethinyl estradiol** (alternative or additional methods of contraception recommended). ↑ levels of **fluticasone** by inhalation; avoid concurrent use.
Drug-Natural Products: Concurrent use with **St. John's wort** may ↓ levels and beneficial effect of lopinavir/ritonavir.

Route/Dosage

PO (Adults and Children >40 kg): 400/100 mg (3 capsules or 5 ml oral solution) twice daily *or* may be given as a single daily dose of 800/200 mg (6 capsules or 10 ml oral solution); single dose approved for adults only.
PO (Children 15–40 kg): 10 mg/kg lopinavir content twice daily.
PO (Children 7–15 kg): 12 mg/kg lopinavir content twice daily.

With Concurrent Efavirenz or Nevirapine

PO (Adults and Children >40 kg): 533/133 mg (4 capsules or 6.5 ml oral solution) twice daily.
PO (Children 15–50 kg): 11 mg/kg lopinavir content twice daily.
PO (Children 7–15 kg): 13 mg/kg lopinavir content twice daily.

Availability

Capsules: 133.3 mg lopinavir/33 mg ritonavir. **Oral solution (cotton candy or vanilla):** 80 mg lopinavir/20 mg ritonavir per ml (contains 42.4% alcohol) in 60-ml bottles.

NURSING IMPLICATIONS

Assessment

- Assess for change in severity of HIV symptoms and for symptoms of opportunistic infections during therapy.
- Assess patient for signs of pancreatitis (nausea, vomiting, abdominal pain, increased serum lipase or amylase) periodically during therapy. May require discontinuation of therapy.
- ***Lab Test Considerations:*** Monitor viral load and CD4 counts regularly during therapy.
- Monitor triglyceride and cholesterol levels prior to initiating therapy and periodically during therapy.
- May cause hyperglycemia.

L

- May cause ↑ serum AST, ALT, GGT, and total bilirubin concentrations.

Potential Nursing Diagnosis

Risk for infection (Indications)
Noncompliance (Patient/Family Teaching)

Implementation

- Do not confuse with Kaletra (lopinavir/ritonavir) with Keppra (levetiracetam).
- Patients taking concurrent didanosine should take didanosine 1 hr before or 2 hr after taking lopinavir/ritonavir.
- **PO:** Administer with food to enhance absorption.
- Oral solution is light yellow to orange.
- Capsules and oral solution are stable if refrigerated until expiration date on label or 2 months at room temperature.

Patient/Family Teaching

- Emphasize the importance of taking lopinavir/ritonavir as directed, at evenly spaced times throughout day. Do not take more than prescribed amount, and do not stop taking this or other antiretrovirals without consulting health care professional. Take missed doses as soon as remembered; do not double doses.
- Instruct patient that lopinavir/ritonavir should not be shared with others.
- Advise patient to avoid taking other medications, Rx, OTC, or herbal products, especially St. John's wort, without consulting health care professional.
- Inform patient that lopinavir/ritonavir does not cure AIDS or prevent associated or opportunistic infections. Lopinavir/ritonavir does not reduce the risk of transmission of HIV to others through sexual contact or blood contamination. Caution patient to use a condom during sexual contact and to avoid sharing needles or donating blood to prevent spreading the AIDS virus to others. Advise patient that the long-term effects of lopinavir/ritonavir are unknown at this time.
- Inform patient that lopinavir/ritonavir may cause hyperglycemia. Advise patient to notify health care professional if increased thirst or hunger; unexplained weight loss; or increased urination occurs.
- Advise patients taking oral contraceptives to use a nonhormonal method of birth control during lopinavir/ritonavir therapy.
- Caution patients taking sildenafil of increased risk of sildenafil-associated side effects (hypotension, visual changes, sustained erection). Notify health care professional promptly if these occur.
- Inform patient that redistribution and accumulation of body fat may occur causing central obesity, dorsocervical fat enlargement (buffalo hump), peripheral wasting, breast enlargement, and cushingoid appearance. The cause and long-term effects are not known.
- Instruct patient to notify health care professional if pregnancy is planned or suspected of if breastfeeding an infant.
- Emphasize the importance of regular follow-up exams and blood counts to determine progress and monitor for side effects.

Evaluation/Desired Outcomes

- Delayed progression of AIDS and decreased opportunistic infections in patients with HIV.
- Decrease in viral load and improvement in CD4 cell counts.

loratadine (lor-**a**-ta-deen)

Alavert, Claritin, Claritin 24–Hour Allergy, Claritin Hives Relief, Children's Loratidine, Claritin Reditabs, Clear-Atadine, Dimetapp Children's ND Non-Drowsy Allergy, Non-Drowsy Allergy Relief for Kids, Tavist ND

Classification
Therapeutic: antihistamines

Pregnancy Category B

Indications

Relief of symptoms of seasonal allergies. Management of chronic idiopathic urticaria. Management of hives.

Action

Blocks peripheral effects of histamine released during allergic reactions. **Therapeutic Effects:** Decreased symptoms of allergic reactions (nasal stuffiness; red, swollen eyes, itching).

Pharmacokinetics

Absorption: Rapidly absorbed after oral administration (80%).
Distribution: Unknown.
Protein Binding: *Loratadine*—97%; *descarboethoxyloratadine*—73–77%.
Metabolism and Excretion: Rapidly and extensively metabolized during first pass through

the liver. Much is converted to descarboethoxyloratadine, an active metabolite.
Half-life: *Loratadine*—7.8–11 hr; *descarboethoxyloratadine*—20 hr.

TIME/ACTION PROFILE (antihistaminic effects)

ROUTE	ONSET	PEAK	DURATION
PO	1–3 hr	8–12 hr	>24 hr

Contraindications/Precautions
Contraindicated in: Hypersensitivity; OB: Lactation.
Use Cautiously in: Patients with hepatic impairment or CCr <30 ml/min (↓ dose to 10 mg every other day); Patients receiving drugs known to affect hepatic metabolism of drugs; Geri: ↑ risk of adverse reactions; OB, Pedi: Pregnancy or children <2 yr (safety not established).

Adverse Reactions/Side Effects
CNS: confusion, drowsiness (rare), paradoxical excitation. **EENT:** blurred vision. **GI:** dry mouth, GI upset. **Derm:** photosensitivity, rash. **Metab:** weight gain.

Interactions
Drug-Drug: The following interactions may occur, but are less likely to occur with loratidine than with more sedating antihistamines. **MAO inhibitors** may intensify and prolong effects of antihistamines. ↑ CNS depression may occur with other **CNS depressants**, including **alcohol**, **antidepressants**, **opioid analgesics**, and **sedative/hypnotics**.
Drug-Natural Products: Kava kava, valerian, or **chamomile** can ↑ CNS depression.

Route/Dosage
PO (Adults and Children ≥6 yr): 10 mg once daily.
PO (Children ≥2–5 yr): 5 mg once daily.

Renal Impairment
PO (Adults): *CCr <30 ml/min*—10 mg every other day.

Hepatic Impairment
PO (Adults): 10 mg every other day.

Availability (generic available)
Rapidly disintegrating tablets (mint): 5 mg, 10 mg[OTC]. **Tablets:** 10 mg[OTC], ♣10 mg. **Chewable tablets:** 5 mg[OTC] (grape flavored). **Syrup (mint, fruit):** 5 mg/5 ml[OTC]. ***In combination with:*** pseudoephedrine (Claritin-D)[OTC]. See Appendix B.

NURSING IMPLICATIONS

Assessment
- Assess allergy symptoms (rhinitis, conjunctivitis, hives) before and periodically during therapy.
- Assess lung sounds and character of bronchial secretions. Maintain fluid intake of 1500–2000 ml/day to decrease viscosity of secretions.
- ***Lab Test Considerations:*** May cause false-negative result on allergy skin testing.

Potential Nursing Diagnoses
Ineffective airway clearance (Indications)
Risk for injury (Adverse Reactions)

Implementation
- **PO:** Administer once daily.
- *For rapidly disintegrating tablets (Alavert, Claritin Reditabs)*—place on tongue. Tablet disintegrates rapidly. May be taken with or without water.

Patient/Family Teaching
- Instruct patient to take medication as directed.
- May cause dizziness or drowsiness. Caution patient to avoid driving or other activities requiring alertness until response to medication is known.
- Caution patient to use sunscreen and protective clothing to prevent photosensitivity reactions.
- Advise patient to avoid taking alcohol or other CNS depressants concurrently with this drug.
- Advise patient that good oral hygiene, frequent rinsing of mouth with water, and sugarless gum or candy may minimize dry mouth. Patient should notify dentist if dry mouth persists >2 wk.
- Instruct patient to contact health care professional immediately if dizziness, fainting, or fast or irregular heartbeat occurs or if symptoms persist.

Evaluation/Desired Outcomes
- Decrease in allergic symptoms.
- Management of chronic idiopathic urticaria.
- Management of hives.

lorazepam (lor-az-e-pam)
Apo-Lorazepam, Ativan, Novo-Lorazem, Nu-Loraz

Classification
Therapeutic: anesthetic adjuncts, antianxiety agents, sedative/hypnotics
Pharmacologic: benzodiazepines

Schedule IV

Pregnancy Category D

Indications
Anxiety disorder (oral). Preoperative sedation (injection). Decreases preoperative anxiety and provides amnesia. **Unlabeled uses: IV:** Antiemetic prior to chemotherapy. Insomnia, panic disorder, as an adjunct with acute mania or acute psychosis.

Action
Depresses the CNS, probably by potentiating GABA, an inhibitory neurotransmitter. **Therapeutic Effects:** Sedation. Decreased anxiety. Decreased seizures.

Pharmacokinetics
Absorption: Well absorbed following oral administration. Rapidly and completely absorbed following IM administration. Sublingual absorption is more rapid than oral and is similar to IM.
Distribution: Widely distributed. Crosses the blood-brain barrier. Crosses the placenta; enters breast milk.
Metabolism and Excretion: Highly metabolized by the liver.
Half-life: Full–term neonates: 18–73 hr; older children: 6–17 hr; adults: 10–16 hr.

TIME/ACTION PROFILE (sedation)

ROUTE	ONSET	PEAK	DURATION
PO	15–60 min	1–6 hr	8–12 hr
IM	30–60 min	1–2 hr†	8–12 hr
IV	15–30 min	15–20 min	8–12 hr

†Amnestic response

Contraindications/Precautions
Contraindicated in: Hypersensitivity; Cross-sensitivity with other benzodiazepines may exist; Comatose patients or those with pre-existing CNS depression; Uncontrolled severe pain; Angle-closure glaucoma; Severe hypotension; Sleep apnea; OB: Use in pregnancy and lactation may cause CNS depression, flaccidity, feeding difficulties, hypothermia, seizures, and respiratory problems in the neonate; Lactation: Recommend to discontinue drug or bottle-feed.
Use Cautiously in: Severe hepatic/renal/pulmonary impairment; Myasthenia gravis; Depression; Psychosis; History of suicide attempt or drug abuse; COPD; Sleep apnea; Pedi: Use cautiously in children under 12 yr. In higher doses, benzyl alcohol in injection may cause potentially fatal "gasping syndrome" in neonates; Geri: Lower doses recommended for geriatric or debilitated patients; Hypnotic use should be short-term; **OVERDOSE:** Administer Flumazenil (do not use with patients with seizure disorder. May induce seizures.

Adverse Reactions/Side Effects
CNS: dizziness, drowsiness, lethargy, hangover, headache, ataxia, slurred speech, forgetfulness, confusion, mental depression, rhythmic myoclonic jerking in pre-term infants, paradoxical excitation. **EENT:** blurred vision. **Resp:** respiratory depression. **CV:** *rapid IV use only*— APNEA, CARDIAC ARREST, bradycardia, hypotension. **GI:** constipation, diarrhea, nausea, vomiting, weight gain (unusual). **Derm:** rashes. **Misc:** physical dependence, psychological dependence, tolerance.

Interactions
Drug-Drug: Additive CNS depression with other **CNS depressants** including **alcohol**, **antihistamines**, **antidepressants**, **opioid analgesics**, **clozapine**, and other **sedative/hypnotics** including other **benzodiazepines.** May ↓ the efficacy of **levodopa**. **Smoking** may ↑ metabolism and ↓ effectiveness. **Valproate** can ↑ serum concentrations and ↓ clearance (↓ dose by 50%). **Probenecid** may ↓ metabolism of lorazepam, enhancing its actions (↓ dose by 50%). **Oral contraceptives** may increase clearance and decrease concentration of lorazepam.
Drug-Natural Products: Concomitant use of **kava kava**, **valerian** or, **chamomile** can ↑ CNS depression.

Route/Dosage
PO (Adults): *Anxiety*—1–3 mg 2–3 times daily (up to 10 mg/day). *Insomnia*—2–4 mg at bedtime.
PO (Geriatric or Debilitated Patients): *Anxiety*—0.5–2 mg/day in divided doses initially. *Insomnia*—0.25–1 mg initially, increased as needed.
PO (Children): *Anxiety/sedation*—0.02–0.1 mg/kg/dose (not to exceed 2 mg) q 4–8 hr.

Preoperative sedation—0.02–0.09 mg/kg/dose.
PO (Infants): *Anxiety/sedation*—0.02–0.1 mg/kg/dose (not to exceed 2 mg) q 4–8 hr. *Preoperative sedation*—0.02–0.09 mg/kg/dose.
SL (Adults and Adolescents >18 yr): *Anxiety*— 2–3 mg/day in divided doses, not to exceed 6 mg/day; *preoperative sedation*—0.05 mg/kg, up to 4 mg total given 1–2 hr before surgery.
SL (Geriatric and Debilitated Patients): 0.5 mg/day, dose may be adjusted as necessary.
IM (Adults): *Preoperative sedation*—50 mcg (0.05 mg)/kg 2 hr before surgery (not to exceed 4 mg).
IM (Children): *Preoperative sedation*—0.02–0.09 mg/kg/dose.
IM (Infants): *Preoperative sedation*—0.02–0.09 mg/kg/dose.
IV (Adults): *Preoperative sedation*—44 mcg (0.044 mg)/kg (not to exceed 2 mg) 15–20 min before surgery. *Operative amnestic effect*—up to 50 mcg/kg (not to exceed 4 mg). *Antiemetic*—2 mg 30 min prior to chemotherapy; may be repeated q 4 hr as needed (unlabeled). *Anticonvulsant*—50 mcg (0.05 mg)/kg, up to 4 mg; may be repeated after 10–15 min (not to exceed 8 mg/12 hr; unlabeled).
IV (Children): *Preoperative sedation*—0.02–0.09 mg/kg/dose; may use smaller doses (0.01–0.03 mg/kg) and repeat q 20 min. *Antiemetic*—Single dose: 0.04–0.08 mg/kg/dose prior to chemotherapy (not to exceed 4 mg). Multiple doses: 0.02–0.05 mg/kg/dose q 6 hr prn (not to exceed 2 mg). *Anxiety/sedation*—0.02–0.1 mg/kg (not to exceed 2 mg) q 4–8 hr. *Status epilepticus*—0.1 mg/kg over 2–5 min (not to exceed 4 mg); may repeat with 0.05 mg/kg if needed.
IV (Infants): *Preoperative sedation*—0.02–0.09 mg/kg/dose; may use smaller doses (0.01–0.03 mg/kg) and repeat q 20 min. *Anxiety/sedation*—0.02–0.1 mg/kg/dose (not to exceed 2 mg) q 4–8 hr. *Status epilepticus*—0.1 mg/kg over 2–5 min (not to exceed 4 mg); may repeat with 0.05 mg/kg if needed.
IV (Neonates): *Status epilepticus*—0.05 mg/kg over 2–5 min; may repeat in 10–15 min.

Availability (generic available)

Tablets: 0.5 mg, 1 mg, 2 mg. **Concentrated oral solution:** 0.5 mg/5 ml, 2 mg/ml. **Sublingual tablets:** ✤0.5 mg, ✤1 mg, ✤2 mg. **Injection:** 2 mg/ml, 4 mg/ml.

NURSING IMPLICATIONS

Assessment

- Conduct regular assessment of continued need for treatment.
- Pedi: Assess neonates for prolonged CNS depression related to inability to metabolize lorazepam.
- Geri: Assess geriatric patients carefully for CNS reactions as they are more sensitive to these effects. Assess falls risk.
- **Anxiety:** Assess degree and manifestations of anxiety and mental status (orientation, mood, behavior) prior to and periodically throughout therapy.
- Prolonged high-dose therapy may lead to psychological or physical dependence. Restrict amount of drug available to patient.
- **Status Epilepticus:** Assess location, duration, characteristics, and frequency of seizures. Institute seizure precautions.
- ***Lab Test Considerations:*** Patients on high-dose therapy should receive routine evaluation of renal, hepatic, and hematologic function.

Potential Nursing Diagnoses

Anxiety (Indications)
Risk for injury (Indications, Side Effects)

Implementation

- Do not confuse Ativan (lorazepam) with Atarax (hydroxyzine).
- Following parenteral administration, keep patient supine for at least 8 hr and observe closely.
- **PO:** Tablet may also be given sublingually (unlabeled) for more rapid onset.
- Take concentrated liquid solution with water, soda, pudding, or applesauce.
- **IM:** Administer IM doses deep into muscle mass at least 2 hr before surgery for optimum effect.

IV Administration

- **Direct IV:** ***Diluent:*** Dilute immediately before use with an equal amount of sterile water for injection, D5W, or 0.9% NaCl for injection. Pedi: To decrease the amount of benzyl alcohol delivered to neonates, dilute the 4 mg/mL injection with preservative-free sterile water for injection to make a 0.4 mg/mL dilution for IV use. Do not use if solution is colored or contains a precipitate. ***Rate:*** Administer at a rate not to exceed 2 mg/min or 0.05 mg/kg over 2–5 min. Rapid IV administration may result in apnea, hypotension, bradycardia, or cardiac arrest.

- **Y-Site Compatibility:** acyclovir, albumin, allopurinol, amifostine, amikacin, amiodarone, amphotericin B cholesteryl sulfate complex, amsacrine, anakinra, argatroban, atracurium, bivalirudin, bumetanide, calcium chloride, calcium gluconate, cefazolin, cefepime, cefotaxime, cefoxitin, ceftazidime, ceftizoxime, ceftriaxone, cefuroxime, chloramphenicol, cimetidine, ciprofloxacin, cisatracurium, clindamycin, cyclosporine, clindamycin, cladribine, clonidine, cyclophosphamide, cytarabine, daptomycin, dexamethasone sodium phosphate, dexmedetomidine, diltiazem, diphenhydramine, dobutamine, docetaxel, dopamine, doxorubicin, doxorubicin liposome, doxycycline, droperidol, enalaprilat, epinephrine, ertapenem, erythromycin lactobionate, esmolol, etomidate, etoposide phosphate, famotidine, fenoldopam, fentanyl, filgrastim, fluconazole, fludarabine, fosphenytoin, furosemide, gemcitabine, gentamicin, granisetron, haloperidol, heparin, hydrocortisone sodium succinate, hydromorphone, hydroxyzine, insulin, isoproterenol, ketorolac, labetalol, levofloxacin, linezolid, magnesium sulfate, melphalan, meropenem, methadone, methotrexate, methylprednisolone sodium succinate, metoclopramide, metoprolol, metronidazole, micafungin, midazolam, milrinone, morphine, nafcillin, nicardipine, nitroglycerin, nitroprusside, norepinephrine, oxaliplatin, paclitaxel, palonosetron, pancuronium, pemetrexed, phenylephrine, piperacillin/tazobactam, potassium chloride, procainamide, prochlorperazine, promethazine, propofol, propranolol, quinupristin/dalfopristin, ranitidine, remifentanil, sodium bicarbonate, tacrolimus, teniposide, thiotepa, ticarcillin/clavulanate, tirofiban, tobramycin, trimethoprim/sulfamethoxazole, vancomycin, vasopressin, vecuronium, verapamil, vinorelbine, voriconazole, zidovudine.
- **Y-Site Incompatibility:** aldesleukin, ampicillin, ampicillin/sulbactam, aztreonam, caspofungin, hydralazine, idarubicin, imipenem/cilastatin, lansoprazole, omeprazole, ondansetron, pantoprazole, phenytoin, potassium phosphate, sargramostim, sufentanil.

Patient/Family Teaching

- Instruct patient to take medication exactly as directed and not to skip or double up on missed doses. If medication is less effective after a few weeks, check with health care professional; do not increase dose.
- Advise patient that lorazepam is usually prescribed for short-term use and does not cure underlying problem.
- Advise patient to taper lorazepam by 0.05 mg q 3 days to decrease withdrawal symptoms; abrupt withdrawal may cause tremors, nausea, vomiting, and abdominal and muscle cramps.
- Teach other methods to decrease anxiety, such as increased exercise, support groups, relaxation techniques. Emphasize that psychotherapy is beneficial in addressing source of anxiety and improving coping skills.
- May cause drowsiness or dizziness. Advise patient to avoid driving or other activities requiring alertness until response to medication is known.
- Caution patient to avoid taking alcohol or other CNS depressants concurrently with this medication.
- Instruct patient to contact health care professional immediately if pregnancy is planned or suspected.
- Emphasize the importance of follow-up exams to determine effectiveness of the medication.

Evaluation/Desired Outcomes

- Increase in sense of well-being.
- Decrease in subjective feelings of anxiety without excessive sedation.
- Reduction of preoperative anxiety.
- Postoperative amnesia.
- Improvement in sleep patterns.

losartan, See ANGIOTENSIN II RECEPTOR ANTAGONISTS.

lovastatin, See HMG-CoA REDUCTASE INHIBITORS (statins).

MAGNESIUM AND ALUMINUM SALTS

magaldrate (with simethicone)
(**mag**-al-drate)
Riopan Plus, ✤Riopan Plus Double Strength

magnesium hydroxide/aluminum hydroxide
(mag-**nee**-zhum hye-**drox**-ide/a-**loo**-mi-num hye-**drox**-ide)
Alamag, ✤Diovol Ex, ✤Gelusil Extra Strength, Maalox, ✤Mylanta, Rulox

Classification
Therapeutic: antiulcer agents
Pharmacologic: antacids

Pregnancy Category C

Indications
Useful in a variety of GI complaints, including: Hyperacidity, Indigestion, GERD, Heartburn.

Action
Neutralize gastric acid following dissolution in gastric contents. Inactivate pepsin if pH is raised to ≥4. **Therapeutic Effects:** Neutralization of gastric acid with healing of ulcers and decrease in associated pain.

Pharmacokinetics
Absorption: During routine use, antacids are nonabsorbable. With chronic use, 15–30% of magnesium and smaller amounts of aluminum may be absorbed.
Distribution: Small amounts absorbed are widely distributed, cross the placenta, and appear in breast milk. Aluminum concentrates in the CNS.
Metabolism and Excretion: Excreted by the kidneys.
Half-life: Unknown.

TIME/ACTION PROFILE (effect on gastric pH)

ROUTE	ONSET	PEAK	DURATION
Aluminum PO	slightly delayed	30 min	30 min–1 hr (empty stomach); 3 hr (after meals)
Magnesium PO	slightly delayed	30 min	30 min–1 hr (empty stomach); 3 hr (after meals)

Contraindications/Precautions
Contraindicated in: Severe abdominal pain of unknown cause, especially if accompanied by fever; Renal failure (CrCl <30 ml/min); Products containing tartrazine or sugar in patients with known intolerance.
Use Cautiously in: Antacids containing magnesium in patients with any degree of renal insufficiency; Decreased bowel motility; Dehydration; Upper GI hemorrhage; Pedi: Children <12 yr (safety not established).

Adverse Reactions/Side Effects
GI: *aluminum salts*— constipation; *magnesium salts*— diarrhea. **F and E:** *magnesium salts*— hypermagnesemia; *aluminum salts*— hypophosphatemia.

Interactions
Drug-Drug: Absorption of **tetracyclines**, **phenothiazines**, **ketoconazole**, **itraconazole**, **iron salts**, **fluoroquinolones**, and **isoniazid** may be ↓ (separate by at least 2 hr).

Route/Dosage

Magaldrate/Simethicone
PO (Adults): 5–10 ml (540–1080 mg) between meals and at bedtime.

Magnesium Hydroxide/Aluminum Hydroxide
PO (Adults and Children ≥12 yr): 5–30 ml or 1–2 tablets 1–3 hr after meals and at bedtime.

Availability

Magaldrate/Simethicone
Suspension: 540 mg magaldrate/20 mg simethicone/5 ml[OTC], 1080 mg magaldrate/40 mg simethicone/5 ml[OTC].

Magnesium Hydroxide/Aluminum Hydroxide
Chewable Tablets: 300 mg aluminum hydroxide/150 mg magnesium hydroxide[OTC]. **Suspension:** 225 mg aluminum hydroxide/200 mg magnesium hydroxide/5 ml[OTC], 500 mg aluminum hydroxide/500 mg magnesium hydroxide/5 ml[OTC]. ***In combination with:*** simethicone[OTC]. See Appendix B.

✤ = Canadian drug name.
* CAPITALS indicates life-threatening; underlines indicate most frequent.

M

NURSING IMPLICATIONS

Assessment

- **Antacid:** Assess for heartburn and indigestion as well as location, duration, character, and precipitating factors of gastric pain.
- ***Lab Test Considerations:*** Monitor serum phosphate, potassium, and calcium levels periodically during chronic use. May cause increased serum calcium and decreased serum phosphate concentrations.

Potential Nursing Diagnoses

Acute pain (Indications)

Implementation

- Magnesium and aluminum are combined as antacids to balance the constipating effects of aluminum with the laxative effects of magnesium.
- **PO:** To prevent tablets from entering small intestine in undissolved form, they must be chewed thoroughly before swallowing. Follow with ½ glass of water.
- Shake suspensions well before administration.
- For an antacid effect, administer 1–3 hr after meals and at bedtime.

Patient/Family Teaching

- Caution patient to consult health care professional before taking antacids for more than 2 wk if problem is recurring, if relief is not obtained, or if symptoms of gastric bleeding (black, tarry stools; coffee-ground emesis) occur.
- Advise patient not to take this medication within 2 hr of taking other medications.
- Pedi: Aluminum- or magnesium-containing medicines can cause serious side effects in children, especially when given to children with renal disease or dehydration. Advise parents or caregivers not to administer OTC antacids to children without a doctor's order.

Evaluation/Desired Outcomes

- Relief of gastric pain and irritation.

magnesium salicylate, **See SALICYLATES.**

MAGNESIUM SALTS (ORAL)

magnesium chloride (12% Mg; 9.8 mEq Mg/g)
(mag-**nee**-zhum **klor**-ide)
Chloromag, Slo-Mag

magnesium citrate (16.2% Mg; 4.4 mEq Mg/g)
(mag-**nee**-zhum **si**-trate)
Citrate of Magnesia, Citroma, ✤Citromag

magnesium gluconate (5.4 % Mg; 4.4 mEq/g)
Almoate, Magtrate, Magonate

magnesium hydroxide (41.7% Mg; 34.3 mEq Mg/g)
(mag-**nee**-zhum hye-**drox**-ide)
Dulcolax Magnesia Tablets, Phillips Magnesia Tablets, Phillips Milk of Magnesia, MOM

magnesium oxide (60.3% Mg; 49.6 mEq Mg/g)
(mag-**nee**-zhum **ox**-ide)
Mag-Ox 400, Maox, Uro-Mag

Classification
Therapeutic: mineral and electrolyte replacements/supplements, laxatives
Pharmacologic: salines

Pregnancy Category UK

Indications

Treatment/prevention of hypomagnesemia. As a: Laxative, Bowel evacuant in preparation for surgical/radiographic procedures. Milk of Magnesia has also been used as an antacid.

Action

Essential for the activity of many enzymes. Play an important role in neurotransmission and muscular excitability. Are osmotically active in GI tract, drawing water into the lumen and causing peristalsis. **Therapeutic Effects:** Replacement in deficiency states. Evacuation of the colon.

Pharmacokinetics

Absorption: Up to 30% may be absorbed orally.
Distribution: Widely distributed. Cross the placenta and are present in breast milk.
Metabolism and Excretion: Excreted primarily by the kidneys.
Half-life: Unknown.

TIME/ACTION PROFILE (laxative effect)

ROUTE	ONSET	PEAK	DURATION
PO	3–6 hr	unknown	unknown

Contraindications/Precautions

Contraindicated in: Hypermagnesemia; Hypocalcemia; Anuria; Heart block; OB: Active labor or within 2 hr of delivery (unless used for preterm labor).
Use Cautiously in: Any degree of renal insufficiency.

Adverse Reactions/Side Effects

GI: diarrhea. **Derm:** flushing, sweating.

Interactions

Drug-Drug: Potentiates **neuromuscular blocking agents**. May ↓ absorption of **fluoroquinolones, nitrofurantoin,** and **tetracyclines** and **penicillamine**.

Route/Dosage

Prevention of Deficiency (in mg of Magnesium)

PO (Adults and Children >10 yr): *Adolescent and adult men*—270–400 mg/day; *adolescent and adult women*—280–300 mg/day; *pregnant women*—320 mg/day; *breastfeeding women*—340–355 mg/day.
PO (Children 7–10 yr): 170 mg/day.
PO (Children 4–6 yr): 120 mg/day.
PO (Children birth–3 yr): 40–80 mg/day.

Treatment of Deficiency (expressed as mg of Magnesium)

PO (Adults): 200–400 mg/day in 3–4 divided doses.
PO (Children 6–11 yr): 3–6 mg/kg/day in 3–4 divided doses.

Laxative

PO (Adults): *Magnesium citrate*—240 ml; *magnesium hydroxide (Milk of Magnesia)*—30–60 ml single or divided dose or 10–20 ml as concentrate.
PO (Children 6–12 yr): *Magnesium citrate*—100 ml; *magnesium hydroxide (Milk of Magnesia)*—15–30 ml single or divided dose.
PO (Children 2–5 yr): *magnesium hydroxide (Milk of Magnesia)*—5–15 ml single or divided dose.

Availability

Magnesium Chloride

Sustained-release tablets: 535 mg (64 mg magnesium)[OTC]. **Enteric-coated tablets:** 833 mg (100 mg magnesium)[OTC].

Magnesium Citrate

Oral solution: 240-, 296-, and 300-ml bottles (77 mEq magnesium/100 ml)[OTC].

Magnesium Gluconate

Tablets: 500 mg[OTC]. **Liquid:** 54 mg/5 ml[OTC].

Magnesium Hydroxide

Liquid: 400 mg/5 ml (164 mg magnesium/5 ml)[OTC]. **Concentrated liquid:** 800 mg/5 ml (328 mg magnesium/5 ml)[OTC]. **Chewable tablets:** 300 mg (130 mg magnesium)[OTC], 600 mg (260 mg magnesium)[OTC].

Magnesium Oxide

Tablets: 400 mg (241.3 mg magnesium)[OTC].
Capsules: 140 mg (84.5 mg magnesium)[OTC].

NURSING IMPLICATIONS

Assessment

- **Laxative:** Assess patient for abdominal distention, presence of bowel sounds, and usual pattern of bowel function.
- Assess color, consistency, and amount of stool produced.
- **Antacid:** Assess for heartburn and indigestion as well as location, duration, character, and precipitating factors of gastric pain.

Potential Nursing Diagnoses

Constipation (Indications)

Implementation

- **PO:** To prevent tablets entering small intestine in undissolved form, they must be chewed thoroughly before swallowing. Follow with ½ glass of water.
- *Magnesium citrate:* Refrigerate solutions to ensure they retain potency and palatability. May be served over ice. Magnesium citrate in an open container will lose carbonation upon standing; this will not affect potency but may reduce palatability.
- *Magnesium hydroxide:* Shake solution well before administration.
- **Antacid:** Administer 1–3 hr after meals and at bedtime.
- Powder and liquid forms are considered more effective than tablets.

M

- **Laxative:** Administer on empty stomach for more rapid results. Follow all oral laxative doses with a full glass of liquid to prevent dehydration and for faster effect. Do not administer at bedtime or late in the day.

Patient/Family Teaching

- Advise patient not to take this medication within 2 hr of taking other medications, especially fluoroquinolones, nitrofurantoin, and tetracyclines.
- **Antacids:** Caution patient to consult health care professional before taking antacids for more than 2 wk if problem is recurring, if relief is not obtained, or if symptoms of gastric bleeding (black, tarry stools; coffee-ground emesis) occur.
- **Laxatives:** Advise patient that laxatives should be used only for short-term therapy. Long-term therapy may cause electrolyte imbalance and dependence.
- Encourage patient to use other forms of bowel regulation, such as increasing bulk in the diet, fluid intake, and mobility. Normal bowel habits are individualized; frequency of bowel movement may vary from 3 times/day to 3 times/wk.
- Advise patient to notify health care professional if unrelieved constipation, rectal bleeding, or symptoms of electrolyte imbalance (muscle cramps or pain, weakness, dizziness) occur.

Evaluation/Desired Outcomes

- Relief of gastric pain and irritation.
- Passage of a soft, formed bowel movement, usually within 3–6 hr.
- Prevention and treatment of magnesium deficiency.

HIGH ALERT

magnesium sulfate (IV, parenteral) (9.9% Mg; 8.1 mEq Mg/g)

(mag-**nee**-zhum **sul**-fate)

Classification
Therapeutic: mineral and electrolyte replacements/supplements
Pharmacologic: minerals/electrolytes

Pregnancy Category D

Indications

Treatment/prevention of hypomagnesemia. Treatment of hypertension. Anticonvulsant associated with severe eclampsia, pre-eclampsia, or acute nephritis. **Unlabeled uses:** Preterm labor. Treatment of Torsade de pointes. Adjunctive treatment for bronchodilation in moderate to severe acute asthma.

Action

Essential for the activity of many enzymes. Plays an important role in neurotransmission and muscular excitability. **Therapeutic Effects:** Replacement in deficiency states. Resolution of eclampsia.

Pharmacokinetics

Absorption: IV administration results in complete bioavailability; well absorbed from IM sites.
Distribution: Widely distributed. Crosses the placenta and is present in breast milk.
Metabolism and Excretion: Excreted primarily by the kidneys.
Half-life: Unknown.

TIME/ACTION PROFILE (anticonvulsant effect)

ROUTE	ONSET	PEAK	DURATION
IM	60 min	unknown	3–4 hr
IV	immediate	unknown	30 min

Contraindications/Precautions

Contraindicated in: Hypermagnesemia; Hypocalcemia; Anuria; Heart block; Active labor or within 2 hr of delivery (unless used for preterm labor).
Use Cautiously in: Any degree of renal insufficiency; Digitalized patients.

Adverse Reactions/Side Effects

CNS: drowsiness. **Resp:** decreased respiratory rate. **CV:** arrhythmias, bradycardia, hypotension. **GI:** diarrhea. **MS:** muscle weakness. **Derm:** flushing, sweating. **Metab:** hypothermia.

Interactions

Drug-Drug: Potentiate **calcium channel blockers** and **neuromuscular blocking agents**.

Route/Dosage

Treatment of Deficiency (expressed as mg of Magnesium)

IM, IV (Adults): *Severe deficiency*—8–12 g/day in divided doses; *mild deficiency*—1 g q 6 hr for 4 doses or 250 mg/kg over 4 hr.

IM, IV (Children >1 month): 25–50 mg/kg/dose q 4–6 hr for 3–4 doses, maximum single dose: 2 g.
IV (Neonates): 25–50 mg/kg/dose q 8–12 hr for 2–3 doses.

Seizures/Hypertension

IM, IV (Adults): 1 g q 6 hr for 4 doses as needed.
IM, IV (Children): 20–100 mg/kg/dose q 4–6 hr as needed, may use up to 200 mg/kg/dose in severe cases.

Torsade de pointes

IV (Infants and Children): 25–50 mg/kg/dose, maximum dose: 2 g.

Bronchodilation

IV (Adults): 2 g single dose.
IV (Children): 25 mg/kg/dose, maximum dose: 2 g.

Eclampsia/Pre-Eclampsia

IV, IM (Adults): 4–5 g by IV infusion, concurrently with up to 5 g IM in each buttock; then 4–5 g IM q 4 hr *or* 4 g by IV infusion followed by 1–2 g/hr continuous infusion (not to exceed 40 g/day or 20 g/48 hr in the presence of severe renal insufficiency).

Part of Parenteral Nutrition

IV (Adults): 4–24 mEq/day.
IV (Children): 0.25–0.5 mEq/kg/day.

Availability (generic available)

Injection: 500 mg/ml (50%). **Premixed infusion:** 1 g/100 ml, 2 g/100 ml, 4 g/50 ml, 4 g/100 ml, 20 g/500 ml, 40 g/1000 ml.

NURSING IMPLICATIONS

Assessment

- **Hypomagnesemia/Anticonvulsant:** Monitor pulse, blood pressure, respirations, and ECG frequently throughout administration of parenteral magnesium sulfate. Respirations should be at least 16/min before each dose.
- Monitor neurologic status before and throughout therapy. Institute seizure precautions. Patellar reflex (knee jerk) should be tested before each parenteral dose of magnesium sulfate. If response is absent, no additional doses should be administered until positive response is obtained.
- Monitor newborn for hypotension, hyporeflexia, and respiratory depression if mother has received magnesium sulfate.
- Monitor intake and output ratios. Urine output should be maintained at a level of at least 100 ml/4 hr.
- ***Lab Test Considerations:*** Monitor serum magnesium levels and renal function periodically throughout administration of parenteral magnesium sulfate.

Potential Nursing Diagnoses

Risk for injury (Indications, Side Effects)

Implementation

- ***High Alert:*** Accidental overdosage of IV magnesium has resulted in serious patient harm and death. Have second practitioner independently double-check original order, dose calculations, and infusion pump settings. Do not confuse milligram (mg), gram (g), or millequivalent (mEq) dosages.
- **IM:** Administer deep IM into gluteal sites. Administer subsequent injections in alternate sides. Dilute to a concentration of 200 mg/ml prior to injection.

IV Administration

- **Direct IV:** ***Diluent:*** 50% solution must be diluted in 0.9% NaCl or D5W to a concentration of ≤20% prior to administration. ***Concentration:*** ≤20%. ***Rate:*** Administer at a rate not to exceed 150 mg/min.
- **Continuous Infusion:** ***Diluent:*** Dilute in D5W, 0.9% NaCl, or LR. ***Concentration:*** 0.5 mEq/ml (60 mg/ml) (may use maximum concentration of 1.6 mEq/ml (200 mg/ml) in fluid-restricted patients). ***Rate:*** Infuse over 2-4 hr. Do not exceed a rate of 1 mEq/kg/hr (125 mg/kg/hr). When rapid infusions are needed (severe asthma or Torsade de pointes) may infuse over 10–20 min.
- **Y-Site Compatibility:** acyclovir, aldesleukin, amifostine, amikacin, ampicillin, atropine, aztreonam, bivalirudin, bumetanide, calcium gluconate, caspofungin, cefazolin, cefotaxime, cefoxitin, ceftazidime, ceftizoxime, chloramphenicol, cimetidine, cisatracurium, clindamycin, daptomycin, cefazolin, cefotaxime dexmedetomidine, digoxin, diltiazem, diphenhydramine, dobutamine, cefazolin, cefotaxime docetaxel, dopamine, cefazolin, cefotaxime, doxorubicin liposome, doxycycline, enalaprilat, epinephrine, cefazo-

M

lin, cefotaxime erythromycin, ertapenem, esmolol, cefazolin, cefotaxime etoposide phosphate, famotidine, fenoldopam, fentanyl, fluconazole, fludarabine, gentamicin, granisetron, heparin, hydromorphone, hydroxyzine, idarubicin, imipenem/cilastatin, insulin, isoproterenol, ketorolac, labetalol, levofloxacin, lidocaine, linezolid, lorazepam, meperidine, metoclopramide, metoprolol, metronidazole, micafungin, midazolam, milrinone, morphine, nafcillin, nicardipine, nitroglycerin, nitroprusside, norepinephrine, ondansetron, oxaliplatin, paclitaxel, palonosetron, pantoprazole, penicillin G potassium, phenylephrine, piperacillin/tazobactam, potassium chloride, procainamide, prochlorperazine, promethazine, propofol, propranolol, protamine, quinupristin/dalfopristin, ranitidine, remifentanil, sargramostim, sodium bicarbonate, tacrolimus, thiotepa, ticarcillin/clavulanate, tirofiban, tobramycin, trimethoprim/sulfamethoxazole, vancomycin, vasopressin, verapamil, vitamin B complex with C, voriconazole.

- **Y-Site Incompatibility:** aminophylline, amphotericin B cholesteryl sulfate complex, calcium chloride, cefepime, ceftriaxone, cefuroxime, ciprofloxacin, dexamethasone sodium phosphate, diazepam, drotrecogin, haloperidol, lansoprazole, methylprednisolone sodium succinate, phenytoin, phytonadione.

Patient/Family Teaching

- Explain purpose of medication to patient and family.

Evaluation/Desired Outcomes

- Normal serum magnesium concentrations.
- Control of seizures associated with toxemias of pregnancy.

mannitol (man-i-tol)

Osmitrol, Resectisol

Classification

Therapeutic: diuretics

Pharmacologic: osmotic diuretics

Pregnancy Category C

Indications

IV: Adjunct in the treatment of: Acute oliguric renal failure, Edema, Increased intracranial or intraocular pressure, Toxic overdose. **GU irrigant:** During transurethral procedures (2.5–5% solution only).

Action

Increases the osmotic pressure of the glomerular filtrate, thereby inhibiting reabsorption of water and electrolytes. Causes excretion of: Water, Sodium, Potassium, Chloride, Calcium, Phosphorus, Magnesium, Urea, Uric acid. **Therapeutic Effects:** Mobilization of excess fluid in oliguric renal failure or edema. Reduction of intraocular or intracranial pressure. Increased urinary excretion of toxic materials. Decreased hemolysis when used as an irrigant after transurethral prostatic resection.

Pharmacokinetics

Absorption: IV administration produces complete bioavailability. Some absorption may follow use as a GU irrigant.

Distribution: Confined to the extracellular space; does not usually cross the blood-brain barrier or eye.

Metabolism and Excretion: Excreted by the kidneys; minimal liver metabolism.

Half-life: 100 min.

TIME/ACTION PROFILE (diuretic effect)

ROUTE	ONSET	PEAK	DURATION
IV	30–60 min	1 hr	6–8 hr

Contraindications/Precautions

Contraindicated in: Hypersensitivity; Anuria; Dehydration; Active intracranial bleeding.

Use Cautiously in: Pregnancy and lactation (safety not established).

Adverse Reactions/Side Effects

CNS: confusion, headache. **EENT:** blurred vision, rhinitis. **CV:** transient volume expansion, chest pain, CHF, pulmonary edema, tachycardia. **GI:** nausea, thirst, vomiting. **GU:** renal failure, urinary retention. **F and E:** dehydration, hyperkalemia, hypernatremia, hypokalemia, hyponatremia. **Local:** phlebitis at IV site.

Interactions

Drug-Drug: Hypokalemia increases the risk of **digoxin** toxicity.

Route/Dosage

IV (Adults): *Edema, oliguric renal failure*—50–100 g as a 5–25% solution; may precede with a test dose of 0.2 g/kg over 3–5 min. *Reduction of intracranial/intraocular pressure*—0.25–2 g/kg as 15–25% solution over 30–60 min (500 mg/kg may be sufficient in

small or debilitated patients). *Diuresis in drug intoxications*—50–200 g as a 5–25% solution titrated to maintain urine flow of 100–500 ml/hr.
IV (Children): *Edema, oliguric renal failure*—0.25–2 g/kg (60 g/m²) as a 15–20% solution over 2–6 hr; may precede with a test dose of 0.2 g/kg over 3–5 min. *Reduction of intracranial/intraocular pressure*—1–2 g/kg (30–60 g/m²) as a 15–20% solution over 30–60 min (500 mg/kg may be sufficient in small or debilitated patients). *Diuresis in drug intoxications*—up to 2 g/kg (60 g/m²) as a 5–10% solution.

Availability (generic available)

IV injection: 5%, 10%, 15%, 20%. **GU irrigant:** 5%. ***In combination with:*** sorbitol for GU irrigation.

NURSING IMPLICATIONS

Assessment

- Monitor vital signs, urine output, CVP, and pulmonary artery pressures (PAP) before and hourly throughout administration. Assess patient for signs and symptoms of dehydration (decreased skin turgor, fever, dry skin and mucous membranes, thirst) or signs of fluid overload (increased CVP, dyspnea, rales/crackles, edema).
- Assess patient for anorexia, muscle weakness, numbness, tingling, paresthesia, confusion, and excessive thirst. Report signs of electrolyte imbalance.
- **Increased Intracranial Pressure:** Monitor neurologic status and intracranial pressure readings in patients receiving this medication to decrease cerebral edema.
- **Increased Intraocular Pressure:** Monitor for persistent or increased eye pain or decreased visual acuity.
- ***Lab Test Considerations:*** Renal function and serum electrolytes should be monitored routinely throughout course of therapy.

Potential Nursing Diagnoses

Excess fluid volume (Indications)
Risk for deficient fluid volume (Side Effects)

Implementation

- Observe infusion site frequently for infiltration. Extravasation may cause tissue irritation and necrosis.
- Do not administer electrolyte-free mannitol solution with blood. If blood must be administered simultaneously with mannitol, add at least 20 mEq NaCl to each liter of mannitol.
- Confer with physician regarding placement of an indwelling Foley catheter (except when used to decrease intraocular pressure).
- **IV:** Administer by IV infusion undiluted. If solution contains crystals, warm bottle in hot water and shake vigorously. Do not administer solution in which crystals remain undissolved. Cool to body temperature. Use an in-line filter for 15%, 20%, and 25% infusions.
- **Test Dose:** Administer over 3–5 min to produce a urine output of 30–50 ml/hr. If urine flow does not increase, administer 2nd test dose. If urine output is not at least 30–50 ml/hr for 2–3 hr after 2nd test dose, patient should be re-evaluated.
- **Oliguria:** Administration rate should be titrated to produce a urine output of 30–50 ml/hr. Administer child's dose over 2–6 hr.
- **Increased Intracranial Pressure:** Infuse dose over 30–60 min in adults and children.
- **Intraocular Pressure:** Administer dose over 30 min. When used preoperatively, administer 60–90 min before surgery.
- **Y-Site Compatibility:** amifostine, aztreonam, fludarabine, fluorouracil, idarubicin, linezolid, melphalan, ondansetron, paclitaxel, piperacillin/tazobactam, sargramostim, teniposide, thiotepa, vinorelbine.
- **Y-Site Incompatibility:** cefepime, filgrastim.
- **Irrigation:** Add contents of two 50-ml vials of 25% mannitol to 900 ml of sterile water for injection for a 2.5% solution for irrigation. Use only clear solutions.

Patient/Family Teaching

- Explain purpose of therapy to patient.

Evaluation/Desired Outcomes

- Urine output of at least 30–50 ml/hr or an increase in urine output in accordance with parameters set by physician.
- Reduction in intracranial pressure.
- Reduction of intraocular pressure.
- Excretion of certain toxic substances.
- Irrigation during transurethral prostate resection.

maraviroc (ma-ra-**vi**-rok)
Selzentry

Classification
Therapeutic: antiretrovirals
Pharmacologic: CCR5 co-receptor antagonists

Pregnancy Category B

Indications
HIV infection (with other antiretrovirals), specifically in patients with only CCR5–tropic HIV-1 detectable, with evidence of viral replication and HIV-1 strains displaying multiple resistance to other antiretrovirals. Use should be determined by treatment history and tropism testing.

Action
Blocks a specific receptor on CD-4 and T-cell surfaces which prevents CCR5–tropic HIV-1 from entering. **Therapeutic Effects:** Decreased invasion of CD-4 and T-cells by CCR5–tropic HIV-1 virus resulting in viral replication.

Pharmacokinetics
Absorption: 2–33% absorbed following oral administration.
Distribution: Unknown.
Metabolism and Excretion: Mostly metabolized by the liver (CYP3A enzyme system); 8% renal excretion as unchanged drug.
Half-life: 14–18 hr.

TIME/ACTION PROFILE (blood levels)

ROUTE	ONSET	PEAK	DURATION
PO	unknown	0.5–4 hr	1–2 hr

Contraindications/Precautions
Contraindicated in: Dual/mixed or CXCR4–tropic HIV-1; OB: Lactation (breastfeeding not recommended for HIV-infected patients).
Use Cautiously in: Pre-existing liver disease including Hepatitis B or C (may ↑ risk of hepatotoxicity; Cardiovascular disease or risk factors (increased risk of cardiovascular events); Hepatic impairment; Renal impairment (if CCr <50 ml/min and using a CYP3A inhibitor use only if necessary); Treatment-naive adults (safety/efficacy not established); Geri: Consider age-related decrease in renal/hepatic function, concurrent drug therapy and concomittant disease; OB: Use only if clearly needed; Pedi: Safe use in children <16 yr not established.

Adverse Reactions/Side Effects
CNS: dizziness. **Resp:** cough, upper respiratory tract infection. **GI:** abdominal pain, appetite disorder, HEPATOTOXICITY. **Derm:** RASH. **MS:** musculoskeletal pain. **Misc:** ALLERGIC REACTIONS, fever, immune reconstitution syndrome, ↑ risk of infection.

Interactions
Drug-Drug: Levels are ↑ by **CYP3A inhibitors** including **protease inhibitors** (excluding tipranavir/ritonavir), **delavirdine**, **ketoconazole**, **lopinavir/ritonavir**, **saquinavir**, and **atazanavir**. Levels are ↓ by **CYP3A inducers** including **efavirenz** and **rifampin**.

Route/Dosage
PO (Adults): *Concurrent CYP3A inhibitors (except tipranavir/ritonavir) or delavirdine*—150 mg twice daily; *Concurrent NRTIs, tipranavir/ritonavir, nevirapine and other drugs that are not strong inhibitors/inducers of CYP3A*—300 mg twice daily; *Concurrent CYP3A inducers including efavirenz*—600 mg twice daily.

Availability
Tablets: 150 mg, 300 mg.

NURSING IMPLICATIONS

Assessment
- Assess patient for change in severity of HIV symptoms and for symptoms of opportunistic infections throughout therapy.
- Assess for signs of hepatitis or allergic reaction (pruritic rash, jaundice, dark urine, vomiting, abdominal pain). If symptoms occur, discontinue maraviroc immediately.
- ***Lab Test Considerations:*** Testing for CCR5–tropic HIV-1 should be obtained prior to initiating therapy.
- Monitor viral load and CD-4 cell count regularly during therapy.
- May cause ↑ AST, ALT, total bilirubin, amylase, and lipase.
- May cause ↓ absolute neutrophil count.

Potential Nursing Diagnoses
Risk for infection (Indications)
Deficient knowledge, related to medication regimen (Patient/Family Teaching)

Implementation
- **PO:** May be administered without regard to food. Tablets should be swallowed whole; do not crush, break, or chew.

Patient/Family Teaching

- Emphasize the importance of taking maraviroc as directed, at the same time each day. Advise patient to read the Patient Information that comes with the medication each time the Rx is refilled. Maraviroc must always be used in combination with other antiretroviral drugs. Do not take more than prescribed amount and do not stop taking without consulting health care professional. If a dose is missed, take as soon as remembered, then return to regular dose schedule. If it is within 6 hr of next dose, omit dose and take next dose at regular time. Do not double doses.
- Instruct patient that maraviroc should not be shared with others.
- Inform patient that maraviroc does not cure AIDS or prevent associated or opportunistic infections. Maraviroc does not reduce the risk of transmission of HIV to others through sexual contact or blood contamination. Caution patient to use a condom and to avoid sharing needles or donating blood to prevent spreading the AIDS virus to others. The long-term effects of maraviroc are unknown at this time. If new symptoms of infection develop after starting maraviroc, notify health care professional.
- Advise patient to discontinue maraviroc and notify health care professional if itchy rash, yellow colored skin or eyes, dark urine, vomiting, or abdominal pain occur.
- May cause dizziness. Caution patient to avoid driving and other activities requiring alertness until response to medication is known.
- Advise patient to make position changes slowly to minimize postural hypotension.
- Instruct patient to consult health care professional before taking any Rx, OTC, or herbal products, especially St. John's Wort; may decrease effectiveness of maraviroc.
- Advise patient to notify health care professional if pregnancy is planned or suspected or if breastfeeding.
- Emphasize the importance of regular follow-up exams and blood counts to determine progress and monitor for side effects.

Evaluation/Desired Outcomes

- Delayed progression of AIDS and decreased opportunistic infections in patients with HIV.
- Decrease in viral load and increase in CD-4 cell counts.

MAST CELL STABILIZERS

cromolyn† (**kroe**-moe-lin)
✤Apo-Cromolyn, Gastrocrom, Intal, NasalCrom

nedocromil† (ne-doe-**kroe**-mil)
Tilade

Classification
Therapeutic: antiasthmatics, allergy, cold, and cough remedies
Pharmacologic: mast cell stabilizers

Pregnancy Category B

†For ophthalmic use, see Appendix C

Indications

Inhalation: Management (long-term control) of asthma; prevention of exercise-induced bronchospasm. **Intranasal (cromolyn only):** Prevention and treatment of seasonal and perennial allergic rhinitis. **Oral (cromolyn only):** Mastocytosis.

Action

Prevents the release of histamine, leukotrienes, and slow-reacting substance of anaphylaxis (SRS-A) from sensitized mast cells. **Therapeutic Effects:** Decreased frequency and intensity of asthmatic episodes, allergic reactions, and mastocytosis.

Pharmacokinetics

Absorption: *Cromolyn*—Poorly absorbed (<1% with oral); action is local. Small amounts may reach systemic circulation after inhalation. *Nedocromil*—poorly absorbed systemically (<2%).
Distribution: Because only small amounts are absorbed, distribution of these agents is not known.
Metabolism and Excretion: Small amounts absorbed are excreted unchanged in urine and bile (urine only for nedocromil).
Half-life: *Cromolyn*—80–90 min; *nedocromil*—1.5 hr.

TIME/ACTION PROFILE (effects on symptoms)

ROUTE	ONSET	PEAK	DURATION
Cromolyn—inhalation	1–2 wk	2–4 wk	unknown
Cromolyn—nasal	1–2 wk	2–4 wk	unknown

M

Cromolyn-oral	1–2 wk	2–6 wk	2–3 wk†
Nedocromil—inhalation	within 2 wk	unknown	unknown

†After treatment discontinued

Contraindications/Precautions
Contraindicated in: Hypersensitivity; Acute attacks of asthma (inhalation products).
Use Cautiously in: Will not relieve and may worsen acute attacks of bronchospasm (inhalation); Will not relieve and may worsen acute attacks of bronchospasm (inhalation); *Cromolyn*—Renal or hepatic dysfunction (oral only); OB, Lactation: Pregnancy and lactation (safety not established); Pedi: *Cromolyn*—Children <2 yr (safety not established); Pedi: *Nedocromil*—Children <6 yr (safety not established).

Adverse Reactions/Side Effects
CNS: dizziness, fatigue, headache. **CV:** chest pain. **EENT:** *intranasal*— nasal irritation, nasal congestion, pharyngitis, rhinitis, sneezing. **Resp:** *inhalation*— cough, cough, irritation of the throat and trachea, bronchospasm. **GI:** unpleasant taste, diarrhea, nausea, vomiting. **Derm:** erythema, rash, urticaria. **Misc:** allergic reactions including ANAPHYLAXIS or worsening of conditions being treated, fever.

Interactions
Drug-Drug: Not known.

Route/Dosage

Cromolyn
Inhaln (Adults and Children ≥2 yr): *Nebulized solution*—One ampule (20 mg) via nebulization 4 times daily. For prevention of bronchospasm, one ampule (20 mg) should be given via nebulization 10–15 min before exposure to known precipitating situation.
Inhaln (Adults and Children ≥5 yr): *Aerosol*—2 inhalations (0.8 mg/inhalation) 4 times daily; ↓ to 2–3 times daily once symptoms are well-controlled. For prevention of bronchospasm, use 2 inhalations 10–15 min before exposure to known precipitating situation.
Intranasal (Adults and Children ≥2 yr): 1 spray (5.2 mg/spray) each nostril 3–4 times daily (up to 6 times daily).
PO (Adults and Children >12 yr): 200 mg 4 times daily.
PO (Children 2–12 yr): 100 mg 4 times daily (not to exceed 40 mg/kg/day).

Nedocromil
Inhaln (Adults and Children ≥6 yr): 2 inhalations (1.75 mg/inhalation) 4 times daily; ↓ to 2–3 times daily once symptoms are well-controlled.

Availability

Cromolyn
Solution for nebulization: 10 mg/ml. **Aerosol for inhalation:** 800 mcg/actuation in 8.1-g (112 actuations) or 14.2-g (200 actuations) containers. **Nasal solution:** 40 mg/ml (5.2 mg/spray) in 13-ml (≥100 sprays) or 26-ml (≥200 sprays) containers[OTC]. **Oral solution:** 100 mg/5 ml.

Nedocromil
Aerosol for inhalation: 1.75 mg/actuation in 16.2-g canister (at least 104 inhalations).

NURSING IMPLICATIONS

Assessment
- **Inhaln:** Evaluate pulmonary function testing before initiating therapy in asthmatics.
- Assess lung sounds and respiratory function before and periodically during therapy.
- **Intranasal:** Assess for symptoms of rhinitis (stuffiness, rhinorrhea).
- **PO:** Assess for symptoms of mastocytosis (diarrhea, flushing, headache, vomiting, urticaria, abdominal pain, nausea, itching).

Potential Nursing Diagnoses
Ineffective airway clearance (Indications)

Implementation
- Reduction in dose of other asthma medications may be possible after 2–4 wk of therapy.
- **Inhaln:** Medication should be used prophylactically, not during acute asthma attacks or status asthmaticus.
- Pretreatment with bronchodilator may be required to increase delivery of inhalation product.
- Do not use nebulizer solution that is cloudy or contains a precipitate.
- **PO:** Cromolyn should be taken 30 min before meals and at bedtime. Dose should be mixed in glass of water. Patient should drink all of the water. Plastic ampules should be stored in foil pouch until ready to use.

Patient/Family Teaching
- Medication must be used routinely and not more frequently than prescribed. Take missed doses as soon as remembered and space other doses at regular intervals. Do not

double doses. Do not discontinue therapy without consulting health care professional, or exacerbation of symptoms may occur.

- Instruct patient not to discontinue concurrent corticosteroid or bronchodilator therapy without consulting health care professional.
- If cromolyn is prescribed before contact with known allergen or exercise, explain that it should be administered 10–15 min, and no earlier than 60 min, in advance.
- **Inhaln:** Instruct patient in the proper use of the metered-dose inhaler. See Appendix D for instructions.
- Caution patient to notify health care professional if asthmatic symptoms do not improve within 4 wk, worsen, or recur.
- **Intranasal:** Instruct patient to clear nasal passages before administration and to inhale through nose during administration.
- Instruct patient to start using product up to 1 wk before coming into contact with allergen and to use every day while in contact with allergen.
- **PO:** Instruct patient that the beneficial effects of cromolyn are dependent upon its use at regular intervals.

Evaluation/Desired Outcomes

- Therapeutic effects, observable within 2–4 wk after beginning therapy, are demonstrated by:
- Reduction in symptoms of asthma.
- Prevention of exercise-induced bronchospasm (cromolyn only).
- Decrease in the symptoms of allergic rhinitis (cromolyn only).
- Reduction in symptoms of mastocytosis (cromolyn only).

meclizine (mek-li-zeen)

Antivert, Antrizine, ✤Bonamine, Bonine, Dramamine Less Drowsy Formula, Meni-D, Vergon

Classification
Therapeutic: antiemetics, antihistamines

Pregnancy Category B

Indications

Management/prevention of: Motion sickness, Vertigo.

Action

Has central anticholinergic, CNS depressant, and antihistaminic properties. Decreases excitability of the middle ear labyrinth and depresses conduction in middle ear vestibular-cerebellar pathways. **Therapeutic Effects:** Decreased motion sickness. Decreased vertigo from vestibular pathology.

Pharmacokinetics

Absorption: Absorbed after oral administration.
Distribution: Unknown.
Metabolism and Excretion: Unknown.
Half-life: 6 hr.

TIME/ACTION PROFILE (antihistaminic effects)

ROUTE	ONSET	PEAK	DURATION
PO	1 hr	unknown	8–24 hr

Contraindications/Precautions

Contraindicated in: Hypersensitivity; Pregnancy.
Use Cautiously in: Prostatic hyperplasia; Angle-closure glaucoma; Geriatric (increased sensitivity; increased risk of adverse reactions); Children or lactation (safety not established).

Adverse Reactions/Side Effects

CNS: drowsiness, fatigue. **EENT:** blurred vision. **GI:** dry mouth.

Interactions

Drug-Drug: Additive CNS depression with other **CNS depressants**, including **alcohol**, other **antihistamines**, **opioid analgesics**, and **sedative/hypnotics**. Additive anticholinergic effects with other **drugs possessing anticholinergic properties**, including some **antihistamines**, **antidepressants**, **atropine**, **haloperidol**, **phenothiazines**, **quinidine**, and **disopyramide**.

Route/Dosage

PO (Adults): *Motion sickness*—25–50 mg 1 hr before exposure; may repeat in 24 hr; *vertigo*—25–100 mg/day in divided doses.

Availability

Tablets: 12.5 mg, 25 mg[Rx, OTC], 50 mg. **Cost:** 12.5 mg $4.09/100, 25 mg $5.40/100, 50 mg $6.99/100. **Chewable tablets:** 25 mg[Rx, OTC]. **Capsules:** 15 mg[OTC], 25 mg, 30 mg[OTC].

NURSING IMPLICATIONS

Assessment

- Assess patient for level of sedation after administration.
- **Motion Sickness:** Assess patient for nausea and vomiting before and 60 min after administration.
- **Vertigo:** Assess degree of vertigo periodically in patients receiving meclizine for labyrinthitis.
- ***Lab Test Considerations:*** May cause false-negative results in skin tests using allergen extracts. Discontinue meclizine 72 hr before testing.

Potential Nursing Diagnoses

Risk for injury (Side Effects)

Implementation

- **PO:** Administer oral doses with food, water, or milk to minimize GI irritation. Chewable tablet may be chewed or swallowed whole.

Patient/Family Teaching

- Instruct patient to take meclizine exactly as directed. If a dose is missed, take as soon as possible unless almost time for next dose. Do not double doses.
- May cause drowsiness. Caution patient to avoid driving or other activities requiring alertness until response to the medication is known.
- Advise patient that frequent mouth rinses, good oral hygiene, and sugarless gum or candy may decrease dryness of mouth.
- Caution patient to avoid concurrent use of alcohol and other CNS depressants with this medication.
- **Motion Sickness:** When used as prophylaxis for motion sickness, advise patient to take medication at least 1 hr before exposure to conditions that may cause motion sickness.

Evaluation/Desired Outcomes

- Prevention and relief of symptoms in motion sickness.
- Prevention and treatment of vertigo due to vestibular pathology.

medroxyPROGESTERone†

(me-**drox**-ee-proe-jess-te-rone)
✤Alti-MPA, Amen, Curretab, Cycrin, Depo-Provera, Depo-Sub Q Provera 104, ✤Gen-Medroxy, ✤Novo-Medrone, Provera, ✤Provera Pak, ✤Ratio-MPA

Classification
Therapeutic: antineoplastics, contraceptive hormones
Pharmacologic: hormones, progestins

Pregnancy Category X

†For contraceptive use see Contraceptives, Hormonal monograph

Indications

To decrease endometrial hyperplasia in postmenopausal women receiving concurrent estrogen (0.625 mg/day conjugated estrogens). Treatment of secondary amenorrhea and abnormal uterine bleeding caused by hormonal imbalance. **IM:** Treatment of advanced unresponsive endometrial or renal carcinoma. Management of endometriosis-associated pain (Depo-Sub Q Provera 104 only). **Unlabeled uses:** Obesity-hypoventilation (pickwickian) syndrome, sleep apnea, hypersomnolence.

Action

A synthetic form of progesterone—actions include secretory changes in the endometrium, increases in basal body temperature, histologic changes in vaginal epithelium, relaxation of uterine smooth muscle, mammary alveolar tissue growth, pituitary inhibition, and withdrawal bleeding in the presence of estrogen. **Therapeutic Effects:** Decreased endometrial hyperplasia in postmenopausal women receiving concurrent estrogen (combination with estrogen decreases vasomotor symptoms and prevents osteoporosis). Restoration of hormonal balance with control of uterine bleeding. Management of endometrial or renal cancer. Prevention of pregnancy.

Pharmacokinetics

Absorption: 0.6–10% absorbed after oral administration.
Distribution: Enters breast milk.
Metabolism and Excretion: Metabolized by the liver.
Half-life: *1st phase*—52 min; *2nd phase*—230 min; *biological*—14.5 hr.

TIME/ACTION PROFILE (IM = antineoplastic effects)

ROUTE	ONSET	PEAK	DURATION
PO	unknown	unknown	unknown
IM	wks–mos	mo	unknown†

SC	unknown	1 wk	3 mo

†Contraceptive effect lasts 3 mo

Contraindications/Precautions

Contraindicated in: Hypersensitivity; Hypersensitivity to parabens (IM suspension only); Pregnancy; Missed abortion; Thromboembolic disease; Cerebrovascular disease; Severe liver disease; Breast or genital cancer; Porphyria.
Use Cautiously in: History of liver disease; Renal disease; Cardiovascular disease; Seizure disorders; Mental depression; Lactation: Lactation (when used as a contraceptive, wait until 6 wk after delivery if breastfeeding).

Adverse Reactions/Side Effects

CNS: depression. **EENT:** retinal thrombosis. **CV:** PULMONARY EMBOLISM, thromboembolism, thrombophlebitis. **GI:** drug-induced hepatitis, gingival bleeding. **GU:** cervical erosions. **Derm:** chloasma, melasma, rashes. **Endo:** amenorrhea, breakthrough bleeding, breast tenderness, changes in menstrual flow, galactorrhea, hyperglycemia, spotting. **F and E:** edema. **Metab:** bone loss. **Misc:** allergic reactions including ANAPHYLAXIS and ANGIOEDEMA, weight gain, weight loss.

Interactions

Drug-Drug: May ↓ effectiveness of **bromocriptine** when used concurrently for galactorrhea/amenorrhea. Contraceptive effectiveness may be ↓ by **carbamazepine**, **phenobarbital**, **phenytoin**, **rifampin**, or **rifabutin**. **Aminoglutethimide** may ↓ oral absorption.

Route/Dosage

Postmenopausal Women Receiving Concurrent Estrogen

PO (Adults): 2.5–5 mg daily concurrently with 0.625 mg conjugated estrogens (monophasic regimen) *or* 5 mg daily on days 15–28 of the cycle with 0.625 mg conjugated estrogens taken daily throughout cycle (biphasic regimen).

Secondary Amenorrhea

PO (Adults): 5–10 mg/day for 5–10 days; start at any time in cycle.

Dysfunctional Uterine Bleeding/Induction of Menses

PO (Adults): 5–10 mg/day for 5–10 days, starting on day 16 or day 21 of menstrual cycle.

Renal or Endometrial Carcinoma

IM (Adults): 400–1000 mg, may be repeated weekly; if improvement occurs, attempt to decrease dosage to 400 mg monthly.

Endometriosis-Associated pain

Subcut (Adults): 104 mg every 12–14 wk (3 mo), beginning on day 5 of normal menses (not recommended for more than 2 years).

Availability (generic available)

Tablets: 2.5 mg, 5 mg, 10 mg, ♣100 mg. **Suspension for depot injection:** ♣50 mg/ml, ♣100 mg/ml, 150 mg/ml, 400 mg/ml. **Suspension for subcutaneous injection (Depo-Sub Q Provera 104):** 104 mg/0.65 ml in single-use syringes. ***In combination with:*** conjugated estrogens as Prempro (single combination tablet of 0.626 mg conjugated estrogens plus 2.5 or 5 mg medroxyprogesterone) or Premphase (0.625 mg conjugated estrogens tablet for 14 days followed by combination tablet of 0.625 mg conjugated estrogens plus 5 mg medroxyprogesterone for days 15–28) in convenience packages. See Appendix B.

NURSING IMPLICATIONS

Assessment

- Monitor blood pressure periodically during therapy.
- Assess patient's usual menstrual history. Administration of drug may begin on any day of cycle in patients with amenorrhea and on day 16 or 21 of cycle in patients with dysfunctional bleeding
- Monitor intake and output ratios and weekly weight. Report significant discrepancies or steady weight gain.
- ***Lab Test Considerations:*** Monitor hepatic function before and periodically during therapy.
- May cause ↑ alkaline phosphatase levels. May ↓ pregnanediol excretion concentrations.
- May cause ↑ serum LDL concentrations or ↓ HDL concentrations.
- May alter thyroid hormone assays.

Potential Nursing Diagnoses

Sexual dysfunction (Indications)
Ineffective tissue perfusion (Side Effects)

M

♣ = Canadian drug name.
* CAPITALS indicates life-threatening; underlines indicate most frequent.

Implementation

- Do not confuse Provera (medroxyprogesterone) with Covera (verapamil).
- Only the 150-mg/ml vial should be used for contraception.
- Injectable medroxyprogesterone may lead to bone loss, especially in women younger than 21 years. Injectable medroxyprogesterone should be used for >2 years only if other methods of contraception are inadequate. If used long term, women should use supplemental calcium and vitamin D, and monitor bone mineral density.
- **Subcut:** Shake vigorously before use to form a uniform suspension. Inject slowly (over 5–7 Seconds) at a 45° angle into fatty area of anterior thigh or abdomen every 12 to 14 wks. If more than 14 wks elapse between injections, rule out pregnancy prior to administration. **Do not rub area after injection**.
- When switching from other hormonal contraceptives, administer within dosing period (7 days after taking last active pill, removing patch or ring, or within the dosing period for IM injection).
- **IM:** Shake vial vigorously before preparing IM dose. Administer deep IM into gluteal or deltoid muscle. If period between injections is >14 wk, determine that patient is not pregnant before administering the drug.
- In patients with cancer, IM dose may initially be required weekly. Once stabilized, IM dose may be required only monthly.

Patient/Family Teaching

- Explain the dose schedule. Instruct patient to take medication at the same time each day. Take missed doses as soon as remembered, but do not double doses.
- Advise patients receiving medroxyprogesterone for menstrual dysfunction to anticipate withdrawal bleeding 3–7 days after discontinuing medication.
- Review patient package insert (PPI) with patient. Emphasize the importance of notifying health care professional if the following side effects occur: visual changes, sudden weakness, incoordination, difficulty with speech, headache, leg or calf pain, shortness of breath, chest pain, changes in vaginal bleeding pattern, yellow skin, swelling of extremities, depression, or rash. Patients receiving medroxyprogesterone for cancer may not receive PPI.
- Advise patient to keep a 1-mo supply of medroxyprogesterone available at all times.
- Instruct patient in correct method of monthly breast self-examination. Increased breast tenderness may occur.
- Advise patient that gingival bleeding may occur. Instruct patient to use good oral hygiene and to receive regular dental care and examinations.
- Instruct patient to notify health care professional if menstrual period is missed or if pregnancy is suspected. Patient should not attempt conception for 3 mo after discontinuing medication in order to decrease risk to fetus.
- Medroxyprogesterone may cause melasma (brown patches of discoloration) on face when patient is exposed to sunlight. Advise patient to avoid sun exposure and to wear sunscreen or protective clothing when outdoors.
- Emphasize the importance of routine follow-up physical exams, including blood pressure; breast, abdomen, and pelvic exams; and Papanicolaou smears every 6–12 mo.
- **IM, Subcut** Advise patient to maintain adequate amounts of dietary calcium and vitamin D to help prevent bone loss.

Evaluation/Desired Outcomes

- Regular menstrual periods.
- Decrease in endometrial hyperplasia in postmenopausal women receiving concurrent estrogen.
- Control of the spread of endometrial or renal cancer.

medroxyprogesterone, See CONTRACEPTIVES, HORMONAL.

megestrol (me-**jess**-trole)

Megace

Classification

Therapeutic: antineoplastics, hormones

Pharmacologic: progestins

Pregnancy Category D (tablets), X (suspension)

Indications

Palliative treatment of endometrial and breast carcinoma, either alone or with surgery or radiation (tablets only). Treatment of anorexia, weight loss, and cachexia associated with AIDS (oral suspension only).

Action

Antineoplastic effect may result from inhibition of pituitary function. **Therapeutic Effects:** Regression of tumor. Increased appetite and weight gain in patients with AIDS.

Pharmacokinetics

Absorption: Well absorbed from the GI tract.
Distribution: Unknown.
Protein Binding: ≥90%.
Metabolism and Excretion: Completely metabolized by the liver.
Half-life: 38 hr (range 13–104 hr).

TIME/ACTION PROFILE (antineoplastic activity)

ROUTE	ONSET	PEAK	DURATION
PO	wk–mos	2 mo	unknown

Contraindications/Precautions

Contraindicated in: Hypersensitivity; OB: Pregnancy, missed abortion, or lactation; Undiagnosed vaginal bleeding; Severe liver disease; Suspension contains alcohol and should be avoided in patients with known intolerance.
Use Cautiously in: Diabetes; Mental depression; Renal disease; History of thrombophlebitis; Cardiovascular disease; Seizure disorders.

Adverse Reactions/Side Effects

CV: THROMBOEMBOLISM, edema. **GI:** GI irritation. **Derm:** alopecia. **Endo:** asymptomatic adrenal suppression (chronic therapy). **Hemat:** thrombophlebitis. **MS:** carpal tunnel syndrome.

Interactions

Drug-Drug: None significant.

Route/Dosage

PO (Adults): *Breast carcinoma*—160 mg/day single dose or divided doses; *endometrial/ovarian carcinoma*—40–320 mg/day in divided doses; *anorexia associated with AIDS*—800 mg day; may decrease to 400 mg/day after 1 mo (range 400–800 mg/day).

Availability (generic available)

Tablets: 20 mg, 40 mg. **Cost:** *Generic*—20 mg $37.99/100, 40 mg $52.99/100. **Oral suspension (lemon-lime flavor):** 40 mg/ml in 10-ml, 20-ml, 240-ml, and 480-ml bottles, 125 mg/ml in 150-ml bottles (Megace ES). **Cost:** *Generic*—40 mg/ml $131.33/240 ml; *Megace ES*—125 mg/ml $526.89/150 ml.

NURSING IMPLICATIONS

Assessment

- Assess patient for swelling, pain, or tenderness in legs. Report these signs of deep vein thrombophlebitis.
- **Anorexia:** Monitor weight, appetite, and nutritional intake in patients with AIDS.

Potential Nursing Diagnoses

Imbalanced nutrition: less than body requirements (Indications)

Implementation

- Because of high dose, suspension is most convenient form for patients with AIDS.
- Do not confuse Megace 800 mg/20 mL with Megace ES 625 mg/5 mL.
- **PO:** May be administered with meals if GI irritation becomes a problem.

Patient/Family Teaching

- Instruct patient to take medication exactly as directed; do not skip or double up on missed doses. Missed doses may be taken as long as it is not right before next dose. Gradually decrease dose prior to discontinuation.
- Advise patient to report to health care professional any unusual vaginal bleeding or signs of deep vein thrombophlebitis.
- Advise patient that this medication may have teratogenic effects. Contraception should be used during therapy and for at least 4 months after therapy is completed.
- Discuss with patient the possibility of hair loss. Explore methods of coping.

Evaluation/Desired Outcomes

- Slowing or arresting the spread of endometrial or breast malignancy. Therapeutic effects usually occur within 2 months of initiating therapy.
- Increased appetite and weight gain in patients with AIDS.

meloxicam (me-lox-i-kam)
Mobic

M

Classification
Therapeutic: nonsteroidal anti-inflammatory agents
Pharmacologic: nonopioid analgesics

Pregnancy Category C

Indications
Relief of signs and symptoms of osteoarthritis and rheumatoid arthritis (including juvenile rheumatoid arthritis).

Action
Inhibits prostaglandin synthesis, probably by inhibiting the enzyme cyclooxygenase. **Therapeutic Effects:** Decreased pain and inflammation associated with osteoarthritis. Also decreases fever.

Pharmacokinetics
Absorption: Well absorbed following oral administration.
Distribution: Unknown.
Protein Binding: 99.4%.
Metabolism and Excretion: Mostly metabolized to inactive metabolites by the liver via the P450 enzyme system; metabolites are excreted in urine and feces.
Half-life: 20.1 hr.

TIME/ACTION PROFILE

ROUTE	ONSET	PEAK*	DURATION
PO	unknown	5–6 hr	24 hr

*Blood levels

Contraindications/Precautions
Contraindicated in: Hypersensitivity; Cross-sensitivity may occur with other NSAIDs, including aspirin; Severe renal impairment (CCr ≤15 ml/min); Concurrent use of aspirin (increased risk of adverse reactions); Peri-operative pain from coronary artery bypass graft (CABG) surgery.
Use Cautiously in: Cardiovascular disease or risk factors for cardiovascular disease (may ↑ risk of serious cardiovascular thrombotic events, myocardial infarction, and stroke, especially with prolonged use). Dehydration (correct deficits before initiating therapy); Geri: Impaired renal function, heart failure, liver dysfunction, geriatric patients (≥65 yr), concurrent ACE inhibitor or diuretic therapy (↑ risk of reversible renal dysfunction); Coagulation disorders or concurrent anticoagulant therapy (may ↑ risk of bleeding); Geri: Geriatric patients (↑ risk of GI bleeding); OB, Pedi: Pregnancy, lactation, or children <2 yr (safety not established; avoid use late in pregnancy).

Adverse Reactions/Side Effects
CV: edema. **GI:** GI BLEEDING, abnormal liver function tests, diarrhea, dyspepsia, nausea. **Derm:** EXFOLIATIVE DERMATITIS, STEVENS-JOHNSON SYNDROME, TOXIC EPIDERMAL NECROLYSIS, pruritus. **Hemat:** anemia, leukopenia, thrombocytopenia.

Interactions
Drug-Drug: May ↓ antihypertensive effects of **ACE inhibitors**. May ↓ diuretic effects of **furosemide** or **thiazide diuretics**. Concurrent use with **aspirin** ↑ meloxicam blood levels and may ↑ risk of adverse reactions. Concurrent use with **cholestyramine** ↓ blood levels. ↑ plasma **lithium** levels (close monitoring recommended when meloxicam is introduced or withdrawn). May ↑ risk of bleeding with **anticoagulants**, including **warfarin**.

Route/Dosage
PO (Adults): 7.5 mg once daily; some patients may require 15 mg/day.
PO (Children 2–17 yr and >12 kg): 0.125 mg/kg once daily up to 7.5mg/day.

Availability (generic available)
Tablets: 7.5 mg, 15 mg. **Cost:** *Generic*—7.5 mg $43.83/90, 15 mg $18.90/90. **Oral suspension (raspberry flavor):** 7.5 mg/5 mL in 100-mL bottles.

NURSING IMPLICATIONS

Assessment
- Patients who have asthma, aspirin-induced allergy, and nasal polyps are at increased risk for developing hypersensitivity reactions. Assess for rhinitis, asthma, and urticaria.
- Assess pain and range of motion prior to and 1–2 hr following administration.
- ***Lab Test Considerations:*** Evaluate BUN, serum creatinine, CBC, and liver function periodically in patients receiving prolonged therapy. May cause anemia, thrombocytopenia, leukopenia, and abnormal liver or renal function tests.
- Bleeding time may be prolonged.

Potential Nursing Diagnoses
Acute pain (Indications)
Impaired physical mobility (Indications)

Implementation
- Administration in higher than recommended doses does not provide increased effective-

ness but may cause increased side effects. Use lowest effective dose for shortest period of time.

- **PO:** May be administered without regard to food.
- Pedi: Use oral suspension to ensure accuracy of dosing in children.

Patient/Family Teaching

- Advise patient to take this medication with a full glass of water and to remain in an upright position for 15–30 min after administration.
- Instruct patient to take medication as directed. Take missed doses as soon as remembered but not if almost time for the next dose. Do not double doses.
- Caution patient to avoid the concurrent use of alcohol, aspirin, acetaminophen, or other OTC medications without consulting health care professional.
- Advise patient to inform health care professional of medication regimen prior to treatment or surgery.
- Advise patient to consult health care professional if rash, itching, visual disturbances, weight gain, edema, black stools, or signs of hepatotoxicity (nausea, fatigue, lethargy, jaundice, upper right quadrant tenderness, flu-like symptoms) occur.

Evaluation/Desired Outcomes

- Relief of pain.
- Improved joint mobility. Patients who do not respond to one NSAID may respond to another.

melphalan (mel-fa-lan)

Alkeran, L-PAM, phenylalanine mustard

Classification

Therapeutic: antineoplastics
Pharmacologic: alkylating agents

Pregnancy Category D

Indications

Alone or with other therapies for: Multiple myeloma, Ovarian cancer. **Unlabeled uses:** Breast cancer. Prostate cancer. Testicular carcinoma. Chronic myelogenous leukemia. Osteogenic sarcoma.

Action

Inhibits DNA and RNA synthesis by alkylation (cell-cycle phase–nonspecific). **Therapeutic Effects:** Death of rapidly replicating cells, particularly malignant ones. Also has immunosuppressive properties.

Pharmacokinetics

Absorption: Incompletely and variably absorbed following oral administration.
Distribution: Rapidly distributed throughout total body water.
Protein Binding: ≤30%.
Metabolism and Excretion: Rapidly metabolized in the bloodstream. Small amounts (10%) excreted unchanged by the kidneys.
Half-life: 1.5 hr.

TIME/ACTION PROFILE (effects on blood counts)

ROUTE	ONSET	PEAK	DURATION
PO	5 days	2–3 wk	5–6 wk

Contraindications/Precautions

Contraindicated in: Hypersensitivity to melphalan or chlorambucil; Pregnancy or lactation.
Use Cautiously in: Patients with childbearing potential; Active infections; Decreased bone marrow reserve; Geri: Geriatric patients or patients with other chronic debilitating illnesses; Impaired renal function (dose reduction recommended if BUN ≥30 mg/dl); Pedi: Children (safety not established).

Adverse Reactions/Side Effects

Resp: bronchopulmonary dysplasia, pulmonary fibrosis. **GI:** diarrhea, hepatitis, nausea, stomatitis, vomiting. **GU:** infertility. **Derm:** alopecia, pruritus, rashes. **Endo:** menstrual irregularities. **Hemat:** leukopenia, thrombocytopenia, anemia. **Metab:** hyperuricemia. **Misc:** allergic reactions, including ANAPHYLAXIS (more common after IV use).

Interactions

Drug-Drug: ↑ bone marrow depression with other **antineoplastics** or **radiation therapy**. May ↓ antibody response to **live-virus vaccines** and ↑ risk of adverse reactions. May ↑ the risk of pulmonary toxicity with **carmustine**. Concurrent IV use with **cyclosporine** may ↑ risk of renal failure. Risk of enterocolitis may be ↑ with concurrent **nalidixic acid**.

M

🍁 = Canadian drug name.
* CAPITALS indicates life-threatening; underlines indicate most frequent.

Route/Dosage

Multiple Myeloma

PO (Adults): 150 mcg (0.15 mg)/kg/day for 7 days, followed by 3-wk rest, then 50 mcg (0.05 mg)/kg/day maintenance dose *or* 100–150 mcg/kg/day or 250 mg (0.25 mg)/kg/day for 4 days followed by 2–4-wk rest, then 2–4 mg/day maintenance dose *or* 7 mg/m² *or* 250 mcg (0.25 mg)/kg daily for 5 days q 5–6 wk.
IV (Adults): 16 mg/m² q 2 wk for 4 doses, then q 4 wk.

Ovarian Carcinoma

PO (Adults): 200 mcg (0.2 mg)/kg/day for 5 days q 4–5 wk.

Availability

Tablets: 2 mg. **Powder for injection:** 50 mg.

NURSING IMPLICATIONS

Assessment

- Assess for signs of infection (fever, chills, sore throat, cough, hoarseness, lower back or side pain, difficult or painful urination). Notify health care professional if these symptoms occur.
- Assess for bleeding (bleeding gums, bruising, petechiae, guaiac stools, urine, and emesis). Avoid IM injections and taking rectal temperatures. Apply pressure to venipuncture sites for 10 min.
- May cause nausea and vomiting. Monitor intake and output, appetite, and nutritional intake. Prophylactic antiemetics may be used. Adjust diet as tolerated.
- Monitor for symptoms of gout (increased uric acid, joint pain, edema). Encourage patient to drink at least 2 L of fluid per day. Allopurinol may be given to decrease uric acid levels.
- Anemia may occur. Monitor for increased fatigue and dyspnea.
- Assess patient for allergy to chlorambucil. Patients may have cross-sensitivity.
- ***Lab Test Considerations:*** Monitor CBC and differential weekly during therapy. The nadir of leukopenia occurs in 2–3 wk. Notify physician if leukocyte count is <3000/mm³. The nadir of thrombocytopenia occurs in 2–3 wk. Notify physician if platelet count is <100,000/mm³. Recovery of leukopenia and thrombocytopenia occurs in 5–6 wk.
- Monitor liver function studies (AST, ALT, LDH, bilirubin) and renal function studies (BUN, creatinine) prior to and periodically during therapy to detect hepatotoxicity and nephrotoxicity.
- May cause ↑ uric acid. Monitor periodically during therapy.
- May cause ↑ 5-hydroxyindoleacetic acid (5-HIAA) concentrations as a result of tumor breakdown.

Potential Nursing Diagnoses

Risk for injury (Side Effects)
Risk for infection (Side Effects)

Implementation

- Solution should be prepared in a biologic cabinet. Wear gloves, gown, and mask while handling medication. Discard IV equipment in specially designated container.
- If solution contacts skin or mucosa, immediately wash skin or mucosa with soap and water.
- **PO:** May be ordered in divided doses or as a single daily dose.

IV Administration

- **Intermittent Infusion:** ***Diluent:*** Reconstitute with 10 ml of diluent supplied for a concentration of 5 mg/ml and shake vigorously until solution is clear. ***Concentration:*** Dilute dose immediately with 0.9% NaCl for a concentration not to exceed 2 mg/ml for central line or 0.45 mg/ml for a peripheral line. Administer within 60 min of reconstitution. ***Rate:*** Administer over at least 15 min (not to exceed 10 mg/min).
- **Y-Site Compatibility:** acyclovir, amikacin, aminophylline, ampicillin, aztreonam, bleomycin, bumetanide, buprenorphine, butorphanol, calcium gluconate, carboplatin, carmustine, cefazolin, cefepime, cefotaxime, ceftazidime, ceftizoxime, ceftriaxone, cefuroxime, cimetidine, cisplatin, clindamycin, cyclophosphamide, cytarabine, dacarbazine, dactinomycin, daunorubicin, dexamethasone, diphenhydramine, doxorubicin, doxycycline, droperidol, enalaprilat, etoposide, famotidine, filgrastim, floxuridine, fluconazole, fludarabine, fluorouracil, furosemide, ganciclovir, gentamicin, haloperidol, heparin, hydrocortisone, hydromorphone, idarubicin, ifosfamide, imipenem/cilastatin, lorazepam, mannitol, mechlorethamine, meperidine, mesna, methotrexate, methylprednisolone, metoclopramide, metronidazole, minocycline, mitomycin, mitoxantrone, morphine, nalbuphine, ondansetron, pentostatin, potassium chloride, prochlorperazine

edisylate, promethazine, ranitidine, sodium bicarbonate, streptozocin, teniposide, thiotepa, ticarcillin/clavulanate, tobramycin, trimethoprim/sulfamethoxazole, vancomycin, vinblastine, vincristine, vinorelbine, zidovudine.

- **Y-Site Incompatibility:** amphotericin B, chlorpromazine.

Patient/Family Teaching

- Instruct patient to take melphalan as directed, even if nausea and vomiting occur. If vomiting occurs shortly after dose is taken, consult health care professional. If a dose is missed, do not take at all.
- Advise patient to notify health care professional if fever; chills; dyspnea; persistent cough; sore throat; signs of infection; bleeding gums; bruising; petechiae; or blood in urine, stool, or emesis occurs. Caution patient to avoid crowds and persons with known infections. Instruct patient to use soft toothbrush and electric razor. Caution patient not to drink alcoholic beverages or take products containing aspirin or other NSAIDs.
- Instruct patient to notify health care professional if rash, itching, joint pain, or swelling occurs.
- Instruct patient to inspect oral mucosa for redness and ulceration. If ulceration occurs, advise patient to use sponge brush and to rinse mouth with water after eating and drinking. Consult health care professional if pain interferes with eating. Stomatitis pain may require treatment with opioid analgesics.
- Advise patient that although fertility may be decreased, contraception should be used during melphalan therapy because of potential teratogenic effects on the fetus.
- Instruct patient not to receive any vaccinations without advice of health care professional.
- Emphasize need for periodic lab tests to monitor for side effects.

Evaluation/Desired Outcomes

- Decrease in size and spread of malignant tissue.

memantine (me-**man**-teen)
Namenda

Classification
Therapeutic: anti-Alzheimer's agents
Pharmacologic:

Pregnancy Category B

Indications

Moderate to severe Alzheimer's dementia.

Action

Binds to CNS N-methyl-D-aspartate (NMDA) receptor sites, preventing binding of glutamate, an excitatory neurotransmitter. **Therapeutic Effects:** Decreased symptoms of dementia. Does not slow progression. Cognitive enhancement. Does not cure disease.

Pharmacokinetics

Absorption: Well absorbed after oral administration.
Distribution: Unknown.
Metabolism and Excretion: 57–82% excreted unchanged in urine by active tubular secretion moderated by pH dependent tubular reabsorption. Remainder metabolized; metabolites are not pharmacologically active.
Half-life: 60–80 hr.

TIME/ACTION PROFILE (blood levels)

ROUTE	ONSET	PEAK	DURATION
PO	unknown	3–7 hr	12 hr

Contraindications/Precautions

Contraindicated in: Severe renal impairment.
Use Cautiously in: Moderate renal impairment (consider ↓ dose); Concurrent use of other NMDA antagonists (amantadine, rimantadine, ketamine, dextromethorphan); Concurrent use of drugs or diets that cause alkaline urine; Conditions that ↑ urine pH including severe urinary tract infections or renal tubular acidosis (lead to ↓ excretion and ↑ levels); OB, Lactation, Pedi: Safety not established. Discontinue drug or bottle-feed.

Adverse Reactions/Side Effects

CNS: dizziness, fatigue, headache, sedation. **CV:** hypertension. **Derm:** rash. **GI:** weight gain. **GU:** urinary frequency. **Hemat:** anemia.

Interactions

Drug-Drug: Medications that ↑ urine pH lead to ↓ excretion and ↑ blood levels (**car-**

M

bonic anhydrase inhibitors, sodium bicarbonate).

Route/Dosage

PO (Adults): 5 mg once daily initially, increased at weekly intervals to 10 mg/day (5 mg twice daily), then 15 mg/day (5 mg once daily, 10 mg once daily as separate doses, then to target dose of 20 mg/day (as 10 mg twice daily).

Availability

Tablets: 5 mg, 10 mg, titration package containing twenty-eight 5-mg tablets and twenty-one 10-mg tablets. **Cost:** 5 mg $458.95/180, 10 mg $435.98/180. **Oral solution, sugar-free, alcohol-free (peppermint):** 2 mg/ml in 360-mL bottles.

NURSING IMPLICATIONS

Assessment

- Assess cognitive function (memory, attention, reasoning, language, ability to perform simple tasks) periodically during therapy.
- ***Lab Test Considerations:*** May cause anemia.

Potential Nursing Diagnoses

Disturbed thought process (Indications)
Risk for injury (Side Effects)
Impaired environmental interpretation syndrome

Implementation

- Dose increases should occur no more frequently than weekly.
- **PO:** May be administered without regard to food.
- Administer oral solution using syringe provided. Do not dilute or mix with other fluids.

Patient/Family Teaching

- Instruct caregivers on how and when to administer memantine and how to titrate dose. Provide caregiver with *Patient Instructions* sheet.
- Caution patient and caregiver that memantine may cause dizziness.
- Teach patient and caregivers that improvement in cognitive functioning may take months; degenerative process is not reversed.

Evaluation/Desired Outcomes

- Improvement in cognitive function (memory, attention, reasoning, language, ability to perform simple tasks) in patients with Alzheimer's disease.

HIGH ALERT

meperidine (me-**per**-i-deen)
Demerol, pethidine

Classification
Therapeutic: opioid analgesics
Pharmacologic: opioid agonists

Schedule II

Pregnancy Category C

Indications

Moderate or severe pain (alone or with nonopioid agents). Anesthesia adjunct. Analgesic during labor. Preoperative sedation. **Unlabeled uses:** Rigors.

Action

Binds to opiate receptors in the CNS. Alters the perception of and response to painful stimuli, while producing generalized CNS depression. **Therapeutic Effects:** Decrease in severity of pain.

Pharmacokinetics

Absorption: 50% from the GI tract; well absorbed from IM sites. Oral doses are about half as effective as parenteral doses.
Distribution: Widely distributed. Crosses the placenta; enters breast milk.
Protein Binding: Neonates: 52%; Infants 3–18 months: 85%; Adults: 60–80%.
Metabolism and Excretion: Mostly metabolized by the liver; some converted to normeperidine, which may accumulate and cause seizures. 5% excreted unchanged by the kidneys.
Half-life: Neonates: 12–39 hr; Infants 3–18 months: 2.3 hr; Children 5–8 yr: 3 hr; Adults: 2.5–4 hr (prolonged in impaired renal or hepatic function [7–11 hr]).

TIME/ACTION PROFILE (analgesia)

ROUTE	ONSET	PEAK	DURATION
PO	15 min	60 min	2–4 hr
IM	10–15 min	30–50 min	2–4 hr
Subcut	10–15 min	40–60 min	2–4 hr
IV	immediate	5–7 min	2–3 hr

Contraindications/Precautions

Contraindicated in: Hypersensitivity; Hypersensitivity to bisulfites (some injectable products); Pregnancy or lactation (chronic use); Recent (14–21 days) MAO inhibitor therapy.
Use Cautiously in: Head trauma; Increased intracranial pressure; Severe renal, hepatic, or

pulmonary disease; Hypothyroidism; Adrenal insufficiency; Alcoholism; Geri: Appears on Beers list. Geriatric patients (morphine recommended); Debilitated patients (dose reduction suggested); Undiagnosed abdominal pain or prostatic hyperplasia; Labor (respiratory depression may occur in the newborn); Patients with renal impairment, or extensive burns; High dose or prolonged therapy (>600 mg/day or >2 days; increased risk of CNS stimulation and seizures due to accumulation of normeperidine); Sickle cell anemia (may require reduced initial doses); Pedi: Neonates (syrup contains benzyl alcohol); Children (increased risk of seizures due to accumulation of normeperidine).

Adverse Reactions/Side Effects

CNS: SEIZURES, confusion, sedation, dysphoria, euphoria, floating feeling, hallucinations, headache, unusual dreams. **EENT:** blurred vision, diplopia, miosis. **Resp:** respiratory depression. **CV:** hypotension, bradycardia. **GI:** constipation, nausea, vomiting. **GU:** urinary retention. **Derm:** flushing, sweating. **Misc:** physical dependence, psychological dependence, tolerance.

Interactions

Drug-Drug: Do not use in patients receiving **MAO inhibitors** or **procarbazine** (may cause fatal reaction—contraindicated within 14–21 days of MAO inhibitor therapy). ↑ CNS depression with **alcohol**, **antihistamines**, and **sedative/hypnotics**. Administration of **agonist/antagonist opioid analgesics** may precipitate opioid withdrawal in physically dependent patients. **Nalbuphine** or **pentazocine** may ↓ analgesia. **Protease inhibitor antiretrovirals** may ↑ effects and adverse reactions (concurrent use should be avoided). **Phenytoin** ↑ metabolism and may ↓ effects. **Chlorpromazine** and **thioridazine** may ↑ the risk of adverse reactions (concurrent use should be avoided). May aggravate side effects of **isoniazid**. **Acyclovir** may ↑ plasma concentrations of meperidine and normeperidine.
Drug-Natural Products: Concomitant use of **kava kava, valerian** or **chamomile** can ↓ CNS depression. **St. John's wort** may increase serious side effects, concurrent use is not recommended.

Route/Dosage

PO, IM, Subcut, IV (Adults): *Analgesia*—50–150 mg q 3–4 hr. *Analgesia during labor*—50–100 mg IM or subcut when contractions become regular; may repeat q 1–3 hr. *Preoperative sedation*—50–100 mg IM or subcut 30–90 min before anesthesia.
PO, IM, Subcut, IV (Children): *Analgesia*—1–1.5 mg/kg q 3–4 hr (should not exceed 100 mg/dose). *Preoperative sedation*—1–2 mg/kg 30–90 min before anesthesia (not to exceed adult dose).
IV (Adults): 15–35 mg/hr as a continuous infusion; *PCA*—10 mg initially; with a range 0f 1–5 mg/incremental dose, recommended lockout interval is 6–10 min (minimum 5 min).
IV (Children): *Continuous infusion*—0.5–1 mg/kg loading dose followed by 0.3 mg/kg/hr, titrate to effect up to 0.5–0.7 mg/kg/hr.

Availability (generic available)

Tablets: 50 mg, 100 mg. **Cost:** 50 mg $99.04/100, 100 mg $188.37/100. **Syrup (banana flavor):** 50 mg/5 ml. **Injection:** ✤ 10 mg/ml, 25 mg/ml, 50 mg/ml, 75 mg/ml, 100 mg/ml. ***In combination with:*** promethazine (Mepergan) and atropine. See Appendix B.

NURSING IMPLICATIONS

Assessment

- Assess type, location, and intensity of pain prior to and 1 hr following PO, subcut, and IM doses and 5 min (peak) following IV administration. When titrating opioid doses, increases of 25–50% should be administered until there is either a 50% reduction in the patient's pain rating on a numerical or visual analogue scale or the patient reports satisfactory pain relief. A repeat dose can be safely administered at the time of the peak if previous dose is ineffective and side effects are minimal.
- An equianalgesic chart (see Appendix J) should be used when changing routes or when changing from one opioid to another.
- Assess blood pressure, pulse, and respirations before and periodically during administration. If respiratory rate is <10/min, assess level of sedation. Dose may need to be decreased by 25–50%. Initial drowsiness will diminish with continued use. Pedi: Neonates and infants are more susceptible to respiratory depression. Assess respiratory rate frequently.

- Assess bowel function routinely. Prevention of constipation should be instituted with increased intake of fluids and bulk and with laxatives to minimize constipating effects. Stimulant laxatives should be administered routinely if opioid use exceeds 2–3 days, unless contraindicated.
- Prolonged use may lead to physical and psychological dependence and tolerance. This should not prevent patient from receiving adequate analgesia. Most patients who receive meperidine for pain do not develop psychological dependence. Progressively higher doses may be required to relieve pain with long-term therapy.
- Monitor patients on chronic or high-dose therapy for CNS stimulation (restlessness, irritability, seizures) due to accumulation of normeperidine metabolite. Risk of toxicity increases with doses >600 mg/24 hr, chronic administration (>2 days), and renal impairment.
- Geri: Meperidine has been reported to cause delirium in the elderly; older adults are at increased risk for normeperidine toxicity. Monitor frequently.
- Pedi: Assess pediatric patient frequently; children are more sensitive to the effects of opioid analgesics and may experience respiratory complications, excitability and restlessness more frequently.
- ***Lab Test Considerations:*** May ↑ plasma amylase and lipase concentrations.
- ***Toxicity and Overdose:*** If an opioid antagonist is required to reverse respiratory depression or coma, naloxone (Narcan) is the antidote. Dilute the 0.4-mg ampule of naloxone in 10 ml of 0.9% NaCl and administer 0.5 ml (0.02 mg) by direct IV push every 2 min. For children and patients weighing <40 kg, dilute 0.1 mg of naloxone in 10 ml of 0.9% NaCl for a concentration of 10 mcg/ml and administer 0.5 mcg/kg every 2 min. Titrate dose to avoid withdrawal, seizures, and severe pain. In patients receiving meperidine chronically, naloxone may precipitate seizures by eliminating the CNS depressant effects of meperidine, allowing the convulsant activity of normeperidine to predominate. Monitor patient closely.

Potential Nursing Diagnoses

Acute pain (Indications)
Disturbed sensory perception (visual, auditory) (Side Effects)
Risk for injury (Side Effects)

Implementation

- ***High Alert:*** Accidental overdose of opioid analgesics has resulted in fatalities. Before administering, clarify all ambiguous orders; have second practitioner independently check original order, dose calculations, and infusion pump settings. Do not confuse with morphine or hydromorphone; fatalities have occurred. Pedi: Medication errors with opioid analgesics are common in the pediatric population and include misinterpretation or miscalculation of doses and use of inappropriate measuring devices.
- Explain therapeutic value of medication prior to administration to enhance the analgesic effect.
- Regularly administered doses may be more effective than prn administration. Analgesic is more effective if given before pain becomes severe.
- Coadministration with nonopioid analgesics may have additive analgesic effects and permit lower doses.
- Oral dose is <50% as effective as parenteral. When changing to oral administration, dose may need to be increased (see Appendix J).
- Medication should be discontinued gradually after long-term use to prevent withdrawal symptoms.
- May be administered via PCA pump.
- **PO:** Doses may be administered with food or milk to minimize GI irritation. Syrup should be diluted in half-full glass of water.
- **IM:** Administration of repeated subcut doses may cause local irritation.

IV Administration

- **Direct IV:** ***Diluent:*** Dilute with sterile water or 0.9% NaCl for injection. ***Concentration:*** ≤10 mg/ml. ***Rate: High Alert:*** Administer slowly over at least 5 min. Rapid administration may lead to increased respiratory depression, hypotension, and circulatory collapse.
- **Intermittent Infusion:** ***Diluent:*** Dilute with D5W, D10W, dextrose/saline combinations, dextrose/Ringer's or lactated Ringer's injection combinations, 0.45% NaCl, 0.9% NaCl, or Ringer's or LR. Administer via infusion pump. ***Concentration:*** 1 mg/ml. ***Rate:*** Administer over 15–30 min.
- **Syringe Compatibility:** atropine, chlorpromazine, cimetidine, dimenhydrinate, diphenhydramine, droperidol, glycopyrrolate, hy-

droxyzine, ketamine, metoclopramide, midazolam, ondansetron, perphenazine, prochlorperazine, promazine, promethazine, ranitidine, scopolamine.
- **Syringe Incompatibility:** heparin, morphine, pantoprazole, pentobarbital.
- **Y-Site Compatibility:** amifostine, amikacin, ampicillin, ampicillin/sulbactam, atenolol, aztreonam bivalirudin, bumetanide, cefazolin, cefotaxime, cefoxitin, ceftazidime, ceftizoxime, ceftriaxone, cefuroxime, chloramphenicol, cisatracurium, cladribine, clindamycin, dexamethasone, dexmedetomidine, digoxin, diltiazem, diphenhydramine, dobutamine, docetaxel, dopamine, doxycycline, droperidol, erythromycin lactobionate, etoposide phosphate, famotidine, fenoldopam, filgrastim, fluconazole, fludarabine, gemcitabine, gentamicin, granisetron, heparin, hydrocortisone sodium succinate, insulin, kanamycin, labetalol, lidocaine, linezolid, magnesium sulfate, melphalan, methyldopate, methylprednisolone, metoclopramide, metoprolol, metronidazole, ondansetron, oxacillin, oxaliplatin, oxytocin, paclitaxel, pemetrexed, penicillin G potassium, piperacillin/tazobactam, potassium chloride, propofol, propranolol, ranitidine, remifentanil, sargramostim, teniposide, thiotepa, ticarcillin/clavulanate, tobramycin, trimethoprim/sulfamethoxazole, vancomycin, verapamil, vinorelbine.
- **Y-Site Incompatibility:** allopurinol, amphotericin B cholesteryl sulfate, cefepime, cefoperazone, doxorubicin liposome, idarubicin, imipenem/cilastatin, lansoprazole.

Patient/Family Teaching
- Instruct patient on how and when to ask for pain medication.
- Instruct patient to take meperidine as directed. If dose is less effective after a few weeks, do not increase dose without consulting health care professional. Pedi: Teach parents or caregivers how to accurately measure liquid medication and to use only the measuring device dispensed with the medication.
- May cause drowsiness or dizziness. Advise patient to call for assistance when ambulating or smoking. Caution patient to avoid driving or other activities requiring alertness until response to medication is known.
- Advise patient to change positions slowly to minimize orthostatic hypotension.
- Instruct patient to avoid concurrent use of alcohol or other CNS depressants.
- Advise ambulatory patients that nausea and vomiting may be decreased by lying down.
- Encourage patient to turn, cough, and breathe deeply every 2 hr to prevent atelectasis.

Evaluation/Desired Outcomes
- Decrease in severity of pain without a significant alteration in level of consciousness or respiratory status.

meropenem
(mer-oh-**pen**-nem)
Merrem

Classification
Therapeutic: anti-infectives
Pharmacologic: carbapenems

Pregnancy Category B

Indications
Treatment of: Intra-abdominal infections, Bacterial meningitis. Skin and skin structure infections. **Unlabeled uses:** Febrile neutropenia. Hospital-acquired pneumonia and sepsis.

Action
Binds to bacterial cell wall, resulting in cell death. Meropenem resists the actions of many enzymes that degrade most other penicillins and penicillin-like anti-infectives. **Therapeutic Effects:** Bactericidal action against susceptible bacteria. **Spectrum:** Active against the following gram-positive organisms: *Staphylococcus aureus*, *Streptococcus pneumoniae*, Viridans group streptococci, *Enterococcus faecalis*. Also active against the following gram-negative pathogens: *Escherichia coli*, *Haemophilus influenzae*, *Klebsiella pneumoniae*, *Neisseria meningitidis*, *Pseudomonas aeruginosa*, *Proteus mirabilis*. Active against the following anaerobes: *Bacteroides fragilis*, *B. fragilis* group, *Peptostreptococcus* species.

Pharmacokinetics
Absorption: IV administration results in complete bioavailability.

Distribution: Widely distributed into body tissues and fluids; enters CSF when meninges are inflamed.
Metabolism and Excretion: 65–83% excreted unchanged by the kidneys.
Half-life: Premature neonates: 3 hr; Term neonates: 2 hr; Infants 3 mo–2 yr: 1.4 hr; Children >2 yr and Adults: 1 hr (increased in renal impairment).

TIME/ACTION PROFILE (blood levels)

ROUTE	ONSET	PEAK	DURATION
IV	rapid	end of infusion	8 hr

Contraindications/Precautions

Contraindicated in: Hypersensitivity to meropenem or imipenem; Serious hypersensitivity to other beta-lactams (penicillins or cephalosporins; cross-sensitivity may occur).
Use Cautiously in: Renal impairment (↑ risk of thrombocytopenia and seizures; dose reduction recommended if CCr <50 ml/min); History of seizures, brain lesions, or meningitis; Pregnancy, lactation, or children <3 mo (safety not established).

Adverse Reactions/Side Effects

CNS: SEIZURES, dizziness, headache. **Resp:** APNEA. **GI:** PSEUDOMEMBRANOUS COLITIS, constipation, diarrhea, glossitis (increased in children), nausea, thrush (increased in children), vomiting. **Derm:** moniliasis (children only), pruritus, rash. **Local:** inflammation at injection site, phlebitis. **Misc:** allergic reactions including ANAPHYLAXIS.

Interactions

Drug-Drug: Probenecid ↓ renal excretion and increases blood levels (coadministration not recommended).

Route/Dosage

IV (Adults): 0.5–1 g q 8 hr. *Meningitis*—2 g q 8 hr.
IV (Children ≥3 mo–12 yr): *Intra-abdominal infections*—20 mg/kg q 8 hr; *meningitis*—40 mg/kg q 8 hr (maximum 2 g q 8 hr).
IV (Neonates <7 days): 20 mg/kg/dose q 12 hr. *Neonates >7 days, 1200–2000 g*—20 mg/kg/dose q 12 hr. *Neonates >7 days, >2000 g*—20 mg/kg/dose q 8 hr.

Renal Impairment

IV (Adults): *CCr 26–50 ml/min*—1 g q 12 hr; *CCr 10–25 ml/min*—500 mg q 12 hr; *CCr <10 ml/min*—500 mg q 24 hr.

Availability

Powder for injection: 500 mg, 1 g.

NURSING IMPLICATIONS

Assessment

- Assess patient for infection (vital signs; appearance of wound, sputum, urine, and stool; WBC) at beginning of and throughout therapy.
- Obtain a history before initiating therapy to determine previous use of and reactions to penicillins. Persons with a negative history of penicillin sensitivity may still have an allergic response.
- Obtain specimens for culture and sensitivity prior to initiating therapy. First dose may be given before receiving results.
- Observe patient for signs and symptoms of anaphylaxis (rash, pruritus, laryngeal edema, wheezing). Discontinue the drug and notify physician immediately if these symptoms occur. Have epinephrine, an antihistamine, and resuscitative equipment close by in the event of an anaphylactic reaction.
- Assess injection site for phlebitis, pain, and swelling periodically during administration.
- ***Lab Test Considerations:*** Monitor hematologic, hepatic, and renal functions periodically during therapy.
- BUN, AST, ALT, LDH, serum alkaline phosphatase, bilirubin, and creatinine may be transiently ↑.
- Hemoglobin and hematocrit concentrations may be ↓.
- May cause positive direct or indirect Coombs' test.

Potential Nursing Diagnoses

Risk for infection (Indications, Side Effects)
Deficient knowledge, related to medication regimen (Patient/Family Teaching)

Implementation

IV Administration

- **Direct IV:** ***Diluent:*** Reconstitute 500-mg and 1-g vials with 10 ml and 20 ml, respectively, of sterile water for injection, 0.9% NaCl, or D5W. Vials reconstituted with sterile water for injection are stable for 2 hr at room temperature and 12 hr if refrigerated; if reconstituted with 0.9% NaCl, stable for 2 hr at room temperature and 18 hr if refrigerated; if reconstituted with D5W, stable for 1 hr at room temperature and 8 hr if refrigerated.

Concentration: 50 mg/ml. ***Rate:*** Administer over 3–5 min.

- **Intermittent Infusion:** ***Diluent:*** Reconstitute 500-mg and 1-g vials with 10 ml and 20 ml, respectively, of sterile water for injection, 0.9% NaCl, or D5W. Further dilute in 0.9% NaCl or D5W to achieve concentration below. Infusions further diluted in 0.9% NaCl are stable for 4 hr at room temperature and 24 hr if refrigerated. Infusions further diluted in D5W are stable for 1 hr at room temperature and 4 hr if refrigerated. ***Concentration:*** Final concentration of infusion should be 1–20 mg/ml. ***Rate:*** Infuse over 15–30 min.
- **Y-Site Compatibility:** aminophylline, anidulafungin, atropine, caspofungin, cimetidine, daptomycin, dexamethasone, digoxin, diltiazem, diphenhydramine, enalaprilat, fluconazole, furosemide, gentamicin, granisetron, heparin, hydromorphone, insulin, linezolid, lorazepam, metoclopramide, milrinone, morphine, norepinephrine, palonosetron, potassium chloride, tacrolimus, tirofiban, vancomycin, vasopressin, voriconazole.
- **Y-Site Incompatibility:** amphotericin B, diazepam, fenoldopam, metronidazole, quinupristin/dalfopristin.

Patient/Family Teaching

- Advise patient to report the signs of superinfection (black, furry overgrowth on the tongue; vaginal itching or discharge; loose or foul-smelling stools) and allergy.
- May cause dizziness. Caution patient to avoid driving or other activities requiring alertness until response to drug is known.
- Caution patient to notify health care professional if fever and diarrhea occur, especially if stool contains blood, pus, or mucus. Advise patient not to treat diarrhea without consulting health care professional. May occur up to several weeks after discontinuation of medication.

Evaluation/Desired Outcomes

- Resolution of the signs and symptoms of infection. Length of time for complete resolution depends on the organism and site of infection.

mesalamine (me-sal-a-meen)

Asacol, Canasa, Lialda, Pentasa, Rowasa, ✤Salofalk

Classification

Therapeutic: gastrointestinal anti-inflammatories—therapeutic

Pregnancy Category B

Indications

Inflammatory bowel diseases including: Ulcerative colitis, Proctitis, Proctosigmoiditis.

Action

Locally acting anti-inflammatory action in the colon, where activity is probably due to inhibition of prostaglandin synthesis. **Therapeutic Effects:** Reduction in the symptoms of inflammatory bowel disease.

Pharmacokinetics

Absorption: 28% absorbed following oral administration; 10–30% absorbed from the colon, depending on retention time, following rectal administration.
Distribution: Unknown.
Metabolism and Excretion: Some metabolism occurs, site unknown; mostly eliminated unchanged in the feces.
Half-life: 12 hr PO (range 2–15 hr); 0.5–1.5 hr rectal.

TIME/ACTION PROFILE (clinical improvement)

ROUTE	ONSET	PEAK	Duration
PO	unknown	unknown	6–8 hr
Extended release	2 hr	9–12 hrs	24 hr
Rectal	3–21 days	unknown	24 hr

Contraindications/Precautions

Contraindicated in: Hypersensitivity reactions to sulfonamides, salicylates, mesalamine, or sulfasalazine; Cross-sensitivity with furosemide, sulfonylurea hypoglycemic agents, or carbonic anhydrase inhibitors may exist; G6PD deficiency; Hypersensitivity to bisulfites (mesalamine enema only); Urinary tract or intestinal obstruction; Porphyria.
Use Cautiously in: Severe hepatic or renal impairment; OB: Pregnancy or lactation (safety not established).

M

Adverse Reactions/Side Effects

CNS: headache, dizziness, malaise, weakness. **EENT:** pharyngitis, rhinitis. **CV:** pericarditis. **GI:** diarrhea, eructation (PO), flatulence, nausea, vomiting. **GU:** interstitial nephritis, pancreatitis, renal failure. **Derm:** hair loss, rash. **Local:** anal irritation (enema, suppository). **MS:** back pain. **Misc:** ANAPHYLAXIS, acute intolerance syndrome, fever.

Interactions

Drug-Drug: May ↓ metabolism and ↑ effects/toxicity of **mercaptopurine** or **thioguanine**.

Route/Dosage

PO (Adults): 800 mg 3 times daily for 6 wk as delayed-release tablets *or* 1 g 4 times daily as controlled-release capsules *or* 2–4 1.2-g tablets once daily with a meal for a total daily dose of 2.4 or 4.8 g of *Lialda*.
Rect (Adults): 4-g enema (60 ml) at bedtime, retained for 8 hr for 3–6 wk *or* 1-g suppository at bedtime.

Availability (generic available)

Delayed-release tablets: ♣250 mg, 400 mg, ♣500 mg, 1.2 g (Lialda). **Cost:** 400 mg $132.01/180, 1.2 g $515.96/120. **Controlled-release capsules:** 250 mg, 500 mg. **Cost:** 250 mg $387.98/480, 500 mg $351.32/240. **Suppositories:** 1 g. **Cost:** $326.96/30. **Rectal suspension:** 4 g/60 ml. **Cost:** *Generic*—$317.69/28 bottles.

NURSING IMPLICATIONS

Assessment

- Assess patient for allergy to sulfonamides and salicylates. Patients allergic to sulfasalazine may take mesalamine or olsalazine without difficulty, but therapy should be discontinued if rash or fever occurs.
- Monitor intake and output ratios. Fluid intake should be sufficient to maintain a urine output of at least 1200–1500 mL daily to prevent crystalluria and stone formation.
- **Inflammatory Bowel Disease:** Assess abdominal pain and frequency, quantity, and consistency of stools at the beginning of and during therapy.
- ***Lab Test Considerations:*** Monitor urinalysis, BUN, and serum creatinine prior to and periodically during therapy. Mesalamine may cause renal toxicity.
- Mesalamine may cause ↑ AST and ALT levels, serum alkaline phosphatase, GGTP, LDH, amylase, and lipase.

Potential Nursing Diagnoses

Acute pain (Indications)
Diarrhea (Indications)

Implementation

- Do not confuse Asacol (mesalamine) with Os-Cal (calcium carbonate).
- **PO:** Administer with a full glass of water. Tablets should be swallowed whole; do not break the outer coating, which is designed to remain intact. Take *Lialda* tablets with a meal. Intact or partially intact tablets may occasionally be found in the stool. If this occurs repeatedly, advise patient to notify health care professional.
- **Rect:** Patient should empty bowel prior to administration of rectal dose forms.
- Avoid excessive handling of *suppository*. Remove foil wrapper and insert pointed end first into rectum with gentle pressure. Suppository should be retained for 1–3 hr or more for maximum benefit.
- Administer 60-mL retention enema once daily at bedtime. Solution should be retained for approximately 8 hr. Prior to administration of *rectal suspension*, shake bottle well and remove the protective cap. Have patient lie on left side with the lower leg extended and the upper leg flexed for support or place the patient in knee-chest position. Gently insert the applicator tip into the rectum, pointing toward the umbilicus. Squeeze the bottle steadily to discharge most of the preparation.

Patient/Family Teaching

- Instruct patient on the correct method of administration. Advise patient to take medication as directed, even if feeling better. Take missed doses as soon as remembered unless almost time for next dose.
- May cause dizziness. Caution patient to avoid driving or other activities that require alertness until response to medication is known.
- Advise patient to notify health care professional if skin rash, sore throat, fever, mouth sores, unusual bleeding or bruising, wheezing, fever, or hives occur.
- Instruct patient to notify health care professional if symptoms do not improve after 1–2 months of therapy.
- Instruct patient to notify health care professional if symptoms worsen or do not improve.

If symptoms of acute intolerance (cramping, acute abdominal pain, bloody diarrhea, fever, headache, rash) occur, discontinue therapy and notify health care professional immediately.

- Inform patient that proctoscopy and sigmoidoscopy may be required periodically during treatment to determine response.
- **Rect:** Instruct patient to use *rectal suspension* at bedtime and retain suspension all night for best results.
- Advise patient not to change brands of mesalamine without consulting health care professional.

Evaluation/Desired Outcomes

- Decrease in diarrhea and abdominal pain.
- Return to normal bowel pattern in patients with inflammatory bowel disease. Effects may be seen within 3–21 days. The usual course of therapy is 3–6 wk.
- Maintenance of remission in patients with inflammatory bowel disease.

mesna (mes-na)

Mesnex, ♣ Uromitexan

Classification

Therapeutic: antidotes

Pharmacologic: ifosfamide detoxifying agents

Pregnancy Category B

Indications

Prevention of ifosfamide-induced hemorrhagic cystitis (see Ifosfamide monograph). **Unlabeled uses:** May also prevent hemorrhagic cystitis from cyclophosphamide.

Action

Binds to the toxic metabolites of ifosfamide in the kidneys. **Therapeutic Effects:** Prevents hemorrhagic cystitis from ifosfamide.

Pharmacokinetics

Absorption: IV administration results in complete bioavailability; 45–79% absorbed after oral administration. Following IV with PO dosing increases systemic exposure.

Distribution: Unknown.

Metabolism and Excretion: Rapidly converted to mesna disulfide, then back to mesna in the kidneys, where it binds to toxic metabolites of ifosfamide (18–26% excreted as free mesna in urine after IV and PO dosing).

Half-life: *Mesna*—0.36 hr (IV); 1.2—8.3 hr (IV followed by PO); *mesna disulfide*—1.17 hr.

TIME/ACTION PROFILE (detoxifying action)

ROUTE	ONSET	PEAK	DURATION
PO, IV	rapid	unknown	4 hr

Contraindications/Precautions

Contraindicated in: Hypersensitivity to mesna or other thiol (rubber) compounds.

Use Cautiously in: Pregnancy or lactation (safety not established).

Adverse Reactions/Side Effects

CNS: dizziness, drowsiness, headache. **GI:** anorexia, diarrhea, nausea, unpleasant taste, vomiting. **Derm:** flushing. **Local:** injection site reactions. **Misc:** flu-like symptoms.

Interactions

Drug-Drug: None significant.

Route/Dosage

IV (Adults): Give a dose of mesna equal to 20% of the ifosfamide dose at the same time as ifosfamide and 4 and 8 hr after.

PO, IV (Adults): Give a dose of IV mesna equal to 20% of the ifosfamide dose at the same time as ifosfamide; then give PO mesna equal to 40% of the ifosfamide dose 2 and 6 hours after ifosfamide (total mesna dose is 100% of ifosfamide dose).

Availability

Tablets: 400 mg. **Injection:** 100 mg/ml in 2-, 4-, and 10-ml ampules. ***In combination with:*** ifosfamide (in a kit).

NURSING IMPLICATIONS

Assessment

- Monitor for development of hemorrhagic cystitis in patients receiving ifosfamide.
- ***Lab Test Considerations:*** Causes a false-positive result when testing urinary ketones.

Potential Nursing Diagnoses

Deficient knowledge, related to medication regimen (Patient/Family Teaching)

Implementation

- Initial IV bolus is to be given at time of ifosfamide administration.

♣ = Canadian drug name.

*CAPITALS indicates life-threatening; underlines indicate most frequent.

- **PO:** If second and third doses are given orally, administer 2 and 6 hours after IV dose.
- If PO mesna is vomited within 2 hr of administration, repeat dose or use IV mesna.

IV Administration

- **Intermittent Infusion:** 2nd IV dose is given 4 hr later, 3rd dose is given 8 hr after initial dose. This schedule must be repeated with each subsequent dose of ifosfamide. ***Diluent:*** Dilute 2-, 4-, and 10-ml ampules, containing a concentration of 100 mg/ml in 8 ml, 16 ml, or 50 ml, respectively, of D5W, 0.9% NaCl, D5/0.9% NaCl, D5/0.2% NaCl, D5/0.33% NaCl, or LR. ***Concentration:*** 20 mg/ml. Refrigerate to store. Use within 6 hr. Discard unused solution. ***Rate:*** Administer over 15–30 min or as a continuous infusion.
- **Syringe Compatibility:** ifosfamide.
- **Y-Site Compatibility:** allopurinol, amifostine, aztreonam, cefepime, docetaxel, doxorubicin liposome, etoposide phosphate, filgrastim, fludarabine, gemcitabine, granisetron, linezolid, melphalan, methotrexate, ondansetron, oxaliplatin, paclitaxel, pemetrexed, piperacillin/tazobactam, sargramostim, sodium bicarbonate, teniposide, thiotepa, vinorelbine.
- **Y-Site Incompatibility:** amphotericin B cholesteryl complex, lansoprazole.
- **Additive Compatibility:** ifosfamide.
- **Additive Incompatibility:** carboplatin, cisplatin.

Patient/Family Teaching

- Inform patient that unpleasant taste may occur during administration.
- Advise patient to notify health care professional if nausea, vomiting, or diarrhea persists or is severe.

Evaluation/Desired Outcomes

- Prevention of hemorrhagic cystitis associated with ifosfamide therapy.

mestranol/norethindrone, See CONTRACEPTIVES, HORMONAL.

metaxalone (me-**tax**-a-lone)

Skelaxin

Classification
Therapeutic: skeletal muscle relaxants (centrally acting)

Pregnancy Category UK

Indications

Muscle spasm associated with acute painful musculoskeletal conditions (with rest and physical therapy).

Action

Skeletal muscle relaxation, probably as a result of CNS depression. **Therapeutic Effects:** Skeletal muscle relaxation.

Pharmacokinetics

Absorption: Well absorbed following oral administration.
Distribution: Unknown.
Metabolism and Excretion: Mostly metabolized by the liver; metabolites excreted in urine.
Half-life: 2–3 hr.

TIME/ACTION PROFILE

ROUTE	ONSET	PEAK	DURATION
PO	1 hr	2 hr	4–6 hr

Contraindications/Precautions

Contraindicated in: Hypersensitivity; Significant hepatic/renal impairment; History of drug-induced hemolytic anemia or other anemia.
Use Cautiously in: History of seizures; Geri: Appears on Beers list. Poorly tolerated due to anticholinergic effects; Pregnancy, lactation, or children ≤12 yr (safety not established; use only in pregnancy/lactation if possible benefits outweigh potential risks).

Adverse Reactions/Side Effects

CNS: drowsiness, dizziness, confusion, headache, irritability, nervousness. **GI:** nausea, anorexia, dry mouth, GI upset, vomiting. **GU:** urinary retention.

Interactions

Drug-Drug: ↑ CNS depression with other **CNS depressants** including **alcohol**, **antihistamines**, **opioid analgesics**, and **sedative/hypnotics**.
Drug-Natural Products: Concomitant use of **kava kava**, **valerian**, or **chamomile** can ↑ CNS depression.

Route/Dosage

PO (Adults): 800 mg 3–4 times daily.

Availability

Tablets: 800 mg. **Cost:** $299.97/100.

NURSING IMPLICATIONS

Assessment

- Assess patient for pain, muscle stiffness, and range of motion before and periodically during therapy.
- Geri: Assess geriatric patients for anticholinergic effects (sedation and weakness).
- ***Lab Test Considerations:*** Monitor hepatic function tests closely in patients with preexisting liver damage.
- May cause false-positive Benedict's tests.

Potential Nursing Diagnoses

Acute pain (Indications)
Impaired bed mobility (Indications)
Risk for injury (Side Effects)

Implementation

- Provide safety measures as indicated. Supervise ambulation and transfer of patients.
- **PO:** Administer 3–4 times daily.

Patient/Family Teaching

- Instruct patient to take medication as directed. Take missed doses within 1 hr; if not, return to regular dosing schedule. Do not double doses.
- Encourage patient to comply with additional therapies prescribed for muscle spasm (rest, physical therapy, heat).
- Medication may cause dizziness, drowsiness, and blurred vision. Advise patient to avoid driving and other activities requiring alertness until response to drug is known.
- Instruct patient to make position changes slowly to minimize orthostatic hypotension.
- Advise patient to avoid concurrent use of alcohol and other CNS depressants while taking this medication.
- Instruct patient to notify health care professional if skin rash or yellowish discoloration of the skin or eyes occurs.
- Emphasize the importance of routine follow-up exams to monitor progress.

Evaluation/Desired Outcomes

- Decreased musculoskeletal pain and muscle spasticity.
- Increased range of motion.

metformin (met-for-min)

Fortamet, Glumetza, Glucophage, Glucophage XR, ✤Novo-Metformin, Riomet

Classification
Therapeutic: antidiabetics
Pharmacologic: biguanides

Pregnancy Category B

Indications

Management of type 2 diabetes mellitus; may be used with diet, insulin, or sulfonylurea oral hypoglycemics.

Action

Decreases hepatic glucose production. Decreases intestinal glucose absorption. Increases sensitivity to insulin. **Therapeutic Effects:** Maintenance of blood glucose.

Pharmacokinetics

Absorption: 50–60% absorbed after oral administration.
Distribution: Enters breast milk in concentrations similar to plasma.
Metabolism and Excretion: Eliminated almost entirely unchanged by the kidneys.
Half-life: 17.6 hr.

TIME/ACTION PROFILE (blood levelse)

ROUTE	ONSET	PEAK	DURATION
PO	unknown	unknown	12 hr
XR	unknown	4–8 hr	24 hr

Contraindications/Precautions

Contraindicated in: Hypersensitivity; Metabolic acidosis; Dehydration, sepsis, hypoxemia, hepatic impairment, excessive alcohol use (acute or chronic); Renal dysfunction (serum creatinine >1.5 mg/dl in men or >1.4 mg/dl in women); Radiographic studies requiring IV iodinated contrast media (withhold metformin); CHF.
Use Cautiously in: Concurrent renal disease; Geri: Geriatric/debilitated patients (↓ doses may be required; avoid in patients >80 yr unless renal function is normal); Chronic alcohol use/abuse; Serious medical conditions (MI, stroke); Patients undergoing stress (infection, surgical procedures); Hypoxia; Pituitary deficiency or hyperthyroidism; OB, Pedi: Pregnancy, lacta-

tion, or children <10 yr (safety not established; extended release for use in patients >17 yr only).

Adverse Reactions/Side Effects

GI: abdominal bloating, diarrhea, nausea, vomiting, unpleasant metallic taste. **Endo:** hypoglycemia. **F and E:** LACTIC ACIDOSIS. **Misc:** decreased vitamin B_{12} levels.

Interactions

Drug-Drug: Acute or chronic **alcohol** ingestion or **iodinated contrast media** ↑ risk of lactic acidosis. **Amiloride**, **digoxin**, **morphine**, **procainamide**, **quinidine**, **ranitidine**, **triamterene**, **trimethoprim**, **calcium channel blockers**, and **vancomycin** may compete for elimination pathways with metformin. Altered responses may occur. **Cimetidine** and **furosemide** may ↑ effects of metformin. **Nifedipine** ↑ absorption and effects.
Drug-Natural Products: Glucosamine may worsen blood glucose control. **Chromium,** and **coenzyme Q-10** may produce ↑ hypoglycemic effects.

Route/Dosage

PO (Adults and Children >17 yr): 500 mg twice daily; may increase by 500 mg at weekly intervals up to 2000 mg/day. If doses >2000 mg/day are required, give in 3 divided doses (not to exceed 2500 mg/day) or 850 mg once daily; may increase by 850 mg at 2-wk intervals (in divided doses) up to 2550 mg/day in divided doses (up to 850 mg 3 times daily); *Extended-release tablets*—500–1000 mg once daily with evening meal, may increase by 500 mg at weekly intervals up to 2500 mg once daily. If 2000 mg once daily is inadequate, 1000 mg twice daily may be used.
PO (Children >10 yr): 500 mg twice daily, may be increased by 500 mg/day at 1-wk intervals, up to 2000 mg/day in 2 divided doses.

Availability (generic available)

Tablets: 500 mg, 850 mg, 1000 mg. **Cost:** 500 mg $86.72/100, 850 mg $149.95/100, 1000 mg $149.95/100. **Extended-release tablets (Fortamet, Glucophage XR, Glumetza):** 500 mg, 750 mg, 1000 mg. **Oral solution (cherry flavor):** 500 mg/5 ml in 120– and 480-ml bottles. ***In combination with:*** glyburide (Glucovance) glipizide (Metaglip), pioglitazone (ACTOplus), rosiglitazone (Avandamet) and sitagliptin (Janumet). See Appendix B.

NURSING IMPLICATIONS

Assessment

- When combined with oral sulfonylureas, observe for signs and symptoms of hypoglycemic reactions (abdominal pain, sweating, hunger, weakness, dizziness, headache, tremor, tachycardia, anxiety).
- Patients who have been well controlled on metformin who develop illness or laboratory abnormalities should be assessed for ketoacidosis or lactic acidosis. Assess serum electrolytes, ketones, glucose, and, if indicated, blood pH, lactate, pyruvate, and metformin levels. If either form of acidosis is present, discontinue metformin immediately and treat acidosis.
- ***Lab Test Considerations:*** Monitor serum glucose and glycosylated hemoglobin periodically during therapy to evaluate effectiveness of therapy. May cause false-positive results for urine ketones.
- Monitor blood glucose concentrations routinely by patient and every 3 mo by health care professional to determine effectiveness of therapy.
- Assess renal function before initiating and at least annually during therapy. Discontinue metformin if renal impairment occurs.
- Monitor serum folic acid and vitamin B_{12} every 1–2 yr in long-term therapy. Metformin may interfere with absorption.

Potential Nursing Diagnoses

Imbalanced nutrition: more than body requirements (Indications)
Noncompliance (Patient/Family Teaching)

Implementation

- Patients stabilized on a diabetic regimen who are exposed to stress, fever, trauma, infection, or surgery may require administration of insulin. Withhold metformin and reinstitute after resolution of acute episode.
- Metformin therapy should be temporarily discontinued in patients requiring surgery involving restricted intake of food and fluids. Resume metformin when oral intake has resumed and renal function is normal.
- Withhold metformin before or at the time of studies requiring IV administration of iodinated contrast media and for 48 hr after study.
- **PO:** Administer metformin with meals to minimize GI effects.
- XR tablets must be swallowed whole; do not crush or chew.

Patient/Family Teaching

- Instruct patient to take metformin at the same time each day, as directed. Take missed doses as soon as possible unless almost time for next dose. Do not double doses.
- Explain to patient that metformin helps control hyperglycemia but does not cure diabetes. Therapy is usually long term.
- Encourage patient to follow prescribed diet, medication, and exercise regimen to prevent hyperglycemic or hypoglycemic episodes.
- Review signs of hypoglycemia and hyperglycemia with patient. If hypoglycemia occurs, advise patient to take a glass of orange juice or 2–3 tsp of sugar, honey, or corn syrup dissolved in water, and notify health care professional.
- Instruct patient in proper testing of blood glucose and urine ketones. These tests should be monitored closely during periods of stress or illness and health care professional notified if significant changes occur.
- Explain to patient the risk of lactic acidosis and the potential need for discontinuation of metformin therapy if a severe infection, dehydration, or severe or continuing diarrhea occurs or if medical tests or surgery is required. Symptoms of lactic acidosis (chills, diarrhea, dizziness, low blood pressure, muscle pain, sleepiness, slow heartbeat or pulse, dyspnea, or weakness) should be reported to health care professional immediately.
- Caution patient to avoid taking other Rx, OTC, herbal products, or alcohol during metformin therapy without consulting health care professional.
- Insulin is the recommended method of controlling blood glucose during pregnancy. Counsel female patients to use a form of contraception other than oral contraceptives and to notify health care professional promptly if pregnancy is planned or suspected.
- Inform patient that metformin may cause an unpleasant or metallic taste that usually resolves spontaneously.
- Inform patients taking XR tablets that inactive ingredients resembling XR tablet may appear in stools.
- Advise patient to inform health care professional of medication regimen before treatment or surgery.
- Advise patient to carry a form of sugar (sugar packets, candy) and identification describing disease process and medication regimen at all times.
- Advise patient to report the occurrence of diarrhea, nausea, vomiting, and stomach pain or fullness to health care professional.
- Emphasize the importance of routine follow-up exams and regular testing of blood glucose, glycosylated hemoglobin, renal function, and hematologic parameters.

Evaluation/Desired Outcomes

- Control of blood glucose levels without the appearance of hypoglycemic or hyperglycemic episodes. Control may be achieved within a few days, but full effect of therapy may be delayed for up to 2 wk. If patient has not responded to metformin after 4 wk of maximum dose therapy, an oral sulfonylurea may be added. If satisfactory results are not obtained with 1–3 months of concurrent therapy, oral agents may be discontinued and insulin therapy instituted.

M

HIGH ALERT

methadone (meth-a-done)
Methadose

Classification
Therapeutic: opioid analgesics
Pharmacologic: opioid agonists

Schedule II

Pregnancy Category C

Indications

Severe pain. Suppresses withdrawal symptoms in opioid detoxification.

Action

Binds to opiate receptors in the CNS. Alters the perception of and response to painful stimuli, while producing generalized CNS depression. **Therapeutic Effects:** Decrease in severity of pain. Suppression of withdrawal symptoms during detoxification and maintenance from heroin and other opioids.

Pharmacokinetics

Absorption: Well absorbed from all sites (50% absorbed following oral administration).

Distribution: Widely distributed. Crosses the placenta; enters breast milk.
Protein Binding: High.
Metabolism and Excretion: Mostly metabolized by the liver; some metabolites are active and may accumulate with chronic administration.
Half-life: 15–25 hr; increases with chronic use.

TIME/ACTION PROFILE (analgesic effect)

ROUTE	ONSET	PEAK	DURATION
PO	30–60 min	90–120 min	4–12 hr
IM, subcut	10–20 min	60–120 min	4–6 hr

Contraindications/Precautions

Contraindicated in: Hypersensitivity; Known alcohol intolerance (some oral solutions); Concurrent MAO inhibitor therapy.
Use Cautiously in: Cardiac hypertrophy, concomitant diuretic use, hypokalemia, hypomagnesemia, history of cardiac conduction abnormalities, concurrent medications affecting cardiac conduction, or other risk factor of arrhythmias; Head trauma; Increased intracranial pressure; Severe renal, hepatic, or pulmonary disease; Hypothyroidism; Adrenal insufficiency; Alcoholism; Undiagnosed abdominal pain; Prostatic hyperplasia or ureteral stricture; OB: Use with addiction control: weigh risk against potential for illicit drug use. Counsel mother about potential harm to fetus; Lactation: Appears in breast milk. Weigh risks against potential for illicit drug use. Counsel mother about potential harm to infant and to wean breastfeeding slowly to prevent abstinence syndrome; Geri: Dose reduction suggested.

Adverse Reactions/Side Effects

CNS: confusion, sedation, dizziness, dysphoria, euphoria, floating feeling, hallucinations, headache, unusual dreams. **EENT:** blurred vision, diplopia, miosis. **Resp:** respiratory depression. **CV:** hypotension, bradycardia, QT prolongation, Torsades de Pointes. **GI:** constipation, nausea, vomiting. **GU:** urinary retention. **Derm:** flushing, sweating. **Misc:** physical dependence, psychological dependence, tolerance.

Interactions

Drug-Drug: Use with extreme caution in patients receiving **MAO inhibitors** (may result in severe, unpredictable reactions—reduce initial dose of methadone to 25% of usual dose). Use with extreme caution with any drug known to potentially prolong QT interval, including **class I and III antiarrhythmics**, some **neuroleptics** and **tricyclic antidepressants**, and **calcium channel blockers**. Concurrent use **laxatives**, **diuretics**, **mineralocorticoids** may ↑ risk of hypomagnesemia or hypokalemia and ↑ risk of arrhythmias. ↑ CNS depression with **alcohol**, **antihistamines**, and **sedative/hypnotics**. Administration of **agonist/antagonist opioids** may precipitate opioid withdrawal in physically dependent patients. **Nalbuphine** or **pentazocine** may ↓ analgesia. **Interferons (alpha)** may ↓ metabolism and ↑ effects. **Nevirapine**, **efavirenz**, **ritonavir**, **ritonavir/lopinavir**, **phenobarbital**, **carbamazepine phenytoin**, and **rifampin** may ↑ metabolism and decrease analgesia; withdrawal may occur. **Fluvoxamine** may increase CNS depression; with **fluvoxamine**, opioid withdrawal may occur. May increase blood levels and effects of **zidovudine** and **desipramine**. May ↓ level and effects of **didanosine** and **stavudine**.
Drug-Natural Products: St. John's Wort ↑ metabolism and ↓ blood levels, concurrent use may result in withdrawal. **Kava kava, valerian,** or **chamomile,** can ↑ CNS depression.

Route/Dosage

Larger doses may be required for analgesia during chronic therapy; interval may be decreased/dose increased if pain recurs.
PO (Adults and Children ≥50 kg): *Analgesic*—20 mg q 6–8 hr. *Opioid detoxification*—15–40 mg once daily or amount needed to prevent withdrawal. Dose may be decreased q 1–2 days; maintenance dose is determined on an individual basis.
PO (Adults and Children <50 kg): *Analgesic*—0.2 mg/kg q 6–8 hr.
IM, Subcut (Adults and Children ≥50 kg): *Analgesic*—10 mg q 6–8 hr. *Opioid detoxification*—15–40 mg once daily or amount needed to prevent withdrawal. Dose may be decreased q 1–2 days; maintenance dose is determined on an individual basis.
IM, Subcut (Adults and Children <50 kg): 0.1 mg/kg mg q 6–8 hr.

Availability (generic available)

Tablets: 5 mg, 10 mg. **Dispersible tablets (diskettes):** 40 mg (available only to licensed detoxification/maintenance programs). **Oral solution (contains alcohol) (citrus):** 5 mg/5 ml, 10 mg/5 ml. **Oral concentrate (cherry and unflavored):** 10 mg/ml.

NURSING IMPLICATIONS

Assessment

- **Pain:** Assess type, location, and intensity of pain prior to and 1–2 hr (peak) following administration. When titrating opioid doses, increases of 25–50% should be administered until there is either a 50% reduction in the patient's pain rating on a numeric or visual analogue scale or the patient reports satisfactory pain relief. A repeat dose can be safely administered at the time of the peak if previous dose is ineffective and side effects are minimal. Cumulative effects of this medication may require periodic dose adjustments.
- Doses of methadone for patients on methadone maintenance prevent only withdrawal symptoms; *no analgesia is provided.* Additional opioid doses are required for treatment of pain.
- An equianalgesic chart (see Appendix J) should be used when changing routes or when changing from one opioid to another.
- Assess blood pressure, pulse, and respirations before and periodically during administration. If respiratory rate is <10/min, assess level of sedation. Dose may need to be decreased by 25–50%. Initial drowsiness will diminish with continued use.
- Assess bowel function routinely. Prevention of constipation should be instituted with increased intake of fluids and bulk and with laxatives to minimize constipating effects. Stimulant laxatives should be administered routinely if opioid use exceeds 2–3 days, unless contraindicated.
- Prolonged use may lead to physical and psychological dependence and tolerance. This should not prevent patient from receiving adequate analgesia. Most patients who receive methadone for pain do not develop psychological dependence. Progressively higher doses may be required to relieve pain with long-term therapy.
- **Opioid Detoxification:** Assess patient for signs of opioid withdrawal (irritability, runny nose and eyes, abdominal cramps, body aches, sweating, loss of appetite, shivering, unusually large pupils, trouble sleeping, weakness, yawning). Methadone maintenance is undertaken only by federally approved treatment centers. This does not preclude maintenance for addicts hospitalized for other conditions and who require temporary maintenance during their care.
- ***Lab Test Considerations:*** May ↑ plasma amylase and lipase levels.
- ***Toxicity and Overdose:*** If an opioid antagonist is required to reverse respiratory depression or coma, naloxone (Narcan) is the antidote. Dilute the 0.4-mg ampule of naloxone in 10 ml of 0.9% NaCl and administer 0.5 ml (0.02 mg) by direct IV push every 2 min. For children and patients weighing <40 kg, dilute 0.1 mg of naloxone in 10 ml of 0.9% NaCl for a concentration of 10 mcg/ml and administer 0.5 mcg/kg every 2 min. Titrate dose to avoid withdrawal, seizures, and severe pain.

Potential Nursing Diagnoses

Acute pain (Indications)
Disturbed sensory perception (visual, auditory) (Side Effects)
Risk for injury (Side Effects)

Implementation

- ***High Alert:*** Accidental overdosage of opioid analgesics has resulted in fatalities. Before administering, clarify all ambiguous orders; have second practitioner independently check original order and dose calculations.
- Explain therapeutic value of medication prior to administration to enhance the analgesic effect.
- Regularly administered doses may be more effective than prn administration. Analgesic is more effective if administered before pain becomes severe. For patients in chronic severe pain, the oral solution containing 5 or 10 mg/5 ml is recommended on a fixed dose schedule.
- Coadministration with nonopioid analgesics may have additive analgesic effects and may permit lower doses.
- Medication should be discontinued gradually after long-term use to prevent withdrawal symptoms.
- Diskettes (dispersible tablets) are to be dissolved and used for detoxification and maintenance treatment only.
- **PO:** Doses may be administered with food or milk to minimize GI irritation.

- Dilute each dose of 10 mg/ml oral concentrate with at least 30 ml of water or other liquid prior to administration.
- **Subcut:**
- **IM:** IM is the preferred parenteral route for repeated doses. Subcut administration may cause tissue irritation.

Patient/Family Teaching

- Instruct patient on how and when to ask for pain medication.
- Instruct patient to take methadone exactly as directed. If dose is less effective after a few weeks, do not increase dose without consulting health care professional.
- May cause drowsiness or dizziness. Advise patient to call for assistance when ambulating or smoking and to avoid driving or other activities requiring alertness until response to medication is known.
- Caution patient notify health care professional if signs of overdose (difficult or shallow breathing, extreme tiredness or sleepiness, blurred vision, inability to think, talk, or walk normally, and feelings of faintness, dizziness, or confusion) occur. Methadone has a prolonged action causing increased risk of overdose.
- Advise patient to change positions slowly to minimize orthostatic hypotension.
- Caution patient to avoid concurrent use of alcohol or other CNS depressants with this medication.
- Encourage patient to turn, cough, and breathe deeply every 2 hr to prevent atelectasis.

Evaluation/Desired Outcomes

- Decrease in severity of pain without a significant alteration in level of consciousness or respiratory status.
- Prevention of withdrawal symptoms in detoxification from heroin and other opioid analgesics.

methimazole (meth-**im**-a-zole)

Tapazole

Classification
Therapeutic: antithyroid agents

Pregnancy Category D

Indications

Palliative treatment of hyperthyroidism. Used as an adjunct to control hyperthyroidism in preparation for thyroidectomy or radioactive iodine therapy.

Action

Inhibits the synthesis of thyroid hormones. **Therapeutic Effects:** Decreased signs and symptoms of hyperthyroidism.

Pharmacokinetics

Absorption: Rapidly absorbed following oral administration.
Distribution: Crosses the placenta and enters breast milk in high concentrations.
Metabolism and Excretion: Mostly metabolized by the liver; <10% eliminated unchanged by the kidneys.
Half-life: 3–5 hr.

TIME/ACTION PROFILE (effect on thyroid function)

ROUTE	ONSET	PEAK	DURATION
PO	1 wk	4–10 wk	wks

Contraindications/Precautions

Contraindicated in: Hypersensitivity; Lactation.
Use Cautiously in: Patients with decreased bone marrow reserve; Patients >40 yr (increased risk of agranulocytosis); Pregnancy (may be used cautiously; however, thyroid problems may occur in the fetus).

Adverse Reactions/Side Effects

CNS: drowsiness, headache, vertigo. **GI:** diarrhea, drug-induced hepatitis, loss of taste, nausea, parotitis, vomiting. **Derm:** rash, skin discoloration, urticaria. **Hemat:** AGRANULOCYTOSIS, anemia, leukopenia, thrombocytopenia. **MS:** arthralgia. **Misc:** fever, lymphadenopathy.

Interactions

Drug-Drug: Additive bone marrow depression with **antineoplastics** or **radiation therapy**. Antithyroid effect may be decreased by **potassium iodide** or **amiodarone**. Increased risk of agranulocytosis with **phenothiazines**. May alter response to **warfarin** and **digoxins**.

Route/Dosage

PO (Adults): *Thyrotoxic crisis*—15–20 mg q 4 hr during the first 24 hr (with other interventions). *Hyperthyroidism*—15–60 mg/day as a single dose or divided doses for 6–8 wk. *Maintenance*—5.30 mg/kg as a single dose or 2 divided doses.
PO (Children): *Initial*—400 mcg (0.4 mg)/kg/day in single dose or 2 divided doses. *Main-*

tenance—200 mcg/kg/day in single dose or 2 divided doses.

Availability
Tablets: 5 mg, 10 mg.

NURSING IMPLICATIONS

Assessment
- Monitor response for symptoms of hyperthyroidism or thyrotoxicosis (tachycardia, palpitations, nervousness, insomnia, fever, diaphoresis, heat intolerance, tremors, weight loss, diarrhea).
- Assess patient for development of hypothyroidism (intolerance to cold, constipation, dry skin, headache, listlessness, tiredness, or weakness). Dosage adjustment may be required.
- Assess patient for skin rash or swelling of cervical lymph nodes. Treatment may be discontinued if this occurs.
- ***Lab Test Considerations:*** Thyroid function studies should be monitored prior to therapy, monthly during initial therapy, and every 2–3 mo throughout therapy.
- WBC and differential counts should be monitored periodically throughout therapy. Agranulocytosis may develop rapidly; it usually occurs during the first 2 mo and is more common in patients over 40 yr and those receiving >40 mg/day. This necessitates discontinuation of therapy.
- May cause increased AST, ALT, LDH, alkaline phosphatase, serum bilirubin, and prothrombin time.

Potential Nursing Diagnoses
Noncompliance (Patient/Family Teaching)

Implementation
- **PO:** Administer at same time in relation to meals every day. Food may either increase or decrease absorption.

Patient/Family Teaching
- Instruct patient to take medication exactly as directed, around the clock. If a dose is missed, take as soon as remembered; take both doses together if almost time for next dose; check with health care professional if more than 1 dose is missed. Consult health care professional prior to discontinuing medication.
- Instruct patient to monitor weight 2–3 times weekly. Notify health care professional of significant changes.
- May cause drowsiness. Caution patient to avoid driving or other activities requiring alertness until response to medication is known.
- Advise patient to consult health care professional regarding dietary sources of iodine (iodized salt, shellfish).
- Advise patient to report sore throat, fever, chills, headache, malaise, weakness, yellowing of eyes or skin, unusual bleeding or bruising, rash, or symptoms of hyperthyroidism or hypothyroidism promptly.
- Instruct patient to consult health care professional before taking any OTC medications.
- Advise patient to carry identification describing medication regimen at all times.
- Advise patient to notify health care professional of medication regimen prior to treatment or surgery.
- Emphasize the importance of routine exams to monitor progress and to check for side effects.

Evaluation/Desired Outcomes
- Decrease in severity of symptoms of hyperthyroidism (lowered pulse rate and weight gain).
- Return of thyroid function studies to normal.
- May be used as short-term adjunctive therapy to prepare patient for thyroidectomy or radiation therapy or may be used in treatment of hyperthyroidism. Treatment from 6 mo to several years may be necessary, usually averaging 1 yr.

M

methocarbamol
(meth-oh-**kar**-ba-mole)
Carbacot, Robaxin

Classification
Therapeutic: skeletal muscle relaxants (centrally acting)

Pregnancy Category C

Indications
Adjunctive treatment of muscle spasm associated with acute painful musculoskeletal conditions (with rest and physical therapy).

Action

Skeletal muscle relaxation, probably as a result of CNS depression. **Therapeutic Effects:** Skeletal muscle relaxation.

Pharmacokinetics

Absorption: Rapidly absorbed from the GI tract.
Distribution: Widely distributed. Crosses the placenta; enters breast milk in small amounts.
Metabolism and Excretion: Metabolized by the liver.
Half-life: 1–2 hr.

TIME/ACTION PROFILE (skeletal muscle relaxation)

ROUTE	ONSET	PEAK	DURATION
PO	30 min	2 hr	unknown
IM	rapid	unknown	unknown
IV	immediate	end of infusion	unknown

Contraindications/Precautions

Contraindicated in: Hypersensitivity; Hypersensitivity to polyethylene glycol (parenteral only); Renal impairment (parenteral form).
Use Cautiously in: Pregnancy, lactation, and children (safety not established); Geri: Appears on Beers list. Poorly tolerated due to anticholinergic effects; Seizure disorders (parenteral form).

Adverse Reactions/Side Effects

CNS: SEIZURES (IV, IM only), dizziness, drowsiness, light-headedness. **EENT:** blurred vision, nasal congestion. **CV:** *IV*—bradycardia, hypotension. **GI:** anorexia, GI upset, nausea. **GU:** brown, black, or green urine. **Derm:** flushing (IV only), pruritus, rashes, urticaria. **Local:** pain at IM site, phlebitis at IV site. **Misc:** allergic reactions including ANAPHYLAXIS (IM, IV use only), fever.

Interactions

Drug-Drug: Additive CNS depression with other **CNS depressants**, including **alcohol**, **antihistamines**, **opioid analgesics**, and **sedative/hypnotics**.
Drug-Natural Products: Concomitant use of **kava kava**, **valerian**, **chamomile**, or **hops** can ↑ CNS depression.

Route/Dosage

PO (Adults): 1.5 g qid initially (up to 8 g/day) for 2–3 days, then 4–4.5 g/day in 3–6 divided doses; may be followed by maintenance dosing of 750 mg q 4 hr or 1 g 4 times daily or 1.5 g 3 times daily.
IM, IV (Adults): 1–3 g/day for not more than 3 days; course may be repeated after a 48-hr rest.

Availability (generic available)

Tablets: 500 mg, 750 mg. **Injection:** ✤100 mg/ml in 10-ml ampules, 100 mg/ml in 10-ml vials. ***In combination with:*** aspirin (Robaxisal). See Appendix B.

NURSING IMPLICATIONS

Assessment

- Assess patient for pain, muscle stiffness, and range of motion before and periodically throughout therapy.
- Monitor pulse and blood pressure every 15 min during parenteral administration.
- Geri: Assess geriatric patients for anticholinergic effects (sedation and weakness).
- Assess patient for allergic reactions (skin rash, asthma, hives, wheezing, hypotension) after parenteral administration. Keep epinephrine and oxygen on hand in the event of a reaction.
- Monitor IV site. Injection is hypertonic and may cause thrombophlebitis. Avoid extravasation.
- ***Lab Test Considerations:*** Monitor renal function periodically during prolonged parenteral therapy (>3 days), because polyethylene glycol 300 vehicle is nephrotoxic.
- May cause falsely increased urinary 5-hydroxyindoleacetic acid (5-HIAA) and vanillylmandelic acid (VMA) determinations.

Potential Nursing Diagnoses

Acute pain (Indications)
Impaired physical mobility (Indications)
Risk for injury (Side Effects)

Implementation

- Provide safety measures as indicated. Supervise ambulation and transfer of patients.
- **PO:** May be administered with food to minimize GI irritation. Tablets may be crushed and mixed with food or liquids to facilitate swallowing. For administration via NG tube, crush tablet and suspend in water or saline.
- **IM:** Do not administer subcut. IM injections should contain no more than 5 ml (500 mg) at a time in the gluteal region.

IV Administration

- **Direct IV:** ***Diluent:*** Administer undiluted. ***Concentration:*** 100 mg/ml. ***Rate:*** Administer at a maximum rate of 180 mg/m²/min but not >3 ml (300 mg)/min.

- **Intermittent Infusion:** ***Diluent:*** Dilute each dose in no more than 250 ml of 0.9% NaCl or D5W for injection. ***Concentration:*** 4 mg/ml for slower infusions. Do not refrigerate after dilution
- Have patient remain recumbent during and for at least 10–15 min after infusion to avoid orthostatic hypotension.

Patient/Family Teaching

- Advise patient to take medication as directed. Take missed doses within 1 hr; if not, return to regular dosing schedule. Do not double doses.
- Encourage patient to comply with additional therapies prescribed for muscle spasm (rest, physical therapy, heat).
- May cause dizziness, drowsiness, and blurred vision. Advise patient to avoid driving and other activities requiring alertness until response to drug is known.
- Instruct patient to change positions slowly to minimize orthostatic hypotension.
- Advise patient to avoid concurrent use of alcohol and other CNS depressants.
- Inform patient that urine may turn black, brown, or green, especially if left standing.
- Instruct patient to notify health care professional if skin rash, itching, fever, or nasal congestion occurs.
- Emphasize the importance of routine follow-up exams to monitor progress.

Evaluation/Desired Outcomes

- Decreased musculoskeletal pain and muscle spasticity.
- Increased range of motion.

HIGH ALERT

methotrexate

(meth-o-**trex**-ate)
amethopterin, Folex, Folex PFS, Rheumatrex, Trexall

Classification
Therapeutic: antineoplastics, antirheumatics (DMARDs), immunosuppressants
Pharmacologic: antimetabolites

Pregnancy Category X

Indications

Alone or with other treatment modalities in the treatment of: Trophoblastic neoplasms (choriocarcinoma, chorioadenoma destruens, hydatidiform mole), Leukemias, Breast carcinoma, Head carcinoma, Neck carcinoma, Lung carcinoma. Treatment of severe psoriasis and rheumatoid arthritis unresponsive to conventional therapy. Treatment of mycosis fungoides (cutaneous T-cell lymphoma).

Action

Interferes with folic acid metabolism. Result is inhibition of DNA synthesis and cell reproduction (cell-cycle S-phase–specific). Also has immunosuppressive activity. **Therapeutic Effects:** Death of rapidly replicating cells, particularly malignant ones, and immunosuppression.

Pharmacokinetics

Absorption: Small doses are well absorbed from the GI tract. Larger doses incompletely absorbed.
Distribution: Actively transported across cell membranes, widely distributed. Does not reach therapeutic concentrations in the CSF. Crosses placenta; enters breast milk in low concentrations. Absorption in children is variable (23–95%) and dose-dependent.
Metabolism and Excretion: Excreted mostly unchanged by the kidneys.
Half-life: *Low dose*—3–10 hr; *high dose*—8–15 hr (increased in renal impairment).

TIME/ACTION PROFILE (effects on blood counts)

ROUTE	ONSET	PEAK	DURATION
PO, IM, IV	4–7 days	7–14 days	21 days

Contraindications/Precautions

Contraindicated in: Hypersensitivity; Pregnancy or lactation; Products containing benzyl alcohol should not be used in neonates.
Use Cautiously in: Renal impairment (CCr must be ≥60 ml/min prior to therapy); Patients with childbearing potential; Active infections; Decreased bone marrow reserve; Geri: Geriatric patients or patients with other chronic debilitating illnesses.

Adverse Reactions/Side Effects

CNS: arachnoiditis (IT use only), dizziness, drowsiness, headaches, malaise. **EENT:** blurred vision, dysarthria transient blindness. **Resp:** PULMONARY FIBROSIS, intestinal pneumonitis. **GI:** anorexia, hepatotoxicity, nausea, stomatitis, vomiting. **GU:** infertility. **Derm:** alopecia, painful plaque erosions (during psoriasis treatment), photosensitivity, pruritus, rashes, skin ulceration, urticaria. **Hemat:** APLASTIC ANEMIA, anemia, leukopenia, thrombocytopenia. **Metab:** hyperuricemia. **MS:** osteonecrosis, stress fracture. **Misc:** nephropathy, chills, fever, soft tissue necrosis.

Interactions

Drug-Drug: The following drugs may ↑ hematologic toxicity of methotrexate: high-dose **salicylates**, **NSAIDs**, **oral hypoglycemic agents (sulfonylureas)**, **phenytoin**, **tetracyclines**, **probenecid**, **trimethoprim/sulfamethoxazole**, **pyrimethamine**, and **chloramphenicol**. ↑ hepatotoxicity with other **hepatotoxic drugs** including **azathioprine**, **sulfasalazine**, and **retinoids**. ↑ nephrotoxicity with other **nephrotoxic drugs**. ↑ bone marrow depression with other **antineoplastics** or **radiation therapy**. **Radiation therapy** ↑ risk of soft tissue necrosis and osteonecrosis. May ↓ antibody response to **live-virus vaccines** and ↑ risk of adverse reactions. ↑ risk of neurologic reactions with **acyclovir** (IT methotrexate only). **Asparaginase** may ↓ effects of methotrexate.

Drug-Natural Products: Concomitant use with **echinacea** and **melatonin** may interfere with immunosuppression. **Caffeine** may ↓ efficacy of methotrexate, similar effect may occur with **guarana.**

Route/Dosage

Trophoblastic Neoplasms

PO, IM (Adults): 15–30 mg/day for 5 days; repeat after 1 or more weeks for 3–5 courses.

Breast Cancer

IV (Adults): 40 mg/m² on days 1 and 8 (with other agents; many regimens are used).

Leukemia

PO (Adults): *Induction*—3.3 mg/m²/day, usually with prednisone.
PO, IM (Adults): *Maintenance*—20–30 mg/m² twice weekly.
IV (Adults): 2.5 mg/kg q 2 wk.
IT (Adults): 12 mg/m² or 15 mg.
IT (Children ≥3 yr): 12 mg.
IT (Children 2 yr): 10 mg.
IT (Children 1 yr): 8 mg.
IT (Children <1 yr): 6 mg.

Osteosarcoma

IV (Adults): 12 g/m² as a 4-hr infusion followed by leucovorin rescue, usually as part of a combination chemotherapeutic regimen (or increase dose until peak serum methotrexate level is 1×10^{-3} M/L but not to exceed 15 g/m²; 12 courses are given starting 4 wk after surgery and repeated at scheduled intervals.

Psoriasis

Therapy may be preceded by a 5–10-mg test dose.
PO (Adults): 2.5–5 mg q 12 hr for 3 doses *or* q 8 hr for 4 doses once weekly (not to exceed 30 mg/wk).
PO, IM, IV (Adults): 10–25 mg/weekly (not to exceed 30 mg/wk).

Arthritis

Therapy may be preceded by a 5–10-mg test dose in adults.
PO (Adults): 7.5 mg weekly (2.5 mg q 12 hr for 3 doses or single dose, not to exceed 20 mg/wk); when response is obtained, dosage should be decreased.
PO (Children): 10 mg/m² once weekly initially, may be increased up to 20–30 mg/m², however response may be better if doses >20 mg/m² are given IM or subcut.

Mycosis Fungoides

PO, IM, Subcut (Adults): 5–50 mg once weekly, if response is poor, dose may be changed to 15–37.5 mg twice weekly.
IM (Adults): 50 mg once weekly or 25 mg twice weekly.

Availability (generic available)

Tablets: 2.5 mg, 5 mg, 7.5 mg, 10 mg, 15 mg. **Injection:** 2.5 mg/ml, 25 mg/ml, 20 mg, 50 mg, 100 mg, 250 mg, 1 g. **Preservative-free injection:** 25 mg/ml.

NURSING IMPLICATIONS

Assessment

- Monitor vital signs periodically during administration. Report significant changes.
- Monitor for abdominal pain, diarrhea, or stomatitis; therapy may need to be discontinued.
- Monitor for bone marrow depression. Assess for bleeding (bleeding gums, bruising, petechiae, guaiac stools, urine, and emesis) and avoid IM injections and taking rectal temperatures if platelet count is low. Apply pressure to venipuncture sites for 10 min. Assess for

signs of infection during neutropenia. Anemia may occur. Monitor for increased fatigue, dyspnea, and orthostatic hypotension.

- Monitor intake and output ratios and daily weights. Report significant changes in totals.
- Monitor for symptoms of pulmonary toxicity, which may manifest early as a dry, nonproductive cough.
- Monitor for symptoms of gout (increased uric acid, joint pain, edema). Encourage patient to drink at least 2 L of fluid each day. Allopurinol and alkalinization of urine may be used to decrease uric acid levels.
- Assess nutritional status. Administering an antiemetic prior to and periodically during therapy and adjusting diet as tolerated may help maintain fluid and electrolyte balance and nutritional status.
- **IT:** Assess for development of nuchal rigidity, headache, fever, confusion, drowsiness, dizziness, weakness, or seizures.
- **Rheumatoid Arthritis:** Assess patient for pain and range of motion prior to and periodically during therapy.
- **Psoriasis:** Assess skin lesions prior to and periodically during therapy.
- ***Lab Test Considerations:*** Monitor CBC and differential prior to and frequently during therapy. The nadir of leukopenia and thrombocytopenia occurs in 7–14 days. Leukocyte and thrombocyte counts usually recover 7 days after the nadirs. Notify health care professional of any sudden drop in values.
- Monitor renal (BUN and creatinine) and hepatic function (AST, ALT, bilirubin, and LDH) prior to and routinely during therapy. Urine pH should be monitored prior to high-dose methotrexate therapy and every 6 hr during leucovorin rescue. Urine pH should be kept above 7.0 to prevent renal damage.
- May cause ↑ serum uric acid concentrations, especially during initial treatment of leukemia and lymphoma.
- ***Toxicity and Overdose:*** Monitor serum methotrexate levels every 12–24 hr during high-dose therapy until levels are <5 × 10 M. This monitoring is essential to plan correct leucovorin dose and determine duration of rescue therapy: With high-dose therapy, patient must receive leucovorin rescue within 24–48 hr to prevent fatal toxicity. In cases of massive overdose, hydration and urinary alkalization may be required to prevent renal tubule damage. Monitor fluid and electrolyte status. Intermittent hemodialysis using a high-flux dialyzer may be used for clearance until levels are <0.05 micromolar.

Potential Nursing Diagnoses

Risk for infection (Adverse Reactions)
Imbalanced nutrition: less than body requirements (Adverse Reactions)

Implementation

- ***High Alert:*** Fatalities have occurred with chemotherapeutic agents. Before administering, clarify all ambiguous orders; double-check single, daily, and course-of-therapy dose limits; have second practitioner independently double-check original order, calculations and infusion pump settings. Methotrexate for non-oncologic use is given at a much lower dose and frequency—often just once a week. Do not confuse non-oncologic dosing regimens with dosing regimens for cancer patients.
- Solutions for injection should be prepared in a biologic cabinet. Wear gloves, gown, and mask while handling medication. Discard equipment in specially designated containers (see Appendix K).

IV Administration

- **Direct IV:** ***Diluent:*** Reconstitute each vial with 25 ml of 0.9% NaCl. Use sterile preservative-free diluents for high-dose regimens to prevent complications from large amounts of benzyl alcohol. Do not use preparations that are discolored or that contain a precipitate. Reconstitute immediately before use. Discard unused portion. ***Concentration:*** <25 mg/ml for direct IV and intermittent/continuous infusions. ***Rate:*** Administer at a rate of 10 mg/min into Y-site of a free-flowing IV.
- **Intermittent/Continuous Infusion:** ***Diluent:*** Doses >100–300 mg/m^2 may also be diluted in D5W, D5/0.9% NaCl, or 0.9% NaCl and infused as intermittent or continuous infusion. ***Rate:*** Administration rates of 4–20 mg/hr have been used.
- **Syringe Compatibility:** bleomycin, cisplatin, cyclophosphamide, doxapram, doxorubicin, fluorouracil, furosemide, heparin, leucovorin, mitomycin, vinblastine, vincristine.
- **Syringe Incompatibility:** droperidol.

- **Y-Site Compatibility:** allopurinol, amifostine, amphotericin B cholesteryl sulfate, asparaginase, aztreonam, bleomycin, cefepime, ceftriaxone, cimetidine, cisplatin, cyclophosphamide, cytarabine, daunorubicin, diphenhydramine, doxorubicin, doxorubicin liposome, etoposide, etoposide phosphate, famotidine, filgrastim, fludarabine, fluorouracil, furosemide, ganciclovir, granisetron, heparin, hydromorphone, imipenem/cilastatin, lansoprazole, leucovorin, linezolid, lorazepam, melphalan, mesna, methylprednisolone sodium succinate, metoclopramide, mitomycin, morphine, ondansetron, oxaliplatin, paclitaxel, piperacillin/tazobactam, prochlorperazine, ranitidine, sargramostim, teniposide, thiotepa, vinblastine, vincristine, vinorelbine.
- **Y-Site Incompatibility:** chlorpromazine, gemcitabine, idarubicin, ifosfamide, midazolam, nalbuphine, promethazine, propofol.
- **Additive Compatibility:** cyclophosphamide, cytarabine, fluorouracil, mercaptopurine, ondansetron, sodium bicarbonate, vincristine.
- **Additive Incompatibility:** bleomycin. **IT:** Reconstitute preservative-free methotrexate with preservative-free 0.9% NaCl, Elliot's B solution, or patient's CSF to a concentration not greater than 2 mg/ml. May be administered via lumbar puncture or Ommaya reservoir. To prevent bacterial contamination, use immediately.

Patient/Family Teaching

- Instruct patient to take medication as directed. If a dose is missed, it should be omitted. Consult health care professional if vomiting occurs shortly after a dose is taken.
- Instruct patient to notify health care professional promptly if fever; chills; cough; hoarseness; sore throat; signs of infection; lower back or side pain; painful or difficult urination; bleeding gums; bruising; petechiae; blood in stools, urine, or emesis; increased fatigue; dyspnea; or orthostatic hypotension occurs. Caution patient to avoid crowds and persons with known infections. Instruct patient to use soft toothbrush and electric razor and to avoid falls. Caution patient not to drink alcoholic beverages or take medication containing aspirin or other NSAIDs; may precipitate gastric bleeding.
- Instruct patient to inspect oral mucosa for erythema and ulceration. If ulceration occurs, advise patient to use sponge brush and to rinse mouth with water after eating and drinking. Topical therapy may be used if mouth pain interferes with eating. Stomatitis pain may require treatment with opioid analgesics.
- Instruct patient to avoid the use of Rx, OTC, or herbal products without first consulting health care professional.
- Advise patient that this medication may have teratogenic effects. Contraception should be used during therapy and for at least 3 mo for men and 1 ovulatory cycle for women after completion of therapy.
- Discuss the possibility of hair loss with patient. Explore methods of coping.
- Instruct patient not to receive any vaccinations without advice of health care professional.
- Caution patient to use sunscreen and protective clothing to prevent photosensitivity reactions.
- Emphasize the need for periodic lab tests to monitor for side effects.

Evaluation/Desired Outcomes

- Improvement of hematopoietic values in leukemia.
- Decrease in symptoms of meningeal involvement in leukemia.
- Decrease in size and spread of non-Hodgkin's lymphomas and other solid cancers.
- Resolution of skin lesions in severe psoriasis.
- Decreased joint pain and swelling.
- Improved mobility in patients with rheumatoid arthritis.
- Regression of lesions in mycosis fungoides.

methyldopa (meth-ill-**doe**-pa)

Aldomet, ✤Apo-Methyldopa, ✤Dopamet, ✤Novamedopa, ✤Nu-Medopa

Classification

Therapeutic: antihypertensives

Pharmacologic: centrally acting antiadrenergics

Pregnancy Category B

Indications

Management of moderate to severe hypertension (with other agents).

Action

Stimulates CNS alpha-adrenergic receptors, producing a decrease in sympathetic outflow to heart, kidneys, and blood vessels. Result is decreased blood pressure and peripheral resistance, a slight decrease in heart rate, and no change in cardiac output. **Therapeutic Effects:** Lowering of blood pressure.

Pharmacokinetics

Absorption: 50% absorbed from the GI tract. Parenteral form, methyldopate hydrochloride, is slowly converted to methyldopa.
Distribution: Crosses the blood-brain barrier. Crosses the placenta; small amounts enter breast milk.
Metabolism and Excretion: Partially metabolized by the liver, partially excreted unchanged by the kidneys.
Half-life: 1.7 hr.

TIME/ACTION PROFILE (antihypertensive effect)

ROUTE	ONSET	PEAK	DURATION
PO	12–24 hr	4–6 hr	24–48 hr
IV	4–6 hr	unknown	10–16 hr

Contraindications/Precautions

Contraindicated in: Hypersensitivity; Active liver disease; Oral suspension contains alcohol and bisulfites and should be avoided in patients with known intolerance.
Use Cautiously in: Previous history of liver disease; Geri: ↑ risk of adverse reactions; consider age-related impairment of hepatic, renal and cardiovascular function as well as other chronic illnesses. Appears on Beers list. May cause bradycardia and exacerbate depression in geriatric patients; OB: Pregnancy (has been used safely); Lactation.

Adverse Reactions/Side Effects

CNS: sedation, decreased mental acuity, depression. **EENT:** nasal stuffiness. **CV:** MYOCARDITIS, bradycardia, edema, orthostatic hypotension. **GI:** DRUG-INDUCED HEPATITIS, diarrhea, dry mouth. **GU:** erectile dysfunction. **Hemat:** eosinophilia, hemolytic anemia. **Misc:** fever.

Interactions

Drug-Drug: Additive hypotension with other **antihypertensives**, acute ingestion of **alcohol**, **anesthesia**, and **nitrates**. **Amphetamines**, **barbiturates**, **tricyclic antidepressants**, **NSAIDs**, and **phenothiazines** may ↓ antihypertensive effect of methyldopa. ↑ effects and risk of psychoses with **haloperidol**. Excess sympathetic stimulation may occur with concurrent use of **MAO inhibitors** or other **adrenergics**. May ↑ effects of **tolbutamide**. May ↑ **lithium** toxicity. Additive hypotension and CNS toxicity with **levodopa**. Additive CNS depression may occur with **alcohol**, **antihistamines**, **sedative/hypnotics**, some **antidepressants**, and **opioid analgesics**. Concurrent use with **nonselective beta blockers** may rarely cause paradoxical hypertension.

Route/Dosage

PO (Adults): 250–500 mg 2–3 times daily (not to exceed 500 mg/day if used with other agents); may be increased q 2 days as needed; usual maintenance dose is 500 mg–2 g/day (not to exceed 3 g/day).
PO (Children): 10 mg/kg/day (300 mg/m²/day); may be increased q 2 days up to 65 mg/kg/day in divided doses (not to exceed 3 g/day).
IV (Adults): 250–500 mg q 6 hr (up to 1 g q 6 hr).
IV (Children): 5–10 mg/kg q 6 hr; up to 65 mg/kg/day in divided doses (not to exceed 3 g/day).

Availability (generic available)

Tablets: 125 mg, 250 mg, 500 mg. **Oral suspension (orange-pineapple flavor, contains bisulfites):** 250 mg/5 ml. **Injection:** 250 mg/5 ml in 5- and 10-ml vials. ***In combination with:*** hydrochlorothiazide (Aldoril) or chlorothiazide (Aldoclor). See Appendix B.

M

NURSING IMPLICATIONS

Assessment

- Monitor blood pressure and pulse frequently during initial dose adjustment and periodically during therapy. Report significant changes.
- Monitor frequency of prescription refills to determine compliance.
- Monitor intake and output ratios and weight and assess for edema daily, especially at beginning of therapy. Report weight gain or edema; sodium and water retention may be treated with diuretics.
- Assess patient for depression or other alterations in mental status. Notify health care pro-

fessional promptly if these symptoms develop.

- Monitor temperature during therapy. Drug fever may occur shortly after initiation of therapy and may be accompanied by eosinophilia and hepatic function changes. Monitor hepatic function test if unexplained fever occurs.
- ***Lab Test Considerations:*** Monitor renal and hepatic function and CBC before and periodically during therapy.
- Monitor direct Coombs' test before and after 6 and 12 mo of therapy. May cause a positive direct Coombs' test, rarely associated with hemolytic anemia.
- May cause ↑ BUN, serum creatinine, potassium, sodium, prolactin, uric acid, AST, ALT, alkaline phosphatase, and bilirubin concentrations.
- May cause prolonged prothrombin times.
- May interfere with serum creatinine and AST measurements.

Potential Nursing Diagnoses

Risk for injury (Side Effects)
Noncompliance (Patient/Family Teaching)

Implementation

- Do not confuse methyldopa with levodopa or L-dopa.
- Fluid retention and expanded volume may cause tolerance to develop within 2–3 mo after initiation of therapy. Diuretics may be added to regimen at this time to maintain control.
- Dose increases should be made with the evening dose to minimize drowsiness.
- When changing from IV to oral forms, dose should remain consistent.
- **PO:** Shake suspension before administration.

IV Administration

- **Intermittent Infusion:*Diluent:*** Dilute in 100 ml of D5W, 0.9% NaCl, D5/0.9% NaCl, 5% sodium bicarbonate, or Ringer's solution. ***Concentration:*** ≤10 mg/ml.***Rate:*** Infuse slowly over 30–60 min.
- **Y-Site Compatibility:** esmolol, heparin, meperidine, morphine, theophylline.

Patient/Family Teaching

- Emphasize the importance of continuing to take this medication, even if feeling well. Instruct patient to take medication at the same time each day; last dose of the day should be taken at bedtime. Take missed doses as soon as remembered but not if almost time for next dose. Do not double doses.
- Encourage patient to comply with additional interventions for hypertension (weight reduction, low-sodium diet, smoking cessation, moderation of alcohol consumption, regular exercise, and stress management). Methyldopa controls but does not cure hypertension.
- Instruct patient and family on proper technique for monitoring blood pressure. Advise them to check blood pressure at least weekly and to report significant changes.
- Inform patient that urine may darken or turn red-black when left standing.
- May cause drowsiness. Advise patient to avoid driving or other activities requiring alertness until response to medication is known. Drowsiness usually subsides after 7–10 days of continuous use.
- Caution patient to avoid sudden changes in position to decrease orthostatic hypotension.
- Advise patient that frequent mouth rinses, good oral hygiene, and sugarless gum or candy may minimize dry mouth. Notify health care professional if dry mouth continues for >2 wk.
- Caution patient to avoid concurrent use of alcohol or other CNS depressants.
- Advise patient to consult health care professional before taking any cough, cold, or allergy remedies.
- Advise patient to notify health care professional of medication regimen before treatment or surgery.
- Instruct patient to notify health care professional if fever, muscle aches, or flu-like syndrome occurs.

Evaluation/Desired Outcomes

- Decrease in blood pressure without appearance of side effects.

methylergonovine

(meth-ill-er-goe-**noe**-veen)
Methergine

Classification
Therapeutic: oxytocic
Pharmacologic: ergot alkaloids

Pregnancy Category C

Indications

Prevention and treatment of postpartum or postabortion hemorrhage caused by uterine atony or subinvolution.

Action
Directly stimulates uterine and vascular smooth muscle. **Therapeutic Effects:** Uterine contraction.

Pharmacokinetics
Absorption: Well absorbed following oral or IM administration.
Distribution: Unknown. Enters breast milk in small quantities.
Metabolism and Excretion: Probably metabolized by the liver.
Half-life: 30–120 min.

TIME/ACTION PROFILE (effects on uterine contractions)

ROUTE	ONSET	PEAK	DURATION
PO	5–15 min	unknown	3 hr
IM	2–5 min	unknown	3 hr
IV	immediate	unknown	45 min–3 hr

Contraindications/Precautions
Contraindicated in: Hypersensitivity; Should not be used to induce labor.
Use Cautiously in: Hypertensive or eclamptic patients (more susceptible to hypertensive and arrhythmogenic side effects); Severe hepatic or renal disease; Sepsis.
Exercise Extreme Caution in: Third stage of labor.

Adverse Reactions/Side Effects
CNS: dizziness, headache. **EENT:** tinnitus. **Resp:** dyspnea. **CV:** HYPOTENSION, arrhythmias, chest pain, hypertension, palpitations. **GI:** nausea, vomiting. **GU:** cramps. **Derm:** diaphoresis. **Misc:** allergic reactions.

Interactions
Drug-Drug: Excessive vasoconstriction may result when used with heavy cigarette smoking (**nicotine**) or other **vasopressors** such as **dopamine**.

Route/Dosage
PO (Adults): 200–400 mcg (0.4–0.6 mg) q 6–12 hr for 2–7 days.
IM, IV (Adults): 200 mcg (0.2 mg) q 2–4 hr for up to 5 doses.

Availability
Tablets: 200 mcg (0.2 mg). **Injection:** 200 mcg (0.2 mg)/ml in 1-ml ampules.

NURSING IMPLICATIONS

Assessment
- Monitor blood pressure, heart rate, and uterine response frequently during medication administration. Notify health care professional promptly if uterine relaxation becomes prolonged or if character of vaginal bleeding changes.
- Assess for signs of ergotism (cold, numb fingers and toes, chest pain, nausea, vomiting, headache, muscle pain, weakness).
- ***Lab Test Considerations:*** If no response to methylergonovine, calcium levels may need to be assessed. Effectiveness of medication is ↓ with hypocalcemia.
- May cause ↓ serum prolactin levels.

Potential Nursing Diagnoses
Acute pain (Side Effects)

Implementation
IV Administration
- **IV:** IV administration is used for emergencies only. Oral and IM routes are preferred.
- **Direct IV:** ***Diluent:*** May be given undiluted or diluted in 5 ml of 0.9% NaCl and administered through Y-site. Do not add to IV solutions. Do not mix in syringe with any other drug. Refrigerate; stable for storage at room temperature for 60 days; deteriorates with age. Use only solution that is clear and colorless and that contains no precipitate. ***Concentration:*** 0.2 mg/ml. ***Rate:*** Administer at a rate of 0.2 mg over at least 1 min.
- **Y-Site Compatibility:** heparin, hydrocortisone sodium succinate, potassium chloride, vitamin B complex with C.

Patient/Family Teaching
- Instruct patient to take medication as directed; do not skip or double up on missed doses. If a dose is missed, omit it and return to regular dose schedule.
- Advise patient that medication may cause menstrual-like cramps.
- Caution patient to avoid smoking, because nicotine constricts blood vessels.
- Instruct patient to notify health care professional if infection develops, as this may cause increased sensitivity to the medication.

Evaluation/Desired Outcomes
- Contractions that maintain uterine tone and prevent postpartum hemorrhage.

M

methylphenidate

(meth-ill-**fen**-i-date)
Concerta, Metadate CD, Metadate ER, Methylin, Methylin ER, ✤ PMS-Methylphenidate, ✤ Riphenidate, Ritalin, Ritalin LA, Ritalin-SR

Classification
Therapeutic: central nervous system stimulants

Schedule II

Pregnancy Category C

Indications

Treatment of ADHD (adjunct). Symptomatic treatment of narcolepsy. **Unlabeled uses:** Management of some forms of refractory depression.

Action

Produces CNS and respiratory stimulation with weak sympathomimetic activity. **Therapeutic Effects:** Increased attention span in ADHD. Increased motor activity, mental alertness, and diminished fatigue in narcoleptic patients.

Pharmacokinetics

Absorption: Slow and incomplete after oral administration; absorption of sustained or extended-release tablet (SR) is delayed and provides continuous release. *Metadate CD, Concerta, Ritalin LA*—provides initial rapid release followed by a second continuous release (biphasic release).
Distribution: Unknown.
Metabolism and Excretion: Mostly metabolized (80%) by the liver.
Half-life: 2–4 hr.

TIME/ACTION PROFILE (CNS stimulation)

ROUTE	ONSET	PEAK	DURATION
PO	unknown	1–3 hr	4–6 hr
PO-ER	unknown	4–7 hr	3–12 hr†

†depends on formulation

Contraindications/Precautions

Contraindicated in: Hypersensitivity; Hyperexcitable states; Hyperthyroidism; Patients with psychotic personalities or suicidal or homicidal tendencies; Tourette's syndrome; Glaucoma; Motor tics; Concurrent use or use within 14 days of MAO inhibitors.

Use Cautiously in: History of cardiovascular disease; Hypertension; Diabetes mellitus; Geriatric or debilitated patients; Continual use (may result in psychological or physical dependence); Pedi: Growth suppression may occur in children with long term use; Seizure disorders (may lower seizure threshold); Concerta product should be used cautiously in patients with esophageal motility disorders or severe GI narrowing (may increase the risk of obstruction); Pregnancy or lactation (safety not established).

Adverse Reactions/Side Effects

CNS: hyperactivity, insomnia, restlessness, tremor, dizziness, headache, irritability. **EENT:** blurred vision. **CV:** hypertension, palpitations, tachycardia, hypotension. **GI:** anorexia, constipation, cramps, diarrhea, dry mouth, metallic taste, nausea, vomiting. **Derm:** rashes. **Neuro:** akathisia, dyskinesia. **Misc:** fever, hypersensitivity reactions, physical dependence, psychological dependence, suppression of weight gain (children), tolerance.

Interactions

Drug-Drug: ↑ sympathomimetic effects with other **adrenergics**, including **vasoconstrictors**, and **decongestants**. Use with **MAO inhibitors** or **vasopressors** may result in hypertensive crisis (concurrent use or use within 14 days of MAO inhibitors is contraindicated). Metabolism of **warfarin**, **phenytoin**, **phenobarbital, primidone, selective serotonin reuptake inhibitors,** and **tricyclic antidepressants** may be ↓ and effects ↑. Avoid concurrent use with **pimozide** (may mask cause of tics). Concurrent use with **clonidine** may result in serious EKG abnormalities (a 40% dose reduction of methylphenidate is necessary).
Drug-Natural Products: Use with **caffeine-containing** herbs (**guarana, tea, coffee**) ↑ stimulant effect. **St. John's Wort** may ↑ serious side effects (concurrent use is NOT recommended).
Drug-Food: Excessive use of **caffeine-containing** foods or beverages (**coffee**, **cola, tea**) may cause ↑ CNS stimulation.

Route/Dosage

PO (Adults): *ADHD*—5–20 mg 2–3 times daily as prompt-release tablets. When maintenance dose is determined, may change to extended-release formulation. *Narcolepsy*—10 mg 2–3 times/day; maximum dose 60 mg/day.
PO (Children >6 yr): *Prompt-release tablets*—0.3 mg/kg/dose or 2.5–5 mg before

breakfast and lunch; increase by 0.1 mg/kg/dose or by 5–10 mg/day at weekly intervals (not to exceed 60 mg/day or 2 mg/kg/day). When maintenance dose is determined, may change to extended-release formulation. *Ritalin SR, Metadate ER*—may be used in place of the Prompt-release tablets when the 8-hour dosage corresponds to the titrated 8-hour dosage of the Prompt-release tablets; *Ritalin LA*—can be used in place of twice daily regimen given once daily at same total dose, or in place of SR product at same dose; *Concerta (patients who have not taken methylphenidate previously)*—18 mg once daily in the morning initially, may be titrated as needed up to 54 mg/day. *Concerta (patients are currently taking other forms of methylphenidate)*—18 mg once daily in the morning if previous dose was 5 mg 2–3 times daily or 20 mg daily as SR product, 36 mg once daily in the morning if previous dose was 10 mg 2–3 times daily or 40 mg daily as SR product, 54 mg once daily in the morning if previous dose was 15 mg 2–3 times daily or 60 mg once daily as SR product. *Metadate CD*—20 mg once daily. Dosage may be adjusted in weekly 20-mg increments to a maximum of 60 mg/day taken once daily in the morning.

Availability (generic available)

Immediate-release tablets: 5 mg, 10 mg, 20 mg. **Cost:** *Generic*—5 mg $37.90/100, 10 mg $52.90/100, 20 mg $74.90/100. **Extended-release tablets (Metadate ER, Methylin ER):** 10 mg, 20 mg. **Extended-release tablets (Concerta):** 18 mg, 27 mg, 36 mg, 54 mg. **Cost:** 18 mg $359.96/90, 27 mg $359.98/90, 36 mg $374.96/90, 54 mg $404.96/90. **Sustained-release tablets (Ritalin SR):** 20 mg. **Cost:** $173.96/90. **Extended-release capsules (Metadate CD):** 10 mg, 20 mg, 30 mg. **Cost:** 10 mg $236.97/90, 20 mg $299.99/90, 30 mg $299.95/90$34.68/30. **Extended-release capsules (Ritalin LA):** 10 mg, 20 mg, 30 mg, 40 mg. **Cost:** 10 mg $299.97/90, 20 mg $299.97/90, 30 mg $299.95/90, 40 mg $299.95/90. **Chewable tablets (Methylin) (grape flavor):** 2.5 mg, 5 mg, 10 mg. **Oral solution (Methylin) (grape flavor):** 5 mg/5 ml, 10 mg/5 ml.

NURSING IMPLICATIONS

Assessment

- Monitor blood pressure, pulse, and respiration before administering and periodically during therapy.
- Pedi: Monitor growth, both height and weight, in children on long-term therapy
- May produce a false sense of euphoria and well-being. Provide frequent rest periods and observe patient for rebound depression after the effects of the medication have worn off.
- Methylphenidate has high dependence and abuse potential. Tolerance to abuse of medication occurs rapidly; do not increase dose.
- **ADHD:** Pedi: Assess children for attention span, impulse control, and interactions with others. Therapy may be interrupted at intervals to determine whether symptoms are sufficient to continue therapy.
- **Narcolepsy:** Observe and document frequency of episodes.
- ***Lab Test Considerations:*** Monitor CBC, differential, and platelet count periodically in patients receiving prolonged therapy.

Potential Nursing Diagnoses

Disturbed thought process (Side Effects)

Implementation

- **PO:** Immediate and sustained-release tablets should be administered on an empty stomach (30–45 min before a meal). Sustained-release tablets should be swallowed whole; do not crush, break, or chew. Metadate CD and Ritalin LA capsules may be opened and sprinkled on cool applesauce; entire mixture should be ingested immediately and followed by a drink of water. Do not store for future use. Concerta may be administered without regard to food, but must be taken with water, milk, or juice.

Patient/Family Teaching

- Instruct patient to take medication as directed. If a dose is missed, take the remaining doses for that day at regularly spaced intervals; do not double doses. Take the last dose before 6 PM to minimize the risk of insomnia. Instruct patient not to alter dose without consulting health care professional. Abrupt cessation of high doses may cause extreme fatigue and mental depression.
- Advise patient to check weight 2–3 times weekly and report weight loss to health care professional.
- May cause dizziness or blurred vision. Caution patient to avoid driving or activities requiring alertness until response to medication is known.

M

- Inform patient and/or parents that shell of Concerta tablet may appear in the stool. This is no cause for concern.
- Advise patient to avoid using caffeine-containing beverages concurrently with this therapy.
- Advise patient to notify health care professional if nervousness, insomnia, palpitations, vomiting, skin rash, or fever occurs.
- Inform patient that health care professional may order periodic holidays from the drug to assess progress and to decrease dependence.
- Emphasize the importance of routine follow-up exams to monitor progress.
- **ADHD:** Pedi: Advise parents to notify school nurse of medication regimen.

Evaluation/Desired Outcomes

- Decreased frequency of narcoleptic symptoms.
- Improved attention span and social interactions in ADHD.

methylPREDNISolone, See CORTICOSTEROIDS (SYSTEMIC).

metoclopramide

(met-oh-**kloe**-pra-mide)

✣ Apo-Metoclop, Clopra, ✣ Emex, ✣ Maxeran, Octamide, Octamide-PFS, Reclomide, Reglan

Classification
Therapeutic: antiemetics

Pregnancy Category B

Indications

Prevention of chemotherapy-induced emesis. Treatment of postsurgical and diabetic gastric stasis. Facilitation of small bowel intubation in radiographic procedures. Management of esophageal reflux. Treatment and prevention of postoperative nausea and vomiting when nasogastric suctioning is undesirable. **Unlabeled uses:** Treatment of hiccups. Adjunct management of migraine headaches.

Action

Blocks dopamine receptors in chemoreceptor trigger zone of the CNS. Stimulates motility of the upper GI tract and accelerates gastric emptying. **Therapeutic Effects:** Decreased nausea and vomiting. Decreased symptoms of gastric stasis. Easier passage of nasogastric tube into small bowel.

Pharmacokinetics

Absorption: Well absorbed from the GI tract, from rectal mucosa, and from IM sites.
Distribution: Widely distributed into body tissues and fluids. Crosses blood-brain barrier and placenta. Enters breast milk in concentrations greater than plasma.
Metabolism and Excretion: Partially metabolized by the liver; 25% eliminated unchanged in the urine.
Half-life: 2.5–6 hr.

TIME/ACTION PROFILE (effects on peristalsis)

ROUTE	ONSET	PEAK	DURATION
PO	30–60 min	unknown	1–2 hr
IM	10–15 min	unknown	1–2 hr
IV	1–3 min	immediate	1–2 hr

Contraindications/Precautions

Contraindicated in: Hypersensitivity; Possible GI obstruction or hemorrhage; History of seizure disorders; Pheochromocytoma; Parkinson's disease.
Use Cautiously in: History of depression; Diabetes (may alter response to insulin); Renal impairment (reduce dose in CCr <50 ml/min); OB, Lactation: Safety not established; Pedi: some syrup products contain benzoate, a metabolite of benzyl alcohol which can cause potentially fatal gasping syndrome in neonates. Prolonged clearance in neonates can result in high serum concentrations and increase the risk for methemoglobinemia. Side effects are more common in children especially extrapyramidal reactions; Geri: More susceptible to oversedation and extrapyramidal reactions.

Adverse Reactions/Side Effects

CNS: <u>drowsiness</u>, <u>extrapyramidal reactions</u>, <u>restlessness</u>, NEUROLEPTIC MALIGNANT SYNDROME, anxiety, depression, irritability, tardive dyskinesia. **CV:** arrhythmias (supraventricular tachycardia, bradycardia), hypertension, hypotension. **GI:** constipation, diarrhea, dry mouth, nausea. **Endo:** gynecomastia. **Hemat:** methemoglobinemia, neutropenia, leukopenia, agranulocytosis.

Interactions

Drug-Drug: Additive CNS depression with other **CNS depressants**, including **alcohol**, **antidepressants**, **antihistamines**, **opioid anal-**

gesics, and **sedative/hypnotics**. May ↑ absorption and risk of toxicity from **cyclosporine**. May affect the GI absorption of other **orally administered drugs** as a result of effect on GI motility. May exaggerate hypotension during **general anesthesia**. ↑ risk of extrapyramidal reactions with agents such as **haloperidol** or **phenothiazines**. **Opioids** and **anticholinergics** may antagonize the GI effects of metoclopramide. Use cautiously with **MAO inhibitors** (causes release of catecholamines). May ↑ neuromuscular blockade from **succinylcholine**. May ↓ effectiveness of **levodopa**. May ↑ **tacrolimus** serum levels.

Route/Dosage

Prevention of Chemotherapy-Induced Vomiting

PO, IV (Adults and Children): 1–2 mg/kg 30 min before chemotherapy. Additional doses of 1–2 mg/kg may be given q 2–4 hr, pretreatment with diphenhydramine will decrease the risk of extrapyramidal reactions to this dosage.

Facilitation of Small Bowel Intubation

IV (Adults and Children >14 yr): 10 mg over 1–2 min.
IV (Children 6–14 yr): 2.5–5 mg (dose should not exceed 0.5 mg/kg) over 1–2 min.
IV (Children <6 yr): 0.1 mg/kg over 1–2 min.

Diabetic Gastroparesis

PO, IV (Adults): 10 mg 30 min before meals and at bedtime for 2–8 weeks.

Gastroesophageal Reflux

PO, IM, IV (Adults): 10–15 mg 30 min before meals and at bedtime (not to exceed 0.5 mg/kg/day). A single dose of 20 mg may be given preventively. Some patients may respond to doses as small as 5 mg.
PO, IM, IV (Neonates, Infants, and Children): 0.4–0.8 mg/kg/day in 4 divided doses.

Postoperative Nausea/Vomiting

IM, IV (Adults and Children >14 yr): 10 mg at the end of surgical procedure, repeat in 6–8 hr if needed.
IM, IV (Children <14 yr): 0.1–0.2 mg/kg/dose, repeat in 6–8 hr if needed.

Treatment of Hiccups

PO, IM (Adults): 10–20 mg 4 times daily PO; may be preceded by a single 10-mg dose IM (unlabeled).

Availability (generic available)

Tablets: 5 mg, 10 mg. **Cost:** *Reglan*—5 mg $50.91/100, 10 mg $80.26/100; *generic*—5 mg $29.77/100, 10 mg $21.12/100. **Concentrated solution:** 10 mg/ml. **Syrup (apricot-peach flavor):** 5 mg/5 ml. **Injection:** 5 mg/ml.

NURSING IMPLICATIONS

Assessment

- Assess patient for nausea, vomiting, abdominal distention, and bowel sounds before and after administration.
- Assess patient for extrapyramidal side effects (*parkinsonian*—difficulty speaking or swallowing, loss of balance control, pill rolling, mask-like face, shuffling gait, rigidity, tremors; and *dystonic*—muscle spasms, twisting motions, twitching, inability to move eyes, weakness of arms or legs) periodically throughout course of therapy. May occur weeks to months after initiation of therapy and are reversible on discontinuation. Dystonic reactions may occur within minutes of IV infusion and stop within 24 hr of discontinuation of metoclopramide. May be treated with 50 mg of IM diphenhydramine or diphenhydramine 1 mg/kg IV may be administered prophylactically 15 min before metoclopramide IV infusion.
- Monitor for tardive dyskinesia (uncontrolled rhythmic movement of mouth, face, and extremities; lip smacking or puckering; puffing of cheeks; uncontrolled chewing; rapid or worm-like movements of tongue). Usually occurs after a year or more of continued therapy. Report immediately; may be irreversible.
- Monitor for neuroleptic malignant syndrome (hyperthermia, muscle rigidity, altered consciousness, irregular pulse or blood pressure, tachycardia, and diaphoresis).
- Assess patient for signs of depression periodically throughout therapy.
- ***Lab Test Considerations:*** May alter hepatic function test results.
- May cause ↑ serum prolactin and aldosterone concentrations.

Potential Nursing Diagnoses

Imbalanced nutrition: less than body requirements (Indications)
Risk for injury (Side Effects)

M

Implementation

- **PO:** Administer doses 30 min before meals and at bedtime.
- **IM:** For prevention of postoperative nausea and vomiting, inject IM near the end of surgery.
- **Rect:** Suppositories may be made by pharmacist. Administer 1 suppository 30–60 min before each meal and at bedtime.

IV Administration

- **Direct IV:** Administer IV dose 30 min before administration of chemotherapeutic agent. ***Rate:*** Doses may be given slowly over 1–2 min. Rapid administration causes a transient but intense feeling of anxiety and restlessness followed by drowsiness.
- **Intermittent Infusion:*****Diluent:*** May be diluted for IV infusion in 50 ml of D5W, 0.9% NaCl, D5/0.45% NaCl, Ringer's solution, or LR. Diluted solution is stable for 48 hr if protected from light or 24 hr under normal light. ***Concentration:*** May dilute to 0.2 mg/ml or give undiluted at 5 mg/ml.***Rate:*** Infuse slowly (maximum rate 5 mg/min) over at least 15–30 min.
- **Syringe Compatibility:** atropine, benztropine, bleomycin, butorphanol, chlorpromazine, cisplatin, cyclophosphamide, cytarabine, dexamethasone, diphenhydramine, doxorubicin, droperidol, fentanyl, fluorouracil, heparin, hydrocortisone, hydromorphone, hydroxyzine, leucovorin, lidocaine, magnesium sulfate, meperidine, methylprednisolone sodium succinate, midazolam, mitomycin, morphine, ondansetron, pentazocine, perphenazine, prochlorperazine, promazine, promethazine, ranitidine, scopolamine, vinblastine, vincristine.
- **Syringe Incompatibility:** furosemide, pantoprazpole.
- **Y-Site Compatibility:** acyclovir, aldesleukin, amifostine, aztreonam, bivalirudin, bleomycin, ciprofloxacin, cisatracurium, cisplatin, cladribine, cyclophosphamide, cytarabine, dexmedetomidine, diltiazem, docetaxel, doxapram, doxorubicin, droperidol, etoposide phosphate, famotidine, fenoldopam, fentanyl, filgrastim, fluconazole, fludarabine, fluorouracil, foscarnet, gemcitabine, granisetron, heparin, hydromorphone, idarubicin, leucovorin, levofloxacin, linezolid, melphalan, meperidine, meropenem, methadone, methotrexate, mitomycin, morphine, ondansetron, oxaliplatin, paclitaxel, pemetrexed, piperacillin/tazobactam, quinupristin/dalfopristin, remifentanil, sargramostim, sufentanil, tacrolimus, teniposide, thiotepa, topotecan, vinblastine, vincristine, vinorelbine, zidovudine.
- **Y-Site Incompatibility:** allopurinol, amphotericin B cholesteryl sulfate complex, amsacrine, cefepime, doxorubicin liposome, furosemide, lansoprazole, propofol.

Patient/Family Teaching

- Instruct patient to take metoclopramide as directed. Take missed doses as soon as remembered if not almost time for next dose.
- Pedi: Unintentional overdose has been reported in infants and children with the use of metoclopramide oral solution. Teach parents how to accurately read labels and administer medication.
- May cause drowsiness. Caution patient to avoid driving or other activities requiring alertness until response to medication is known.
- Advise patient to avoid concurrent use of alcohol and other CNS depressants while taking this medication.
- Advise patient to notify health care professional immediately if involuntary movement of eyes, face, or limbs occurs.

Evaluation/Desired Outcomes

- Prevention or relief of nausea and vomiting.
- Decreased symptoms of gastric stasis.
- Facilitation of small bowel intubation.
- Decreased symptoms of esophageal reflux.

metolazone (me-**tole**-a-zone)

Zaroxolyn

Classification

Therapeutic: antihypertensives, diuretics

Pharmacologic: thiazide-like diuretics

Pregnancy Category B

Indications

Mild to moderate hypertension. Edema associated with CHF or the nephrotic syndrome.

Action

Increases excretion of sodium and water by inhibiting sodium reabsorption in the distal tubule. Promotes excretion of chloride, potassium, magnesium, and bicarbonate. May produce arteriolar dilation. **Therapeutic Effects:** Lowering of blood pressure in hypertensive patients.

Diuresis with subsequent mobilization of edema. Effect may continue in renal impairment.

Pharmacokinetics

Absorption: Absorption is variable.
Distribution: Unknown.
Metabolism and Excretion: Excreted mainly unchanged by the kidneys.
Half-life: 8 hr.

TIME/ACTION PROFILE (diuretic effect†)

ROUTE	ONSET	PEAK	DURATION
PO	1 hr	2 hr	12–24 hr

†Full antihypertensive effect may take days–weeks

Contraindications/Precautions

Contraindicated in: Hypersensitivity; Cross-sensitivity with other sulfonamides may exist; Anuria; OB: Lactation.
Use Cautiously in: Severe hepatic impairment; Geri: Increased sensitivity; OB, Pedi: Pregnancy or children (safety not established; children may be more susceptible to diuretic and hypokalemic effects).

Adverse Reactions/Side Effects

CNS: drowsiness, lethargy. **CV:** chest pain, hypotension, palpitations. **GI:** anorexia, bloating, cramping, drug-induced hepatitis, nausea, vomiting. **Derm:** photosensitivity, rashes. **Endo:** hyperglycemia. **F and E:** hypokalemia, dehydration, hypercalcemia, hypochloremic alkalosis, hypomagnesemia, hyponatremia, hypophosphatemia, hypovolemia. **Hemat:** blood dyscrasias. **Metab:** hyperuricemia. **MS:** muscle cramps. **Misc:** chills, pancreatitis.

Interactions

Drug-Drug: ↑ risk of hypotension with **nitrates**, acute ingestion of **alcohol**, or other **antihypertensives**. ↑ risk of hypokalemia with **corticosteroids**, **amphotericin B**, **piperacillin**, or **ticarcillin**. May ↑ the risk of **digoxin** toxicity. ↓ the excretion of **lithium**; may cause toxicity. May ↓ the effectiveness of **methenamine**. **Stimulant laxatives** (including **aloe, senna)** may ↑ risk of potassium depletion.
Drug-Food: Food may ↑ extent of absorption.

Route/Dosage

PO (Adults): *Hypertension*—2.5–5 mg/day; *edema*—5–20 mg/day.

Availability (generic available)

Tablets: 2.5 mg, 5 mg, 10 mg. **Cost:** *Generic*—2.5 mg $99.99/90, 5 mg $110.09/90, 10 mg $121.97/90.

NURSING IMPLICATIONS

Assessment

- Monitor blood pressure, intake and output, and daily weight, and assess feet, legs, and sacral area for edema daily.
- Assess patient, especially if taking digoxin, for anorexia, nausea, vomiting, muscle cramps, paresthesia, and confusion. Notify physician or other health care professional if these signs of electrolyte imbalance occur. Patients taking digoxin are at risk of digoxin toxicity because of the potassium-depleting effect of the diuretic.
- Assess patient for allergy to sulfonamides.
- **Hypertension:** Monitor blood pressure before and periodically during therapy.
- Monitor frequency of prescription refills to determine compliance.
- ***Lab Test Considerations:*** Monitor electrolytes (especially potassium), blood glucose, BUN, and serum creatinine and uric acid levels before and periodically during therapy.
- May cause ↑ in serum and urine glucose in diabetic patients.
- May cause an ↑ in serum bilirubin, calcium, creatinine, and uric acid, and a ↓ in serum magnesium, potassium, and sodium and urinary calcium concentrations.
- May cause ↓ serum protein-bound iodine (PBI) concentrations.
- May cause ↑ serum cholesterol, low-density lipoprotein, and triglyceride concentrations.

Potential Nursing Diagnoses

Excess fluid volume (Indications)
Risk for deficient fluid volume (Side Effects)

Implementation

- Administer in the morning to prevent disruption of sleep cycle.
- Intermittent dose schedule may be used for continued control of edema.
- **PO:** May give with food or milk to minimize GI irritation.

Patient/Family Teaching

- Instruct patient to take metolazone at the same time each day. Take missed doses as

M

soon as remembered but not just before next dose is due. Do not double doses.

- Instruct patient to monitor weight biweekly and notify health care professional of significant changes.
- Caution patient to change positions slowly to minimize orthostatic hypotension; may be potentiated by alcohol.
- Advise patient to use sunscreen and protective clothing in the sun to prevent photosensitivity reactions.
- Instruct patient to discuss dietary potassium requirements with health care professional (see Appendix L).
- Instruct patient to notify health care professional of medication regimen before treatment or surgery.
- Advise patient to report muscle weakness, cramps, nausea, vomiting, diarrhea, or dizziness to health care professional.
- Emphasize the importance of routine follow-up exams.
- **Hypertension:** Advise patient to continue taking the medication even if feeling better. Medication controls but does not cure hypertension.
- Encourage patient to comply with additional interventions for hypertension (weight reduction, low-sodium diet, regular exercise, smoking cessation, moderation of alcohol consumption, and stress management).
- Instruct patient and family in correct technique for monitoring weekly blood pressure.
- Advise patient to consult health care professional before taking OTC medication, especially cough or cold preparations, concurrently with this therapy.

Evaluation/Desired Outcomes

- Decrease in blood pressure.
- Increase in urine output.
- Decrease in edema.

HIGH ALERT

metoprolol (me-**toe**-proe-lole)

✤Beloc, ✤Beloc-ZOK, ✤Betaloc Durules, ✤Betaloc-ZOK, ✤Lopresor, ✤Lopresor SR, Lopressor, ✤Metoprol, ✤Novo-metoprol, ✤Seloken-ZOK, Toprol-XL

Classification
Therapeutic: antianginals, antihypertensives
Pharmacologic: beta blockers

Pregnancy Category C

Indications

Hypertension. Angina pectoris. Prevention of MI and decreased mortality in patients with recent MI. Management of stable, symptomatic (class II or III) heart failure due to ischemic, hypertensive or cardiomyopathc origin (may be used with ACE inhibitors, diuretics and/or digoxin; Toprol XL 25 mg only). **Unlabeled uses:** Ventricular arrhythmias/tachycardia. Migraine prophylaxis. Tremors. Aggressive behavior. Drug-induced akathisia. Anxiety.

Action

Blocks stimulation of $beta_1$ (myocardial)-adrenergic receptors. Does not usually affect $beta_2$ (pulmonary, vascular, uterine)-adrenergic receptor sites. **Therapeutic Effects:** Decreased blood pressure and heart rate. Decreased frequency of attacks of angina pectoris. Decreased rate of cardiovascular mortality and hospitalization in patients with heart failure.

Pharmacokinetics

Absorption: Well absorbed after oral administration.
Distribution: Crosses the blood-brain barrier, crosses the placenta; small amounts enter breast milk.
Metabolism and Excretion: Mostly metabolized by the liver.
Half-life: 3–7 hr.

TIME/ACTION PROFILE (cardiovascular effects)

ROUTE	ONSET	PEAK	DURATION
PO†	15 min	unknown	6–12 hr
PO–ER	unknown	6–12 hr	24 hr
IV	immediate	20 min	5–8 hr

†Maximal effects on BP (chronic therapy) may not occur for 1 wk. Hypotensive effects may persist for up to 4 wk after discontinuation

Contraindications/Precautions

Contraindicated in: Uncompensated CHF; Pulmonary edema; Cardiogenic shock; Bradycardia or heart block.
Use Cautiously in: Renal impairment; Hepatic impairment; Geri: Geriatric patients (↑ sensitivity to beta blockers; initial dose reduction rec-

ommended); Pulmonary disease (including asthma; $beta_1$ selectivity may be lost at higher doses); Diabetes mellitus (may mask signs of hypoglycemia); Thyrotoxicosis (may mask symptoms); Patients with a history of severe allergic reactions (intensity of reactions may be increased); OB: Pregnancy, lactation, or children (safety not established; all agents cross the placenta and may cause fetal/neonatal bradycardia, hypotension, hypoglycemia, or respiratory depression).

Adverse Reactions/Side Effects

CNS: fatigue, weakness, anxiety, depression, dizziness, drowsiness, insomnia, memory loss, mental status changes, nervousness, nightmares. **EENT:** blurred vision, stuffy nose. **Resp:** bronchospasm, wheezing. **CV:** BRADYCARDIA, CHF, PULMONARY EDEMA, hypotension, peripheral vasoconstriction. **GI:** constipation, diarrhea, drug-induced hepatitis, dry mouth, flatulence, gastric pain, heartburn, increased liver function studies, nausea, vomiting. **GU:** erectile dysfunction, decreased libido, urinary frequency. **Derm:** rashes. **Endo:** hyperglycemia, hypoglycemia. **MS:** arthralgia, back pain, joint pain. **Misc:** drug-induced lupus syndrome.

Interactions

Drug-Drug: General anesthesia, **IV phenytoin**, and **verapamil** may cause ↑ myocardial depression. ↑ bradycardia may occur with **digoxin**. ↑ hypotension may occur with other **antihypertensives**, acute ingestion of **alcohol**, or **nitrates**. Concurrent use with **amphetamines**, **cocaine**, **ephedrine**, **epinephrine**, **norepinephrine**, **phenylephrine**, or **pseudoephedrine** may result in unopposed alpha-adrenergic stimulation (excessive hypertension, bradycardia). Concurrent administration of **thyroid** administration may ↓ effectiveness. May alter the effectiveness of **insulins** or **oral hypoglycemic agents** (dosage adjustments may be necessary). May ↓ the effectiveness of **theophylline**. May ↓ the beneficial $beta_1$-cardiovascular effects of **dopamine** or **dobutamine**. Use cautiously within 14 days of **MAO inhibitor** therapy (may result in hypertension).

Route/Dosage

PO (Adults): *Antihypertensive/antianginal*—25–100 mg/day as a single dose initially or 2 divided doses; may be increased q 7 days as needed up to 450 mg/day (for angina, give in divided doses). Extended-release products are given once daily. *MI*—25–50 mg (starting 15 min after last IV dose) q 6 hr for 48 hr, then 100 mg twice daily for a minimum of 3 mo. *Heart failure*—12.5–25 mg once daily, can be doubled every 2 wk up to 200 mg/day. *Migraine prevention*—50–100 mg 2–4 times daily (unlabeled).

IV (Adults): *MI*—5 mg q 2 min for 3 doses, followed by oral dosing.

Availability (generic available)

Tablets (tartrate): 25 mg, 50 mg, 100 mg. **Cost:** *Generic*—25 mg $28.37/180, 50 mg $27.00/180, 100 mg $22.99/180. **Extended-release tablets (succinate; Toprol XL):** 25 mg, 50 mg, 100 mg, 200 mg. **Cost:** *Generic*—25 mg $66.97/90, 50 mg $73.97/90, 100 mg $99.92/90, 200 mg $176.98/90. **Injection:** 1 mg/ml. ***In combination with:*** hydrochlorothiazide (Lopressor HCT). See Appendix B.

M

NURSING IMPLICATIONS

Assessment

- Monitor blood pressure, ECG, and pulse frequently during dose adjustment and periodically during therapy.
- Monitor frequency of prescription refills to determine compliance.
- Monitor vital signs and ECG every 5–15 min during and for several hours after parenteral administration. If heart rate <40 bpm, especially if cardiac output is also decreased, administer atropine 0.25–0.5 mg IV.
- Monitor intake and output ratios and daily weights. Assess routinely for signs and symptoms of CHF (dyspnea, rales/crackles, weight gain, peripheral edema, jugular venous distention).
- **Angina:** Assess frequency and characteristics of anginal attacks periodically during therapy.
- ***Lab Test Considerations:*** May cause ↑ BUN, serum lipoprotein, potassium, triglyceride, and uric acid levels.
- May cause ↑ ANA titers.
- May cause ↑ in blood glucose levels.
- May cause ↑ serum alkaline phosphatase, LDH, AST, and ALT levels.

Potential Nursing Diagnoses

Decreased cardiac output (Side Effects)

Noncompliance (Patient/Family Teaching)

Implementation

- ***High Alert:*** IV vasoactive medications are inherently dangerous. Before administering intravenously, have second practitioner independently check original order and dose calculations.
- ***High Alert:*** Do not confuse metoprolol with misoprostol. Do not confuse Toprol-XL (metoprolol) with Topomax (topiramate) or Tegretol (carbamazepine).
- **PO:** Take apical pulse before administering. If <50 bpm or if arrhythmia occurs, withhold medication and notify health care professional.
- Administer metoprolol with meals or directly after eating.
- Extended-release tablets should be swallowed whole; do not crush, break, or chew.

IV Administration

- **Direct IV:** ***Diluent:*** Administer undiluted. ***Concentration:*** 1 mg/ml. ***Rate:*** Administer over 1 min.
- **Y-Site Compatibility:** abciximab, acyclovir, alteplase, amikacin, aminophylline, argatroban, atropine, aztreonam, bivalirudin, bumetanide, calcium chloride, calcium gluconate, caspofungin, cefazolin, cefotaxime, cefoxitin, ceftazidime, ceftizoxime, ceftriaxone, cefuroxime, chloramphenicol, cimetidine, clindamycin, cyclosporine, daptomycin, dexamethasone sodium phosphate, digoxin, diltiazem, diphenhydramine, dobutamine, dopamine, doxycycline, enalaprilat, epinephrine, eptifibatide, esmolol, famotidine, fenoldopam, fentanyl, fluconazole, furosemide, ganciclovir, gentamicin, granisetron, heparin, hydrocortisone sodium succinate, hydromorphone, hydroxyzine, imipenem/cilastatin, insulin, isoproterenol, ketorolac, labetalol, lidocaine, linezolid, lorazepam, magnesium sulfate, meperidine, methylprednisolone sodium succinate, metoclopramide, metronidazole, midazolam, morphine, nafcillin, nesiritide, nitroglycerin, nitroprusside, norepinephrine, ondansetron, palonosetron, penicillin G potassium, phenylephrine, phytonadione, piperacillin/tazobactam, potassium chloride, procainamide, prochlorperazine, promethazine, propranolol, protamine, quinupristin/dalfopristin, ranitidine, sodium bicarbonate, tacrolimus, ticarcillin/clavulanate, tirofiban, tobramycin, vancomycin, vasopressin, verapamil, voriconazole.
- **Y-Site Incompatibility:** amphotericin B cholesteryl sulfate complex, diazepam, pantoprazole, phenytoin, trimethoprim/sulfamethoxazole.

Patient/Family Teaching

- Instruct patient to take medication as directed, at the same time each day, even if feeling well; do not skip or double up on missed doses. Take missed doses as soon as possible up to 8 hr before next dose. Abrupt withdrawal may precipitate life-threatening arrhythmias, hypertension, or myocardial ischemia.
- Teach patient and family how to check pulse daily and blood pressure biweekly and to report significant changes to health care professional.
- May cause drowsiness. Caution patient to avoid driving or other activities that require alertness until response to the drug is known.
- Advise patient to change positions slowly to minimize orthostatic hypotension.
- Caution patient that this medication may increase sensitivity to cold.
- Instruct patient to consult health care professional before taking any OTC medications or herbal products, especially cold preparations, concurrently with this medication. Patients on antihypertensive therapy should also avoid excessive amounts of caffeinated coffee, tea, and cola.
- Diabetics should closely monitor blood glucose, especially if weakness, malaise, irritability, or fatigue occurs. Medication does not block sweating as a sign of hypoglycemia.
- Advise patient to notify health care professional if slow pulse, difficulty breathing, wheezing, cold hands and feet, dizziness, light-headedness, confusion, depression, rash, fever, sore throat, unusual bleeding, or bruising occurs.
- Instruct patient to inform health care professional of medication regimen before treatment or surgery.
- Advise patient to carry identification describing disease process and medication regimen at all times.
- **Hypertension:** Reinforce the need to continue additional therapies for hypertension (weight loss, sodium restriction, stress reduction, regular exercise, moderation of alcohol consumption, and smoking cessation). Medication controls but does not cure hypertension.

Evaluation/Desired Outcomes
- Decrease in blood pressure.
- Reduction in frequency of anginal attacks.
- Increase in activity tolerance.
- Prevention of MI.

metronidazole
(me-troe-**ni**-da-zole)
♣Apo-Metronidazole, Flagyl, Flagyl ER, Metric 21, MetroCream, MetroGel, MetroGel-Vaginal, MetroLotion, Metro IV, Metryl, ♣Nidagel, Noritate, ♣Novonidazol, Protostat, ♣Trikacide

Classification
Therapeutic: anti-infectives, antiprotozoals, antiulcer agents

Pregnancy Category B

Indications
PO, IV: Treatment of the following anaerobic infections: Intra-abdominal infections (may be used with a cephalosporin), Gynecologic infections, Skin and skin structure infections, Lower respiratory tract infections, Bone and joint infections, CNS infections, Septicemia, Endocarditis. **IV:** Perioperative prophylactic agent in colorectal surgery. **PO:** Amebicide in the management of amebic dysentery, amebic liver abscess, and trichomoniasis. Treatment of peptic ulcer disease caused by *Helicobacter pylori*. **Topical:** Treatment of acne rosacea. **Vag:** Management of bacterial vaginosis. **Unlabeled uses:** Treatment of giardiasis. Treatment of anti-infective associated pseudomembranous colitis.

Action
Disrupts DNA and protein synthesis in susceptible organisms. **Therapeutic Effects:** Bactericidal, trichomonacidal, or amebicidal action. **Spectrum:** Most notable for activity against anaerobic bacteria, including: *Bacteroides*, *Clostridium*. In addition, is active against: *Trichomonas vaginalis*, *Entamoeba histolytica*, *Giardia lamblia*, *H. pylori*, *Clostridium difficile*.

Pharmacokinetics
Absorption: 80% absorbed after oral administration. Minimal absorption after topical or vaginal application.
Distribution: Widely distributed into most tissues and fluids, including CSF. Crosses the placenta and enters fetal circulation rapidly; enters breast milk in concentrations equal to plasma levels.
Metabolism and Excretion: Partially metabolized by the liver (30–60%), partially excreted unchanged in the urine, 6–15% eliminated in the feces.
Half-life: Neonates: 25–75 hr; Children and adults: 6–12 hr.

TIME/ACTION PROFILE (PO, IV = blood levels; topical = improvement in rosacea)

ROUTE	ONSET	PEAK	DURATION
PO	rapid	1–3 hr	8 hr
PO-ER	rapid	unknown	up to 24 hr
IV	rapid	end of infusion	6–8 hr
Topical	3 wk	9 wk	12 hr
Vaginal	unknown	6–12 hr	12 hr

Contraindications/Precautions
Contraindicated in: Hypersensitivity; Hypersensitivity to parabens (topical only); First trimester of pregnancy.
Use Cautiously in: History of blood dyscrasias; History of seizures or neurologic problems; Severe hepatic impairment (dose reduction suggested); Pregnancy (although safety not established, has been used to treat trichomoniasis in 2nd- and 3rd-trimester pregnancy—but not as single-dose regimen); Lactation (if needed, use single dose and interrupt nursing for 24 hr thereafter); Patients receiving corticosteroids or predisposed to edema (injection contains 28 mEq sodium/g metronidazole).

Adverse Reactions/Side Effects
CNS: SEIZURES, dizziness, headache. **EENT:** tearing (topical only). **GI:** abdominal pain, anorexia, nausea, diarrhea, dry mouth, furry tongue, glossitis, unpleasant taste, vomiting. **Derm:** rashes, urticaria; *topical only*— burning, mild dryness, skin irritation, transient redness. **Hemat:** leukopenia. **Local:** phlebitis at IV site. **Neuro:** peripheral neuropathy. **Misc:** superinfection, disulfiram-type reaction with alcohol.

Interactions
Drug-Drug: Cimetidine may ↓ the metabolism of metronidazole. **Phenobarbital** and **rifampin** ↑ metabolism and may ↓ effectiveness. Metronidazole ↑ the effects of

♣ = Canadian drug name.
* CAPITALS indicates life-threatening; underlines indicate most frequent.

phenytoin, lithium, and **warfarin**. Disulfiram-like reaction may occur with **alcohol** ingestion. May cause acute psychosis and confusion with **disulfiram**. ↑ risk of leukopenia with **fluorouracil** or **azathioprine**.

Route/Dosage

PO (Adults): *Anaerobic infections*—7.5 mg/kg q 6 hr (not to exceed 4 g/day). *Trichomoniasis*—250 mg q 8 hr for 7 days *or* single 2-g dose *or* 1 g bid for 1 day. *Amebiasis*—500–750 mg q 8 hr for 5–10 days. *H. pylori*—250 mg 4 times daily *or* 500 mg twice daily for 1–2 wk (with other agents). *Bacterial vaginoses*—750 mg once daily as ER tablets for 7 days. *Antibiotic associated pseudomembranous colitis*—250–500 mg 3–4 times/day for 10–14 days.

PO (Infants and Children): *Anaerobic infections* —30 mg/kg/day divided q 6 hr, maximum dose: 4 g/day. *Trichomoniasis*—15–30 mg/kg/day divided q 8 hr for 7–10 days. *Amebiasis*—35–50 mg/kg/day divided q 8 hr for 5–10 days (not to exceed 750 mg/dose). *Antibiotic associated pseudomembranous colitis*—30 mg/kg/day divided q 6 hr for 7–10 days. *H. pylori*—15–20 mg/kg/day divided twice daily for 4 weeks.

IV, PO (Neonates 0–4 weeks, <1200 g): 7.5 mg/kg q 48 hr. *Postnatal age <7 days, 1200–2000 g* –7.5 mg/kg/day q 24 hr. *Postnatal age <7 days, >2000 g*—15 mg/kg/day divided q 12 hr. *Postnatal age >7 days, 1200–2000 g*—15 mg/kg/day divided q 12 hr. *Postnatal age >7 days, >2000 g*—30 mg/kg/day divided q 12 hr.

IV (Adults): *Anaerobic infections*—Initial dose 15 mg/kg, then 7.5 mg/kg q 6–8 hr *or* 500 mg q 6–8 hr (not to exceed 4 g/day). *Perioperative prophylaxis*—Initial dose 15 mg/kg 1 hr before surgery, then 7.5 mg/kg 6 and 12 hr later. *Amebiasis*—500–750 mg q 8 hr for 5–10 days.

IV (Children): *Anaerobic infections*—30 mg/kg/day divided q 6 hr, maximum dose: 4 g/day.

Topical (Adults): *Acne rosacea*—apply thin film to affected area bid.

Vag (Adults): *Bacterial vaginosis*—One applicatorful (5 g) 2 times daily for 5 days.

Availability (generic available)

Tablets: 250 mg, 500 mg. **Cost:** *Generic*—250 mg $16.99/30, 500 mg $9.99/30. **Extended-release (ER) tablets:** 750 mg. **Cost:** $297.98/30. **Capsules:** 375 mg, ✤ 500 mg. **Premixed injection:** 500 mg/100 ml RTU (ready to use). **Topical gel:** 0.75% in 45-g and 60-g tubes. **Cost:** $132.99/60 g. **Topical cream:** 0.75% in 45-g tubes, 1% in 60-g tubes. **Cost:** *Generic*—$59.99/45 g. **Topical lotion:** 0.75% in 59-ml bottle. **Cost:** *Generic*—$79.99/59 ml. **Vaginal gel:** 0.75% (37.5 mg/5 g applicatorful) in 70-g tubes. **Cost:** $32.22/70 g. ***In combination with:*** bismuth subsalicylate tablets and tetracycline capsules (Helidac) as part of a compliance package; bismuth subcitrate potassium and tetracycline (Pylera). See Appendix B.

NURSING IMPLICATIONS

Assessment

- Assess patient for infection (vital signs; appearance of wound, sputum, urine, and stool; WBC) at beginning of and throughout therapy.
- Obtain specimens for culture and sensitivity before initiating therapy. First dose may be given before receiving results
- Monitor neurologic status during and after IV infusions. Inform physician if numbness, paresthesia, weakness, ataxia, or seizures occur
- Monitor intake and output and daily weight, especially for patients on sodium restriction. Each 500 mg of Flagyl IV for dilution contains 5 mEq of sodium; each 500 mg of Flagyl RTU contains 14 mEq of sodium.
- **Giardiasis:** Monitor three stool samples taken several days apart, beginning 3–4 wk after treatment.
- ***Lab Test Considerations:*** May alter results of serum AST, ALT, and LDH tests.

Potential Nursing Diagnoses

Risk for infection (Indications)
Diarrhea (Indications)

Implementation

- **PO:** Administer on an empty stomach, or may administer with food or milk to minimize GI irritation. Tablets may be crushed for patients with difficulty swallowing.

IV Administration

- **Intermittent Infusion:** ***Diluent:*** Flagyl IV RTU is prediluted and ready to use. Do not refrigerate. Once taken out of overwrap, premixed infusion stable for 30 days at room temperature. ***Concentration:*** 5 mg/ml. ***Rate:*** Infuse over 30–60 min.
- **Y-Site Compatibility:** acyclovir, anidulafungin, bivalirudin, cefepime, cisatracurium, diltiazem, dopamine, enalaprilat, ertapenam,

esmolol, fenoldopam, fluconazole, granisetron, heparin, hydromorphone, labetalol, levofloxacin, linezolid, lorazepam, magnesium sulfate, meperidine, methylprednisolone, midazolam, milrinone, morphine, nicardipine, palonosetron, piperacillin/tazobactam, tacrolimus, theophylline, tirofiban, vasopressin, voriconazole.

- **Y-Site Incompatibility:** amphotericin B cholesteryl sulfate, aztreonam, caspofungin, daptomycin, filgrastim, lansoprazole, pantoprazole.
- **Topical:** Cleanse affected area before application. Apply and rub in a thin film twice daily, morning and evening. Avoid contact with eyes.

Patient/Family Teaching

- Instruct patient to take medication exactly as directed with evenly spaced times between doses, even if feeling better. Do not skip doses or double up on missed doses. Take missed doses as soon as remembered if not almost time for next dose.
- Advise patients treated for trichomoniasis that sexual partners may be asymptomatic sources of reinfection and should be treated concurrently. Patient should also refrain from intercourse or use a condom to prevent reinfection.
- Caution patient to avoid intake of alcoholic beverages or preparations containing alcohol during and for at least 1 day after treatment with metronidazole, including vaginal gel. May cause a disulfiram-like reaction (flushing, nausea, vomiting, headache, abdominal cramps).
- May cause dizziness or light-headedness. Caution patient to avoid driving or other activities requiring alertness until response to medication is known.
- Inform patient that medication may cause an unpleasant metallic taste.
- Advise patient not to take OTC medications concurrently without consulting health care professional.
- Advise patient that frequent mouth rinses, good oral hygiene, and sugarless gum or candy may minimize dry mouth. Notify health care professional if dry mouth persists for more than 2 wk.
- Advise patient to inform health care professional if pregnancy is suspected before taking this medication.
- Inform patient that medication may cause urine to turn dark.
- Advise patient to consult health care professional if no improvement in a few days or if signs and symptoms of superinfection (black, furry overgrowth on tongue; vaginal itching or discharge; loose or foul-smelling stools) develop.
- **Vag:** Instruct patient in correct technique for intravaginal instillation. Advise patient to avoid intercourse during treatment with vaginal gel.
- **Topical:** Instruct patient on correct technique for application of topical gel. Cosmetics may be used after application of gel.

Evaluation/Desired Outcomes

- Resolution of the signs and symptoms of infection. Length of time for complete resolution depends on organism and site of infection.
- Significant results should be seen within 3 wk of application of topical gel. Application may be continued for 9 wk.

mexiletine (mex-il-e-teen)

Mexitil

Classification

Therapeutic: antiarrhythmics (class IB)

Pregnancy Category C

Indications

Prophylaxis/treatment of serious ventricular arrhythmias, including VT and PVCs. **Unlabeled uses:** Management of chronic neuropathic pain.

Action

Decreases the duration of the action potential and effective refractory period in cardiac conduction tissue by altering transport of sodium across myocardial cell membranes. Has little or no effect on heart rate. **Therapeutic Effects:** Control of ventricular arrhythmias.

Pharmacokinetics

Absorption: Well absorbed from the GI tract.

Distribution: Enters breast milk in concentrations similar to plasma.

Metabolism and Excretion: Mostly metabolized by the liver; 10% excreted unchanged by the kidneys.
Half-life: 10–12 hr.

TIME/ACTION PROFILE (antiarrhythmic effects†)

ROUTE	ONSET	PEAK	DURATION
PO	30 min–2 hr	2–3 hr	8–12 hr

†Provided a loading dose has been given

Contraindications/Precautions

Contraindicated in: Hypersensitivity; Cardiogenic shock; 2nd- or 3rd-degree heart block (if a pacemaker has not been inserted); Lactation.
Use Cautiously in: Sinus node or intraventricular conduction abnormalities; Hypotension; CHF; Severe hepatic impairment (dosage reduction suggested); Pregnancy or children (safety not established).

Adverse Reactions/Side Effects

CNS: dizziness, nervousness, confusion, fatigue, headache, sleep disorder. **EENT:** blurred vision, tinnitus. **Resp:** dyspnea. **CV:** ARRHYTHMIAS, chest pain, edema, palpitations. **GI:** HEPATIC NECROSIS, heartburn, nausea, vomiting. **Derm:** rashes. **Hemat:** blood dyscrasias. **Neuro:** tremor, coordination difficulties, paresthesia.

Interactions

Drug-Drug: Opioid analgesics, **atropine**, and **antacids** may slow absorption. **Metoclopramide** may speed absorption. **Phenytoin**, **rifampin**, **cigarette smoking**, or **phenobarbital** may ↑ metabolism and ↓ effectiveness. **Cimetidine** may ↑ or ↓ mexiletine levels. May ↑ blood levels and risk of toxicity from **theophylline**. Additive cardiac effects may occur with other **antiarrhythmics**. **Drugs that drastically alter urine pH** may alter blood levels (alkalinization ↑ reabsorption and blood levels; acidification ↑ excretion and ↓ blood levels).
Drug-Food: Foods that drastically alter urine pH may alter blood levels. Alkalinization ↑ reabsorption and ↑ blood levels. Acidification ↑ excretion and may ↓ effectiveness (see Appendix L).

Route/Dosage

PO (Adults): 400-mg loading dose initially, then 200 mg 8 hr later, then 200–400 mg q 8 hr; dosage alterations of 50–100 mg may be made q 2–3 days. If controlled on ≤300 mg q 8 hr, can give same daily dose at 12-hr intervals (not to exceed 1200 mg/day). Some patients may require q 6 hr dosing.

Availability

Capsules: ✤ 100 mg, 150 mg, 200 mg, 250 mg.

NURSING IMPLICATIONS

Assessment

- Monitor pulse, blood pressure, and ECG periodically throughout therapy. Continuous Holter monitoring and chest x-ray examinations may be necessary to determine efficacy and aid in dosage adjustment.
- **Pain:** Assess type, location, and severity of pain prior to and periodically throughout therapy.
- ***Lab Test Considerations:*** May occasionally cause a positive ANA test result.
- May cause a transient increase in AST concentrations.
- May cause thrombocytopenia within a few days after initiation of therapy. Blood counts usually return to normal within 1 mo after discontinuation of therapy.
- ***Toxicity and Overdose:*** Serum mexiletine concentrations may be determined during dosage adjustment. Incidence of side effects is greater with concentrations >2 mcg/ml.

Potential Nursing Diagnoses

Decreased cardiac output (Indications)
Deficient knowledge, related to medication regimen (Patient/Family Teaching)

Implementation

- When changing from other antiarrhythmic therapy, give the 1st dose of mexiletine 6–12 hr after the last dose of quinidine, 3–6 hr after last dose of procainamide, or 8–12 hr after last dose of tocainide. When changing from parenteral lidocaine, decrease lidocaine dose or discontinue lidocaine 1–2 hr after administration of mexiletine or administer lower initial doses of mexiletine.
- Transfer of patients with life-threatening arrhythmias from other antiarrhythmics to mexiletine should be managed in the hospital.
- **PO:** Administer with food or antacids to minimize GI irritation.

Patient/Family Teaching

- Advise patient to take medication exactly as directed, at evenly spaced intervals, even if feeling well. Missed doses should be taken within 4 hr or omitted. Do not skip or double up on missed doses.

- Teach patients to monitor pulse. Advise patient to contact health care professional if pulse rate is <50 bpm or becomes irregular.
- May cause dizziness and light-headedness. Caution patient to avoid driving and other activities requiring alertness until response to medication is known.
- Instruct patient to avoid changes in diet that may drastically acidify or alkalinize the urine (see Appendix L for foods included).
- Advise patient to notify health care professional of disease process and medication regimen prior to treatment or surgery.
- Advise patient to notify health care professional if general tiredness, yellowing of the skin or eyes, fever, sore throat, or persistent side effects occur.
- Patient should carry identification describing disease process and medication regimen at all times.

Evaluation/Desired Outcomes

- Decrease in frequency or resolution of serious ventricular arrhythmias.
- Decrease in severity of chronic neurogenic pain.

micafungin (my-ka-fun-gin)

Mycamine

Classification

Therapeutic: antifungals

Pharmacologic: echinocandins

Pregnancy Category C

Indications

Esophageal candidiasis. Prophylaxis of *Candida* infections during hematopoetic stem cell transplantation.

Action

Inhibits synthesis of glucan required for the formation of fungal cell wall. **Therapeutic Effects:** Death of susceptible fungi. **Spectrum:** Active against the following *Candida* spp: *C. albicans*, *C. glabrata*, *C. krusei*, *C. parapsilosis*, *C. tropicalis*.

Pharmacokinetics

Absorption: IV administration results in complete bioavailability.

Distribution: Unknown.

Protein Binding: >99 %.

Metabolism and Excretion: Mostly metabolized; 71% fecal elimination.

Half-life: 15 hr.

TIME/ACTION PROFILE

ROUTE	ONSET	PEAK	DURATION
IV	rapid	end of infusion	24 hr

Contraindications/Precautions

Contraindicated in: Hypersensitivity.

Use Cautiously in: Severe hepatic impairment; Lactation or children (safety not established), pregnancy (use only if clearly needed).

Adverse Reactions/Side Effects

GI: worsening hepatic function/hepatitis. **GU:** renal impairment. **Hemat:** hemolysis/hemolytic anemia. **Local:** injection site reactions. **Misc:** allergic reactions including ANAPHYLAXIS (rare).

Interactions

Drug-Drug: ↑ blood levels and risk of toxicity with **sirolimus** and **nifedipine** (dose adjustments may be necessary).

Route/Dosage

IV (Adults): *Esophageal candidiasis*—150 mg/day for 15 days (range 10–30 days); *prevention of Candida infections in stem cell transplantation*—50 mg/day.

Availability

Lyophilized powder for injection: 50 mg/vial, 100 mg/vial.

NURSING IMPLICATIONS

Assessment

- Assess symptoms of esophageal candidiasis (dysphagia, odynophagia, retrosternal pain) prior to and during therapy.
- Monitor for signs of anaphylaxis (rash, pruritus, wheezing, laryngeal edema, abdominal pain). Discontinue micafungin and notify physician or health care professional immediately if these occur.
- Assess for injection site reactions (phlebitis, thrombophlebitis) during therapy. These occur more frequently in patients receiving micafungin via peripheral IV infusion.
- ***Lab Test Considerations:*** May cause ↑ serum alkaline phosphatase, bilirubin, ALT,

M

AST, and LDH levels. If elevations occur, monitor for worsening liver function; may require discontinuation of therapy.

- May cause ↑ BUN and serum creatinine.
- May cause leukopenia, neutropenia, thrombocytopenia, and anemia. Monitor for worsening levels; may require discontinuation of therapy.
- May cause hypokalemia, hypocalcemia, and hypomagnesemia.

Potential Nursing Diagnoses

Risk for infection (Indications)

Implementation

IV Administration

- **Intermittent Infusion:** ***Diluent:*** Reconstitute each 50-mg vial with 5 ml of 0.9% NaCl or D5W to achieve concentration of 10 mg/ml. Reconstitute each 100-mg vial with 5 ml of 0.9% NaCl or D5w to achieve concentration of 20 mg/ml. Dissolve by gently swirling vial; do not shake vigorously. Directions for further dilution based on indication for use. For prophylaxis of *Candida* infections, add 50 mg of micafungin to 100 ml of 0.9% NaCl or D5W. For treatment of esophageal candidiasis, add 150 mg of micafungin to 100 ml of 0.9% NaCl or D5W. Reconstituted vials and infusion are stable for 24 hr at room temperature. Protect diluted solution from light. ***Concentration:*** 0.5–1.5 mg/ml. ***Rate:*** Flush line with 0.9% NaCl prior to administration. Infuse over 1 hr. More rapid infusions may result in more frequent histamine mediated reactions.
- **Y-Site Compatibility:** aminophylline, bumetanide, calcium chloride, calcium gluconate, cyclosporine, dopamine, eptifibatide, esmolol, fenoldopam, furosemide, heparin, hydromorphone, lidocaine, lorazepam, magnesium sulfate, milrinone, nitroglycerin, nitroprusside, norepinephrine, phenylephrine, potassium chloride, potassium phosphate, tacrolimus, vasopressin.
- **Y-Site Incompatibility:** amiodarone, cisatracurium, diltiazem, dobutamine, epinephrine, insulin, labetalol, meperidine, midazolam, morphine, mycophenolate mofetil, nesiritide, nicardipine, octreotide, ondansetron, phenytoin, vecuronium.

Patient/Family Teaching

- Inform patient of the purpose of micafungin.
- Advise patient to notify health care professional immediately if signs of anaphylaxis occur.

Evaluation/Desired Outcomes

- Resolution of signs and symptoms of esophageal candidiasis.
- Prevention of *Candida* infections during hematopoetic stem cell transplantation.

---

miconazole, See ANTIFUNGALS (TOPICAL), ANTIFUNGALS (VAGINAL).

HIGH ALERT

midazolam (mid-ay-zoe-lam)

Versed

Classification

Therapeutic: antianxiety agents, sedative/hypnotics

Pharmacologic: benzodiazepines

Schedule IV

Pregnancy Category D

Indications

PO: Preprocedural sedation and anxiolysis in pediatric patients. **IM, IV:** Preoperative sedation/anxiolysis/amnesia. **IV:** Provides sedation/anxiolysis/amnesia during therapeutic, diagnostic, or radiographic procedures (conscious sedation). Aids in the induction of anesthesia and as part of balanced anesthesia. As a continuous infusion, provides sedation of mechanically ventilated patients during anesthesia or in a critical care setting, Status epilepticus.

Action

Acts at many levels of the CNS to produce generalized CNS depression. Effects may be mediated by GABA, an inhibitory neurotransmitter. **Therapeutic Effects:** Short-term sedation. Postoperative amnesia.

Pharmacokinetics

Absorption: Rapidly absorbed following oral and nasal administration; undergoes substantial intestinal and first-pass hepatic metabolism. Well absorbed following IM administration; IV administration results in complete bioavailability.

Distribution: Crosses the blood-brain barrier and placenta.

Protein Binding: 97%.

Metabolism and Excretion: Almost exclusively metabolized by the liver, resulting in conversion to hydroxymidazolam, an active metabolite, and 2 other inactive metabolites (metabolized by cytochrome P450 3A4 enzyme system); metabolites are excreted in urine.
Half-life: Preterm neonates: 2.6–17.7 hr; Neonates: 4–12 hr; Children: 3–7 hr; Adults: 2–6 hr (increased in renal impairment, CHF, or cirrhosis).

TIME/ACTION PROFILE (sedation)

ROUTE	ONSET	PEAK	DURATION
IN	5 min	10 min	30–60 min
IM	15 min	30–60 min	2–6 hr
IV	1.5–5 min	rapid	2–6 hr

Contraindications/Precautions
Contraindicated in: Hypersensitivity; Cross-sensitivity with other benzodiazepines may occur; Shock; Comatose patients or those with pre-existing CNS depression; Uncontrolled severe pain; Products containing benzyl alcohol should not be used in neonates; Pregnancy; Acute angle-closure glaucoma.
Use Cautiously in: Pulmonary disease; CHF; Renal impairment; Severe hepatic impairment; Obese pediatric patients (calculate dose on the basis of ideal body weight); Geriatric or debilitated patients (especially patients >70 yr) more susceptible to cardiorespiratory depressant effects; dosage reduction required; Lactation (safety not established).

Adverse Reactions/Side Effects
CNS: agitation, drowsiness, excess sedation, headache. **EENT:** blurred vision. **Resp:** APNEA, LARYNGOSPASM, RESPIRATORY DEPRESSION, bronchospasm, coughing. **CV:** CARDIAC ARREST, arrhythmias. **GI:** hiccups, nausea, vomiting. **Derm:** rashes. **Local:** phlebitis at IV site, pain at IM site.

Interactions
Drug-Drug: ↑ CNS depression with **alcohol**, **antihistamines**, **opioid analgesics**, and other **sedative/hypnotics** (↓ midazolam dose by 30–50% if used concurrently). ↑ risk of hypotension with **antihypertensives**, **opioid analgesics**, acute ingestion of **alcohol**, or **nitrates**. Midazolam is metabolized by the cytochrome P450 3A4 enzyme system; drugs that induce or inhibit this system may be expected to alter the effects of midazolam. **Carbamazepine**, **phenytoin**, **rifampin**, **rifabutin**, and **phenobarbital** ↓ levels of midazolam. The following agents ↓ midazolam metabolism and may ↑ its effects: **erythromycin**, **cimetidine**, **ranitidine**, **diltiazem**, **verapamil**, **fluconazole**, **itraconazole**, and **ketoconazole**.
Drug-Natural Products: Concomitant use of **kava kava**, **valerian**, or **chamomile** can ↑ CNS depression. Long-term use of **St. John's wort** may significantly decrease serum concentrations of oral midazolam.
Drug-Food: Grapefruit juice ↓ metabolism and may ↑ effects of midazolam.

Route/Dosage
Dose must be individualized, taking caution to reduce dose in geriatric patients and in those who are already sedated.

Preoperative Sedation/Anxiolysis/Amnesia
PO (Children 6 mo–16 yr): 0.25–0.5 mg/kg, may require up to 1 mg/kg (dose should not exceed 20 mg); *patients with cardiac/respiratory compromise or concurrent CNS depressants*—0.25 mg/kg.
IM (Adults Otherwise Healthy and <60 yr): 0.07–0.08 mg/kg 1 hr before surgery (usual dose 5 mg).
IM (Adults ≥60 yr, Debilitated or Chronically Ill): 0.02–0.03 mg/kg 1 hr before surgery (usual dose 1–3 mg).
IM (Children): 0.1–0.15 mg/kg up to 0.5 mg/kg 30–60 min prior to procedure; not to exceed 10 mg/dose.

Conscious Sedation for Short Procedures
IV (Adults and Children Otherwise Healthy >12 yr and <60 yr): 1–1.5 mg initially; dose may be increased further as needed. Total doses >3.5 mg are rarely needed (reduce dose by 30% if other CNS depressants are used). Maintenance doses of 25% of the dose required for initial sedation may be given as necessary.
IV (Children 6–12 yr): 0.025–0.05 mg/kg initially, then titrate dose carefully, may need up to 0.4 mg/kg total, maximum dose 10 mg.
IV (Children 6 mo–5 yr): 0.05 mg/kg initially, then titrate dose carefully, may need up to 0.6 mg/kg total, maximum dose 6 mg.
IV (Geriatric Patients ≥60 yr, Debilitated or Chronically Ill): 1–2.5 mg initially; dosage may be increased further as needed. Total doses

M

>5 mg are rarely needed (reduce dose by 50% if other CNS depressants are used). Maintenance doses of 25% of the dose required for initial sedation may be given as necessary.
Intranasal (Children): 0.2–0.3 mg/kg, may repeat in 5–15 min.

Status Epilepticus

IV (Children >2 months): 0.15 mg/kg load followed by a continuous infusion of 1 mcg/kg/min. Titrate dose upward q 5 min until seizure controlled, range: 1–18 mcg/kg/min.

Induction of Anesthesia (Adjunct)

May give additional dose of 25% of initial dose if needed
IV (Adults Otherwise Healthy and <55 yr): 300–350 mcg/kg initially (up to 600 mcg/kg total). If patient is premedicated, initial dose should be further reduced.
IV (Geriatric Patients >55 yr): 150–300 mcg/kg as initial dose. If patient is premedicated, initial dose should be further reduced.
IV (Adults—Debilitated): 150–250 mcg/kg initial dose. If patient is premedicated, initial dose should be further reduced.

Sedation in Critical Care Settings

IV (Adults): 0.01–0.05 mg/kg (0.5–4 mg in most adults) initially if a loading dose is required; may repeat q 10–15 min until desired effect is obtained; may be followed by infusion at 0.02–0.1 mg/kg/hr (1–7 mg/hr in most adults).
IV (Children): *Intubated patients only*—0.05–0.2 mg/kg initially as a loading dose; follow with infusion at 0.06–0.12 mg/kg/min (1–2 mcg/kg/min), titrate to effect, range:0.4–6 mcg/kg/min.
IV (Neonates >32 wk): *Intubated patients only*—0.06 mg/kg/hr (1 mcg/kg/min).
IV (Neonates <32 wk): *Intubated patients only*—0.03 mg/kg/hr (0.5 mcg/kg/min).

Availability (generic available)

Injection: 1 mg/ml, 5 mg/ml. **Syrup (cherry flavor):** 2 mg/ml.

NURSING IMPLICATIONS

Assessment

- Assess level of sedation and level of consciousness throughout and for 2–6 hr following administration.
- Monitor blood pressure, pulse, and respiration continuously during IV administration. Oxygen and resuscitative equipment should be immediately available.
- ***Toxicity and Overdose:*** If overdose occurs, monitor pulse, respiration, and blood pressure continuously. Maintain patent airway and assist ventilation as needed. If hypotension occurs, treatment includes IV fluids, repositioning, and vasopressors. The effects of midazolam can be reversed with flumazenil (Romazicon).

Potential Nursing Diagnoses

Ineffective breathing pattern (Adverse Reactions)
Risk for injury (Side Effects)

Implementation

- ***High Alert:*** Accidental overdose of oral midazolam syrup in children has resulted in serious harm and death. Do not accept orders prescribed by volume (5 mL or 1 tsp); instead, request dose be expressed in milligrams. Have second practitioner independently check original order and dose calculations. Midazolam syrup should only be administered by health care professionals authorized to administer conscious sedation. Do not confuse Versed (midazolam) with VePesid (etoposide).
- **PO:** To use the *Press-in Bottle Adaptor (PIBA),* remove the cap and push bottle adaptor into neck of bottle. Close bottle tightly with cap. Solution is a clear red to purplish-red cherry-flavored syrup. Then remove cap and insert tip of oral dispenser in bottle adaptor. Push the plunger completely down toward tip of oral dispenser and insert firmly into bottle adaptor. Turn entire unit (bottle and oral dispenser) upside down. Pull plunger out slowly until desired amount of medication is withdrawn into oral dispenser. Turn entire unit right side up and slowly remove oral dispenser from the bottle. Tip of dispenser may be covered with tip of cap until time of use. Close bottle with cap after each use.
- Dispense directly into mouth. Do not mix with any liquid prior to dispensing.
- **Intranasal:** Administer using a 1-ml needleless syringe into the nares over 15 sec. Using the 5 mg/ml injection, administer half dose into each nare.
- **IM:** Administer IM doses deep into muscle mass, maximum concentration 1 mg/ml.

IV Administration

- **Direct IV:** ***Diluent:*** Administer undiluted or diluted with D5W or 0.9% NaCl. ***Concentration:*** Undiluted: 1 mg/ml or 5 mg/ml. Diluted: 0.03–3 mg/ml. ***Rate:*** Administer slowly over at least 2–5 min. Titrate dose to patient response. Rapid injection, especially in neonates, has caused severe hypotension.

- **Continuous Infusion: *Diluent:*** Dilute with 0.9% NaCl or D5W. ***Concentration:*** 0.5–1 mg/ml. ***Rate:*** Based on patient's weight (see Route/Dosage section). Titrate to desired level of sedation. Assess sedation at regular intervals and adjust rate up or down by 25–50% as needed. Dose should also be decreased by 10–25% every few hours to find minimum effective infusion rate, which prevents accumulation of midazolam and provides more rapid recovery upon termination.
- **Y-Site Compatibility:** abciximab, amikacin, amiodarone, anidulafungin, argatroban, atropine, aztreonam, bivalirudin, calcium gluconate, caspofungin, cefazolin, cefotaxime, cefoxitin, ceftizoxime, ceftriaxone, cimetidine, ciprofloxacin, cisatracurium, cyclosporine, daptomycin, digoxin, diltiazem, diphenhydramine, dopamine, doxycycline, enalaprilat, epinephrine, eptifibatide, erythromycin lactobionate, esmolol, etomidate, famotidine, fenoldopam, fentanyl, fluconazole, gentamicin, granisetron, heparin, hydromorphone, hydroxyzine, isoproterenol, labetalol, levofloxacin, lidocaine, linezolid, lorazepam, magnesium sulfate, meperidine, methylprednisolone, metoclopramide, metoprolol, metronidazole, milrinone, morphine, nicardipine, nitroglycerin, nitroprusside, norepinephrine, ondansetron, palonosetron, pancuronium, penicillin G potassium, phenylephrine, phytonadione, potassium chloride, procainamide, promethazine, propranolol, protamine, quinupristin/dalfopristin, ranitidine, rifampin, tobramycin, vancomycin, vecuronium.
- **Y-Site Incompatibility:** acyclovir, amphotericin B cholesteryl sulfate, aminophylline, ampicillin, ampicillin/sulbactam, bumetanide, cefepime, ceftazidime, cefuroxime, chloramphenicol, dexamethasone sodium phosphate, diazepam, ertapenem, furosemide, ganciclovir, ketorolac, lansoprazole, micafungin, pantoprazole, phenytoin, piperacillin/tazobactam, prochlorperazine, sodium bicarbonate, thiopental, trimethoprim/sulfamethoxazole.

Patient/Family Teaching

- Inform patient that this medication will decrease mental recall of the procedure.
- May cause drowsiness or dizziness. Advise patient to request assistance prior to ambulation and transfer and to avoid driving or other activities requiring alertness for 24 hr following administration.
- Instruct patient to inform health care professional prior to administration if pregnancy is suspected.
- Advise patient to avoid alcohol or other CNS depressants for 24 hr following administration of midazolam.

Evaluation/Desired Outcomes

- Sedation during and amnesia following surgical, diagnostic, and radiologic procedures.
- Sedation and amnesia for mechanically ventilated patients in a critical care setting.

mifepristone

(mi-fe-**priss**-tone)
Mifeprex

Classification
Therapeutic: abortifacients
Pharmacologic: antiprogestational agents

Pregnancy Category UK

Indications

Medical termination of intrauterine pregnancy up to day 49 of pregnancy.

Action

Antagonizes endometrial and myometrial effects of progesterone. Sensitizes the myometrium to contraction-inducing activity of prostaglandins. **Therapeutic Effects:** Termination of pregnancy.

Pharmacokinetics

Absorption: Rapidly absorbed following oral administration (69% bioavailability).
Distribution: Unknown.
Protein Binding: 98%.
Metabolism and Excretion: Mostly metabolized by the liver (cytochrome CYP450 3A4 [CY P450 3A4] enzyme system).
Half-life: 18 hr.

TIME/ACTION PROFILE (termination of pregnancy)

ROUTE	ONSET	PEAK	DURATION
PO	unknown	within 2 days	unknown

Contraindications/Precautions

Contraindicated in: Presence of an intrauterine device (IUD); Confirmed or suspected ectopic pregnancy; Undiagnosed adnexal mass; Chronic adrenal failure; Concurrent long-term corticosteroid therapy; Bleeding disorders or concurrent anticoagulant therapy; Inherited porphyrias.
Use Cautiously in: Chronic medical conditions such as cardiovascular, hypertensive, hepatic, renal, or respiratory disease (safety and efficacy not established); Women >35 yrs old or who smoke ≥10 cigarettes/day.

Adverse Reactions/Side Effects

CNS: dizziness, fainting, headache, weakness.
GI: abdominal pain, diarrhea, nausea, vomiting.
GU: uterine bleeding, uterine cramping, ruptured ectopic pregnancy, pelvic pain.

Interactions

Drug-Drug: Blood levels and therapeutic effectiveness may be ↑ by **ketoconazole**, **itraconazole**, and **erythromycin**. Blood levels and effects may be ↓ by **rifampin**, **dexamethasone**, **phenytoin**, **phenobarbital**, and **carbamazepine**. Mifepristone may ↓ metabolism and ↑ effects of other **drugs metabolized by the CYP 450 3A4 enzyme system**, including **some agents used during general anesthesia**.
Drug-Natural Products: Blood levels and effects may be ↓ by **St. John's wort**.
Drug-Food: Blood levels and effects may be ↑ by **grapefruit juice**.

Route/Dosage

PO (Adults): *Day 1*—600 mg (given as three 200 mg tablets) as a single dose, followed on *day 3* by 400 mcg misoprostol (Cytotec), unless abortion has occurred and has been confirmed by clinical or ultrasonographic examination (see misoprostol monograph).

Availability

Tablets: 200 mg.

NURSING IMPLICATIONS

Assessment

- Determine duration of pregnancy. Pregnancy is dated from the first day of the last menstrual period in a presumed 28-day cycle with ovulation occurring at mid-cycle and can be determined by menstrual history and clinical examination; use ultrasound if duration is uncertain or if ectopic pregnancy is suspected.
- Assess amount of bleeding and cramping during treatment. Determine if termination is complete on day 14.
- ***Lab Test Considerations:*** Decrease in hemoglobin, hematocrit, and RBCs may occur in women who bleed heavily.
- Changes in quantitative human chorionic gonadotropin (hCG) levels are not accurate until at least 10 days after mifepristone administration; complete termination of pregnancy must be confirmed by clinical examination.

Potential Nursing Diagnoses

Acute pain (Side Effects)

Implementation

- Mifepristone should be administered only by health care professionals who have read and understood the prescribing information, are able to assess gestational age of an embryo and diagnose ectopic pregnancies, and who are able to provide surgical intervention in cases of incomplete abortion or severe bleeding.
- Any IUD should be removed prior to mifepristone adminstration.
- Measures to prevent rhesus immunization, similar to those of surgical abortion, should be taken.
- **PO:** On *day 1*, after the patient has read the Medication Guide and signed the Patient Agreement, administer three 200-mg tablets of mifepristone as a single dose. On *day 3*, unless abortion has occurred and been confirmed by clinical examination or ultrasound, administer two 200-mcg tablets of misoprostol. On *day 14*, confirm that termination of pregnancy has occurred by clinical examination or ultrasound.

Patient/Family Teaching

- Advise patient of the treatment and its effects. Patients must be given a copy of the Medication Guide and Patient Agreement. Patient must understand the necessity of completing the treatment schedule of three office visits (day 1, day 3, and day 14).
- Inform patient that vaginal bleeding and uterine cramping will probably occur and that prolonged or heavy vaginal bleeding is not

proof of complete expulsion. Bleeding or spotting occurs for an average of 9–16 days; but may continue for more than 30 days. Advise patient that if the treatment fails, there is a risk of fetal malformation; medical abortion failures are managed by surgical termination.

- Caution patient to notify health care professional immediately if she develops weakness, nausea, vomiting, diarrhea, with or without abdominal pain or fever more than 24 hr after taking misoprostol; may indicate life-threatening sepsis.
- Instruct patient in the steps to take in an emergency situation, including precise instructions and a telephone number to call if she has problems or concerns.
- May cause dizziness or fainting. Caution patient to avoid driving or other activities requiring alertness until response to medication is known.
- Caution patient that pregnancy can occur following termination of pregnancy and before resumption of normal menses. Contraception can be initiated as soon as pregnancy termination is confirmed or before sexual intercourse is resumed.
- Advise patient to notify health care professional if she smokes at least 10 cigarettes a day.

Evaluation/Desired Outcomes

- Termination of an intrauterine pregnancy of less than 49 days' duration.

miglitol (mi-gli-tole)
Glyset

Classification
Therapeutic: antidiabetics
Pharmacologic: alpha-glucosidase inhibitors

Pregnancy Category B

Indications
Management of non–insulin-dependent diabetes mellitus (type 2) in conjunction with dietary therapy; may be used concurrently with sulfonylurea oral hypoglycemic agents.

Action
Lowers blood glucose by inhibiting the enzyme alpha-glucosidase in the GI tract, resulting in delayed glucose absorption. **Therapeutic Effects:** Lowering of blood glucose in diabetic patients, especially postprandial hyperglycemia.

Pharmacokinetics
Absorption: Completely absorbed at lower doses (25 mg); 50–70% absorbed at higher doses (100 mg).
Distribution: Distributes primarily into extracellular fluid; small amounts enter breast milk.
Metabolism and Excretion: Not metabolized; action is primarily local in the GI tract; amounts that are absorbed are excreted mostly unchanged in urine.
Half-life: 2 hr.

TIME/ACTION PROFILE (effect on glucose absorption)

ROUTE	ONSET	PEAK	DURATION
PO	rapid	within 1 hr	unknown

Contraindications/Precautions
Contraindicated in: Hypersensitivity; Diabetic ketoacidosis; Inflammatory bowel disease or other chronic intestinal conditions resulting in impaired absorption or predisposition to obstruction; Lactation.
Use Cautiously in: Patients with fever, infection, trauma, or stress (may cause hyperglycemia requiring alternate therapy); Renal impairment (use not recommended if creatinine >2 mg/dl); Pregnancy or children (safety not established).

Adverse Reactions/Side Effects
GI: abdominal pain, diarrhea, flatulence. **Hemat:** low serum iron.

Interactions
Drug-Drug: May decrease absorption of **ranitidine** and **propranolol**. Effects may be decreased by **intestinal adsorbents** (such as **charcoal**) and **digestive enzyme products**; concurrent use should be avoided.
Drug-Food: Concurrent **carbohydrates** may increase diarrhea.

Route/Dosage
PO (Adults): 25 mg 3 times daily; may begin with 25 mg once daily; may be increased up to 100 mg 3 times daily.

Availability
Tablets: 25 mg, 50 mg, 100 mg.

M

NURSING IMPLICATIONS

Assessment

- Observe patient for signs and symptoms of hypoglycemic reactions (sweating, hunger, weakness, dizziness, tremor, tachycardia, anxiety), especially when taking concurrently with other oral hypoglycemic agents.
- ***Lab Test Considerations:*** Serum glucose and glycosylated hemoglobin levels should be monitored periodically throughout therapy to evaluate effectiveness of therapy.
- ***Toxicity and Overdose:*** Symptoms of overdose are transient increase in flatulence, diarrhea, and abdominal discomfort. Miglitol alone does not cause hypoglycemia; however, other concurrently administered hypoglycemic agents may produce hypoglycemia requiring treatment. Mild hypoglycemia may be treated with administration of oral glucose.

Potential Nursing Diagnoses

Imbalanced nutrition: more than body requirements (Indications)
Noncompliance (Patient/Family Teaching)

Implementation

- Patients stabilized on a diabetic regimen who are exposed to stress, fever, trauma, infection, or surgery may require administration of insulin.
- Does not cause hypoglycemia when taken while fasting but may increase hypoglycemic effect of other hypoglycemic agents.
- **PO:** Administer miglitol 3 times daily with the first bite of each meal. Dose may be started lower and increased gradually to minimize GI effects.

Patient/Family Teaching

- Instruct patient to take miglitol at the same time each day, exactly as directed.
- Explain to patient that miglitol helps control hyperglycemia but does not cure diabetes. Therapy is usually long term.
- Encourage patient to follow prescribed diet, medication, and exercise regimen to prevent hyperglycemic or hypoglycemic episodes.
- Review signs of hypoglycemia and hyperglycemia with patient. If hypoglycemia occurs, advise patient to take a glass of orange juice, 2–3 tsp of sugar, honey, or corn syrup dissolved in water, and notify health care professional.
- Instruct patient in proper testing of blood glucose or urine ketones. These tests should be monitored closely during periods of stress or illness and health care professional notified of significant changes.
- Insulin is the recommended method of controlling blood glucose during pregnancy. Counsel female patients to use a form of contraception other than oral contraceptives and to notify health care professional promptly if pregnancy is planned or suspected.
- Advise patient to inform health care professional of medication regimen prior to treatment or surgery.
- Advise patient to carry a form of oral glucose (dextrose, D-glucose) and identification describing disease process and medication regimen at all times.
- Emphasize the importance of routine follow-up exams and regular testing of blood glucose and glycosylated hemoglobin.

Evaluation/Desired Outcomes

- Control of blood glucose levels without the appearance of hypoglycemic or hyperglycemic episodes.

HIGH ALERT

milrinone (mill-ri-none)

Primacor

Classification
Therapeutic: inotropics

Pregnancy Category C

Indications

Short-term treatment of CHF unresponsive to conventional therapy with digoxin, diuretics, and vasodilators.

Action

Increases myocardial contractility. Decreases preload and afterload by a direct dilating effect on vascular smooth muscle. **Therapeutic Effects:** Increased cardiac output (inotropic effect).

Pharmacokinetics

Absorption: IV administration results in complete bioavailability.
Distribution: Unknown.
Metabolism and Excretion: 80–90% excreted unchanged by the kidneys.
Half-life: 2.3 hr (increased in renal impairment).

TIME/ACTION PROFILE (hemodynamic effects)

ROUTE	ONSET	PEAK	DURATION
IV	5–15 min	unknown	3–6 hr

Contraindications/Precautions

Contraindicated in: Hypersensitivity; Severe aortic or pulmonic valvular heart disease; Hypertrophic subaortic stenosis (may increase outflow tract obstruction).

Use Cautiously in: History of arrhythmias, electrolyte abnormalities, abnormal digoxin levels, or insertion of vascular catheters (↑ risk of ventricular arrhythmias); Renal impairment (reduced infusion rate recommended if CCr is <50 ml/min); Pregnancy, lactation, or children (safety not established).

Adverse Reactions/Side Effects

CNS: headache, tremor. **CV:** VENTRICULAR ARRHYTHMIAS, angina pectoris, chest pain, hypotension, supraventricular arrhythmias. **CV:** skin rash. **GI:** liver function abnormalities. **F and E:** hypokalemia. **Hemat:** thrombocytopenia.

Interactions

Drug-Drug: None significant.

Route/Dosage

IV (Adults): *Loading dose*—50 mcg/kg followed by *infusion* at 0.50 mcg/kg/min (range 0.375–0.75 mcg/kg/min).

Availability

Injection: 1 mg/ml in 10-, 20-, and 50-ml vials. **Premixed infusion:** 20 mg/100 ml, 40 mg/200 ml.

NURSING IMPLICATIONS

Assessment

- Monitor heart rate and blood pressure continuously during administration. Milrinone should be slowed or discontinued if blood pressure drops excessively.
- Monitor intake and output and daily weight. Assess patient for resolution of signs and symptoms of CHF (peripheral edema, dyspnea, rales/crackles, weight gain) and improvement in hemodynamic parameters (increase in cardiac output and cardiac index, decrease in pulmonary capillary wedge pressure). Correct effects of previous aggressive diuretic therapy to allow for optimal filling pressure.
- Monitor ECG continuously during infusion. Arrhythmias are common and may be life threatening. The risk of ventricular arrhythmias is increased in patients with a history of arrhythmias, electrolyte abnormalities, abnormal digoxin levels, or insertion of vascular catheters.
- ***Lab Test Considerations:*** Monitor electrolytes and renal function frequently during administration. Hypokalemia should be corrected prior to administration to decrease the risk of arrhythmias.
- Monitor platelet count during therapy.
- ***Toxicity and Overdose: High Alert:*** Overdose manifests as hypotension. Dose should be decreased or discontinued. Supportive measures may be necessary.

Potential Nursing Diagnoses

Decreased cardiac output (Indications)

Implementation

- ***High Alert:*** Accidental overdose of milrinone can cause patient harm or death. Have second practitioner independently check original order, dose calculations, and infusion pump settings.

IV Administration

- **Direct IV:** ***Diluent:*** Loading dose may be administered undiluted. May also be diluted in 0.9% NaCl, 0.45% NaCl, or D5W for ease of administration. ***Concentration:*** 1 mg/ml. ***Rate:*** Administer the loading dose over 10 min.
- **Continuous Infusion:** ***Diluent:*** Milrinone drawn from vials must be diluted. Dilute 10 mg (10 ml) of milrinone in 40 ml of diluent or 20 mg (20 ml) of milrinone in 80 ml of diluent. Compatible diluents include 0.45% NaCl, 0.9% NaCl, and D5W. Premixed infusions are already diluted and ready to use. Admixed solutions are stable for 72 hr at room temperature. Stability of premixed infusions based on manufacturer's expiration date. Do not use solutions that are discolored or contain particulate matter. ***Concentration:*** 200-mcg/ml. ***Rate:*** Based on patient's weight (see Route/Dosage section). Titrate according to hemodynamic and clinical response.

- **Y-Site Compatibility:** acyclovir, amikacin, amiodarone, ampicillin, argatroban, bivalirudin, bumetanide, calcium chloride, calcium gluconate, caspofungin, cefazolin, cefepime, cefotaxime, ceftazidime, cefuroxime, cimetidine, ciprofloxacin, clindamycin, daptomycin, dexamethasone sodium phosphate, digoxin, diltiazem, dobutamine, dopamine, epinephrine, ertapenem, fenoldopam, fentanyl, furosemide, gentamicin, granisetron, heparin, hydromorphone, insulin, isoproterenol, labetalol, levofloxacin, linezolid, lorazepam, magnesium sulfate, meropenem, methylprednisolone sodium succinate, metronidazole, micafungin, midazolam, morphine, nesiritide, nicardipine, nitroglycerin, nitroprusside, norepinephrine, palonosetron, pancuronium, piperacillin/tazobactam, potassium chloride, propofol, propranolol, quinupristin/dalfopristin, ranitidine, rocuronium, sodium bicarbonate, tacrolimus, theophylline, thiopental, tirofiban, tobramycin, torsemide, vancomycin, vasopressin, vecuronium, voriconazole.
- **Y-Site Incompatibility:** imipenem/cilastatin, lansoprazole, pantoprazole, procainamide.

Patient/Family Teaching

- Inform patient and family of reasons for administration. Milrinone is not a cure but is a temporary measure to control the symptoms of CHF.

Evaluation/Desired Outcomes

- Decrease in the signs and symptoms of CHF.
- Improvement in hemodynamic parameters.

minocycline, See TETRACYCLINES.

mirtazapine (meer-**taz**-a-peen)

Remeron, Remeron Soltabs

Classification

Therapeutic: antidepressants

Pharmacologic: tetracyclic antidepressants

Pregnancy Category C

Indications

Major Depressive Disorder. **Unlabeled uses:** Panic Disorder. Generalized Anxiety Disorder (GAD). Post-Traumatic Stress Disorder (PTSD).

Action

Potentiates the effects of norepinephrine and serotonin. **Therapeutic Effects:** Antidepressant action, which may develop only after several weeks.

Pharmacokinetics

Absorption: Well absorbed but rapidly metabolized, resulting in 50% bioavailability.
Distribution: Unknown.
Protein Binding: 85%.
Metabolism and Excretion: Extensively metabolized by the liver (P450 2D6, 1A2 and 3A enzymes involved); metabolites excreted in urine (75%) and feces (15%).
Half-life: 20–40 hr.

TIME/ACTION PROFILE (antidepressant effect)

ROUTE	ONSET	PEAK	DURATION
PO	1–2 wk	6 wk or more	unknown

Contraindications/Precautions

Contraindicated in: Hypersensitivity; Concurrent MAO inhibitor therapy.
Use Cautiously in: History of seizures; History of suicide attempt; May ↑ risk of suicide attempt/ideation especially during early treatment or dose adjustment; History of mania/hypomania; Patients with hepatic or renal impairment; OB: Safety not established; Lactation: Discontinue drug or bottle-feed; Pedi: Safety not established. Suicide risk may be greater in chilren or adolscents; Geri: ↑ sensitivity to CNS effects and oversedation. Begin at lower doses and titrate carefully.

Adverse Reactions/Side Effects

CNS: drowsiness, abnormal dreams, abnormal thinking, agitation, anxiety, apathy, confusion, dizziness, malaise, weakness. **EENT:** sinusitis. **Resp:** dyspnea, increased cough. **CV:** edema, hypotension, vasodilation. **GI:** constipation, dry mouth, increased appetite, abdominal pain, anorexia, elevated liver enzymes, nausea, vomiting. **GU:** urinary frequency. **Derm:** pruritus, rash. **F and E:** increased thirst. **Hemat:** AGRANULOCYTOSIS. **Metab:** weight gain, hypercholesterolemia, increased triglycerides. **MS:** arthralgia, back pain, myalgia. **Neuro:** hyperkinesia, hypesthesia, twitching. **Misc:** flu-like syndrome.

Interactions

Drug-Drug: May cause hypertension, seizures, and death when used with **MAO inhibitors**; do

not use within 14 days of MAO inhibitor therapy. ↑ CNS depression with other **CNS depressants**, including **alcohol** and **benzodiazepines**. **Drugs affecting P450 enzymes, CYP2D6**, **CYP1A2**, and **CYP3A4** may alter the effects of mirtazapine.
Drug-Natural Products: Concomitant use of **kava kava**, **valerian**, **skullcap**, **chamomile**, or **hops** can ↑ CNS depression. ↑ risk of serotinergic side effects including serotonin syndrome with **St. John's wort** and **SAMe**.

Route/Dosage

PO (Adults): 15 mg/day as a single bedtime dose initially; may be increased q 1–2 wk up to 45 mg/day.

Availability (generic available)

Tablets: 15 mg, 30 mg, 45 mg. **Cost:** *Generic*—15 mg $50.00/30, 30 mg $45.99/30, 45 mg $45.99/30. **Orally disintegrating tablets (orange flavor):** 15 mg, 30 mg, 45 mg. **Cost:** *Generic*—15 mg $70.38/30, 30 mg $65.99/30, 45 mg $71.49/30.

NURSING IMPLICATIONS

Assessment

- Assess mental status (orientation, mood, behavior) frequently. Assess for suicidal tendencies, especially during early therapy. Restrict amount of drug available to patient.
- Assess weight and BMI initially and throughout therapy.
- Monitor blood pressure and pulse rate periodically during initial therapy. Report significant changes.
- For overweight/obese individuals, obtain BFS and cholesterol levels. Refer as appropriate for nutritional/weight management and medical management.
- Monitor for seizure activity in patients with a history of seizures or alcohol abuse. Institute seizure precautions.
- ***Lab Test Considerations:*** Assess CBC and hepatic function before and periodically during therapy.

Potential Nursing Diagnoses

Ineffective coping (Indications)
Anxiety (Indications)
Imbalanced nutrition: risk for more than body requirements (Side Effects)

Implementation

- May be given as a single dose at bedtime to minimize excessive drowsiness or dizziness.
- May be taken without regard to food.
- For *orally disintegrating tablets*, do not attempt to push through foil backing; with dry hands, peal back backing and remove tablet. Immediately place tablet on tongue; tablet will dissolve in seconds, then swallow with saliva. Administration with liquid is not necessary.

Patient/Family Teaching

- Instruct patient to take mirtazapine as directed. Take missed doses as soon as remembered; if almost time for next dose, skip missed dose and return to regular schedule. If single bedtime dose regimen is used, do not take missed dose in morning, but consult health care professional. Do not discontinue abruptly; gradual dose reduction may be required.
- May cause drowsiness and dizziness. Caution patient to avoid driving and other activities requiring alertness until response to drug is known.
- Caution patient to change positions slowly to minimize orthostatic hypotension.
- Advise patient to avoid alcohol or other CNS depressant drugs during and for at least 3–7 days after therapy has been discontinued.
- Advise patient to notify health care professional if dry mouth, urinary retention, or constipation occurs. Frequent rinses, good oral hygiene, and sugarless candy or gum may diminish dry mouth. An increase in fluid intake, fiber, and exercise may prevent constipation.
- Inform patient of need to monitor dietary intake. Increase in appetite may lead to undesired weight gain.
- Advise patient to consult health care professional before taking any OTC cold remedies or herbal products with this medication.
- Advise patient to notify health care professional of medication regimen before treatment or surgery.
- Therapy for depression may be prolonged. Emphasize the importance of follow-up exam to monitor effectiveness and side effects.

Evaluation/Desired Outcomes

- Resolution of the symptoms of depression.
- Increased sense of well-being.

M

- Renewed interest in surroundings.
- Increased appetite.
- Improved energy level.
- Improved sleep.
- Therapeutic effects may be seen within 1 wk, although several wks are usually necessary before improvement is observed.

misoprostol

(mye-soe-**prost**-ole)
Cytotec

Classification
Therapeutic: antiulcer agents, cytoprotective agents
Pharmacologic: prostaglandins

Pregnancy Category X

Indications
Prevention of gastric mucosal injury from NSAIDs, including aspirin, in high-risk patients (geriatric patients, debilitated patients, or those with a history of ulcers). With mifepristone for termination of pregnancy. **Unlabeled uses:** Treatment of duodenal ulcers.

Action
Acts as a prostaglandin analogue, decreasing gastric acid secretion (antisecretory effect) and increasing the production of protective mucus (cytoprotective effect). Causes uterine contractions. **Therapeutic Effects:** Prevention of gastric ulceration from NSAIDs. With mifepristone terminates pregnancy of less than 49 days.

Pharmacokinetics
Absorption: Well absorbed following oral administration and rapidly converted to its active form (misoprostol acid).
Distribution: Unknown.
Protein Binding: 85%.
Metabolism and Excretion: Undergoes some metabolism and is then excreted by the kidneys.
Half-life: 20–40 min.

TIME/ACTION PROFILE (effect on gastric acid secretion)

ROUTE	ONSET	PEAK	DURATION
PO	30 min	unknown	3–6 hr

Contraindications/Precautions
Contraindicated in: Hypersensitivity to prostaglandins; Pregnancy or lactation (when used to prevent NSAID-induced gastric injury).
Use Cautiously in: Patients with childbearing potential; Children <18 yr (safety not established).
Exercise Extreme Caution in: When used for cervical ripening (unlabeled use) may cause uterine rupture; risk factors are late trimester pregnancy, previous cesarian section or uterine surgery or ≥5 previous pregnancies.

Adverse Reactions/Side Effects
CNS: headache. **GI:** abdominal pain, diarrhea, constipation, dyspepsia, flatulence, nausea, vomiting. **GU:** miscarriage, menstrual disorders.

Interactions
Drug-Drug: Increased risk of diarrhea with **magnesium-containing antacids**.

Route/Dosage
PO (Adults): *Antiulcer*—200 mcg 4 times daily with or after meals and at bedtime, *or* 400 mcg twice daily, with the last dose at bedtime. If intolerance occurs, dosage may be decreased to 100 mcg 4 times daily. *Termination of Pregnancy*—400 mcg single dose two days after mifepristone if abortion has not occurred.

Availability (generic available)
Tablets: 100 mcg (0.1 mg), 200 mcg (0.2 mg). ***In combination with:*** 50 mg diclofenac/200 mcg misoprostol and 75 mg diclofenac/200 mcg misoprostol (Arthrotec). See Appendix B.

NURSING IMPLICATIONS

Assessment
- Assess patient routinely for epigastric or abdominal pain and for frank or occult blood in the stool, emesis, or gastric aspirate.
- Assess women of childbearing age for pregnancy. Misoprostol is usually begun on 2nd or 3rd day of menstrual period following a negative pregnancy test result.

Potential Nursing Diagnoses
Acute pain (Indications)

Implementation
- Do not confuse Cytotec (misoprostol) with Cytoxan (cyclophosphamide).
- Misoprostol therapy should be started at the onset of treatment with NSAIDs.
- **PO:** Administer medication with meals and at bedtime to reduce severity of diarrhea.
- Antacids may be administered before or after misoprostol for relief of pain. Avoid those containing magnesium, because of increased diarrhea with misoprostol.

Patient/Family Teaching

- Instruct patient to take medication as directed for the full course of therapy, even if feeling better. Take missed doses as soon as possible unless almost time for next dose; do not double doses. Emphasize that sharing of this medication may be dangerous.
- Inform patient that misoprostol will cause spontaneous abortion. Women of childbearing age must be informed of this effect through verbal and written information and must use contraception throughout therapy. If pregnancy is suspected, the woman should stop taking misoprostol and immediately notify her health care professional.
- Inform patient that diarrhea may occur. Health care professional should be notified if diarrhea persists for more than 1 wk. Also advise patient to report onset of black, tarry stools or severe abdominal pain.
- Advise patient to avoid alcohol and foods that may cause an increase in GI irritation.

Evaluation/Desired Outcomes

- The prevention of gastric ulcers in patients receiving chronic NSAID therapy.

mitomycin (mye-toe-**mye**-sin)

MitoExtra, Mutamycin

Classification

Therapeutic: antineoplastics

Pharmacologic: antitumor antibiotics

Pregnancy Category UK

Indications

Used with other agents in the management of disseminated adenocarcinoma of the stomach or pancreas. **Unlabeled uses:** Palliative treatment of: Carcinoma of the colon or breast, Head and neck tumors, Advanced biliary, lung, and cervical squamous cell carcinomas.

Action

Primarily inhibits DNA synthesis by causing cross-linking; also inhibits RNA and protein synthesis (cell-cycle phase–nonspecific but is most active in S and G phases). **Therapeutic Effects:** Death of rapidly replicating cells, particularly malignant ones.

Pharmacokinetics

Absorption: IV administration results in complete bioavailability.

Distribution: Widely distributed, concentrates in tumor tissue. Does not enter CSF.

Metabolism and Excretion: Mostly metabolized by the liver. Small amounts (<10%) excreted unchanged by the kidneys and in bile.

Half-life: 50 min.

TIME/ACTION PROFILE (effects on blood counts)

ROUTE	ONSET	PEAK	DURATION
IV	3–8 wk	4–8 wk	up to 3 mo

Contraindications/Precautions

Contraindicated in: Hypersensitivity; Pregnancy or lactation.

Use Cautiously in: Patients with childbearing potential; Active infections; Decreased bone marrow reserve; Geri: Geriatric patients or patients with other chronic debilitating illnesses; Impaired liver function; History of pulmonary problems.

Adverse Reactions/Side Effects

Resp: PULMONARY TOXICITY. **CV:** edema. **GI:** nausea, vomiting, anorexia, stomatitis. **GU:** infertility, renal failure. **Derm:** alopecia, desquamation. **Hemat:** leukopenia, thrombocytopenia, anemia. **Local:** phlebitis at IV site. **Misc:** HEMOLYTIC UREMIC SYNDROME, fever, prolonged malaise.

Interactions

Drug-Drug: Additive bone marrow depression with other **antineoplastics** or **radiation therapy**. May ↓ antibody response to **live-virus vaccines** and ↑ risk of adverse reactions. Concurrent or sequential use with **vinca alkaloids** may result in respiratory toxicity.

Route/Dosage

IV (Adults): 20 mg/m^2 every 6–8 wk.

Availability

Injection: 5-mg, 20-mg, and 40-mg vials.

NURSING IMPLICATIONS

Assessment

- Monitor vital signs periodically during administration.
- Monitor for bone marrow depression. Assess for bleeding (bleeding gums, bruising, petechiae, guaiac stools, urine, and emesis) and avoid IM injections and taking rectal temperatures if platelet count is low. Apply pressure

♣ = Canadian drug name.

* CAPITALS indicates life-threatening; underlines indicate most frequent.

to venipuncture sites for 10 min. Assess for signs of infection during neutropenia. Anemia may occur. Monitor for increased fatigue, dyspnea, and orthostatic hypotension.

- Monitor intake and output, appetite, and nutritional intake. Nausea and vomiting usually occur within 1–2 hr. Vomiting may stop within 3–4 hr; nausea may persist for 2–3 days. Antiemetics may be administered prophylactically. Adjust diet as tolerated to help maintain fluid and electrolyte balance and nutritional status.
- Assess respiratory status and chest x-ray examination prior to and periodically throughout course of therapy. Cough, bronchospasm, hemoptysis, or dyspnea usually occurs after several doses and may be indicative of pulmonary toxicity, which may be life threatening.
- Monitor for potentially fatal hemolytic uremic syndrome in patients receiving long-term therapy. Symptoms include microangiopathic hemolytic anemia, thrombocytopenia, renal failure, and hypertension.
- ***Lab Test Considerations:*** Monitor CBC with differential, platelet count, and observation for fragmented RBCs on peripheral blood smears prior to and periodically throughout therapy and for several months following therapy.
- The nadirs of leukopenia and thrombocytopenia occur in 4–8 wk. Notify physician if leukocyte count is $<4000/mm^3$ or if platelet count is $<150,000/mm^3$ or is progressively declining. Recovery from leukopenia and thrombocytopenia occurs within 10 wk after cessation of therapy. Myelosuppression is cumulative and may be irreversible. Repeat courses of therapy are held until leukocyte count is $>4000/mm^3$ and platelet count is $>100,000/mm^3$.
- Monitor liver function studies (AST, ALT, LDH, bilirubin) and renal function studies (BUN, creatinine) prior to and periodically throughout therapy to detect hepatotoxicity and nephrotoxicity. Notify physician if creatinine is >1.7 mg/dl.

Potential Nursing Diagnoses

Risk for injury (Side Effects)
Risk for infection (Side Effects)
Disturbed body image (Side Effects)

Implementation

- Solution should be prepared in a biologic cabinet. Wear gloves, gown, and mask while handling medication. Discard equipment in designated containers.
- Ensure patency of IV. Extravasation may cause severe tissue necrosis. If patient complains of discomfort at IV site, discontinue immediately and restart infusion at another site. Promptly notify physician of extravasation.

IV Administration

- **Direct IV:** ***Diluent:*** Reconstitute 5-mg vial with 10 ml and 10-mg vial with 40 ml of sterile water for injection or 0.9% NaCl. Shake the vial; may need to stand at room temperature for additional time to dissolve. Final solution is blue-gray. Reconstituted solution is stable for 7 days at room temperature, 14 days if refrigerated. ***Concentration:*** Dilute drug in vial to a concentration of 0.5–1 mg/ml and then may further dilute to 20–40 mcg/ml for administration. ***Rate:*** May be administered IV push over 5–10 min through free-flowing IV of 0.9% NaCl or D5W.
- **Y-Site Compatibility:** amifostine, bleomycin, cisplatin, cyclophosphamide, doxorubicin, droperidol, fluorouracil, furosemide, granisetron, heparin, leucovorin, melphalan, methotrexate, metoclopramide, ondansetron, teniposide, thiotepa, vinblastine, vincristine.
- **Y-Site Incompatibility:** aztreonam, cefepime, etoposide phosphate, filgrastim, gemcitabine, piperacillin/tazobactam, sargramostim, topotecan, vinorelbine.

Patient/Family Teaching

- Instruct patient to notify health care professional promptly if fever; chills; cough; hoarseness; sore throat; signs of infection; lower back or side pain; painful or difficult urination; bleeding gums; bruising; petechiae; blood in stools, urine, or emesis; increased fatigue; dyspnea; or orthostatic hypotension occurs. Caution patient to avoid crowds and persons with known infections. Instruct patient to use soft toothbrush and electric razor and to avoid falls. Caution patient not to drink alcoholic beverages or take medication containing aspirin or NSAIDs; may precipitate gastric bleeding.
- Instruct patient to notify health care professional if decreased urine output, edema in lower extremities, shortness of breath, skin ulceration, or persistent nausea occurs.
- Instruct patient to inspect oral mucosa for redness and ulceration. If ulceration occurs,

advise patient to use sponge brush and rinse mouth with water after eating and drinking. Topical agents may be used if pain interferes with eating. Stomatitis pain may require treatment with opioid analgesics.
- Discuss with patient the possibility of hair loss. Explore coping strategies.
- Advise patient that, although mitomycin may cause infertility, contraception during therapy is necessary because of teratogenic effects.
- Instruct patient not to receive any vaccinations without advice of health care professional.
- Emphasize need for periodic lab tests to monitor for side effects.

Evaluation/Desired Outcomes
- Decrease in size and spread of malignant tissue.

mitoxantrone
(mye-toe-**zan**-trone)
Novantrone

Classification
Therapeutic: antineoplastics
Pharmacologic: antitumor antibiotics

Pregnancy Category D

Indications
Acute nonlymphocytic leukemia (ANLL) in adults (with other antineoplastics). Initial chemotherapy for patients with pain associated with advanced hormone-refractory prostate cancer. Secondary (chronic) progressive, progressive relapsing, or worsening relapsing-remitting multiple sclerosis (MS). **Unlabeled uses:** Breast cancer, liver cancer, and non-Hodgkin's lymphoma.

Action
Inhibits DNA synthesis (cell-cycle phase–nonspecific). **Therapeutic Effects:** Death of rapidly replicating cells, particularly malignant ones. Decreased pain in patients with advanced prostate cancer. Decreased disability and slowed progression of MS.

Pharmacokinetics
Absorption: IV administration results in complete bioavailability.
Distribution: Widely distributed; limited penetration of CSF.
Metabolism and Excretion: Mostly eliminated by hepatobiliary clearance; <10% excreted unchanged by the kidneys.
Half-life: 5.8 days.

TIME/ACTION PROFILE (effects on blood counts)

ROUTE	ONSET	PEAK	DURATION
IV	unknown	10 days	21 days

Contraindications/Precautions
Contraindicated in: Hypersensitivity; OB: Pregnancy or lactation.
Use Cautiously in: Previous cardiac disease; OB: Patients with childbearing potential; Active infections; Depressed bone marrow reserve; Previous mediastinal radiation; Geriatric patients or patients with other chronic debilitating illness; Pedi: Children (safety not established); Impaired hepatobiliary function or decreased blood counts (dose reduction required).

Adverse Reactions/Side Effects
CNS: SEIZURES, headache. **EENT:** blue-green sclera, conjunctivitis. **Resp:** cough, dyspnea. **CV:** CARDIOTOXICITY, arrhythmias, ECG changes. **GI:** abdominal pain, diarrhea, hepatic toxicity, nausea, stomatitis, vomiting. **GU:** blue-green urine, gonadal suppression, renal failure. **Derm:** alopecia, rashes. **Hemat:** anemia, leukopenia, secondary leukemia, thrombocytopenia. **Metab:** hyperuricemia. **Misc:** fever, hypersensitivity reactions.

Interactions
Drug-Drug: ↑ bone marrow depression with other **antineoplastics** or **radiation therapy**. Risk of cardiomyopathy ↑ by previous **anthracycline antineoplastics** (**daunorubicin**, **doxorubicin**, **idarubicin**) or **mediastinal radiation**. May ↓ antibody response to **live-virus vaccines** and ↑ risk of adverse reactions.

Route/Dosage

Acute Nonlymphatic Leukemia
IV (Adults): *Induction*—12 mg/m²/day for 3 days (usually given with cytosine arabinoside 100 mg/m²/day for 7 days); if incomplete remission occurs, a 2nd induction may be given. *Consolidation*—12 mg/m²/day for 2 days (usually given with cytosine arabinoside 100 mg/m²/day

for 5 days), given 6 wk after induction with another course 4 wk later.

Advanced Prostate Cancer

IV (Adults): 12–14 mg/m^2 single dose as a short infusion (with corticosteroids).

Multiple Sclerosis

IV (Adults): 12 mg/m^2 q 3 mo.

Availability

Injection: 2 mg/ml in 10-, 12.5-, and 15-ml vials.

NURSING IMPLICATIONS

Assessment

- Monitor for hypersensitivity reaction (rash, urticaria, bronchospasm, tachycardia, hypotension). If these occur, stop infusion and notify physician. Keep epinephrine, an antihistamine, and resuscitation equipment close by in the event of an anaphylactic reaction.
- Monitor for bone marrow depression. Assess for bleeding (bleeding gums, bruising, petechiae, guaiac stools, urine, and emesis) and avoid IM injections and taking rectal temperatures if platelet count is low. Apply pressure to venipuncture sites for 10 min. Assess for signs of infection during neutropenia. Anemia may occur. Monitor for increased fatigue, dyspnea, and orthostatic hypotension.
- Monitor intake and output, appetite, and nutritional intake. Assess patient for nausea and vomiting. Antiemetics may be administered prophylactically. Adjust diet as tolerated to help maintain fluid and electrolyte balance and nutritional status.
- Monitor chest x-ray, ECG, echocardiography or MUGA, and radionuclide angiography to determine ejection fraction prior to and periodically during therapy. Multiple sclerosis patients with baseline left ventricular ejection fraction (LVEF) <50% should not receive mitoxantrone. May cause cardiotoxicity, especially in patients who have received daunorubicin or doxorubicin. Assess for rales/crackles, dyspnea, edema, jugular vein distention, ECG changes, arrhythmias, and chest pain. Monitor LVEF with echocardiogram or MUGA if signs of CHF occur and prior to each dose in patients with multiple sclerosis. Potentially fatal CHF may occur during or for months or years after therapy. Risk is greater in patients receiving a cumulative dose >140 mg/m^2.
- Monitor for symptoms of gout (↑ uric acid levels and joint pain and swelling). Encourage patient to drink at least 2 L of fluid per day. Allopurinol may be given to decrease serum uric acid levels.
- **Multiple sclerosis:** Assess frequency of exacerbations of symptoms of multiple sclerosis periodically during therapy.
- ***Lab Test Considerations:*** Monitor CBC with differential and platelet count prior to and periodically during therapy. The nadir of leukopenia usually occurs within 10 days, and recovery usually occurs within 21 days.
- Monitor liver function studies (AST, ALT, LDH, bilirubin) and renal function studies (BUN, creatinine) prior to and periodically during therapy to detect hepatotoxicity and nephrotoxicity.
- May cause ↑ uric acid concentrations. Monitor periodically during therapy.

Potential Nursing Diagnoses

Risk for injury (Side Effects)
Risk for infection (Side Effects)
Disturbed body image (Side Effects)

Implementation

- Solution should be prepared in a biologic cabinet. Wear gloves, gown, and mask while handling medication. Discard equipment in designated containers.
- Avoid contact with skin. Use Luer-Lok tubing to prevent accidental leakage. If contact with skin occurs, immediately wash skin with soap and water.
- Clean all spills with an aqueous solution of calcium hypochlorite. Mix solution by adding 5.5 parts (per weight) of calcium hypochlorite to 13 parts water.

IV Administration

- **IV:** Monitor IV site. If extravasation occurs, discontinue IV and restart at another site. Mitoxantrone is not a vesicant
- **Direct IV:** ***Diluent:*** Dilute dark blue mitoxantrone solution in at least 50 ml of 0.9% NaCl or D5W. Discard unused solution appropriately. ***Rate:*** Administer slowly over at least 3 min into the tubing of a free-flowing IV of 0.9% NaCl or D5W.
- **Intermittent Infusion:** May be further diluted in D5W, 0.9% NaCl, or D5/0.9% NaCl and used immediately. ***Concentration:*** 0.02-0.5 mg/ml. ***Rate:*** Administer over 15–30 min.

- **Y-Site Compatibility:** allopurinol, amifostine, cladribine, etoposide, etoposide phosphate, filgrastim, fludarabine, gemcitabine, granisetron, linezolid, melphalan, ondansetron, oxaliplatin, sargramostim, teniposide, thiotepa, vinorelbine.
- **Y-Site Incompatibility:** amphotericin B cholesteryl sulfate, aztreonam, cefepime, doxorubicin liposome, lansoprazole, paclitaxel, pemetrexed, piperacillin/tazobactam, propofol.
- **Additive Compatibility:** cyclophosphamide, cytarabine, etoposide, fluorouracil, hydrocortisone sodium succinate, potassium chloride.
- **Additive Incompatibility:** heparin.

Patient/Family Teaching

- Instruct patient to notify health care professional promptly if fever; chills; cough; hoarseness; sore throat; signs of infection; lower back or side pain; painful or difficult urination; bleeding gums; bruising; petechiae; blood in stools, urine, or emesis; increased fatigue; dyspnea; or orthostatic hypotension occurs. Caution patient to avoid crowds and persons with known infections. Instruct patient to use soft toothbrush and electric razor and to avoid falls. Caution patient not to drink alcoholic beverages or take medication containing aspirin or NSAIDS; may precipitate gastric bleeding.
- Instruct patient to notify health care professional if abdominal pain, yellow skin, cough, diarrhea, or decreased urine output occurs.
- Inform patient that medication may cause the urine and sclera to turn blue-green.
- Instruct patient to inspect oral mucosa for redness and ulceration. If mouth sores occur, advise patient to use sponge brush and rinse mouth with water after eating and drinking. Topical agents may be used if pain interferes with eating. Stomatitis pain may require treatment with opioid analgesics.
- Discuss with patient the possibility of hair loss. Explore coping strategies.
- Advise patient that, although mitoxantrone may cause infertility, contraception during therapy is necessary because of possible teratogenic effects.
- Instruct patient not to receive any vaccinations without advice of health care professional.
- Emphasize need for periodic lab tests to monitor for side effects.

Evaluation/Desired Outcomes

- Decrease in the production and spread of leukemic cells.
- Decreased pain in patients with prostate cancer.
- Decrease in the frequency of relapse (neurologic dysfunction) in patients with relapsing-remitting multiple sclerosis.

modafinil (mo-**daf**-i-nil)

Provigil

Classification

Therapeutic: central nervous system stimulants

Pregnancy Category C

Indications

To improve wakefulness in patients with excessive daytime drowsiness due to narcolepsy, obstructive sleep apnea, or shift work sleep disorder.

Action

Produces CNS stimulation. **Therapeutic Effects:** Decreased daytime drowsiness in patients with narcolepsy and obstructive sleep apnea. Decreased drowsiness during work in patients with shift work sleep disorder.

Pharmacokinetics

Absorption: Rapidly absorbed; bioavailability unknown.
Distribution: Well distributed; moderately (60%) bound to plasma proteins.
Metabolism and Excretion: Highly (90%) metabolized by the liver; <10% eliminated unchanged.
Half-life: 15 hr.

TIME/ACTION PROFILE (blood levels)

ROUTE	ONSET	PEAK	DURATION
PO	rapid	2–4 hr	24 hr

Contraindications/Precautions

Contraindicated in: Hypersensitivity; History of left ventricular hypertrophy or ischemic ECG changes, chest pain, arrhythmia, or other significant manifestations of mitral valve prolapse in association with CNS stimulant use.

Use Cautiously in: History of MI or unstable angina; Severe hepatic impairment with or without cirrhosis (dosage reduction recommended); Concurrent use of MAO inhibitors; Geriatric patients (lower doses may be necessary); Pregnancy, lactation, or children <16 yr (safety not established).

Adverse Reactions/Side Effects

CNS: headache, amnesia, anxiety, cataplexy, confusion, depression, dizziness, insomnia, nervousness. **EENT:** rhinitis, abnormal vision, amblyopia, epistaxis, pharyngitis. **Resp:** dyspnea, lung disorder. **CV:** arrhythmias, chest pain, hypertension, hypotension, syncope, vasodilation. **GI:** nausea, abnormal liver function, anorexia, diarrhea, gingivitis, mouth ulcers, thirst, vomiting. **GU:** abnormal ejaculation, albuminuria, urinary retention. **Derm:** dry skin, herpes simplex. **Endo:** hyperglycemia. **Hemat:** eosinophilia. **MS:** joint disorder, neck pain. **Neuro:** ataxia, dyskinesia, hypertonia, paresthesia, tremor. **Misc:** infection.

Interactions

Drug-Drug: May decrease the metabolism and increase the effects of **diazepam**, **phenytoin**, **propranolol**, or **tricyclic antidepressants** (dosage adjustments may be necessary). May increase metabolism and decrease effects of **hormonal contraceptives**, **cyclosporine**, and **theophylline** (dosage adjustments or additional methods of contraception may be necessary).

Drug-Natural Products: Use with **caffeine-containing** herbs (**cola nut**, **guarana**, **mate**, **tea**, **coffee**) may increase stimulant effect.

Route/Dosage

PO (Adults): 200 mg/day as a single dose.

Hepatic Impairment

PO (Adults): *Severe hepatic impairment*—100 mg/day as a single dose.

Availability

Tablets: 100 mg, 200 mg. **Cost:** 100 mg $176.99/30, 200 mg $269.97/30.

NURSING IMPLICATIONS

Assessment

- Observe and document frequency of narcoleptic episodes.
- ***Lab Test Considerations:*** May cause elevated liver enzymes.

Potential Nursing Diagnoses

Disturbed thought process (Side Effects)
Deficient knowledge, related to medication regimen (Patient/Family Teaching)

Implementation

- **PO:** Administer as a single dose in the morning for patients with narcolepsy or obstructive sleep apnea. Administer 1 hour before the start of work shift for patients with shift work sleep disorder.

Patient/Family Teaching

- Instruct patient to take medication as directed.
- Medication may impair judgment. Advise patient to use caution when driving or during other activities requiring alertness.
- Nonhormonal methods of contraception should be used during and for 1 month following discontinuation of therapy. Instruct patient to notify health care professional promptly if pregnancy is planned or suspected or if breastfeeding.
- Instruct patient to avoid taking other prescription or OTC medication without consulting health care professional. If alcohol is used during therapy, intake should be limited to moderate amounts.
- Instruct patient to notify physician if rash, hives, or other allergic reactions occur.

Evaluation/Desired Outcomes

- Decrease in narcoleptic symptoms and an enhanced ability to stay awake.

moexipril, See ANGIOTENSIN-CONVERTING ENZYME (ACE) INHIBITORS.

mometasone, See CORTICOSTEROIDS (INHALATION), CORTICOSTEROIDS (NASAL), CORTICOSTEROIDS (TOPICAL/LOCAL).

MONOAMINE OXIDASE (MAO) INHIBITORS

isocarboxazid
(eye-soe-kar-**boks**-a-zid)
Marplan

phenelzine (**fen**-el-zeen)
Nardil

tranylcypromine
(tran-ill-**sip**-roe-meen)
Parnate

Classification
Therapeutic: antidepressants
Pharmacologic: monamine oxidase (MAO) inhibitors

Pregnancy Category C

Indications

Depression in patients who have failed other modes of therapy (tricyclic antidepressants, SSRIs, SSNRIs, or electroconvulsive therapy). **Unlabeled uses:** Treatment-resistant depression, panic disorder, social anxiety disorder (social phobia).

Action

Inhibit the enzyme monoamine oxidase, resulting in an accumulation of various neurotransmitters (dopamine, epinephrine, norepinephrine, and serotonin) in the body. **Therapeutic Effects:** Improved mood in depressed patients.

Pharmacokinetics

Absorption: *Phenelzine*—well absorbed from the GI tract; *isocarboxazid* and *tranylcypromine*—unknown.
Distribution: *Phenelzine* and *tranylcypromine*—cross the placenta and enter breast milk; *isocarboxazid*—unknown.
Metabolism and Excretion: *Phenelzine*—metabolized by the liver and excreted in urine as metabolites and unchanged drug; *isocarboxazid* and *tranylcypromine*—unknown.
Half-life: *Phenelzine*—12 hr; *tranylcypromine*—90–190 min; *isocarboxazid*—unknown.

TIME/ACTION PROFILE (antidepressant effect)

ROUTE	ONSET	PEAK	DURATION
Isocarboxazid	unknown	3–6 wk	unknown
Phenelzine	2–4 wk	3–6 wk	2 wk
Tranylcypromine	2 days–3 wk	2–3 wk	3–5 days

Contraindications/Precautions

Contraindicated in: Hypersensitivity; Liver disease; Severe renal disease; Cardiovascular disease; Uncontrolled hypertension; Cerebrovascular disease; Pheochromocytoma; CHF; History of severe or frequent headache; Patients undergoing elective surgery requiring anesthesia (should be discontinued at least days before surgery); Concurrent meperidine, SSRI antidepressants, SSNRI antidepressants, tricyclic antidepressants, tetracyclic antidepressants, nefazodone, trazodone, procarbazine, selegilene, linezolid, carbamazepine, cyclobenzaprine, bupropion, buspirone, sympathomimetics, dextromethorphan, narcotics, alcohol, anesthetics, diuretics, tryptophan, or antihistamines; Excessive consumption of caffeine; Concurrent use of food containing high concentrations of tyramine (see Appendix L); Lactation: Safety not established; Pedi: Children <16 yr (isocarboxazid only; safety and effectiveness not established).
Use Cautiously in: Patients who may be suicidal or have a history of drug dependency; Schizophrenia; Bipolar disorder; Diabetes mellitus (↑ risk of hypoglycemia); Hyperthyroidism; Seizure disorders; OB, Lactation: Safety not established. Discontinue drug or bottle-feed.; Pedi: Safe use in children/adolescents not established. May ↑ risk of suicide attempt/ideation especially during first early treatment or dose adjustments; risk may be greater in children or adolescents. Geri: ↑ risk of adverse reactions.

Adverse Reactions/Side Effects

CNS: SEIZURES, dizziness, headache, anxiety, ataxia, confusion, drowsiness, euphoria, insomnia, restlessness, tremor, weakness. **EENT:** blurred vision, glaucoma, nystagmus. **CV:** HYPERTENSIVE CRISIS, arrhythmias, edema, orthostatic hypotension. **GI:** diarrhea, weight gain, abdominal pain, anorexia, constipation, dry mouth, liver enzyme elevation, nausea, vomiting. **GU:** dysuria, sexual dysfunction, urinary incontinence, urinary retention. **Derm:** pruritis, rashes. **Endo:** hypoglycemia. **MS:** arthralgia. **Neuro:** paresthesia.

Interactions

Drug-Drug: Serious, potentially fatal adverse reactions may occur with concurrent use of other **antidepressants (SSRIs, SSNRIs, buproprion, tricyclics, tetracyclics, nefazodone, trazodone)**, **carbamazepine**, **cyclobenzaprine**, **sibutramine**, **linezolid**, **procarbazine**, or **selegiline**. Avoid using within 2 wk of each other (wait 5 wk from end of **fluoxetine** therapy). Hypertensive crisis may occur with

M

amphetamines, **methyldopa**, **levodopa**, **dopamine**, **epinephrine**, **norepinephrine**, **methylphenidate**, **reserpine**, or **vasoconstrictors**. Hypertension or hypotension, coma, seizures, respiratory depression, and death may occur with **meperidine** (avoid using within 2–3 wk of MAO inhibitor therapy). Concurrent use with **dextromethorphan** may produce psychosis or bizarre behavior. Hypertension may occur with concurrent use of **buspirone**; avoid using within 10 days of each other. Additive hypotension may occur with **antihypertensives**, **spinal anesthesia**, **opioids**, or **barbiturates**. Additive hypoglycemia may occur with **insulins** or **oral hypoglycemic agents**. Risk of seizures may be ↑ with **tramadol**.

Drug-Natural Products: Serious, potentially fatal adverse effects (serotonin syndrome) may occur with concomitant use of **St. John's wort** and **SAMe**. Hypertensive crises may occur with large amounts of **caffeine**-containing herbs (**cola nut**, **guarana**, **malt**, **coffee**, **tea**). Insomnia, headache, tremor, hypomania may occur with **ginseng**. Hypertensive crises, disorientation, and memory impairment may occur with **tryptophan** or supplements containing **tyrosine** or **phenylalanine**.

Drug-Food: Hypertensive crisis may occur with ingestion of foods containing high concentrations of **tyramine** (see Appendix L). Consumption of foods or beverages with high **caffeine** content increases the risk of hypertension and arrhythmias.

Route/Dosage

Isocarboxazid

PO (Adults and Children ≥16 yr): 10 mg twice daily; may be ↑ every 2–4 days by 10 mg, up to 40 mg/day by the end of the first wk, then may ↑ by up to 20 mg every wk, up to 60 mg/day in 2–4 divided doses. After optimal response is obtained, dose should be slowly decreased to lowest effective amount (40 mg/day or less).

Phenelzine

PO (Adults): 15 mg 3 times daily; ↑ to 60–90 mg/day in divided doses; after maximal benefit achieved, gradually reduce to smallest effective dose (15 mg/day or every other day).

Tranylcypromine

PO (Adults): 30 mg/day in 2 divided doses (morning and afternoon); after 2 wk can ↑ by 10 mg/day, at 1–3 wk intervals, up to 60 mg/day.

Availability

Isocarboxazid

Tablets: 10 mg.

Phenelzine

Tablets: 15 mg.

Tranylcypromine

Tablets: 10 mg.

NURSING IMPLICATIONS

Assessment

- Assess mental status (orientation, mood, behavior) and anxiety level frequently. Assess for suicidal tendencies, especially during early therapy. Restrict amount of drug available to patient.
- Monitor blood pressure and pulse before and frequently during therapy. Report significant changes promptly. Headache is often first symptom of a hypertensive crisis.
- Monitor intake and output ratios and daily weight. Assess patient for urinary retention.
- Monitor weight and BMI initially and throughout treatment.
- For overweight/obese individuals, moitor fasting blood sugar and cholesterol levels.
- ***Lab Test Considerations:*** Assess hepatic function periodically during prolonged or high-dose therapy.
- Monitor serum glucose closely in diabetic patients; hypoglycemia may occur.
- ***Toxicity and Overdose:*** Concurrent ingestion of tyramine-rich foods and many medications may result in a life-threatening hypertensive crisis. Signs and symptoms of hypertensive crisis include chest pain, tachycardia, severe headache, nausea, vomiting, photosensitivity, neck stiffness, sweating, and enlarged pupils. Treatment includes IV phentolamine or a single dose of oral calcium channel blocker (nifedipine). Symptoms of overdose include anxiety, irritability, tachycardia, hypertension or hypotension, respiratory distress, dizziness, drowsiness, hallucinations, confusion, seizures, sluggish reflexes, fever, and diaphoresis. Treatment includes induction of vomiting or gastric lavage and supportive therapy as symptoms arise.

Potential Nursing Diagnoses

Ineffective coping (Indications)

Ineffective therapeutic regimen management (Patient/Family Teaching)
Risk for falls (Side Effects)
Imbalanced nutrition: more than body requirements (Side Effects)
Sexual dysfunction (Side Effects)
Impaired oral mucous membrane (Side Effects)

Implementation

- Do not administer these medications in the evening because the psychomotor stimulating effects may cause insomnia or other sleep disturbances.
- **PO:** Tablets may be crushed and mixed with food or fluids for patients with difficulty swallowing.

Patient/Family Teaching

- Instruct patient to take medication as directed. Take missed doses if remembered within 2 hr; otherwise, omit and return to regular dosage schedule. Do not discontinue abruptly as withdrawal symptoms (nausea, vomiting, malaise, nightmares, agitation, psychosis, seizures) may occur.
- Caution patient to avoid alcohol, CNS depressants, OTC drugs, and foods or beverages containing tyramine (see Appendix L) or excessive caffeine during and for at least 2 wk after therapy has been discontinued; they may precipitate a hypertensive crisis. Instruct patient to notify health care professional immediately if symptoms of hypertensive crisis (e.g. severe headache, palpitations, chest or throat tightness, sweating, dizziness, neck stiffness, nausea, or vomiting) develop.
- Instruct parents or guardians of children to contact health care professional if child exhibits any suicidal thoughts or behaviors (e.g. worsening depression, new or worsening anxiety, agitation, panic attacks, insomnia, new or worsening irritability, violent behavior, impulsive actions, excessive talking, unusual changes in mood or behavior).
- May cause dizziness or drowsiness. Caution patient to avoid driving and other activities requiring alertness until response to medication is known.
- Caution patient to change positions slowly to minimize orthostatic hypotension. Geriatric patients are at increased risk for this side effect.
- Instruct patient to consult with health care professional before taking any new Rx, OTC, or herbal product.
- Advise patient to notify health care professional if dry mouth, urinary retention, or constipation occurs. Frequent rinses, good oral hygiene, and sugarless candy or gum may diminish dry mouth. An increase in fluid intake, fiber, and exercise may prevent constipation.
- Advise patient to notify health care professional of medication regimen before treatment or surgery. If possible, therapy should be discontinued at least 2 wk before surgery.
- Instruct patient to carry identification describing medication regimen at all times.
- Emphasize the importance of participation in psychotherapy to improve coping skills. Refer for ophthalmic testing periodically during long-term therapy.
- Advise patient of possibility of weight gain and cholesterol elevation and recommend appropriate nutritional, weight, or medical management.
- Refer patient/family to local support group.

Evaluation/Desired Outcomes

- Improved mood in depressed patients.
- Increased sense of well-being.
- Decreased anxiety.
- Increased appetite.
- Improved energy level.
- Improved sleep.
- Patients may require 3–6 wk of therapy before therapeutic effects of medication are seen.

M

montelukast

(mon-te-**loo**-kast)
Singulair

Classification
Therapeutic: allergy, cold, and cough remedies, bronchodilators
Pharmacologic: leukotriene antagonists

Pregnancy Category B

Indications

Prevention and chronic treatment of asthma. Management of seasonal allergic rhinitis. Prevention of exercise-induced bronchoconstriction in patients 15 yr and older.

Action
Antagonizes the effects of leukotrienes, which mediate the following: Airway edema, Smooth muscle constriction, Altered cellular activity. Result is decreased inflammatory process, which is part of asthma and allergic rhinitis. **Therapeutic Effects:** Decreased frequency and severity of acute asthma attacks. Decreased severity of allergic rhinitis. Decreased attacks of exercise-induced bronchoconstriction.

Pharmacokinetics
Absorption: Rapidly absorbed (63–73%) following oral administration.
Distribution: Unknown.
Protein Binding: 99%.
Metabolism and Excretion: Mostly metabolized by the liver (by P450 3A4 and 2C9 enzyme systems); metabolites eliminated in feces via bile; negligible renal excretion.
Half-life: 2.7–5.5 hr.

TIME/ACTION PROFILE (improved symptoms of asthma)

ROUTE	ONSET	PEAK†	DURATION
PO (swallow)	within 24 hr	3–4 hr	24 hr
PO (chew)	within 24 hr	2–2.5 hr	24 hr

†Blood levels

Contraindications/Precautions
Contraindicated in: Hypersensitivity; Lactation.
Use Cautiously in: Acute attacks of asthma; Phenylketonuria (chewable tablets contain aspartame); Hepatic impairment (may need lower doses); Reduction of corticosteroid therapy (may increase the risk of eosinophilic conditions); Pregnancy, lactation, or children <1 yr (safety not established).

Adverse Reactions/Side Effects
CNS: fatigue, headache, weakness. **EENT:** otitis (children), sinusitis (children). **Resp:** cough, rhinorrhea. **GI:** abdominal pain, diarrhea (children), dyspepsia, nausea (children), increased liver enzymes. **Derm:** rash. **Misc:** eosinophilic conditions (including CHURG-STRAUSS SYNDROME), fever.

Interactions
Drug-Drug: Drugs which induce the CYP450 enzyme system (**phenobarbital** and **rifampin**) may decrease the effects of montelukast.

Route/Dosage
Asthma and Allergic Rhinitis
PO (Adults and Children ≥14 yr): 10 mg once daily.
PO (Children 6–14 yr): 5 mg once daily (as chewable tablet).
PO (Children 2–5 yr): 4 mg once daily (as chewable tablet or granules).
PO (Children 6–23 months): 4 mg once daily (as oral granules).

Exercise-Induced Bronchoconstriction (EIB)
PO (Adults and Children ≥15 yrs): 10 mg at least 2 hrs before exercise. Do not take within 24 hrs of another dose; if taking daily doses, do not take dose for EIB.

Availability
Tablets: 10 mg. **Cost:** $302.99/90. **Chewable tablets (cherry flavor):** 4 mg, 5 mg. **Cost:** 4 mg $294.97/90, 5 mg $305.97/90. **Oral granules:** 4 mg/packet in 30-packet cartons. **Cost:** $110.00/carton.

NURSING IMPLICATIONS

Assessment
- Assess lung sounds and respiratory function prior to and periodically throughout therapy.
- Assess allergy symptoms (rhinitis, conjunctivitis, hives) before and periodically throughout therapy.
- ***Lab Test Considerations:*** May cause ↑ AST and ALT concentrations.

Potential Nursing Diagnoses
Ineffective airway clearance (Indications)

Implementation
- Doses of inhaled corticosteroids may be gradually decreased with supervision of health care professional; do not discontinue abruptly.
- **PO:** For asthma, administer once daily in the evening. For allergic rhinitis, may be administered at any time of day.
- Administer granules directly into mouth or mixed in a spoonful of cold or room temperature foods (use only applesauce, mashed carrots, rice, or ice cream). Do not open packet until ready to use. After opening packet, administer full dose within 15 min. Do not store mixture. Discard unused portion. Do not dissolve granules in fluid, but fluid may be taken following administration. Granules may be administered without regard to meals.

Patient/Family Teaching

- Instruct patient to take medication daily in the evening, even if not experiencing symptoms of asthma. Do not double doses. Do not discontinue therapy without consulting health care professional.
- Instruct patient not to discontinue or reduce other asthma medications without consulting health care professional.
- Advise patient that montelukast is not used to treat acute asthma attacks, but may be continued during an acute exacerbation. Patient should carry rapid-acting therapy for bronchospasm at all times. Advise patient to notify health care professional if more than the maximum number of short-acting bronchodilator treatments prescribed for a 24-hr period are needed.

Evaluation/Desired Outcomes

- Prevention of and reduction in symptoms of asthma.
- Decrease in severity of allergic rhinitis.
- Prevention of exercise-induced bronchoconstriction.

HIGH ALERT

morphine (mor-feen)

Astramorph, Astramorph PF, Avinza, Duramorph, DepoDur, ✤ Epimorph, Infumorph, Kadian, ✤ M-Eslon, ✤ Morphine H.P, ✤ Morphitec, ✤ M.O.S, ✤ M.O.S.-S.R, MS, MS Contin, ✤ MS•IR, MSIR, MSO_4, OMS Concentrate, Oramorph SR, RMS, Roxanol, Roxanol Rescudose, Roxanol-T, ✤ Statex

Classification

Therapeutic: opioid analgesics
Pharmacologic: opioid agonists

Schedule II

Pregnancy Category C

Indications

Severe pain. Pulmonary edema. Pain associated with MI.

Action

Binds to opiate receptors in the CNS. Alters the perception of and response to painful stimuli while producing generalized CNS depression.
Therapeutic Effects: Decrease in severity of pain.

Pharmacokinetics

Absorption: Variably absorbed (about 30%) following oral administration. More reliably absorbed from rectal, subcut, and IM sites. Following epidural administration, systemic absorption and absorption into the intrathecal space via the meninges occurs.
Distribution: Widely distributed. Crosses the placenta; enters breast milk in small amounts.
Protein Binding: Premature infants: <20%; Adults: 35%.
Metabolism and Excretion: Mostly metabolized by the liver. Active metabolites excreted renally.
Half-life: Premature neonates: 10–20 hr; Neonates: 7.6 hr; Infants 1–3 mo: 6.2 hr; Children 6 mo–2.5 yr: 2.9 hr; Children 3–6 yr: 1–2 hr; Children 6–19 yr with sickle cell disease: 1.3 hr; Adults: 2–4 hr.

TIME/ACTION PROFILE (analgesia)

ROUTE	ONSET	PEAK	DURATION
PO	unknown	60 min	4–5 hr
PO-ER, SR	unknown	3–4 hr	8–24 hr
IM	10–30 min	30–60 min	4–5 hr
Subcut	20 min	50–90 min	4–5 hr
Rect	unknown	20–60 min	3–7 hr
IV	rapid	20 min	4–5 hr
Epidural	6–30 min	1 hr	up to 24 hr (48 hr for liposomal injection)
IT	rapid (min)	unknown	up to 24 hr

Contraindications/Precautions

Contraindicated in: Hypersensitivity; Some products contain tartrazine, bisulfites, or alcohol and should be avoided in patients with known hypersensitivity.
Use Cautiously in: Head trauma; Increased intracranial pressure; Severe renal, hepatic, or pulmonary disease; Hypothyroidism; Adrenal insufficiency; History of substance abuse; Geri: Geriatric or debilitated patients (dose reduction suggested); Undiagnosed abdominal pain; Prostatic hyperplasia; Patients undergoing procedures that rapidly decrease pain (cordotomy, radiation); long-acting agents should be discontinued 24 hr before and replaced with short-acting agents; OB: Pregnancy or lactation (avoid

chronic use; has been used during labor but may cause respiratory depression in the newborn); Pedi: Children <18 yr (epidural liposomal injection only-not recommended); Neonates and infants <3 mo (more susceptible to respiratory depression); Neonates (oral solution contains sodium benzoate which can cause potentially fatal gasping syndrome).

Adverse Reactions/Side Effects

CNS: confusion, sedation, dizziness, dysphoria, euphoria, floating feeling, hallucinations, headache, unusual dreams. **EENT:** blurred vision, diplopia, miosis. **Resp:** RESPIRATORY DEPRESSION. **CV:** hypotension, bradycardia. **GI:** constipation, nausea, vomiting. **GU:** urinary retention. **Derm:** flushing, itching, sweating. **Misc:** physical dependence, psychological dependence, tolerance.

Interactions

Drug-Drug: Use with **extreme caution** in patients receiving **MAO inhibitors** within 14 days prior (may result in unpredictable, severe reactions— ↓ initial dose of morphine to 25% of usual dose). ↑ CNS depression with **alcohol**, **sedative/hypnotics**, **clomipramine**, **barbiturates**, **tricyclic antidepressants**, and **antihistamines**. Administration of **partial-antagonist opioid analgesics** may precipitate opioid withdrawal in physically dependent patients. **Buprenorphine**, **nalbuphine**, **butorphanol**, or **pentazocine** may ↓ analgesia. May ↑ the anticoagulant effect of **warfarin**. **Cimetidine** ↓ metabolism and may ↑ effects. Epidural test dose of lidocaine/epinephrine may alter release of liposomal injection.
Drug-Natural Products: Concomitant use of **kava kava**, **valerian** or **chamomile** can ↑ CNS depression.

Route/Dosage

Larger doses may be required during chronic therapy.
PO, Rect (Adults ≥50 kg): *Usual starting dose for moderate to severe pain in opioid-naive patients*—30 mg q 3–4 hr initially *or* once 24-hr opioid requirement is determined, convert to controlled, extended *or* sustained-release morphine by administering total daily oral morphine dose every 24 hr (as *Kadian* or *Avinza*), 50% of the total daily oral morphine dose every 12 hr (as *Oramorph SR, Kadian, MS Contin*), or 33% of the total daily oral morphine dose every 8 hr (as *MS Contin*). See equianalgesic chart, Appendix J. *Avinza* dose should not exceed 1600 mg/day because of fumaric acid in formulation.
PO, Rect (Adults and Children <50 kg): *Usual starting dose for moderate to severe pain in opioid-naive patients*—0.3 mg/kg q 3–4 hr initially.
PO (Children >1 mo): *Prompt-release tablets and solution*—0.2–0.5 mg/kg/dose q 4–6 hr as needed. *Controlled-release tablet*—0.3–0.6 mg/kg/dose q 12 hr.
IM, IV, Subcut (Adults ≥50 kg): *Usual starting dose for moderate to severe pain in opioid-naive patients*—4–10 mg q 3–4 hr. *MI*—8–15 mg, for very severe pain additional smaller doses may be given every 3–4 hr.
IM, IV, Subcut (Adults and Children <50 kg): *Usual starting dose for moderate to severe pain in opioid-naive patients*—0.05–0.2 mg/kg q 3–4 hr, maximum: 15 mg/dose.
IM, IV, Subcut (Neonates): 0.05 mg/kg q 4–8 hr, maximum dose: 0.1 mg/kg. Use preservative-free formulation.
IV, Subcut (Adults): *Continuous infusion*—0.8–10 mg/hr; may be preceded by a bolus of 15 mg (infusion rates vary greatly; up to 400 mg/hr have been used).
IV, Subcut (Children >1 mo): *Continuous infusion, postoperative pain*—0.01–0.04 mg/kg/hr. *Continuous infusion, sickle cell or cancer pain*—0.02–2.6 mg/kg/hr.
IV (Neonates): *Continuous infusion*—0.01–0.03 mg/kg/hr.
Epidural: (Adults): *Intermittent injection*—5 mg/day (initially); if relief is not obtained at 60 min, 1–2 mg increments may be made; (total dose not to exceed 10 mg/day. *Continuous infusion*—2–4 mg/24 hr; may increase by 1–2 mg/day (up to 30 mg/day); *single-dose extended-release liposomal injection*—lower extremity orthopedic surgery: 15 mg, lower abdominal/pelvic surgery: 10–15 mg, cesarean section:10 mg. Use preservative-free formulation.
Epidural: (Children >1 mo): 0.03–0.05 mg/kg, maximum dose: 0.1 mg/kg or 5 mg/24 hr. Use preservative-free formulation.
IT (Adults): 0.2–1 mg. Use preservative-free formulation.

Availability (generic available)

Soluble tablets: 10 mg, 15 mg, 30 mg. **Tablets:** 15 mg, 30 mg. **Cost:** *MSIR*—15 mg $18.32/100, 30 mg $31.22/100. **Extended (controlled, sustained)-release tablets:** 15 mg, 30 mg, 60 mg, 100 mg, 200 mg. **Cost:** *MS*

Contin—15 mg $99.63/100, 30 mg $189.34/100, 60 mg $369.44/100, 100 mg $546.99/100, 200 mg $1001.71/100; *Oramorph SR*—15 mg $90.03/100, 30 mg $171.09/100, 60 mg $333.83/100, 100 mg $511.24/100. **Sustained-release capsules (Kadian):** 10 mg, 20 mg, 30 mg, 50 mg, 60 mg, 80 mg, 200 mg. **Cost:** *Kadian*—20 mg $105.49/60, 30 mg $119.00/60, 50 mg $223.05/60, 60 mg $227.39/60, 100 mg $383.80/60. **Extended-release capsules (Avinza):** 30 mg, 60 mg, 90 mg, 120 mg. **Cost:** *Avinza*—30 mg $231.00/100, 60 mg $445.00/100, 90 mg $675.00/100, 120 mg $790.00/100. **Oral solution (Roxanol-T—20 mg/ml fruit and mint flavor; also unflavored):** 10 mg/5 ml, 20 mg/5 ml, 100 mg/5 ml, ♣ 2 mg/ml, ♣ 4 mg/ml, 20 mg/ml (concentrate). **Cost:** *Roxanol*—20 mg/ml $20.76/30 ml. **Rectal suppositories:** 5 mg, 10 mg, 20 mg, 30 mg. **Solution for IM, subcut, IV injection:** 1 mg/ml, 2 mg/ml, 4 mg/ml, 5 mg/ml, 8 mg/ml, 10 mg/ml, 15 mg/ml, 25 mg/ml, 50 mg/ml. **Solution for epidural, IV injection (preservative-free):** 0.5 mg/ml, 1 mg/ml. **Solution for epidural or IT use (continuous microinfusion device; preservative-free):** 10 mg/ml in 20-ml vial, 25 mg/ml in 20-ml vial. **Extended-release liposome injection for epidural use:** 10 mg/ml in 1–, 2.5– and 2-ml vials. **Solution for IV injection (PCA device):** 1 mg/ml, 2 mg/ml, 3 mg/ml, 5 mg/ml.

NURSING IMPLICATIONS

Assessment

- Assess type, location, and intensity of pain prior to and 1 hr following PO, subcut, IM, and 20 min (peak) following IV administration. When titrating opioid doses, increases of 25–50% should be administered until there is either a 50% reduction in the patient's pain rating on a numerical or visual analogue scale or the patient reports satisfactory pain relief. When titrating doses of short-acting morphine, a repeat dose can be safely administered at the time of the peak if previous dose is ineffective and side effects are minimal.
- Patients on a continuous infusion should have additional bolus doses provided every 15–30 min, as needed, for breakthrough pain. The bolus dose is usually set to the amount of drug infused each hour by continuous infusion.
- Patients taking sustained-release morphine may require additional short-acting opioid doses for breakthrough pain. Doses should be equivalent to 10–20% of 24 hr total and given every 2 hr as needed.
- An equianalgesic chart (see Appendix J) should be used when changing routes or when changing from one opioid to another.
- ***High Alert:*** Assess level of consciousness, blood pressure, pulse, and respirations before and periodically during administration. If respiratory rate is <10/min, assess level of sedation. Physical stimulation may be sufficient to prevent significant hypoventilation. Subsequent doses may need to be decreased by 25–50%. Initial drowsiness will diminish with continued use. Geri: Assess geriatric patients frequently; older adults are more sensitive to the effects of opioid analgesics and may experience side effects and respiratory complications more frequently. Pedi: Assess pediatric patient frequently; children are more sensitive to the effects of opioid analgesics and may experience respiratory complications, excitability and restlessness more frequently.
- Prolonged use may lead to physical and psychological dependence and tolerance. This should not prevent patient from receiving adequate analgesia. Most patients who receive morphine for pain do not develop psychological dependence. Progressively higher doses may be required to relieve pain with long-term therapy.
- Assess bowel function routinely. Institute prevention of constipation with increased intake of fluids and bulk and with laxatives to minimize constipating effects. Administer stimulant laxatives routinely if opioid use exceeds 2–3 days, unless contraindicated.
- ***Lab Test Considerations:*** May ↑ plasma amylase and lipase levels.
- ***Toxicity and Overdose:*** If an opioid antagonist is required to reverse respiratory depression or coma, naloxone (Narcan) is the antidote. Dilute the 0.4-mg ampule of naloxone in 10 ml of 0.9% NaCl and administer 0.5 ml (0.02 mg) by direct IV push every 2 min. For children and adults weighing <40 kg, dilute 0.1 mg of naloxone in 10 ml of 0.9% NaCl

M

for a concentration of 10 mcg/ml and administer 0.5 mcg/kg every 2 min. Titrate dose to avoid withdrawal, seizures, and severe pain.

Potential Nursing Diagnoses

Acute pain (Indications)
Disturbed sensory perception (visual, auditory) (Side Effects)
Risk for injury (Side Effects)

Implementation

- ***High Alert:*** Do not confuse morphine with hydromorphone or meperidine—errors have resulted in death. Other errors associated with morphine include overdose and infusion pump miscalculations. Consider patients' previous analgesic use and current requirements, but clarify doses that greatly exceed normal range. Have second practitioner independently check original order, dose calculations and infusion pump settings. Pedi: Use only preservative-free formulations in neonates, and for epidural and intrathecal routes in all patients. Medication errors with opioid analgesics are common in the pediatric population and include misinterpretation or miscalculation of doses and use of inappropriate measuring devices.
- Explain therapeutic value of medication prior to administration to enhance the analgesic effect.
- Regularly administered doses may be more effective than prn administration. Analgesic is more effective if given before pain becomes severe.
- Coadministration with nonopioid analgesics may have additive analgesic effects and may permit lower doses.
- When transferring from other opioids or other forms of morphine to extended-release tablets, administer a total daily dose of oral morphine equivalent to previous daily dose (see Appendix J) and divided every 8 hr (MS Contin), every 12 hr (Kadian, MS Contin, Oramorph SR), every 24 hr (Kadian or Avinza).
- Morphine should be discontinued gradually to prevent withdrawal symptoms after long-term use.
- **PO:** Doses may be administered with food or milk to minimize GI irritation.
- Administer oral solution with properly calibrated measuring device; may be diluted in a glass of fruit juice just prior to administration to improve taste.
- Extended-release and controlled-release tablets should be swallowed whole; do not crush, break, dissolve or chew (could result in rapid release and absorption of a potentially toxic dose).
- *Kadian and Avinza* capsules may be opened and the pellets sprinkled onto applesauce immediately prior to administration. Patients should rinse mouth and swallow to assure ingestion of entire dose. Pellets should not be chewed, crushed, or dissolved. *Kadian* capsules may also be opened and sprinkled on approximately 10 ml of water and flushed while swirling through a pre-wetted 16 French gastrostomy tube fitted with a funnel at the port end. Additional water should be used to transfer and flush any remaining pellets. *Kadian* should not be administered via a nasogastric tube.
- **Rect:** *MS Contin* and *Oramorph SR* have been administered rectally.
- **IM, Subcut:** Use IM route for repeated doses, because morphine is irritating to subcut tissues.

IV Administration

- **IV:** Solution is colorless; do not administer discolored solution.
- **Direct IV:** ***Diluent:*** Dilute with at least 5 ml of sterile water or 0.9% NaCl for injection. ***Concentration:*** 0.5–5 mg/ml. ***Rate: High Alert:*** Administer 2.5–15 mg over 5 min. Rapid administration may lead to increased respiratory depression, hypotension, and circulatory collapse.
- **Continuous Infusion:** ***Diluent:*** May be added to D5W, D10W, 0.9% NaCl, 0.45% NaCl, Ringer's or LR, dextrose/saline solution, or dextrose/Ringer's or LR. ***Concentration:*** 0.1–1 mg/ml or greater for continuous infusion. ***Rate:*** Administer via infusion pump to control the rate. Dose should be titrated to ensure adequate pain relief without excessive sedation, respiratory depression, or hypotension. May be administered via patient-controlled analgesia (PCA) pump.
- **Syringe Compatibility:** atropine, bupivacaine, cimetidine, diphenhydramine, droperidol, glycopyrrolate, hydroxyzine, ketamine, metoclopramide, midazolam, milrinone, ondansetron, perphenazine, ranitidine, scopolamine.
- **Syringe Incompatibility:** pantoprazole, thiopental.
- **Y-Site Compatibility:** aldesleukin, allopurinol, amifostine, amikacin, aminophylline, amiodarone, ampicillin, ampicillin/sulbac-

tam, amsacrine, argatroban, atenolol, atracurium, atropine, aztreonam, bivalirudin, bumetanide, calcium chloride, cefazolin, cefotaxime, cefoxitin, ceftazidime, ceftizoxime, ceftriaxone, cefuroxime, chloramphenicol, cisatracurium, cisplatin, cladribine, clindamycin, cyclophosphamide, cytarabine, dexamethasone sodium phosphate, diazepam, digoxin, diltiazem, diphenhydramine, dobutamine, docetaxel, dopamine, doxorubicin, doxycycline, enalaprilat, epinephrine, erythromycin lactobionate, esmolol, etomidate, etoposide phosphate, famotidine, fenoldopam, fentanyl, filgrastim, fluconazole, fludarabine, foscarnet, gemcitabine, gentamicin, granisetron, haloperidol, heparin, hydrocortisone sodium succinate, hydromorphone, insulin, kanamycin, ketorolac, labetalol, levofloxacin, lidocaine, linezolid, lorazepam, magnesium sulfate, melphalan, meropenem, methotrexate, methyldopate, methylprednisolone, metoclopramide, metoprolol, metronidazole, midazolam, milrinone, nicardipine, nitroglycerin, nitroprusside, norepinephrine, ondansetron, oxaliplatin, oxytocin, paclitaxel, pancuronium, pantoprazole, pemetrexed, penicillin G potassium, phenobarbital, piperacillin/tazobactam, potassium chloride, propranolol, ranitidine, scopolamine, sodium bicarbonate, tacrolimus, teniposide, thiotepa, ticarcillin/clavulanate, tirofiban, tobramycin, trimethoprim/sulfamethoxazole, vancomycin, vecuronium, vinorelbine, vitamin B complex with C, warfarin, zidovudine.

- **Y-Site Incompatibility:** amphotericin B cholesteryl sulfate, azithromycin, doxorubicin liposome, lansoprazole, phenytoin, sargramostim.
- **Epidural:** Invert vial gently to re-suspend liposomal product immediately prior to administration; do not shake. Administer undiluted. If a lidocaine test dose is administered, flush catheter with 0.9% NaCl and wait 15 min before administration of *DepoDur*. Do not use an in-lint filter. Do not admix or administer other medications in epidural space for 48 hr after administration. Administer within 4 hr after removing from vial. Store in refrigerator; do not freeze.

Patient/Family Teaching

- Instruct patient how and when to ask for pain medication.
- ***High Alert:*** Instruct family not to administer PCA doses to the sleeping patient. Overmedication, sedation, and respiratory depression can result.
- May cause drowsiness or dizziness. Caution patient to call for assistance when ambulating or smoking and to avoid driving or other activities requiring alertness until response to medication is known.
- Advise patient to change positions slowly to minimize orthostatic hypotension.
- Caution patient to avoid concurrent use of alcohol or other CNS depressants with this medication.
- Encourage patients who are immobilized or on prolonged bedrest to turn, cough, and breathe deeply every 2 hr to prevent atelectasis.
- **Home Care Issues: *High Alert:*** Explain to patient and family how and when to administer morphine and how to care for infusion equipment properly. Pedi: Teach parents or caregivers how to accurately measure liquid medication and to use only the measuring device dispensed with the medication.
- Emphasize the importance of aggressive prevention of constipation with the use of morphine.

Evaluation/Desired Outcomes

- Decrease in severity of pain without a significant alteration in level of consciousness or respiratory status.
- Decrease in symptoms of pulmonary edema.

moxifloxacin, See FLUOROQUINOLONES.

mupirocin (myoo-**peer**-oh-sin)

Bactroban, Bactroban Nasal

Classification
Therapeutic: anti-infectives

Pregnancy Category B

Indications

Topical: Treatment of: Impetigo, Secondarily infected traumatic skin lesions (up to 10 cm in length or 100 cm^2 area) caused by *Staphylococcus aureus* and *Streptococcus pyogenes*. **Intranasal:** Eradicates nasal colonization with methicillin-resistant *S. aureus*.

Action

Inhibits bacterial protein synthesis. **Therapeutic Effects:** Inhibition of bacterial growth and reproduction. **Spectrum:** Greatest activity against gram-positive organisms, including: *S. aureus*, Beta-hemolytic streptococci. Resolution of impetigo. Eradication of *S. aureus* carrier state.

Pharmacokinetics

Absorption: Minimal systemic absorption.
Distribution: Remains in the stratum corneum after topical use for prolonged periods of time (72 hr).
Metabolism and Excretion: Metabolized in the skin, removed by desquamation.
Half-life: 17–36 min.

TIME/ACTION PROFILE (anti-infective effect)

ROUTE	ONSET	PEAK	DURATION
Nasal	unknown	unknown	12 hr
Topical†	unknown	3–5 days	72 hr

†Resolution of lesions

Contraindications/Precautions

Contraindicated in: Hypersensitivity to mupirocin or polyethylene glycol.
Use Cautiously in: Pregnancy or lactation (safety not established); Impaired renal function; Burn patients.

Adverse Reactions/Side Effects

CNS: *nasal only*— headache. **EENT:** *nasal only*— cough, itching, pharyngitis, rhinitis, upper respiratory tract congestion. **GI:** nausea; *nasal only*— altered taste. **Derm:** *topical only*— burning, itching, pain, stinging.

Interactions

Drug-Drug: Nasal mupirocin should not be used concurrently with other **nasal products**.

Route/Dosage

Topical (Adults and Children ≥2 mo): *Ointment:*—Apply 3–5 times daily for 5–14 days.
Topical (Adults and Children ≥3 mo): *Cream:*—Apply small amount 3 times/day for 10 days.
Intranasal (Adults and Children ≥1 yr): Apply small amount nasal ointment to each nostril 2–4 times/day for 5–14 days.

Availability (generic available)

Ointment: 2% in 0.9-g, 15-g, 22-g, and 30-g tubes, ✤2% in 15- and 30-g tubes[OTC]. **Cost:** *Generic*—$34.99/22 g. **Cream:** 2% in 15- and 30-g tubes. **Cost:** $47.99/15 g, $77.13/30 g. **Nasal ointment:** 2% in 1-g single-use tubes.

NURSING IMPLICATIONS

Assessment

- Assess lesions before and daily during therapy.

Potential Nursing Diagnoses

Impaired skin integrity (Indications)
Risk for infection (Indications, Patient/Family Teaching)

Implementation

- **Topical:** Wash affected area with soap and water and dry thoroughly. Apply a small amount of mupirocin to the affected area 3 times daily and rub in gently. Treated area may be covered with gauze if desired.
- **Nasal:** Apply one half of the ointment from the single-use tube to each nostril twice daily (morning and evening) for 5 days. After application, close nostrils by pressing together and releasing sides of the nose repeatedly for 1 min.

Patient/Family Teaching

- Instruct patient on the correct application of mupirocin. Advise patient to apply medication exactly as directed for the full course of therapy. If a dose is missed, apply as soon as possible unless almost time for next dose. Avoid contact with eyes.
- **Topical:** Teach patient and family appropriate hygienic measures to prevent spread of impetigo.
- Instruct parents to notify school nurse for screening and prevention of transmission.
- Patient should consult health care professional if symptoms have not improved in 3–5 days.

Evaluation/Desired Outcomes

- Healing of skin lesions. If no clinical response is seen in 3–5 days, condition should be re-evaluated.
- Eradication of methicillin-resistant *S. aureus* carrier state in patients and health care workers during institutional outbreaks.

muromonab-CD3

(myoo-roe-**moe**-nab CD3)
Orthoclone OKT3

Classification
Therapeutic: immunosuppressants
Pharmacologic: monoclonal antibodies

Pregnancy Category C

Indications
Acute renal allograft rejection reactions in transplant patients that have occurred despite conventional antirejection therapy. Acute corticosteroid-resistant hepatic or cardiac allograft rejection reactions.

Action
A purified immunoglobulin antibody that acts as an immunosuppressant by interfering with normal T-cell function. **Therapeutic Effects:** Reversal of graft rejection in transplant patients.

Pharmacokinetics
Absorption: Administered IV only, resulting in complete bioavailability.
Distribution: Unknown.
Metabolism and Excretion: Eliminated by binding to T lymphocytes.
Half-life: 18 hr.

TIME/ACTION PROFILE (noted as levels of circulating CD3-positive T cells)

ROUTE	ONSET	PEAK	DURATION
IV	mins	2–7 days	1 wk

Contraindications/Precautions
Contraindicated in: Hypersensitivity to muromonab-CD3, murine (mouse) proteins, or polysorbate; Previous muromonab therapy; Fluid overload; Fever >37.8°C or 100°F; Chickenpox or recent exposure to chickenpox; Herpes zoster.
Use Cautiously in: Active infections; Depressed bone marrow reserve; Chronic debilitating illnesses; CHF; Pregnancy, lactation, or children <2 yr (safety not established).

Adverse Reactions/Side Effects
CNS: tremor, aseptic meningitis, dizziness. **Resp:** PULMONARY EDEMA, dyspnea, shortness of breath, wheezing. **CV:** chest pain. **GI:** diarrhea, nausea, vomiting. **Misc:** CYTOKINE RELEASE SYNDROME, INFECTIONS, chills, fever, hypersensitivity reactions, increased risk of lymphoma.

Interactions
Drug-Drug: Additive immunosuppression with other **immunosuppressives**. Concurrent **prednisone** and **azathioprine** dosages should be reduced during muromonab therapy (↑ risk of infection and lymphoproliferative disorders). **Cyclosporine** should be reduced or discontinued during muromonab-CD3 therapy (↑ risk of infection and lymphoproliferative disorders). ↑ risk of adverse CNS reactions with **indomethacin**. May ↓ antibody response to and ↑ risk of adverse reactions from **live-virus vaccines**.
Drug-Natural Products: Concommitant use with **astragalus**, **echinacea**, and **melatonin** may interfere with immunosuppression.

Route/Dosage
IV (Adults): 5 mg/day for 10–14 days (pretreatment with corticosteroids, acetaminophen, and/or antihistamines recommended).
IV (Children): 0.1 mg (100 mcg)/kg/day for 10–14 days.

Availability
Solution for injection: 1 mg/ml in 5-ml ampules.

NURSING IMPLICATIONS

Assessment
- Assess for fluid overload (monitor weight and intake and output, assess for edema and rales/crackles). Notify physician if patient has experienced 3% or more weight gain in the previous week. Chest x-ray examination should be obtained within 24 hr before beginning therapy. Fluid-overloaded patients are at high risk of developing pulmonary edema. Monitor vital signs and breath sounds closely.
- Assess for cytokine release syndrome (CRS), usually manifested by high fever and chills, headache, tremor, nausea and vomiting, chest pain, muscle and joint pain, generalized weakness, shortness of breath, dizziness, abdominal pain, malaise, diarrhea, and trembling of hands, but may occasionally cause a severe, life-threatening, shock-like reaction. The severity of this reaction is greatest with initial dose. Reaction occurs within 30–48 hr

M

and may persist for up to 6 hr. Acetaminophen and antihistamines may be used to treat early reactions. Patient temperature should be maintained below 37.8°C (100°F) at administration of each dose. Manifestations of CRS may be prevented or minimized by pretreatment with methylprednisolone sodium succinate 8 mg/kg IV given 1–4 hr before 1st dose of muromonab-CD3. Hydrocortisone 100 mg IV may also be given 30 min after the 1st and possibly 2nd dose to control respiratory side effects. Serious symptoms of CRS may require oxygen, IV fluids, corticosteroids, vasopressors, antihistamines, and intubation.

- Monitor for signs of anaphylactic or hypersensitivity reactions at each dose. Resuscitation equipment should be readily available.
- Monitor for infection (fever, chills, rash, sore throat, purulent discharge, dysuria). Notify physician immediately if these symptoms occur; may necessitate discontinuation of therapy.
- Monitor for development of aseptic meningitis. Onset is usually within 3 days of beginning therapy. Assess for fever, headache, nuchal rigidity, and photophobia.
- ***Lab Test Considerations:*** Monitor CBC with differential and platelet count before and periodically throughout therapy.
- Monitor assays of T cells (CD3, CD4, CD8); target CD3 is <25 cells/mm^3 or plasma levels as determined by ELISA daily; target levels should be ≥800 mg/ml.
- Monitor BUN, serum creatinine, and hepatic enzymes (AST, ALT, alkaline phosphatase, bilirubin), especially during the first 1–3 days of therapy. May cause transient ↑.

Potential Nursing Diagnoses

Risk for infection (Side Effects)
Excess fluid volume (Side Effects)

Implementation

- Physician will reduce dose of corticosteroids and azathioprine and discontinue cyclosporine during 10–14-day course of muromonab-CD3. Cyclosporine may be resumed 3 days before end of therapy.
- Initial dose is administered during hospitalization; patient should be monitored closely for 48 hr. Subsequent doses may be administered on outpatient basis.
- Keep medication refrigerated at 2–8°C. Do not shake vial. Solution may contain a few fine translucent particles that do not affect potency. Discard unused portion.

IV Administration

- **Direct IV:** Draw solution into syringe via low-protein-binding 0.2- or 0.22-micrometer filter to ensure removal of translucent protein particles that may be present. Discard filter and attach 20-gauge needle for IV administration. ***Concentration:*** 1 mg/ml (undiluted). ***Rate:*** Administer IV push over <1 min. Do not administer as an infusion. **Compatibility:** Do not admix; do not administer in IV line containing other medications. If line must be used for other medications, flush with 0.9% NaCl before and after muromonab-CD3.

Patient/Family Teaching

- Explain purpose of medication to patient. Inform patient of possible initial-dose side effects, which are markedly reduced in subsequent doses. Explain that patient will need to resume lifelong therapy with other immunosuppressive drugs after completion of muromonab-CD3 course.
- Inform patient of potential for CRS. Describe reportable symptoms.
- Instruct patient to continue to avoid crowds and persons with known infections, as this drug also suppresses the immune system.
- Advise patient to notify health care professional at first sign of rash, urticaria, tachycardia, dyspnea, or difficulty swallowing.
- May cause dizziness. Caution patient to avoid driving or other activities requiring alertness until response is known.
- Instruct patient not to receive any vaccinations and to avoid contact with persons receiving oral polio vaccine without advice of health care professional.

Evaluation/Desired Outcomes

- Reversal of the symptoms of acute organ rejection.

mycophenolate mofetil

(mye-koe-**fee**-noe-late **moe**-fe-til)
CellCept

mycophenolic acid

(mye-koe-**fee**-noe-lik)
Myfortic

Classification
Therapeutic: immunosuppressants

Pregnancy Category C (mycophenolic acid), D (mycophenolate mofetil)

Indications

Mycophenolate mofetil: Prevention of rejection in allogenic renal, hepatic, and cardiac transplantation (used concurrently with cyclosporine and corticosteroids). **Mycophenolic acid:** Prevention of rejection in allogenic renal transplantation (used concurrently with cyclosporine and corticosteroids).

Action

Inhibits the enzyme inosine monophosphate dehydrogenase, which is involved in purine synthesis. This inhibition results in suppression of T- and B-lymphocyte proliferation. **Therapeutic Effects:** Prevention of heart, kidney, or liver transplant rejection.

Pharmacokinetics

Absorption: Following oral and IV administration, mycophenolate mofetil is rapidly hydrolyzed to mycophenolic acid (MPA), the active metabolite. Absorption of enteric-coated mycophenolic acid (Myfortic) is delayed compared to mycophenolate mofetil (CellCept).
Distribution: Cross the placenta and enter breast milk.
Protein Binding: *MPA*—97%.
Metabolism and Excretion: MPA is extensively metabolized; <1% excreted unchanged in urine. Some enterohepatic recirculation of MPA occurs.
Half-life: *MPA*—8–18 hr.

TIME/ACTION PROFILE (blood levels of MPA)

ROUTE	ONSET	PEAK	DURATION
mycophenolate mofetil-PO	rapid	0.25–1.25 hr	N/A
mycophenolic acid	rapid	1.5–2.75 hr	N/A

Contraindications/Precautions

Contraindicated in: Hypersensitivity; Hypersensitivity to polysorbate 80 (for IV mycophenolate mofetil); OB: Pregnancy or lactation.
Use Cautiously in: Active serious pathology of the GI tract (including history of ulcer disease or GI bleeding); Phenylketonuria (oral suspension contains aspartame); Severe chronic renal impairment (dose not to exceed 1 g twice daily (CellCept) if CCr <25 ml/min/1.73 m^2); careful monitoring recommended; Delayed graft function following transplantation (observe for increased toxicity); Geri: Increased risk of adverse reactions related to immunosuppression; OB: Pregnancy or patients with childbearing potential; Lactation: Lactation (safety not established); Pedi: Children (mycophenolate mofetil approved in children ≥3 mo for renal transplant; mycophenolic acid approved in children ≥5 yr for renal transplant; safety not established for other age groups).

Adverse Reactions/Side Effects

CNS: anxiety, dizziness, headache, insomnia, paresthesia, tremor. **CV:** edema, hypertension, hypotension, tachycardia. **Derm:** rashes. **Endo:** hypercholesterolemia, hyperglycemia, hyperkalemia, hypocalcemia, hypokalemia, hypomagnesemia. **GI:** GI BLEEDING, anorexia, constipation, diarrhea, nausea, vomiting, abdominal pain. **GU:** renal dysfunction. **Hemat:** leukocytosis, leukopenia, thrombocytopenia, anemia. **Resp:** cough, dyspnea. **Misc:** fever, infection, increased risk of malignancy.

Interactions

Drug-Drug: Combined use with **azathioprine** is not recommended (effects unknown). **Acyclovir** and **ganciclovir** compete with MPA for renal excretion and, in patients with renal dysfunction, may ↑ each other's toxicity. **Magnesium** and **aluminum hydroxide** antacids ↓ the absorption of MPA (avoid simultaneous administration). **Cholestyramine** and **colestipol** ↓ the absorption of MPA (avoid concurrent use). May interfere with the action of **oral contraceptives** (additional contraceptive method should be used). May ↓ the antibody response to and ↑ risk of adverse reactions from **live-virus vaccines**, although influenza vaccine may be useful.
Drug-Food: When administered with food, peak blood levels of MPA are significantly ↓ (should be administered on an empty stomach).

Route/Dosage

Mycophenolate Mofetil (CellCept)
Renal Transplantation

PO, IV (Adults): 1 g twice daily; IV should be started ≤24 hr after transplantation and

M

🍁 = Canadian drug name.
*CAPITALS indicates life-threatening; underlines indicate most frequent.

switched to PO as soon as possible (IV not recommended for ≥14 days).
PO (Children 3 mo–18 yr): 600 mg/m^2 twice daily (not to exceed 2 g/day).

Hepatic Transplantation

PO, IV (Adults): 1 g twice daily IV, or 1.5 g twice daily PO. IV should be started ≤24 hr after transplantation and switched to PO as soon as possible (IV not recommended for ≥14 days).

Cardiac Transplantation

PO, IV (Adults): 1.5 g twice daily; IV should be started ≤24 hr after transplantation and switched to PO as soon as possible (IV not recommended for ≥14 days).

Renal Impairment

PO, IV (Adults): *CCr <25 ml/min*—daily dose should not exceed 2 g.

Mycophenolic Acid (Myfortic)

Mycophenolate mofetil and mycophenolic acid should not be used interchangeably without the advice of a health care professional

Renal Transplantation

PO (Adults): 720 mg twice daily.
PO (Children 5–16 yr and ≥1.19 m^2): 400 mg/m^2 twice daily (not to exceed 720 mg twice daily).

Availability

Mycophenolate Mofetil (Cellcept)

Capsules: 250 mg. **Tablets:** 500 mg. **Oral suspension (fruit flavor):** 200 mg/ml in 225 ml bottles. **Powder for injection:** 500 mg vial.

Mycophenolic acid (Myfortic)

Delayed-release tablets (Myfortic): 180 mg, 360 mg.

NURSING IMPLICATIONS

Assessment

- Assess for symptoms of organ rejection throughout therapy.
- ***Lab Test Considerations:*** Monitor CBC with differential weekly during the 1st month, twice monthly for the 2nd and 3rd month of therapy, and then monthly during the 1st yr. Neutropenia occurs most frequently from 31–180 days post-transplant. If ANC is <1000/mm^3, dose should be reduced or discontinued.
- Monitor hepatic and renal status and electrolytes periodically during therapy. May cause ↑ serum alkaline phosphatase, AST, ALT, LDH, BUN, and creatinine. May also cause hyperkalemia, hypokalemia, hypocalcemia, hypomagnesemia, hyperglycemia, and hyperlipidemia.

Potential Nursing Diagnoses

Risk for infection (Adverse Reactions)

Implementation

- The initial dose of mycophenolate (usually IV) should be given within 24 hr of transplant.
- Women of childbearing years should have a negative serum or urine pregnancy test within 1 wk prior to initiation of therapy.
- **PO:** Administer on an empty stomach, 1 hr before or 2 hr after meals. Capsules and delayed-release tablets should be swallowed whole; do not open, crush, or chew. Mycophenolate may be teratogenic; contents of capsules should not be inhaled or come in contact with skin or mucous membranes.
- Do not administer mycophenolate concurrently with antacids containing magnesium or aluminum.

IV Administration

- **IV:** IV route should only be used for patients unable to take oral medication and should be switched to oral dose form as soon as patient can tolerate capsules or tablets
- **Intermittent Infusion:** ***Diluent:*** Reconstitute each vial with 14 ml of D5W. Shake gently to dissolve. Solution is slightly yellow; discard if solution is discolored or contains particulate matter. Dilute contents of 2 vials (1-g dose) further with 140 ml of D5W or 3 vials (1.5-g dose) with 210 ml of D5W. ***Concentration:*** 6 mg/ml. Solution is stable for 4 hr. ***Rate:*** Administer via slow IV infusion over 2 hr.
- **Y-Site Incompatibility:** Do not admix or administer mycophenolate in same catheter as other medications.

Patient/Family Teaching

- Instruct patient to take medication as directed, at the same time each day. Do not skip or double up on missed doses. Do not discontinue without consulting health care professional.
- Reinforce the need for lifelong therapy to prevent transplant rejection. Review symptoms of rejection for the transplanted organ, and stress need to notify health care professional immediately if signs of rejection or infection occur.

- Inform female patients of the importance of simultaneously using two reliable forms of contraception, unless abstinence is the chosen method, prior to beginning, during, and for 6 wk following discontinuation of therapy.
- Advise patient to avoid contact with persons with contagious diseases.
- Inform patient of the increased risk of lymphoma and other malignancies. Advise patient to use sunscreen and wear protective clothing to decrease risk of skin cancer.
- Advise patient to consult health care professional prior to taking other medications concurrently with mycophenolate.
- Emphasize the importance of routine follow-up laboratory tests.

Evaluation/Desired Outcomes

- Prevention of rejection of transplanted organs.

nabumetone
(na-**byoo**-me-tone)
Relafen

Classification
Therapeutic: antirheumatics, nonsteroidal anti-inflammatory agents

Pregnancy Category C

Indications
Symptomatic management of rheumatoid arthritis and osteoarthritis.

Action
Inhibits prostaglandin synthesis. **Therapeutic Effects:** Suppression of pain and inflammation.

Pharmacokinetics
Absorption: Nabumetone (a prodrug) is 80% absorbed after oral administration; 35% is rapidly converted to 6-methoxy-2-naphthylacetic acid (6-MNA), which is the active drug.
Distribution: Unknown.
Protein Binding: >99%.
Metabolism and Excretion: 6-MNA is metabolized by the liver to inactive compounds.
Half-life: 24 hr (increased in severe renal impairment).

TIME/ACTION PROFILE (analgesia/anti-inflammatory effects)

ROUTE	ONSET	PEAK	DURATION
PO	1–2 days	few days–2 wk	12–24 hr

Contraindications/Precautions
Contraindicated in: Hypersensitivity; Use with other NSAIDs, including aspirin; cross-sensitivity may occur; Active GI bleeding or ulcer disease; Perioperative pain from coronary artery bypass graft (CABG) surgery.
Use Cautiously in: Severe renal, or hepatic disease; History of ulcer disease; Pregnancy, lactation, or children (safety not established; avoid using during 2nd half of pregnancy).

Adverse Reactions/Side Effects
CNS: agitation, anxiety, confusion, depression, dizziness, drowsiness, fatigue, headache, insomnia, malaise, weakness. **EENT:** abnormal vision, tinnitus. **Resp:** dyspnea, hypersensitivity pneumonitis. **CV:** edema, fluid retention, vasculitis. **GI:** GI BLEEDING, abdominal pain, diarrhea, abnormal liver function tests, anorexia, constipation, dry mouth, dyspepsia, flatulence, gastritis, gastroenteritis, increased appetite, nausea, stomatitis, vomiting. **GU:** albuminuria, azotemia, interstitial nephritis. **Derm:** EXFOLIATIVE DERMATITIS, STEVENS-JOHNSON SYNDROME, TOXIC EPIDERMAL NECROLYSIS, increased sweating, photosensitivity, pruritus, rash. **Hemat:** prolonged bleeding time. **Metab:** weight gain. **Neuro:** paresthesia, tremor. **Misc:** allergic reactions including ANAPHYLAXIS, ANGIONEUROTIC EDEMA.

Interactions
Drug-Drug: ↑ adverse GI effects with **aspirin**, other **NSAIDs**, **potassium supplements**, **corticosteroids**, or **alcohol**. Chronic use with **acetaminophen** may ↑ risk of adverse renal reactions. May ↓ effectiveness of **diuretics** or **antihypertensives**. May ↑ hypoglycemic effects of **insulins** or **oral hypoglycemic agents**. ↑ risk of toxicity from **methotrexate**. ↑ risk of bleeding with **cefotetan**, **cefoperazone**, **valproic acid**, **anticoagulants**, **ticlopidine**, **clopidogrel**, **eptifibatide**, **tirofiban**, or **thrombolytic agents**. ↑ risk of adverse hematologic reactions with **antineoplastics** or **radiation therapy**. Concurrent use with **cyclosporine** may ↑ risk of renal toxicity.

Route/Dosage
PO (Adults): 1000 mg/day as a single dose or divided dose twice daily; may be increased up to 2000 mg/day; use lowest effective dose during chronic therapy.

Availability
Tablets: 500 mg, 750 mg.

NURSING IMPLICATIONS

Assessment
- Patients who have asthma, aspirin-induced allergy, and nasal polyps are at increased risk for developing hypersensitivity reactions. Monitor for rhinitis, asthma, and urticaria.
- Assess pain and range of motion before and periodically throughout therapy.
- ***Lab Test Considerations:*** Evaluate BUN, serum creatinine, CBC, and liver function periodically in patients receiving prolonged therapy.
- Serum potassium, BUN, serum creatinine, alkaline phosphatase, LDH, AST, and ALT tests

may show ↑ levels. Blood glucose, hemoglobin, and hematocrit concentrations, leukocyte and platelet counts, and CCr may be ↓.

- May cause prolonged bleeding time.

Potential Nursing Diagnoses

Acute pain (Indications)
Impaired physical mobility (Indications)

Implementation

- Administration in higher than recommended doses does not provide increased effectiveness but may cause increased side effects. Geri: Use lowest effective dose for shortest period of time.
- **PO:** Administer with meals or antacids to decrease GI irritation and increase absorption.

Patient/Family Teaching

- Advise patient to take this medication with a full glass of water and to remain in an upright position for 15–30 min after administration.
- Instruct patient to take medication as directed. Take missed doses as soon as remembered but not if almost time for the next dose. Do not double doses.
- May cause drowsiness, dizziness, or visual disturbances. Advise patient to avoid driving or other activities requiring alertness until response to the medication is known.
- Advise patient to use sunscreen and protective clothing to prevent photosensitivity reactions.
- Caution patient to avoid the concurrent use of alcohol, aspirin, acetaminophen, or other OTC medications without consulting health care professional.
- Advise patient to inform health care professional of medication regimen before treatment or surgery.
- Advise patient to consult health care professional if rash, itching, visual disturbances, tinnitus, weight gain, edema, black stools, persistent headache, or influenza-like syndrome (chills, fever, muscle aches, pain) occurs.

Evaluation/Desired Outcomes

- Decreased pain and improved joint mobility. Partial arthritic relief is usually seen within 1 wk, but maximum effectiveness may require 2 wk or more of continuous therapy. Patients who do not respond to one NSAID may respond to another.

nadolol (nay-doe-lole)

Corgard, ✤Syn-Nadolol

Classification
Therapeutic: antianginals, antihypertensives
Pharmacologic: beta blockers

Pregnancy Category C

Indications

Management of hypertension. Management of angina pectoris. **Unlabeled uses:** Arrhythmias. Migraine prophylaxis. Tremors (essential, lithium-induced, parkinsonian). Aggressive behavior. Antipsychotic-associated akathisia. Situational anxiety. Esophageal varices. Reduction of intraocular pressure.

Action

Blocks stimulation of $beta_1$ (myocardial) and $beta_2$ (pulmonary, vascular, and uterine) receptor sites. **Therapeutic Effects:** Decreased heart rate and blood pressure.

Pharmacokinetics

Absorption: 30% absorbed after oral administration.
Distribution: Minimal penetration of the CNS. Crosses the placenta and enters breast milk.
Metabolism and Excretion: 70% excreted unchanged by the kidneys.
Half-life: 10–24 hr (increased in renal impairment).

TIME/ACTION PROFILE (anithypertensive effects)

ROUTE	ONSET	PEAK	DURATION
PO†	up to 5 days	6–9 days	24 hr

†With chronic dosing

Contraindications/Precautions

Contraindicated in: Uncompensated CHF; Pulmonary edema; Cardiogenic shock; Bradycardia or heart block.
Use Cautiously in: Renal impairment (CCr <50 ml/min); Hepatic impairment; Geriatric patients (increased sensitivity to beta blockers; initial dosage reduction recommended); Pulmonary disease (including asthma); Diabetes mellitus (may mask signs of hypoglycemia); Thyrotoxicosis (may mask symptoms); Patients with a history of severe allergic reactions (intensity of reactions may be increased); Pregnancy, lactation, or children (safety not established; crosses the placenta and may cause fetal/neonatal bradycardia, hypotension, hypoglycemia, or respiratory depression).

Adverse Reactions/Side Effects

CNS: fatigue, weakness, anxiety, depression, dizziness, drowsiness, insomnia, memory loss, mental status changes, nightmares. **EENT:** blurred vision, dry eyes, nasal stuffiness. **Resp:** bronchospasm, wheezing. **CV:** ARRHYTHMIAS, BRADYCARDIA, CHF, PULMONARY EDEMA, orthostatic hypotension, peripheral vasoconstriction. **GI:** constipation, diarrhea, nausea. **GU:** erectile dysfunction, decreased libido. **Derm:** itching, rashes. **Endo:** hyperglycemia, hypoglycemia. **MS:** arthralgia, back pain, muscle cramps. **Neuro:** paresthesia. **Misc:** drug-induced lupus syndrome.

Interactions

Drug-Drug: General anesthesia, **IV phenytoin**, **diltiazem**, and **verapamil** may cause additive myocardial depression. Additive bradycardia may occur with **digoxin**. Additive hypotension may occur with other **antihypertensives**, acute ingestion of **alcohol**, or **nitrates**. Concurrent use with **amphetamines**, **cocaine**, **ephedrine**, **epinephrine**, **norepinephrine**, **phenylephrine**, or **pseudoephedrine** may result in unopposed alpha-adrenergic stimulation (excessive hypertension, bradycardia). Concurrent use with **clonidine** increases hypotension and bradycardia. Concurrent **thyroid** administration may ↓ effectiveness. May alter the effectiveness of **insulins** or **oral hypoglycemic agents** (dosage adjustments may be necessary). May ↓ the effectiveness of **theophylline**. May ↓ the beneficial beta cardiovascular effects of **dopamine** or **dobutamine**. Use cautiously within 14 days of **MAO inhibitor therapy** (may result in hypertension). Concurrent **NSAIDs** may ↓ antihypertensive action.

Route/Dosage

PO (Adults): *Antianginal*—40 mg once daily initially; may increase by 40–80 mg/day q 3–7 days as needed (up to 240 mg/day). *Antihypertensive*—40 mg once daily initially; may increase by 40–80 mg/day q 7 days as needed (up to 320 mg/day).

Renal Impairment

PO (Adults): *CCr 31–50 ml/min*—increase dosing interval to 24–36 hr; *CCr 10–30 ml/min*—increase dosing interval to 24–48 hr; *CCr <10 ml/min*—increase dosing interval to 40–60 hr.

Availability (generic available)

Tablets: 20 mg, 40 mg, 80 mg, 120 mg, 160 mg. ***In combination with:*** bendroflumethiazide (Corzide). See Appendix B.

NURSING IMPLICATIONS

Assessment

- Monitor blood pressure and pulse frequently during dose adjustment and periodically during therapy. Assess for orthostatic hypotension when assisting patient up from supine position.
- Monitor intake and output ratios and daily weight. Assess patient routinely for evidence of fluid overload (peripheral edema, dyspnea, rales/crackles, fatigue, weight gain, jugular venous distention).
- **Hypertension:** Check frequency of refills to determine compliance.
- **Angina:** Assess frequency and characteristics of angina periodically during therapy.
- ***Lab Test Considerations:*** May cause increased BUN, serum lipoprotein, potassium, triglyceride, and uric acid levels.
- May cause increased ANA titers.
- May cause increase in blood glucose levels.
- ***Toxicity and Overdose:*** Monitor patients receiving beta blockers for signs of overdose (bradycardia, severe dizziness or fainting, severe drowsiness, dyspnea, bluish fingernails or palms, seizures). Notify health care professional immediately if these signs occur.

Potential Nursing Diagnoses

Decreased cardiac output (Side Effects)
Noncompliance (Patient/Family Teaching)

Implementation

- Discontinuation of concurrent clonidine should be done gradually, with beta blocker discontinued first; then, after several days, discontinue clonidine.
- **PO:** Take apical pulse before administering. If <50 bpm or if arrhythmia occurs, withhold medication and notify health care professional.
- May be administered with food or on an empty stomach.
- Tablets may be crushed and mixed with food.

Patient/Family Teaching

- Instruct patient to take medication exactly as directed, at the same time each day, even if

N

feeling well; do not skip or double up on missed doses. Take missed doses as soon as possible up to 8 hr before next dose. Abrupt withdrawal may precipitate life-threatening arrhythmias, hypertension, or myocardial ischemia.

- Advise patient to ensure that enough medication is available for weekends, holidays, and vacations. A written prescription may be kept in wallet for emergencies.
- Teach patient and family how to check pulse and blood pressure. Instruct them to check pulse daily and blood pressure biweekly. Advise patient to hold dose and contact health care professional if pulse is <50 bpm or if blood pressure changes significantly.
- May cause drowsiness or dizziness. Caution patients to avoid driving or other activities that require alertness until response to the drug is known.
- Advise patients to make position changes slowly to minimize orthostatic hypotension, especially during initiation of therapy or when dose is increased.
- Caution patient that this medication may increase sensitivity to cold.
- Instruct patient to consult health care professional before taking any OTC medications, especially cold preparations, concurrently with this medication.
- Patients with diabetes should closely monitor blood glucose, especially if weakness, malaise, irritability, or fatigue occurs. Medication may mask some signs of hypoglycemia, but dizziness and sweating may still occur.
- Advise patient to notify health care professional if slow pulse, difficulty breathing, wheezing, cold hands and feet, dizziness, confusion, depression, rash, fever, sore throat, unusual bleeding, or bruising occurs.
- Instruct patient to inform health care professional of medication regimen before treatment or surgery.
- Advise patient to carry identification describing disease process and medication regimen at all times.
- **Hypertension:** Reinforce the need to continue additional therapies for hypertension (weight loss, sodium restriction, stress reduction, regular exercise, moderation of alcohol consumption, and smoking cessation). Medication controls but does not cure hypertension.
- **Angina:** Caution patient to avoid overexertion with decrease in chest pain.

Evaluation/Desired Outcomes

- Decrease in blood pressure.
- Reduction in frequency of angina.
- Increase in activity tolerance. May require up to 5 days before therapeutic effects are seen.

nafarelin (na-fare-e-lin)

Synarel

Classification

Therapeutic: hormones

Pharmacologic: gonadotropin-releasing hormones

Pregnancy Category X

Indications

Management of endometriosis. Management of central precocious puberty (gonadotropin-dependent) in children.

Action

Acts as a synthetic analogue of gonadotropin-releasing hormone (GnRH). Initially increases pituitary production of luteinizing hormone (LH) and follicle-stimulating hormone (FSH), which cause ovarian steroid production. Chronic administration leads to decreased production of gonadotropins. Endometriotic lesions are sensitive to ovarian hormones. **Therapeutic Effects:** Reduction in lesions and associated pain in endometriosis. Arrest and regression of puberty in children with central precocious puberty.

Pharmacokinetics

Absorption: Well absorbed following intranasal administration.

Distribution: Unknown.

Metabolism and Excretion: 20–40% excreted in feces; 3% excreted unchanged by the kidneys.

Half-life: 3 hr.

TIME/ACTION PROFILE (decreased ovarian steroid production)

ROUTE	ONSET	PEAK	DURATION
Intranasal	within 4 wk	3–4 wk	3–6 mo†

†Relief of symptoms of endometriosis following discontinuation

Contraindications/Precautions

Contraindicated in: Hypersensitivity to GnRH, its analogues, or sorbitol; Pregnancy or lactation.

Use Cautiously in: Rhinitis.

Adverse Reactions/Side Effects

CNS: emotional instability, headaches, depression, insomnia. **EENT:** nasal irritation. **CV:** edema. **GU:** vaginal dryness. **Derm:** acne, hirsutism, seborrhea. **Endo:** cessation of menses, impaired fertility, reduced breast size. **MS:** decreased bone density, myalgia. **Misc:** decreased libido, hot flashes, hypersensitivity reactions, weight gain.

Interactions

Drug-Drug: Concurrent **topical nasal decongestants** may reduce absorption of nafarelin (administer decongestant at least 2 hr after nafarelin).

Route/Dosage

Intranasal (Adults): *Endometriosis*—1 spray (200 mcg) in 1 nostril in the morning and 1 spray in the other nostril in the evening (400 mcg/day). May be increased to 1 spray in each nostril in the morning and evening (800 mcg/day).

Intranasal (Children): *Central precocious puberty*—2 sprays in each nostril in the morning and in the evening (1600-mcg/day); may be increased up to 1800 mcg/day (3 sprays in alternating nostrils 3 times daily).

Availability

Nasal spray: 2 mg/ml 10-ml bottle (200 mcg/spray).

NURSING IMPLICATIONS

Assessment

- **Endometriosis:** Assess patient for endometriotic pain periodically throughout therapy.
- **Central Precocious Puberty:** Prior to therapy, a complete physical and endocrinologic examination including height, weight, hand and wrist x-ray, total sex steroid level (estradiol or testosterone), adrenal steroid level, beta-human chorionic gonadotropin level, GnRH stimulation test, pelvic/adrenal/testicular ultrasound, and CTof the head must be performed. These parameters are monitored after 6–8 wk and every 3–6 mo during therapy.
- Assess patient for signs of precocious puberty (menses, breast development, testicular growth) periodically throughout therapy
- Nafarelin is discontinued when the onset of normal puberty is desired. Monitor the onset of normal puberty and assess menstrual cycle, reproductive function, and final adult height.

Potential Nursing Diagnoses

Acute pain (Indications)
Sexual dysfunction (Indications, Side Effects)

Implementation

- **Endometriosis:** Treatment should be started between days 2 and 4 of the menstrual cycle and continued for up to 6 mo.

Patient/Family Teaching

- Instruct patient on the correct technique for nasal spray: The head should be tilted back slightly; wait 30 sec between sprays.
- Advise patient to consult health care professional if rhinitis occurs during therapy. If a topical decongestant is needed, do not use decongestant until 2 hr after nafarelin dosing. If possible, avoid sneezing during and immediately after nafarelin dose.
- **Endometriosis:** Inform patient that 1 spray should be administered into 1 nostril in the morning and 1 spray into the other nostril in the evening for the 400 mcg/day dose. If dose is increased to 800 mcg/day, administer 1 spray to each nostril (2 sprays) morning and evening; 1 bottle should provide a 30-day supply at the 400 mcg/day dose.
- Advise patient to use a form of contraception other than oral contraceptives during therapy. Inform patient that amenorrhea is expected. Instruct patient to notify health care professional if regular menstruation persists or if successive doses are missed.
- Advise patient that medication may cause hot flashes. Notify health care professional if these become bothersome.
- **Central Precocious Puberty:** Instruct patient on correct timing and number of sprays. The 1600 mcg/day dose is achieved by 2 sprays to each nostril in the morning (4 sprays) and 2 sprays to each nostril in the evening (4 sprays), for a total of 8 sprays. The 1800 mcg/day dose is achieved by 3 sprays into alternating nostrils 3 times per day, for a total of 9 sprays. Inform patient and parents that if doses are not taken as directed pubertal process may be reactivated. One bottle

N

should provide a 7-day supply at the 1600-mcg/day dose.

- Advise patient and parents that during 1st mo of therapy some signs of puberty (vaginal bleeding, breast enlargement) may occur. These should resolve after the 1st mo of therapy. If these signs persist after the 2nd mo of therapy, notify health care professional.

Evaluation/Desired Outcomes

- Reduction in lesions and associated pain in endometriosis.
- Resolution of the signs of precocious puberty.

nafcillin, See PENICILLINS, PENICILLINASE RESISTANT.

naftifine, See ANTIFUNGALS (TOPICAL).

HIGH ALERT

nalbuphine (nal-byoo-feen)

Nubain

Classification

Therapeutic: opioid analgesics

Pharmacologic: opioid agonists/analgesics

Pregnancy Category C

Indications

Moderate to severe pain. Also provides: Analgesia during labor, Sedation before surgery, Supplement to balanced anesthesia.

Action

Binds to opiate receptors in the CNS. Alters the perception of and response to painful stimuli while producing generalized CNS depression. In addition, has partial antagonist properties, which may result in opioid withdrawal in physically dependent patients. **Therapeutic Effects:** Decreased pain.

Pharmacokinetics

Absorption: Well absorbed after IM and subcut administration.

Distribution: Probably crosses the placenta and enters breast milk.

Metabolism and Excretion: Mostly metabolized by the liver and eliminated in the feces via biliary excretion. Minimal amounts excreted unchanged by the kidneys.

Half-life: 5 hr.

TIME/ACTION PROFILE (analgesia)

ROUTE	ONSET	PEAK	DURATION
IM	<15 min	60 min	3–6 hr
Subcut	<15 min	unknown	3–6 hr
IV	2–3 min	30 min	3–6 hr

Contraindications/Precautions

Contraindicated in: Hypersensitivity to nalbuphine or bisulfites; Patients who are physically dependent on opioids and have not been detoxified (may precipitate withdrawal).

Use Cautiously in: Head trauma; Increased intracranial pressure; Severe renal, hepatic, or pulmonary disease; Hypothyroidism; Adrenal insufficiency; Alcoholism; Geriatric or debilitated patients (dose reduction suggested); Undiagnosed abdominal pain; Prostatic hyperplasia; Patients who have recently received opioid agonists; OB: Pregnancy (has been used during labor but may cause respiratory depression in the newborn); Lactation or children (safety not established).

Adverse Reactions/Side Effects

CNS: dizziness, headache, sedation, confusion, dysphoria, euphoria, floating feeling, hallucinations, unusual dreams. **EENT:** blurred vision, diplopia, miosis (high doses). **Resp:** respiratory depression. **CV:** hypertension, orthostatic hypotension, palpitations. **GI:** dry mouth, nausea, vomiting, constipation, ileus. **GU:** urinary urgency. **Derm:** clammy feeling, sweating. **Misc:** physical dependence, psychological dependence, tolerance.

Interactions

Drug-Drug: Use with extreme caution in patients receiving **MAO inhibitors** (may result in unpredictable, severe reactions—reduce initial dose of nalbuphine to 25% of usual dose). Additive CNS depression with **alcohol**, **antihistamines**, and **sedative/hypnotics**. May precipitate withdrawal in patients who are physically dependent on **opioid agonists**. Avoid concurrent use with other **opioid analgesic agonists** (may diminish analgesic effect).

Drug-Natural Products: Concomitant use of **kava kava, valerian, skullcap, chamomile,** or **hops** can ↑ CNS depression.

Route/Dosage

Analgesia

IM, Subcut, IV (Adults): Usual dose is 10 mg q 3–6 hr (single dose not to exceed 20 mg; total daily dose not to exceed 160 mg).

Supplement to Balanced Anesthesia

IV (Adults): *Initial*—0.3–3 mg/kg over 10–15 min. *Maintenance*—0.25–0.5 mg/kg as needed.

Availability (generic available)

Injection: 10 mg/ml in 1- and 10-ml vials, 20 mg/ml in 1- and 10-ml vials and 1-ml preloaded syringes.

NURSING IMPLICATIONS

Assessment

- Assess type, location, and intensity of pain before and 1 hr after IM or 30 min (peak) after IV administration. When titrating opioid doses, increases of 25–50% should be administered until there is either a 50% reduction in the patient's pain rating on a numeric or visual analogue scale or the patient reports satisfactory pain relief. A repeat dose can be safely administered at the time of the peak if previous dose is ineffective and side effects are minimal. Patients requiring doses higher than 20 mg should be converted to an opioid agonist. Nalbuphine is not recommended for prolonged use or as first-line therapy for acute or cancer pain.
- An equianalgesic chart (see Appendix J) should be used when changing routes or when changing from one opioid to another.
- Assess blood pressure, pulse, and respirations before and periodically during administration. If respiratory rate is <10/min, assess level of sedation. Physical stimulation may be sufficient to prevent significant hypoventilation. Dose may need to be decreased by 25–50%. Nalbuphine produces respiratory depression, but this does not markedly increase with increased doses.
- Assess previous analgesic history. Antagonistic properties may induce withdrawal symptoms (vomiting, restlessness, abdominal cramps, and increased blood pressure and temperature) in patients physically dependent on opioids.
- Although this drug has a low potential for dependence, prolonged use may lead to physical and psychological dependence and tolerance. This should not prevent patient from receiving adequate analgesia. Most patients who receive nalbuphine for pain do not develop psychological dependence. If tolerance develops, changing to an opioid agonist may be required to relieve pain.
- ***Lab Test Considerations:*** May cause ↑ serum amylase and lipase concentrations.
- ***Toxicity and Overdose:*** If an opioid antagonist is required to reverse respiratory depression or coma, naloxone (Narcan) is the antidote. Dilute the 0.4-mg ampule of naloxone in 10 ml of 0.9% NaCl and administer 0.5 ml (0.02 mg) by direct IV push every 2 min. For children and patients weighing <40 kg, dilute 0.1 mg of naloxone in 10 ml of 0.9% NaCl for a concentration of 10 mcg/ml and administer 0.5 mcg/kg every 2 min. Titrate dose to avoid withdrawal, seizures, and severe pain.

Potential Nursing Diagnoses

Acute pain (Indications)
Risk for injury (Side Effects)
Disturbed sensory perception (visual, auditory) (Side Effects)

Implementation

- ***High Alert:*** Accidental overdose of opioid analgesics has resulted in fatalities. Before administering, clarify all ambiguous orders; have second practitioner independently check original order, dose calculations, and infusion pump settings.
- Explain therapeutic value of medication before administration to enhance the analgesic effect.
- Regularly administered doses may be more effective than prn administration. Analgesic is more effective if administered before pain becomes severe.
- Coadministration with nonopioid analgesics may have additive effects and permit lower opioid doses.
- **IM:** Administer deep into well-developed muscle. Rotate sites of injections.

IV Administration

- **Direct IV:** May give IV undiluted. ***Concentration:*** 10–20 mg/ml. ***Rate:*** Administer slowly, each 10 mg over 3–5 min.
- **Syringe Compatibility:** atropine, cimetidine, diphenhydramine, droperidol, glycopyrrolate, hydroxyzine, lidocaine, midazolam, prochlorperazine, ranitidine, scopolamine.
- **Syringe Incompatibility:** diazepam, ketorolac, pentobarbital.

- **Y-Site Compatibility:** amifostine, aztreonam, bivalirudin, cisatracurium, cladribine, dexmedetomidine, etoposide phosphate, fenoldopam, filgrastim, fludarabine, gemcitabine, granisetron, lansoprazole, linezolid, melphalan, oxaliplatin, paclitaxel, propofol, remifentanil, teniposide, thiotepa, vinorelbine.
- **Y-Site Incompatibility:** allopurinol, amphotericin B cholesteryl sulfate complex, cefepime, docetaxel, methotrexate, pemetrexed, piperacillin/tazobactam, sargramostim, sodium bicarbonate.

Patient/Family Teaching

- Instruct patient on how and when to ask for pain medication.
- May cause drowsiness or dizziness. Advise patient to call for assistance when ambulating and to avoid driving or other activities requiring alertness until response to the medication is known.
- Caution patient to change positions slowly to minimize orthostatic hypotension.
- Advise patient that frequent mouth rinses, good oral hygiene, and sugarless gum or candy may decrease dry mouth.
- Encourage patient to turn, cough, and breathe deeply every 2 hr to prevent atelectasis.
- Advise patient to avoid concurrent use of alcohol or other CNS depressants with this medication.

Evaluation/Desired Outcomes

- Decrease in severity of pain without significant alteration in level of consciousness or respiratory status.

naloxone (nal-**ox**-one)

Narcan

Classification

Therapeutic: antidotes (for opioids)
Pharmacologic: opioid antagonists

Pregnancy Category B

Indications

Reversal of CNS depression and respiratory depression because of suspected opioid overdose. **Unlabeled uses:** Opioid-induced pruritus (low dose IV infusion). Management of refractory circulatory shock.

Action

Competitively blocks the effects of opioids, including CNS and respiratory depression, without producing any agonist (opioid-like) effects. **Therapeutic Effects:** Reversal of signs of opioid excess.

Pharmacokinetics

Absorption: Well absorbed after IM or subcut administration.
Distribution: Rapidly distributed to tissues. Crosses the placenta.
Metabolism and Excretion: Metabolized by the liver.
Half-life: 60–90 min (up to 3 hr in neonates).

TIME/ACTION PROFILE (reversal of opioid effects)

ROUTE	ONSET	PEAK	DURATION
IV	1–2 min	unknown	45 min
IM, Subcut	2–5 min	unknown	>45 min

Contraindications/Precautions

Contraindicated in: Hypersensitivity.
Use Cautiously in: Cardiovascular disease; Patients physically dependent on opioids (may precipitate severe withdrawal); Pregnancy (may cause withdrawal in mother and fetus if mother is opioid dependent); Lactation (safety not established); Neonates of opioid-dependent mothers.

Adverse Reactions/Side Effects

CV: hypertension, hypotension, ventricular fibrillation, ventricular tachycardia. **GI:** nausea, vomiting.

Interactions

Drug-Drug: Can precipitate withdrawal in patients physically dependent on **opioid analgesics**. Larger doses may be required to reverse the effects of **buprenorphine**, **butorphanol**, **nalbuphine**, **pentazocine**, or **propoxyphene**. Antagonizes postoperative **opioid analgesics**.

Route/Dosage

Postoperative Opioid-Induced Respiratory Depression

IV (Adults): 0.02–0.2 mg q 2–3 min until response obtained; repeat q 1–2 hr if needed.
IV (Children): 0.01 mg/kg; may repeat q 2–3 min until response obtained. Additional doses may be given q 1–2 hr if needed.
IM, IV, Subcut (Neonates): 0.01 mg/kg; may repeat q 2–3 min until response obtained. Additional doses may be given q 1–2 hr if needed.

Opioid-Induced Respiratory Depression During Chronic (>1 wk) Opioid Use
IV, IM, Subcut (Adults >40 kg): 20–40 mcg (0.02–0.04 mg) given as small, frequent (q min) boluses or as an infusion titrated to improve respiratory function without reversing analgesia.
IV, IM, Subcut (Adults and Children <40 kg): 0.005–0.02 mg/dose given as small, frequent (q min) boluses or as an infusion titrated to improve respiratory function without reversing analgesia.

Overdose of Opioids
IV, IM, Subcut (Adults): *Patients not suspected of being opioid dependent*—0.4 mg (10 mcg/kg); may repeat q 2–3 min (IV route is preferred). Some patients may require up to 2 mg. *Patients suspected to be opioid dependent*—Initial dose should be decreased to 0.1–0.2 mg q 2–3 min. May also be given by IV infusion at rate adjusted to patient's response.
IV, IM, Subcut (Children >5 yr or >20 kg): 2 mg/dose, may repeat q 2–3 min.
IV, IM, Subcut (Infants up to 5 yr or 20 kg): 0.1 mg/kg, may repeat q 2–3 min.

Opioid-induced Pruritus
IV (Children): 2 mcg/kg/hr continuous infusion, may increase by 0.5 mcg/kg/hr every few hours if pruritus continues.

Availability (generic available)
Injection: 0.4 mg/ml in 1-ml prefilled syringes and 10-ml vials, 1 mg/ml in 2-ml prefilled syringes. ***In combination with:*** pentazocine (Talwin NX). See Appendix B.

NURSING IMPLICATIONS

Assessment
- Monitor respiratory rate, rhythm, and depth; pulse, ECG, blood pressure; and level of consciousness frequently for 3–4 hr after the expected peak of blood concentrations. After a moderate overdose of a short half-life opioid, physical stimulation may be enough to prevent significant hypoventilation. The effects of some opioids may last longer than the effects of naloxone, and repeat doses may be necessary.
- Patients who have been receiving opioids for >1 wk are extremely sensitive to the effects of naloxone. Dilute and administer carefully.
- Assess patient for level of pain after administration when used to treat postoperative respiratory depression. Naloxone decreases respiratory depression but also reverses analgesia.
- Assess patient for signs and symptoms of opioid withdrawal (vomiting, restlessness, abdominal cramps, increased blood pressure, and temperature). Symptoms may occur within a few minutes to 2 hr. Severity depends on dose of naloxone, the opioid involved, and degree of physical dependence.
- Lack of significant improvement indicates that symptoms are caused by a disease process or other non-opioid CNS depressants not affected by naloxone.
- ***Toxicity and Overdose:*** Naloxone is a pure antagonist with no agonist properties and minimal toxicity.

Potential Nursing Diagnoses
Ineffective breathing pattern (Indications)
Ineffective coping (Indications)
Acute pain

Implementation
- Larger doses of naloxone may be necessary when used to antagonize the effects of buprenorphine, butorphanol, nalbuphine, pentazocine, and propoxyphene.
- Resuscitation equipment, oxygen, vasopressors, and mechanical ventilation should be available to supplement naloxone therapy as needed.
- Doses should be titrated carefully in postoperative patients to avoid interference with control of postoperative pain.

IV Administration
- **Direct IV:** ***Diluent:*** Administer undiluted for *suspected opioid overdose*. For *opioid-induced respiratory depression*, dilute with sterile water for injection. For children or adults weighing <40 kg, dilute 0.1 mg of naloxone in 10 mL of sterile water or 0.9% NaCl for injection. ***Concentration:*** 0.4 mg/ml, 1 mg/ml, or 10 mcg/mL (depending on preparation used). ***Rate:*** Administer over 30 seconds for patients with a *suspected opioid overdose*. For patients who develop *opioid-induced respiratory depression*, administer dilute solution of 0.4 mg/10 mL at a rate of 0.5 mL (0.02 mg) direct IV every 2 min. Titrate to avoid withdrawal and severe pain. Ex-

cessive dose in postoperative patients may cause excitement, pain, hypotension, hypertention, pulmonary edema, ventricular tachycardia and fibrillation, and seizures. For children and adults weighing <40 kg, administer 10 mcg/mL solution at a rate of 0.5 mcg/kg every 1–2 min.

- **Continuous Infusion:** ***Diluent:*** Dilute 2 mg of naloxone in 500 ml of 0.9% NaCl or D5W. Infusion is stable for 24 hr. ***Concentration:*** 4 mcg/ml. ***Rate:*** Titrate dose according to patient response.
- **Y-Site Compatibility:** acyclovir, amikacin, aminophylline, atropine, aztreonam, bumetanide, calcium chloride, calcium gluconate, caspofungin, cefazolin, cefotaxime, cefoxitin, ceftazidime, ceftizoxime, ceftriaxone, cefuroxime, chloramphenicol, cimetidine, clindamycin, cyclosporine, daptomycin, dexamethasone sodium phosphate, digoxin, diltiazem, diphenhydramine, dobutamine, dopamine, doxycycline, enalaprilat, epinephrine, ertapenem, erythromycin, esmolol, famotidine, fenoldopam, fentanyl, fluconazole, furosemide, ganciclovir, gentamicin, granisetron, heparin, hydrocortisone sodium succinate, hydroxyzine, imipenem/cilastatin, insulin, isoproterenol, ketorolac, labetalol, levofloxacin, lidocaine, linezolid, lorazepam, methylprednisolone sodium succinate, metoclopramide, metoprolol, metronidazole, midazolam, nafcillin, nitroglycerin, nitroprusside, norepinephrine, ondansetron, palonosetron, penicillin G potassium, phenylephrine, phytonadione, piperacillin/tazobactam, potassium chloride, procainamide, prochlorperazine, promethazine, propofol, propranolol, protamine, quinupristin/dalfopristin, ranitidine, sodium bicarbonate, tacrolimus, ticarcillin/clavulanate, tirofiban, tobramycin, vancomycin, vasopressin, verapamil, voriconazole.
- **Y-Site Incompatibility:** diazepam, lansoprazole, pantoprazole, phenytoin, trimethoprim/sulfamethoxazole.
- **Additive Incompatibility:** Incompatible with preparations containing bisulfite, sulfite, and solutions with an alkaline pH.

Patient/Family Teaching

- As medication becomes effective, explain purpose and effects of naloxone to patient.

Evaluation/Desired Outcomes

- Adequate ventilation.
- Alertness without significant pain or withdrawal symptoms.

naproxen (na-prox-en)

Aleve, Anaprox, Anaprox DS, ✤Apo-Napro-Na, Apo-Napro-Na DS, ✤Apo-Naproxen, EC-Naprosyn, Naprelan, Napron X, Naprosyn, ✤Naprosyn-E, ✤Naprosyn-SR, ✤Naxen, ✤Novo-Naprox, ✤Novo-Naprox Sodium DS, ✤Nu-Naprox, ✤Synflex, ✤Synflex DS

Classification

Therapeutic: nonopioid analgesics, nonsteroidal anti-inflammatory agents, antipyretics

Pregnancy Category B (first trimester)

Indications

Mild to moderate pain. Dysmenorrhea. Fever. Inflammatory disorders, including: Rheumatoid arthritis (adults and children), Osteoarthritis.

Action

Inhibits prostaglandin synthesis. **Therapeutic Effects:** Decreased pain. Reduction of fever. Suppression of inflammation.

Pharmacokinetics

Absorption: Completely absorbed from the GI tract. Sodium salt (Anaprox) is more rapidly absorbed.
Distribution: Crosses the placenta; enters breast milk in low concentrations.
Protein Binding: >99%.
Metabolism and Excretion: Mostly metabolized by the liver.
Half-life: Children <8 yr: 8–17 hr; Children 8–14 yr: 8–10 hr; Adults: 10–20 hr.

TIME/ACTION PROFILE

ROUTE	ONSET	PEAK	DURATION
PO (analgesic)	1 hr	unknown	8–12 hr
PO (anti-inflammatory)	14 days	2–4 wk	unknown

Contraindications/Precautions

Contraindicated in: Hypersensitivity; Cross-sensitivity may occur with other NSAIDs, including aspirin; Active GI bleeding; Ulcer disease; Lactation: Passes into breast milk and should not be used by nursing mothers.

Use Cautiously in: Severe cardiovascular, renal, or hepatic disease; History of ulcer disease or any other history of gastrointestinal bleeding (may increase the risk of GI bleeding); Underlying cardiovascular disease (may increase the risk of MI or stroke); Chronic alcohol use/abuse; Geri: Increased risk of adverse reactions; OB: Avoid using during third trimester of pregnancy; may cause premature closure of the ductus arteriosis; Pedi: Children <2 yr (safety not established).

Adverse Reactions/Side Effects

CNS: dizziness, drowsiness, headache. **EENT:** tinnitus, visual disturbances. **Resp:** dyspnea. **CV:** edema, palpitations, tachycardia. **GI:** DRUG-INDUCED HEPATITIS, GI BLEEDING, constipation, dyspepsia, nausea, anorexia, diarrhea, discomfort, flatulence, vomiting. **GU:** cystitis, hematuria, renal failure. **Derm:** photosensitivity, rashes, sweating, pseudoporphyria (12% incidence in children with juvenile rheumatoid arthritis—discontinue therapy if this occurs). **Hemat:** blood dyscrasias, prolonged bleeding time. **Misc:** allergic reactions including ANAPHYLAXIS and STEVENS-JOHNSON SYNDROME.

Interactions

Drug-Drug: Concurrent use with **aspirin** ↓ naproxen blood levels and may ↓ effectiveness. ↑ risk of bleeding with **anticoagulants**, **thrombolytic agents**, **eptifibatide**, **tirofiban**, **cefotetan**, **cefoperazone**, **valproic acid**, **clopidogrel**, and **ticlopidine**. Additive adverse GI side effects with **aspirin**, **corticosteroids**, and other **NSAIDs**. **Probenecid** ↑ blood levels and may ↑ toxicity. ↑ risk of photosensitivity with other **photosensitizing agents**. May ↑ the risk of toxicity from **methotrexate**, **antineoplastics**, or **radiation therapy**. May ↑ serum levels and risk of toxicity from **lithium**. ↑ risk of adverse renal effects with **cyclosporine** or chronic use of **acetaminophen**. May ↓ response to **ACE Inhibitors**, **angiotensin II antagonists**, or **furosemide**. May ↑ risk of hypoglycemia with **insulin** or **oral hypoglycemic agents Oral potassium supplements** may ↑ GI adverse effects.

Drug-Natural Products: ↑ anticoagulant effect and bleeding risk with **anise**, **arnica**, **chamomile**, **clove**, **dong quai**, **feverfew**, **garlic**, **ginger**, **ginkgo**, **Panax ginseng**, **licorice**, and others.

Route/Dosage

275 mg naproxen sodium is equivalent to 250 mg naproxen.

Anti-inflammatory/Analgesic/Antidysmenorrheal

PO (Adults): *Naproxen*—250–500 mg bid (up to 1.5 g/day). *Delayed-release naproxen*—375–500 mg twice daily. *Naproxen sodium*—275–550 mg twice daily (up to 1.65 g/day).

PO (Children >2 yr): *Analgesia:* 5–7 mg/kg/dose every 8–12 hr. *Inflammatory disease:* 10–15 mg/kg/day divided q 12 hr, maximum: 1000 mg/day.

Antigout

PO (Adults): *Naproxen*—750 mg naproxen initially, then 250 mg q 8 hr. *Naproxen sodium*—825 mg initially, then 275 mg q 8 hr.

OTC Use (naproxen sodium)

PO (Adults): 200 mg q 8–12 hr or 400 mg followed by 200 mg q 12 hr (not to exceed 600 mg/24 hr).

PO (Geriatric Patients >65 yr): Not to exceed 200 mg q 12 hr.

Availability

Naproxen

Tablets (Naprosyn, {Apo-Naproxen, Naxen, Novo-Naprox, Nu-Naprox}): ✤125 mg, 250 mg, 375 mg, 500 mg. **Controlled-release tablets (Naprelan):** 375 mg, 500 mg. **Delayed-release tablets (EC-Naprosyn, Naprosyn-E):** ✤250 mg, 375 mg, 500 mg. **Extended-release tablets (Naprosyn-SR):** ✤750 mg. **Oral suspension (Naprosyn):** 125 mg/5 ml. **Suppositories (Naprosyn, Naxen):** ✤500 mg.

Naproxen Sodium

Tablets (Aleve, Anaprox, Anaprox DS, Apo-Napro-Na, Novo-Naprox Sodium, Novo-Naprox Sodium DS, Synaflex, Synaflex DS): 220 mg^{OTC}, 275 mg, 550 mg. ***In combination with:*** lansoprazole in a combination package (Prevacid NapraPac), pseudoephedrine (Aleve Cold and Sinus Tablets, Aleve Sinus and Headache Tablets). See Appendix B.

N

✤ = Canadian drug name.

*CAPITALS indicates life-threatening; underlines indicate most frequent.

NURSING IMPLICATIONS

Assessment

- Patients who have asthma, aspirin-induced allergy, and nasal polyps are at increased risk for developing hypersensitivity reactions. Assess for rhinitis, asthma, and urticaria.
- **Pain:** Assess pain (note type, location, and intensity) prior to and 1–2 hr following administration.
- **Arthritis:** Assess pain and range of motion prior to and 1–2 hr following administration.
- **Fever:** Monitor temperature; note signs associated with fever (diaphoresis, tachycardia, malaise).
- ***Lab Test Considerations:*** Evaluate BUN, serum creatinine, CBC, and liver function tests periodically in patients receiving prolonged therapy.
- May ↑ serum potassium, BUN, serum creatinine, alkaline phosphatase, LDH, AST, and ALT tests levels. May ↓ blood glucose, hemoglobin, and hematocrit concentrations, leukocyte and platelet counts, and CCr.
- Bleeding time may be prolonged up to 4 days following discontinuation of therapy.
- May alter test results for urine 5-HIAA and urine steroid determinations.

Potential Nursing Diagnoses

Acute pain (Indications)
Impaired physical mobility (Indications)

Implementation

- Administration in higher than recommended doses does not provide increased effectiveness but may cause increased side effects.
- Coadministration with opioid analgesics may have additive analgesic effects and may permit lower opioid doses.
- Analgesic is more effective if given before pain becomes severe.
- **PO:** For rapid initial effect, administer 30 min before or 2 hr after meals. May be administered with food, milk, or antacids to decrease GI irritation. Food slows but does not reduce the extent of absorption. Do not mix suspension with antacid or other liquid prior to administration.
- **Dysmenorrhea:** Administer as soon as possible after the onset of menses. Prophylactic treatment has not been shown to be effective.

Patient/Family Teaching

- Advise patient to take this medication with a full glass of water and to remain in an upright position for 15–30 min after administration.
- Instruct patient to take medication as directed. Take missed doses as soon as remembered but not if almost time for the next dose. Do not double doses.
- May cause drowsiness or dizziness. Advise patient to avoid driving or other activities requiring alertness until response to the medication is known.
- Caution patient to avoid the concurrent use of alcohol, aspirin, acetaminophen, or other OTC medications without consulting health care professional. Use of naproxen with 3 or more glasses of alcohol per day may increase risk of GI bleeding.
- Advise patient to inform health care professional of medication regimen prior to treatment or surgery.
- Caution patient to wear sunscreen and protective clothing to prevent photosensitivity reactions (especially in children with juvenile rhumatoid arthritis [JRA]).
- Instruct patients not to take OTC naproxen preparations for more than 3 days for fever and to consult health care professional if symptoms persist or worsen.
- Advise patient to consult health care professional if rash, itching, visual disturbances, tinnitus, weight gain, edema, black stools, persistent headache, or influenza-like syndrome (chills, fever, muscle aches, pain) occurs.

Evaluation/Desired Outcomes

- Relief of pain.
- Improved joint mobility. Partial arthritic relief is usually seen within 2 wk, but maximum effectiveness may require 2–4 wk of continuous therapy. Patients who do not respond to one NSAID may respond to another.
- Reduction of fever.

naratriptan (nar-a-**trip**-tan)

Amerge

Classification

Therapeutic: vascular headache suppressants

Pharmacologic: 5-HT_1 agonists

Pregnancy Category C

Indications

Acute treatment of migraine headache.

Action
Acts as an agonist at specific 5-HT_1 receptor sites in intracranial blood vessels and sensory trigeminal nerves. **Therapeutic Effects:** Cranial vessel vasoconstriction with resultant decrease in migraine headache.

Pharmacokinetics
Absorption: Well absorbed (70%) following oral administration.
Distribution: Unknown.
Metabolism and Excretion: 60% excreted unchanged in urine; 30% metabolized by the liver.
Half-life: 6 hr (increased in renal impairment).

TIME/ACTION PROFILE (decreased migraine pain)

ROUTE	ONSET	PEAK	DURATION
PO	30–60 min	2–3 hr†	up to 24 hr

†3–4 hr during migraine attack

Contraindications/Precautions
Contraindicated in: Hypersensitivity; Geriatric patients; Ischemic cardiovascular, cerebrovascular, or peripheral vascular syndromes; History of significant cardiovascular disease; Uncontrolled hypertension; Severe renal impairment (CCr <15 ml/min); Severe hepatic impairment; Should not be used within 24 hr of other 5-HT_1 agonists or ergot-type compounds (dihydroergotamine).
Use Cautiously in: Mild to moderate renal or hepatic impairment (dose should not exceed 2.5 mg/24 hr; initial dose should be decreased); Pregnancy, lactation, or children (safety not established).
Exercise Extreme Caution in: Cardiovascular risk factors (hypertension, hypercholesterolemia, cigarette smoking, obesity, diabetes, strong family history, menopausal women or men >40 yr); use only if cardiovascular status has been evaluated and determined to be safe and 1st dose is administered under supervision.

Adverse Reactions/Side Effects
CNS: dizziness, drowsiness, malaise/fatigue. **CV:** CORONARY ARTERY VASOSPASM, MI, VENTRICULAR FIBRILLATION, VENTRICULAR TACHYCARDIA, myocardial ischemia. **GI:** nausea. **Neuro:** paresthesia. **Misc:** pain/pressure sensation in throat/neck.

Interactions
Drug-Drug: Concurrent use with **SSRI antidepressants** may result in weakness, hyper-reflexia, and incoordination. **Cigarette smoking** ↑ the metabolism of naratriptan. Blood levels and effects are ↑ by **hormonal contraceptives**. Avoid concurrent use (within 24 hr of each other) with **ergot-containing drugs (dihydroergotamine)** may result in prolonged vasospastic reactions. Avoid concurrent (within 2 wk) use with **MAO inhibitors**; produces increased systemic exposure and risk of adverse reactions to naratriptan. Serotonin syndrome may occur with **sibutramine**.
Drug-Natural Products: ↑ risk of serotinergic side effects including serotonin syndrome with **St. John's wort** and **SAMe**.

Route/Dosage
PO (Adults): 1 or 2.5 mg; dose may be repeated in 4 hr if response is inadequate (not to exceed 5 mg/24 hr or treatment of more than 4 headaches/mo).

Availability
Tablets: 1 mg, 2.5 mg. **Cost:** 1 mg $210.69/9, 2.5 mg $210.97/9.

NURSING IMPLICATIONS

Assessment
- Assess pain location, character, intensity, and duration and associated symptoms (photophobia, phonophobia, nausea, vomiting) during migraine attack.

Potential Nursing Diagnoses
Acute pain (Indications)

Implementation
- **PO:** Tablets may be administered at any time after the headache starts.

Patient/Family Teaching
- Inform patient that naratriptan should be used only during a migraine attack. It is meant to be used for relief of migraine attacks but not to prevent or reduce the number of attacks.
- Instruct patient to administer naratriptan as soon as symptoms of a migraine attack appear, but it may be administered any time during an attack. If migraine symptoms return, a 2nd dose may be used. Allow at least 4 hr between doses, and do not use more than

N

2 tablets in any 24-hr period. Do not use to treat more than 4 headaches per month.

- Advise patient that lying down in a darkened room following naratriptan administration may further help relieve headache.
- Caution patient not to use naratriptan if she is pregnant, suspects she is pregnant, or plans to become pregnant. Adequate contraception should be used during therapy.
- Advise patient to notify health care professional prior to next dose of naratriptan if pain or tightness in the chest occurs during use. If pain is severe or does not subside, notify health care professional immediately. If wheezing; heart throbbing; swelling of eyelids, face, or lips; skin rash; skin lumps; or hives occur, notify health care professional immediately and do not take more naratriptan without approval of health care professional. If feelings of tingling, heat, flushing, heaviness, pressure, drowsiness, dizziness, tiredness, or sickness develop, discuss with health care professional at next visit.
- Instruct patient not to take additional naratriptan if no response is seen with initial dose without consulting health care professional. There is no evidence that 5 mg provides greater relief than 2.5-mg dose. Additional naratriptan doses are not likely to be effective and alternative medications, as previously discussed with health care professional, may be used.
- Naratriptan may cause dizziness or drowsiness. Caution patient to avoid driving or other activities requiring alertness until response to medication is known.
- Advise patient to avoid alcohol, which aggravates headaches, during naratriptan use.

Evaluation/Desired Outcomes

- Relief of migraine attack.

nateglinide (na-**teg**-li-nide)

Starlix

Classification

Therapeutic: antidiabetics

Pharmacologic: meglitinides

Pregnancy Category C

Indications

To improve glycemic control in patients with type 2 diabetes (with diet and exercise); may also be used with metformin or a thiazolidinedione (pioglitazone, rosiglitazole).

Action

Stimulates the release of insulin from pancreatic beta cells by closing potassium channels, which results in the opening of calcium channels in beta cells. This is followed by release of insulin. Requires functioning pancreatic beta cells. **Therapeutic Effects:** Lowering of blood glucose.

Pharmacokinetics

Absorption: Well absorbed (73%) following oral administration; absorption is rapid.
Distribution: Unknown.
Protein Binding: 98%.
Metabolism and Excretion: Mostly metabolized by the liver (cytochrome P2 C9 and P3 A4 [CYP2 C9 and CYP3 A4] enzyme systems); 16% excreted unchanged in urine.
Half-life: 1.5 hr.

TIME/ACTION PROFILE (effect on blood glucose)

ROUTE	ONSET	PEAK	DURATION
PO	within 20 min	1 hr	4 hr

Contraindications/Precautions

Contraindicated in: Hypersensitivity; OB: Pregnancy or lactation (insulin recommended to control diabetes during pregnancy); Diabetic ketoacidosis; Type 1 diabetes.
Use Cautiously in: Geri: Elderly patients, malnourished patients, patients with pituitary or adrenal insufficiency (increased susceptibility to hypoglycemia); Strenuous physical exercise, insufficient caloric intake (increased risk of hypoglycemia); Autonomic neuropathy (hypoglycemia may be masked); Moderate to severe liver impairment; Fever, infection, trauma, or surgery (may lead to transient loss of glycemic control; insulin may be required); Pedi: Children (safety not established).

Adverse Reactions/Side Effects

CNS: dizziness. **Resp:** bronchitis, coughing, upper respiratory infection. **GI:** diarrhea. **Endo:** HYPOGLYCEMIA. **MS:** arthropathy, back pain. **Misc:** flu symptoms.

Interactions

Drug-Drug: Concurrent use with **beta blockers** may mask hypoglycemia. **Alcohol**, combination with other **antidiabetics**, **NSAIDs**, **MAO inhibitors**, **nonselective beta blockers** may ↑ the risk of hypoglycemia. Hypogly-

cemic effects may be ↓ by **thiazide diuretics**, **corticosteroids**, **thyroid supplements**, or **sympathomimetic (adrenergic) agents**.
Drug-Food: Blood levels and effects are significantly ↓ when administered prior to a **liquid meal**.

Route/Dosage

PO (Adults): 120 mg 3 times daily before meals; patients who are approaching glycemic control may be started at 60 mg 3 times daily.

Availability

Tablets: 60 mg, 120 mg.

NURSING IMPLICATIONS

Assessment

- Observe for signs and symptoms of hypoglycemic reactions (sweating, hunger, weakness, dizziness, tremor, tachycardia, anxiety).
- ***Lab Test Considerations:*** Monitor serum glucose and HbA_{1c} periodically during therapy to evaluate effectiveness.
- May cause ↑ uric acid levels.
- ***Toxicity and Overdose:*** Overdose is manifested by symptoms of hypoglycemia. Mild hypoglycemia may be treated with administration of oral glucose. Severe hypoglycemia should be treated with IV D50W followed by continuous IV infusion of more dilute dextrose solution at a rate sufficient to keep serum glucose at approximately 100 mg/dl.

Potential Nursing Diagnoses

Imbalanced nutrition: more than body requirements (Indications)
Noncompliance (Patient/Family Teaching)

Implementation

- Patients stabilized on a diabetic regimen who are exposed to stress, fever, trauma, infection, or surgery may require administration of insulin.
- **PO:** Administer 1–30 min prior to meals.
- May be administered concurrently with metformin, pioglitazone, or rosiglitazole.

Patient/Family Teaching

- Instruct patient to take medication at same time each day. Take missed doses as soon as remembered unless almost time for next dose. Do not take if unable to eat.
- Explain to patient that this medication controls hyperglycemia but does not cure diabetes. Therapy is long term.
- Review signs of hypoglycemia and hyperglycemia with patient. If hypoglycemia occurs, advise patient to take a glass of orange juice or 2–3 tsp of sugar, honey, or corn syrup dissolved in water and notify health care professional.
- Encourage patient to follow prescribed diet, medication, and exercise regimen to prevent hypoglycemic or hyperglycemic episodes.
- Instruct patient in proper testing of serum glucose and ketones. These tests should be closely monitored during periods of stress or illness and health care professional notified if significant changes occur.
- May occasionally cause dizziness. Caution patient to avoid driving or other activities requiring alertness until response to medication is known.
- Caution patient to avoid other medications, especially aspirin and alcohol, while on this therapy without consulting health care professional.
- Insulin is the recommended method of controlling blood glucose during pregnancy. Counsel female patients to use a form of contraception other than oral contraceptives and to notify health care professional promptly if pregnancy is planned or suspected.
- Advise patient to inform health care professional of medication regimen prior to treatment or surgery.
- Advise patient to carry a form of sugar (sugar packets, candy) and identification describing disease process and medication regimen at all times.
- Emphasize the importance of routine follow-up exams.

Evaluation/Desired Outcomes

- Control of blood glucose levels without the occurrence of hypoglycemic or hyperglycemic episodes.

---

nedocromil, See MAST CELL STABILIZERS.

---

nefazodone (neff-**a**-zoe-done)
Serzone

N

Classification
Therapeutic: antidepressants

Pregnancy Category C

Indications
Major depression. **Unlabeled uses:** Panic disorder, post-traumatic stress disorder (PSTD).

Action
Inhibits the reuptake of serotonin and norepinephrine by neurons. Antagonizes alpha$_1$-adrenergic receptors. **Therapeutic Effects:** Antidepressant action, which may develop only after several weeks.

Pharmacokinetics
Absorption: Well absorbed but undergoes extensive and variable first-pass hepatic metabolism (bioavailability about 20%).
Distribution: Widely distributed; enters the CNS.
Protein Binding: ≥99%.
Metabolism and Excretion: Extensively metabolized. One metabolite (hydroxynefazodone) has antidepressant activity.
Half-life: *Nefazodone*—2–4 hr; *hydroxynefazodone*—1.5–4 hr.

TIME/ACTION PROFILE (antidepressant action)

ROUTE	ONSET	PEAK	DURATION
PO	days–wks	several wk	unknown

Contraindications/Precautions
Contraindicated in: Hypersensitivity; Concurrent MAO inhibitor therapy; Active liver disease or baseline elevated serum transaminases.
Use Cautiously in: May ↑ risk of suicide attempt/ideation especially during early treatment or dose adjustment; History of suicide attempt or drug abuse; Underlying cardiovascular or cerebrovascular disease; History of mania; OB: Safety not established; Lactation: Discontinue drug or bottle-feed; Pedi: Safety not established in children; suicide risk may be greater in children and adolescents; Geri: Iinitiate therapy at lower doses.

Adverse Reactions/Side Effects
CNS: <u>dizziness</u>, <u>insomnia</u>, <u>somnolence</u>, agitation, confusion, weakness. **EENT:** abnormal vision, blurred vision, eye pain, tinnitus. **Resp:** dyspnea. **CV:** bradycardia, hypotension. **GI:** HEPATIC FAILURE, HEPATOTOXICITY, <u>constipation</u>, <u>dry mouth</u>, <u>nausea</u>, gastroenteritis. **GU:** erectile dysfunction. **Derm:** rashes. **Hemat:** decreased hematocrit.

Interactions
Drug-Drug: Serious, potentially fatal reactions may occur during concurrent use with **MAO inhibitors** (do not use concurrently or within 2 wk of MAO inhibitors; discontinue nefazodone at least 14 days before starting MAO inhibitor therapy). ↑ CNS depression with other CNS depressants including **alcohol**, **antihistamines**, **opioid analgesics**, and **sedative/hypnotics**. May ↑ blood levels and effects of **alprazolam** or **triazolam**. May increase serum **digoxin** levels. Additive hypotension may occur with **antihypertensives**, **nitrates**, or acute ingestion of **alcohol**. May ↑ risk of myopathy with **HMG-CoA reductase inhibitors**. ↓ **antidepressant** action with concomitant use of **carabazepine**. May ↓ clearance of **haloperidol**, so **haloperidol** dose may need to be decreased.
Drug-Natural Products: ↑ risk of seritonergic side effects including serotonin syndrome with **St. John's wort** and **SAMe. Kava kava, valerian,** or **chamomile** can ↑ CNS depression.

Route/Dosage
PO (Adults): 100 mg twice daily initially; may be increased weekly up to 600 mg/day in 2 divided doses.
PO (Geriatric Patients): 50 mg twice daily initially; may be increased weekly as tolerated.

Availability (generic available)
Tablets: 50 mg, 100 mg, 150 mg, 200 mg, 250 mg.

NURSING IMPLICATIONS

Assessment
- Assess mental status (orientation, mood, behavior) frequently. Inform health care professional if patient demonstrates significant increase in anxiety, nervousness, or insomnia.
- Assess suicidal tendencies, especially in early therapy. Restrict amount of drug available to patient.
- Monitor blood pressure and pulse before and periodically during therapy.
- Monitor liver function tests prior to and routinely during therapy. Obtain LFTs at first sign of hepatic dysfunction (nausea, vomiting, abdominal pain, fatigue, anorexia, dark urine).

- Assess for sexual dysfunction throughout treatment.
- ***Lab Test Considerations:*** May cause decrease in hematocrit and leukopenia.
- Monitor liver function periodically. If serum AST or ALT levels are >3 times the upper limit of normal discontinue nefazodone.
- May also cause hypercholesterolemia and hypoglycemia.

Potential Nursing Diagnoses

Ineffective coping (Indications)
Risk for injury (Side Effects)

Implementation

- Do not confuse Serzone (nefazodone) with Seroquel (quetiapine).
- Discontinue nefazodone prior to elective surgery to prevent potential interactions with general anesthesia.
- **PO:** Administer doses twice daily.

Patient/Family Teaching

- Instruct patient to take medication as directed. Several weeks may be required to obtain a full antidepressant response. Once response is obtained, therapy should be continued for at least 6 mo. If a dose is missed, take as soon as possible unless almost time for next dose. Do not double doses.
- May cause drowsiness or dizziness. Caution patient to avoid driving or other activities requiring alertness until response to the drug is known.
- Advise patient to make position changes slowly to minimize orthostatic hypotension.
- Caution patient to avoid taking alcohol or other CNS depressant drugs during therapy and not to take other prescription, OTC medications, or herbal products without consulting health care professional.
- Advise patient to notify health care professional immediately if signs of liver dysfunction (jaundice, anorexia, GI complaints, malaise, dark urine) occur.
- Inform patient that frequent mouth rinses, good oral hygiene, and sugarless gum or candy may minimize dry mouth. If dry mouth persists for more than 2 wk, consult health care professional regarding use of saliva substitute.
- Instruct female patient to inform health care professional if pregnancy is planned or suspected or if breastfeeding.
- Instruct patient to notify health care professional of signs of allergy (rash, hives) or if agitation, blurriness or other changes in vision, confusion, dizziness, unsteadiness, difficult or frequent urination, difficulty concentrating, or memory problems occur.
- Emphasize the importance of follow-up examinations to monitor progress. Encourage patient participation in psychotherapy.
- Refer to local support group.
- Inform patient that some side effects may go away with time.

Evaluation/Desired Outcomes

- Increased sense of well-being.
- Renewed interest in surroundings. May require several weeks of therapy to obtain full response. Need for therapy should be periodically reassessed. Therapy is usually continued for 6 months or more.

neomycin, See AMINOGLYCOSIDES.

neostigmine

(nee-oh-**stig**-meen)
Prostigmin

Classification
Therapeutic: antimyasthenics
Pharmacologic: cholinergics

Pregnancy Category C

Indications

Improvement in muscle strength in symptomatic treatment of myasthenia gravis. Prevention and treatment of postoperative bladder distention and urinary retention or ileus. Reversal of nondepolarizing neuromuscular blockers.

Action

Inhibits the breakdown of acetylcholine so that it accumulates and has a prolonged effect. Effects include miosis, increased intestinal and skeletal muscle tone, bronchial and ureteral constriction, bradycardia, increased salivation, lacrimation, and sweating. **Therapeutic Effects:** Improved muscular function in patients with myasthenia gravis, improved bladder-emptying in patients with urinary retention, or reversal of nondepolarizing neuromuscular blockers.

Pharmacokinetics

Absorption: Poorly absorbed following oral administration, necessitating large oral doses compared with parenteral doses.

Distribution: Probably does not cross the placenta or enter breast milk.

Metabolism and Excretion: Metabolized by plasma cholinesterases and the liver.

Half-life: *PO, IV*—40–60 min; *IM*—50–90 min.

TIME/ACTION PROFILE (cholinergic effects, increased muscle tone)

ROUTE	ONSET	PEAK	DURATION
PO	45–75 min	unknown	2–4 hr
IM	10–30 min	20–30 min	2–4 hr
IV	10–30 min	20–30 min	2–4 hr

Contraindications/Precautions

Contraindicated in: Hypersensitivity; Mechanical obstruction of the GI or GU tract.

Use Cautiously in: History of asthma; Ulcer disease; Cardiovascular disease; Epilepsy; Hyperthyroidism; OB: Pregnancy (may cause uterine irritability after IV administration near term; newborns may display muscle weakness); Lactation.

Adverse Reactions/Side Effects

CNS: SEIZURES, dizziness, weakness. **EENT:** lacrimation, miosis. **Resp:** bronchospasm, excess secretions. **CV:** bradycardia, hypotension. **GI:** abdominal cramps, diarrhea, excess salivation, nausea, vomiting. **Derm:** sweating, rashes.

Interactions

Drug-Drug: Action may be antagonized by **drugs possessing anticholinergic properties**, including **antihistamines**, **antidepressants**, **atropine**, **haloperidol**, **phenothiazines**, **quinidine**, and **disopyramide**. Prolongs action of **depolarizing muscle-relaxing agents (succinylcholine, decamethonium)**.

Route/Dosage

Myasthenia Gravis

PO (Adults): 15 mg q 3–4 hr initially; increase at daily intervals until optimal response is achieved. Usual maintenance dose is 150 mg/day (up to 375 mg/day may be needed).

PO (Children): 2 mg/kg/day (60 mg/m^2) in 6–8 divided doses.

Subcut, IM (Adults): 0.5 mg.

Subcut, IM (Children): 10–40 mcg/kg q 2–3 hr; may give with 10 mcg/kg atropine.

Bladder Atony, Abdominal Distention: Prevention

IM, Subcut (Adults): 250 mcg q 4–6 hr for 2–3 days.

Bladder Atony, Abdominal Distention: Treatment

IM, Subcut (Adults): 500 mcg as needed; may repeat q 3 hr for 5 doses after bladder has been emptied for bladder atony.

Antidote for Nondepolarizing Neuromuscular Blockers

IV (Adults): 0.5–2 mg slowly; pretreat with 0.6–1.2 mg atropine IV (may be repeated to a total dose of 5 mg).

IV (Children): 40 mcg/kg with 20 mcg/kg atropine.

Availability (generic available)

Tablets: 15 mg. **Injection:** 1:1000 in 10-ml vials, 1:2000 in 1-ml ampules and 10-ml vials, 1:4000 in 1-ml ampules. **In combination with:** atropine (Neostigmine Methylsulfate Min-I-Mix).

NURSING IMPLICATIONS

Assessment

- Assess pulse, respiratory rate, and blood pressure prior to administration. Report significant changes in heart rate.
- **Myasthenia Gravis:** Assess neuromuscular status, including vital capacity, ptosis, diplopia, chewing, swallowing, hand grasp, and gait, prior to administering and at peak effect. Patients with myasthenia gravis may be advised to keep a daily record of their condition and the effects of this medication.
- Assess patient for overdose and underdose or resistance. Both have similar symptoms (muscle weakness, dyspnea, dysphagia), but symptoms of overdose usually occur within 1 hr of administration, whereas underdose symptoms occur 3 or more hr after administration. Overdose (cholinergic crisis) symptoms may also include increased respiratory secretions and saliva, bradycardia, nausea, vomiting, cramping, diarrhea, and diaphoresis. A Tensilon test (edrophonium chloride) may be used to distinguish between overdose and underdose.
- **Postoperative Ileus:** Monitor abdominal status (assess for distention, auscultate bowel sounds). A rectal tube may be inserted to facilitate expulsion of flatus.

- **Postoperative Urinary Retention:** Assess for bladder distention. Monitor intake and output. If patient is unable to void within 1 hr of neostigmine administration, consider catheterization.
- **Antidote to Nondepolarizing Neuromuscular Blocking Agents:** Monitor reversal of effects of neuromuscular blocking agents with a peripheral nerve stimulator. Recovery usually occurs consecutively in the following muscles: diaphragm, intercostal muscles, muscles of the glottis, abdominal muscles, limb muscles, muscles of mastication, and levator muscles of the eyelids. Closely observe the patient for residual muscle weakness and respiratory distress throughout the recovery period. Maintain airway patency and ventilation until recovery of normal respiration occurs.
- ***Toxicity and Overdose:*** If overdose occurs, atropine is the antidote.

Potential Nursing Diagnoses

Impaired physical mobility (Indications)
Ineffective breathing pattern (Indications)

Implementation

- Oral and parenteral doses are not interchangeable.
- When used as an antidote to nondepolarizing neuromuscular blocking agents, atropine may be used prior to or concurrently with neostigmine to prevent or treat bradycardia.
- **PO:** Administer with food or milk to minimize side effects. For patients who have difficulty chewing, neostigmine may be taken 30 min before meals.

IV Administration

- **Direct IV:** Administer doses undiluted. May be given through Y-site of an IV of D5W, 0.9% NaCl, Ringer's solution, or LR. ***Concentration:*** 0.5–1 mg/ml. ***Rate:*** Administer each 0.5 mg over 1 min.
- **Syringe Compatibility:** glycopyrrolate, heparin, ondansetron, pentobarbital, thiopental.
- **Y-Site Compatibility:** heparin, hydrocortisone sodium succinate, potassium chloride, vitamin B complex with C.

Patient/Family Teaching

- Instruct patient to take medication exactly as directed. Do not skip or double up on missed doses. Patients with a history of dysphagia should have a nonelectric or battery-operated backup alarm clock to remind them of exact dosage time. Patients with dysphagia may not be able to swallow the medication if the dose is not taken exactly on time. Taking the dose late may result in myasthenic crisis. Taking the dose early may result in cholinergic crisis. Patients with myasthenia gravis must continue this regimen as lifelong therapy.
- Instruct patient with myasthenia gravis to space activities to avoid fatigue.
- Advise patient to carry identification describing disease and medication regimen at all times.

Evaluation/Desired Outcomes

- Relief of ptosis and diplopia.
- Improved chewing, swallowing, extremity strength, and breathing without the appearance of cholinergic symptoms in myasthenia gravis.
- Relief or prevention of postoperative gastrointestinal ileus.
- Relief of nonobstructive postoperative urinary retention.
- Reversal of nondepolarizing neuromuscular blocking agents in general anesthesia.

HIGH ALERT

nesiritide (ne-**sir**-i-tide)

Natrecor

Classification
Therapeutic: none assigned
Pharmacologic: vasodilators (human B-type natriuretic peptide)

Pregnancy Category C

Indications

Acutely decompensated CHF in hospitalized patients who have dyspnea at rest or with minimal activity; has been used with digoxin, diuretics, and ACE inhibitors. Should not be used for intermittent outpatient infusion, scheduled repetitive use, as a diuretic, or to improve renal function.

Action

Binds to guanyl cyclase receptors in vascular smooth muscle and endothelial cells, producing increased intracellular guanosine 3′5′-cyclic monophosphate (cGMP) and smooth muscle cell relaxation. cGMP acts as a "second messenger" to dilate veins and arteries. **Therapeutic Effects:** Dose-dependent reduction in pulmonary capillary wedge pressure (PCWP) and systemic arterial pressure in patients with heart failure with resultant decrease in dyspnea.

Pharmacokinetics

Absorption: IV administration results in complete bioavailability.
Distribution: Unknown.
Metabolism and Excretion: Cleared from circulation by binding to cell surface clearance receptors resulting in cellular internalization and proteolysis, proteolytic breakdown by endopeptidases, and renal filtration.
Half-life: 18 min.

TIME/ACTION PROFILE (effects on cardiovascular parameters)

ROUTE	ONSET	PEAK	DURATION
IV	15 min	1 hr	60 min†

†Longer with higher than recommended doses

Contraindications/Precautions

Contraindicated in: Hypersensitivity; Cardiogenic shock; Systolic blood pressure <90 mm Hg; Low cardiac filling pressure, significant valvular stenosis, restrictive/subtractive cardiomyopathy, constrictive pericarditis/cardiac tamponade, or other conditions in which cardiac output is dependent on venous return.
Use Cautiously in: Heart failure where renal function is dependent on activity of the renin/angiotensin/aldosterone system (may cause azotemia); BP <90 mm Hg (increased risk of hypotension); Geri: Geriatric patients (some may be more sensitive to effects); Cardiogenic shock (should not be used as primary therapy); OB: Pregnancy, lactation; Pedi: Children (safety not established).

Adverse Reactions/Side Effects

CNS: anxiety, confusion, dizziness, headache, hypotension (dose related), insomnia, drowsiness. **EENT:** amblyopia. **Resp:** APNEA, cough, hemoptysis. **CV:** <u>hypotension</u>, arrhythmias, bradycardia. **GI:** abdominal pain, nausea, vomiting. **GU:** ↑ creatinine, renal failure. **Derm:** itching, rash, sweating. **Hemat:** anemia. **Local:** injection site reactions. **MS:** back pain, leg cramps. **Neuro:** paresthesia, tremor. **Misc:** fever.

Interactions

Drug-Drug: None reported.

Route/Dosage

IV (Adults): 2 mcg/kg bolus followed by 0.01 mcg/kg/min as a continuous infusion. May increase by 0.005 mcg/kg/min every 3 hr up to a maximum infusion rate of 0.03 mcg/kg/min (based on response).

Availability

Lyophilized powder for injection (requires reconstitution): 1.5 mg/vial.

NURSING IMPLICATIONS

Assessment

- Monitor blood pressure, pulse, ECG, respiratory rate, cardiac index, PCWP, and central venous pressure frequently during administration. May cause hypotension, especially in patients with a BP <100 mm Hg. Reduce dose or discontinue nesiritide if patient develops hypotension. Hypotension may cause renal compromise. Use IV fluids and changes in body position to support blood pressure if symptomatic hypotension occurs. Nesiritide may be restarted at a dose reduced by 30% with no bolus administration once patient is stabilized. Hypotension may be prolonged for hours, requiring a period of monitoring prior to restarting administration.
- Monitor intake and output and weigh daily. Assess for decrease in signs of CHF (dyspnea, rales/crackles, peripheral edema, weight gain).
- ***Lab Test Considerations:*** Monitor BUN and serum creatinine. May cause ↑ in serum creatinine; ↑ serum creatinine may be dose-related.

Potential Nursing Diagnoses

Decreased cardiac output (Indications)
Activity intolerance (Indications)
Excess fluid volume (Indications)

Implementation

- ***High Alert:*** Intravenous vasoactive medications have an increased potential for causing harm. Have second practitioner independently check original order, dose calculations, and infusion pump settings. Administer only in settings where blood pressure can be closely monitored.
- Prime the IV tubing with an infusion of 25 ml prior to connecting to the patient's vascular access port and prior to administering bolus or infusion. Flush catheter between administration of nesiritide and other medications. Do not administer through a central heparin-

coated catheter as nesiritide binds to heparin. Concomitant administration of a heparin infusion through a separate catheter is acceptable.

IV Administration

- **Direct IV:** ***Diluent:*** Reconstitute 1.5-mg vial of nesiritide by adding 5 ml of diluent removed from a prefilled 250-ml plastic IV bag containing D5W, 0.9% NaCl, D5/0.45% NaCl, or D5/0.2% NaCl. Do not shake vial; rock gently so all surfaces including stopper are in contact with diluent to ensure complete reconstitution. Withdraw entire content of reconstituted vial and add back to 250-ml plastic IV bag. Invert IV bag several times to ensure complete mixing of solution. Infusion stable for 24 hr. After preparation of infusion bag, withdraw bolus volume from infusion bag. To calculate amount: bolus volume (ml) = 0.33 × patient weight (kg). ***Concentration:*** 6 mcg/ml. ***Rate:*** Administer bolus over 60 seconds through a port in the IV tubing.
- **Intermittent Infusion:** ***Diluent:*** See Diluent section under Direct IV section above for preparation instructions for infusion bag. Immediately follow bolus with infusion. ***Concentration:*** 6 mcg/ml. ***Rate:*** Based on patient's weight (see Route/Dosage section).
- **Y-Site Compatibility:** amiodarone, argatroban, digoxin, diltiazem, metoprolol, milrinone, nicardipine, nitroglycerin, nitroprusside, palonosetron, propranolol, tirofiban, torsemide, verapamil.
- **Y-Site Incompatibility:** bumetanide, daptomycin, enalaprilat, ethacrynic acid, furosemide, heparin, hydralazine, insulin, micafungin.

Patient/Family Teaching

- Explain purpose of nesiritide to patient and family.

Evaluation/Desired Outcomes

- Improvement in dyspnea and reduction in mean PCWP in patients with decompensated CHF.

nevirapine (ne-**veer**-a-peen)

Viramune

Classification
Therapeutic: antiretrovirals
Pharmacologic: non-nucleoside reverse transcriptase inhibitors

Pregnancy Category C

Indications

Management of HIV infection in combination with a nucleoside analogue.

Action

Binds to the enzyme reverse transcriptase, which results in disruption of DNA synthesis. **Therapeutic Effects:** Slowed progression of HIV infection and decreased occurrence of sequelae.

Pharmacokinetics

Absorption: >90% absorbed after oral administration.
Distribution: Crosses placenta and enters breast milk; CSF levels are 45% of those in plasma.
Metabolism and Excretion: Mostly metabolized by the liver (CYP3A4 enzyme system); minor amounts excreted unchanged in urine.
Half-life: 25–30 hr (during multiple dosing).

TIME/ACTION PROFILE (blood levels)

ROUTE	ONSET	PEAK	DURATION
PO	rapid	4 hr	12 hr

Contraindications/Precautions

Contraindicated in: Hypersensitivity; Concurrent ketoconazole or rifampin; Women with CD4+ cell counts >250 cells/mm^3 (↑ risk of liver toxicity).
Use Cautiously in: Women (↑ risk of liver toxicity); Hepatic or renal impairment; Concurrent clarithromycin, fluconazole, methadone or rifabutin (careful monitoring required; alternative therapy should be considered); OB, Pedi: Pregnancy, lactation, or children (safety not established; breastfeeding not recommended in HIV-infected patients).

Adverse Reactions/Side Effects

Reflects combination therapy.
CNS: headache. **GI:** HEPATOTOXICITY, elevated liver enzyme levels, nausea, abdominal pain, diarrhea, hepatitis, ulcerative stomatitis. **Derm:** RASH (MAY PROGRESS TO TOXIC EPIDERMAL NECROLYSIS). **Hemat:** granulocytopenia (increased in children).

MS: myalgia. **Neuro:** paresthesia, peripheral neuropathy. **Misc:** STEVENS-JOHNSON SYNDROME, fever.

Interactions

Drug-Drug: Nevirapine induces the hepatic CYP3A4 enzyme system and can affect the behavior of drugs metabolized by this system. Significantly ↓ **ketoconazole** levels (concurrent use contraindicated). May induce **methadone** withdrawal within 2 weeks of starting therapy in patients physically dependent on methadone. May ↓ levels and effectiveness **hormonal contraceptives** (concurrent use of hormonal contraceptives should be avoided). **Rifampin** significantly ↓ levels and effectiveness of nevirapine (concurrent use contraindicated). ↓ levels and effectiveness of **clarithromycin** (consider other agents). Also may ↓ levels and effectiveness of the following: **lopinavir, saquinavir, nelfnavir, indinavir, efavirenz, amiodarone, disopyramide, lidocaine, itraconazole, carbamazepine, clonazepam, ethosuximide, diltiazem, nifedipine, verapamil, cyclosporine, tacrolimus, sirolimus, cyclophosphamide, ergotamine, fentanyl, rifabutin** (use together only with careful monitoring). **Fluconazole** ↑ nevirapine levels and risk of toxcity. May ↑ risk of bleeding with **warfarin**. Use of **prednisone** during first 2 wk of therapy may ↑ risk of rash. Initiating other **drugs that often cause rash**, including **trimethoprim/sulamethoxazole** and **abacavir** simultaneously with nevirapine may ↑ risk of rash.
Drug-Natural Products: St. John's wort may ↓ efficacy.

Route/Dosage

PO (Adults): 200 mg daily for the first 2 wk, then 200 mg twice daily (in combination with a nucleoside analogue antiretroviral).
PO (Children ≥8 yr): 4 mg/kg once daily for first 2 wk, then 4 mg/kg twice daily.
PO (Children 2 mo–8 yr): 4 mg/kg once daily for first 2 wk, then 7 mg/kg twice daily.

Availability

Tablets: 200 mg. **Oral suspension:** 50 mg/5 ml.

NURSING IMPLICATIONS

Assessment

- Assess for change in severity of HIV symptoms and for symptoms of opportunistic infections throughout therapy.
- Assess for rash (mild to moderate rash = erythema or maculopapular rash; urticaria, pruritic raised rash with welts; constitutional symptoms—fever, blistering, oral erosive lesions, conjunctivitis, facial edema, myalgia, arthralgia), especially during 1st 6 wks of therapy. If rash is severe (extensive erythematous or maculopapular rash with moist desquamation or angioedema) or accompanied by systemic symptoms (serum sickness-like reaction, Stevens-Johnson syndrome, toxic epidermal necrolysis), therapy must be discontinued immediately. Prednisone and antihistamines are not effective in preventing or treating the rash. Nevirapine may be continued if rash is mild to moderate without constitutional symptoms or increased ALT or AST, but should not be restarted if stopped. If rash is severe or accompanied by constitutional symptoms, organ dysfunction, or increased AST or ALT, nevirapine should be permanently discontinued.
- ***Lab Test Considerations:*** Monitor viral load and CD4 cell count regularly during therapy.
- Monitor for liver function at baseline and frequently during the first 18 wks for toxicity, especially during first 6 wks of therapy. May be asymptomatic with ↑ AST and ALT without clinical signs or symptoms, or symptomatic with ↑ liver enzymes and at least one symptom (rash, flu-like symptoms, fever). May progress to liver failure and dealth. If signs of liver toxicity occur, permanently discontinue nevirapine.
- Assess patient for hepatitis B and C. Patients with HBV and/or HCV are at risk for liver toxicity.

Potential Nursing Diagnoses

Risk for infection (Indications)
Noncompliance (Patient/Family Teaching)

Implementation

- Do not confuse nevirapine (Viramune) with nelfinavir (Viracept).
- **PO:** May be administered with or without food.
- Shake oral solution prior to administration. Use an oral dosing syringe for amounts <5 ml. Rinse syringe or cup and readminister to ensure patient receives full dose.
- If therapy is interrupted for more than 7 days, restart therapy at 200 mg daily for 14 days, then increase dose to 200 mg twice daily.

Patient/Family Teaching

- Emphasize the importance of taking nevirapine as directed, at evenly spaced times throughout day. Instruct patient to read the *Medication Guide* prior to initiating therapy and with each Rx refill. Do not take more than prescribed amount and do not stop taking without consulting health care professional. Take missed doses as soon as remembered; do not double doses.
- Instruct patient not to share nevirapine with others.
- Advise patient to avoid taking other Rx, OTC, and herbal products without consulting health care professional.
- Inform patient that nevirapine does not cure AIDS or prevent associated or opportunistic infections. Nevirapine does not reduce the risk of transmission of HIV to others through sexual contact or blood contamination. Caution patient to use a condom and avoid sharing needles or donating blood to prevent spreading the AIDS virus to others. Advise patient that the long-term effects of nevirapine are unknown at this time.
- Advise patients taking oral contraceptives to use a nonhormonal method of birth control during nevirapine therapy.
- Instruct patient to notify health care professional immediately if signs and symptoms of hepatitis (flu-like symptoms, tiredness, nausea, lack of appetite, yellow skin or eyes, dark urine, pale stools, pain or sensitivity to touch on right side below ribs), or skin reactions with symptoms (flu-like symptoms, fever, muscle aches, conjunctivitis, blisters, mouth sores, swelling of face, tiredness) occur. Nevirapine should be discontinued immediately.
- Emphasize the importance of regular follow-up exams and blood counts to determine progress and monitor for side effects.

Evaluation/Desired Outcomes

- Delayed progression of AIDS and decreased opportunistic infections in patients with HIV.
- Decrease in viral load and increase in CD4 cell counts.

niacin (nye-a-sin)

Edur-Acin, Nia-Bid, Niac, Niacels, Niacor, Niaspan, Nicobid, Nico-400, Nicolar, Nicotinex, nicotinic acid, ✤Novo-Niacin, Slo-Niacin, vitamin B

niacinamide (nye-a-**sin**-a-mide)

nicotinamide

Classification

Therapeutic: lipid-lowering agents, vitamins

Pharmacologic: water-soluble vitamins

Pregnancy Category C

Indications

Treatment and prevention of niacin deficiency (pellagra). Adjunctive therapy in certain hyperlipidemias (niacin only).

Action

Required as coenzymes (for lipid metabolism, glycogenolysis, and tissue respiration). Large doses decrease lipoprotein and triglyceride synthesis by inhibiting the release of free fatty acids from adipose tissue and decreasing hepatic lipoprotein synthesis (niacin only). Causes peripheral vasodilation in large doses (niacin only). **Therapeutic Effects:** Decreased blood lipids (niacin only). Supplementation in deficiency states.

Pharmacokinetics

Absorption: Well absorbed following oral administration.

Distribution: Widely distributed following conversion to niacinamide. Enters breast milk.

Metabolism and Excretion: Amounts required for metabolic processes are converted to niacinamide. Large doses of niacin are excreted unchanged in the urine.

Half-life: 45 min.

TIME/ACTION PROFILE (effects on blood lipids)

ROUTE	ONSET	PEAK	DURATION
PO (cholesterol)	several days	unknown	unknown
PO (triglycerides)	several hr	unknown	unknown

Contraindications/Precautions

Contraindicated in: Hypersensitivity to niacin; Some products may contain tartrazine and should be avoided in patients with known hyper-

✤ = Canadian drug name.

* CAPITALS indicates life-threatening; underlines indicate most frequent.

sensitivity; Alcohol intolerance (Nicotinex only).
Use Cautiously in: Liver disease; Arterial bleeding; History of peptic ulcer disease; Gout; Glaucoma; Diabetes mellitus.

Adverse Reactions/Side Effects

Adverse reactions and side effects refer to IV administration or doses used to treat hyperlipidemias.
CNS: nervousness, panic. **EENT:** blurred vision, loss of central vision, proptosis, toxic amblyopia. **CV:** orthostatic hypotension. **GI:** HEPATOTOXICITY (ER oral form only), GI upset, bloating, diarrhea, dry mouth, flatulence, heartburn, hunger pains, nausea, peptic ulceration. **Derm:** flushing of the face and neck, pruritus, burning, dry skin, hyperpigmentation, increased sebaceous gland activity, rashes, stinging or tingling of skin. **Metab:** glycosuria, hyperglycemia, hyperuricemia.

Interactions

Drug-Drug: ↑ risk of myopathy with concurrent use of **HMG-CoA reductase inhibitors**. Additive hypotension with **ganglionic blocking agents (guanadrel)**. Large doses may ↓ uricosuric effects of **probenecid** or **sulfinpyrazone**.

Route/Dosage

PO (Adults and Children): *Dietary supplement*—10–20 mg/day. *Dietary deficiency*—Up to 500 mg/day in divided doses. *Hyperlipidemias–Niacin only*—100–500 mg/day initially; increase slowly up to 1–2 g tid (up to 8 g/day).
PO (Children 7–10 yr): *Prevention of deficiency*—13 mg/day.
PO (Children 4–6 yr): *Prevention of deficiency*—12 mg/day.
PO (Children birth–3 yr): *Prevention of deficiency*—5–9 mg/day.

Availability

Niacin

Tablets: 25 mg^{OTC}, 50 mg^{OTC}, 100 mg^{OTC}, 125 mg^{OTC}, 250 mg^{OTC}, 400 mg^{OTC}, 500 mg$^{Rx, OTC}$. **Extended-release tablets:** 125 mg$^{Rx, OTC}$, 250 mg$^{Rx, OTC}$, 400 mg^{OTC}, 500 mg$^{Rx, OTC}$, 750 mg$^{Rx, OTC}$, 1000 mg^{OTC}. **Cost:** 500 mg $184.97/90, 750 mg $255.96/90, 1000 mg $331.97/90. **Extended-release capsules:** 125 mg$^{Rx, OTC}$, 250 mg$^{Rx, OTC}$, 300 mg$^{Rx, OTC}$, 400 mg$^{Rx, OTC}$, 500 mg$^{Rx, OTC}$. **Elixir:** 50 mg/5 ml in pints and gallons^{OTC}. ***In combination with:*** lovastatin (Advicor) See Appendix B.

Niacinamide

Tablets: 50 mg^{OTC}, 100 mg^{OTC}, 125 mg^{OTC}, 250 mg^{OTC}, 500 mg$^{Rx, OTC}$.

NURSING IMPLICATIONS

Assessment

- **Vitamin Deficiency:** Assess patient for signs of niacin deficiency (*pellagra*—dermatitis, stomatitis, glossitis, anemia, nausea and vomiting, confusion, memory loss, and delirium) prior to and periodically throughout therapy.
- **Hyperlipidemia:** Obtain a diet history, especially with regard to fat consumption.
- ***Lab Test Considerations:*** Serum glucose and uric acid levels and hepatic function tests should be monitored periodically during prolonged high-dose therapy. Notify physician or other health care professional if AST, ALT, or LDH becomes elevated. May increase prothrombin times and decrease serum albumin.
- High-dose therapy may cause elevated serum glucose and uric acid levels.
- When niacin is used as a lipid-lowering agent, serum cholesterol and triglyceride levels should be monitored prior to and periodically throughout course of therapy.

Potential Nursing Diagnoses

Imbalanced nutrition: less than body requirements (Indications)
Noncompliance (Patient/Family Teaching)

Implementation

- Because of infrequency of single B-vitamin deficiencies, combinations are commonly administered.
- **PO:** Administer with meals or milk to minimize GI irritation.
- Timed-release tablets and capsules should be swallowed whole, without crushing, breaking, or chewing. Use calibrated measuring device to ensure accurate dosage of solution.

Patient/Family Teaching

- Inform patient that cutaneous flushing and a sensation of warmth, especially in the face, neck, and ears; itching or tingling; and headache may occur within the first 2 hr after taking the drug. These effects are usually transient and subside with continued therapy. If flushing is distressing or persistent, aspirin 300 mg given 30 min before each dose or slow upward titration of dose may decrease flushing.
- Advise patient to change positions slowly to minimize orthostatic hypotension.

- Instruct patients taking long-term extended-release niacin to report signs of hepatotoxicity (darkening of urine, light gray–colored stool, loss of appetite, severe stomach pain, yellow eyes or skin) to health care professional.
- Emphasize the importance of follow-up examinations to evaluate progress.
- **Vitamin Deficiency:** Encourage patient to comply with dietary recommendations of health care professional. Explain that the best source of vitamins is a well-balanced diet with foods from the four basic food groups.
- Foods high in niacin include meats, eggs, milk, and dairy products; little is lost during ordinary cooking.
- Patients self-medicating with vitamin supplements should be cautioned not to exceed RDA. The effectiveness of megadoses for treatment of various medical conditions is unproved and may cause side effects.
- **Hyperlipidemia:** Advise patient that this medication should be used in conjunction with dietary restrictions (fat, cholesterol, carbohydrates, alcohol), exercise, and cessation of smoking.

Evaluation/Desired Outcomes

- Prevention and treatment of niacin deficiency.
- Decrease in serum cholesterol and triglyceride levels.

niCARdipine (nye-kar-di-peen)

Cardene, Cardene SR, Cardene IV

Classification

Therapeutic: antianginals, antihypertensives

Pharmacologic: calcium channel blockers

Pregnancy Category C

Indications

Management of: Hypertension, Angina pectoris, Vasospastic (Prinzmetal's) angina. **Unlabeled uses:** Management of CHF.

Action

Inhibits the transport of calcium into myocardial and vascular smooth muscle cells, resulting in inhibition of excitation-contraction coupling and subsequent contraction. **Therapeutic Effects:** Systemic vasodilation resulting in decreased blood pressure. Coronary vasodilation resulting in decreased frequency and severity of attacks of angina.

Pharmacokinetics

Absorption: Well absorbed following oral administration but extensively metabolized, resulting in decreased bioavailability.

Distribution: Unknown.

Metabolism and Excretion: Mostly metabolized by the liver; ≤10% excreted unchanged by kidneys.

Half-life: 2–4 hr.

TIME/ACTION PROFILE (cardiovascular effects)

ROUTE	ONSET	PEAK	DURATION
PO	20 min	0.5–2 hr	8 hr
PO-ER	unknown	unknown	12 hr
IV	within min	45 min	50 hr†

†Following discontinuation

Contraindications/Precautions

Contraindicated in: Hypersensitivity; Sick sinus syndrome; 2nd- or 3rd-degree AV block (unless an artificial pacemaker is in place); BP <90 mm Hg; Advanced aortic stenosis.

Use Cautiously in: Severe hepatic impairment (dose reduction recommended); Geri: Geriatric patients (dose reduction/slower IV infusion rates recommended for most agents; increased risk of hypotension); Severe renal impairment (dose reduction may be necessary); History of serious ventricular arrhythmias or CHF; OB, Lactation, Pedi: Pregnancy, lactation, or children (safety not established).

Adverse Reactions/Side Effects

CNS: abnormal dreams, anxiety, confusion, dizziness, drowsiness, headache, jitteriness, nervousness, psychiatric disturbances, weakness. **EENT:** blurred vision, disturbed equilibrium, epistaxis, tinnitus. **Resp:** cough, dyspnea, shortness of breath. **CV:** ARRHYTHMIAS, CHF, peripheral edema, bradycardia, chest pain, hypotension, palpitations, syncope, tachycardia. **GI:** abnormal results in liver function studies, anorexia, constipation, diarrhea, dry mouth, dysgeusia, dyspepsia, nausea, vomiting. **GU:** dysuria, nocturia, polyuria, sexual dysfunction, urinary frequency. **Derm:** dermatitis, erythema multiforme, flushing, increased sweating, photosensitivity, pruritus/urticaria, rash. **Endo:** gynecomastia, hyperglycemia. **Hemat:** anemia, leukopenia, thrombocytopenia. **Metab:** weight gain. **MS:** joint stiffness, muscle cramps. **Neuro:** paresthesia, tremor. **Misc:** STEVENS-JOHNSON SYNDROME, gingival hyperplasia.

Interactions

Drug-Drug: Additive hypotension may occur when used concurrently with **fentanyl**, other **antihypertensives**, **nitrates**, acute ingestion of **alcohol**, or **quinidine**. Antihypertensive effects may be ↓ by concurrent use of **NSAIDs**. Concurrent use with **beta blockers**, **digoxin**, **disopyramide**, or **phenytoin** may result in bradycardia, conduction defects, or CHF. **Cimetidine** and **propranolol** may ↓ metabolism and increase the risk of toxicity. May ↓ the metabolism of and ↑ risk of toxicity from **cyclosporine**, **prazosin**, **quinidine**, or **carbamazepine**.

Drug-Food: Grapefruit and **grapefruit juice** ↑ serum levels and effect.

Route/Dosage

PO (Adults): 20 mg 3 times daily, may increase q 3 days (range 20–40 mg 3 times daily); or 30 mg twice daily as sustained-release form (up to 60 mg twice daily).

IV (Adults): *To replace PO use*—0.5–2.2 mg/hr continuous infusion. *For acute hypertensive episodes*—5 mg/hr titrated as needed (up to 15 mg/hr).

Availability (generic available)

Capsules: 20 mg, 30 mg. **Sustained-release capsules:** 30 mg, 45 mg, 60 mg. **Injection:** 2.5 mg/ml in 10-ml amps.

NURSING IMPLICATIONS

Assessment

- Monitor blood pressure and pulse prior to therapy, during dosage titration, and periodically throughout therapy. Monitor ECG periodically during prolonged therapy.
- Monitor intake and output ratios and daily weight. Assess for signs of CHF (peripheral edema, rales/crackles, dyspnea, weight gain, jugular venous distention).
- **Angina:** Assess location, duration, intensity, and precipitating factors of patient's anginal pain.
- ***Lab Test Considerations:*** Total serum calcium concentrations are not affected by calcium channel blockers.
- Monitor serum potassium periodically. Hypokalemia ↑ risk of arrhythmias; should be corrected.
- Monitor renal and hepatic functions periodically during long-term therapy. Several days of therapy may cause increase in hepatic enzymes, which return to normal upon discontinuation of therapy.

Potential Nursing Diagnoses

Decreased cardiac output (Indications)
Acute pain (Indications)

Implementation

- Do not confuse nicardipine with nifedipine or nimodipine. Do not confuse Cardene (nicardipine) with Cardura (doxazosin), codeine, or Cardizem (diltiazem).
- To transfer from IV nicardipine infusion to oral therapy with other antihypertensive, start oral therapy simultaneously with discontinuation of nicardipine infusion. If transferring to oral nicardipine therapy, administer first dose of a 3-times-a-day regimen 1 hr prior to discontinuation of infusion.
- Dosage adjustments of nicardipine should be made no more frequently than every 3 days.
- **PO:** May be administered without regard to meals. May be administered with meals if GI irritation becomes a problem.
- Do not open, crush, break, or chew sustained-release capsules.

IV Administration

- **Continuous Infusion:** ***Diluent:*** Dilute each 25-mg ampule with 240 ml of D5W, D5/0.45% NaCl, D5/0.9% NaCl, 0.45% NaCl, or 0.9% NaCl. Infusion is stable for 24 hr at room temperature. ***Concentration:*** 0.1 mg/ml. ***Rate:*** Titrate rate according to blood pressure response.
- **Y-Site Compatibility:** amikacin, aminophylline, aztreonam, calcium gluconate, caspofungin, cefazolin, ceftizoxime, chloramphenicol, cimetidine, clindamycin, daptomycin, diltiazem, dobutamine, dopamine, enalaprilat, epinephrine, ertapenem, erythromycin, famotidine, fenoldopam, fentanyl, gentamicin, hydrocortisone sodium succinate, hydromorphone, labetalol, lidocaine, linezolid, lorazepam, magnesium sulfate, methylprednisolone sodium succinate, metronidazole, midazolam, milrinone, morphine, nafcillin, nesiritide, nitroglycerin, nitroprusside, norepinephrine, palonosetron, penicillin G potassium, potassium chloride,

potassium phosphate, quinupristin/dalfopristin, ranitidine, tacrolimus, tirofiban, tobramycin, trimethoprim/sulfamethoxazole, vancomycin, vecuronium, voriconazole.
- **Y-Site Incompatibility:** amphotericin B liposome, ampicillin, ampicillin/sulbactam, cefepime, furosemide, lansoprazole, micafungin, pantoprazole.

Patient/Family Teaching
- Advise patient to take medication exactly as directed, even if feeling well. Take missed doses as soon as possible unless almost time for next dose; do not double doses. May need to be discontinued gradually.
- Instruct patient on technique for monitoring pulse. Instruct patient to contact health care professional if heart rate is <50 bpm.
- Advise patient to avoid grapefruit and grapefruit juice during therapy.
- Caution patient to change positions slowly to minimize orthostatic hypotension.
- May cause drowsiness or dizziness. Advise patient to avoid driving or other activities requiring alertness until response to the medication is known.
- Instruct patient to avoid concurrent use of alcohol or OTC medications, especially cold preparations, without consulting health care professional.
- Advise patient to notify health care professional if irregular heartbeat, dyspnea, swelling of hands and feet, pronounced dizziness, nausea, constipation, or hypotension occurs or if headache is severe or persistent.
- Caution patient to wear protective clothing and to use sunscreen to prevent photosensitivity reactions.
- **Angina:** Instruct patient on concurrent nitrate or beta-blocker therapy to continue taking both medications as directed and to use SL nitroglycerin as needed for anginal attacks.
- Advise patient to contact health care professional if chest pain does not improve, worsens after therapy, or occurs with diaphoresis; if shortness of breath; or if persistent headache occurs.
- Caution patient to discuss exercise restrictions with health care professional prior to exertion.
- **Hypertension:** Encourage patient to comply with other interventions for hypertension (weight reduction, low-sodium diet, smoking cessation, moderation of alcohol consumption, regular exercise, and stress management). Medication controls but does not cure hypertension.
- Instruct patient and family in proper technique for monitoring blood pressure. Advise patient to take blood pressure weekly and to report significant changes to health care professional.

Evaluation/Desired Outcomes
- Decrease in blood pressure.
- Decrease in frequency and severity of anginal attacks.
- Decrease in need for nitrate therapy.
- Increase in activity tolerance and sense of well-being.

NICOTINE (nik-o-teen)

nicotine chewing gum
Nicorette, Thrive

nicotine inhaler
Nicotrol Inhaler

nicotine lozenge
Commit

nicotine nasal spray
Nicotrol NS

nicotine transdermal
Nicoderm CQ

Classification
Therapeutic:

Pregnancy Category D

Indications
Adjunct therapy (with behavior modification) in the management of nicotine withdrawal in patients desiring to give up cigarette smoking.

Action
Provides a source of nicotine during controlled withdrawal from cigarette smoking. **Therapeutic Effects:** Lessened sequelae of nicotine withdrawal (irritability, insomnia, somnolence, headache, and increased appetite).

Pharmacokinetics
Absorption: *Gum, lozenge*—Slowly absorbed from buccal mucosa during chewing/sucking.

Inhaler—50% of dose is systemically absorbed; most of nicotine released from inhaler is deposited in the mouth; absorption from buccal mucosa is slow. *Nasal spray*—53% absorbed from nasal mucosa. *Transdermal*—70% of nicotine released from the patch is absorbed through the skin.
Distribution: Enters breast milk.
Metabolism and Excretion: Mostly metabolized by the liver. Small amounts are metabolized by kidneys and lungs; 10–20% excreted unchanged by kidneys.
Half-life: 1–2 hr.

TIME/ACTION PROFILE (nicotine blood levels)

ROUTE	ONSET	PEAK	DURATION
gum	rapid	15–30 min	unknown
inhaler	slow	within 15 min	unknown
lozenge	unknown	unknown	unknown
nasal spray	rapid	4–15 min	unknown
transdermal	rapid	2–4 hr	unknown

Contraindications/Precautions

Contraindicated in: Hypersensitivity; Recent history of MI (inhaler or nasal spray); Arrhythmias (inhaler or nasal spray); Severe or worsening angina (inhaler or nasal spray); Severe cardiovascular disease; Children; OB: Pregnancy or lactation.
Use Cautiously in: Cardiovascular disease including hypertension; Recent history of MI (gum, lozenge, patch); Arrhythmias (gum, lozenge, patch); Severe or worsening angina (gum, lozenge, patch); Diabetes mellitus; Pheochromocytoma; Peripheral vascular diseases; Hyperthyroidism; Diabetes; Continued smoking; Peptic ulcer disease; Hepatic disease; Bronchospastic lung disease (inhaler or nasal spray).

Adverse Reactions/Side Effects

CNS: headache, insomnia, abnormal dreams, dizziness, drowsiness, impaired concentration, nervousness, weakness. **EENT:** sinusitus; *gum*— pharyngitis; *nasal spray*— nasopharyngeal irritation, sneezing, watering eyes, change in smell, earache, epistaxis, eye irritation, hoarseness; *inhaler*— local mouth/throat irritation. **Resp:** *Nasal spray, inhaler*— cough, dyspnea. **CV:** tachycardia, chest pain, hypertension. **GI:** abdominal pain, abnormal taste, constipation, diarrhea, dry mouth, dyspepsia, hiccups, nausea, vomiting; *gum*— belching, increased appetite, increased salivation, oral injury, sore mouth. **Derm:** *transdermal*— burning at patch site, erythema, pruritus, cutaneous hypersensitivity, rash, sweating. **Endo:** dysmenorrhea. **MS:** arthralgia, back pain, myalgia; *gum*— jaw muscle ache. **Neuro:** paresthesia. **Misc:** allergy.

Interactions

Drug-Drug: Effects of **acetaminophen**, **caffeine**, **imipramine**, **insulin**, **oxazepam**, **pentazocine**, **propranolol**, or other **beta blockers**, **adrenergic antagonists (prazosin**, **labetalol)**, and **theophylline** may be ↑ during smoking cessation because of ↓ metabolism; dosage ↓ at cessation may be necessary. Doses of adrenergic agonists (e.g. **isoproterenol**, **phenylephrine**) may need to be ↑ because of lower levels of circulating catecholamines at cessation of smoking. Concurrent treatment with **bupropion** may cause treatment-emergent hypertension.

Route/Dosage

Gum (Adults): If patient smokes <25 cigarettes/day start with 2-mg gum, if patient smokes ≥25 cigarettes/day start with 4-mg gum; Patients should chew one piece of gum every 1–2 hr for 6 wk, then one piece of gum every 2–4 hr for 2 wk, then one piece of gum every 4–8 hr for 2 wk, then discontinue. Should not exceed 24 pieces of gum/day.
Lozenge (Adults): If first cigarette is desired >30 min after awakening, start with 2-mg lozenge, if first cigarette is desired <30 min after awakening, start with 4-mg lozenge. Patients should use one lozenge every 1–2 hr for 6 wk, then one lozenge every 2–4 hr for 2 wk, then one lozenge every 4–8 hr for 2 wk, then discontinue. Should not exceed 20 lozenges/day or more than 5 lozenges in 6 hr.
Intranasal (Adults): One spray in each nostril 1–2 times/hr (up to 5 times/hr); may be ↑ up to maximum of 40 times/day (should not exceed 3 mo of therapy).
Inhaln (Adults): Patients are encouraged to use at least 6 cartridges/day for first 3–6 wk, with additional cartridges as necessary (up to 16/day) for 12 wk. Patients are self-titrated to level of nicotine they require (usual usage 6–16 cartridges/day) followed by gradual withdrawal over 6–12 wk (maximum duration of use = 6 mo).
Transdermal (Adults): *Patients smoking >10 cigarettes/day*—Begin with Step 1 (21 mg/day) for 6 wk, followed by Step 2 (14 mg/day) for 2 wk, and then Step 3 (7 mg/day) for 2 wk, then stop (total of 10 wk) (new patch

should be applied every 24 hr); *Patients smoking ≤10 cigarettes/day*—Begin with Step 2 (14 mg/day) for 6 wk, followed by Step 3 (7 mg/day) for 2 wk, then stop (total of 8 wk) (new patch should be applied every 24 hr).

Availability (generic available)

Chewing gum (mint, orange, and fruit chill flavors): 2 mg[OTC], 4 mg[OTC]. **Inhalation:** each system contains 168 cartridges, each containing 10 mg of nicotine (deliver 4 mg). **Lozenge:** 2 mg[OTC], 4 mg[OTC]. **Nasal spray:** 10 mg/ml (0.5 mg/spray) in 10-ml bottles (200 sprays). **Transdermal patch:** 7 mg/day[OTC], 14 mg/day[OTC], 21 mg/day[OTC].

NURSING IMPLICATIONS

Assessment

- Prior to therapy, assess smoking history (number of cigarettes smoked daily, smoking patterns, nicotine content of preferred brand, degree to which patient inhales smoke).
- Assess patient for symptoms of smoking withdrawal (irritability, drowsiness, fatigue, headache, nicotine craving) periodically during nicotine replacement therapy (NRT)
- Evaluate progress in smoking cessation periodically during therapy.
- ***Toxicity and Overdose:*** Monitor for nausea, vomiting, diarrhea, increased salivation, abdominal pain, headache, dizziness, auditory and visual disturbances, weakness, dyspnea, hypotension, and irregular pulse.

Potential Nursing Diagnoses

Ineffective coping (Indications)

Implementation

- **Gum:** Protect gum from light; exposure to light causes gum to turn brown.
- **Lozenge:** Lozenge should be allowed to dissolve slowly in the mouth; it should not be chewed or swallowed.
- **Transdermal:** Patch can be worn for 16 or 24 hr; the patch can be removed before the patient goes to bed (especially if patient has vivid dreams or sleep distrubances) or can remain on while the patient sleeps (especially if patient craves cigarettes upon awakening).
- **Nasal Spray and Inhaler:** Regular use of the spray or inhaler during the first week of therapy may help patient adjust to irritant effects of the spray.

Patient/Family Teaching

- Explain to patient the necessity of immediate cessation of smoking upon initiation and throughout therapy.
- Encourage patient to participate in a smoking cessation program while using this product.
- Review the patient instruction sheet enclosed in the package.
- Instruct patient in proper method of disposal of unit. Emphasize need to keep out of the reach of children or pets.
- Nicotine in any form can be harmful to a pregnant woman and/or the fetus. Assist patient in determining risk/benefit of NRT and harm to the fetus versus the likelihood of stopping smoking without NRT.
- Emphasize the importance of regular visits to health care professional to monitor progress of smoking cessation.
- **Gum:** Explain purpose of nicotine gum to patient. The patient should chew 1 piece of gum whenever a craving for nicotine occurs or according to a fixed schedule (every 1–2 hr while awake) as directed. The gum should be chewed slowly until a tingling sensation is felt (about 15 chews). Then, patient should stop chewing and store the gum between the cheek and gums until the tingling sensation disappears (about 1 min). The process of stopping, then resuming chewing should be repeated for approximately 30 min until most of the tingle has disappeared. Rapid, vigorous chewing may result in side effects similar to those of smoking too many cigarettes (headache, dizziness, nausea, increased salivation, heartburn, and hiccups).
- Inform patient that the gum has a slight tobacco/pepper-like taste. Many patients initially find it unpleasant and slightly irritating to the mouth. This usually resolves after several days of therapy.
- Advise patient to carry gum at all times during therapy.
- Advise patient to avoid eating or drinking for 15 min before and during chewing of nicotine gum; these interfere with buccal absorption of nicotine.
- The gum usually can be chewed by denture wearers. Contact dentist if the gum adheres to bridgework.
- Inform patient that they should stop using the gum at the end of 12 wk; if they still feel the

N

need to use the gum after this time period, advise them to contact a health care professional.

- Instruct patient not to swallow gum.
- Dispose of the gum by wrapping in wrapper to prevent ingestion by children and animals. Call the poison control center, emergency department, or health care professional immediately if a child ingests the gum.
- Emphasize the need to discontinue the gum and to inform health care professional if pregnancy occurs.
- **Transdermal:** Instruct patient in application and use of patch. Apply patch at the same time each day. Keep patch in sealed pouch until ready to apply. Apply to clean, dry skin of upper arm or torso free of oil, hair, scars, cuts, burns, or irritation. Press patch firmly in place with palm for 10 sec, making sure there is good contact, especially around the edges. Keep patch in place during showering, bathing, or swimming; replace patches that have fallen off. Wash hands with soap and water after handling patches. Do not trim or cut patch. No more than 1 patch should be worn at a time. Alternate application sites. Dispose of used patches by folding adhesive sides together and replacing in protective pouch or aluminum foil; keep out of reach of children.
- Advise patient that redness, itching, and burning at application site usually subside within 1 hr. Instruct patient to notify health care professional and not apply new patch if signs of allergic reaction (urticaria, generalized rash, hives) or persistent local skin reactions (severe erythema, pruritus, edema) occur.
- May cause drowsiness or dizziness. Caution patient to avoid driving or other activities requiring alertness until response to medication is known.
- **Nasal Spray:** Instruct patient in proper use of spray. Tilt head back slightly. Do not sniff, swallow, or inhale through nose as spray is being administered. Patients who have successfully stopped smoking should continue to use the same dose for up to 8 wk, after which the spray should be discontinued over the next 4–6 wk.
- Discontinue nasal spray by using ½ dose (1 spray at a time), using the spray less frequently, skipping a dose by not using every hour, or setting a planned stop date for use of the spray.
- Treatment should be discontinued in patients who are unable to stop smoking by the 4th wk of therapy (patient is unlikely to quit on that attempt).
- Patients who fail to stop smoking should be given a therapy holiday before another attempt.
- Instruct patient to replace childproof cap after using and before disposal.
- **Inhalation:** Inhalation regimens should consist of frequent, continuous puffing for 20 minutes.
- Treatment should be discontinued in patients who are unable to stop smoking by the 4th wk of therapy (patient is unlikely to quit on that attempt).
- Patients who fail to stop smoking should be given a therapy holiday before another attempt.
- **Lozenge:** Instruct patient to place lozenge in mouth and allow it to slowly dissolve (20–30 min). Minimize swallowing; advise patient not to chew or swallow lozenge. May cause a warm tingling sensation in mouth. Advise patient to occasionally move lozenge from side to side of mouth until completely dissolved. Instruct patient not to eat or drink 15 min before or while lozenge is in mouth. For best chances of quitting, use at least 9 lozenges/day during 1st 6 wks. Do not use more than 1 lozenge at a time or use continuously one after the another. Lozenge should not be used after 12 wks without consulting health care professional.

Evaluation/Desired Outcomes

- Smoking cessation.

NIFEdipine (nye-**fed**-i-peen)

Adalat, Adalat CC, ✤Adalat PA, ✤Adalat XL, Afeditab CR, ✤Apo-Nifed, Nifedical XL, ✤Novo-Nifedin, ✤Nu-Nifed, Procardia, Procardia XL

Classification

Therapeutic: antianginals, antihypertensives

Pharmacologic: calcium channel blockers

Pregnancy Category C

Indications

Management of: Hypertension (extended-release only), Angina pectoris, Vasospastic

(Prinzmetal's) angina. **Unlabeled uses:** Prevention of migraine headache. Management of CHF or cardiomyopathy.

Action

Inhibits calcium transport into myocardial and vascular smooth muscle cells, resulting in inhibition of excitation-contraction coupling and subsequent contraction. **Therapeutic Effects:** Systemic vasodilation, resulting in decreased blood pressure. Coronary vasodilation, resulting in decreased frequency and severity of attacks of angina.

Pharmacokinetics

Absorption: Well absorbed after oral administration, but large amounts are rapidly metabolized (primarily by CYP3A4 enzyme system), resulting in decreased bioavailability (45–70%); bioavailability is increased (80%) with long-acting (CC, PA, XL) forms.
Distribution: Unknown.
Protein Binding: 92–98%.
Metabolism and Excretion: Mostly metabolized by the liver.
Half-life: 2–5 hr.

TIME/ACTION PROFILE

ROUTE	ONSET	PEAK	DURATION
PO	20 min	unknown	6–8 hr
PO–PA	unknown	4 hr	12 hr
PO–CC, PA, XL	unknown	6 hr	24 hr

Contraindications/Precautions

Contraindicated in: Hypersensitivity; Sick sinus syndrome; 2nd- or 3rd-degree AV block (unless an artificial pacemaker is in place); Blood pressure <90 mm Hg; Coadministration with grapefruit juice.
Use Cautiously in: Severe hepatic impairment (↓ dose recommended); History of porphyria; Geri: Short-acting forms appear on Beers list due to increased risk of hypotension and constipation in geriatric patients (↓ dose recommended). Is also associated with increased incidence of falls; Severe renal impairment (↓ dose may be necessary); History of serious ventricular arrhythmias or CHF; OB, Lactation, Pedi: Pregnancy, lactation, or children (safety not established).

Adverse Reactions/Side Effects

CNS: headache, abnormal dreams, anxiety, confusion, dizziness, drowsiness, jitteriness, nervousness, psychiatric disturbances, weakness. **EENT:** blurred vision, disturbed equilibrium, epistaxis, tinnitus. **Resp:** cough, dyspnea, shortness of breath. **CV:** ARRHYTHMIAS, CHF, peripheral edema, bradycardia, chest pain, hypotension, palpitations, syncope, tachycardia. **GI:** abnormal liver function studies, anorexia, constipation, diarrhea, dry mouth, dysgeusia, dyspepsia, nausea, vomiting. **GU:** dysuria, nocturia, polyuria, sexual dysfunction, urinary frequency. **Derm:** flushing, dermatitis, erythema multiforme, increased sweating, photosensitivity, pruritus/urticaria, rash. **Endo:** gynecomastia, hyperglycemia. **Hemat:** anemia, leukopenia, thrombocytopenia. **Metab:** weight gain. **MS:** joint stiffness, muscle cramps. **Neuro:** paresthesia, tremor. **Misc:** STEVENS-JOHNSON SYNDROME, gingival hyperplasia.

Interactions

Drug-Drug: Additive hypotension may occur when used concurrently with **fentanyl**, other **antihypertensives**, **nitrates**, acute ingestion of **alcohol**, or **quinidine**. Antihypertensive effects may be ↓ by concurrent use of **NSAIDs**. May ↑ serum levels and risk of toxicity from **digoxin**. Concurrent use with **beta blockers**, **digoxin**, **disopyramide**, or **phenytoin** may result in bradycardia, conduction defects, or CHF. **Cimetidine** and **propranolol** may ↓ metabolism and ↑ risk of toxicity. May ↓ metabolism of and ↑ risk of toxicity from **cyclosporine**, **prazosin**, **quinidine**, or **carbamazepine**.
Drug-Food: Grapefruit and **grapefruit juice** ↑ serum levels and effect.

Route/Dosage

PO (Adults): 10–30 mg 3 times daily (not to exceed 180 mg/day), *or* 10–20 mg twice daily as PA form, *or* 30–90 mg once daily as sustained-release (CC, XL) form (not to exceed 90–120 mg/day).

Availability (generic available)

Capsules: ✤5 mg, 10 mg, 20 mg. **Cost:** *Generic*—10 mg $62.99/90, 20 mg $104.97/90. **Tablets:** ✤10 mg. **Extended-release tablets, (Adalat CC, Afeditab CR, Nifedical XL, Procardia XL):** ✤10 mg, ✤20 mg, 30 mg, 60 mg, 90 mg. **Cost:** *Generic*—30 mg $94.00/90, 60 mg $164.99/90, 90 mg $174.99/90.

NURSING IMPLICATIONS

Assessment

- Monitor blood pressure and pulse before therapy, during dose titration, and periodically during therapy. Monitor ECG periodically during prolonged therapy.
- Monitor intake and output ratios and daily weight. Assess for signs of CHF (peripheral edema, rales/crackles, dyspnea, weight gain, jugular venous distention).
- Geri: Assess fall risk and institute fall prevention strategies.
- Patients receiving digoxin concurrently with nifedipine should have routine tests of serum digoxin levels and be monitored for signs and symptoms of digoxin toxicity.
- **Angina:** Assess location, duration, intensity, and precipitating factors of patient's anginal pain.
- ***Lab Test Considerations:*** Total serum calcium concentrations are not affected by calcium channel blockers.
- Monitor serum potassium periodically. Hypokalemia increases risk of arrhythmias; should be corrected.
- Monitor renal and hepatic functions periodically during long-term therapy. Several days of therapy may cause increase in hepatic enzymes, which return to normal upon discontinuation of therapy.
- Nifedipine may cause positive ANA and direct Coombs' test results.

Potential Nursing Diagnoses

Decreased cardiac output (Indications)
Acute pain (Indications)

Implementation

- **PO:** May be administered without regard to meals. May be administered with meals if GI irritation becomes a problem.
- Do not open, crush, break, or chew extended-release tablets. Empty tablets that appear in stool are not significant.
- Avoid administration with grapefruit juice.
- Sublingual use is not recommended due to serious adverse drug reactions.

Patient/Family Teaching

- Advise patient to take medication exactly as directed, even if feeling well. Take missed doses as soon as possible unless almost time for next dose; do not double doses. May need to be discontinued gradually.
- Instruct patient on technique for monitoring pulse. Instruct patient to contact health care professional if heart rate is <50 bpm.
- Advise patient to avoid grapefruit and grapefruit juice during therapy.
- Caution patient to change positions slowly to minimize orthostatic hypotension.
- May cause drowsiness or dizziness. Advise patient to avoid driving or other activities requiring alertness until response to the medication is known.
- Geri: Teach patients and family about risk for falls and how to reduce risk in the home.
- Instruct patient on importance of maintaining good dental hygiene and seeing dentist frequently for teeth cleaning to prevent tenderness, bleeding, and gingival hyperplasia (gum enlargement).
- Instruct patient to avoid concurrent use of alcohol or OTC medications and natural/herbal products, especially cold preparations, without consulting health care professional.
- Advise patient to notify health care professional if irregular heartbeat, dyspnea, swelling of hands and feet, pronounced dizziness, nausea, constipation, or hypotension occurs or if headache is severe or persistent.
- Caution patient to wear protective clothing and use sunscreen to prevent photosensitivity reactions.
- **Angina:** Instruct patient on concurrent nitrate or beta-blocker therapy to continue taking both medications as directed and use SL nitroglycerin as needed for anginal attacks.
- Inform patient that anginal attacks may occur 30 min after administration because of reflex tachycardia. This is usually temporary and is not an indication for discontinuation.
- Advise patient to contact health care professional if chest pain does not improve, worsens after therapy, or occurs with diaphoresis; if shortness of breath occurs; or if persistent headache occurs.
- Caution patient to discuss exercise restrictions with health care professional before exertion.
- **Hypertension:** Encourage patient to comply with other interventions for hypertension (weight reduction, low-sodium diet, smoking cessation, moderation of alcohol consumption, regular exercise, and stress manage-

ment). Medication controls but does not cure hypertension.

- Instruct patient and family in proper technique for monitoring blood pressure. Advise patient to take blood pressure weekly and to report significant changes to health care professional.

Evaluation/Desired Outcomes

- Decrease in blood pressure.
- Decrease in frequency and severity of anginal attacks.
- Decrease in need for nitrate therapy.
- Increase in activity tolerance and sense of well-being.

nilutamide (nye-**loot**-a-mide)

✱Anandron, Nilandron

Classification

Therapeutic: antineoplastics

Pharmacologic: antiandrogens

Pregnancy Category C

Indications

Management of metastatic prostate cancer (with surgical castration).

Action

Blocks the effects of androgen (testosterone) at the cellular level. **Therapeutic Effects:** Decreased spread of prostate cancer.

Pharmacokinetics

Absorption: Rapidly and completely absorbed following oral administration.

Distribution: Unknown.

Metabolism and Excretion: Extensively metabolized by the liver; two metabolites have antiandrogenic activity; <2% excreted unchanged in urine.

Half-life: 41–49 hr.

TIME/ACTION PROFILE (antiandrogenic effects)

ROUTE	ONSET	PEAK	DURATION
PO	rapid	unknown	24 hr

Contraindications/Precautions

Contraindicated in: Hypersensitivity; Severe hepatic impairment; Severe respiratory insufficiency.

Use Cautiously in: History of liver disease or alcoholism; History of respiratory problems; Pregnancy, lactation, or children (safety not established).

Adverse Reactions/Side Effects

CNS: dizziness. **EENT:** impaired adaptation to darkness, abnormal vision. **Resp:** interstitial pneumonitis. **CV:** hypertension. **GI:** HEPATOTOXICITY, constipation, hepatitis, increased liver enzymes, nausea. **Derm:** hot flashes, hair loss, sweating.

Interactions

Drug-Drug: May increase the effects of **warfarin, phenytoin**, and **theophylline**. May cause **alcohol** intolerance.

Route/Dosage

PO (Adults): 300 mg once daily for 30 days; then 150 mg once daily.

Availability

Tablets: 150 mg, ✱100 mg.

NURSING IMPLICATIONS

Assessment

- Patients should have a chest x-ray prior to initiation of therapy. Assess patient for symptoms of interstitial pneumonitis (dyspnea or worsening of pre-existing dyspnea). If symptoms occur, nilutamide should be discontinued until cause can be determined. Pneumonitis usually occurs during the first 3 mo of therapy and is almost always reversible when treatment is discontinued.
- ***Lab Test Considerations:*** Monitor hepatic function prior to and every 3 mo throughout therapy. If AST or ALT is elevated more than 2–3 times normal, treatment should be discontinued.
- May cause hyperglycemia; increased serum alkaline phosphatase, BUN, and creatinine; and leukopenia.

Potential Nursing Diagnoses

Risk for injury (Side Effects)

Implementation

- **PO:** May be taken without regard to food.

Patient/Family Teaching

- Instruct patient to take nilutamide exactly as directed. If a dose is missed, take as soon as possible unless almost time for next dose. Do not double doses.

- Caution patient that adaptation to darkness may be impaired and may cause difficulty driving at night or through tunnels. Wearing tinted glasses may minimize this effect.
- Advise patient to notify physician immediately if dark urine, fatigue, abdominal pain, yellow eyes or skin, or unexplained GI symptoms occur. Hepatotoxicity usually resolves when nilutamide is discontinued but may be progressive and fatal; requires immediate medical attention.

Evaluation/Desired Outcomes

- Decrease in the spread of prostate cancer.

nimodipine (nye-moe-di-peen)
Nimotop

Classification
Therapeutic: subarachnoid hemorrhage therapy agents
Pharmacologic: calcium channel blockers

Pregnancy Category C

Indications
Management of subarachnoid hemorrhage.

Action
Inhibits the transport of calcium into vascular smooth muscle cells, resulting in inhibition of excitation-contraction coupling and subsequent contraction. Potent peripheral vasodilator. **Therapeutic Effects:** Prevention of vascular spasm after subarachnoid hemorrhage, resulting in decreased neurologic impairment.

Pharmacokinetics
Absorption: Well absorbed following oral administration but extensively metabolized, resulting in decreased bioavailability.
Distribution: Crosses the blood-brain barrier; remainder of distribution unknown.
Protein Binding: >95%.
Metabolism and Excretion: Mostly metabolized by the liver; ≤10% excreted unchanged by kidneys.
Half-life: 1–2 hr.

TIME/ACTION PROFILE (vasodilation)

ROUTE	ONSET	PEAK	DURATION
PO	unknown	1 hr	4 hr

Contraindications/Precautions
Contraindicated in: Hypersensitivity; Sick sinus syndrome; 2nd- or 3rd-degree AV block (unless an artificial pacemaker is in place); BP <90 mm Hg.
Use Cautiously in: Severe hepatic impairment (dose reduction recommended); Geri: Geriatric patients (dose reduction recommended; increased risk of hypotension); Severe renal impairment; History of serious ventricular arrhythmias or CHF; OB, Lactation, Pedi: Pregnancy, lactation, or children (safety not established).

Adverse Reactions/Side Effects
CNS: abnormal dreams, anxiety, confusion, dizziness, drowsiness, headache, nervousness, psychiatric disturbances, weakness. **EENT:** blurred vision, disturbed equilibrium, epistaxis, tinnitus. **Resp:** cough, dyspnea. **CV:** ARRHYTHMIAS, CHF, bradycardia, chest pain, hypotension, palpitations, peripheral edema, syncope, tachycardia. **GI:** abnormal liver function studies, anorexia, constipation, diarrhea, dry mouth, dysgeusia, dyspepsia, nausea, vomiting. **GU:** dysuria, nocturia, polyuria, sexual dysfunction, urinary frequency. **Derm:** dermatitis, erythema multiforme, flushing, increased sweating, photosensitivity, pruritus/urticaria, rash. **Endo:** gynecomastia, hyperglycemia. **Hemat:** anemia, leukopenia, thrombocytopenia. **Metab:** weight gain. **MS:** joint stiffness, muscle cramps. **Neuro:** paresthesia, tremor. **Misc:** STEVENS-JOHNSON SYNDROME, gingival hyperplasia.

Interactions
Drug-Drug: Additive hypotension may occur when used concurrently with **fentanyl**, other **antihypertensives**, **nitrates**, acute ingestion of **alcohol**, or **quinidine**. Concurrent use with **beta blockers**, **digoxin**, **disopyramide**, or **phenytoin** may result in bradycardia, conduction defects, or CHF.
Drug-Natural Products: Grapefruit and **grapefruit juice** ↑ serum levels and effect.

Route/Dosage
PO (Adults): 60 mg q 4 hr for 21 days; therapy should be started within 96 hr of subarachnoid hemorrhage.

Hepatic Impairment
PO (Adults): 30 mg q 4 hr for 21 days; therapy should be started within 96 hr of subarachnoid hemorrhage.

Availability
Capsules: 30 mg.

NURSING IMPLICATIONS

Assessment
- Assess patient's neurologic status (level of consciousness, movement) prior to and periodically following administration.

- Monitor blood pressure and pulse prior to therapy and periodically throughout therapy.
- Monitor intake and output ratios and daily weight. Assess for signs of CHF (peripheral edema, rales/crackles, dyspnea, weight gain, jugular venous distention).
- ***Lab Test Considerations:*** Total serum calcium concentrations are not affected by calcium channel blockers.
- Monitor serum potassium periodically. Hypokalemia increases risk of arrhythmias; should be corrected.
- Monitor renal and hepatic functions periodically. Several days of therapy may cause increase in hepatic enzymes, which return to normal upon discontinuation of therapy.
- May occasionally cause decreased platelet count.

Potential Nursing Diagnoses
Ineffective tissue perfusion (Indications)

Implementation
- Do not confuse nimodipine with nicardipine or nifedipine.
- Begin administration within 96 hr of subarachnoid hemorrhage and continue every 4 hr for 21 consecutive days.
- **PO:** If patient is unable to swallow capsule, make a hole in both ends of the capsule with a sterile 18-gauge needle and extract the contents into a syringe. Empty contents into water or nasogastric tube and flush with 30 ml normal saline.

Patient/Family Teaching
- Advise patient to take medication exactly as directed, even if feeling well. If a dose is missed, take as soon as possible unless almost time for next dose; do not double doses. May need to be discontinued gradually.
- Advise patient to avoid grapefruit or grapefruit juice during therapy.
- Caution patient to change positions slowly to minimize orthostatic hypotension.
- May cause drowsiness or dizziness. Advise patient to avoid driving or other activities requiring alertness until response to the medication is known.
- Instruct patient to avoid concurrent use of alcohol or OTC medications, especially cold preparations, without consulting health care professional.
- Advise patient to notify health care professional if irregular heartbeats, dyspnea, swelling of hands and feet, pronounced dizziness, nausea, constipation, or hypotension occurs or if headache is severe or persistent.
- Caution patient to wear protective clothing and use sunscreen to prevent photosensitivity reactions.

Evaluation/Desired Outcomes
- Improvement in neurologic deficits due to vasospasm following subarachnoid hemorrhage.

nisoldipine (nye-**sole**-di-peen)
Sular

Classification
Therapeutic: antihypertensives
Pharmacologic: calcium channel blockers

Pregnancy Category C

Indications
Management of hypertension.

Action
Inhibits the transport of calcium into vascular smooth muscle cells, resulting in inhibition of vasoconstriction and dilation of arterioles. **Therapeutic Effects:** Systemic vasodilation, resulting in decreased blood pressure.

Pharmacokinetics
Absorption: Well absorbed (87%) following oral administration but rapidly and extensively metabolized in the gut wall, resulting in 5% bioavailability.
Distribution: Unknown.
Metabolism and Excretion: Highly metabolized CYP3A4 enzyme system.
Half-life: 7–12 hr.

TIME/ACTION PROFILE (antihypertensive effects)

ROUTE	ONSET	PEAK	DURATION
PO	unknown	6–12 hr	24 hr

Contraindications/Precautions
Contraindicated in: Hypersensitivity; Cross-sensitivity with calcium channel blockers may occur; Concurrent phenytoin use.
Use Cautiously in: CHF/left ventricular dysfunction; Hepatic impairment (dose reduction

may be necessary); Geri: Geriatric patients (dose reduction may be necessary); Coronary artery disease (may precipitate angina); OB, Lactation, Pedi: Pregnancy, lactation, or children (safety not established).

Adverse Reactions/Side Effects

CNS: headache, dizziness. **EENT:** pharyngitis, sinusitis. **CV:** peripheral edema, chest pain, hypotension, palpitations. **GI:** nausea. **Derm:** rash. **Endo:** gynecomastia.

Interactions

Drug-Drug: Additive hypotension may occur with other **antihypertensives**, acute ingestion of **alcohol**, or **nitrates**. Antihypertensive effects may be decreased by concurrent use of **NSAIDs**. **Phenytoin** or **other CYP3A4 inducers** decrease blood levels and effectiveness (avoid concurrent use).
Drug-Food: Grapefruit and **grapefruit juice** ↑ serum levels and effect. Blood levels are increased by concurrent ingestion of a **high-fat meal** and should be avoided.

Route/Dosage

PO (Adults): 20 mg/day as a single dose initially; may be increased by 10 mg/day q 7 days, up to 60 mg/day (usual range 20–40 mg/day).

Availability

Extended-release tablets: 10 mg, 20 mg, 30 mg, 40 mg. **Cost:** 10 mg $179.98/90, 20 mg $225.97/90, 30 mg $239.99/90, 40 mg $240.32/90.

NURSING IMPLICATIONS

Assessment

- Monitor blood pressure and pulse prior to therapy, during dosage titration, and periodically throughout therapy. Monitor ECG periodically during prolonged therapy.
- Monitor intake and output ratios and daily weight. Assess for signs of CHF (peripheral edema, rales/crackles, dyspnea, weight gain, jugular venous distention).
- ***Lab Test Considerations:*** Total serum calcium concentrations are not affected by calcium channel blockers.

Potential Nursing Diagnoses

Decreased cardiac output (Indications)

Implementation

- **PO:** Avoid administration within 1 hr of high-fat meals or grapefruit products.
- Do not crush, break, or chew tablets.

Patient/Family Teaching

- Advise patient to take medication exactly as directed, even if feeling well. If a dose is missed, take as soon as possible unless almost time for next dose; do not double doses. May need to be discontinued gradually.
- Advise patient to avoid grapefruit or grapefruit juice during therapy.
- Encourage patient to comply with other interventions for hypertension (weight reduction, low-sodium diet, smoking cessation, moderation of alcohol consumption, regular exercise, and stress management). Medication controls but does not cure hypertension.
- Instruct patient and family in proper technique for monitoring blood pressure. Advise patient to take blood pressure weekly and to report significant changes to health care professional.
- Caution patient to change positions slowly to minimize orthostatic hypotension.
- May cause dizziness. Advise patient to avoid driving or other activities requiring alertness until response to the medication is known.
- Instruct patient to avoid concurrent use of alcohol or OTC medications, especially cold preparations, without consulting health care professional.
- Advise patient to notify health care professional if irregular heartbeat, dyspnea, swelling of hands and feet, pronounced dizziness, nausea, constipation, or hypotension occurs or if headache is severe or persistent.

Evaluation/Desired Outcomes

- Decrease in blood pressure.

nitrofurantoin

(nye-troe-fyoor-**an**-toyn)
✤Apo-Nitrofurantoin, Furadantin, Macrobid, Macrodantin

Classification
Therapeutic: anti-infectives

Pregnancy Category B

Indications

Prevention and treatment of urinary tract infections caused by susceptible organisms; not effective in systemic bacterial infections.

Action

Interferes with bacterial enzymes. **Therapeutic Effects:** Bactericidal or bacteriostatic action against susceptible organisms. **Spectrum:** Many gram-negative and some gram-positive organisms, specifically: *Citrobacter*, *Corynebacterium*, *Enterobacter*, *Escherichia coli*, *Klebsiella*, *Neisseria*, *Salmonella*, *Shigella*, *Staphylococcus aureus*, *S. epidermidis*, *Enterococcus*.

Pharmacokinetics

Absorption: Readily absorbed after oral administration. Absorption is slower but more complete with macrocrystals (Macrodantin).
Distribution: Crosses placenta; enters breast milk.
Protein Binding: 40%.
Metabolism and Excretion: Partially metabolized by the liver; 30–50% excreted unchanged by the kidneys.
Half-life: 20 min (increased in renal impairment).

TIME/ACTION PROFILE (urine levels)

ROUTE	ONSET	PEAK	DURATION
PO	unknown	30 min	6–12 hr

Contraindications/Precautions

Contraindicated in: Hypersensitivity; Hypersensitivity to parabens (suspension); Oliguria, anuria, or significant renal impairment (CCr <60 ml/min); G6PD deficiency; Infants <1 mo and pregnancy near term (increased risk of hemolytic anemia in newborn).
Use Cautiously in: Patients with diabetes or debilitated patients (neuropathy may be more common); Lactation, OB: Safety not established but has been used safely in pregnant women. May cause hemolysis in G6PD-deficient infants who are breastfed; Geri: Appears on Beers list. Geriatric patients may increase risk for renal, hepatic, and pulmonary reactions.

Adverse Reactions/Side Effects

CNS: dizziness, drowsiness, headache. **EENT:** nystagmus. **Resp:** pneumonitis. **CV:** chest pain. **GI:** PSEUDOMEMBRANOUS COLITIS, anorexia, nausea, vomiting, abdominal pain, diarrhea, drug-induced hepatitis. **GU:** rust/brown discoloration of urine. **Derm:** photosensitivity. **Hemat:** blood dyscrasias, hemolytic anemia. **Neuro:** peripheral neuropathy. **Misc:** hypersensitivity reactions.

Interactions

Drug-Drug: Probenecid and **sulfinpyrazone** prevent high urinary concentrations; may ↓ effectiveness. **Antacids** may decrease absorption. ↑ risk of neurotoxicity with **neurotoxic drugs**. ↑ risk of hepatotoxicity with **hepatotoxic drugs**. ↑ risk of pneumonitis with **drugs having pulmonary toxicity**.

Route/Dosage

PO (Adults): *Treatment of active infection*—50–100 mg q 6–8 hr *or* 100 mg q 12 hr as extended-release product. *Chronic suppression*—50–100 mg single evening dose.
PO (Children >1 mo): *Treatment of active infection*—5–7 mg/kg/day divided q 6 hr; maximum dose: 400 mg/day. *Chronic suppression*—1–2 mg/kg/day as a single dose at bedtime; maximum dose: 100 mg/day (unlabeled).

Availability (generic available)

Tablets: 50 mg, 100 mg. **Oral suspension:** 25 mg/5 ml. **Capsules:** 25 mg, 50 mg, 100 mg. **Extended-release capsules:** 100 mg.

N

NURSING IMPLICATIONS

Assessment

- Assess for signs and symptoms of urinary tract infection (frequency, urgency, pain, and burning on urination; fever; cloudy or foul-smelling urine) before and periodically during therapy.
- Obtain specimens for culture and sensitivity before and during drug administration.
- Monitor intake and output ratios. Report significant discrepancies in totals.
- ***Lab Test Considerations:*** Monitor CBC routinely with patients on prolonged therapy.
- May cause ↑ serum glucose, bilirubin, alkaline phosphatase, BUN, and creatinine.

Potential Nursing Diagnoses

Risk for infection (Indications)

Implementation

- **PO:** Administer with food or milk to minimize GI irritation, to delay and increase absorption, to increase peak concentration, and to prolong duration of therapeutic concentration in the urine.
- Do not crush tablets or open capsules.
- Administer liquid preparations with calibrated measuring device. Shake well before administration. Oral suspension may be mixed

with water, milk, fruit juices, or infant formula. Rinse mouth with water after administration of oral suspension to avoid staining teeth.

Patient/Family Teaching

- Instruct patient to take medication around the clock, as directed. Take missed doses as soon as remembered and space next dose 2–4 hr apart. Do not skip or double up on missed doses.
- May cause dizziness or drowsiness. Caution patient to avoid driving or other activities requiring alertness until response to medication is known.
- Inform patient that medication may cause a rust-yellow to brown discoloration of urine, which is not significant.
- Advise patient to notify health care professional if fever, chills, cough, chest pain, dyspnea, skin rash, numbness or tingling of the fingers or toes, or intolerable GI upset occurs. Signs of superinfection (milky, foul-smelling urine; perineal irritation; dysuria) should also be reported.
- Instruct patient to notify health care professional if fever and diarrhea develop, especially if stool contains blood, pus, or mucus. Advise patient not to treat diarrhea without consulting health care professional.
- Instruct patient to consult health care professional if no improvement is seen within a few days after initiation of therapy.

Evaluation/Desired Outcomes

- Resolution of the signs and symptoms of infection. Therapy should be continued for a minimum of 7 days and for at least 3 days after the urine has become sterile.
- Decrease in the frequency of infections in chronic suppressive therapy.

nitroglycerin

(nye-tro-**gli**-ser-in)

extended-release capsules
Nitrocot, NitroglynE-R, Nitro-par, Nitro-Time

extended-release tablets
Nitrong

extended-release buccal tablets
Nitrogard, ✤Nitrogard SR

intravenous
Nitro-Bid IV, Tridil

translingual spray
Nitrolingual

ointment
Nitro-Bid, Nitrol

sublingual
Nitrostat, NitroQuick

transdermal system
Deponit, Minitran, Nitrek, Nitro-disc, Nitro-Dur, Transderm-Nitro

Classification
Therapeutic: antianginals
Pharmacologic: nitrates

Pregnancy Category C

Indications

Acute (**translingual and SL**) and long-term prophylatic (**oral, buccal, transdermal**) management of angina pectoris. **PO:** Adjunct treatment of CHF. **IV:** Adjunct treatment of acute MI. Production of controlled hypotension during surgical procedures. Treatment of CHF associated with acute MI. **Unlabeled uses:** Management of chronic CHF.

Action

Increases coronary blood flow by dilating coronary arteries and improving collateral flow to ischemic regions. Produces vasodilation (venous greater than arterial). Decreases left ventricular end-diastolic pressure and left ventricular end-diastolic volume (preload). Reduces myocardial oxygen consumption. **Therapeutic Effects:** Relief or prevention of anginal attacks. Increased cardiac output. Reduction of blood pressure.

Pharmacokinetics

Absorption: Well absorbed after oral, buccal, and sublingual administration. Also absorbed through skin. Orally administered nitroglycerin is rapidly metabolized, leading to decreased bioavailability.
Distribution: Unknown.
Metabolism and Excretion: Undergoes rapid and almost complete metabolism by the liver; also metabolized by enzymes in bloodstream.
Half-life: 1–4 min.

TIME/ACTION PROFILE (cardiovascular effects)

ROUTE	ONSET	PEAK	DURATION
SL	1–3 min	unknown	30–60 min
Buccal-ER	unknown	unknown	5 hr

PO-ER	40–60 min	unknown	8–12 hr
TD-Oint	20–60 min	unknown	4–8 hr
TD-Patch	40–60 min	unknown	8–24 hr
IV	immediate	unknown	several min

Contraindications/Precautions

Contraindicated in: Hypersensitivity; Severe anemia; Pericardial tamponade; Constrictive pericarditis; Alcohol intolerance (large IV doses only); Concurrent use of sildenafil.

Use Cautiously in: Head trauma or cerebral hemorrhage; Glaucoma; Hypertrophic cardiomyopathy; Severe liver impairment; Malabsorption or hypermotility (PO); Hypovolemia (IV); Normal or decreased pulmonary capillary wedge pressure (IV); Cardioversion (remove transdermal patch before procedure); OB: Pregnancy (may compromise maternal/fetal circulation); Pedi, Lactation: Children or lactation (safety not established).

Adverse Reactions/Side Effects

CNS: dizziness, headache, apprehension, restlessness, weakness. **EENT:** blurred vision. **CV:** hypotension, tachycardia, syncope. **GI:** abdominal pain, nausea, vomiting. **Derm:** contact dermatitis (transdermal or ointment). **Misc:** alcohol intoxication (large IV doses only), cross-tolerance, flushing, tolerance.

Interactions

Drug-Drug: Concurrent use of nitrates in any form with **sildenafil**, **tadalafil**, and **vardenafil** ↑ risk of serious and potentially fatal hypotension; concurrent use is contraindicated. Additive hypotension with **antihypertensives**, acute ingestion of **alcohol**, **beta blockers**, **calcium channel blockers**, **haloperidol**, or **phenothiazines**. **Agents having anticholinergic properties (tricyclic antidepressants, antihistamines, phenothiazines)** may ↓ absorption of lingual, sublingual, or buccal nitroglycerin.

Route/Dosage

SL (Adults): 0.3–0.6 mg; may repeat q 5 min for 15 min for acute attack. Lingual Spray (Adults) 1–2 sprays; may be repeated q 5 min for 15 min. May also be used prophylactically 5–10 min before activities that may precipitate an acute attack.

Buccal (Adults): 1 mg q 5 hr; dosage and frequency may be increased as needed.

PO (Adults): *Extended-release capsules*—2.5–9 mg q 8–12 hr. *Extended-release tablets*—1.3–6.5 mg q 8–12 hr.

IV (Adults): 5 mcg/min; increase by 5 mcg/min q 3–5 min to 20 mcg/min, then increase by 10–20 mcg/min q 3–5 min (dosing determined by hemodynamic parameters).

Transdermal (Adults): *Ointment*—(1 in. = 15 mg) 1–2 in. q 8 hr (up to 5 in. q 4 hr). *Transdermal patch*—0.1–0.6 mg/hr, up to 0.8 mg/hr. Patch should be worn 12–14 hr/day.

Availability (generic available)

Extended-release tablets: 2.6 mg, 6.5 mg, 9 mg. **Extended-release capsules:** 2.5 mg, 6.5 mg, 9 mg. **Sublingual tablets:** 0.3 mg, 0.4 mg, 0.6 mg. **Cost:** *NitroQuick*—0.3 mg $6.82/100, 0.4 mg $6.82/100, 0.6 mg $6.82/100; *Nitrostat*—0.3 mg $9.09/100, 0.4 mg $9.09/100, 0.6 mg $9.09/100. **Translingual spray (Nitrolingual):** 400 mcg/spray in 14.5-g canister (200 doses), NitroMist 400 mcg/spray in 8.5-g canister (230 doses). **Extended-release buccal tablets:** 1 mg, 2 mg, 3 mg, ✤5 mg. **Transdermal systems:** 0.1 mg/hr, 0.2 mg/hr, 0.3 mg/hr, 0.4 mg/hr, 0.6 mg/hr, 0.8 mg/hr. **Transdermal ointment:** 2%. **Injection:** 5 mg/ml. **Injection solution:** 25 mg/250 ml, 50 mg/250 ml, 50 mg/500 ml, 100 mg/250 ml, 200 mg/500 ml.

NURSING IMPLICATIONS

Assessment

- Assess location, duration, intensity, and precipitating factors of patient's anginal pain.
- Monitor blood pressure and pulse before and after administration. Patients receiving IV nitroglycerin require continuous ECG and blood pressure monitoring. Additional hemodynamic parameters may be monitored.
- ***Lab Test Considerations:*** May cause ↑ urine catecholamine and urine vanillylmandelic acid concentrations.
- Excessive doses may cause ↑ methemoglobin concentrations.
- May cause falsely ↑ serum cholesterol levels.

Potential Nursing Diagnoses

Acute pain (Indications)
Ineffective tissue perfusion (Indications)

Implementation

- **PO:** Administer dose 1 hr before or 2 hr after meals with a full glass of water for faster absorption. Sustained-release preparations should be swallowed whole; do not crush, break, or chew. **SL:** Tablet should be held under tongue until dissolved. Avoid eating, drinking, or smoking until tablet is dissolved. **Buccal:** Place tablet under upper lip or between cheek and gum. Onset of action may be increased by touching the tablet with the tongue or by drinking hot liquids.

IV Administration

- **IV:** Doses must be diluted and administered as an infusion. Standard infusion sets made of polyvinyl chloride (PVC) plastic may absorb up to 80% of the nitroglycerin in solution. Use glass bottles only and special tubing provided by manufacturer
- **Continuous Infusion:** ***Diluent:*** Vials must be diluted in D5W or 0.9% NaCl. Premixed infusions already diluted in D5W and are ready to be administered (no further dilution needed). Admixed solutions stable for 48 hr at room temperature or 7 days if refrigerated. Stability of premixed solutions based on manufacturer's expiration date. ***Concentration:*** Should not exceed 400 mcg/ml. ***Rate:*** See Route/Dosage section. Administer via infusion pump to ensure accurate rate. Titrate rate according to patient response.
- **Y-Site Compatibility:** amiodarone, amphotericin B cholesteryl sulfate complex, cisatracurium, diltiazem, dobutamine, dopamine, epinephrine, eptifibatide, esmolol, famotidine, fentanyl, fluconazole, furosemide, haloperidol, heparin, hydralazine, hydromorphone, insulin, labetalol, lidocaine, linezolid, lorazepam, midazolam, morphine, nesiritide, norepinephrine, nitroprusside, pancuronium, propofol, ranitidine, tacrolimus, theophylline, thiopental, tirofiban, vecuronium, warfarin.
- **Y-Site Incompatibility:** alteplase, diazepam, lansoprazole, levofloxacin, phenytoin, trimethoprim/sulfamethoxazole.
- **Additive Incompatibility:** Manufacturer recommends that nitroglycerin not be admixed with other medications.
- **Topical:** Sites of topical application should be rotated to prevent skin irritation. Remove patch or ointment from previous site before application.
- Doses may be increased to the highest dose that does not cause symptomatic hypotension.
- Apply ointment by using dose-measuring application papers supplied with ointment. Squeeze ointment onto measuring scale printed on paper. Use paper to spread ointment onto nonhairy area of skin (chest, abdomen, thighs; avoid distal extremities) in a thin, even layer, covering a 2–3-in. area. Do not allow ointment to come in contact with hands. Do not massage or rub in ointment; this will increase absorption and interfere with sustained action. Apply occlusive dressing if ordered.
- Transdermal patches may be applied to any hairless site (avoid distal extremities or areas with cuts or calluses). Apply firm pressure over patch to ensure contact with skin, especially around edges. Apply a new dosage unit if the first one becomes loose or falls off. Units are waterproof and not affected by showering or bathing. Do not cut or trim system to adjust dosage. Do not alternate between brands of transdermal products; dosage may not be equivalent. Remove patches before cardioversion or defibrillation to prevent patient burns. Patch may be worn for 12–14 hr and removed for 10–12 hr at night to prevent development of tolerance.

Patient/Family Teaching

- Instruct patient to take medication exactly as directed, even if feeling better. Take missed doses as soon as remembered unless next dose is scheduled within 2 hr (6 hr with extended-release preparations). Do not double doses. Do not discontinue abruptly; gradual dosage reduction may be necessary to prevent rebound angina.
- Caution patient to change positions slowly to minimize orthostatic hypotension. First dose should be taken while in a sitting or reclining position, especially in geriatric patients.
- Advise patient to avoid concurrent use of alcohol with this medication. Patient should also consult health care professional before taking OTC medications while taking nitroglycerin.
- Inform patient that headache is a common side effect that should decrease with continuing therapy. Aspirin or acetaminophen may be ordered to treat headache. Notify health care professional if headache is persistent or severe.

- Advise patient to notify health care professional if dry mouth or blurred vision occurs.
- **Acute Anginal Attacks:** Advise patient to sit down and use medication at first sign of attack. Relief usually occurs within 5 min. Dose may be repeated if pain is not relieved in 5–10 min. Call health care professional or go to nearest emergency room if anginal pain is not relieved by 3 tablets in 15 min.
- **SL:** Inform patient that tablets should be kept in original glass container or in specially made metal containers, with cotton removed to prevent absorption. Tablets lose potency in containers made of plastic or cardboard or when mixed with other capsules or tablets. Exposure to air, heat, and moisture also causes loss of potency. Instruct patient not to open bottle frequently, handle tablets, or keep bottle of tablets next to body (i.e., shirt pocket) or in automobile glove compartment. Advise patient that tablets should be replaced 6 mo after opening to maintain potency.
- **Lingual Spray:** Instruct patient to lift tongue and spray dose under tongue (*Nitrolingual, NitroMist*) or on tongue (*NitroMist*).

Evaluation/Desired Outcomes

- Decrease in frequency and severity of anginal attacks.
- Increase in activity tolerance. During long-term therapy, tolerance may be minimized by intermittent administration in 12–14 hr or 10–12 hr off intervals.
- Controlled hypotension during surgical procedures.

nitroprusside

(nye-troe-**pruss**-ide)
Nitropress

Classification
Therapeutic: antihypertensives
Pharmacologic: vasodilators

Pregnancy Category C

Indications

Hypertensive crises. Controlled hypotension during anesthesia. Cardiac pump failure or cardiogenic shock (alone or with dopamine).

Action

Produces peripheral vasodilation by a direct action on venous and arteriolar smooth muscle. **Therapeutic Effects:** Rapid lowering of blood pressure. Decreased cardiac preload and afterload.

Pharmacokinetics

Absorption: IV administration results in complete bioavailability.
Distribution: Unknown.
Metabolism and Excretion: Rapidly metabolized in RBCs and tissues to cyanide and subsequently by the liver to thiocyanate.
Half-life: 2 min.

TIME/ACTION PROFILE (hypotensive effect)

ROUTE	ONSET	PEAK	DURATION
IV	immediate	rapid	1–10 min

Contraindications/Precautions

Contraindicated in: Hypersensitivity; Decreased cerebral perfusion.
Use Cautiously in: Renal disease (↑ risk of thiocyanate accumulation); Hepatic disease (↑ risk of cyanide accumulation); Geriatric patients (↑ sensitivity); Hypothyroidism; Hyponatremia; Vitamin B deficiency; Pregnancy or lactation (safety not established).

Adverse Reactions/Side Effects

CNS: <u>dizziness</u>, <u>headache</u>, restlessness. **EENT:** blurred vision, tinnitus. **CV:** dyspnea, hypotension, palpitations. **GI:** <u>abdominal pain</u>, <u>nausea</u>, vomiting. **F and E:** acidosis. **Local:** phlebitis at IV site. **Misc:** CYANIDE TOXICITY, thiocyanate toxicity.

Interactions

Drug-Drug: ↑ hypotensive effect with **ganglionic blocking agents**, **general anesthetics**, and other **antihypertensives**. **Estrogens** and **sympathomimetics** may ↓ the response to nitroprusside.

Route/Dosage

IV (Adults and Children): 0.3 mcg/kg/min initially; may be increased as needed up to 10 mcg/kg/min (usual dose is 3 mcg/kg/min; not to exceed 10 min of therapy at 10 mcg/kg/min infusion rate).

Availability (generic available)

Injection: 25 mg/ml in 2-ml vials.

N

NURSING IMPLICATIONS

Assessment

- Monitor blood pressure, heart rate, and ECG frequently throughout therapy; continuous monitoring is preferred. Consult physician for parameters. Monitor for rebound hypertension following discontinuation of nitroprusside.
- Pulmonary capillary wedge pressure (PCWP) may be monitored in patients with MI or CHF.
- ***Lab Test Considerations:*** May cause ↓ bicarbonate concentrations, PCO_2, and pH.
- May cause ↑ lactate concentrations.
- May cause ↑ serum cyanide and thiocyanate concentrations.
- Monitor serum methemoglobin concentrations in patients receiving >10 mg/kg and exhibiting signs of impaired oxygen delivery despite adequate cardiac output and arterial PCO_2 (blood is chocolate brown without change on exposure to air). Treatment of methemoglobinemia is 1–2 mg/kg of methylene blue IV administered over several minutes.
- ***Toxicity and Overdose:*** If severe hypotension occurs, drug effects are quickly reversed, within 1–10 min, by decreasing rate or temporarily discontinuing infusion. May place patient in Trendelenburg position to maximize venous return: Monitor plasma thiocyanate levels daily in patients receiving prolonged infusions at a rate >3 mcg/kg/min or 1 mcg/kg/min in patients with anuria. Thiocyanate levels should not exceed 1 millimole/liter. Signs and symptoms of thiocyanate toxicity include tinnitus, toxic psychoses, hyperreflexia, confusion, weakness, seizures, and coma, Cyanide toxicity may manifest as lactic acidosis, hypoxemia, tachycardia, altered consciousness, seizures, and characteristic breath odor similar to almonds. Acute treatment of cyanide toxicity includes 4–6 mg/kg of *sodium nitrite* (as a 3% solution) over 2–4 min. This acts as a buffer for cyanide by converting 10% of hemoglobin to methemoglobin. If administration of sodium nitrite is delayed, inhalation of crushed ampule (vaporole, aspirole) of *amyl nitrite* for 15–30 sec of every minute should be started until sodium nitrite is running. Following completion of sodium nitrite infusion, administer *sodium thiosulfate* 150–200 mcg/kg (available as 25% and 50% solutions). This will convert cyanide to thiocyanate, which may then be eliminated. If required, entire regimen may be repeated in 2 hr at 50% of the initial doses.

Potential Nursing Diagnoses

Ineffective tissue perfusion (Indications)

Implementation

- If infusion of 10 mcg/kg/min for 10 min does not produce adequate reduction in blood pressure, manufacturer recommends nitroprusside be discontinued.
- May be administered in left ventricular CHF concurrently with an inotropic agent (dopamine, dobutamine) when effective doses of nitroprusside restore pump function and cause excessive hypotension.

IV Administration

- **Continuous Infusion: *Diluent:*** Dilute 50 mg of nitroprusside in 250–1000 ml of D5W. Wrap infusion in aluminum foil to protect from light; administration-set tubing need not be covered. Amber plastic bags do not offer sufficient protection from light; wrap must be opaque. Freshly prepared solution has a slight brownish tint; discard if solution is dark brown, orange, blue, green, or dark red. Solution must be used within 24 hr of preparation. ***Concentration:*** 50–200 mcg/ml. ***Rate:*** Based on patient's weight (see Route/Dosage section). Administer via infusion pump to ensure accurate dosage rate.
- **Y-Site Compatibility:** amikacin, aminophylline, argatroban, atropine, aztreonam, bivalirudin, bumetanide, calcium chloride, calcium gluconate, cefazolin, cefotaxime, cefoxitin, ceftizoxime, ceftriaxone, cefuroxime, chloramphenicol, cimetidine, clindamycin, cyclosporine, daptomycin, dexamethasone sodium phosphate, digoxin, diltiazem, dopamine, doxycycline, enalaprilat, epinephrine, ertapenem, esmolol, famotidine, fenoldopam, fentanyl, fluconazole, furosemide, ganciclovir, gentamicin, granisetron, heparin, hydrocortisone sodium succinate, hydromorphone, insulin, isoproterenol, ketorolac, labetalol, lidocaine, linezolid, lorazepam, magnesium sulfate, meperidine, methylprednisolone sodium succinate, metoclopramide, metoprolol, metronidazole, micafungin, midazolam, milrinone, morphine, nafcillin, nesiritide, nicardipine, nitroglycerin, norepinephrine, ondansetron, palonosetron, pancuronium, pantoprazole, penicillin G potassium, phenylephrine, phytonadione, pi-

peracillin/tazobactam, potassium chloride, potassium phosphate, procainamide, propofol, propranolol, protamine, ranitidine, sodium bicarbonate, tacrolimus, ticarcillin/clavulanate, tirofiban, tobramycin, vancomycin, vasopressin, verapamil.

- **Y-Site Incompatibility:** acyclovir, ampicillin, caspofungin, ceftazidime, diazepam, diphenhydramine, erythromycin, hydralazine, hydroxyzine, levofloxacin, phenytoin, prochlorperazine, promethazine, quinupristin/dalfopristin, trimethoprim/sulfamethoxazole, voriconazole.

Patient/Family Teaching

- Advise patient to report the onset of tinnitus, dyspnea, dizziness, headache, or blurred vision immediately.

Evaluation/Desired Outcomes

- Decrease in blood pressure without the appearance of side effects.
- Treatment of cardiac pump failure or cardiogenic shock.

nizatidine, See HISTAMINE H_2 ANTAGONISTS.

norethindrone, norethindrone/ethinyl acetate, See CONTRACEPTIVES, HORMONAL.

norfloxacin, See FLUOROQUINOLONES.

nortriptyline (nor-**trip**-ti-leen)

Aventyl, Pamelor

Classification

Therapeutic: antidepressants

Pharmacologic: tricyclic antidepressants

Pregnancy Category D

Indications

Various forms of depression. **Unlabeled uses:** Management of chronic neurogenic pain.

Action

Potentiates the effect of serotonin and norepinephrine. Has significant anticholinergic properties. **Therapeutic Effects:** Antidepressant action that develops slowly over several weeks.

Pharmacokinetics

Absorption: Well absorbed after oral administration.

Distribution: Widely distributed. Enters breast milk in small amounts; probably crosses the placenta.

Protein Binding: 92%.

Metabolism and Excretion: Extensively metabolized by the liver, much of it on its first pass. Some is converted to active compounds. Undergoes enterohepatic recirculation and secretion into gastric juices.

Half-life: 18–28 hr.

TIME/ACTION PROFILE (antidepressant effect)

ROUTE	ONSET	PEAK	DURATION
PO	2–3 wk	6 wk	unknown

Contraindications/Precautions

Contraindicated in: Hypersensitivity; Angle-closure glaucoma; Alcohol intolerance (solution only).

Use Cautiously in: Pre-existing cardiovascular disease; History of seizures; Asthma; May ↑ risk of suicide attempt/ideation especially during early treatment or dose adjustment; risk may be greater in children and adolescents; OB: Use only if clearly needed and maternal benefits outweigh risk to fetus; Lactation: May result in sedation in infant; discontinue drug or bottle-feed; Pedi: Safety not established; Geri: More susceptible to adverse reactions; dose reduction recommended). Pre-existing cardiovascular disease. Geriatric men with prostatic hyperplasia may be more susceptible to urinary retention.

Adverse Reactions/Side Effects

CNS: drowsiness, fatigue, lethargy, agitation, confusion, extrapyramidal reactions, hallucinations, headache, insomnia. **EENT:** blurred vision, dry eyes, dry mouth. **CV:** ARRHYTHMIAS, hypotension, ECG changes. **GI:** constipation, nausea, paralytic ileus, unpleasant taste, weight gain. **GU:** urinary retention. **Derm:** photosensitivity. **Endo:** gynecomastia. **Hemat:** blood dyscrasias.

Interactions

Drug-Drug: May cause hypertension, hyperpyrexia, seizures, and death when used with **MAO inhibitors** (avoid concurrent use—dis-

✤ = Canadian drug name.

*CAPITALS indicates life-threatening; underlines indicate most frequent.

continue 2 wk before starting nortriptyline). May prevent the therapeutic response to most **antihypertensives**. Hypertensive crisis may occur with **clonidine**. ↑ CNS depression with other **CNS depressants**, including **alcohol**, **antihistamines**, **opioids**, and **sedative/hypnotics**. Adrenergic effects may be ↑ with other **adrenergic agents**, including **vasoconstrictors** and **decongestants**. ↑ anticholinergic effects with other **drugs possessing anticholinergic properties**, including **antihistamines**, **antidepressants**, **atropine**, **haloperidol**, **phenothiazines**, **quinidine**, and **disopyramide**. **Cimetidine**, **fluoxetine**, or **hormonal contraceptives** ↑ blood levels and risk of toxicity. ↑ risk of agranulocytosis with **antithyroid agents**.

Drug-Natural Products: Concomitant use of **kava kava**, **valerian**, or **chamomile** can ↑ CNS depression. **St. John's wort** may ↓ serum concentrations and efficacy. ↑ anticholinergic effects with **jimson weed** and **scopolia**.

Route/Dosage

PO (Adults): 25 mg 3–4 times daily, up to 150 mg/day.

PO (Geriatric Patients or adolescents): 30–50 mg/day in divided doses or as a single dose.

Availability (generic available)

Capsules: 10 mg, 25 mg, 50 mg, 75 mg. **Oral solution:** 10 mg/5 ml.

NURSING IMPLICATIONS

Assessment

- Monitor mental status (orientation, mood, behavior). Assess for suicidal tendencies, especially during early therapy. Restrict amount of drug available to patient.
- Assess weight and BMI initially and throughout treatment
- Monitor blood pressure and pulse rate before and during initial therapy. Report significant decreases in blood pressure or a sudden increase in pulse rate
- Monitor baseline and periodic ECGs in geriatric patients or patients with heart disease. May cause prolonged PR and QT intervals and may flatten T waves
- For overweight/obese individuals, monitor FBS and cholesterol levels.
- **Pain:** Assess type, location, and severity of pain before and periodically during therapy. Use pain scale to monitor effectiveness of medication.
- ***Lab Test Considerations:*** Assess leukocyte and differential blood counts, liver function, and serum glucose periodically. May cause ↑ serum bilirubin and alkaline phosphatase. May cause bone marrow depression. Serum glucose may be ↑ or ↓.
- Serum levels may be monitored in patients who fail to respond to usual therapeutic dose. Therapeutic plasma concentration range is 50–150 mg/ml.
- May cause alterations in blood glucose levels.
- ***Toxicity and Overdose:*** Symptoms of acute overdose include disturbed concentration, confusion, restlessness, agitation, seizures, drowsiness, mydriasis, arrhythmias, fever, hallucinations, vomiting, and dyspnea: Treatment of overdose includes gastric lavage, activated charcoal, and a stimulant cathartic. Maintain respiratory and cardiac function (monitor ECG for at least 5 days) and temperature. Medications may include digoxin for CHF, antiarrhythmics, and anticonvulsants.

Potential Nursing Diagnoses

Ineffective coping (Indications)
Risk for injury (Side Effects)
Chronic pain (Indications)
Sexual dysfunction (Side Effects)

Implementation

- Do not confuse nortriptyline with desipramine.
- Taper to avoid withdrawal effects. Reduce dose 50% for 3 days, then by 50% for 3 more days, then discontinue.
- **PO:** Administer medication with meals to minimize gastric irritation.
- May be given as a single dose at bedtime to minimize sedation during the day. Dose increases should be made at bedtime because of sedation.

Patient/Family Teaching

- Instruct patient to take medication as directed. Take missed doses as soon as possible unless almost time for next dose; if regimen is a single dose at bedtime, do not take in the morning because of side effects. Advise patient that drug effects may not be noticed for at least 2 wk. Abrupt discontinuation may cause nausea, vomiting, diarrhea, headache, trouble sleeping with vivid dreams, and irritability.

- May cause drowsiness and blurred vision. Caution patient to avoid driving and other activities requiring alertness until response to drug is known.
- Instruct patient to notify health care professional if visual changes occur. Inform patient that periodic glaucoma testing may be required during long-term therapy.
- Caution patient to make position changes slowly to minimize orthostatic hypotension. (This side effect is less pronounced with this medication than with other tricyclic antidepressants.).
- Advise patient to avoid alcohol or other CNS depressant drugs during therapy and for at least 3–7 days after therapy has been discontinued.
- Instruct patient to notify health care professional if urinary retention occurs or if dry mouth or constipation persists. Sugarless candy or gum may diminish dry mouth, and an increase in fluid intake or bulk may prevent constipation. If symptoms persist, dose reduction or discontinuation may be necessary. Consult health care professional if dry mouth persists for more than 2 wk.
- Caution patient to use sunscreen and protective clothing to prevent photosensitivity reactions.
- Alert patient that urine may turn blue-green in color.
- Inform patient of need to monitor dietary intake. Increase in appetite may lead to undesired weight gain. Refer as appropriate for nutritional, weight, or medical management.
- May have teratogenic effects. Instruct patient to notify health care professional immediately if pregnancy is planned or suspected.
- Advise patient to notify health care professional of medication regimen before treatment or surgery.
- Therapy for depression is usually prolonged. Emphasize the importance of follow-up exams and participation in prescribed psychotherapy to improve coping skills.
- Refer to local support group.

Evaluation/Desired Outcomes

- Increased sense of well-being.
- Renewed interest in surroundings.
- Increased appetite.
- Improved energy level.
- Improved sleep.
- Decrease in severity of chronic neurogenic pain. Patients may require 2–6 wk of therapy before full therapeutic effects of medication are seen.

nystatin (nye-**stat**-in)
Mycostatin, ✤Nadostine, Nilstat, Nystex, ✤PMS-Nystatin

Classification
Therapeutic: antifungals (topical/local)

Pregnancy Category B

For other nystatin dosage forms, see antifungals (topical) and antifungals (vaginal)

Indications

Lozenges, oral suspension: Local treatment of oropharyngeal candidiasis. Treatment of intestinal candidiasis.

Action

Binds to fungal cell membrane, allowing leakage of cellular contents. **Therapeutic Effects:** Fungistatic or fungicidal action. **Spectrum:** Active against most pathogenic *Candida* species, including *C. albicans*.

Pharmacokinetics

Absorption: Poorly absorbed; action is primarily local.
Distribution: Unknown.
Metabolism and Excretion: Excreted unchanged in the feces after oral administration.
Half-life: Unknown.

TIME/ACTION PROFILE (antifungal effects)

ROUTE	ONSET	PEAK	DURATION
Top	rapid	unknown	2 hr†

†Maintenance of saliva levels required to inhibit growth of Candida species after oral dissolution of 2 lozenges

Contraindications/Precautions

Contraindicated in: Hypersensitivity; Some products may contain ethyl alcohol or benzyl alcohol—avoid use in patients who may be hypersensitive to or intolerant of these additives.
Use Cautiously in: Denture wearers (dentures require soaking in nystatin suspension); Pedi: Children <5 yr (lozenges, pastilles, troches).

N

Adverse Reactions/Side Effects

GI: diarrhea, nausea, stomach pain (large doses), vomiting. **Derm:** contact dermatitis, Stevens-Johnson syndrome.

Interactions

Drug-Drug: None significant.

Route/Dosage

PO (Adults and Children): 400,000–600,000 units 4 times daily as oral suspension or 200,000–400,000 units 4–5 times daily as pastilles (lozenges).
PO (Infants): 200,000 units 4 times daily or 100,000 units to each side of the mouth 4 times daily.
PO (Neonates, Premature and Low Birth Weight): 100,000 units 4 times daily or 50,000 units to each side of the mouth 4 times a day.

Availability (generic available)

Oral suspension: 100,000 units/ml in 5-, 60-, and 480-ml containers. **Oral pastilles (lozenges, troches):** 200,000 units/troche. **Powder for oral suspension:** ⅛ tsp = 500,000 units in 50-, 150-, and 500-million, 1-, 2-, and 5-billion-unit containers. **Oral tablets:** 500,000 units.

NURSING IMPLICATIONS

Assessment

- Inspect oral mucous membranes before and frequently throughout therapy. Increased irritation of mucous membranes may indicate need to discontinue medication.

Potential Nursing Diagnoses

Risk for impaired skin integrity (Indications)
Risk for infection (Indications)

Implementation

- **PO:** Suspension should be administered by placing ½ of dose in each side of mouth. Patient should hold suspension in mouth or swish throughout mouth for several minutes before swallowing, then gargle and swallow. Use calibrated measuring device for liquid doses. Shake well before administration. Pedi: For neonates and infants, paint suspension into recesses of the mouth.
- To prepare oral solution from powder, add ⅛ tsp (approximately 500,000 units) to 120 ml of water and stir well. Prepare immediately before use; contains no preservatives.
- Lozenges (pastilles) should be allowed to dissolve slowly and completely in mouth; do not chew or swallow whole. Nystatin vaginal tablets can be administered orally for treatment of oral candidiasis.

Patient/Family Teaching

- Instruct patient to take medication as directed. If a dose is missed, take as soon as remembered but not if almost time for next dose. Do not double doses. Therapy should be continued for at least 2 days after symptoms subside.
- Pedi: Instruct parents or caregivers of infants and children on correct dosage and administration. Remind them to use only the measuring devise dispensed with the product.
- Advise patient to report increased irritation of mucous membranes or lack of therapeutic response to health care professional.

Evaluation/Desired Outcomes

- Decrease in stomatitis.
- To prevent relapse after oral therapy, therapy should be continued for 48 hr after symptoms have disappeared and cultures are negative.
- Therapy for a period of 2 wk is usually sufficient, but more prolonged therapy may be necessary.

nystatin, See ANTIFUNGALS (TOPICAL), ANTIFUNGALS (VAGINAL).

octreotide (ok-tree-oh-tide)
Sandostatin, Sandostatin LAR

Classification
Therapeutic: antidiarrheals, hormones

Pregnancy Category B

Indications
Treatment of severe diarrhea and flushing episodes in patients with GI endocrine tumors, including metastatic carcinoid tumors and vasoactive intestinal peptide tumors (VIPomas). **Unlabeled uses:** Relief of symptoms and suppressed tumor growth in patients with pituitary tumors associated with acromegaly. Management of diarrhea in AIDS patients or patients with fistulas.

Action
Suppresses secretion of serotonin and gastroenterohepatic peptides. Increases absorption of fluid and electrolytes from the GI tract and increases transit time. Decreases levels of serotonin metabolites. Also suppresses growth hormone, insulin, and glucagon. **Therapeutic Effects:** Control of severe flushing and diarrhea associated with GI endocrine tumors.

Pharmacokinetics
Absorption: Well absorbed following subcut administration and IM administration of depot form.
Distribution: Unknown.
Protein Binding: 65%.
Metabolism and Excretion: 32% excreted unchanged in urine.
Half-life: 1.5 hr.

TIME/ACTION PROFILE (control of symptoms)

ROUTE	ONSET	PEAK	DURATION
Subcut, IV	unknown	unknown	up to 12 hr
IM (LAR)	unknown	2 wk	up to 4 wk

Contraindications/Precautions
Contraindicated in: Hypersensitivity.
Use Cautiously in: Gallbladder disease (↑ risk of stone formation); Renal impairment (dose reduction may be necessary); Hyperglycemia or hypoglycemia (changes in blood glucose may occur); Fat malabsorption (may be aggravated); OB: Pregnancy or lactation (safety not established).

Adverse Reactions/Side Effects
CNS: dizziness, drowsiness, fatigue, headache, weakness. **EENT:** visual disturbances. **CV:** edema, orthostatic hypotension, palpitations. **GI:** abdominal pain, cholelithiasis, diarrhea, fat malabsorption, nausea, vomiting. **Derm:** flushing. **Endo:** hyperglycemia, hypoglycemia. **Local:** injection-site pain.

Interactions
Drug-Drug: May alter requirements for **insulin** or **oral hypoglycemic agents**. May ↓ blood levels of **cyclosporine**.

Route/Dosage

Carcinoid Tumors
Subcut, IV (Adults): *Sandostatin*—100–600 mcg/day in 2–4 divided doses during first 2 wk of therapy (range 50–1500 mcg/day).
IM (Adults): *Sandostatin LAR*—20 mg q 4 wk for 2 mo; dose may be further adjusted.

VIPomas
Subcut, IV (Adults): *Sandostatin*—200–300 mcg/day in 2–4 divided doses during first 2 wk of therapy (range 150–750 mcg/day).
IM (Adults): *Sandostatin LAR*—20 mg q 2 wk for 2 mo; dose may be further adjusted.

Suppression of Growth Hormone (Acromegaly)
Subcut, IV (Adults): *Sandostatin*—50–100 mcg 2–3 times daily.
IM (Adults): *Sandostatin LAR*—20 mg q 4 wk for 3 mo, then adjusted on the basis of growth hormone levels.

Antidiarrheal (AIDS Patients)
Subcut, IV (Adults): 100–1800 mcg/day (unlabeled).

Availability (generic available)
Injection: 0.05 mg/ml in 1-ml ampules, 0.1 mg/ml in 1-ml ampules, 0.2 mg/ml in 5-ml vials, 0.5 mg/ml in 1-ml ampules, 1 mg/ml in 5-ml vials. **Depot injection:** 10 mg, 20 mg, 30 mg.

NURSING IMPLICATIONS

Assessment
- Assess frequency and consistency of stools and bowel sounds throughout therapy.

- Monitor pulse and blood pressure prior to and periodically during therapy.
- Assess patient's fluid and electrolyte balance and skin turgor for dehydration.
- Monitor diabetic patients for signs of hypoglycemia. May require reduction in requirements for insulin and sulfonylureas and treatment with diazoxide.
- Assess for gallbladder disease; assess for pain and monitor ultrasound examinations of gallbladder and bile ducts prior to and periodically during prolonged therapy.
- ***Lab Test Considerations:*** Monitor 5-HIAA (urinary 5-hydroxyindoleacetic acid), plasma serotonin, and plasma substance P in patients with carcinoid; plasma vasoactive intestinal peptide (VIP) in patients with VIPoma; and free T_4 and serum glucose concentrations prior to and periodically during therapy in all patients taking octreotide.
- Monitor quantitative 72-hr fecal fat and serum carotene determinations periodically for possible drug-induced aggravations of fat malabsorption.
- May cause a slight ↑ in liver enzymes.
- May cause ↓ serum thyroxine (T_4) concentrations.

Potential Nursing Diagnoses

Diarrhea (Indications)

Implementation

- Do not use solution that is discolored or contains particulate matter. Ampules should be refrigerated but may be stored at room temperature for the days they will be used. Discard unused solution.
- **Subcut:** Administer the smallest volume needed to achieve required dose to prevent pain at injection site. Rotate injection sites; avoid multiple injections in same site within short periods of time. Preferred injection sites are the hip, thigh, or abdomen.
- Administer injections between meals and at bedtime to avoid GI side effects.
- Allow medication to reach room temperature prior to injection to minimize local reactions at injection site.
- **IM:** Mix IM solution by adding diluent included in kit. Administer immediately after mixing into the gluteal muscle. Avoid using deltoid site due to pain of injection.
- Patients with carcinoid tumors and VIPomas should continue to receive subcut dose for 2 wk following switch to IM depot form to maintain therapeutic level.

IV Administration

- **Direct IV:** ***Diluent:*** May be administered undiluted. ***Rate:*** Administer over 3 min.
- **Intermittent Infusion:** ***Diluent:*** Dilute in 50–200 ml of 0.9% NaCl or D5W. ***Concentration:*** 1.5–250 mcg/ml. ***Rate:*** Infuse over 15–30 min.
- **Y-Site Compatibility:** acyclovir, ondansetron, tirofiban.
- **Y-Site Incompatibility:** micafungin.

Patient/Family Teaching

- May cause dizziness, drowsiness, or visual disturbances. Caution patient to avoid driving or other activities requiring alertness until response to medication is known.
- Advise patient to change positions slowly to minimize orthostatic hypotension.
- **Home Care Issues:** Instruct patients administering octreotide at home on correct technique for injection, storage, and disposal of equipment.
- Instruct patient to administer octreotide exactly as directed. If a dose is missed, administer as soon as possible, then return to regular schedule. Do not double doses.

Evaluation/Desired Outcomes

- Decrease in severity of diarrhea and improvement of electrolyte imbalances in patients with carcinoid or VIP-secreting tumors.
- Relief of symptoms and suppressed tumor growth in patients with pituitary tumors associated with acromegaly.
- Management of diarrhea in patients with AIDS.

ofloxacin, See FLUOROQUINOLONES.

olanzapine (oh-lan-za-peen)

Zyprexa, Zyprexa Zydis

Classification

Therapeutic: antipsychotics, mood stabilizers

Pharmacologic: thienobenzodiazepines

Pregnancy Category C

Indications

Psychotic disorders: Acute manic episodes associated with bipolar disorder (may be used with lithium or valproate), long-term maintenance therapy of bipolar disorder, long-term treatment/maintenance of schizophrenia, agitation due to schizophrenia or mania (IM). **Unlabeled uses:** Management of anorexia nervosa. Treatment of nausea and vomiting related to highly emetogenic chemotherapy.

Action

Antagonizes dopamine and serotonin type 2 in the CNS. Also has anticholinergic, antihistaminic, and anti–$alpha_1$-adrenergic effects. **Therapeutic Effects:** Decreased manifestations of psychoses.

Pharmacokinetics

Absorption: Well absorbed but rapidly metabolized by first-pass effect, resulting in 60% bioavailability. Conventional tablets and orally disintegrating tablets (Zydis) are bioequivalent. IM administration results in significantly higher blood levels (5 times that of oral).
Distribution: Extensively distributed.
Protein Binding: 93%.
Metabolism and Excretion: Highly metabolized (mostly by the hepatic P450 CYP 1A2 system); 7% excreted unchanged in urine.
Half-life: 21–54 hr.

TIME/ACTION PROFILE (antipsychotic effects)

ROUTE	ONSET	PEAK*	DURATION
PO	unknown	6 hr	unknown
IM	rapid	15–45 min	2–4 hr

*Blood levels

Contraindications/Precautions

Contraindicated in: Hypersensitivity; Lactation: Discontinue drug or bottle feed; **Orally disintegrating tablets only:** Phenylketonuria (orally disintegrating tablets contain aspartame).
Use Cautiously in: Patients with hepatic impairment; Patients at risk for aspiration; Cardiovascular or cerebrovascular disease; History of seizures; History of attempted suicide; Diabetes or risk factors for diabetes (may worsen glucose control); Prostatic hyperplasia; Angle-closure glaucoma; History of paralytic ileus; Dysphagia and aspiration have been associated with antipsychotic drug use; use with caution in patients at risk for aspiration; OB, Pedi: Safety not established; Geri: Geriatric patients (may require ↓ doses; inappropriate use for dementia is associated with ↑ mortality).

Adverse Reactions/Side Effects

CNS: NEUROLEPTIC MALIGNANT SYNDROME, SEIZURES, agitation, dizziness, headache, restlessness, sedation, weakness, dystonia, insomnia, mood changes, personality disorder, speech impairment, tardive dyskinesia. **EENT:** amblyopia, rhinitis, increased salivation, pharyngitis. **CV:** orthostatic hypotension (↑ with IM). **Resp:** cough, dyspnea. **CV:** orthostatic hypotension, tachycardia, chest pain. **GI:** constipation, dry mouth, abdominal pain, increased appetite, weight loss or gain, nausea, increased thirst. **GU:** decreased libido, urinary incontinence. **Derm:** photosensitivity. **Endo:** hyperglycemia, goiter. **Metab:** dyslipidema. **MS:** hypertonia, joint pain. **Neuro:** tremor. **Misc:** fever, flu-like syndrome.

Interactions

Drug-Drug: Effects may be ↓ by concurrent **carbamazepine**, **omeprazole**, or **rifampin**. ↑ hypotension may occur with **antihypertensives**. ↑ CNS depression may occur with concurrent use of **alcohol** or other **CNS depressants**. May antagonize the effects of **levodopa** or other **dopamine agonists**. **Nicotine** can decrease olanzapine levels.

Route/Dosage

PO (Adults—Most Patients): *Schizophrenia*—5–10 mg/day initially; may increase at weekly intervals by 5 mg/day (not to exceed 20 mg/day). *Bipolar mania*—10–15 mg/day initially; may increase every 24 hr by 5 mg/day (not to exceed 20 mg/day).
PO (Adults—Debilitated or Nonsmoking Female Patients ≥65 yr): Initiate therapy at 5 mg/day.
IM (Adults): *Acute agitation*—5–10 mg, may repeat in 2 hr, then 4 hr later.

Availability

Tablets: 2.5 mg, 5 mg, 7.5 mg, 10 mg, 15 mg, 20 mg. **Cost:** 2.5 mg $556.93/90, 5 mg $645.82/90, 7.5 mg $805.91/90, 10 mg $1,007.96/90, 15 mg $1,475.96/90, 20 mg $1,860.77/90. **Orally disintegrating tablets (Zydis):** 5 mg, 10 mg, 15 mg, 20 mg. **Cost:** 5 mg $765.95/90, 10 mg $1,139.83/90, 15 mg $1,648.53/90, 20 mg $2,163.23/90. **Powder for injection:** 10 mg/vial. ***In combination with:*** fluoxetine (Symbyax; see Appendix B).

O

🍁 = Canadian drug name.
* CAPITALS indicates life-threatening; underlines indicate most frequent.

NURSING IMPLICATIONS

Assessment

- Assess mental status (orientation, mood, behavior) before and periodically during therapy.
- Monitor blood pressure (sitting, standing, lying), ECG, pulse, and respiratory rate before and frequently during dose adjustment
- Assess weight and BMI initially and throughout therapy
- Assess fasting blood glucose and cholesterol levels initially and throughout therapy
- Observe patient carefully when administering medication to ensure that medication is taken and not hoarded or cheeked
- Assess fluid intake and bowel function. Increased bulk and fluids in the diet may help minimize constipation
- Monitor patient for onset of akathisia (restlessness or desire to keep moving) and extrapyramidal side effects (*parkinsonian*—difficulty speaking or swallowing, loss of balance control, pill rolling of hands, mask-like face, shuffling gait, rigidity, tremors; and *dystonic*—muscle spasms, twisting motions, twitching, inability to move eyes, weakness of arms or legs) every 2 mo during therapy and 8–12 wk after therapy has been discontinued. Report these symptoms if they occur, as reduction in dose or discontinuation of medication may be necessary. Trihexyphenidyl or benztropine may be used to control symptoms
- Monitor for tardive dyskinesia (uncontrolled rhythmic movement of mouth, face, and extremities; lip smacking or puckering; puffing of cheeks; uncontrolled chewing; rapid or worm-like movements of tongue, excessive blinking of eyes). Report immediately; may be irreversible
- Monitor for development of neuroleptic malignant syndrome (fever, respiratory distress, tachycardia, seizures, diaphoresis, hypertension or hypotension, pallor, tiredness, severe muscle stiffness, loss of bladder control). Notify health care professional immediately if these symptoms occur.
- ***Lab Test Considerations:*** Evaluate CBC, liver function tests, and ocular examinations periodically during therapy. May cause ↓ platelets. May cause ↑ bilirubin, AST, ALT, GGT, CPK, and alkaline phosphatase.
- Monitor blood glucose prior to and periodically during therapy.

Potential Nursing Diagnoses

Disturbed thought process (Indications)
Impaired oral mucous membrane (Side Effects)
Sexual dysfunction (Side Effects)

Implementation

- Do not confuse Zyprexa (olanzapine) with Celexa (citalopram) or Zyrtec (cetirizine).
- **PO:** May be administered without regard to meals.
- For orally disintegrating tablets, peel back foil on blister, do not push tablet through foil. Using dry hands, remove from foil and place entire tablet in mouth. Tablet will disintegrate with or without liquid.
- **IM:** Reconstitute with 2.1 mL of sterile water for injection for a concentration of 5 mg/mL. Solution should be clear and yellow; do not administer solutions that are discolored or contain particulate matter. Inject slowly, deep into muscle. Do not administer IV or subcutaneously. Administer within 1 hr of reconstitution. Discard unused solution.

Patient/Family Teaching

- Advise patient to take medication as directed and not to skip doses or double up on missed doses. May need to discontinue gradually.
- Inform patient of possibility of extrapyramidal symptoms and tardive dyskinesia. Instruct patient to report these symptoms immediately to health care professional.
- Advise patient to change positions slowly to minimize orthostatic hypotension.
- Medication may cause drowsiness. Caution patient to avoid driving or other activities requiring alertness until response to the medication is known.
- Caution patient to avoid taking alcohol and to notify health care professional prior to taking other Rx, OTC, or herbal products concurrently with this medication.
- Advise patient to use sunscreen and protective clothing when exposed to the sun. Extremes of temperature (exercise, hot weather, hot baths or showers) should also be avoided; this drug impairs body temperature regulation.
- Instruct patient to use saliva substitute, frequent mouth rinses, good oral hygiene, and sugarless gum or candy to minimize dry mouth. Consult dentist if dry mouth continues for >2 wk.
- Advise patient to notify health care professional of medication regimen before treatment or surgery.

- Instruct patient to notify health care professional promptly if sore throat, fever, unusual bleeding or bruising, rash, weakness, tremors, visual disturbances, dark-colored urine, or clay-colored stools occur.
- Advise patient to notify health care professional if pregnancy is planned or suspected, or if breastfeeding or planning to breastfeed.
- Emphasize the importance of routine follow-up exams and continued participation in psychotherapy to improve coping skills.

Evaluation/Desired Outcomes

- Decrease in excitable, manic behavior.
- Decrease in positive symptoms (delusions, hallucinations) of schizophrenia.
- Decrease in negative symptoms (social withdrawal; flat, blunted affect) of schizophrenia.

olmesartan, See ANGIOTENSIN II RECEPTOR ANTAGONISTS.

olsalazine (ole-**sal**-a-zeen)

Dipentum

Classification

Therapeutic: gastrointestinal anti-inflammatories—therapeutic

Pregnancy Category C

Indications

Ulcerative colitis (when patients cannot tolerate sulfasalazine).

Action

Locally acting anti-inflammatory action in the colon, where activity is probably due to inhibition of prostaglandin synthesis. **Therapeutic Effects:** Reduction in the symptoms of inflammatory bowel disease.

Pharmacokinetics

Absorption: Acts locally in colon, where 98–99% is converted to mesalamine (5-aminosalicylic acid).

Distribution: Action is primarily local and remains in the colon.

Metabolism and Excretion: 2% absorbed into systemic circulation is rapidly metabolized; mostly eliminated as mesalamine in the feces.

Half-life: 0.9 hr.

TIME/ACTION PROFILE (levels)

ROUTE	ONSET	PEAK	DURATION
PO	unknown	1 hr; 4–8 hr	12 hr

Contraindications/Precautions

Contraindicated in: Hypersensitivity reactions to salicylates; Cross-sensitivity with furosemide, sulfonylurea hypoglycemic agents, or carbonic anhydrase inhibitors may exist; G6PD deficiency; Urinary tract or intestinal obstruction; Pedi: Children <2 yr (safe use not established); Porphyria.

Use Cautiously in: Severe hepatic or renal impairment; OB: Pregnancy; Geri: Geriatric patients (consider ↓ body mass, hepatic/renal/cardiac function, intercurrent illness and drug therapies; Renal impairment (↑ risk of renal tubular damage); Lactation: Lactation (safety not established).

Adverse Reactions/Side Effects

CNS: ataxia, confusion, dizziness, drowsiness, headache, mental depression, psychosis, restlessness. **GI:** diarrhea, abdominal pain, anorexia, exacerbation of colitis, drug-induced hepatitis, nausea, vomiting. **Derm:** itching, rash. **Hemat:** blood dyscrasias.

Interactions

Drug-Drug: ↑ risk of bleeding after neuraxial anesthesia with **low molecular weight heparins** and **heparinoids**; discontinue osalazine before initiation of therapy or monitor closely if discontinuation not possible. May ↓ metabolism, and ↑ effects/toxicity of **mercaptopurine** or **thioguanine** with and ↑ risk of myelosuppression (use lowest possible dose and monitor closely). ↑ risk of developing Reye's syndrome; avoid osalazine during 6 wks after **varicella vaccine**.

Route/Dosage

PO (Adults): 500 mg twice daily.

Availability

Capsules: 250 mg.

NURSING IMPLICATIONS

Assessment

- Assess patient for allergy to sulfonamides and salicylates. Patients allergic to sulfasalazine may take mesalamine or olsalazine without

difficulty, but therapy should be discontinued if rash or fever occur.
- Monitor intake and output ratios. Fluid intake should be sufficient to maintain a urine output of at least 1200–1500 ml daily to prevent crystalluria and stone formation.
- **Inflammatory Bowel Disease:** Assess abdominal pain and frequency, quantity, and consistency of stools at the beginning of and throughout therapy.
- ***Lab Test Considerations:*** Monitor urinalysis, BUN, and serum creatinine prior to and periodically during therapy.
- Olsalazine may cause ↑ AST and ALT levels.
- ***Lab Test Considerations:*** Monitor CBC prior to and every 3–6 mo during prolonged therapy. Discontinue olsalazine if blood dyscrasias occur.

Potential Nursing Diagnoses
Acute pain (Indications)
Diarrhea (Indications)

Implementation
- **PO:** Administer with food in evenly divided doses every 12 hr.

Patient/Family Teaching
- Instruct patient to take medication as directed, even if feeling better. Take missed doses as soon as remembered unless almost time for next dose.
- May cause dizziness. Caution patient to avoid driving or other activities that require alertness until response to medication is known.
- Advise patient to notify health care professional if skin rash, sore throat, fever, mouth sores, unusual bleeding or bruising, wheezing, fever, or hives occurs.
- Instruct patient to notify health care professional if symptoms do not improve after 1–2 mo of therapy.
- Instruct patient to notify health care professional if symptoms worsen or do not improve. If symptoms of acute intolerance (cramping, acute abdominal pain, bloody diarrhea, fever, headache, rash) occur, discontinue therapy and notify health care professional immediately.
- Inform patient that proctoscopy and sigmoidoscopy may be required periodically during treatment to determine response.

Evaluation/Desired Outcomes
- Decrease in diarrhea and abdominal pain.
- Return to normal bowel pattern in patients with inflammatory bowel disease. Effects may be seen within 3–21 days. The usual course of therapy is 3–6 wk.
- Maintenance of remission in patients with inflammatory bowel disease.
- Decrease in pain and inflammation, and increase in mobility in patients with rheumatoid arthritis.

omalizumab (o-ma-**liz**-u-mab)
Xolair

Classification
Therapeutic: antiasthmatics
Pharmacologic: monoclonal antibodies

Pregnancy Category B

Indications
Moderate to severe asthma not controlled by inhaled corticosteroids.

Action
Inhibits binding of IgE to receptors on mast cells and eosinophils; preventing the release of mediators of the allergic response. Also decreases amount of IgE receptors on basophils. **Therapeutic Effects:** Decreased incidence of exacerbations of asthma.

Pharmacokinetics
Absorption: 62% absorbed slowly from subcut sites.
Distribution: Enters breast milk.
Metabolism and Excretion: Degraded similarly to IgG via binding degradation, reticuloendothelial system and the liver.
Half-life: 26 days.

TIME/ACTION PROFILE (effects on IgE levels)

ROUTE	ONSET	PEAK	DURATION
Subcut	within 1 hr	unknown	up to 1 yr

Contraindications/Precautions
Contraindicated in: Hypersensitivity; Acute bronchospasm.
Use Cautiously in: Chronic use of inhaled corticosteroids; Pregnancy, lactation or children <12 yr (safety not established, use in pregnancy only if clearly needed).

Adverse Reactions/Side Effects
Local: injection site reactions. **Misc:** allergic reactions including ANAPHYLAXIS, ↑ risk of malignancy.

Interactions

Drug-Drug: None noted.

Route/Dosage

Subcut (Adults and Children >12 yr): 150–375 mg every 2–4 wk (determined by pretreatment serum IgE level and body weight).

Availability

Sterile powder for subcut injection (requires reconstitution): 150 mg/vial.

NURSING IMPLICATIONS

Assessment

- Assess lung sounds and respiratory function prior to and periodically during therapy.
- Assess allergy symptoms (rhinitis, conjunctivitis, hives) before and periodically throughout therapy.
- Assess for allergic reactions (urticaria, tongue and/or throat edema) within 2 hr of first and subsequent injections. Observe patient following injection. Epinephrine, diphenhydramine, and corticosteroids should be available in case of anaphylaxis.
- Monitor for injection site reactions (bruising, redness, warmth, burning, stinging, itching, hives, pain, induration, mass, inflammation). Usually occur within 1 hr of injection, last <8 days, and decrease in frequency with subsequent dosing.
- ***Lab Test Considerations:*** Serum IgE levels will ↑ following administration and may persist for up to 1 year following discontinuation. Serum total IgE levels obtained <1 year following discontinuation may not reflect steady state free IgE levels and should not be used to reassess the dosing regimen.

Potential Nursing Diagnoses

Ineffective airway clearance

Implementation

- Doses of inhaled corticosteroids may be gradually decreased with supervision of health care professional; do not discontinue abruptly.
- **Subcut:** To reconstitute, draw 1.4 ml of sterile water for injection into a 3-cc syringe with a 1-in 18-gauge needle. With the vial upright on a flat surface, inject the sterile water into vial. Keep vial upright and gently swirl for approximately 1 min to evenly wet powder. Do not shake. Lyophilized omalizumab takes 15–20 min to dissolve. Gently swirl vial for 5–10 seconds every 5 min to dissolve any remaining particles. Solution should be clear or slightly opalescent and may have small bubbles or foam around edge of vial. Do not use if particles are visible or if contents do not dissolve completely within 40 min. Invert vial for 15 seconds to allow solution to drain toward stopper. Solution may be somewhat viscous. In order to obtain full 1.2 ml dose, all of solution must be withdrawn from the vial using a new 3-cc syringe with an 18-gauge needle, before expelling any air or excess solution from syringe. Administer within 8 hr if refrigerated or within 4 hr if stored at room temperature. Discard unused solution.
- Replace the 18-gauge needle with a 25-gauge needle for subcut injection. Because solution is slightly viscous, injection may take 5–10 seconds to administer. Divide doses >150 mg into 2 injection sites.

Patient/Family Teaching

- Explain purpose of medication to patient. Inform patient that they may not see immediate results from omalizumab therapy.
- Instruct patient not to discontinue or reduce other asthma medications, especially inhaled corticosteroids, without consulting health care professional.

Evaluation/Desired Outcomes

- Decreased incidence of exacerbations of asthma.

omega-3-acid ethyl esters

(oh-**me**-ga three **as**-id **eth**-il **es**-ters)

Lovaza

Classification

Therapeutic: lipid-lowering agents

Pharmacologic: fatty acids

Pregnancy Category C

Indications

Hypertriglyceridemia (triglycerides ≥500 mmg/dL) in adults; used with specific diet.

Action

Inhibits synthesis of triglycerides. **Therapeutic Effects:** Lowering of triglycerides.

O

Pharmacokinetics

Absorption: Well absorbed.
Distribution: Unknown.
Metabolism and Excretion: Incorporated into phospholipids.
Half-life: Unknown.

TIME/ACTION PROFILE (lowering of triglycerides)

ROUTE	ONSET	PEAK	DURATION
PO	unknown	2 mo	unknown

Contraindications/Precautions

Contraindicated in: Hypersensitivity.
Use Cautiously in: Allery/hypersensitivity to fish; OB: Use only if maternal benefit justifies fetal risk during pregnancy; use cautiously during lactation; Pedi: safety in children <18 yr not established.

Adverse Reactions/Side Effects

GI: altered taste, eructation. **Derm:** rash.

Interactions

Drug-Drug: Beta-blockers, **thiazide diuretics**, and **estrogens** may ↑ triglycerides and should be discontinued prior to therapy.

Route/Dosage

PO (Adults): 4 g/day; may be given as a single dose or 2 g twice daily.

Availability

Gelatin capsules (oil-filled): 1 g.

NURSING IMPLICATIONS

Assessment

- Obtain a diet history, especially with regard to fat consumption.
- ***Lab Test Considerations:*** Monitor serum triglyceride levels prior to and periodically during therapy.
- Monitor serum ALT periodically during therapy. May cause ↑ serum ALT without concurrent ↑ in AST levels.
- Monitor serum LDL cholesterol levels periodically during therapy. May cause ↑ in serum LDL levels.

Potential Nursing Diagnoses

Noncompliance (Patient/Family Teaching)

Implementation

- An appropriate lipid-lowering diet should be followed before therapy and should continue during therapy.
- **PO:** May be taken as a single 4-g dose or as 2 g twice daily. May be administered with meals.

Patient/Family Teaching

- Instruct patient to take medication as directed, not to skip doses or double up on missed doses. Medication helps control but does not cure elevated serum triglyceride levels.
- Advise patient that this medication should be used in conjunction with diet restrictions (fat, cholesterol, carbohydrates, alcohol), exercise, weight loss in overweight patients, and control of medical problems (such as diabetes mellitus and hypothyroidism) that may contribute to hypertriglyceridemia.
- Emphasize the importance of follow-up exams to determine effectiveness.

Evaluation/Desired Outcomes

- Lowering of serum triglyceride levels. Patients who do not have an adequate response after 2 mo of treatment should be withdrawn from therapy.

omeprazole (o-**mep**-ra-zole)

✤Losec, Prilosec, Prilosec OTC, Zegerid

Classification
Therapeutic: antiulcer agents
Pharmacologic: proton-pump inhibitors

Pregnancy Category C

Indications

GERD/maintenance of healing in erosive esophagitis. Duodenal ulcers (with or without anti-infectives for *Helicobacter pylori*). Short-term treatment of active benign gastric ulcer. Pathologic hypersecretory conditions, including Zollinger-Ellison syndrome. Reduction of risk of GI bleeding in critically ill patients. **OTC:** Heartburn occurring ≥twice/wk.

Action

Binds to an enzyme on gastric parietal cells in the presence of acidic gastric pH, preventing the final transport of hydrogen ions into the gastric lumen. **Therapeutic Effects:** Diminished accumulation of acid in the gastric lumen with lessened gastroesophageal reflux. Healing of duodenal ulcers.

Pharmacokinetics

Absorption: Rapidly absorbed following oral administration; immediate-release formulation

contains bicarbonate to prevent acid degradation.
Distribution: Good distribution into gastric parietal cells.
Protein Binding: 95%.
Metabolism and Excretion: Extensively metabolized by the liver.
Half-life: 0.5–1 hr (increased in liver disease to 3 hr).

TIME/ACTION PROFILE (antisecretory effects)

ROUTE	ONSET	PEAK	DURATION
PO-delayed release	within 1 hr	within 2 hr	72–96 hr
PO-immediate release	rapid	30 min	24 hr

Contraindications/Precautions
Contraindicated in: Hypersensitivity; Metabolic alkalosis and hypocalcemia (Zegerid only).
Use Cautiously in: Liver disease (dosage reduction may be necessary); Geri: Increased risk of hip fractures in patients using high-doses for >1 year; Bartter's syndrome, hypokalemia, and respiratory alkalosis (Zegerid only); Pregnancy, lactation, or children <2 yr (safety not established).

Adverse Reactions/Side Effects
CNS: dizziness, drowsiness, fatigue, headache, weakness. **CV:** chest pain. **GI:** abdominal pain, acid regurgitation, constipation, diarrhea, flatulence, nausea, vomiting. **Derm:** itching, rash. **Misc:** allergic reactions.

Interactions
Drug-Drug: Omeprazole is metabolized by the CYP450 enzyme system and may compete with other agents metabolized by this system. ↓ metabolism and may ↑ effects of Rx **antifungal agents**, **atazanavir**, **diazepam**, **digoxin**, **flurazepam**, **triazolam**, **cyclosporine**, **disulfiram**, **phenytoin**, **tacrolimus**, and **warfarin**. May interfere with absorption of drugs requiring acidic gastric pH, including esters of **ampicillin**, **iron salts**, **digoxin**, **cyanocobalamine**, and **ketoconazole**. Has been used safely with **antacids**. May ↑ risk of bleeding with **warfarin** (monitor INR/PT).

Route/Dosage
PO (Adults): *GERD/erosive esophagitis*—20 mg once daily. *Duodenal ulcers associated with* H. pylori—40 mg daily in the morning with clarithromycin for 2 wk, then 20 mg once daily for 2 wk *or* 20 mg twice daily with clarithromycin 500 mg twice daily and amoxicillin 1000 mg twice daily for 10 days (if ulcer is present at beginning of therapy, continue omeprazole 20 mg daily for 18 more days); has also been used with clarithromycin and metronidazole. *Gastric ulcer*—40 mg once daily for 4–6 wk. *Reduction of the risk of GI bleeding in critically ill patients*—40 mg initially, then another 40 mg 6–8 hr later, followed by 40 mg once daily for up to 14 days. *Gastric hypersecretory conditions*—60 mg once daily initially; may be increased up to 120 mg 3 times daily (doses >80 mg/day should be given in divided doses); *OTC*—20 mg once daily for up to 14 days.
PO (Children >2 yr and <20 kg): 10 mg once daily.
PO (Children >2 yr and ≥20 kg): 20 mg once daily.
PO (Children): *Alternative dosing*—1 mg/kg/day given once or divided twice daily (range of doses in the literature: 0.2—3.5 mg/kg/day); *Adjunctive therapy of duodenal ulcers associated with H. pylori*—15–30 kg: 10 mg BID; >30 kg: 20 mg BID.

Availability (generic available)
Delayed-release capsules: 10 mg, 20 mg[Rx, OTC], 40 mg. **Immediate-release powder for oral suspension (peach-mint):** 20-mg packet, 40-mg packet. ***In combination with:*** metronidazole and clarithromycin in a compliance package (Losec 1-2-3 M); with amoxicillin and clarithromycin in a compliance package (Losec 1-2-3A) (in Canada only; see Appendix B).

NURSING IMPLICATIONS

Assessment
- Assess patient routinely for epigastric or abdominal pain and frank or occult blood in the stool, emesis, or gastric aspirate.
- ***Lab Test Considerations:*** Monitor CBC with differential periodically during therapy.
- May cause ↑ AST, ALT, alkaline phosphatase, and bilirubin.

O

- May cause serum gastrin concentrations to ↑ during first 1–2 wk of therapy. Levels return to normal after discontinuation of omeprazole.
- Monitor INR and prothrombin time in patients taking warfarin.

Potential Nursing Diagnoses
Acute pain (Indications)

Implementation
- Do not confuse Prilosec (omeprazole) with Prinivil (lisinopril).
- **PO:** Administer doses before meals, preferably in the morning. Capsules should be swallowed whole; do not crush or chew. Capsules may be opened and sprinkled on cool applesauce, entire mixture should be ingested immediately and followed by a drink of water. Do not store for future use.
- *Powder for oral suspension:* Administer on empty stomach, as least 1 hr before a meal. For patients with nasogastric or enteral feeding, suspend feeding for 3 hr before and 1 hr after administration. Empty packet contents into a small cup containing 1–2 tablespoons of water. **Do not use other liquids or foods.** If administered through a nasogastric tube, suspend in 20 ml of water. Stir well and drink immediately. Refill cup with water and drink again.
- May be administered concurrently with antacids.

Patient/Family Teaching
- Instruct patient to take medication as directed for the full course of therapy, even if feeling better. Take missed doses as soon as remembered but not if almost time for next dose. Do not double doses.
- May cause occasional drowsiness or dizziness. Caution patient to avoid driving or other activities requiring alertness until response to medication is known.
- Advise patient to consult health care professional before taking any Rx, OTC, or herbal products with omeprazole.
- Advise patient to avoid alcohol, products containing aspirin or NSAIDs, and foods that may cause an increase in GI irritation.
- Advise patient to report onset of black, tarry stools; diarrhea; abdominal pain; or persistent headache to health care professional promptly.

Evaluation/Desired Outcomes
- Decrease in abdominal pain or prevention of gastric irritation and bleeding. Healing of duodenal ulcers can be seen on x-ray examination or endoscopy.
- Decrease in symptoms of GERD. Therapy is continued for 4–8 wk after initial episode.

ondansetron (on-**dan**-se-tron)
Zofran

Classification
Therapeutic: antiemetics
Pharmacologic: 5-HT_3 antagonists

Pregnancy Category B

Indications
Prevention of nausea and vomiting associated with chemotherapy or radiation therapy. **IM, IV:** Prevention and treatment of postoperative nausea and vomiting.

Action
Blocks the effects of serotonin at 5-HT_3–receptor sites (selective antagonist) located in vagal nerve terminals and the chemoreceptor trigger zone in the CNS. **Therapeutic Effects:** Decreased incidence and severity of nausea and vomiting following chemotherapy or surgery.

Pharmacokinetics
Absorption: IV administration results in complete bioavailability; 50% absorbed following oral administration.
Distribution: Unknown.
Metabolism and Excretion: Extensively metabolized by the liver; 5% excreted unchanged by the kidneys.
Half-life: 3.5–5.5 hr.

TIME/ACTION PROFILE (antiemetic effect)

ROUTE	ONSET	PEAK	DURATION
PO, IV	rapid	15–30 min	4 hr–8 hr
IM	rapid	40 min	unknown

Contraindications/Precautions
Contraindicated in: Hypersensitivity; Orally disintegrating tablets contain aspartame and should not be used in patients with phenylketonuria.
Use Cautiously in: Liver impairment (daily dose not to exceed 8 mg); Abdominal surgery (may mask ileus); OB, Pedi: Pregnancy, lactation, or children ≤3 yr (safety not established).

Adverse Reactions/Side Effects

CNS: headache, dizziness, drowsiness, fatigue, weakness. **GI:** constipation, diarrhea, abdominal pain, dry mouth, increased liver enzymes. **Neuro:** extrapyramidal reactions.

Interactions

Drug-Drug: May be affected by **drugs altering the activity of liver enzymes.**

Route/Dosage

PO (Adults and Children ≥12 yr): *Prevention of chemotherapy-induced nausea/vomiting*—8 mg 30 min prior to chemotherapy and repeated 8 hr later; 8 mg q 12 hr may be given for 1–2 days following chemotherapy. *Prevention of radiation-induced nausea/vomiting*—8 mg 1–2 hr prior to radiation; may be repeated q 8 hr, depending on type, location, and extent of radiation. *Prevention of postoperative nausea/vomiting*—16 mg 1 hr before induction of anesthesia.

PO (Children 4–11 yr): *Prevention of chemotherapy-induced nausea/vomiting*—4 mg 30 min prior to chemotherapy and repeated 4 and 8 hr later; 4 mg q 8 hr may be given for 1–2 days following chemotherapy.

IV (Adults): *Prevention of chemotherapy-induced nausea/vomiting*—0.15 mg/kg 15–30 min prior to chemotherapy, repeated 4 and 8 hr later, or 32-mg single dose 30 min prior to chemotherapy (lower doses have been used).

IM, IV (Adults): *Prevention of postoperative nausea/vomiting*—4 mg before induction of anesthesia or postoperatively.

IV (Children 4–18 yr): *Prevention of chemotherapy-induced nausea/vomiting*—0.15 mg/kg 15–30 min prior to chemotherapy, repeated 4 and 8 hr later.

IV (Children 2–12 yr and ≤40 kg): *Prevention of postoperative nausea/vomiting*—0.15 mg/kg.

IV (Children >40 kg): *Prevention of postoperative nausea/vomiting*—4 mg.

Hepatic Impairment

PO, IM, IV (Adults): Not to exceed 8 mg/day.

Availability (generic available)

Orally disintegrating tablets (contain aspartame) (strawberry flavor): 4 mg, 8 mg. **Cost:** *Generic*—4 mg $549.00/30. **Tablets:** 4 mg, 8 mg, 24 mg. **Cost:** *Generic*—4 mg $569.99/30, 8 mg $1,048.95/30. **Oral solution (strawberry flavor):** 4 mg/5 ml. **Solution for injection:** 2 mg/ml in 2- and 20-ml vials. **Premixed injection:** 32 mg/50 ml D5W.

NURSING IMPLICATIONS

Assessment

- Assess patient for nausea, vomiting, abdominal distention, and bowel sounds prior to and following administration.
- Assess patient for extrapyramidal effects (involuntary movements, facial grimacing, rigidity, shuffling walk, trembling of hands) periodically during therapy.
- ***Lab Test Considerations:*** May cause transient ↑ in serum bilirubin, AST, and ALT levels.

Potential Nursing Diagnoses

Imbalanced nutrition: less than body requirements (Indications)
Diarrhea (Side Effects)
Constipation (Side Effects)

Implementation

- Do not confuse Zofran (ondansetron) with Zosyn (piperacillin/tazobactam).
- First dose is administered prior to emetogenic event.
- **PO:** For orally disintegrating tablets, do not attempt to push through foil backing; with dry hands, peel back backing and remove tablet. Immediately place tablet on tongue; tablet will dissolve in seconds, then swallow with saliva. Administration of liquid is not necessary.

IV Administration

- **Direct IV:** Administer undiluted (2 mg/ml) immediately before induction of anesthesia or postoperatively if nausea and vomiting occur shortly after surgery. ***Rate:*** Administer over at least 30 sec and preferably over 2–5 min.
- **Intermittent Infusion: *Diluent:*** Dilute doses for prevention of nausea and vomiting associated with chemotherapy in 50 ml of D5W, 0.9% NaCl, D5/0.9% NaCl, D5/0.45% NaCl. Solution is clear and colorless. Stable for 7 days at room temperature following dilution. ***Concentration:*** 1 mg/ml. ***Rate:*** Administer each dose over 15 min.
- **Syringe Compatibility:** alfentanil, atropine, fentanyl, glycopyrrolate, meperidine, metoclopramide, midazolam, morphine, naloxone, neostigmine, propofol.

- **Syringe Incompatibility:** droperidol.
- **Y-Site Compatibility:** aldesleukin, amifostine, amikacin, azithromycin, aztreonam, bleomycin, carboplatin, carmustine, cefazolin, cefotaxime, cefoxitin, ceftazidime, ceftizoxime, cefuroxime, chlorpromazine, cimetidine, cisatracurium, cisplatin, cladribine, clindamycin, cyclophosphamide, cytarabine, dacarbazine, dactinomycin, daunorubicin, dexamethasone sodium phosphate, dexmedetomidine, diphenhydramine, docetaxel, dopamine, doxorubicin, doxorubicin liposome, doxycycline, droperidol, etoposide, etoposide phosphate, famotidine, fenoldopam, filgrastim, floxuridine, fluconazole, fludarabine, gemcitabine, gentamicin, haloperidol, heparin, hydrocortisone sodium succinate, hydrocortisone sodium phosphate, hydromorphone, ifosfamide, imipenem/cilastatin, linezolid, magnesium sulfate, mannitol, mechlorethamine, melphalan, meperidine, mesna, methotrexate, metoclopramide, mitomycin, mitoxantrone, morphine, oxaliplatin, paclitaxel, pentostatin, piperacillin/tazobactam, potassium chloride, promethazine, prochlorperazine edisylate, ranitidine, remifentanil, sodium acetate, streptozocin, teniposide, thiotepa, ticarcillin/clavulanate, topotecan, vancomycin, vinblastine, vincristine, vinorelbine, zidovudine.
- **Y-Site Incompatibility:** acyclovir, allopurinol, aminophylline, amphotericin B, amphotericin B cholesteryl sulfate, ampicillin, ampicillin/sulbactam, amsacrine, cefepime, cefoperazone, furosemide, ganciclovir, lansoprazole, lorazepam, methylprednisolone sodium succinate, pemetrexed, sargramostim, sodium bicarbonate.

Patient/Family Teaching

- Instruct patient to take ondansetron as directed.
- Advise patient to notify health care professional immediately if involuntary movement of eyes, face, or limbs occurs.

Evaluation/Desired Outcomes

- Prevention of nausea and vomiting associated with initial and repeat courses of emetogenic cancer chemotherapy.
- Prevention of postoperative nausea and vomiting.
- Prevention of nausea and vomiting due to radiation therapy.

oprelvekin (o-**prell**-ve-kin)

Neumega

Classification

Therapeutic: colony-stimulating factors

Pharmacologic: interleukins, thrombopoetic growth factors

Pregnancy Category C

Indications

Prevention of severe thrombocytopenia and reduction of the need for platelet transfusions following myelosuppressive chemotherapy in patients with nonmyeloid malignancies at risk for thrombocytopenia.

Action

Stimulates production of megakaryocytes and platelets. **Therapeutic Effects:** Increased platelet count.

Pharmacokinetics

Absorption: >80% absorbed following subcut administration.

Distribution: Unknown.

Metabolism and Excretion: Appears to be mostly metabolized, with metabolites eliminated by kidneys.

Half-life: 6.9 hr.

TIME/ACTION PROFILE (increase in platelet count)

ROUTE	ONSET	PEAK	DURATION
Subcut	5–9 days	unknown	7–14 days†

†Counts continue to rise for 7 days following discontinuation and then return to baseline by 14 days

Contraindications/Precautions

Contraindicated in: Hypersensitivity; Lactation.

Use Cautiously in: Any condition in which sodium and water retention would pose problems (CHF, renal disease); Pre-existing pericardial effusion or ascites (may be exacerbated); History of atrial arrhythmias (especially if receiving cardiac medications or previous doxorubicin therapy); Pre-existing papilledema or tumors of the CNS; OB, Pedi: Pregnancy or children (safety not established).

Adverse Reactions/Side Effects

These effects occurred in patients who had recently received myelosuppressive chemotherapy.

CNS: dizziness, headache, insomnia, nervousness, weakness. **EENT:** conjunctival hemorrhage, blurred vision, changes in visual acuity, blindness, papilledema, pharyngitis, rhinitis. **Resp:** cough, dyspnea, pleural effusions. **CV:** atrial fibrillation, edema, palpitations, syncope, tachycardia, vasodilation, ventricular arrhythmias. **GI:** anorexia, constipation, diarrhea, dyspepsia, mucositis, nausea, oral moniliasis, vomiting, abdominal pain. **Derm:** alopecia, ecchymoses, rash. **F and E:** sodium and water retention. **Local:** injection site reactions. **MS:** bone pain, myalgia. **Misc:** chills, fever, infection, pain.

Interactions

Drug-Drug: None significant.

Route/Dosage

Subcut (Adults): 50 mcg/kg once daily for 10–21 days.

Availability

Powder for injection: 5-mg vial.

NURSING IMPLICATIONS

Assessment

- Assess patient for signs of fluid retention (dyspnea on exertion, peripheral edema) during therapy. Fluid retention is a common side effect that usually resolves within several days following discontinuation of oprelvekin.
- ***Lab Test Considerations:*** Monitor platelet count prior to and periodically during therapy, especially at expected nadir. Therapy is continued until postnadir platelet count is ≥50,000 cells/ml.
- CBC should be monitored prior to and at regular intervals during therapy. Decrease in hemoglobin concentration, hematocrit, and RBC count may occur because of increased plasma volume (dilutional anemia); usually begins within 3–5 days of therapy and is reversible within a week of discontinuation of therapy.
- Monitor electrolyte concentrations in patients receiving chronic diuretic therapy. Hypokalemia may be fatal.
- May cause an ↑ in plasma fibrinogen.

Potential Nursing Diagnoses

Excess fluid volume (Side Effects)

Implementation

- Therapy should be started within 6–24 hr after completion of chemotherapy and continued for 10–21 days.
- Treatment should be discontinued at least 2 days prior to next planned chemotherapy cycle.
- **Subcut:** Reconstitute with 1 ml of sterile water for injection without preservatives for a concentration of 5 mg/ml. Direct diluent to sides of vial and swirl gently. Solution is clear and colorless. Do not administer solutions that are discolored or contain particulate matter. Do not shake or agitate vigorously. Do not freeze. Do not reuse vials. Administer within 3 hr of reconstitution as a single injection in abdomen, hip, thigh, or upper arm.

Patient/Family Teaching

- Instruct patient in proper technique for preparation and administration of medication. Provide a puncture-resistant container for disposal of needles.
- May cause transient blurred vision or dizziness. Caution patient to avoid driving or other activities requiring alertness until response to medication is known.
- Advise patient to notify health care professional if pregnancy is planned or suspected.
- Inform patient of side effects and advise patient to notify health care professional if chest pain, shortness of breath, fatigue, blurred vision, or irregular heartbeat persists.

Evaluation/Desired Outcomes

- Increase in postnadir platelet count to ≥50,000 cells/ml.

orlistat (or-li-stat)

Xenical

Classification

Therapeutic: weight control agents

Pharmacologic: lipase inhibitors

Pregnancy Category B

Indications

Obesity management (weight loss and maintenance) when used in conjunction with a reduced-calorie diet in patients with an initial BMI ≥30 kg/m^2 or ≥27 kg/m^2 in the presence of additional risk factors (diabetes, hypertension, hyperlipidemia). Reduces the risk of weight regain after prior loss. May delay onset of type 2 diabetes in prediabetic patients.

O

Action
Decreases the absorption of dietary fat by reversibly inhibiting enzymes (lipases), which are necessary for the breakdown and subsequent absorption of fat. **Therapeutic Effects:** Weight loss and maintenance in obese patients. Delayed onset of type 2 diabetes.

Pharmacokinetics
Absorption: Minimal systemic absorption.
Distribution: Action is local, within the GI tract.
Protein Binding: Minimally absorbed drug is >99% bound to plasma proteins.
Metabolism and Excretion: Major route is fecal elimination of unabsorbed drug.
Half-life: 1–2 hr.

TIME/ACTION PROFILE (effects on fecal fat)

ROUTE	ONSET	PEAK	DURATION
PO	24–48 hr	unknown	48–72 hr†

†Following discontinuation

Contraindications/Precautions
Contraindicated in: Hypersensitivity; Chronic malabsorption syndrome or cholestasis; OB: Pregnancy or lactation.
Use Cautiously in: Pedi: Children <16 (safety not established).

Adverse Reactions/Side Effects
With initial use; incidence decreases with prolonged use.
GI: fecal urgency, flatus with discharge, increased defecation, oily evacuation, oily spotting, fecal incontinence.

Interactions
Drug-Drug: Reduces the absorption of some **fat-soluble vitamins** and **beta-carotene**.

Route/Dosage
PO (Adults and adolescents ≥16 yr): 60–120 mg three times daily with each meal containing fat.

Availability
Capsules: 120 mg, 60 mg[OTC].

NURSING IMPLICATIONS

Assessment
- Monitor patients for weight loss and adjust concurrent medications (antihypertensives, antidiabetics, lipid-lowering agents) as needed.

Potential Nursing Diagnoses
Disturbed body image (Indications)
Imbalanced nutrition: more than body requirements (Indications)

Implementation
- **PO:** Administer one capsule 3 times daily with or up to 1 hour after a meal. If a meal is missed or contains no fat, dose of orlistat can be omitted.
- A supplemental multivitamin containing vitamins D, E, K, and beta-carotene should be taken daily, at least 2 hr before or after orlistat dose.
- Psyllium 6 g with each dose or 12 g at bedtime may decrease GI side effects.

Patient/Family Teaching
- Instruct patient to take orlistat with meals as directed. If a meal is missed or contains no fat, orlistat dose can be omitted. Do not take more than recommended dose; does not improve benefit.
- Instruct patient to adhere to a reduced-calorie diet. Daily intake of fat should be distributed over three main meals. Meals should contain no more than 30% fat. Taking orlistat with a meal high in fat may increase the GI side effects.
- Advise patient that regular physical activity, approved by a health care professional, should be used in conjunction with orlistat and diet.
- Inform patient of common GI side effects (oily spotting, gas with discharge, urgent need to go to the bathroom, oily or fatty stools, an oily discharge, increased number of bowel movements, inability to control bowel movements). Oil in bowel movement may be clear or have orange or brown colorations. GI side effects usually occur in first weeks of treatment and are more increased following a meal high in fat. May lessen or disappear, or may continue for 6 mo or longer.
- Advise patient to notify health care professional prior to taking any Rx, OTC, or herbal product.
- Advise patient to notify health care professional if pregnancy is planned or suspected.

Evaluation/Desired Outcomes
- Slow, consistent weight loss when combined with a reduced-calorie diet.
- Delayed onset of type 2 diabetes.

orphenadrine

(or-**fenn**-a-dreen)

Antiflex, Banflex, ♣Disipal, Flexoject, Flexon, Mio-Rel, Myolin, Myotrol, Norflex, Orfro, Orphenate

Classification

Therapeutic: skeletal muscle relaxants (centrally acting)

Pharmacologic: diphenhydramine analogues

Pregnancy Category C

Indications

Adjunct to rest and physical therapy in the treatment of muscle spasm associated with acute painful musculoskeletal conditions. Adjunct therapy of Parkinson's disease (Canadian labeling only).

Action

Skeletal muscle relaxation, probably due to CNS depression. **Therapeutic Effects:** Skeletal muscle relaxation, with decreased discomfort.

Pharmacokinetics

Absorption: Readily absorbed after oral and IM administration; IV administration results in complete bioavailability.

Distribution: Unknown.

Metabolism and Excretion: Mostly metabolized by the liver.

Half-life: 14 hr.

TIME/ACTION PROFILE (skeletal muscle effects)

ROUTE	ONSET	PEAK	DURATION
PO-ER	within 1 hr	6–8 hr	12 hr
IM	5 min	30 min	12 hr
IV	immediate	unknown	12 hr

Contraindications/Precautions

Contraindicated in: Hypersensitivity; Bladder neck obstruction, prostatic hyperplasia, glaucoma, myasthenia gravis, peptic ulcer disease, GI obstruction.

Use Cautiously in: Underlying cardiovascular disease; Impaired renal function; Geri: Appears on Beers list. Geriatric patients are more susceptible to sedation and anticholinergic effects; OB, Pedi: Pregnancy, lactation, or children (safety not established).

Adverse Reactions/Side Effects

CNS: CNS excitation, confusion, dizziness, drowsiness. **EENT:** blurred vision, dry eyes. **CV:** orthostatic hypotension, tachycardia. **GI:** constipation, dry mouth. **GU:** urinary retention.

Interactions

Drug-Drug: Concurrent use of other **anticholinergics** ↑ risk of anticholinergic side effects. ↑ risk of CNS depression with other **CNS depressants** including **alcohol**, **antihistamines**, **antidepressants**, **sedative/hypnotics**, or **opioid analgesics**.

Drug-Natural Products: Kava kava, **valerian**, **chamomile**, or **hops** can ↑ CNS depression.

Route/Dosage

Skeletal muscle relaxation

PO (Adults): 100 mg twice daily.

IV, IM (Adults): 60 mg q 12 hr.

Adjunctive therapy of Parkinson's disease

PO (Adults): 50 mg 3 times daily (lower doses if used with other agents).

Availability (generic available)

Tablets: ♣50 mg[OTC]. **Extended-release tablets:** 100 mg. **Injection:** 30 mg/ml.

NURSING IMPLICATIONS

Assessment

- Geri: Assess geriatric patients for anticholinergic adverse effects (delirium, acute confusion, dizziness, dry mouth, blurred vision, urinary retention, constipation, tachycardia) and sedation.
- **Skeletal Muscle Relaxant:** Assess patient for pain, muscle stiffness, and range of motion before and periodically throughout therapy.
- **Parkinson's Disease:** Assess parkinsonian and extrapyramidal symptoms (restlessness or desire to keep moving, rigidity, tremors, pill rolling, mask-like face, shuffling gait, muscle spasms, twisting motions, difficulty speaking or swallowing, loss of balance control) prior to and throughout therapy.
- ***Lab Test Considerations:*** Monitor CBC and renal and hepatic function tests periodically during prolonged therapy.

Potential Nursing Diagnoses

Acute pain (Indications)

O

Impaired physical mobility (Indications)
Risk for injury (Side Effects)

Implementation

- Do not confuse Norflex (orphenadrine) with norfloxacin (Noroxin).
- Provide safety measures as indicated. Supervise ambulation and transfer of patients.
- **PO:** Do not break, crush or chew extended-release tablets.

IV Administration

- **Direct IV:** May be administered undiluted. ***Concentration:*** 30 mg/ml.

Patient/Family Teaching

- Advise patient to take medication as directed. Take missed doses within 1 hr; if not, return to regular dosing schedule. Do not double doses.
- Encourage patient to comply with additional therapies prescribed for muscle spasm (rest, physical therapy, heat).
- Medication may cause dizziness, drowsiness, and blurred vision. Advise patient to avoid driving and other activities requiring alertness until response to drug is known.
- Instruct patient to make position changes slowly to minimize orthostatic hypotension.
- Advise patient to avoid concurrent use of alcohol and other CNS depressants while taking this medication.
- Emphasize the importance of routine follow-up exams to monitor progress.

Evaluation/Desired Outcomes

- Decreased musculoskeletal pain and muscle spasticity,
- Increased range of motion.
- Decrease in tremors and rigidity and an improvement in gait and balance.

oseltamivir (o-sel-**tam**-i-vir)

Tamiflu

Classification
Therapeutic: antivirals
Pharmacologic: neuramidase inhibitors

Pregnancy Category C

Indications

Uncomplicated acute illness due to influenza infection in adults and children >1 yr who have had symptoms for ≤2 days. Prevention of influenza in patients ≥1 yr.

Action

Inhibits the enzyme neuramidase, which may alter virus particle aggregation and release.
Therapeutic Effects: Reduced duration of flu-related symptoms.

Pharmacokinetics

Absorption: Rapidly absorbed from the GI tract and converted by the liver to the active form, oseltamivir carboxylate. 75% reaches systemic circulation as the active drug.
Distribution: Unknown.
Metabolism and Excretion: Rapidly metabolized by the liver to oseltamivir carboxylate, the active drug. Oseltamivir is >99% excreted unchanged in urine.
Half-life: *Oseltamivir carboxylate*—6–10 hr.

TIME/ACTION PROFILE (blood levels)

ROUTE	ONSET	PEAK	DURATION
PO	unknown	unknown	12 hr

Contraindications/Precautions

Contraindicated in: Hypersensitivity; Pedi: Children <1 yr.
Use Cautiously in: OB, Lactation: Safety not established; use only if potential benefits outweigh possible risks.

Adverse Reactions/Side Effects

CNS: insomnia, vertigo, confusion, self-injurious behavior. **Resp:** bronchitis. **GI:** nausea, vomiting.

Interactions

Drug-Drug: None significant.

Route/Dosage

Treatment of Influenza

PO (Adults and Children >40kg): 75 mg twice daily for 5 days.
PO (Children 23–40 kg): 60 mg twice daily.
PO (Children 15–23 kg): 45 mg twice daily.
PO (Children ≤15 kg and ≥1 yr): 30 mg twice daily.

Renal Impairment

PO (Adults): *CCr <30 ml/min*—75 mg once daily for 5 days.

Influenza Prevention

PO (Adults and Children ≥13 yrs): 75 mg once daily for at least 10 days.
PO (Children >40 kg): 75 mg once daily for 10 days.
PO (Children 23–40 kg): 60 mg once daily for 10 days.

PO (Children 15–23 kg): 45 mg once daily for 10 days.
PO (Children ≤15 kg and ≥1 yr): 30 mg once daily.

Renal Impairment
PO (Adults and Children ≥13 yrs): *CCr 10–30 ml/min*—75 mg every other day *or* 30 mg every day.

Availability
Capsules: 30 mg, 45 mg, 75 mg. **Cost:** 75 mg $84.99/10. **Oral suspension (tutti-frutti flavor):** 12 mg/ml in 25-ml bottle.

NURSING IMPLICATIONS

Assessment
- Monitor influenza symptoms (sudden onset of fever, cough, headache, fatigue, muscular weakness, sore throat). Additional supportive treatment may be indicated to treat symptoms.

Potential Nursing Diagnoses
Risk for infection (Indications)

Implementation
- Treatment with oseltamivir should be started as soon as possible from the first sign of flu symptoms.
- **PO:** May be administered with food or milk to minimize GI irritation.
- To prepare oral solution, tap closed bottle to loosen powder. Add total amount of water for constitution and shake closed bottle for 15 seconds. Remove childproof cap and push bottle adaptor into neck of bottle. Close bottle with childproof top tightly, assuring proper seating of bottle adaptor and childproof status. Shake well before use. Use within 10 days of constitution. If oral suspension is not available, capsules can be opened and mixed with sweetened liquids, such as regular or sugar-free chocolate syrup.

Patient/Family Teaching
- Instruct patient to take oseltamivir as soon as influenza symptoms appear and to continue to take it as directed, for the full course of therapy, even if feeling better. Take missed doses as soon as remembered unless within 2 hr of next dose. Do not double doses.
- Caution patient that oseltamivir should not be shared with anyone, even if they have the same symptoms.
- Advise patient that oseltamivir is not a substitute for a flu shot. Patients should receive annual flu shot according to immunization guidelines.
- Advise patient to consult health care professional before taking other medications concurrently with oseltamivir.

Evaluation/Desired Outcomes
- Reduction of the duration of flu symptoms.

oxacillin, See PENICILLINS, PENICILLINASE RESISTANT.

oxaliplatin (ox-a-li-pla-tin)
Eloxatin

Classification
Therapeutic: antineoplastics

Pregnancy Category D

O

Indications
Used in combination with 5–Fluorouracil and leucovorin in the treatment of advanced or metastatic colon or rectal cancer. **Unlabeled uses:** Treatment of ovarian cancer that has progressed despite treatment with other agents.

Action
Inhibits DNA replication and transcription by incorporating platinum into normal cross-linking (cell-cycle nonspecific). **Therapeutic Effects:** Death of rapidly replicating cells, particularly malignant ones.

Pharmacokinetics
Absorption: IV administration results in complete bioavailability.
Distribution: Extensive tissue distribution.
Protein Binding: >90% (platinum).
Metabolism and Excretion: Undergoes rapid and extensive nonenzymatic biotransformation; excreted mostly by the kidneys.
Half-life: 391 hours.

TIME/ACTION PROFILE

ROUTE	ONSET	PEAK	DURATION
IV	unknown	unknown	unknown

Contraindications/Precautions
Contraindicated in: Hypersensitivity; Hypersensitivity to other platinum compounds; Pregnancy or lactation.

Use Cautiously in: Renal impairment; Geri: Geriatric patients (increased risk of adverse reactions); Pedi: Children (safety not established).

Adverse Reactions/Side Effects

Adverse reactions are noted for the combination of oxaliplatin, 5–FU and leucovorin.

CNS: fatigue. **CV:** chest pain, edema, thromboembolism. **Resp:** PULMONARY FIBROSIS, coughing, dyspnea. **GI:** diarrhea, nausea, vomiting, abdominal pain, anorexia, gastroesophageal reflux, stomatitis. **F and E:** dehydration, hypokalemia. **Hemat:** leukopenia, NEUTROPENIA, THROMBOCYTOPENIA, anemia. **Local:** injection site reactions. **MS:** back pain. **Neuro:** neurotoxicity. **Misc:** ANAPHYLAXIS/ANAPHYLACTOID REACTIONS, fever.

Interactions

Drug-Drug: Concurrent use of **nephrotoxic agents** may ↑ toxicity.

Route/Dosage

IV (Adults): *Day 1*—85 mg/m² with leucovorin 200 mg/m² at the same time over 2 hr, followed by 5-FU 400 mg/m² bolus over 2–4 min, then 5–FU 600 mg/m² as a 22-hr infusion. *Day 2*—leucovorin 200 mg/m² over 2 hr, followed by 5-FU 400 mg/m² bolus over 2–4 min, then 5-FU 600 mg/m² as a 22-hr infusion. Cycle is repeated every 2 wk. Dosage reduction/alteration may be required for neurotoxicity or other serious adverse effects.

Availability

Solution for injection: 5 mg/mL in 10-mL vials (50 mg), 5 mg/mL in 20-mL vials (100 mg).

NURSING IMPLICATIONS

Assessment

- Assess for peripheral sensory neuropathy. *Acute onset* occurs within hrs to 1–2 days of dosing, resolves within 14 days, and frequently recurs with further dosing (transient paresthesia, dysesthesia and hypothesia of hands, feet, perioral area, or throat). Symptoms may be precipitated or exacerbated by exposure to cold or cold objects. May also cause jaw spasm, abnormal tongue sensation, dysarthria, eye pain, and a feeling of chest pressure. *Persistent* (>14 days) causes paresthesias, dysethesias, and hypoesthesias, but may also include deficits in proprioception that may interfere with daily activities (walking, writing, swallowing). Persistent neuropathy may occur without prior acute neuropathy and may improve upon discontinuation of oxaliplatin.
- Assess for signs of pulmonary fibrosis (nonproductive cough, dyspnea, crackles, radiological; infiltrates). May be fatal. Discontinue oxaliplatin if pulmonary fibrosis occurs.
- Monitor for signs of anaphylaxis (rash, hives, swelling or lips or tongue, sudden cough). Epinephrine, corticosteroids, and antihistamines should be readily available.
- ***Lab Test Considerations:*** Monitor WBC with differential, hemoglobin, platelet count, and blood chemistries (ALT, AST, bilirubin, and creatinine) before each oxaliplatin cycle.

Potential Nursing Diagnoses

Nausea (Adverse Reactions)

Implementation

- Extravasation may result in local pain and inflammation that may be severe and lead to necrosis.
- Premedicate patient with antiemetics with or without dexamethasone. Prehydration is not required.

IV Administration

- **Intermittent Infusion:** Protect concentrated solution from light; do not freeze. ***Diluent:*** Must be further diluted with 250–500 ml of D5W. Do not use 0.9% NaCl or any other chloride-containing solution for final solution. Do not use aluminum needles or administration sets containing aluminum parts; aluminum may cause degradation of platinum compounds. May be stored in refrigerator for 24 hr or 6 hr at room temperature. Diluted solution is not light-sensitive. Do not administer solutions that are discolored or contain particulate matter. ***Concentration:*** 0.2–0.6 mg/ml. ***Rate:*** Administer oxaliplatin simultaneously with leucovorin in separate bags via Y-line over 120 min. Prolonging infusion time to 6 hr may decrease acute toxicities. Infusion times for fluorouracil and leucovorin do not need to change.
- **Y-Site Compatibility:** bumetanide, buprenorphine, butorphanol, calcium gluconate, carboplatin, chlorpromazine, cimetidine, cyclophosphamide, dexamethasone sodium phosphate, dobutamine, docetaxel, dolasetron, dopamine, doxorubicin, droperidol, enalaprilat, epirubicin, etoposide phosphate, famotidine, fentanyl, furosemide, gemcita-

bine, granisetron, haloperidol, heparin, hydrocortisone sodium succinate, hydromorphone, ifosfamide, irinotecan, leucovorin, lorazepam, magnesium sulfate, mannitol, meperidine, mesna, methotrexate, methylprednisolone sodium succinate, metoclopramide, mitoxantrone, morphine, nalbuphine, ondansetron, paclitaxel, palonosetron, potassium chloride, prochlorperazine, promethazine, ranitidine, theophylline, topotecan, verapamil, vincristine, vinorelbine.

- **Y-Site Incompatibility:** diazepam, alkaline solutions, chloride-containing solutions. Infusion line should be flushed with D5W prior to administration of other solutions or medications.

Patient/Family Teaching

- Inform patients and caregivers of potential for peripheral neuropathy and potentiation by exposure to cold or cold objects. Advise patient to avoid cold drinks, use of ice in drinks or as ice packs, and to cover exposed skin prior to exposure to cold temperature or cold objects. Caution patients to cover themselves with a blanket during infusion, do not breathe deeply when exposed to cold air, wear warm clothing, and cover mouth and nose with a scarf or pull-down ski cap to warm the air that goes to their lungs, do not take things from the freezer or refrigerator without wearing gloves, drink fluids warm or at room temperature, always drink through a straw, do not use ice chips for nausea, be aware that most metals (car doors, mailbox) are cold; wear gloves to touch, do not run air conditioning at high levels in house or car, if hands get cold wash them with warm water. Advise health care professional of how you did since last treatment before next infusion.
- Instruct patient to notify health care professional immediately if signs of low blood cell counts (fever, persistent diarrhea, infection) or if persistent vomiting, signs of dehydration, cough or breathing difficulty, thirst, dry mouth, dizziness, decreased urination or signs of allergic reactions occur.

Evaluation/Desired Outcomes

- Decrease in size and spread of malignancies.

oxaprozin (ox-a-**proe**-zin)

Daypro

Classification

Therapeutic: antirheumatics, nonsteroidal anti-inflammatory agents

Pregnancy Category B, C (first trimester), UK (second and third trimester)

Indications

Rheumatoid arthritis and osteoarthritis.

Action

Inhibits prostaglandin synthesis. **Therapeutic Effects:** Suppression of pain and inflammation.

Pharmacokinetics

Absorption: Well absorbed following oral administration (80%); 35% is rapidly converted to an active metabolite.
Distribution: Unknown.
Protein Binding: 99.9%.
Metabolism and Excretion: The active metabolite is metabolized by the liver to inactive compounds.
Half-life: 42–50 hr.

TIME/ACTION PROFILE (antirheumatic action)

ROUTE	ONSET	PEAK	DURATION
PO	within 7 days	unknown	unknown

Contraindications/Precautions

Contraindicated in: Hypersensitivity; Cross-sensitivity may exist with other NSAIDs, including aspirin; Active GI bleeding or ulcer disease; Perioperative pain from coronary artery bypass graft (CABG) surgery.
Use Cautiously in: Cardiovascular disease or risk factors for cardiovascular disease (may ↑ risk of serious cardiovascular thrombotic events, myocardial infarction, and stroke, especially with prolonged use); Severe hepatic disease; Renal impairment (lower initial dose may be necessary); History of ulcer disease; Geri: Appears on Beers list. Geriatric patients are at ↑ risk of GI bleeding. May require dose adjustments due to age-related decrease in renal function); Pedi: Pregnancy, lactation, or children (safety not established; not recommended for use during the second half of pregnancy).

O

Adverse Reactions/Side Effects

CNS: agitation, anxiety, confusion, depression, dizziness, drowsiness, fatigue, headache, insomnia, malaise, weakness. **EENT:** abnormal vision, tinnitus. **Resp:** dyspnea, hypersensitivity pneumonitis. **CV:** edema, vasculitis. **GI:** GI BLEEDING, abdominal pain, diarrhea, dyspepsia, abnormal liver function tests, anorexia, cholestatic jaundice, constipation, dry mouth, duodenal ulcer, flatulence, gastritis, increased appetite, nausea, stomatitis, vomiting. **GU:** albuminuria, azotemia, interstitial nephritis. **Derm:** EXFOLIATIVE DERMATITIS, STEVENS-JOHNSON SYNDROME, TOXIC EPIDERMAL NECROLYSIS, increased sweating, photosensitivity, pruritus, rash. **Hemat:** prolonged bleeding time. **Metab:** weight gain. **Neuro:** paresthesia, tremor. **Misc:** allergic reactions including ANAPHYLAXIS, ANGIONEUROTIC EDEMA.

Interactions

Drug-Drug: ↑ adverse GI effects and toxicity with **aspirin**, other **NSAIDs**, **potassium supplements**, **corticosteroids**, or **alcohol**. Chronic use with **acetaminophen** may ↑ risk of adverse renal reactions. May ↓ effectiveness of **diuretics** or **antihypertensive** therapy. May ↑ hypoglycemic effects of **insulin** or **oral hypoglycemic agents**. ↑ risk of toxicity from **methotrexate**. ↑ risk of bleeding with **cefotetan**, **cefoperazone**, **thrombolytic agents**, **anticoagulants**, **ticlopidine**, **clopidogrel**, **eptifibatide**, or **tirofiban**. ↑ risk of adverse hematologic reactions with **antineoplastics** or **radiation therapy**.
Drug-Natural Products: ↑ anticoagulant effect and bleeding risk with **arnica**, **chamomile**, **clove**, **feverfew**, **garlic**, **ginger**, **ginkgo**, **Panax ginseng**, and others.

Route/Dosage

PO (Adults): 1200 mg once daily; onset may be more rapid with an initial 1800-mg dose. Patients with low body weight, mild disease, or renal impairment may be started at 600 mg/day (not to exceed 1800 mg/day or 26 mg/kg/day). Daily doses >1200 mg should be given in 2–3 divided doses. Consideration should be given to decreasing dose to lowest effective amount.

Availability (generic available)

Tablets: 600 mg.

NURSING IMPLICATIONS

Assessment

- Patients who have asthma, aspirin-induced allergy, and nasal polyps are at increased risk for developing hypersensitivity reactions. Monitor for rhinitis, asthma, and urticaria.
- Assess pain and range of motion prior to and periodically during therapy.
- ***Lab Test Considerations:*** May cause prolonged bleeding time, which may persist for up to 2 wk following discontinuation of therapy.
- Evaluate BUN, serum creatinine, CBC, and liver function tests periodically in patients receiving prolonged therapy. Serum potassium, BUN, serum creatinine, alkaline phosphatase, LDH, AST, and ALT tests may show ↑ levels. Blood glucose, hemoglobin, and hematocrit concentrations, leukocyte and platelet counts, and CCr may be ↓.

Potential Nursing Diagnoses

Acute pain (Indications)

Implementation

- Administration in higher than recommended doses does not provide increased effectiveness but may cause increased side effects. Use lowest effective dose for shortest period of time.
- **PO:** Administer with food or antacids to decrease GI irritation.

Patient/Family Teaching

- Advise patient to take oxaprozin with a full glass of water and to remain in an upright position for 15–30 min after administration.
- Instruct patient to take medication as directed. Take missed doses as soon as remembered but not if almost time for the next dose. Do not double doses.
- May cause drowsiness and dizziness. Advise patient to avoid driving or other activities requiring alertness until response to the medication is known.
- Caution patient to avoid the concurrent use of alcohol, aspirin, acetaminophen, and other OTC or herbal products without consulting health care professional.
- Advise patient to notify health care professional of medication regimen prior to treatment or surgery. Oxaprozin should be discontinued 2 wk prior to surgery.
- Caution patient to use sunscreen and protective clothing to prevent photosensitivity reactions.
- Advise patient to consult health care professional if rash, itching, visual disturbances, tinnitus, weight gain, edema, black stools, persistent headache, or influenza-like syn-

drome (chills, fever, muscle aches, pain) occurs.

Evaluation/Desired Outcomes

- Decreased pain and improved joint mobility. Maximum effectiveness may require 2 wk or more of continuous therapy. Patients who do not respond to one NSAID may respond to another.

oxazepam (ox-az-e-pam)

✤Apo-Oxazepam, ✤Novoxapam, Serax

Classification

Therapeutic: antianxiety agents, sedative/hypnotics

Pharmacologic: benzodiazepines

Schedule IV

Pregnancy Category D

Indications

Management of anxiety, anxiety associated with depression. Symptomatic treatment of alcohol withdrawal.

Action

Depresses the CNS, probably by potentiating GABA, an inhibitory neurotransmitter. **Therapeutic Effects:** Decreased anxiety. Diminished symptoms of alcohol withdrawal.

Pharmacokinetics

Absorption: Well absorbed following oral administration. Absorption is slower than with other benzodiazepines.

Distribution: Widely distributed. Crosses the blood-brain barrier. May cross the placenta and enter breast milk. Recommend to discontinue drug or bottle feed.

Metabolism and Excretion: Metabolized by the liver to inactive compounds.

Protein Binding: 97%.

Half-life: 5–15 hr.

TIME/ACTION PROFILE (sedation)

ROUTE	ONSET	PEAK	DURATION
PO	45–90 min	unknown	6–12 hr

Contraindications/Precautions

Contraindicated in: Hypersensitivity; Cross-sensitivity with other benzodiazepines may exist; Comatose patients or those with pre-existing CNS depression; Uncontrolled severe pain; Angle-closure glaucoma; Pregnancy and lactation; Some products contain tartrazine and should be avoided in patients with known intolerance.

Use Cautiously in: Hepatic dysfunction (may be preferred over some benzodiazepines due to short half-life); History of suicide attempt or drug abuse; Debilitated patients (initial dosage reduction recommended); Severe chronic obstructive pulmonary disease; Myasthenia gravis; Geri: Elderly patients have increased sensitivity to benzodiazepines. Appears on Beers list and is associated with increased risk of falls (↓ dose required).

Adverse Reactions/Side Effects

CNS: dizziness, drowsiness, confusion, hangover, headache, impaired memory, mental depression, paradoxical excitation, slurred speech. **EENT:** blurred vision. **Resp:** respiratory depression. **CV:** tachycardia. **GI:** constipation, diarrhea, drug-induced hepatitis, nausea, vomiting, weight gain (unusual). **GU:** urinary problems. **Derm:** rashes. **Hemat:** leukopenia. **Misc:** physical dependence, psychological dependence, tolerance.

Interactions

Drug-Drug: Additive CNS depression with other **CNS depressants**, including **alcohol**, **antihistamines**, **antidepressants**, **opioid analgesics**, and other **sedative/hypnotics** (including other **benzodiazepines**). May ↓ the therapeutic effectiveness of **levodopa**. **Hormonal contraceptives** or **phenytoin** may ↓ effectiveness. **Theophylline** may ↓ sedative effects of oxazepam.

Drug-Natural Products: Concomitant use of **kava kava, valerian, skullcap, chamomile**, or **hops** can increase CNS depression.

Route/Dosage

PO (Adults): *Antianxiety agent*—10–30 mg 3–4 times daily. *Sedative/hypnotic/management of alcohol withdrawal*—15–30 mg 3–4 times daily.

PO (Geriatric Patients): 5 mg 1–2 times daily initially or 10 mg 3 times daily; may be increased as needed.

Availability (generic available)

Capsules: 10 mg, 15 mg, 30 mg. **Tablets:** ✤10 mg, 15 mg, ✤30 mg.

✤ = Canadian drug name.

*CAPITALS indicates life-threatening; underlines indicate most frequent.

NURSING IMPLICATIONS

Assessment

- Assess patient for anxiety and orientation, mood and behavior.
- Assess level of sedation (ataxia, dizziness, slurred speech) periodically throughout therapy.
- Assess regularly for continued need for treatment.
- Prolonged high-dose therapy may lead to psychological or physical dependence. Restrict the amount of drug available to patient.
- Geri: Assess CNS effects and risk of falls. Institute falls prevention strategies.
- ***Lab Test Considerations:*** Monitor CBC and liver function tests periodically during prolonged therapy.
- May cause decreased thyroidal uptake of sodium iodide ^{123}I and ^{131}I.

Potential Nursing Diagnoses

Anxiety (Indications)
Ineffective coping (Indications)
Risk for injury (Side Effects)

Implementation

- Medication should be tapered at the completion of therapy (taper by 0.5 mg q 3 days). Sudden cessation of medication may lead to withdrawal (insomnia, irritability, nervousness, tremors).
- **PO:** Administer with food if GI irritation becomes a problem.

Patient/Family Teaching

- Instruct patient to take oxazepam exactly as directed. Missed doses should be taken within 1 hr; if remembered later, omit and return to regular dosing schedule. Do not double or increase doses. If dose is less effective after a few weeks, notify health care professional.
- Inform patient that oxazepam is usually prescribed for short-term use. Encourage patient to participate in psychotherapy to address source of anxiety and improve coping skills.
- Encourage patient to participate in psychotherapy to address source of anxiety and improve coping skills.
- Teach other methods to decrease anxiety, such as increased exercise, support group, relaxation techniques.
- May cause drowsiness or dizziness. Caution patient to avoid driving or other activities requiring alertness until response to medication is known.
- Advise patient to avoid the use of alcohol and to consult health care professional prior to the use of OTC preparations that contain antihistamines or alcohol.
- Advise patient to inform health care professional if pregnancy is planned or suspected.
- Advise patient to notify health care professional of medication regimen prior to treatment or surgery.
- Emphasize the importance of follow-up exams to monitor effectiveness of medication.
- Geri: Instruct patient and family how to reduce falls risk at home.

Evaluation/Desired Outcomes

- Decreased sense of anxiety.
- Increased ability to cope.
- Prevention or relief of acute agitation, tremor, and hallucinations during alcohol withdrawal.

oxcarbazepine

(ox-kar-**baz**-e-peen)
Trileptal

Classification
Therapeutic: anticonvulsants
Pharmacologic: carbamazepine analogues

Pregnancy Category C

Indications

Monotherapy or adjunctive therapy of partial seizures in adults and children 4 yrs and older with epilepsy. Adjunctive therapy in patients 2–16 yr with epilepsy. **Unlabeled uses:** Management of trigeminal neuralgia.

Action

Blocks sodium channels in neural membranes, stabilizing hyperexcitable states, inhibiting repetitive neuronal firing, and decreasing propagation of synaptic impulses. **Therapeutic Effects:** Decreased incidence of seizures.

Pharmacokinetics

Absorption: Rapidly absorbed after oral administration and rapidly converted to the active 10-hydroxy metabolite (MHD).
Distribution: Enters breast milk in significant amounts.
Metabolism and Excretion: Extensively converted to MHD, which is then primarily excreted by the kidneys.
Half-life: *Oxcarbazepine*—2 hr; *MHD*—9 hr.

TIME/ACTION PROFILE (blood levels)

ROUTE	ONSET	PEAK	DURATION
PO 12 hr	PO	rapid	4.5 hr†

†Steady-state levels of MHD are reached after 2–3 days during twice-daily dosing

Contraindications/Precautions

Contraindicated in: Hypersensitivity; cross-sensitivity with carbamazepine may occur; OB: Lactation.
Use Cautiously in: Renal impairment (dose reduction recommended if CCr <30 ml/min); OB: Pregnancy (use only if potential benefit justifies the potential risk to the fetus); Pedi: Children <4 yr (safety not established).

Adverse Reactions/Side Effects

CNS: dizziness/vertigo, drowsiness/fatigue, headache, cognitive symptoms. **EENT:** abnormal vision, diplopia, nystagmus. **GI:** abdominal pain, dyspepsia, nausea, vomiting, thirst. **Derm:** acne, rash, urticaria. **F and E:** hyponatremia. **Neuro:** ataxia, gait disturbances, tremor. **Misc:** allergic reactions, hypersensitivity reactions including STEVENS-JOHNSON SYNDROME and MULTIORGAN REACTIONS, lymphadenopathy.

Interactions

Drug-Drug: Oxcarbazepine may inhibit the CYP 2C19 enzyme system drugs and would be expected to alter the effects of other drugs that are metabolized by this system. Oxcarbazepine and MHD induce the P450 3A4/5 enzyme systems and would be expected to alter the effects of other drugs that are metabolized by this system. This may result in decreased levels and effectiveness of **hormonal contraceptives**, **felodipine**, **isradipine**, **nicardipine**, **nifedipine**, and **nimodipine**. In addition, oxcarbazepine itself is metabolized by cytochrome P450 drugs system and other **drugs that alter the activity of this system**. ↑ CNS depression may occur with other CNS depressants, including **alcohol**, **antihistamines**, **antidepressants**, **sedative/hypnotics**, and **opioids**. **Carbamazepine**, **phenobarbital**, **phenytoin**, **valproic acid** and **verapamil** ↓ levels. May ↑ serum levels and effects of **phenytoin** (dosage reduction of phenytoin may be required).

Route/Dosage

(Tablets and oral suspension can be interchanged at equal doses).
PO (Adults): *Adjunctive therapy*—300 mg twice daily, may be increased by up to 600 mg/day at weekly intervals up to 1200 mg/day (up to 2400 mg/day may be needed); *conversion to monotherapy*—300 mg twice daily; may be increased by 600 mg/day at weekly intervals, whereas other antiepileptic drugs are tapered over 3–6 wk; dose of oxcarbazepine should be increased up to 2400 mg/day over a period of 2–4 wk; *initiation of monotherapy*—300 mg twice daily, increase by 300 mg/day every third day, up to 1200 mg/day. Maximum maintenance dose should be achieved over 2–4 wks.
PO (Children 2–16 yr): *Adjunctive therapy*—4–5 mg/kg twice daily (up to 600 mg/day), increased over 2 wk to achieve 900 mg/day in patients 20–29 kg, 1200 mg/day in patients 29.1–39 kg and 1800 mg/day in patients >39 kg (range 6–51 mg/kg/day). In patients <20 kg, initial dose of 16–20 mg/kg/day may be used not to exceed 60 mg/kg/day; *conversion to monotherapy*—8–10 mg/kg/day given twice daily; may be increased by 10 mg/kg/day at weekly intervals, whereas other antiepileptic drugs are tapered over 3–6 wk; dose of oxcarbazepine should be increased up to 600–900 mg/day in patient ≤20 kg, 900–1200 mg/day in patients 25–30 kg, 900–1500 mg/day in patients 35–40 kg. 1200–1500 mg/day in patients 45 kg, 1200–1800 mg/day in patients 50–55 kg, 1200–2100 mg/day in patients 60–65 kg, and 1500–2100 mg/day in patients 70 kg. Maximum maintenance dose should be achieved over 2–4 wks.

Renal Impairment

PO (Adults): *CCr<30 ml/min*—Initiate therapy at 300 mg/day and increase slowly to achieve desired response.

Availability (generic available)

Tablets: 150 mg, 300 mg, 600 mg. **Cost:** *Generic*—150 mg $53.79/100, 300 mg $375.97/180, 600 mg $742.97/180, 150 mg $96.21/100, 300 mg $175.70/100, 600 mg $322.94/100. **Oral suspension:** 60 mg/ml in 250-ml bottle. **Cost:** $155.23/250 ml.

NURSING IMPLICATIONS

Assessment

- **Seizures:** Assess frequency, location, duration, and characteristics of seizure activity.

Hyponatremia may increase frequency and severity of seizures.
- Monitor patient for CNS changes. May manifest as cognitive symptoms (psychomotor slowing, difficulty with concentration, speech or language problems), somnolence or fatigue, or coordination abnormalities (ataxia, gait disturbances).
- ***Lab Test Considerations:*** Monitor ECG and serum electrolytes before and periodically during therapy. May cause hyponatremia. Usually occurs during the first 3 months of therapy. May require dose reduction, fluid restriction, or discontinuation of therapy. Sodium levels return to normal within a few days of discontinuation.

Potential Nursing Diagnoses
Risk for injury (Indications, Side Effects)

Implementation
- Implement seizure precautions as indicated.
- **PO:** Administer twice daily with or without food.
- Shake oral suspension well and prepare dose immediately after. Withdraw using oral dosing syringe supplied by manufacturer. May be mixed in a small glass of water just prior to administration or swallowed directly from syringe. Rinse syringe with warm water and allow to dry.

Patient/Family Teaching
- Instruct patient to take oxcarbazepine in equally spaced doses, as directed. Take missed doses as soon as possible but not just before next dose; do not double doses. Notify health care professional if more than one dose is missed. Medication should be gradually discontinued to prevent seizures.
- May cause dizziness, drowsiness, or CNS changes. Advise patients to avoid driving or other activities requiring alertness until response to medication is known. Do not resume driving until physician gives clearance based on control of seizure disorder.
- Advise patient not to take alcohol or other CNS depressants concurrently with this medication.
- Advise female patients to use an additional nonhormonal method of contraception during therapy and until next menstrual period. Instruct patient to notify health care professional if pregnancy is planned or suspected.
- Instruct patient to notify health care professional of medication regimen before treatment or surgery.
- Advise patients to carry identification describing disease and medication regimen at all times.

Evaluation/Desired Outcomes
- Absence or reduction of seizure activity.

---

oxiconazole, **See ANTIFUNGALS (TOPICAL).**

OXYBUTYNIN (ox-i-**byoo**-ti-nin)

oxybutynin (oral)
Ditropan, Ditropan XL

oxybutynin (transdermal)
Oxytrol

Classification
Therapeutic: urinary tract antispasmodics
Pharmacologic: anticholinergics

Pregnancy Category B

Indications
Urinary symptoms that may be associated with neurogenic bladder including: Frequent urination, Urgency, Nocturia, Urge incontinence. Overactive bladder with symptoms of urge incontinence, urgency, and frequency.

Action
Inhibits the action of acetylcholine at postganglionic receptors. Has direct spasmolytic action on smooth muscle, including smooth muscle lining the GU tract, without affecting vascular smooth muscle. **Therapeutic Effects:** Increased bladder capacity. Delayed desire to void. Decreased urge incontinence, urinary urgency, and frequency and decreased number of urinary accidents associated with overactive bladder.

Pharmacokinetics
Absorption: Rapidly absorbed following oral administration, but undergoes extensive first-pass metabolism; XL tablets provide extended release. Transdermal absorption occurs by passive diffusion through intact skin and bypasses the first-pass effect.
Distribution: Widely distributed.
Metabolism and Excretion: Extensively metabolized by the liver (CYP3A4 enzyme system);

one metabolite is pharmacologically active; metabolites are renally excreted with negligible (<0.1%) excretion of unchanged drug.
Half-life: 7–8 hr.

TIME/ACTION PROFILE (urinary spasmolytic effect)

ROUTE	ONSET	PEAK	DURATION
PO	30–60 min	3–6 hr	6–10 hr (up to 24 hr with XL tablet)
Transdermal	within 24 hr	36 hr	3–4 days

Contraindications/Precautions

Contraindicated in: Hypersensitivity; Uncontrolled angle-closure glaucoma; Intestinal obstruction or atony; Urinary retention.
Use Cautiously in: Hepatic/renal impairment; Bladder outflow obstruction; Ulcerative colitis; Benign prostatic hyperplasia; Cardiovascular disease; Reflux esophagitis or gastrointestinal osbstructive disorders; Myasthenia gravis; OB: Pregnancy and lactation (safety not established); Geri: Appears on Beers list. Poorly tolerated due to anticholinergic effects; Pedi: Pregnancy or children <5 yr (safety not established).

Adverse Reactions/Side Effects

CNS: dizziness, drowsiness, headache. **EENT:** blurred vision. **CV:** tachycardia. **GI:** constipation, dry mouth, nausea, abdominal pain, diarrhea. **GU:** urinary retention. **Derm:** decreased sweating, *transdermal only:* application site reactions. **Metab:** hyperthermia.

Interactions

Drug-Drug: ↑ anticholinergic effects with other **agents having anticholinergic properties**, including **amantadine**, **antidepressants**, **phenothiazines**, **disopyramide**, and **haloperidol**. Additive CNS depression with other **CNS depressants**, including **alcohol**, **antihistamines**, **antidepressants**, **opioids**, and **sedative/hypnotics**. **Ketoconazole**, **itraconazole**, **erythromycin**, and **clarithromycin** may ↑ effects.

Route/Dosage

PO (Adults): *Immediate-release tablets*—5 mg 2–3 times daily (not to exceed 5 mg 4 times daily) (may start with 2.5 mg 2–3 times daily in elderly). *Extended-release tablets*—5–10 mg once daily; may ↑, as needed, (in 5-mg increments) up to maximum dose of 30 mg/day.
PO (Children >5 yr): *Immediate-release tablets*—5 mg 2–3 times daily (not to exceed 15 mg/day). *Extended-release tablets (children ≥6 yr)*—5 mg once daily; may ↑, as needed, (in 5-mg increments) up to maximum dose of 20 mg/day.
Transdermal (Adults): One 3.9-mg system applied twice week-ly (every 3–4 days).

Availability (generic available)

Tablets: 5 mg. **Cost:** *Generic*—$29.97/180. **Extended-release tablets:** 5 mg, 10 mg, 15 mg. **Cost:** *Generic*—5 mg $260.98/90, 10 mg $262.80/90, 15 mg $269.99/90. **Syrup:** 5 mg/5 ml. **Cost:** *Generic*—$35.95/480 ml. **Transdermal system:** 3.9-mg/day system. **Cost:** $106.50/8 patches.

NURSING IMPLICATIONS

Assessment

- Monitor voiding pattern and intake and output ratios, and assess abdomen for bladder distention prior to and periodically during therapy. Catheterization may be used to assess postvoid residual. Cystometry, to diagnose type of bladder dysfunction, is usually performed prior to prescription of oxybutynin.
- Geri: Assess geriatric patients for anticholinergic effects (sedation and weakness).

Potential Nursing Diagnoses

Impaired urinary elimination (Indications)
Acute pain (Indications)

Implementation

- Do not confuse Ditropan (oxybutynin) with diazepam.
- **PO:** May be administered on an empty stomach or with meals or milk to prevent gastric irritation.
- **Transdermal:** Apply patch on same two days each week (Sunday/Wednesday, Monday/Thursday) to hip, abdomen, or buttock in an area that is clean, dry, and without irritation. Patch should be worn continuously.

Patient/Family Teaching

- Instruct patient to take oxybutinin as directed. Take missed doses as soon as remembered unless almost time for next dose.
- May cause drowsiness or blurred vision. Advise patient to avoid driving and other activi-

O

✤ = Canadian drug name.
*CAPITALS indicates life-threatening; underlines indicate most frequent.

ties requiring alertness until response to medication is known.
- Advise patient to avoid concurrent use of alcohol and other CNS depressants while taking this medication.
- Instruct patient that frequent rinsing of mouth, good oral hygiene, and sugarless gum or candy may decrease dry mouth. Health care professional should be notified if mouth dryness persists >2 wk.
- Inform patient that oxybutynin decreases the body's ability to perspire. Avoid strenuous activity in a warm environment because overheating may occur.
- Advise patient to notify health care professional if urinary retention occurs or if constipation persists. Discuss methods of preventing constipation, such as increasing dietary bulk, increasing fluid intake, and increasing mobility.
- Discuss need for continued medical follow-up. Periodic cystometry may be used to evaluate effectiveness. Ophthalmic exams should be performed periodically to detect glaucoma, especially in patients over 40 yr of age.
- **Transdermal:** Instruct patient on correct application and disposal of patch. Open pouch by tearing along arrows; apply immediately. Apply ½ patch to skin by removing ½ protective cover and applying firmly to skin. Apply second half by bending in half and rolling patch onto skin while removing protective liner. Press patch firmly in place.
- Remove slowly; fold in half, sticky sides together, and discard. Wash site with mild soap and water or a small amount of baby oil.

Evaluation/Desired Outcomes
- Relief of bladder spasm and associated symptoms (frequency, urgency, nocturia, and incontinence) in patients with a neurogenic or overactive bladder.

HIGH ALERT

oxycodone (ox-i-**koe**-done)
Endocodone, M-Oxy, Oxycontin, OxyFAST, OxyIR, Percolone, Roxicodone, ✤Supeudol

oxycodone/acetaminophen†
Endocet, Magnacet, Oxycet, Percocet, Roxicet, Roxilox, Tylox

oxycodone/aspirin†
Endodan, ✤Oxycodan, Percodan

Classification
Therapeutic: opioid analgesics
Pharmacologic: opioid agonists, opioid agonists/nonopioid analgesic combinations

Schedule II

Pregnancy Category C (oxycodone alone)

†See also acetaminophen and salicylates monographs

Indications
Moderate to severe pain.

Action
Binds to opiate receptors in the CNS. Alters the perception of and response to painful stimuli, while producing generalized CNS depression. **Therapeutic Effects:** Decreased pain.

Pharmacokinetics
Absorption: Well absorbed from the GI tract.
Distribution: Widely distributed. Crosses the placenta; enters breast milk.
Metabolism and Excretion: Mostly metabolized by the liver.
Half-life: 2–3 hr.

TIME/ACTION PROFILE (analgesic effects)

ROUTE	ONSET	PEAK	DURATION
PO	10–15 min	60–90 min	3–6 hr
PO-CR	10–15 min	3 hr	12 hr

Contraindications/Precautions
Contraindicated in: Hypersensitivity; Pregnancy or lactation (avoid chronic use); Some products contain alcohol or bisulfites and should be avoided in patients with known intolerance or hypersensitivity.
Use Cautiously in: Head trauma; Increased intracranial pressure; Severe renal, hepatic, or pulmonary disease; Hypothyroidism; Adrenal insufficiency; Alcoholism; Geriatric or debilitated patients (initial dosage reduction recommended); Undiagnosed abdominal pain; Prostatic hyperplasia.

Adverse Reactions/Side Effects
CNS: confusion, sedation, dizziness, dysphoria, euphoria, floating feeling, hallucinations, headache, unusual dreams. **EENT:** blurred vision, diplopia, miosis. **Resp:** RESPIRATORY DEPRESSION. **CV:** orthostatic hypotension. **GI:** constipation, dry mouth, nausea, vomiting. **GU:** urinary retention. **Derm:** flushing, sweating. **Misc:** physical

dependence, psychological dependence, tolerance.

Interactions

Drug-Drug: Use with caution in patients receiving **MAO inhibitors** (may result in unpredictable reactions—decrease initial dose of oxycodone to 25% of usual dose). ↑ CNS depression with **alcohol**, **antihistamines**, and **sedative/hypnotics**. Administration of **partial-antagonist opioid analgesics** may precipitate withdrawal in physically dependent patients. **Nalbuphine**, **buprenorphine**, or **pentazocine** may decrease analgesia.
Drug-Natural Products: Concomitant use of **kava kava**, **valerian**, or **chamomile** can ↑ CNS depression.

Route/Dosage

Larger doses may be required during chronic therapy. Consider cumulative effects of additional acetaminophen/aspirin; if toxic levels are exceeded, change to pure oxycodone product.
PO (Adults ≥50 kg): 5–10 mg q 3–4 hr initially, as needed. Controlled-release tablets (Oxycontin) may be given q 12 hr after careful consideration as to dose, indication, and previous analgesic use/abuse history.
PO (Adults <50 kg or Children 6–12 years): 1.25 mg every 6 hr as needed or 0.2 mg/kg q 3–4 hr initially, as needed.
PO (Children >12): 2.5 mg every 6 hr as needed.
Rect (Adults): 10–40 mg 3–4 times daily initially, as needed.

Availability (generic available)

Oxycodone

Tablets (Percolone, Roxicodone): 5 mg, 15 mg, 30 mg. **Cost:** *Generic*—5 mg $24.99/30, 15 mg $26.99/30, 30 mg $36.99/30. **Immediate-release capsules (OxyIR):** 5 mg. **Cost:** *Generic*—$13.99/30. **Controlled-release tablets (Oxycontin):** 10 mg, 20 mg, 40 mg, 80 mg. **Cost:** *Generic*—10 mg $43.99/30, 20 mg $79.99/30, 40 mg $139.99/30, 80 mg $250.01/30. **Oral solution (Roxicodone) (burgundy cherry):** 5 mg/5 ml in 500-ml bottle. **Concentrated oral solution (Roxicodone Intensol, OxyFAST):** 20 mg/ml in 30-ml bottle with dropper. **Cost:** *Generic*—$33.99/30 ml. **Suppositories:** ✤10 mg, ✤20 mg.

Oxycodone/Acetaminophen

Tablets (Endocet, Oxycet, Percocet, Roxicet): 2.5 mg oxycodone with 325 mg acetaminophen, 2.5 mg oxycodone with 400 mg acetaminophen (Magnacet), 5 mg oxycodone with 325 mg acetaminophen, 5 mg oxycodone with 400 mg acetaminophen (Magnacet), 7.5 mg oxycodone with 325 mg acetaminophen (Percocet 7.5/325), 7.5 mg oxycodone with 400 mg acetaminophen (Magnacet), 7.5 mg oxycodone with 500 mg acetaminophen, 10 mg oxycodone with 325 mg acetaminophen, 10 mg oxycodone with 400 mg acetaminophen (Magnacet), 10 mg oxycodone with 650 mg acetaminophen. **Cost:** *Generic*—5/325 mg $16.99/30, 7.5/325 mg $47.99/30, 10/325 mg $60.99/30, 10/650 mg $49.99/30. **Capsules (Roxilox, Tylox):** 5 mg oxycodone with 500 mg acetaminophen. **Cost:** *Generic*—$23.99/30. **Caplets (Roxicet 5/500):** 5 mg oxycodone with 500 mg acetaminophen. **Oral solution (Roxicet) (mint):** 5 mg oxycodone with 325 mg acetaminophen/5 ml in 500-ml bottles. **Cost:** $43.43/500 ml.

Oxycodone/Aspirin

Tablets (Endodan, Percodan): 4.88 mg oxycodone with 325 mg aspirin).

NURSING IMPLICATIONS

Assessment

- Assess type, location, and intensity of pain prior to and 1 hr (peak) after administration. When titrating opioid doses, increases of 25–50% should be administered until there is either a 50% reduction in the patient's pain rating on a numerical or visual analogue scale or the patient reports satisfactory pain relief. A repeat dose can be safely administered at the time of the peak if previous dose is ineffective and side effects are minimal.
- Patients taking controlled-release tablets may require additional short-acting opioid doses for breakthrough pain. Doses should be equivalent to 10–20% of 24 hr total and given every 2 hr as needed.
- An equianalgesic chart (see Appendix J) should be used when changing routes or when changing from one opioid to another.
- Assess blood pressure, pulse, and respirations before and periodically during administration. If respiratory rate is <10/min, assess level of sedation. Physical stimulation may be

sufficient to prevent significant hypoventilation. Dose may need to be decreased by 25–50%. Initial drowsiness will diminish with continued use.

- Prolonged use may lead to physical and psychological dependence and tolerance. This should not prevent patient from receiving adequate analgesia. Most patients who receive oxycodone for pain do not develop psychological dependence. Progressively higher doses may be required to relieve pain with long-term therapy.
- Assess bowel function routinely. Prevention of constipation should be instituted with increased intake of fluids and bulk, and laxatives to minimize constipating effects. Stimulant laxatives should be administered routinely if opioid use exceeds 2–3 days, unless contraindicated.
- ***Lab Test Considerations:*** May ↑ plasma amylase and lipase levels.
- ***Toxicity and Overdose:*** If an opioid antagonist is required to reverse respiratory depression or coma, naloxone (Narcan) is the antidote. Dilute the 0.4-mg ampule of naloxone in 10 ml of 0.9% NaCl and administer 0.5 ml (0.02 mg) by direct IV push every 2 min. For children and patients weighing <40 kg, dilute 0.1 mg of naloxone in 10 ml of 0.9% NaCl for a concentration of 10 mcg/ml and administer 0.5 mcg/kg every 2 min. Titrate dose to avoid withdrawal, seizures, and severe pain.

Potential Nursing Diagnosis

Acute pain (Indications)
Disturbed sensory perception (visual, auditory) (Side Effects)
Risk for injury (Side Effects)

Implementation

- ***High Alert:*** Accidental overdosage of opioid analgesics has resulted in fatalities. Before administering, clarify all ambiguous orders; have second practitioner independently check original order and dose calculations. Do not confuse oxycodone with OxyContin. Do not confuse Percocet with Percodan.
- Regularly administered doses may be more effective than prn administration. Analgesic is more effective if given before pain becomes severe.
- Coadministration with nonopioid analgesics may have additive analgesic effects and may permit lower doses. Medication should be discontinued gradually after long-term use to prevent withdrawal symptoms.
- **PO:** May be administered with food or milk to minimize GI irritation.
- Administer solution with properly calibrated measuring device.
- Controlled-release tablets should be swallowed whole; do not crush, break, or chew. Taking broken, chewed, or crushed controlled-release tablets leads to rapid release and absorption of a potentially fatal dose of oxycodone.
- **Controlled Release:** Dose should be based on 24-hr opioid requirement determined with short-acting opioids then converted to controlled-release form.

Patient/Family Teaching

- Instruct patient on how and when to ask for pain medication. Caution patient not to increase the dose of controlled-release oxycodone without consulting health care professional.
- Caution patient that controlled-release oxycodone is a potential drug of abuse. Medication should be protected from theft and never given to anyone other than the individual for whom it was prescribed.
- Medication may cause drowsiness or dizziness. Advise patient to call for assistance when ambulating or smoking. Caution patient to avoid driving and other activities requiring alertness until response to medication is known.
- Advise patients taking Oxycontin tablets that empty matrix tablets may appear in stool.
- Advise patient to make position changes slowly to minimize orthostatic hypotension.
- Advise patient to avoid concurrent use of alcohol or other CNS depressants with this medication.
- Encourage patient to turn, cough, and breathe deeply every 2 hr to prevent atelectasis.

Evaluation/Desired Outcomes

- Decrease in severity of pain without a significant alteration in level of consciousness or respiratory status.

HIGH ALERT

oxymorphone (ox-i-**mor**-fone)
Opana, Opana ER

Classification
Therapeutic: opioid analgesics
Pharmacologic: opioid agonists

Schedule II

Pregnancy Category UK

Indications
Management of moderate to severe pain. Extended-release tablets should only be used in patients who require continuous 24-hr management of chronic pain. Supplement in balanced anesthesia.

Action
Binds to opiate receptors in the CNS. Alters the perception of and response to painful stimuli, while producing generalized CNS depression.
Therapeutic Effects: Decrease in pain.

Pharmacokinetics
Absorption: 10% absorbed following oral administration. Food and alcohol significantly ↑ absorption (38%). Well absorbed following IM, subcut, or rectal administration.
Distribution: Widely distributed; crosses placenta, enters breast milk.
Metabolism and Excretion: Mostly metabolized by the liver; at least 2 metabolites are pharmacologically active, <1% excreted unchanged in urine.
Half-life: 2.6–4 hr.

TIME/ACTION PROFILE (analgesic effects)

ROUTE	ONSET	PEAK	DURATION
PO	unknown	unknown	4–6 hr
PO ER	unknown	unknown	12 hr
IM	10–15 min	30–90 min	3–6 hr
IV	5–10 min	15–30 min	3–6 hr
Subcut	10–20 min	unknown	3–4 hr

Contraindications/Precautions
Contraindicated in: Hypersensitivity; Concurrent alcohol; Moderate/severe hepatic impairment; Respiratory depression (unless monitoring and resuscitative equipment are readily available); Known/suspected paralytic ileus.
Use Cautiously in: Acute alcoholism or delirium tremens or other toxic psychoses; Mild hepatic impairment; Head injury/increased intracranial pressure (may obscure neurologic signs and further increase pressure); Volume depletion or drugs that may cause hypotension including diuretics and phenothiazines (may increase the risk of severe hypotension); Geri: Blood levels are ↑, dose accordingly; Circulatory shock (may increase the risk of severe hypotension); Adrenocortical insufficiency; Hypothyroidism; Prostatic hypertrophy or ureteral stricture; Severe pulmonary or renal impairment; Biliary tract disease or pancreatitis; OB: Use only in pregnancy if maternal benefit outweighs fetal risk; may enter breast milk and increase the risk of sedation/respiratory depression in infant.
Exercise Extreme Caution in: Conditions association with hypoxia, hypercapnea, decreased respiratory reserve (including asthma, COPD, cor pulmonale, morbid obesity, sleep apnea, myxedema, kyphoscoliosis, CNS depression, and coma).

Adverse Reactions/Side Effects
CNS: <u>confusion</u>, <u>sedation</u>, dizziness, dysphoria, euphoria, floating feeling, hallucinations, headache, unusual dreams. **EENT:** blurred vision, diplopia, miosis. **Resp:** RESPIRATORY DEPRESSION. **CV:** orthostatic hypotension. **GI:** <u>constipation</u>, dry mouth, nausea, vomiting. **GU:** urinary retention. **Derm:** flushing, sweating. **Misc:** physical dependence, psychological dependence, tolerance.

Interactions
Drug-Drug: Use with caution in patients receiving **MAO inhibitors** (may result in unpredictable reactions—decrease initial dose of oxymorphone to 25% of usual dose). ↑ risk of CNS depression, hypotension and respiratory depression with **alcohol**, other **opioids** or **CNS depressants** including **sedatives**, **hypnotics**, **general anesthetics**, **phenothiazines**, **tranquilizers**, **skeletal muscle relaxants** or **sedating antihistamines**; may initiate therapy with 1/2 to 1/2 usual starting dose. **Drugs that may cause volume depletion or hypotension** including **diuretics** and **phenothiazines** may ↑ risk of severe hypotension. Administration of **partial-antagonist opioid analgesics** may precipitate withdrawal in physically dependent patients. **Nalbuphine**,

buprenorphine, or **pentazocine** ↓ analgesia.
Drug-Natural Products: Concomitant use of **kava kava**, **valerian**, or **chamomile** can ↑ CNS depression.

Route/Dosage

Larger doses may be required during chronic therapy.
PO (Adults): *Opioid-naive patients*—10–20 mg every 4–6 hr, some patients may require initial dose of 5 mg, not to exceed 20 mg. Once optimal analgesia is obtained, chronic pain patients may be converted to an equivalent 24-hour dose given as extended release tablets every 12 hr.
Subcut, IM (Adults): 1–1.5 mg q 3–6 hr as needed. *Analgesia during labor*—0.5–1 mg.
IV (Adults): 0.5 mg q 3–6 hr as needed; increase as needed.

Availability

Tablets (Opana): 5 mg, 10 mg. **Extended-release tablets (Opana ER):** 5 mg, 10 mg, 20 mg, 40 mg. **Injection:** 1 mg/ml in 1-ml ampules, 1.5 mg/ml in 1-ml ampules and 10-ml vials.

NURSING IMPLICATIONS

Assessment

- Assess type, location, and intensity of pain prior to and 1 hr following IM and 15–30 min (peak) following IV administration. When titrating opioid doses, increases of 25–50% should be administered until there is either a 50% reduction in the patient's pain rating on a numerical or visual analogue scale or the patient reports satisfactory pain relief. A repeat dose can be safely administered at the time of the peak if previous dose is ineffective and side effects are minimal.
- Patients taking controlled-release tablets should also be given supplemental short-acting opioid doses for breakthrough pain.
- An equianalgesic chart (see Appendix J) should be used when changing routes or when changing from one opioid to another.
- Assess blood pressure, pulse, and respirations before and periodically during administration. If respiratory rate is <10/min, assess level of sedation. Physical stimulation may be sufficient to prevent significant hypoventilation. Dose may need to be decreased by 25–50%. Initial drowsiness will diminish with continued use.
- Prolonged use may lead to physical and psychological dependence and tolerance. This should not prevent patient from receiving adequate analgesia. Most patients who receive oxymorphone for pain do not develop psychological dependence. Progressively higher doses may be required to relieve pain with long-term therapy.
- Assess bowel function routinely. Prevention of constipation should be instituted with increased intake of fluids and bulk, and laxatives. Stimulant laxatives should be administered routinely if opioid use exceeds 2–3 days, unless contraindicated.
- ***Lab Test Considerations:*** May ↑ plasma amylase and lipase levels.
- ***Toxicity and Overdose:*** If an opioid antagonist is required to reverse respiratory depression or coma, naloxone (Narcan) is the antidote. Dilute the 0.4-mg ampule of naloxone in 10 ml of 0.9% NaCl and administer 0.5 ml (0.02 mg) by direct IV push every 2 min. For children and patients weighing <40 kg, dilute 0.1 mg of naloxone in 10 ml of 0.9% NaCl for a concentration of 10 mcg/ml and administer 0.5 mcg/kg every 2 min. Titrate dose to avoid withdrawal, seizures, and severe pain.

Potential Nursing Diagnoses

Acute pain (Indications)
Disturbed sensory perception (visual, auditory) (Side Effects)
Risk for injury (Side Effects)

Implementation

- ***High Alert:*** Accidental overdose of opioid analgesics has resulted in fatalities. Before administering, clarify all ambiguous orders; have second practitioner independently check original order, dose calculations, and infusion pump settings.
- Explain therapeutic value of medication prior to administration to enhance the analgesic effect.
- Regularly administered doses may be more effective than prn administration. Analgesic is more effective if given before pain becomes severe.
- Coadministration with nonopioid analgesics may have additive analgesic effects and may permit lower doses.
- Medication should be discontinued gradually after long-term use to prevent withdrawal symptoms.

- **PO:** Administer at least 1 hr prior to or 2 hrs after eating.
- Controlled-release tablets should be swallowed whole; do not crush, break, or chew.
- **Controlled Release:** Patients should be titrated to mild to no pain with the regular use of no more than 2 doses of supplemental analgesia (rescue) per 24 hrs. Dose should be based on 24-hr opioid requirement determined with short-acting opioids then converted to controlled-release form.
- If patient is opioid-naive, start with 5 mg every 12 hrs, then titrate in increments of 5–10 mg every 12 hrs every 3–7 days to a level that provides adequate analgesia with minimal side effects.
- If converting from *Opana* to *Opana ER*, administer half the patient's total daily dose of *Opana* as *Opana ER* every 12 hrs.
- If converting from parenteral oxymorphone, administer 10 times the patient's total daily parenteral oxymorphone dose as *Opana ER* in two equally divided doses every 12 hrs.
- If converting from other opioids, 10 mg of oral oxymorphone is equianalgesic to hydrocodone 20 mg, oxycodone 20 mg, methadone 20 mg, and morphine 30 mg orally.

IV Administration

- **Direct IV:** Administer undiluted. ***Concentration:*** 1–1.5 mg/ml. ***Rate:*** Give over 2–3 min.
- **Syringe Compatibility:** glycopyrrolate, hydroxyzine, ranitidine.

Patient/Family Teaching

- Instruct patient on how and when to ask for pain medication.
- Instruct patient to take oxymorphone as directed and not to adjust dose without consulting health care professional. Take missed doses as soon as possible. If almost time for next dose, skip dose and return to regular schedule. Do not double doses unless advised by health care professional. Do not stop taking oxymorphone abruptly, may cause withdrawal symptoms. Discontinue gradually under supervision of health care professional. Caution patient to keep medication out of reach of children and pets.
- Caution patient not to share this medication; may cause harm or death and is against the law.
- Medication may cause drowsiness or dizziness. Advise patient to call for assistance when ambulating or smoking. Caution patient to avoid driving and other activities requiring alertness until response to medication is known.
- Advise patient to make position changes slowly to minimize orthostatic hypotension.
- Advise patient to avoid concurrent use of alcohol or other CNS depressants with this medication.
- Caution patient not to take any new Rx, OTC, or herbal products without notifying health care professional.
- Encourage patient to turn, cough, and breathe deeply every 2 hr to prevent atelectasis.
- OB: Advise patient to notify health care professional if pregnancy is planned or suspected.

Evaluation/Desired Outcomes

- Decrease in severity of pain without a significant alteration in level of consciousness or respiratory status.

oxytocin (ox-i-**toe**-sin)

Pitocin, Syntocinon

Classification

Therapeutic: hormones

Pharmacologic: oxytocics

Pregnancy Category X (intranasal), UK (IV, IM)

Indications

IV: Induction of labor at term. Facilitation of uterine contractions at term. Facilitation of threatened abortion. Postpartum control of bleeding after expulsion of the placenta. **Intranasal:** Used to promote milk letdown in lactating women. **Unlabeled uses:** Evaluation of fetal competence (fetal stress test).

Action

Stimulates uterine smooth muscle, producing uterine contractions similar to those in spontaneous labor. Stimulates mammary gland smooth muscle, facilitating lactation. Has vasopressor and antidiuretic effects. **Therapeutic Effects:** Induction of labor (IV). Milk letdown (intranasal).

Pharmacokinetics

Absorption: Well absorbed from the nasal mucosa.
Distribution: Widely distributed in extracellular fluid. Small amounts reach fetal circulation.
Metabolism and Excretion: Rapidly metabolized by liver and kidneys.
Half-life: 3–9 min.

TIME/ACTION PROFILE (IV = uterine contractions; intranasal = milk letdown)

ROUTE	ONSET	PEAK	DURATION
IV	immediate	unknown	1 hr
IM	3–5 min	unknown	30–60 min
Intranasal	few min	unknown	20 min

Contraindications/Precautions

Contraindicated in: Hypersensitivity; Anticipated nonvaginal delivery; Pregnancy (intranasal).
Use Cautiously in: First and second stages of labor.

Adverse Reactions/Side Effects

Maternal adverse reactions are noted for IV use only.

CNS: *maternal*— COMA, SEIZURES; *fetal*—INTRACRANIAL HEMORRHAGE. **Resp:** *fetal*—ASPHYXIA, hypoxia. **CV:** *maternal*—hypotension; *fetal*—arrhythmias. **F and E:** *maternal*—hypochloremia, hyponatremia, water intoxication. **Misc:** *maternal*— increased uterine motility, painful contractions, abruptio placentae, decreased uterine blood flow, hypersensitivity.

Interactions

Drug-Drug: Severe hypertension may occur if oxytocin follows administration of **vasopressors**. Concurrent use with **cyclopropane** anesthesia may result in excessive hypotension.

Route/Dosage

Induction/Stimulation of Labor

IV (Adults): 0.5–2 milliunits/min; increase by 1–2 milliunits/min q 15–60 min until pattern established (usually 5–6 milliunits/min; maximum 20 milliunits/min), then decrease dose.

Postpartum Hemorrhage

IV (Adults): 10 units infused at 20–40 milliunits/min.
IM (Adults): 10 units after delivery of placenta.

Incomplete/Inevitable Abortion

IV (Adults): 10 units at a rate of 20–40 milliunits/min.

Promotion of Milk Letdown

Intranasal (Adults): 1 spray in 1 or both nostrils 2–3 min before breastfeeding or pumping breasts.

Fetal Stress Test

IV (Adults): 0.5 milliunits/min; may be doubled q 20 min until 3 moderate contractions occur in one 10-min period (usually 5–6 milliunits/min) to a maximum of 20 milliunits/min with maternal/fetal monitoring.

Availability (generic available)

Solution for injection: 10 units/ml in 0.5- and 1-ml ampules, 1-ml prefilled syringes, 1- and 10-ml vials. **Nasal spray:** 40 units/ml in 2- and 5-ml containers.

NURSING IMPLICATIONS

Assessment

- Fetal maturity, presentation, and pelvic adequacy should be assessed prior to administration of oxytocin for induction of labor.
- Assess character, frequency, and duration of uterine contractions; resting uterine tone; and fetal heart rate frequently throughout administration. If contractions occur <2 min apart and are >50–65 mm Hg on monitor, if they last 60–90 sec or longer, or if a significant change in fetal heart rate develops, stop infusion and turn patient on her left side to prevent fetal anoxia. Notify health care professional immediately.
- Monitor maternal blood pressure and pulse frequently and fetal heart rate continuously throughout administration.
- This drug occasionally causes water intoxication. Monitor patient for signs and symptoms (drowsiness, listlessness, confusion, headache, anuria) and notify physician or other health care professional if they occur.
- ***Lab Test Considerations:*** Monitor maternal electrolytes. Water retention may result in hypochloremia or hyponatremia.

Potential Nursing Diagnoses

Deficient knowledge, related to medication regimen (Patient/Family Teaching)

Implementation

- Do not confuse Pitocin (oxytocin) with Pitressin (vasopressin).
- Do not administer oxytocin simultaneously by more than one route.

IV Administration

- **Continuous Infusion:** Rotate infusion container to ensure thorough mixing. Store solution in refrigerator, but do not freeze.
- Infuse via infusion pump for accurate dose. Oxytocin should be connected via Y-site injection to an IV of 0.9% NaCl for use during adverse reactions.
- Magnesium sulfate should be available if needed for relaxation of the myometrium.
- **Induction of Labor:** ***Diluent:*** Dilute 1 ml (10 units) in 1 L of compatible infusion fluid (0.9% NaCl, D5W, or LR). ***Concentration:*** 10 milliunits/ml. ***Rate:*** Begin infusion at 0.5–2 milliunits/min (0.05–0.2 ml); increase in increments of 1–2 milliunits/min at 15–30-min intervals until contractions simulate normal labor.
- **Postpartum Bleeding:** ***Diluent:*** For control of postpartum bleeding, dilute 1–4 ml (10–40 units) in 1 L of compatible infusion fluid. ***Concentration:*** 10–40 milliunits/ml. ***Rate:*** Begin infusion at a rate of 20–40 milliunits/min to control uterine atony. Adjust rate as indicated.
- **Incomplete or Inevitable Abortion:** ***Diluent:*** For incomplete or inevitable abortion, dilute 1 ml (10 units) in 500 ml of 0.9% NaCl or D5W. ***Concentration:*** 20 milliunits/ml. ***Rate:*** Infuse at a rate of 20–40 milliunits/min.
- **Y-Site Compatibility:** heparin, hydrocortisone sodium succinate, insulin, meperidine, morphine, potassium chloride, vitamin B complex with C, warfarin, zidovudine.
- **Solution Compatibility:** dextrose/Ringer's or lactated Ringer's combinations, dextrose/saline combinations, Ringer's or lactated Ringer's injection, D5W, D10W, 0.45% NaCl, 0.9% NaCl.
- **Intranasal:** Hold squeeze bottle upright while patient is in sitting position. Patient should clear nasal passages prior to administration.

Patient/Family Teaching

- Advise patient to expect contractions similar to menstrual cramps after administration has started.
- **Nasal Spray:** Advise patient to administer nasal spray 2–3 min prior to planned breastfeeding. Patient should notify health care professional if milk drips from non-nursed breast or if uterine cramps occur.

Evaluation/Desired Outcomes

- Onset of effective contractions.
- Increase in uterine tone.
- Effective letdown reflex.

O

paclitaxel (pak-li-tax-el)
Onxol, Taxol

paclitaxel protein-bound particles (albumin-bound)
Abraxane

Classification
Therapeutic: antineoplastics
Pharmacologic: taxoids

Pregnancy Category D

Indications
Paclitaxel: Advanced ovarian cancer (with cisplatin). Non-small cell lung cancer when potentially curative surgery and/or radiation therapy is not an option. Metastatic breast cancer unresponsive to other therapy. Node-positive breast cancer when administered sequentially to standard combination chemotherapy that includes doxorubicin. Treatment of AIDS-related Kaposi's sarcoma. **Paclitaxel (albumin-bound):** Metastatic breast cancer after treatment failure or relapse where therapy included an anthracycline.

Action
Interferes with the normal cellular microtubule function that is required for interphase and mitosis. **Therapeutic Effects:** Death of rapidly replicating cells, particularly malignant ones.

Pharmacokinetics
Absorption: IV administration results in complete bioavailability.
Distribution: Cross the placenta.
Protein Binding: 89–98%.
Metabolism and Excretion: Highly metabolized by the liver, <10% excreted unchanged in urine.
Half-life: *Paclitaxel*—13–52 hr; *Paclitaxel protein-bound particles (albumin-bound)* 27 hr.

TIME/ACTION PROFILE (effect on WBCs)

ROUTE	ONSET	PEAK	DURATION
IV	unknown	11 days	3 wk

Contraindications/Precautions
Contraindicated in: Hypersensitivity to paclitaxel or to castor oil (non-protein-bound vehicle contains polyoxyethylated castor oil); Known alcohol intolerance; OB: Pregnancy or lactation; ANC ≤1500/mm^3 in patients with ovarian, lung, or breast cancer; ANC ≤1000/mm^3 in patients with AIDS-related Kaposi's sarcoma.
Use Cautiously in: Severe hepatic impairment; Geri: ↑ risk of neuropathy, myelosuppression, and cardiovascular events; OB: Childbearing potential; Active infection; Decreased bone marrow reserve; Pedi: Children (safety and effectiveness not established).

Adverse Reactions/Side Effects
CV: ECG changes, hypotension, hypotension, bradycardia. **GI:** abnormal liver function tests, diarrhea, mucositis, nausea, vomiting. **Derm:** alopecia. **Hemat:** anemia, neutropenia, thrombocytopenia. **MS:** arthralgia, myalgia. **Neuro:** peripheral neuropathy. **Resp:** cough, dyspnea. **Local:** injection site reactions. **Misc:** hypersensitivity reactions including ANAPHYLAXIS and STEVENS-JOHNSON SYNDROME, TOXIC EPIDERMAL NECROLYSIS.

Interactions
Drug-Drug: Ketoconazole, verapamil, quinidine, cyclosporine, diazepam, dexamethasone, teniposide, etoposide, or vincristine may ↓ metabolism and ↑ risk of serious toxicity; concurrent use should be undertaken with caution. ↑ risk of myelosuppression with other **antineoplastics** or **radiation therapy**. Myelosuppression ↑ when given after **cisplatin**. May ↑ levels and toxicity of **doxorubicin**. May ↓ antibody response to and ↑ risk of adverse reactions from **live-virus vaccines**.

Route/Dosage
Many other regimens are used.

PACLITAXEL
Ovarian Cancer
IV (Adults): *Previously untreated patients*—175 mg/m^2 over 3 hr every 3 wk, or 135 mg/m^2 over 24 hr every 3 wk, followed by cisplatin; *Previously treated patients*—135 mg/m^2 or 175 mg/m^2 over 3 hr every 3 wk.

Breast Cancer
IV (Adults): *Adjuvant treatment of node-positive breast cancer*—175 mg/m^2 over 3 hr every 3 wk for 4 courses administered sequentially to doxorubicin-containing combination chemotherapy; *Failure of initial therapy for metastatic disease or relapse within 6 mo of adjuvant therapy*—175 mg/m^2 over 3 hr every 3 wk.

Non-Small Cell Lung Cancer

IV (Adults): 135 mg/m² over 24 hr every 3 wk, followed by cisplatin.

AIDS-Related Kaposi's Sarcoma

IV (Adults): 135 mg/m² over 3 hr every 3 wk or 100 mg/m² over 3 hr every 2 wk (dose reduction/adjustment may be necessary in patients with advanced HIV infection).

PACLITAXEL PROTEIN-BOUND PARTICLES (albumin-bound)

IV (Adults): 260 mg/m² over 30 min every 3 wk.

Availability

Paclitaxel

Solution for injection: 6 mg/ml in 5-ml, 16.7-ml, 25-ml, and 50-ml vials.

Paclitaxel protein-bound particles (albumin-bound)

Powder for injection: 100 mg/vial.

NURSING IMPLICATIONS

Assessment

- Monitor vital signs frequently, especially during first hr of the infusion.
- Monitor cardiovascular status especially during first 3 hr of infusion. Hypotension and bradycardia are common but usually do not require treatment. Continuous ECG monitoring is recommended only for patients with serious underlying conduction abnormalities.
- Monitor for bone marrow depression. Assess for bleeding (bleeding gums, bruising, petechiae, guaiac stools, urine, and emesis) and avoid IM injections and taking rectal temperatures if platelet count is low. Apply pressure to venipuncture sites for 10 min. Assess for signs of infection during neutropenia. Anemia may occur. Monitor for increased fatigue, dyspnea, and orthostatic hypotension. Granulocyte-colony stimulating factor (G-CSF) may be used if necessary.
- Assess for development of peripheral neuropathy. If severe symptoms occur, subsequent dose should be reduced by 20%.
- Monitor intake and output, appetite, and nutritional intake. Paclitaxel causes nausea and vomiting in 50% of patients. Prophylactic antiemetics may be used. Adjust diet as tolerated to help maintain fluid and electrolyte balance and nutritional status.
- Assess patient for arthralgia and myalgia, which usually begin 2–3 days after therapy and resolve within 5 days. Pain is usually relieved by nonopioid analgesics but may be severe enough to require treatment with opioid analgesics.
- **Paclitaxel:** Monitor for hypersensitivity reactions continuously during the first 30 min and frequently thereafter. These occur frequently (19%), usually during the first 10 min of paclitaxel infusion, after the first or second dose. Pretreatment is recommended for **all** patients and should include dexamethasone 20 mg PO (10 mg for patients with advanced HIV disease) 12 and 6 hours prior to paclitaxel, diphenhydramine 50 mg IV 30–60 min prior to paclitaxel, and cimetidine 300 mg or ranitidine 50 mg IV 30–60 min prior to paclitaxel. Most common manifestations are dyspnea, flushing, tachycardia, rash, hypotension, and chest pain. If these occur, stop infusion and notify physician. Treatment may include bronchodilators, epinephrine, antihistamines, and corticosteroids. Keep these agents and resuscitative equipment close by in the event of an anaphylactic reaction. Other manifestations of hypersensitivity reactions include flushing and rash.
- No premedication for hypersensitivty is required for paclitaxel protein-bound (albumin-bound).
- ***Lab Test Considerations:*** Monitor CBC and differential prior to and periodically during therapy. The nadir of leukopenia occurs in 11 days, with recovery by days 15–21. Notify physician if the leukocyte count is $<1500/mm^3$ ($1000/mm^3$ in AIDS-related Kaposi's sarcoma) or if the platelet count is $<100,000/mm^3$. Subsequent doses are usually held until leukocyte count is $>1500/mm^3$ ($1000/mm^3$ in AIDS-related Kaposi's sarcoma) and platelet count is $>100,000/mm^3$.
- Monitor liver function studies (AST, ALT, LDH, bilirubin) prior to and periodically during therapy to detect hepatotoxicity.

Potential Nursing Diagnoses

Risk for infection (Adverse Reactions)
Risk for injury (Adverse Reactions)

Implementation

- Do not confuse Taxol (paclitaxel) with Taxotere (docetaxel). Do not confuse paclitaxel with Paxil (paroxetine).

Paclitaxel

IV Administration

- **Continuous Infusion:** Paclitaxel must be diluted prior to injection. ***Diluent:*** Dilute contents of 5-ml (30-mg) vials with the following diluents: 0.9% NaCl, D5W, D5/0.9% NaCl, or dextrose in Ringer's solution. ***Concentration:*** 0.3–1.2 mg/ml. Although haziness in the solution is normal, inspect for particulate matter or discoloration before use. Use an in-line filter of not >0.22-micron pore size. Solutions are stable for 27 hr at room temperature and lighting. Do not use PVC containers or administration sets. ***Rate:*** Dose for *breast cancer or AIDS-related Kaposi's sarcoma* is administered over 3 hr. Dose for *ovarian cancer* is administered as a 24-hr infusion.

- **Y-Site Compatibility:** acyclovir, amikacin, aminophylline, ampicillin/sulbactam, bleomycin, butorphanol, calcium chloride, carboplatin, cefepime, ceftazidime, ceftriaxone, cimetidine, cisplatin, cladribine, cyclophosphamide, cytarabine, dacarbazine, dexamethasone sodium phosphate, diphenhydramine, doxorubicin, droperidol, etoposide, etoposide phosphate, famotidine, floxuridine, fluconazole, fluorouracil, furosemide, ganciclovir, gemcitabine, gentamicin, granisetron, haloperidol, heparin, hydrocortisone, hydromorphone, ifosfamide, lansoprazole, linezolid, lorazepam, magnesium sulfate, mannitol, meperidine, mesna, methotrexate, metoclopramide, morphine, nalbuphine, ondansetron, oxaliplatin, palonosetron, pemetrexed, pentostatin, potassium chloride, prochlorperazine edisylate, propofol, ranitidine, sodium bicarbonate, thiotepa, topotecan, vancomycin, vinblastine, vincristine, zidovudine.
- **Y-Site Incompatibility:** amphotericin B, amphotericin B cholesteryl sulfate, chlorpromazine, doxorubicin liposome, methylprednisolone sodium succinate, mitoxantrone.

Paclitaxel Protein-Bound Particles (Albumin-Bound)

IV Administration

- **Intermittent Infusion:** Reconstitute by slowly adding 20 mL to each vial over at least 1 min for a concentration of 5 mg/mL. Direct solution to inside wall of vial to prevent foaming. Allow vial to sit for at least 5 min to ensure proper wetting of cake/powder. Gently swirl or invert vial for at least 2 min until powder is completely dissolved; avoid foaming. If foaming or clumping occurs, allow vial to stand for 15 min until foaming dissolves. Solution should be milky and homogenous without visible particles. If particles or settling are visible, gently invert vial to resuspend. Inject appropriate amount into sterile PVC IV bag. Do not use an in-line filter during administration. Do not administer solutions that are discolored or contain particulate matter. Reconstituted solution should be administered immediately but is stable for 8 hr if refrigerated. Discard unused portion. ***Rate:*** Administer over no more than 30 min. Monitor infusion site closely for infiltration.

Patient/Family Teaching

- Instruct patient to notify health care professional promptly if fever; chills; cough; hoarseness; sore throat; signs of infection; lower back or side pain; painful or difficult urination; bleeding gums; bruising; petechiae; blood in stools, urine, or emesis; increased fatigue; dyspnea; or orthostatic hypotension occurs. Caution patient to avoid crowds and persons with known infections. Instruct patient to use soft toothbrush and electric razor and to avoid falls. Caution patient not to drink alcoholic beverages or to take medication containing aspirin or NSAIDs; may precipitate gastric bleeding.
- Instruct patient to notify health care professional if abdominal pain, yellow skin, weakness, paresthesia, gait disturbances, or joint or muscle aches occur.
- Instruct patient to inspect oral mucosa for redness and ulceration. If mouth sores occur, advise patient to use sponge brush and rinse mouth with water after eating and drinking. Stomatitis usually resolves in 5–7 days.
- Discuss with patient the possibility of hair loss. Complete hair loss usually occurs between days 14 and 21 and is reversible after discontinuation of therapy. Explore coping strategies.
- Advise patient to use a nonhormonal method of contraception. Advise male patients not to father a child while receiving paclitaxel.
- Instruct patient not to receive any vaccinations without advice of health care professional.
- Emphasize the need for periodic lab tests to monitor for side effects.

P

Evaluation/Desired Outcomes

- Decrease in size or spread of malignancy.

palifermin (pa-**liff**-er-min)
Kepivance

Classification
Therapeutic: cytoprotective agents
Pharmacologic: keratinocyte growth factors (rDNA)

Pregnancy Category C

Indications

To decrease incidence/duration of severe oral mucositis associated with myelotoxic therapy requiring stem cell support for hematologic malignancies.

Action

Enhances proliferation of epithelial cells. **Therapeutic Effects:** Decreased incidence/duration of mucositis.

Pharmacokinetics

Absorption: IV administration results in complete bioavailability.
Distribution: Distributes into extravascular space.
Metabolism and Excretion: Unknown.
Half-life: 4.5 hr.

TIME/ACTION PROFILE (levels)

ROUTE	ONSET	PEAK	DURATION
IV	unknown	end of dose	unknown

Contraindications/Precautions

Contraindicated in: Hypersensitivity to palifermin or other *E. coli*–derived proteins.
Use Cautiously in: OB: Pregnancy (use only if maternal benefit outweighs fetal risk); Pedi: Children, lactation (safety not established).

Adverse Reactions/Side Effects

Derm: skin toxicity. **GI:** oral toxicity. **Metab:** ↑ amylase, ↑ lipase. **MS:** arthralgia. **Neuro:** dysesthesia.

Interactions

Drug-Drug: Binds to and inactivates **heparin** (flush tubing between use). Administration within 24 hr after **myelotoxic therapy (chemotherapy/radiation)** ↑ severity and duration of mucositis.

Route/Dosage

IV (Adults): 60 mcg/kg/day for 3 days before and 3 days after myelotoxic therapy.

Availability

Powder for injection: 6.25 mg/vial.

NURSING IMPLICATIONS

Assessment

- Assess level of oral mucositis prior to and periodically during therapy.
- ***Lab Test Considerations:*** May cause ↑ serum lipase and amylase; usually reversible.
- May cause proteinuria.

Potential Nursing Diagnoses

Acute pain (Indications)
Impaired oral mucous membrane (Indications)

Implementation

- Do not administer palifermin within 24 hrs before, during infusion, or 24 hr after infusion of myelotoxic chemotherapy.
- Administer doses for 3 consecutive days before (third dose 24–48 hrs prior to chemotherapy) and 3 consecutive days after myelotoxic chemotherapy (fourth dose on same days as hematopoietic stem cells infusion and at least 4 days after most recent palifermin administration) for a total of 6 doses.

IV Administration

- **Direct IV:** ***Diluent:*** Reconstitute palifermin powder by slowly injecting 1.2 mL of sterile water for injection aseptically. ***Concentration:*** 5 mg/mL. Swirl gently; do not shake or vigorously agitate. Solution should be clear and colorless; do not administer solution that is discolored or contains particulate matter. Dissolution usually takes less than 3 minutes. Administer immediately after reconstitution or refrigerate and administer within 24 hrs. Do not freeze. Allow to reach room temperature for up to 1 hr. Protect from light. Discard palifermin after expiration date or if left at room temperature for more than 1 hr. ***Rate:*** Administer via bolus injection. Do not use a filter.
- **Y-Site Incompatibility:** heparin. If heparin solution is used to maintain IV line, flush with 0.9% NaCl prior to and after use of palifermin.

Patient/Family Teaching

- Inform patient of evidence of tumor growth and stimulation in cell culture and animal models.
- Advise patient to notify health care professional if rash, erythema, edema, pruritus, oral/perioral dysesthesia, tongue discolora-

tion, tongue thickening, alteration of taste occur.

Evaluation/Desired Outcomes

- Decrease in incidence and duration of oral mucositis in patients receiving myelotoxic therapy requiring hematopoietic stem cell support.

paliperidone (pa-li-**per**-i-done)

Invega

Classification
Therapeutic: antipsychotics
Pharmacologic: benzisoxazoles

Pregnancy Category C

Indications

Schizophrenia.

Action

May act by antagonizing dopamine and serotonin in the CNS. Paliperidone is the active metabolite of risperidone. **Therapeutic Effects:** Decreased manifestations of schizophrenia.

Pharmacokinetics

Absorption: 28% absorbed following oral administration; food increases absorption.
Distribution: Unknown.
Metabolism and Excretion: 59% excreted unchanged in urine; 32% excreted in urine as metabolites.
Half-life: 23 hr.

TIME/ACTION PROFILE (blood levels)

ROUTE	ONSET	PEAK	DURATION
PO	unknown	24 hr	24 hr

Contraindications/Precautions

Contraindicated in: Hypersensitivity to paliperidone or risperidone; Concurrent use of drugs known to cause QTc prolongation (including quinidine, procainamide, sotalol, amiodarone, chlorpromazine, thioridazine, moxofloxacin); History of congenital QTc prolongation or other cardiac arrhythmias; Bradycardia, hypokalemia, hypomagnesemia (increased risk of QTc prolongation); Pre-existing severe GI narrowing (due to nature of tablet formulation); Lactation: Discontinue drug or bottle feed.

Use Cautiously in: Patients with Parkinson's Disease or Dementia with Lewy Bodies (increased sensitivity to effects of antipsychotics); History of suicide attempt; Patients at risk for aspiration pneumonia; History of seizures; Conditions which may increase body temperature (strenuous exercise, exposure to extreme heat, concurrent anticholinergics or risk of dehydration); Decreased GI transit time (may increase blood levels); May mask symptoms of some drug overdoses, intestinal obstruction, Reye's Syndrome or brain tumor (due to antiemetic effect); Diabetes mellitus; Severe hepatic impairment; Renal impairment (dose reduction recommended if CCr <80 ml/min); OB: Safe use not established; use only if maternal benefit outweighs fetal risk; Pedi: Safety not established; Geri: Increased risk of death when used to treat dementia-related psychoses; consider age-related decrease in renal function.

Adverse Reactions/Side Effects

CNS: NEUROLEPTIC MALIGNANT SYNDROME, drowsiness, headache, anxiety, confusion, dizziness, extrapyramidal disorders (dose related), fatigue, Parkinsonism (dose related), syncope, tardive dyskinesia, weakness. **EENT:** blurred vision. **Resp:** dyspnea, cough. **CV:** palpitations, tachycardia (dose related), bradycardia, orthostatic hypotension, ↑ QTc interval. **GI:** abdominal pain, dry mouth, dyspepsia, nausea, swollen tongue. **Endo:** hyperglycemia. **MS:** back pain, dystonia (dose related). **Neuro:** akithisia, dyskinesia, tremor (dose related). **Misc:** fever.

Interactions

Drug-Drug: ↑ risk of CNS depression with other **CNS depressants** including **alcohol**, **antihistamines**, **sedative/hypnotics**, or **opioid analgesics**. May antagonize the effects of **levodopa** or other **dopamine agonists**. ↑ risk of orthostatic hypotension with **antihypertensives**, **nitrates**, or other **agents that lower blood pressure**.

Route/Dosage

PO (Adults): 6 mg/day; may be titrated as needed (range 3–12 mg/day)

Renal Impairment

PO (Adults): *CCr 50–80 ml/min*—dose should not exceed 6 mg/day; *CCr 10–<50 ml/min*—dose should not exceed 3 mg/day.

Availability
Extended-release tablets: 3 mg, 6 mg, 9 mg.

NURSING IMPLICATIONS

Assessment
- Monitor patient's mental status (orientation, mood, behavior) before and periodically during therapy.
- Assess for suicidal tendencies, especially during early therapy. Restrict amount of drug available to patient.
- Assess weight and BMI initially and throughout therapy.
- Monitor blood pressure (sitting, standing, lying down) and pulse before and periodically during therapy. May cause prolonged QT interval, tachycardia, and orthostatic hypotension.
- Observe patient when administering medication to ensure that medication is actually swallowed and not hoarded or cheeked.
- Monitor patient for onset of extrapyramidal side effects (*akathisia*—restlessness; *dystonia*—muscle spasms and twisting motions; or *pseudoparkinsonism*—mask-like face, rigidity, tremors, drooling, shuffling gait, dysphagia). Report these symptoms; reduction of dose or discontinuation of medication may be necessary.
- Monitor for tardive dyskinesia (involuntary rhythmic movement of mouth, face, and extremities). Report immediately; may be irreversible.
- Monitor for development of neuroleptic malignant syndrome (fever, respiratory distress, tachycardia, seizures, diaphoresis, hypertension or hypotension, pallor, tiredness). Discontinue paliperidone and notify physician or other health care professional immediately if these symptoms occur.
- ***Lab Test Considerations:*** Monitor fasting blood glucose and cholesterol levels before and periodically during therapy.
- May cause ↑ serum prolactin levels.

Potential Nursing Diagnoses
Risk for self-directed violence (Indications)
Risk for other-directed violence (Indications)
Disturbed thought process (Indications)
Risk for injury (Side Effects)
Sexual dysfunction (Side Effects)
Impaired oral mucous membrane (Side Effects)
Risk for constipation (Side Effects)
Imbalanced nutrition: risk for more than body requirements (Side Effects)
Disturbed sensory perception: (specify: visual, auditory, kinesthetic, gustatory, tactile, olfactory) (Indications)

Implementation
- **PO:** Administer once daily in the morning without regard to food. Tablets should be swallowed whole; do not crush, break or chew.
- May administer Brief Psychiatric Rating Scale (BPRS) to evaluate treatment response to medication.

Patient/Family Teaching
- Instruct patient to take medication exactly as directed. Advise patient that appearance of tablets in stool is normal and not of concern.
- Inform patient of the possibility of extrapyramidal symptoms. Instruct patient to report these symptoms immediately to health care professional.
- Advise patient to change positions slowly to minimize orthostatic hypotension.
- May cause drowsiness. Caution patient to avoid driving or other activities requiring alertness until response to medication is known.
- Advise patient to use sunscreen and protective clothing when exposed to the sun to prevent photosensitivity reactions. Extremes in temperature should also be avoided; this drug impairs body temperature regulation.
- Caution patient to avoid concurrent use of alcohol, other CNS depressants, and Rx, OTC, or herbal products without consulting health care professional.
- Advise patient to seek nutritional, weight, or medical management as needed for weight gain or cholesterol elevation.
- Advise female patients to notify health care professional if pregnancy is planned or suspected, or if breastfeeding or planning to breastfeed.
- Advise patient to notify health care professional of medication regimen before treatment or surgery.
- Instruct patient to notify health care professional promptly if sore throat, fever, unusual bleeding or bruising, rash, or tremors occur.
- Emphasize the importance of routine follow-up exams to monitor side effects and continued participation in psychotherapy to improve coping skills.
- Refer to local support group.

Evaluation/Desired Outcomes

- Decrease in excited, manic behavior.
- Decrease in positive symptoms (delusions, hallucinations) of schizophrenia.
- Decrease in negative symptoms (social withdrawal, flat, blunted affect) of schizophrenia.

palonosetron

(pa-lone-**o**-se-tron)
Aloxi

Classification
Therapeutic: antiemetics
Pharmacologic: $5\text{-}HT_3$ antagonists

Pregnancy Category B

Indications

Prevention of acute and delayed nausea and vomiting caused by initial or repeat courses of moderate or highly emetogenic chemotherapy.

Action

Blocks the effects of serotonin at receptor sites (selective antagonist) located in vagal nerve terminals and in the chemoreceptor trigger zones in the CNS. **Therapeutic Effects:** Decreased incidence and severity of nausea and vomiting following emetogenic chemotherapy.

Pharmacokinetics

Absorption: IV administration results in complete bioavailability.
Distribution: Unknown.
Metabolism and Excretion: 50% metabolized; 40% excreted unchanged in urine.
Half-life: 40 hr.

TIME/ACTION PROFILE

ROUTE	ONSET	PEAK	DURATION
IV	within 30 min	unknown	7 days

Contraindications/Precautions

Contraindicated in: Hypersensitivity; cross sensitivity with other $5\text{-}HT_3$ antagonists may occur; Lactation.
Use Cautiously in: Hereditary or acquired QTc prolongation, hypokalemia, hypomagnesemia, concurrent diuretic or antiarrhythmic therapy or history of high cumulative anthracycline therapy (may ↑ risk of arrhythmias); OB, Pedi: Pregnancy or children (safety not established).

Adverse Reactions/Side Effects

CNS: dizziness, headache. **GI:** constipation, diarrhea,.

Interactions

Drug-Drug: Concurrent **diuretic** or **antiarrhythmic** therapy or history of high cumulative **anthracycline** therapy may ↑ risk of arrhythmias.

Route/Dosage

IV (Adults): 0.25 mg 30 min before start of chemotherapy.

Availability

Solution for IV injection: 0.25mg/5-ml vials.

NURSING IMPLICATIONS

Assessment

- Assess patient for nausea, vomiting, abdominal distention, and bowel sounds prior to and following administration.
- ***Lab Test Considerations:*** May cause transient ↑ in serum bilirubin, AST, and ALT levels.

Potential Nursing Diagnoses

Imbalanced nutrition: less than body requirements (Indications)
Diarrhea (Side Effects)
Constipation (Side Effects)

Implementation

- First dose is administered prior to emetogenic event.
- Repeated dose within a 7 day period is not recommended.

IV Administration

- **Direct IV:** Administer dose undiluted 30 min prior to chemotherapy. Flush line prior to and after administration with 0.9% NaCl. Do not administer solutions that are discolored or contain particulate matter. ***Concentration:*** 0.05 mg/ml. ***Rate:*** Administer over 30 seconds.
- **Syringe Compatibility:** dexamethasone sodium phosphate.
- **Y-Site Compatibility:** carboplatin, cisplatin, docetaxel, irinotecan, lorazepam, midazolam, oxaliplatin, paclitaxel, topotecan.

Patient/Family Teaching

- Inform patient of purpose of medication.
- Advise patient to notify health care professional if nausea or vomiting occur.

P

Evaluation/Desired Outcomes

- Prevention of nausea and vomiting associated with initial and repeat courses of emetogenic cancer chemotherapy.

pamidronate

(pa-**mid**-roe-nate)
Aredia

Classification
Therapeutic: bone resorption inhibitors
Pharmacologic: biphosphonates, hypocalcemics

Pregnancy Category D

Indications

Moderate to severe hypercalcemia associated with malignancy. Osteolytic bone lesions associated with multiple myeloma or breast cancer. Moderate to severe Paget's disease.

Action

Inhibits resorption of bone. **Therapeutic Effects:** Decreased serum calcium. Decreased skeletal destruction in multiple myeloma or breast cancer. Decreased skeletal complications in Paget's disease.

Pharmacokinetics

Absorption: IV administration results in complete bioavailability.
Distribution: Rapidly absorbed by bone. Reaches high concentrations in bone, liver, spleen, teeth, and tracheal cartilage. Approximately 50% of a dose is retained by bone and then slowly released.
Metabolism and Excretion: 50% is excreted unchanged in the urine.
Half-life: Elimination half-life from plasma is biphasic—1st phase 1.6 hr, 2nd phase 27.2 hr. Elimination half-life from bone is 300 days.

TIME/ACTION PROFILE (effect on serum calcium)

ROUTE	ONSET	PEAK	DURATION
IV	24 hr	7 days	unknown

Contraindications/Precautions

Contraindicated in: Hypersensitivity to pamidronate, other biphosphonates, or mannitol.
Use Cautiously in: Underlying cardiovascular disease, especially CHF (initiate saline hydration cautiously); Concurrent dental surgery; Renal impairment (dosage reduction recommended); Pregnancy, lactation, or children (safety not established).

Adverse Reactions/Side Effects

CNS: fatigue. **EENT:** conjunctivitis, blurred vision, eye pain/inflammation, rhinitis. **Resp:** rales. **CV:** arrhythmias, hypertension, syncope, tachycardia. **GI:** nausea, abdominal pain, anorexia, constipation, vomiting. **F and E:** hypocalcemia, hypokalemia, hypomagnesemia, hypophosphatemia, fluid overload. **Hemat:** leukopenia, anemia. **Local:** phlebitis at injection site. **Metab:** hypothyroidism. **MS:** muscle stiffness, bone pain, osteonecrosis of the jaw. **Misc:** fever, generalized pain.

Interactions

Drug-Drug: Hypokalemia and hypomagnesemia may ↑ risk of **digoxin** toxicity. **Calcium** and **vitamin D** will antagonize the beneficial effects of pamidronate.

Route/Dosage

Single doses should not exceed 90 mg.

Hypercalcemia of Malignancy

IV (Adults): *Moderate hypercalcemia*—30–90 mg; may be repeated after 7 days.

Osteolytic Lesions from Multiple Myeloma

IV (Adults): 90 mg monthly.

Osteolytic Lesions from Metastatic Breast Cancer

IV (Adults): 90 mg q 3–4 wk.

Paget's Disease

IV (Adults): 90–180 mg/treatment; may be given as 30 mg daily for 3 days up to 30 mg/wk for 6 wk. Single doses of 60–90 mg may also be effective.

Availability (generic available)

Injection: 30 mg/vial, 60 mg/vial, 90 mg/vial.

NURSING IMPLICATIONS

Assessment

- Monitor intake/output ratios and blood pressure frequently during therapy. Assess for signs of fluid overload (edema, rales/crackles).
- Monitor symptoms of hypercalcemia (nausea, vomiting, anorexia, weakness, constipation, thirst, and cardiac arrhythmias).
- Observe for evidence of hypocalcemia (paresthesia, muscle twitching, laryngospasm, and Chvostek's or Trousseau's sign). Protect

symptomatic patients by elevating and padding side rails; keep bed in low position.
- Monitor IV site for phlebitis (pain, redness, swelling). Symptomatic treatment should be used if this occurs.
- Assess for bone pain. Treatment with non-opioid or opioid analgesics may be necessary.
- ***Lab Test Considerations:*** Monitor serum electrolytes (including calcium, phosphate, potassium, and magnesium), hemoglobin, and creatinine closely. Monitor CBC and platelet count during the first 2 wk of therapy.

Potential Nursing Diagnoses
Acute pain (Indications, Side Effects)
Risk for injury (Indications)

Implementation
- Initiate a vigorous saline hydration, maintaining a urine output of 2000 ml/24 hr, concurrently with pamidronate therapy. Patients should be adequately hydrated, but avoid overhydration. Use caution in patients with underlying cardiovascular disease, especially CHF. Do not use diuretics prior to treatment of hypovolemia.
- Patients with severe hypercalcemia should be started at the 90-mg dose.
- **IV:** Reconstitute by adding 10 ml of sterile water for injection to each vial for a concentration of 30 mg/10 ml, 60 mg/ml, or 90 mg/ml. Allow drug to dissolve before withdrawing. Solution is stable for 24 hr if refrigerated.
- **Hypercalcemia:** Dilute further in 1000 ml of 0.45% NaCl, 0.9% NaCl, or D5W. Solution is stable for 24 hr at room temperature. ***Rate:*** Administer 60-mg infusion over at least 4 hr and 90-mg infusion over 24 hr.
- **Multiple Myeloma:** Dilute reconstituted solution in 500 ml of 0.45% NaCl, 0.9% NaCl, or D5W. ***Rate:*** Administer over 4 hr.
- **Paget's Disease:** Dilute reconstituted solution in 500 ml of 0.45% NaCl, 0.9% NaCl, or D5W. ***Rate:*** Administer over 4 hr.
- **Additive Incompatibility:** Calcium-containing solutions, such as Ringer's solution.

Patient/Family Teaching
- Advise patient to report signs of hypercalcemic relapse (bone pain, anorexia, nausea, vomiting, thirst, lethargy) or eye problems (pain, inflammation, blurred vision, conjunctivitis) to health care professional promptly.
- Advise patient to notify nurse of pain at the infusion site.
- Encourage patient to comply with dietary recommendations. Diet should contain adequate amounts of calcium and vitamin D.
- Advise patient to notify health care professional if bone pain is severe or persistent.
- Caution patients to avoid dental surgery during treatment; recovery may be prolonged.
- Emphasize the need for keeping follow-up exams to monitor progress, even after medication is discontinued, to detect relapse.

Evaluation/Desired Outcomes
- Lowered serum calcium levels.
- Decreased pain from lytic lesions.

pancrelipase (pan-kre-**li**-pase)
Cotazym, ✤Cotazym-65 B, Cotazym E.C.S. 8, Cotazym E.C.S. 20, Cotazym-S, Creon 10, Creon 25, Enzymase-16, Ilozyme, Ku-Zyme HP, Lipram-PN16, Lipram-CR20, Lipram-UL12, Lipram-PN10, Lipram-UL18, Lipram,-UL20, Pancoate, Pancrease, Pancrease MT 4, Pancrease MT 10, Pancrease MT 16, Pancrease MT 20, Pancrebarb MS-8, Protilase, Ultrase MT 12, Ultrase MT 20, Viokase, Zymase

Classification
Therapeutic: digestive agents
Pharmacologic: pancreatic enzymes

Pregnancy Category C

P

Indications
Pancreatic insufficiency associated with: Chronic pancreatitis, Pancreatectomy, Cystic fibrosis, GI bypass surgery, Ductal obstruction secondary to tumor.

Action
Contains lipolytic, amylolytic, and proteolytic activity. **Therapeutic Effects:** Increased digestion of fats, carbohydrates, and proteins in the GI tract.

Pharmacokinetics
Absorption: Unknown.
Distribution: Unknown.

Metabolism and Excretion: Unknown.
Half-life: Unknown.

TIME/ACTION PROFILE (digestant effects)

ROUTE	ONSET	PEAK	DURATION
PO	rapid	unknown	unknown

Contraindications/Precautions

Contraindicated in: Hypersensitivity to hog proteins.
Use Cautiously in: Pregnancy or lactation (safety not established).

Adverse Reactions/Side Effects

EENT: nasal stuffiness. **Resp:** dyspnea, shortness of breath, wheezing. **GI:** abdominal pain (high doses only), diarrhea, nausea, stomach cramps, oral irritation. **GU:** hematuria. **Derm:** hives, rash. **Metab:** hyperuricemia. **Misc:** allergic reactions.

Interactions

Drug-Drug: Antacids **calcium carbonate** or **magnesium hydroxide** may ↓ effectiveness of pancrelipase. May ↓ the absorption of concurrently administered **iron supplements**.
Drug-Food: Alkaline foods destroy coating on enteric-coated products.

Route/Dosage

PO (Adults): 1–3 capsule(s) before or with meals; dosage may be increased as needed (up to 8 capsules may be needed), *or* 1–2 delayed-release capsule(s), *or* 0.7 g powder.
PO (Children): 1–3 capsule(s) before or with meals; dosage may be increased as needed, *or* 1–2 delayed-release capsule(s), *or* 0.7 g powder.

Availability (generic available)

Capsules: 8000 units lipase/30,000 units protease and amylase. **Delayed-release capsules:** 4000 units lipase/12,000 units protease and amylase, 4000 units lipase/25,000 units protease/20,000 units amylase, 5000 units lipase/20,000 units protease and amylase, ✤8000 units lipase/30,000 units protease and amylase, 10,000 units lipase/30,000 units protease and amylase, 12,000 units lipase/24,000 units protease and amylase, 12,000 units lipase/39,000 units protease and amylase, 16,000 units lipase/48,000 units protease and amylase, ✤20,000 units lipase/55,000 units protease and amylase, 20,000 units lipase/65,000 units protease and amylase, 24,000 units lipase/78,000 units protease and amylase. **Powder:** 16,800 units lipase/70,000 units protease and amylase.

NURSING IMPLICATIONS

Assessment

- Assess patient's nutritional status (height, weight, skin-fold thickness, arm muscle circumference, and lab values) prior to and periodically throughout therapy.
- Monitor stools for high fat content (steatorrhea). Stools will be foul-smelling and frothy.
- Assess patient for allergy to pork; sensitivity to pancrelipase may exist.
- ***Lab Test Considerations:*** May cause elevated serum and urine uric acid concentrations.

Potential Nursing Diagnoses

Imbalanced nutrition: less than body requirements (Indications)

Implementation

- **PO:** Administer immediately before or with meals and snacks.
- Capsules may be opened and sprinkled on foods. Capsules filled with enteric-coated beads should not be chewed (sprinkle on soft foods that can be swallowed without chewing, such as applesauce or Jell-O).
- Pancrelipase is destroyed by acid. Concurrent sodium bicarbonate or aluminum-containing antacids may be used with nonenteric-coated preparations to neutralize gastric pH. Enteric-coated beads are designed to withstand the acid pH of the stomach. These medications should not be chewed or mixed with alkaline foods prior to ingestion or coating will be destroyed.

Patient/Family Teaching

- Encourage patients to comply with diet recommendations of health care professional (generally high-calorie, high-protein, low-fat). Dosage should be adjusted for fat content of diet. Usually 300 mg of pancrelipase is necessary to digest every 17 g of dietary fat. If a dose is missed, it should be omitted.
- Instruct patient not to chew tablets and to swallow them quickly with plenty of liquid to prevent mouth and throat irritation. Patient should be sitting upright to enhance swallowing. Eating immediately after taking medication helps further ensure that the medication is swallowed and does not remain in contact with mouth and esophagus for a prolonged period. Patient should avoid sniffing powdered contents of capsules, as sensitization of nose and throat may occur (nasal stuffiness or respiratory distress).

- Instruct patient to notify health care professional if joint pain, swelling of legs, gastric distress, or rash occurs.

Evaluation/Desired Outcomes

- Improved nutritional status in patients with pancreatic insufficiency.
- Normalization of stools in patients with steatorrhea.

HIGH ALERT

pancuronium

(pan-cure-**oh**-nee-yum)
Pavulon

Classification
Therapeutic: neuromuscular blocking agents—nondepolarizing

Pregnancy Category C

Indications

Induction of skeletal muscle paralysis and facilitation of intubation after induction of anesthesia in surgical procedures. Facilitation of compliance during mechanical ventilation.

Action

Prevents neuromuscular transmission by blocking the effect of acetylcholine at the myoneural junction. Has no analgesic or anxiolytic properties. **Therapeutic Effects:** Skeletal muscle paralysis.

Pharmacokinetics

Absorption: Following IV administration, absorption is essentially complete.
Distribution: Rapidly distributes into extracellular fluid; small amounts cross the placenta.
Metabolism and Excretion: Excreted mostly unchanged by the kidneys; small amounts are eliminated in bile.
Half-life: 2 hr.

TIME/ACTION PROFILE (neuromuscular blockade)

ROUTE	ONSET	PEAK	DURATION
IV	30–45 sec	3–4.5 min	40–60 min

Contraindications/Precautions

Contraindicated in: Hypersensitivity; Hypersensitivity to bromides; Products containing benzyl alcohol should be avoided in neonates.
Use Cautiously in: Patients with underlying cardiovascular disease (increased risk of arrhythmias); Dehydration or electrolyte abnormalities (should be corrected); Situations in which histamine release would be problematic; Fractures or muscle spasm; Geriatric patients or patients with impaired renal function (decreased elimination); Hyperthermia (increased duration/intensity of paralysis); Patients with significant hepatic impairment (altered response); Shock; Extensive burns (may be more resistant to effects of cisatracurium); Low plasma pseudocholinesterase levels (may be seen in association with anemia, dehydration, cholinesterase inhibitors/insecticides, severe liver disease, pregnancy, or hereditary predisposition); Obese patients; Neonates (contains benzyl alcohol which can cause potentially fatal gasping syndrome); Pregnancy or lactation (safety not established for some agents; most agents have been used safely in pregnant women undergoing cesarean section).
Exercise Extreme Caution in: Patients with neuromuscular diseases such as myasthenia gravis (small test dose may be used to assess response).

Adverse Reactions/Side Effects

Resp: bronchospasm. **CV:** hypertension, tachycardia. **GI:** excessive salivation. **Derm:** rash. **Misc:** allergic reactions including ANAPHYLAXIS.

Interactions

Drug-Drug: Intensity and duration of paralysis may be prolonged by pretreatment with **succinylcholine**, **general anesthesia** (inhalation), **aminoglycosides**, **vancomycin**, **tetracyclines**, **polymyxin B**, **colistin**, **cyclosporine**, **calcium channel blockers** , **clindamycin**, **lidocaine**, and other **local anesthetics**, **lithium**, **quinidine**, **procainamide**, **beta blockers**, **potassium-losing diuretics**, or **magnesium**. **Inhalation anesthetics** including **enflurane**, **isoflurane**, **halothane**, **desflurane**, **sevoflurane** may enhance effects. Higher infusion rates may be required and duration of action may be shortened in patients receiving long-term **carbamazepine**, **steroids (chronic)**, **azathioprine** or **phenytoin**.

Route/Dosage

IV (Adults and Children >12 yrs): 0.15 mg/kg initially; incremental doses of 0.15 mg/kg may be given q 20–60 min as needed to main-

P

tain paralysis or as a continuous infusion of 0.02–0.04 mg/kg/hr or 0.4–0.6 mcg/kg/min.
IV (Children >1 yr): 0.15 mg/kg q 30–60 min as needed or as a continuous infusion of 0.03–0.1 mg/kg/hr or 0.5–1.7 mcg/kg/min.
IV (Neonates and Infants): 0.1 mg/kg q 30–60 min as needed or as a continuous infusion of 0.02–0.04 mg/kg/hr or 0.4–0.6 mcg/kg/min.

Availability
Injection: 1 mg/ml in 10-ml vials, 2 mg/ml in 2- and 5-ml vials.

NURSING IMPLICATIONS

Assessment
- Assess respiratory status continuously throughout therapy with neuromuscular blocking agents. These medications should be used only to facilitate intubation or in patients already intubated.
- Neuromuscular response should be monitored with a peripheral nerve stimulator intraoperatively. Paralysis is initially selective and usually occurs sequentially in the following muscles: levator muscles of eyelids, muscles of mastication, limb muscles, abdominal muscles, muscles of the glottis, intercostal muscles, and the diaphragm. Recovery of muscle function usually occurs in reverse order.
- Monitor ECG, heart rate, and blood pressure throughout administration.
- Observe the patient for residual muscle weakness and respiratory distress during the recovery period.
- Monitor infusion site frequently. If signs of tissue irritation or extravasation occur, discontinue and restart in another vein.
- ***Toxicity and Overdose:*** If overdose occurs, use peripheral nerve stimulator to determine the degree of neuromuscular blockade. Maintain airway patency and ventilation until recovery of normal respirations occurs: Administration of anticholinesterase agents (neostigmine, pyridostigmine) may be used to antagonize the action of neuromuscular blocking agents once the patient has demonstrated some spontaneous recovery from neuromuscular block. Atropine is usually administered prior to or concurrently with anticholinesterase agents to counteract the muscarinic effects. Administration of fluids and vasopressors may be necessary to treat severe hypotension or shock.

Potential Nursing Diagnoses
Ineffective breathing pattern (Indications)
Impaired verbal communication (Side Effects)
Fear (Side Effects)

Implementation
- ***High Alert:*** Unintended administration of a neuromuscular blocking agent instead of administration of the intended medication or administration of a neuromuscular blocking agent in the absence of ventilatory support has resulted in serious harm or death. Confusing similarities in packaging and insufficiently controlled access to these medications are often implicated in these medication errors. Store these products in a separate, locked container.
- Dose is titrated to patient response.
- Neuromuscular blocking agents have *no* effect on consciousness or pain threshold. Adequate anesthesia/analgesia should *always* be used when neuromuscular blocking agents are used as an adjunct to surgical procedures or when painful procedures are performed. Benzodiazepines and/or analgesics should be administered concurrently when prolonged neuromuscular blocker therapy is used for ventilator patients, because patient is awake and able to feel all sensations.
- If eyes remain open throughout prolonged administration, protect corneas with artificial tears.
- Store pancuronium in refrigerator. To prevent absorption by plastic, pancuronium should not be stored in plastic syringes. May be administered in plastic syringes.
- Most neuromuscular blocking agents are incompatible with barbiturates and sodium bicarbonate. Do not admix.

IV Administration
- **Direct IV:** ***Diluent:*** May be administered undiluted. ***Concentration:*** 1 mg/ml (10-ml vial); 2-mg/ml (2-ml or 5-ml vial). ***Rate:*** Administer over 1–2 min.
- **Intermittent Infusion:** ***Diluent:*** Add 100 mg of pancuroniuum to 250 ml of D5W, 0.9% NaCl, D5/0.9% NaCl, or LR. ***Concentration:*** 0.4 mg/ml. ***Rate:*** Based on patient's weight (see Route/Dosage section).
- **Y-Site Compatibility:** aminophylline, cefazolin, cefuroxime, cimetidine, daptomycin, diltiazem, dobutamine, dopamine, epinephrine, ertapenem, esmolol, etomidate, fenoldopam, fentanyl, fluconazole, gentamicin, granisetron, heparin, hydrocortisone sodium

succinate, hydromorphone, isoproterenol, levofloxacin, linezolid, lorazepam, midazolam, morphine, nitroglycerin, nitroprusside, palonosetron, piperacillin/tazobactam, quinupristin/dalfopristin, ranitidine, trimethoprim/sulfamethoxazole, tacrolimus, tirofiban, vancomycin, voriconazole.

- **Y-Site Incompatibility:** caspofungin, diazepam, pantoprazole, thiopental.

Patient/Family Teaching

- Explain all procedures to patient receiving neuromuscular blocker therapy without general anesthesia, because consciousness is not affected by neuromuscular blocking agents alone.
- Reassure patient that communication abilities will return as the medication wears off.

Evaluation/Desired Outcomes

- Adequate suppression of the twitch response when tested with peripheral nerve stimulation and subsequent muscle paralysis.
- Improved compliance during mechanical ventilation.

panitumumab

(pan-i-**tu**-mu-mab)

Vectibix

Classification

Therapeutic: antineoplastics

Pharmacologic: monoclonal antibodies

Pregnancy Category C

Indications

Treatment of metastatic colorectal cancer that expresses EGFR (epidermal growth factor receptor) and has failed conventional treatments.

Action

Binds to EGFR resulting in inactivation of kinases that regulate proliferation and transformation. **Therapeutic Effects:** Decreased progression of colorectal cancer.

Pharmacokinetics

Absorption: IV administration results in complete bioavailability.

Distribution: Monoclonal antibodies cross the placenta and enter breast milk.

Metabolism and Excretion: Unknown.

Half-life: 7.5 days.

TIME/ACTION PROFILE

ROUTE	ONSET	PEAK	DURATION
IV	unknown	end of infusion	unknown

Contraindications/Precautions

Contraindicated in: Concurrent leucovorin; OB: Pregnancy or lactation.

Use Cautiously in: Pedi: Safe use in children not established.

Adverse Reactions/Side Effects

CNS: fatigue. **EENT:** OCULAR TOXICITY, eyelash growth. **Resp:** PULMONARY FIBROSIS, cough. **GI:** abdominal pain, constipation, diarrhea, nausea, vomiting, stomatitis. **Derm:** DERMATOLOGIC TOXICITY, paromychia, photosensitivity. **F and E:** edema, hypocalcemia, hypomagnesemia. **Misc:** INFUSION REACTIONS.

Interactions

Drug-Drug: None noted.

Route/Dosage

IV (Adults): 6 mg/kg as a 60-min infusion every 14 days; decreased infusion rates and dose modifications are recommended for infusion reactions and other serious toxicities.

Availability

Solution for IV administration (requires dilution): 20 mg/mL in 5-ml vials (100 mg/vial).

NURSING IMPLICATIONS

Assessment

- Assess for dermatologic toxicity (dermatitis acneiform, pruritus, erythema, rash, skin exfoliation, paronychia, dry skin, skin fissures). If severe, may lead to infection (sepsis, septic death, abscesses requiring incision and drainage). With severe reactions, withhold panitumumab and monitor for inflammatory or infectious sequelae.
- Monitor for severe infusion reactions (anaphylactic reaction, bronchospasm, fever, chills, hypotension). If severe reaction occurs, stop panitumumab; may require permanent discontinuation.
- Assess for pulmonary fibrosis (cough, wheezing, exertional dyspnea, interstitial lung disease, pneumonitis, lung infiltrates). Perma-

P

nently discontinue panitumumab if these signs occur.

- Monitor for diarrhea during therapy.
- ***Lab Test Considerations:*** Monitor electrolyte levels periodically during and for 8 wks after completion of therapy. May cause hypomagnesemia and hypocalcemia.

Potential Nursing Diagnoses

Risk for impaired skin integrity (Adverse Reactions)

Impaired gas exchange (Adverse Reactions)

Implementation

- **Intermittent Infusion:** Withdraw necessary amount of panitumumab. Dilute to a volume of 100 mL with 0.9% NaCl; dilute doses >1000 mg with 150 mL for a concentration of 10 mg/mL. Mix by inverting gently; do not shake. Administer via infusion pump using a low-protein binding 0.2 mcg or 0.22 mcg in-line filter. Solution is colorless and may contain a small amount of visible translucent to white, amorphous, proteinaceous particles. Do not administer solutions that are discolored or contain particulate matter. Store in refrigerator; do not freeze. Use diluted solution within 6 hr of preparation if stored at room temperature or within 24 hr if refrigerated. ***Rate:*** Administer over 60 min every 14 days. Administer doses >1000 mg over 90 min.
- If mild to moderate infusion reaction (Grade 1 or 2) occurs decrease infusion rate by 50% If severe reaction (Grade 3 or 4) occurs, immediately and permanently discontinue panitumumab.
- If severe dermatologic toxicities (Grade 3 or higher) or those considered intolerable occur, withhold panitumumab. If toxicity does not improve to ≤grade 2 within 1 month, discontinue permanently. If toxicity improves to ≤grade 2 and patient improves symptomatically after withholding no more than 2 doses, resume therapy at 50% dose. If toxicities recur, permanently discontinue panitumumab. If toxicities do not recur, increase subsequent doses in 25% increments of the original dose until recommended dose of 6 mg/kg is reached.
- **Y-Site Incompatibility:** Flush line before and after administration with 0.9% NaCl. Do not mix with other medications or solutions.

Patient/Family Teaching

- May cause photosensitivity. Caution patient to wear sunscreen and hats and to limit sun exposure.
- Advise patient that panitumumab may cause fertility impairment and may have teratogenic effects. Caution women of childbearing years to use contraception during and for at least 6 months after the last dose and not to breast feed during and for at least 2 months after the last dose of panitumumab.
- Inform patient of potential for dermatologic toxicity, infusion reactions, pulmonary fibrosis and impairment of fertility. Advise patient to notify health care professional if skin or ocular changes or dyspnea occur. Advise patient that periodic electrolyte monitoring is required.

Evaluation/Desired Outcomes

- Decreased progression of colorectal cancer.

pantoprazole

(pan-**toe**-pra-zole)

✱Pantoloc, Protonix, Protonix I.V

Classification

Therapeutic: antiulcer agents

Pharmacologic: proton-pump inhibitors

Pregnancy Category B

Indications

Erosive esophagitis associated with GERD. Decrease relapse rates of daytime and nighttime heartburn symptoms on patients with GERD. Pathologic gastric hypersecretory conditions. **Unlabeled uses:** Adjunctive treatment of duodenal ulcers associated with *Helicobacter pylori*.

Action

Binds to an enzyme in the presence of acidic gastric pH, preventing the final transport of hydrogen ions into the gastric lumen. **Therapeutic Effects:** Diminished accumulation of acid in the gastric lumen, with lessened acid reflux. Healing of duodenal ulcers and esophagitis. Decreased acid secretion in hypersecretory conditions.

Pharmacokinetics

Absorption: Tablet is enteric-coated; absorption occurs only after tablet leaves the stomach.

Distribution: Unknown.

Protein Binding: 98%.

Metabolism and Excretion: Mostly metabolized by the liver via the cytochrome P450 (CYP) system; inactive metabolites are excreted in urine (71%) and feces (18%).
Half-life: 1 hr.

TIME/ACTION PROFILE (effect on acid secretion)

ROUTE	ONSET†	PEAK	DURATION†
PO	2.5 hr	unknown	1 wk
IV	15–30 min	2 hr	unknown

†Onset = 51% inhibition; duration = return to normal following discontinuation

Contraindications/Precautions

Contraindicated in: Hypersensitivity; OB: Should be used during pregnancy only if clearly needed; Lactation: Discontinue breastfeeding due to potential for serious adverse reactions in infants.
Use Cautiously in: Pedi: Safety not established.

Adverse Reactions/Side Effects

CNS: headache. **GI:** abdominal pain, diarrhea, eructation, flatulence. **Endo:** hyperglycemia.

Interactions

Drug-Drug: May alter the bioavailability and effects of **drugs for which absorption is pH dependent**. May ↑ risk of bleeding with **warfarin** (monitor INR/PT).

Route/Dosage

PO (Adults): *GERD*—40 mg once daily; *Gastric hypersecretory conditions*—40 mg twice daily, up to 120 mg twice daily.
PO (Children): 0.5–1 mg/kg/day.
IV (Adults): *GERD*—40 mg once daily for 7–10 days. *Gastric hypersecretory conditions*—80 mg q 12 hr (up to 240 mg/day).

Availability

Delayed-release tablets: 20 mg, 40 mg. **Cost:** 20 mg $353.61/90, 40 mg $351.97/90. **Powder for injection:** 40 mg/vial.

NURSING IMPLICATIONS

Assessment

- Assess patient routinely for epigastric or abdominal pain and for frank or occult blood in stool, emesis, or gastric aspirate.
- ***Lab Test Considerations:*** May cause abnormal liver function tests, including ↑ AST, ALT, alkaline phosphatase, and bilirubin.

Potential Nursing Diagnoses

Acute pain (Indications)

Implementation

- Patients receiving pantoprazole IV should be converted to PO dosing as soon as possible.
- **PO:** May be administered with or without food. Do not break, crush, or chew tablets.
- Antacids may be used concurrently.

IV Administration

- **IV:** ***Diluent:*** Reconstitute each vial with 10 mL of 0.9% NaCl. Reconstituted solution is stable for 6 hr at room temperature
- **Direct IV:** ***Concentration:*** Administer the 4 mg/mL solution undiluted. ***Rate:*** Administer over at least 2 min.
- **Intermittent Infusion:** Dilute further with D5W, 0.9% NaCl, or LR. ***Concentration:*** 0.4–0.8 mg/ml. Diluted solution is stable for 24 hr at room temperature. ***Rate:*** Administer over 15 min at a rate of <3 mg/min.
- **Y-Site Compatibility:** ampicillin, cefazolin, ceftriaxone, dopamine, furosemide, epinephrine, insulin, morphine, nitroglycerin, potassium chloride, vasopressin.
- **Y-Site Incompatibility:** dobutamine, esmolol, mannitol, midazolam, multivitamins, solutions containing zinc.

Patient/Family Teaching

- Instruct patient to take medication as directed for the full course of therapy, even if feeling better.
- Advise patient to avoid alcohol, products containing aspirin or NSAIDs, and foods that may cause an increase in GI irritation.
- Advise patient to report onset of black, tarry stools; diarrhea; or abdominal pain to health care professional promptly.

Evaluation/Desired Outcomes

- Healing in patients with erosive esophagitis. Therapy is continued for up to 8 wk.

paricalcitol, See VITAMIN D COMPOUNDS.

paroxetine hydrochloride
(par-**ox**-e-teen)
Paxil, Paxil CR

P

paroxetine mesylate
Pexeva

Classification
Therapeutic: antianxiety agents, antidepressants
Pharmacologic: selective serotonin reuptake inhibitors (SSRIs)

Pregnancy Category D

Indications
Paxil, Paxil CR, Pexeva. Major depressive disorder, panic disorder. Paxil, Pexeva. Obsessive compulsive disorder (OCD), generalized anxiety disorder (GAD). Paxil, Paxil CRSocial anxiety disorder. Paxil. Post-traumatic stress disorder (PTSD). Paxil CRPremenstrual dysphoric disorder (PMDD).

Action
Inhibits neuronal reuptake of serotonin in the CNS, thus potentiating the activity of serotonin; has little effect on norepinephrine or dopamine.
Therapeutic Effects: Antidepressant action. Decreased frequency of panic attacks, OCD, or anxiety. Improvement in manifestations of post-traumatic stress disorder. Decreased dysphoria prior to menses.

Pharmacokinetics
Absorption: Completely absorbed following oral administration. Controlled-release tablets are enteric-coated and control medication release over 4–5 hr.
Distribution: Widely distributed throughout body fluids and tissues, including the CNS; cross the placenta and enter breast milk.
Protein Binding: 95%.
Metabolism and Excretion: Highly metabolized by the liver (partly by P450 2D6 enzyme system); 2% excreted unchanged in urine.
Half-life: 21 hr.

TIME/ACTION PROFILE (antidepressant action)

ROUTE	ONSET	PEAK	DURATION
PO	1–4 wk	unknown	unknown

Contraindications/Precautions
Contraindicated in: Hypersensitivity; Concurrent MAO inhibitor, thioridazine, or pimozide therapy.
Use Cautiously in: Risk of suicide (may ↑ risk of suicide attempt/ ideation especially during early treatment or dose adjustment); History of seizures; History of bipolar disorder; OB: Use during the first trimester may be associated with an increased risk of cardiac malformations—consider fetal risk/ maternal benefit; use during third trimester may result in neonatal serotonin syndrome requiring prolonged hospitalization, respiratory and nutritional support; Lactation: Safety not established; discontinue drug or bottle feed; Pedi: May ↑ risk of suicide attempt/ideation especially during early treatment or dose adjustment may be greater in children and adolescents (safety in children/adolescents not established); Geri: Severe renal hepatic impairment; geriatric or debilitated patients (daily dose should not exceed 40 mg); History of mania/ risk of suicide.

Adverse Reactions/Side Effects
CNS: anxiety, dizziness, drowsiness, headache, insomnia, weakness, agitation, amnesia, confusion, emotional lability, hangover, impaired concentration, malaise, mental depression, suicidal behavior, syncope. **EENT:** blurred vision, rhinitis. **Resp:** cough, pharyngitis, respiratory disorders, yawning. **CV:** chest pain, edema, hypertension, palpitations, postural hypotension, tachycardia, vasodilation. **GI:** constipation, diarrhea, dry mouth, nausea, abdominal pain, decreased appetite, dyspepsia, flatulence, increased appetite, taste disturbances, vomiting. **GU:** ejaculatory disturbance, decreased libido, genital disorders, urinary disorders, urinary frequency. **Derm:** sweating, photosensitivity, pruritus, rash. **Metab:** weight gain, weight loss. **MS:** back pain, myalgia, myopathy. **Neuro:** paresthesia, tremor. **Misc:** chills, fever.

Interactions
Drug-Drug: Serious, potentially fatal reactions (hyperthermia, rigidity, myoclonus, autonomic instability, with fluctuating vital signs and extreme agitation, which may proceed to delirium and coma) may occur with concurrent **MAO inhibitor** therapy. MAO inhibitors should be stopped at least 14 days prior to paroxetine therapy. Paroxetine should be stopped at least 14 days prior to MAO inhibitor therapy. May ↓ metabolism and ↑ effects of certain **drugs that are metabolized by the liver**, including other **antidepressants**, **phenothiazines**, **class IC antiarrhythmics**, **risperidone**, **atomoxetine**, **theophylline**, **procyclidine**, and **quinidine**. Concurrent use should be undertaken with caution. Concurrent use with **pimozide** or **thioridazine** may ↑ risk of QT inter-

val prolongation and torsades de pointes. Concurrent use is contraindicated. **Cimetidine** ↑ blood levels. **Phenobarbital** and **phenytoin** may ↓ effectiveness. Concurrent use with **alcohol** is not recommended. May ↓ the effectiveness of **digoxin**. May ↑ risk of bleeding with **warfarin**, **aspirin**, or **NSAIDs**. Concurrent use with **5-HT$_1$ agonists** (**frovatriptan**, **naratriptan**, **rizatriptan**, **sumatriptan**, **zolmitriptan**), **linezolid**, **lithium**, or **tramadol** may result in increased serotonin levels and lead to serotonin syndrome.

Drug-Natural Products: ↑ risk of serotonergic side effects including serotonin syndrome with **St. John's wort**, **SAMe**, and **tryptophan**.

Route/Dosage

Depression

PO (Adults): 20 mg as a single dose in the morning; may be ↑ by 10 mg/day at weekly intervals (not to exceed 50 mg/day). *Controlled-release tablets*—25 mg once daily initially. May ↑ at weekly intervals by 12.5 mg (not to exceed 62.5 mg/day).

PO (Geriatric Patients or Debilitated Patients): 10 mg/day initially; may be slowly ↑ (not to exceed 40 mg/day). *Controlled-release tablets*—12.5 mg once daily initially; may be slowly ↑ (not to exceed 50 mg/day).

Obsessive-Compulsive Disorder

PO (Adults): 20 mg/day initially; ↑ by 10 mg/day at weekly intervals up to 40 mg (not to exceed 60 mg/day).

Panic Disorder

PO (Adults): 10 mg/day initially; ↑ by 10 mg/day at weekly intervals up to 40 mg (not to exceed 60 mg/day). *Controlled-release tablets*—12.5 mg/day initially; ↑ by 12.5 mg/day at weekly intervals (not to exceed 75 mg/day).

Social Anxiety Disorder

PO (Adults): 20 mg/day. *Controlled-release tablets*—12.5 mg/day initially; may ↑ by 12.5 mg/day weekly intervals (not to exceed 37.5 mg/day).

Generalized Anxiety Disorder

PO (Adults): 20 mg once daily initially; ↑ by 10 mg/day at weekly intervals (not to exceed 50 mg/day).

Post-traumatic Stress Disorder

PO (Adults): 20 mg/day initially; may be ↑ by 10 mg/day at weekly intervals (not to exceed 50 mg/day).

Premenstrual Dysphoric Disorder

PO (Adults): *Controlled-release tablets*—12.5 mg once daily throughout menstrual cycle or during luteal phase of menstrual cycle only; may be ↑ to 25 mg/day after one week.

Hepatic Impairment

PO (Adults): *Severe hepatic impairment*—10 mg/day initially; may be slowly ↑ (not to exceed 40 mg/day). *Controlled-release tablets*—12.5 mg once daily initially; may be slowly ↑ (not to exceed 50 mg/day).

Renal Impairment

PO (Adults): *Severe renal impairment*—10 mg/day initially; may be slowly ↑ (not to exceed 40 mg/day). *Controlled-release tablets*—12.5 mg once daily initially; may be slowly ↑ increased (not to exceed 50 mg/day).

Availability (generic available)

Paroxetine hydrochloride tablets: 10 mg, 20 mg, 30 mg, 40 mg. **Cost:** *Generic*—10 mg $89.96/90, 20 mg $28.99/90, 30 mg $101.97/90, 40 mg $110.96/90. **Paroxetine hydrochloride controlled-release tablets:** 12.5 mg, 25 mg, 37.5 mg. **Cost:** 12.5 mg $297.99/90, 25 mg $303.95/90, 37.5 mg $317.99/90. **Paroxetine hydrochloride oral suspension (orange flavor):** 10 mg/5 ml. **Cost:** $166.90/250 ml. **Paroxetine mesylate tablets:** 10 mg, 20 mg, 30 mg, 40 mg. **Cost:** 20 mg $352.95/90, 30 mg $256.21/90, 40 mg $383.97/90.

NURSING IMPLICATIONS

Assessment

- Monitor appetite and nutritional intake. Weigh weekly. Notify health care professional of continued weight loss. Adjust diet as tolerated to support nutritional status.
- **Depression:** Monitor mental status (orientation, mood, behavior). Inform health care professional if patient demonstrates significant increase in anxiety, nervousness, or insomnia.
- Assess for suicidal tendencies, especially during early therapy. Restrict amount of drug available to patient.

P

- **OCD:** Assess patient for frequency of obsessive-compulsive behaviors. Note degree to which these thoughts and behaviors interfere with daily functioning.
- **Panic Attacks:** Assess frequency and severity of panic attacks.
- **Social Anxiety Disorder:** Assess frequency and severity of episodes of anxiety.
- **Post-traumatic Stress Disorder:** Assess manifestations of post-traumatic stress disorder periodically during therapy.
- **Premenstrual Dysphoria:** Assess symptoms of premenstrual distress prior to and during therapy.
- ***Lab Test Considerations:*** Monitor CBC and differential periodically during therapy. Report leukopenia or anemia.

Potential Nursing Diagnoses

Ineffective coping (Indications)
Risk for injury (Side Effects)

Implementation

- Do not confuse paroxetine (Paxil) with paclitaxel (Taxol).
- Paroxetine mesylate (Pexeva) cannot be substituted with paroxetine (Paxil or Paxil CR) or generic paroxetine.
- Periodically reassess dose and continued need for therapy.
- **PO:** Administer as a single dose in the morning. May administer with food to minimize GI irritation.
- Tablets should be swallowed whole. Do not crush, break, or chew.
- Taper to avoid potential withdrawal reactions.

Patient/Family Teaching

- Instruct patient to take paroxetine as directed. Take missed doses as soon as possible and return to regular dosing schedule. Do not double doses. Caution patient to consult health care professional before discontinuing paroxetine. Daily doses should be decreased slowly. Abrupt withdrawal may cause dizziness, sensory disturbances, agitation, anxiety, nausea, and sweating.
- May cause drowsiness or dizziness. Caution patient to avoid driving and other activities requiring alertness until response to the drug is known.
- Advise patient to avoid alcohol or other CNS-depressant drugs during therapy and to consult with health care professional before taking other medications or herbal products with paroxetine.
- Inform patient that frequent mouth rinses, good oral hygiene, and sugarless gum or candy may minimize dry mouth. Saliva substitute may be used. Consult dentist if dry mouth persists for more than 2 wk.
- Instruct female patient to inform health care professional if pregnancy is planned or suspected or if she is breastfeeding.
- Advise patient to notify health care professional if headache, weakness, nausea, anorexia, anxiety, or insomnia persists.
- Emphasize the importance of follow-up exams to monitor progress. Encourage patient participation in psychotherapy to improve coping skills.
- Refer patient to local support group.

Evaluation/Desired Outcomes

- Increased sense of well-being.
- Renewed interest in surroundings. May require 1–4 wk of therapy to obtain antidepressant effects.
- Decrease in obsessive-compulsive behaviors.
- Decrease in frequency and severity of panic attacks.
- Decrease in frequency and severity of episodes of anxiety.
- Improvement in manifestations of post-traumatic stress disorder.
- Decreased dysphoria prior to menses.

pegaspargase

(peg-ass-**par**-jase)
Oncaspar, PEG-L-asparaginase

Classification
Therapeutic: antineoplastics
Pharmacologic: enzymes

Pregnancy Category C

Indications

Treatment (usually with other agents) of acute lymphoblastic leukemia (ALL) in patients who have had a previous hypersensitivity reaction to native asparaginase.

Action

Consists of L-asparaginase bound to polyethylene glycol (PEG). This compound depletes asparagine, which leukemic cells cannot synthesize. Normal cells are able to produce their own asparagine and are less susceptible to the effects of asparaginase. Binding to PEG renders asparaginase less antigenic and therefore less likely to induce hypersensitivity reactions. **Therapeutic Effects:** Death of leukemic cells.

Pharmacokinetics

Absorption: IV administration results in complete bioavailability.
Distribution: Unknown.
Metabolism and Excretion: Metabolized by serum proteases and in the reticuloendothelial system.
Half-life: 5.7 days (less in patients with previous hypersensitivity to native L-asparaginase).

TIME/ACTION PROFILE (hematologic effects)

ROUTE	ONSET	PEAK	DURATION
IV	rapid	unknown	14 days

Contraindications/Precautions

Contraindicated in: Pancreatitis or history of pancreatitis; History of previous hemorrhagic reaction to asparaginase therapy; Previous hypersensitivity reactions to pegaspargase.
Use Cautiously in: History of previous hypersensitivity reactions to other drugs; Patients with childbearing potential; OB: Pregnancy or lactation (safety not established).

Adverse Reactions/Side Effects

CNS: SEIZURES, headache, malaise. **GI:** PANCREATITIS, abdominal pain, abnormal liver function tests, anorexia, diarrhea, lip edema, nausea, vomiting. **Derm:** jaundice. **Endo:** hyperglycemia. **F and E:** peripheral edema. **Hemat:** decreased fibrinogen, disseminated intravascular coagulation, hemolytic anemia, increased thromboplastin, leukopenia, pancytopenia, thrombocytopenia. **Local:** injection site hypersensitivity, injection site pain, thrombosis. **MS:** arthralgia, myalgia, pain in extremities. **Neuro:** paresthesia. **Misc:** chills, hypersensitivity reactions, night sweats.

Interactions

Drug-Drug: May alter response to **anticoagulants** or **antiplatelet agents**. May alter the response to other **drugs that are metabolized by the liver**.

Route/Dosage

IM, IV (Adults up to 21 yr, and Children with Body Surface Area ≥0.6 m²): 2500 IU/m² q 14 days (usually in combination with other agents).
IM, IV (Children with Body Surface Area <0.6 m²): 82.5 IU/kg q 14 days (usually in combination with other agents).

Availability

Injection: 750 IU/ml.

NURSING IMPLICATIONS

Assessment

- Assess patient for previous hypersensitivity reactions to native L-asparaginase. Monitor for hypersensitivity reaction (urticaria, diaphoresis, facial swelling, joint pain, hypotension, bronchospasm). Epinephrine and resuscitation equipment should be readily available. Reaction may occur up to 2 hr after administration.
- Monitor for development of bone marrow depression. Assess for fever, sore throat, and signs of infection. Monitor platelet count throughout therapy. Assess for bleeding (bleeding gums, bruising, petechiae, guaiac test stools, urine, and emesis). Avoid giving IM injections and taking rectal temperatures. Apply pressure to venipuncture sites for 10 min. Anemia may occur. Monitor for increased fatigue, dyspnea, and orthostatic hypotension.
- Monitor patient frequently for signs of pancreatitis (nausea, vomiting, abdominal pain).
- Assess nausea, vomiting, and appetite. Weigh patient weekly. Prophylactic antiemetics may be used prior to administration.
- ***Lab Test Considerations:*** Monitor CBC prior to and periodically throughout therapy. May alter coagulation studies. Fibrinogen may be decreased; PT and partial thromboplastin time (PTT) may be ↑.
- Monitor serum amylase frequently to detect pancreatitis.
- Monitor blood glucose; may cause hyperglycemia.
- May cause elevated BUN and serum creatinine.
- Hepatotoxicity may be manifested by increased AST, ALT, or bilirubin. Liver function tests usually return to normal after therapy.
- May cause ↓ serum calcium.
- May cause elevated serum and urine uric acid and hyponatremia.

P

Potential Nursing Diagnoses

Risk for infection (Adverse Reactions)

Implementation

- Do not confuse pegaspargase with asparaginase.
- IM is the preferred route because of a lower incidence of adverse reactions.
- Solutions should be prepared in a biologic cabinet. Wear gloves, gown, and mask while handling medication. Discard equipment in specially designated containers.
- **IM:** Limit single injection volume to 2 ml. If volume of injection is >2 ml, use multiple injection sites.

IV Administration

- **Intermittent Infusion:** ***Diluent:*** Dilute each dose in 100 ml of 0.9% NaCl or D5W. Do not shake or agitate. Do not use if solution is cloudy or has formed a precipitate
- Use only 1 dose per vial; do not re-enter the vial. Discard unused portions.
- Keep refrigerated but do not freeze. Freezing destroys activity but does not change the appearance of pegaspargase. ***Rate:*** Administer over 1–2 hr via Y-site through an infusion that is already running.
- **Additive Incompatibility:** Information unavailable. Do not admix with other medications or solutions.

Patient/Family Teaching

- Inform patient of the possibility of hypersensitivity reactions, including anaphylaxis.
- Advise patient that concurrent use of other medications may increase the risk of bleeding and the toxicity of pegaspargase. Consult health care professional before taking any other medications, including OTC drugs.
- Instruct patient to notify health care professional if abdominal pain, severe nausea and vomiting, jaundice, fever, chills, sore throat, bleeding or bruising, excess thirst or urination, or mouth sores occur. Caution patient to avoid crowds and persons with known infections. Instruct patient to use soft toothbrush, electric razor, and to be especially careful to avoid falls. Patients should also be cautioned not to drink alcoholic beverages or take medications containing aspirin or NSAIDs because these may precipitate gastric bleeding.
- Instruct patient not to receive any vaccinations without advice of health care professional. Advise parents that this may alter child's immunization schedule.
- Emphasize the need for periodic lab tests to monitor for side effects.

Evaluation/Desired Outcomes

- Improvement of hematologic status in patients with leukemia.

pegfilgrastim

(peg-fil-**gra**-stim)
Neulasta

Classification
Therapeutic: colony-stimulating factors

Pregnancy Category C

Indications

To decrease the incidence of infection (febrile neutropenia) in patients with nonmyeloid malignancies receiving myelosuppressive antineoplastics associated with a high risk of febrile neutropenia.

Action

Filgrastim is a glycoprotein that binds to and stimulates neutrophils to divide and differentiate. Also activates mature neutrophils. Binding to a polyethylene glycol molecule prolongs its effects. **Therapeutic Effects:** Decreased incidence of infection in patients who are neutropenic from chemotherapy.

Pharmacokinetics

Absorption: Well absorbed following subcut administration.
Distribution: Unknown.
Metabolism and Excretion: Unknown.
Half-life: 15–80 hr.

TIME/ACTION PROFILE

ROUTE	ONSET	PEAK	DURATION
subcut	unknown	unknown	unknown

Contraindications/Precautions

Contraindicated in: Hypersensitivity to filgrastim or *Escherichia coli*-derived proteins.
Use Cautiously in: Patients with sickle cell disease (increased risk of sickle cell crisis); Concurrent use of lithium; Malignancy with myeloid characteristics; Pregnancy, lactation, or children (safety not established; 6 mg fixed dose should not be used in infants, children, and smaller adolescents weighing <45 kg; use in pregnancy only if potential benefits to mother justifies potential risk to the fetus).

Adverse Reactions/Side Effects

Resp: ADULT RESPIRATORY DISTRESS SYNDROME (ARDS). **GI:** SPLENIC RUPTURE. **Hemat:** SICKLE CELL CRISIS, leukocytosis. **MS:** medullary bone pain. **Misc:** allergic reaction including ANAPHYLAXIS.

Interactions

Drug-Drug: Simultaneous use with **antineoplastics** may have adverse effects on rapidly proliferating neutrophils; avoid use for 24 hr before and 24 hr following chemotherapy. **Lithium** may potentiate the release of neutrophils; concurrent use should be undertaken cautiously.

Route/Dosage

Subcut (Adults): 6 mg per chemotherapy cycle.

Availability

Solution for subcut injection: 6 mg/0.6 ml in prefilled syringes.

NURSING IMPLICATIONS

Assessment

- Assess patient for bone pain throughout therapy. Pain is usually mild to moderate and controllable with nonopioid analgesics, but may require opioid analgesics.
- Assess patient periodically for signs of ARDS (fever, lung infiltration, respiratory distress). If ARDS occurs, treat condition and discontinue pegfilgrastim and/or withold until symptoms resolve.
- ***Lab Test Considerations:*** Obtain CBC and platelet count before chemotherapy. Monitor hematocrit and platelet count regularly.
- May cause elevated LDH, alkaline phosphatase, and uric acid.

Potential Nursing Diagnoses

Risk for infection (Indications)
Acute pain (Side Effects)

Implementation

- Pegfilgrastim should not be administered between 14 and 24 days after administration of cytotoxic chemotherapy.
- Keep patients with sickle cell disease receiving pegfilgrastim well hydrated and monitor for sickle cell crisis.
- **Subcut:** Administer subcut once per chemotherapy cycle. Do not administer solutions that are discolored or contain particulate matter. Do not shake. Store refrigerated; may be allowed to reach room temperature for a maximum of 48 hr, but protect from light.
- Supplied in prefilled syringes. Following administration, activate UltraSafe Needle Guard to prevent needle sticks by placing hands behind needle, grasping guard with one hand, and sliding guard forward until needle is completely covered and guard clicks into place. If audible click is not heard, guard may not be completely activated. Dispose of by placing entire prefilled syringe with guard activated into puncture-proof container.

Patient/Family Teaching

- Advise patient to notify health care professional immediately if signs of allergic reaction (shortness of breath, hives, rash, pruritus, laryngeal edema) or signs of splenic rupture (left upper abdominal or shoulder tip pain) occur.
- Emphasize the importance of compliance with therapy and regular monitoring of blood counts.
- **Home Care Issues:** Instruct patient on correct disposal technique for home administration. Caution patient not to reuse needle, syringe, or drug product. Provide patient with a puncture-proof container for disposal of prefilled syringe.

Evaluation/Desired Outcomes

- Decreased incidence of infection in patients who receive bone marrow–depressing antineoplastics.

---

peginterferon alpha-2b/2a, See INTERFERONS, ALFA.

---

pemetrexed (pe-me-**trex**-ed)
Alimta

Classification
Therapeutic: antineoplastics
Pharmacologic: antimetabolites, folate antagonists

Pregnancy Category D

Indications

Malignant pleural mesothelioma (with cisplatin) when tumor is unresectable or patient is not a candidate for surgery. Local advanced or metastatic non-small cell lung cancer in previously treated patients.

Action

Disrupts folate dependent metabolic processes involved in thymidine and purine synthesis. Converted intracellularly to polyglutamate form which increases duration of action. **Therapeutic Effects:** Decreases growth and spread of mesothelioma.

Pharmacokinetics

Absorption: IV administration results in complete bioavailability.
Distribution: Unknown.
Metabolism and Excretion: Minimal metabolism; 70–90% excreted unchanged in urine.
Half-life: 3.5 hr (normal renal function).

TIME/ACTION PROFILE (hematologic effects)

ROUTE	ONSET	PEAK	DURATION
IV	unknown	8–15 days	21 days

Contraindications/Precautions

Contraindicated in: Hypersensitivity; CCr <45 ml/min; OB: Pregnancy, lactation.
Use Cautiously in: Concurrent use of NSAIDs (avoid those with short half-lives); CCr 45–80 ml/min; Third space fluid accumulation (ascites, pleural effusions); consider drainage prior to therapy; Hepatic impairment (dosage alteration recommended); Pedi: Children (safety not established).

Adverse Reactions/Side Effects

Resp: pharyngitis. **CV:** chest pain. **GI:** constipation, nausea, stomatitis, vomiting, anorexia, diarrhea, esophagitis, mouth pain. **Derm:** desquamation, rash. **Hemat:** anemia, leukopenia, thrombocytopenia. **Neuro:** neuropathy. **Misc:** fever, infection.

Interactions

Drug-Drug: NSAIDs, especially those with short half-lives, ↑ blood levels and risk of toxicity; avoid for 2 days before, day of and 2 days after treatment. **Probenecid** ↑ blood levels. Concurrent use of **nephrotoxic agents** ↑ risk of nephrotoxicity.

Route/Dosage

IV (Adults): *Mesothelioma*—500 mg/m^2 on day 1 of each 21 day cycle (with cisplatin); concurrent hydration, folic acid, vitamin B_{12}, pretreatment with dexamethasone required. Dose adjustments for hematologic, non-hematologic toxicities and neurotoxicity recommended. *Non–small cell lung cancer* 500 mg/m^2 on day 1 of each 21 day cycle (pretreatment with corticosteroids, folic acid and vitamin B_{12} recommended). Dose adjustments for hematologic, non-hematologic toxicities and neurotoxicity recommended.

Availability

Lyophilized powder for IV infusion: 500 mg/vial.

NURSING IMPLICATIONS

Assessment

- Monitor for rash during therapy. Pretreatment with dexamethasone 4 mg orally twice daily the day before, the day of, and the day after administration reduces incidence and severity or reaction.
- Monitor for hematologic and GI (mucositis, diarrhea) toxicities. If any Grade 3 or 4 toxicities, except mucositis or diarrhea, requiring hospitalization occur, decrease doses of pemetrexed and cisplatin by 75%. If Grade 3 or 4 mucositis occurs decrease pemetrexed dose by 50% and cisplatin by 100% of previous dose.
- Monitor for bone marrow depression. Assess for bleeding (bleeding gums, bruising, petechiae, guaiac stools, urine, and emesis) and avoid IM injections and taking rectal temperatures if platelet count is low. Apply pressure to venipuncture sites for 10 min. Assess for signs of infection during neutropenia. Anemia may occur; monitor for increased fatigue, dyspnea, and orthostatic hypotension.
- Assess for neurotoxicity during therapy. If Grade 0–1 neurotoxicity occurs, decrease pemetrexed and cisplatin doses by 100% of previous dose. If Grade 2 neurotoxicity occurs, decrease pemetrexed dose by 100% and cisplatin dose by 50% of previous dose. If Grade 3 or 4 neurotoxicity occurs, discontinue therapy.
- ***Lab Test Considerations:*** Monitor CBC and platelet counts for nadir and recovery, before each dose and on days 8 and 15 of each cycle and chemistry for renal and liver functions periodically. May cause neutropenia, thrombocytopenia, leukopenia, and anemia. A new cycle should not be started unless the ANC is at least 1500 cells/mm^3, platelet count is at least 100,000 cells/mm^3, and creatinine clearance is at least 45 mL/min. If nadir of ANC is less than 500/mm^3 and nadir of

platelets are at least 50,000/mm³ decrease doses of pemetrexed and cisplatin by 75%. If nadir of platelets is less than 50,000/mm³ regardless of ANC nadir decrease pemetrexed and cisplatin doses by 50%.

Potential Nursing Diagnoses

Risk for injury (Adverse Reactions)

Implementation

- Pemetrexed should be administered under supervision of a physician experienced in the use of chemotherapeutic agents.
- Solution should be prepared in a biologic cabinet. Wear gloves, gown, and mask while handling medication. Discard equipment in designated containers.
- To reduce toxicity, at least 5 mg of folic acid must be taken daily for 7 days preceding first dose of pemetrexed and should continue during and for 21 days after last dose. Patients must also receive an injection of vitamin B_{12} 1000 mcg during the week preceding first dose of pemetrexed and every 3 cycles thereafter. Subsequent doses of vitamin B_{12} may be given on same day as pemetrexed.

IV Administration

- **Intermittent Infusion:** Calculate number of pemetrexed 500-mg vials needed; vials contain excess to facilitate delivery. ***Diluent:*** Reconstitute 500 mg with 20 mL of preservative–free 0.9% NaCl for a solution containing 25 mg/mL. Swirl gently until powder is completely dissolved. Solution is clear and colorless to yellow or green-yellow. Do not administer if discolored or containing particulate matter. Dilute further to 100 mL with preservative–free 0.9% NaCl. Solution is stable at room temperature or if refrigerated for up to 24 hr. ***Rate:*** Administer over 10 min.
- **Y-Site Compatibility:** acyclovir, amifostine, amikacin, ampicillin, amipicillin/sulbactam, aztreonam, bumetanide, buprenorphine, butorphanol, carboplatin, ceftizoxime, ceftriaxone, cefuroxime, cimetidine, cisplatin, clindamycin, cyclophosphamide, cytarabine, dexamethasone sodium phosphate, dexrazoxane, diphenhydramine, docetaxel, dopamine, enalaprilat, famotidine, fluconazole, fluorouracil, ganciclovir, granisetron, haloperidol, heparin, hydromoorphone, ifosfamide, leucovorin, lorazepam, mannitol, meperidine, mesna, methylprednisolone sodium succinate, metoclopramide, morphine, paclitaxel, potassium chloride, promethazine, ranitidine, sodium bicarbonate, ticarcillin/clavulanate, trimethoprim/sulfamethoxazole, vancomycin, vinblastine, vincristine, zidoudine.
- **Y-Site Incompatibility:** amphotericin B, cefazolin, cefotaxime, cefoxitin, ceftazidime, chlorpromazine, ciprofloxacin, dobutamine, doxorubicin, doxycycline, droperidol, gemcitabine, gentamicin, irinotecan, metronidazole, mitoxantrone, nalbuphine, ondansetron, prochlorperazine, tobramycin, topotecan.
- **Additive Incompatibility:** Solutions containing calcium, including Lactated Ringer's and Ringer's solution.

Patient/Family Teaching

- Emphasize the importance of taking prophylactic folic acid and vitamin B_{12} to reduce treatment-related hematologic and GI toxicity.
- OB: Advise patient to avoid becoming pregnant during therapy. If pregnancy is planned or suspected notify health care professional promptly.

Evaluation/Desired Outcomes

- Decreased growth and spread of mesothelioma or non-small cell lung cancer.

penciclovir

(pen-**sye**-kloe-veer)
Denavir

Classification
Therapeutic: antivirals (topical)

Pregnancy Category B

Indications

Recurrent herpes labialis (cold sores).

Action

Inhibits viral DNA synthesis and replication. **Therapeutic Effects:** Death of herpes virus. Decreased lesion duration and pain. Active against herpes viruses.

Pharmacokinetics

Absorption: Not absorbed following topical use.
Distribution: Unknown.

P

Metabolism and Excretion: Converted intracellularly to active triphosphate form; excreted in urine.
Half-life: 2–2.5 hr.

TIME/ACTION PROFILE

ROUTE	ONSET	PEAK	DURATION
topical	unknown	unknown	unknown

Contraindications/Precautions
Contraindicated in: Hypersensitivity to penciclovir or other components of the formulation.
Use Cautiously in: Pregnancy, lactation, or children (safety not established).

Adverse Reactions/Side Effects
CNS: headache. **Local:** application site reactions.

Interactions
Drug-Drug: None significant.

Route/Dosage
PO (Adults): Apply 1% cream q 2 hr for 4 days while awake.

Availability
Cream: 1% in 2-g tubes.

NURSING IMPLICATIONS

Assessment
- Assess lesions prior to and daily during therapy.

Potential Nursing Diagnoses
Risk for impaired skin integrity (Indications)
Risk for infection (Indications, Patient/Family Teaching)
Deficient knowledge, related to medication regimen (Patient/Family Teaching)

Implementation
- Do not confuse Denavir (penciclovir) with indinivir.
- Begin treatment as early as possible, during prodrome or when lesions appear.
- **Topical:** Apply to lesions every 2 hr for 4 days while awake.
- Apply to lips and face only; avoid application to mucous membranes or near the eyes.

Patient/Family Teaching
- Advise patient to apply medication exactly as directed for the full course of therapy. If a dose is missed, apply as soon as possible but not just before next dose is due; do not double doses. Penciclovir should not be used more frequently or longer than prescribed.
- Advise patients that the additional use of OTC creams, lotions, and ointments may delay healing and may cause spreading of lesions.

Evaluation/Desired Outcomes
- More rapid healing of lesions and relief of pain in herpes labialis.

PENICILLINS (pen-i-**sill**-ins)

penicillin G
Pfizerpen

penicillin V
✤Apo-Pen VK, ✤Crystapen, ✤Novo-Pen-VK, ✤Nu-Pen-VK, ✤Penicilline V

procaine penicillin G
Wycillin

benzathine penicillin G
Bicillin L-A, Permapen

Classification
Therapeutic: anti-infectives
Pharmacologic: penicillins

Pregnancy Category B

Indications
Treatment of a wide variety of infections including: Pneumococcal pneumonia, Streptococcal pharyngitis, Syphilis, Gonorrhea strains. Treatment of enterococcal infections (requires the addition of an aminoglycoside). Prevention of rheumatic fever. Should not be used as a single agent to treat anthrax. **Unlabeled uses:** Treatment of Lyme disease. Prevention of recurrent *Streptococcal pneumoniae* septicemia in children with sickle-cell disease.

Action
Bind to bacterial cell wall, resulting in cell death. **Therapeutic Effects:** Bactericidal action against susceptible bacteria. **Spectrum:** Active against: Most gram-positive organisms, including many streptococci (*Streptococcus pneumoniae*, group A beta-hemolytic streptococci), staphylococci (non–penicillinase-producing strains) and *Bacillus anthracis*. Some gram-negative organisms, such as *Neisseria meningitidis* and *Neisseria gonorrhoeae* (only penicillin susceptible strains). Some anaerobic bacteria and spirochetes including *Borellia burgdorferi*.

Pharmacokinetics

Absorption: Variably absorbed from the GI tract. *Penicillin V*—resists acid degradation in the GI tract. *Procaine and benzathine penicillin*—IM absorption is delayed and prolonged and results in sustained therapeutic blood levels.
Distribution: Widely distributed, although CNS penetration is poor in the presence of uninflamed meninges. Cross the placenta and enter breast milk.
Metabolism and Excretion: Minimally metabolized by the liver, excreted mainly unchanged by the kidneys.
Half-life: 30–60 min.

TIME/ACTION PROFILE (blood levels)

ROUTE	ONSET	PEAK	DURATION
penicillin V PO	rapid	0.5–1 hr	4–6 hr
penicillin G IM	rapid	0.25–0.5 hr	4–6 hr
benzathine penicillin IM	delayed	12–24 hr	3 wk
procaine penicillin IM	delayed	1–4 hr	12 hr
penicillin G IV	rapid	end of infusion	4–6 hr

Contraindications/Precautions

Contraindicated in: Previous hypersensitivity to penicillins (cross-sensitivity may exist with cephalosporins and other beta-lactams); Hypersensitivity to procaine or benzathine (procaine and benzathine preparations only); Some products may contain tartrazine and should be avoided in patients with known hypersensitivity.
Use Cautiously in: Geri: Geriatric patients (consider decreased body mass, age-related decrease in renal/hepatic/cardiac function, intercurrent diseases and drug therapy); Severe renal insufficiency (dose reduction recommended); OB: Pregnancy (although safety not established, has been used safely); Lactation (safety not established).

Adverse Reactions/Side Effects

CNS: SEIZURES. **GI:** diarrhea, epigastric distress, nausea, vomiting, pseudomembranous colitis. **GU:** interstitial nephritis. **Derm:** rashes, urticaria. **Hemat:** eosinophilia, hemolytic anemia, leukopenia. **Local:** pain at IM site, phlebitis AT IV SITE. **Misc:** allergic reactions including ANAPHYLAXIS and SERUM SICKNESS, superinfection.

Interactions

Drug-Drug: Penicillin may ↓ effectiveness of oral contraceptive agents. **Probenecid** ↓ renal excretion and ↑ blood levels of penicillin (therapy may be combined for this purpose). **Neomycin** may ↓ absorption of penicillin V. ↓ elimination of **methotrexate** and ↑ risk of serious toxicity.

Route/Dosage

Penicillin G (aqueous)

IM, IV (Adults): *Most infections*—1–5 million units q 4–6 hr.
IM, IV (Children): 8333–16,667 units/kg q 4 hr; 12,550–25,000 units/kg q 6 hr; up to 250,000 units/kg/day in divided doses, some infections may require up to 300,000 units/kg/day.
IV (Infants >7 days): 25,000 units/kg q 8 hr; *meningitis*—50,000–75,000 units/kg q 6 hr.
IV (Infants <7 days): 25,000 units/kg q 12 hr; *Streptococcus B meningitis*—100,000–150,000 units/kg/day in divided doses.

Penicillin V

PO (Adults and Children ≥12 yr): *Most infections*—125–500 mg q 6–8 hr. *Rheumatic fever prevention*—125–250 mg q 12 hr.
PO (Children <12 yr): *Lyme disease*—12.5 mg/kg q 6 hr (unlabeled); prevention of *Streptococcus pneumoniae* sepsis in children with sickle cell disease—125 mg twice daily.

Benzathine Penicillin G

IM (Adults): *Streptococcal infections/erysipeloid*—1.2 million units single dose. *Primary, secondary, and early latent syphilis*—2.4 million units single dose. *Tertiary and late latent syphilis (not neurosyphilis)*—2.4 million units once weekly for 3 wk. *Prevention of rheumatic fever*—1.2 million units q 3–4 wk.
IM (Children >27 kg): *Streptococcal infections/erysipeloid*—900,000–1.2 million units (single dose). *Primary, secondary, and early latent syphilis*—up to 2.4 million units single dose. *Late latent or latent syphilis of undetermined duration*—50,000 units/kg weekly for 3 wk. *Prevention of rheumatic fever*—1.2 million units q 2–3 wk.
IM (Children <27 kg): *Streptococcal infections/erysipeloid*—300,000–600,000 units

single dose. *Primary, secondary, and early latent syphilis*—up to 2.4 million units single dose. *Late latent or latent syphilis of undetermined duration*—50,000 units/kg weekly for 3 wk. *Prevention of rheumatic fever*—1.2 million units q 2–3 wk.

Procaine Penicillin G

IM (Adults): *Moderate or severe infections*—600,000–1.2 million units/day as a single dose or in 2 divided doses. *Neurosyphilis*—2.4 million units/day with 500 mg probenecid PO 4 times daily for 10–14 days.
IM (Children): *Congenital syphilis*—50,000 units/kg/day for 10–14 days.

Availability

Penicillin G Potassium

Powder for injection: 5 million units/vial, 20 million units/vial. **Premixed (frozen) solution for injection:** 1 million units/50 ml, 2 million units/50 ml, 3 million units/50 ml.

Penicillin G Sodium

Powder for injection: 5 million units/vial.

Penicillin V Potassium

Tablets: 250 mg, 500 mg. **Oral solution:** 125 mg/5 ml, 250 mg/5 ml.

Procaine Penicillin G

Suspension for IM injection: 600,000 units/ml in 1-ml and 2-ml prefilled syringes.

Benzathine Penicillin G

Suspension for IM injection: 600,000 units/ml in 1-, 2-, and 4-ml prefilled syringes.

NURSING IMPLICATIONS

Assessment

- Assess for infection (vital signs; appearance of wound, sputum, urine, and stool; WBC) at beginning of and during therapy.
- Obtain a history to determine previous use of and reactions to penicillins, cephalosporins, or other beta-lactam antibiotics. Persons with a negative history of penicillin sensitivity may still have an allergic response.
- Obtain specimens for culture and sensitivity before initiating therapy. First dose may be given before receiving results.
- Observe patient for signs and symptoms of anaphylaxis (rash, pruritus, laryngeal edema, wheezing). Discontinue drug and health care professional immediately if these symptoms occur. Keep epinephrine, an antihistamine, and resuscitation equipment close by in case of an anaphylactic reaction.
- ***Lab Test Considerations:*** May cause positive direct Coombs' test results.
- Hyperkalemia may develop after large doses of penicillin G potassium.
- Monitor serum sodium concentrations in patient with hypertension or CHF. Hypernatremia may develop after large doses of penicillin sodium.
- May cause ↑ AST, ALT, LDH, and serum alkaline phosphatase concentrations.
- May cause leukopenia and neutropenia, especially with prolonged therapy or hepatic impairment.

Potential Nursing Diagnoses

Risk for infection (Indications, Side Effects)
Noncompliance (Patient/Family Teaching)

Implementation

- Do not confuse penicillin with penicillamine. Do not confuse penicillin G aqueous (potassium or sodium salt) with penicillin G procaine.
- **PO:** Administer around the clock. Penicillin V may be administered without regard for meals.
- Use calibrated measuring device for liquid preparations. Solution is stable for 14 days if refrigerated.
- **IM:** Reconstitute according to manufacturer's directions with sterile water for injection, D5W, or 0.9% NaCl.
- **IM:** Shake medication well before injection. Inject penicillin deep into a well-developed muscle mass at a slow, consistent rate to prevent blockage of the needle. Massage well. Accidental injury near or into a nerve can result in severe pain and dysfunction.
- Penicillin G potassium or sodium may be diluted with lidocaine (without epinephrine) 1% or 2% to minimize pain from IM injection.
- Never give penicillin G benzathine or penicillin G procaine suspensions IV. May cause embolism or toxic reactions.

IV Administration

- **IV:** Change IV sites every 48 hr to prevent phlebitis
- Administer slowly and observe patient closely for signs of hypersensitivity.
- **Intermittent Infusion:** ***Diluent:*** Doses of 3 million units or less should be diluted in at least 50 ml of D5W or 0.9% NaCl; doses of more than 3 million units should be diluted with 100 ml. ***Concentration:*** 100,000–

500,000 units/ml (50,000 units/ml in neonates). ***Rate:*** Infuse over 1–2 hr in adults or 15–30 min in children.
- **Continuous Infusion:** Doses of 10 million units or more may be diluted in 1 or 2 L. ***Rate:*** Infuse over 24 hr.

Penicillin G Potassium
- **Y-Site Compatibility:** acyclovir, amiodarone, cyclophosphamide, diltiazem, enalaprilat, esmolol, fluconazole, foscarnet, heparin, hydromorphone, labetalol, magnesium sulfate, meperidine, morphine, nicardipine, perphenazine, potassium chloride, tacrolimus, theophylline, verapamil, vitamin B complex with C.
- **Y-Site Incompatibility:** If aminoglycosides and penicillins must be administered concurrently, administer in separate sites at least 1 hr apart.
- **Additive Incompatibility:** Incompatible with aminoglycosides; do not admix.

Penicillin G Sodium
- **Y-Site Compatibility:** levofloxacin.
- **Y-Site Incompatibility:** If aminoglycosides and penicillins must be administered concurrently, administer in separate sites at least 1 hr apart.
- **Additive Incompatibility:** Incompatible with aminoglycosides; do not admix.

Patient/Family Teaching
- Instruct patient to take medication around the clock and to finish drug completely as directed, even if feeling better. Advise patient that sharing this medication may be dangerous.
- Advise patient to report signs of superinfection (black, furry overgrowth on tongue; vaginal itching or discharge; loose or foul-smelling stools) and allergy.
- Instruct patient to notify health care professional if fever and diarrhea develop, especially if stool contains blood, pus, or mucus. Advise patient not to treat diarrhea without consulting health care professional.
- Instruct patient to notify health care professional if symptoms do not improve.
- Advise patient taking oral contraceptives to use an additional nonhormonal method of contraception during therapy with penicillin and until next menstrual period.
- Patient with an allergy to penicillin should be instructed to always carry an identification card with this information.

Evaluation/Desired Outcomes
- Resolution of signs and symptoms of infection. Length of time for complete resolution depends on the organism and site of infection.

PENICILLINS, PENICILLINASE RESISTANT

cloxacillin (klox-a-**sill**-in)
✤Apo-Cloxi, Cloxapen, ✤Novo-Cloxin, ✤Nu-Cloxi

dicloxacillin (dye-klox-a-**sill**-in)

nafcillin (naf-**sill**-in)

oxacillin (ox-a-**sill**-in)
Bactocill

Classification
Therapeutic: anti-infectives
Pharmacologic: penicillinase–resistant penicillins

Pregnancy Category B

Indications
Treatment of the following infections due to penicillinase-producing staphylococci: Respiratory tract infections, Sinusitis, Skin and skin structure infections. **Dicloxacillin:** Osteomyelitis. **Nafcillin, oxacillin:** Are also used to treat: Bone and joint infections, Urinary tract infections, Endocarditis, Septicemia, Meningitis.

Action
Bind to bacterial cell wall, leading to cell death. Not inactivated by penicillinase enzymes. **Therapeutic Effects:** Bactericidal action. **Spectrum:** Active against most gram-positive aerobic cocci but less so than penicillin. Spectrum is notable for activity against: Penicillinase-producing strains of *Staphylococcus aureus*, *Staphylococcus epidermidis*. Not active against methicillin-resistant staphylococci.

Pharmacokinetics
Absorption: *Cloxacillin*—Moderately absorbed (50%) following oral administration. *Dicloxacillin*—Rapidly but incompletely (35–76%) absorbed from the GI tract. *Nafcillin and*

oxacillin—Completely absorbed following IV administration; well absorbed from IM sites.
Distribution: Widely distributed; penetration into CSF is minimal, but sufficient in the presence of inflamed meninges; cross the placenta and enter breast milk.
Metabolism and Excretion: *Cloxacillin*—Some metabolism by the liver (9–22%) and some renal excretion of unchanged drug (30–45%). *Dicloxacillin*—Some metabolism by the liver (6–10%) and some renal excretion of unchanged drug (60%); small amounts eliminated in the feces via the bile. *Nafcillin, oxacillin*—Partially metabolized by the liver (nafcillin 60%, oxacillin 49%), partially excreted unchanged by the kidneys.
Half-life: *Cloxacillin and dicloxacillin*—0.5–1.1 hr (↑ in severe hepatic and renal dysfunction); *nafcillin*—Neonates: 1–5 hr; Children 1 month–14 yr: 0.75–1.9 hr; Adults: 0.5–1.5 hr (↑ in renal impairment); *oxacillin*—Neonates: 1.6 hr; Children up to 2 yr: 0.9–1.8 hr; Adults: 0.3–0.8 hr (↑ in severe hepatic impairment).

TIME/ACTION PROFILE (blood levels)

ROUTE	ONSET	PEAK	DURATION
cloxacillin PO	30 min	30–120 min	6 hr
dicloxacillin PO	30 min	30–120 min	6 hr
nafcillin IM	30 min	60–120 min	4–6 hr
nafcillin IV	rapid	end of infusion	4–6 hr
oxacillin IM	rapid	30 min	4–6 hr
oxacillin IV	rapid	end of infusion	4–6 hr

Contraindications/Precautions

Contraindicated in: Hypersensitivity to penicillins (cross-sensitivity with cephalosporins may exist).
Use Cautiously in: Severe renal or hepatic impairment; OB: Pregnancy or lactation (safety not established).

Adverse Reactions/Side Effects

CNS: SEIZURES (high doses). **GI:** PSEUDOMEMBRANOUS COLITIS, diarrhea, nausea, vomiting, drug-induced hepatitis. **GU:** interstitial nephritis. **Derm:** rashes, urticaria. **Hemat:** eosinophilia, leukopenia. **Local:** pain at IM sites, phlebitis at IV sites. **Misc:** allergic reactions including ANAPHYLAXIS and SERUM SICKNESS, superinfection.

Interactions

Drug-Drug: Probenecid ↓ renal excretion and ↑ blood levels (treatment may be combined for this purpose). May ↓ effectiveness of **oral contraceptive agents**. May ↓ elimination of **methotrexate** and ↑ risk of serious toxicity.

Route/Dosage

Cloxacillin

PO (Adults): 250–500 mg q 6 hr.
PO (Children >1 mo): 12.5–25 mg/kg q 6 hr up to a maximum of 4 g/day.

Dicloxacillin

PO (Adults and Children ≥40 kg): 125–250 mg q 6 hr (up to 2 g/day).
PO (Children <40 kg): 6.25–12.5 mg/kg q 6 hr; (up to 12.25 mg/kg q 6 hr has been used for osteomyelitis), maximum: 2 g/day.

Nafcillin

IM (Adults): 500-mg q 4–6 hr.
IM, IV (Children and Infants): 50–200 mg/kg/day divided q 4–6 hr, maximum: 12 g/day.
IM, IV (Neonates 0–4 weeks, <1200 g): 25 mg/kg q 12 hr.
IM, IV (Neonates 1.2–2 kg):—25 mg/kg q 12 hr for the first 7 days of life, then 25 mg/kg q 8 hr.
IM, IV (Neonates >2 kg):—25 mg/kg q 8 hr for the first 7 days of life, then 25 mg/kg q 6 hr.
IV (Adults): 500–2000 mg q 4–6 hr.

Oxacillin

IM, IV (Adults and Children ≥40 kg): 250–2000 mg q 4–6 hr (up to 12 g/day).
IM, IV (Children <40 kg): 100–200 mg/kg/day divided q 4–6 hr, maximum: 12 g/day.
IM, IV (Neonates <1200 g):—25 mg/kg q 12 hr.
IM, IV (Neonates ≥2 kg):—25 mg/kg q 8 hr for the first 7 days of life, then 25 mg/kg q 6 hr.
IM, IV (Neonates 1.2–2 kg):—25 mg/kg q 12 hr for the first 7 days of life, then 25 mg/kg q 8 hr.

Availability

Cloxacillin

Capsules: 250 mg, 500 mg. **Oral solution:** 125 mg/5 ml. **Powder for injection:** ✤500-mg vial, ✤1-g vial, ✤2-g vial.

Dicloxacillin

Capsules: 250 mg, 500 mg. **Oral suspension:** 62.5 mg/5 ml.

Nafcillin

Powder for injection: 500-mg vial, 1-g vial, 2-g vial, 10-g vial.

Oxacillin

Powder for injection: 250-mg vial, 500-mg vial, 1-g vial, 2-g vial, 4-g vial, 10-g vial.

NURSING IMPLICATIONS

Assessment

- Assess patient for infection (vital signs; appearance of wound, sputum, urine, and stool; WBC) at beginning of and throughout therapy.
- Obtain a history before initiating therapy to determine previous use of and reactions to penicillins, cephalosporins, or other beta-lactam antibiotics. Persons with a negative history of penicillin sensitivity may still have an allergic response.
- Obtain specimens for culture and sensitivity prior to initiating therapy. First dose may be given before receiving results.
- Observe patient for signs and symptoms of anaphylaxis (rash, pruritus, laryngeal edema, wheezing, abdominal pain). Discontinue the drug and notify the physician or other health care professional immediately if these occur. Keep epinephrine, an antihistamine, and resuscitation equipment close by in the event of an anaphylactic reaction.
- Assess vein for signs of irritation and phlebitis. Change IV site every 48 hr to prevent phlebitis.
- ***Lab Test Considerations:*** May cause leukopenia and neutropenia, especially with prolonged therapy or hepatic impairment.
- May cause positive direct Coombs' test result.
- May cause ↑ AST, ALT, LDH, and serum alkaline phosphatase concentrations.

Potential Nursing Diagnoses

Risk for infection (Indications, Side Effects)
Noncompliance (Patient/Family Teaching)

Implementation

- **PO:** Administer around the clock on an empty stomach at least 1 hr before or 2 hr after meals. Take with a full glass of water; acidic juices may decrease absorption of penicillins.
- Use calibrated measuring device for liquid preparations. Shake well. Solution is stable for 14 days if refrigerated.

Nafcillin

IV Administration

- **IV, IM:** To reconstitute, add 3.4 ml to each 1-g vial or 6.8 ml to each 2-g vial, for a concentration of 250 mg/ml. Stable for 2–7 days if refrigerated.
- **Direct IV: *Diluent:*** Dilute reconstituted solution with 15–30 ml of sterile water, 0.45% NaCl, or 0.9% NaCl for injection. ***Concentration:*** 100 mg/ml. ***Rate:*** Administer over 5–10 min.
- **Intermittent Infusion: *Diluent:*** Dilute with sterile water for injection, 0.9% NaCl, D5W, D10W, D5/0.25% NaCl, D5/0.45% NaCl, D5/0.9% NaCl, D5/LR, Ringer's or LR. Stable for 24 hr at room temperature, 96 hr if refrigerated. ***Concentration:*** 2–40 mg/ml. ***Rate:*** Infuse over at least 30–60 min to avoid vein irritation.
- **Y-Site Compatibility:** acyclovir, atropine, cyclophosphamide, diazepam, enalaprilat, esmolol, famotidine, fentanyl, fluconazole, foscarnet, heparin, hydromorphone, magnesium sulfate, morphine, nicardipine, perphenazine, propofol, theophylline, zidovudine.
- **Y-Site Incompatibility:** droperidol, insulin, labetalol, midazolam, nalbuphine, pentazocine, verapamil. If penicillins and aminoglycosides must be administered concurrently, administer at separate sites.

Oxacillin

IV Administration

- **IV, IM:** To reconstitute for IM or IV use, add 1.4 ml of sterile water for injection to each 250-mg vial, 2.7 ml to each 500-mg vial, 5.7 ml to each 1-g vial, 11.5 ml to each 2-g vial, and 23 ml to each 4-g vial, for a concentration of 250 mg/1.5 ml. Stable for 3 days at room temperature or 7 days if refrigerated.
- **Direct IV: *Diluent:*** Further dilute each reconstituted 250-mg or 500-mg vial with 5 ml of sterile water or 0.9% NaCl for injection, 10 ml for each 1-g vial, 20 ml for each 2-g vial, and 40 ml for each 4-g vial. ***Concentration:*** 100 mg/ml. ***Rate:*** Administer slowly over 10 min.
- **Intermittent Infusion: *Diluent:*** Dilute with 0.9% NaCl, D5W, D5/0.9% NaCl, or LR. ***Concentration:*** 0.5–40 mg/ml. ***Rate:*** May be infused for up to 6 hr.

P

- **Y-Site Compatibility:** acyclovir, cyclophosphamide, diltiazem, doxapram, famotidine, fluconazole, foscarnet, heparin, hydrocortisone sodium succinate, hydromorphone, labetalol, levofloxacin, magnesium sulfate, meperidine, methotrexate, milrinone, morphine, perphenazine, potassium chloride, tacrolimus, vitamin B complex with C, zidovudine.
- **Y-Site Incompatibility:** sodium bicarbonate, verapamil. If penicillins and aminoglycosides must be administered concurrently, administer at separate sites.

Patient/Family Teaching

- Instruct patient to take medication around the clock and to finish the drug completely as directed, even if feeling better. Missed doses should be taken as soon as remembered. Advise patient that sharing of this medication may be dangerous.
- Advise patient to report signs of superinfection (black, furry overgrowth on the tongue; vaginal itching or discharge; loose or foul-smelling stools) and allergy.
- Instruct patient to notify health care professional if fever and diarrhea develop, especially if stool contains blood, pus, or mucus. Advise patient not to treat diarrhea without consulting health care professional.
- Instruct patient to notify health care professional if symptoms do not improve.

Evaluation/Desired Outcomes

- Resolution of the signs and symptoms of infection. Length of time for complete resolution depends on the organism and site of infection.

pentamidine (pen-**tam**-i-deen)

NebuPent, Pentam 300, ✤Pentacarinat, ✤Pneumopent

Classification

Therapeutic: antiprotozoals

Pregnancy Category C

Indications

IV: Treatment of *Pneumocystis carinii* pneumonia (PCP). **Inhaln:** Prevention of PCP in AIDS or HIV-positive patients who have had PCP or who have a peripheral CD4 lymphocyte count of ≤200/mm^3. **Unlabeled uses: Inhaln:** Treatment of PCP.

Action

Appears to disrupt DNA or RNA synthesis in protozoa. Also has a direct toxic effect on pancreatic islet cells. **Therapeutic Effects:** Death of susceptible protozoa.

Pharmacokinetics

Absorption: Minimal systemic absorption occurs following inhalation.
Distribution: Widely and extensively distributed but does not cross the blood-brain barrier. Concentrates in liver, kidneys, lungs, and spleen, with prolonged storage in some tissues.
Metabolism and Excretion: 1–30% excreted unchanged by the kidneys. Remainder of metabolic fate unknown.
Half-life: 6.4–9.4 hr (increased in renal impairment).

TIME/ACTION PROFILE (blood levels)

ROUTE	ONSET	PEAK	DURATION
IV	unknown	end of infusion	24 hr
Inhaln	unknown	unknown	unknown

Contraindications/Precautions

Contraindicated in: History of previous anaphylactic reaction to pentamidine.
Use Cautiously in: Hypotension; Hypertension; Hypoglycemia; Hyperglycemia; Hypocalcemia; Leukopenia; Thrombocytopenia; Anemia; Renal impairment (dose reduction required); Diabetes mellitus; Liver impairment; Cardiovascular disease; Bone marrow depression, previous antineoplastic therapy, or radiation therapy; OB: Pregnancy or lactation (safety not established during pregnancy; breastfeeding not recommended).

Adverse Reactions/Side Effects

For parenteral form, unless otherwise indicated.
CNS: anxiety, headache, confusion, dizziness, hallucinations. **EENT:** *inhalation*— burning in throat. **Resp:** *inhalation*— bronchospasm, cough. **CV:** ARRHYTHMIAS, HYPOTENSION. **GI:** PANCREATITIS, abdominal pain, anorexia, drug-induced hepatitis, nausea, unpleasant metallic taste, vomiting. **GU:** nephrotoxicity. **Derm:** pallor, rash. **Endo:** HYPOGLYCEMIA, hyperglycemia. **F and E:** hyperkalemia, hypocalcemia. **Hemat:** anemia, leukopenia, thrombocytopenia. **Local: IV:**—phlebitis, pruritus, urticaria at IV site. **IM:**—sterile abscesses at IM sites. **Misc:** allergic reactions including ANAPHYLAXIS, STEVENS-JOHNSON SYNDROME, chills, fever.

Interactions

Interactions listed for parenteral administration

Drug-Drug: Concurrent use with **erythromycin** IV may ↑ risk of potentially fatal arrhythmias. Additive nephrotoxicity with other **nephrotoxic agents**, including **aminoglycosides**, **amphotericin B**, and **vancomycin**. Additive bone marrow depression with **antineoplastics** or previous **radiation therapy**. ↑ risk of pancreatitis with **didanosine**. ↑ risk of nephrotoxicity, hypocalcemia, and hypomagnesemia with **foscarnet**.

Route/Dosage

IV (Adults and Children): 4 mg/kg once daily for 14–21 days (longer treatment may be required in AIDS patients; some patients may respond to 3 mg/kg/day).

Inhaln (Adults): *NebuPent, Pentacarinat*—300 mg q 4 wk, using a Respirgard II jet nebulizer (150 mg q 2 wk has also been used). *Pneumopent*—60 mg q 24–72 hr for 5 doses over a 2-wk period, then q 2 wk using a Fisoneb ultrasonic nebulizer.

Inhaln (Children >5 yr): *NebuPent, Pentacarinat*—300 mg q 4 wk, using a Respirgard II jet nebulizer (for patients who cannot tolerate trimethoprim/sulfamethoxazole; unlabeled).

Availability (generic available)

Injection: 300 mg/vial. **Solution for aerosol use (NebuPent, Pentacarinat):** 300 mg/vial. **Solution for aerosol use (Pneumopent):** ✤60 mg/vial.

NURSING IMPLICATIONS

Assessment

- Assess patient for infection (vital signs, sputum, WBC) and monitor respiratory status (rate, character, lung sounds, dyspnea, sputum) at beginning of and throughout therapy.
- Obtain specimens for culture and sensitivity prior to initiating therapy. First dose may be given before receiving results.
- **IV, IM:** Monitor blood pressure frequently during and following IM or IV administration of pentamidine. Patient should be lying down during administration. Sudden, severe hypotension may occur following a single dose. Resuscitation equipment should be immediately available.
- Assess patient for signs of hypoglycemia (anxiety; chills; diaphoresis; cold, pale skin; headache; increased hunger; nausea; nervousness; shakiness) and hyperglycemia (drowsiness; flushed, dry skin; fruit-like breath odor; increased thirst; increased urination; loss of appetite), which may occur up to several months after therapy is discontinued.
- Pulse and ECG should be monitored prior to and periodically during course of therapy. Fatalities due to cardiac arrhythmias, tachycardia, and cardiotoxicity have been reported.
- **Inhaln:** A tuberculin skin test, chest x-ray, and sputum culture should be performed prior to administration to rule out tuberculosis.
- ***Lab Test Considerations:*** *IM, IV*—Monitor blood glucose concentrations prior to, daily during, and for several months following therapy. Severe hypoglycemia and permanent diabetes mellitus have occurred.
- Monitor BUN and serum creatinine prior to and daily during therapy to monitor for nephrotoxicity. Concentrations may be ↑.
- Monitor CBC and platelet count prior to and every 3 days during therapy. Pentamidine may cause leukopenia, anemia, and thrombocytopenia.
- May cause ↑ serum bilirubin, alkaline phosphatase, AST, and ALT concentrations. Monitor liver function tests prior to and every 3 days during therapy.
- Monitor serum calcium and magnesium concentrations prior to and every 3 days during therapy; may cause hypocalcemia and hypomagnesemia.
- May cause ↑ serum potassium concentrations.

Potential Nursing Diagnoses

Risk for infection (Indications, Side Effects)

Implementation

- Pentamidine must be given on a regular schedule for the full course of therapy. Administer missed doses as soon as remembered. If almost time for the next dose, skip the missed dose and return to the regular schedule. Do not double doses.
- **IM:** Dilute 300 mg of pentamidine with 3 ml of sterile water for injection for a concentration of 100 mg/ml. IM administration should be used only for patients with adequate muscle mass and given deep IM via Z-track technique. May cause sterile abscesses.

P

✤ = Canadian drug name.

*CAPITALS indicates life-threatening; underlines indicate most frequent.

IV Administration

- **Intermittent Infusion:** ***Diluent:*** To reconstitute, add 3–5 ml of sterile water for injection or D5W to each 300-mg vial for a concentration of 100, 75, or 60 mg/ml, respectively. Withdraw dose and dilute further in 50–250 ml of D5W. Solution is stable for 48 hr at room temperature. Discard unused portions. ***Concentration:*** Not to exceed 6 mg/ml for administration. ***Rate:*** Administer slowly over 1–2 hr.
- **Y-Site Compatibility:** diltiazem, zidovudine.
- **Y-Site Incompatibility:** aldesleukin, cefazolin, cefotaxime, cefoxitin, ceftazidime, ceftriaxone, fluconazole, foscarnet, lansoprazole, linezolid. **Inhaln:** If using inhalation bronchodilator, administer bronchodilator 5–10 min prior to pentamidine administration.
- Administer in a well-ventilated area.
- Administration with patient in supine or recumbent position appears to provide a more uniform distribution of pentamidine.
- *NebuPent* or *Pentacarinat:* Dilute 300 or 600 mg (for prophylaxis or treatment, respectively) in 6 ml of sterile water for injection. Place reconstituted solution into Respirgard II nebulizer. Do not dilute with 0.9% NaCl or admix with other medications, as solution will form a precipitate. Do not use Respirgard II nebulizer for other medications.
- Administer inhalation dose through nebulizer until chamber is empty, approximately 30–45 min.
- *Pneumopent:* Remove rubber stopper and set upside down on a clean surface for use later. Add 3–5 ml of sterile water for inhalation or preservative-free water for injection to vial and replace rubber stopper. Do not use tap water or 0.9% NaCl. Powder should dissolve immediately; if not, shake gently to mix. Solution should be clear and colorless; do not use if cloudy. Solution is stable for 24 hr at room temperature or 48 hr if refrigerated. Place entire reconstituted contents into Fisoneb ultrasonic nebulizer.
- Administer with the flow rate of the nebulizer at the midflow mark over approximately 15 min until the chamber is empty.

Patient/Family Teaching

- Inform patient of the importance of completing the full course of pentamidine therapy, even if feeling better.
- **IV:** Instruct patient to notify health care professional promptly if fever; sore throat; signs of infection; bleeding of gums; unusual bruising; petechiae; or blood in stool, urine, or emesis occurs. Caution patient to avoid crowds and persons with known infections. Instruct patient to use soft toothbrush and electric razor and to avoid falls. Patient should not be given IM injections or rectal thermometers. Patient should be cautioned not to drink alcoholic beverages or take medication containing aspirin or NSAIDs, as these may precipitate gastric bleeding.
- Caution patient to make position changes slowly to minimize orthostatic hypotension.
- **Inhaln:** Advise patient that an unpleasant metallic taste may occur with pentamidine administration but is not significant.
- Inform patients who continue to smoke that bronchospasm and coughing during therapy are more likely.

Evaluation/Desired Outcomes

- Prevention or resolution of the signs and symptoms of PCP in HIV-positive patients.

HIGH ALERT

pentazocine (pen-**taz**-oh-seen)

Talwin, Talwin NX

Classification

Therapeutic: opioid analgesics

Pharmacologic: opioid agonists/antagonists

Schedule IV

Pregnancy Category C

Indications

Moderate to severe pain. Also used for: Analgesia during labor; Sedation prior to surgery; Supplemention in balanced anesthesia.

Action

Binds to opiate receptors in the CNS. Alters perception of and response to painful stimuli, while producing generalized CNS depression. Has partial antagonist properties, which may result in opioid withdrawal in physically dependent patients. **Therapeutic Effects:** Decrease in moderate to severe pain.

Pharmacokinetics

Absorption: Well absorbed following oral, IM, and subcut administration. Small amount (0.5

mg) of naloxone in tablets included to prevent parenteral abuse.
Distribution: Widely distributed. Crosses the placenta.
Metabolism and Excretion: Mostly metabolized by the liver. Small amounts excreted unchanged by the kidneys.
Half-life: 2–3 hr.

TIME/ACTION PROFILE (analgesia)

ROUTE	ONSET	PEAK	DURATION
PO	15–30 min	60–90 min	3 hr
IM, subcut	15–20 min	30–60 min	2–3 hr
IV	2–3 min	15–30 min	2–3 hr

Contraindications/Precautions

Contraindicated in: Hypersensitivity; Patients who are physically dependent on opioids (may precipitate withdrawal).
Use Cautiously in: Head trauma; History of drug abuse; Increased intracranial pressure; Severe renal, hepatic, or pulmonary disease; Hypothyroidism; Adrenal insufficiency; Alcoholism; Debilitated patients or patients with severe liver impairment (dose reduction recommended); Geri: Appears on Beers list and is associated with increase risk of falls. Geriatric patients are more susceptible to adverse CNS effects; dose reduction recommended; Undiagnosed abdominal pain; Prostatic hyperplasia; Patients who have recently received opioid agonists; OB: Pregnancy (has been used during labor but may cause respiratory depression in the newborn); Lactation or children (safety not established).

Adverse Reactions/Side Effects

CNS: dizziness, euphoria, hallucinations, headache, sedation, confusion, dysphoria, floating feeling, unusual dreams. **EENT:** blurred vision, diplopia, miosis (high doses). **Resp:** respiratory depression. **CV:** hypertension, hypotension, palpitations. **GI:** nausea, constipation, dry mouth, ileus, vomiting. **GU:** urinary retention. **Derm:** clammy feeling, sweating. **Local:** severe tissue damage at subcut sites. **Misc:** physical dependence, psychological dependence, tolerance.

Interactions

Drug-Drug: Use with caution in patients receiving **MAO inhibitors** (may result in unpredictable reactions—decrease initial dose of pentazocine to 25% of usual dose). Additive CNS depression with **alcohol**, **antihistamines**, and **sedative/hypnotics**. May precipitate withdrawal in patients who are physically dependent on **opioid analgesic agonists**. May ↓ analgesic effects of other **opioids**.
Drug-Natural Products: Concomitant use of **kava kava, valerian, or chamomile can ↑ CNS depression.**

Route/Dosage

PO (Adults): 50–100 mg q 3–4 hr (not to exceed 600 mg/day).
Subcut, IV, IM (Adults): 30 mg q 3–4 hr (not to exceed 30 mg/dose IV or 60 mg/dose IM or subcut; not to exceed 360 mg/day subcut, IV, or IM). *Obstetrical use*—20 mg IV or 30 mg IM when contractions become regular, may repeat q 2–3 hr for 2–3 doses.

Availability

Tablets: 50 mg (with 0.5 mg naloxone), ✤50 mg. **Injection:** 30 mg/ml. ***In combination with:*** acetaminophen (Talacen) or aspirin (Talwin compound). See Appendix B.

NURSING IMPLICATIONS

Assessment

- Assess type, location, and intensity of pain prior to and 1 hr following PO, subcut, or IM and 15–30 min (peak) following IV administration. When titrating opioid doses, increases of 25–50% should be administered until there is either a 50% reduction in the patient's pain rating on a numeric or visual analogue scale or the patient reports satisfactory pain relief. A repeat dose can be safely administered at the time of the peak if previous dose is ineffective and side effects are minimal. Patients requiring doses higher than 100 mg should be converted to an opioid agonist. Pentazocine is not recommended for prolonged use or as first-line therapy for acute or cancer pain.
- An equianalgesic chart (see Appendix J) should be used when changing routes or when changing from one opioid to another.
- Assess blood pressure, pulse, and respirations before and periodically during administration. If respiratory rate is <10/min, assess level of sedation. Physical stimulation may be sufficient to prevent significant hypoventilation. Dose may need to be decreased by 25–50%. Pentazocine produces respiratory de-

P

✤ = Canadian drug name.

* CAPITALS indicates life-threatening; underlines indicate most frequent.

pression, but this does not markedly increase with increased doses.

- Assess prior analgesic history. Antagonistic properties may induce withdrawal symptoms (vomiting, restlessness, abdominal cramps, and increased blood pressure and temperature) in patients physically dependent on opioids.
- Although this drug has a low potential for dependence, prolonged use may lead to physical and psychological dependence and tolerance. This should not prevent patient from receiving adequate analgesia. Most patients receiving pentazocine for pain do not develop psychological dependence. If tolerance develops, changing to an opioid agonist may be required to relieve pain.
- Geri: Assess falls risk and implement prevention strategies. Assess for adverse CNS effects.
- ***Lab Test Considerations:*** May cause ↑ serum amylase and lipase levels.
- ***Toxicity and Overdose:*** If an opioid antagonist is required to reverse respiratory depression or coma, naloxone (Narcan) is the antidote. Dilute the 0.4-mg ampule of naloxone in 10 ml of 0.9% NaCl and administer 0.5 ml (0.02 mg) by direct IV push every 2 min. For patients weighing <40 kg, dilute 0.1 mg of naloxone in 10 ml of 0.9% NaCl for a concentration of 10 mcg/ml and administer 0.5 mcg/kg every 2 min. Titrate dose to avoid withdrawal, seizures, and severe pain.

Potential Nursing Diagnoses

Acute pain (Indications)
Risk for injury (Side Effects)
Disturbed sensory perception (visual, auditory) (Side Effects)

Implementation

- ***High Alert:*** Accidental overdose of opioid analgesics has resulted in fatalities. Before administering, clarify all ambiguous orders; have second practitioner independently check original order and dose calculations.
- Explain therapeutic value of medication prior to administration to enhance the analgesic effect.
- Regularly administered doses may be more effective than prn administration. Analgesic is more effective if administered before pain becomes severe.
- Coadministration with nonopioid analgesics may have additive effects and may permit lower opioid doses.
- **PO:** Talwin NX contains 0.5 mg of naloxone, which has no pharmacologic activity when administered orally. If the product is abused by injection, naloxone antagonizes pentazocine. Parenteral use of oral pentazocine may lead to severe, potentially fatal reactions (pulmonary emboli, vascular occlusion, ulceration and abscess, and withdrawal symptoms in opioid-dependent individuals).
- **IM, Subcut:** Administer IM injections deep into well-developed muscle. Rotate sites of injections. Subcut route may cause tissue damage with repeated injections.

IV Administration

- **Direct IV:** ***Diluent:*** Manufacturer recommends diluting each 5 mg with at least 1 ml of sterile water for injection. ***Concentration:*** 5 mg/ml. ***Rate:*** Administer slowly, each 5 mg over at least 1 min.
- **Syringe Compatibility:** atropine, chlorpromazine, cimetidine, dimenhydrinate, diphenhydramine, droperidol, hydroxyzine, metoclopramide, perphenazine, prochlorperazine edisylate, promazine, promethazine, ranitidine, scopolamine.
- **Syringe Incompatibility:** glycopyrrolate, heparin, pentobarbital.
- **Y-Site Compatibility:** heparin, hydrocortisone sodium succinate, potassium chloride, vitamin B complex with C.
- **Y-Site Incompatibility:** nafcillin.

Patient/Family Teaching

- Instruct patient on how and when to ask for pain medication.
- Medication may cause drowsiness, dizziness, or hallucinations, particularly in geriatric patients. Advise patient to call for assistance when ambulating and to avoid driving or other activities requiring alertness until response to medication is known. Institute fall prevention strategies and teach patient or family how to prevent falls at home.
- Caution patient to change positions slowly to minimize orthostatic hypotension.
- Advise patient to avoid concurrent use of alcohol and other CNS depressants.
- Encourage patient to turn, cough, and breathe deeply every 2 hr to prevent atelectasis.
- Advise patient that frequent mouth rinses, good oral hygiene, and sugarless gum or candy may decrease dry mouth.

Evaluation/Desired Outcomes

- Decrease in severity of pain without a significant alteration in level of consciousness or respiratory status.

pentoxifylline (pen-tox-if-i-lin)
Trental

Classification
Therapeutic: blood viscosity reducing agents

Pregnancy Category C

Indications
Management of symptomatic peripheral vascular disease (intermittent claudication).

Action
Increases the flexibility of RBCs by increasing levels of cyclic adenosine monophosphate (cAMP). Decreases blood viscosity by inhibiting platelet aggregation and decreasing fibrinogen. **Therapeutic Effects:** Increased blood flow.

Pharmacokinetics
Absorption: Well absorbed following oral administration.
Distribution: Bound to RBC membrane. Enters breast milk.
Metabolism and Excretion: Metabolized by RBCs and the liver.
Half-life: 25–50 min.

TIME/ACTION PROFILE (improvement in blood flow)

ROUTE	ONSET	PEAK	DURATION
PO	2–4 wk	8 wk	8 hr

Contraindications/Precautions
Contraindicated in: Hypersensitivity; Intolerance to other xanthine derivatives (caffeine and theophylline).
Use Cautiously in: Coronary artery or cerebrovascular disease; Renal disease (lower doses may be used); Geriatric patients (increased risk of adverse reactions); Pregnancy, lactation, or children (safety not established).

Adverse Reactions/Side Effects
CNS: agitation, dizziness, drowsiness, headache, insomnia, nervousness. **EENT:** blurred vision. **Resp:** dyspnea. **CV:** angina, arrhythmias, edema, flushing, hypotension. **GI:** abdominal discomfort, belching, bloating, diarrhea, dyspepsia, flatus, nausea, vomiting. **Neuro:** tremor.

Interactions
Drug-Drug: Additive hypotension may occur with **antihypertensives** and **nitrates**. May increase the risk of bleeding with **warfarin, heparin, aspirin, NSAIDs, cefoperazone, cefotetan, valproic acid, clopidogrel, ticlopidine, eptifibatide, tirofiban,** or **thrombolytic agents**. May increase the risk of **theophylline** toxicity. **Smoking** may decrease the beneficial effects of pentoxifylline.
Drug-Natural Products: Increased bleeding risk with **anise, arnica, asafoetida, chamomile, clove, dong quai, fenugreek, feverfew, garlic, ginger, ginkgo, Panax ginseng, licorice,** and others.

Route/Dosage
PO (Adults): 400 mg 3 times daily; if GI or CNS side effects occur, decrease dose to 400 mg twice daily.

Availability (generic available)
Controlled-release tablets: 400 mg. **Extended-release tablets:** 400 mg.

NURSING IMPLICATIONS

Assessment
- Assess patient for intermittent claudication prior to and periodically throughout therapy.
- Monitor blood pressure periodically in patients on concurrent antihypertensive therapy.

Potential Nursing Diagnoses
Acute pain (Indications)
Activity intolerance (Indications)

Implementation
- **PO:** Administer with meals to minimize GI irritation. Tablets should be swallowed whole; do not crush, break, or chew.
- If GI and CNS side effects occur, decrease dose to twice daily. Discontinue if side effects persist.

Patient/Family Teaching
- Instruct patient to take medication exactly as directed. If a dose is missed, it should be taken as soon as remembered unless almost time for next dose. Consult health care professional before discontinuing medication,

P

because several weeks of therapy may be required before effects are seen.

- May cause dizziness and blurred vision. Caution patient to avoid driving and other activities requiring alertness until response to medication is known.
- Advise patient to avoid smoking, because nicotine constricts blood vessels.
- Instruct patient to notify health care professional if nausea, vomiting, GI upset, drowsiness, dizziness, or headache persists.

Evaluation/Desired Outcomes

- Relief from cramping in calf muscles, buttocks, thighs, and feet during exercise.
- Improvement in walking endurance. Therapeutic effects may be seen in 2–4 wk, but therapy should be continued for ≥8 wk.

perindopril, See ANGIOTENSIN-CONVERTING ENZYME (ACE) INHIBITORS.

permethrin (per-**meth**-rin)

Acticin, Elimite, Nix

Classification
Therapeutic: pediculocides

Pregnancy Category B

Indications

1% lotion: Eradication of *Pediculus humanus capitis* (head lice and their eggs): Prevention of infestation of head lice during epidemics. **5% cream:** Eradication of *Sarcoptes scabiei* (scabies).

Action

Causes repolarization and paralysis in lice by disrupting sodium transport in normal nerve cells. **Therapeutic Effects:** Death of parasites.

Pharmacokinetics

Absorption: Small amounts (<2%) systemically absorbed. Remains on hair for 10 days.
Distribution: Unknown.
Metabolism and Excretion: Rapidly inactivated by enzymes.
Half-life: Unknown.

TIME/ACTION PROFILE (pediculocidal action)

ROUTE	ONSET	PEAK	DURATION
topical	10 min	unknown	14 days

Contraindications/Precautions

Contraindicated in: Hypersensitivity to permethrin, pyrethrins (insecticides or veterinary pesticides), chrysanthemums, or isopropyl alcohol.
Use Cautiously in: Pregnancy or lactation; Children <2 yr (1% lotion); Children <2 mo (5% cream).

Adverse Reactions/Side Effects

Derm: burning, itching, rash, redness, stinging, swelling. **Neuro:** numbness, tingling.

Interactions

Drug-Drug: No significant interactions.

Route/Dosage

Head Lice (Treatment and Prevention)

Topical (Adults and Children >2 yr): 1% lotion applied to the hair, left on for 10 min, then rinsed, for 1 application.

Scabies

Topical (Adults and Children): Massage 5% cream into all skin surfaces. Leave on for 8–14 hr, then wash off.
Topical (Infants >2 mo): Massage 5% cream into hairline, scalp, neck, temple, and forehead. Leave on for 8–14 hr, then wash off.

Availability (generic available)

Liquid cream rinse (lotion): 1% in 60-ml containers[OTC]. **Cream:** 5% in 60-g tube.

NURSING IMPLICATIONS

Assessment

- **Head Lice:** Assess scalp for presence of lice and their ova (nits) prior to and 1 wk after application of permethrin.
- **Scabies:** Assess skin for scabies prior to and following therapy.

Potential Nursing Diagnoses

Impaired home maintenance (Indications)
Bathing/hygiene self-care deficit (Indications)

Implementation

- **Topical:** For topical application only.

Patient/Family Teaching

- Instruct patient to notify health care professional if scalp itching, numbness, redness, or rash occurs.

- Instruct patient to avoid getting Elimite cream in eyes. If this occurs, eyes should be flushed thoroughly with water. Health care professional should be contacted if eye irritation persists.
- Advise patient that others residing in the home should also be checked for lice.
- Instruct patient on methods of preventing reinfestation. All clothes, including outdoor apparel and household linens, should be machine-washed using very hot water and dried for at least 20 min in a hot dryer. Dry-clean nonwashable clothes. Brushes and combs should be soaked in hot (130°F), soapy water for 5–10 min. Remind patient that brushes and combs should not be shared. Wigs and hairpieces should be shampooed. Rugs and upholstered furniture should be vacuumed. Toys should be washed in hot, soapy water. Items that cannot be washed should be sealed in a plastic bag for 2 wk.
- If patient is a child, instruct parents to notify school nurse or day care center so that classmates and playmates can be checked.
- **Head Lice:** Instruct patient to wash hair with regular shampoo, rinse, and towel dry. Each container holds enough medication for one treatment. Shake the container well. Thoroughly wet scalp and hair with the lotion. The patient should use as much of the solution as needed to coat entire head of hair, then discard remainder of solution. Allow lotion to remain on hair for 10 min, then thoroughly rinse hair and towel dry with a clean towel. Comb hair with a fine-toothed comb to remove dead lice and eggs (not necessary but may be desired for cosmetic effects). Products are available for removal of nits (Rid Lice Egg Loosener Gel®Step 2). Schools usually require children to be nit-free prior to returning to school.
- Explain to patient that permethrin will protect from reinfestation for 2 wk. These effects continue even when the patient resumes regular shampooing.
- **Scabies:** Instruct patient to massage thoroughly into the skin from head to soles of feet. Treat infants on the hairline, neck, scalp, temple, and forehead. Remove the cream by washing after 8–14 hr. Usually 30 g (½ tube) is sufficient for adults. One application is curative.

Evaluation/Desired Outcomes

- The absence of lice and eggs 1 wk after therapy. A second application is indicated if lice are detected at this time.
- Prevention of infestation of head lice during epidemics.
- Eradication of scabies following one application.
- If resistance to permethrin develops, malathion may be used.

phenazopyridine

(fen-az-oh-**peer**-i-deen)

Azo-Standard, Baridium, Geridium, ✤Phenazo, Prodium, Pyridiate, Pyridium, Pyridium Plus, Urodine, Urogesic, UTI Relief

Classification

Therapeutic: nonopioid analgesics

Pharmacologic: urinary tract analgesics

Pregnancy Category B

Indications

Provides relief from the following urinary tract symptoms, which may occur in association with infection or following urologic procedures: Pain, Itching, Burning, Urgency, Frequency.

Action

Acts locally on the urinary tract mucosa to produce analgesic or local anesthetic effects. Has no antimicrobial activity. **Therapeutic Effects:** Diminished urinary tract discomfort.

Pharmacokinetics

Absorption: Appears to be well absorbed following oral administration.

Distribution: Unknown. Small amounts cross the placenta.

Metabolism and Excretion: Rapidly excreted unchanged in the urine.

Half-life: Unknown.

TIME/ACTION PROFILE (urinary analgesia)

ROUTE	ONSET	PEAK	DURATION
PO	unknown	5–6 hr	6–8 hr

Contraindications/Precautions

Contraindicated in: Hypersensitivity; Glomerulonephritis; Severe hepatitis, uremia, or renal failure; Renal insufficiency; G6PD deficiency.

✤ = Canadian drug name.

* CAPITALS indicates life-threatening; underlines indicate most frequent.

Use Cautiously in: Hepatitis; Pregnancy or lactation (safety not established).

Adverse Reactions/Side Effects

CNS: headache, vertigo. **GI:** hepatotoxicity, nausea. **GU:** bright-orange urine, renal failure. **Derm:** rash. **Hemat:** hemolytic anemia, methemoglobinemia.

Interactions

Drug-Drug: None significant.

Route/Dosage

PO (Adults): 200 mg 3 times daily for 2 days.
PO (Children): 4 mg/kg 3 times daily for 2 days.

Availability (generic available)

Tablets: 95 mg[OTC], 100 mg, ✦100 mg[OTC], ✦200 mg[OTC], 200 mg.

NURSING IMPLICATIONS

Assessment

- Assess patient for urgency, frequency, and pain on urination prior to and throughout therapy.
- ***Lab Test Considerations:*** Renal function should be monitored periodically during course of therapy.
- Interferes with urine tests based on color reactions (glucose, ketones, bilirubin, steroids, protein).

Potential Nursing Diagnoses

Acute pain (Indications)
Impaired urinary elimination (Indications)

Implementation

- Medication should be discontinued after pain or discomfort is relieved (usually 2 days for treatment of urinary tract infection). Concurrent antibiotic therapy should continue for full prescribed duration.
- **PO:** Administer medication with or following meals to decrease GI irritation. Do not crush, break, or chew tablet.

Patient/Family Teaching

- Instruct patient to take medication exactly as directed. If a dose is missed, take as soon as remembered unless almost time for next dose.
- Advise patient that while phenazopyridine administration is stopped once pain or discomfort is relieved, concurrent antibiotic therapy must be continued for full duration of therapy. Do not save unused portion of phenazopyridine without consulting health care professional.
- Inform patient that drug causes reddish-orange discoloration of urine that may stain clothing or bedding. Sanitary napkin may be worn to avoid clothing stains. May also cause staining of soft contact lenses.
- Instruct patient to notify health care professional if rash, skin discoloration, or unusual tiredness occurs.

Evaluation/Desired Outcomes

- Decrease in pain and burning on urination.

---

phenelzine, See **MONOAMINE OXIDASE (MAO) INHIBITORS.**

---

phenobarbital

(fee-noe-**bar**-bi-tal)
✦Ancalixir, Luminal, Solfoton

Classification
Therapeutic: anticonvulsants, sedative/hypnotics
Pharmacologic: barbiturates

Schedule IV

Pregnancy Category D

Indications

Anticonvulsant in tonic-clonic (grand mal), partial, and febrile seizures in children. Preoperative sedative and in other situations in which sedation may be required. Hypnotic (short-term). **Unlabeled uses:** Prevention/treatment of hyperbilirubinemia in neonates.

Action

Produces all levels of CNS depression. Depresses the sensory cortex, decreases motor activity, and alters cerebellar function. Inhibits transmission in the nervous system and raises the seizure threshold. Capable of inducing (speeding up) enzymes in the liver that metabolize drugs, bilirubin, and other compounds. **Therapeutic Effects:** Anticonvulsant activity. Sedation.

Pharmacokinetics

Absorption: Absorption is slow but relatively complete (70–90%).
Distribution: Unknown.
Metabolism and Excretion: 75% metabolized by the liver, 25% excreted unchanged by the kidneys.

Half-life: Neonates: 1.8–8.3 days; Infants: 0.8–5.5 days; Children: 1.5–3 days; Adults: 2–6 days.

TIME/ACTION PROFILE (sedation†)

ROUTE	ONSET	PEAK	DURATION
PO	30–60 min	unknown	>6 hr
IM, subcut	10–30 min	unknown	4–6 hr
IV	5 min	30 min	4–6 hr

†Full anticonvulsant effects occur after 2–3 wk of chronic dosing unless a loading dose has been used

Contraindications/Precautions

Contraindicated in: Hypersensitivity; Comatose patients or those with pre-existing CNS depression; Severe respiratory disease with dyspnea or obstruction; Uncontrolled severe pain; Known alcohol intolerance (elixir only); Lactation: Discontinue drug or bottle feed.
Use Cautiously in: Hepatic dysfunction; Severe renal impairment; History of suicide attempt or drug abuse; Hypnotic use should be short-term. Chronic use may lead to dependence; OB: Chronic use during pregnancy results in drug dependency in the infant; may result in coagulation defects and fetal malformation; acute use at term may result in respiratory depression in the newborn; Geri: Iinitial dose reduction recommended; Hypnotic use should be short-term. Chronic use may lead to dependence.

Adverse Reactions/Side Effects

CNS: hangover, delirium, depression, drowsiness, excitation, lethargy, vertigo. **Resp:** respiratory depression; *IV*— LARYNGOSPASM, bronchospasm. **CV:** *IV*— hypotension. **GI:** constipation, diarrhea, nausea, vomiting. **Derm:** photosensitivity, rashes, urticaria. **Local:** phlebitis at IV site. **MS:** arthralgia, myalgia, neuralgia. **Misc:** hypersensitivity reactions including ANGIOEDEMA and SERUM SICKNESS, physical dependence, psychological dependence.

Interactions

Drug-Drug: Additive CNS depression with other **CNS depressants**, including **alcohol, antihistamines, opioid analgesics**, and other **sedative/hypnotics**. May induce hepatic enzymes that metabolize other drugs, ↓ their effectiveness, including **hormonal contraceptives, warfarin, chloramphenicol, cyclosporine, dacarbazine, corticosteroids, tricyclic antidepressants, felodipine, clonazepam, carbamazepine, verapamil, theophylline, metronidazole,** and **quinidine**. May ↑ risk of hepatic toxicity of **acetaminophen**. **MAO inhibitors, valproic acid**, or **divalproex** may ↓ metabolism of phenobarbital, ↑ sedation. **Rifampin** may ↑ metabolism of and ↓ effects of phenobarbital. May ↑ risk of hematologic toxicity with **cyclophosphamide**.
Drug-Natural Products: Concomitant use of **kava kava, valerian, chamomile,** or **hops** can ↑ CNS depression. **St. John's wort** may ↓ effects.

Route/Dosage

Status Epilepticus

IV (Adults and Children >1 month): 15–18 mg/kg in a single or divided dose, maximum loading dose 20 mg/kg.
IV (Neonates): 15–20 mg/kg in a single or divided dose.

Maintenance Anticonvulsant

IV, PO (Adults and Children >12 yrs): 1–3 mg/kg/day as a single dose or 2 divided doses.
IV, PO (Children 5–12 yr): 4–6 mg/kg/day in 1–2 divided doses.
IV, PO (Children 1–5 yr): 6–8 mg/kg/day in 1–2 divided doses.
IV, PO (Infants): 5–6 mg/kg/day in 1–2 divided doses.
IV, PO (Neonates): 3–4 mg/kg/day once daily, may need to increase up to 5 mg/kg/day by 2nd week of therapy.

Sedation

PO, IM (Adults): 30–120 mg/day in 2–3 divided doses. *Preoperative sedation*—100–200 mg IM 1–1.5 hours before the procedure.
PO (Children): 2 mg/kg 3 times daily. *Preoperative sedation*—1–3 mg/kg PO/IM/IV 1–1.5 hours before the procedure.

Hypnotic

PO, Subcut, IV, IM (Adults): 100–320 mg at bedtime.
IV, IM, Subcut (Children): 3–5 mg/kg at bedtime.

Hyperbilirubinemia

PO (Adults): 90–180 mg/day in 2–3 divided doses.

P

PO (Children <12 yr): 3–8 mg/kg/day in 2–3 divided doses, doses up to 12 mg/kg/day have been used.

Availability (generic available)

Tablets: 8 mg, 15 mg, 30 mg, 60 mg, 100 mg. **Capsules:** 15 mg. **Elixir:** 20 mg/5 ml. **Injection:** 30 mg/ml in 1-ml prefilled syringes, 60 mg/ml in 1-ml prefilled syringes, 65 mg/ml in 1-ml vials, 130 mg/ml in 1-ml prefilled syringes, 1-ml vials, and 1-ml ampules. ***In combination with:*** phenytoin. See Appendix B.

NURSING IMPLICATIONS

Assessment

- Monitor respiratory status, pulse, and blood pressure frequently in patients receiving phenobarbital IV. Equipment for resuscitation and artificial ventilation should be readily available. Respiratory depression is dose-dependent.
- Prolonged therapy may lead to psychological or physical dependence. Restrict amount of drug available to patient, especially if depressed, suicidal, or with a history of addiction.
- Geri: Elderly patients may react to phenobarbital with marked excitement, depression, and confusion. Monitor for these adverse reactions.
- **Seizures:** Assess location, duration, and characteristics of seizure activity.
- **Sedation:** Assess level of consciousness and anxiety when used as a preoperative sedative.
- Assess postoperative patients for pain with a pain scale. Phenobarbital may increase sensitivity to painful stimuli.
- ***Lab Test Considerations:*** Patients on prolonged therapy should have hepatic and renal function and CBC evaluated periodically.
- Monitor serum folate concentrations periodically during therapy because of increased folate requirements of patients on long-term anticonvulsant therapy with phenobarbital.
- May cause ↓ serum bilirubin concentrations in neonates, in patients with congenital nonhemolytic unconjugated hyperbilirubinemia, and in epileptics.
- ***Toxicity and Overdose:*** Serum phenobarbital levels may be monitored when used as an anticonvulsant. Therapeutic blood levels are 10–40 mcg/ml. Symptoms of toxicity include confusion, drowsiness, dyspnea, slurred speech, and staggering.

Potential Nursing Diagnoses

Risk for injury (Indications, Side Effects)
Acute confusion (Side Effects)

Implementation

- Do not confuse phenobarbital with pentobarbital.
- Supervise ambulation and transfer of patients following administration. Two side rails should be raised and call bell within reach at all times. Keep bed in low position. Institute seizure and fall precautions.
- When changing from phenobarbital to another anticonvulsant, gradually decrease phenobarbital dose while concurrently increasing dose of replacement medication to maintain anticonvulsant effects.
- **PO:** Tablets may be crushed and mixed with food or fluids (do not administer dry) for patients with difficulty swallowing. Oral solution may be taken undiluted or mixed with water, milk, or fruit juice. Use calibrated measuring device for accurate measurement of liquid doses.
- **IM:** Injections should be given deep into the gluteal muscle to minimize tissue irritation. Do not inject >5 ml into any one site, because of tissue irritation.

IV Administration

- **IV:** Doses may require 15–30 min to reach peak concentrations in the brain. Administer minimal dose and wait for effectiveness before administering 2nd dose to prevent cumulative barbiturate-induced depression.
- **Direct IV:** ***Diluent:*** Reconstitute sterile powder for IV dose with a minimum of 3 ml of sterile water for injection. Dilute further with 10 ml of sterile water. Do not use solution that is not absolutely clear within 5 min after reconstitution or that contains a precipitate. Discard powder or solution that has been exposed to air for longer than 30 min.
- Solution is highly alkaline; avoid extravasation, which may cause tissue damage and necrosis. If extravasation occurs, injection of 5% procaine solution into affected area and application of moist heat may be ordered. ***Concentration:*** 130 mg/ml (undiluted). ***Rate:*** Do not inject IV faster than 1 mg/kg/min with a maximum of 30 mg over 1 min in infants and children and 60 mg over 1 min in adults. Titrate slowly for desired response. Rapid administration may result in respiratory depression.
- **Y-Site Compatibility:** doxapram, enalaprilat, fentanyl, fosphenytoin, levofloxacin, line-

zolid, meropenem, methadone, morphine, propofol, sufentanil.

- **Y-Site Incompatibility:** amphotericin B cholesteryl sulfate complex, lansoprazole.

Patient/Family Teaching

- Advise patient to take medication as directed. Take missed doses as soon as remembered if not almost time for next dose; do not double doses.
- Advise patients on prolonged therapy not to discontinue medication without consulting health care professional. Abrupt withdrawal may precipitate seizures or status epilepticus.
- Medication may cause daytime drowsiness. Caution patient to avoid driving and other activities requiring alertness until response to medication is known. Do not resume driving until physician gives clearance based on control of seizure disorder.
- Caution patient to avoid taking alcohol or other CNS depressants concurrently with this medication.
- Advise female patients using oral contraceptives to use an additional nonhormonal contraceptive during therapy and until next menstrual period. Instruct patient to contact health care professional immediately if pregnancy is planned or suspected.
- Advise patient to notify health care professional if fever, sore throat, mouth sores, unusual bleeding or bruising, nosebleeds, or petechiae occur.
- Teach sleep hygiene techniques (dark room, quiet, bedtime ritual, limit daytime napping, avoid nicotine and caffeine).
- Pedi: Advise parents or caregivers that child may experience irritability, hyperactivity and/or sleep disturbances, which may diminish in a few days to a few weeks or may persist until drug is stopped. An alternative medication can be considered. Instruct parents to monitor for skin rash occurring 7–20 days after treatment begins and to contact a health care provider if rash occurs. Teach family about symptoms of toxicity (staggering, drowsiness, slurred speech).

Evaluation/Desired Outcomes

- Decrease or cessation of seizure activity without excessive sedation. Several weeks may be required to achieve maximum anticonvulsant effects.
- Preoperative sedation.
- Improvement in sleep patterns.
- Decrease in serum bilirubin levels.

phentolamine

(fen-**tole**-a-meen)

Regitine, ✤Rogitine

Classification

Therapeutic: agents for pheochromocytoma

Pharmacologic: alpha-adrenergic blockers

Pregnancy Category C

Indications

IV: Control of blood pressure during surgical removal of a pheochromocytoma. **IV, Infiltration:** Prevention and treatment of dermal necrosis and sloughing following extravasation of norepinephrine, phenylephrine, or dopamine. **Unlabeled uses: IM, IV:** Treatment of hypertension associated with pheochromocytoma or adrenergic (sympathetic) excess, such as administration of phenylephrine, tyramine-containing foods in patients on MAO inhibitor therapy, or clonidine withdrawal.

Action

Produces incomplete and short-lived blockade of alpha-adrenergic receptors located primarily in smooth muscle and exocrine glands. Induces hypotension by direct relaxation of vascular smooth muscle and by alpha blockade. **Therapeutic Effects:** Reduction of blood pressure in situations in which hypertension is due to adrenergic (sympathetic) excess. When infiltrated locally, reverses vasoconstriction caused by norepinephrine or dopamine.

Pharmacokinetics

Absorption: Well absorbed following IM administration.

Distribution: Unknown.

Metabolism and Excretion: 10% excreted unchanged by kidneys.

Half-life: Unknown.

TIME/ACTION PROFILE (alpha-adrenergic blockade)

ROUTE	ONSET	PEAK	DURATION
IM	unknown	20 min	30–45 min
IV	immediate	2 min	15–30 min

P

Contraindications/Precautions

Contraindicated in: Hypersensitivity; Coronary or cerebral arteriosclerosis; Renal impairment.

Use Cautiously in: Peptic ulcer disease; Geri: Geriatric patients (more susceptible to hypotensive effects; dose reduction recommended); OB, Geri: Pregnancy or lactation (safety not established).

Adverse Reactions/Side Effects

With parenteral use. **CNS:** CEREBROVASCULAR SPASM, dizziness, weakness. **EENT:** nasal stuffiness. **CV:** HYPOTENSION, MI, angina, arrhythmias, tachycardia. **GI:** abdominal pain, diarrhea, nausea, vomiting, aggravation of peptic ulcer. **Derm:** flushing.

Interactions

Drug-Drug: Antagonizes the effects of **alpha-adrenergic stimulants**. May ↓ pressor response to **ephedrine** or **phenylephrine**. Severe hypotension may occur with concurrent use of **epinephrine** or **methoxamine**. Use with **guanadrel** may result in exaggerated hypotension and bradycardia. ↓ peripheral vasoconstriction from high doses of **dopamine**.

Route/Dosage

Hypertension Associated with Pheochromocytoma—Before/During Surgery

IV (Adults): 5 mg given 1–2 hr preop, repeated as necessary. May be infused at a rate of 0.5–1 mg/min during surgery.

IV, IM (Children): 1 mg or 0.1 mg/kg (3 mg/m^2) given 1–2 hr preop, repeated IV as necessary during surgery.

Prevention of Dermal Necrosis during Infusion of Norepinephrine, Phenylephrine, or Dopamine

IV (Adults): Add 10 mg phentolamine to every 1000 ml of fluid containing norepinephrine.

Treatment of Dermal Necrosis Following Extravasation of Norepinephrine, Phenylephrine, or Dopamine

Infiltrate **(Adults):** 5–10 mg.

Infiltrate **(Children):** 0.1–0.2 mg/kg (up to 10 mg).

Availability (generic available)

Powder for injection: 5 mg/vial.

NURSING IMPLICATIONS

Assessment

- Monitor blood pressure, pulse, and ECG every 2 min until stable during IV administration. If hypotensive crisis occurs, epinephrine is contraindicated and may cause paradoxic further decrease in blood pressure; norepinephrine may be used.

Potential Nursing Diagnoses

Ineffective tissue perfusion (Indications)
Risk for injury (Indications)

Implementation

- Patient should remain supine throughout parenteral administration.

IV Administration

- **IV:** ***Diluent:*** Reconstitute each 5 mg with 1 ml of sterile water for injection or 0.9% NaCl. Discard unused solution. ***Concentration:*** 5 mg/ml. ***Rate:*** Inject each 5 mg over 1 min.
- **Continuous Infusion:** Dilute 5–10 mg in 500 ml of D5W. ***Rate:*** Titrate infusion rate according to patient response.
- May also add 10 mg to every 1000 ml of fluid containing norepinephrine for prevention of dermal necrosis and sloughing. Does not affect pressor effect of norepinephrine.
- **Syringe Compatibility:** papaverine.
- **Y-Site Compatibility:** amiodarone.
- **Additive Compatibility:** dobutamine, norepinephrine.
- **Infiltration:** Dilute 5–10 mg of phentolamine in 10 ml of 0.9% NaCl. For children, use 0.1–0.2 mg/kg up to a maximum of 10 mg. Infiltrate site of extravasation promptly. Must be given within 12 hr of extravasation to be effective.

Patient/Family Teaching

- Advise patient to change positions slowly to minimize orthostatic hypotension.
- Instruct patient to notify health care professional if chest pain occurs during IV infusion.

Evaluation/Desired Outcomes

- Decrease in blood pressure.
- Prevention of dermal necrosis and sloughing in extravasation of norepinephrine, dopamine, and phenylephrine.

phenytoin (fen-i-toyn)
Dilantin, Phenytek

Classification
Therapeutic: antiarrhythmics (group IB), anticonvulsants
Pharmacologic: hydantoins

Pregnancy Category D

Indications
Treatment/prevention of tonic-clonic (grand mal) seizures and complex partial seizures. **Unlabeled uses:** As an antiarrhythmic, particularly for ventricular arrhythmias associated with digoxin toxicity, prolonged QT interval, and surgical repair of congenital heart diseases in children. Management of neuropathic pain, including trigeminal neuralgia.

Action
Limits seizure propagation by altering ion transport. May also decrease synaptic transmission. Antiarrhythmic properties as a result of shortening the action potential and decreasing automaticity. **Therapeutic Effects:** Diminished seizure activity. Termination of ventricular arrhythmias.

Pharmacokinetics
Absorption: Absorbed slowly from the GI tract. Bioavailability differs among products; the Dilantin and Phenytek preparations are considered to be "extended" products. Other products are considered to be prompt release.
Distribution: Distributes into CSF and other body tissues and fluids. Enters breast milk; crosses the placenta, achieving similar maternal/fetal levels. Preferentially distributes into fatty tissue.
Protein Binding: Adults 90–95%; decreased protein binding in neonates (up to 20% free fraction available), infants (up to 15% free), and patients with hyperbilirubinemia, hypoalbuminemia, severe renal dysfunction or uremia.
Metabolism and Excretion: Mostly metabolized by the liver; minimal amounts excreted in the urine.
Half-life: 22 hr (range 7–42 hr).

TIME/ACTION PROFILE (anticonvulsant effect)

ROUTE	ONSET	PEAK	DURATION
PO	2–24 hr (1 wk)*	1.5–3 hr	6–12 hr
PO-ER	2–24 hr (1 wk)	4–12 hr	12–36 hr
IV	0.5–1 hr (1 wk)	rapid	12–24 hr

*() = time required for onset of action without a loading dose

Contraindications/Precautions
Contraindicated in: Hypersensitivity; Hypersensitivity to propylene glycol (phenytoin injection only); Alcohol intolerance (phenytoin injection and liquid only); Sinus bradycardia, sinoatrial block, 2nd- or 3rd-degree heart block, or Stokes-Adams syndrome (phenytoin injection only).
Use Cautiously in: Hepatic or renal disease (↑ risk of adverse reactions; dose reduction recommended for hepatic impairment); Patients with severe cardiac or respiratory disease (use of IV phenytoin may result in an ↑ risk of serious adverse reactions); OB: Safety not established; may result in fetal hydantoin syndrome if used chronically or hemorrhage in the newborn if used at term; Lactation: Safety not established; Pedi: Suspension contains sodium benzoate, a metabolite of benzyl alcohol that can cause potentially fatal gasping syndrome in neonates; Geri: Use of IV phenytoin may result in an ↑ risk of serious adverse reactions.

P

Adverse Reactions/Side Effects
Most listed are for chronic use of phenytoin.
CNS: ataxia, agitation, confusion, dizziness, drowsiness, dysarthria, dyskinesia, extrapyramidal syndrome, headache, insomnia, weakness. **EENT:** diplopia, nystagmus. **CV:** hypotension (↑ with IV phenytoin), tachycardia. **GI:** gingival hyperplasia, nausea, constipation, drug-induced hepatitis, vomiting. **Derm:** hypertrichosis, rash, exfoliative dermatitis, pruritus. **Hemat:** AGRANULOCYTOSIS, APLASTIC ANEMIA, leukopenia, megaloblastic anemia, thrombocytopenia. **MS:** osteomalacia. **Misc:** allergic reactions including STEVENS-JOHNSON SYNDROME, fever, lymphadenopathy.

Interactions
Drug-Drug: Disulfiram, acute ingestion of **alcohol, amiodarone, ethosuximide, isoniazid, chloramphenicol, sulfonamides, fluoxetine, gabapentin, H2 antagonists, benzodiazepines, omeprazole, ketoconazole, fluconazole, estrogens, succinamides, halothane, methylphenidate, phenothiazines, salicylates, ticlopidine, tolbutamide, topiramate, trazodone, felbamate**, and **cimetidine** may ↑ phenytoin blood levels. **Barbiturates, carbamazepine, reserpine**, and chronic ingestion of **alcohol** may ↓ phenytoin blood levels. Phenytoin may

↓ the effects of **amiodarone**, **benzodiazepines**, **carbamazepine**, **chloramphenicol**, **corticosteroids**, **disopyramide**, **warfarin**, **felbamate**, **doxycycline**, **lamotrigine**, **oral contraceptives**, **paroxetine**, **propafenone**, **rifampin**, **ritonavir**, **quinidine**, **tacrolimus**, **theophylline**, **topiramate**, **tricyclic antidepressants**, **zonisamide**, **methadone**, **cyclosporine**, and **estrogens**. IV phenytoin and **dopamine** may cause additive hypotension. Additive CNS depression with other **CNS depressants**, including **alcohol**, **antihistamines**, **antidepressants**, **opioids**, and **sedative/hypnotics**. **Antacids** may ↓ absorption of orally administered phenytoin. ↑ systemic clearance of antileukemic drugs **teniposide** and **methotrexate** which has been associated with a worse event free survival, phenytoin use is not recommended in children undergoing chemotherapy for acute lymphocytic leukemia. **Calcium** and **sucralfate** ↓ phenytoin absorption.
Drug-Food: Phenytoin may ↓ absorption of **folic acid**. Concurrent administration of **enteral tube feedings** may ↓ phenytoin absorption.

Route/Dosage

IM administration is not recommended due to erratic absorption and pain on injection.

Anticonvulsant

PO (Adults): Loading dose of 15–20 mg/kg as extended capsules in 3 divided doses given every 2–4 hr; maintenance dose 5–6 mg/kg/day given in 1–3 divided doses; usual dosing range = 200–1200 mg/day.
PO (Children 10–16 yr): 6–7 mg/kg/day in 2–3 divided doses.
PO (Children 7–9 yr): 7–8 mg/kg/day in 2–3 divided doses.
PO (Children 4–6 yr): 7.5–9 mg/kg/day in 2–3 divided doses.
PO (Children 0.5–3 yr): 8–10 mg/kg/day in 2–3 divided doses.
PO (Neonates up to 6 months): 5–8 mg/kg/day in 2 divided doses, may require q 8 hr dosing.
IV (Adults): *Status epilepticus loading dose*—15–20 mg/kg. Rate not to exceed 25–50 mg/min. *Maintenance dose*—same as PO dosing above.
IV (Children): *Status epilepticus loading dose*—15–20 mg/kg at 1–3 mg/kg/min. *Maintenance dose*—same as PO dosing above.

Antiarrhythmic

IV (Adults): 50–100 mg q 10–15 min until arrhythmia is abolished, or a total of 15 mg/kg has been given, or toxicity occurs.
PO (Adults): Loading dose: 250 mg QID for 1 day, then 250 mg BID for 2 days, then maintenance at 300–400 mg/day in divided doses 1–4 times/day.
IV (Children): 1.25 mg/kg q 5 min, may repeat up to total loading dose of 15 mg/kg. *Maintenance dose*—5–10 mg/kg/day in 2–3 divided doses IV or PO.

Availability (generic available)

Chewable tablets: 50 mg^{Rx}. **Cost:** \$41.99/90. **Oral suspension:** 125 mg/5 ml^{Rx}. **Cost:** *Generic*—\$28.99/237 ml. **Extended-release capsules:** 30 mg^{Rx}, 100 mg^{Rx}, 200 mg^{Rx}, 300 mg^{Rx}. **Cost:** *Dilantin*—30 mg \$34.99/90; *Phenytek*—200 mg \$65.97/90, 300 mg \$95.27/90; *Generic*—100 mg \$23.18/90. **Injection:** 50 mg/ml^{Rx}.

NURSING IMPLICATIONS

Assessment

- Assess oral hygiene. Vigorous cleaning beginning within 10 days of initiation of phenytoin therapy may help control gingival hyperplasia.
- Assess patient for phenytoin hypersensitivity syndrome (fever, skin rash, lymphadenopathy). Rash usually occurs within the first 2 wk of therapy. Hypersensitivity syndrome usually occurs at 3–8 wk but may occur up to 12 wk after initiation of therapy. May lead to renal failure, rhabdomyolysis, or hepatic necrosis; may be fatal.
- **Seizures:** Assess location, duration, frequency, and characteristics of seizure activity. EEG may be monitored periodically throughout therapy.
- Monitor blood pressure, ECG, and respiratory function continuously during administration of IV phenytoin and throughout period when peak serum phenytoin levels occur (15–30 min after administration).
- **Arrhythmias:** Monitor ECG continuously during treatment of arrhythmias.
- ***Lab Test Considerations:*** Monitor CBC, serum calcium, albumin, and hepatic function tests prior to and monthly for the first several months, then periodically throughout therapy.
- May cause ↑ serum alkaline phosphatase, GGT, and glucose levels.

- Monitor serum folate concentrations periodically during prolonged therapy.
- ***Toxicity and Overdose:*** Monitor serum phenytoin levels routinely. Therapeutic blood levels are 10–20 mcg/ml (8–15 mcg/ml in neonates) in patients with normal serum albumin and renal function. In patients with altered protein binding (neonates, patients with renal failure, hypoalbuminemia, acute trauma), free phenytoin serum concentrations should be monitored. Therapeutic serum free phenytoin levels are 1–2 mcg/ml: Progressive signs and symptoms of phenytoin toxicity include nystagmus, ataxia, confusion, nausea, slurred speech, and dizziness.

Potential Nursing Diagnoses

Risk for injury (Indications)
Impaired oral mucous membrane (Side Effects)

Implementation

- Implement seizure precautions.
- When transferring from phenytoin to another anticonvulsant, dosage adjustments are made gradually over several weeks.
- When substituting *fosphenytoin* for oral *phenytoin* therapy, the same total daily dose may be given as a single dose. Unlike parenteral phenytoin, fosphenytoin may be given safely by the IM route.
- **PO:** Administer with or immediately after meals to minimize GI irritation. Shake liquid preparations well before pouring. Use a calibrated measuring device for accurate dose. Chewable tablets must be crushed or chewed well before swallowing. Capsules may be opened and mixed with food or fluids for patients with difficulty swallowing. To prevent direct contact of alkaline drug with mucosa, have patient swallow a liquid first, follow with mixture of medication, then follow with a full glass of water or milk or with food.
- If patient is receiving enteral tube feedings, 2 hr should elapse between feeding and phenytoin administration. If phenytoin is administered via nasogastric tube, flush tube with 2–4 oz water before and after administration.
- Do not interchange chewable phenytoin tablets with phenytoin sodium capsules, because they are not bioequivalent.
- Capsules labeled "extended" may be used for once-a-day dose (Dilantin Kapseals only); those labeled "prompt" may result in toxic serum levels if used for once-a-day dose.

IV Administration

- **IV:** Slight yellow color will not alter solution potency. If refrigerated, may form precipitate, which dissolves after warming to room temperature. Discard solution that is not clear
- To prevent precipitation and minimize local venous irritation, follow infusion with 0.9% NaCl through the same needle or catheter. Avoid extravasation; phenytoin is caustic to tissues.
- **Direct IV:** Administer undiluted. ***Rate:*** Administer at a rate not to exceed 50 mg over 1 min in adults or 1–3 mg/kg/min in neonates. Rapid administration may result in severe hypotension, cardiovascular collapse, or CNS depression.
- **Intermittent Infusion:** Administer by mixing with no more than 50 ml of 0.9% NaCl in a concentration of 1–10 mg/ml. Administer immediately following admixture. Use tubing with a 0.45- to 0.22-micron in-line filter. ***Rate:*** Complete infusion within 1 hr at a rate not to exceed 50 mg/min. In patients who may develop hypotension, patients with cardiovascular disease, or geriatric patients maximum rate of 25 mg/min [may be as low as 5–10 mg/min]. Monitor cardiac function and blood pressure throughout infusion.
- **Y-Site Compatibility:** esmolol, famotidine, fluconazole, foscarnet, tacrolimus.
- **Y-Site Incompatibility:** amphotericin B cholesteryl sulfate, cefepime, ceftazidime, ciprofloxacin, diltiazem, enalaprilat, fenoldopam, fentanyl, heparin, hydrocortisone sodium succinate, hydromorphone, lansoprazole, linezolid, methadone, morphine, potassium chloride, propofol, sufentanil, theophylline, vitamin B complex with C.
- **Additive Incompatibility:** Do not admix with other solutions or medications, especially dextrose, because precipitation will occur.

Patient/Family Teaching

- Instruct patient to take medication as directed, at the same time each day. If a dose is missed from a once-a-day schedule, take as soon as possible and return to regular dosing schedule. If taking several doses a day, take missed dose as soon as possible within 4 hr of next scheduled dose; do not double doses.

P

Consult health care professional if doses are missed for 2 consecutive days. Abrupt withdrawal may lead to status epilepticus.

- May cause drowsiness or dizziness. Caution patient to avoid driving or other activities requiring alertness until response to medication is known. Do not resume driving until physician gives clearance based on control of seizure disorder.
- Caution patient to avoid taking alcohol, OTC medications, or herbal medications concurrently with phenytoin without consulting health care professional.
- Instruct patient on importance of maintaining good dental hygiene and seeing dentist frequently for teeth cleaning to prevent tenderness, bleeding, and gingival hyperplasia. Institution of oral hygiene program within 10 days of initiation of phenytoin therapy may minimize growth rate and severity of gingival enlargement. Patients under 23 yr of age and those taking doses >500 mg/day are at increased risk for gingival hyperplasia.
- Advise patient that brands of phenytoin may not be equivalent. Check with health care professional if brand or dosage form is changed.
- Advise diabetic patients to monitor blood glucose carefully and to notify health care professional of significant changes.
- Instruct patient to notify health care professional of medication regimen prior to treatment or surgery.
- Advise patient not to take phenytoin within 2–3 hr of antacids.
- Advise female patients to use an additional nonhormonal method of contraception during therapy. Instruct patient to notify health care professional if pregnancy is planned or suspected.
- Advise patient to carry identification describing disease process and medication regimen at all times.
- Advise patient to notify health care professional if skin rash, severe nausea or vomiting, drowsiness, slurred speech, unsteady gait, swollen glands, bleeding or tender gums, yellow skin or eyes, joint pain, fever, sore throat, unusual bleeding or bruising, or persistent headache occurs.
- Emphasize the importance of routine exams to monitor progress. Patient should have routine physical exams, especially monitoring skin and lymph nodes, and EEG testing.

Evaluation/Desired Outcomes

- Decrease or cessation of seizures without excessive sedation.
- Suppression of arrhythmias.
- Relief of pain due to neuralgia.

phosphate/biphosphate

(**foss**-fate/bye-**foss**-fate)

Fleet Enema, Fleet Phospho-Soda, Visicol

Classification

Therapeutic: laxatives (saline)

Pregnancy Category C (Visicol)

Indications

Preparation of the bowel prior to surgery or radiologic studies. Intermittent treatment of chronic constipation. **Visicol:** Cleansing of the bowel as a preparation for colonoscopy in adults 18 years of age or older.

Action

Osmotically active in the lumen of the GI tract. Produces laxative effect by causing water retention and stimulation of peristalsis. Stimulates motility and inhibits fluid and electrolyte absorption from the small intestine. **Therapeutic Effects:** Relief of constipation. Emptying of the bowel.

Pharmacokinetics

Absorption: 1–20% of rectally administered sodium and phosphate may be absorbed; some absorption follows oral administration.
Distribution: Unknown.
Metabolism and Excretion: Excreted by the kidneys.
Half-life: Unknown.

TIME/ACTION PROFILE (laxative effect)

ROUTE	ONSET	PEAK	DURATION
PO	0.5–3 hr	unknown	unknown
rect	2–5 min	unknown	unknown

Contraindications/Precautions

Contraindicated in: Hypersensitivity; Abdominal pain, nausea, or vomiting, especially when associated with fever or other signs of an acute abdomen; Severe renal or cardiovascular disease; Intestinal obstruction; Pregnancy (at term); *Visicol*—CHF, ascites, unstable angina, acute colitis, toxic megacolon, or hypomotility syndrome.

Use Cautiously in: Excessive or chronic use (may lead to dependence); Renal or cardiovascular disease, dehydration or concurrent use of diuretics or other drugs known to alter electrolytes (correct abnormalities prior to administration); Pregnancy (may cause sodium retention and edema); *Visicol tablets*—use cautiously within 3 mos of MI, cardiac surgery, in patients with acute exacerbations of inflammatory bowel disease.

Adverse Reactions/Side Effects

CNS: *Visicol*— dizziness, headache. **CV:** ARRHYTHMIAS. **GI:** cramping, nausea, colonic aphtous ulcerations; *Visicol*— abdominal bloating, abdominal pain, vomiting. **F and E:** hyperphosphatemia, hypocalcemia, hypokalemia, sodium retention.

Interactions

Drug-Drug: *Visicol*—Concurrently administered oral medications may not be absorbed due to rapid peristalsis and diarrhea.

Route/Dosage

Each Fleet Enema contains 4.4 g sodium/118 ml. Each 20 ml of Fleet Phospho-Soda oral solution contains 96.4 mEq sodium.

PO (Adults): 20–30 ml Phospho-Soda; *Visicol*—evening before colonoscopy: 3 tablets every 15 min (with at least 8 oz of water), last dose will be 2 tablets (total of 20 tablets), on morning of colonoscopy starting 3–5 hr before procedure, 3 tablets every 15 min (with at least 8 oz of clear liquids), last dose will be 2 tablets (total of 20 tablets); should not be repeated in less than 7 days.

PO (Children): 5–15 ml Phospho-Soda.

Rect (Adults and Children >12 yr): 118 ml Fleet Enema.

Rect (Children >2 yr): ½ of the adult dose.

Availability (generic available)

Oral solution: 18 g sodium phosphate and 48 g sodium biphosphate/100 ml in 45-, 90-, and 237-ml containers[OTC]. **Enema:** 7 g sodium phosphate and 19 g sodium biphosphate/118 ml in 67.5- and 133-ml containers[OTC]. **Tablets (Visicol):** 2 g (40 tablets/bottle).

NURSING IMPLICATIONS

Assessment

- Assess patient for fever, abdominal distention, presence of bowel sounds, and usual pattern of bowel function.
- Assess color, consistency, and amount of stool produced.
- May rarely cause arrhythmias. Monitor patients with underlying cardiovascular disease, renal disease, bowel perforation, misuse or overdose.
- ***Lab Test Considerations:*** May cause increased serum sodium and phosphorus levels, decreased serum calcium and potassium levels, and acidosis. Electrolyte changes are transient, self-limiting, do not require treatment and are not usually associated with adverse clinical events.

Potential Nursing Diagnoses

Constipation (Indications)

Implementation

- Do not administer at bedtime or late in the day.
- **PO:** Administer on an empty stomach for more rapid results. Mix dose in at least ½ glass cold water. May be followed by carbonated beverage or fruit juice to improve flavor.
- See Route and Dose section for dosing of Visicol. Undigested Visicol tablets may appear in the stool or be visualized during colonoscopy.
- **Rect:** Position patient on left side with knee slightly flexed. Insert prelubricated tip about 2 in. into rectum, aiming toward the umbilicus. Gently squeeze bottle until empty. Discontinue if resistance is met, because perforation may occur if contents are forced into rectum.

Patient/Family Teaching

- Advise patient that laxatives should be used only for short-term therapy. Long-term therapy may cause electrolyte imbalance and dependence.
- Caution patient on sodium restriction that this product has a high sodium content.
- Advise patient not to take oral form of this medication within 2 hr of other medications.
- Encourage patient to use other forms of bowel regulation, such as increasing bulk in the diet, fluid intake, and mobility. Normal bowel habits may vary from 3 times/day to 3 times/wk.
- Advise patient to notify health care professional if unrelieved constipation, rectal bleeding, or symptoms of electrolyte imbal-

P

ance (muscle cramps or pain, weakness, dizziness, and so forth) occur.

Evaluation/Desired Outcomes

- Soft, formed bowel movement.
- Evacuation of the bowel.

phytonadione

(fye-toe-na-**dye**-one)
AquaMEPHYTON, Mephyton, vitamin K

Classification
Therapeutic: antidotes, vitamins
Pharmacologic: fat-soluble vitamins

Pregnancy Category UK

Indications

Prevention and treatment of hypoprothrombinemia, which may be associated with: Excessive doses of oral anticoagulants, Salicylates, Certain anti-infective agents, Nutritional deficiencies, Prolonged total parenteral nutrition. Prevention of hemorrhagic disease of the newborn.

Action

Required for hepatic synthesis of blood coagulation factors II (prothrombin), VII, IX, and X. **Therapeutic Effects:** Prevention of bleeding due to hypoprothrombinemia.

Pharmacokinetics

Absorption: Well absorbed following oral, IM, or subcut administration. Oral absorption requires presence of bile salts. Some vitamin K is produced by bacteria in the GI tract.
Distribution: Crosses the placenta; does not enter breast milk.
Metabolism and Excretion: Rapidly metabolized by the liver.
Half-life: Unknown.

TIME/ACTION PROFILE

ROUTE	ONSET	PEAK†	DURATION‡
PO	6–12 hr	unknown	unknown
IM, subcut	1–2 hr	3–6 hr	12–14 hr
IV	1–2 hr	3–6 hr	12 hr

†Control of hemorrhage
‡Normal PT achieved

Contraindications/Precautions

Contraindicated in: Hypersensitivity; Hypersensitivity or intolerance to benzyl alcohol (injection only).
Use Cautiously in: Impaired liver function.
Exercise Extreme Caution in: Severe life-threatening reactions have occurred following IV administration, use other routes unless risk is justified.

Adverse Reactions/Side Effects

GI: gastric upset, unusual taste. **Derm:** flushing, rash, urticaria. **Hemat:** hemolytic anemia. **Local:** erythema, pain at injection site, swelling. **Misc:** allergic reactions, hyperbilirubinemia (large doses in very premature infants), kernicterus.

Interactions

Drug-Drug: Large doses will counteract the effect of **warfarin**. Large doses of **salicylates** or broad-spectrum **anti-infectives** may increase vitamin K requirements. **Bile acid sequestrants**, **mineral oil**, and **sucralfate** may decrease vitamin K absorption from the GI tract.

Route/Dosage

IV use of phytonadione should be reserved for emergencies, subcutaneous route is preferred.

Treatment of Hypoprothrombinemia due to Vitamin K Deficiency

Subcut, IM, IV (Adults): 10 mg.
PO (Adults): 2.5–25 mg/day.
Subcut, IM, IV (Children >1 month): 1–2-mg single dose.
PO (Children >1 month): 2.5–5 mg/day.

Prevention of Hypoprothrombinemia during Total Parenteral Nutrition

IM, IV (Adults): 5–10 mg once weekly.
IM, IV (Children): 2–5 mg once weekly.

Oral Anticoagulant Overdose

Subcut, IV (Adults): 2.5–10 mg/dose (rarely up to 25–50 mg has been used); may repeat 12–48 hr after with oral route.
Subcut, IV (Children >1 month): 0.5–5 mg.

Prevention of Hemorrhagic Disease of Newborn

IM (Neonates): 0.5–1 mg, within 1 hr of birth, may repeat in 6–8 hrs if needed. May be repeated in 2–3 wk if mother received previous anticonvulsant/anticoagulant/anti-infective/antitubercular therapy. 1–5 mg may be given IM to mother 12–24 hr before delivery.

Treatment of Hemorrhagic Disease of Newborn

IM, Subcut (Neonates): 1–2 mg/day.

Availability

Tablets: 5 mg. **Injection:** 2 mg/ml in 0.5-ml ampules, 10 mg/ml in 1-ml ampules.

NURSING IMPLICATIONS

Assessment

- Monitor for frank and occult bleeding (guaiac stools, Hematest urine, and emesis). Monitor pulse and blood pressure frequently; notify physician immediately if symptoms of internal bleeding or hypovolemic shock develop. Inform all personnel of patient's bleeding tendency to prevent further trauma. Apply pressure to all venipuncture sites for at least 5 min; avoid unnecessary IM injections.
- Pedi: Monitor for side effects and adverse reactions. Children may be especially sensitive to the effects and side effects of vitamin K. Neonates, especially premature neonates, may be more sensitive than older children.
- ***Lab Test Considerations:*** Monitor prothrombin time (PT) prior to and throughout vitamin K therapy to determine response to and need for further therapy.

Potential Nursing Diagnoses

Imbalanced nutrition: less than body requirements (Indications)
Ineffective tissue perfusion (Indications)

Implementation

- The parenteral route is preferred for phytonadione therapy but, because of severe, potentially fatal hypersensitivity reactions, IV vitamin K is not recommended.
- Administration of whole blood or plasma may also be required in severe bleeding because of the delayed onset of this medication.
- Phytonadione is an antidote for warfarin overdose but does not counteract the anticoagulant activity of heparin.

IV Administration

- **Intermittent Infusion:** ***Diluent:*** Dilute in 0.9% NaCl, D5W, or D5/0.9% NaCl. ***Rate:*** Administer over 30–60 min. Rate should not exceed 1 mg/min.
- **Y-Site Compatibility:** amikacin, aminophylline, atropine, aztreonam, bumetanide, calcium chloride, calcium gluconate, cefazolin, cefotaxime, cefoxitin, ceftazidime, ceftizoxime, ceftriaxone, cefuroxime, chloramphenicol, cimetidine, clindamycin, cyclosporine, dexamethasone sodium phosphate, digoxin, diphenhydramine, dopamine, doxycycline, enalaprilat, epinephrine, erythromycin, esmolol, famotidine, fentanyl, fluconazole, furosemide, ganciclovir, gentamicin, heparin, hydrocortisone sodium succinate, hydroxyzine, imipenem/cilastatin, insulin, isoproterenol, ketorolac, labetalol, lidocaine, meperidine, metoclopramide, metoprolol, metronidazole, midazolam, morphine, nafcillin, nitroglycerin, nitroprusside, norepinephrine, ondansetron, penicillin G potassium, piperacillin, potassium chloride, procainamide, prochlorperazine, propranolol, ranitidine, sodium bicarbonate, ticarcillin/clavulanate, tobramycin, tolazoline, vancomycin, vasopressin, verapamil, vitamin B with C.
- **Y-Site Incompatibility:** diazepam, dobutamine, magnesium sulfate, phenytoin, trimethoprim/sulfamethoxazole.

Patient/Family Teaching

- Instruct patient to take this medication as directed. Take missed doses as soon as remembered unless almost time for next dose. Notify health care professional of missed doses.
- Cooking does not destroy substantial amounts of vitamin K. Patient should not drastically alter diet while taking vitamin K. See Appendix L for foods high in vitamin K.
- Caution patient to avoid IM injections and activities leading to injury. Use a soft toothbrush, do not floss, and shave with an electric razor until coagulation defect is corrected.
- Advise patient to report any symptoms of unusual bleeding or bruising (bleeding gums; nosebleed; black, tarry stools; hematuria; excessive menstrual flow).
- Patients receiving vitamin K therapy should be cautioned not to take OTC medications without advice of health care professional.
- Advise patient to inform health care professional of medication regimen prior to treatment or surgery.
- Advise patient to carry identification at all times describing disease process.
- Emphasize the importance of frequent lab tests to monitor coagulation factors.

Evaluation/Desired Outcomes

- Prevention of spontaneous bleeding or cessation of bleeding in patients with hypopro-

thrombinemia secondary to impaired intestinal absorption or oral anticoagulant, salicylate, or anti-infective therapy.
- Prevention of hemorrhagic disease in the newborn.

pilocarpine (oral)†
(pye-loe-**kar**-peen)
Salagen

Classification
Therapeutic: none assigned
Pharmacologic: cholinergics

Pregnancy Category C

†For ophthalmic use of pilocarpine, see Appendix C

Indications
Management of xerostomia, which may occur as a consequence of radiation therapy for cancer of the head and neck. Treatment of dry mouth in patients with Sjögren's syndrome.

Action
Stimulates cholinergic receptors, resulting in primarily muscarinic action, including stimulation of exocrine glands. Other effects include: Increased sweating, gastric secretions, Increased bronchial secretions, Increased tone and motility of the urinary tract, gallbladder, and biliary duct smooth muscle. **Therapeutic Effects:** Increased salivary gland secretion.

Pharmacokinetics
Absorption: Well absorbed after oral administration.
Distribution: Unknown.
Metabolism and Excretion: Inactivated at neuronal synapses and in plasma. Some unchanged pilocarpine and metabolites are excreted in urine.
Half-life: *After 5-mg dose for 2 days*—0.8 hr; *after 10-mg dose for 2 days*—1.3 hr.

TIME/ACTION PROFILE

ROUTE	ONSET	PEAK	DURATION
PO	20 min	1 hr	3–5 hr

Contraindications/Precautions
Contraindicated in: Hypersensitivity; Uncontrolled asthma; Angle-closure glaucoma; Iritis.
Use Cautiously in: History of pulmonary disease (asthma, bronchitis, or chronic obstructive pulmonary disease); Biliary tract disease or cholelithiasis; Cardiovascular disease; Retinal disease; Nephrolithiasis; History of psychiatric or cognitive disorders; OB: Pregnancy, lactation, or children (safety not established).

Adverse Reactions/Side Effects
CNS: dizziness, headache, weakness. **EENT:** amblyopia, epistaxis, rhinitis. **CV:** edema, hypertension, tachycardia. **GI:** nausea, vomiting, dyspepsia, dysphagia. **GU:** urinary frequency. **Derm:** flushing, sweating. **Neuro:** tremors. **Misc:** chills, voice change.

Interactions
Drug-Drug: Concurrent use of **anticholinergics** will ↓ the effectiveness of pilocarpine. Concurrent use of **bethanechol** or **ophthalmic cholinergics** may result in ↑ cholinergic effects. Concurrent use with **beta blockers** may ↑ the risk of adverse cardiovascular reactions (conduction disturbances).

Route/Dosage

Head and Neck Cancer Patients
PO (Adults): 5 mg three times daily initially, then titrated to need/response, usual range 15–30 mg/day (no single should exceed 10 mg).

Patients with Sjögren's Syndrome
PO (Adults): 5 mg four times daily.

Availability
Tablets: 5 mg, 7.5 mg.

NURSING IMPLICATIONS

Assessment
- Assess oral mucosa for dryness and ulceration periodically during therapy.

Potential Nursing Diagnoses
Impaired oral mucous membrane (Indications)

Implementation
- **PO:** Use lowest dose that is tolerated and effective for maintenance.

Patient/Family Teaching
- Instruct patient to take medication as directed.
- Caution patient that pilocarpine may cause visual changes, especially at night; avoid driving or other activities requiring alertness until effects of medication are known.
- Advise patient to drink adequate daily fluids (1500–2000 ml/day), especially if sweating occurs. Less than adequate fluid intake may lead to dehydration.

Evaluation/Desired Outcomes

- Increased salivary gland secretion in patients with xerostomia.
- Decrease in dry mouth in patients with Sjögren's syndrome. Full effects in cancer patients may not be seen for up to 12 weeks or 6 weeks in patients with Sjögren's syndrome.

pimecrolimus

(pi-me-**cro**-li-mus)
Elidel

Classification
Therapeutic: immunosuppressants (topical)

Indications

Short-term and intermittent long-term management of mild to moderate atopic dermatitis unresponsive to or in patients intolerant of conventional treatment.

Action

Inhibits T-cell and mast cell activation by interfering with production of inflammatory cytokines. **Therapeutic Effects:** Decreased severity of atopic dermatatis.

Pharmacokinetics

Absorption: Minimally absorbed through intact skin.
Distribution: Local distribution after topical administration.
Metabolism and Excretion: Systemic metabolism and excretion is negligible with local application.
Half-life: Not applicable.

TIME/ACTION PROFILE (improvement in symptoms)

ROUTE	ONSET	PEAK	DURATION
topical	within 6 days	unknown	unknown

Contraindications/Precautions

Contraindicated in: Hypersensitivity; Should not be applied to areas of active cutaneous viral infections (increased risk of dissemination); Concurrent use of occlusive dressings; Netherton's syndrome (increased absorption of pimecrolimus); Lactation: Discontinue breast-feeding.

Use Cautiously in: Possible risk of cancer. Do not use as first-line therapy; Clinical infection at treatment site (infection should be treated/cleared prior to use); Skin papillomas (warts); allow treatment/resolution prior to use; Natural/artificial sunlight (minimize exposure); OB: Use only if clearly needed; Pedi: Use only if other treatments have failed; safety not established in children <2 yr.

Adverse Reactions/Side Effects

Local: burning. **Misc:** increased risk of lymphoma/skin cancer.

Interactions

Drug-Drug: None significant as systemic absorption is negligible.

Route/Dosage

Topical (Adults and Children ≥2 yr): Apply thin film twice daily; rub in gently and completely.

Availability

Cream: 1% in 30-g, 60-g, and 100-g tubes. **Cost:** $75.99/30 g, $141.58/60 g, $220.98/100 g.

P

NURSING IMPLICATIONS

Assessment

- Assess skin lesions prior to and periodically during therapy. Discontinue therapy after signs and symptoms of atopic dermatitis have resolved. Resume treatment at the first signs and symptoms of recurrence.

Potential Nursing Diagnoses

Impaired skin integrity (Indications)

Implementation

- **Topical:** Apply a thin layer to affected area twice daily and rub in gently and completely. May be used on all skin areas including head, neck, and intertriginous areas. Do not use with occlusive dressings.

Patient/Family Teaching

- Instruct patient on correct technique for application. Apply only as directed to external areas. Wash hands following application, unless hands are areas of application.
- Caution patient to avoid exposure to natural or artificial sunlight, including tanning beds, while using cream.
- Advise patient that pimecrolimus may cause skin burning. This occurs most commonly

during first few days of application, is of mild to moderate severity, and improves within 5 days or as atopic dermatitis resolves.
- Advise patient to notify health care provider if no improvement is seen following 6 wk of treatment or at any time if condition worsens.

Evaluation/Desired Outcomes
- Resolution of signs and symptoms of atopic dermatitis.

pioglitazone (pi-o-**glit**-a-zone)
Actos

Classification
Therapeutic: antidiabetics (oral)
Pharmacologic: thiazolidinediones

Pregnancy Category C

Indications
Management of type 2 diabetes mellitus; may also be used with a sulfonylurea, metformin, or insulin when the combination of diet, exercise, and metformin does not achieve glycemic control.

Action
Improves sensitivity to insulin by acting as an agonist at receptor sites involved in insulin responsiveness and subsequent glucose production and utilization. Requires insulin for activity. **Therapeutic Effects:** Decreased insulin resistance, resulting in glycemic control without hypoglycemia.

Pharmacokinetics
Absorption: Well absorbed following oral administration.
Distribution: Unknown.
Protein Binding: >99% bound to plasma proteins. Active metabolites are also highly (>99 %) bound.
Metabolism and Excretion: Extensively metabolized by the liver; at least two metabolites have pharmacologic activity. Minimal renal excretion of unchanged drug.
Half-life: *Pioglitazone*—3–7 hr; *total pioglitazone (pioglitazone plus metabolites)*—16–24 hr.

TIME/ACTION PROFILE (effects on blood glucose)

ROUTE	ONSET	PEAK	DURATION
PO	30 min	2–4 hr	24 hr

Contraindications/Precautions
Contraindicated in: Hypersensitivity; Diabetic ketoacidosis; Clinical evidence of active liver disease or increased ALT (>2.5 times upper limit of normal); OB: Pregnancy or lactation (not recommended for use during pregnancy or lactation; insulin should be used); Pedi: Children <18 yr or type 1 diabetes (requires insulin for activity).
Use Cautiously in: Edema; CHF (avoid use in moderate to severe CHF); Hepatic impairment; Women (may increase distal upper and lower limb fractures); Women with childbearing potential (may restore ovulation and risk of pregnancy).

Adverse Reactions/Side Effects
CV: edema. **GI:** hepatitis, ↑ liver enzymes. **Hemat:** anemia. **Misc:** fractures (arm, hand, foot) in female patients.

Interactions
Drug-Drug: May ↓ efficacy of **hormonal contraceptives**. Pioglitazone is metabolized by the **CYP450 3A4** enzyme system. Concurrent use of drugs that alter the activity of this system may result in drug-drug interactions. **Ketoconazole** may ↑ effects of pioglitazone. Concurrent use with **insulin** may ↑ risk of CHF (consider predisposing factors).
Drug-Natural Products: Glucosamine may worsen blood glucose control. Chromium, and coenzyme Q-10 may produce ↑ hypoglycemic effects.

Route/Dosage
PO (Adults): 15–30 mg once daily, may be increased to 45 mg/day if needed. Doses greater than 30 mg have not been evaluated in combination with insulin and other antidiabetics.

Availability
Tablets: 15 mg, 30 mg, 45 mg. **Cost:** 15 mg $329.97/90, 30 mg $505.97/90, 45 mg $549.97/90. ***In combination with:*** Metformin (Actoplus Met), glimepride (Duetact); see Appendix B.

NURSING IMPLICATIONS

Assessment
- Observe patient taking concurrent insulin for signs and symptoms of hypoglycemic reac-

tions (sweating, hunger, weakness, dizziness, tremor, tachycardia, anxiety).
- ***Lab Test Considerations:*** Monitor serum glucose and Hb A_{1c} periodically during therapy to evaluate effectiveness.
- Monitor CBC with differential periodically during therapy. May cause ↓ in hemoglobin and hematocrit, usually during the first 4–12 wk of therapy; then levels stabilize.
- Monitor serum ALT levels before starting therapy and periodically thereafter or if jaundice or symptoms of hepatic dysfunction occur. Pioglitazone should not be started in patients with active liver disease or ALT levels >2.5 times the upper limit of normal. Patients with mild ALT ↑ should have more frequent monitoring. If ALT ↑ to >3 times the upper limit of normal, recheck ALT promptly. Discontinue pioglitazone if ALT remains >3 times normal.
- May cause transient ↑ in CPK levels.

Potential Nursing Diagnoses

Imbalanced nutrition: more than body requirements (Indications)
Noncompliance (Patient/Family Teaching)

Implementation

- Patients stabilized on a diabetic regimen who are exposed to stress, fever, trauma, infection, or surgery may require administration of insulin.
- **PO:** May be administered with or without meals.

Patient/Family Teaching

- Instruct patient to take medication as directed. If dose for 1 day is missed, do not double dose the next day.
- Explain to patient that this medication controls hyperglycemia but does not cure diabetes. Therapy is long-term.
- Review signs of hypoglycemia and hyperglycemia with patient. If hypoglycemia occurs, advise patient to take a glass of orange juice or 2–3 tsp of sugar, honey, or corn syrup dissolved in water and notify health care professional.
- Encourage patient to follow prescribed diet, medication, and exercise regimen to prevent hypoglycemic or hyperglycemic episodes.
- Instruct patient in proper testing of serum glucose and ketones. These tests should be closely monitored during periods of stress or illness, and health care professional should be notified if significant changes occur.
- Advise patient to notify health care professional immediately if signs of hepatic dysfunction (nausea, vomiting, abdominal pain, fatigue, anorexia, dark urine, jaundice) or CHF (edema, shortness of breath, rapid weight gain) occur.
- Insulin is the preferred method of controlling blood glucose during pregnancy. Counsel female patients that higher doses of oral contraceptives or a form of contraception other than oral contraceptives may be required and to notify health care professional promptly if pregnancy is planned or suspected.
- Advise patient to inform health care professional of medication regimen before treatment or surgery.
- Advise patient to carry a form of sugar (sugar packets, candy) and identification describing disease process and medication regimen at all times.
- Emphasize the importance of routine follow-up exams.

Evaluation/Desired Outcomes

- Control of blood glucose levels.

piperacillin/tazobactam

(pi-**per**-a-sill-in/tay-zoe-**bak**-tam)
Zosyn

Classification
Therapeutic: anti-infectives
Pharmacologic: extended spectrum penicillins

Pregnancy Category B

Indications

Appendicitis and peritonitis. Skin and skin structure infections. Gynecologic infections. Community-acquired and nosocomial pneumonia caused by piperacillin-resistant, beta-lactamase–producing bacteria.

Action

Piperacillin binds to bacterial cell wall membrane, causing cell death. Spectrum is extended compared with other penicillins. Tazobactam inhibits beta-lactamase, an enzyme that can destroy penicillins. **Therapeutic Effects:** Death of susceptible bacteria. **Spectrum:** Active

P

against piperacillin-resistant, beta-lactamase–producing: *Bacteroides fragilis*, *E. coli*, *Acinetobacter baumanii*, *Klebsiella pneumoniae*, *Pseudomonas aeruginosa*, *Staphylococcus aureus*, *Haemophilus influenzae*.

Pharmacokinetics

Absorption: Piperacillin is well absorbed (80%) from IM sites.
Distribution: Widely distributed. Enter CSF well only when meninges are inflamed. Cross the placenta and enter breast milk in low concentrations.
Metabolism and Excretion: Piperacillin (68%) and tazobactam (80%) are mostly excreted unchanged by the kidneys.
Half-life: 0.7–1.2 hr.

TIME/ACTION PROFILE (piperacillin blood levels)

ROUTE	ONSET	PEAK	DURATION
IV	rapid	end of infusion	4–6 hr

Contraindications/Precautions

Contraindicated in: Hypersensitivity to penicillins, beta-lactams, cephalosporins, or tazobactam (cross-sensitivity may occur).
Use Cautiously in: Renal impairment (dosage reduction or increased interval recommended if CCr <40 ml/min); Sodium restriction; Pedi: Children (safety and efficacy not established); OB: Pregnancy and lactation (safety not established).

Adverse Reactions/Side Effects

CNS: SEIZURES (higher doses), confusion, dizziness, headache, insomnia, lethargy. **GI:** PSEUDOMEMBRANOUS COLITIS, diarrhea, constipation, drug-induced hepatitis, nausea, vomiting. **GU:** interstitial nephritis. **Derm:** rashes (↑ in cystic fibrosis patients), urticaria. **Hemat:** bleeding, leukopenia, neutropenia, thrombocytopenia. **Local:** pain, phlebitis at IV site. **Misc:** hypersensitivity reactions, including ANAPHYLAXIS and SERUM SICKNESS, fever (↑ in cystic fibrosis patients), superinfection.

Interactions

Drug-Drug: Probenecid ↓ renal excretion and ↑ blood levels. May alter excretion of **lithium**. **Potassium-losing diuretics**, **corticosteroids**, or **amphotericin B** may ↑ risk of hypokalemia. ↑ risk of hepatotoxicity with other **hepatotoxic agents**. May ↓ half-life of **aminoglycosides** in patients with renal impairment. May ↑ levels and risk of toxicity from **methotrexate**.

Route/Dosage

Contains 2.79 mEq (64 mg) sodium/g of piperacillin; dose below expressed as combined piperacillin/tazobactam content.
IV (Adults): *Most infections*—3.375 g q 6 hr. *Nosocomial pneumonia*—4,5 g q 6 hr.

Renal Impairment

IV (Adults): *CCr 20–40 ml/min*—2.25 g q 6 hr (3.375 g q 6 hr for nosocomial pneumonia); *CCr <20 ml/min*—2.25 g q 8 hr (2.25 g q 6 hr for nosocomial pneumonia); *Hemodialysis*—2.25 g q 12 h (2.25 g q 8 hr for nosocomial pneumonia).

Availability

Powder for injection: 2-g piperacillin/0.25-g tazobactam vials and 50-g ml premixed frozen containers, 3-g piperacillin/0.375-g tazobactam vials and 50-ml premixed frozen containers, 4-g piperacillin/0.5-g tazobactam vials and 50-ml premixed frozen containers, 36-g piperacillin/4.5-g tazobactam bulk vials.

NURSING IMPLICATIONS

Assessment

- Assess patient for infection (vital signs; appearance of wound, sputum, urine, and stool; WBC) at beginning of and during therapy.
- Obtain a history before initiating therapy to determine previous use of and reactions to penicillins or cephalosporins. Persons with a negative history of penicillin sensitivity may still have an allergic response.
- Obtain specimens for culture and sensitivity prior to initiating therapy. First dose may be given before receiving results.
- Observe patient for signs and symptoms of anaphylaxis (rash, pruritus, laryngeal edema, wheezing). Discontinue the drug and notify the physician or other health care professional immediately if these occur. Keep epinephrine, an antihistamine, and resuscitation equipment close by in the event of an anaphylactic reaction.
- ***Lab Test Considerations:*** Evaluate renal and hepatic function, CBC, serum potassium, and bleeding times prior to and routinely during therapy.
- May cause positive direct Coombs' test result.
- May cause ↑ BUN, creatinine, AST, ALT, serum bilirubin, alkaline phosphatase, and LDH.

- May cause leukopenia and neutropenia, especially with prolonged therapy or hepatic impairment.
- May cause prolonged prothrombin and partial thromboplastin time.
- May cause ↓ hemoglobin and hematocrit and thrombocytopenia, eosinophilia, leukopenia, and neutropenia. It also may cause proteinuria; hematuria; pyuria; hyperglycemia; ↓ total protein or albumin; and abnormalities in sodium, potassium, and calcium levels.

Potential Nursing Diagnosis

Risk for infection (Indications, Side Effects)
Deficient knowledge, related to medication regimen (Patient/Family Teaching)

Implementation

- Do not confuse Zosyn (piperacillin/tazobactam) with Zofran (ondansetron).

IV Administration

- **Intermittent Infusion:** ***Diluent:*** Reconstitute each 1 g of piperacillin with at least 5 ml of 0.9% NaCl, sterile water for injection, or D5W. Dilute further in 50–100 ml of 0.9% NaCl, D5W, D5/0.9% NaCl, or LR. Reconstituted vials stable for 24 hr at room temperature or 48 hr if refrigerated. Infusion stable for 24 hr at room temperature or 7 days if refrigerated. ***Rate:*** Infuse over 30 min.
- **Y-Site Compatibility:** amikacin, aminophylline, anidulafungin, aztreonam, bivalirudin, bleomycin, bumetanide, buprenorphine, butorphanol, carboplatin, carmustine, calcium chloride, calcium gluconate, cefepime, chloramphenicol, cimetidine, clindamycin, cyclosporine, cytarabine, daptomycin, dexamethasone sodium phosphate, dexmedetomidine, diazepam, digoxin, diphenhydramine, docetaxel, dopamine, enalaprilat, epinephrine, erythromycin, esmolol, etoposide, etoposide phosphate, fenoldopam, fentanyl, floxuridine, fluconazole, fludarabine, fluorouracil, furosemide, granisetron, heparin, hydrocortisone sodium succinate, hydromorphone, ifosfamide, isoproterenol, ketorolac, lansoprazole, leucovorin, lidocaine, linezolid, lorazepam, magnesium sulfate, mannitol, meperidine, mesna, methotrexate, methylprednisolone sodium succinate, metoclopramide, metoprolol, metronidazole, milrinone, morphine, nitroglycerin, nitroprusside, norepinephrine, ondansetron, palonosetron, pancuronium, pantoprazole, phenylephrine, potassium chloride, procainamide, ranitidine, remifentanil, sargramostim, sodium bicarbonate, tacrolimus, thiotepa, trimethoprim/sulfamethoxazole, tigecycline, tirofiban, vasopressin, vinblastine, vincristine, voriconazole, zidovudine.
- **Y-Site Incompatibility:** acyclovir, amiodarone, amphotericin B, amphotericin b cholesteryl sulfate complex, azithromycin, caspofungin, chlorpromazine, ciprofloxacin, cisplatin, dacarbazine, daunorubicin, diltiazem, dobutamine, doxorubicin, doxorubicin liposome, doxycycline, droperidol, drotrecogin, famotidine, ganciclovir, gemcitabine, haloperidol, hydralazine, hydroxyzine, idarubicin, insulin, labetalol, levofloxacin, midazolam, mitomycin, mitoxantrone, nalbuphine, phenytoin, prochlorperazine, promethazine, propranolol, quinupristin/dalfopristin, thiotepa, tobramycin, vecuronium, verapamil.

P

Patient/Family Teaching

- Advise patient to report signs of superinfection (black furry overgrowth on tongue, vaginal itching or discharge, loose or foul-smelling stools) and allergy.
- Caution patient to notify health care professional if fever and diarrhea occur, especially if stool contains blood, pus, or mucus. Advise patient not to treat diarrhea without consulting health care professional. May occur up to several weeks after discontinuation of medication.

Evaluation/Desired Outcomes

- Resolution of the signs and symptoms of infection. Length of time for complete resolution depends on the organism and site of infection.

piroxicam (peer-**ox**-i-kam)

♣Apo-Piroxicam, Feldene, ♣Novo-Pirocam, ♣Nu-Pirox, ♣PMS-Piroxicam

Classification

Therapeutic: antirheumatics, nonsteroidal anti-inflammatory agents

Pregnancy Category C

Indications

Management of inflammatory disorders, including: Rheumatoid arthritis, Osteoarthritis. **Unlabeled uses:** Management of dysmenorrhea.

Action

Inhibits prostaglandin synthesis. **Therapeutic Effects:** Suppression of pain and inflammation.

Pharmacokinetics

Absorption: Well absorbed from the GI tract.
Distribution: Unknown. Enters breast milk in small amounts.
Metabolism and Excretion: Mostly metabolized by the liver. Minimal amounts excreted unchanged by the kidneys.
Half-life: 50 hr.

TIME/ACTION PROFILE

ROUTE	ONSET	PEAK	DURATION
PO (analgesic effect)	1 hr	unknown	48–72 hr
PO (anti-inflammatory effect)	7–12 days	2–3 wk†	unknown

†May take up to 12 wk

Contraindications/Precautions

Contraindicated in: Hypersensitivity; Cross-sensitivity may exist with other NSAIDs, including aspirin; Active GI bleeding or ulcer disease; OB: Lactation; Peri-operative pain from coronary artery bypass graft (CABG) surgery.
Use Cautiously in: Cardiovascular disease or risk factors for cardiovascular disease (may ↑ risk of serious cardiovascular thrombotic events, myocardial infarction, and stroke, especially with prolonged use); Severe hepatic disease; History of ulcer disease; Geri: Appears on Beers list. Geriatric patients are at increased risk for GI bleeding, edema, renal failure; Renal impairment (dosage reduction recommended); OB, Pedi: Pregnancy or children (safety not established; avoid use during 2nd half of pregnancy).

Adverse Reactions/Side Effects

CNS: drowsiness, headache, dizziness. **EENT:** blurred vision, tinnitus. **CV:** edema. **GI:** DRUG-INDUCED HEPATITIS, GI BLEEDING, discomfort, dyspepsia, nausea, vomiting, anorexia, constipation, diarrhea, flatulence. **GU:** renal failure. **Derm:** EXFOLIATIVE DERMATITIS, STEVENS-JOHNSON SYNDROME, TOXIC EPIDERMAL NECROLYSIS, rashes. **Hemat:** blood dyscrasias, prolonged bleeding time. **Misc:** allergic reactions including ANAPHYLAXIS.

Interactions

Drug-Drug: Concurrent use with **aspirin** ↓ piroxicam blood levels and may ↓ effectiveness. ↑ risk of bleeding with **anticoagulants**, **cefoperazone**, **cefotetan**, **heparin**, **ticlopidine**, **clopidogrel**, **eptifibatide**, **tirofiban**, **thrombolytic agents**, **valproic acid**. ↑ adverse GI side effects with **aspirin**, **corticosteroids**, and other **NSAIDs**. **Probenecid** ↑ blood levels and may increase toxicity. May ↓ response to **antihypertensives** or **diuretics**. May ↑ serum levels and risk of toxicity from **lithium**. May ↑ risk of hypoglycemia from **insulin** or **oral hypoglycemic agents**. ↑ risk of adverse renal effects with **gold compounds**, **cyclosporine**, or chronic use of **acetaminophen**. May ↑ risk of hematologic toxicity from **antineoplastics** or **radiation therapy**.
Drug-Natural Products: Increased anticoagulant effect and bleeding risk with **arnica**, **chamomile**, **clove**, **dong quai**, **fenugreek**, **feverfew**, **garlic**, **ginger**, **ginkgo**, **Panax ginseng**, and others.

Route/Dosage

PO (Adults): *Anti-inflammatory*—10–20 mg/day; may be given as single dose or 2 divided doses. *Antidysmenorrheal*—40 mg initially, then 20 mg/day.
PO (Geriatric Patients): 10 mg/day initially.

Availability (generic available)

Capsules: 10 mg, 20 mg. **Suppositories:** ✤10 mg, ✤20 mg.

NURSING IMPLICATIONS

Assessment

- Patients who have asthma, aspirin-induced allergy, and nasal polyps are at increased risk for developing hypersensitivity reactions. Monitor for rhinitis, asthma, and urticaria.
- **Arthritis:** Assess pain and range of motion prior to and 1–2 hr following administration.
- ***Lab Test Considerations:*** Bleeding time may be prolonged for up to 2 wk following discontinuation of therapy.
- May cause ↓ hemoglobin, hematocrit, leukocyte, and platelet counts.
- Monitor liver function tests periodically during therapy. May cause ↑ serum alkaline phosphatase, LDH, AST, and ALT concentrations.
- Monitor BUN, serum creatinine, and electrolytes periodically during therapy. May cause ↑ BUN, serum creatinine, and electrolyte

concentrations and ↓ urine electrolyte concentrations.

Potential Nursing Diagnoses

Acute pain (Indications)
Impaired physical mobility (Indications)

Implementation

- Administration in higher than recommended doses does not provide increased effectiveness but may cause increased side effects, especially in geriatric patients. Use lowest effective dose for shortest period of time.
- **PO:** Administer after meals or with food or an antacid containing aluminum or magnesium to minimize gastric irritation.
- Administer as soon as possible after the onset of menses. Prophylactic use has not been proved effective.

Patient/Family Teaching

- Advise patient to take this medication with a full glass of water and to remain in an upright position for 15–30 min after administration.
- Instruct patient to take medication as directed. Take missed doses as soon as remembered but not if almost time for the next dose. Do not double doses.
- May cause drowsiness or dizziness. Advise patient to avoid driving or other activities requiring alertness until response to the medication is known.
- Caution patient to avoid the concurrent use of alcohol, aspirin, acetaminophen, or other OTC or herbal products without consulting health care professional.
- Advise patient to inform health care professional of medication regimen prior to treatment or surgery.
- Caution patient to use sunscreen and protective clothing to prevent photosensitivity reaction (rare).
- Advise patient to consult health care professional if rash, itching, visual disturbances, tinnitus, weight gain, edema, black stools, persistent headache, or influenza-like syndrome (chills, fever, muscle aches, pain) occurs.

Evaluation/Desired Outcomes

- Decreased pain and improved joint mobility. Partial arthritic relief is usually seen within 2 wk, but maximum effectiveness may require up to 12 wk of continuous therapy. Patients who do not respond to one NSAID may respond to another.

polyethylene glycol

(po-lee-**eth**-e-leen **glye**-kole)
MiraLax

Classification
Therapeutic: laxatives
Pharmacologic: osmotics

Pregnancy Category C

Indications

Treatment of occasional constipation.

Action

Polyethylene glycol (PEG) in solution acts as an osmotic agent, drawing water into the lumen of the GI tract. **Therapeutic Effects:** Evacuation of the GI tract without water or electrolyte imbalance.

Pharmacokinetics

Absorption: Nonabsorbable.
Distribution: Unknown.
Metabolism and Excretion: Excreted in fecal contents.
Half-life: Unknown.

TIME/ACTION PROFILE (bowel movement)

ROUTE	ONSET	PEAK	DURATION
PO	unknown	2–4 days	unknown

Contraindications/Precautions

Contraindicated in: GI obstruction; Gastric retention; Toxic colitis; Megacolon.
Use Cautiously in: Abdominal pain of uncertain cause, particularly if accompanied by fever; Pregnancy or children (safety not established).

Adverse Reactions/Side Effects

GI: abdominal bloating, cramping, flatulence, nausea.

Interactions

Drug-Drug: None significant.

Route/Dosage

PO (Adults): 17 g (heaping tablespoon) in 8 oz of water; may be used for up to 2 wk.

Availability (generic available)

Powder: 14-oz, 16-oz, 24-oz, and 26-oz containers, 17-g packets.

NURSING IMPLICATIONS

Assessment

- Assess patient for abdominal distention, presence of bowel sounds, and usual pattern of bowel function.
- Assess color, consistency, and amount of stool produced.

Potential Nursing Diagnoses

Constipation (Indications)
Diarrhea (Side Effects)

Implementation

- **PO:** Dissolve powder in 8 oz of water prior to administration.

Patient/Family Teaching

- Inform patient that 2–4 days may be required to produce a bowel movement. PEG should not be used for more than 2 wk. Prolonged, frequent, or excessive use may result in electrolyte imbalance and laxative dependence.
- Advise patient to notify health care professional if unusual cramps, bloating, or diarrhea occurs.

Evaluation/Desired Outcomes

- A soft, formed bowel movement.

polyethylene glycol/ electrolyte

(po-lee-**eth**-e-leen **glye**-kole/e-**lek**-troe-lite)
Colovage, Colyte, GoLYTELY, ✤Klean-Prep, NuLytely, OCL, Peglyte, TriLyte

Classification
Therapeutic: laxatives
Pharmacologic: osmotics

Pregnancy Category C

Indications

Bowel cleansing in preparation for GI examination. **Unlabeled uses:** Treatment of acute iron overdose in children.

Action

Polyethylene glycol (PEG) in solution acts as an osmotic agent, drawing water into the lumen of the GI tract. **Therapeutic Effects:** Evacuation of the GI tract without water or electrolyte imbalance.

Pharmacokinetics

Absorption: Ions in the solution are nonabsorbable.
Distribution: Unknown.
Metabolism and Excretion: Solution is excreted in fecal contents.
Half-life: Unknown.

TIME/ACTION PROFILE

ROUTE	ONSET	PEAK	DURATION
PO	1 hr	unknown	4 hr

Contraindications/Precautions

Contraindicated in: GI obstruction; Gastric retention; Toxic colitis; Megacolon.
Use Cautiously in: Patients with absent or diminished gag reflex; Unconscious or semicomatose states, in which administration is via NG tube; History of ulcerative colitis (increased risk of hypoglycemia, dehydration, and hypokalemia); Barium enema using double-contrast technique (may not allow proper barium coating of mucosa); Abdominal pain of uncertain cause, particularly if accompanied by fever; Geri: May be more sensitive to effects; Pedi: Children (safety not established; children <2 yr more prone to hypoglycemia, dehydration, and hypokalemia).

Adverse Reactions/Side Effects

GI: abdominal fullness, diarrhea, bloating, cramps, nausea, vomiting. **Misc:** allergic reactions (rare).

Interactions

Drug-Drug: Interferes with the absorption of **orally administered medications** by decreasing transit time (do not administer within 1 hr of start of therapy).

Route/Dosage

PO (Adults): 240 ml q 10 min (up to 4 L) until fecal discharge appears clear and has no solid material; may be given through NG tube at 20–30 ml/min (up to 4 L).
PO (Children ≥6 mo): 25 ml/kg/hr until fecal discharge is clear and has no solid material; may also be given through a NG tube (unlabeled).

Availability

Oral solution: OCL—1500-ml 3-pack. **Powder for oral solution (regular, pineapple, citrus berry, lemon lime, cherry flavor):** CoLyte—powder in bottles for reconstitution, GoLYTLEY—powder in packets and disposable jugs for reconstitution, NuLytely—powder in disposable jugs for reconstitution.

NURSING IMPLICATIONS

Assessment

- Assess patient for abdominal distention, presence of bowel sounds, and usual pattern of bowel function.
- Assess color, consistency, and amount of stool produced.
- Monitor semiconscious or unconscious patients closely for regurgitation when administering via NG tube.

Potential Nursing Diagnoses

Diarrhea (Side Effects)

Implementation

- Do not add extra flavorings or additional ingredients to solution prior to administration.
- Patient should fast for 3–4 hr prior to administration and should never have solid food within 2 hr of administration.
- Patient should be allowed only clear liquids after administration.
- May be administered on the morning of the examination as long as time is allotted to drink solution (3 hr) and evacuate bowel (1 additional hr). For barium enema, administer solution early evening (6 PM) prior to exam to allow proper mucosal coating by barium.
- **PO:** Solution may be reconstituted with tap water. Shake vigorously until powder is dissolved.
- May be administered via NG tube at a rate of 20–30 ml/min.

Patient/Family Teaching

- Instruct patient to drink 240 ml every 10 min until 4 L have been consumed or fecal discharge is clear and free of solid matter. Rapidly drinking each 240 ml is preferred over drinking small amounts continuously.

Evaluation/Desired Outcomes

- Diarrhea, which cleanses the bowel within 4 hr. The first bowel movement usually occurs within 1 hr of administration.

posaconazole

(po-sa-**kon**-a-zole)
Noxafil

Classification
Therapeutic: antifungals
Pharmacologic: triazoles

Pregnancy Category C

Indications

Prevention of invasive Aspergillus and Candida infections in severely immunocompromised patients. Treatment of orpharyngeal candidiasis (including candidiasis unresponsive to itraconazole or fluconazole).

Action

Blocks ergosterol synthesis, a major component of fungal cell wall. **Therapeutic Effects:** Fungistatic/fungicidal action against susceptible fungi.

Pharmacokinetics

Absorption: Well absorbed following oral administration; absorption is optimized by food.
Distribution: Extensive extravascular distribution and penetration into body tissues.
Protein Binding: >98%.
Metabolism and Excretion: Some metabolism via UDP glucuronidation; 66% eliminated unchanged in feces, 13% in urine (mostly as metabolites).
Half-life: 35 hr.

TIME/ACTION PROFILE (blood levels)

ROUTE	ONSET	PEAK	DURATION
PO	unknown	3–5 hr	8 hr

Contraindications/Precautions

Contraindicated in: Hypersensitivity; Concurrent use of pimozide or quinidine (↑ risk of serious arrhythmias); Concurrent use of ergot alkaloids (↑ risk of ergotism).
Use Cautiously in: History of/predisposition to QTc prolongation including congenital QTc prolongation, concurrent medications which prolong QTc, high cumulative anthracycline history or electrolyte abnormalities (hypokalemia, hypomagnesemia); correct pre-existing abnormalities prior to administration; Hypersensitivity to other azole antifungals; Hepatic impairment; Severe diarrhea, vomiting, or renal impairment (monitor for breakthrough fungal infections); OB: Use only in pregnancy or lactation if maternal benefit outweighs risk to child;

Pedi: Safe use in children <13 yr not established.

Adverse Reactions/Side Effects

GI: HEPATOCELLULAR DAMAGE, diarrhea, nausea, vomiting. **Endo:** adrenal insufficiency. **Metab:** ALLERGIC RECTIONS.

Interactions

Drug-Drug: Posaconazole inhibits the CYP3A4 enzyme systems and should be expected to interact with other drugs affected by this system. **Rifabutin**, **phenytoin**, **cimetidine** ↓ levels and may ↓ antifungal effectiveness; avoid concurrent use. ↑ **cyclosporine**, **sirolimus**, and **tacrolimus** levels and risk of toxicity, decrease dose initially and monitor levels frequently. ↑ **rifabutin** levels; avoid concurrent use of **phenytoin**, and **midazolam**; monitor for excess clinical effect and dose accordingly. ↑ levels and risk of toxicity from **ergot alkaloids**, including **ergotamine** and **dihydroergotamine**; concurrent administration is contraindicated. ↑ levels and risk of neurotoxicity of **vinca alkaloids**, including **vincristine** and **vinblastine**; consider dose adjustment. ↑ levels and risk of toxicity of **HMG CoA reductase inhibitors (statins)**; consider ↓ statin dose. May ↑ levels and risk of adverse cardiovascular reactions to **calcium channel blockers**; consider dosage reduction.

Route/Dosage

PO (Adults): 200 mg three times daily.

Availability

Oral suspension (cherry): 40 mg/ml in 105-ml bottles.

NURSING IMPLICATIONS

Assessment

- Assess for signs and symptoms of fungal infection.
- ***Lab Test Considerations:*** Monitor liver function tests prior to and periodically during therapy. May cause ↑ ALT, ↑ AST, ↑ alkaline phosphatase and ↑ total bilirubin levels; generally reversible on discontinuation. Discontinue posaconazole if clinical signs and symptoms of liver disease develop.

Potential Nursing Diagnoses

Risk for infection (Indications)

Implementation

- **PO:** Shake suspension well before use. Administer 200 mg (5-mL dose) with a full meal or liquid nutritional supplement to enhance absorption. Rinse spoon for administration with water after each use. Alternative therapy or close monitoring for breakthrough fungal infections should be considered for patients unable to eat a full meal or tolerate a nutritional supplement.

Patient/Family Teaching

- Advise patient to notify health care professional if severe diarrhea or vomiting occur; may decrease posaconazole blood levels and allow breakthrough fungal infections.
- Instruct patient to consult health care professional prior to taking Rx, OTC, or herbal products during posaconazole therapy.
- Advise patient to notify health care professional of pregnancy is planned or suspected or if breastfeeding.

Evaluation/Desired Outcomes

- Resolution of clinical and laboratory indications of fungal infections. Duration of therapy is based on recovery from neutropenia or immunosuppression.

potassium and sodium phosphates

(po-**tas**-e-um/**soe**-dee-yum **foss**-fates)

K-Phos M.F, K-Phos Neutral, K-Phos No. 2, Neutra-Phos, Uro-KP Neutral

Classification

Therapeutic: antiurolithics, mineral and electrolyte replacements/supplements

Pregnancy Category C

Indications

Treatment and prevention of phosphate depletion in patients who are unable to ingest adequate dietary phosphate. Adjunct therapy of urinary tract infections with methenamine hippurate or mandelate. Prevention of calcium urinary stones. Phosphate salts of potassium may be used in hypokalemic patients with metabolic acidosis or coexisting phosphorus deficiency.

Action

Phosphate is present in bone and is involved in energy transfer and carbohydrate metabolism. Serves as a buffer for the excretion of hydrogen ions by the kidneys. Dibasic potassium phosphate is converted in renal tubule to monobasic salt, resulting in urinary acidification, which is required for methenamine hippurate or mandelate to be active as urinary anti-infectives. Acidification of urine increases solubility of calcium, decreasing calcium stone formation. **Therapeutic Effects:** Replacement of phosphorus in deficiency states. Urinary acidification. Increased efficacy of methenamine. Decreased formation of calcium urinary tract stones.

Pharmacokinetics

Absorption: Well absorbed following oral administration. Vitamin D promotes GI absorption of phosphates.
Distribution: Phosphates enter extracellular fluids and are then actively transported to sites of action.
Metabolism and Excretion: Excreted mainly (>90%) by the kidneys.
Half-life: Unknown.

TIME/ACTION PROFILE (effects on serum phosphate levels)

ROUTE	ONSET	PEAK	DURATION
PO	unknown	unknown	unknown

Contraindications/Precautions

Contraindicated in: Hyperkalemia (potassium salts); Hyperphosphatemia; Hypocalcemia; Severe renal impairment; Untreated Addison's disease (potassium salts).
Use Cautiously in: Hyperparathyroidism; Cardiac disease; Hypernatremia (sodium phosphate only); Hypertension (sodium phosphate only); Renal impairment.

Adverse Reactions/Side Effects

Related to hyperphosphatemia, unless otherwise indicated.
CNS: confusion, dizziness, headache, weakness. **CV:** ARRHYTHMIAS, CARDIAC ARREST, bradycardia, ECG changes (absent P waves, widening of the QRS complex with biphasic curve, peaked T waves), edema. **GI:** diarrhea, abdominal pain, nausea, vomiting. **F and E:** hyperkalemia, hypernatremia, hyperphosphatemia, hypocalcemia, hypomagnesemia. **MS:** *hypocalcemia*, *hyperkalemia*—muscle cramps. **Neuro:** flaccid paralysis, heaviness of legs, paresthesias, tremors.

Interactions

Drug-Drug: Concurrent use of **potassium-sparing, diuretics, ACE inhibitors**, or **angiotensin II receptor blockers** with potassium phosphates may result in hyperkalemia. Concurrent use of **corticosteroids** with sodium phosphate may result in hypernatremia. Concurrent administration of **calcium-, magnesium-**, or **aluminum-containing compounds** ↓ absorption of phosphates by formation of insoluble complexes. **Vitamin D** enhances the absorption of phosphates.
Drug-Food: Oxalates (in spinach and rhubarb) and **phytates** (in bran and whole grains) may ↓ absorption of phosphates by binding them in the GI tract.

Route/Dosage

Phosphorous Supplementation

PO (Adults and Children >4 yr): 250–500 mg (8–16 mmol) phosphorus (1–2 packets) 4 times daily.
PO (Children <4 yr): 250 mg (8 mmol) phosphorus (1 packet) 4 times daily.

Urinary Acidification

PO (Adults): 2 tablets 4 times/day.

Maintenance Phosphorus

PO (Adults): 50–150 mmol/day in divided doses.
PO (Children): 2–3 mmol/kg/day in divided doses.

Availability

Potassium and Sodium Phosphates

Tablets (K-Phos MF): elemental phosphorus 125.6 mg (4 mmol), sodium 67 mg (2.9 mEq), and potassium 44.5 mg (1.1 mEq). **Tablets (K-Phos Neutral):** elemental phosphorus 250 mg (8 mmol), sodium 298 mg (13 mEq), and potassium 45 mg (1.1 mEq). **Tablets (K-Phos No.2):** elemental phosphorus 250 mg (8 mmol), sodium 134 mg (5.8 mEq), and potassium 88 mg (2.3 mEq). **Tablets (Uro-KP Neutral):** elemental phosphorus 258 mg, sodium 262.4 mg (10.8 mEq), and potassium 49.4 mg (1.3 mEq). **Powder for oral solution (Neutra-Phos):** elemental phosphorus 250 mg (8 mmol), sodium 164 mg (7.1 mEq), and potassium 278 mg (7.1 mEq)/packet.

NURSING IMPLICATIONS

Assessment

- Assess patient for signs and symptoms of hypokalemia (weakness, fatigue, arrhythmias,

P

presence of U waves on ECG, polyuria, polydipsia) and hypophosphatemia (anorexia, weakness, decreased reflexes, bone pain, confusion, blood dyscrasias) throughout therapy.
- Monitor intake and output ratios and daily weight. Report significant discrepancies.
- ***Lab Test Considerations:*** Monitor serum phosphate, potassium, sodium, and calcium levels prior to and periodically throughout therapy. Increased phosphate may cause hypocalcemia.
- Monitor renal function studies prior to and periodically throughout therapy.
- Monitor urinary pH in patients receiving potassium and sodium phosphate as a urinary acidifier.

Potential Nursing Diagnoses

Imbalanced nutrition: less than body requirements (Indications)

Implementation

- **PO:** Tablets should be dissolved in a full glass of water. Allow mixture to stand for 2–5 min to ensure it is fully dissolved. Solutions prepared by pharmacy should not be further diluted.
- Medication should be administered after meals to minimize gastric irritation and laxative effect.
- Do not administer simultaneously with antacids containing aluminum, magnesium, or calcium.

Patient/Family Teaching

- Explain to the patient the purpose of the medication and the need to take as directed. Take missed doses as soon as remembered unless within 1 or 2 hr of the next dose. Explain that the tablets should not be swallowed whole. Tablets should be dissolved in water.
- Instruct patients in low-sodium diet (see Appendix L).
- Advise patient of the importance of maintaining a high fluid intake (drinking at least one 8-oz glass of water each hr) to prevent kidney stones.
- Instruct the patient to promptly report diarrhea, weakness, fatigue, muscle cramps, unexplained weight gain, swelling of lower extremities, shortness of breath, unusual thirst, or tremors.

Evaluation/Desired Outcomes

- Prevention and correction of serum phosphate and potassium deficiencies.
- Maintenance of acid urine.
- Decreased urine calcium, which prevents formation of renal calculi.

---

potassium iodide, **See IODINE, IODIDE.**

HIGH ALERT

POTASSIUM SUPPLEMENTS

(poe-**tass**-ee-um)

potassium acetate

potassium bicarbonate
K+Care ET, K-Electrolyte, K-Ide, Klor-Con/EF, K-Lyte, K-Vescent

potassium bicarbonate/potassium chloride
K-Lyte/Cl, ✤Neo-K, ✤Potassium Sandoz

potassium bicarbonate/potassium citrate
Effer-K, K-Lyte DS

potassium chloride
✤Apo-K, Cena-K, Gen-K, K+ Care, K+ 10, ✤Kalium Durules, Kaochlor, Kaochlor S-F, Kaon-Cl, Kay Ciel, KCl, K-Dur, K-Lease, ✤K-Long, K-Lor, Klor-Con, Klorvess Liquid, Klotrix, K-Lyte/Cl Powder, K-Med, K-Norm, K-Sol, K-Tab, Micro-K, Micro-K ExtenCaps, Micro-LS, Potasalan, Roychlor, Rum-K, Slow-K, Ten-K

potassium chloride/potassium bicarbonate/potassium citrate
Kaochlor Eff

potassium gluconate
Kaon, Kaylixir, K-G Elixir, ✤Potassium-Rougier

potassium gluconate/potassium chloride
Kolyum

potassium gluconate/potassium citrate
Twin-K

trikates (potassium acetate/potassium bicarbonate/potassium citrate)
Tri-K

Classification
Therapeutic: mineral and electrolyte replacements/supplements

Pregnancy Category C

Indications
PO, IV: Treatment/prevention of potassium depletion. **IV:** Arrhythmias due to digoxin toxicity.

Action
Maintain acid-base balance, isotonicity, and electrophysiologic balance of the cell. Activator in many enzymatic reactions; essential to transmission of nerve impulses; contraction of cardiac, skeletal, and smooth muscle; gastric secretion; renal function; tissue synthesis; and carbohydrate metabolism. **Therapeutic Effects:** Replacement. Prevention of deficiency.

Pharmacokinetics
Absorption: Well absorbed following oral administration.
Distribution: Enters extracellular fluid; then actively transported into cells.
Metabolism and Excretion: Excreted by the kidneys.
Half-life: Unknown.

TIME/ACTION PROFILE (increase in serum potassium levels)

ROUTE	ONSET	PEAK	DURATION
PO	unknown	1–2 hr	unknown
IV	rapid	end of infusion	unknown

Contraindications/Precautions
Contraindicated in: Hyperkalemia; Severe renal impairment; Untreated Addison's disease; Severe tissue trauma; Hyperkalemic familial periodic paralysis; Some products may contain tartrazine (FDC yellow dye #5) or alcohol; avoid using in patients with known hypersensitivity or intolerance; Potassium acetate injection contains aluminum, which may become toxic with prolonged use to high risk groups (renal impairment, premature neonates).

Use Cautiously in: Cardiac disease; Renal impairment; Diabetes mellitus (liquids may contain sugar); Hypomagnesemia (may make correction of hypokalemia more difficult); GI hypomotility including dysphagia or esophageal compression from left atrial enlargement (tablets, capsules); Patients receiving potassium-sparing drugs.

Adverse Reactions/Side Effects
CNS: confusion, restlessness, weakness. **CV:** ARRHYTHMIAS, ECG changes. **GI:** abdominal pain, diarrhea, flatulence, nausea, vomiting; *tablets, capsules only*—GI ulceration, stenotic lesions. **Local:** irritation at IV site. **Neuro:** paralysis, paresthesia.

Interactions
Drug-Drug: Use with **potassium-sparing diuretics** or **ACE inhibitors** or **angiotensin II receptor antagonists** may lead to hyperkalemia. **Anticholinergics** may ↑ GI mucosal lesions in patients taking wax-matrix potassium chloride preparations.

Route/Dosage
Expressed as mEq of potassium. Potassium acetate contains 10.2 mEq/g; potassium bicarbonate contains 10 mEq potassium/g; potassium chloride contains 13.4 mEq potassium/g; potassium gluconate contains 4.3 mEq/g.

Normal Daily Requirements
PO, IV (Adults): 40–80 mEq/day.
PO, IV (Children): 2–3 mEq/kg/day.
PO, IV (Neonates): 2–6 mEq/kg/day.

Prevention of Hypokalemia During Diuretic Therapy
PO (Adults): 20–40 mEq/day in 1–2 divided doses; single dose should not exceed 20 mEq.
PO (Neonates, Infants and Children): 1–2 mEq/kg/day in 1–2 divided doses.

Treatment of Hypokalemia
PO (Adults): 40–100 mEq/day in divided doses.
PO (Neonates, Infants and Children): 2–5 mEq/kg/day in divided doses.
IV (Adults): *Serum potassium >2.5 mEq/L*—Up to 20 mEq/day as an infusion (not to exceed 10 mEq/hr) or a concentration of 40 mEq/L via peripheral line (up to 100 mEq/L have been used via central line [unlabeled]). *Serum potassium <2 mEq/L with symptoms*—Up to 40

mEq/day as an infusion (rate should generally not exceed 20 mEq/hr).
IV (Neonates, Infants and Children): 0.5–1 mEq/kg/dose (maximum 30 mEq/dose) as an infusion to infuse at 0.3–0.5 mEq/kg/hr (maximum infusion rate 1 mEq/kg/hr).

Availability

Potassium Acetate
Concentrate for injection (contains aluminum): 2 mEq/ml in 20-, 50-, and 100-ml vials, 4 mEq/ml in 50-ml vials.

Potassium Bicarbonate
Tablets for effervescent oral solution: 25 mEq.

Potassium Bicarbonate/Potassium Chloride
Packets for effervescent oral solution: 20 mEq/2.8-g packet. **Tablets for effervescent oral solution:** ✤12 mEq, 20 mEq, 25 mEq, 50 mEq.

Potassium Bicarbonate/Potassium Citrate
Tablets for effervescent oral solution: 25 mEq, 50 mEq. **Cost:** 25 mEq $122.98/90, 50 mEq $213.97/90.

Potassium Chloride
Extended-release tablets: 8 mEq, 10 mEq, 20 mEq. **Cost:** *Generic*—10 mEq $22.49/90, 20 mEq $32.97/90. **Extended-release capsules:** 8 mEq, 10 mEq. **Cost:** *Generic*—10 mEq $24.74/90. **Oral solution:** 20 mEq/15 ml, 40 mEq/15 ml. **Cost:** *Generic*—20 mEq/15 ml $8.99/473 ml, 40 mEq/15 ml $19.97/480 ml. **Powder/packets for oral solution:** 20-mEq/1.5-g packet, 25-mEq/1.8-g packet. **Packets for oral suspension:** 20-mEq/1.5-g packet. **Concentrate for injection:** 0.1 mEq/ml in 10-mEq ampules and vials, 0.2 mEq/ml in 10- and 20-mEq ampules and vials, 0.3 mEq/ml in 30-mEq ampules and vials, 0.4 mEq/ml in 20- and 40-mEq ampules and vials, 1.5 mEq/ml, 2 mEq/ml, 3 mEq/ml. **Solution for IV infusion:** 10 mEq/L in various dextrose and saline solutions in 250-, 500-, and 100-ml containers, 20 mEq/L in dextrose/saline/LRs in 250-, 500-, and 100-ml containers, 30 mEq/L in various dextrose and saline solutions in 250-, 500-, and 100-ml containers, 40 mEq/L in various dextrose and saline solutions in 250-, 500-, and 100-ml containers.

Potassium Chloride/Potassium Bicarbonate/Potassium Citrate
Tablets for effervescent oral solution: 20 mEq.

Potassium Gluconate
Tablets: 2 mEq, 5 mEq. **Elixir:** 20 mEq/15 ml.

Potassium Gluconate/Potassium Chloride
Oral solution: 20 mEq/15 ml. **Powder for oral solution:** 20 mEq/5-g packet.

Potassium Gluconate/Potassium Citrate
Oral solution: 20 mEq/15 ml.

Trikates (Potassium Acetate/Potassium Bicarbonate/Potassium Citrate)
Oral solution: 15 mEq/5 ml.

NURSING IMPLICATIONS

Assessment
- Assess for signs and symptoms of hypokalemia (weakness, fatigue, U wave on ECG, arrhythmias, polyuria, polydipsia) and hyperkalemia (see Toxicity and Overdose).
- Monitor pulse, blood pressure, and ECG periodically during IV therapy.
- ***Lab Test Considerations:*** Monitor serum potassium before and periodically during therapy. Monitor renal function, serum bicarbonate, and pH. Determine serum magnesium level if patient has refractory hypokalemia; hypomagnesemia should be corrected to facilitate effectiveness of potassium replacement. Monitor serum chloride because hypochloremia may occur if replacing potassium without concurrent chloride.
- ***Toxicity and Overdose:*** Symptoms of toxicity are those of hyperkalemia (slow, irregular heartbeat; fatigue; muscle weakness; paresthesia; confusion; dyspnea; peaked T waves; depressed ST segments; prolonged QT segments; widened QRS complexes; loss of P waves; and cardiac arrhythmias): Treatment includes discontinuation of potassium, administration of sodium bicarbonate to correct acidosis, dextrose and insulin to facilitate passage of potassium into cells, calcium salts to reverse ECG effects (in patients who are not receiving digoxin), sodium polystyrene used as an exchange resin, and/or dialysis for patient with impaired renal function.

Potential Nursing Diagnoses
Imbalanced nutrition: less than body requirements (Indications)

Implementation
- ***High Alert:*** Medication errors involving too rapid infusion or bolus IV administration of potassium chloride have resulted in fatalities. See IV administration guidelines below.

- Do not confuse K-Dur with Imdur (isosorbide mononitrate). Do not confuse Micro-K with micronase (glyburide).
- For most purposes, potassium chloride should be used, except for renal tubular acidoses (hyperchloremic acidosis), in which other salts are more appropriate (potassium bicarbonate, potassium citrate, or potassium gluconate).
- If hypokalemia is secondary to diuretic therapy, consideration should be given to decreasing the dose of diuretic, unless there is a history of significant arrhythmias or concurrent digitalis glycoside therapy.
- **PO:** Administer with or after meals to decrease GI irritation.
- Use of tablets and capsules should be reserved for patients who cannot tolerate liquid preparations.
- Dissolve effervescent tablets in 3–8 oz of cold water. Ensure that effervescent tablet is fully dissolved. Powders and solutions should be diluted in 3–8 oz of cold water or juice (do not use tomato juice if patient is on sodium restriction). Instruct patient to drink slowly over 5–10 min.
- Tablets and capsules should be taken with a meal and full glass of water. Do not chew or crush enteric-coated or extended-release tablets or capsules. Micro-K ExtenCaps capsules can be opened and sprinkled on soft food (pudding, applesauce) and swallowed immediately with a glass of cool water or juice.
- **IV:** Assess for extravasation; severe pain and tissue necrosis may occur.

High Alert: Never administer potassium IV push or bolus.

Potassium Acetate

- **Continuous Infusion: *High Alert:*** Do not administer undiluted. Each single dose *must* be diluted and thoroughly mixed in 100–1000 ml of dextrose, saline, Ringer's or LR, dextrose/saline, dextrose/Ringer's, or LR combinations. Usually limited to 80 mEq/L via peripheral line (200 mEq/L via central line). ***Rate: High Alert:*** Infuse slowly, at a rate up to 10 mEq/hr in adults or 0.5 mEq/kg/hr in children on general care areas. Check hospital policy for maximum infusion rates (maximum rate in monitored setting 40 mEq/hr in adults or 1 mEq/kg/hr in children).
- **Y-Site Compatibility:** ciprofloxacin.

Potassium Chloride

- **Continuous Infusion: *High Alert:*** Do not administer concentrations of ≥1.5 mEq/ml undiluted; fatalities have occurred. Concentrated products have black caps on vials or black stripes above constriction on ampules and are labeled with a warning about dilution requirement. Each single dose must be diluted and thoroughly mixed in 100–1000 ml of IV solution. Usually limited to 80 mEq/L via peripheral line (200 mEq/L via central line).
- Concentrations of 0.1 and 0.4 mEq/ml are intended for administration via calibrated infusion device and do not require dilution. ***Rate: High Alert:*** Infuse slowly, at a rate up to 10 mEq/hr in adults or 0.5 mEq/kg/hr in children in general care areas. Check hospital policy for maximum infusion rates (maximum rate in monitored setting 40 mEq/hr in adults or 1 mEq/kg/hr in children). Use an infusion pump.
- **Solution Compatibility:** May be diluted in dextrose, saline, Ringer's solution, LR, dextrose/saline, dextrose/Ringer's solution, and dextrose/LR combinations. Commercially available premixed with many of the above IV solutions.
- **Y-Site Compatibility:** acyclovir, allopurinol, amifostine, aminophylline, amiodarone, ampicillin, atropine, aztreonam, betamethasone, bivalirudin, calcium gluconate, chlordiazepoxide, chlorpromazine, ciprofloxacin, cisatracurium, cladribine, cyanocobalamin, dexamethasone sodium phosphate, dexmedetomidine, digoxin, diltiazem, diphenhydramine, dobutamine, docetaxel, dopamine, doxorubicin liposome, droperidol, drotrecogin, edrophonium, enalaprilat, epinephrine, ertapenem, esmolol, conjugated estrogens, ethacrynate sodium, etoposide phosphate, famotidine, fenoldopam, fentanyl, filgrastim, fludarabine, fluorouracil, furosemide, gemcitabine, granisetron, heparin, hydralazine, idarubicin, inamrinone, indomethacin, insulin, isoproterenol, kanamycin, labetalol, lidocaine, linezolid, lorazepam, magnesium sulfate, melphalan, menadiol, meperidine, meropenem, methoxamine, methylergono-

vine, midazolam, milrinone, morphine, neostigmine, nicardipine, nitroprusside, norepinephrine, ondansetron, oxacillin, oxaliplatin, oxytocin, paclitaxel, pantoprazole, pemetrexed, penicillin G potassium, pentazocine, phytonadione, piperacillin/tazobactam, procainamide, prochlorperazine, propofol, propranolol, pyridostigmine, quinupristin/dalfopristin, remifentanil, sargramostim, scopolamine, sodium bicarbonate, succinylcholine, tacrolimus, teniposide, theophylline, thiotepa, tirofiban, vinorelbine, warfarin, zidovudine.

- **Y-Site Incompatibility:** amphotericin B cholesteryl sulfate complex, azithromycin, diazepam, ergotamine tartrate, lansoprazole, phenytoin.
- **Additive Compatibility:** calcium gluconate, cimetidine, dobutamine, dopamine, furosemide, heparin, hydrocortisone, hydromorphone, lidocaine, ranitidine, sodium bicarbonate, vitamin B complex with C.

Patient/Family Teaching

- Explain to patient purpose of the medication and the need to take as directed, especially when concurrent digoxin or diuretics are taken. Take missed doses as soon as remembered within 2 hr; if not, return to regular dose schedule. Do not double dose.
- Emphasize correct method of administration. GI irritation or ulceration may result from chewing enteric-coated tablets or insufficient dilution of liquid or powder forms.
- Some extended-release tablets are contained in a wax matrix that may be expelled in the stool. This occurrence is not significant.
- Instruct patient to avoid salt substitutes or low-salt milk or food unless approved by health care professional. Patient should be advised to read all labels to prevent excess potassium intake.
- Advise patient regarding sources of dietary potassium (see Appendix L). Encourage compliance with recommended diet.
- Instruct patient to report dark, tarry, or bloody stools; weakness; unusual fatigue; or tingling of extremities. Notify health care professional if nausea, vomiting, diarrhea, or stomach discomfort persists. Dosage may require adjustment.
- Emphasize the importance of regular follow-up exams to monitor serum levels and progress.

Evaluation/Desired Outcomes

- Prevention and correction of serum potassium depletion.
- Cessation of arrhythmias caused by digoxin toxicity.

pramipexole (pra-mi-**pex**-ole)

Mirapex

Classification

Therapeutic: antiparkinson agents

Pharmacologic: dopamine agonists

Pregnancy Category C

Indications

Management of idiopathic Parkinson's disease. Restless leg syndrome.

Action

Stimulates dopamine receptors in the striatum of the brain. **Therapeutic Effects:** Decreased tremor and rigidity in Parkinson's disease. Decreased leg restlessness.

Pharmacokinetics

Absorption: >90% absorbed following oral administration.

Distribution: Widely distributed.

Metabolism and Excretion: 90% excreted unchanged in urine.

Half-life: 8 hr (increased in geriatric patients and patients with renal impairment).

TIME/ACTION PROFILE (blood levels)

ROUTE	ONSET	PEAK	DURATION
PO	unknown	2 hr	8 hr

Contraindications/Precautions

Contraindicated in: Hypersensitivity.

Use Cautiously in: Geri: Geriatric patients (increased risk of hallucinations); Renal impairment (increased dosing interval recommended if CCr <60 ml/min); OB, Pedi, Geri: Pregnancy, lactation, or children (safety not established).

Adverse Reactions/Side Effects

CNS: SLEEP ATTACKS, amnesia, dizziness, drowsiness, hallucinations, weakness, abnormal dreams, confusion, dyskinesia, extrapyramidal syndrome, headache, insomnia. **CV:** postural hypotension. **GI:** constipation, dry mouth, dyspepsia, nausea, tooth disease. **GU:** urinary frequency. **MS:** leg cramps. **Neuro:** hypertonia, unsteadiness/falling.

Interactions

Drug-Drug: Concurrent **levodopa** increases the risk of hallucinations and dyskinesia. Effectiveness may be increased by **cimetidine**. Effectiveness may be decreased by **dopamine antagonists**, including **butyrophenones**, **metoclopramide**, **phenothiazines**, or **thioxanthenes**.

Route/Dosage

PO (Adults): *Parkinson's disease*—0.125 mg 3 times daily initially; may be increased q 5–7 days (range 1.5–4.5 mg/day in 3 divided doses). *Restless Leg Syndrome*—0.125 mg once daily 1–3 hrs before bedtime. May be increased at 4–7 day intervals to 0.25 mg, then up to 0.5 mg.

Renal Impairment

PO (Adults): *Parkinson's disease—CCr 35–59 ml/min*—0.125 mg twice daily initially, may be increased q 5–7 days up to 1.5 mg twice daily; *CCr 15–34 ml/min*—0.125 mg once daily initially, may be increased q 5–7 days up to 1.5 mg once daily. *Restless Leg Syndrome*—0.125 mg once daily 1–3 hrs before bedtime. May be increased at 14 day intervals to 0.25 mg, then up to 0.5 mg.

Availability

Tablets: 0.125 mg, 0.25 mg, 0.5 mg, 0.75 mg, 1 mg, 1.5 mg. **Cost:** 0.125 mg $517.05/270, 0.25 mg $491.97/270, 0.5 mg $605.96/270, 1 mg $574.97/270, 1.5 mg $605.96/270.

NURSING IMPLICATIONS

Assessment

- Assess patient for confusion or hallucinations. Notify physician or other health care professional if these occur.
- Monitor ECG and blood pressure frequently during dosage adjustment and periodically throughout therapy.
- Assess patient for drowsiness and sleep attacks. Drowsiness is a common side effect of pramipexole, but sleep attacks or episodes of falling asleep during activities that require active participation may occur without warning. Assess patient for concomitant medications that have sedating effects or may increase serum pramipexole levels (see Interactions). May require discontinuation of therapy.
- **Parkinson's Disease:** Assess patient for signs and symptoms of Parkinson's disease (tremor, muscle weakness and rigidity, ataxia) before and throughout therapy.
- **Restless Leg Syndrome:** Assess sleep patterns and frequency of restless leg disturbances.

Potential Nursing Diagnoses

Impaired physical mobility (Indications)
Risk for injury (Indications, Side Effects)

Implementation

- **PO:** An attempt to reduce the dose of levodopa/carbidopa may be made cautiously during pramipexole therapy.
- Administer with meals to minimize nausea; usually resolves with continued therapy.

Patient/Family Teaching

- Instruct patient to take medication exactly as directed. Missed doses should be taken as soon as remembered if it is not almost time for next dose. Do not double doses. Consult health care professional before reducing dose or discontinuing medication.
- May cause drowsiness and unexpected episodes of falling asleep. Caution patient to avoid driving or other activities requiring alertness until response to medication is known. Advise patient to notify health care professional if episodes of falling asleep occur.
- Advise patient to change position slowly to minimize orthostatic hypotension. May occur more frequently during initial therapy.
- Advise female patient to notify health care professional if pregnancy is planned or suspected or if currently breastfeeding or planning to breastfeed.

Evaluation/Desired Outcomes

- Decreased tremor and rigidity in Parkinson's disease.
- Decrease in restless legs and improved sleep.

HIGH ALERT

pramlintide (pram-lin-tide)
Symlin

Classification
Therapeutic: antidiabetics
Pharmacologic: hormones

Pregnancy Category C

P

♣ = Canadian drug name.
* CAPITALS indicates life-threatening; underlines indicate most frequent.

Indications
Used with mealtime insulin in the management of diabetics whose blood sugar cannot be controlled by optimal insulin therapy; can be used with other agents (sulfonylureas, metformin).

Action
Acts as a synthetic analogue of amylin, an endogenous pancreatic hormone that helps to control postprandial hyperglycemia; effects include slowed gastric emptying, suppression of glucagon secretion and regulation of food intake.
Therapeutic Effects: Improved control of postprandial hyperglycemia.

Pharmacokinetics
Absorption: 30–40% absorbed following subcutaneous administration.
Distribution: Does not appear to significantly cross the placenta.
Metabolism and Excretion: metabolized by the kidneys; major metabolite has pharmacologic properties similar to the parent compound.
Half-life: 48 min.

TIME/ACTION PROFILE (effect on blood sugar)*

ROUTE	ONSET	PEAK	DURATION
subcut	rapid	20 min	3 hr

*Blood level

Contraindications/Precautions
Contraindicated in: Hypersensitivty; Inability to identify hypoglycemia; Gastroparesis or need for medications to stimulate gastric motility; Poor compliance with current insulin regimen or self-monitoring; HbA1c >9%; Recurring severe hypoglycemia within the last 6 mo, requiring treatment; Pedi: Children.
Use Cautiously in: OB: Pregnancy/lactation (use only if maternal benefit outweighs potential risks to fetus/newborn).

Adverse Reactions/Side Effects
Noted for concurrent use with insulin.
CNS: dizziness, fatigue, headache. **Resp:** cough. **GI:** nausea, abdominal pain, anorexia, vomiting. **Endo:** HYPOGLYCEMIA. **Derm:** local allergy. **MS:** arthralgia. **Misc:** systemic allergic reactions.

Interactions
Drug-Drug: ↑ likelihood of hypoglycemia with short-acting **insulin**; reduce dose of short-acting pre-meal insulin by 50%. Avoid concurrent use with other agents that ↓ GI motility, including **atropine** and other **anticholinergics**. Avoid concurrent use with other agents that ↓ GI absorption of nutrients, including **α-glucosidase inhibitors** including **acarbose** and **miglitol**. May delay oral absorption of concurrently administered drugs; if prompt absorption is desired, administer 1 hr before or 2 hr after pramlintide.

Route/Dosage

Insulin-using Type 2 Diabetes
Subcut (Adults): 60 mcg, immediately prior to major meals initially, if no significant nausea occurs, dose may be increased to 120 mcg.

Type 1 Diabetes
Subcut (Adults): 15 mcg, immediately prior to major meals initially, if no significant nausea occurs, dose may be increased by 15 mcg every 3 days up to 60 mcg.

Availability
Injection: 0.6 mg/ml in 5-mL vials.

NURSING IMPLICATIONS

Assessment
- Assess hemoglobin A1c, recent blood glucose monitoring data, history of insulin-induced hypoglycemia, current insulin regimen, and body weight prior to initiation of therapy.
- Assess for signs and symptoms of hypoglycemia (hunger, headache, sweating, tremor, irritability, difficulty concentrating, loss of consciousness, coma, seizure), occurs within 3 hr of injection. Pramlintide alone does not cause hypoglycemia, may increase risk when administered with insulin.
- ***Lab Test Considerations:*** Monitor blood glucose frequently, including pre- and post-meals and at bedtime.

Potential Nursing Diagnoses
Noncompliance (Patient/Family Teaching)

Implementation
- ***High Alert:*** Dose errors are a potential problem with administration of pramlintide. Pramlintide is available in a concentration of 0.6 mg/ml, dosing is in mcg, and insulin syringe for administration is in units. Carefully review dosing and conversion table prior to administration.
- Administer pramlintide and insulin as separate injections; do not mix.

- Adjust insulin doses to optimize glycemic control once target dose of pramlintide is achieved and nausea has subsided.
- **Subcut:** Administer immediately prior to major meals ≥250 kcal or containing ≥30 g of carbohydrate. Reduce preprandial rapid-acting, short-acting, and fixed-mix insulin doses by 50%. Use a U-100 syringe (preferably a 0.3 ml size) for optimal accuracy. Administer into abdomen or thigh, rotating injection sites. Do not administer solutions that are cloudy. Store unopened vials in refrigerator. Opened vials may be refrigerated or kept at room temperature for up to 28 days.

Patient/Family Teaching

- Instruct patient in proper use of pramlintide (injection technique, timing of doses, storage, and disposal of equipment). Make sure patient understands dosing and preparation of correct dose. Emphasize importance of adherence to meal planning, physical activity, recognition and management of hypoglycemia and hyperglycemia, and assessment of diabetes complications. Advise patient to read the Medication Guide before use and with each refill for new information.
- Review with patient how to handle illness or stress, inadequate or omitted insulin dose, inadvertent administration of increased dose of insulin or pramlintide, inadequate food intake or missed meals. If a dose is missed, wait until the next meal and take usual dose; do not give an additional injection.
- Instruct patient to contact health care professional at least once a week until target dose of pramlintide is achieved, pramlintide is well-tolerated, and blood glucose concentrations are stable.
- May cause difficulty concentrating. Caution patient to avoid driving or other activities requiring alertness until response to medication is known.
- Inform patient that signs of local allergy (redness, swelling, itching at site of injection) usually resolve within a few days to a few weeks; may be related to pramlintide, irritants in skin cleansing agent or improper injection technique.
- Advise patient to contact health care professional if recurrent nausea or hypoglycemia occur; may lead to increased risk of severe hypoglycemia. Discontinue pramlintide therapy if recurrent unexplained hypoglycemia requiring medical assistance, persistent clinically significant nausea, or noncompliance with self-monitoring of blood glucose concentrations, insulin dose adjustments, or scheduled health care professional contacts or recommended clinic visits occur.
- Advise patient to contact health care professional before taking other Rx, OTC, vitamins, or herbal products with pramlintide and to avoid concurrent alcohol use.
- Advise female patients to notify health care professional if pregnancy is planned or suspected or if breastfeeding.

Evaluation/Desired Outcomes

- Reduction in postprandial glucose concentrations.

---

pravastatin, See HMG-CoA REDUCTASE INHIBITORS (statins).

---

prazosin (pra-zoe-sin)
Minipress

Classification
Therapeutic: antihypertensives
Pharmacologic: peripherally acting anti-adrenergics

Pregnancy Category C

Indications
Mild to moderate hypertension. **Unlabeled uses:** Management of urinary outflow obstruction in patients with benign prostatic hyperplasia.

Action
Dilates both arteries and veins by blocking postsynaptic alpha$_1$-adrenergic receptors. Decreases contractions in smooth muscle of prostatic capsule. **Therapeutic Effects:** Lowering of blood pressure. Decreased cardiac preload and afterload. Decreased symptoms of prostatic hyperplasia (urinary urgency, urinary hesitancy, nocturia).

Pharmacokinetics
Absorption: 60% absorbed following oral administration.
Distribution: Widely distributed.

Protein Binding: 97%.
Metabolism and Excretion: Extensively metabolized by the liver. Minimal (5–10%) renal excretion of unchanged drug.
Half-life: 2–3 hr.

TIME/ACTION PROFILE (antihypertensive effects)

ROUTE	ONSET	PEAK	DURATION
PO	2 hr	2–4 hr†	10 hr

†Following single dose; maximal antihypertensive effects occur after 3–4 wk of chronic dosing

Contraindications/Precautions
Contraindicated in: Hypersensitivity.
Use Cautiously in: Renal insufficiency (increased sensitivity to effects; dosage reduction may be required); Pregnancy, lactation, or children (safety not established); Angina pectoris; When adding diuretics (reduce dose of prazosin).

Adverse Reactions/Side Effects
CNS: dizziness, headache, weakness, drowsiness, mental depression, syncope. **EENT:** blurred vision. **CV:** first-dose orthostatic hypotension, palpitations, angina, edema. **GI:** abdominal cramps, diarrhea, dry mouth, nausea, vomiting. **GU:** erectile dysfunction, priapism.

Interactions
Drug-Drug: Additive hypotension with acute ingestion of **alcohol**, other **antihypertensives**, or **nitrates**. Antihypertensive effects may be decreased by **NSAIDs**.

Route/Dosage

Hypertension
PO (Adults): 1 mg 2–3 times daily (give first dose at bedtime) for initial 3 days of therapy, then increase gradually to maintenance dose of 6–15 mg/day in 2–3 divided doses (not to exceed 20–40 mg/day).
PO (Children): 50–400 mcg (0.05–0.4 mg)/kg/day in 2–3 divided doses (not to exceed 7 mg/dose or 15 mg/day).

Benign Prostatic Hyperplasia
PO (Adults): 1–5 mg twice daily.

Availability (generic available)
Capsules: 1 mg, 2 mg, 5 mg. **Cost:** *Generic*—1 mg $35.96/180, 2 mg $43.00/180, 5 mg $93.98/180. **Tablets:** ✤1 mg, ✤2 mg, ✤5 mg. ***In combination with:*** polythiazide (Minizide). See Appendix B.

NURSING IMPLICATIONS

Assessment
- Monitor intake and output ratios and daily weight and assess for edema daily, especially at beginning of therapy. Report significant weight gain or edema.
- **Hypertension:** Monitor blood pressure and pulse frequently during initial dosage adjustment and periodically throughout therapy. Report significant changes.
- Monitor frequency of prescription refills to determine compliance.
- **Benign Prostatic Hyperplasia:** Assess patient for urinary symptoms (retention, dribbling, hesitancy, urgency) periodically during therapy.
- ***Lab Test Considerations:*** May cause elevated serum sodium levels.
- May cause increased vanillylmandelic acid (VMA) concentrations; false-positive results may occur in screening tests for pheochromocytoma.

Potential Nursing Diagnoses
Risk for injury (Side Effects)
Noncompliance (Patient/Family Teaching)

Implementation
- Following initial dose, patient may develop first-dose orthostatic hypotensive reaction, which most frequently occurs 30–90 min after initial dose and may be manifested by dizziness, weakness, and syncope. Observe patient closely during this period, and take precautions to prevent injury. The first dose may be given at bedtime to minimize this reaction.
- Commonly administered concurrently with a thiazide diuretic or a beta blockers for treatment of hypertension.

Patient/Family Teaching
- Emphasize the importance of continuing to take this medication, even if feeling well. Instruct patient to take medication at the same time each day. If a dose is missed, take as soon as remembered unless almost time for next dose. Do not double doses.
- Encourage patient to comply with additional interventions for hypertension (weight reduction, low-sodium diet, smoking cessation, moderation of alcohol consumption, regular exercise, stress management).
- Instruct patient and family on proper technique for blood pressure monitoring. Advise

them to check blood pressure at least weekly and to report significant changes.

- May cause drowsiness or dizziness. Advise patient to avoid driving or other activities requiring alertness until response to medication is known.
- Caution patient to change positions slowly to decrease orthostatic hypotension.
- Advise patient to consult health care professional before taking any OTC medications, especially cough, cold, or allergy remedies.
- Emphasize the importance of follow-up visits to determine effectiveness of therapy.

Evaluation/Desired Outcomes

- Decrease in blood pressure without appearance of side effects.
- Decrease in symptoms of prostatic hyperplasia.

---

prednicarbate, See CORTICOSTEROIDS (TOPICAL/LOCAL).

---

prednisoLONE, See CORTICOSTEROIDS (SYSTEMIC).

---

predniSONE, See CORTICOSTEROIDS (SYSTEMIC).

---

pregabalin (pre-**gab**-a-lin)

Lyrica

Classification

Therapeutic: analgesics, anticonvulsants

Pharmacologic: gamma aminobutyric acid (GABA) analogues, nonopioid analgesics

Schedule V

Pregnancy Category C

Indications

Pain due to: diabetic peripheral neuropathy, postherpetic neuralgia, fibromyalgia. Adjunctive therapy of partial-onset seizures in adults.

Action

Binds to calcium channels in CNS tissues which regulate neurotransmitter release. Does not bind to opioid receptors. **Therapeutic Effects:** Decreased neuropathic or post-herpetic pain. Decreased partial-onset seizures.

Pharmacokinetics

Absorption: Well absorbed (90%) following oral administration.

Distribution: Probably crosses the blood-brain barrier.

Metabolism and Excretion: Minimally metabolized, 90% excreted unchanged in urine.

Half-life: 6 hr.

TIME/ACTION PROFILE (decreased post–herpetic pain)

ROUTE	ONSET	PEAK	DURATION
PO	unknown	2–4 wk	unknown

Contraindications/Precautions

Contraindicated in: Myopathy (known/suspected); OB: Lactation.

Use Cautiously in: Renal impairment (dose alteration recommended for CCr <60 ml/min); Geri: Elderly patients (consider age-related decrease in renal function; CHF; History of drug dependence/drug-seeking behavior; Pedi: Children (safety not established); OB: Use only if maternal benefit outweighs fetal risk; may also have ↑ risk of male-mediated teratogenicity).

Adverse Reactions/Side Effects

CNS: dizziness, drowsiness, impaired attention/concentration/thinking. **CV:** edema. **EENT:** blurred vision. **GI:** dry mouth, abdominal pain, constipation, ↑ appetite, vomiting. **Hemat:** ↓ platelet count. **Metab:** weight gain. **Misc:** allergic reactions, fever.

Interactions

Drug-Drug: Concurrent use with **thiazolidinediones (pioglitazone, rosiglitazone)** may ↑ risk of fluid retention. ↑ risk of CNS depression with other **CNS depressants** including **opioids, alcohol, benzodiazepines**, or other **sedatives/hypnotics**.

Route/Dosage

PO (Adults): *Diabetic neuropathic pain*—50 mg three times daily, increased over 7 days up to 100 mg three times daily; *Partial onset seizures*—150 mg/day initially in 2–3 divided doses, may be gradually increased to 600 mg/day; *Post-herpetic neuralgia*—75 mg twice daily or 50 mg three times daily initially, may be increased over 7 days to 300 mg/day in 2–3 divided doses, after 2–4 wk may be increased to 600 mg/day in 2–3 divided doses; Fibromyalgia- 75 mg twice daily initially, may be increased to 150 mg twice daily within 1 wk based on efficacy and tolerability. May be increased to 225 twice daily.

Renal Impairment

PO (Adults): *CCr 30–60 ml/min*— 75–300 mg/day in 2–3 divided doses; *CCr 15–30 ml/min*—25–150 mg/day in 1–2 divided doses; *CCr <15 ml/min*—25–75 mg/day as a single daily dose.

Availability

Capsules: 25 mg, 50 mg, 75 mg, 100 mg, 150 mg, 200 mg, 225 mg, 300 mg. **Cost:** 25 mg $335.95/180, 50 mg $335.95/180, 75 mg $335.95/180, 100 mg $335.95/180, 150 mg $335.95/180, 200 mg $343.94/180, 225 mg $337.01/180, 300 mg $351.92/180.

NURSING IMPLICATIONS

Assessment

- **Diabetic Peripheral Neuropathy, Postherpetic Neuralgia, and Fibromylagia:** Assess location, characteristics, and intensity of pain periodically during therapy.
- **Seizures:** Assess location, duration, and characteristics of seizure activity.
- ***Lab Test Considerations:*** May cause ↑ creatine kinase levels.
- May cause ↓ platelet count.

Potential Nursing Diagnoses

Risk for injury (Adverse Reactions)

Implementation

- Pregabalin should be discontinued gradually over at least 1 wk. Abrupt discontinuation may cause insomnia, nausea, headache, and diarrhea when used for pain and may cause increase in seizure frequency when treating seizures.
- **PO:** May be administered without regard to meals.

Patient/Family Teaching

- Instruct patient to take medication as directed. Do not discontinue abruptly; may cause insomnia, nausea, headache, or diarrhea or increase in frequency of seizures. Advise patient to read the *Patient Information Leaflet* prior to taking pregabalin.
- May cause dizziness, drowsiness, and blurred vision. Caution patient to avoid driving or activities requiring alertness until response to medication is known. Advise patient to notify health care professional if changes in vision occur. Seizure patients should not resume driving until physician gives clearance based on control of seizure disorder.
- Instruct patient to promptly report unexplained muscle pain, tenderness, or weakness, especially if accompanied by malaise or fever. Discontinue therapy if myopathy is diagnosed or suspected or if markedly elevated creatine kinase levels occur.
- Inform patient that pregabalin may cause edema and weight gain.
- Caution patient to avoid alcohol or other CNS depressants with pregabalin.
- Advise female patient to notify health care professional if pregnancy is planned or suspected or if she intends to breastfeed or is breastfeeding an infant. Inform male patients who plan to father a child of the potential risk of male-mediated teratogenicity.
- Instruct patient to notify health care professional of medication regimen before treatment or surgery.
- Advise patient to carry identification describing disease process and medication regimen at all times.

Evaluation/Desired Outcomes

- Decrease in intensity of chronic pain.
- Decrease in the frequency or cessation of seizures.

probenecid (proe-**ben**-e-sid)

✤Benuryl, Probalan

Classification

Therapeutic: antigout agents, uricosurics

Pregnancy Category B

Indications

Prevention of recurrences of gouty arthritis. Treatment of hyperuricemia secondary to thiazide therapy. Used to increase and prolong serum levels of penicillin and related anti-infectives.

Action

Inhibits renal tubular reabsorption of uric acid, thus promoting its renal excretion. **Therapeutic Effects:** Reduction of serum uric acid levels.

Pharmacokinetics

Absorption: Well absorbed following oral administration.

Distribution: Crosses the placenta.
Protein Binding: 75–95%.
Metabolism and Excretion: Mostly metabolized by the liver; 10% excreted unchanged in the urine.
Half-life: 4–17 hr.

TIME/ACTION PROFILE (effects on serum uric acid levels)

ROUTE	ONSET	PEAK	DURATION
PO	30 min	2–4 hr	8 hr

Contraindications/Precautions

Contraindicated in: Hypersensitivity; Chronic high-dose salicylate therapy; Children <2 yr.
Use Cautiously in: Peptic ulcer; Blood dyscrasias; Uric acid kidney stones; Renal impairment (dosage reduction recommended; may not be effective if CCr ≤30 ml/min); Pregnancy or lactation (has been used safely during pregnancy; safety during lactation not established).

Adverse Reactions/Side Effects

CNS: headache, dizziness. **GI:** nausea, vomiting, abdominal pain, diarrhea, drug-induced hepatitis, sore gums. **GU:** uric acid stones, urinary frequency. **Derm:** flushing, rashes. **Hemat:** APLASTIC ANEMIA, anemia.

Interactions

Drug-Drug: Increases blood levels of **acyclovir, allopurinol, barbiturates, benzodiazepines, cephalosporins, clofibrate, dapsone, dyphylline, methotrexate, NSAIDs, pantothenic acid, penicillamine, penicillins, rifampin, sulfonamides, sulfonylurea oral hypoglycemic agents**, or **zidovudine**. Large doses of **salicylates** may decrease uricosuric activity.

Route/Dosage

PO (Adults and Children >50 kg): *Hyperuricemia*—250 mg bid for 1 wk; increase to 500 mg twice daily, then may increase by 500 mg/day every 4 wk (not to exceed 3 g/day). *Augmentation of penicillin/cephalosporins*—500 mg 4 times daily. *Single-dose therapy of gonorrhea*—1 g with amoxicillin or penicillin.
PO (Children 2–14 yr and ≤50 kg): 25 mg/kg (700 mg/m^2) initially; then 10 mg/kg (300 mg/m^2) 4 times daily.

Availability

Tablets: 0.5 g.

NURSING IMPLICATIONS

Assessment

- **Gout:** Assess involved joints for pain, mobility, and edema throughout course of therapy.
- Monitor intake and output ratios. Fluids should be encouraged to prevent urate stone formation (2000–3000 ml/day). Alkalinization of the urine with sodium bicarbonate, potassium citrate, or acetazolamide may also be used for this purpose.
- ***Lab Test Considerations:*** CBC, serum uric acid levels, and renal function should be monitored routinely during long-term therapy.
- Serum and urine uric acid determinations may be measured periodically when probenecid is used to treat hyperuricemia.

Potential Nursing Diagnoses

Acute pain (Indications)
Impaired physical mobility (Indications)
Deficient knowledge, related to medication regimen (Patient/Family Teaching)

Implementation

- Probenecid therapy is not used to treat gouty arthritis but, rather, to prevent it. If acute attacks occur during therapy, probenecid is usually continued at full dose along with colchicine or NSAIDs.
- **PO:** Administer with food or antacid to minimize gastric irritation.
- Gradual dosage reduction should be attempted if uric acid levels remain stable following 6 mo of therapy.

Patient/Family Teaching

- Instruct patient to take medication exactly as directed, not to discontinue without consulting health care professional. Irregular dosage schedules may cause elevation of uric acid levels and precipitate an acute gout attack.
- Explain purpose of the medication to patients taking probenecid with penicillin.
- Advise patient to follow recommendations of health care professional regarding weight loss, diet, and alcohol consumption.
- Caution patient not to take aspirin or other salicylates, because they decrease the effects of probenecid.
- Instruct patient to report nausea, vomiting, loss of appetite, abdominal pain, unusual bleeding

P

or bruising, sore throat, fatigue, malaise, or yellowing of the skin or eyes promptly.

Evaluation/Desired Outcomes

- Decrease in pain and swelling in affected joints and subsequent decrease in frequency of gout attacks. May require several months of continuous therapy for maximum effects.
- Decrease in serum uric acid levels.
- Prolonged serum levels of penicillins and other related antibiotics.

procainamide

(proe-**kane**-ah-mide)

Pronestyl

Classification

Therapeutic: antiarrhythmics (class IA)

Pregnancy Category C

Indications

Treatment of a wide variety of ventricular and atrial arrhythmias, including: Atrial premature contractions, Premature ventricular contractions, Ventricular tachycardia, Paroxysmal atrial tachycardia. Maintenance of normal sinus rhythm after conversion from atrial fibrillation or flutter.

Action

Decreases myocardial excitability. Slows conduction velocity. May depress myocardial contractility. **Therapeutic Effects:** Suppression of arrhythmias.

Pharmacokinetics

Absorption: Well absorbed (75–90%) following IM administration. Sustained-release oral preparation is more slowly absorbed.
Distribution: Rapidly and widely distributed.
Metabolism and Excretion: Converted by the liver to *N*-acetylprocainamide (NAPA), an active antiarrhythmic compound. Remainder (40–70%) excreted unchanged by the kidneys.
Half-life: 2.5–4.7 hr (NAPA—7 hr); prolonged in renal impairment.

TIME/ACTION PROFILE (antiarrhythmic effects)

ROUTE	ONSET	PEAK	DURATION
IV	immediate	25–60 min	3–4 hr
IM	10–30 min	15–60 min	3–4 hr

Contraindications/Precautions

Contraindicated in: Hypersensitivity; AV block; Myasthenia gravis; Hypersensitivity to tartrazine (FDC yellow dye #5; present in some oral products).
Use Cautiously in: MI or cardiac glycoside toxicity; CHF, renal or hepatic insufficiency, geriatric patients (dose reduction or increased dosing intervals recommended); Pregnancy, lactation, or children (safety not established).

Adverse Reactions/Side Effects

CNS: SEIZURES, confusion, dizziness. **CV:** ASYSTOLE, HEART BLOCK, VENTRICULAR ARRHYTHMIAS, hypotension. **GI:** diarrhea, anorexia, bitter taste, nausea, vomiting. **Derm:** rashes. **Hemat:** AGRANULOCYTOSIS, eosinophilia, leukopenia, thrombocytopenia. **Misc:** chills, drug-induced systemic lupus syndrome, fever.

Interactions

Drug-Drug: May have additive or antagonistic effects with other **antiarrhythmics**. Additive neurologic toxicity (confusion, seizures) with **lidocaine**. **Antihypertensives** and **nitrates** may potentiate hypotensive effect. Potentiates **neuromuscular blocking agents**. May partially antagonize the therapeutic effects of **anticholinesterase agents** in myasthenia gravis. ↑ risk of arrhythmias with **pimozide**. Additive anticholinergic effects with other **drugs possessing anticholinergic properties**, including **antihistamines**, **antidepressants**, **atropine**, **haloperidol**, and **phenothiazines**. Effects of procainamide may be ↑ by **cimetidine**, **quinidine**, or **trimethoprim**.

Route/Dosage

IM (Adults): 50 mg/kg/day in divided doses q 3–6 hr.
IV (Adults): 100 mg q 5 min until arrhythmia is abolished or 1000 mg have been given; wait at least 10 min until further dosing *or* loading infusion of 500–600 mg over 30–60 min followed by maintenance infusion of 1–4 mg/min.

Availability

Injection: 100 mg/ml in 10-ml vials, 500 mg/ml in 2-ml vials.

NURSING IMPLICATIONS

Assessment

- Monitor ECG, pulse, and blood pressure continuously throughout IV administration. Parameters should be monitored periodically during oral administration. IV administration is usually discontinued if any of the following occur: arrhythmia is resolved, QRS complex widens by 50%, PR interval is prolonged, blood pressure drops >15 mm Hg, or toxic side effects develop. Patient should remain supine throughout IV administration to minimize hypotension.

- ***Lab Test Considerations:*** Monitor CBC every 2 wk during the first 3 mo of therapy. May cause ↓ leukocyte, neutrophil, and platelet counts. Therapy may be discontinued if leukopenia occurs. Blood counts usually return to normal within 1 mo of discontinuation of therapy.
- Monitor ANA periodically during prolonged therapy or if symptoms of lupus-like reaction occur. Therapy is discontinued if a steady increase in ANA titer occurs.
- May cause ↑ AST, ALT, alkaline phosphatase, LDH, bilirubin, and a positive Coombs' test result.
- ***Toxicity and Overdose:*** Serum procainamide and *N*-acetylprocainamide levels may be monitored periodically during dosage adjustment. Therapeutic blood level of procainamide is 4–8 mcg/ml: Toxicity may occur with procainamide blood levels of 8–16 mcg/ml or greater, Signs of toxicity include confusion, dizziness, drowsiness, decreased urination, nausea, vomiting, and tachyarrhythmias.

Potential Nursing Diagnoses

Decreased cardiac output (Indications)

Implementation

- **IM:** Used only when oral and IV routes are not feasible.

IV Administration

- **Direct IV:** (only to be used for life-threatening arrhythmias) ***Diluent:*** Dilute each 100 mg of procainamide with 10 ml of 0.9% NaCl. ***Rate:*** Administer at a rate not to exceed 25 mg/min. Rapid administration may cause ventricular fibrillation or asystole.
- **Intermittent Infusion:** (preferred route of administration). ***Diluent:*** Add 2 g of procainamide to 250 ml of 0.9% NaCl. ***Concentration:*** 8 mg/ml. ***Rate:*** Administer initial infusion over 30–60 min. Administer maintenance infusion at rate of 1–4 mg/min to maintain control of arrhythmia.
- **Y-Site Compatibility:** amikacin, aminophylline, amiodarone, atropine, aztreonam, bivalirudin, bumetanide, calcium chloride, calcium gluconate, caspofungin, cefazolin, cefotaxime, cefoxitin, ceftazidime, ceftriaxone, cefuroxime, cimetidine, cisatracurium, clindamycin, cyclosporine, daptomycin, dexamethasone sodium phosphate, dexmedetomidine, digoxin, diphenhydramine, dobutamine, dopamine, doxycycline, enalaprilat, epinephrine, ertapenem, erythromycin, esmolol, famotidine, fenoldopam, fentanyl, fluconazole, furosemide, gentamicin, granisetron, heparin, hydrocortisone sodium succinate, hydromorphone, insulin, isoproterenol, ketorolac, labetalol, lidocaine, linezolid, lorazepam, magnesium sulfate, meperidine, methylprednisolone sodium succinate, metoclopramide, metoprolol, midazolam, morphine, nafcillin, nitroglycerin, nitroprusside, norepinephrine, ondansetron, palonosetron, pantoprazole, penicillin G potassium, phenylephrine, piperacillin, piperacillin/tazobactam, potassium chloride, prochlorperazine, promethazine, propranolol, protamine, quinupristin/dalfopristin, ranitidine, remifentanil, sodium bicarbonate, tacrolimus, ticarcillin/clavulanate, tirofiban, tobramycin, vancomycin, vasopressin, verapamil, vitamin B complex with C, voriconazole.
- **Y-Site Incompatibility:** acyclovir, ceftizoxime, chloramphenicol, diazepam, ganciclovir, hydralazine, lansoprazole, metronidazole, milrinone, phenytoin trimethoprim/sulfamethoxazole.

Patient/Family Teaching

- Instruct patient or family member on how to take pulse. Advise patient to report changes in pulse rate or rhythm to health care professional.
- May cause dizziness. Caution patient to avoid driving or other activities requiring alertness until response to medication is known.
- Advise patient to notify health care professional immediately if signs of drug-induced lupus syndrome (fever, chills, joint pain or swelling, pain with breathing, skin rash), leukopenia (sore throat, mouth, or gums), or thrombocytopenia (unusual bleeding or bruising) occur. Medication may be discontinued if these occur.
- Caution patient not to take OTC medications with procainamide without consulting health care professional.

- Advise patient to inform health care professional of medication regimen prior to treatment or surgery.
- Advise patient to carry identification at all times describing disease process and medication regimen.
- Emphasize the importance of routine follow-up exams to monitor progress.

Evaluation/Desired Outcomes

- Resolution of cardiac arrhythmias without detrimental side effects.

procaine penicillin G, See PENICILLINS.

procarbazine

(proe-**kar**-ba-zeen)
Matulane, ✱Natulan

Classification
Therapeutic: antineoplastics
Pharmacologic: alkylating agents

Pregnancy Category D

Indications

Treatment of Hodgkin's disease (with other treatment modalities). **Unlabeled uses:** Other lymphomas. Brain and lung tumors. Multiple myeloma. Malignant melanoma. Polycythemia vera.

Action

Appears to inhibit DNA, RNA, and protein synthesis (cell-cycle S-phase–specific). **Therapeutic Effects:** Death of rapidly replicating cells, particularly malignant ones.

Pharmacokinetics

Absorption: Well absorbed following oral administration.
Distribution: Widely distributed; crosses the blood-brain barrier.
Metabolism and Excretion: Metabolized by the liver; <5% excreted unchanged by the kidneys; some respiratory elimination as methane and carbon dioxide.
Half-life: 1 hr.

TIME/ACTION PROFILE (effects on blood counts)

ROUTE	ONSET	PEAK	DURATION
PO	14 days	2–8 wk	28 days or more (up to 6 wk)

Contraindications/Precautions

Contraindicated in: Hypersensitivity; Pregnancy or lactation; Alcoholism; Severe renal or liver impairment; Pheochromocytoma; CHF.
Use Cautiously in: Patients with childbearing potential; Infections; Decreased bone marrow reserve; Other chronic debilitating illnesses; Headaches; Psychiatric illness; Liver impairment; Cardiovascular disease.

Adverse Reactions/Side Effects

CNS: SEIZURES, confusion, dizziness, drowsiness, hallucinations, headache, mania, mental depression, nightmares, psychosis, syncope, tremor. **EENT:** nystagmus, photophobia, retinal hemorrhage. **Resp:** cough, pleural effusions. **CV:** edema, hypotension, tachycardia. **GI:** nausea, vomiting, anorexia, diarrhea, dry mouth, dysphagia, hepatic dysfunction, stomatitis. **GU:** gonadal suppression. **Derm:** alopecia, photosensitivity, pruritus, rashes. **Endo:** gynecomastia. **Hemat:** anemia, leukopenia, thrombocytopenia. **Neuro:** neuropathy, paresthesia. **Misc:** ascites, secondary malignancy.

Interactions

Drug-Drug: Concurrent use with **sympathomimetics** including **methylphenidate** may produce life-threatening hypertension (avoid concurrent use during and for 14 days following procarbazine). Deep coma and death may result from concurrent use of **opioid analgesics**; avoid **meperidine**. Use small incremental doses of other agents and titrate to effect. ↑ bone marrow depression may occur with other **antineoplastics** or **radiation therapy**. Seizures and hyperpyrexia may occur with concurrent use of **MAO inhibitors**, **tricyclic antidepressants**, **SSRI antidepressants** (should not be used within 5 wk of **fluoxetine**), or **carbamazepine**. May ↓ serum **digoxin** levels. Concurrent use with **levodopa** may result in flushing and hypertension. ↑ CNS depression with other **CNS depressants**, including **alcohol**, **antidepressants**, **antihistamines**, **opioid analgesics**, **phenothiazines**, and **sedative/hypnotics**. Disulfiram-like reaction

may occur with **alcohol**. **Cigarette smoking** may ↑ the risk of secondary lung cancer.
Drug-Food: Ingestion of foods high in **tyramine** content (see Appendix L) may result in hypertension. Ingestion of foods high in **caffeine** content may result in arrhythmias.

Route/Dosage

PO (Adults): 2–4 mg/kg/day as a single dose or in divided doses for 1 wk, then 4–6 mg/kg/day until response is obtained; then maintenance dose of 1–2 mg/kg/day. Dosage should be rounded off to the nearest 50 mg.
PO (Children): 50 mg/m²/day for 7 days, then 100 mg/m²/day, maintenance dose of 50 mg/m²/day.

Availability

Capsules: 50 mg.

NURSING IMPLICATIONS

Assessment

- Monitor blood pressure, pulse, and respiratory rate periodically during therapy. Report significant changes to health care professional.
- Assess nutritional status (appetite, intake and output ratios, weight, frequency and amount of emesis). Anorexia and weight loss can be decreased by feeding light, frequent meals. Nausea and vomiting can be minimized by administering an antiemetic at least 1 hr prior to receiving medication. Phenothiazine antiemetics should be avoided.
- Monitor for bone marrow depression. Assess for bleeding (bleeding gums, bruising, petechiae, guaiac stools, urine, and emesis) and avoid IM injections and taking rectal temperatures if platelet count is low. Apply pressure to venipuncture sites for 10 min. Assess for signs of infection during neutropenia. Anemia may occur. Monitor for increased fatigue, dyspnea, and orthostatic hypotension.
- Concurrent ingestion of tyramine-rich foods and many medications may result in life-threatening hypertensive crisis. Signs and symptoms of hypertensive crisis include chest pain, severe headache, nausea and vomiting, photosensitivity, and enlarged pupils. Treatment includes IV phentolamine.
- Procarbazine should be discontinued until side effects clear and then resumed at a lower dose if leukopenia, thrombocytopenia, hypersensitivity reaction, stomatitis (first small ulceration or persistent soreness), diarrhea, hemorrhage, or bleeding tendencies occur.
- ***Lab Test Considerations:*** Monitor hemoglobin, hematocrit, WBC, differential, reticulocytes, and platelet count prior to and every 3–4 days during therapy. Notify physician if WBC <4000/mm³ or platelet count <100,000/mm³. Therapy should be discontinued and resumed at a lower dose when counts improve. The nadir of leukopenia and thrombocytopenia occurs in approximately 2–8 wk, and recovery usually occurs in about 6 wk. Anemia also may occur.
- Assess hepatic and renal function prior to therapy. Monitor urinalysis, AST, ALT, alkaline phosphatase, and BUN at least weekly during therapy.
- Closely monitor serum glucose in diabetic patients. Oral hypoglycemics or insulin dosage may need to be reduced, because hypoglycemic effects are enhanced.
- Bone marrow aspiration studies are recommended prior to initiation of therapy and at time of maximum hematologic response to ensure adequate bone marrow reserve.

Potential Nursing Diagnoses

Risk for infection (Adverse Reactions)
Imbalanced nutrition: less than body requirements (Adverse Reactions)

Implementation

- **PO:** Administer with food or fluids if GI irritation occurs. Confer with pharmacist regarding opening of capsules if patient has difficulty swallowing.

Patient/Family Teaching

- Emphasize the need to take medication as directed. Take missed doses as soon as remembered within a few hours but not if several hours have passed or if almost time for next dose. Health care professional should be consulted if vomiting occurs shortly after a dose is taken.
- Instruct patient to notify health care professional promptly if signs of infection (fever, sore throat, chills, cough, thickened bronchial secretions, hoarseness, pain in lower back or side, difficult or painful urination); bleeding gums; bruising; petechiae; or blood in stool, urine, or emesis occurs. Caution patient to avoid crowds and persons with known

P

infections. Instruct patient to use soft toothbrush and electric razor and to avoid falls. Patient should not receive IM injections or rectal temperatures. Caution patient not to drink alcoholic beverages or take medication containing aspirin or NSAIDs; may precipitate gastric bleeding.

- Caution patient to avoid alcohol, caffeinated beverages, CNS depressants, OTC drugs, and foods or beverages containing tyramine (see Appendix L for foods included) during therapy and for at least 2 wk after therapy has been discontinued, because they may precipitate a hypertensive crisis.
- Advise patient that an additional interaction of alcohol with procarbazine is a disulfiram-like reaction (flushing, nausea, vomiting, headache, abdominal cramps).
- Instruct patient to inspect oral mucosa for erythema and ulceration. If ulceration occurs, advise patient to notify health care professional and to use sponge brush and rinse mouth with water after eating and drinking. Topical agents may be used if mouth pain interferes with eating. Stomatitis pain may require treatment with opioid analgesics.
- May cause drowsiness or dizziness. Caution patient to avoid driving or other activities that require alertness until response to medication is known.
- Advise patient that this medication may have teratogenic effects. Contraception should be practiced during therapy and for at least 4 mo after therapy is concluded.
- Discuss the possibility of hair loss with patient. Explore methods of coping.
- Caution patient to use sunscreen and protective clothing to prevent photosensitivity reactions.
- Instruct patient not to receive any vaccinations without advice of health care professional.
- Advise patient to notify health care professional of medication regimen prior to treatment or surgery. This therapy usually should be withdrawn at least 2 wk prior to surgery.
- Instruct patient to inform health care professional if muscle or joint pain, nausea, vomiting, sweating, tiredness, weakness, constipation, headache, difficulty swallowing, or loss of appetite becomes pronounced.
- Advise patient to carry identification describing medication regimen at all times.
- Emphasize the need for periodic lab tests to monitor for side effects.

Evaluation/Desired Outcomes

- Decrease in size and spread of malignant tissue in Hodgkin's disease.

prochlorperazine

(proe-klor-**pair**-a-zeen)

Compazine, ✤Stemetil, Ultrazine

Classification

Therapeutic: antiemetics, antipsychotics

Pharmacologic: phenothiazines

Pregnancy Category C

Indications

Management of nausea and vomiting. Treatment of psychoses. Treatment of anxiety.

Action

Alters the effects of dopamine in the CNS. Possesses significant anticholinergic and alpha-adrenergic blocking activity. Depresses the chemoreceptor trigger zone (CTZ) in the CNS.
Therapeutic Effects: Diminished nausea and vomiting. Diminished signs and symptoms of psychoses or anxiety.

Pharmacokinetics

Absorption: Absorption from tablet is variable; may be better with oral liquid formulations. Well absorbed after IM administration.
Distribution: Widely distributed, high concentrations in the CNS. Crosses the placenta and probably enters breast milk.
Protein Binding: ≥90%.
Metabolism and Excretion: Highly metabolized by the liver and GI mucosa. Converted to some compounds with antipsychotic activity.
Half-life: Unknown.

TIME/ACTION PROFILE (antiemetic effect)

ROUTE	ONSET	PEAK	DURATION
PO	30–40 min	unknown	3–4 hr
PO-ER	30–40 min	unknown	10–12 hr
rect	60 min	unknown	3–4 hr
IM	10–20 min	10–30 min	3–4 hr
IV	rapid (min)	10–30 min	3–4 hr

Contraindications/Precautions

Contraindicated in: Hypersensitivity; Cross-sensitivity with other phenothiazines may exist; Angle-closure glaucoma; Bone marrow depression; Severe liver or cardiovascular disease; Hypersensitivity to bisulfites or benzyl alcohol

(some parenteral products); Pedi: Children <2 yr or 9.1 kg.
Use Cautiously in: Geri: Geriatric or debilitated patients (dose reduction recommended); Diabetes mellitus; Respiratory disease; Prostatic hypertrophy; CNS tumors; Epilepsy; Intestinal obstruction; Geri: Pregnancy or lactation (safety not established).

Adverse Reactions/Side Effects

CNS: NEUROLEPTIC MALIGNANT SYNDROME, extrapyramidal reactions, sedation, tardive dyskinesia. **EENT:** blurred vision, dry eyes, lens opacities. **CV:** ECG changes, hypotension, tachycardia. **GI:** constipation, dry mouth, anorexia, drug-induced hepatitis, ileus. **GU:** pink or reddish-brown discoloration of urine, urinary retention. **Derm:** photosensitivity, pigment changes, rashes. **Endo:** galactorrhea. **Hemat:** AGRANULOCYTOSIS, leukopenia. **Metab:** hyperthermia. **Misc:** allergic reactions.

Interactions

Drug-Drug: Additive hypotension with **antihypertensives**, **nitrates**, or acute ingestion of **alcohol**. Additive CNS depression with other **CNS depressants**, including **alcohol**, **antidepressants**, **antihistamines**, **opioid analgesics**, **sedative/hypnotics**, or **general anesthetics**. Additive anticholinergic effects with other **drugs possessing anticholinergic properties**, including **antihistamines**, some **antidepressants**, **atropine**, **haloperidol**, and other **phenothiazines**. **Lithium** ↑ risk of extrapyramidal reactions. May mask early signs of **lithium** toxicity. ↑ risk of agranulocytosis with **antithyroid agents**. ↓ beneficial effects of **levodopa**. **Antacids** may ↓ absorption.
Drug-Natural Products: Concomitant use of **kava kava**, **valerian**, **chamomile**, or **hops** can ↑ CNS depression. ↑ anticholinergic effects with **angel's trumpet**, **jimson weed**, and **scopolia**.

Route/Dosage

Pediatric dose should not exceed 10 mg on the 1st day and then should not exceed 20 mg/day in children 2–5 yr or 25 mg/day in children 6–12 yr.

Antiemetic

PO (Adults and Children ≥12 yr): 5–10 mg 3–4 times daily; may also be given as 15–30 mg once daily *or* 10 mg twice daily as ER capsules (up to 40 mg/day).
PO (Children 18–39 kg): 2.5 mg 3 times daily *or* 5 mg twice daily (not to exceed 15 mg/day).
PO (Children 14–17 kg): 2.5 mg 2–3 times daily (not to exceed 10 mg/day).
PO (Children 9–13 kg): 2.5 mg 1–2 times daily (not to exceed 7.5 mg/day).
IM (Adults and Children ≥12 yr): 5–10 mg q 3–4 hr as needed. *Nausea/vomiting associated with surgery*—5–10 mg; may be repeated once.
IM (Children 2–12 yr): 132 mcg (0.132 mg)/kg; usually only 1 dose is required.
IV (Adults and Children ≥12 yr): 2.5–10 mg (not to exceed 40 mg/day). *Nausea/vomiting associated with surgery*—5–10 mg; may be repeated once.
Rect (Adults): 25 mg twice daily.
Rect (Children 18–39 kg): 2.5 mg 3 times daily or 5 mg twice daily (not to exceed 15 mg/day).
Rect (Children 14–17 kg): 2.5 mg 2–3 times daily (not to exceed 10 mg/day).
Rect (Children 9–13 kg): 2.5 mg 1–2 times daily (not to exceed 7.5 mg/day).

Antipsychotic

PO (Adults and Children ≥12 yr): 5–10 mg 3–4 times daily; may be increased q 2–3 days (up to 150 mg/day).
PO (Children 2–12 yr): 2.5 mg 2–3 times daily.
IM (Adults): 10–20 mg q 2–4 hr for up to 4 doses, then 10–20 mg q 4–6 hr (up to 200 mg/day).
IM (Children 2–12 yr): 132 mcg (0.132 mg)/kg (not to exceed 10 mg/dose).
IV (Adults and Children ≥12 yr): 2.5–10 mg (up to 40 mg/day).
Rect (Adults): 10 mg 3–4 times daily; may be increased by 5–10 mg q 2–3 days as needed.

Antianxiety

PO (Adults and Children ≥12 yr): 5 mg 3–4 times daily (not to exceed 20 mg/day or longer than 12 wk); may also be given as 15 mg once daily or 10 mg twice daily as ER capsules.
IM (Adults and Children ≥12 yr): 5–10 mg q 3–4 hr as needed (up to 40 mg/day).
IM (Children 2–12 yr): 132 mcg (0.132 mg)/kg.

P

IV (Adults): 2.5–10 mg (up to 40 mg/day).

Availability (generic available)

Tablets: 5 mg, 10 mg, 25 mg. **Syrup (fruit flavor):** 5 mg/5 ml (edisylate), ✤5 mg/5 ml (mesylate). **Extended-release capsules:** 10 mg, 15 mg, 30 mg. **Injection:** 5 mg/ml (edisylate), ✤5 mg/ml (mesylate). **Suppositories:** 2.5 mg, 5 mg, 25 mg.

NURSING IMPLICATIONS

Assessment

- Monitor blood pressure (sitting, standing, lying down), ECG, pulse, and respiratory rate before and frequently during the period of dosage adjustment. May cause Q-wave and T-wave changes in ECG.
- Assess patient for level of sedation after administration
- Monitor patient for onset of akathisia (restlessness or desire to keep moving) and extrapyramidal side effects (*parkinsonian*—difficulty speaking or swallowing, loss of balance control, pill rolling, mask-like face, shuffling gait, rigidity, tremors; and *dystonic*—muscle spasms, twisting motions, twitching, inability to move eyes, weakness of arms or legs) every 2 mo during therapy and 8–12 wk after therapy has been discontinued. Report these symptoms; reduction in dosage or discontinuation may be necessary. Trihexyphenidyl or diphenhydramine may be used to control these symptoms
- Monitor for tardive dyskinesia (uncontrolled rhythmic movement of mouth, face, and extremities; lip smacking or puckering; puffing of cheeks; uncontrolled chewing; rapid or worm-like movements of tongue). Report immediately; may be irreversible
- Monitor for development of neuroleptic malignant syndrome (fever, respiratory distress, tachycardia, seizures, diaphoresis, hypertension or hypotension, pallor, tiredness, severe muscle stiffness, loss of bladder control). Notify physician or other health care professional immediately if these symptoms occur.
- **Antiemetic:** Assess patient for nausea and vomiting before and 30–60 min after administration.
- **Antipsychotic:** Monitor patient's mental status (orientation to reality and behavior) before and periodically throughout therapy.
- Observe patient carefully when administering oral medication to ensure that medication is actually taken and not hoarded
- Assess fluid intake and bowel function. Increased bulk and fluids in the diet may help minimize constipation.
- **Anxiety:** Assess degree and manifestations of anxiety and mental status before and periodically during therapy.
- ***Lab Test Considerations:*** CBC and liver function tests should be evaluated periodically throughout course of therapy. May cause blood dyscrasias, especially between wks 4 and 10 of therapy. Hepatotoxicity is more likely to occur between wks 2 and 4 of therapy. May recur if medication is restarted. Liver function abnormalities may require discontinuation of therapy.
- May cause false-positive or false-negative pregnancy test results and false-positive urine bilirubin test results.
- May cause increased serum prolactin levels.

Potential Nursing Diagnoses

Deficient fluid volume (Indications)
Disturbed thought process (Indications)

Implementation

- Do not confuse prochlorperazine with chlorpromazine.
- To prevent contact dermatitis, avoid getting solution on hands.
- Phenothiazines should be discontinued 48 hr before and not resumed for 24 hr after myelography; they lower seizure threshold.
- **PO:** Do not crush or chew extended-release capsules. Administer with food, milk, or a full glass of water to minimize gastric irritation.
- Dilute syrup in citrus or chocolate-flavored drinks.
- Do not open, crush, or chew extended-release capsules.
- **IM:** Do not inject subcut. Inject slowly, deep into well-developed muscle. Keep patient recumbent for at least 30 min after injection to minimize hypotensive effects. Slight yellow color will not alter potency. Do not administer solution that is markedly discolored or that contains a precipitate.

IV Administration

- **Direct IV:** ***Concentration:*** Dilute to a concentration of 1 mg/ml. ***Rate:*** Administer at a rate of 1 mg/min; not to exceed 5 mg/min.
- **Intermittent Infusion:** ***Diluent:*** Dilute 20 mg in up to 1 L dextrose, saline, Ringer's or LR, dextrose/saline, dextrose/Ringer's, or lactated Ringer's combinations

- **Continuous Infusion:** Has been used as infusion with 20 mg/L of compatible solution.
- **Syringe Incompatibility:** Manufacturer does not recommend mixing prochlorperazine with other medications in syringe.
- **Y-Site Compatibility:** amsarcine, calcium gluconate, cisatracurium, cisplatin, cladribine, cyclophosphamide, cytarabine, dexmedetomidine, doxorubicin, doxorubicin liposome, fluconazole, granisetron, heparin, hydrocortisone sodium succinate, linezolid, melphalan, methotrexate, ondansetron, oxaliplatin, paclitaxel, potassium chloride, propofol, remifentanil, sargramostim, sufentanil, teniposide, thiotepa, topotecan, vinorelbine, vitamin B complex with C.
- **Y-Site Incompatibility:** aldesleukin, allopurinol, amifostine, amphotericin B cholesteryl, amifostine, aztreonam, bivalirudin, cefepime, etoposide phosphate, fenoldopam, filgrastim, fludarabine, foscarnet, gemcitabine, lansoprazole, pemetrexed, piperacillin/tazobactam.

Patient/Family Teaching

- Instruct patient to take medication as directed, not to skip doses or double up on missed doses. If a dose is missed, it should be taken as soon as remembered unless almost time for next dose. If more than 2 doses are scheduled each day, missed dose should be taken within about 1 hr of the ordered time. Abrupt withdrawal may lead to gastritis, nausea, vomiting, dizziness, headache, tachycardia, and insomnia.
- Inform patient of possibility of extrapyramidal symptoms and tardive dyskinesia. Instruct patient to report these symptoms immediately to health care professional.
- Advise patient to change positions slowly to minimize orthostatic hypotension.
- May cause drowsiness. Caution patient to avoid driving or other activities requiring alertness until response to medication is known.
- Caution patient to avoid taking alcohol or other CNS depressants concurrently with this medication.
- Advise patient to use sunscreen and protective clothing when exposed to the sun to prevent photosensitivity reactions. Extremes in temperature should also be avoided, because this drug impairs body temperature regulation.
- Instruct patient to use frequent mouth rinses, good oral hygiene, and sugarless gum or candy to minimize dry mouth. Consult health care professional if dry mouth continues for >2 wk.
- Advise patient not to take prochlorperazine within 2 hr of antacids or antidiarrheal medication.
- Advise patient that increasing bulk and fluids in the diet and exercise may help minimize the constipating effects of this medication.
- Inform patient that this medication may turn urine pink to reddish-brown.
- Advise patient to notify health care professional of medication regimen before treatment or surgery.
- Instruct patient to notify health care professional promptly if sore throat, fever, unusual bleeding or bruising, skin rashes, weakness, tremors, visual disturbances, dark-colored urine, or clay-colored stools are noted.
- Emphasize the importance of routine follow-up exams to monitor response to medication and detect side effects. Periodic ocular exams are indicated. Encourage continued participation in psychotherapy as ordered by health care professional.

Evaluation/Desired Outcomes

- Relief of nausea and vomiting.
- Decrease in excitable, paranoic, or withdrawn behavior when used as an antipsychotic.
- Decrease in feelings of anxiety.

progesterone

(proe-**jess**-te-rone)

Crinone, Endometrin, Prochieve, Prometrium

Classification

Therapeutic: hormones

Pharmacologic: progestins

Pregnancy Category D

Indications

Secondary amenorrhea and abnormal uterine bleeding due to hormonal imbalance. **Prometrium:** Prevention of cell overgrowth in the uterine lining in postmenopausal women who have not had a hysterectomy (with estrogen). Part of assisted reproductive technology (ART) in the management of infertility (4% and 8% vaginal gel). **Endometrin:** Support of embryo implantation and early pregnancy. **Unlabeled uses:** Corpus luteum dysfunction.

Action

Produces: Secretory changes in the endometrium, Increase in basal body temperature, Histologic changes in vaginal epithelium, Relaxation of uterine smooth muscle, Mammary alveolar tissue growth, Pituitary inhibition, Withdrawal bleeding in the presence of estrogen. **Therapeutic Effects:** Restoration of hormonal balance with control of uterine bleeding. Successful outcome in assisted reproduction.

Pharmacokinetics

Absorption: Micronization increases oral and vaginal absorption.
Distribution: Enters breast milk.
Protein Binding: ≥90%.
Metabolism and Excretion: Metabolized by the liver; 50–60% eliminated by kidneys; 10% eliminated in feces.
Half-life: Several minutes.

TIME/ACTION PROFILE (blood levels)

ROUTE	ONSET	PEAK	DURATION
PO	unknown	2–4 hr	unknown
vaginal	unknown	34.8–55 hr	unknown
IM	unknown	19.6–28 hr	unknown

Contraindications/Precautions

Contraindicated in: Hypersensitivity; Hypersensitivity to parabens or sesame oil (IM suspension only); Thromboembolic disease; Cerebrovascular disease; Severe liver disease; Breast or genital cancer; Porphyria; Missed abortion; OB: Pregnancy (except corpus luteum dysfunction).

Use Cautiously in: History of liver disease; Renal disease; Cardiovascular disease; Seizure disorders; Mental depression.

Adverse Reactions/Side Effects

CNS: depression. **EENT:** retinal thrombosis. **CV:** PULMONARY EMBOLISM, THROMBOEMBOLISM, thrombophlebitis. **GI:** gingival bleeding, hepatitis. **GU:** cervical erosions. **Derm:** chloasma, melasma, rashes. **Endo:** amenorrhea, breakthrough bleeding, breast tenderness, changes in menstrual flow, galactorrhea, spotting. **F and E:** edema. **Local:** irritation or pain at IM injection site. **Misc:** allergic reactions including ANAPHYLAXIS and ANGIOEDEMA, weight gain, weight loss.

Interactions

Drug-Drug: May ↓ effectiveness of **bromocriptine** when used concurrently for galactorrhea and amenorrhea.

Route/Dosage

PO (Adults): *Secondary amenorrhea*—400 mg once daily in the evening for 10 days; *prevention of postmenopausal estrogen-induced endometrial hyperplasia*—200 mg once daily at bedtime for 14 days on days 8–21 of a 28-day cycle or on days 12–25 of a 30-day cycle; if patient currently receives ≥1.25 mg/day of estrogen, then a daily of dose of 300 mg of progesterone as 100 mg 2 hr after breakfast and 200 mg at bedtime is used; further adjustments may be required.

Vag (Adults): *Secondary amenorrhea*—45 mg (1 applicatorful of 4% gel) once every other day for up to 6 doses, may be increased to 90 mg (1 applicatorful of 8% gel) once every other day for up to 6 doses; *Corpus luteum insufficiency or assisted reproduction technology*—For luteal phase support: 90 mg (1 applicatorful of 8% gel) once daily; for *in vitro* fertilization: 90 mg (1 applicatorful of 8% gel) once daily beginning within 24 hr of embryo transfer and continued through day 30 post-transfer (if pregnancy occurs, treatment may be continued for up to 10–12 wk); *partial or complete ovarian failure*—90 mg (1 applicatorful of 8% gel) twice daily while undergoing donor oocyte transfer (if pregnancy occurs, treatment may be continued for up to 10–12 wk).—*Support of embryo implantation and early pregnancy*—100 mg insert 2 or 3 times daily for up to 10 wks.

IM (Adults): *Secondary amenorrhea*—100–150 mg (single dose) or 5–10 mg daily for 6–8 days given 8–10 days before expected menstrual period. *Dysfunctional uterine bleeding*—5–10 mg daily for 6 days. *Corpus luteum insufficiency*—12.5 mg/day at onset of ovulation for 2 wk; may continue until 11th wk of gestation (unlabeled).

Availability (generic available)

Micronized capsules (Prometrium): 100 mg, 200 mg. **Cost:** 100 mg $48.99/30, 200 mg $85.99/30. **Bioadhesive vaginal gel (Crinone, Prochieve):** 4%, 8%. **Vaginal tablets (Endometrin):** 100 mg. **Injection:** 50 mg/ml in 10-ml vials.

NURSING IMPLICATIONS

Assessment

- Blood pressure be monitored periodically during therapy.
- Monitor intake and output ratios and weekly weight. Report significant discrepancies or steady weight gain.
- **Amenorrhea:** Assess patient's usual menstrual history. Administration of drug usually begins 8–10 days before anticipated menstruation. Withdrawal bleeding usually occurs 48–72 hr after course of therapy. Therapy should be discontinued if menses occur during injection series.
- **Dysfunctional Bleeding:** Monitor pattern and amount of vaginal bleeding (pad count). Bleeding should end by sixth day of therapy. Therapy should be discontinued if menses occur during injection series.
- ***Lab Test Considerations:*** Monitor hepatic function before and periodically during therapy.
- May cause ↑ plasma amino acid and alkaline phosphatase levels.
- May ↓ pregnanediol excretion concentrations.
- May cause ↑ serum concentrations of LDL and ↓ concentrations of HDL.
- High doses may ↑ sodium and chloride excretion.
- May alter thyroid function test results.

Potential Nursing Diagnoses

Sexual dysfunction (Indications)

Implementation

- **IM:** Shake vial before preparing IM dose. Administer deep IM. Rotate sites.
- **Vag:** Vaginal gel and insert are administered with disposable applicator provided by manufacturer.
- If dose increase is required from 4% gel to 8% gel, doubling the volume of the 4% gel will not accomplish dose increase; changing to 8% gel is required.

Patient/Family Teaching

- Advise patient to report signs and symptoms of fluid retention (swelling of ankles and feet, weight gain), thromboembolic disorders (pain, swelling, tenderness in extremities, headache, chest pain, blurred vision), mental depression, or hepatic dysfunction (yellowed skin or eyes, pruritus, dark urine, light-colored stools) to health care professional.
- Instruct patient to notify health care professional if change in vaginal bleeding pattern or spotting occurs.
- Instruct patient to stop taking medication and notify health care professional if pregnancy is suspected.
- Caution patient to use sunscreen and protective clothing to prevent photosensitivity reactions.
- Advise patient to notify health care professional of medication regimen before treatment or surgery.
- Emphasize the importance of routine follow-up physical exams, including blood pressure; breast, abdomen, and pelvic examinations; and Pap smears.
- **Vag:** Instruct patient not use vaginal gel concurrently with other vaginal agents. If these agents must be used concurrently, administer at least 6 hr before or after vaginal gel.

Evaluation/Desired Outcomes

- Development of normal cyclic menses.
- Successful outcome in assisted reproduction.

P

promethazine

(proe-**meth**-a-zeen)

Antinaus, ✤Histanil, Pentazine, Phenadoz, Phenergan, Promacot, Promet, Prorex

Classification

Therapeutic: antiemetics, antihistamines, sedative/hypnotics

Pharmacologic: phenothiazines

Pregnancy Category C

Indications

Treatment of various allergic conditions and motion sickness. Preoperative sedation. Treatment and prevention of nausea and vomiting. Adjunct to anesthesia and analgesia.

Action

Blocks the effects of histamine. Has inhibitory effect on the chemoreceptor trigger zone in the medulla, resulting in antiemetic properties. Alters the effects of dopamine in the CNS. Possesses significant anticholinergic activity. Produces CNS depression by indirectly decreased

✤ = Canadian drug name.

*CAPITALS indicates life-threatening; underlines indicate most frequent.

stimulation of the CNS reticular system. **Therapeutic Effects:** Relief of symptoms of histamine excess usually seen in allergic conditions. Diminished nausea or vomiting. Sedation.

Pharmacokinetics

Absorption: Well absorbed after oral (88%) and IM administration; rectal administration may be less reliable.
Distribution: Widely distributed; crosses the blood-brain barrier and the placenta.
Protein Binding: 65–90%.
Metabolism and Excretion: Metabolized by the liver.
Half-life: 9–16 hr.

TIME/ACTION PROFILE (noted as antihistaminic effects; sedative effects last 2–8 hr)

ROUTE	ONSET	PEAK	DURATION
PO, IM	20 min	unknown	4–12 hr
rectal	20 min	unknown	4–12 hr
IV	3–5 min	unknown	4–12 hr

Contraindications/Precautions

Contraindicated in: Hypersensitivity; Comatose patients; Prostatic hypertrophy; Bladder neck obstruction; Some products contain alcohol or bisulfites and should be avoided in patients with known intolerance; Angle-closure glaucoma; Pedi: May cause fatal respiratory depression in children <2 yr.
Use Cautiously in: IV administration, may cause severe injury to tissue; Hypertension; Cardiovascular disease; Impaired liver function; Prostatic hypertrophy; Glaucoma; Asthma; Sleep apnea; Epilepsy; Underlying bone marrow depression; Pedi: For children >2 yr, use lowest effective dose, avoid concurrent respiratory depressants; OB: Has been used safely during labor; avoid chronic use during pregnancy; Lactation: Safety not established; may cause drowsiness in infant. Geri: Appears on Beers list. Geriatric patients are sensitive to anticholinergic effects and have increased risk for side effects.

Adverse Reactions/Side Effects

CNS: NEUROLEPTIC MALIGNANT SYNDROME, confusion, disorientation, sedation, dizziness, extrapyramidal reactions, fatigue, insomnia, nervousness. **EENT:** blurred vision, diplopia, tinnitus. **CV:** bradycardia, hypertension, hypotension, tachycardia. **GI:** constipation, drug-induced hepatitis, dry mouth. **Derm:** photosensitivity, severe tissue necrosis upon infiltration at IV site, rashes. **Hemat:** blood dyscrasias.

Interactions

Drug-Drug: Additive CNS depression with other **CNS depressants**, including **alcohol**, other **antihistamines**, **opioid analgesics**, and other **sedative/hypnotics**. Neuroleptic malignant syndrome can occur when used concurrently with **antipsychotics**. Additive anticholinergic effects with other **drugs possessing anticholinergic properties**, including other **antihistamines**, **antidepressants**, **atropine**, **haloperidol**, other **phenothiazines**, **quinidine**, and **disopyramide**. May precipitate seizures when used with **drugs that lower seizure threshold**. Concurrent use with **MAO inhibitors** may result in ↑ sedation and anticholinergic side effects.

Route/Dosage

Antihistamine

PO (Adults): 6.25–12.5 mg 3 times/day and 25 mg at bedtime.
PO (Children ≥2 yr): 0.1 mg/kg/dose (not to exceed 12.5 mg) q 6 hr during the day and 0.5 mg/kg/dose (not to exceed 25 mg) at bedtime.
IM, IV, Rect (Adults): 25 mg; may repeat in 2 hr.
Rect (Children ≥2 yr): 0.125 mg/kg q 4–6 hr *or* 0.5 mg/kg at bedtime.

Antivertigo (Motion Sickness)

PO (Adults): 25 mg 30–60 min before departure; may be repeated in 8–12 hr.
PO, Rect (Children ≥2 yr): 0.5 mg/kg (not to exceed 25 mg) 30–60 min before departure; may be given q 12 hr as needed.

Sedation

PO, Rect, IM, IV (Adults): 25–50 mg; may repeat q 4–6 hr if needed.
PO, Rect, IM (Children >2 yr): 0.5–1 mg/kg (not to exceed 50 mg) q 6 hr as needed.

Sedation during Labor

IM, IV (Adults): 50 mg in early labor; when labor is established, additional doses of 25–75 mg may be given 1–2 times at 4-hr intervals (24-hr dose should not exceed 100 mg).

Antiemetic

PO, Rect, IM, IV (Adults): 12.5–25 mg q 4 hr as needed; initial PO dose should be 25 mg.
PO, Rect, IM, IV (Children ≥2 yr): 0.25–1 mg/kg (not to exceed 25 mg) q 4–6 hr.

Availability (generic available)

Tablets: 10 mg[OTC], 12.5 mg, ✱12.5 mg[OTC], 25 mg, ✱25 mg[OTC], 50 mg, ✱50 mg[OTC]. **Syrup**

(cherry flavor): 3.25 mg/120 ml, 6.25 mg/5 ml, ♣10 mg/5 ml[OTC], 25 mg/5 ml. **Injection:** 25 mg/ml in 1-ml ampules and 1- and 10-ml vials, 50 mg/ml in 1-ml ampules and 10-ml vials. **Suppositories:** 2.5 mg, 5 mg, 12.5 mg, 25 mg. ***In combination with:*** codeine, dextromethorphan, phenylephrine, and/or pseudoephedrine in a variety of cough and cold preparations. See Appendix B.

NURSING IMPLICATIONS

Assessment

- Monitor blood pressure, pulse, and respiratory rate frequently in patients receiving IV doses.
- Assess patient for level of sedation after administration. Risk of sedation and respiratory depression are increased when administered concurrently with other drugs that cause CNS depression
- Monitor patient for onset of extrapyramidal side effects (*akathisia*—restlessness; *dystonia*—muscle spasms and twisting motions; *pseudoparkinsonism*—mask-like face, rigidity, tremors, drooling, shuffling gait, dysphagia). Notify physician or other health care professional if these symptoms occur.
- Geri: Assess for adverse anticholinergic effects (delirium, acute confusion, dizziness, dry mouth, blurred vision, urinary retention, constipation, tachycardia).
- **Allergy:** Assess allergy symptoms (rhinitis, conjunctivitis, hives) before and periodically throughout course of therapy.
- **Antiemetic:** Assess patient for nausea and vomiting before and after administration.
- **IV:** If administered IV, assess for burning and pain at IV site; may cause severe tissue injury. Avoid IV administration, if possible. If pain occurs, discontinue administration immediately.
- ***Lab Test Considerations:*** May cause false-positive or false-negative pregnancy test results.
- CBC should be evaluated periodically during chronic therapy; blood dyscrasias may occur.
- May cause increased serum glucose.
- May cause false-negative results in skin tests using allergen extracts. Promethazine should be discontinued 72 hr before the test.

Potential Nursing Diagnoses

Deficient fluid volume (Indications)
Risk for injury (Side Effects)

Implementation

- When administering promethazine concurrently with opioid analgesics, supervise ambulation closely to prevent injury from increased sedation.
- **PO:** Administer with food, water, or milk to minimize GI irritation. Tablets may be crushed and mixed with food or fluids for patients with difficulty swallowing.
- **IM:** Administer deep into well-developed muscle. Subcut or inadvertent intra-arterial administration may cause severe tissue necrosis.

IV Administration

- **Direct IV:** ***Diluent:*** Dilute with 0.9% NaCl or D5W. ***Concentration:*** Doses should not exceed a concentration of 25 mg/ml. Administer through a large-bore vein through a running IV line into the most distal port. Slight yellow color does not alter potency. Do not use if precipitate is present. ***Rate:*** Administer each 25 mg slowly, over at least 10–15 min. Rapid administration may produce a transient fall in blood pressure.
- **Solution Compatibility:** dextrose, saline, Ringer's or LR, dextrose/saline, dextrose/Ringer's, lactated Ringer's combinations.
- **Syringe Compatibility:** atropine, butorphanol, cimetidine, droperidol, fentanyl, glycopyrrolate, hydromorphone, meperidine, metoclopramide, midazolam, pentazocine, ranitidine, scopolamine.
- **Syringe Incompatibility:** heparin, ketorolac, pentobarbital, thiopental.
- **Y-Site Compatibility:** amifostine, amsacrine, aztreonam, bivalirudin, ciprofloxacin, cisatracurium, cisplatin, cladribine, cyclophosphamide, cytarabine, dexmedetomidine, docetaxel, doxorubicin, etoposide, fenoldopam, filgrastim, fluconazole, fludarabine, gemcitabine, granisetron, linezolid, melphalan, ondansetron, oxaliplatin, pemetrexed, remifentanil, sargramostim, teniposide, thiotepa, vinorelbine.
- **Y-Site Incompatibility:** aldesleukin, allopurinol, amphotericin B cholesteryl, cefepime, cefotetan, doxorubicin liposome, fos-

P

carnet, lansoprazole, methotrexate, piperacillin/tazobactam.

Patient/Family Teaching

- Review dose schedule with patient. If medication is ordered regularly and a dose is missed, take as soon as remembered unless time for next dose Pedi: Caution caregivers to use only the measuring device accompanying the liquid medication and not to use household measuring devices.
- May cause drowsiness. Caution patient to avoid driving or other activities requiring alertness until response to medication is known.
- Advise patient that frequent mouth rinses, good oral hygiene, and sugarless gum or candy may decrease dry mouth. Health care professional should be notified if dry mouth persists >2 wk.
- Caution patient to use sunscreen and protective clothing to prevent photosensitivity reactions.
- Advise patient to change positions slowly to minimize orthostatic hypotension. Geri: Geriatric patients are at increased risk.
- Caution patient to avoid concurrent use of alcohol and other CNS depressants with this medication.
- Instruct patient to notify health care professional if sore throat, fever, jaundice, or uncontrolled movements are noted.
- Geri: Teach patient and family about anticholinergic effects and to contact a health care professional if such effects persist.
- **Motion Sickness:** When used as prophylaxis for motion sickness, advise patient to take medication at least 30 min and preferably 1–2 hr before exposure to conditions that may cause motion sickness.

Evaluation/Desired Outcomes

- Relief from allergic symptoms.
- Prevention of motion sickness.
- Sedation.
- Relief from nausea and vomiting.

propafenone

(proe-**paff**-e-nown)
Rythmol

Classification
Therapeutic: antiarrhythmics (class IC)

Pregnancy Category C

Indications

Treatment of life-threatening ventricular arrhythmias, including ventricular tachycardia. Prolongs the time to recurrence of symptomatic paroxysmal atrial arrhythmias, including paroxysmal atrial fibrillation/flutter (PAF) and paroxysmal supraventricular tachycardia (PSVT). **Unlabeled uses:** Single dose treatment for atrial fibrillation.

Action

Slows conduction in cardiac tissue by altering transport of ions across cell membranes. **Therapeutic Effects:** Suppression of ventricular arrhythmias.

Pharmacokinetics

Absorption: Although well absorbed following oral administration, undergoes rapid hepatic metabolism (bioavailability 3–11%).
Distribution: Widely distributed; crosses the placenta.
Metabolism and Excretion: Extensively metabolized by the liver (CYP1A2, CYP2D6, and CYP3A4 enzyme systems), some metabolites have antiarrhythmic activity. >90% of patients are considered extensive metabolizers. Others metabolize propafenone more slowly.
Half-life: 2–10 hr in extensive metabolizers, 10–32 hr in slow metabolizers.

TIME/ACTION PROFILE (antiarrhythmic effects)

ROUTE	ONSET	PEAK	DURATION
PO	hrs–days	4–5 days†	hrs

†Chronic dosing

Contraindications/Precautions

Contraindicated in: Hypersensitivity; Cardiogenic shock; Conduction disorders including sick sinus syndrome and AV block (without a pacemaker); Bradycardia; Severe hypotension; Concurrent quinidine or amiodarone; Nonallergic bronchospasm; Electrolyte disturbances; Uncontrolled CHF.
Use Cautiously in: Severe hepatic or renal impairment (dose reduction may be necessary); Geri: Lower doses may be necessary due to age-related decrease in renal/hepatic/cardiovascular function, concurrent chronic illnesses and medications); OB, Pedi: Pregnancy, lactation, or children (safety not established).

Adverse Reactions/Side Effects

CNS: dizziness, shaking, weakness. **EENT:** blurred vision. **CV:** SUPRAVENTRICULAR ARRHYTHMIA,

VENTRICULAR ARRHYTHMIAS, conduction disturbances, angina, bradycardia, hypotension. **GI:** altered taste, constipation, nausea, vomiting, diarrhea, dry mouth. **Derm:** rash. **MS:** joint pain.

Interactions

Drug-Drug: Any **inhibitors of the CYP1A2, CYP2D6 or CYP3A4 enzyme systems** may ↑ levels, including **desipramine**, **paroxetine**, **ritonavir**, **sertraline**, **ketoconazole**, **saquinavir**, **erythromycin** (blood level monitoring recommended). **Quinidine** is a strong inhibitor of CYP2D6 and significantly ↑ levels of propafenone; concurrent use is not recommended. Propafenone is also an inhibitor of CYP2D6 and may ↑ levels of **desipramine**, **imipramine**, **haloperidol**, and **venlafaxine**. Significantly ↑ serum **digoxin** levels (blood level monitoring recommended, ↓ dose may be required). ↑ blood levels of **metoprolol** and **propranolol** (↓ dose may be required). Concurrent use of **local anesthetics** may ↑ risk of CNS adverse reactions. ↑ effects of **warfarin** (↓ warfarin dose if necessary, monitor prothrombin time). Concurrent with **amiodarone** can adversely effect conduction/repolarization and should be avoided. May ↑ risk of CNS adverse reactions with **lidocaine**. May ↑ **cyclosporine** through blood levels and risk of nephrotoxicity. **Rifampin** may ↓ serum levels and effectiveness of propafenone. **Cimetidine** may ↑ serum levels.
Drug-Food: Grapefruit juice may ↑ levels.

Route/Dosage

PO (Adults): 150 mg q 8 hr; may be gradually increased at 3–4-day intervals as required up to 300 mg q 8–12 hr. *Single dose treatment of atrial fibrillation (unlabeled)*— 450 or 600 mg.

Availability (generic available)

Tablets: 150 mg, 225 mg, 300 mg. **Cost:** *Generic*—150 mg $316.95/270, 225 mg $355.00/270, 300 mg $593.95/270.

NURSING IMPLICATIONS

Assessment

- Monitor ECG or use Holter monitor prior to and periodically during therapy. May cause PR and QT prolongation.
- Monitor blood pressure and pulse periodically during therapy.
- Monitor intake and output ratios and daily weight. Assess patients for signs of CHF (peripheral edema, rales/crackles, dyspnea, weight gain, jugular venous distention). May require reduction or discontinuation of therapy.
- ***Lab Test Considerations:*** May cause ↑ ANA titer, which is usually asymptomatic and reversible.
- Monitor prothrombin level in patients taking warfarin; may ↑ effects of warfarin.
- ***Toxicity and Overdose:*** Signs of toxicity include hypotension, excessive drowsiness, and decreased or abnormal heart rate. Notify physician or other health care professional if these signs occur.

Potential Nursing Diagnoses

Decreased cardiac output (Indications)

Implementation

- **PO:** Propafenone therapy should be initiated in a hospital with facilities for cardiac rhythm monitoring. Most serious proarrhythmic effects are seen in the first 2 wk of therapy.
- Previous antiarrhythmic therapy should be withdrawn 2–5 half-lives before starting propafenone.
- Dose adjustments should be at least 3–4 days apart because of the long half-life of propafenone.
- Correct pre-existing hypokalemia or hyperkalemia prior to instituting therapy.

Patient/Family Teaching

- Instruct patient to take medication around the clock as directed, even if feeling better. Take missed doses as soon as remembered if within 4 hr; omit if remembered later. Gradual dosage reduction may be necessary.
- May cause dizziness. Caution patient to avoid driving and other activities requiring alertness until response to medication is known.
- Advise patient to notify health care professional of medication regimen prior to treatment or surgery.
- Instruct patient to notify health care professional if fever, sore throat, chills, or unusual bleeding or bruising occurs or if chest pain, shortness of breath, diaphoresis, palpitations, or visual changes become bothersome.
- Advise patient to carry identification describing disease process and medication regimen at all times.

P

- Emphasize the importance of follow-up exams to monitor progress.

Evaluation/Desired Outcomes

- Decrease in frequency of ventricular arrhythmias.
- Prolonged time to recurrence of symptomatic paroxysmal atrial arrhythmias, including paroxysmal atrial fibrillation/flutter and PSVT.

propofol (proe-poe-fol)

Diprivan, Disoprofol

Classification

Therapeutic: general anesthetics

Pregnancy Category B

Indications

Induction of general anesthesia in children >3 yr and adults. Maintenance of balanced anesthesia when used with other agents in children >2 months and adults. Initiation and maintenance of monitored anesthesia care (MAC). Sedation of intubated, mechanically ventilated patients in intensive care units (ICUs).

Action

Short-acting hypnotic. Mechanism of action is unknown. Produces amnesia. Has no analgesic properties. **Therapeutic Effects:** Induction and maintenance of anesthesia.

Pharmacokinetics

Absorption: Administered IV only, resulting in complete absorption.
Distribution: Rapidly and widely distributed. Crosses the blood-brain barrier well; rapidly redistributed to other tissues. Crosses the placenta and enters breast milk.
Protein Binding: 95–99%.
Metabolism and Excretion: Rapidly metabolized by the liver.
Half-life: 3–12 hr (blood-brain equilibration half-life 2.9 min).

TIME/ACTION PROFILE (loss of consciousness)

ROUTE	ONSET	PEAK	DURATION†
IV	40 sec	unknown	3–5 min

†Time to recovery is 8 min (up to 19 min if opioid analgesics have been used)

Contraindications/Precautions

Contraindicated in: Hypersensitivity to propofol, soybean oil, egg lecithin, or glycerol; Labor and delivery.
Use Cautiously in: Cardiovascular disease; Lipid disorders (emulsion may have detrimental effect); Increased intracranial pressure; Cerebrovascular disorders; Geriatric (>60 yr), debilitated, or hypovolemic patients (lower induction and maintenance dosage reduction recommended); Children <3 yr (for induction of anesthesia), children <2 mos (maintenance of anesthesia), or lactation (safety not established).

Adverse Reactions/Side Effects

CNS: dizziness, headache. **Resp:** APNEA, cough. **CV:** bradycardia, hypotension, hypertension. **GI:** abdominal cramping, hiccups, nausea, vomiting. **Derm:** flushing. **Local:** burning, pain, stinging, coldness, numbness, tingling at IV site. **MS:** involuntary muscle movements, perioperative myoclonia. **GU:** discoloration of urine (green). **Misc:** fever.

Interactions

Drug-Drug: Additive CNS and respiratory depression with **alcohol**, **antihistamines**, **opioid analgesics**, and **sedative/hypnotics** (dosage reduction may be required). **Theophylline** may antagonize the CNS effects of propofol. Propofol may increase the serum concentrations of **alfentanil**. Cardiorespiratory instability can occur when used with **acetazolamide**. Serious bradycardia can occur with concurrent use of **fentanyl** in children. Increased risk of hypertriglyceridemia with **intravenous fat emulsion**.

Route/Dosage

General Anesthesia

IV (Adults <55 yr): *Induction*—40 mg q 10 sec until induction achieved (2–2.5 mg/kg total). *Maintenance*—100–200 mcg/kg/min. Rates of 150–200 mcg/kg/min are usually required during first 10–15 min after induction, then decreased by 30–50% during first 30 min of maintenance. Rates of 50–100 mcg/kg/min are associated with optimal recovery time. May also be given intermittently in increments of 25–50 mg.
IV (Geriatric Patients, Cardiac Patients, Debilitated Patients, or Hypovolemic Patients): *Induction*—20 mg q 10 sec until induction achieved (1–1.5 mg/kg total). *Maintenance*—50–100 mcg/kg/min (dose in cardiac anesthesia ranges from 50–150 mcg/kg/min depending on concurrent use of opioid).
IV (Adults Undergoing Neurosurgical Procedures): *Induction*—20 mg q 10 sec until

induction achieved (1–2 mg/kg total). *Maintenance*—100–200 mcg/kg/min.
IV (Children ≥3 yr–16 yr): *Induction*—2.5–3.5 mg/kg, use lower dose for children ASA III or IV.
IV (Children 2 mos–16 yr): *Maintenance*—200–300 mcg/kg/min (following first 30 min of maintenance, rate should be decreased to 125–150 mcg/kg/min if possible), younger children may require larger infusion rates compared to older children.

Monitored Anesthesia Care (MAC) Sedation

IV (Adults <55 yr): *Initiation*—100–150 mcg/kg/min infusion *or* 0.5 mg/kg as slow injection. *Maintenance*—25–75 mcg/kg/min infusion or incremental boluses of 10–20 mg.
IV (Geriatric Patients, Debilitated Patients, or ASA III/IV Patients): *Initiation*—Use slower infusion or injection rates. *Maintenance*—20% less than the usual adult infusion dose; rapid/repeated bolus dosing should be avoided.

ICU Sedation

IV (Adults): 5 mcg/kg/min for a minimum of 5 min. Additional increments of 5–10 mcg/kg/min over 5–10 min may be given until desired response is obtained. (Range 5–50 mcg/kg/min.) Dose should be reassessed every 24 hr.

Availability (generic available)

Injection: 10 mg/ml in 20-, 50-, and 100-ml infusion vials.

NURSING IMPLICATIONS

Assessment

- Assess respiratory status, pulse, and blood pressure continuously throughout propofol therapy. Frequently causes apnea lasting ≥60 sec. Maintain patent airway and adequate ventilation. Propofol should be used only by individuals experienced in endotracheal intubation, and equipment for this procedure should be readily available.
- Assess level of sedation and level of consciousness throughout and following administration.
- When using for ICU sedation, wake-up and assessment of CNS function should be done daily throughout maintenance to determine minimum dose required for sedation. Maintain a light level of sedation during these assessments; do not discontinue. Abrupt discontinuation may cause rapid awakening with anxiety, agitation, and resistance to mechanical ventilation.
- ***Toxicity and Overdose:*** If overdose occurs, monitor pulse, respiration, and blood pressure continuously. Maintain patent airway and assist ventilation as needed. If hypotension occurs, treatment includes IV fluids, repositioning, and vasopressors.

Potential Nursing Diagnoses

Ineffective breathing pattern (Adverse Reactions)
Risk for injury (Side Effects)

Implementation

- Do not confuse Diprivan (propofol) with Diflucan (fluconazole).
- Dose is titrated to patient response.
- Propofol has no effect on the pain threshold. Adequate analgesia should *always* be used when propofol is used as an adjunct to surgical procedures.

IV Administration

- **Direct IV:** ***Diluent:*** Usually administered undiluted. If dilution is necessary, use only D5W. Shake well before use. Solution is opaque, making detection of contaminants difficult. Do not use if separation of the emulsion is evident. Contains no preservatives; maintain sterile technique and administer immediately after preparation. ***Concentration:*** Undiluted: 10 mg/ml. If dilution is necessary, dilute to concentration ≥2 mg/ml.
- Discard unused portions and IV lines at the end of anesthetic procedure or within 6 hr. For ICU sedation, discard after 12 hr if administered directly from vial or after 6 hr if transferred to a syringe or other container. Do not administer via filter <5–micron pore size.
- Aseptic technique is essential. Solution is capable of rapid growth of bacterial contaminants. Infections and subsequent deaths have been reported. ***Rate:*** Administer over 3–5 min. Titrate to desired level of sedation. Frequently causes pain, burning, and stinging at injection site; use larger veins of the forearm, antecubital fossa, or a dedicated IV catheter. Lidocaine 10–20 mg IV may be administered prior to injection to minimize pain. Pedi: In-

P

duction doses may be administered over 20–30 seconds. Intermittent/Continuous Infusion ***Diluent:*** Administer undiluted. ***Concentration:*** 10 mg/ml. ***Rate:*** Based on patient's weight (see Route/Dosage section).

- **Solution Compatibility:** D5W, LR, D5/LR, D5/0.45% NaCl, D5/0.2% NaCl.
- **Y-Site Compatibility:** acyclovir, alfentanil, aminophylline, ampicillin, aztreonam, bumetanide, buprenorphine, butorphanol, calcium gluconate, carboplatin, cefazolin, cefepime, cefotaxime, cefoxitin, ceftizoxime, ceftriaxone, cefuroxime, chlorpromazine, cimetidine, cisplatin, clindamycin, cyclophosphamide, cyclosporine, cytarabine, dexamethasone sodium phosphate, dexmedetomidine, diphenhydramine, dobutamine, dopamine, doxycycline, droperidol, enalaprilat, epinephrine, esmolol, famotidine, fenoldopam, fentanyl, fluconazole, fluorouracil, furosemide, ganciclovir, glycopyrrolate, granisetron, haloperidol, heparin, hydrocortisone sodium succinate, hydromorphone, ifosfamide, imipenem/cilastatin, inamrinone, insulin, isoproterenol, ketamine, labetalol, levorphanol, lidocaine, lorazepam, magnesium sulfate, mannitol, meperidine, milrinone, nafcillin, nalbuphine, naloxone, nitroglycerin, nitroprusside, norepinephrine, paclitaxel, pentobarbital, phenobarbital, piperacillin, potassium chloride, prochlorperazine, propranolol, ranitidine, scopolamine, sodium bicarbonate, succinylcholine, sufentanil, thiopental, ticarcillin/clavulanate, vecuronium.
- **Y-Site Incompatibility:** amikacin, amphotericin B, calcium chloride, ciprofloxacin, diazepam, digoxin, doxorubicin, gentamicin, levofloxacin, methotrexate, methylprednisolone sodium succinate, metoclopramide, mitoxantrone, phenytoin, tobramycin, verapamil.

Patient/Family Teaching

- Inform patient that this medication will decrease mental recall of the procedure.
- May cause drowsiness or dizziness. Advise patient to request assistance prior to ambulation and transfer and to avoid driving or other activities requiring alertness for 24 hr following administration.
- Advise patient to avoid alcohol or other CNS depressants without the advice of a health care professional for 24 hr following administration.

Evaluation/Desired Outcomes

- Induction and maintenance of anesthesia.
- Amnesia.
- Sedation in mechanically ventilated patients in an intensive care setting.

PROPOXYPHENE

propoxyphene hydrochloride
(pro-**pox**-i-feen hye-droe-**klor**-ide)
Darvon

propoxyphene hydrochloride/aspirin/caffeine
Darvon Compound-65, Darvon Compound-32

propoxyphene napsylate
(pro-**pox**-i-feen **nap**-si-late)
Darvon N

propoxyphene napsylate/acetaminophen
Darvon A500, Darvocet-N, Propacet, Propoxyphene with APAP, Wygesic

propoxyphene napsylate/aspirin
✤Darvon-N with ASA

propoxyphene/aspirin/caffeine
✤Darvon-N Compound, ✤692

Classification
Therapeutic: opioid analgesics
Pharmacologic: opioid agonists, opioid agonists/nonopioid analgesic combinations

Pregnancy Category C

See also Acetaminophen monograph and Salicylates monograph

Indications

Mild to moderate pain.

Action

Binds to opiate receptors in the CNS. Alters the perception of and response to painful stimuli, while producing generalized CNS depression. **Therapeutic Effects:** Decrease in mild to moderate pain.

Pharmacokinetics

Absorption: Well absorbed following oral administration. Napsylate salt is more slowly absorbed.

Distribution: Widely distributed. Probably crosses the placenta. Enters breast milk in small amounts.
Metabolism and Excretion: Mostly metabolized by the liver. Some conversion to norpropoxyphene, a toxic metabolite. This metabolite accumulates in elderly patients and patients with decreased renal function.
Half-life: 6–12 hr.

TIME/ACTION PROFILE (analgesic effect)

ROUTE	ONSET	PEAK	DURATION
PO	15–60 min	2–3 hr	4–6 hr

Contraindications/Precautions

Contraindicated in: Hypersensitivity; OB: Pregnancy or lactation (avoid chronic use); Pedi: Children.
Use Cautiously in: Head trauma; Increased intracranial pressure; Severe renal, hepatic, or pulmonary disease; Hypothyroidism; Adrenal insufficiency; Alcoholism; Geri: Appears on Beers list. Elderly or debilitated patients require reduced dosages.; Undiagnosed abdominal pain; Prostatic hyperplasia; OB: Lactation (has been used safely).

Adverse Reactions/Side Effects

CNS: dizziness, weakness, dysphoria, euphoria, headache, insomnia, paradoxical excitement, sedation. **EENT:** blurred vision. **CV:** hypotension. **GI:** nausea, abdominal pain, constipation, vomiting. **Derm:** rashes. **Misc:** physical dependence, psychological dependence, tolerance.

Interactions

Drug-Drug: Use with extreme caution in patients receiving **MAO inhibitors** (may result in unpredictable, severe, and potentially fatal reactions—decrease initial dose to 25% of usual dose). ↑ CNS depression with **alcohol, antidepressants**, and **sedative/hypnotics**. **Smoking** ↑ metabolism and may decrease analgesic effectiveness. Administration of **partial-antagonist opioid analgesics** may precipitate withdrawal in physically dependent patients. **Nalbuphine**, **buprenorphine**, or **pentazocine** may ↓ analgesia.
Drug-Natural Products: Concomitant use of **kava kava, valerian, or chamomile can** ↑ **CNS depression.**

Route/Dosage

Consider cumulative effects of additional acetaminophen/aspirin; if toxic levels are exceeded, change to pure propoxyphene product.
PO (Adults): 65 mg q 4 hr (hydrochloride—Darvon) or 100 mg q 4 hr (napsylate—Darvon-N) as needed (not to exceed 390 mg/day as hydrochloride or 600 mg/day as napsylate). 100 mg propoxyphene napsylate = 65 mg propoxyphene hydrochloride.

Availability (generic available)

Propoxyphene Hydrochloride
Capsules: 65 mg. **Tablets:** ♣65 mg.

Propoxyphene Napsylate
Capsules: ♣100 mg. **Tablets:** 50 mg, 100 mg.

Propoxyphene Hydrochloride/Acetaminophen
Tablets: propoxyphene 65 mg/acetaminophen 650 mg.

Propoxyphene Napsylate/Acetaminophen
Tablets: propoxyphene 50 mg/acetaminophen 325 mg, propoxyphene 100 mg/acetaminophen 650 mg, propoxyphene 100 mg/acetaminophen 500 mg.

Propoxyphene Hydrochloride/Aspirin/Caffeine
Capsules: propoxyphene 32 mg, aspirin 389 mg, caffeine 32.4 mg, propoxyphene 65 mg, aspirin 389 mg, caffeine 32.4 mg. **Tablets:** ♣propoxyphene 65 mg, aspirin 375 mg, caffeine 30 mg.

Propoxyphene Napsylate/Aspirin
Tablets: ♣propoxyphene 100 mg/aspirin 325 mg.

Propoxyphene Napsylate/Aspirin/Caffeine
Tablets: ♣propoxyphene 100 mg/aspirin 375 mg/caffeine 30 mg.

NURSING IMPLICATIONS

Assessment

- Assess type, location, and intensity of pain prior to and 2 hr (peak) following administration. When titrating opioid doses, increases of 25–50% should be administered until there is either a 50% reduction in the patient's pain rating on a numeric or visual analogue scale or the patient reports satisfactory pain relief. A repeat dose can be safely administered at the time of the peak if previ-

P

ous dose is ineffective and side effects are minimal.

- Use an equianalgesic chart (see Appendix J) when changing routes or when changing from one opioid to another.
- Prolonged, high-dose therapy may lead to physical and psychological dependence and tolerance. This should not prevent patient from receiving adequate analgesia. Most patients who receive propoxyphene for pain do not develop psychological dependence. Progressively higher doses or change to a stronger opioid may be required to relieve pain with long-term therapy.
- Assess blood pressure, pulse, and respirations before and periodically during administration. If respiratory rate is <10/min, assess level of sedation. Physical stimulation may be sufficient to prevent significant hypoventilation. Dose may need to be decreased by 25–50%. Initial drowsiness will diminish with continued use.
- Assess bowel function routinely. Prevention of constipation should be instituted with increased intake of fluids and bulk, and laxatives to minimize constipating effects. Stimulant laxatives should be administered routinely if opioid use exceeds 2–3 days, unless contraindicated.
- Geri: Geriatric patients may be more sensitive to CNS effects; monitor closely and assess falls risk.
- ***Lab Test Considerations:*** May cause ↑ serum amylase and lipase levels.
- May cause ↑ AST, ALT, serum alkaline phosphatase, LDH, and bilirubin concentrations.
- ***Toxicity and Overdose:*** If an opioid antagonist is required to reverse respiratory depression or coma, naloxone (Narcan) is the antidote. Dilute the 0.4-mg ampule of naloxone in 10 ml of 0.9% NaCl and administer 0.5 ml (0.02 mg) by direct IV push every 2 min. For patients weighing <40 kg, dilute 0.1 mg of naloxone in 10 ml of 0.9% NaCl for a concentration of 10 mcg/ml and administer 0.5 mcg/kg every 2 min. Titrate dose to avoid withdrawal, seizures, and severe pain.

Potential Nursing Diagnosis

Acute pain (Indications)
Disturbed sensory perception (visual, auditory) (Side Effects)
Risk for injury (Side Effects)

Implementation

- Explain therapeutic value of medication prior to administration, to enhance the analgesic effect.
- Regularly administered doses may be more effective than prn administration. Analgesic is more effective if given before pain becomes severe.
- Coadministration with nonopioid analgesics may have additive analgesic effects and may permit lower opioid doses.
- Medication should be discontinued gradually after long-term use to prevent withdrawal symptoms.
- **PO:** Doses may be administered with food or milk to minimize GI irritation.

Patient/Family Teaching

- Advise patient to take medication as directed and not to take more than the recommended amount. Severe and permanent liver damage may result from prolonged use or high doses of acetaminophen. Renal damage may occur with prolonged use of acetaminophen or aspirin. Doses of nonopioid agents should not exceed the maximum recommended daily dose.
- Instruct patient on how and when to ask for pain medication.
- May cause drowsiness or dizziness. Caution patient to avoid driving and other activities requiring alertness until response to the drug is known.
- Geri: Advise geriatric patients of increased risk for CNS effects and potential for falls.
- Advise patient to change positions slowly to minimize orthostatic hypotension.
- Caution patient to avoid concurrent use of alcohol or other CNS depressants with this medication.
- Encourage patient to turn, cough, and breathe deeply every 2 hr to prevent atelectasis.
- Advise patient that good oral hygiene, frequent mouth rinses, and sugarless gum or candy may decrease dry mouth.

Evaluation/Desired Outcomes

- Decrease in severity of pain without a significant alteration in level of consciousness.

HIGH ALERT

propranolol

(proe-**pran**-oh-lole)
✤Apo-Propranolol, ✤Betachron E-R, Inderal, Inderal LA, InnoPran

XL, ✤Novopranol, ✤pms Propranolol

Classification
Therapeutic: antianginals, antiarrhythmics (Class II), antihypertensives, vascular headache suppressants
Pharmacologic: beta blockers

Pregnancy Category C

Indications

Management of hypertension, angina, arrhythmias, hypertrophic cardiomyopathy, thyrotoxicosis, essential tremors, pheochromocytoma. Also used in the prevention and management of MI, and the prevention of vascular headaches. **Unlabeled uses:** Also used to manage alcohol withdrawal, aggressive behavior, antipsychotic-associated akathisia, situational anxiety, and esophageal varices. Post-traumatic stress disorder (PTSD) (Ongoing clinical trials at National Institute for Mental Health [NIMH].)

Action

Blocks stimulation of $beta_1$ (myocardial) and $beta_2$ (pulmonary, vascular, and uterine)-adrenergic receptor sites. **Therapeutic Effects:** Decreased heart rate and blood pressure. Suppression of arrhythmias. Prevention of MI.

Pharmacokinetics

Absorption: Well absorbed but undergoes extensive first-pass hepatic metabolism.
Distribution: Moderate CNS penetration. Crosses the placenta; enters breast milk.
Protein Binding: 93%.
Metabolism and Excretion: Almost completely metabolized by the liver.
Half-life: 3.4–6 hr.

TIME/ACTION PROFILE (cardiovascular effects)

ROUTE	ONSET	PEAK	DURATION
PO	30 min	60–90 min†	6–12 hr
PO–ER	unknown	6 hr	24 hr
IV	immediate	1 min	4–6 hr

†Following single dose, full effect not seen until several weeks of therapy

Contraindications/Precautions

Contraindicated in: Uncompensated CHF; Pulmonary edema; Cardiogenic shock; Bradycardia or heart block.

Use Cautiously in: Renal or hepatic impairment; pulmonary disease (including asthma); diabetes mellitus (may mask signs of hypoglycemia); thyrotoxicosis (may mask symptoms); history of severe allergic reactions (may ↑ intensity of response); OB: Crosses the placenta and may cause fetal/neonatal bradycardia, hypotension, hypoglycemia, or respiratory depression. May also ↓ blood supply to the placenta, increase the risk for premature birth or fetal death, and cause intrauterine growth retardation. May ↑ risk of cardiac and pulmonary complications in the infant during the neonatal time frame. Lactation: Appears in breast milk; use formula if propranolol must be taken; Pedi: ↑ risk of hypoglycemia, especially during periods of fasting such as before surgery, during prolonged exertion, or with coexisting renal insufficiency; Geri: ↑ sensitivity to all beta blockers; initial dose reduction and careful titration recommended.

Adverse Reactions/Side Effects

CNS: <u>fatigue</u>, <u>weakness</u>, anxiety, dizziness, drowsiness, insomnia, memory loss, mental depression, mental status changes, nervousness, nightmares. **EENT:** blurred vision, dry eyes, nasal stuffiness. **Resp:** bronchospasm, wheezing. **CV:** ARRHYTHMIAS, BRADYCARDIA, CHF, PULMONARY EDEMA, orthostatic hypotension, peripheral vasoconstriction. **GI:** constipation, diarrhea, nausea. **GU:** <u>erectile dysfunction</u>, decreased libido. **Derm:** itching, rashes. **Endo:** hyperglycemia, hypoglycemia (increased in children). **MS:** arthralgia, back pain, muscle cramps. **Neuro:** paresthesia. **Misc:** drug-induced lupus syndrome.

Interactions

Drug-Drug: General anesthesia, **IV phenytoin**, and **verapamil** may cause additive myocardial depression. Additive bradycardia may occur with **digoxin**. Additive hypotension may occur with other **antihypertensives**, acute ingestion of **alcohol**, or **nitrates**. Concurrent use with **amphetamines**, **cocaine**, **ephedrine**, **epinephrine**, **norepinephrine**, **phenylephrine**, or **pseudoephedrine** may result in unopposed alpha-adrenergic stimulation (excessive hypertension, bradycardia). Concurrent **thyroid** administration may decrease effectiveness. May alter the effectiveness of **insulin** or **oral hypoglycemics** (dose ad-

P

justments may be necessary). May ↓ effectiveness of **beta-adrenergic bronchodilators** and **theophylline**. May ↓ beneficial beta cardiovascular effects of **dopamine** or **dobutamine**. Use cautiously within 14 days of **MAO inhibitor** therapy (may result in hypertension). **Cimetidine** may ↑ blood levels and toxicity. Concurrent **NSAIDs** may ↓ antihypertensive action. **Smoking** ↑ metabolism and ↓ effects; smoking cessation may ↑ effects.

Route/Dosage

PO (Adults): *Antianginal*—80–320 mg/day in 2–4 divided doses or once daily as extended/sustained-release capsules. *Antihypertensive*—40 mg twice daily initially; may be increased as needed (usual range 120–240 mg/day; doses up to 1 g/day have been used); *or* 80 mg once daily as extended/sustained-release capsules, increased as needed up to 120 mg. *InnoPran XL* dosing form is designed to be given once daily at bedtime. *Antiarrhythmic*—10–30 mg 3–4 times daily. *Prevention of MI*—180–240 mg/day in divided doses. *Hypertrophic cardiomyopathy*—20–40 mg 3–4 times daily. *Adjunct therapy of pheochromocytoma*—20 mg 3 times daily to 40 mg 3–4 times daily concurrently with alpha-blocking therapy, started 3 days before surgery is planned. *Vascular headache prevention*—20 mg 4 times daily *or* 80 mg/day as extended/sustained-release capsules; may be increased as needed up to 240 mg/day. *Management of tremor*—40 mg twice daily; may be increased up to 120 mg/day (up to 320 mg have been used).

PO (Children): *Antihypertensive/antiarrhythmic*—0.5–1 mg/kg/day in 2–4 divided doses; may be increased as needed (usual range for maintenance dose is 2–4 mg/kg/day in 2 divided doses).

IV (Adults): *Antiarrhythmic*—1–3 mg; may be repeated after 2 min and again in 4 hr if needed.

IV (Children): *Antiarrhythmic*—10–100 mcg (0.01–0.1 mg)/kg (up to 1 mg/dose); may be repeated q 6–8 hr if needed.

Availability (generic available)

Oral solution: 4 mg/ml, 8 mg/ml. **Cost:** *Generic*—4 mg/ml $38.54/480 ml. **Tablets:** 10 mg, 20 mg, 40 mg, 60 mg, 80 mg. **Cost:** *Generic*—10 mg $8.99/100, 20 mg $7.99/100, 40 mg $12.22/100, 60 mg $86.65/100, 80 mg $15.59/100. **Sustained-release capsules (Inderal LA):** 60 mg, 80 mg, 120 mg, 160 mg. **Cost:** 60 mg $132.98/90, 80 mg $141.97/90, 120 mg $176.80/90, 120 mg $230.05/90. **Extended-release capsules:** 60 mg, 80 mg, 120 mg, 160 mg. **Cost:** *Generic*—60 mg $99.99/90, 80 mg $141.97/90, 120 mg $176.80/90, 160 mg $230.05/90. **Injection:** 1 mg/ml. ***In combination with:*** hydrochlorothiazide (Inderide). See Appendix B.

NURSING IMPLICATIONS

Assessment

- Monitor blood pressure and pulse frequently during dose adjustment period and periodically during therapy.
- Abrupt withdrawal of propranolol may precipitate life-threatening arrhythmias, hypertension, or myocardial ischemia. Drug should be tapered over a 2 week period before discontinuation. Assess patient carefully during tapering and after medication is discontinued. Consider that patients taking propranolol for non-cardiac indications may have undiagnosed cardiac disease. Abrupt discontinuation or withdrawal over too-short a period of time (less than 9 days) should be avoided
- Pedi: Assess pediatric patients for signs and symptoms of hypoglycemia, particularly when oral foods and fluids are restricted.
- Patients receiving **propranolol IV** must have continuous ECG monitoring and may have pulmonary capillary wedge pressure (PCWP) or central venous pressure (CVP) monitoring during and for several hours after administration.
- Assess for orthostatic hypotension when assisting patient up from supine position.
- Monitor intake and output ratios and daily weight. Assess patient routinely for evidence of fluid overload (peripheral edema, dyspnea, rales/crackles, fatigue, weight gain, jugular venous distention).
- **Angina:** Assess frequency and characteristics of anginal attacks periodically during therapy.
- **Vascular Headache Prophylaxis:** Assess frequency, severity, characteristics, and location of vascular headaches periodically during therapy.
- **PTSD:** Assess frequency of symptoms (flashbacks, nightmares, efforts to avoid thoughts or activities that may trigger memories of the trauma, and hypervigilance) periodically throughout therapy.

- ***Lab Test Considerations:*** May cause ↑ BUN, serum lipoprotein, potassium, triglyceride, and uric acid levels.
- May cause ↑ ANA titers.
- May cause ↓ or ↑ in blood glucose levels. In labile diabetic patients, hypoglycemia may be accompanied by precipitous ↑ of blood pressure.
- ***Toxicity and Overdose:*** Monitor patients receiving beta blockers for signs of overdose (bradycardia, severe dizziness or fainting, severe drowsiness, dyspnea, bluish fingernails or palms, seizures). Notify physician or other health care professional immediately if these signs occur: Hypotension may be treated with modified Trendelenburg position and IV fluids unless contraindicated. Vasopressors (epinephrine, norepinephrine, dopamine, dobutamine) may also be used. Hypotension does not respond to beta agonists, Glucagon has been used to treat bradycardia and hypotension.

Potential Nursing Diagnoses

Decreased cardiac output (Side Effects)
Noncompliance (Patient/Family Teaching)

Implementation

- ***High Alert:*** IV vasoactive medications are inherently dangerous. Before administering intravenously, have second practitioner independently check the original order, dose calculations, and infusion pump settings. Also, patient harm or fatalities have occurred when switching from oral to IV *propranolol*; oral and parenteral doses are not interchangeable. IV dose is 1/10 of the oral dose. Change to oral therapy as soon as possible. Do not confuse propranolol with pravachol. Do not confuse Inderal (a brand name of propranolol) with Adderall (an amphetamine/dextroamphetamine combination drug).
- **PO:** Take apical pulse prior to administering. If <50 bpm or if arrhythmia occurs, withhold medication and notify physician or other health care professional.
- Administer with meals or directly after eating to enhance absorption.
- Extended-release capsules should be swallowed whole; do not crush, open, or chew. *Propranolol tablets* may be crushed and mixed with food.
- Mix propranolol oral solution with liquid or semisolid food (water, juices, applesauce, puddings). To ensure entire dose is taken, rinse glass with more liquid or have patient consume all of the applesauce or pudding. Do not store after mixing.

IV Administration

- **Direct IV: *Diluent:*** Administer undiluted or dilute each 1 mg in 10 ml of D5W for injection. ***Concentration:*** Undiluted: 1 mg/ml. Diluted in 10 ml of D5W: 0.1 mg/ml. ***Rate:*** Administer at 0.5 mg/min for adults to avoid hypotension and cardiac arrest; do not exceed 1 mg/min. Pedi: Administer over 10 min.
- **Intermittent Infusion: *Diluent:*** May be diluted in 50 ml of 0.9% NaCl, D5W, D5/0.45% NaCl, D5/0.9% NaCl, or lactated Ringer's injection. ***Concentration:*** Depends on dose. ***Rate:*** Infuse over 10–15 min.
- **Syringe Compatibility:** inamrinone, milrinone.
- **Syringe Incompatibility:** pantoprazole.
- **Y-Site Compatibility:** alteplase, fenoldopam, heparin, hydrocortisone sodium succinate, inamrinone, linezolid, meperidine, milrinone, morphine, potassium chloride, propofol, tacrolimus, vitamin B complex with C.
- **Y-Site Incompatibility:** amphotericin B cholesteryl sulfate complex, diazoxide, lansoprazole.

Patient/Family Teaching

- Instruct patient to take medication as directed, at the same time each day, even if feeling well; do not skip or double up on missed doses. Take missed doses as soon as possible up to 4 hr before next dose (8 hr with extended-release propranolol). Inform patient that abrupt withdrawal can cause life-threatening arrhythmias, hypertension, or myocardial ischemia.
- Advise patient to make sure enough medication is available for weekends, holidays, and vacations. A written prescription may be kept in wallet in case of emergency.
- Teach patient and family how to check pulse daily and blood pressure biweekly. Advise patient to hold dose and contact health care professional if pulse is <50 bpm or blood pressure changes significantly.

P

- May cause drowsiness or dizziness. Caution patients to avoid driving or other activities that require alertness until response to the drug is known.
- Advise patients to change positions slowly to minimize orthostatic hypotension, especially during initiation of therapy or when dose is increased.
- Caution patient that this medication may increase sensitivity to cold.
- Instruct patient to ask a health care professional before taking any OTC medications or herbal products, especially cold preparations, when taking this medication.
- Diabetic patients should closely monitor blood glucose, especially if weakness, malaise, irritability, or fatigue occurs. May mask tachycardia and increased blood pressure as signs of hypoglycemia, but dizziness and sweating may still occur.
- Advise patient to notify health care professional if slow pulse, difficulty breathing, wheezing, cold hands and feet, dizziness, light-headedness, confusion, depression, rash, fever, sore throat, unusual bleeding, or bruising occurs.
- Instruct patient to inform health care professional of medication regimen prior to treatment or surgery.
- Advise patient to carry identification describing disease process and medication regimen at all times.
- **Hypertension:** Reinforce the need to continue additional therapies for hypertension (weight loss, sodium restriction, stress reduction, regular exercise, moderation of alcohol consumption, and smoking cessation). Medication controls but does not cure hypertension.
- **Angina:** Caution patient to avoid overexertion with decrease in chest pain.
- **Vascular Headache Prophylaxis:** Caution patient that sharing this medication may be dangerous.
- **PTSD:** Advise patient that medication may relieve distressing symptoms but that psychotherapy is the primary treatment for the disorder. Refer patient and family to a PTSD support group.

Evaluation/Desired Outcomes

- Decrease in blood pressure.
- Control of arrhythmias without appearance of detrimental side effects.
- Reduction in frequency of anginal attacks.
- Increase in activity tolerance.
- Prevention of MI.
- Prevention of vascular headaches.
- Management of thyrotoxicosis.
- Management of pheochromocytoma.
- Decrease in tremors.
- Management of hypertrophic cardiomyopathy.
- Decrease in symptoms associated with PTSD.

propylthiouracil

(proe-pill-thye-oh-**yoor**-a-sill)

✤Propyl-Thyracil, PTU

Classification

Therapeutic: antithyroid agents

Pregnancy Category D

Indications

Palliative treatment of hyperthyroidism. Adjunct in the control of hyperthyroidism in preparation for thyroidectomy or radioactive iodine therapy.

Action

Inhibits the synthesis of thyroid hormones. **Therapeutic Effects:** Decreased signs and symptoms of hyperthyroidism.

Pharmacokinetics

Absorption: Rapidly absorbed from the GI tract.

Distribution: Concentrates in the thyroid gland; crosses the placenta and enters breast milk in low concentrations.

Metabolism and Excretion: Metabolized by the liver.

Half-life: 1–2 hr.

TIME/ACTION PROFILE (effects on clinical thyroid status)

ROUTE	ONSET	PEAK	DURATION
PO	10–21 days†	6–10 wk	wks

†Effects on serum thyroid hormone concentration may occur within 60 min of a single dose

Contraindications/Precautions

Contraindicated in: Hypersensitivity.

Use Cautiously in: Decreased bone marrow reserve; Pregnancy (may be used safely; however, fetus may develop thyroid problems); Lactation (safety not established).

Adverse Reactions/Side Effects

CNS: drowsiness, headache, vertigo. **GI:** nausea, vomiting, diarrhea, drug-induced hepatitis, loss of taste. **Derm:** rash, skin discoloration, urticaria. **Endo:** hypothyroidism. **Hemat:** AGRANULOCYTOSIS, leukopenia, thrombocytopenia. **MS:** arthralgia. **Misc:** fever, lymphadenopathy, parotitis.

Interactions

Drug-Drug: Additive bone marrow depression with **antineoplastics** or **radiation therapy**. Additive antithyroid effects with **lithium**, **potassium iodide**, or **sodium iodide**. Increased risk of agranulocytosis with **phenothiazines**.

Route/Dosage

PO (Adults): *Thyrotoxic crisis*—200–400 mg q 4 hr during the first 24 hr. *Hyperthyroidism*—300–900 mg once daily or in 2–4 divided doses initially (up to 1.2 g/day); maintenance dose 50–600 mg/day once daily or in 2–4 divided doses.
PO (Children >10 yr): 50–300 mg/day given once daily or in 2–4 divided doses.
PO (Children 6–10 yr): 50–150 mg/day given once daily or in 2–4 divided doses.
PO (Neonates): 10 mg/kg/day in divided doses.

Availability (generic available)

Tablets: 50 mg, ✤100 mg.

NURSING IMPLICATIONS

Assessment

- Monitor response of symptoms of hyperthyroidism or thyrotoxicosis (tachycardia, palpitations, nervousness, insomnia, fever, diaphoresis, heat intolerance, tremors, weight loss, diarrhea).
- Assess patient for development of hypothyroidism (intolerance to cold, constipation, dry skin, headache, listlessness, tiredness, or weakness). Dosage adjustment may be required.
- Assess patient for skin rash or swelling of cervical lymph nodes. Treatment may be discontinued if this occurs.
- ***Lab Test Considerations:*** Thyroid function studies should be monitored prior to therapy, monthly during initial therapy, and every 2–3 mo throughout therapy.
- WBC and differential counts should be monitored periodically throughout course of therapy. Agranulocytosis may develop rapidly and usually occurs during first 2 mo. This necessitates discontinuation of therapy.
- May cause increased AST, ALT, LDH, alkaline phosphatase, serum bilirubin, and prothrombin time.

Potential Nursing Diagnoses

Deficient knowledge, related to medication regimen (Patient/Family Teaching)
Noncompliance (Patient/Family Teaching)

Implementation

- Can be compounded by pharmacist into enema or suppository.
- **PO:** Administer at same time in relation to meals every day. Food may either increase or decrease absorption.

Patient/Family Teaching

- Instruct patient to take medication exactly as directed, around the clock. If a dose is missed, take as soon as remembered; take both doses together if almost time for next dose; check with health care professional if more than 1 dose is missed. Consult health care professional prior to discontinuing medication.
- Instruct patient to monitor weight 2–3 times weekly. Report significant changes.
- May cause drowsiness. Caution patient to avoid driving or other activities requiring alertness until response to medication is known.
- Advise patient to consult health care professional regarding dietary sources of iodine (iodized salt, shellfish).
- Advise patient to report sore throat, fever, chills, headache, malaise, weakness, yellowing of eyes or skin, unusual bleeding or bruising, symptoms of hyperthyroidism or hypothyroidism, or rash to health care professional promptly.
- Instruct patient to consult health care professional before taking any OTC medications containing iodine concurrently with this medication.
- Advise patient to carry identification describing medication regimen at all times and to notify health care professional of medication regimen prior to treatment or surgery.
- Emphasize the importance of routine exams to monitor progress and to check for side effects.

P

Evaluation/Desired Outcomes

- Decrease in severity of symptoms of hyperthyroidism (lowered pulse rate and weight gain).
- Return of thyroid function studies to normal.
- May be used as short-term adjunctive therapy to prepare patient for thyroidectomy or radiation therapy or may be used in treatment of hyperthyroidism. Treatment of 6 mo to several years may be necessary, usually averaging 1 yr.

protamine sulfate
(**proe**-ta-meen)

Classification
Therapeutic: antidotes
Pharmacologic: antiheparins

Pregnancy Category C

Indications
Acute management of severe heparin overdosage. Used to neutralize heparin received during dialysis, cardiopulmonary bypass, and other procedures. **Unlabeled uses:** Management of overdose of heparin-like compounds.

Action
A strong base that forms a complex with heparin (an acid). **Therapeutic Effects:** Inactivation of heparin.

Pharmacokinetics
Absorption: Administered IV only, resulting in complete bioavailability.
Distribution: Unknown.
Metabolism and Excretion: Metabolic fate not known. Protamine-heparin complex eventually degrades.
Half-life: Unknown.

TIME/ACTION PROFILE (reversal of heparin effect)

ROUTE	ONSET	PEAK	DURATION
IV	30 sec–1 min	unknown	2 hr†

†Depends on body temperature

Contraindications/Precautions
Contraindicated in: Hypersensitivity to protamine or fish.
Use Cautiously in: Patients who have received previous protamine-containing insulin or vasectomized men (increased risk of hypersensitivity reactions); Pregnancy, lactation, and children (safety not established).

Adverse Reactions/Side Effects
Resp: dyspnea. **CV:** bradycardia, hypertension, hypotension, pulmonary hypertension. **GI:** nausea, vomiting. **Derm:** flushing, warmth. **Hemat:** bleeding. **MS:** back pain. **Misc:** hypersensitivity reactions, including ANAPHYLAXIS, ANGIOEDEMA, and PULMONARY EDEMA.

Interactions
Drug-Drug: None significant.

Route/Dosage
IV (Adults and Children): *Heparin overdose*—1 mg/100 units of heparin. If given >30 min after heparin, give 0.5 mg/100 units of heparin (not to exceed 100 mg/2 hr). Further doses should be determined by coagulation tests. If heparin was administered subcutaneously, use 1–1.5 mg protamine per 100 units of heparin, give 25–50 mg of the protamine dose slowly followed by a continuous infusion over 8–16 hours. *Enoxaparin overdose*—1 mg/each mg of enoxaparin to be neutralized (unlabeled). *Dalteparin overdose*—1 mg/100 anti-Xa IU of dalteparin. If required, a second dose of 0.5 mg/100 anti-Xa IU of dalteparin may be given 2–4 hr later if laboratory assessment indicates need (unlabeled).

Availability (generic available)
Injection: 10 mg/ml in 5- and 25-ml vials.

NURSING IMPLICATIONS

Assessment

- Assess for bleeding and hemorrhage throughout therapy. Hemorrhage may recur 8–9 hr after therapy because of rebound effects of heparin. Rebound may occur as late as 18 hr after therapy in patients heparinized for cardiopulmonary bypass.
- Assess for allergy to fish (salmon), previous reaction to or use of protamine insulin or protamine sulfate. Vasectomized and infertile men also have higher risk of hypersensitivity reaction.
- Observe patient for signs and symptoms of hypersensitivity reaction (hives, edema, coughing, wheezing). Keep epinephrine, an antihistamine, and resuscitative equipment close by in the event of anaphylaxis.
- Assess for hypovolemia before initiation of therapy. Failure to correct hypovolemia may result in cardiovascular collapse from pe-

ripheral vasodilating effects of protamine sulfate.

- ***Lab Test Considerations:*** Monitor clotting factors, activated clotting time (ACT), activated partial thromboplastin time (aPTT), and thrombin time (TT) 5–15 min after therapy and again as necessary.

Potential Nursing Diagnoses

Risk for injury (Indications)
Ineffective tissue perfusion (Indications)

Implementation

- Discontinue heparin infusion. In milder cases, overdosage may be treated by heparin withdrawal alone.
- In severe cases, fresh frozen plasma or whole blood may also be required to control bleeding.
- Dose varies with type of heparin, route of heparin therapy, and amount of time elapsed since discontinuation of heparin.
- Do not administer >100 mg in 2 hr without rechecking clotting studies, as protamine sulfate has its own anticoagulant properties.

IV Administration

- **Direct IV: *Diluent:*** May be administered undiluted. If further dilution is desired, D5W or 0.9% NaCl may be used. ***Concentration:*** 10 mg/ml. ***Rate:*** Administer by slow IV push over 1–3 min. Rapid infusion rate may result in hypotension, bradycardia, flushing, or feeling of warmth. If these symptoms occur, stop infusion and notify physician. No more than 50 mg should be administered within a 10–min period.
- **Y-Site Compatibility:** amikacin, aminophylline, atropine, aztreonam, bumetanide, calcium chloride, calcium gluconate, cimetidine, clindamycin, cyclosporine, digoxin, diphenhydramine, doxycycline, enalaprilat, epinephrine, erythromycin, esmolol, famotidine, fentanyl, fluconazole, ganciclovir, gentamicin, hydroxyzine, imipenem/cilastatin, isoproterenol, labetalol, lidocaine, meperidine, metoclopramide, metoprolol, metronidazole, midazolam, morphine, nitroglycerin, nitroprusside, norepinephrine, ondansetron, phenylephrine, potassium chloride, procainamide, prochlorperazine, promethazine, propranolol, ranitidine, sodium bicarbonate, tobramycin, vancomycin, verapamil.
- **Y-Site Incompatibility:** ampicillin, ampicillin/sulbactam, cefazolin, cefotaxime, cefoxitin, ceftazidime, cefuroxime, chloramphenicol, dexamethasone sodium phosphate, diazepam, furosemide, hydrocortisone sodium succinate, insulin, ketorolac, methylprednisolone sodium succinate, nafcillin, penicillin G potassium, phenytoin, ticarcillin/clavulanate, trimethoprim/sulfamethoxazole.

Patient/Family Teaching

- Explain purpose of the medication to patient. Instruct patient to report recurrent bleeding immediately.
- Advise patient to avoid activities that may result in bleeding (shaving, brushing teeth, receiving injections or rectal temperatures, or ambulating) until risk of hemorrhage has passed.

Evaluation/Desired Outcomes

- Control of bleeding.
- Normalization of clotting factors in heparinized patients.

P

pseudoephedrine

(soo-doe-e-**fed**-rin)

♣Balminil Decongestant Syrup, Cenafed, Congestaid, Decofed, Dimetapp Maximum Strength 12–Hour Non-Drowsy Extentabs, Dimetapp Decongestant Pediatric, Drixoral 12 Hour Non-Drowsy Formula, Efidac 24, ♣Eltor 120, Genafed, Halofed, Kid Kare, Medi-First Sinus Decongestant, Pedia-Care Infants' Decongestant Drops, Pediatric Nasal Decongestant, Simply Stuffy, Sinustop, ♣Robidrine, Silfedrine, Sudafed, Sudafed Childrens's Non-Drowsy, Sudafed 12 Hour, Sudafed Non-Drowsy Maximum Strength, Sudodrin, Triaminic Allergy Congestion Softchews, Unifed

Classification

Therapeutic: allergy, cold, and cough remedies, nasal drying agents/decongestants

Pregnancy Category B

Indications

Symptomatic management of nasal congestion associated with acute viral upper respiratory tract infections. Used in combination with antihistamines in the management of allergic conditions. Used to open obstructed eustachian tubes in chronic otic inflammation or infection.

Action

Stimulates alpha- and beta-adrenergic receptors. Produces vasoconstriction in the respiratory tract mucosa (alpha-adrenergic stimulation) and possibly bronchodilation (beta$_2$-adrenergic stimulation). **Therapeutic Effects:** Reduction of nasal congestion, hyperemia, and swelling in nasal passages.

Pharmacokinetics

Absorption: Well absorbed after oral administration.
Distribution: Appears to enter the CSF; probably crosses the placenta and enters breast milk.
Metabolism and Excretion: Partially metabolized by the liver. 55–75% excreted unchanged by the kidneys (depends on urine pH).
Half-life: Children: 3.1 hr; Adults: 9–16 hr (depends on urine pH).

TIME/ACTION PROFILE (decongestant effects)

ROUTE	ONSET	PEAK	DURATION
PO	15–30 min	unknown	4–6 hr
PO-ER	60 min	unknown	12 hr

Contraindications/Precautions

Contraindicated in: Hypersensitivity to sympathomimetic amines; Hypertension, severe coronary artery disease; Concurrent MAO inhibitor therapy; Known alcohol intolerance (some liquid products).
Use Cautiously in: Hyperthyroidism; Diabetes mellitus; Prostatic hyperplasia; Ischemic heart disease; Glaucoma; Neonates (some products contain a metabolite of benzyl alcohol, avoid use); Pregnancy or lactation (safety not established).

Adverse Reactions/Side Effects

CNS: SEIZURES, anxiety, nervousness, dizziness, drowsiness, excitability, fear, hallucinations, headache, insomnia, restlessness, weakness. **Resp:** respiratory difficulty. **CV:** CARDIOVASCULAR COLLAPSE, palpitations, hypertension, tachycardia. **GI:** anorexia, dry mouth. **GU:** dysuria. **Misc:** diaphoresis.

Interactions

Drug-Drug: Concurrent use with **MAO inhibitors** may cause hypertensive crisis. Additive adrenergic effects with other **adrenergics**. Concurrent use with **beta blockers** may result in hypertension or bradycardia. **Drugs that acidify the urine** may decrease effectiveness. **Phenothiazines** and **tricyclic antidepressants** potentiate pressor effects. **Drugs that alkalinize the urine (sodium bicarbonate, high-dose antacid therapy)** may intensify effectiveness.
Drug-Food: Foods that acidify the urine may decrease effectiveness. **Foods that alkalinize the urine** may intensify effectiveness (see lists in Appendix L).

Route/Dosage

PO (Adults and Children >12 yr): 60 mg q 6 hr as needed (not to exceed 240 mg/day) *or* 120 mg of extended-release preparation q 12 hr *or* 240 mg extended-release preparation q 24 hr.
PO (Children 6–12 yr): 30 mg q 6 hr as needed (not to exceed 120 mg/day).
PO (Children 2–5 yr): 15 mg q 6 hr (not to exceed 60 mg/day).
PO (Children <2 yr): 4 mg/kg/day in divided doses q 6 hr.

Availability (generic available)

Tablets: 30 mg[OTC], 60 mg[OTC]. **Extended-release tablets:** 120 mg[OTC]. **Controlled-release tablets:** 240 mg[OTC]. **Capsules:** 🍁 60 mg[OTC]. **Extended-release capsules:** 🍁 240 mg[OTC]. **Softgel capsules:** 30 mg[OTC]. **Liquid (grape and others):** 15 mg/5 ml[OTC], 30 mg/5 ml[OTC]. **Drops (cherry and fruit flavor):** 7.5 mg/0.8 ml[OTC]. ***In combination with:*** antihistamines, acetaminophen, cough suppressants, and expectorants[OTC]. See Appendix B.

NURSING IMPLICATIONS

Assessment

- Assess congestion (nasal, sinus, eustachian tube) before and periodically during therapy.
- Monitor pulse and blood pressure before beginning therapy and periodically during therapy.
- Assess lung sounds and character of bronchial secretions. Maintain fluid intake of 1500–2000 ml/day to decrease viscosity of secretions.

Potential Nursing Diagnoses

Ineffective airway clearance (Indications)

Implementation

- Administer pseudoephedrine at least 2 hr before bedtime to minimize insomnia.
- **PO:** Extended-release tablets and capsules should be swallowed whole; do not crush, break, or chew. Contents of the capsule can be mixed with jam or jelly and swallowed without chewing for patients with difficulty swallowing.

Patient/Family Teaching

- Instruct patient to take medication as directed and not to take more than recommended. Take missed doses within 1 hr; if remembered later, omit. Do not double doses.
- **Instruct patient to notify health care professional if nervousness, slow or fast heart rate, breathing difficulties, hallucinations, or seizures occur, because these symptoms may indicate overdose.**
- Instruct patient to contact health care professional if symptoms do not improve within 7 days or if fever is present.

Evaluation/Desired Outcomes

- Decreased nasal, sinus, or eustachian tube congestion.

psyllium (sill-i-yum)

Alramucil, Cillium, Effer-Syllium, Fiberall, Fibrepur, Hydrocil, ✤Karacil, Konsyl, Metamucil, Modane Bulk, Mylanta Natural Fiber Supplement, Naturacil Caramels, ✤Natural Source Fibre Laxative, Perdiem, ✤Prodiem, Pro-Lax, Reguloid Natural, Serutan, Siblin, Syllact, Vitalax, V-Lax

Classification

Therapeutic: laxatives

Pharmacologic: bulk-forming agents

Pregnancy Category UK

Indications

Management of simple or chronic constipation, particularly if associated with a low-fiber diet. Useful in situations in which straining should be avoided (after MI, rectal surgery, prolonged bed rest). Used in the management of chronic watery diarrhea.

Action

Combines with water in the intestinal contents to form an emollient gel or viscous solution that promotes peristalsis and reduces transit time. **Therapeutic Effects:** Relief and prevention of constipation.

Pharmacokinetics

Absorption: Not absorbed from the GI tract.
Distribution: No distribution occurs.
Metabolism and Excretion: Excreted in feces.
Half-life: Unknown.

TIME/ACTION PROFILE (laxative effect)

ROUTE	ONSET	PEAK	DURATION
PO	12–24 hr	2–3 days	unknown

Contraindications/Precautions

Contraindicated in: Hypersensitivity; Abdominal pain, nausea, or vomiting (especially when associated with fever); Serious adhesions; Dysphagia.
Use Cautiously in: Some dosage forms contain sugar, aspartame, or excessive sodium and should be avoided in patients on restricted diets; Pregnancy and lactation (has been used safely).

Adverse Reactions/Side Effects

Resp: bronchospasm. **GI:** cramps, intestinal or esophageal obstruction, nausea, vomiting.

Interactions

Drug-Drug: May decrease the absorption of **warfarin**, **salicylates**, or **digoxins**.

Route/Dosage

PO (Adults): 1–2 tsp/packet/wafer (3–6 g psyllium) in or with a full glass of liquid 2–3 times daily. Up to 30 g daily in divided doses.
PO (Children >6 yr): 1 tsp/packet/wafer (1.5–3 g psyllium) in or with 4–8 ozglass of liquid 2–3 times daily. Up to 15 g daily in divided doses.

Availability (generic available)

Powder: 3.3–3.5 g/dose or packet[OTC]. **Effervescent powder:** 3–3.5 g/dose or packet[OTC]. **Granules:** 2.5 g/dose[OTC]. **Wafers:** 3.4 g/dose[OTC].

NURSING IMPLICATIONS

Assessment

- Assess patient for abdominal distention, presence of bowel sounds, and usual pattern of bowel function.

- Assess color, consistency, and amount of stool produced.
- ***Lab Test Considerations:*** May cause elevated blood glucose levels with prolonged use of preparations containing sugar.

Potential Nursing Diagnoses

Constipation (Indications)

Implementation

- Packets are not standardized for volume, but each contains 3–3.5 g of psyllium.
- **PO:** Administer with a full glass of water or juice, followed by an additional glass of liquid. Solution should be taken immediately after mixing; it will congeal. Do not administer without sufficient fluid and do not chew granules.

Patient/Family Teaching

- Encourage patient to use other forms of bowel regulation, such as increasing bulk in the diet, increasing fluid intake, and increasing mobility. Normal bowel habits are individualized and may vary from 3 times/day to 3 times/wk.
- May be used for long-term management of chronic constipation.
- Instruct patients with cardiac disease to avoid straining during bowel movements (Valsalva maneuver).
- Advise patient not to use laxatives when abdominal pain, nausea, vomiting, or fever is present.

Evaluation/Desired Outcomes

- A soft, formed bowel movement, usually within 12–24 hr. May require 3 days of therapy for results.

pyrazinamide

(peer-a-**zin**-a-mide)

✤PMS Pyrazinamide, ✤Tebrazid

Classification

Therapeutic: antituberculars

Pregnancy Category C

Indications

Used in combination with other agents in the treatment of active tuberculosis.

Action

Mechanism not known. **Therapeutic Effects:** Bacteriostatic action against susceptible mycobacteria. **Spectrum:** Active against mycobacteria only.

Pharmacokinetics

Absorption: Well absorbed after oral administration.

Distribution: Widely distributed. Reaches high concentrations in the CNS (same as plasma). Excreted in breast milk.

Metabolism and Excretion: Mostly metabolized by the liver. Metabolite (pyrazinoic acid) has antimycobacterial activity; 3–4% excreted unchanged by the kidneys.

Half-life: *Pyrazinamide*—9.5 hr. *Pyrazinoic acid*—12 hr. Both are prolonged in renal impairment.

TIME/ACTION PROFILE (blood levels)

ROUTE	ONSET	PEAK	DURATION
PO	unknown	1–2 hr (4–5 hr†)	24 hr

†For pyrazinoic acid

Contraindications/Precautions

Contraindicated in: Hypersensitivity; Cross-sensitivity with ethionamide, isoniazid, niacin, or nicotinic acid may exist; Severe liver impairment; Concurrent use with rifampin.

Use Cautiously in: Gout; Diabetes mellitus; Acute intermittent porphyria; Pregnancy (safety not established).

Adverse Reactions/Side Effects

GI: HEPATOTOXICITY, anorexia, diarrhea, nausea, vomiting. **GU:** dysuria. **Derm:** acne, itching, photosensitivity, skin rash. **Hemat:** anemia, thrombocytopenia. **Metab:** hyperuricemia. **MS:** arthralgia, gouty arthritis.

Interactions

Drug-Drug: Concurrent use with **rifampin** may result in life-threatening hepatoxicity and should be avoided. May ↓ blood levels and effectiveness of **cyclosporine**. May ↓ effectiveness of **antigout agents**.

Route/Dosage

PO (Adults and Children): 15–30 mg/kg/day as a single dose. Up to 60 mg/kg/day has been used in isoniazid-resistant tuberculosis (not to exceed 2 g/day as a single dose or 3 g/day in divided doses). May also be given as 50–70 mg/kg 2–3 times weekly (not to exceed 2 g/dose on daily regimen, 3 g/dose for 3-times-weekly regimen, or 4 g/dose for twice-weekly regimen). *Patients with HIV*—20–30 mg/kg/day for first

2 mo of therapy; further dosing depends on regimen employed.

Availability (generic available)

Tablets: 500 mg.

NURSING IMPLICATIONS

Assessment

- Perform mycobacterial studies and susceptibility tests before and periodically during therapy to detect possible resistance.
- ***Lab Test Considerations:*** Evaluate hepatic function before and every 2–4 wk during therapy. Increased AST and ALT may not be predictive of clinical hepatitis and may return to normal levels during treatment. Patients with impaired liver function should receive pyrazinamide therapy only if crucial to treatment.
- Monitor serum uric acid concentrations during therapy. May cause ↑ resulting in precipitation of acute gout.
- May interfere with urine ketone determinations.

Potential Nursing Diagnoses

Risk for infection (Indications)
Noncompliance (Patient/Family Teaching)

Implementation

- May be given concurrently with isoniazid.

Patient/Family Teaching

- Advise patient to take medication as directed and not to skip doses or double up on missed doses. Take missed doses as soon as remembered unless almost time for next dose. Emphasize the importance of continuing therapy even after symptoms have subsided. Length of therapy depends on regimen being used and underlying disease states.
- Inform diabetic patients that pyrazinamide may interfere with urine ketone measurements.
- Advise patients to notify health care professional if no improvement is noticed after 2–3 wk of therapy or if fever, anorexia, malaise, nausea, vomiting, darkened urine, yellowish discoloration of the skin and eyes, pain, or swelling of the joints occurs.
- Advise patients to use sunscreen and protective clothing to prevent photosensitivity reactions.
- Emphasize the importance of regular follow-up exams to monitor progress and check for side effects.

Evaluation/Desired Outcomes

- Resolution of signs and symptoms of tuberculosis.
- Negative sputum cultures.

pyridostigmine

(peer-id-oh-**stig**-meen)
Mestinon, ✤Mestinon SR, Mestinon Timespan, Regonol

Classification
Therapeutic: antimyasthenics
Pharmacologic: cholinergics

Pregnancy Category C

Indications

Used to increase muscle strength in the symptomatic treatment of myasthenia gravis. Reversal of nondepolarizing neuromuscular blocking agents. Prophylaxis of lethal effects of poisoning with the nerve agent soman.

Action

Inhibits the breakdown of acetylcholine and prolongs its effects (anticholinesterase). Effects include: Miosis, Increased intestinal and skeletal muscle tone, Bronchial and ureteral constriction, Bradycardia, Increased salivation, Lacrimation, Sweating. **Therapeutic Effects:** Improved muscular function in patients with myasthenia gravis. Reversal of paralysis from nondepolarizing neuromuscular blocking agents. Prevention of Soman nerve gas toxicity.

Pharmacokinetics

Absorption: Poorly absorbed after oral administration, necessitating large oral doses compared with parenteral doses.
Distribution: Appears to cross the placenta.
Metabolism and Excretion: Metabolized by plasma cholinesterases and the liver.
Half-life: *PO*—3.7 hr; *IV*—1.9 hr.

TIME/ACTION PROFILE (cholinergic effects)

ROUTE	ONSET	PEAK	DURATION
PO	30–35 min	unknown	3–6 hr
PO-SR	30–60 min	unknown	6–12 hr
IM	15 min	unknown	2–4 hr
IV	2–5 min	unknown	2–3 hr

Contraindications/Precautions

Contraindicated in: Hypersensitivity to pyridostigmine or bromides; Mechanical obstruc-

P

tion of the GI or GU tract; Known alcohol intolerance (syrup only).
Use Cautiously in: History of asthma; Ulcer disease; Cardiovascular disease; Epilepsy; Hyperthyroidism; OB: Pregnancy or lactation (may cause uterine irritability after IV administration near term; 20% of newborns display transient muscle weakness).

Adverse Reactions/Side Effects

CNS: SEIZURES, dizziness, weakness. **EENT:** lacrimation, miosis. **Resp:** bronchospasm, excessive secretions. **CV:** bradycardia, hypotension. **GI:** abdominal cramps, diarrhea, excessive salivation, nausea, vomiting. **Derm:** sweating, rashes.

Interactions

Drug-Drug: Cholinergic effects may be antagonized by other **drugs possessing anticholinergic properties**, including **antihistamines**, **antidepressants**, **atropine**, **haloperidol**, **phenothiazines**, **procainamide**, **quinidine**, or **disopyramide**. Prolongs the action of **depolarizing muscle-relaxing agents** and **cholinesterase inhibitors** (**succinylcholine, decamethonium**). ↑ toxicity with other **cholinesterase inhibitors**, including **demecarium**, **echothiophate**, and **isoflurophate**. Antimyasthenic effects may be ↓ by concurrent **guanadrel**.

Route/Dosage

Myasthenia Gravis

PO (Adults): *Tablets/syrup*—30–60 mg q 3–4 hr initially; then adjusted as required; usual maintenance dose is 600 mg/day in divided doses (range 60–1500 mg/day). *Extended-release tablets*—180–540 mg 1–2 times daily (dosing interval should be at least 6 hr; may be associated with increased risk of cholinergic crisis; concurrent immediate-release products may be required).
PO (Children): 7 mg/kg (200 mg/m²)/day in 5–6 divided doses.
IM, IV (Adults): 2 mg (1/30 of oral dose); may be repeated q 2–3 hr. *During labor/delivery*—1 mg before second stage of labor is complete.
IM (Neonates Born to Myasthenic Mothers): 50–150 mcg/kg q 4–6 hr.

Antidote for Nondepolarizing Neuromuscular Blocking Agents

IV (Adults): 10–20 mg; pretreat with 0.6–1.2 mg atropine IV.

Prevention of Soman Nerve Gas Effects

PO (Adults): 30 mg every 8 hr before exposure, stopped on exposure to gas.

Availability (generic available)

Tablets: 30 mg[Rx], 60 mg. **Extended-release tablets:** 180 mg. **Syrup:** 60 mg/5 ml. **Injection:** 5 mg/ml in 2-ml ampules and 5-ml vials.

NURSING IMPLICATIONS

Assessment

- Assess pulse, respiratory rate, and blood pressure before administration. Report significant changes in heart rate.
- **Myasthenia Gravis:** Assess neuromuscular status, including vital capacity, ptosis, diplopia, chewing, swallowing, hand grasp, and gait before administering and at peak effect. Patients with myasthenia gravis may be advised to keep a daily record of their condition and the effects of this medication.
- Assess patient for overdose, underdose, or resistance. Both have similar symptoms (muscle weakness, dyspnea, dysphagia), but symptoms of overdosage usually occur within 1 hr of administration, whereas symptoms of underdose occur ≥3 hr after administration. Overdose (cholinergic crisis) symptoms may also include increased respiratory secretions and saliva, bradycardia, nausea, vomiting, cramping, diarrhea, and diaphoresis. A Tensilon test (edrophonium chloride) may be used to differentiate between overdosage and underdosage.
- **Antidote to Nondepolarizing Neuromuscular Blocking Agents:** Monitor reversal of effect of neuromuscular blocking agents with a peripheral nerve stimulator. Recovery usually occurs consecutively in the following muscles: diaphragm, intercostal muscles, muscles of the glottis, abdominal muscles, limb muscles, muscles of mastication, and levator muscles of eyelids. Closely observe patient for residual muscle weakness and respiratory distress throughout the recovery period. Maintain airway patency and ventilation until recovery of normal respirations occurs.
- ***Toxicity and Overdose:*** Atropine is the antidote.

Potential Nursing Diagnoses

Impaired physical mobility (Indications)
Ineffective breathing pattern (Indications)

Implementation

- For patients who have difficulty chewing, pyridostigmine may be administered 30 min before meals.
- Oral dose is not interchangeable with IV dose. Parenteral form is 30 times more potent.
- When used as an antidote to nondepolarizing neuromuscular blocking agents, atropine may be ordered before or currently with large doses of pyridostigmine to prevent or to treat bradycardia and other side effects.
- **PO:** Administer with food or milk to minimize side effects. Extended-release tablets should be swallowed whole; do not crush, break, or chew. Regular tablets or syrup may be administered with extended-release tablets for optimum control of symptoms. Mottled appearance of sustained-release tablet does not affect potency.

IV Administration

- **Direct IV:** Administer undiluted. Do not add to IV solutions. May be given through Y-site of infusion of D5W, 0.9% NaCl, LR, D5/Ringer's solution, or D5/LR. ***Concentration:*** 5 mg/ml. ***Rate:*** For myasthenia gravis, administer each 0.5 mg over 1 min. For reversal of nondepolarizing neuromuscular blocking agents, administer each 5 mg over 1 min.
- **Syringe Compatibility:** glycopyrrolate.
- **Y-Site Compatibility:** heparin, hydrocortisone sodium succinate, potassium chloride, vitamin B complex with C.

Patient/Family Teaching

- Instruct patient to take medication as directed. Do not skip or double up on missed doses. Patients with a history of dysphagia should have a nonelectric or battery-operated back-up alarm clock to remind them of exact dose time. Patients with dysphagia may not be able to swallow medication if the dose is not taken exactly on time. Taking dose late may result in myasthenic crisis. Taking dose early may result in cholinergic crisis. Patients with myasthenia gravis must continue this regimen as a life-long therapy.
- Advise patient to carry identification describing disease and medication regimen at all times.
- Instruct patient to space activities to avoid fatigue.

Evaluation/Desired Outcomes

- Relief of ptosis and diplopia; improved chewing, swallowing, extremity strength, and breathing without the appearance of cholinergic symptoms.
- Reversal of nondepolarizing neuromuscular blocking agents in general anesthesia.
- Prevention of Soman nerve gas toxicity.

pyridoxine (peer-i-**dox**-een)

Beesix, Doxine, Nestrex, Pyri, Rodex, Vitabee 6, vitamin B_6

Classification
Therapeutic: vitamins
Pharmacologic: water soluble vitamins

Pregnancy Category A

Indications

Treatment and prevention of pyridoxine deficiency (may be associated with poor nutritional status or chronic debilitating illnesses). Treatment of pyridoxine-dependent seizures in infants. Treatment and prevention of neuropathy, which may develop from isoniazid, penicillamine, or hydralazine therapy. Management of isoniazid overdose >10 g.

Action

Required for amino acid, carbohydrate, and lipid metabolism. Used in the transport of amino acids, formation of neurotransmitters, and synthesis of heme. **Therapeutic Effects:** Prevention of pyridoxine deficiency. Prevention or reversal of neuropathy associated with hydralazine, penicillamine, or isoniazid therapy.

Pharmacokinetics

Absorption: Well absorbed from the GI tract.
Distribution: Stored in liver, muscle, and brain. Crosses the placenta and enters breast milk.
Metabolism and Excretion: Converted in RBCs to pyridoxal phosphate and another active metabolite. Amounts in excess of requirements are excreted unchanged by the kidneys.
Half-life: 15–20 days.

P

TIME/ACTION PROFILE

ROUTE	ONSET	PEAK	DURATION
PO, IM, IV	unknown	unknown	unknown

Contraindications/Precautions

Contraindicated in: Hypersensitivity to pyridoxine or any component.

Use Cautiously in: Parkinson's disease (treatment with levodopa only); Pregnancy (chronic ingestion of large doses may produce pyridoxine-dependency syndrome in newborn).

Adverse Reactions/Side Effects

Adverse reactions listed are seen with excessive doses only. **Neuro:** sensory neuropathy, paresthesia. **Misc:** pyridoxine-dependency syndrome.

Interactions

Drug-Drug: Interferes with the therapeutic response to **levodopa** when used without carbidopa. Requirements are increased by **isoniazid**, **hydralazine**, **chloramphenicol**, **penicillamine**, **estrogens**, and **immunosuppressants**. Decreases serum levels of **phenobarbital** and **phenytoin**.

Route/Dosage

Prevention of Deficiency (Recommended Daily Allowance)

PO (Adults and Children >14 yr): 1.2–1.7 mg/day (larger doses required with cycloserine, ethionamide, hydralazine, immunosuppressants, isoniazid, penicillamine, and estrogen-containing oral contraceptives).

PO (Children 9–13 yr): 1 mg/day (larger doses required with cycloserine, ethionamide, hydralazine, immunosuppressants, isoniazid, and penicillamine).

PO (Children 1–8 yr): 0.5–0.6 mg/day (larger doses required with cycloserine, ethionamide, hydralazine, immunosuppressants, isoniazid, and penicillamine).

PO (Infants 6–12 months): 0.3 mg/day.

PO (Infants <6 months): 0.1 mg/day.

Treatment of Deficiency

PO (Adults): 2.5–10 mg/day until clinical signs are corrected, then 2–5 mg/day.

PO (Children): 5–25 mg/day for 3 weeks, then 1.5–2.5 mg/day.

Pyridoxine-Dependent Seizures

PO, IM, IV (Neonates and Infants): 10–100 mg initially then 50–100 mg/day orally.

Drug-Induced Neuritis

PO (Adults): Treatment—100–300 mg/day; Prophylaxis—25–100 mg/day.

PO (Children): Treatment—10–50 mg/day; Prophylaxis—1–2 mg/kg/day.

Isoniazid Overdose (>10 g)

IM, IV (Adults and Children): Amount in mg equal to amount of isoniazid ingested given as 1–4 g IV, then 1 g IM q 30 min.

Availability (generic available)

Tablets: 20 mg^{OTC}, 25 mg^{OTC}, 50 mg^{OTC}, 100 mg^{OTC}, 250 mg^{OTC}, 500 mg^{OTC}. **Extended-release tablets:** 100 mg^{OTC}, 200 mg^{OTC}, 500 mg^{OTC}. **Extended-release capsules:** 150 mg^{OTC}. **Injection:** 100 mg/ml in 10- and 30-ml vials. ***In combination with:*** vitamins, minerals, and trace elements in a variety of multivitamin preparations^{OTC}.

NURSING IMPLICATIONS

Assessment

- Assess patient for signs of vitamin B_6 deficiency (anemia, dermatitis, cheilosis, irritability, seizures, nausea, and vomiting) before and periodically throughout therapy. Institute seizure precautions in pyridoxine-dependent infants.
- ***Lab Test Considerations:*** May cause false elevations in urobilinogen concentrations.

Potential Nursing Diagnoses

Imbalanced nutrition: less than body requirements (Indications)

Implementation

- Because of infrequency of single B-vitamin deficiencies, combinations are commonly administered.
- Administration of parenteral vitamin B_6 is limited to patients who are NPO or who have nausea and vomiting or malabsorption syndromes.
- Protect parenteral solution from light; decomposition will occur.
- **PO:** Extended-release capsules and tablets should be swallowed whole, without crushing, breaking, or chewing. For patients unable to swallow capsule, contents of capsules may be mixed with jam or jelly.
- **IM:** Rotate sites; burning or stinging at site may occur.
- **IV:** May be administered slowly by direct IV or as infusion in standard IV solutions. Moni-

tor respiratory rate, heart rate, and blood pressure when administering large IV doses.
- Pyridoxine-dependent seizures should cease within 2–3 min of IV administration. ***Rate:*** Infusion rates of 15–30 min and up to 3 hr have been used.
- **Additive Incompatibility:** alkaline solutions, riboflavin.

Patient/Family Teaching
- Instruct patient to take medication as directed. If a dose is missed, it may be omitted because an extended period of time is required to become deficient in vitamin B_6.
- Encourage patient to comply with diet recommended by health care professional. Explain that the best source of vitamins is a well-balanced diet with foods from the four basic food groups. Foods high in vitamin B_6 include bananas, whole-grain cereals, potatoes, lima beans, and meats.
- Patients self-medicating with vitamin supplements should be cautioned not to exceed RDA. The effectiveness of megadoses for treatment of various medical conditions is unproved and may cause side effects, such as unsteady gait, numbness in feet, and difficulty with hand coordination.
- Emphasize the importance of follow-up exams to evaluate progress.

Evaluation/Desired Outcomes
- Decrease in the symptoms of vitamin B_6 deficiency.

pyrimethamine
(peer-i-**meth**-a-meen)
Daraprim

Classification
Therapeutic: antimalarials, antiprotozoals

Pregnancy Category C

Indications
Used in combination with other antimalarials in the treatment of chloroquine-resistant malaria. Used in combination with a sulfonamide in the treatment of toxoplasmosis. **Unlabeled uses:** Used in combination with other agents (sulfonamides, dapsone) in the treatment of *Pneumocystis carinii* pneumonia.

Action
Binds to an enzyme in the protozoa, which results in depletion of folic acid. **Therapeutic Effects:** Death and arrested growth of susceptible organisms (protozoa).

Pharmacokinetics
Absorption: Well absorbed after oral administration.
Distribution: Widely distributed with high concentrations achieved in blood cells, kidneys, lungs, liver, and spleen. Some enters CSF (13–26% of serum levels). Crosses the placenta and enters breast milk.
Metabolism and Excretion: Mostly metabolized by the liver. 20–30% excreted unchanged by the kidneys.
Half-life: 4 days (shortened in patients with AIDS).

TIME/ACTION PROFILE (blood levels)

ROUTE	ONSET	PEAK	DURATION
PO	unknown	3 hr	2 wk†

†Suppressive levels

Contraindications/Precautions
Contraindicated in: Hypersensitivity; First 14–16 wk of pregnancy; Megaloblastic anemia caused by folate deficiency; Concurrent folate antagonist therapy (because of risk of megaloblastic anemia); Tablets contain lactose and potato starch and should be avoided in patients with known hypersensitivity/intolerance.
Use Cautiously in: History of seizures (high doses); Underlying anemia or bone marrow depression; Impaired liver function; G6PD deficiency; OB: Pregnancy >16 wk (may require concurrent leucovorin); OB: Lactation (large doses to mother may cause folic acid deficiency in infant).

Adverse Reactions/Side Effects
CNS: SEIZURES (high doses), headache, insomnia, light-headedness, malaise, mental depression. **Resp:** dry throat, pulmonary eosinophilia. **CV:** ARRHYTHMIAS (large doses). **GI:** atrophic glossitis (high doses), anorexia, diarrhea, nausea. **GU:** hematuria. **Derm:** abnormal pigmentation, dermatitis. **Hemat:** megaloblastic anemia (HIGH DOSES), pancytopenia, thrombocytopenia. **Misc:** fever.

P

🍁 = Canadian drug name.
*CAPITALS indicates life-threatening; underlines indicate most frequent.

Interactions

Drug-Drug: ↑ risk of bone marrow depression with other **bone marrow depressants**, including **antineoplastics**, **proguanil**, or **radiation therapy**. ↑ risk of megaloblastic anemia with folate antagonists (**methotrexate**); concurrent use should be avoided.

Route/Dosage

Treatment of Malaria

PO (Adults and Children >10 yr): 50 mg/day for 2 days, then 25 mg once weekly in combination with other agents.
PO (Children 4–10 yr): 25 mg daily for 2 days, then 12.5 mg once weekly in combination with other agents.

Toxoplasmosis

PO (Adults): 50–200 mg/day for 1–2 days, followed by 25–50 mg/day for 2–6 wk; given with a sulfonamide.
PO (Children): 1 mg/kg/day for 1–3 days, then 0.5 mg/kg/day for 4–6 wk; given with a sulfonamide.

Toxoplasmosis in AIDS Patients

PO (Adults): 100–200 mg/day for 1–2 days, followed by 50–100 mg/day for 3–6 wk, then 25–50 mg/day for life; given with clindamycin or sulfadiazine.

Availability

Tablets: 25 mg. ***In combination with:*** sulfadoxine (Fansidar)[Rx]. See Appendix B.

NURSING IMPLICATIONS

Assessment

- Assess patient for improvement in signs and symptoms of infection daily during therapy.
- ***Lab Test Considerations:*** Monitor CBC and platelet count periodically during therapy; semiweekly in patients with toxoplasmosis. May cause ↓ WBC and platelet counts.

Potential Nursing Diagnoses

Risk for infection (Indications)

Implementation

- Leucovorin may be administered concurrently to prevent folic acid deficiency and restore normal hematopoiesis.
- **PO:** Administer with milk or meals to minimize GI distress.
- Tablets may be crushed and mixed with saline or with other vehicles by pharmacist for patients with difficulty swallowing.

Patient/Family Teaching

- Instruct patient to take medication as directed on a regular schedule and continue full course of therapy, even if feeling better. Take missed doses as soon as remembered unless almost time for next dose; do not double doses.
- Advise patient to notify health care professional promptly if sore throat, pallor, purpura, or glossitis occurs. Instruct patient to stop taking pyrimethamine and notify health care professional immediately at the first sign of a skin rash or if no improvement is seen within a few days.
- Emphasize the importance of lab tests at scheduled intervals, especially in patients taking high doses. Tests should not be delayed or missed.

Evaluation/Desired Outcomes

- Improvement in the signs and symptoms of malaria.
- Improvement in signs and symptoms of toxoplasmosis.

quetiapine (kwet-eye-a-peen)

Seroquel, Seroquel XR

Classification

Therapeutic: antipsychotics, mood stabilizers

Pregnancy Category C

Indications

Schizophrenia. Depressive episodes with bipolar disorder. Bipolar mania associated with Bipolar I as monotherapy or with lithium or divalproex.

Action

Probably acts by serving as an antagonist of dopamine and serotonin. Also antagonizes histamine H_1 receptors and $alpha_1$-adrenergic receptors. **Therapeutic Effects:** Decreased manifestations of psychoses, depression, or acute mania.

Pharmacokinetics

Absorption: Well absorbed after oral administration.

Distribution: Widely distributed.

Metabolism and Excretion: Extensively metabolized by the liver (mostly by P450 CYP3A4 enyzme system); <1% excreted unchanged in the urine.

Half-life: 6 hr.

TIME/ACTION PROFILE (antipsychotic effects)

ROUTE	ONSET	PEAK	DURATION
PO	unknown	unknown	8–12 hr
PO-XR	unknown	unknown	unknown

Contraindications/Precautions

Contraindicated in: Hypersensitivity; Lactation: Discontinue drug or bottle feed.

Use Cautiously in: Cardiovascular disease, cerebrovascular disease, dehydration or hypovolemia (increased risk of hypotension); History of seizures, Alzheimer's dementia; Pedi: May ↑ risk of suicide attempt/ideation especially during early treatment or dose adjustment; risk may be greater in children or adolescents; Hepatic impairment (dose reduction may be necessary); Hypothyroidism (may be exacerbated); History of suicide attempt; OB, Pedi: Pregnancy or children (safety not established); Geri: May require ↓ doses; inappropriate use for dementia is associated with ↑ mortality.

Adverse Reactions/Side Effects

CNS: NEUROLEPTIC MALIGNANT SYNDROME, SEIZURES, dizziness, cognitive impairment, extrapyramidal symptoms, sedation, tardive dyskinesia. **EENT:** ear pain, rhinitis, pharyngitis. **Resp:** cough, dyspnea. **CV:** palpitations, peripheral edema, postural hypotension. **GI:** anorexia, constipation, dry mouth, dyspepsia. **Derm:** sweating. **Hemat:** leukopenia. **Metab:** weight gain. **Misc:** flu-like syndrome.

Interactions

Drug-Drug: ↑ CNS depression may occur with **alcohol**, **antihistamines**, **opioid analgesics**, and **sedative/hypnotics**. ↑ risk of hypotension with acute ingestion of **alcohol** or **antihypertensives**. **Phenytoin** and **thioridazine** ↑ clearance and ↓ effectiveness of quetiapine (dose change may be necessary); similar effects may occur with **carbamazepine**, **barbiturates**, **rifampin**, or **corticosteroids**. Effects may be ↑ by **ketoconazole**, **itraconazole**, **fluconazole**, or **erythromycin**, as well as by other **agents that inhibit the cytochrome P450 CYP3A4 enzyme**.

Route/Dosage

PO (Adults): *Schizophrenia*—25 mg twice daily initially, increased by 25–50 mg 2–3 times daily over 3 days, up to 300–400 mg/day in 2–3 divided doses by the 4th day (not to exceed 800 mg/day); or 300 mg once daily as XR tablets, increased by 300 mg/day, up to 400–800 mg/day (not to exceed 800 mg/day). Elderly patients or patients with hepatic impairment should be started on immediate-release product and converted to extended-release product once effective dose is reached. *Bipolar mania*—100 mg/day in two divided doses on day 1, increase dose by 100 mg/day up to 400 mg/day by day 4, then may increase in 200 mg/day increments up to 800 mg/day on day 6 if required. *Depressive Bipolar Disorder*- once daily at bedtime to reach 300 mg by Day 4 with the following schedule: Day 1—50 mg; Day 2—100 mg; Day 3—200 mg; Day 4—300 mg. *Bipolar Manic Disorder*—Initially 50 mg twice daily, increasing to 400 mg/day by Day 4 in increments of up to 100 mg/day in divided doses. Further dose adjustments up to 800 mg/day should be made in increments of no >200 mg/day in divided doses.

Q

🍁 = Canadian drug name.

*CAPITALS indicates life-threatening; underlines indicate most frequent.

Availability

Tablets: 25 mg, 50 mg, 100 mg, 200 mg, 300 mg, 400 mg. **Cost:** 25 mg $360.95/180, 50 mg $604.78/180, 100 mg $610.97/180, 200 mg $1,142.96/180, 300 mg $1,579.93/180, 400 mg $1,787.40/180. **Extended-release Tablets:** 200 mg, 300 mg, 400 mg. **Cost:** 200 mg $395.00/60, 300 mg $510.00/60, 400 mg $595.00/60.

NURSING IMPLICATIONS

Assessment

- Monitor mental status (mood, orientation, behavior) before and periodically during therapy.
- Assess for suicidal tendencies, especially during early therapy. Restrict amount of drug available to patient.
- Assess weight and BMI initially and throughout therapy.
- Monitor blood pressure (sitting, standing, lying) and pulse before and frequently during initial dose titration. If hypotension occurs during dose titration, return to the previous dose.
- Observe patient carefully when administering to ensure medication is swallowed and not hoarded or cheeked.
- Monitor for onset of extrapyramidal side effects (*akathisia*—restlessness; *dystonia*—muscle spasms and twisting motions; or *pseudoparkinsonism*—mask-like faces, rigidity, tremors, drooling, shuffling gait, dysphagia). Report these symptoms; reduction of dose or discontinuation may be necessary. Trihexyphenidyl or benztropine may be used to control these symptoms.
- Monitor for tardive dyskinesia (involuntary rhythmic movement of mouth, face, and extremities). Report immediately; may be irreversible.
- Monitor for development of neuroleptic malignant syndrome (fever, respiratory distress, tachycardia, seizures, diaphoresis, hypertension or hypotension, pallor, tiredness). Notify health care professional immediately if these symptoms occur.
- ***Lab Test Considerations:*** May cause asymptomatic ↑ in AST and ALT.
- May also cause anemia, thrombocytopenia, leukocytosis, and leukopenia.
- May cause ↑ total cholesterol and triglycerides.
- Obtain fasting blood glucose and cholestol levels initially and throughout therapy.

Potential Nursing Diagnoses

Risk for self-directed violence (Indications)
Disturbed thought process (Indications)
Risk for injury (Side Effects)
Imbalanced nutrition: risk for more than body requirements (Side Effects)

Implementation

- Do not confuse Seroquel (quetiapine) with Serzone (nefazodone).
- If therapy is reinstituted after an interval of ≥1 wk off, follow initial titration schedule.
- **PO:** May be administered without regard to food. Extended-release tablets should be swallowed whole, do not crush, break, or chew.

Patient/Family Teaching

- Instruct patient to take medication as directed.
- Inform patient of the possibility of extrapyramidal symptoms. Instruct patient to report symptoms immediately to health care professional.
- Advise patient to change positions slowly to minimize orthostatic hypotension.
- May cause drowsiness. Caution patient to avoid driving or other activities requiring alertness until response to medication is known.
- Advise patient to avoid extremes in temperature; this drug impairs body temperature regulation.
- Caution patient to avoid concurrent use of alcohol, other CNS depressants, and OTC or herbal medications without consulting health care professional.
- Advise female patients to notify health care professional if pregnancy is planned or suspected or if they are breastfeeding or planning to breastfeed.
- Refer patient for nutritional, weight or medical management of dyslipidemia as indicated.
- Advise patient to notify health care professional of medication regimen before treatment or surgery.
- Instruct patient to notify health care professional promptly of sore throat, fever, unusual bleeding or bruising, or rash.
- Emphasize importance of routine follow-up exams to monitor side effects and continued participation in psychotherapy as indicated to improve coping skills. Ophthalmologic

exams should be performed before and every 6 months during therapy.
- Refer to local support group.

Evaluation/Desired Outcomes
- Decrease in excited, manic, behavior.
- Decrease in signs of depression in patients with bipolar disorder.
- Decrease in manic episodes in patients with bipolar I disorder.
- Decrease in positive symptoms (delusions, hallucinations) of schizophrenia.
- Decrease in negative symptoms (social withdrawal, flat, blunt affect) of schizophrenia.

quinapril, See ANGIOTENSIN-CONVERTING ENZYME (ACE) INHIBITORS.

QUINIDINE (kwin-i-deen)

quinidine gluconate
✤Apo-Quin-G

quinidine sulfate
✤Apo-Quinidine

Classification
Therapeutic: antiarrhythmics (class IA)

Pregnancy Category C

Indications
Restoration and maintenance of sinus rhythm in patients with atrial fibrillation or flutter. Prevention of recurrent ventricular arrhythmias. Treatment of malaria.

Action
Decrease myocardial excitability. Slow conduction velocity. **Therapeutic Effects:** Suppression of arrhythmias.

Pharmacokinetics
Absorption: Bioavailability of oral formulations is 70–80%. Extended-release preparations are absorbed slowly following oral administration.
Distribution: Widely distributed. Cross the placenta; enter breast milk.
Metabolism and Excretion: Metabolized by the liver; 5–20% excreted unchanged by the kidneys.
Half-life: 6–8 hr (increased in CHF or severe liver impairment).

TIME/ACTION PROFILE (antiarrhythmic effects)

ROUTE	ONSET	PEAK	DURATION
PO (sulfate)	30 min	1–1.5 hr	6–8 hr
PO (sulfate-ER)	unknown	4 hr	8–12 hr
PO (gluconate)	unknown	3–4 hr	6–8 hr
IV	1–5 min	rapid	6–8 hr

Contraindications/Precautions
Contraindicated in: Hypersensitivity; Conduction defects (in the absence of a pacemaker); Myasthenia gravis.
Use Cautiously in: CHF (dose reduction recommended); Severe liver disease (dose reduction recommended); Hypokalemia or hypomagnesemia (↑ risk of torsades de pointes); Bradycardia (↑ risk of torsades de pointes); Renal impairment; OB, Lactation, Pedi: Safety not established; extended-release preparations should not be used in children.

Adverse Reactions/Side Effects
CNS: <u>dizziness</u>, confusion, fatigue, headache, syncope, vertigo. **EENT:** blurred vision, diplopia, mydriasis, photophobia, tinnitus. **CV:** HYPOTENSION, TORSADES DE POINTES, arrhythmias, palpitations, tachycardia. **GI:** <u>anorexia</u>, <u>abdominal cramping</u>, <u>diarrhea</u>, <u>nausea</u>, <u>vomiting</u>, drug-induced hepatitis. **Derm:** rash. **Hemat:** AGRANULOCYTOSIS, hemolytic anemia, thrombocytopenia. **Neuro:** ataxia, tremor. **Misc:** fever.

Interactions
Drug-Drug: May ↑ risk of QT interval prolongation when used with **tricyclic antidepressants**, **erythromycin**, **clarithromycin**, **haloperidol**, **sotalol**, or **fluoroquinolones**. ↑ serum **digoxin** levels and may cause toxicity (dose reduction recommended). **Phenytoin**, **phenobarbital**, **carbamazepine** or **rifampin** may ↑ metabolism and ↓ effectiveness. **Cimetidine**, **diltiazem**, **verapamil**, **amiodarone**, **ketoconazole**, **itraconazole**, and **protease inhibitors** ↓ metabolism and may ↑ blood levels. Excretion is delayed and effects ↑ by drugs that alkalinize the urine, including **carbonic anhydrase inhibitors**, **thiazide diuretics**, and **sodium bicarbonate**. Potentiates the effects of **neuromuscular blocking**

✤ = Canadian drug name.
*CAPITALS indicates life-threatening; <u>underlines</u> indicate most frequent.

agents and **warfarin**. Additive hypotension with **antihypertensives**, **nitrates**, and acute ingestion of **alcohol**. May increase **procainamide**, **haloperidol**, **mexiletine** or **tricyclic antidepressant** levels and risk of toxicity. May antagonize **anticholinesterase therapy** in patients with myasthenia gravis. Additive anticholinergic effects may occur with **agents having anticholinergic properties** (including **antihistamines**, **tricyclic antidepressants**). **Drug-Food: Grapefruit juice** ↑ serum levels and effect (avoid concurrent use). **Foods that alkalinize the urine** (see Appendix L) may ↑ serum quinidine levels and the risk of toxicity.

Route/Dosage

Quinidine Gluconate (62% Quinidine)

PO (Adults): 324–972 mg q 8–12 hr.
IV (Adults): 200–400 mg given at a rate ≤10 mg/min until arrhythmia is suppressed, QRS complex widens, bradycardia or hypotension occurs.

Quinidine Sulfate (83% Quinidine)

PO (Adults): *Atrial/ventricular arrhythmias*—200–400 mg q 4–6 hr; may be ↑ to achieve therapeutic response (not to exceed 3–4 g/day).
PO (Children): 6 mg/kg 4–5 times daily.

Availability (generic available)

Quinidine Gluconate

Extended-release tablets: 324 mg. **Solution for Injection:** 80 mg/ml in 10-ml vials.

Quinidine Sulfate

Tablets: 200 mg, 300 mg. **Extended-release tablets:** 300 mg.

NURSING IMPLICATIONS

Assessment

- Monitor ECG, pulse, and blood pressure continuously throughout IV administration and periodically during oral administration. IV administration is usually discontinued if any of the following occur: arrhythmia is resolved, QRS complex widens by 50%, PR or QT intervals are prolonged, or frequent ventricular ectopic beats or tachycardia, bradycardia, or hypotension develops. Patient should remain supine throughout IV administration to minimize hypotension.
- ***Lab Test Considerations:*** Monitor hepatic and renal function, CBC, and serum potassium and magnesium levels periodically during prolonged therapy.
- ***Toxicity and Overdose:*** Serum quinidine levels may be monitored periodically during dose adjustment. Therapeutic serum concentrations are 2–6 mcg/ml. Toxic effects usually occur at concentrations >8 mcg/ml: Signs and symptoms of toxicity or cinchonism include tinnitus, hearing loss, visual disturbances, headache, nausea, and dizziness. These may occur after a single dose, Cardiac signs of toxicity include QRS widening, cardiac asystole, ventricular ectopic beats, idioventricular rhythms (ventricular tachycardia, ventricular fibrillation), paradoxical tachycardia, and torsades de pointes.

Potential Nursing Diagnoses

Decreased cardiac output (Indications)

Implementation

- Do not confuse quinidine with quinine.
- **PO:** Administer with a full glass of water on an empty stomach either 1 hr before or 2 hr after meals for faster absorption. If GI irritation becomes a problem, may be administered with or immediately after meals. Extended-release preparations should be swallowed whole; do not break, crush, or chew.

IV Administration

- **IV:** Use only clear, colorless solution
- **Intermittent Infusion:** ***Diluent:*** Dilute 800 mg of quinidine gluconate (10 ml) in 50 ml of D5W. Infusion is stable for 24 hr at room temperature or 48 hr if refrigerated. ***Concentration:*** 16 mg/ml. ***Rate:*** Administer quinidine gluconate at a rate not to exceed 0.25 mg/kg/min. Administer via infusion pump to ensure accurate dose. Rapid administration may cause peripheral vascular collapse and severe hypotension.
- **Y-Site Compatibility:** amikacin, atropine, bumetanide, calcium gluconate, caspofungin, cimetidine, cyclosporine, digoxin, diltiazem, diphenhydramine, dobutamine, dopamine, doxycycline, enalaprilat, epinephrine, erythromycin, esmolol, famotidine, fenoldopam, fentanyl, fluconazole, gentamicin, granisetron, hydromorphone, imipenem, isoproterenol, labetalol, lidocaine, linezolid, lorazepam, meperidine, metoclopramide, metoprolol, milrinone, morphine, nesiritide, nitroglycerin, norepinephrine, ondansetron, palonosetron, phenylephrine, phytonadione, potassium chloride, procainamide, prochlorperazine, promethazine, propranolol, protamine, ranitidine, succinylcholine, tacrolimus,

tirofiban, tobramycin, vancomycin, vasopressin, verapamil, voriconazole.

- **Y-Site Incompatibility:** acyclovir, aminophylline, ampicillin, ampicillin/sulbactam, aztreonam, cefazolin, cefotaxime, cefoxitin, ceftazidime, ceftizoxime, ceftriaxone, cefuroxime, chloramphenicol, clindamycin, daptomycin, dexamethasone, ertapenem, furosemide, ganciclovir, hydrocortisone sodium succinate, insulin, ketorolac, methylprednisolone sodium succinate, metronidazole, nafcillin, nitroprusside, pantoprazole, penicillin G potassium, phenytoin, piperacillin/tazobacatam, sodium bicarbonate, sulfamethoxazole/trimethoprim, ticarcillin/clavulanate.

Patient/Family Teaching

- Instruct patient to take medication around the clock, exactly as directed, even if feeling well. Take missed doses as soon as remembered if within 2 hr; if remembered later, omit. Do not double doses.
- Instruct patient or family member on how to take pulse. Advise patient to report changes in pulse rate or rhythm to health care professional.
- May cause dizziness or blurred vision. Caution patient to avoid driving or other activities requiring alertness until response to medication is known.
- Inform patient that quinidine may cause increased sensitivity to light. Dark glasses may minimize this effect.
- Advise patient to inform health care professional of medication regimen prior to treatment or surgery.
- Instruct patient not to take Rx, OTC, or herbal products with quinidine without consulting health care professional.
- Advise patient to consult health care professional if symptoms of cinchonism, rash, or dyspnea occur or if diarrhea is severe or persistent.
- Advise patient to carry identification at all times describing disease process and medication regimen.
- Emphasize the importance of routine follow-up exams to monitor progress.

Evaluation/Desired Outcomes

- Decrease or cessation of cardiac arrhythmiass.
- Resolution of malarial infection.

quinine (kwi-nine)

Qualaquin

Classification

Therapeutic: antimalarials

Pregnancy Category C

Indications

Chloroquine-resistant falciparum malaria (alone or with pyrimethamine and a sulfonamide or with a tetracycline; has also be used with clindamycin and mefloquine depending on origin of illness). **Unlabeled uses:** Leg cramps (not recommended due to cardiac side effects.

Action

Disrupts metabolism of the erythrocytic phase of *Plasmodium falciparum*. Increases the refractory period of skeletal muscle, increases the distribution of calcium within muscle fibers, decreases the excitability of motor end-plate regions, resulting in decreased response to repetitive nerve stimulation and acetylcholine. **Therapeutic Effects:** Death of *P. falciparum*.

Pharmacokinetics

Absorption: Rapidly and almost completely (80%) absorbed following oral administration.
Distribution: Varies with condition and patient; does not enter CSF well. Crosses the placenta and enters breast milk.
Protein Binding: >90% in patients with cerebral malaria, pregnant women and children, 85–90% in patients with uncomplicated malaria, 70% in healthy adults.
Metabolism and Excretion: >80% metabolized by the liver; metabolites have less activity than quinine; metabolites excreted in urine. 20% excreted unchanged in urine. Excretion increased in acidic urine.
Half-life: 11 hr (increased in patients with malaria).

TIME/ACTION PROFILE (antimalarial blood levels)

ROUTE	ONSET	PEAK	DURATION
PO	unknown	3.2–5.9 hr	8 hr

Contraindications/Precautions

Contraindicated in: Hypersensitivity to quinine, quinidine or mefloquine; History of previous serious adverse reaction to quinine including thrombotic thrombocytopenic purpura, thrombocytopenia, acute intravascular hemolysis, hemoglobinuria or hemoglobinemia; QTc prolongation or conditions predisposing to QTc prolongation including hypokalemia and bradycardia; Concurrent use of Class IA or Class III antiarrhythmics, mefloquine, pimozide, or macrolide anti-infectives (↑ risk of arrhythmias); G6PD deficiency; Myasthenia gravis; Optic neuritis; OB: Use only if potential maternal benefit outweighs fetal risk; consider alternative therapies); Lactation: Discontinue drug or breastfeeding; Geri: Avoid if possible (↑ risk of arrhythmias).

Use Cautiously in: Recurrent or interrupted malaria therapy; History of arrhythmias, especially QTc prolongation; Atrial fibrillation/flutter (may cause paradoxical increase in ventricular response); Hypoglycemia; History of thrombocytopenic purpura; Pedi: Safety not established for children <16 yr.

Adverse Reactions/Side Effects

CV: CARDIAC ARRHYTHMIAS. **GI:** abdominal cramps/pain, diarrhea, nausea, vomiting, hepatotoxicity. **Derm:** rash. **Endo:** hypoglycemia (↑ in pregnancy). **Hemat:** bleeding, blood dyscrasias, thrombotic thrombocytopenic pupura, thrombocytopenia. **Misc:** cinchonism, hypersensitivity reactions including fever and ANAPHYLAXIS, HEMOLYTIC UREMIC SYNDROME, STEVENS-JOHNSON SYNDROME.

Interactions

Drug-Drug: Concurrent use of Class IA antiarrhythmics (**quinidine procainamide disopyramide** or Class III antiarrhythmics, mefloquine, pimozide, or macrolide anti-infectives ↑ risk of arrhythmias and should be avoided. **Antacids** ↓ absorption. **Cimetidine** ↓ metabolism and may ↑ effects. **Rifampin** and **rifabutin** ↑ metabolism and may ↓ effects; concurrent use with rifampin should be avoided. May ↑ effects of **neuromuscular blocking agents**. May ↑ serum **digoxin** levels; dose adjustments may be necessary. May ↑ risk of hemolytic, ototoxic, or neurotoxic reactions when used concurrently with **agents sharing these toxicities**. Concurrent use with **quinidine** may ↑ risk of adverse cardiovascular reactions. May ↑ risk of bleeding with **warfarin**. Concurrent use with **mefloquine** ↑ risk of seizures and adverse cardiovascular reactions. **Urinary alkalinizers** including **acetazolamide** and **sodium bicarbonate** may ↑ blood levels. Quinine inhibits the CYP3A4 and CYP2D6 enzyme systems and can ↑ levels of **carbamazepine phenobarbital** and **phenytoin**. A similar effect may occur with **dextromethorphan metoprolol flecainide** and **paroxetine**. **Carbamazepine phenobarbital** and **phenytoin** induce metabolism and ↓ levels of quinine; frequent monitoring recommended.

Route/Dosage

PO (Adults): *Malaria*—648 mg every 8 hr for seven days

Renal Impairment

PO (Adults): *Severe chronic renal failure*—648 mg initially, then 324 mg every 12 hr for 7 days.

Availability

Capsules: 325 mg. **Tablets:** 324 mg.

NURSING IMPLICATIONS

Assessment

- **Malaria:** Assess patient for improvement in signs and symptoms of condition daily during therapy.
- ***Lab Test Considerations:*** May cause ↑ urinary 17-ketogenic steroids when metyrapone or Zimmerman method is used.
- ***Toxicity and Overdose:*** Plasma quinine levels of >10 mcg/ml may cause tinnitus and impaired hearing: Signs of toxicity or cinchonism include tinnitus, headache, nausea, and slightly disturbed vision; usually disappear rapidly upon discontinuing quinine.

Potential Nursing Diagnoses

Risk for infection (Indications)

Implementation

- **PO:** Administer with or after meals to minimize GI distress. Aluminum-containing antacids will decrease and delay absorption; avoid concurrent use.

Patient/Family Teaching

- Instruct patient to take medication as directed and continue full course of therapy, even if feeling better. Take missed doses as soon as remembered, unless almost time for the next dose. If more than 4 hr has elapsed since missed dose, wait and take the next dose as scheduled. Do not double doses or take more than recommended. Advise patient to read the "Patient Information" leaflet prior to starting therapy and with each Rx refill.
- Review methods of minimizing exposure to mosquitoes with patients receiving quinine

(use insect repellent, wear long-sleeved shirt and long trousers, use screen or netting).
- Quinine may cause visual changes. Caution patient to avoid driving or other activities requiring alertness until response to medication is known.
- May cause diarrhea, nausea, stomach cramps or pain, vomiting, or ringing in the ears. Advise patient to notify health care professional promptly if these become pronounced.
- Advise patient to stop quinine and notify health care professional of any evidence of allergy (flushing, itching, rash, fever, facial swelling, stomach pain, difficult breathing, ringing in the ears, visual problems).
- Instruct patient to consult health care professional before taking any Rx, OTC, or herbal products with quinine.
- Advise patient to notify health care professional if pregnancy is planned or suspected or if breastfeeding.

Evaluation/Desired Outcomes
- Prevention of or improvement in signs and symptoms of malaria.

quinupristin/dalfopristin
(kwin-oo-**pris**-tin/dal-foe-**pris**-tin)
Synercid

Classification
Therapeutic: anti-infectives
Pharmacologic: streptogramins

Pregnancy Category B

Indications
Treatment of serious or life-threatening infections associated with vancomycin-resistant *Enterococcus faecium* (VREF). Complicated skin/skin structure infections caused by *Staphylococcus aureus* (methicillin, susceptible) or *Streptococcus pyogenes*.

Action
Quinupristin inhibits the late phase of protein synthesis at the level of the bacterial ribosome; dalfopristin inhibits the early phase. **Therapeutic Effects:** Bacteriostatic effect against susceptible organisms. **Spectrum:** Active against vancomycin-resistant and multidrug-resistant strains of *E. faecium*, *S. aureus* (methicillin-susceptible), and *S. pyogenes*. Not active against *E. faecalis*.

Pharmacokinetics
Absorption: IV administration results in complete bioavailability.
Distribution: Unknown.
Protein Binding: Moderate.
Metabolism and Excretion: Both are converted to compounds with additional anti-infective activity; parent drugs and metabolites are mostly excreted in feces (75–77%); 15% of quinupristin and 17% of dalfopristin excreted in urine.
Half-life: *Quinupristin*—0.85 hr; *dalfopristin*—0.7 hr.

TIME/ACTION PROFILE

ROUTE	ONSET	PEAK	DURATION
IV	rapid	end of infusion	8–12 hr

Contraindications/Precautions
Contraindicated in: Hypersensitivity.
Use Cautiously in: Concurrent use of other drugs metabolized by the cytochrome P450 3A4 enzyme system (serious interactions may occur; see Drug-Drug Interactions); Hepatic impairment (dose adjustment may be necessary); Patients with a history of GI disease, especially colitis; Pregnancy, lactation, or children <16 yr (safety not established).

Adverse Reactions/Side Effects
CNS: headache. **CV:** thrombophlebitis. **GI:** PSEUDOMEMBRANOUS COLITIS, diarrhea, nausea, vomiting. **Derm:** pruritus, rash. **Local:** edema/inflammation/pain at infusion site, infusion site reactions. **Misc:** allergic reactions including ANAPHYLAXIS, pain.

Interactions
Drug-Drug: Inhibits the cytochrome P450 3A4 drug metabolizing enzyme system; inhibits metabolism of **cyclosporine**, **midazolam**, and **nifedipine** and ↑ risk of toxicity (careful monitoring required). Similar effects may be expected with concurrent use of **delavirdine**, **nevirapine**, **indinavir**, **ritonavir**, **vinca alkaloids**, **docetaxel**, **paclitaxel**, **diazepam**, **verapamil**, **diltiazem**, **HMG CoA reductase inhibitors**, **tacrolimus**, **methylprednisolone**, **carbamazepine**, **quinidine**, **lidocaine**, and **disopyramide**.

Route/Dosage

IV (Adults): *Vancomycin-resistant E. faecium*—7.5 mg/kg q 8 hr for at least 7 days; *complicated skin/skin structure infections*—7.5 mg/kg q 12 hr for at least 7 days.

Availability

Powder for injection: 500 mg (150 mg quinupristin and 350 mg dalfopristin in 10-ml vials), 600 mg (180 mg quinupristin and 420 mg dalfopristin in 10-ml vials).

NURSING IMPLICATIONS

Assessment

- Assess patient for infection (vital signs; appearance of wound, sputum, urine, and stool; WBC) at beginning of and throughout therapy.
- Obtain specimens for culture and sensitivity before initiating therapy. First dose may be given before receiving results.
- Monitor patient for pain or inflammation at the infusion site frequently throughout infusion. Increasing the volume of diluent from 250 ml to 500 ml or 750 ml or infusing via a peripherally inserted central catheter or central venous catheter may be required.
- Observe patient for signs and symptoms of anaphylaxis (rash, pruritus, laryngeal edema, wheezing). Discontinue drug and notify physician or other health care professional immediately if these problems occur. Keep epinephrine, an antihistamine, and resuscitation equipment close by in case of an anaphylactic reaction.
- Assess patient for myalgia and arthralgia after infusion. May be severe. Reducing dose frequency to every 12 hr may decrease pain. Symptoms usually resolve upon discontinuation of medication.
- ***Lab Test Considerations:*** May cause ↑ serum total bilirubin concentrations.

Potential Nursing Diagnoses

Risk for infection (Indications, Side Effects)
Diarrhea (Adverse Reactions)

Implementation

IV Administration

- **Intermittent Infusion:** ***Diluent:*** Reconstitute the 500-mg vial with 5 ml and the 600 mg vial with 6 mL of D5W or sterile water for injection, respectively, for a concentration of 100 mg/ml. Avoid shaking to prevent foam formation. Allow solution to sit until all foam has disappeared. Dilute further with 250 ml of D5W (100 ml can be used for central line administration). May dilute in 500 ml or 750 ml of D5W if severe venous irritation occurs after peripheral administration. Reconstituted vials should be used within 30 min. Infusion is stable for 5 hr at room temperature or 54 hr if refrigerated. ***Rate:*** Infuse over 60 min. Flush line before and after infusion with D5W.
- **Y-Site Compatibility:** amikacin, amiodarone, anidulafungin, aztreonam, caspofungin, cimetidine, ciprofloxacin, cyclosporine, daptomycin, diltiazem, diphenhydramine, dolasetron, doxycycline, droperidol, enalaprilat, epinephrine, esmolol, fenoldopam, fentanyl, fluconazole, granisetron, haloperidol, hydromorphone, hydroxyzine, isoproterenol, labetalol, levofloxacin, lidocaine, linezolid, lorazepam, meperidine, metoclopramide, metoprolol, midazolam, milrinone, morphine, nicardipine, nitroglycerin, ondansetron, palonosetron, pancuronium, phenylephrine, potassium chloride, procainamide, prochlorperazine, promethazine, propranolol, tacrolimus, tirofiban, tobramycin, verapamil, voriconazole.
- **Y-Site Incompatibility:** acyclovir, aminophylline, ampicillin, ampicillin/sulbacatam, azithromycin, bumetanide, calcium chloride, calcium gluconate, cefazolin, cefepime, cefotaxime, ceftazidime, ceftizoxime, ceftriaxone, cefuroxime, clindamycin, dexamethasone sodium phosphate, diazepam, digoxin, ertapenem, furosemide, ganciclovir, heparin, hydrocortisone sodium succinate, imipenem/cilastatin, insulin, ketorolac, meropenem, methylprednisolone sodium succinate, nitroprusside, pantoprazole, phenytoin, piperacillin/tazobactam, potassium phosphate, ranitidine, sodium bicarbonate, trimethoprim/sulfamethoxazole, ticarcillin/clavulanate.
- **Solution Incompatibility:** 0.9% NaCl.

Patient/Family Teaching

- Instruct patient to notify health care professional if fever and diarrhea develop, especially if stool contains blood, pus, or mucus. Advise patient not to treat diarrhea without consulting health care professional.

Evaluation/Desired Outcomes

- Resolution of signs and symptoms of infection. Length of time for complete resolution depends on the organism and site of infection.

rabeprazole (ra-bep-ra-zole)
Aciphex, ♣Pariet

Classification
Therapeutic: antiulcer agents
Pharmacologic: proton-pump inhibitors

Pregnancy Category B

Indications
Gastroesophageal reflux disease (GERD). Duodenal ulcers (including combination therapy with clarithromycin and amoxicillin to eradicate *h. pylori* and prevent recurrence). Pathological hypersecretory conditions, including Zollinger-Ellison syndrome.

Action
Binds to an enzyme in the presence of acidic gastric pH, preventing the final transport of hydrogen ions into the gastric lumen. **Therapeutic Effects:** Diminished accumulation of acid in the gastric lumen, with lessened acid reflux. Healing of duodenal ulcers and esophagitis. Decreased acid secretion in hypersecretory conditions.

Pharmacokinetics
Absorption: Delayed-release tablet is designed to allow rabeprazole, which is not stable in gastric acid, to pass through the stomach intact. Subsequently 52% is absorbed after oral administration.
Distribution: Unknown.
Protein Binding: 96.3%.
Metabolism and Excretion: Mostly metabolized by the liver (hepatic cytochrome P450 3A and 2C19 enzyme systems); 10% excreted in feces; remainder excreted in urine as inactive metabolites.
Half-life: 1–2 hr.

TIME/ACTION PROFILE (acid suppression)

ROUTE	ONSET	PEAK	DURATION
PO	within 1 hr	unknown	24 hr†

†Suppression continues to increase over the first week of therapy

Contraindications/Precautions
Contraindicated in: Hypersensitivity to rabeprazole or related drugs (benzimidazoles).
Use Cautiously in: Severe hepatic impairment (dosage reduction may be necessary); Geri: Increased risk of hip fractures in patients using high-doses for >1 year; Pregnancy, lactation, or children (breastfeeding not recommended; use in pregnancy only if needed; safety not established).

Adverse Reactions/Side Effects
CNS: dizziness, headache, malaise. **GI:** abdominal pain, constipation, diarrhea, nausea. **Derm:** photosensitivity, rash. **MS:** neck pain. **Misc:** allergic reactions, chills, fever.

Interactions
Drug-Drug: Rabeprazole is metabolized by the CYP450 enzyme system and may interact with other drugs metabolized by this sytem. ↓ blood levels of **ketoconazole**. ↑ blood levels of **digoxin**. May alter the effects of **drugs whose absorption is pH dependent**. May increase the risk of bleeding with **warfarin** (monitor INR/PT).

Route/Dosage
PO (Adults): *GERD, duodenal ulcers*—20 mg once daily; *prevention of duodenal ulcer recurrence*—20 mg twice daily for 7 days with amoxicillin 1000 mg twice daily for 7 days and clarithromycin 500 mg twice daily for 7 days; *hypersecretory conditions*—60 mg once daily initially, may be adjusted as needed and continued as necessary; doses up to 100 mg daily or 60 mg twice daily have been used.

Availability
Delayed-release tablets: 20 mg. **Cost:** 20 mg $419.97/90.

NURSING IMPLICATIONS

Assessment
- Assess routinely for epigastric or abdominal pain and frank or occult blood in the stool, emesis, or gastric aspirate.
- ***Lab Test Considerations:*** Monitor CBC with differential periodically during therapy.

Potential Nursing Diagnoses
Acute pain (Indications)

Implementation
- **PO:** Administer doses before meals, preferably in the morning. Tablets should be swallowed whole; do not crush, break, or chew.

Patient/Family Teaching
- Instruct patient to take medication as directed for the full course of therapy, even if feel-

ing better. Take missed doses as soon as remembered but not if almost time for next dose. Do not double doses.

- May cause occasional drowsiness or dizziness. Caution patient to avoid driving or other activities requiring alertness until response to medication is known.
- Advise patient to avoid alcohol, products containing aspirin or NSAIDs, and foods that may cause an increase in GI irritation.
- Caution patients to wear sunscreen and protective clothing to prevent photosensitivity reactions.
- Advise patient to report onset of black, tarry stools; diarrhea; abdominal pain; or persistent headache to health care professional promptly.

Evaluation/Desired Outcomes

- Decrease in abdominal pain or prevention of gastric irritation and bleeding. Healing of duodenal ulcers can be seen on x-ray examination or endoscopy.
- Decrease in symptoms of GERD. Therapy is continued for 4–8 wk after initial episode.

raloxifene (ra-lox-i-feen)

Evista

Classification

Therapeutic: bone resorption inhibitors

Pharmacologic: selective estrogen receptor modulators

Pregnancy Category X

Indications

Treatment and prevention of osteoporosis in postmenopausal women. Reduction of the risk of breast cancer in postmenopausal women with osteoporosis and those at high risk for invasive breast cancer.

Action

Binds to estrogen receptors, producing estrogen-like effects on bone, resulting in reduced resorption of bone and decreased bone turnover. **Therapeutic Effects:** Prevention of osteoporosis in patients at risk. Decreased risk of breast cancer.

Pharmacokinetics

Absorption: Although well absorbed (>60%), after oral administration, extensive first-pass metabolism results in 2% bioavailability.

Distribution: Highly bound to plasma proteins; remainder of distribution unknown.

Protein Binding: Highly bound to plasma proteins.

Metabolism and Excretion: Extensively metabolized by the liver; undergoes enterohepatic cycling; excreted primarily in feces.

Half-life: 27.7 hr.

TIME/ACTION PROFILE (effects on bone turnover)

ROUTE	ONSET	PEAK	DURATION
PO	unknown	3 mo	unknown

Contraindications/Precautions

Contraindicated in: Hypersensitivity; History of thromboembolic events; OB: Women with childbearing potential; OB, Pedi: Pregnancy, lactation, or children.

Use Cautiously in: Potential immobilization (increased risk of thromboembolic events); History of stroke or transient ischemic attack; Atrial fibrillation; Hypertension; Cigarette smoking.

Adverse Reactions/Side Effects

CV: STROKE, deep vein thrombosis, pulmonary embolism, retinal vein thrombosis. **MS:** leg cramps. **Misc:** hot flashes.

Interactions

Drug-Drug: Cholestyramine ↓ absorption (avoid concurrent use). May alter effects of **warfarin** and other **highly protein-bound drugs**. Concurrent systemic **estrogen** therapy is not recommended.

Route/Dosage

PO (Adults): 60 mg once daily.

Availability

Tablets: 60 mg. **Cost:** $269.96/90.

NURSING IMPLICATIONS

Assessment

- Assess patient for bone mineral density with x-ray, serum, and urine bone turnover markers (bone-specific alkaline phosphatase, osteocalcin, and collagen breakdown products) before and periodically during therapy.
- ***Lab Test Considerations:*** May cause ↑ apolipoprotein A-I and reduced serum total cholesterol, LDL cholesterol, fibrinogen, apolipoprotein B, and lipoprotein.
- May cause ↑ hormone-binding globulin (sex steroid-binding globulin, thyroxine-

binding globulin, corticosteroid-binding globulin) with ↑ total hormone concentrations.
- May cause small ↓ in serum total calcium, inorganic phosphate, total protein, and albumin.
- May also cause slight decrease in platelet count.

Potential Nursing Diagnoses
Risk for injury (Indications)

Implementation
- **PO:** May be administered without regard to meals.
- Calcium supplementation should be added to diet if daily intake is inadequate.

Patient/Family Teaching
- Instruct patient to take raloxifene as directed. Discuss the importance of adequate calcium and vitamin D intake or supplementation. Advise patient to discontinue smoking and alcohol consumption.
- Emphasize the importance of regular weight-bearing exercise. Advise patient that raloxifene should be discontinued at least 72 hr before and during prolonged immobilization (recovery from surgery, prolonged bedrest). Instruct patient to avoid prolonged restrictions of movement during travel because of the increased risk of venous thrombosis.
- Advise patient that raloxifene will not reduce hot flashes or flushes associated with estrogen deficiency and may cause hot flashes.
- OB: Advise patient that raloxifene may have teratogenic effects. Instruct patient to notify health care provider immediately if pregnancy is planned or suspected.
- Instruct patient to read the patient package insert when initiating therapy and again with each prescription refill.

Evaluation/Desired Outcomes
- Prevention of osteoporosis in postmenopausal women.
- Reduced risk of breast cancer in postmenopausal women with osteoporosis and those at high risk for invasive breast cancer.

ramelteon (ra-**mel**-tee-on)
Rozerem

Classification
Therapeutic: sedative/hypnotics
Pharmacologic: melatonin receptor agonists

Pregnancy Category C

Indications
Treatment of insomnia characterized by difficult sleep onset.

Action
Activates melatonin receptors, which promotes maintenance of circadian rhythm, a part of the sleep-wake cycle. **Therapeutic Effects:** Easier onset of sleep.

Pharmacokinetics
Absorption: Well absorbed (84%), but bioavailability is low (1.8%) due to extensive first pass liver metabolism. Absorption in increased by a high fat meal.
Distribution: Widely distributed to body tissues.
Metabolism and Excretion: Extensively metabolized by the liver; mainly by CYP1A2 enzyme system. Metabolites are excreted mostly in urine (88%); 4% excreted in feces.
Half-life: 1–2.6 hr.

TIME/ACTION PROFILE (blood levels)

ROUTE	ONSET	PEAK	DURATION
PO	rapid	30–90 min	unknown

Contraindications/Precautions
Contraindicated in: Hypersensitivity; Severe hepatic impairment; Concurrent fluvoxamine; OB: lactation; Pedi: safety not established.
Use Cautiously in: Depression or history of suicidal ideation; Moderate hepatic impairment; Concurrent use of CYP3A4 inhibitors, such as ketoconazole; Concurrent use of CYP2C9 inhibitors, such as fluconazole; OB: use only if maternal benefit outweighs fetal risk.

Adverse Reactions/Side Effects
CNS: abnormal thinking, behavior changes, dizziness, fatigue, hallucinations, headache, insomnia (worsened), sleep–driving. **GI:** nausea. **Endo:** ↑ prolactin levels, ↓ testosterone levels.

Interactions
Drug-Drug: Blood levels and effects are ↑ by **fluvoxamine**, potent inhibitor of the CYP1A2

R

enzyme system; concurrent use is contraindicated. Levels and effects may be ↓ by Id **rifampin**, an inducer of CYP enzymes. Concurrent use of CYP3A4 inhibitors, such as **ketoconazole** may ↑ levels and effects; use cautiously. Concurrent use of CYP2C9 inhibitors, such as **fluconazole** may ↑ levels and effects; use cautiously. ↑ risk of excessive CNS depression with other CNS depressants including **alcohol**, **benzodiazepines**, **opioids**, and other **sedative/hypnotics**.

Route/Dosage

PO (Adults): 8 mg within 30 min of going to bed.

Availability

Tablets: 8 mg.

NURSING IMPLICATIONS

Assessment

- Assess sleep patterns before and periodically throughout therapy.

Potential Nursing Diagnoses

Insomnia (Indications)
Risk for injury (Side Effects)

Implementation

- Do not administer with or immediately after a high fat meal.
- Before administering, reduce external stimuli and provide comfort measures to increase effectiveness of medication.
- **PO:** Administer within 30 min prior to going to bed.

Patient/Family Teaching

- Instruct patient to take ramelteon as directed, within 30 minutes of going to bed and to confine activities to those necessary to prepare for bed.
- Causes drowsiness. Caution patient to avoid driving and other activities requiring alertness until response to medication is known.
- Caution patient to avoid concurrent use of alcohol or other CNS depressants.

Evaluation/Desired Outcomes

- Relief of insomnia.

---

ramipril, See ANGIOTENSIN-CONVERTING ENZYME (ACE) INHIBITORS.

---

ranitidine, See HISTAMINE H_2 ANTAGONISTS.

---

ranolazine (ra-nole-a-zeen)

Ranexa

Classification
Therapeutic: antianginals

Pregnancy Category C

Indications

Chronic angina pectoris not adequately controlled by conventional antianginals (amlodipine, beta blockers, nitrates).

Action

Does not decrease blood pressure or heart rate; remainder of mechanism is not known. **Therapeutic Effects:** Decreased frequency of angina.

Pharmacokinetics

Absorption: Highly variable.
Distribution: Unknown.
Metabolism and Excretion: Metabolized in the gut (P-glycoprotein) and by the liver (primarily CYP3A and less by CYP2D6); <5% excreted unchanged in urine and feces.
Half-life: 7 hr

TIME/ACTION PROFILE (blood levels)

ROUTE	ONSET	PEAK	DURATION
PO	unknown	2–5 hr	12 hr

Contraindications/Precautions

Contraindicated in: Hypersensitivity; Pre-existing QTc prolongation or concurrent use of other medications causing QTc prolongation; Potent inhibitors of CYP3A (ketoconazole, verapamil, diltiazem); Hepatic impairment; Lactation.
Use Cautiously in: Geri: Patients >75 yr (↑ risk of adverse reactions; Severe renal impairment (may ↑ blood pressure); OB: Pregnancy (use only when use outweighs risk to fetus); Pedi: Children (safety not established).

Adverse Reactions/Side Effects

CNS: dizziness, headache. **EENT:** tinnitus. **CV:** palpitations, QTc prolongation. **GI:** abdominal pain, constipation, dry mouth, nausea, vomiting.

Interactions

Drug-Drug: ↑ blood levels of **simvastatin** and its active metabolite. Partially inhibits

CYP2D6 enzyme system; may ↓ metabolism and increase effects of **tricyclic antidepressants** and **antipsychotics**, dosage adjustments may be necessary. Inhibits P-glycoprotein (P-gp) which may lead to ↑ **digoxin** levels; dosage adjustment may be required.

Route/Dosage

PO (Adults): 500 mg twice daily initially, may be increased to 1000 mg twice daily.

Availability

Extended-release tablet: 500 mg.

NURSING IMPLICATIONS

Assessment

- Assess location, duration, intensity, and precipitating factors of anginal pain.
- Monitor ECG at baseline and periodically during therapy to evaluate effects on QT interval.
- ***Lab Test Considerations:*** May cause ↑ serum creatinine. Usually has a rapid onset, but does not progress during therapy and is reversible with discontinuation of ranolazine.
- May cause transient eosinophilia.
- May cause small mean ↓ in hematocrit.

Potential Nursing Diagnoses

Ineffective tissue perfusion (Indications, Indications)
Activity intolerance (Indications)

Implementation

- Ranolazine should be used in combination with amlodipine, beta blockers, or nitrates.
- Do not administer with grapefruit juice or grapefruit products.
- **PO:** May be administered without regard to food. Tablets should be swallowed whole; do not crush, break, or chew.

Patient/Family Teaching

- Instruct patient to take ranolazine as directed. If a dose is missed, take the usual dose at the next scheduled time; do not double doses. Explain to patient that ranolazine is used for chronic therapy and will not help an acute angina episode.
- Advise patient to avoid grapefruit juice and grapefruit products when taking ranolazine.
- May cause dizziness and light-headedness. Caution patient to avoid driving and other activities requiring alertness until response to medication is known.
- Inform patient that ranolazine may cause changes in the ECG. Patient should inform health care professional if they have a personal or family history of QTc prolongation, congenital long QT syndrome, or proarrhythmic conditions such as hypokalemia.
- Advise patient to consult health care professional prior to taking other Rx, OTC, or herbal products.

Evaluation/Desired Outcomes

- Decrease in frequency of angina attacks.

rasagiline (raza-ji-leen)

Azilect

Classification
Therapeutic: antiparkinson agents
Pharmacologic: monoamine oxidase type B inhibitors

Pregnancy Category C

Indications

Parkinson's disease (monotherapy and adjunctive to levodopa).

Action

Irreversibly inactivates monoamine oxidase (MAO) by binding to it at type B (brain sites); inactivation of MAO leads to increased amounts of dopamine available in the CNS. Differs from selegiline by its nonamphetamine characteristics. **Therapeutic Effects:** Improvement in symptoms of Parkinson's disease, allowing increase in function.

Pharmacokinetics

Absorption: 36% absorbed following oral administration.
Distribution: Readily crosses the blood-brain barrier.
Metabolism and Excretion: Extensively metabolized by the liver (CYP1A2 enzyme) to an inactive metabolite); less than 1% excreted in urine.
Half-life: 1.3 hr; does not correlate with duration of MAO-B inhibition.

TIME/ACTION PROFILE

ROUTE	ONSET	PEAK	DURATION
PO	rapid	1 hr	40 days*

*Recovery of MAO-B function.

Contraindications/Precautions

Contraindicated in: Hypersensitivity; Concurrent meperidine, tramadol, propoxyphene, methadone, sympathomimetic amines, dextromethorphan, mirtazapine, cyclobenzaprine, cocaine or St. John's wort; Moderate to severe hepatic impairment; Elective surgery requiring general anesthesia; allow 14 days after discontinuation; Pheochromocytoma.

Use Cautiously in: Mild hepatic impairment (↑ blood levels); OB: Pregnancy and lactation, use only if maternal benefit outweighs fetal risk; may inhibit lactation; Pedi: Safety in children has not been established.

Adverse Reactions/Side Effects

CNS: depression, dizziness, hallucinations, malaise, vertigo. **EENT:** conjunctivitis, rhinitis. **Resp:** asthma. **CV:** chest pain, postural hypotension (may ↑ levodopa-induced hypotension), syncope. **GI:** anorexia, dizziness, dyspepsia, gastroenteritis, vomiting. **GU:** albuminuria, ↓ libido. **Derm:** alopecia, ecchymosis, ↑ melanoma risk, rash. **Endo:** weight loss. **Hemat:** leukopenia. **MS:** arthralgia, arthritis, neck pain. **Neuro:** dyskinesia (may ↑ levodopa-induced dyskinesia), paresthesia. **Misc:** allergic reactions, flu-like syndrome, ↑ fall risk, fever.

Interactions

Drug-Drug: ciprofloxacin and other **inhibitors of the CYP1A2 enzyme** ↑ rasagiline levels; dose adjustment is recommended. **Meperidine** has resulted in life-threatening reactions when used with other MAO inhibitors; wait at least 14 days after discontinuation of rasagiline to initiate meperidine. Similar reactions may occur with **tramadol**, **methadone**, **propoxyphene**; concurrent use should be avoided. Concurrent use with **dextromethorphan** may result in psychosis/bizarre behavior and should be avoided. Risk of adverse reactions in ↑ with **mirtazapine** and **cyclobenzapine**; concurrent use should be avoided. Hypertensive crisis may occur with **sympathomimetic amines** including **amphetamines**, **cold products**, and some **weight loss products** containing **vasoconstrictors** such as **pseudoephedrine**, **phenylephrine**, or **ephedrine**; avoid concurrent use. Risk of CNS toxicity is ↑ with **tricyclic antidepressants**, **SSRI antidepressants**, **NSRI antidepressants**, and other **MAO inhibitors**; rasagiline should be discontinued at least 14 days prior to initiation of antidepressants (**fluoxetine** should be discontinued at least 5 weeks prior to rasagiline therapy). Hypertensive crisis may also occur when rasagiline is used with **other MAO inhibitors**; allow at least 14 days between usage.

Drug-Natural Products: Risk of toxicity is ↑ with **St. John's wort.**

Drug-Food: Ingestion of **tyramine-rich foods or beverages** may result in life-threatening hypertensive crisis.

Route/Dosage

PO (Adults): *Monotherapy*—1 mg daily; *adjunct therapy*—0.5 mg daily, may be increased to 1 mg daily; *concurrent ciprofloxacin or other CYP1A2 inhibitors*—0.5 mg daily.

Hepatic Impairment

PO (Adults): *Mild hepatic impairment*—1 mg daily; *adjunct therapy*—0.5 mg daily, may be increased to 1 mg daily.

Availability

Tablets: 0.5 mg, 1 mg.

NURSING IMPLICATIONS

Assessment

- Assess signs and symptoms of Parkinson's disease (tremor, muscle weakness and rigidity, ataxic gait) prior to and during therapy.
- Monitor blood pressure periodically during therapy.
- Assess skin for melanomas periodically during therapy.
- ***Lab Test Considerations:*** May cause albuminuria, leukopenia, and abnormal liver function tests.
- ***Toxicity and Overdose:*** Concurrent ingestion of tyramine-rich foods and many medications may result in a life-threatening hypertensive crisis. Signs and symptoms of hypertensive crisis include chest pain, tachycardia or bradycardia, severe headache, neck stiffness or soreness, nausea and vomiting, sweating, photosensitivity, and enlarged pupils.

Potential Nursing Diagnoses

Impaired physical mobility (Indications)
Risk for injury (Indications, Side Effects)

Implementation

- If used in combination with levodopa, a reduction in levodopa dose may be considered based on individual results.
- **PO:** Administer once daily.

Patient/Family Teaching

- Instruct patient to take rasagiline as directed. Missed doses should be omitted and next dose taken at usual time the following day. Do not double doses.

- Caution patient to avoid alcohol, CNS depressants, and foods or beverages containing tyramine (see Appendix L) during and for at least 2 wk after therapy has been discontinued; they may precipitate a hypertensive crisis. Contact health care professional immediately if symptoms of hypertensive crisis develop.
- Instruct patient to consult health care professional before taking any Rx, OTC, or herbal products. Caution patient to avoid use of St. John's Wort and the analgesics meperidine, propoxyphene, tramadol, or methadone during therapy.
- Caution patient to avoid elective surgery requiring general anesthesia, cocaine, or local anesthesia containing sympathomimetic vasoconstrictors within 14 days of discontinuing rasagiline. If surgery is necessary sooner, benzodiazepines, mivacurium, rapacuronium, fentanyl, morphine, and codeine may be used cautiously.
- May cause dizziness or drowsiness. Caution patient to avoid driving and other activities requiring alertness until response to medication is known.
- Caution patient to change positions slowly to minimize orthostatic hypotension. Geriatric patients are at increased risk for this side effect.
- Advise patient to monitor for melanomas frequently and on a regular basis.
- Advise patient to notify health care professional immediately if severe headache, neck stiffness, heart racing or palpitations, occur.

Evaluation/Desired Outcomes

- Improvement in symptoms of Parkinson's disease, allowing increase in function.

rasburicase (ras-**byoor**-i-case)

Elitek

Classification

Therapeutic: antigout agents, antihyperuricemics

Pharmacologic: enzymes

Pregnancy Category C

Indications

Initial management of increased uric acid levels in children with leukemia, lymphoma or other malignancies who are being treated with antineoplastics which are expected to produce hyperuricemia.

Action

An enzyme which promotes the conversion of uric acid to allantoin, an inactive, water-soluble compound. Produced by recombinant DNA technology. **Therapeutic Effects:** Decreased sequelae of hyperuricemia (nephropathy, arthropathy).

Pharmacokinetics

Absorption: IV administration results in complete bioavailability.

Distribution: Unknown.

Metabolism and Excretion: Unknown.

Half-life: 18 hr.

TIME/ACTION PROFILE (decrease in uric acid)

ROUTE	ONSET	PEAK	DURATION
IV	rapid	unknown	4–24 hr

Contraindications/Precautions

Contraindicated in: G6–PD deficiency; Previous allergic reaction, hemolysis or methemoglobinemia from rasburicase; Lactation.

Use Cautiously in: OB: Pregnancy (use only if clearly needed).

Adverse Reactions/Side Effects

CNS: headache. **Resp:** respiratory distress. **GI:** abdominal pain, constipation, diarrhea, nausea, vomiting, mucositis. **Derm:** rash. **Hemat:** HEMOLYSIS, METHEMOGLOBINEMIA, neutropenia. **Misc:** hypersensitivity reactions including ANAPHYLAXIS, fever, sepsis.

Interactions

Drug-Drug: None known.

Route/Dosage

IV (Children): 0.15 or 0.2 mg/kg daily as a single dose for 5 days.

Availability

lyophilized powder for reconstitution: 1.5 mg/vial in cartons of 3 vials with specific diluent[Rx].

NURSING IMPLICATIONS

Assessment

- Monitor patients for signs of allergic reactions and anaphylaxis (chest pain, dyspnea, hypotension, urticaria). If these signs occur, rasburicase should be immediately and permanently discontinued.
- ***Lab Test Considerations:*** Monitor patients for hemolysis. Screen patients at higher risk for G6PD deficiency (patients of African American or Mediterranean ancestry) prior to therapy. If hemolysis occurs, discontinue and do not restart rasburicase.
- Monitor patients for methemoglobinemia. Discontinue rasburicase and do not restart in patients who develop methemoglobinemia.
- May cause spuriously low uric acid levels in blood samples left at room temperature. Collect blood for uric acid levels in pre-chilled tubes containing heparin and immediately immerse and maintain in an ice water bath. Uric acid must be analyzed in plasma. Plasma samples must be assayed within 4 hr of collection.

Potential Nursing Diagnoses

Deficient knowledge, related to medication regimen (Patient/Family Teaching)

Implementation

- Chemotherapy is initiated 4–24 hr after first dose of rasburicase.

IV Administration

- **Intermittent Infusion:** Determine number of vials of rasburicase needed based on patient's weight and dose/kg. ***Diluent:*** Reconstitute in diluent provided. Add 1 ml of diluent provided to each vial and mix by swirling very gently. Do not shake or vortex. Solution should be clear and colorless. Do not use solutions that are discolored or contain particulate matter. ***Concentration:*** Remove dose from reconstituted vials and inject into infusion bag of 0.9% NaCl for a final total volume of 50 ml. Administer within 24 hr of reconstitution. Store reconstituted or diluted solution in refrigerator for up to 24 hr. ***Rate:*** Administer over 30 min. Do not administer as a bolus.
- **Y-Site Incompatibility:** Infuse through a separate line. Do not use a filter with infusion. If separate line is not possible, flush line with at least 15 ml of 0.9% NaCl prior to rasburicase infusion.

Patient/Family Teaching

- Inform patient and family of purpose of rasburicase infusion.

Evaluation/Desired Outcomes

- Decrease in plasma uric acid levels in pediatric patients receiving antineoplastics expected to result in tumor lysis and subsequent elevation of plasma uric acid levels.

repaglinide (re-pag-gli-nide)

✱Gluconorm, Prandin

Classification
Therapeutic: antidiabetics
Pharmacologic: meglitinides

Pregnancy Category C

Indications

Type 2 diabetes mellitus, with diet and exercise; may be used with metformin, rosigliazone, or pioglitazone.

Action

Stimulates the release of insulin from pancreatic beta cells by closing potassium channels, which results in the opening of calcium channels in beta cells. This is followed by release of insulin. **Therapeutic Effects:** Lowering of blood glucose levels.

Pharmacokinetics

Absorption: Well absorbed (56%) following oral administration.
Distribution: Unknown.
Protein Binding: >98%.
Metabolism and Excretion: Mostly metabolized by the liver; metabolites are excreted primarily in feces.
Half-life: 1 hr.

TIME/ACTION PROFILE

ROUTE	ONSET	PEAK	DURATION
PO	within 30 min	60–90 min	<4 hr

Contraindications/Precautions

Contraindicated in: Hypersensitivity; Lactation; Diabetic ketoacidosis; Insulin-dependent diabetes.
Use Cautiously in: Impaired liver function (longer dosing intervals may be necessary); Severe renal impairment (dosage reduction recommended); Geri: Consider age-related decrease in renal/hepatic/cardiovascular function; OB, Pedi: Pregnancy and children

(safety not established; insulin recommended to control diabetes during pregnancy).

Adverse Reactions/Side Effects

CV: angina, chest pain. **Endo:** HYPOGLYCEMIA, hyperglycemia.

Interactions

Drug-Drug: Ketoconazole, **miconazole**, **gemofibrozil**, **itraconazole**, and **erythromycin** may ↓ metabolism and ↑ risk of hypoglycemia. Effects may also be ↑ by **NSAIDs**, **hormonal contraceptives**, **simvastatin**, **sulfonamides**, **chloramphenicol**, **warfarin**, **probenecid**, **MAO inhibitors**, and **beta blockers**. Effects may be ↓ by **corticosteroids**, **phenothiazines**, **thyroid preparations**, **estrogens**, **hormonal contraceptives**, **phenytoin**, **nicotinic acid**, **sympathomimetics**, **isoniazid**, and **calcium channel blockers**.

Drug-Natural Products: Glucosamine may worsen blood glucose control. **Chromium** and **coenzyme Q-10** may produce ↑ hypoglycemic effects.

Route/Dosage

PO (Adults): 0.5–4 mg taken before meals (not to exceed 16 mg/day)

Renal Impairment

PO (Adults): *Severe renal impairment*—start with 0.5 mg/day and titrate carefully.

Availability

Tablets: 0.5 mg, 1 mg, 2 mg. **Cost:** 0.5 mg $385.64/270, 1 mg $377.70/270, 2 mg $377.97/270.

NURSING IMPLICATIONS

Assessment

- Observe patient for signs and symptoms of hypoglycemic reactions (abdominal pain, sweating, hunger, weakness, dizziness, headache, tremor, tachycardia, anxiety). Hypoglycemia may be difficult to recognize in geriatric patients and in patients taking beta blockers. Hypoglycemia is more likely to occur with insufficient caloric intake, following intense prolonged exercise, or when alcohol or more than one hypoglycemic agent is used.
- ***Lab Test Considerations:*** Monitor fasting serum glucose and glycosylated hemoglobin periodically during therapy to evaluate effectiveness.

Potential Nursing Diagnoses

Imbalanced nutrition: more than body requirements (Indications)
Noncompliance (Patient/Family Teaching)

Implementation

- Patients stabilized on a diabetic regimen who are exposed to stress, fever, trauma, infection, or surgery may require administration of insulin. Withhold repaglinide and reinstitute after resolution of acute episode.
- Repaglinide therapy should be temporarily discontinued from patients requiring surgery involving restricted intake of food and fluids.
- There is no fixed dose of repaglinide. Dose is based on periodic monitoring of blood glucose and long-term response is based on glycolysated hemoglobin levels. If adequate response is not achieved, metformin may be added to regimen. If combination therapy is unsuccessful, oral hypoglycemic therapy may need to be discontinued and replaced with insulin.
- When replacing other oral hypoglycemic agents, repaglinide may be started on the day following discontinuation of the other agent. Monitor blood glucose closely. Discontinuation of long-acting oral hypoglycemics may require monitoring for a week or more.
- Short-term repaglinide therapy may be used for patients well controlled with diet experiencing transient loss of control.
- **PO:** Administer up to 30 min before meals. Patients who skip a meal or add an extra meal should skip or add a dose, respectively, for that meal.

Patient/Family Teaching

- Instruct patient to take repaglinide before each meal, exactly as directed.
- Explain to patient that repaglinide helps control hyperglycemia but does not cure diabetes. Therapy is usually long term.
- Encourage patient to follow prescribed diet, medication, and exercise regimen to prevent hyperglycemic or hypoglycemic episodes.
- Review signs of hypoglycemia and hyperglycemia with patient. If hypoglycemia occurs, advise patient to take a glass of orange juice or 2–3 tsp of sugar, honey, or corn syrup dissolved in water, and notify health care professional.

R

- Instruct patient in proper testing of blood glucose. These tests should be monitored closely during periods of stress or illness and a health care professional notified if significant changes occur.
- Caution patient to avoid taking other Rx, OTC or herbal products, or alcohol during repaglinide therapy without consulting health care professional.
- Insulin is the recommended method of controlling blood glucose during pregnancy. Counsel female patients to use a form of contraception other than oral contraceptives and to notify health care professional promptly if pregnancy is planned or suspected.
- Advise patient to inform health care professional of medication regimen prior to treatment or surgery.
- Advise patient to carry a form of sugar (sugar packets, candy) and identification describing disease process and medication regimen at all times.
- Emphasize the importance of routine follow-up exams and regular testing of blood glucose and glycosylated hemoglobin.

Evaluation/Desired Outcomes

- Control of blood glucose levels without the appearance of hypoglycemic or hyperglycemic episodes.

reteplase, See THROMBOLYTIC AGENTS.

Rh_0(D) IMMUNE GLOBULIN

(arr aych oh dee im-**yoon** **glob**-yoo-lin)

Rh_0(D) immune globulin standard dose IM
HyperRHO S/D Full Dose, RhoGAM

Rh_0(D) immune globulin microdose IM
HyperRHO S/D Mini-Dose, MICRhoGAM, Mini-Gamulin R

Rh_0(D) immune globulin IV
WinRho SDF

Rh_0(D) immune globulin microdose IM, IV
Rhophylac

Classification
Therapeutic: vaccines/immunizing agents
Pharmacologic: immune globulins

Pregnancy Category C

Indications

IM, IV: Administered to Rh_0(D)-negative patients who have been exposed to Rh_0(D)-positive blood by: Pregnancy or delivery of a Rh_0(D)-positive infant, Abortion of a Rh_0(D)-positive fetus, Fetal-maternal hemorrhage due to amniocentesis, other obstetrical manipulative procedure, or intra-abdominal trauma while carrying a Rh_0(D)-positive fetus, Transfusion of Rh_0(D)-positive blood or blood products to a Rh_0(D)-negative patient. **IV:** Management of immune thrombocytopenic purpura (ITP).

Action

Prevent production of anti-Rh_0(D) antibodies in Rh_0(D)-negative patients who were exposed to Rh_0(D)-positive blood. Increase platelet counts in patients with ITP. **Therapeutic Effects:** Prevention of antibody response and hemolytic disease of the newborn (erythroblastosis fetalis) in future pregnancies of women who have conceived a Rh_0(D)-positive fetus. Prevention of Rh_0(D) sensitization following transfusion accident. Decreased bleeding in patients with ITP.

Pharmacokinetics

Absorption: Completely absorbed with IV administration. Well absorbed from IM sites.
Distribution: Unknown.
Metabolism and Excretion: Unknown.
Half-life: approximately 25–30 days.

TIME/ACTION PROFILE (blood levels)

ROUTE	ONSET	PEAK	DURATION
IM	rapid	5–10 days	unknown
IV†	unknown	2 hr	unknown

†When given for ITP, platelet counts start to rise in 1–2 days, peak after 5–7 days, and last for 30 days

Contraindications/Precautions

Contraindicated in: Prior hypersensitivity reaction to human immune globulin; Rh_0(D)- or Du-positive patients.
Use Cautiously in: ITP patients with pre-existing anemia (decrease dose if Hgb <10 g/dl). May also cause disseminated intravascular coagulation in ITP patients.

Adverse Reactions/Side Effects

CNS: dizziness, headache. **CV:** hypertension, hypotension. **Derm:** rash. **GI:** diarrhea, nausea, vomiting. **Hemat:** *ITP*— anemia, intravascular hemolysis. **MS:** arthralgia, myalgia. **Local:** pain at injection site. **Misc:** fever.

Interactions

Drug-Drug: May decrease antibody response to some **live-virus vaccines (measles, mumps, rubella)**.

Route/Dosage

Rh_0(D) Immune Globulin (for IM use only)

Following Delivery

IM (Adults): *HyperRHO S/D Full Dose, RhoGAM*—1 vial standard dose (300 mcg) within 72 hr of delivery.

Before Delivery

IM (Adults): *HyperRHO S/D Full Dose, RhoGAM*—1 vial standard dose (300 mcg) at 26–28 wk.

Termination of Pregnancy (<13 wk Gestation)

IM (Adults): *HyperRHO S/D Mini-Dose, MICRhoGAM*—1 vial of microdose (50 mcg) within 72 hr.

Termination of Pregnancy (>13 wk Gestation)

IM (Adults): *RhoGAM*—1 vial standard dose (300 mcg) within 72 hr.

Large Fetal-Maternal Hemorrhage (>15 ml)

IM (Adults): *RhoGAM*—20 mcg/ml of Rh_0(D)-positive fetal RBCs.

Transfusion Accident

IM (Adults): *HyperRHO S/D Full Dose, RhoGAM*—(Volume of Rh-positive blood administered × Hct of donor blood)/15 = number of vials of standard dose (300 mcg) preparation (round to next whole number of vials).

Rh_0(D) Immune Globulin IV (for IM or IV Use)

Following Delivery

IM, IV (Adults): *WinRho SDF*—600 IU (120 mcg) within 72 hr of delivery. *Rhophylac*—1500 IU (300 mcg) within 72 hr of delivery.

Prior to Delivery

IM, IV (Adults): *WinRho SDF, Rhophylac*—1500 IU (300 mcg) at 28 wk; if initiated earlier in pregnancy, repeat q 12 wk.

Following Amniocentesis or Chorionic Villus Sampling

IM, IV (Adults): *WinRho SDF (before 34 wk gestation)*—1500 IU (300 mcg) immediately; repeat q 12 wk during pregnancy. *Rhophylac*—1500 IU (300 mcg) within 72 hr of procedure.

Termination of Pregnancy, Amniocentesis, or Any Other Manipulation

IM, IV (Adults): *WinRho SDF*—600 IU (120 mcg) within 72 hr after event.

Large Fetal-Maternal Hemorrhage/Transfusion Accident

IM (Adults): *WinRho SDF*—6000 IU (1200 mcg) q 12 hr until total dose is given (total dose determined by amount of blood loss/hemorrhage).

IV (Adults): 3000 IU (600 mcg) q 8 hr until total dose is given (total dose determined by amount of blood loss/hemorrhage).

Immune Thrombocytopenic Purpura

IV (Adults and Children): *WinRho SDF, Rhophylac*—50 mcg (250 IU)/kg initially (if Hgb <10 g/dl, ↓ dose to 25–40 mcg [125–200 IU]/kg); further dosing/frequency determined by clinical response (range 25–60 mcg [125–300 IU]/kg). Each dose may be given as a single dose or in 2 divided doses on separate days.

Availability

Rh_0(D) Immune Globulin (for IM Use)

Injection: 50 mcg/vial (microdose - MICRhoGAM, HyperRHO S/D Mini-Dose), 300 mcg/vial (standard dose—RhoGAM, HyperRHO S/D Full Dose).

Rh_0(D) Immune Globulin Intravenous (for IM or IV Use)

Injection: 600 IU (120 mcg)/vial, 1500 IU (300 mcg)/vial, 2500 IU (500 mcg)/vial, 5000 IU (1000 mcg)/vial, 15000 IU (3000 mcg)/vial. **Prefilled syringes:** 1500 IU (300 mcg/2 ml).

NURSING IMPLICATIONS

Assessment

- **IV:** Assess vital signs periodically during therapy in patients receiving IV Rh_0(D) immune globulin.
- **ITP:** Monitor patient for signs and symptoms of intravascular hemolysis (IVH) (back pain, shaking chills, fever, hemoglobinuria), anemia, and renal insufficiency. If transfusions

are required, use Rh_0(D) negative packed red blood cells to prevent exacerbation of IVH.

- ***Lab Test Considerations:*** *Pregnancy:* Type and crossmatch of mother and newborn's cord blood must be performed to determine need for medication. Mother must be Rh_0(D)-negative and Du-negative. Infant must be Rh_0(D)-positive. If there is doubt regarding infant's blood type or if father is Rh_0(D)-positive, medication should be given.
- An infant born to a woman treated with Rh_0(D) immune globulin antepartum may have a weakly positive direct Coombs' test result on cord or infant blood.
- *ITP:* Monitor platelet counts, RBC counts, hemoglobin, and reticulocyte levels to determine effectiveness of therapy.

Potential Nursing Diagnoses

Deficient knowledge, related to medication regimen (Patient/Family Teaching)

Implementation

- Do not give to infant, to Rh_0(D)-positive individual, or to Rh_0(D)-negative individual previously sensitized to the Rh_0(D) antigen. However, there is no more risk than when given to a woman who is not sensitized. When in doubt, administer Rh_0(D) immune globulin.
- Do not confuse IM and IV formulations. Rh immune globulin for IV administration is labeled 'Rh Immune Globulin Intravenous.' Rh Immune Globulin Intravenous may be given IM; however, Rh Immune Globulin (microdose and standard dose) is for IM use only and cannot be given IV.
- When using prefilled syringes, allow solution to reach room temperature before administration.
- **IM:** Reconstitute Rh_0(D) immune globulin IV for IM use immediately before use with 1.25 ml of 0.9% NaCl. Inject diluent onto inside wall of vial and wet pellet by gently swirling until dissolved. Do not shake.
- Administer into the deltoid muscle. Dose should be given within 3 hr but may be given up to 72 hr after delivery, miscarriage, abortion, or transfusion.

IV Administration

- **Direct IV:** Reconstitute Rh_0(D) immune globulin IV for IV administration immediately before use with 2.5 ml of 0.9% NaCl. Inject diluent onto inside wall of vial and wet pellet by gently swirling until dissolved. Do not shake. ***Rate:*** Administer over 3–5 min.

Patient/Family Teaching

- **Pregnancy:** Explain to patient that the purpose of this medication is to protect future Rh_0(D)-positive infants.
- **ITP:** Explain purpose of medication to patient.

Evaluation/Desired Outcomes

- Prevention of erythroblastosis fetalis in future Rh_0(D)-positive infants.
- Prevention of Rh_0(D) sensitization following incompatible transfusion.
- Decreased bleeding episodes in patients with ITP.

ribavirin (rye-ba-**vye**-rin)

Copegus, Rebetol, Virazole

Classification

Therapeutic: antivirals

Pharmacologic: nucleoside analogues

Pregnancy Category X

Indications

Inhaln: Treatment of severe lower respiratory tract infections caused by the respiratory syncytial virus (RSV) in infants and young children. **PO:** *Rebetol*—with interferon alfa-2b (*Intron A*) or peginterferon alfa-2b (*PEG-Intron*) in the treatment of chronic hepatitis C in patients who have failed previous therapy. **PO:** *Copegus*—with peginterferon alfa-2a (Pegasys) in the treatment of chronic hepatitis C in patients who have failed previous therapy. **Unlabeled uses:** Early (within 24 hr of symptoms) secondary treatment of influenza A or B in young adults.

Action

Inhibits viral DNA and RNA synthesis and subsequent replication. Must be phosphorylated intracellularly to be active. **Therapeutic Effects:** **Inhaln:** Virustatic action. **PO:** Decreased progression and sequelae of chronic hepatitis C.

Pharmacokinetics

Absorption: Systemic absorption occurs following nasal and oral inhalation. Rapidly and extensively absorbed following oral administration, but undergoes first-pass hepatic metabolism (64% bioavailability).

Distribution: 70% of inhaled drug is deposited in the respiratory tract. Appears to concentrate in the respiratory tract and red blood cells. Enters breast milk.

Metabolism and Excretion: Eliminated from the respiratory tract by distribution across membranes, macrophages, and ciliary motion. Metabolized primarily by the liver; metabolites are renally excreted.
Half-life: *Inhaln*—9.5 hr (40 days in RBCs); *oral*—43.6 hr (single dose); 12 days (multiple dose).

TIME/ACTION PROFILE (blood levels)

ROUTE	ONSET	PEAK	DURATION
Inhaln	unknown	end of inhaln	unknown
PO	unknown	1.7–3 hr	12 hr

Contraindications/Precautions

Contraindicated in: Hypersensitivity; **Inhalation** Patients receiving mechanically assisted ventilation; **Oral** OB: Pregnancy or lactation; OB: Male partners of pregnant patients; CCr <50 ml/min; Significant/unstable cardiovascular disease; Hemoglobinopathies; Autoimmune hepatitis or hepatic decompensation before/during treatment (for combined therapy with interferon alfa-2b or peginterferon alfa-2a); Concurrent use of didanosine, stavudine or zidovudine.
Use Cautiously in: PO: Sarcoidosis (may exacerbate condition; Anemia (dose reduction/discontinuation may be required); Any pre-existing cardiac disease; OB: Patients with childbearing potential.

Adverse Reactions/Side Effects

Inhalation **CNS:** dizziness, faintness. **EENT:** blurred vision, conjunctivitis, erythema of the eyelids, ocular irritation, photosensitivity. **CV:** CARDIAC ARREST, hypotension. **Derm:** rash. **Hemat:** <u>hemolytic anemia (with interferon alpha 2b)</u>, reticulocytosis.
Oral (may reflect combination with interferon). **CNS:** emotional lability (↑ in children), fatigue (↓ in children), impaired concentration (↓ in children), insomnia (↓ in children), irritability (↓ in children). **EENT:** dry mouth. **Resp:** dyspnea (↓ in children). **GI:** anorexia (↑ in children), dyspepsia (↓ in children), vomiting (↑ in children). **Hemat:** <u>hemolytic anemia.</u> **Derm:** pruritus (↓ in children). **MS:** arthralgia (↓ in children). **Misc:** fever (↑ in children).

Interactions

Drug-Drug: Oral. May ↓ the antiretroviral action of **stavidine** and **zidovudine**. May ↑ hematologic toxicity of **zidovudine**. May ↑ blood levels and risk of toxicity of **didanosine**. Although used together in the management of hepatitis, concurrent use with **interferon alpha 2b** ↑ risk of hemolytic anemia.

Route/Dosage

Inhaln (Infants and Young Children): 300 ml of 20 mg/ml solution delivered via mist for 12–18 hr/day.

Rebetol (with interferon alfa-2b or peginterferon alfa-2b)

PO (Adults >75 kg): 600 mg in the morning, then 600 mg in the evening for 6 mo.
PO (Adults ≤75 kg and Children >61 kg): 400 mg in the morning, then 600 mg in the evening for 6 mo.
PO (Children 50–61 kg): 400 mg in the morning and evening.
PO (Children 37–49 kg): 200 mg in the morning and 400 mg in the evening.
PO (Children 25–36 kg): 200 mg in the morning and evening.

Copegus—viral genotype 1 or 4 (with peginterferon alfa-2a)

PO (Adults ≥75 kg): 600 mg twice daily for 48 wk.
PO (Adults <75 kg): 500 mg twice daily for 48 wk.

Copegus—viral genotype 2 or 4 (with peginterferon alfa-2a)

PO (Adults): 400 mg twice daily for 24 wk.

Availability

Powder for reconstitution for aerosol use: 6 g/vial. **Capsules (Rebetol):** 200 mg. **Tablets (Copegus):** 200 mg, 400 mg. ***In combination with:*** Rebetrol with interferon alfa-2b (Intron A) as combination therapy for chronic hepatitis C (Rebetron). See Appendix B; *Copegus* is intended for combined therapy with pegylated interferon alfa-2a (*Pegasys*).

NURSING IMPLICATIONS

Assessment

- **RSV:** Assess patient for infection (vital signs, sputum, WBC) at beginning and during therapy.

R

- Obtain specimens for culture and sensitivity prior to initiating therapy. First dose may be given before receiving results
- Assess respiratory (lung sounds, quality and rate of respirations) and fluid status prior to and frequently throughout therapy.
- **Chronic Hepatitis C:** Monitor symptoms of hepatitis during therapy.
- Assess patient for signs of depression during therapy.
- Assess patient for cardiovascular disorders (pulse, blood pressure, chest pain). May cause myocardial infarction
- Assess patients for signs of colitis (abdominal pain, bloody diarrhea, fever) and pancreatitis (nausea, vomiting, abdominal pain) during therapy. Discontinue therapy if these occur; may be fatal
- Assess pulmonary status (lung sounds, respirations) periodically during therapy. May require discontinuation.
- ***Lab Test Considerations:*** **Chronic Hepatitis C:** Monitor CBC with differential and platelet count prior to initiation, at week 2, and week 4, and regularly during therapy. If hemoglobin <10 g/dl in patients with no history of cardiac disease or ↓ more than 2 g/dl in any 4 wk treatment period in patients with history of stable cardiac disease, decrease ribavirin dose to 600 mg (200 mg in AM and 400 mg in PM). If hemoglobin <8.5 g/dl in patients with no history of cardiac disease or <12 g/dl despite dose reduction in patients with history of stable cardiac disease, discontinue combination therapy permanently.
- Monitor liver function tests and thyroid stimulating hormone prior to and periodically during therapy.
- OB: Monitor pregnancy tests prior to, monthly during and for 6 mo following discontinuation of therapy in women of childbearing age. Ribavarin should be started following a negative pregnancy test.
- May cause ↑ serum bilirubin and uric acid levels.

Potential Nursing Diagnoses

Risk for infection (Indications, Side Effects)
Impaired gas exchange (Indications)

Implementation

Inhaln: Infants requiring assisted ventilation should be suctioned every 1–2 hr and pulmonary pressures monitored every 2–4 hr.

- Ribavirin treatment should begin within the first 3 days of RSV infection to be effective.
- Ribavirin aerosol should be administered using the Viratek SPAG model SPAG-2 only. Do not administer via other aerosol-generating devices. Usually administered using an infant oxygen hood attached to the SPAG-2 aerosol generator. Administration by face mask may be used if the oxygen hood cannot be used.
- Reconstitute ribavirin 6-g vial with preservative-free sterile water for injection or inhalation. Transfer to clean, sterilized Erlenmeyer flask of the SPAG-2 reservoir and dilute to a final volume of 300 ml. This recommended concentration (20 mg/ml) in the reservoir provides a concentration of aerosol ribavirin of 190 mcg/liter of air over a 12-hr period. Solution should be discarded and replaced every 24 hr.
- Aerosol treatments should be administered continuously 12–18 hr/day for 3–7 days.
- **PO:** Administer with food. Capsules should be swallowed whole; do not open, crush, or chew.

Patient/Family Teaching

- **RSV:** Explain the purpose and route of treatment to the patient and parents.
- Inform patient and parents that ribavirin may cause blurred vision and photosensitivity.
- **Chronic Hepatitis C:** Instruct patient to take ribavirin for the full course of therapy Emphasize the importance of routine lab test to monitor for side effects.
- Advise patient to brush teeth twice daily, have regular dental examinations, and rinse mouth thoroughly after vomiting to prevent dental and periodontal disorders.
- Inform patient about teratogenic effects of ribavirin. Instruct women with childbearing potential, and men, to use 2 forms of effective contraception during and for at least 6 mo following conclusion of therapy. Men must use a condom.
- May cause dizziness. Caution patient to avoid driving or other activities requiring alertness until response to medication is known.
- Inform patient that ribavirin may not reduce the risk of transmission of HCV to others or prevent cirrhosis, liver failure, or liver cancer.

Evaluation/Desired Outcomes

- Resolution of the signs and symptoms of RSV.
- Decreased progression and sequelae of chronic hepatitis C.

rifabutin (riff-a-**byoo**-tin)
Mycobutin

Classification
Therapeutic: agents for atypical mycobacterium

Pregnancy Category B

Indications
Prevention of disseminated *Mycobacterium avium* complex (MAC) disease in patients with advanced HIV infection. **Unlabeled uses:** Treatment of *Helicobacter pylori* ulcer disease which has failed on other regimens (with pantoprazole and amoxicillin).

Action
Appears to inhibit DNA-dependent RNA polymerase in susceptible organisms. **Therapeutic Effects:** Antimycobacterial action against susceptible organisms. **Spectrum:** Active against *M. avium* and most strains of *M. tuberculosis*.

Pharmacokinetics
Absorption: Well absorbed following oral administration (50–85%). Absorption is decreased in HIV-positive patients (20%).
Distribution: Widely distributed to body tissues and fluids.
Metabolism and Excretion: Mostly metabolized by the liver; <5% excreted unchanged by the kidneys.
Half-life: 45 hr.

TIME/ACTION PROFILE (blood levels)

ROUTE	ONSET	PEAK	DURATION
PO	rapid	2–4 hr	24 hr

Contraindications/Precautions
Contraindicated in: Hypersensitivity. Cross-sensitivity with other rifamycins (rifampin) may occur; Active tuberculosis; Concurrent ritonavir or delavirdine.
Use Cautiously in: Pregnancy, lactation, or children (safety not established).

Adverse Reactions/Side Effects
EENT: brown-orange discoloration of tears, ocular disturbances. **Resp:** dyspnea. **CV:** chest pain, chest pressure. **GI:** brown-orange discoloration of saliva, altered taste, drug-induced hepatitis. **GU:** brown-orange discoloration of urine. **Derm:** rash, skin discoloration. **Hemat:** hemolysis, neutropenia, thrombocytopenia. **MS:** arthralgia, myositis. **Misc:** brown-orange discoloration of body fluids, flu-like syndrome.

Interactions
Drug-Drug: Increases metabolism and may decrease the effectiveness of other drugs, including **amprenavir**, **efavirenz**, **indinavir**, **nelfinavir**, **nevirapine**, **saquinavir**, (dosage adjustment may be necessary), **delavirdine**, (concurrent use should be avoided), **corticosteroids**, **disopyramide**, **quinidine**, **opioid analgesics**, **oral hypoglycemic agents**, **warfarin**, **estrogens**, **estrogen-containing contraceptives**, **phenytoin**, **verapamil**, **fluconazole**, **quinidine**, **tocainide**, **theophylline**, **zidovudine**, and **chloramphenicol**. **Ritonavir** increases blood levels of rifabutin (concurrent use is contraindicated), similar effects occur with **efavirenz** and **nevirapine**.

Route/Dosage
PO (Adults): 300 mg once daily. If GI upset occurs, may give as 150 mg twice daily with food. *H. pylori*—300 mg/day (unlabeled).

Availability
Capsules: 150 mg.

NURSING IMPLICATIONS

Assessment
- Monitor patient for signs of active tuberculosis (purified protein derivative [PPD], chest x-ray, sputum culture, blood culture, urine culture, biopsy of suspicious lymph nodes) prior to and throughout therapy. Rifabutin must not be administered to patients with active tuberculosis.
- ***Lab Test Considerations:*** Monitor CBC periodically throughout therapy. May cause neutropenia and thrombocytopenia.

Potential Nursing Diagnoses
Risk for infection (Indications)
Noncompliance (Patient/Family Teaching)

Implementation
- Do not confuse rifabutin with rifampin.
- **PO:** May be administered without regard to meals. High-fat meals slow rate but not extent of absorption. May be mixed with foods such as applesauce. If GI upset occurs, administer with food.

R

♣ = Canadian drug name.
* CAPITALS indicates life-threatening; underlines indicate most frequent.

Patient/Family Teaching

- Advise patient to take medication exactly as directed. Do not skip doses or double up on missed doses. Emphasize the importance of continuing therapy even if asymptomatic.
- Advise patient to notify health care professional promptly if signs and symptoms of neutropenia (sore throat, fever, signs of infection), thrombocytopenia (unusual bleeding or bruising), or hepatitis (yellow eyes and skin, nausea, vomiting, anorexia, unusual tiredness, weakness) occur.
- Caution patient to avoid the use of alcohol during this therapy, because this may increase the risk of hepatotoxicity.
- Instruct patient to report symptoms of myositis (myalgia, arthralgia) or uveitis (intraocular inflammation) to health care professional promptly.
- Inform patient that saliva, sputum, sweat, tears, urine, and feces may become red-orange to red-brown and that soft contact lenses may become permanently discolored.
- Advise patient that this medication has teratogenic properties and may decrease the effectiveness of oral contraceptives. Counsel patient to use a nonhormonal form of contraception throughout therapy.
- Emphasize the importance of regular follow-up exams to monitor progress and to check for side effects.

Evaluation/Desired Outcomes

- Prevention of disseminated MAC in patients with advanced HIV infection.

rifampin (rif-am-pin)

Rifadin, Rimactane, ♣Rofact

Classification
Therapeutic: antituberculars
Pharmacologic: rifamycins

Pregnancy Category C

Indications

Active tuberculosis (with other agents). Elimination of meningococcal carriers. **Unlabeled uses:** Prevention of disease caused by *Haemophilus influenzae* type B in close contacts.

Action

Inhibits RNA synthesis by blocking RNA transcription in susceptible organisms. **Therapeutic Effects:** Bactericidal action against susceptible organisms. **Spectrum:** Broad spectrum notable for activity against: *Mycobacterium* spp, *Staphylococcus aureus*, *H. influenzae*, *Legionella pneumophila*, *Neisseria meningitidis*.

Pharmacokinetics

Absorption: Well absorbed following oral administration.
Distribution: Widely distributed; enters CSF. Crosses placenta; enters breast milk.
Metabolism and Excretion: Mostly metabolized by the liver; 60% eliminated in feces via biliary elimination.
Half-life: 3 hr.

TIME/ACTION PROFILE (blood levels)

ROUTE	ONSET	PEAK	DURATION
PO	rapid	2–4 hr	12–24 hr
IV	rapid	end of infusion	12–24 hr

Contraindications/Precautions

Contraindicated in: Hypersensitivity; Concurrent indinavir, nelfinavir, pyrazinamide, or saquinavir.
Use Cautiously in: History of liver disease; Concurrent use of other hepatotoxic agents; Pregnancy or lactation.

Adverse Reactions/Side Effects

CNS: ataxia, confusion, drowsiness, fatigue, headache, weakness. **EENT:** red discoloration of tears. **GI:** abdominal pain, diarrhea, flatulence, heartburn, nausea, vomiting, drug-induced hepatitis, red discoloration of saliva. **GU:** red discoloration of urine. **Hemat:** hemolytic anemia, thrombocytopenia. **MS:** arthralgia, myalgia. **Misc:** red discoloration of all body fluids, flu-like syndrome.

Interactions

Drug-Drug: ↑ risk of hepatotoxicity with other **hepatotoxic agents**, including **alcohol**, **ketoconazole isoniazid**, **pyrazinamide** (concurrent use with **pyrazinamide** may result in potentially fatal hepatotoxicity and should be avoided). Rifampin significantly ↓ blood levels of **delavirdine**, **indinavir**, **nelfinavir**, and **saquinavir**; concurrent use is contraindicated. Rifampin stimulates liver enzymes, which may ↑ metabolism and ↓ effectiveness of other drugs, including **ritonavir**, **nevirapine**, and **efavirenz** (dosage adjustment may be necessary), **corticosteroids**, **disopyramide**, **quinidine**, **opioid analgesics**, **oral hypoglycemic agents**, **warfarin**, **estrogens**,

phenytoin, **verapamil**, **fluconazole**, **ketoconazole**, **itraconazole**, **quinidine**, **tocainide**, **theophylline**, **chloramphenicol**, and **hormonal contraceptive agents**.

Route/Dosage

Tuberculosis

PO, IV (Adults): 600 mg/day or 10 mg/kg/day (up to 600 mg/day) single dose; may also be given 2–3 times weekly.

PO, IV (Children): 10–20 mg/kg/day single dose (not to exceed 600 mg/day); may also be given 2–3 times weekly.

Asymptomatic Carriers of Meningococcus

PO, IV (Adults): 600 mg q 12 hr for 2 days.

PO, IV (Children ≥1 mo): 10 mg/kg q 12 hr for 2 days.

PO (Infants <1 mo): 5 mg/kg q 12 hr for 2 days.

Prevention of *H. influenzae* Type B Infection

PO (Adults): 600 mg/day for 4 days.

PO (Children): 20 mg/kg/day for 4 days.

Availability (generic available)

Capsules: 150 mg, 300 mg. **Powder for injection:** 600 mg/vial. ***In combination with:*** isoniazid (Rifamate); isoniazid and pyrazinamide (Rifater). See Appendix B.

NURSING IMPLICATIONS

Assessment

- Perform mycobacterial studies and susceptibility tests prior to and periodically during therapy to detect possible resistance.
- Assess lung sounds and character and amount of sputum periodically during therapy.
- ***Lab Test Considerations:*** Evaluate renal function, CBC, and urinalysis periodically and during therapy.
- Monitor hepatic function at least monthly during therapy. May cause ↑ BUN, AST, ALT, and serum alkaline phosphatase, bilirubin, and uric acid concentrations.
- May cause false-positive direct Coombs' test results. May interfere with folic acid and vitamin B assays.
- May interfere with dexamethasone suppression test results; discontinue rifampin 15 days prior to test.
- May interfere with methods for determining serum folate and vitamin B levels and with urine tests based on color reaction.
- May delay hepatic uptake and excretion of sulfobromophthalein (SBP) during SBP uptake and excretion tests; perform test prior to daily dose of rifampin.

Potential Nursing Diagnoses

Risk for infection (Indications)

Noncompliance (Patient/Family Teaching)

Implementation

- Do not confuse rifampin with rifabutin.
- **PO:** Administer medication on an empty stomach at least 1 hr before or 2 hr after meals with a full glass (240 ml) of water. If GI irritation becomes a problem, may be administered with food. Antacids may also be taken 1 hr prior to administration. Capsules may be opened and contents mixed with applesauce or jelly for patients with difficulty swallowing.
- Pharmacist can compound a syrup for patients unable to swallow solids.

IV Administration

- **Intermittent Infusion:** ***Diluent:*** Reconstitute each 600-mg vial with 10 ml of sterile water for injection for a concentration of 60 mg/ml. Dilute further in 100 ml or 500 ml of D5W or 0.9% NaCl. Reconstituted vials are stable for 24 hr at room temperature. Infusion is stable at room temperature for 4 hr (in D5W or 24 hr (in 0.9% NaCl). ***Concentration:*** Final concentration of infusion should not exceed 6 mg/ml. ***Rate:*** Administer solutions diluted in 100 ml over 30 min and solutions diluted in 500 ml over 3 hr.
- **Y-Site Compatibility:** amiodarone, bumetanide, midazolam, pantoprazole, vancomycin.
- **Y-Site Incompatibility:** diltiazem.

Patient/Family Teaching

- Advise patient to take medication once daily (unless biweekly regimens are used), as directed, and not to skip doses or double up on missed doses. Emphasize the importance of continuing therapy even after symptoms have subsided. Length of therapy for tuberculosis depends on regimen being used and underlying disease states. Patients on short-term prophylactic therapy should also be advised of the importance of compliance with therapy.

R

- Advise patient to notify health care professional promptly if signs and symptoms of hepatitis (yellow eyes and skin, nausea, vomiting, anorexia, unusual tiredness, weakness) or of thrombocytopenia (unusual bleeding or bruising) occur.
- Caution patient to avoid the use of alcohol during this therapy, because this may increase the risk of hepatotoxicity.
- Instruct patient to report the occurrence of flu-like symptoms (fever, chills, myalgia, headache) promptly.
- Rifampin may occasionally cause drowsiness. Caution patient to avoid driving or other activities requiring alertness until response to medication is known.
- Inform patient that saliva, sputum, sweat, tears, urine, and feces may become red-orange to red-brown and that soft contact lenses may become permanently discolored.
- Advise patient that this medication has teratogenic properties and may decrease the effectiveness of oral contraceptives. Counsel patient to use a nonhormonal form of contraception throughout therapy.
- Emphasize the importance of regular follow-up exams to monitor progress and to check for side effects.

Evaluation/Desired Outcomes

- Decreased fever and night sweats.
- Diminished cough and sputum production.
- Negative sputum cultures.
- Increased appetite.
- Weight gain.
- Reduced fatigue.
- Sense of well-being in patients with tuberculosis.
- Prevention of meningococcal meningitis.
- Prevention of *H. influenzae* type B infection. Prophylactic course is usually short-term.

rifaximin (ri-fax-i-min)

Xifaxan

Classification

Therapeutic: anti-infectives

Pharmacologic: rifamycins

Pregnancy Category C

Indications

Travelers' diarrhea due to noninvasive strains of *Escherichia coli*.

Action

Inhibits bacterial RNA synthesis by binding to bacterial DNA-dependent RNA polymerase. **Therapeutic Effects:** Decreased severity of travelers' diarrhea. **Spectrum:** *Escherichia coli* (enterotoxigenic and enteroaggregative strains).

Pharmacokinetics

Absorption: Poorly absorbed (<0.4%), action is primarily in GI tract.
Distribution: 80–90% concentrated in gut.
Metabolism and Excretion: Almost exclusively excreted unchanged in feces.
Half-life: 6 hr.

TIME/ACTION PROFILE

ROUTE	ONSET	PEAK	DURATION
PO	unknown	unknown	unknown

Contraindications/Precautions

Contraindicated in: Hypersensitivity to rifaximin or other rifamycins; Diarrhea with fever or bloody stools; Diarrhea caused by other infections agents; Lactation.
Use Cautiously in: Pregnancy (use only benefits outweigh risk to fetus); Children <12 yr (safety not established).

Adverse Reactions/Side Effects

CNS: dizziness. **GI:** PSEUDOMEMBRANOUS COLITIS.

Interactions

Drug-Drug: Although rifaximin induces the CYP3A4 enzyme system, since it is not absorbed, drug interactions are unlikely.

Route/Dosage

PO (Adults and Children ≥12 yr): 200 mg three times daily for 3 days.

Availability

Tablets: 200 mg.

NURSING IMPLICATIONS

Assessment

- Assess frequency and consistency of stools and bowel sounds prior to and during therapy.
- Assess fluid and electrolyte balance and skin turgor for dehydration.
- ***Lab Test Considerations:*** May cause lymphocytosis, monocytosis, and neutropenia.

Potential Nursing Diagnoses

Diarrhea (Indications)
Risk for deficient fluid volume (Indications)

Implementation

- **PO:** Administer with or without food, 3 times daily for 3 days.

Patient/Family Teaching

- Instruct patient to take rifaximin as directed and to complete therapy, even if feeling better. Caution patient to stop taking rifaximin if diarrhea symptoms get worse, persist more than 24–48 hr, or are accompanied by fever or blood in the stool. Consult health care professional if these occur.
- May cause dizziness. Caution patient to avoid driving and other activities requiring alertness until response to medication is known.
- Advise female patients to notify health care professional if pregnant or if pregnancy is suspected.

Evaluation/Desired Outcomes

- Decreased severity of travelers' diarrhea.

risedronate (riss-**ed**-roe-nate)

Actonel

Classification

Therapeutic: bone resorption inhibitors
Pharmacologic: biphosphonates

Pregnancy Category C

Indications

Prevention and treatment of postmenopausal and corticosteroid-induced osteoporosis. Management of Paget's disease of bone in patients who: have a serum alkaline phosphatase level of at least twice normal, have symptoms, are at risk for complications. Increase bone mass in men with osteoporosis.

Action

Inhibits bone resorption by binding to bone hydroxyapatite, which inhibits osteoclast activity.
Therapeutic Effects: Reversal of the progression of osteoporosis with decreased fractures and other sequelae. Reduced bone turnover and resorption; normalization of serum alkaline phosphatase with reduced complications of Paget's disease.

Pharmacokinetics

Absorption: Rapidly but poorly absorbed following oral administration (0.63% bioavailability).
Distribution: 60% of absorbed dose distributes to bone.
Metabolism and Excretion: 40% of absorbed dose is excreted unchanged by kidneys; unabsorbed drug is excreted in feces.
Half-life: *Initial*—1.5 hr; *terminal*—220 hr (reflects dissociation from bone).

TIME/ACTION PROFILE (effects on serum alkaline phosphatase)

ROUTE	ONSET	PEAK	DURATION
PO	within days	30 days	up to 16 mo

Contraindications/Precautions

Contraindicated in: Hypersensitivity; Hypocalcemia; Lactation; Severe renal impairment (CCr <30 ml/min).
Use Cautiously in: History of upper GI disorders; Other disturbances of bone or mineral metabolism (correct abnormalities before initiating therapy); Dietary deficiencies (supplemental vitamin D and calcium may be required); OB, Pedi: Pregnancy or children (safety not established; use in pregnancy only if potential benefit justifies potential risks).

Adverse Reactions/Side Effects

CNS: weakness. **EENT:** amblyopia, conjunctivitis, dry eyes, eye pain/inflammation, tinnitus. **CV:** chest pain, edema. **GI:** abdominal pain, diarrhea, belching, colitis, constipation, dysphagia, esophagitis, esophageal ulcer, gastric ulcer, nausea. **Derm:** rash. **MS:** arthralgia, bone pain, leg cramps, myasthenia. **Misc:** flu-like syndrome.

Interactions

Drug-Drug: Concurrent use with **NSAIDs** or **aspirin** ↑ risk of GI irritation. Absorption is ↓ by **calcium supplements** or **antacids**.
Drug-Food: Food decreases absorption (administer at least 30 min before breakfast).

Route/Dosage

PO (Adults): *Postmenopausal Osteoporosis*—5 mg once daily; taken 30 min before breakfast *or* 35 mg once weekly; *or* 75 mg taken on two consecutive days for a total of 2 tablets each month; *Osteoporosis in Men*—35 mg once weekly; *Glucocorticoid-induced Osteoporosis*—5 mg daily; *Paget's disease*—30 mg once daily for 2 mo; taken 30 min before breakfast. Retreatment may be considered after 2 mo off therapy.

R

✤ = Canadian drug name.
* CAPITALS indicates life-threatening; underlines indicate most frequent.

Availability

Tablets: 5 mg, 30 mg, 35mg, 75 mg. **Cost:** 5 mg $272.31/90, 30 mg $1,282.24/90, 35 mg $90.97/4, 75 mg $97.47/2. ***In combination with:*** **calcium carbonate**.

NURSING IMPLICATIONS

Assessment

- **Osteoporosis:** Assess patients via bone density study for low bone mass before and periodically during therapy.
- **Paget's disease:** Assess for symptoms of Paget's disease (bone pain, headache, decreased visual and auditory acuity, increased skull size).
- ***Lab Test Considerations:*** *Osteoporosis:* Assess serum calcium before and periodically during therapy. Hypocalcemia and vitamin D deficiency should be treated before initiating alendronate therapy. May cause mild, transient ↑ of calcium and phosphate.
- *Paget's disease:* Monitor alkaline phosphatase prior to and periodically during therapy to monitor effectiveness of therapy.

Potential Nursing Diagnoses

Risk for injury (Indications)

Implementation

- **PO:** Administer first thing in the morning with 6–8 oz of plain water, 30 min prior to other medications, beverages, or food.
- Calcium-, magnesium-, or aluminum-containing agents may interfere with absorption of risedronate and should be taken at a different time of day with food.

Patient/Family Teaching

- Instruct patient on the importance of taking exactly as directed, first thing in the morning, 30 min prior to other medications, beverages, or food. Waiting longer than 30 min will improve absorption. Risedronate should be taken with 6–8 oz of plain water (mineral water, orange juice, coffee, and other beverages decrease absorption). If a dose is missed, skip dose and resume the next morning; do not double doses or take later in the day. Do not discontinue without consulting health care professional.
- Caution patients to remain upright for 30 min following dose to facilitate passage to stomach and minimize risk of esophageal irritation.
- Advise patient to eat a balanced diet and consult health care professional about the need for supplemental calcium and vitamin D.
- Encourage patient to participate in regular exercise and to modify behaviors that increase the risk of osteoporosis (stop smoking, reduce alcohol consumption).
- Advise female patients to notify health care professional if pregnancy is planned or suspected or if she is nursing.

Evaluation/Desired Outcomes

- Reversal of the progression of osteoporosis with decreased fractures and other sequelae.
- Decrease in serum alkaline phosphatase and the progression of Paget's disease.

risperidone (riss-**per**-i-done)

Risperdal, Risperdal M-TAB, Risperdal Consta

Classification

Therapeutic: antipsychotics, mood stabilizers

Pharmacologic: benzisoxazoles

Pregnancy Category C

Indications

Schizophrenia in adults and adolescents age 13–17 yrs. Bipolar mania (oral only) in adults and children 10–17 yrs in adults and children 10–17 yrs; can be used with lithium or valproate (adults only). Treatment of irritability associated with autistic disorder in children age 5–16 yrs.

Action

May act by antagonizing dopamine and serotonin in the CNS. **Therapeutic Effects:** Decreased symptoms of psychoses, bipolar mania, or autism.

Pharmacokinetics

Absorption: 70% after administration of tablets, solution or orally disintegrating tablets. Following IM administration, small initial release of drug, followed by 3-wk lag; the rest of release starts at 3 wk and lasts 4–6 wk.

Distribution: Unknown.

Metabolism and Excretion: Extensively metabolized by the liver. Metabolism is genetically determined; extensive metabolizers (most patients) convert risperidone to 9-hydroxyrisperidone rapidly. Poor metabolizers (6–8% of whites) convert it more slowly. The 9-hydroxy-

risperidone is an antipsychotic compound. Risperidone and its active metabolite are renally eliminated.
Half-life: *Extensive metabolizers*—3 hr for risperidone, 21 hr for 9-hydroxyrisperidone. *Poor metabolizers*—20 hr for risperidone and 30 hr for 9-hydroxyrisperidone.

TIME/ACTION PROFILE (clinical effects)

ROUTE	ONSET	PEAK	DURATION
PO	1–2 wk	unknown	up to 6 wk†
IM	3 wk	4–6 wk	up to 6 wk†

†After discontinuation

Contraindications/Precautions

Contraindicated in: Hypersensitivity; Lactation: Discontinue drug or bottle feed.
Use Cautiously in: Debilitated patients, patients with renal or hepatic impairment (initial dose reduction recommended); Underlying cardiovascular disease (may be more prone to arrhythmias and hypotension); History of seizures; History of suicide attempt or drug abuse; Diabetes or risk factors for diabetes (may worsen glucose control); Patients at risk for aspiration; OB, Pedi: Safety not established; Geri: Initial dosage reduction recommended. ↑ cardiovascular morbidity/mortality in elderly patients with dementia-related psychoses.

Adverse Reactions/Side Effects

CNS: NEUROLEPTIC MALIGNANT SYNDROME, aggressive behavior, dizziness, extrapyramidal reactions, headache, increased dreams, increased sleep duration, insomnia, sedation, fatigue, impaired temperature regulation, nervousness, tardive dyskinesia. **EENT:** pharyngitis, rhinitis, visual disturbances. **Resp:** cough, dyspnea. **CV:** arrhythmias, orthostatic hypotension, tachycardia. **GI:** constipation, diarrhea, dry mouth, nausea, abdominal pain, anorexia, dyspepsia, increased salivation, vomiting, weight gain, weight loss, polydipsia. **GU:** decreased libido, dysmenorrhea/menorrhagia, difficulty urinating, polyuria. **Derm:** itching/skin rash, dry skin, increased pigmentation, increased sweating, photosensitivity, seborrhea. **Endo:** galactorrhea, hyperglycemia. **MS:** arthralgia, back pain.

Interactions

Drug-Drug: May ↓ the antiparkinsonian effects of **levodopa** or other **dopamine agonists**. **Carbamazepine**, **phenytoin**, **rifampin**, **phenobarbital**, and other **enzyme inducers** ↑ metabolism and may ↓ effectiveness; dose adjustments may be necessary. **Fluoxetine** and paroxetine ↑ blood levels and may ↑ effects; dose adjustments may be necessary. **Clozapine** ↓ metabolism and may ↑ effects of risperidone. ↑ CNS depression may occur with other **CNS depressants**, including **alcohol**, **antihistamines**, **sedative/hypnotics**, or **opioid analgesics**.
Drug-Natural Products: Kava kava, valerian or chamomile can ↑ CNS depression.

Route/Dosage

Schizophrenia

PO (Adults): 1 mg twice daily, increased by 1–2 mg/day no more frequently than every 24 hrs to 4–8 mg daily.
PO (Children 13–17 yrs): 0.5 mg once daily, increased by 0.5–1.0 mg no more frequently than every 24 hr to 3 mg daily. May administer half the daily dose twice daily if drowsiness persists.
IM (Adults): 25 mg every 2 wk; some patients may require larger dose of 37.5 or 50 mg every 2 wks.

R

Bipolar Mania

PO (Adults): 2–3 mg/day as a single daily dose, dose may be increased at 24–hr intervals by 1 mg (range 1–5 mg/day).
PO (Children 13–17 yrs): 0.5 mg once daily, increased by 0.5–1.0 mg no more frequently than every 24 hr to 2.5mg daily. May administer half the daily dose twice daily if drowsiness persists.
PO (Geriatric Patients or Debilitated Patients): Start with 0.5 mg twice daily; increase by 0.5 mg twice daily, up to 1.5 mg twice daily; then increase at weekly intervals if necessary. May also be given as a single daily dose after initial titration.

Irritability Associated with Autistic Disorder

PO (Children 5–16 yrs weighing <20 kg): 0.25 mg/day initially. After at least 4 days of therapy, may increase to 0.50 mg/day. Dose increases in increments of 0.25 mg/day may be considered at 2 wk or longer intervals. May be as a single or divided dose.
PO (Children 5–16 yrs weighing >20 kg): 0.50 mg/day initially. After at least 4 days of ther-

apy, may increase to 1.0 mg/day. Dose increases in increments of 0.5 mg/day may be considered at 2 wk or longer intervals. May be as a single or divided dose.

Renal Impairment
Hepatic Impairment

PO (Adults): Start with 0.5 mg twice daily; increase by 0.5 mg twice daily, up to 1.5 mg twice daily; then increase at weekly intervals if necessary. May also be given as a single daily dose after initial titration.

Availability

Tablets: 0.25 mg, 0.5 mg, 1 mg, 2 mg, 3 mg, 4 mg. **Cost:** 0.25 mg $605.97/180, 0.5 mg $671.96/180, 1 mg $751.93/180, 2 mg $1,219.95/180, 3 mg $1,489.95/180, 4 mg $1,831.84/180. **Orally disintegrating tablets (Risperdal M-Tabs):** 0.5 mg, 1 mg, 2 mg, 3 mg, 4 mg. **Cost:** 0.5 mg $122.93/28, 1 mg $138.95/28, 2 mg $130.68/28, 3 mg $148.49/28, 4 mg $194.02/28. **Oral solution:** 1 mg/ml in 30-ml bottles. **Cost:** $136.66/30 ml. **Microspheres for injection (Risperdal Consta) (requires specific diluent for suspension):** 12.5 mg/vial kit, 25 mg/vial kit, 37.5 mg/vial kit, 50 mg/vial kit.

NURSING IMPLICATIONS

Assessment

- Monitor patient's mental status (orientation, mood, behavior) before and periodically during therapy.
- Assess weight and BMI initially and throughout therapy. Obtain fasting blood glucose and cholesterol levels initially and throughout therapy.
- Monitor mood changes. Assess for suicidal tendencies, especially during early therapy. Restrict amount of drug available to patient.
- Monitor blood pressure (sitting, standing, lying down) and pulse before and frequently during initial dose titration. May cause prolonged QT interval, tachycardia, and orthostatic hypotension. If hypotension occurs, dose may need to be decreased.
- Observe patient when administering medication to ensure medication is swallowed and not hoarded or cheeked.
- Monitor patient for onset of extrapyramidal side effects (*akathisia*—restlessness; *dystonia*—muscle spasms and twisting motions; or *pseudoparkinsonism*—mask-like face, rigidity, tremors, drooling, shuffling gait, dysphagia). Report these symptoms; reduction of dose or discontinuation may be necessary. Trihexyphenidyl or benztropine may be used to control symptoms.
- Monitor for tardive dyskinesia (involuntary rhythmic movement of mouth, face, and extremities). Report immediately; may be irreversible.
- Monitor for development of neuroleptic malignant syndrome (fever, respiratory distress, tachycardia, seizures, diaphoresis, hypertension or hypotension, pallor, tiredness). Notify health care professional immediately if these symptoms occur.
- ***Lab Test Considerations:*** May cause ↑ serum prolactin levels.
- May cause ↑ AST and ALT.
- May also cause anemia, thrombocytopenia, leukocytosis, and leukopenia.

Potential Nursing Diagnoses

Risk for self-directed violence (Indications)
Disturbed thought process (Indications)
Risk for injury (Side Effects)
Risk for aspiration (Side Effects)

Implementation

- Do not confuse risperidone with reserpine.
- When switching from other antipsychotics, discontinue previous agents when starting risperidone and minimize the period of overlapping antipsychotic agents.
- If therapy is reinstituted after an interval off risperidone, follow initial titration schedule.
- For IM use, establish tolerance with oral dosing before IM use and continue oral dosing for 3 wk following initial IM injection. Do not increase dose more frequently than every 4 wks.
- **PO:** Daily doses can be taken in the morning or evening.
- For orally disintegrating tablets, open blister pack by pealing back foil to expose tablet; do not try to push tablet through foil. Use dry hands to remove tablet from blister and immediately place entire tablet on tongue. Tablets disintegrate in mouth within seconds and can be swallowed with or without liquid. Do not attempt to split or chew tablet. Do not try to store tablets once removed from blister.
- Oral solution can be mixed with water, coffee, orange juice, or low fat milk; do not mix with cola or tea.
- **IM:** Reconstitute with 2 ml of diluent provided by manufacturer. Administer via deep gluteal injection using enclosed safety needle; al-

ternate buttocks with each injection. Allow solution to warm to room temperature prior to injection. Administer immediately after mixed with diluent; shake well to mix suspension. Must be administered within 6 hr of reconstitution. Store dose pack in refrigerator.
- Do not combine dose strengths in a single injection.

Patient/Family Teaching

- Instruct patient to take medication exactly as directed.
- Inform patient of the possibility of extrapyramidal symptoms. Instruct patient to report these symptoms immediately to health care professional.
- Advise patient to change positions slowly to minimize orthostatic hypotension.
- May cause drowsiness. Caution patient to avoid driving or other activities requiring alertness until response to medication is known.
- Advise patient to use sunscreen and protective clothing when exposed to the sun to prevent photosensitivity reactions. Extremes in temperature should also be avoided; this drug impairs body temperature regulation.
- Caution patient to avoid concurrent use of alcohol, other CNS depressants, and OTC medications or herbal products without consulting health care professional.
- Refer as appropriate for nutrition/weight management and medical management.
- Advise female patients to notify health care professional if pregnancy is planned or suspected, or if breastfeeding or planning to breastfeed.
- Advise patient to notify health care professional of medication regimen before treatment or surgery.
- Instruct patient to notify health care professional promptly if sore throat, fever, unusual bleeding or bruising, rash, or tremors occur.
- Emphasize the importance of routine follow up exams to monitor side effects and continued participation in psychotherapy to improve coping skills.
- Refer to local support group.

Evaluation/Desired Outcomes

- Decrease in excited, manic behavior.
- Decrease in positive symptoms (delusions, hallucinations) of schizophrenia.
- Decreased aggression toward others, deliberate self—injury, temper tantrums, and mood changes in children with autism.
- Decrease in negative symptoms (social withdrawal, flat, blunted affects) of schizophrenia.

ritonavir (ri-toe-na-veer)

Norvir

Classification

Therapeutic: antiretrovirals

Pharmacologic: protease inhibitors

Pregnancy Category B

Indications

HIV infection (with other antiretrovirals).

Action

Inhibits the action of HIV protease and prevents the cleavage of viral polyproteins. **Therapeutic Effects:** Increased CD4 cell counts and decreased viral load with subsequent slowed progression of HIV infection and its sequelae.

Pharmacokinetics

Absorption: Appears to be well absorbed after oral administration.

Distribution: Poor CNS penetration.

Protein Binding: 98–99%.

Metabolism and Excretion: Highly metabolized by the liver (by P450 CYP3A and CYP2D6 enzymes); one metabolite has antiretroviral activity; 3.5% excreted unchanged in urine.

Half-life: 3–5 hr.

TIME/ACTION PROFILE (blood levels)

ROUTE	ONSET	PEAK	DURATION
PO	rapid	4 hr*	12 hr

*Nonfasting

Contraindications/Precautions

Contraindicated in: Hypersensitivity; Concurrent use of alprazolam, alfuzosin, amiodarone, bupropion, clorazepate, clozapine, diazepam, dihydroergotamine, encainide, ergotamine, estazolam, flecainide, flurazepam, fluticasone (inhalation), meperidine, midazolam, pimozide, piroxicam, propafenone, propoxyphene, quinidine, rifabutin, triazolam, or zolpidem; Hypersensitivity or intolerance to alcohol or castor oil (present in capsules and liquid).

Use Cautiously in: Impaired hepatic function, history of hepatitis; Diabetes mellitus; Hemophilia (increased risk of bleeding); OB, Pedi: Pregnancy, lactation, or children <12 yr (safety not established; breast feeding not recommended in HIV-infected patients).

Adverse Reactions/Side Effects

CNS: SEIZURES, abnormal thinking, weakness, dizziness, headache, malaise, somnolence, syncope. **EENT:** pharyngitis, throat irritation. **Resp:** ANGIOEDEMA, bronchospasm. **CV:** orthostatic hypotension, vasodilation. **GI:** abdominal pain, altered taste, anorexia, diarrhea, nausea, vomiting, constipation, dyspepsia, flatulence. **GU:** renal insufficiency. **Derm:** rash, skin eruptions, sweating, urticaria. **Endo:** hyperglycemia. **F and E:** dehydration. **Metab:** hyperlipidemia. **MS:** increased creatine phosphokinase, myalgia. **Neuro:** circumoral paresthesia, peripheral paresthesia. **Misc:** hypersensitivity reactions including STEVENS-JOHNSON SYNDROME and ANAPHYLAXIS, fat redistribution, fever.

Interactions

Drug-Drug: Produces large ↑ in blood levels and effects of **amiodarone**, **alfuzosin**, **bupropion**, **clozapine**, **encainide**, **flecainide**, **fluticasone (inhalation)**, **meperidine**, **piroxicam**, **propafenone**, **propoxyphene**, **quinidine**, and **rifabutin**; because of the increased risk of serious arrhythmias, hematologic toxicity, hypotension, corticosteroid effects or seizures, these agents should not be used with ritonavir. Ergot toxicity may occur with concurrent use of **ergotamine** or **dihydroergotamine**; concurrent use should be avoided. Should not be used with **pimozide**. ↑ blood levels and the risk of excessive sedation and/or respiratory depression from **alprazolam**, **clorazepate**, **diazepam**, **estazolam**, **flurazepam**, **midazolam**, **triazolam**, and **zolpidem**; concurrent use should be avoided. May also increase blood levels and effects of some **opioid analgesics (alfentanil, fentanyl, hydrocodone, oxycodone)**, **tramadol**; some **NSAIDs (diclofenac, ibuprofen, indomethacin)**; some **antiarrhythmics (disopyramide, lidocaine, mexiletine)**; some **anti-infectives (clarithromycin, erythromycin)**; many **antidepressants (amitriptyline, clomipramine, desipramine, imipramine, nortriptyline, nefazodone, sertraline, trazodone, fluoxetine, paroxetine, venlafaxine)**; some **antiemetics (dronabinol, ondansetron)**; some **beta blockers (metoprolol, pindolol, propranolol, timolol)**; many **calcium channel blockers (amlodipine, diltiazem, felodipine, isradipine, nicardipine, nifedipine, nimodipine, nisoldipine, verapamil)**; some **antineoplastics (etoposides, paclitaxel, tamoxifen, vinblastine, vincristine)**; some **corticosteroids (dexamethasone, prednisone)**, most **HMG CoA reductase inhibitors**; some **immunosuppressants (cyclosporine, tacrolimus)**; some **antipsychotics (chlorpromazine, haloperidol, perphenazine, risperidone, thioridazine)**; and also **quinidine**, **saquinavir**, **methamphetamine**, and **warfarin**. Dosage ↓ may be necessary. ↓ blood levels and effects of **hormonal contraceptives**, **zidovudine**, and **theophylline**; dose alteration or alternative therapy may be necessary. Levels may be ↑ by **clarithromycin** or **fluoxetine**.
Drug-Natural Products: St. John's wort decreases levels and may promote resistance.
Drug-Food: Food ↑ absorption.

Route/Dosage

PO (Adults): 300 mg twice daily for 1 day, then 400 mg twice daily for 3 days, then 500 mg twice daily for 1 day, then 600 mg twice daily as maintenance.
PO (Children): 250 mg/m^2 twice daily initially; increase by 50 mg/m^2 twice daily q 2–3 days up to 400 mg/m^2 twice daily (if unable to get up to 400 mg/m^2 twice daily, additional antiretroviral therapy is required).

Availability

Capsules: 100 mg. **Oral solution:** 600 mg/7.5 ml (80 mg/ml) in 240-ml bottles.

NURSING IMPLICATIONS

Assessment

- Assess patient for change in severity of HIV symptoms and for symptoms of opportunistic infections during therapy.
- ***Lab Test Considerations:*** Monitor viral load and CD4 counts regularly during therapy.
- May cause hyperglycemia.
- May cause ↑ serum AST, ALT, GGT, total bilirubin, CPK, triglycerides, and uric acid concentrations.

Potential Nursing Diagnoses

Risk for infection (Indications)
Noncompliance (Patient/Family Teaching)

Implementation

- Do not confuse with Retrovir (zidovudine).
- **PO:** Administer with a meal or light snack.
- Oral powder may be mixed with chocolate milk, Ensure, or Advera within 1 hr of dosing to improve taste. Capsules should be stored in the refrigerator and protected from light. Use calibrated oral dosing syringe for oral solution. Oral solution does not require refrigeration if used within 30 days and stored below 77°F in the original container. Keep cap tightly closed.
- If nausea occurs on dose of 600 mg twice daily, may titrate by 300 mg twice daily for 1 day, then 400 mg twice daily for 2 days, then 500 mg twice daily for 1 day, then 600 mg twice daily thereafter.
- Patients initiating concurrent therapy with nucleoside analogues may have less GI intolerance by initiating ritonavir for 2 wk and then adding the nucleoside analogue.

Patient/Family Teaching

- Emphasize the importance of taking ritonavir exactly as directed, at evenly spaced times throughout day. Do not take more than prescribed amount and do not stop taking without consulting health care professional. Take missed doses as soon as remembered; do not double doses.
- Instruct patient that ritonavir should not be shared with others.
- Advise patient to avoid taking other medications, prescription or OTC, without consulting health care professional.
- Inform patient that ritonavir does not cure AIDS or prevent associated or opportunistic infections. Ritonavir does not reduce the risk of transmission of HIV to others through sexual contact or blood contamination. Caution patient to use a condom during sexual contact and to avoid sharing needles or donating blood to prevent spreading the AIDS virus to others. Advise patient that the long-term effects of ritonavir are unknown at this time.
- Inform patient that ritonavir may cause hyperglycemia. Advise patient to notify health care professional if increased thirst or hunger; unexplained weight loss; increased urination; fatigue; or dry, itchy skin occurs.
- Advise patients taking oral contraceptives to use a nonhormonal method of birth control during ritonavir therapy.
- Inform patient that redistribution and accumulation of body fat may occur, causing central obesity, dorsocervical fat enlargement (buffalo hump), peripheral wasting, breast enlargement, and cushingoid appearance. The cause and long-term effects are not known.
- Emphasize the importance of regular follow-up exams and blood counts to determine progress and monitor for side effects.

Evaluation/Desired Outcomes

- Delayed progression of AIDS and decreased opportunistic infections in patients with HIV.
- Decrease in viral load and improvement in CD4 cell counts.

rituximab (ri-**tux**-i-mab)

Rituxan

Classification

Therapeutic: antineoplastics

Pharmacologic: monoclonal antibodies

Pregnancy Category C

R

Indications

Treatment of low-grade or follicular, CD20-positive, B-cell non-Hodgkin's lymphoma alone, with, or following treatment with cyclophosphamide, vincristine, and prednisolone (CVP). Moderately to severely active rheumatoid arthritis with methotrexate in patients who have had an inadequate response to one of more TNF antagonist therapies.

Action

Binds to the CD20 antigen on the surface of lymphoma cells, preventing the activation process for cell cycle initiation and differentiation. **Therapeutic Effects:** Death of lymphoma cells. Reduced signs and symptoms of rheumatoid arthritis.

Pharmacokinetics

Absorption: IV administration results in complete bioavailability.
Distribution: Binds specifically to CD20 binding sites on lymphoma cells.
Metabolism and Excretion: Unknown.
Half-life: 59.8–174 hr (depending on tumor burden).

TIME/ACTION PROFILE (B-cell depletion)

ROUTE	ONSET	PEAK	DURATION
IV	within 14 days	3–4 wk	6–9 mo†

†Duration of depletion after 4 wk of treatment

Contraindications/Precautions

Contraindicated in: Hypersensitivity to murine (mouse) proteins; OB: Can pass placental barrier potentially causing fetal B-cell depletion. Give only if clearly needed; Lactation: Potential for immunosuppresion in infant. Discontinue nursing.

Use Cautiously in: Pre-existing bone marrow depression; Hepatitis B infection (may reactivate infection during and for several months after treatment); Systemic lupus erythematosus (may cause fatal progressive multifocal leukoencephalopathy); HIV infection (may increase risk of HIV-associated lymphoma); Pedi: Safety not established.

Adverse Reactions/Side Effects

CNS: headache. **Resp:** bronchospasm, cough, dyspnea. **CV:** ARRHYTHMIAS, hypotension, peripheral edema. **GI:** abdominal pain, altered taste, dyspepsia. **Derm:** MUCOCUTANEOUS SKIN REACTIONS, flushing, urticaria. **Endo:** hyperglycemia. **F and E:** hypocalcemia. **Hemat:** ANEMIA, NEUTROPENIA, THROMBOCYTOPENIA. **MS:** arthralgia, back pain. **Misc:** allergic reactions including ANAPHYLAXIS and ANGIOEDEMA, infections, INFUSION REACTIONS, TUMOR LYSIS SYNDROME, fever/chills/rigors (infusion related).

Interactions

Drug-Drug: None known.

Route/Dosage

Relapsed or refractory, low-grade or follicular, CD20–positive, B-cell Non-hogkins lymphoma

IV (Adults): 375 mg/m² once weekly for 4–8 doses.

Retreatment Therapy

IV (Adults): 375 mg/m² once weekly for 4 doses.

Previously untreated follicular, CD20–positive, B-cell Non-hogkins lymphoma

IV (Adults): 375 mg/m² given on Day 1 of each cycle of CVP for up to 8 doses.

Previously untreated low-grade, CD20–positive, B-cell Non-hogkins lymphoma

IV (Adults): For patients who have not progressed following 6–8 cycles of CVP chemotherapy, 375 mg/m² given once weekly for 4 doses given every 6 months for up to 16 doses.

Diffuse Large B-cell Non-hogkins lymphoma

IV (Adults): 375 mg/m² given on Day 1 of each cycle of CVP for up to 8 infusions.

Rheumatoid Arthritis

IV (Adults): Two 1000 mg separated by 2 wks.

Availability

Solution for injection (requires dilution): 10 mg/ml in 100 mg and 500-mg vials.

NURSING IMPLICATIONS

Assessment

- Monitor patient for fever, chills/rigors, nausea, urticaria, fatigue, headache, pruritus, bronchospasm, dyspnea, sensation of tongue or throat swelling, rhinitis, vomiting, hypotension, flushing, and pain at disease sites. These infusion-related events occur frequently within 30 min–2 hr of beginning first infusion and may resolve with slowing or discontinuing infusion and treatment with IV saline, diphenhydramine, and acetaminophen. Patients with increased risk (females, patients with pulmonary infiltrates, chronic lymphocytic leukemia, or mantle cell leukemia) may have more severe reactions, which may be fatal. Signs of severe reactions include hypotension, angioedema, hypoxia, or bronchospasm and may require interruption of infusion. May result in pulmonary infiltrates, adult respiratory distress syndrome, MI, ventricular fibrillation, and cardiogenic shock. Monitor closely. Incidence decreases with subsequent infusions.
- Monitor patient for tumor lysis syndrome due to rapid reduction in tumor volume (acute renal failure, hyperkalemia, hypocalcemia, hyperuricemia, or hypophosphatemia) usually occurring 12–24 hr after first infusion. Risks are higher in patients with greater tumor burden; may be fatal. Correct electrolyte abnormalities, monitor renal function and fluid balance, and administer supportive care, including dialysis, as indicated.
- Assess patient for hypersensitivity reactions (hypotension, bronchospasm, angioedema)

during administration. May respond to decrease in infusion rate. Premedication with diphenhydramine and acetaminophen is recommended. Treatment includes diphenhydramine, acetaminophen, bronchodilators, or IV saline as indicated. Epinephrine, antihistamines, and corticosteroids should be readily available in the event of a severe reaction. If severe reactions occur, discontinue infusion; may be resumed at 50% of the rate when symptoms have resolved completely.

- Monitor ECG during and immediately after infusion in patients with pre-existing cardiac conditions (arrhythmias, angina) or patients who have developed arrhythmias during previous infusions of rituximab. Life-threatening arrhythmias may occur.
- ***Lab Test Considerations:*** Monitor CBC and platelet count regularly during therapy and frequently in patients with blood dyscrasias. May cause anemia, thrombocytopenia, or neutropenia.
- Frequently causes B-cell depletion with an associated ↓ in serum immunoglobulins in a minority of patients; does not appear to cause an increased incidence of infection.

Potential Nursing Diagnoses

Risk for infection (Side Effects)

Implementation

- Transient hypotension may occur during infusion; antihypertensive medications may be held for 12 hr before infusion.
- **Rheumatoid Arthritis:** Administer 100 mg methylprednisolone Iv or equivalent 30 min prior to each infusion to minimize infusion reactions.

IV Administration

- **Intermittent Infusion: *Diluent:*** Dilute with 0.9% NaCl or D5W. ***Concentration:*** 1–4 mg/ml. Gently invert bag to mix. Solution is clear and colorless; do not administer solutions that are discolored or contain particulate matter. Discard unused portion remaining in vial. Solution is stable for 12 hr at room temperature and for 24 hr if refrigerated. ***Rate:*** Do not administer as an IV push or bolus.
- ***First infusion:*** Administer at an initial rate of 50 mg/hr. If hypersensitivity or infusion-related events do not occur, rate may be escalated in 50 mg/hr increments every 30 min to a maximum of 400 mg/hr.
- ***Subsequent infusions:*** May be administered at an initial rate of 100 mg/hr and increased by 100-mg/hr increments at 30-min intervals to a maximum of 400 mg/hr.
- **Additive Incompatibility:** Do not admix with other medications.

Patient/Family Teaching

- Inform patient of the purpose of the medication.
- Advise patient to report infusion-related events or symptoms of hypersensitivity reactions immediately.
- Instruct patient to notify health care professional promptly if fever; chills; cough; hoarseness; sore throat; signs of infection; lower back or side pain; painful or difficult urination; bleeding gums; bruising; petechiae; blood in stools, urine, or emesis; increased fatigue; dyspnea; or orthostatic hypotension occurs. Caution patient to avoid crowds and persons with known infections. Instruct patient to use soft toothbrush and electric razor and to avoid falls. Caution patient not to drink alcoholic beverages or take medication containing aspirin or NSAIDs; may precipitate gastric bleeding.
- Instruct patient to use contraception throughout therapy.
- Advise patient to consult health care professional prior to receiving any vaccinations.

Evaluation/Desired Outcomes

- Decrease in spread of malignancy.
- Reduced signs and symptoms of rheumatoid arthritis.

rivastigmine

(rye-va-**stig**-meen)

Exelon, Exelon Patch

Classification

Therapeutic: anti-Alzheimer's agents

Pharmacologic: cholinergics (cholinesterase inhibitors)

Pregnancy Category B

Indications

PO: Mild to moderate dementia associated with Alzheimer's disease. **Transdermal:** Treatment

R

of mild to moderate dementia associated with Alzheimer's disease and Parkinson's disease.

Action

Enhances cholinergic function by reversible inhibition of cholinesterase. Does not cure the disease. **Therapeutic Effects:** Decreased dementia (temporary) associated with Alzheimer's disease and Parkinson's disease. Enhanced cognitive ability.

Pharmacokinetics

Absorption: Well absorbed following oral administration. Transdermal patch is slowly absorbed over 8 hrs.

Distribution: Widely distributed.

Metabolism and Excretion: Rapidly and extensively metabolized by the liver; metabolites are excreted by the kidneys.

Half-life: *PO*—1.5 hr; *Transdermal*—24 hr.

TIME/ACTION PROFILE (improvement in dementia)

ROUTE	ONSET	PEAK	DURATION
PO	within 2 wk	up to 12 wk	unknown
transdermal	unknown	unknown	unknown

Contraindications/Precautions

Contraindicated in: Hypersensitivity to rivastigmine or other carbamates.

Use Cautiously in: History of asthma or obstructive pulmonary disease; History of GI bleeding; Sick sinus syndrome or other supraventricular cardiac conduction abnormalities; **Transdermal:** Patients weighing <50 kg; at risk for ↑ adverse reactions; OB, Pedi: Pregnancy, lactation, or children (safety not established).

Adverse Reactions/Side Effects

CNS: weakness, dizziness, drowsiness, headache, sedation (unusual). **CV:** edema, heart failure, hypotension. **GI:** anorexia, dyspepsia, nausea, vomiting, abdominal pain, diarrhea, flatulence, weight gain (unusual). **Neuro:** tremor. **Misc:** fever, weight loss.

Interactions

Drug-Drug: Nicotine use may increase metabolism and decrease blood levels.

Route/Dosage

PO (Adults): 1.5 mg twice daily initially; after at least 2 weeks, dose may be increased to 3 mg twice daily. Further increments may be made at 2-week intervals up to 6 mg twice daily.

Transdermal (Adults): *Initial Dose*—One patch 4.6 mg/24 hr intially. After a minimum of 4 wks; *Maintenance Dose*—With good tolerability, may increase to one patch 9.5 mg/24.

Availability

Capsules: 1.5 mg, 3 mg, 4.5 mg, 6 mg. **Oral Solution:** 2 mg/ml in 120-ml bottle. **Transdermal Patch:** 4.6 mg/24 hr, 9.5 mg/24 hr.

NURSING IMPLICATIONS

Assessment

- Assess cognitive function (memory, attention, reasoning, language, ability to perform simple tasks) periodically throughout therapy.
- Monitor patient for nausea, vomiting, anorexia, and weight loss. Notify health care professional if these side effects occur.

Potential Nursing Diagnoses

Disturbed thought process (Indications)
Impaired environmental interpretation syndrome (Indications)
Imbalanced nutrition: less than body requirements (Side Effects)

Implementation

- Rivastigmine oral solution and capsules may be interchanged at equal doses.
- Patients switching from oral doses of <6 mg to transdermal doses should use 4.6 mg/24 hr patch. Patients taking oral doses of 6 mg–12 mg may be converted directly to 9.5 mg/24 hr patch. Apply patch on the day following the last oral dose.
- **PO:** Administer in the morning and evening with food.
- Oral solution may be administered directly from syringe provided or mixed with a small glass of water, cold fruit juice, or soda. Mixture should be stirred prior to drinking. Ensure patient drinks entire mixture. Oral solution is stable for 4 hours at room temperature when mixed with cold fruit juice or soda. Do not mix with other solutions. **Transdermal:** Apply patch to clean, dry, hairless area that will not be rubbed by tight clothing. Upper or lower back is recommended, may also use upper arm or chest. Do not apply to red, irritated or cut skin. Rotate sites to prevent irritation, do not use same site within 14 days. Remove adhesive liner and apply by pressing patch firmly until edges stick well. May be worn during bathing and hot weather. Each 24 hrs, remove old patch and discard by folding in half and apply new patch to a new area.

Patient/Family Teaching

- **PO:** Emphasize the importance of taking rivastigmine at regular intervals as directed.
- Explain to patient and caregiver how to use oral dosing syringe provided with oral solution. Remove syringe from protective case and push down and twist child resistant closure to open bottle. Insert syringe into opening in white stopper in bottle. Hold the syringe and pull plunger to the level corresponding to the prescribed dose. Before removing syringe from bottle, push out larger bubbles (small bubbles will not alter dose) by moving plunger up and down a few times. After large bubbles are gone, move plunger to level of dose. Remove syringe from bottle.
- **Transdermal:** Instruct patient and caregiver on the correct application, rotation, and discarding of patch. Patch should be folded in half and discarded out of reach of children and pets; medication remains in discarded patch. Replace missed doses immediately and apply next patch at usual time. Advise patient and caregiver to avoid contact with eyes and to wash hands after applying patch. Avoid exposure to heat sources (excessive sunlight, saunas, heating pads) for long periods.
- Caution patient and caregiver that rivastigmine may cause dizziness. Caution patient to avoid driving or other activities requiring alertness until response to medication is known.
- Advise patient and caregiver to notify health care professional if nausea, vomiting, anorexia, or weight loss occur. If adverse effects become intolerable during treatment with *transdermal patch,* instruct patient to discontinue patches for several days and then restart at same or next lower dose level. If treatment is interrupted for more than several days, lowest dose level should be used when restarting and titrate according to Route and Dosage section.
- Advise patient and caregiver to notify health care professional of medication regimen prior to treatment or surgery.
- Inform patient and caregivers that improvement in cognitive functioning may take weeks to months and that the degenerative process is not reversed.
- Advise patient to notify health care professional if pregnancy is planned or suspected or if breastfeeding.

Evaluation/Desired Outcomes

- Temporary improvement in cognitive function (memory, attention, reasoning, language, ability to perform simple tasks) in patients with Alzheimer's disease.
- Improvement in cognitive function and overall functioning in patients with Parkinson's disease.

rizatriptan (riz-a-**trip**-tan)

Maxalt, Maxalt-MLT

Classification

Therapeutic: vascular headache suppressants

Pharmacologic: 5-HT_1 agonists

Pregnancy Category C

Indications

Acute treatment of migraine headache.

Action

Acts as an agonist at specific 5-HT_1 receptor sites in intracranial blood vessels and sensory trigeminal nerves. **Therapeutic Effects:** Cranial vessel vasoconstriction with associated decrease in release of neuropeptides and resultant decrease in migraine headache.

Pharmacokinetics

Absorption: Completely absorbed after oral administration, but first-pass metabolism results in 45% bioavailability.

Distribution: Unknown.

Metabolism and Excretion: Primarily metabolized by monoamine oxidase-A (MAO-A); minor conversion to an active compound; 14% excreted unchanged in urine.

Half-life: 2–3 hr.

TIME/ACTION PROFILE (blood levels)

ROUTE	ONSET	PEAK	DURATION
PO	30 min	1–1.5 hr	unknown

Contraindications/Precautions

Contraindicated in: Hypersensitivity; Ischemic or vasospastic cardiovascular, cerebrovascular, or peripheral vascular syndromes; History of significant cardiovascular disease;

Uncontrolled hypertension; Should not be used within 24 hr of other 5-HT_1 agonists or ergot-type compounds (dihydroergotamine); Basilar or hemiplegic migraine; Concurrent MAO-A inhibitor therapy or within 2 wk of discontinuing MAO-A inhibitor therapy; Phenylketonuria (orally disintegrating tablet contains aspartame).
Use Cautiously in: Severe renal impairment, especially in patients on dialysis; Moderate hepatic impairment; Pregnancy, lactation, or children <18 yr (safety not established).
Exercise Extreme Caution in: Cardiovascular risk factors (hypertension, hypercholesterolemia, cigarette smoking, obesity, diabetes, strong family history, menopausal women or men >40 yr); use only if cardiovascular status has been evaluated and determined to be safe and first dose is administered under supervision.

Adverse Reactions/Side Effects

CNS: dizziness, drowsiness, weakness. **CV:** CORONARY ARTERY VASOSPASM, MI, VENTRICULAR FIBRILLATION, VENTRICULAR TACHYCARDIA, chest pain, myocardial ischemia. **GI:** dry mouth, nausea. **Misc:** hypersensitivity reactions including ANGIOEDEMA, toxic epidermal necrolysis, pain.

Interactions

Drug-Drug: Concurrent use with **MAO-A inhibitors** ↑ blood levels and adverse reactions (concurrent use or use within 2 wk or MAO inhibitor is contraindicated). Concurrent use with other **5-HT agonists** or **ergot-type compounds (dihydroergotamine)** may result in ↑ vasoactive properties (avoid use within 24 hr of each other). **Propranolol** ↑ blood levels and risk of adverse reactions (dosage reduction recommended). Concurrent use with **SSRI antidepressants** may result in weakness, hyperreflexia, and incoordination.
Drug-Natural Products: Increased risk of serotinergic side effects including serotonin syndrome with **St. John's wort** and **SAMe**.

Route/Dosage

PO (Adults): 5–10 mg (use 5-mg dose in patients receiving propranolol); may be repeated in 2 hr; not to exceed 3 doses/24 hr. Dose is same for both types of tablets.

Availability

Tablets: 5 mg, 10 mg. **Cost:** 5 mg $107.44/6, 10 mg $231.99/12. **Orally disintegrating tablets (Maxalt-MLT) (peppermint flavor):** 5 mg, 10 mg. **Cost:** 5 mg $116.58/6, 10 mg $113.99/6.

NURSING IMPLICATIONS

Assessment

- Assess pain location, character, intensity, and duration and associated symptoms (photophobia, phonophobia, nausea, vomiting) during migraine attack.

Potential Nursing Diagnoses

Acute pain (Indications)

Implementation

- **PO:** Tablets should be swallowed whole with liquid.
- Orally disintegrating tablets should be left in the package until use. Remove from the blister pouch. Do not push tablet through the blister; peel open the blister pack with dry hands and place tablet on tongue. Tablet will dissolve rapidly and be swallowed with saliva. No liquid is needed to take the orally disintegrating tablet.

Patient/Family Teaching

- Inform patient that rizatriptan should be used only during a migraine attack. It is meant to be used for relief of migraine attacks but not to prevent or reduce the number of attacks.
- Instruct patient to administer rizatriptan as soon as symptoms of a migraine attack appear, but it may be administered at any time during an attack. If migraine symptoms return, a second dose may be used. Allow at least 2 hr between doses, and do not use more than 30 mg in any 24-hr period.
- If first dose does not relieve headache, additional rizatriptan doses are not likely to be effective; notify health care professional.
- Caution patient not to take rizatriptan within 24 hr of other vascular headache suppressants.
- Advise patient that lying down in a darkened room after rizatriptan administration may further help relieve headache.
- Caution patient not to use rizatriptan if she is pregnant, suspects she is pregnant, plans to become pregnant, or is breastfeeding. Adequate contraception should be used during therapy.
- Advise patient to notify health care professional before next dose of rizatriptan if pain or tightness in the chest occurs during use. If pain is severe or does not subside, notify health care professional immediately. If feelings of tingling, heat, flushing, heaviness, pressure, drowsiness, dizziness, tiredness, or

sickness develop, discuss with health care professional at next visit.

- May cause dizziness or drowsiness. Caution patient to avoid driving or other activities requiring alertness until response to medication is known.
- Advise patient to avoid alcohol, which aggravates headaches, during rizatriptan use.

Evaluation/Desired Outcomes

- Relief of migraine attack.

ropinirole (roe-**pin**-i-role)

Requip

Classification

Therapeutic: antiparkinson agents

Pharmacologic: dopamine agonists

Pregnancy Category C

Indications

Management of signs and symptoms of idiopathic Parkinson's disease. Restless legs syndrome.

Action

Stimulates dopamine receptors in the brain. **Therapeutic Effects:** Decreased tremor and rigidity in Parkinson's disease. Decreased leg restlessness.

Pharmacokinetics

Absorption: 55% absorbed following oral administration.

Distribution: Widely distributed.

Metabolism and Excretion: Extensively metabolized by the liver (by cytochrome P450 CYP1A2 enzyme system); <10% excreted unchanged in urine.

Half-life: 6 hr.

TIME/ACTION PROFILE

ROUTE	ONSET	PEAK	DURATION
PO	unknown	unknown	8 hr

Contraindications/Precautions

Contraindicated in: Hypersensitivity.

Use Cautiously in: Geri: ↑ risk of hallucinations in patients >65 yr; Hepatic impairment (slower titration may be required); Severe cardiovascular disease; OB, Pedi: Pregnancy, lactation, or children (safety not established; may inhibit lactation).

Adverse Reactions/Side Effects

CNS: SLEEP ATTACKS, <u>dizziness</u>, <u>syncope</u>, confusion, drowsiness, fatigue, hallucinations, headache, increased dyskinesia, weakness. **EENT:** abnormal vision. **CV:** orthostatic hypotension, peripheral edema. **GI:** constipation, dry mouth, dyspepsia, nausea, vomiting. **Derm:** increased sweating.

Interactions

Drug-Drug: Drugs that alter the activity of cytochrome P450 CYP1A2 enzyme system may affect the activity of ropinirole. Effects may be ↑ by **estrogens**. Effects may be ↓ by **phenothiazines**, **butyrophenones**, **thioxanthenes**, or **metoclopramide**. May ↑ effects of **levodopa** (may allow dose reduction of levodopa).

Route/Dosage

PO (Adults): *Parkinson's disease*—0.25 mg 3 times daily for 1 wk, then 0.5 mg 3 times daily for 1 wk, then 0.75 mg 3 times daily for 1 wk, then 1 mg 3 times daily for 1 wk; then may increase by 1.5 mg/day every wk, up to 9 mg/day; then may increase by up to 3 mg/day every wk up to 24 mg/day. *Restless legs syndrome*—0.25 mg once daily initially, 1 to 3 hours before bedtime. After 2 days, increase to 0.5 mg once daily and to 1 mg once daily by the end of first week of dosing, then increase by 0.5 mg weekly, up to 4 mg/day as needed/tolerated.

Availability

Tablets: 0.25 mg, 0.5 mg, 1 mg, 2 mg, 3 mg, 4 mg, 5 mg. **Cost:** 0.25 mg $569.92/270, 0.5 mg $569.92/270, 1 mg $568.84/270, 2 mg $575.94/270, 3 mg $638.87/270, 4 mg $638.87/270, 5 mg $639.98/270.

NURSING IMPLICATIONS

Assessment

- Assess blood pressure periodically during therapy.
- Assess patient for drowsiness and sleep attacks. Drowsiness is a common side effect of ropinirole, but sleep attacks or episodes of falling asleep during activities that require active participation may occur without warning. Assess patient for concomitant medications that have sedating effects or may increase serum ropinirole levels (see Interactions). May require discontinuation of therapy.

R

- **Parkinson's Disease:** Assess patient for signs and symptoms of Parkinson's disease (tremor, muscle weakness and rigidity, ataxic gait) prior to and during therapy.
- **Restless Leg Syndrome:** Assess sleep patterns and frequency of restless leg disturbances.
- ***Lab Test Considerations:*** May cause ↑ BUN.

Potential Nursing Diagnoses

Impaired physical mobility (Indications)
Risk for injury (Indications, Side Effects)

Implementation

- **PO:** May be administered with or without food. Administration with food may decrease nausea.

Patient/Family Teaching

- Instruct patient to take medication exactly as directed. Missed doses should be taken as soon as possible, but not if almost time for next dose. Do not double doses.
- Caution patient to change positions slowly to minimize orthostatic hypotension.
- May cause drowsiness and unexpected episodes of falling asleep. Caution patient to avoid driving or other activities requiring alertness until response to medication is known. Advise patient to notify health care professional if episodes of falling asleep occur.
- Advise patient to avoid alcohol and other CNS depressants concurrently with ropinirole.
- Advise patient that increasing fluids, sugarless gum or candy, ice, or saliva substitutes may help minimize dry mouth. Consult health care professional if dry mouth continues for >2 wk.

Evaluation/Desired Outcomes

- Decreased tremor and rigidity in Parkinson's disease.
- Decrease in restless legs and improved sleep.

ropivacaine, See EPIDURAL LOCAL ANESTHETICS.

rosiglitazone

(roe-zi-**glit**-a-zone)
Avandia

Classification
Therapeutic: antidiabetics
Pharmacologic: thiazolidinediones

Pregnancy Category C

Indications

Type 2 diabetes mellitus (with diet and exercise); may be used with metformin, sulfonylureas or insulin.

Action

Improves sensitivity to insulin by acting as an agonist at receptor sites involved in insulin responsiveness and subsequent glucose production and utilization. Requires insulin for activity. **Therapeutic Effects:** Decreased insulin resistance, resulting in glycemic control without hypoglycemia.

Pharmacokinetics

Absorption: Well absorbed (99%) following oral administration.
Distribution: Unknown.
Protein Binding: 99.8% bound to plasma proteins.
Metabolism and Excretion: Entirely metabolized by the liver.
Half-life: 3.2–3.6 hr (increased in liver disease).

TIME/ACTION PROFILE (effects on blood glucose)

ROUTE	ONSET	PEAK	DURATION
PO	unknown	unknown	12–24 hr

Contraindications/Precautions

Contraindicated in: Hypersensitivity; Diabetic ketoacidosis; Clinical evidence of active liver disease or increased ALT (>2.5 times upper limit of normal); Renal disease or dysfunction (creatinine over 1.5 mg/dL in males or 1.4 mg/dL in females; OB, Lactation: Potential for fetal or infant harm. Insulin monotherapy should be used.; Pedi: Safety and effectiveness not established.

Use Cautiously in: Edema; CHF (avoid use in moderate to severe CHF unless benefits outweigh risks); Concurrent use with insulin (may increase risk of adverse cardiovascular reactions); Hepatic impairment; OB: May restore ovulation and risk of pregnancy in premenopausal women; Geri: Dose reduction and careful titration recommended due to age-related decline in renal function. Avoid maximum dose. Should not be given to patients older than 80 yr.

Adverse Reactions/Side Effects

CV: CHF, edema. **EENT:** new onset and worsening diabetic macular edema. **Derm:** urticaria. **GI:** hepatitis, ↑ liver enzymes. **Hemat:** anemia. **Metab:** LACTIC ACIDOSIS, ↑ total cholesterol, LDL and HDL, weight gain. **Misc:** ANGIOEDEMA (rare), fractures (arm, hand, foot) in female patients.

Interactions

Drug-Drug: Concurrent use with **rifampin** ↓ levels and may ↓ effectiveness. **Gemfibrozil** ↑ levels and may ↑ risk of hypoglycemia (↓ dose of rosiglitazone).

Drug-Natural Products: Glucosamine may worsen blood glucose control. **Chromium** and **coenzyme Q-10** may produce additive hypoglycemic effects.

Route/Dosage

PO (Adults): 4 mg as a single dose once daily or 2 mg twice daily; after 8 weeks, may be increased if necessary to 8 mg once daily or 4 mg twice daily.

Availability

Tablets: 2 mg, 4 mg, 8 mg. **Cost:** 2 mg $218.99/90, 4 mg $338.96/90, 8 mg $575.95/90. ***In combination with:*** metformin (Avandamet), glimepiride (Avandaryl). See Appendix B.

NURSING IMPLICATIONS

Assessment

- Observe patient taking concurrent insulin for signs and symptoms of hypoglycemia (sweating, hunger, weakness, dizziness, tremor, tachycardia, anxiety).
- Assess patient for edema and signs of CHF (dyspnea, rales/crackles, peripheral edema, weight gain, jugular venous distension). May require discontinuation of rosiglitazone.
- Assess patient for signs of lactic acidosis (malaise, myalgias, respiratory distress, somnolence, nonspecific abdominal distress).
- ***Lab Test Considerations:*** Monitor serum glucose and glycosylated hemoglobin periodically during therapy to evaluate effectiveness.
- Monitor CBC with differential periodically during therapy. May cause ↓ in hemoglobin, hematocrit, and WBC, usually during the first 4–8 wk of therapy; then levels stabilize.
- Monitor AST and ALT prior to initiating therapy and periodically thereafter or if jaundice or symptoms of hepatic dysfunction occur. May cause irreversible ↑ in AST and ALT or hepatic failure (rare). If ALT increases to >3 times the upper limit of normal, recheck ALT promptly. Discontinue rosiglitazone if ALT remains >3 times normal.
- May cause ↑ in total cholesterol, LDL, and HDL and ↓ in free fatty acids.
- Monitor renal function tests prior to initiating therapy and periodically thereafter (BUN, creatinine, creatinine clearance), especially in older adults.

Potential Nursing Diagnoses

Imbalanced nutrition: more than body requirements (Indications)

Implementation

- Patients stabilized on a diabetic regimen who are exposed to stress, fever, trauma, infection, or surgery may require administration of insulin.
- **PO:** May be administered with or without meals.

Patient/Family Teaching

- Instruct patient to take medication as directed. If dose for 1 day is missed, do not double dose the next day.
- Explain to patient that this medication controls hyperglycemia but does not cure diabetes. Therapy is long term.
- Review signs of hypoglycemia and hyperglycemia with patient. If hypoglycemia occurs, advise patient to take a glass of orange juice or 2–3 tsp of sugar, honey, or corn syrup dissolved in water and notify health care professional.
- Encourage patient to follow prescribed diet, medication, and exercise regimen to prevent hypoglycemic or hyperglycemic episodes.
- Instruct patient in proper testing of serum glucose and ketones. These tests should be closely monitored during periods of stress or illness and health care professional notified if significant changes occur.
- Advise patient to notify health care professional immediately if signs of hepatic dysfunction (nausea, vomiting, abdominal pain, fatigue, anorexia, dark urine, jaundice), CHF,

or lactic acidosis (malaise, myalgias, respiratory distress, somnolence, nonspecific abdominal distress, hypothermia, hypotension, and bradyarrhythmias) occur.
- Advise patient to inform health care professional of medication regimen prior to treatment, studies using IV contrast, or surgery.
- Advise patient to carry a form of sugar (sugar packets, candy) and identification describing disease process and medication regimen at all times.
- Emphasize the importance of routine follow-up exams.
- OB: Insulin is the preferred method of controlling blood glucose during pregnancy. Counsel female patients that higher doses of oral contraceptives or a form of contraception other than oral contraceptives may be required and to notify health care professional promptly if pregnancy is planned or suspected.

Evaluation/Desired Outcomes
- Control of blood glucose levels.

rosuvastatin, See HMG-CoA REDUCTASE INHIBITORS (statins).

rotigotine transdermal system (ro-ti-go-teen)
Neupro

Classification
Therapeutic: antiparkinson agents
Pharmacologic: dopamine agonists

Pregnancy Category C

Indications
Symptomatic management of early-stage idiopathic Parkinson's disease.

Action
Acts as an agonist of dopamine in the CNS, primarily at D2 receptor sites. **Therapeutic Effects:** Improvement in symptoms of Parkinson's disease.

Pharmacokinetics
Absorption: 45% absorbed from patch over 24 hr.
Distribution: Unknown.
Metabolism and Excretion: Mostly metabolized and excreted in urine as metabolites (71%); 11% excreted in feces.
Half-life: Biphasic: initial half-life 3 hr; terminal half-life 5–7 hr.

TIME/ACTION PROFILE

ROUTE	ONSET	PEAK	DURATION
transdermal	1–3 hr	15–18 hr (rage 4–27 hr)	24 hr

Contraindications/Precautions
Contraindicated in: Hypersensitivity to rotigotine or sulfites; OB: Lactation.
Use Cautiously in: Severe cardiovascular disease (may increase risk of postural hypotension); Severe hepatic impairment; Geri: Skin changes in patients >80 yr may result in higher blood levels; OB: use only if maternal benefits outweigh risk to fetus; Pedi: Safe use in children not established.

Adverse Reactions/Side Effects
CNS: DROWSINESS, insomnia, confusion, dizziness, hallucinations, headache, malaise, sudden sleep attacks. **CV:** peripheral edema, postural hypotension, syncope. **GI:** nausea, vomiting, anorexia, dry mouth, dyspepsia, ↑ liver enzymes. **GU:** urinary incontinence. **Derm:** application site reactions, ↑ risk of melanoma, ↑ sweating, pruritus, purpura. **Metab:** weight gain. **MS:** leg pain. **Neuro:** abnormal gait, ataxia, dyskinesia, hypertonia, hypoesthesia, neuralgia, paresthesia. **Misc:** fever.

Interactions
Drug-Drug: Concurrent use of **dopamine antagonists** including some **antipsychotics** or **metoclopramide** may ↓ effectiveness.

Route/Dosage
Transdermal (Adults): 2 mg/24 hr initially, may increase by 2 mg/24 hr weekly, up to 6 mg/24 hr.

Availability
Transdermal system: 2 mg/24 hr (contains 4.5 mg rotigotine/10 cm^2), 4 mg/24 hr (contains 9 mg rotigotine/20 cm^2), 6 mg/24 hr (contains 13.5 mg rotigotine/30 cm^2).

NURSING IMPLICATIONS

Assessment
- Assess for allergy to sulfite, may be more common in asthmatics.
- Assess frequently for drowsiness, a common side effect of rotigotine. Episodes of falling asleep during activities that require active participation may occur without warning. Pa-

tients may not acknowledge drowsiness unless directly questioned about drowsiness during specific activities. May occur as late as 1 year after initiation of therapy. Assess patient for concomitant medications that have sedating effects. May require discontinuation of therapy.

- Monitor blood pressure, sitting and standing, periodically during therapy, especially during dose escalation. May also cause syncope.
- Assess for application site reactions (erythema, edema, pruritus). If persistent, (more than a few days), increasing in severity, or spreading outside application site, determine risk/benefit ratio. If generalized skin reaction (allergic macular-papular rash) occurs, discontinue rotigotine.
- Assess for hallucinations. May require discontinuation.
- Monitor for weight gain; usually associated with peripheral edema.
- Assess for development of new or increased gambling urges, sexual urges, or other urges during therapy.
- ***Lab Test Considerations:*** May cause ↓ hemoglobin and serum albumin and glucose levels.
- May cause ↑ BUN and GGT levels.

Potential Nursing Diagnoses

Impaired physical mobility (Indications)
Risk for injury (Adverse Reactions)

Implementation

Transdermal: Apply once daily to clean, dry, intact skin on abdomen, thigh, hip, flank, shoulder, or upper arm. Hold in place for 20–30 seconds to make sure of good contact, especially around edges. If applied to hairy area, shave area at least 3 days prior to application. Do not apply to areas that could be rubbed by tight clothing, are under a waistband, or to skin folds. Do not apply to skin that is red, irritated, or impaired. Do not apply creams, lotions, ointments, oils, or powders to skin areas where patch will be placed. Wash hands following application to remove any drug and do not touch eyes. Rotate patch site daily; do not use same application site more than once every 14 days. Do not cut or damage patch. Remove patch slowly and carefully to avoid irritation. Fold over so it sticks to itself and discard. Wash application site with soap and water to remove drug or adhesive. May use baby or mineral oil to remove excess residue. Avoid using alcohol or other solvents, may cause skin irritation. If therapy is discontinued, decrease gradually by 2 mg/24 hrs every other day until complete withdrawal.

Patient/Family Teaching

- Instruct patient on proper method of patch application. Advise patient to wear patch continuously for 24 hrs and to apply system at the same time each day; if patch change is missed, apply as soon as possible and replace at usual time the following day. Patients may bathe, shower or swim with patch on. If patch falls off, apply a new on immediately to a different site and change according to regular schedule. Do not stop therapy without consulting health care professional. withdrawal.
- May cause drowsiness and unexpected episodes of falling asleep. Caution patient to avoid driving and other activities requiring alertness until response to medication is known. Advise patient to notify health care professional if episodes of falling asleep occur.
- Advise patient to notify health care professional if application site reaction occurs.
- Inform patient that rotigotine may cause hallucinations.
- Advise patient to remove rotigotine patch prior to magnetic resonance imaging or cardioversion.
- Caution patient to avoid exposing patch to external heat (heating pad, electric blanket, heat lamp, sauna, hot tub, heated water bed, prolonged direct sunlight).
- Advise patient to consult health care professional porior to taking other Rx, OTC, or herbal products or alcohol.
- Advise female patients to notify health care professional if pregnancy is planned or suspected or if breastfeeding.
- Advise patient to notify health care professional if they experience new or increased gambling, sexual or other intense urges during therapy. May require discontinuation.
- Advise patient to have health care professional check their skin for skin cancer regularly due to increase risk of melanoma.

Evaluation/Desired Outcomes

- Improvement in signs and symptoms of early-stage Parkinson's disease.

R

SALICYLATES

aspirin (**as**-pir-in)
✤Apo-ASA, ✤Apo-ASEN, ✤Arthrinol, ✤Arthrisin, ✤Artria S.R, ASA, ✤Asaphen, Ascriptin, Aspercin, Aspergum, Aspirtab, ✤Astrin, Bayer Aspirin, Bufferin, ✤Coryphen, Easprin, Ecotrin, ✤Entrophen, Genacote, Halfprin, ✤Headache Tablets, Healthprin, ✤Novasen, ✤PMS-ASA, ✤Rivasa, St. Joseph Adult Chewable Aspirin, ZORprin

choline salicylate
(**koe**-leen sal-**i**-sil-ate)
Arthropan

choline and magnesium salicylates
(**koe**-leen mag-**neez**-ee-um sal-**i**-sil-ates)
CMT, Tricosal, Trilisate

magnesium salicylate
(mag-**neez**-ee-um sal-**i**-sil-ate)
✤Doan's Backache Pills, Doan's Regular Strength Tablets, Magan, Mobidin

salsalate (**sal**-sa-late)
Amigesic, Anaflex, Disalcid, Marthritic, Mono-Gesic, Salflex, Salgesic, Salsitab

sodium salicylate
(**soe**-dee-yum sal-**i**-sil-ate)
✤Dodd's Extra Strength, ✤Dodd's Pills, ✤Gin Pain Pills

Classification
Therapeutic: antipyretics, nonopioid analgesics
Pharmacologic: salicylates

Pregnancy Category D (aspirin–first trimester), C (magnesium salicylate, salsalate–first trimester)

Indications

Inflammatory disorders including: Rheumatoid arthritis, Osteoarthritis. Mild to moderate pain. Fever. **Aspirin:** Prophylaxis of transient ischemic attacks and MI.

Action

Produce analgesia and reduce inflammation and fever by inhibiting the production of prostaglandins. Aspirin Only Decreases platelet aggregation. **Therapeutic Effects:** Analgesia. Reduction of inflammation. Reduction of fever. Aspirin. Decreased incidence of transient ischemic attacks and MI.

Pharmacokinetics

Absorption: *Aspirin*—Well absorbed from the upper small intestine; absorption from enteric-coated preparations may be unreliable; rectal absorption is slow and variable. *Choline and magnesium salicylates*—Well absorbed after oral administration. *Salsalate*—Splits into 2 molecules of salicylic acid after oral administration; absorbed in the small intestine.
Distribution: All salicylates are rapidly and widely distributed; cross the placenta and enter breast milk.
Metabolism and Excretion: Extensively metabolized by the liver; inactive metabolites excreted by the kidneys. Amount excreted unchanged by the kidneys depends on urine pH; as pH increases, amount excreted unchanged increases from 2–3% up to 80%.
Half-life: 2–3 hr for low doses; up to 15–30 hr with larger doses because of saturation of liver metabolism.

TIME/ACTION PROFILE (analgesia/fever reduction†)

ROUTE	ONSET	PEAK	DURATION
aspirin–PO	5–30 min	1–3 hr	3–6 hr
aspirin–PO-ER	5–30 min	2–4 hr	8–12 hr
aspirin–Rect	1–2 hr	4–5 hr	7 hr
all other salicylates–PO	5–30 min	1–3 hr	3–6 hr

†Antirheumatic effect may take 2–3 wk of chronic dosing

Contraindications/Precautions

Contraindicated in: Hypersensitivity to aspirin, tartrazine (FDC yellow dye #5), or other salicylates; Cross-sensitivity with other NSAIDs may exist (less with nonaspirin salicylates); Bleeding disorders or thrombocytopenia (more important with aspirin); Children or adolescents with viral infections (may increase the risk of Reye's syndrome); **Salsalate:** Peri-operative

S

pain from coronary artery bypass graft (CABG) surgery.

Use Cautiously in: History of GI bleeding or ulcer disease; Chronic alcohol use/abuse; Severe renal disease (magnesium toxicity may occur with magnesium salicylate); Severe hepatic disease; Salsalate. Cardiovascular disease or risk factors for cardiovascular disease (may ↑ risk of serious cardiovascular thrombotic events, myocardial infarction, and stroke, especially with prolonged use); Geri: Geriatric patients (↑ risk of adverse reactions especially GI bleeding; more sensitive to toxic levels); OB: Pregnancy; salicylates may have adverse effects on fetus and mother and in general should be avoided during pregnancy, especially during the 3rd trimester; Lactation: Lactation (safety not established).

Adverse Reactions/Side Effects

EENT: tinnitus. **GI:** GI BLEEDING, dyspepsia, epigastric distress, nausea, abdominal pain, anorexia, hepatotoxicity, vomiting. **Derm:** *salsalate*— EXFOLIATIVE DERMATITIS, STEVENS-JOHNSON SYNDROME, TOXIC EPIDERMAL NECROLYSIS. **Hemat:** *aspirin*— anemia, hemolysis, increased bleeding time. **Misc:** allergic reactions including ANAPHYLAXIS and LARYNGEAL EDEMA.

Interactions

Drug-Drug: Aspirin may ↑ the risk of bleeding with **warfarin**, **heparin**, **heparin-like agents**, **thrombolytic agents**, **ticlopidine**, **clopidogrel**, **abciximab**, **tirofiban**, or **eptifibatide**, although these agents are frequently used safely in combination and in sequence. Ibuprofen may negate the cardioprotective antiplatelet effects of low-dose aspirin. Aspirin may ↑ risk of bleeding with **cefoperazone**, **cefotetan**, and **valproic acid**. May ↑ activity of **penicillins**, **phenytoin**, **methotrexate**, **valproic acid**, **oral hypoglycemic agents**, and **sulfonamides**. May ↓ beneficial effects of **probenecid** or **sulfinpyrazone**. **Corticosteroids** may ↓ serum salicylate levels. **Urinary acidification** ↑ reabsorption and may ↑ serum salicylate levels. **Alkalinization of the urine** or the ingestion of large amounts of **antacids** ↑ excretion and ↓ serum salicylate levels. May blunt the therapeutic response to **diuretics**, and **antihypertensives**. ↑ risk of GI irritation with **NSAIDs**.

Drug-Natural Products: ↑ anticoagulant effect and bleeding risk when using aspirin with **arnica**, **chamomile**, **clove**, **feverfew**, **garlic**, **ginger**, **ginkgo**, **Panax ginseng**, and others.

Drug-Food: Foods capable of acidifying the urine (see Appendix L) may ↑ serum salicylate levels.

Route/Dosage

Aspirin

Pain/Fever

PO, Rect (Adults): 325–1000 mg q 4–6 hr (not to exceed 4 g/day). *Extended-release tablets*—650 mg q 8 hr or 800 mg q 12 hr.

PO, Rect (Children 2–11 yr): 10–15 mg/kg q 4–6 hr (not to exceed 4 g/day).

Inflammation

PO (Adults): 2.4 g/day initially; increased to maintenance dose of 3.6–5.4 g/day in divided doses (up to 7.8 g/day for acute rheumatic fever).

PO (Children): 60–100 mg/kg/day in divided doses (up to 130 mg/kg/day for acute rheumatic fever).

Prevention of Transient Ischemic Attacks

PO (Adults): 50–325 mg once daily.

Prevention of Myocardial Infarction

PO (Adults): 80–325 mg once daily.

PO (Children): 3–10 mg/kg once daily (round dose to a convenient amount.

Kawasaki Disease

PO (Children): 80–100 mg/kg/day in 4 divided doses until fever resolves; may be followed by maintenance dose of 3–5 mg/kg/day as a single dose for up to 8 wk.

Choline Salicylate

435 mg of choline salicylate is equivalent to 325 mg of aspirin

PO (Adults): *Analgesic/antipyretic*—435–669 mg ($^1/_2$–$^3/_4$ tsp) q 3 hr or 425–870 mg ($^1/_2$–1 tsp) q 4 hr or 870–1305 mg (1–1$^1/_2$ tsp) q 6 hr as needed. *Anti-inflammatory*—4.8–7.2 g/day in divided doses.

PO (Children): *Pain/fever*—2 g/m^2/day in 4–6 divided doses. *Inflammation*—107–133 mg/kg/day in 4–6 divided doses (up to 174 mg/kg).

Magnesium Salicylate

PO (Adults): 304 mg q 4 hr or 467 mg q 6 hr.

Choline and Magnesium Salicylates

5 ml of liquid equivalent to 500 mg salicylate or 650 mg of aspirin. Tablet strength expressed in mg of salicylate: 500-mg tablet equivalent to 650 mg of aspirin, 750-mg tablet equivalent to 975

mg of aspirin, 1000-mg tablet equivalent to 1.3 g of aspirin

PO (Adults): *Anti-inflammatory*—3 g/day of salicylate at bedtime or in 2–3 divided doses (not to exceed 4.5 g/day).

PO (Children >37 kg): 2.25 g of salicylate/day in 2 divided doses.

PO (Children <37 kg): 50 mg of salicylate/kg/day in 2 divided doses.

Salsalate

PO (Adults): 1 g 3 times daily initially; further titration may be required.

Sodium Salicylate

PO (Adults): *Pain/fever*—325–650 mg q 4 hr. *Inflammation*—3.6–5.4 g/day in divided doses.

PO (Children): *Pain/fever*—1.5 g/m^2/day in 4–6 divided doses. *Inflammation*—80–100 mg/kg/day in 4–6 divided doses.

Availability

Aspirin

Tablets: 81 mg[OTC], 162.5 mg[OTC], 325 mg[OTC], 500 mg[OTC], 650 mg[OTC], ✤975 mg[OTC]. **Chewable tablets:** ✤80 mg[OTC], 81 mg[OTC]. **Chewing gum:** 227 mg[OTC]. **Dispersible tablets:** 325 mg[OTC], 500 mg[OTC]. **Enteric-coated (delayed-release) tablets:** 80 mg[OTC], 165 mg[OTC], ✤300 mg[OTC], 325 mg[OTC], 500 mg[OTC], ✤600 mg[OTC], 650 mg[OTC], 975 mg[OTC]. **Extended-release tablets:** ✤325 mg[OTC], 650 mg[OTC], 800 mg. **Delayed-release capsules:** ✤325 mg[OTC], ✤500 mg[OTC]. **Suppositories:** 60 mg[OTC], 120 mg[OTC], 125 mg[OTC], 130 mg[OTC], ✤150 mg[OTC], ✤160 mg[OTC], 195 mg[OTC], 200 mg[OTC], 300 mg[OTC], ✤320 mg[OTC], 325 mg[OTC], 600 mg[OTC], ✤640 mg[OTC], 650 mg[OTC], 1.2 g[OTC]. ***In combination with:*** antihistamines, decongestants, cough suppressants[OTC], and opioids. See Appendix B.

Choline Salicylate

Oral solution: 870 mg/5 ml[OTC].

Magnesium Salicylate

Tablets: 304 mg[OTC], 467 mg[OTC], 545 mg, 600 mg, 650 mg.

Choline and Magnesium Salicylates (listed as salicylate content)

Tablets: 500 mg, 750 mg, 1000 mg. **Liquid:** 500 mg/5 ml.

Salsalate

Tablets: 500 mg, 750 mg. **Cost:** *Disalcid*—500 mg $22.90/20, 750 mg $41.87/30; *generic*—500 mg $32.74/100, 750 mg $41.04/100.

Sodium Salicylate

Tablets: 325 mg[OTC], 650 mg[OTC]. **Delayed-release tablets:** 324 mg[OTC], 325 mg[OTC], 650 mg[OTC].

NURSING IMPLICATIONS

Assessment

- Patients who have asthma, allergies, and nasal polyps or who are allergic to tartrazine are at an increased risk for developing hypersensitivity reactions.
- **Pain:** Assess pain and limitation of movement; note type, location, and intensity before and at the peak (see Time/Action Profile) after administration.
- **Fever:** Assess fever and note associated signs (diaphoresis, tachycardia, malaise, chills).
- ***Lab Test Considerations:*** Monitor hepatic function before antirheumatic therapy and if symptoms of hepatotoxicity occur; more likely in patients, especially children, with rheumatic fever, systemic lupus erythematosus, juvenile arthritis, or pre-existing hepatic disease. May cause ↑ serum AST, ALT, and alkaline phosphatase, especially when plasma concentrations exceed 25 mg/100 ml. May return to normal despite continued use or dose reduction. If severe abnormalities or active liver disease occurs, discontinue and use with caution in future.
- Monitor serum salicylate levels periodically with prolonged high-dose therapy to determine dose, safety, and efficacy, especially in children with Kawasaki disease.
- *Aspirin:* Prolongs bleeding time for 4–7 days and, in large doses, may cause prolonged prothrombin time. Monitor hematocrit periodically in prolonged high-dose therapy to assess for GI blood loss.
- ***Toxicity and Overdose:*** Monitor patient for the onset of tinnitus, headache, hyperventilation, agitation, mental confusion, lethargy, diarrhea, and sweating. If these symptoms appear, withhold medication and notify physician or other health care professional immediately.

Potential Nursing Diagnoses

Acute pain (Indications)
Impaired physical mobility (Indications)

Implementation

- Use lowest effective dose for shortest period of time.
- **PO:** Administer after meals or with food or an antacid to minimize gastric irritation. Food slows but does not alter the total amount absorbed.
- Do not crush or chew enteric-coated tablets. Do not take antacids within 1–2 hr of enteric-coated tablets. Chewable tablets may be chewed, dissolved in liquid, or swallowed whole. Some extended-release tablets may be broken or crumbled but must not be ground up before swallowing. See manufacturer's prescribing information for individual products.

Patient/Family Teaching

- Instruct patient to take salicylates with a full glass of water and to remain in an upright position for 15–30 min after administration.
- Advise patient to report tinnitus; unusual bleeding of gums; bruising; black, tarry stools; or fever lasting longer than 3 days.
- Caution patient to avoid concurrent use of alcohol with this medication to minimize possible gastric irritation; 3 or more glasses of alcohol per day may increase the risk of GI bleeding. Caution patient to avoid taking concurrently with acetaminophen or NSAIDs for more than a few days, unless directed by health care professional to prevent analgesic nephropathy.
- Teach patients on a sodium-restricted diet to avoid effervescent tablets or buffered-aspirin preparations.
- Tablets with an acetic (vinegar-like) odor should be discarded.
- Advise patients on long-term therapy to inform health care professional of medication regimen before surgery. Aspirin may need to be withheld for 1 wk before surgery.
- Pedi: Centers for Disease Control and Prevention warns against giving aspirin to children or adolescents with varicella (chickenpox) or influenza-like or viral illnesses because of a possible association with Reye's syndrome.
- **Transient Ischemic Attacks or MI:** Advise patients receiving aspirin prophylactically to take only prescribed dose. Increasing the dose has not been found to provide additional benefits.

Evaluation/Desired Outcomes

- Relief of mild to moderate discomfort.
- Increased ease of joint movement. May take 2–3 wk for maximum effectiveness.
- Reduction of fever.
- Prevention of transient ischemic attacks.
- Prevention of MI.

salmeterol (sal-**me**-te-role)

Serevent

Classification

Therapeutic: bronchodilators
Pharmacologic: adrenergics

Pregnancy Category C

Indications

Long-term control of reversible airway obstruction due to asthma and for maintenance treatment of asthma and prevention of bronchospasm. Prevention of exercise-induced asthma. Maintenance treatment to prevent bronchospasm in COPD including chronic bronchitis and emphysema.

Action

Produces accumulation of cyclic adenosine monophosphate (cAMP) at $beta_2$-adrenergic receptors. Relatively specific for beta (pulmonary) receptors. **Therapeutic Effects:** Bronchodilation.

Pharmacokinetics

Absorption: Minimal systemic absorption follows inhalation.
Distribution: Action is primarily local.
Metabolism and Excretion: Unknown.
Half-life: 3–4 hr.

TIME/ACTION PROFILE (bronchodilation)

ROUTE	ONSET	PEAK	DURATION
inhalation	10–25 min	3–4 hr	12 hr†

†9 hr in adolescents

Contraindications/Precautions

Contraindicated in: Hypersensitivity; Acute attack of asthma (onset of action is delayed).
Use Cautiously in: Cardiovascular disease (including angina and hypertension); Convulsive disorders; Diabetes; Glaucoma; Hyperthyroidism; Pheochromocytoma; Excessive use (may lead to tolerance and paradoxical bronchospasm); Pregnancy, lactation, or children <4 yr (dry powder inhalation may be used in children 4–12 yr; aerosol inhalation may be used in chil-

dren >12 yr; may inhibit contractions during labor).

Adverse Reactions/Side Effects

CNS: headache, nervousness. **CV:** palpitations, tachycardia. **GI:** abdominal pain, diarrhea, nausea. **MS:** muscle cramps/soreness. **Neuro:** trembling. **Resp:** paradoxical bronchospasm, cough.

Interactions

Drug-Drug: Beta blockers may ↓ therapeutic effects of salmeterol. **MAO inhibitors** and **tricyclic antidepressants** potentiate cardiovascular effects.
Drug-Natural Products: Use with caffeine-containing herbs **(cola nut, guarana, mate, tea, coffee) ↑ stimulant effect.**

Route/Dosage

Inhaln (Adults and Children ≥4 yr): Diskus—50 mcg (one inhalation as dry powder) twice daily (approximately 12 hr apart); Inhaler 42 mcg (2 puffs) twice daily, 12 hours apart. *Exercise-induced bronchospasm*—Inhaler—42 mcg (two puffs) 30–60 min before exercise.

Availability

Powder for inhalation (Serevent Diskus): 50 mcg/blister. **Aerosol for oral inhalation (Serevent Inhaler):** 25 mcg/actuation (delivers 21 mcg/inhalation) 6.5 g (60 inhalations), 13 g (120 inhalations). ***In combination with:*** fluticasone (Advair Diskus, see Appendix B).

NURSING IMPLICATIONS

Assessment

- Assess lung sounds, pulse, and blood pressure before administration and periodically during therapy.
- Monitor pulmonary function tests before initiating therapy and periodically during course to determine effectiveness.
- Observe for paradoxical bronchospasm (wheezing, dyspnea, tightness in chest) and hypersensitivity reaction (rash; urticaria; swelling of the face, lips, or eyelids). Frequently occurs with first use of new canister or vial. If condition occurs, withhold medication and notify physician or other health care professional immediately.
- ***Lab Test Considerations:*** May cause ↑ serum glucose concentrations; occurs rarely with recommended doses and is more pronounced with frequent use of high doses.
- May cause ↓ serum potassium concentrations, which are usually transient and dose related; rarely occurs at recommended doses and is more pronounced with frequent use of high doses.
- ***Toxicity and Overdose:*** Symptoms of overdose include persistent agitation, chest pain or discomfort, decreased blood pressure, dizziness, hyperglycemia, hypokalemia, seizures, tachyarrhythmias, persistent trembling, and vomiting: Treatment includes discontinuing salmeterol and other beta-adrenergic agonists and providing symptomatic, supportive therapy. Cardioselective beta blockers are used cautiously because they may induce bronchospasm.

Potential Nursing Diagnoses

Ineffective airway clearance (Indications)

Implementation

- Do not confuse salmeretol with Salbutamol (albuterol). **Inhaln:** Once removed from foil overwrap, discard discus when every blister has been used or 6 wk have passed, whichever comes first.
- Do not use a spacer with powder for inhalation.

Patient/Family Teaching

- Instruct patient on proper technique for use of powder for inhalation and advise patient to take salmeterol as directed. Do not use more than the prescribed dose. If a regularly scheduled dose is missed, use as soon as possible and resume regular schedule. Do not double doses. If symptoms occur before next dose is due, use a rapid-acting inhaled bronchodilator.
- Instruct patient using *powder for inhalation* never to exhale into diskus device and always to hold device in a level horizontal position. Mouthpiece should be kept dry; never wash.
- Caution patient not to use salmeterol to treat acute symptoms. A rapid-acting inhaled beta-adrenergic bronchodilator should be used for relief of acute asthma attacks.
- Advise patients on chronic therapy not to use additional salmeterol to prevent exercise-induced bronchospasm. Patients using salmeterol for prevention of exercise-induced bronchospasm should not use additional doses of

salmeterol for 12 hr after prophylactic administration.

- Advise patient to notify health care professional immediately if difficulty in breathing persists after use of salmeterol, if condition worsens, if more inhalations of rapid-acting bronchodilator than usual are needed to relieve an acute attack, or if using 4 or more inhalations of a rapid-acting bronchodilator for 2 or more consecutive days or more than 1 canister in an 8-wk period.
- Salmeterol is often used with inhaled corticosteroids and is not a substitute for corticosteroids or adrenergic bronchodilators. Advise patients using inhalation or systemic corticosteroids to consult health care professional before stopping or reducing therapy.
- Emphasize the importance of regular follow-up exams to determine progress during therapy.

Evaluation/Desired Outcomes

- Prevention of bronchospasm or reduction of frequency of acute asthma attacks in patients with chronic asthma.
- Prevention of exercise-induced asthma.

saquinavir (sa-**kwin**-a-vir)

Invirase

Classification
Therapeutic: antiretrovirals
Pharmacologic: protease inhibitors

Pregnancy Category B

Indications

HIV infection with ritonavir (may also add other antiretrovirals).

Action

Inhibits the action of HIV protease and prevents the cleavage of viral polyproteins. **Therapeutic Effects:** Slowing of the progression of HIV infection and its sequelae. Increased CD4 cell counts and decreased viral load.

Pharmacokinetics

Absorption: Incompletely absorbed after oral administration; rapidly undergoes extensive first-pass hepatic metabolism. Absorption of Invirase and Fortovase is not the same; products are not interchangeable.
Distribution: Distributes into tissues, but CNS penetration is poor.
Protein Binding: 98%.
Metabolism and Excretion: Mostly metabolized by the liver. <1% excreted unchanged in urine.
Half-life: 13 hr.

TIME/ACTION PROFILE (blood levels)

ROUTE	ONSET	PEAK	DURATION
PO	unknown	unknown	8 hr

Contraindications/Precautions

Contraindicated in: Hypersensitivity; Concurrent dihydroergotamine (or other ergot derivatives), midazolam, rifabutin, rifampin, lovastatin, simvastatin, and triazolam; OB: Lactation (breast-feeding not recommended in HIV-infection).
Use Cautiously in: Diabetes mellitus (may exacerbate hyperglycemia; hyperglycemia may progress to ketoacidosis); Hemophilia (increased risk of bleeding); Hepatic impairment (may exacerbate liver dysfunction caused by hepatitis B or C or other causes); OB, Pedi: Pregnancy or children <16 yr (safety not established).

Adverse Reactions/Side Effects

CNS: SEIZURES, confusion, headache, mental depression, psychic disorders, weakness. **CV:** thrombophlebitis. **GI:** <u>abdominal discomfort</u>, <u>diarrhea</u>, <u>increased liver enzymes</u>, <u>jaundice</u>, <u>nausea</u>. **Derm:** photosensitivity, severe cutaneous reactions. **Endo:** hyperglycemia. **Hemat:** acute myeloblastic leukemia, hemolytic anemia, thrombocytopenia. **Neuro:** ataxia. **Misc:** STEVENS-JOHNSON SYNDROME.

Interactions

Drug-Drug: Rifampin and **rifabutin** significantly ↓ saquinavir levels; concurrent use is contraindicated. **Dihydroergotamine** and **ergotamine** (↑ risk of vasoconstriction); **midazolam** and **triazolam** (↑ CNS depression); **lovastatin** and **simvastatin** (↑ risk of myopathy); concurrent use is contraindicated. Coadministration with **clarithromycin** significantly ↑ saquinavir levels and ↓ clarithromycin levels. Saquinavir levels are also significantly ↑ by **indinavir**, **delavirdine**, **nelfinavir**, **ritonavir**, and **ketoconazole** (dose adjustments may be necessary). **Carbamazepine**, **phenobarbital**, **phenytoin**, **nevirapine**, and **dexamethasone** may ↓ saquinavir levels. Concurrent use with proton pump inhibitors may ↑ saquinavir levels. May ↑ serum cortisol levels

with **fluticasone**. May ↑ serum **trazodone** levels.
Drug-Natural Products: St. John's wort ↓ levels and effectiveness; may promote development of drug resistance.
Drug-Food: Grapefruit juice ↑ serum levels and effects. Food significantly increases ↑ the absorption of saquinavir. **Garlic** can significantly ↓ levels.

Route/Dosage

Invirase

PO (Adults): 600 mg 3 times daily within 2 hr of a meal *or* 1000 mg twice daily.

Availability

Invirase

Capsules: 200 mg. **Tablets:** 500 mg.

NURSING IMPLICATIONS

Assessment

- Assess for change in severity of symptoms of HIV and for symptoms of opportunistic infections during therapy.
- ***Lab Test Considerations:*** Monitor viral load and CD4 count regularly during therapy.
- May cause hyperglycemia, which may result in diabetic ketoacidosis.
- Monitor hematologic and hepatic function before and periodically during therapy. May cause anemia, thrombocytopenia, and ↑ liver enzymes. Use with rifampin greatly ↑ risk of hepatitis and ↑ serum transaminases.

Potential Nursing Diagnoses

Risk for infection (Indications, Side Effects)

Implementation

- **PO:** Administer within 2 hr after a full meal to increase effectiveness. Taking without food causes decreased blood concentrations and may result in no antiviral activity.
- Capsules are stable until expiration date if refrigerated or for 3 months when brought to room temperature.

Patient/Family Teaching

- Instruct patient to take saquinavir as directed at the same time each day, within 2 hr after a full meal. Take missed doses as soon as possible if not almost time for next dose; do not double doses. Do not discontinue without consulting health care professional. Changes from Invirase to Fortovase should be made under supervision of health care professional.
- Instruct patient that saquinavir should not be shared with others.
- Inform patient that saquinavir does not cure HIV or prevent associated or opportunistic infections. Saquinavir does not reduce the risk of transmission of HIV to others through sexual contact or blood contamination. Caution patient to use a condom during sexual contact and to avoid sharing needles or donating blood to prevent spreading HIV to others. Advise patient that the long-term effects of saquinavir are unknown at this time.
- Advise patient not to take other medications, prescription or OTC, or herbal products concurrently without consulting health care professional.
- Inform patient that saquinavir may cause hyperglycemia. Advise patient to notify health care professional if increased thirst or hunger; unexplained weight loss; increased urination; fatigue; or dry, itchy skin occurs. Rare but serious bullous skin eruptions with polyarthritis may also occur.
- Inform patient that long-term effects of saquinavir are unknown at this time.
- Emphasize the importance of regular follow-up exams and blood tests to determine progress and monitor for side effects.

Evaluation/Desired Outcomes

- Slowing of the progression of HIV infection and its sequelae.
- Decrease in viral load and improvement in CD4 cell counts.

sargramostim

(sar-**gram**-oh-stim)
Leukine, rHu GM-CSF (recombinant human granulocyte/macrophage colony-stimulating factor)

Classification
Therapeutic: colony-stimulating factors
Pharmacologic: biologic response modifiers

Pregnancy Category C

Indications

Acceleration of bone marrow recovery after: Autologous bone marrow transplantation in pa-

S

tients with non-Hodgkin's lymphoma, acute lymphoblastic leukemia, or Hodgkin's disease, Allogenic bone marrow transplantation from HLA-matched donors. Management of bone marrow transplant failure or engraftment delay. After induction chemotherapy for acute myelogenous leukemia (AML) in patients ≥55 yr. Mobilization and after transplant of autologous peripheral blood progenitor cells (PBPCs); increases harvest by leukapheresis.

Action

Consists of a glycoprotein produced by recombinant DNA technique that is capable of binding to and stimulating the production, division, differentiation, and activation of granulocytes and macrophages. **Therapeutic Effects:** Accelerated recovery of bone marrow after autologous bone marrow transplantation, resulting in decreased risk of infection and other complications.

Pharmacokinetics

Absorption: After IV administration, absorption is essentially complete. Well absorbed after subcut administration.
Distribution: Unknown.
Metabolism and Excretion: Unknown.
Half-life: Unknown.

TIME/ACTION PROFILE (noted as effects on blood counts)

ROUTE	ONSET	PEAK	DURATION
subcut, IV	rapid	unknown	3–7 days

Contraindications/Precautions

Contraindicated in: Presence of ≥10% leukemic myeloid blast cells in bone marrow or peripheral blood; Hypersensitivity to granulocyte macrophage colony-stimulating factor (GM-CSF), yeast products, or additives (mannitol, tromethamine, or sucrose); Products containing benzyl alcohol should not be used in newborns.
Use Cautiously in: Pre-existing fluid retention, CHF, or pulmonary infiltrates; Pre-existing cardiac disease; Myeloid malignancies; Previous extensive radiation or chemotherapy (response may be limited); OB: Pregnancy (use only if clearly needed); Lactation or children (safety not established).

Adverse Reactions/Side Effects

CNS: headache, malaise, weakness. **Resp:** dyspnea. **CV:** pericardial effusion, peripheral edema, transient supraventricular tachycardia. **GI:** diarrhea. **Derm:** itching, rash. **MS:** arthralgia, bone pain, myalgia. **Misc:** chills, fever, first-dose reaction.

Interactions

Drug-Drug: Lithium or **corticosteroids** may potentiate myeloproliferative effects of sargramostim (concurrent use should be undertaken cautiously).

Route/Dosage

After Bone Marrow Transplantation

IV (Adults): 250 mcg/m²/day for 21 days.

Failure/Delay of Engraftment after Bone Marrow Transplantation

IV (Adults): 250 mcg/m²/day for 14 days; may be repeated after a 7-day rest between courses; if results are inadequate, a 3rd course at 500 mcg/m²/day for 14 days may be given after a 7-day rest.

After Chemotherapy for AML

IV (Adults): 250 mcg/m²/day started around day 11 or 4 days after induction if day 10 bone marrow is hypoplastic with <5% blast cells and continued until absolute neutrophil count (ANC) >1500 cells/mm³ for 3 consecutive days (not to exceed 42 days); if adverse reactions occur, decrease dose by 50% or temporarily discontinue.

Mobilization of PBPCs

IV, Subcut (Adults): 250 mcg/m²/day continued throughout collection of PBPCs.

After PBPC Transplantation

IV, Subcut (Adults): 250 mcg/m²/day continued until ANC >1500 cells/mm³ for 3 consecutive days.

Availability

Powder for injection: 250 mcg/vial, 500 mcg/vial.

NURSING IMPLICATIONS

Assessment

- Monitor heart rate, blood pressure, and respiratory status during and immediately after infusion. If dyspnea develops, slow infusion rate by half. Reassess; medication may need to be discontinued. Assess for peripheral edema daily throughout therapy. Capillary leak syndrome (swelling of feet or lower legs, sudden weight gain, dyspnea) and pleural or pericardial effusion may occur, usually at doses >32 mcg/kg/day.

- Monitor for first-dose reaction (flushing, hypotension, syncope, weakness). Does not recur with first dose of each course but may occur with first dose of more than 1 course.
- Assess patient for fever daily during therapy. Usually mild and dose related and resolves with discontinuation or administration of antipyretics.
- Assess patient for arthralgias and myalgias, usually in lower extremities, which tend to occur when granulocyte counts are returning to normal. May also cause mild to moderate bone pain, possibly from bone marrow expansion. Usually occurs over a 1–3-day period before myeloid recovery and occurs in the sternum, spine, pelvis, and long bones. Treat with analgesics.
- ***Lab Test Considerations:*** Obtain a CBC with differential and platelet count before chemotherapy and twice weekly during therapy to avoid leukocytosis. Monitor ANC; may increase rapidly. If ANC >20,000/mm³ or 10,000/mm³ after the nadir has occurred or if platelet count >500,000/mm³, interrupt administration and reduce dose by half or discontinue. Excessive blood levels usually return to baseline 3–7 days after discontinuation of therapy. If blast cells appear, sargramostim should be discontinued.
- Monitor renal and hepatic function before and biweekly throughout therapy in patients with renal or hepatic dysfunction. May cause ↑ BUN, creatinine, and hepatic enzymes.
- May cause ↓ serum albumin concentrations.

Potential Nursing Diagnoses

Risk for infection (Indications)

Implementation

- Do not confuse Leukine (sargramostim) with leukeran (chlorambucil) or leucovorin.
- Administer 2–4 hr after bone marrow transplant and no earlier than 24 hr after cytotoxic chemotherapy or 12 hr after last dose of radiotherapy.
- Refrigerate but do not freeze powder, reconstituted solution, or diluted solution. Reconstitute with 1 ml of sterile water without preservatives injected toward side of vial. Swirl gently to avoid foaming. Do not shake. Solution should be clear and colorless. Discard if left at room temperature for >6 hr. Vial is for 1-time use only.
- **Subcut:** Administer reconstituted solution without further dilution.

IV Administration

- **Intermittent Infusion: *Diluent:*** Dilute in 0.9% NaCl. ***Concentration:*** If final concentration is <10 mcg/ml, add 1 mg human albumin per 1 ml of 0.9% NaCl before addition of sargramostim to prevent absorption of the components of the drug delivery system. Do not administer with an in-line filter. ***Rate:*** Usually infused over 2–4 hr. Has been administered over 30–60 min, over 5–12 hr, and as a continuous infusion over 24 hr.
- *After bone marrow transplantation or failure of engraftment:* Administer over 2 hr.
- *Chemotherapy for AML:* Administer over 4 hr.
- *Mobilization of PBPCs or PBPC transplant:* Administer as a continuous infusion over 24 hr.
- **Y-Site Compatibility:** amikacin, aminophylline, aztreonam, bleomycin, butorphanol, calcium gluconate, carboplatin, carmustine, cefazolin, cefepime, cefotaxime, ceftizoxime, ceftriaxone, cefuroxime, cimetidine, cisplatin, clindamycin, cyclophosphamide, cyclosporine, cytarabine, dacarbazine, dactinomycin, dexamethasone sodium phosphate, diphenhydramine, dopamine, doxorubicin, doxycycline, droperidol, etoposide, famotidine, fentanyl, floxuridine, fluconazole, fluorouracil, furosemide, gentamicin, granisetron, heparin, idarubicin, ifosfamide, immune globulin, magnesium sulfate, mannitol, mechlorethamine, meperidine, mesna, methotrexate, metoclopramide, metronidazole, mitoxantrone, pentostatin, piperacillin/tazobactam, potassium chloride, prochlorperazine, promethazine, ranitidine, teniposide, ticarcillin/clavulanate, trimethoprim/sulfamethoxazole, vinblastine, vincristine, zidovudine.
- **Y-Site Incompatibility:** acyclovir, ampicillin, ampicillin/sulbactam, chlorpromazine, ganciclovir, haloperidol, hydrocortisone, hydromorphone, imipenem/cilastatin, lorazepam, methylprednisolone sodium succinate, mitomycin, morphine, nalbuphine, ondansetron, sodium bicarbonate, tobramycin.

S

- **Additive Incompatibility:** Do not admix with other medications.

Patient/Family Teaching

- Instruct patient to notify nurse or physician if dyspnea or palpitations occur.

Evaluation/Desired Outcomes

- Acceleration of bone marrow recovery and decreased incidence of infection in patients after autologous and allogenic bone marrow transplantation, bone marrow transplant failure or engraftment delay, chemotherapy for AML, and PBPC transplantation.

scopolamine

(scoe-**pol**-a-meen)
Isopto Hyoscine, Transderm-Scop, ✤Transderm-V

Classification
Therapeutic: antiemetics
Pharmacologic: anticholinergics

Pregnancy Category C

Indications

Transdermal: Prevention of motion sickness. Management of nausea and vomiting associated with opioid analgesia or general anesthesia/recovery from anesthesia. **IM, IV, Subcut** Preoperatively to produce amnesia and to decrease salivation and excessive respiratory secretions.

Action

Inhibits the muscarinic activity of acetylcholine. Corrects the imbalance of acetylcholine and norepinephrine in the CNS, which may be responsible for motion sickness. **Therapeutic Effects:** Reduction of nausea and vomiting. Preoperative amnesia and decreased secretions.

Pharmacokinetics

Absorption: Well absorbed following IM, subcut, and transdermal administration.
Distribution: Crosses the placenta and blood-brain barrier.
Metabolism and Excretion: Mostly metabolized by the liver.
Half-life: 8 hr.

TIME/ACTION PROFILE (antiemetic, sedative properties)

ROUTE	ONSET	PEAK	DURATION
PO, IM, subcut	30 min	1 hr	4–6 hr
IV	10 min	1 hr	2–4 hr
transdermal	4 hr	unknown	72 hr

Contraindications/Precautions

Contraindicated in: Hypersensitivity; Hypersensitivity to bromides (injection only); Angle-closure glaucoma; Acute hemorrhage; Tachycardia secondary to cardiac insufficiency or thyrotoxicosis.
Use Cautiously in: OB, Geri: Geriatric patients, infants, and children (increased risk of adverse reactions); Possible intestinal obstruction; Prostatic hyperplasia; Chronic renal, hepatic, pulmonary, or cardiac disease; OB: Pregnancy or lactation (safety not established); to minimize exposure to fetus, apply 1 hr prior to cesarean section.

Adverse Reactions/Side Effects

CNS: drowsiness, confusion. **EENT:** blurred vision, mydriasis, photophobia. **CV:** tachycardia, palpitations. **GI:** dry mouth, constipation. **GU:** urinary hesitancy, urinary retention. **Derm:** decreased sweating.

Interactions

Drug-Drug: ↑ anticholinergic effects with **antihistamines**, **antidepressants**, **quinidine**, or **disopyramide**. ↑ CNS depression with **alcohol**, **antidepressants**, **antihistamines**, **opioid analgesics**, or **sedative/hypnotics**. May alter the absorption of other **orally administered drugs** by slowing motility of the GI tract. May ↑ GI mucosal lesions in patients taking oral **wax-matrix potassium chloride preparations**.
Drug-Natural Products: ↑ anticholinergic effects with **jimson weed and scopolia.**

Route/Dosage

Transdermal (Adults): *Motion sickness*—1.5 mg. Transderm-Scop system delivers 1 mg over 72 hr; apply 4 hr prior to travel (US product); *Recovery from anesthesia/surgery*—1.5 mg. Transderm-Scop system delivers 1 mg over 72 hr; apply evening before surgery or 1 hr prior to cesarean section.
IM, IV, Subcut (Adults): *Antiemetic/anticholinergic*—0.3–0.6 mg; *antisecretory effect*—0.2–0.6 mg; *amnestic effect*—0.32–0.65 mg; *sedation*—0.6 mg 3–4 times daily.
IM, IV, Subcut (Children): *Antiemetic/anticholinergic*—6 mcg/kg or 0.2 mg/m^2.
IM (Children 8–12 yr): *Antisecretory*—0.3 mg.
IM (Children 3–8 yr): *Antisecretory*—0.2 mg.

IM (Children 7 mo–3 yr): *Antisecretory*—0.15 mg.
IM (Children 4–7 mo): *Antisecretory*—0.1 mg.

Availability (generic available)

Transdermal therapeutic system: Transderm-Scop—1.5 mg scopolamine/patch releases 0.5 mg scopolamine over 3 days in packs of 4 units, ✤Transderm-V—1.5 mg scopolamine/patch releases 1 mg scopolamine over 3 days. **Injection:** 0.3 mg/ml in 1-ml vials, 0.4 mg/ml in 0.5-ml ampules and 1-ml vials, 0.86 mg/ml in 0.5-ml ampules, 1 mg/ml in 1-ml vials.

NURSING IMPLICATIONS

Assessment

- Assess patient for signs of urinary retention periodically during therapy.
- Monitor heart rate periodically during parenteral therapy.
- Assess patient for pain prior to administration. Scopolamine may act as a stimulant in the presence of pain, producing delirium if used without morphine or meperidine.
- **Antiemetic:** Assess patient for nausea and vomiting periodically during therapy.

Potential Nursing Diagnoses

Impaired oral mucous membrane (Indications, Side Effects)
Risk for injury (Side Effects)

Implementation

IV Administration

- **Direct IV:** ***Diluent:*** Scopolamine should be diluted with sterile water for injection prior to IV administration. ***Concentration:*** Dilute dose with an equal volume of diluent. ***Rate:*** Inject slowly over 2–3 min.
- **Syringe Compatibility:** butorphanol, chlorpromazine, cimetidine, diphenhydramine, droperidol, fentanyl, hydromorphone, meperidine, metoclopramide, midazolam, morphine, nalbuphine, pentazocine, pentobarbital, perphenazine, prochlorperazine, promethazine, ranitidine, sufentanil, thiopental.
- **Y-Site Compatibility:** fentanyl, heparin, hydrocortisone sodium succinate, hydromorphone, methadone, morphine, potassium chloride, propofol, sufentanil, vitamin B complex with C.

Patient/Family Teaching

- Instruct patient to take medication as directed. Take missed doses as soon as remembered. Do not double doses.
- Medication may cause drowsiness or blurred vision. Caution patient to avoid driving or other activities requiring alertness until response to medication is known.
- Patient should use caution when exercising and in hot weather; overheating may result in heatstroke.
- Advise patient to avoid concurrent use of alcohol and other CNS depressants with this medication.
- Inform patient that frequent mouth rinses, good oral hygiene, and sugarless gum or candy may minimize dry mouth.
- **Transdermal:** Instruct patient on application of transdermal patches. Apply at least 4 hr (US product) before exposure to travel to prevent motion sickness. Wash hands and dry thoroughly before and after application. Apply to hairless, clean, dry area behind ear; avoid areas with cuts or irritation. Apply pressure over system to ensure contact with skin. System is effective for 3 days. If system becomes dislodged, replace with a new system on another site behind the ear. System is waterproof and not affected by bathing or showering.
- Instruct patient to remove patch and notify health care professional immediately if symptoms of acute angle-closure glaucoma (pain or reddening of the eyes with pupil dilation) occur.
- Caution patients engaging in underwater sports of potentially distorting effects of scopolamine.
- For *perioperative nausea and vomiting*, apply patch the night before surgery, or 1 hr prior to Cesarean section to minimize exposure to infant. Keep patch in place for 24 hrs, then remove and discard.

Evaluation/Desired Outcomes

- Decrease in salivation and respiratory secretion preoperatively.
- Postoperative amnesia.
- Prevention of motion sickness.
- Prevention and treatment of opioid- or anesthesia-induced nausea and vomiting.

selegiline (se-le-ji-leen)
Apo-Selegiline, Carbex, Eldepryl, Gen-Selegiline, Nu-Selegiline, ✤Novo-Selegiline, SD-Deprenyl, Zelapar

Classification
Therapeutic: antiparkinson agents
Pharmacologic: monoamine oxidase type B inhibitors

Pregnancy Category C

Indications
Management of Parkinson's disease (with levodopa or levodopa/carbidopa) in patients who fail to respond to levodopa/carbidopa alone.

Action
Following conversion by MAO to its active form, selegiline inactivates MAO by irreversibly binding to it at type B (brain) sites. Inactivation of MAO leads to increased amounts of dopamine available in the CNS. **Therapeutic Effects:** Increased response to levodopa/dopamine therapy in Parkinson's disease.

Pharmacokinetics
Absorption: Appears to be well absorbed following oral administration.
Distribution: Widely distributed.
Metabolism and Excretion: Metabolism involves some conversion to amphetamine and methamphetamine. 45% excreted in urine as metabolites.
Half-life: Unknown; orally disintegrating tablets 1.3 hr.

TIME/ACTION PROFILE (onset of beneficial effects in Parkinson's disease)

ROUTE	ONSET	PEAK	DURATION
PO	2–3 days	40–90 min	unknown
orally disintegrating	5 min	10–15 min	unknown

Contraindications/Precautions
Contraindicated in: Hypersensitivity; Concurrent meperidine or opioid analgesic therapy (possible fatal reactions); Concurrent use of SSRIs or tricyclic antidepressants.
Use Cautiously in: Doses >10 mg/day (↑ risk of hypertensive reactions with tyramine-containing foods and some medications); History of peptic ulcer disease.

Adverse Reactions/Side Effects
CNS: confusion, dizziness, fainting, hallucinations, insomnia, vivid dreams. **GI:** nausea, abdominal pain, dry mouth.

Interactions
Drug-Drug: Concurrent use with **meperidine** or other **opioid analgesics** may possibly result in a potentially fatal reaction (excitation, sweating, rigidity, and hypertension; or hypotension and coma). Serotonin syndrome (confusion, agitation, hyperpyrexia, hypertension, seizures) may occur with concurrent use of **nefazolone** or **SSRI antidepressants** (fluoxetine should be discontinued 5 wk prior to selegiline, **venlafaxine** should be discontinued 7 days before selegiline, other agents should be discontinued 2 wk before selegiline). Selegiline should be discontinued 2 wk before **SSRIs** are initiated. Concurrent use with **tricyclic antidepressants** may result in asystole, diaphoresis, hypertension, syncope, behavioral changes, altered consciousness, hyperpyrexia, tremors, muscle rigidity, and seizures (avoid concurrent use; discontinue selegiline 2 wk before initiating tricyclic antidepressant therapy). May initially ↑ risk of side effects of **levodopa/carbidopa** (dosage of levodopa/carbidopa may need to be ↓ by 10–30%).
Drug-Food: Doses >10 mg/day may produce hypertensive reactions with **tyramine-containing foods** (see Appendix L).

Route/Dosage
PO (Adults): 5 mg bid, with breakfast and lunch (some patients may require further dividing of doses—2.5 mg 4 times daily).
PO (Adults): *Orally disintegrating tablets*—1.25 mg once daily for at least 6 wks. After 6 wks, may increase to 2.5 mg if effect not achieved and patient is tolerating medication.

Availability (generic available)
Capsules: 5 mg. **Tablets:** 5 mg. **Orally disintegrating tablets:** 1.25 mg.

NURSING IMPLICATIONS

Assessment
- Assess patient for signs and symptoms of Parkinson's disease (tremor, muscle weakness and rigidity, ataxic gait) prior to and during therapy.
- Assess blood pressure periodically during therapy.

Potential Nursing Diagnoses

Impaired physical mobility (Indications)
Risk for injury (Indications, Side Effects)

Implementation

- Do not confuse selegiline with sertraline.
- An attempt to reduce the dose of levodopa/carbidopa by 10–30% may be made after 2–3 days of selegiline therapy.
- **PO:** Administer 5-mg tablet with breakfast and lunch.
- Administer *orally disintegrating tablets* in the morning, before breakfast and without liquid. Remove tablet gently from blister pack with clean dry hands immediately before administering. Do not attempt to push tablet through backing. Tablet will disintegrate within seconds when placed on tongue. Avoid food or liquid within 5 min of administering orally disintegrating tablets.

Patient/Family Teaching

- Instruct patient to take medication as directed. Take missed doses as soon as possible, but not if late afternoon or evening or almost time for next dose. Do not double doses. Caution patient that taking more than the prescribed dose may increase side effects and place patient at risk for hypertensive crisis if foods containing tyramine are consumed (see Appendix L).
- Advise patients taking selegiline ≥20 mg/day to avoid large amounts of tyramine-containing foods (see Appendix L), alcoholic beverages, large quantities of caffeine-containing beverages, or OTC or herbal cough or cold medications.
- Inform patient and family of the signs and symptoms of MAO inhibitor–induced hypertensive crisis (severe headache, chest pain, nausea, vomiting, photosensitivity, enlarged pupils). Advise patient to notify health care professional immediately if severe headache or any other unusual symptom occurs.
- Caution patient to change positions slowly to minimize orthostatic hypotension.
- Advise patient that increasing fluids, sugarless gum or candy, ice, or saliva substitutes may help minimize dry mouth. Consult health care professional if dry mouth continues for >2 wk.
- Inform patient that selegiline may cause hallucinations.

Evaluation/Desired Outcomes

- Improved response to levodopa/carbidopa in patients with Parkinson's disease.

selegiline transdermal

(se-**le**-ji-leen)
Emsam

Classification
Therapeutic: antidepressants
Pharmacologic: monoamine oxidase type B inhibitors

Pregnancy Category C

Indications

Major depressive disorder.

Action

Following conversion by MAO to its active form, selegiline inactivates MAO by irreversibly binding to it at type B (brain) sites; this results in higher levels of monoamine neurotransmitters in the brain (dopamine, serotonin, norepinephrine). **Therapeutic Effects:** Decreased symptoms of depression.

Pharmacokinetics

Absorption: 25–30% of patch content is transdermally absorbed, blood levels are higher than those following oral administration because there is less first pass hepatic metabolism.
Distribution: Rapidly distributes to all body tissues; crosses the blood brain barrier.
Metabolism and Excretion: Mostly metabolized by the liver, primarily by the CYP2A6, CYP2C9 and CYP3A4/5 enzyme systems. 10% excreted in urine as metabolites, 2% in feces; negligible renal excretion of unchanged drug.
Half-life: 18–25 hr.

TIME/ACTION PROFILE

ROUTE	ONSET	PEAK	DURATION
transdermal	unknown	2 or more weeks	2 wk (after discontinuation)

Contraindications/Precautions

Contraindicated in: Hypersensitivity; Pheochromocytoma; Concurrent selective serotonin re-uptake inhibitors (fluoxetine, paroxetine citalopram, escitalopram and others), non-selective serotonin re-uptake inhibitors (venlafaxine,

S

duloxetine), tricyclic antidepressants (amitriptyline, imipramine and others), carbamazepine, oxcarbazepine, amphetamines, vasoconstrictors (ephedrine, pseudoephedrine), bupropion, meperidine, tramadol, methadone, propoxyphene, dextromethorphan, mirtazapine cyclobenzaprine, other MAO inhibitors (isocarboxazid, phenelzine, tranylcypromine) oral selegiline, sympathomimetic amines, amphetamines, cocaine or local anesthetics with vasoconstrictors; St. John's wort; Alcohol.
Use Cautiously in: Elective surgery within 10 days; benzodiazepines, mivacurium, rapacuronium, fentanyl, morphine and codeine may be used cautiously; May ↑ risk of suicide attempt/ideation especially during early treatment or dose adjustment; risk may be greater in children or adolescents (safe use in children <8 yr not established); History of mania; Dosing at 9 mg/24 hr or 12 mg/24 hr requires dietary modification (avoid foods containing large amounts of tyramine); Geri: Patients ≥65 yr may be more susceptible to orthostatic hypotension; OB: Pregnancy; use only if benefit outweighs risk to the fetus; OB: Lactation; safety not established; Pedi: Safe use in children and adolescents not established.

Adverse Reactions/Side Effects

CNS: insomnia, abnormal thinking, agitation, amnesia, worsening of mania/hypomania. **EENT:** tinnitus. **Resp:** ↑ cough. **CV:** HYPERTENSIVE CRISIS, chest pain, orthostatic hypotension, peripheral edema. **GI:** diarrhea, altered taste, anorexia, constipation, flatulence, gastroenteritis, vomiting. **GU:** dysmenorrhea, metrorrhagia, urinary frequency. **Derm:** application site reactions, acne, ecchymoses, pruritus, sweating. **MS:** mylagia, neck pain, pathologic fracture. **Neuro:** paresthesia.

Interactions

Drug-Drug: Concurrent **selective serotonin re-uptake inhibitors (fluoxetine, paroxetine, citalopram, escitalopram** and others), **non-selective serotonin re-uptake inhibitors (venlafaxine, duloxetine), tricyclic antidepressants (amitriptyline, imipramine**, and others), **carbamazepine, oxcarbazepine, amphetamines, vasoconstrictors (ephedrine, pseudoephedrine, phenylprolanolamine), bupropion, meperidine, tramadol, methadone, propoxyphene, dextromethorphan, mirtazapine, cyclobenzaprine**, other MAO inhibitors (**isocarboxazid, phenelzine, tranylcypromine**) oral **selegiline, sympathomimetic amines, amphetamines, cocaine**, or **local anesthetics with vasoconstrictors**; these may all ↑ risk of hypertensive crisis. (**Fluoxetine** should not be used within 2 wks of initiating therapy).
Drug-Natural Products: St. John's wort may ↑ risk of hypertensive crisis.

Route/Dosage

Transdermal (Adults): 6 mg/24 hr, if necessary, may be increased at 2 wk intervals in increments of 3 mg, up to 12 mg/24 hr.

Availability

Transdermal patch: 6 mg/24 hr, 9 mg/24 hr, 12 mg/24 hr.

NURSING IMPLICATIONS

Assessment

- Assess mental status, mood changes, and anxiety level frequently. Assess for suicidal tendencies, agitation, irritability, and unusual changes in behavior especially during early therapy. Monitor pediatric patients face-to-face weekly during first 4 wks, every other week for 4 wks, at 12 weeks, and as clinically indicated during therapy. Restrict amount of drug available to patient.
- Monitor blood pressure and pulse rate before and frequently during therapy. Report significant changes promptly.
- ***Toxicity and Overdose:*** Concurrent ingestion of tyramine-rich foods and many medications may result in a life-threatening hypertensive crisis. Signs and symptoms of hypertensive crisis include chest pain, tachycardia or bradycardia, severe headache, neck stiffness or soreness, nausea and vomiting, sweating, photosensitivity, and enlarged pupils. If hypertensive crisis occurs, discontinue selegiline transdermal and administer phentolamine 5 mg or labetalol 20 mg slowly IV to control hypertension. Manage fever with external cooling. Monitor patient closely until symptoms have stabilized.

Potential Nursing Diagnoses

Ineffective coping (Indications)
Noncompliance (Patient/Family Teaching)

Implementation

Transdermal: Apply system to dry, intact skin on the upper torso such as chest, back, upper thigh, or outer surface of the upper arm once every 24 hr at the same time each day. Avoid areas that are hairy, oily, irritated, broken, scarred, or calloused. Wash area gently with soap and warm water, rinse thoroughly. Allow skin to dry completely before application. Apply immediately after removing from package. Do not alter the system (i.e., cut) in any way before application. Remove liner from adhesive layer and press firmly in place with palm of hand for 30 sec, especially around the edges, to make sure contact is complete. Remove used system and fold so that adhesive edges are together. Only one selegiline patch should be worn at a time. Dispose away from children and pets. Apply new system to a different site. Wash hands thoroughly with soap and water to remove any medicine that may have gotten on them.

Patient/Family Teaching

- Instruct patient to apply patch as directed. Advise patients and caregivers to read the *Medication Guide about Using Antidepressants in Children and Teenagers*. Inform patient that improvement may be noticed after one to several weeks of therapy. Advise patient not to discontinue therapy without consulting health care professional.
- Caution patient to avoid alcohol and CNS depressants during and for at least 2 wk after therapy has been discontinued; they may precipitate a hypertensive crisis. Contact health care professional immediately if symptoms of hypertensive crisis develop. Patients taking 9 mg/24 hr or 12 mg/24 hr must avoid foods or beverages containing tyramine (see Appendix L) from the first day of the increased dose through 2 wks after discontinuation of selegiline transdermal therapy.
- Advise patient to avoid exposing application site to external sources of direct heat such as heating pads, electric blankets, heat lamps, saunas, hot tubs, heated water beds, and prolonged direct sunlight.
- May cause dizziness or drowsiness. Caution patient to avoid driving and other activities requiring alertness until response to medication is known.
- Caution patient to change positions slowly to minimize orthostatic hypotension. Geriatric patients are at increased risk for this side effect.
- Advise patients and caregivers to notify health care professional if severe headache, neck stiffness, heart racing or palpitations, anxiety, agitation, panic attacks, insomnia, irritability, hostility, agressiveness, impulsivity, akathisia, hypomania, mania, change in behavior, worsening of depression, or suicidal ideation occur, especially during initial therapy or during changes in dose.
- Instruct patient to consult health care professional before taking any Rx, OTC, or herbal products. Caution patient to avoid use of St. John's Wort and the analgesics meperidine, propoxyphene, tramadol, or methadone during therapy.
- Advise patient to notify health care professional of medication regimen before treatment or surgery. If possible, therapy should be discontinued at least 2 wk before surgery.
- Advise patient to notify health care professional if pregnancy is planned or suspected or if breastfeeding.

Evaluation/Desired Outcomes

- Improved mood in depressed patients.
- Decreased anxiety.
- Increased appetite.
- Improved energy level.
- Improved sleep. Evaluate effectiveness of therapy periodically.

sennosides (sen-oh-sides)

Black-Draught, Ex-Lax, Ex-Lax Chocolated, Fletchers' Castoria, Maximum Relief Ex-Lax, Sena-Gen, Senexon, Senokot, Senokot-XTRA

Classification
Therapeutic: laxatives
Pharmacologic: stimulant laxatives

Pregnancy Category C

Indications

Treatment of constipation, particularly when associated with: Slow transit time, Constipating drugs, Irritable or spastic bowel syndrome, Neurologic constipation.

Action

Active components of senna (sennosides) alter water and electrolyte transport in the large intestine, resulting in accumulation of water and increased peristalsis. **Therapeutic Effects:** Laxative action.

Pharmacokinetics

Absorption: Minimally absorbed following oral administration.
Distribution: Unknown.
Metabolism and Excretion: Unknown.
Half-life: Unknown.

TIME/ACTION PROFILE (laxative effect)

ROUTE	ONSET	PEAK	DURATION
PO	6–12 hr†	unknown	3–4 days

†May take as long as 24 hr

Contraindications/Precautions

Contraindicated in: Hypersensitivity; Abdominal pain of unknown cause, especially if associated with fever; Rectal fissures; Ulcerated hemorrhoids; Known alcohol intolerance (some liquid products).
Use Cautiously in: Chronic use (may lead to laxative dependence); Possible intestinal obstruction; Pregnancy or lactation (safety not established; may be used safely during breastfeeding).

Adverse Reactions/Side Effects

GI: <u>cramping</u>, <u>diarrhea</u>, nausea. **GU:** pink-red or brown-black discoloration of urine. **F and E:** electrolyte abnormalities (chronic use or dependence). **Misc:** laxative dependence.

Interactions

Drug-Drug: May decrease absorption of other **orally administered drugs** because of decreased transit time.

Route/Dosage

Larger doses have been used to treat/prevent opioid-induced constipation. Consult labeling of individual OTC products for more speceific dosing information.
PO (Adults and Children >12 yr): 12–50 mg 1–2 times daily.
PO (Children 6–12 yr): 6–25 mg 1–2 times daily.
PO (Children 2–6 yr): 3–12.5 mg 1–2 times daily.

Availability (generic available)

Noted as sennoside content **Tablets:** 6 mg^OTC, 8.6 mg^OTC, 15 mg^OTC, 17 mg^OTC, 25 mg^OTC. **Granules:** 15 mg/5 ml^OTC, 20 mg/5 ml^OTC. **Syrup:** 8.8 mg/5 ml^OTC. **Liquid:** 25 mg/15 ml^OTC, 33.3 mg/ml senna concentrate^OTC. ***In combination with:*** psyllium and docusate^OTC. See Appendix B.

NURSING IMPLICATIONS

Assessment

- Assess patient for abdominal distention, presence of bowel sounds, and usual pattern of bowel function.
- Assess color, consistency, and amount of stool produced.

Potential Nursing Diagnoses

Constipation (Indications)
Diarrhea (Side Effects)

Implementation

- **PO:** Take with a full glass of water. Administer at bedtime for evacuation 6–12 hr later. Administer on an empty stomach for more rapid results.
- Shake oral solution well before administering.
- Granules should be dissolved or mixed in water or other liquid before administration.

Patient/Family Teaching

- Advise patient that laxatives should be used only for short-term therapy. Long-term therapy may cause electrolyte imbalance and dependence.
- Encourage patient to use other forms of bowel regulation, such as increasing bulk in the diet, increasing fluid intake, and increasing mobility. Normal bowel habits are individualized and may vary from 3 times/day to 3 times/wk.
- Inform patient that this medication may cause a change in urine color to pink, red, violet, yellow, or brown.
- Instruct patients with cardiac disease to avoid straining during bowel movements (Valsalva maneuver).
- Advise patient not to use laxatives when abdominal pain, nausea, vomiting, or fever is present.

Evaluation/Desired Outcomes

- A soft, formed bowel movement.

sertaconazole

(ser-ta-**kon**-a-zole)
Ertaczo

Classification
Therapeutic: antifungals
Pharmacologic: imidazoles

Indications

Topical treatment of interdigital tinea pedis in immunocompetent patients >12 yr.

Action

Inhibits synthesis of ergosterol, a component of fungal cell membrane, resulting in cytoplasmic leakage and fungal cell death. **Therapeutic Effects:** Resolution of fungal infection. **Spectrum:** Active against *Trichophyton rubrum*, *Trichophyton mentagrophytes*, *Epidermophyton floccosum*.

Pharmacokinetics

Absorption: Minimal systemic absorption.
Distribution: Unknown.
Metabolism and Excretion: Unknown.
Half-life: Unknown.

TIME/ACTION PROFILE

ROUTE	ONSET	PEAK	DURATION
top	within 2 wk	unknown	unknown

Contraindications/Precautions

Contraindicated in: Hypersensitivity to sertaconazole or other imidazoles.

Use Cautiously in: Children <12 yr, lactation (safety not established); Pregnancy (use only if clearly needed).

Adverse Reactions/Side Effects

Derm: application site reactions, burning, contact dermatitis, dry skin, tenderness.

Interactions

Drug-Drug: None noted.

Route/Dosage

Topical (Adults and Children >12 yr): Apply twice daily for 4 wk.

Availability

2% cream: 15 g tube, 30 g tube.

NURSING IMPLICATIONS

Assessment

- Inspect involved areas of skin and mucous membranes before and frequently during therapy. Increased skin irritation may indicate need to discontinue medication.

Potential Nursing Diagnoses

Impaired skin integrity (Indications)
Risk for infection (Indications)

Implementation

- **Topical:** Apply small amount to cover affected areas between the toes and the immediately surrounding healthy skin. Dry affected area well if applied after bathing. Avoid the use of occlusive wrappings or dressings unless directed by health care professional.

Patient/Family Teaching

- Instruct patient to apply medication as directed for full course of therapy, even if symptoms have improved. Emphasize the importance of avoiding the eyes, nose, mouth, and other mucous membranes. Do not use for disorders other than for which it was prescribed.
- Patients with athlete's foot should be taught to wear well-fitting, ventilated shoes and to change shoes and socks at least once a day.
- Advise patient to report increased skin irritation, redness, itching, burning, blistering, swelling, oozing or lack of response to therapy to health care professional.

Evaluation/Desired Outcomes

- Decrease in skin irritation and resolution of infection. If no clinical improvement is seen in 2 wks, diagnosis should be reviewed. Recurrent fungal infections may be a sign of systemic illness.

sertraline (ser-tra-leen)

Zoloft

Classification

Therapeutic: antidepressants
Pharmacologic: selective serotonin reuptake inhibitors (SSRIs)

Pregnancy Category C

Indications

Major Depressive Disorder. Panic disorder. Obsessive-compulsive disorder (OCD). Post-traumatic stress disorder (PTSD). Socal anxiety disorder (social phobia). Premenstrual dysphoric disorder (PMDD). **Unlabeled uses:** Geralized anxiety disorder (GAD).

Action

Inhibits neuronal uptake of serotonin in the CNS, thus potentiating the activity of serotonin. Has little effect on norepinephrine or dopamine. **Therapeutic Effects:** Antidepressant action.

Decreased incidence of panic attacks. Decreased obsessive and compulsive behavior. Decreased feelings of intense fear, helplessness, or horror. Decreased social anxiety. Decrease in premenstrual dysphoria.

Pharmacokinetics

Absorption: Appears to be well absorbed after oral administration.
Distribution: Extensively distributed throughout body tissues.
Protein Binding: 98%.
Metabolism and Excretion: Extensively metabolized by the liver; one metabolite has some antidepressant activity; 14% excreted unchanged in feces.
Half-life: 24 hr.

TIME/ACTION PROFILE (antidepressant effect)

ROUTE	ONSET	PEAK	DURATION
PO	within 2–4 wk	unknown	unknown

Contraindications/Precautions

Contraindicated in: Hypersensitivity; Concurrent MAO inhibitor therapy (may result in serious, potentially fatal reactions); Concurrent pimozide; Oral concentrate contains alcohol and should be avoided in patients with known intolerance.
Use Cautiously in: Severe hepatic or renal impairment; Patients with a history of mania; Patients at risk of suicide; Pregnancy or lactation; Children (increased incidence of adverse CNS reactions).

Adverse Reactions/Side Effects

CNS: dizziness, drowsiness, fatigue, headache, insomnia, agitation, anxiety, confusion, emotional lability, impaired concentration, manic reaction, nervousness, weakness, yawning. **EENT:** pharyngitis, rhinitis, tinnitus, visual abnormalities. **CV:** chest pain, palpitations. **GI:** diarrhea, dry mouth, nausea, abdominal pain, altered taste, anorexia, constipation, dyspepsia, flatulence, increased appetite, vomiting. **GU:** sexual dysfunction, menstrual disorders, urinary disorders, urinary frequency. **Derm:** increased sweating, hot flashes, rash. **MS:** back pain, myalgia. **Neuro:** tremor, hypertonia, hypoesthesia, paresthesia, twitching. **Misc:** fever, thirst.

Interactions

Drug-Drug: Serious, potentially fatal reactions (hyperthermia, rigidity, myoclonus, autonomic instability, with fluctuating vital signs and extreme agitation, which may proceed to delirium and coma) may occur with concurrent **MAO inhibitors**. MAO inhibitors should be stopped at least 14 days before sertraline therapy. Sertraline should be stopped at least 14 days before MAO inhibitor therapy. May ↑ **pimozide** levels and the risk of potentially life-threatening cardiovascular reactions. May ↑ sensitivity to **adrenergics** and ↑ the risk of serotonin syndrome. Concurrent use with **alcohol** is not recommended. May ↑ levels/effects of **warfarin, phenytoin, tricyclic antidepressants** some **benzodiazepines (alprazolam), cloazapine** or **tolbutamide**. **Cimetidine** ↑ blood levels and effects.
Drug-Natural Products: ↑ risk of serotinergic side effects including serotonin syndrome with **St. John's wort** and **SAMe**.

Route/Dosage

Depression/OCD

PO (Adults): 50 mg/day as a single dose in the morning or evening initially; after several weeks may be increased at weekly intervals up to 200 mg/day, depending on response.
PO (Children 13–17 yr): *OCD*—50 mg once daily.
PO (Children 6–12 yr): *OCD*—25 mg once daily.

Panic Disorder

PO (Adults): 25 mg/day initially, may increase after 1 wk to 50 mg/day.

PTSD

PO (Adults): 25 mg once daily for 7 days, then increase to 50 mg once daily; may then be increased if needed at intervals of at least 7 days (range 50–200 mg once daily).

Social Anxiety Disorder

PO (Adults): 25 mg once daily initially, then 50 mg once daily; may be increased at weekly intervals up to 200 mg/day.

Premenstrual Dysphoric Disorder

PO (Adults): 50 mg/day initially either daily or daily during luteal phase of cycle. Daily dosing may be titrated upward in 50 mg increments at the beginning of a cycle. In luteal phase-only dosing a 50 mg/day titration step for three days at the beginning of each luteal phase dosing period should be used (range 50–150 mg/day).

Availability (generic available)

Tablets: 25 mg, 50 mg, 100 mg. **Cost:** *Generic*—25 mg $87.98/90, 50 mg $89.98/90, 100 mg $99.96/90. **Capsules:** ✤50 mg, ✤100 mg. **Oral concentrate (12% alcohol):** 20 mg/ml in 60-ml bottles. **Cost:** $65.28/60 ml.

NURSING IMPLICATIONS

Assessment

- Monitor appetite and nutritional intake. Weigh weekly. Notify health care professional of continued weight loss. Adjust diet as tolerated to support nutritional status.
- **Depression:** Monitor mood changes. Inform physician or other health care professional if patient demonstrates significant increase in anxiety, nervousness, or insomnia.
- Assess for suicidal tendencies, especially during early therapy. Restrict amount of drug available to patient.
- **OCD:** Assess patient for frequency of obsessive-compulsive behaviors. Note degree to which these thoughts and behaviors interfere with daily functioning.
- **Panic Attacks:** Assess frequency and severity of panic attacks.
- **PTSD:** Assess patient for feelings of fear, helplessness, and horror. Determine effect on social and occupational functioning.
- **Social Anxiety Disorder:** Assess patient for symptoms of social anxiety disorder (blushing, sweating, trembling, tachycardia during interactions with new people, people in authority, or groups) periodically during therapy.
- **Premenstrual Dysphoric Disorder:** Assess patient for symptoms of premenstrual dysphoric disorder (feeling angry, tense, or tired; crying easily, feeling sad or hopeless; arguing with family or friends for no reason; difficulty sleeping or paying attention; feeling out of control or unable to cope; having cramping, bloating, food craving, or breast tenderness) periodically during therapy.

Potential Nursing Diagnoses

Ineffective coping (Indications)
Risk for injury (Side Effects)
Sexual dysfunction (Side Effects)

Implementation

- Do not confuse sertraline with selegiline.
- Periodically reassess dose and continued need for therapy.
- **PO:** Administer as a single dose in the morning or evening.

Patient/Family Teaching

- Instruct patient to take sertraline as directed. Take missed doses as soon as possible and return to regular dosing schedule. Do not double doses.
- May cause drowsiness or dizziness. Caution patient to avoid driving and other activities requiring alertness until response to the drug is known.
- Advise patient to avoid alcohol or other CNS depressant drugs during therapy and to consult with health care professional before taking other medications with sertraline.
- Inform patient that frequent mouth rinses, good oral hygiene, and sugarless gum or candy may minimize dry mouth. If dry mouth persists for more than 2 wk, consult health care professional regarding use of saliva substitute.
- Advise patient to wear sunscreen and protective clothing to prevent photosensitivity reactions.
- Instruct female patient to inform health care professional if pregnancy is planned or suspected or if she is breastfeeding.
- Advise patient to notify health care professional if headache, weakness, nausea, anorexia, anxiety, or insomnia persists.
- Emphasize the importance of follow-up exams to monitor progress. Encourage patient participation in psychotherapy to improve coping skills.
- Refer patient/family to local support group.

Evaluation/Desired Outcomes

- Increased sense of well-being.
- Renewed interest in surroundings. May require 1–4 wk of therapy to obtain antidepressant effects.
- Decrease in obsessive-compulsive behaviors.
- Decrease in frequency and severity of panic attacks.
- Decrease in symptoms of PTSD.
- Decrease in social anxiety disorder.
- Decrease in symptoms of premenstrual dysphoric disorder.

sevelamer (se-**vel**-a-mer)
Renagel

Classification
Therapeutic: electrolyte modifiers
Pharmacologic: phosphate binders

Pregnancy Category C

Indications
Reduction of serum phosphate levels in patients with hyperphosphatemia associated with end-stage renal disease.

Action
A polymer that binds phosphate in the GI tract, preventing its absorption. **Therapeutic Effects:** Decreased serum phosphate levels and reduction in the consequences of hyperphosphatemia (ectopic calcification, secondary hyperparathyroidism with osteitis fibrosa).

Pharmacokinetics
Absorption: Not absorbed; action is local (in GI tract).
Distribution: Unknown.
Metabolism and Excretion: Eliminated in feces.
Half-life: Unknown.

TIME/ACTION PROFILE (decrease in serum phosphate levels)

ROUTE	ONSET	PEAK	DURATION
PO	5 days	2 wks	unknown

Contraindications/Precautions
Contraindicated in: Hypersensitivity; Hypophosphatemia; Bowel obstruction.
Use Cautiously in: Dysphagia, swallowing disorders, severe GI motility disorders, or major GI tract surgery; OB, Pedi: Pregnancy, lactation, or children (safety not established).

Adverse Reactions/Side Effects
GI: diarrhea, dyspepsia, vomiting, constipation, flatulence, nausea.

Interactions
Drug-Drug: Concurrent **anticonvulsants** or **antiarrhythmics**; sevelamer may affect absorption; administer 1 hr before or 3 hr after. May ↓ absorption of other drugs and ↓ effectiveness, especially **drugs whose efficacy is dependent on tightly controlled blood levels**.

Route/Dosage
PO (Adults): 800–1600 mg with each meal.

Availability
Tablets: 400 mg, 800 mg.

NURSING IMPLICATIONS

Assessment
- Assess patient for GI side effects periodically during therapy.
- ***Lab Test Considerations:*** Monitor serum phosphorous, calcium, bicarbonate, and chloride levels periodically during therapy.

Potential Nursing Diagnoses
Deficient knowledge, related to medication regimen (Patient/Family Teaching)

Implementation
- Doses of concurrent medications, especially antiarrhythmics, should be spaced at least 1 hr before or 3 hr after sevelamer.
- **PO:** Administer with meals. Do not break, chew, or crush tablets; contents expand in water.

Patient/Family Teaching
- Instruct patient to take sevelamer with meals as directed and to adhere to prescribed diet. Do not break, crush or chew tablets.
- Caution patient to space concurrent medications at least 1 hr before or 3 hr after sevelamer.
- Advise patient to notify health care professional if GI effects are severe or prolonged.

Evaluation/Desired Outcomes
- Decrease in serum phosphorous concentration to ≤6 mg/dl. Dose adjustment is based on serum phosphorous concentrations.

sibutramine
(si-**byoo**-tra-meen)
Meridia

Classification
Therapeutic: weight control agents
Pharmacologic: appetite suppressants

Schedule IV

Pregnancy Category C

Indications
Treatment of obesity in patients with body mass index ≥30 kg/m^2 (or ≥27 kg/m^2 in patients with diabetes, hypertension, or other risk factors) in conjunction with other interventions (dietary restriction, exercise); used to produce and maintain weight loss.

Action
Acts as an inhibitor of the reuptake of serotonin, norepinephrine, and dopamine; increases the satiety-producing effects of serotonin. **Therapeutic Effects:** Decreased hunger with resultant weight loss in obese patients.

Pharmacokinetics
Absorption: 77% absorbed, then rapidly undergoes extensive first-pass hepatic metabolism (via the P450 3A4 metabolic pathway) to active metabolites (M1 and M2).
Distribution: Widely and rapidly distributed; high concentrations in liver and kidneys.
Metabolism and Excretion: Active metabolites are extensively metabolized to inactive metabolites that are mostly excreted by the kidneys.
Half-life: *M1 metabolite*—14 hr; *M2 metabolite*—16 hr.

TIME/ACTION PROFILE (appetite suppression/weight loss)

ROUTE	ONSET	PEAK	DURATION
PO	days	4 wk	unknown

Contraindications/Precautions
Contraindicated in: Hypersensitivity; Anorexia nervosa; Concurrent use of other centrally acting appetite suppressants, MAO inhibitors, SSRIs, sumatriptan, naratriptan, zolmitriptan, dihydroergotamine, dextromethorphan, meperidine, pentazocine, fentanyl, lithium, or tryptophan; Organic causes of obesity (untreated hypothyroidism); Severe hepatic/renal impairment; Uncontrolled/poorly controlled hypertension; History of coronary artery disease, CHF, arrhythmias, or stroke; Excessive consumption of alcohol; Pregnancy or lactation.
Use Cautiously in: History of seizures; Angle-closure glaucoma; Geriatric patients; Children <16 yr (safety not established).

Adverse Reactions/Side Effects
CNS: SEIZURES, headache, insomnia, CNS stimulation, dizziness, drowsiness, emotional lability, nervousness. **EENT:** laryngitis/pharyngitis, rhinitis, sinusitis. **CV:** hypertension, palpitations, tachycardia, vasodilation. **GI:** anorexia, constipation, dry mouth, altered taste, dyspepsia, increased appetite, nausea. **GU:** dysmenorrhea. **Derm:** increased sweating, rash.

Interactions
Drug-Drug: Concurrent use of **other centrally acting appetite suppressants, MAO inhibitors, SSRIs, naratriptan, frovatriptan, rizatriptan, zolmitriptan, sumatriptan, dihydroergotamine, dextromethorphan, meperidine, pentazocine, fentanyl, lithium,** or **tryptophan** may result in potentially fatal "serotonin syndrome" (avoid concurrent use; allow 2 wk between use of MAO inhibitors and sibutramine). Concurrent use of **decongestants** may increase the risk of hypertension. **Drugs that affect the P450 3A4 enzyme system** may alter the effects of sibutramine. **Ketoconazole**, **cimetidine**, and **erythromycin** decrease metabolism and may increase blood levels and effects.

Route/Dosage
PO (Adults): 10 mg once daily; may be increased to 15 mg/day after 4 wk. Patients who do not tolerate an initial dose of 10 mg/day may be started on 5 mg/day.

Availability
Capsules: 5 mg, 10 mg, 15 mg.

NURSING IMPLICATIONS

Assessment
- Monitor patients for weight loss and adjust concurrent medications (antihypertensives, antidiabetics, lipid-lowering agents) as needed.
- Monitor blood pressure and heart rate regularly during therapy. Increases in blood pressure or heart rate, especially during early therapy, may require decrease in dose or discontinuation of sibutramine.

Potential Nursing Diagnoses
Disturbed body image (Indications)
Imbalanced nutrition: more than body requirements (Indications)
Deficient knowledge, related to medication regimen (Patient/Family Teaching)

Implementation
- **PO:** Capsules should be taken once daily without regard to meals.

Patient/Family Teaching
- Instruct patient to take medication as directed and not to exceed dose recommended. Medication may need to be discontinued gradually.

S

- Caution patient to avoid using other CNS depressants or excessive amounts of alcohol with this medication.

Evaluation/Desired Outcomes

- Slow, consistent weight loss when combined with a reduced-calorie diet. If this does not occur, therapy should be re-evaluated. Loss of at least 10% of initial body weight should occur within 1 yr.

sildenafil (sil-den-a-fil)

Revatio, Viagra

Classification

Therapeutic: erectile dysfunction agents

Pharmacologic: phosphodiesterase type 5 inhibitors

Pregnancy Category B

Indications

Viagra: Erectile dysfunction. Revatio: Pulmonary hypertension.

Action

Viagra: Enhances effects of nitric oxide released during sexual stimulation. Nitric oxide activates guanylate cyclase, which produces increased levels of cyclic guanosine monophosphate (cGMP). cGMP produces smooth muscle relaxation of the corpus cavernosum, which promotes increased blood flow and subsequent erection. Sildenafil inhibits the enzyme phosphodiesterase type 5 (PDE5), PDE5 inactivates cGMP. *Revatio:* Produces vasodilation of the pulmonary vascular bed. **Therapeutic Effects:** *Viagra:* Enhanced blood flow to the corpus cavernosum and erection sufficient to allow sexual intercourse. Requires sexual stimulation. *Revatio:* Improved exercise tolerance.

Pharmacokinetics

Absorption: Rapidly absorbed (40%) after oral administration.

Distribution: Widely distributed to tissues; negligible amount in semen.

Protein Binding: 96%.

Metabolism and Excretion: Mostly metabolized by the liver (by P450 3A4 enzyme system); one metabolite is active and accounts for 20% or more of drug effect. Metabolites excreted mostly (80%) in feces; 13% excreted in urine.

Half-life: 4 hr (for sildenafil and active metabolite).

TIME/ACTION PROFILE (vasodilation, ability to produce erection)

ROUTE	ONSET	PEAK	DURATION
PO	within 1 hr	30–120 min	up to 4 hr

Contraindications/Precautions

Contraindicated in: Hypersensitivity; Concurrent organic nitrate therapy (nitroglycerin, isosorbide mononitrate, isosorbide dinitrate), ritonavir, ketoconazole and itraconazole; Pulmonary veno-occlusive disease; **Viagra** OB, Pedi: Newborns, women, children.

Use Cautiously in: Serious underlying cardiovascular disease (including history of MI, stroke, or serious arrhythmia within 6 mo), cardiac failure, or coronary artery disease with unstable angina; History of CHF, coronary artery disease, uncontrolled hypertension (BP >170/110 mm Hg) or hypotension (BP <90/50 mm Hg), dehydration, autonomic dysfunction, or severe left ventricular outflow obstruction; Concurrent treatment with antihypertensives or glipizide; Renal impairment (CCr 30 ml/min, hepatic impairment; all result in ↑ blood levels; ↓ dose required); Anatomic penile deformity (angulation, cavernosal fibrosis, Peyronie's disease); Conditions associated with priapism (sickle cell anemia, multiple myeloma, leukemia); Bleeding disorders or active peptic ulceration; History of sudden severe vision loss or non arteritic ischemic optic neuropathy (NAION); may ↑ risk of recurrence; Retinitis pigmentosa; Concurrent bosentan, erythromycin, or saquinavir (↓ dose recommended); Geri: Elderly have ↑ blood levels and may require lower doses; consider age-related decrease in cardiac, hepatic and renal function as well as concurrent drug therapy and chronic disease states; OB: Lactation; Pedi: ***Revatio;*** Safe use in pediatric patients with pulmonary hypertension not established; May ↑ risk of bleeding with **warfarin**.

Adverse Reactions/Side Effects

CNS: <u>headache</u>, dizziness, insomnia. **EENT:** abnormal vision (color tinge to vision, increased sensitivity to light, blurred vision), epistaxis, nasal congestion. **CV:** MI, SUDDEN DEATH, CARDIOVASCULAR COLLAPSE. **GI:** <u>dyspepsia</u>, diarrhea. **GU:** priapism, urinary tract infection. **Derm:** <u>flushing</u>, rash. **MS:** mylagia. **Neuro:** paresthesias.

Interactions

Drug-Drug: ↑ risk of hypotension with **nitrates** in any form or **ritonavir**; concurrent use is contraindicated because of the risk of serious and potentially fatal hypotension. Blood levels and effects, including the risk of hypotension may be ↑ by **enzyme inhibitors** including **cimetidine**, **erythromycin**, **tacrolimus ketoconazole**, **itraconazole** and **protease inhibitor antiretrovirals** including **nelfinavir**, **indinavir**, **saquinavir** (initial dose of sildenafil for erectile dysfunction should be decreased to 25 mg). Increased risk of hypotension with **antihypertensives** (especially **alpha-blockers**) or substantial **alcohol**. **Rifampin**, **bosentan**, **barbiturates**, **carbamazepine**, **phenytoin**, **efavirenz**, **nevirapine**, **rifampin** or **rifabutin** may ↓ blood levels and effects; dose adjustments may be necessary in the treatment of pulmonary arterial hypertension. ↑ levels of **bosentan**. Use cautiously with **glipizide**.

Route/Dosage

Revatio (for pulmonary arterial hypertension)

PO (Adults): 20 mg three times daily; dose adjustments may be necessary for concurrent bosentan, barbiturates, carbamazepine, phenytoin, efavirenz, nevirapine, rifampin or rifabutin.

Viagra (for erectile dysfunction)

PO (Adults): 50 mg taken 1 hr before sexual activity (range 25–100 mg taken 30 min–4 hr before sexual activity); not more than once daily; *Concurrent use with alpha-blocker antihypertensives*—do not use 50–100 mg dose within 4 hr of alpha-blocker, 25 mg dose may be taken anytime.

PO (Geriatric Patients ≥65 yr or with concurrent enzyme inhibitors): 25 mg taken 1 hr before sexual activity (range 25–100 mg taken 30 min–4 hr before sexual activity); not more than once daily.

Hepatic/Renal Impairment

PO (Adults): 25 mg taken 1 hr before sexual activity (range 25–100 mg taken 30 min–4 hr before sexual activity); not more than once daily.

Availability

Tablets (Viagra): 25 mg, 50 mg, 100 mg. **Cost:** All strengths $115.99/10. **Tablets (Revatio):** 20 mg. **Cost:** $1,091.58/90.

NURSING IMPLICATIONS

Assessment

- **Viagra:** Determine erectile dysfunction before administration. Sildenafil has no effect in the absence of sexual stimulation.
- **Revatio:** Monitor hemodynamic parameters and exercise tolerance prior to and periodically during therapy.

Potential Nursing Diagnoses

Sexual dysfunction (Indications)
Risk for activity intolerance (Indications)

Implementation

- **PO:** Dose for *erectile dysfunction* is usually administered 1 hr before sexual activity. May be administered 30 min to 4 hr before sexual activity.
- Dose for *pulmonary hypertension* is administered 3 times daily without regard to food. Doses should be spaced 4–6 hr apart.

Patient/Family Teaching

- Instruct patient to take sildenafil as directed. For *erectile dysfunction*, take approximately 1 hr before sexual activity and not more than once per day.
- Advise patient that *Viagra* is not indicated for use in women.
- Caution patient not to take sildenafil concurrently with nitrates. Advise patient taking sildenafil for pulmonary hypertension to consult health care professional prior to taking other Rx, OTC, or herbal products.
- Instruct patient to notify health care professional promptly if erection lasts longer than 4 hr or if they experience sudden or decreased vision loss in one or both eyes.
- Inform patient that sildenafil offers no protection against sexually transmitted diseases. Counsel patient that protection against sexually transmitted diseases and HIV infection should be considered.

Evaluation/Desired Outcomes

- Male erection sufficient to allow intercourse.
- Increased exercise tolerance.

simethicone (si-**meth**-i-kone)
Degas, Extra Strength Gas-X,
✤Extra Strength Maalox GRF Gas
Re-

S

lief Formula, Flatulex, Gas-X, Genasyme, ✤Maalox GRF Gas Relief Formula, Maximum Strength Mylanta Gas, Mylanta Gas, Mylicon, ✤Ovol, ✤Ovol-40, Phazyme

Classification
Therapeutic: antiflatulents

Pregnancy Category UK

Indications
Relief of painful symptoms of excess gas in the GI tract that may occur postoperatively or as a consequence of: Air swallowing, Dyspepsia, Peptic ulcer, Diverticulitis.

Action
Causes the coalescence of gas bubbles. Does not prevent the formation of gas. **Therapeutic Effects:** Passage of gas through the GI tract by belching or passing flatus.

Pharmacokinetics
Absorption: No systemic absorption occurs.
Distribution: Not systemically distributed.
Metabolism and Excretion: Excreted unchanged in the feces.
Half-life: Unknown.

TIME/ACTION PROFILE (antiflatulent effect)

ROUTE	ONSET	PEAK	DURATION
PO	immediate	unknown	3 hr

Contraindications/Precautions
Contraindicated in: Not recommended for infant colic.
Use Cautiously in: Abdominal pain of unknown cause, especially when accompanied by fever; Has been used safely during pregnancy and lactation.

Adverse Reactions/Side Effects
None significant.

Interactions
Drug-Drug: None significant.

Route/Dosage
PO (Adults): 40–125 mg qid, after meals and at bedtime (up to 500 mg/day).
PO (Children 2–12 yr): 40 mg 4 times daily.
PO (Children <2 yr): 20 mg 4 times daily (up to 240 mg/day).

Availability (generic available)
Chewable tablets: 40 mg^OTC^, 80 mg^OTC^, 125 mg^OTC^, 150 mg^OTC^. **Tablets:** 60 mg^OTC^, 80 mg^OTC^, 95 mg^OTC^. **Capsules:** ✤95 mg^OTC^, 125 mg^OTC^. **Drops:** 40 mg/0.6 ml^OTC^, ✤40 mg/1 ml^OTC^, ✤95 mg/1.425 ml^OTC^. ***In combination with:*** antacids^OTC^. See Appendix B.

NURSING IMPLICATIONS

Assessment
- Assess patient for abdominal pain, distention, and bowel sounds prior to and periodically throughout course of therapy. Frequency of belching and passage of flatus should also be assessed.

Potential Nursing Diagnoses
Acute pain (Indications)

Implementation
- **PO:** Administer after meals and at bedtime for best results. Shake liquid preparations well prior to administration. Chewable tablets should be chewed thoroughly before swallowing, for faster and more complete results.
- Drops can be mixed with 30 ml of cool water, infant formula, or other liquid as directed. Shake well before using.

Patient/Family Teaching
- Explain to patient the importance of diet and exercise in the prevention of gas. Also explain that this medication does not prevent the formation of gas.
- Advise patient to notify health care professional if symptoms are persistent.

Evaluation/Desired Outcomes
- Decrease in abdominal distention and discomfort.

simvastatin, See HMG-CoA REDUCTASE INHIBITORS (statins).

sirolimus (sir-**oh**-li-mus)
Rapamune

Classification
Therapeutic: immunosuppressants

Pregnancy Category C

Indications
Prevention of organ rejection in allogenic kidney transplantation (with corticosteroids and cyclosporine). Sirolimus is also eluted from the Cypher coronary stent used in angioplasty procedures.

Action
Inhibits T-lymphocyte activation/proliferation, which occurs as a response to antigenic and cy-

tokine stimulation; antibody production is also inhibited. **Therapeutic Effects:** Decreased incidence and severity of organ rejection.

Pharmacokinetics

Absorption: Rapidly absorbed following oral administration (14% bioavailability).
Distribution: Concentrates in erythrocytes; distributes to heart, intestines, kidneys, liver, lungs, muscle, spleen, and testes in high concentrations.
Protein Binding: 92%.
Metabolism and Excretion: Extensively metabolized (some metabolism by P450 3A4 system); 91% excreted in feces.
Half-life: 62 hr.

TIME/ACTION PROFILE (blood levels)

ROUTE	ONSET	PEAK	DURATION
PO	rapid	1–2 hr	24 hr

Contraindications/Precautions

Contraindicated in: Hypersensitivity; Alcohol intolerance/sensitivity (solution contains ethanol); Concurrent ketoconazole, voriconazole, itraconazole, erythromycin, telithromycin, clarithromycin, rifampin, rifabutin or grapefruit juice; Severe hepatic impairment; OB: Pregnancy and lactation.
Use Cautiously in: Mild to moderate hepatic impairment; OB: Women with childbearing potential; Pedi: Children <13 yr (safety not established).

Adverse Reactions/Side Effects

Reflects combined therapy with corticosteroids and cyclosporine. **CNS:** insomnia. **Resp:** interstitial lung disease. **CV:** edema, hypotension. **GI:** hepatic toxicity. **GU:** renal impairment. **Derm:** acne, rash, thrombocytopenic purpura. **F and E:** hypokalemia. **Hemat:** leukopenia, thrombocytopenia, anemia. **Metab:** hyperlipidemia. **MS:** arthralgias. **Neuro:** tremor. **Misc:** ↑ risk of infection, ↑ risk of lymphoma, ↑ risk of lymphocele, mucosal herpes simplex infections, ↓ wound healing, lymphocele.

Interactions

Drug-Drug: Cyclosporine (modified) greatly ↑ blood levels (administer sirolimus 4 hr after cyclosporine). Drugs which inhibit the CYP3A4 enzyme system may be expected to ↑ blood levels and the risk of adverse reactions. **Ketoconazole**, **voriconazole**, **itraconazole**, **clarithromycin**, **erythromycin**, **telithromycin** significantly ↑ blood levels (concurrent use is contraindicated). Blood levels are also ↑ by **diltiazem** and **verapamil** (monitor sirolimus levels and adjust dose as necessary) and may be ↑ by **nicardipine**, **verapamil**, **clotrimazole**, **fluconazole**, **troleandomycin**, **metoclopramide**, **cimetidine**, **danazol**, and **protease inhibitor antiretrovirals**. **Rifampin** and **rifabutin** ↑ metabolism by stimulating the CYP3A4 enzyme systemand significantly ↓ blood levels. Blood levels may also be ↓ by **carbamazepine**, **phenobarbital**, **phenytoin**, and **rifapentine**. Risk of renal impairment may be ↑ by concurrent use of other **nephrotoxic agents**. Concurrent use with **tacrolimus** and **corticosteroids** in lung transplantation may ↑ risk of anastamotic dehiscence; fatalites have been reported (not approved for this use). Concurrent use with **tacrolimus** and **corticosteroids** in liver transplantation may ↑ risk of hepatic artery thrombosis; fatalites have been reported (not approved for this use). May ↓ antibody response to and ↑ risk of adverse reactions to **live-virus vaccines** (avoid vaccination).
Drug-Natural Products: Concomitant use with **echinacea and melatonin** may interfere with immunosuppression. **St. John's wort may ↑ blood levels and the risk of toxicity.**
Drug-Food: Grapefruit juice ↓ CYP3A4 metabolism and ↑ levels; do not use as a diluent and avoid concurrent ingestion.

Route/Dosage

PO (Adults and Children ≥13 yr): 6-mg loading dose, followed by 2 mg/day maintenance dose. *Dosing following cyclosporine withdrawal*—Patients at low to moderate risk for rejection after transplantation may be withdrawn from cyclosporine over 4–8 wk beginning 2–4 mo after transplant. Thereafter, sirolimus dose should be titrated upward to maintain a whole blood trough level of 12–14 mg/ml. Clinical assessment should also be used to gauge dose. Dose changes can be made at 7–14 day intervals. The following formula may also be used: sirolimus maintenance dose = current dose x (target concentration/current concentration). If a large increase is needed, a loading dose may be given and blood levels reassessed 3–4 days later. Loading dose may be calculated by the following formula: sirolimus loading dose = 3 x (new maintenance dose-current mainte-

S

nance dose). Loading doses >40 mg should be spread over 2 days.

PO (Adults and Children ≥13 yr and <40 kg): 3 mg/m² loading dose, followed by 1 mg/m²/day maintenance dose. *See adjustments above for doses following cyclosporine withdrawal.*

Hepatic Impairment

PO (Adults and Children ≥13 yr and <40 kg): Decrease maintenance dose by 33%; loading dose is unchanged.

Availability

Tablet: 1 mg, 2 mg. **Cost:** 1 mg $246.98/30. **Oral solution:** 1 mg/ml in 60-ml bottles (with oral syringes). **Cost:** $480.95/60 ml.

NURSING IMPLICATIONS

Assessment

- Monitor blood pressure closely during therapy. Hypertension is a common complication of sirolimus therapy and should be treated.
- ***Lab Test Considerations:*** Monitor sirolimus blood levels in patients likely to have altered drug metabolism, patients ≥13 yr who weigh <40 kg, patients with hepatic impairment, and during concurrent administration of drugs that may interact with sirolimus. Trough concentrations of ≥15 mg/ml are associated with an ↑ in adverse effects.
- Monitor patients for hyperlipidemia. May require additional interventions to treat hyperlipidemia.
- May cause anemia, leukopenia, thrombocytopenia, and hypokalemia.

Potential Nursing Diagnoses

Risk for infection (Adverse Reactions)

Implementation

- Therapy with sirolimus should be started as soon as possible post-transplant. Concurrent therapy with cyclosporine and corticosteroids is recommended. Sirolimus should be taken 4 hr after cyclosporine (MODIFIED, Neoral).
- Sirolimus should be ordered only by physicians skilled in immunosuppressive therapy, with the staff and facilities to manage renal transplant patients.
- Antimicrobial prophylaxis for *Pneumocystis carinii* pneumonia for 1 year and for cytomegalovirus protection for 3 months post-transplant are recommended.
- **PO:** Administer consistently with or without food. Do not administer with or mix with grapefruit juice.
- To dilute from bottle, use amber oral dose syringe to withdraw prescribed amount. Empty sirolimus from syringe into a glass or plastic container holding at least 2 oz (60 ml) of water or orange juice; do not use other liquids. Stir vigorously and drink at once. Refill container with at least 4 oz of additional liquid, stir vigorously, and drink at once.
- If using the pouch, empty entire contents of pouch into at least 2 oz of water or orange juice; do not use other liquids. Stir vigorously and drink at once. Refill container with at least 4 oz of additional liquid, stir vigorously, and drink at once.
- Store bottles and pouches in refrigerator. Solution may develop a slight haze when refrigerated; allow to stand at room temperature and shake gently until haze disappears. Sirolimus may remain in syringe at room temperature or refrigerated for up to 24 hr. Discard syringe after 1 use.

Patient/Family Teaching

- Instruct patient to take sirolimus at the same time each day, as directed. Do not skip or double up on missed doses. Do not discontinue medication without advice of health care professional.
- Reinforce the need for lifelong therapy to prevent transplant rejection. Review symptoms of rejection for transplanted organ and stress need to notify health care professional immediately if they occur.
- Emphasize the importance of repeated lab tests during sirolimus therapy.
- Advise patient of the risk of taking sirolimus during pregnancy. Caution women of child-bearing years to use effective contraception prior to, during, and for 12 weeks following therapy.

Evaluation/Desired Outcomes

- Prevention of transplanted kidney rejection.

sitagliptin (sit-a-**glip**-tin)

Januvia

Classification

Therapeutic: antidiabetics

Pharmacologic: enzyme inhibitors

Pregnancy Category B

Indications

Adjunct to diet and exercise to improve glycemic control in patients with type 2 diabetes mellitus; may be used at monotherapy or combination therapy with metformin and a thiazolidinodione and/or a sulfonurea (glimepride).

Action

Inhibits the enzyme dipeptidyl peptidase-4 (DPP-4), which slows the inactivation of incretin hormones, resulting in increased levels of active incretin hormones. These hormones are released by the intestine throughout the day, and are involved in regulation of glucose homeostasis. Increased/prolonged incretin levels, increase insulin release and decrease glucagon levels. **Therapeutic Effects:** Improved control of blood glucose.

Pharmacokinetics

Absorption: 87% absorbed following oral administration.
Distribution: Unknown.
Metabolism and Excretion: 79% excreted unchanged in urine, minor metabolism.
Half-life: 12.4 hr.

TIME/ACTION PROFILE

ROUTE	ONSET	PEAK	DURATION
PO	rapid	1–4 hr	24 hr

Contraindications/Precautions

Contraindicated in: Type 1 diabetes mellitus; Diabetic ketoacidosis; hypersensitivity.
Use Cautiously in: Renal impairment (dose reduction required for CCr <50 ml/min; Geri: Consider age-related decrease in renal function when determining dose; OB: Use in pregnancy only if clearly needed; use cautiously in lactation; Pedi: Safe use in children not established.

Adverse Reactions/Side Effects

CNS: headache. **GI:** nausea, diarrhea. **Resp:** upper respiratory tract infection, nasopharyngitis. **Misc:** hypersensitivity reactions including anaphylaxis, angioedema, and exfoliative skin conditions (Stevens-Johnson syndrome), rash, urticaria.

Interactions

Drug-Drug: May slightly ↑ serum digoxin levels; monitoring recommended.

Route/Dosage

PO (Adults): 100 mg once daily

Renal Impairment

PO (Adults): *CCr 30–<50 ml/min*—50 mg once daily; *CCr <30 ml/min*—25 mg once daily.

Availability

Tablets: 25 mg, 50 mg, 100 mg. ***In combination with:*** metformin (Janumet). See Appendix B.

NURSING IMPLICATIONS

Assessment

- Observe patient for signs and symptoms of hypoglycemic reactions (abdominal pain, sweating, hunger, weakness, dizziness, headache, tremor, tachycardia, anxiety).
- ***Lab Test Considerations:*** Monitor hemoglobin A1C prior to and periodically during therapy.
- Monitor renal function prior to and periodically during therapy.

Potential Nursing Diagnoses

Imbalanced nutrition: more than body requirements (Indications)
Noncompliance (Patient/Family Teaching)

Implementation

- Patients stabilized on a diabetic regimen who are exposed to stress, fever, trauma, infection, or surgery may require administration of insulin.
- **PO:** May be administered without regard to food.

Patient/Family Teaching

- Instruct patient to take sitagliptin as directed. Take missed doses as soon as remembered, unless it is almost time for next dose; do not double doses.
- Explain to patient that sitagliptin helps control hyperglycemia but does not cure diabetes. Therapy is usually long term.
- Instruct patient not to share this medication with others, even if they have the same symptoms; it may harm them.
- Encourage patient to follow prescribed diet, medication, and exercise regimen to prevent hyperglycemic or hypoglycemic episodes.
- Review signs of hypoglycemia and hyperglycemia with patient. If hypoglycemia occurs, advise patient to take a glass of orange juice or 2–3 tsp of sugar, honey, or corn syrup dissolved in water, and notify health care professional.

S

- Instruct patient in proper testing of blood glucose and urine ketones. These tests should be monitored closely during periods of stress or illness and health care professional notified if significant changes occur.
- Instruct patient to notify health care professional prior to taking any Rx, OTC, and herbal products.
- Advise patient to notify health care professional if pregnancy is planned or suspected or if breastfeeding.

Evaluation/Desired Outcomes

- Improved hemoglobin A1C, fasting plasma glucose and 2-hr post-prandial glucose levels.

sodium bicarbonate

(**soe**-dee-um bye-**kar**-boe-nate)
Baking Soda, Bell-Ans, Citrocarbonate, Neut, Soda Mint

Classification
Therapeutic: antiulcer agents
Pharmacologic: alkalinizing agents

Pregnancy Category C

Indications

PO, IV: Management of metabolic acidosis. **PO, IV:** Used to alkalinize urine and promote excretion of certain drugs in overdosage situations (phenobarbital, aspirin). **PO:** Antacid.

Action

Acts as an alkalinizing agent by releasing bicarbonate ions. Following oral administration, releases bicarbonate, which is capable of neutralizing gastric acid. **Therapeutic Effects:** Alkalinization. Neutralization of gastric acid.

Pharmacokinetics

Absorption: Following oral administration, excess bicarbonate is absorbed and results in metabolic alkalosis and alkaline urine.
Distribution: Widely distributed into extracellular fluid.
Metabolism and Excretion: Sodium and bicarbonate are excreted by the kidneys.
Half-life: Unknown.

TIME/ACTION PROFILE (PO = antacid effect; IV = alkalinization)

ROUTE	ONSET	PEAK	DURATION
PO	immediate	30 min	1–3 hr
IV	immediate	rapid	unknown

Contraindications/Precautions

Contraindicated in: Metabolic or respiratory alkalosis; Hypocalcemia; Excessive chloride loss; As an antidote following ingestion of strong mineral acids; Patients on sodium-restricted diets (oral use as an antacid only); Renal failure (oral use as an antacid only); Severe abdominal pain of unknown cause, especially if associated with fever (oral use as an antacid only).
Use Cautiously in: CHF; Renal insufficiency; Concurrent corticosteroidtherapy; Pedi: Children with diabetic ketoacidosis (may ↑ risk of cerebral edema); Chronic use as an antacid (may cause metabolic alkalosis and possible sodium overload).

Adverse Reactions/Side Effects

CV: edema. **GI:** *PO*— flatulence, gastric distention. **F and E:** metabolic alkalosis, hypernatremia, hypocalcemia, hypokalemia, sodium and water retention. **Local:** irritation at IV site. **Neuro:** tetany.

Interactions

Drug-Drug: Following oral administration, may ↓ absorption of **ketoconazole**. Concurrent use with **calcium-containing antacids** may lead to milk-alkali syndrome. Urinary alkalinization may result in ↓ **salicylate** or **barbiturate** blood levels; ↑ blood levels of **quinidine**, **mexiletine**, **flecainide**, or **amphetamines**; ↑ risk of crystalluria from **fluoroquinolones**; ↓ effectiveness of **methenamine**. May negate the protective effects of **enteric-coated products** (do not administer within 1–2 hr of each other).

Route/Dosage

Contains 12 mEq of sodium/g.

Alkalinization of Urine

PO (Adults): 48 mEq (4 g) initially. Then 12–24 mEq (1–2 g) q 4 hr (up to 48 mEq q 4 hr) or 1 tsp of powder q 4 hr as needed.
PO (Children): 1–10 mEq/kg (12–120 mg/kg) per day in divided doses.
IV (Adults and Children): 2–5 mEq/kg as a 4–8 hr infusion.

Antacid

PO (Adults): *Tablets/powder*—325 mg–2 g 1–4 times daily or ½ tsp q 2 hr as needed. *Effervescent powder*—3.9–10 g in water after meals; patients >60 yr should receive 1.9–3.9 g after meals.
PO (Children 6–12 yr): 520 mg; may repeat in 30 min.

Systemic Alkalinization/Cardiac Arrest
IV (Adults and Children): *Cardiac arrest/urgent situations*—1 mEq/kg; may repeat 0.5 mEq/kg q 10 min. *Less urgent situations*—2–5 mEq/kg as a 4–8 hr infusion.

Availability (generic available)

Oral powder: (20.9 mEq Na/½ tsp) in 120-, 240-, 480-, and 2400-g containers^OTC. **Tablets:** 325 mg (3.9 mEq Na/tablet)^OTC, ✤500 mg (6.0 mEq Na/tablet^OTC, 520 mg (6.2 mEq Na/tablet)^OTC, 650 mg (7.7 mEq Na/tablet)^OTC. **Solution for injection:** 4.2% (0.5 mEq/ml) in 2.5-, 5-, and 10-ml prefilled syringes, 5% (0.6 mEq/ml) in 500-ml containers, 7.5% (0.9 mEq/ml) in 50-ml vials and prefilled syringes and 200-ml vials, 8.4% (1 mEq/ml) in 10- and 50-ml vials and prefilled syringes. **Neutralizing additive solution for injection:** 4% (0.48 mEq/ml) in 5-ml vials, 4.2% (0.5 mEq/ml) in 6-ml vials.

NURSING IMPLICATIONS

Assessment

- **IV:** Assess fluid balance (intake and output, daily weight, edema, lung sounds) throughout therapy. Report symptoms of fluid overload (hypertension, edema, dyspnea, rales/crackles, frothy sputum) if they occur.
- Assess patient for signs of acidosis (disorientation, headache, weakness, dyspnea, hyperventilation), alkalosis (confusion, irritability, paresthesia, tetany, altered breathing pattern), hypernatremia (edema, weight gain, hypertension, tachycardia, fever, flushed skin, mental irritability), or hypokalemia (weakness, fatigue, U wave on ECG, arrhythmias, polyuria, polydipsia) throughout therapy
- Observe IV site closely. Avoid extravasation, as tissue irritation or cellulitis may occur. If infiltration occurs, confer with physician or other health care professional regarding warm compresses and infiltration of site with lidocaine or hyaluronidase.
- **Antacid:** Assess patient for epigastric or abdominal pain and frank or occult blood in the stool, emesis, or gastric aspirate.
- ***Lab Test Considerations:*** Monitor serum sodium, potassium, calcium, bicarbonate concentrations, serum osmolarity, acid-base balance, and renal function prior to and periodically throughout therapy.
- Obtain arterial blood gases (ABGs) frequently in emergency situations and during parenteral therapy.
- Monitor urine pH frequently when used for urinary alkalinization.
- Antagonizes effects of pentagastrin and histamine during gastric acid secretion test. Avoid administration during the 24 hr preceding the test.

Potential Nursing Diagnoses

Impaired gas exchange (Indications)
Excess fluid volume (Side Effects)

Implementation

- This medication may cause premature dissolution of enteric-coated tablets in the stomach.
- **PO:** Tablets must be taken with a full glass of water.
- When used in treatment of peptic ulcers, may be administered 1 and 3 hr after meals and at bedtime.

IV Administration

- **Direct IV:** Used in cardiac arrest or urgent situations. ***Diluent:*** Use premeasured ampules or prefilled syringes to ensure accurate dose. ***Rate:*** Administer by rapid bolus. Flush IV line before and after administration to prevent incompatible medications used in arrest management from precipitating.
- **Continuous Infusion:** ***Diluent:*** May be diluted in dextrose, saline, and dextrose/saline combinations. Premixed infusions are already diluted and ready to use. ***Rate:*** May be administered over 4–8 hr.
- **Y-Site Compatibility:** acyclovir, amifostine, amikacin, aminophylline, asparaginase, atropine, aztreonam, bivalirudin, bumetanide, cefazolin, cefepime, ceftazidime, ceftizoxime, ceftriaxone, chloramphenicol, cimetidine, cladribine, clindamycin, cyclophosphamide, cyclosporine, cytarabine, daptomycin, daunorubicin, dexamethasone sodium phosphate, dexmedetomidine, digoxin, docetaxel, doxorubicin, enalaprilat, ertapenem, erythromycin, esmolol, etoposide, etoposide phosphate, famotidine, fentanyl, filgrastim, fluconazole, fludarabine, furosemide, gallium nitrate, gemcitabine, gentamicin, granisetron, heparin, hydrocortisone sodium succinate, ifosfamide, indomethacin, insulin, ketorolac, labetalol, levofloxacin, lidocaine,

S

linezolid, lorazepam, magnesium sulfate, melphalan, mesna, meperidine, methylprednisolone sodium succinate, metoclopramide, metoprolol, metronidazole, milrinone, morphine, nafcillin, nitroglycerin, nitroprusside, paclitaxel, palonosetron, pantoprazole, pemetrexed, penicillin G potassium, phenylephrine, phytonadione, piperacillin/tazobactam, potassium chloride, procainamide, propranolol, propofol, protamine, ranitidine, remifentanil, tacrolimus, teniposide, thiotepa, ticarcillin/clavulanate, tirofiban, tobramycin, tolazoline, vasopressin, vitamin B complex with C, voriconazole.

- **Y-Site Incompatibility:** allopurinol, amiodarone, amphotericin B, amphotericin B cholesteryl sulfate complex, ampicillin, anidulafungin, calcium chloride, calcium gluconate, caspofungin, cefotaxime, cefoxitin, cefuroxime, diazepam, diphenhydramine, dobutamine, doxorubicin liposome, doxycycline, epinephrine, fenoldopam, ganciclovir, haloperidol, hydroxyzine, idarubicin, imipenem/cilastatin, inamrinone, isoproterenol, lansoprazole, leucovorin, midazolam, nalbuphine, norepinephrine, ondansetron, phenytoin, prochlorperazine, promethazine, quinupristin/dalfopristin, sargramostim, trimethoprim/sulfamethoxazole, verapamil, vincristine, vinorelbine.
- **Solution Incompatibility:** Do not add to Ringer's solution, LR, or Ionosol products, as compatibility varies with concentration.

Patient/Family Teaching

- Instruct patient to take medication as directed. Take missed doses as soon as remembered unless almost time for next dose.
- Review symptoms of electrolyte imbalance with patients on chronic therapy; instruct patient to notify health care professional if these symptoms occur.
- Advise patient not to take milk products concurrently with this medication. Renal calculi or hypercalcemia (milk-alkali syndrome) may result.
- Emphasize the importance of regular follow-up examinations to monitor serum electrolyte levels and acid-base balance and to monitor progress.
- **Antacid:** Advise patient to avoid routine use of sodium bicarbonate for indigestion. Dyspepsia that persists >2 wk should be evaluated by a health care professional.
- Advise patient on sodium-restricted diet to avoid use of baking soda as a home remedy for indigestion.
- Instruct patient to notify health care professional if indigestion is accompanied by chest pain, difficulty breathing, or diaphoresis or if stools become dark and tarry.

Evaluation/Desired Outcomes

- Increase in urinary pH.
- Clinical improvement of acidosis.
- Enhanced excretion of selected overdoses and poisonings.
- Decreased gastric discomfort.

sodium ferric gluconate complex, See IRON SUPPLEMENTS.

HIGH ALERT

sodium chloride (IV/oral)

(**soe**-dee-um **klor**-ide)

Slo-Salt

Classification

Therapeutic: mineral and electrolyte replacements/supplements

Pregnancy Category C

Indications

IV: Hydration and provision of NaCl in deficiency states. Maintenance of fluid and electrolyte status in situations in which losses may be excessive (excess diuresis or severe salt restriction). 0.45% ("half-normal saline") solution is most commonly used for hydration and the treatment of hyperosmolar diabetes (hypotonic). 0.9% ("normal saline") solution is used for: Replacement, Treatment of metabolic alkalosis, A priming fluid for hemodialysis, To begin and end blood transfusions. Small volumes of 0.9% NaCl (preservative-free or bacteriostatic) are used to reconstitute or dilute other medications. Hypertonic solution (3%, 5%) may be required in situations in which rapid replacement of sodium is necessary: Hyponatremia, Hypochloremia, Renal failure, Heart failure. **PO:** Prevention of or management of volume depletion due to salt restriction or heat prostration when excessive sweating occurs during exposures to high temperatures. **Irrigating Solutions:** 0.9% and 0.45% may be used as irrigating solutions. **Concentrated Sodium Chloride:** Used as an additive to parenteral fluid therapy in very specific situations.

Action

Sodium is a major cation in extracellular fluid and helps maintain water distribution, fluid and electrolyte balance, acid-base equilibrium, and osmotic pressure. Chloride is the major anion in extracellular fluid and is involved in maintaining acid-base balance. Solutions of NaCl resemble extracellular fluid. Reduces corneal edema by an osmotic effect. **Therapeutic Effects: IV, PO:** Replacement in deficiency states and maintenance of homeostasis.

Pharmacokinetics

Absorption: Well absorbed following oral administration. Replacement solutions of NaCl are administered IV only.
Distribution: Rapidly and widely distributed.
Metabolism and Excretion: Excreted primarily by the kidneys.
Half-life: Unknown.

TIME/ACTION PROFILE (various clinical effects†)

ROUTE	ONSET	PEAK	DURATION
PO	unknown	unknown	unknown
IV	rapid (min)	end of infusion	unknown

†PO, IV = electrolyte effects

Contraindications/Precautions

Contraindicated in: IV solution: Hypertonic (3%, 5%) solutions should not be used in patients with elevated, slightly decreased, or normal serum sodium, Fluid retention or hypernatremia.
Use Cautiously in: IV: Patients prone to metabolic, acid-base, or fluid and electrolyte abnormalities, including: Geriatric patients, Those with nasogastric suctioning, Vomiting, Diarrhea, Diuretic therapy, Glucocorticoid therapy, Fistulas, CHF, Severe renal failure, Severe liver diseases (additional electrolytes may be required); NaCl preserved with benzyl alcohol should not be used in neonates; **PO:** Inadequate hydration (water and other electrolytes must be replaced).

Adverse Reactions/Side Effects

Seen primarily during PO and IV use **CV:** CHF, PULMONARY EDEMA, edema. **F and E:** hypernatremia, hypervolemia, hypokalemia. **Local:** *IV*— extravasation, irritation at IV site.

Interactions

Drug-Drug: Excessive amounts of NaCl may partially antagonize the effects of **antihypertensives**. Use with **corticosteroids** may result in excess sodium retention.

Route/Dosage

IV (Adults): *0.9% NaCl (isotonic)*—1 L (contains 150 mEq sodium/L), rate and amount determined by condition being treated. *0.45% NaCl (hypotonic)*—1–2 L (contains 75 mEq sodium/L), rate and amount determined by condition being treated. *3%, 5% NaCl (hypertonic)*—100 ml over 1 hr (3% contains 50 mEq sodium per 100 ml; 5% contains 83.3 mEq sodium per 100 ml).
PO (Adults): 1–2 g 3 times daily.

Availability (generic available)

IV solutions: 0.45%, 0.9%, 3%, 5%. **Diluents:** 0.9%. **Concentrate for dilution:** 14.6%, 23.4%. **Tablets:** 650 mg[OTC]. ***In combination with:*** potassium (Slo-Salt-K), dextrose, electrolytes.

NURSING IMPLICATIONS

S

Assessment

- Assess fluid balance (intake and output, daily weight, edema, lung sounds) throughout therapy.
- Assess patient for symptoms of hyponatremia (headache, tachycardia, lassitude, dry mucous membranes, nausea, vomiting, muscle cramps) or hypernatremia (edema, weight gain, hypertension, tachycardia, fever, flushed skin, mental irritability) throughout therapy. Sodium is measured in relation to its concentration to fluid in the body, and symptoms may change based on patient's hydration status.
- ***Lab Test Considerations:*** Monitor serum sodium, potassium, bicarbonate, and chloride concentrations and acid-base balance periodically for patients receiving prolonged therapy with sodium chloride.
- Monitor serum osmolarity in patients receiving hypertonic saline solutions.

Potential Nursing Diagnoses

Deficient fluid volume (Indications)
Excess fluid volume (Side Effects)

Implementation

- ***High Alert:*** Accidental administration of hypertonic sodium chloride solutions (greater than 0.9%) have resulted in serious electrolyte imbalances. Do not confuse vials of concentrated sodium chloride (23.4%) with vials of sodium chloride flush solution (0.9%).
- Dose of NaCl depends on patient's age, weight, condition, fluid and electrolyte balance, and acid-base balance.
- Do not administer bacteriostatic NaCl containing benzyl alcohol as a preservative to neonates. This should not be used to reconstitute or to dilute solutions or to flush intravascular catheters in neonates.
- Infusion of 0.45% NaCl is hypotonic, 0.9% NaCl is isotonic, and 3% and 5% NaCl are hypertonic.

IV Administration

- **Intermittent Infusion:** Administer 3% or 5% NaCl via a large vein and prevent infiltration. After the first 100 ml, sodium, chloride, and bicarbonate concentrations should be re-evaluated to determine the need for further administration. ***Rate:*** Rate of hypertonic NaCl solutions should not exceed 100 ml/hr or 1 mEq/kg/hr.
- **Solution Compatibility:** D5W, D10W, Ringer's and lactated Ringer's injection, dextrose/Ringer's solution combinations, dextrose/LR combinations, dextrose/saline combinations, ⅙ M sodium lactate.

Patient/Family Teaching

- Explain to patient the purpose of the infusion.
- Advise patients at risk for dehydration due to exposure to extreme temperatures when and how to take NaCL tablets. Inform patients that undigested tablets may be passed in the stool; oral electrolyte solutions are preferable.

Evaluation/Desired Outcomes

- Prevention or correction of dehydration.
- Normalization of serum sodium and chloride levels.
- Prevention of heat prostration during exposure to high temperatures.

sodium salicylate, See SALICYLATES.

sodium citrate and citric acid

(**soe**-dee-um **sye**-trate and **sit**-rik **as**-id)

Bicitra, Oracit, ✦PMS-Dicitrate, Shohl's Solution modified

Classification

Therapeutic: antiurolithics, mineral and electrolyte replacements/supplements

Pharmacologic: alkalinizing agents

Pregnancy Category C

Indications

Management of chronic metabolic acidosis associated with chronic renal insufficiency or renal tubular acidosis. Alkalinization of urine. Prevention of cystine and urate urinary calculi. Prevention of aspiration pneumonitis during surgical procedures. Used as a neutralizing buffer.

Action

Converted to bicarbonate in the body, resulting in increased blood pH. As bicarbonate is renally excreted, urine is also alkalinized, increasing the solubility of cystine and uric acid. Neutralizes gastric acid. **Therapeutic Effects:** Provision of bicarbonate in metabolic acidosis. Alkalinization of the urine. Prevention of cystine and urate urinary calculi. Prevention of aspiration pneumonitis.

Pharmacokinetics

Absorption: Well absorbed following oral administration.

Distribution: Rapidly and widely distributed.

Metabolism and Excretion: Rapidly oxidized to bicarbonate, which is excreted primarily by the kidneys. Small amounts (<5%) excreted unchanged by the lungs.

Half-life: Unknown.

TIME/ACTION PROFILE (effects on serum pH)

ROUTE	ONSET	PEAK	DURATION
PO	rapid (min–hr)	unknown	4–6 hr

Contraindications/Precautions

Contraindicated in: Severe renal insufficiency; Severe sodium restriction; CHF, untreated hypertension, edema, or toxemia of pregnancy.

Use Cautiously in: Pregnancy or lactation (safety not established).

Adverse Reactions/Side Effects
GI: diarrhea. **F and E:** fluid overload, hypernatremia (severe renal impairment), hypocalcemia, metabolic alkalosis (large doses only). **MS:** tetany.

Interactions
Drug-Drug: May partially antagonize the effects of **antihypertensives**. Urinary alkalinization may result in decreased **salicylate** or **barbiturate** blood levels or increased blood levels of **quinidine**, **flecainide**, or **amphetamines**.

Route/Dosage
Adjust dosage according to urine pH. Contains 1 mEq sodium and 1 mEq bicarbonate/ml solution.

Alkalinizer
PO (Adults): 10–30 ml solution diluted in water qid.
PO (Children): 5–15 ml solution diluted in water qid.

Antiurolithic
PO (Adults): 10–30 ml solution diluted in water qid.

Neutralizing Buffer
PO (Adults): 15–30 ml solution diluted in 15–30 ml of water.

Availability
Oral solution: 500 mg sodium citrate/334 mg citric acid/5 ml (Bicitra, PMS-Dicitrate), 490 mg sodium citrate/640 mg citric acid/5 ml (Oracit).

NURSING IMPLICATIONS

Assessment
- Assess patient for signs of alkalosis (confusion, irritability, paresthesia, tetany, altered breathing pattern) or hypernatremia (edema, weight gain, hypertension, tachycardia, fever, flushed skin, mental irritability) throughout therapy.
- Monitor patients with renal dysfunction for fluid overload (discrepancy in intake and output, weight gain, edema, rales/crackles, and hypertension).
- ***Lab Test Considerations:*** Prior to and every 4 mo throughout chronic therapy, monitor hematocrit, hemoglobin, electrolytes, pH, creatinine, urinalysis, and 24-hr urine for citrate.
- Monitor urine pH if used to alkalinize urine.

Potential Nursing Diagnoses
Deficient knowledge, related to medication regimen (Patient/Family Teaching)

Implementation
- **PO:** Solution is more palatable if chilled. Administer with 30–90 ml of chilled water. Administer 30 min after meals or as bedtime snack to minimize saline laxative effect.
- When used as preanesthetic, administer 15–30 ml of sodium citrate with 15–30 ml of chilled water.

Patient/Family Teaching
- Instruct patient to take as directed. Missed doses should be taken within 2 hr. Do not double doses.
- Instruct patients receiving chronic sodium citrate on correct method of monitoring urine pH, maintenance of alkaline urine, and the need to increase fluid intake to 3000 ml/day. When treatment is discontinued, pH begins to fall toward pretreatment levels.
- Advise patients receiving long-term therapy on need to avoid salty foods.

Evaluation/Desired Outcomes
- Correction of metabolic acidosis.
- Maintenance of alkaline urine with resulting decreased stone formation.
- Buffering the pH of gastric secretions, thereby preventing aspiration pneumonitis associated with intubation and anesthesia.

S

sodium polystyrene sulfonate
(**soe**-dee-um po-lee-**stye**-reen **sul**-fon-ate)
Kayexalate, ✤K-Exit, ✤PMS-Sodium Polystyrene Sulfonate, SPS

Classification
Therapeutic: hypokalemics, electrolyte modifiers
Pharmacologic: cationic exchange resins

Pregnancy Category C

Indications
Mild to moderate hyperkalemia (if severe, more immediate measures such as sodium bicarbon-

✤ = Canadian drug name.
* CAPITALS indicates life-threatening; underlines indicate most frequent.

ate IV, calcium, or glucose/insulin infusion should be instituted).

Action

Exchanges sodium ions for potassium ions in the intestine (each 1 g is exchanged for 1 mEq potassium). **Therapeutic Effects:** Reduction of serum potassium levels.

Pharmacokinetics

Absorption: Distributed throughout the intestine but is nonabsorbable.
Distribution: Not distributed.
Metabolism and Excretion: Eliminated in the feces.
Half-life: Unknown.

TIME/ACTION PROFILE (decrease in serum potassium)

ROUTE	ONSET	PEAK	DURATION
PO	2–12 hr	unknown	6–24 hr
rectal	2–12 hr	unknown	4–6 hr

Contraindications/Precautions

Contraindicated in: Life-threatening hyperkalemia (other, more immediate measures should be instituted); Hypersensitivity to saccharin or parabens (some products); Ileus; Known alcohol intolerance (suspension only).
Use Cautiously in: Geriatric patients; CHF, hypertension, edema; Sodium restriction; Constipation.

Adverse Reactions/Side Effects

GI: constipation, fecal impaction, anorexia, gastric irritation, nausea, vomiting. **F and E:** hypocalcemia, hypokalemia, sodium retention, hypomagnesemia.

Interactions

Drug-Drug: Administration with **calcium** or **magnesium-containing antacids** may decrease resin-exchanging ability and increase risk of systemic alkalosis. Hypokalemia may enhance **digoxin** toxicity.

Route/Dosage

4 level tsp = 15 g (4.1 mEq sodium/g).
PO (Adults): 15 g 1–4 times daily in water or sorbitol (up to 40 g 4 times daily).
Rect (Adults): 30–50 g as a retention enema; repeat as needed q 6 hr.
PO, Rect (Children): 1 g/kg/dose q 6 hr.

Availability (generic available)

Suspension: 15 g sodium polystyrene sulfonate with 20 g sorbitol/60 ml, 15 g sodium polystyrene sulfonate with 14.1 g sorbitol/60 ml. **Powder:** 15 g/4 level tsp.

NURSING IMPLICATIONS

Assessment

- Monitor response of symptoms of hyperkalemia (fatigue, muscle weakness, paresthesia, confusion, dyspnea, peaked T waves, depressed ST segments, prolonged QT segments, widened QRS complexes, loss of P waves, and cardiac arrhythmias). Assess for development of hypokalemia (weakness, fatigue, arrhythmias, flat or inverted T waves, prominent U waves).
- Monitor intake and output ratios and daily weight. Assess for symptoms of fluid overload (dyspnea, rales/crackles, jugular venous distention, peripheral edema). Concurrent low-sodium diet may be ordered for patients with CHF (see Appendix L).
- In patients receiving concurrent digoxin, assess for symptoms of digitalis toxicity (anorexia, nausea, vomiting, visual disturbances, arrhythmias).
- Assess abdomen and note character and frequency of stools. Concurrent sorbitol or laxatives may be ordered to prevent constipation or impaction. Some products contain sorbitol to prevent constipation. Patient should ideally have 1–2 watery stools each day during course of therapy.
- ***Lab Test Considerations:*** Monitor serum potassium daily during therapy. Notify physician or other health care professional when potassium decreases to 4–5 mEq/L.
- Monitor renal function and electrolytes (especially sodium, calcium, bicarbonate, and magnesium) prior to and periodically throughout therapy.

Potential Nursing Diagnoses

Constipation (Side Effects)

Implementation

- Solution is stable for 24 hr when refrigerated.
- Consult physician or other health care professional regarding discontinuation of medications that may increase serum potassium (angiotensin-converting enzyme inhibitors, potassium-sparing diuretics, potassium supplements, salt substitutes).
- **PO:** An osmotic laxative (sorbitol) is usually administered concurrently to prevent constipation.

- For oral administration, shake commercially-available suspension well before use. When using powder, add prescribed amount to 3–4 ml water/g of powder. Shake well. Syrup may be ordered to improve palatability. Resin cookie or candy recipes are available; discuss with pharmacist or dietitian.
- **Retention Enema:** Precede retention enema with cleansing enema. Administer solution via rectal tube or 28-French Foley catheter with 30-ml balloon. Insert tube at least 20 cm and tape in place.
- For retention enema, add powder to 100 ml of prescribed solution (usually sorbitol or 20% dextrose in water). Shake well to dissolve powder thoroughly; should be of liquid consistency. Position patient on left side and elevate hips on pillow if solution begins to leak. Follow administration of medication with additional 50–100 ml of diluent to ensure administration of complete dose. Encourage patient to retain enema as long as possible, at least 30–60 min.
- After retention period, irrigate colon with 1–2 L of non–sodium-containing solution. Y-connector with tubing may be attached to Foley or rectal tube; cleansing solution is administered through one port of the Y and allowed to drain by gravity through the other port.

Patient/Family Teaching

- Explain purpose and method of administration of medication to patient.
- Inform patient of need for frequent lab tests to monitor effectiveness.

Evaluation/Desired Outcomes

- Normalization of serum potassium levels.

solifenacin (so-li-**fen**-a-sin)

VESIcare

Classification

Therapeutic: urinary tract antispasmodics
Pharmacologic: anticholinergics

Pregnancy Category C

Indications

Overactive bladder with symptoms (urge incontinence, urgency, frequency).

Action

Acts as a muscarinic (cholinergic) receptor antagonist; antagonizes bladder smooth muscle contraction. **Therapeutic Effects:** Decreased symptoms of overactive bladder.

Pharmacokinetics

Absorption: Well absorbed (90%).
Distribution: Unknown.
Protein Binding: 98%.
Metabolism and Excretion: Extensively metabolized by the CYP3A4 enzyme system. 69% excreted in urine as mebolites, 22% in feces.
Half-life: 45–68 hr.

TIME/ACTION PROFILE

ROUTE	ONSET	PEAK	DURATION
oral	unknown	3–8 hr	24 hr

Contraindications/Precautions

Contraindicated in: Hypersensitivity; Urinary retention; Gastric retention; Uncontrolled angle-closure glaucoma; Severe hepatic impairment; Lactation.
Use Cautiously in: Concurrent use of CYP3A4 inhibitors (use lower dose/clinical monitoring may be necessary); Moderate hepatic impairment (lower dose recommended); Renal impairment (dose should not exceed 5 mg/day if CCr <30 ml/min); Bladder outflow obstruction; GI obstructive disorders, severe constipation or ulcerative colitis; Myasthenia gravis; Angle-closure glaucoma; Children (safety not established); Pregnancy (use only if maternal benefit outweighs fetal risk).

Adverse Reactions/Side Effects

EENT: blurred vision. **GI:** constipation, dry mouth, dyspepsia, nausea.

Interactions

Drug-Drug: Drugs that induce or inhibit the CYP3A4 enzyme system may significantly alter blood levels of solifenacin; **ketoconazole** ↑ blood levels and risk of toxicity (do not exceed 5 mg/day).

Route/Dosage

PO (Adults): 5 mg once daily, may be ↑ to 10 mg once daily; ***hepatic impairment/severe renal impairment, concurrent use of ketoconazole or other inhibitors of CYP3A4***—dose should not exceed 5 mg/day.

Availability

Tablets: 5 mg, 10 mg.

NURSING IMPLICATIONS

Assessment

- Monitor voiding pattern and assess symptoms of overactive bladder (urinary urgency, urinary incontinence, urinary frequency) to and periodically during therapy.

Potential Nursing Diagnoses

Impaired urinary elimination (Indications)

Implementation

- **PO:** Administer once daily without regard to food. Tablets must be swallowed whole; do not break, crush, or chew.

Patient/Family Teaching

- Instruct patient to take solifenacin as directed. Advise patient to read the *Patient Information* before starting therapy and with each prescription refill. If a dose is missed, skip dose and take next day; do not take 2 doses in same day.
- Do not share solifenacin with others; may be dangerous.
- Inform patient of potential anticholinergic side effects (constipation, urinary retention, blurred vision, heat prostration in a hot environment).
- May cause dizziness and blurred vision. Caution patient to avoid driving and other activities that require alertness until response to medication is known.
- Advise patient to consult health care professional prior to taking Rx, OTC, or herbal products with solifenacin.

Evaluation/Desired Outcomes

- Decrease in symptoms of overactive bladder (urge urinary incontinence, urgency, frequency).

---

somatropin, See GROWTH HORMONES.

---

sotalol (soe-ta-lole)

Betapace, Betapace AF, Sorine, ✤Sotacor

Classification

Therapeutic: antiarrhythmics (classes II and III)

Pharmacologic: beta blockers

Pregnancy Category B

Indications

Management of life-threatening ventricular arrhythmias. **Betapace AF:** Maintenance of normal sinus rhythm in patients with highly symptomatic atrial fibrillation/atrial flutter (AFIB/AFL) who are currently in sinus rhythm.

Action

Blocks stimulation of $beta_1$ (myocardial) and $beta_2$ (pulmonary, vascular, and uterine) -adrenergic receptor sites. **Therapeutic Effects:** Suppression of arrhythmias.

Pharmacokinetics

Absorption: Well absorbed following oral administration.

Distribution: Crosses the placenta; enters breast milk.

Metabolism and Excretion: Elimination is mostly renal.

Half-life: 12 hr (increased in renal impairment).

TIME/ACTION PROFILE (antiarrhythmic effects)

ROUTE	ONSET	PEAK	DURATION
PO	hrs	2–3 days	8–12 hr

Contraindications/Precautions

Contraindicated in: Hypersensitivity; Uncompensated CHF; Pulmonary edema; Asthma; Cardiogenic shock; Congenital or acquired long QT syndromes; Sinus bradycardia, 2nd- and 3rd-degree AV block (unless a functioning pacemaker is present); CCr <40 ml/min in patients who are being treated with Betapace AF.

Use Cautiously in: Renal impairment (increased dosing interval recommended if CCr ≤60 ml/min for patients with ventricular arrhythmias); Hepatic impairment; Hypokalemia (increased risk of serious arrhythmias); Geriatric patients (increased sensitivity to beta blockers; initial dosage reduction recommended); Other pulmonary pathology; Diabetes mellitus (may mask signs of hypoglycemia); Thyrotoxicosis (may mask symptoms); Patients with a history of severe allergic reactions (intensity of reactions may be increased); Pregnancy, lactation, or children (safety not established; may cause fetal/neonatal bradycardia, hypotension, hypoglycemia, or respiratory depression).

Adverse Reactions/Side Effects

CNS: fatigue, weakness, anxiety, dizziness, drowsiness, insomnia, memory loss, mental depression, mental status changes, nervousness, nightmares. **EENT:** blurred vision, dry eyes, nasal stuffiness. **Resp:** bronchospasm, wheezing. **CV:** ARRHYTHMIAS, BRADYCARDIA, CHF, PULMONARY EDEMA, orthostatic hypotension, peripheral vasoconstriction. **GI:** constipation, diarrhea, nausea. **GU:** erectile dysfunction, decreased libido. **Derm:** itching, rashes. **Endo:** hyperglycemia, hypoglycemia. **MS:** arthralgia, back pain, muscle cramps. **Neuro:** paresthesia. **Misc:** drug-induced lupus syndrome.

Interactions

Drug-Drug: Concurrent use with other **class 1A antiarrhythmics** is not recommended due to increased risk of arrhythmias. **General anesthesia**, **IV phenytoin**, and **verapamil** may cause additive myocardial depression. Concurrent use with other **calcium channel blockers** may increase the risk of adverse cardiovascular reactions. Additive bradycardia may occur with **digoxin**. Additive hypotension may occur with other **antihypertensives**, acute ingestion of **alcohol**, or **nitrates**. Concurrent use with **amphetamines**, **cocaine**, **ephedrine**, **epinephrine**, **norepinephrine**, **phenylephrine**, or **pseudoephedrine** may result in unopposed alpha-adrenergic stimulation (excessive hypertension, bradycardia). Concurrent **thyroid** administration may decrease effectiveness. May alter the effectiveness of **insulin** or **oral hypoglycemic agents** (dosage adjustments may be necessary). May decrease the effectiveness of **beta-adrenergic bronchodilators** and **theophylline**. May decrease the beneficial $beta_1$ cardiovascular effects of **dopamine** or **dobutamine**. Discontinuation of **clonidine** in patients receiving sotalol may result in excessive rebound hypertension. Use cautiously within 14 days of **MAO inhibitors** (may result in hypertension).

Route/Dosage

Ventricular arrhythmias

PO (Adults): 80 mg twice daily; may be gradually increased (usual maintenance dose is 160–320 mg/day in 2–3 divided doses; some patients may require up to 480–640 mg/day).

Renal Impairment

PO (Adults): *CCr 30–59 ml/min*—initial dose of 80 mg, with subsequent doses given q 24 hr; *CCr <10 ml/min–29 ml/min*—initial dose of 80 mg, with subsequent doses given q 36–48 hr.

Atrial fibrillation/atrial flutter

PO (Adults): 80 mg twice daily, may be increased during careful monitoring to 120 mg twice daily if necessary

Renal Impairment

PO (Adults): *CCr 40–60 ml/min*—80 mg once daily.

Availability (generic available)

Tablets: 80 mg, 120 mg, 160 mg, 240 mg. **Cost:** *Generic*—80 mg $204.95/180, 120 mg $304.99/180, 160 mg $359.41/180, 240 mg $366.44/180. **Tablets (Betapace AF):** 80 mg, 120 mg, 160 mg.

NURSING IMPLICATIONS

Assessment

- Monitor blood pressure and pulse frequently during dosage adjustment period and periodically throughout therapy. Assess for orthostatic hypotension when assisting patient up from supine position.
- Monitor intake and output ratios and daily weight. Assess patient routinely for evidence of fluid overload (peripheral edema, dyspnea, rales/crackles, fatigue, weight gain, jugular venous distention).
- ***Lab Test Considerations:*** May cause increased BUN, serum lipoprotein, potassium, triglyceride, and uric acid levels.
- May cause increased ANA titers.
- May cause increase in blood glucose levels.
- ***Toxicity and Overdose:*** Monitor patients receiving beta blockers for signs of overdose (bradycardia, severe dizziness or fainting, severe drowsiness, dyspnea, bluish fingernails or palms, seizures). Notify physician or other health care professional immediately if these signs occur: Glucagon has been used to treat bradycardia and hypotension.

Potential Nursing Diagnoses

Decreased cardiac output (Side Effects)
Noncompliance (Patient/Family Teaching)

S

Implementation

- Patients should be hospitalized and monitored for arrhythmias during initiation of therapy and dose increases.
- Do not substitute Betapace for Betapace AF. Make sure patients transfered from Betapace to Betapace AF have enough Betapace AF upon leaving the hospital to allow for uninterrupted therapy until Betapace AF prescription can be filled.
- **PO:** Take apical pulse prior to administering. If <50 bpm or if arrhythmia occurs, withhold medication and notify physician or other health care professional.
- Administer on an empty stomach, 1 hr before or 2 hr after meals. Administration with food, especially milk or milk products, reduces absorption by approximately 20%.
- Avoid administering antacids containing aluminum or magnesium within 2 hr before administration of sotalol.

Patient/Family Teaching

- Instruct patient to take medication exactly as directed, at the same time each day, even if feeling well; do not skip or double up on missed doses. If a dose is missed, it should be taken as soon as possible up to 8 hr before next dose. Abrupt withdrawal may precipitate life-threatening arrhythmias, hypertension, or myocardial ischemia.
- Advise patient to make sure enough medication is available for weekends, holidays, and vacations. A written prescription may be kept in wallet in case of emergency.
- Teach patient and family how to check pulse and blood pressure. Instruct them to check pulse daily and blood pressure biweekly. Advise patient to hold dose and contact physician or other health care professional if pulse is <50 bpm or if blood pressure changes significantly.
- May cause drowsiness or dizziness. Caution patients to avoid driving or other activities that require alertness until response to the drug is known.
- Advise patients to change positions slowly to minimize orthostatic hypotension, especially during initiation of therapy or when dose is increased.
- Caution patient that this medication may increase sensitivity to cold.
- Instruct patient to consult health care professional before taking any OTC medications, especially cold preparations, concurrently with this medication.
- Diabetic patients should closely monitor blood glucose, especially if weakness, malaise, irritability, or fatigue occurs. Medication may mask tachycardia and increased blood pressure as signs of hypoglycemia, but dizziness and sweating may still occur.
- Advise patient to notify health care professional if slow pulse, difficulty breathing, wheezing, cold hands and feet, dizziness, confusion, depression, rash, fever, sore throat, unusual bleeding, or bruising occurs.
- Instruct patient to inform health care professional of medication regimen prior to treatment or surgery.
- Advise patient to carry identification describing disease process and medication regimen at all times.

Evaluation/Desired Outcomes

- Control of arrhythmias without appearance of detrimental side effects.

---

spironolactone, See DIURETICS (POTASSIUM-SPARING).

---

streptokinase, See THROMBOLYTIC AGENTS.

---

streptomycin, See AMINOGLYCOSIDES.

---

sucralfate (soo-**kral**-fate)

Carafate, ✤Sulcrate

Classification
Therapeutic: antiulcer agents
Pharmacologic: GI protectants

Pregnancy Category B

Indications

Short-term management of duodenal ulcers. Maintenance (preventive) therapy of duodenal ulcers. **Unlabeled uses:** Management of gastric ulcer or gastroesophageal reflux. Prevention of gastric mucosal injury caused by high-dose aspirin or other NSAIDs in patients with rheumatoid arthritis or in high-stress situations (e.g., intensive care unit). **Suspension:** Mucositis/stomatitis/rectal or oral ulcerations from various etiologies.

Action

Aluminum salt of sulfated sucrose reacts with gastric acid to form a thick paste, which selectively adheres to the ulcer surface. **Therapeutic Effects:** Protection of ulcers, with subsequent healing.

Pharmacokinetics

Absorption: Systemic absorption is minimal (<5%).
Distribution: Unknown.
Metabolism and Excretion: >90% is eliminated in the feces.
Half-life: 6–20 hr.

TIME/ACTION PROFILE (mucosal protectant effect)

ROUTE	ONSET	PEAK	DURATION
PO	1–2 hr	unknown	6 hr

Contraindications/Precautions

Contraindicated in: Hypersensitivity.
Use Cautiously in: Renal failure (accumulation of aluminum can occur).

Adverse Reactions/Side Effects

CNS: dizziness, drowsiness. **GI:** constipation, diarrhea, dry mouth, gastric discomfort, indigestion, nausea. **Derm:** pruritus, rashes.

Interactions

Drug-Drug: May decrease the absorption of **phenytoin**, **fat-soluble vitamins**, or **tetracycline**. Concurrent **antacids**, **cimetidine** or **ranitidine** decrease the effectiveness of sucralfate. Decreases absorption of **fluoroquinolones** (separate administration by 2 hours).

Route/Dosage

Treatment of Ulcers

PO (Adults): 1 g qid, 1 hr before meals and at bedtime; or 2 g twice daily, on waking and at bedtime.

Prevention of Ulcers

PO (Adults): 1 g twice daily, 1 hr before a meal.

Gastroesophageal Reflux

PO (Adults): 1 g qid, 1 hr before meals and at bedtime (unlabeled).
PO (Children): 40–80 mg/kg/day divided q 6 hr, 1 hr before meals and at bedtime (unlabeled).

Stomatitis

PO (Adults and Children): 5–10 ml of suspension swish and spit or swish and swallow 4 times/day.

Proctitis

Rect (Adults): 2 g of suspension given as an enema once or twice daily.

Availability (generic available)

Tablets: 1 g. **Oral suspension:** 500 mg/5 ml.

NURSING IMPLICATIONS

Assessment

- Assess patient routinely for abdominal pain and frank or occult blood in the stool.

Potential Nursing Diagnoses

Acute pain (Indications)
Constipation (Side Effects)
Deficient knowledge, related to medication regimen (Patient/Family Teaching)

Implementation

- Do not confuse Carafate (sucralfate) with Cafergot (ergotamine/caffeine).
- **PO:** Administer on an empty stomach, 1 hr before meals and at bedtime. Tablet may be broken or dissolved in water before ingestion. Shake suspension well before administration.
- If nasogastric administration is required, consult pharmacist; protein-binding properties of sucralfate have resulted in formation of a bezoar when administered with enteral feedings and other medications.
- If antacids are also required for pain, administer 30 min before or after sucralfate dosage.

Patient/Family Teaching

- Advise patient to continue with course of therapy for 4–8 wk, even if feeling better, to ensure ulcer healing. If a dose is missed, take as soon as remembered unless almost time for next dose; do not double doses.
- Advise patient that increase in fluid intake, dietary bulk, and exercise may prevent drug-induced constipation.
- Emphasize the importance of routine examinations to monitor progress.

S

Evaluation/Desired Outcomes

- Decrease in abdominal pain.
- Prevention and healing of duodenal ulcers, seen by x-ray examination and endoscopy.

sulconazole, See ANTIFUNGALS (TOPICAL).

sulfasalazine

(sul-fa-**sal**-a-zeen)

Azulfidine, Azulfidine EN-tabs, ✤PMS-Sulfasalazine, ✤Salazopyrin, ✤S.A.S

Classification

Therapeutic: antirheumatics (DMARD), gastrointestinal anti-inflammatories—therapeutic

Pregnancy Category B

Indications

Inflammatory bowel diseases including: Ulcerative colitis, Proctitis, Proctosigmoiditis. Rheumatoid arthritis unresponsive or intolerant to salicylates and/or NSAIDs.

Action

Locally acting anti-inflammatory action in the colon, where activity is probably a result of inhibition of prostaglandin synthesis. **Therapeutic Effects:** Reduction in the symptoms of inflammatory bowel disease.

Pharmacokinetics

Absorption: 10–15% absorbed after oral administration.
Distribution: Widely distributed; crosses the placenta and enters breast milk.
Protein Binding: 99%.
Metabolism and Excretion: Split by intestinal bacteria into sulfapyridine and 5-aminosalicylic acid. Some absorbed sulfasalazine is excreted by bile back into intestines; 15% excreted unchanged by the kidneys. Sulfapyridine also excreted mostly by the kidneys.
Half-life: 6 hr.

TIME/ACTION PROFILE (blood levels)

ROUTE	ONSET	PEAK	DURATION
PO	1 hr	1.5–6 hr	6–12 hr

Contraindications/Precautions

Contraindicated in: Hypersensitivity reactions to sulfonamides, salicylates, or sulfasalazine; Cross-sensitivity with furosemide, sulfonylurea hypoglycemic agents, or carbonic anhydrase inhibitors may exist; G6PD deficiency; Hypersensitivity to bisulfites (mesalamine enema only); Urinary tract or intestinal obstruction; Porphyria; Children <2 yr.
Use Cautiously in: Severe hepatic or renal impairment; Renal impairment; History of porphyria; Pregnancy (has been used safely); Lactation (safety not established).

Adverse Reactions/Side Effects

CNS: headache. **Resp:** pneumonitis. **GI:** anorexia, diarrhea, nausea, vomiting, drug-induced hepatitis. **GU:** crystalluria, oligospermia, orange-yellow discoloration of urine. **Derm:** rashes, exfoliative dermatitis, photosensitivity, yellow discoloration. **Hemat:** AGRANULOCYTOSIS, APLASTIC ANEMIA, blood dyscrasias, eosinophilia, megaloblastic anemia, thrombocytopenia. **Neuro:** peripheral neuropathy. **Misc:** *hypersensitivity reactions including*— SERUM SICKNESS and STEVENS-JOHNSON SYNDROME, fever.

Interactions

Drug-Drug: May ↑ action/risk of toxicity from **oral hypoglycemic agents**, **phenytoin**, **methotrexate**, **zidovudine**, or **warfarin**. ↑ risk of drug-induced hepatitis with other **hepatotoxic agents**. ↑ risk of crystalluria with **methenamine**. May ↓ metabolism and increase effects/toxicity of **mercaptopurine** or **thioguanine**.
Drug-Food: May decrease **iron** and **folic acid** absorption.

Route/Dosage

Inflammatory bowel disease

PO (Adults): *Inflammatory bowel disease*—1 g q 6–8 hr (may start with 500 mg q 6–12 hr), followed by maintenance dose of 500 mg q 6 hr.
PO (Children >2 yr): *Initial*—6.7–10 mg/kg q 4 hr *or* 10–15 mg/kg q 6 hr *or* 13.3–20 mg/kg q 8 hr. *Maintenance*—7.5 mg/kg q 6 hr (not to exceed 2 g/day).

Rheumatoid arthritis

PO (Adults): 500 mg–1 g/day (as delayed-release tablets) for 1 wk, then increase by 500 mg/day q wk up to 2 g/day in 2 divided doses; if no benefit seen after 12 wk, increase to 3 g/day in 2 divided doses.
PO (Children ≥6 yr): 30–50 mg/kg/day in 2 divided doses (as delayed-release tablets); initiate therapy at 1/4–1/3 of planned maintenance

dose and increase q 7 days until maintenance dose is reached (not to exceed 2 g/day).

Availability (generic available)

Tablets: 500 mg. **Delayed-release (enteric-coated) tablets (Azulfidine EN-tabs):** 500 mg. **Oral suspension:** ✤ 250 mg/5 ml. **Rectal suspension:** ✤ 3 g.

NURSING IMPLICATIONS

Assessment

- Assess patient for allergy to sulfonamides and salicylates. Therapy should be discontinued if rash or fever occurs.
- Monitor intake and output ratios. Fluid intake should be sufficient to maintain a urine output of at least 1200–1500 ml daily to prevent crystalluria and stone formation.
- **Inflammatory Bowel Disease:** Assess abdominal pain and frequency, quantity, and consistency of stools at the beginning of and during therapy.
- **Rheumatoid Arthritis:** Assess range of motion and degree of swelling and pain in affected joints before and periodically during therapy.
- ***Lab Test Considerations:*** Monitor urinalysis, BUN, and serum creatinine before and periodically during therapy. May cause crystalluria and urinary cell calculi formation.
- ***Lab Test Considerations:*** Monitor CBC before and every 3–6 mo during prolonged therapy. Discontinue sulfasalazine if blood dyscrasias occur.

Potential Nursing Diagnoses

Acute pain (Indications)
Diarrhea (Indications)

Implementation

- Do not confuse sulfasalazine with sulfisoxazole.
- Varying dosing regimens of sulfasalazine may be used to minimize GI side effects.
- **PO:** Administer after meals or with food to minimize GI irritation, with a full glass of water. Do not crush or chew enteric-coated tablets. Shake oral suspension well before administration. Use a calibrated measuring device to measure liquid preparations.
- **Rect:** Patient should empty bowel before administration of rectal dose forms.
- Administer 60-ml retention enema once daily at bedtime. Solution should be retained for approximately 8 hr. Before administration of *rectal suspension,* shake bottle well and remove the protective cap. Have patient lie on left side with the lower leg extended and the upper leg flexed for support or place the patient in knee-chest position. Gently insert the applicator tip into the rectum, pointing toward the umbilicus. Squeeze the bottle steadily to discharge most of the preparation.

Patient/Family Teaching

- Instruct patient on the correct method of administration. Advise patient to take medication as directed, even if feeling better. Take missed doses as soon as remembered unless almost time for next dose.
- May cause dizziness. Caution patient to avoid driving or other activities that require alertness until response to medication is known.
- Advise patient to notify health care professional if skin rash, sore throat, fever, mouth sores, unusual bleeding or bruising, wheezing, fever, or hives occur.
- Caution patient to use sunscreen and protective clothing to prevent photosensitivity reactions.
- Inform patient that this medication may cause orange-yellow discoloration of urine and skin, which is not significant. May permanently stain contact lenses yellow.
- Instruct patient to notify health care professional if symptoms worsen or do not improve. If symptoms of acute intolerance (cramping, acute abdominal pain, bloody diarrhea, fever, headache, rash) occur, discontinue therapy and notify health care professional immediately.
- Inform patient that proctoscopy and sigmoidoscopy may be required periodically during treatment to determine response.
- Instruct patient to notify health care professional if symptoms do not improve after 1–2 mo of therapy.
- **Rect:** Instruct patient to use *rectal suspension* at bedtime and retain suspension all night for best results.

Evaluation/Desired Outcomes

- Decrease in diarrhea and abdominal pain.
- Return to normal bowel pattern in patients with inflammatory bowel disease. Effects may

S

be seen within 3–21 days. The usual course of therapy is 3–6 wk.

- Maintenance of remission in patients with inflammatory bowel disease.
- Decrease in pain and inflammation, and increase in mobility in patients with rheumatoid arthritis.

sulindac (soo-lin-dak)

✤Apo-Sulin, Clinoril, ✤Novo-Sundac

Classification

Therapeutic: antirheumatics, nonsteroidal anti-inflammatory agents

Pregnancy Category UK

Indications

Management of inflammatory disorders, including: Rheumatoid arthritis, Osteoarthritis, Acute gouty arthritis, Bursitis.

Action

Inhibits prostaglandin synthesis. **Therapeutic Effects:** Suppression of pain and inflammation.

Pharmacokinetics

Absorption: Well absorbed from the GI tract after oral administration.

Distribution: Unknown. Enters breast milk in small amounts.

Metabolism and Excretion: Converted by the liver to active drug. Minimal amounts excreted unchanged by the kidneys.

Half-life: 7.8 hr (16.4 hr for active metabolite).

TIME/ACTION PROFILE

ROUTE	ONSET	PEAK	DURATION
PO (analgesic)	1–2 days	unknown	12 hr
PO (anti-inflammatory)	few days–1 wk	2 wk or more	unknown

Contraindications/Precautions

Contraindicated in: Hypersensitivity; Cross-sensitivity may occur with other NSAIDs, including aspirin; Active GI bleeding or ulcer disease; Peri-operative pain from coronary artery bypass graft (CABG) surgery.

Use Cautiously in: Cardiovascular disease or risk factors for cardiovascular disease (may ↑ risk of serious cardiovascular thrombotic events, myocardial infarction, and stroke, especially with prolonged use); Severe renal, or hepatic disease (dosage modification recommended); Geri: Geriatric patients (increased risk of GI bleeding); History of ulcer disease; Pedi, OB: Pregnancy, lactation, or children (use not recommended).

Adverse Reactions/Side Effects

CNS: dizziness, headache, drowsiness. **EENT:** blurred vision, tinnitus. **CV:** edema. **GI:** GI BLEEDING, DRUG-INDUCED HEPATITIS, constipation, diarrhea discomfort, dyspepsia, nausea, vomiting, anorexia, flatulence, pancreatitis. **GU:** renal failure. **Derm:** EXFOLIATIVE DERMATITIS, STEVENS-JOHNSON SYNDROME, TOXIC EPIDERMAL NECROLYSIS, rashes, photosensitivity. **Hemat:** blood dyscrasias, prolonged bleeding time. **Misc:** allergic reactions including ANAPHYLAXIS and HYPERSENSITIVITY SYNDROME.

Interactions

Drug-Drug: Concurrent use of **aspirin** may ↓ effectiveness. ↑ risk of bleeding with **anticoagulants**, **thrombolytic agents**, **tirofiban eptifibatide**, **clopidogrel**, **ticlopidine**, **cefoperazone**, **cefotetan**, or **valproic acid**. ↑ adverse GI side effects with **aspirin**, **corticosteroids**, and other **NSAIDs**. May ↓ response to **antihypertensives** or **diuretics**. May ↑ serum levels and risk of toxicity from **lithium**. May ↑ risk of hematologic toxicity from **antineoplastics** or **radiation therapy**. ↑ risk of adverse renal effects with **gold compounds**, **cyclosporine**, or chronic use of **acetaminophen**. **Antacids** ↓ blood levels and decrease effectiveness of sulindac. ↑ risk of photosensitivity reactions with other **photosensitizing medications**. ↑ risk of hypoglycemia with **insulins** or **oral hypoglycemic agents**. Should not be used concurrently with **dimethyl sulfoxide** because of ↑ risk of peripheral neuropathy and ↓ levels of sulindac and its metabolite.

Route/Dosage

PO (Adults): 150–200 mg bid (not to exceed 400 mg/day).

Availability (generic available)

Tablets: 150 mg, 200 mg.

NURSING IMPLICATIONS

Assessment

- Patients who have asthma, aspirin-induced allergy, and nasal polyps are at increased risk for developing hypersensitivity reactions. Monitor for rhinitis, asthma, and urticaria.

- Assess pain and range of movement before and after 1–2 wk of therapy.
- ***Lab Test Considerations:*** Evaluate BUN, serum creatinine, CBC, and liver function periodically in patients receiving prolonged therapy.
- Serum potassium, glucose, alkaline phosphatase, AST, and ALT may show ↑ levels.
- Bleeding time may be prolonged for 1 day after discontinuation of therapy.

Potential Nursing Diagnoses
Acute pain (Indications)
Impaired physical mobility (Indications)

Implementation
- Do not confuse Clinoril (sulindac) with Clozaril (clozapine).
- Administration in higher than recommended doses does not provide increased effectiveness but may cause increased side effects. Use lowest effective dose for shortest period of time.
- **PO:** May be administered with food, milk, or antacids to decrease GI irritation. Food slows but does not reduce the extent of absorption. Tablets may be crushed and mixed with fluids or food.

Patient/Family Teaching
- Advise patient to take this medication with a full glass of water and to remain in an upright position for 15–30 min after administration.
- Instruct patient to take medication as directed. Take missed doses as soon as remembered but not if almost time for the next dose. Do not double doses.
- May cause dizziness. Advise patient to avoid driving or other activities requiring alertness until response to the medication is known.
- Caution patient to avoid the concurrent use of alcohol, aspirin, NSAIDs, acetaminophen, or other OTC medications without consulting health care professional.
- Advise patient to inform health care professional of medication regimen before treatment or surgery.
- Advise patient to inform health care professional if pregnancy is planned or suspected.
- Advise patient to use sunscreen and protective clothing to prevent photosensitivity reactions.
- Advise patient to consult health care professional if rash, itching, visual disturbances, tinnitus, weight gain, edema, black stools, persistent headache, or influenza-like syndrome (chills, fever, muscle aches, pain) occurs.

Evaluation/Desired Outcomes
- Decreased pain and improved joint mobility. Partial arthritic relief may be seen within 7 days, but maximum effectiveness may require 2–3 wk of continuous therapy. Patients who do not respond to one NSAID may respond to another.

sumatriptan (soo-ma-**trip**-tan)
Imitrex, Imitrex STATdose

Classification
Therapeutic: vascular headache suppressants
Pharmacologic: 5-HT_1 agonists

Pregnancy Category C

Indications
Acute treatment of migraine attacks. **Subcut:** Acute treatment of cluster headache episodes.

Action
Acts as a selective agonist of 5-HT_1 at specific vascular serotonin receptor sites, causing vasoconstriction in large intracranial arteries. **Therapeutic Effects:** Relief of acute attacks of migraine.

Pharmacokinetics
Absorption: Well absorbed (97%) after subcut administration. Absorption after oral administration is incomplete and significant amounts undergo substantial hepatic metabolism, resulting in poor bioavailability (14%). Well absorbed after intranasal administration.
Distribution: Does not cross the blood-brain barrier. Remainder of distribution not known.
Metabolism and Excretion: Mostly metabolized (80%) by the liver.
Half-life: 2 hr.

TIME/ACTION PROFILE (relief of migraine)

ROUTE	ONSET	PEAK	DURATION
PO	within 30 min	2–4 hr	up to 24 hr
subcut	30 min	up to 2 hr	up to 24 hr
nasal	within 60 min	2 hr	unknown

Contraindications/Precautions
Contraindicated in: Hypersensitivity; Patients with ischemic heart disease or signs and symp-

toms of ischemic heart disease, Prinzmetal's angina, or uncontrolled hypertension; Concurrent MAO inhibitor therapy; Geri: Excessive risk of cardiovascular complications.
Use Cautiously in: Patients with childbearing potential; OB, Lactation, Pedi: Safety not established.
Exercise Extreme Caution in: Cardiovascular risk factors (hypertension, hypercholesterolemia, smoking, obesity, diabetes, family history, menopausal women or men >40 yr); use only if cardiovascular status has been evaluated and determined to be safe and first dose is administered under supervision.

Adverse Reactions/Side Effects
All adverse reactions are less common after oral administration.
CNS: dizziness, vertigo, anxiety, drowsiness, fatigue, feeling of heaviness, feeling of tightness, headache, malaise, strange feeling, tight feeling in head, weakness. **EENT:** alterations in vision, nasal sinus discomfort, throat discomfort. **CV:** MI, angina, chest pressure, chest tightness, coronary vasospasm, ECG changes, transient hypertension. **GI:** abdominal discomfort, dysphagia. **Derm:** tingling, warm sensation, burning sensation, cool sensation, flushing. **Local:** injection site reaction. **MS:** jaw discomfort, muscle cramps, myalgia, neck pain, neck stiffness. **Neuro:** numbness.

Interactions
Drug-Drug: The risk of vasospastic reactions may be increased by concurrent use of **ergotamine** or **dihydroergotamine** (avoid within 24 hr of each other). Concurrent use with **lithium**, **MAO inhibitors** (do not use within 2 wk of discontinuing MAO inhibitor), or **SSRI antidepressants** (may cause weakness, hyperreflexia and incoordination). Increased serotonin levels and serotonin syndrome may occur when used concurrently with **SSRI and SNRI antidepressants**.
Drug-Natural Products: Increased risk of serotinergic side effects including serotonin syndrome with **St. John's wort** and **SAMe**.

Route/Dosage
PO (Adults): 25 mg initially; if response is inadequate at 2 hr, up to 100 mg may be given (initial doses of 25–50 mg may be more effective than 25 mg). If headache recurs, doses may be repeated q 2 hr (not to exceed 300 mg/day). If PO therapy is to follow subcut injection, additional PO sumatriptan may be taken q 2 hr (not to exceed 200 mg/day).
Subcut (Adults): 6 mg; may repeat after 1 hr (not to exceed 12 mg in 24 hr).
Intranasal (Adults): Single dose of 5, 10, or 20 mg in one nostril; may be repeated in 2 hr, not to exceed 40 mg/24 hr or treatment of >5 episodes/mo.

Hepatic Impairment
PO (Adults): 25 mg initially; if response is inadequate at 2 hr, up to 50 mg may be given (initial doses of 25–50 mg may be more effective than 25 mg). If headache recurs, doses may be repeated q 2 hr (not to exceed 300 mg/day). If PO therapy is to follow subcut injection, additional PO sumatriptan may be taken q 2 hr (not to exceed 200 mg/day); no single oral dose should exceed 50 mg.

Availability
Tablets: 25 mg, 50 mg, 100 mg. **Cost:** 25 mg $202.97/9, 50 mg $188.98/9, 100 mg $188.98/9. **Injection:** 4 mg/0.5-ml prefilled syringes (for use in STAT dose system), 6 mg/0.5-ml prefilled syringes (for use in STAT dose system) or vials. **Cost:** 6 mg $117.15/2 prefilled syringes. **Nasal spray:** 5 mg/nasal spray device (delivers 5 mg/spray) (box of 6), 20 mg/nasal spray device (delivers 20 mg/spray) (box of 6). **Cost:** 5 mg $188.73/box, 20 mg $191.55/box.

NURSING IMPLICATIONS

Assessment
- Assess pain location, intensity, duration, and associated symptoms (photophobia, phonophobia, nausea, vomiting) during migraine attack.
- Give initial subcut dose under observation to patients with potential for coronary artery disease including postmenopausal women, men >40 years, patients with risk factors for coronary artery disease such as hypertension, hypercholesterolemia, obesity, diabetes, smoking, or family history. Monitor blood pressure before and for 1 hr after initial injection. If angina occurs, monitor ECG for ischemic changes.

Potential Nursing Diagnoses
Acute pain (Indications)

Implementation
- Do not confuse sumatriptan with zolmitriptan.
- **PO:** Tablets should be swallowed whole; do not crush, break, or chew. Tablets are film-

coated to prevent contact with tablet contents, which have an unpleasant taste and may cause nausea and vomiting.

- **Subcut:** Administer as a single injection just below the skin.
- **Intranasal:** 10-mg dose may be administered as 2 sprays of 5 mg in one nostril or 1 spray in each nostril.

Patient/Family Teaching

- Inform patient that sumatriptan should be used only during a migraine attack. It is meant to be used for relief of migraine attacks but not to prevent or reduce the number of attacks.
- Instruct patient to administer sumatriptan as soon as symptoms of a migraine attack appear, but it may be administered at any time during an attack. If migraine symptoms return, a 2nd injection may be used. Allow at least 1 hr between doses, and do not use more than 2 injections in any 24-hr period.
- Advise patient that lying down in a darkened room after sumatriptan administration may further help relieve headache.
- OB: Caution patient not to use sumatriptan if pregnant, suspects pregnancy, or plans to become pregnant. Adequate contraception should be used during therapy.
- Advise patient to notify health care professional before next dose of sumatriptan if pain or tightness in the chest occurs during use. If pain is severe or does not subside, notify health care professional immediately. If wheezing; heart throbbing; swelling of eyelids, face, or lips; skin rash; skin lumps; or hives occur, notify health care professional immediately and do not take more sumatriptan without approval of health care professional. Additional sumatriptan doses are not likely to be effective and alternative medications, as previously discussed with health care professional, may be used. If usual dose fails to relieve 3 consecutive headaches or if frequency and/or severity increases, notify health care professional. If feelings of tingling, heat, flushing, heaviness, pressure, drowsiness, dizziness, tiredness, or sickness develop, discuss with health care professional at next visit.
- Sumatriptan may cause dizziness or drowsiness. Caution patient to avoid driving or other activities requiring alertness until response to medication is known.
- Advise patient to avoid alcohol, which aggravates headaches, during sumatriptan use.
- Advise patient to consult health care professional before taking other medications, OTC medications, or herbal products concurrently with sumatriptan.
- **Subcut:** Instruct patient on the proper technique for loading, administering, and discarding the auto-injector. Patient information pamphlet is provided. Instructional video is available from the manufacturer.
- Inform patient that pain or redness at the injection site usually lasts less than 1 hr.
- **Intranasal:** Instruct patient in proper technique for intranasal administration. Usual dose is a single spray in one nostril. If headache returns, a 2nd dose may be administered in ≥2 hr. Do not administer 2nd dose if no relief was provided by 1st dose without consulting health care professional.

Evaluation/Desired Outcomes

- Relief of migraine attack.

sunitinib (su-**ni**-ti-nib)

Sutent

Classification

Therapeutic: antineoplastics

Pharmacologic: kinase inhibitors

Pregnancy Category D

Indications

Gastrointestinal stromal tumor which has progressed on or intolerance to imatinib. Advanced renal cell carcinoma.

Action

Inhibits multiple receptor tyrosine kinases, which are enzymes implicated in tumor growth, abnormal vascular growth and tumor metastases. **Therapeutic Effects:** Decreased tumor spread.

Pharmacokinetics

Absorption: Well absorbed following oral administration.

Distribution: Unknown.

Protein Binding: *Sunitinib*—95%; *primary active metabolite*—90%.

S

Metabolism and Excretion: Metabolized by the CYP3A4 enzyme system to its primary active metabolite. This metabolite is further metabolized by CYP3A4. Excretion is primarily fecal.
Half-life: *Sunitinib*—40–60 hr; *primary active metabolite*—80–110 hr.

TIME/ACTION PROFILE (sblood levels)

ROUTE	ONSET	PEAK	DURATION
PO	unknown	6–12 hr	24 hr

Contraindications/Precautions

Contraindicated in: Hypersensitivity; OB: Pregnancy, lactation; Concurrent use of ketoconazole or St. John's wort.
Use Cautiously in: Hepatic/renal impairment; OB: Child—bearing potential; Pedi: Children (safety not established).

Adverse Reactions/Side Effects

CNS: fatigue, dizziness, headache. **CV:** CHF, hypertension, peripheral edema, thromboembolic events. **GI:** diarrhea, dyspepsia, nausea, stomatitis, vomiting, altered taste, anorexia, constipation, ↑ lipase/amylase, ↑ liver enzymes, oral pain. **Derm:** alopecia, hand-foot syndrome, hair color change, rash, skin discoloration. **Endo:** adrenal insufficiency, hypothyroidism. **F and E:** dehydration, hypophosphatemia. **Hemat:** HEMORRHAGE, anemia, lymphopenia, neutropenia, thrombocytopenia. **Metab:** hyperuricemia. **MS:** arthralgia, back pain, limb pain, myalgia. **Misc:** fever.

Interactions

Drug-Drug: Ketoconazole and other **inhibitors of the CYP3A4 enzyme system** may ↑ levels and the risk of toxicity; dosage may need to be decreased (avoid ketoconazole). **Rifampin** and other **inducers of the CYP3A4 enzyme system** may ↓ levels and effectiveness; dose may need to be increased.
Drug-Natural Products: St. John's wort may ↓ levels and effectiveness; avoid concurrent use.

Route/Dosage

PO (Adults): 50 mg once daily for 4 wk, followed by 2 week rest, alteration of dose is based on safety/tolerability and is made in 12.5 mg increments/decrements.

Availability

Capsules: 12.5 mg, 25 mg, 50 mg.

NURSING IMPLICATIONS

Assessment

- Monitor for signs of CHF (dyspnea, edema, jugular venous distension) during therapy. Assess left ventricular ejection fraction (LVEF) at baseline and periodically during therapy in patients with cardiac events in the previous 12 mo and a baseline ejection fraction in patients without cardiovascular risk factors. Discontinue sunitinib if signs of CHF occur.
- Monitor for hypertension and treat with standard antihypertensive therapy. If sever hypertension occurs, may discontinue sunitinib until controlled.
- ***Lab Test Considerations:*** Monitor CBC with platelet count and serum chemistries including phosphate at the beginning of each treatment cycle. May cause neutropenia, lymphopenia, anemia, and thrombocytopenia. May cause ↑ creatinine, hypokalemia, hyperuricemia, and ↑ uric acid.
- May cause ↑ AST, ALT, alkaline phosphatase, total and indirect bilirubin, amylase and lipase.
- Monitor thyroid function in patients with symptoms of hypothyroidism. May be treated with standard medical practice.

Potential Nursing Diagnoses

Diarrhea (Adverse Reactions)
Nausea (Adverse Reactions)

Implementation

- **PO:** Administer once daily with or without food for 4 wks, then 2 wks off therapy.

Patient/Family Teaching

- Instruct patient to take sunitinib as directed for 4 wks, followed by 2 wks off.
- Advise patient that GI disorders (diarrhea, nausea, stomatitis, dyspepsia, vomiting) are common and may require antiemetic and antidiarrheal medications.
- Inform patient that sunitinib may cause discoloration (yellow) of skin and depigmentation of hair or skin.
- Advise women of childbearing potential to avoid becoming pregnant while receiving sunitinib.
- Advise patient to consult health care professional before taking other Rx, OTC, or herbal products during sunitinib therapy.

Evaluation/Desired Outcomes

- Decrease in tumor spread.

tacrine (tak-rin)
Cognex

Classification
Therapeutic: anti-Alzheimer's agents
Pharmacologic: cholinergics (cholinesterase inhibitors)

Pregnancy Category C

Indications
Mild to moderate dementia associated with Alzheimer's disease.

Action
Increases levels of acetylcholine in the CNS by inhibiting its breakdown. **Therapeutic Effects:** Improved cognitive function in patients with mild to moderate Alzheimer's disease. Does not cure the disease.

Pharmacokinetics
Absorption: Rapidly absorbed following oral administration, although bioavailability is low (17%).
Distribution: Unknown.
Metabolism and Excretion: Highly metabolized by the liver (mostly by the P450 enzyme system).
Half-life: 2–4 hr.

TIME/ACTION PROFILE (improvement in cognitive function)

ROUTE	ONSET	PEAK	DURATION
PO	within 6 wk	18–24 wk	unknown

Contraindications/Precautions
Contraindicated in: Hypersensitivity to tacrine or other acridines; Jaundice associated with previous courses of tacrine therapy.
Use Cautiously in: Patients with a history or risk of GI bleeding, including current therapy with NSAIDs.

Adverse Reactions/Side Effects
CNS: dizziness, headache. **CV:** bradycardia. **GI:** GI BLEEDING, anorexia, diarrhea, drug-induced hepatitis, dyspepsia, nausea, vomiting.

Interactions
Drug-Drug: Metabolized by the cytochrome P450 enzyme system; levels and effects may be altered by other drugs which increase/inhibit this system or drugs that may compete for this metabolic pathway. Increases **theophylline** levels and risk of toxicity (blood level monitoring recommended; dosage reduction may be required). Potentiates the effects of **succinylcholine** (increases neuromuscular blockade) during anesthesia; also potentiates the effects of other **cholinesterase inhibitors**. May potentiate the action of **cholinergics (bethanechol)**. **Fluvoxamine** significantly increases blood levels and the risk of adverse reactions. **Cigarette smoking** decreases blood levels of tacrine. **Cimetidine** increases tacrine levels. May interfere with the action of **anticholinergics**. Concurrent use of **NSAIDs** may increase the risk of GI bleeding.
Drug-Food: Food decreases absorption of tacrine by 30–40%.

Route/Dosage
PO (Adults): 10 mg 4 times daily for 4 wk. If ALT remains unchanged, increase dose to 20 mg 4 times daily. Further increments may be made at 4-wk intervals as tolerated, up to 160 mg/day.

Availability
Capsules: 10 mg, 20 mg, 30 mg, 40 mg. **Cost:** 10 mg $147.01/120, 20 mg $147.01/120, 30 mg $147.01/120, 40 mg $147.01/120.

NURSING IMPLICATIONS

Assessment
- Assess cognitive function (memory, attention, reasoning, language, ability to perform simple tasks) periodically throughout therapy.
- Monitor heart rate periodically during therapy. May cause bradycardia.
- ***Lab Test Considerations:*** May cause ALT elevations; monitor levels every other wk for the first 16 wk of therapy, monthly for 2 mo, and then every 3 mo throughout therapy. Biweekly monitoring should be resumed for at least 6 wk after any dose increase. If ALT levels are <3 times the upper limit of normal, continue dose titration; if levels are >3 to <5 times the upper limit of normal, decrease the dose of tacrine by 40 mg/day and resume dose titration when ALT returns to normal. Tacrine should be discontinued if ALT levels are >5 times the upper limit of normal. Levels usually return to normal 4–6 wk after discontinuation of therapy.
- Tacrine should be permanently discontinued and a new trial should not be attempted in pa-

T

tients with clinical jaundice and a total bilirubin >3 mg/dl.

Potential Nursing Diagnoses

Disturbed thought process (Indications)
Risk for injury (Indications)
Impaired environmental interpretation syndrome (Indications)

Implementation

- **PO:** Administer at regular intervals between meals on an empty stomach. If GI upset occurs, may be administered with meals; however, plasma levels may be reduced by 30–40%.
- Tacrine capsules may be dissolved in any aqueous solution for patients with difficulty swallowing (orange juice best masks the bitter taste). Place intact capsule in liquid to avoid loss of medication by spillage.

Patient/Family Teaching

- Emphasize the importance of taking tacrine at regular intervals as directed. If a dose is missed, take as soon as possible unless within 2 hr of next dose; do not double doses or discontinue without consulting health care professional. Abrupt discontinuation of doses >80 mg/day may cause a decline in cognitive function and behavioral disturbances.
- Caution patient and caregiver that tacrine may cause dizziness, unsteadiness, and clumsiness.
- Advise patient and caregiver to notify health care professional if nausea, vomiting, diarrhea, rash, jaundice, or changes in the color of the stool occur or if new symptoms occur or previously noted symptoms increase in severity.
- Advise patient to notify health care professional of medication regimen prior to treatment or surgery.

Evaluation/Desired Outcomes

- Improvement in cognitive function (memory, attention, reasoning, language, ability to perform simple tasks) in patients with Alzheimer's disease.

TACROLIMUS

tacrolimus (oral, IV)
(ta-**kroe**-li-mus)
Prograf

tacrolimus (topical)
Protopic

Classification
Therapeutic: immunosuppressants

Pregnancy Category C

Indications

PO, IV: Prevention of organ rejection in patients who have undergone allogenic liver, kidney, or heart transplantation (used concurrently with corticosteroids). **Topical:** Moderate to severe atopic dermatitis in patients who do not respond to or cannot tolerate alternative, conventional therapies.

Action

Inhibit T-lymphocyte activation. **Therapeutic Effects:** Prevention of transplanted organ rejection. Improvement in signs/symptoms of atopic dermatitis.

Pharmacokinetics

Absorption: Absorption following oral administration is erratic and incomplete (bioavailability ranges from 5–67%); minimal amounts absorbed following topical use.
Distribution: Cross the placenta and enter breast milk.
Protein Binding: 99%.
Metabolism and Excretion: 99% metabolized by the liver; <1% excreted unchanged in the urine.
Half-life: *Liver transplant patients*—11.7 hr; *healthy volunteers*—21.2 hr.

TIME/ACTION PROFILE (immunosuppression)

ROUTE	ONSET	PEAK	DURATION
PO	rapid	1.3–3.2 hr*	12 hr
IV	rapid	unknown	8–12 hr
topical†	unknown	1–2 wk	unknown

*Blood level
†Improvement in atopic dermatitis

Contraindications/Precautions

Contraindicated in: Hypersensitivity to tacrolimus or to castor oil (a component in the injection); Concurrent use with cyclosporine should be avoided; Lactation: Breastfeeding should be avoided; **Topical:** Weakened/compromised immune system; Malignant or premalignant skin condition; Children <2 yr (safety not established).
Use Cautiously in: Renal or hepatic impairment (dosage reduction may be required; if oliguria occurs, wait 48 hr before initiating tacrolimus); Exposure to sunlight/UV light (may ↑

risk of malignant skin changes); OB: Hyperkalemia and renal impairment may occur in the newborn; use only if benefit to mother justifies risk to the fetus; Pedi: Higher end of dosing range required to maintain adequate blood levels); **Topical:** Superficial skin infections.

Adverse Reactions/Side Effects

Noted primarily for PO and IV use.

CNS: SEIZURES, dizziness, headache, insomnia, tremor, abnormal dreams, agitation, anxiety, confusion, depression, emotional lability, hallucinations, psychoses, somnolence. **EENT:** abnormal vision, amblyopia, sinusitis, tinnitus. **Resp:** cough, pleural effusion, asthma, bronchitis, pharyngitis, pneumonia, pulmonary edema. **CV:** hypertension, peripheral edema, QTc prolongation. **GI:** GI BLEEDING, abdominal pain, anorexia, ascites, constipation, diarrhea, dyspepsia, liver function test elevation, nausea, vomiting, cholangitis, cholestatic jaundice, dysphagia, flatulence, increased appetite, oral thrush, peritonitis. **GU:** nephrotoxicity, urinary tract infection. **Derm:** pruritus, rash, alopecia, herpes simplex, hirsutism, photosensitivity, sweating. **Endo:** hyperglycemia, hyperlipidemia. **F and E:** hyperkalemia, hypomagnesemia, hyperphosphatemia, hypocalcemia, hyponatremia, hypophosphatemia, metabolic acidosis, metabolic alkalosis. **Hemat:** anemia, leukocytosis, leukopenia, thrombocytopenia, coagulation defects. **Local:** *topical*—burning, stinging. **MS:** arthralgia, hypertonia, leg cramps, muscle spasm, myalgia, myasthenia, osteoporosis. **Neuro:** paresthesia, neuropathy. **Misc:** allergic reactions including ANAPHYLAXIS, generalized pain, abnormal healing, chills, fever, increased risk of lymphoma/skin cancer (topical).

Interactions

Noted primarily for PO and IV use, but should be considered for topical use

Drug-Drug: Risk of nephrotoxicity is ↑ by concurrent use of **aminoglycosides, amphotericin B, cisplatin**, or **cyclosporine** (allow 24 hr to pass after stopping cyclosporine before starting tacrolimus). Concurrent use of **potassium-sparing diuretics, ACE inhibitors**, or **angiotensin II receptor blockers** ↑ risk of hyperkalemia. The following drugs ↑ tacrolimus blood levels: **azole antifungals, bromocriptine, calcium channel blockers, chloramphenicol, cimetidine, lansoprazole, clarithromycin, cyclosporine, danazol, erythromycin, magnesium/aluminum hydroxide methylprednisolone, omeprazole, nefazodone**, and **metoclopramide, protease inhibitors**, and **voriconazole. Phenobarbital, phenytoin, caspofungin, sirolimus carbamazepine**, and **rifamycins** may ↓ tacrolimus blood levels. **Vaccinations** may be less effective if given concurrently with tacrolimus (avoid use of live-virus vaccines).

Drug-Natural Products: Concomitant use with **astragalus, echinacea, and melatonin** may interfere with immunosuppression. **St. John's wort** may ↓ tacrolimus blood levels.

Drug-Food: Food decreases the rate and extent of GI absorption. **Grapefruit juice** increases absorption.

Route/Dosage

Because of the potential risk for anaphylaxis, the IV route of administration should be reserved for those patients unable to take the drug orally.

Kidney Transplantation

PO (Adults): *Initial dose*—0.2 mg/kg/day in 2 divided doses; titrate to achieve recommended blood concentration.

PO (Children): 0.15–0.4 mg/kg/day in 2 divided doses.

IV (Adults): *Initial dose*—0.03–0.1 mg/kg/day as a continuous infusion; titrate dose to achieve recommended blood concentration.

IV (Children): 0.03–0.15 mg/kg/day.

Liver Transplantation

PO (Adults): *Initial dose*—0.1–0.15 mg/kg/day in 2 divided doses; titrate to achieve recommended blood concentration.

PO (Children): *Initial dose*—0.15–0.2 mg/kg/day in 2 divided doses; titrate to achieve recommended blood concentration.

IV (Adults and Children): Same as for kidney transplant.

Heart Transplantation

PO (Adults): *Initial dose*—0.075 mg/kg/day in 2 divided doses; titrate to achieve recommended blood concentration.

IV (Adults): *Initial dose*—0.01 mg/kg/day as a continuous infusion; titrate dose to achieve recommended blood concentration.

T

Atopic Dermatitis

Topical (Adults): Apply 0.03% or 0.1% ointment twice daily. Discontinue when signs/symptoms of atopic dermatitis resolve.

Topical (Children ≥2–15 yr): Apply 0.03% ointment twice daily. Discontinue when signs/symptoms of atopic dermatitis resolve.

Availability

Capsules: 0.5 mg, 1 mg, 5 mg. **Cost:** 0.5 mg $359.96/180, 1 mg $694.46/180, 5 mg $3,645.61/180. **Injection:** 5 mg/ml. **Ointment:** 0.03% in 30-g, 60-g, and 100-g tubes, 0.1% in 30-g, 60-g, and 100-g tubes.

NURSING IMPLICATIONS

Assessment

- **Prevention of Organ Rejection:** Monitor blood pressure closely during therapy. Hypertension is a common complication of tacrolimus therapy and should be treated.
- Observe patients receiving IV tacrolimus for the development of anaphylaxis (rash, pruritus, laryngeal edema, wheezing) for at least 30 min and frequently thereafter. If signs develop, stop infusion and initiate treatment.
- **Atopic Dermatitis:** Assess skin lesions prior to and periodically during therapy.
- Use only for short time, not continuously, and in the minimum dose possible to decrease risk of developing skin cancer.
- ***Lab Test Considerations:*** Tacrolimus blood level monitoring may be helpful in the evaluation of rejection and toxicity, dose adjustments, and assessment of compliance. For liver transplantation, most patients are stable when tacrolimus trough whole blood concentrations are maintained between 5–20 mg/ml. For kidney transplantation, during the first 3 mo, most patients maintained tacrolimus whole blood concentrations between 7–20 mg/ml and then between 5–15 mg/ml through 1 yr. For heart transplantation, from wk 1 to 3 mo, most patients maintained tacrolimus trough whole blood concentrations between 8–20 mg/ml and then between 6–18 mg/ml from 3–18 mo post-transplant.
- Monitor serum creatinine, potassium, and glucose closely. ↑ serum creatinine and ↓ urine output may indicate nephrotoxicity. May also cause insulin-dependent post-transplant diabetes mellitus (incidence is higher in African American and Hispanic patients).
- May also cause hyperuricemia, hypokalemia, hyperkalemia, hypomagnesemia, metabolic acidosis, metabolic alkalosis, hyperlipidemia, hyperphosphatemia, hypophosphatemia, hypocalcemia, and hyponatremia.
- Monitor CBC. May cause anemia, leukocytosis, and thrombocytopenia.

Potential Nursing Diagnoses

Risk for infection (Adverse Reactions)

Implementation

- Therapy with tacrolimus should be started no sooner than 6 hr post-transplantation. Concurrent therapy with corticosteroids is recommended in the early postoperative period.
- Tacrolimus should not be used concomitantly with cyclosporine. Tacrolimus or cyclosporine should be discontinued at least 24 hr before starting the other.
- Oral therapy is preferred because of the risk of anaphylactic reactions with IV tacrolimus. IV therapy should be replaced with oral therapy as soon as possible.
- Adults should be started at the lower end of the dose range; children require ahigher doses to maintain blood trough concentrations similar to adults.
- **PO:** Oral doses can be initiated 8–12 hr after discontinuation of IV doses.
- **Topical:** Do not use continuously for a long time.

IV Administration

- **Continuous Infusion:** ***Diluent:*** Dilute in 0.9% NaCl or D5W. ***Concentration:*** 0.004–0.02 mg/ml. May be stored in polyethylene or glass containers for 24 hr following dilution. Do not store in PVC containers. ***Rate:*** Administer daily dose as a continuous infusion over 24 hr.
- **Y-Site Compatibility:** aminophylline, amphotericin B, ampicillin, ampicillin/sulbactam, benztropine, calcium gluconate, cefazolin, cefotetan, ceftazidime, ceftriaxone, cefuroxime, chloramphenicol, cimetidine, ciprofloxacin, clindamycin, dexamethasone sodium phosphate, digoxin, diphenhydramine, dobutamine, dopamine, doxycycline, erythromycin lactobionate, esmolol, fluconazole, furosemide, gentamicin, haloperidol, heparin, hydrocortisone sodium succinate, hydromorphone, imipenem/cilastatin, insulin, isoproterenol, leucovorin, lorazepam, methylprednisolone, metoclopramide, metronidazole, morphine, multivitamins, nitroprusside, nitroglycerin, oxacillin, penicillin G potassium, perphenazine, phenytoin, piperacillin, potassium, propranolol, ranitidine, so-

dium bicarbonate, tobramycin, trimethoprim/sulfamethoxazole, vancomycin.
- **Y-Site Incompatibility:** acyclovir, ganciclovir.

Patient/Family Teaching

- Instruct patient to take tacrolimus at the same time each day, as directed. Do not skip or double up on missed doses. Do not discontinue medication without advice of health care professional.
- Reinforce the need for lifelong therapy to prevent transplant rejection. Review symptoms of rejection for transplanted organ and stress need to notify health care professional immediately if they occur.
- Emphasize the importance of repeated lab tests during tacrolimus therapy.
- Advise patient to avoid eating raw oysters or other shellfish; make sure they are fully cooked before eating.
- Advise patient to wear protective clothing and sunscreen to avoid photosensitivity reactions.
- Instruct patient to avoid exposure to chicken pox, measles, mumps, and rubella. If exposed, see health care professional for prophylactic therapy.
- OB: Advise patient of the risk of taking tacrolimus during pregnancy.
- Inform patient of the risk of lymphoma or skin cancer with tacrolimus therapy.
- **Topical:** Advise patients to contact health care professional if their symptoms do not improve after 6 wk of therapy, if their symptoms worsen, or they develop a skin infection.
- Instruct patient to use ointment only on areas of skin with atopic dermatitis.
- Advise patient to stop using the ointment when the signs/symptoms of atopic dermatitis go away.
- Advise patient to limit sun exposure during treatment.

Evaluation/Desired Outcomes

- Prevention of transplanted organ rejection.
- Management of atopic dermatitis.

tadalafil (ta-**da**-la-fil)

Cialis

Classification
Therapeutic: erectile dysfunction agents
Pharmacologic: phosphodiesterase type 5 inhibitors

Pregnancy Category B

Indications

Erectile dysfunction.

Action

Increases cyclic guanosine monophosphate (cGMP) levels by inhibiting phosphodiesterase type 5 (PDE5) an enzyme responsible for the breakdown of cGMP. cGMP produces smooth muscle relaxation of the corpus cavernosum, which in turn promotes increased blood flow and subsequent erection. **Therapeutic Effects:** Enhanced blood flow to the corpus cavernosum and erection sufficient to allow sexual intercourse. Requires sexual stimulation.

Pharmacokinetics

Absorption: Well absorbed following oral administration.
Distribution: Extensive tissue distribution; penetrates semen.
Protein Binding: 94%.
Metabolism and Excretion: Mostly metabolized by the liver (mainly CYP3A4 enzyme system); metabolites are excreted in feces (61%) and urine (36%).
Half-life: 17.5 hr.

TIME/ACTION PROFILE (improved erectile function)

ROUTE	ONSET	PEAK	DURATION
PO	rapid	0.5–6 hr	36

Contraindications/Precautions

Contraindicated in: Hypersensitivity; Concurrent use of nitrates, nitric oxide donors, alpha adrenergic blockers (except tamsulosin 0.4 mg once daily); Unstable angina, recent history of stroke, life-threatening heart failure within 6 months, uncontrolled hypertension, arrhythmias, stroke within 6 months or MI within 90 days; Any other cardiovascular pathology precluding sexual activity; Known hereditary degenerative retinal disorders; Severe hepatic impairment; Congenital or acquired QT prolongation or concurrent use of Class IA or III antiarrhythmics; Women, children or newborns.

Use Cautiously in: Left ventricular outflow obstruction; Penile deformity; Underlying conditions predisposing to priapism including sickle cell anemia, multiple myeloma or leukemia; Bleeding disorders or active peptic ulcer disease; Strong inhibitors of the CYP3A4 enzyme system; History of sudden severe vision loss or non arteritic ischemic optic neuropathy (NAION); may ↑ risk of recurrence; Geri: Patients >65 yr have ↑ blood levels and may experience more side effects.

Adverse Reactions/Side Effects

CNS: headache. **EENT:** nasal congestion. **CV:** hypotension. **GI:** dyspepsia. **GU:** priapism. **Derm:** flushing. **MS:** back pain, limb pain, myalgia.

Interactions

Drug-Drug: Concurrent use of **nitrates** or **alpha adrenergic blockers** may cause serious, life threatening hypotension and is contraindicated except for tamsulosin 0.4 mg once daily. ↑ risk of hypotension with acute ingestion of **alcohol**. Strong inhibitors of CYP3A4 including **ritonavir**, **ketoconazole**, **itraconazole** ↑ effects and the risk of adverse reactions (dosage adjustments recommended). Similar effects may be expected of other **inhibitors of CY3A4**.

Route/Dosage

PO (Adults): 10 mg prior to sexual activity (range 5–20 mg; not to exceed one dose/24 hr); *concurrent use of CYP3A4 inhibitors including itraconazole, ketoconazole and ritonavir*—single dose should not exceed 10 mg in any 72 hour period.

Renal Impairment

PO (Adults): *CCr 31–50 ml/min*—Initial dose should not exceed 5 mg/day; maximum dose should not exceed 10 mg in 48 hr; *CCr <30 ml/min*—maximum dose 5 mg.

Hepatic Impairment

PO (Adults): *Mild or moderate hepatic impairment (Child–Pugh class A or B)*—Daily dose should not exceed 10 mg.

Availability

Tablets: 5 mg, 10 mg, 20 mg. **Cost:** 5 mg $357.97/30, 10 mg $356.97/30, 20 mg $365.97/30.

NURSING IMPLICATIONS

Assessment

- Determine erectile dysfunction before administration. Tadalafil has no effect in the absence of sexual stimulation.

Potential Nursing Diagnoses

Sexual dysfunction (Indications)

Implementation

- **PO:** Administer at least 30 min prior to sexual activity; effectiveness may continue for 36 hrs.
- May be administered without regard to food.

Patient/Family Teaching

- Instruct patient to take tadalafil at least 30 min before sexual activity and not more than once per day. Inform patient that sexual stimulation is required for an erection to occur after taking tadalafil.
- Advise patient that tadalafil is not indicated for use in women.
- Caution patient not to take tadalafil concurrently with nitrates or alpha adrenergic blockers. If chest pain occurs after taking tadalafil, instruct patient to seek immediate medical attention.
- Advise patient to avoid excess alcohol intake (≥5 units) in combination with tadalafil; may increase risk of orthostatic hypotension, increased heart rate, decreased standing blood pressure, dizziness, headache.
- Instruct patient to notify health care professional promptly if erection lasts longer than 4 hr, if they are not satisfied with their sexual performance or develop unwanted side effects or if they experience sudden or decreased vision loss in one or both eyes.
- Advise patient to consult health care professional before taking other Rx or OTC medications or herbal supplements that may interact with tadalafil.
- Inform patient that tadalafil offers no protection against sexually transmitted diseases. Counsel patient that protection against sexually transmitted diseases and HIV infection should be considered.

Evaluation/Desired Outcomes

- Male erection sufficient to allow intercourse.

tamoxifen (ta-**mox**-i-fen)
✤Alpha-Tamoxifen, ✤Med Tamoxifen, ✤Nolvadex-D, ✤Novo-Tamoxifen, Soltamox, ✤Tamofen, ✤Tamone, ✤Tamoplex

Classification
Therapeutic: antineoplastics
Pharmacologic: antiestrogens

Pregnancy Category D

Indications
Adjuvant therapy of breast cancer after surgery and radiation (delays recurrence). Palliative or adjunctive treatment of advanced breast cancer. Prevention of breast cancer in high-risk patients. Treatment of ductal carcinoma *in situ* following breast surgery and radiation. McCune-Albright syndrome with precocious puberty in girls 2–10 yr.

Action
Competes with estrogen for binding sites in breast and other tissues. Reduces DNA synthesis and estrogen response. **Therapeutic Effects:** Suppression of tumor growth. Reduced incidence of breast cancer in high-risk patients. Delayed puberty in McCune-Albright syndrome.

Pharmacokinetics
Absorption: Absorbed after oral administration.
Distribution: Widely distributed.
Metabolism and Excretion: Mostly metabolized by the liver. Slowly eliminated in the feces. Minimal amounts excreted in the urine.
Half-life: 7 days.

TIME/ACTION PROFILE (tumor response)

ROUTE	ONSET	PEAK	DURATION
PO	4–10 wk	several mo	several wk

Contraindications/Precautions
Contraindicated in: Hypersensitivity; Concurrent warfarin therapy with history of deep vein thrombosis (patients at high risk for breast cancer only); Pregnancy or lactation.
Use Cautiously in: Decreased bone marrow reserve; Women with childbearing potential.

Adverse Reactions/Side Effects
CNS: confusion, depression, headache, weakness. **EENT:** blurred vision. **CV:** PULMONARY EMBOLISM, STROKE, edema. **GI:** nausea, vomiting. **GU:** UTERINE MALIGNANCIES, vaginal bleeding. **F and E:** hypercalcemia. **Hemat:** leukopenia, thrombocytopenia. **Metab:** hot flashes. **MS:** bone pain. **Misc:** tumor flare.

Interactions
Drug-Drug: Estrogens and **aminoglutethimide** may ↓ effectiveness of concurrently administered tamoxifen. Blood levels are ↑ by **bromocriptine**. May ↑ the anticoagulant effect of **warfarin**. Risk of thromboembolic events is ↑ by concurrent use of other **antineoplastics**.

Route/Dosage

Treatment of Breast Cancer
PO (Adults): 10–20 mg twice daily; doses of 20 mg/day may be taken as a single dose.

Prevention of Breast Cancer/Ductal Carcinoma *in situ*
PO (Adults): 20 mg once daily for 5 yr.

McCune-Albright Syndrome
PO (Children [girls] 2–10 yr): 20 mg once daily for up to one year.

Availability (generic available)
Tablets: 10 mg, 20 mg. **Cost:** *Generic*—10 mg $39.97/90, 20 mg $49.97/90. **Enteric-coated tablets:** ✤ 20 mg. **Oral Solution (Soltamox) (sugar-free licorice and aniseed taste and smell):** 10 mg/5 mL.

NURSING IMPLICATIONS

Assessment
- Assess for an increase in bone or tumor pain. Confer with physician or other health care professional regarding analgesics. This transient pain usually resolves despite continued therapy.
- ***Lab Test Considerations:*** Monitor CBC, platelets, and calcium levels before and during therapy. May cause transient hypercalcemia in patients with metastases to the bone. An estrogen receptor assay should be assessed before initiation of therapy.
- Monitor serum cholesterol and triglyceride concentrations in patients with pre-existing hyperlipidemia. May cause ↑ concentrations.
- Monitor hepatic function tests and thyroxine (T_4) periodically during therapy. May cause ↑ serum hepatic enzyme and thyroxine concentrations.
- Gynecologic examinations should be performed regularly; may cause variations in Papanicolaou and vaginal smears.

T

Potential Nursing Diagnoses

Deficient knowledge, related to medication regimen (Patient/Family Teaching)

Implementation

- **PO:** Administer with food or fluids if GI irritation becomes a problem. Consult physician or other health care professional if patient vomits shortly after administration of medication to determine need for repeat dose.
- Do not crush, break, chew, or administer an antacid within 1–2 hr of enteric-coated tablet.
- Store oral solution in original bottle to protect from light. Do not refrigerate or freeze. Use within 3 months.

Patient/Family Teaching

- Instruct patient to take medication as directed. If a dose is missed, it should be omitted.
- If skin lesions are present, inform patient that lesions may temporarily increase in size and number and may have increased erythema.
- Advise patient to report bone pain to health care professional promptly. This pain may be severe. Inform patient that this may be an indication of the drug's effectiveness and will resolve over time. Analgesics should be ordered to control pain.
- Instruct patient to monitor weight weekly. Weight gain or peripheral edema should be reported to health care professional.
- This medication may induce ovulation and may have teratogenic properties. Advise patient to use a nonhormonal method of contraception during and for 1 mo after the therapy.
- Advise patient that medication may cause hot flashes. Notify health care professional if these become bothersome.
- Instruct patient to notify health care professional promptly if pain or swelling of legs, shortness of breath, weakness, sleepiness, confusion, nausea, vomiting, weight gain, dizziness, headache, loss of appetite, or blurred vision occurs. Patient should also report menstrual irregularities, vaginal bleeding, pelvic pain or pressure.

Evaluation/Desired Outcomes

- Decrease in the size or spread of breast cancer. Observable effects of therapy may not be seen for 4–10 wk after initiation.
- Delayed puberty in McCune-Albright syndrome.

tamsulosin (tam-**soo**-loe-sin)

Flomax

Classification

Therapeutic: none assigned

Pharmacologic: peripherally acting anti-adrenergics

Pregnancy Category B

Indications

Management of outflow obstruction in male patients with prostatic hyperplasia.

Action

Decreases contractions in smooth muscle of the prostatic capsule by preferentially binding to alpha$_1$-adrenergic receptors. **Therapeutic Effects:** Decreased symptoms of prostatic hyperplasia (urinary urgency, hesitancy, nocturia).

Pharmacokinetics

Absorption: Slowly absorbed after oral administration.

Distribution: Widely distributed.

Protein Binding: 94–99%.

Metabolism and Excretion: Extensively metabolized by the liver; <10% excreted unchanged in urine.

Half-life: 14 hr.

TIME/ACTION PROFILE (increase in urine flow)

ROUTE	ONSET	PEAK	DURATION
PO	unknown	2 wk	unknown

Contraindications/Precautions

Contraindicated in: Hypersensitivity.

Use Cautiously in: Patients at risk for prostate carcinoma (symptoms may be similar).

Adverse Reactions/Side Effects

CNS: dizziness, headache. **EENT:** rhinitis. **CV:** orthostatic hypotension. **GU:** retrograde/diminished ejaculation.

Interactions

Drug-Drug: Cimetidine may increase blood levels and the risk of toxicity. Increased risk of hypotension with other peripherally acting anti-adrenergics (**doxazosin**, **prazosin**, **terazosin**); concurrent use should be avoided.

Route/Dosage

PO (Adults): 0.4 mg once daily after a meal; may be increased after 2–4 wk to 0.8 mg/day.

Availability

Capsules: 0.4 mg. **Cost:** $233.98/90.

NURSING IMPLICATIONS

Assessment

- Assess patient for symptoms of prostatic hyperplasia (urinary hesitancy, feeling of incomplete bladder emptying, interruption of urinary stream, impairment of size and force of urinary stream, terminal urinary dribbling, straining to start flow, dysuria, urgency) before and periodically throughout therapy.
- Assess patient for first-dose orthostatic hypotension and syncope. Incidence may be dose related. Observe patient closely during this period and take precautions to prevent injury.
- Monitor intake and output ratios and daily weight, and assess for edema daily, especially at beginning of therapy. Report weight gain or edema.

Potential Nursing Diagnoses

Risk for injury (Side Effects)
Impaired urinary elimination (Indications)

Implementation

- Do not confuse Flomax (tamsulosin) with Fosamax (alendronate) or Volmax (albuterol).
- **PO:** Administer daily dose 30 min after the same meal each day.
- If dose is interrupted for several days at either the 0.4-mg or 0.8-mg dose, restart therapy with the 0.4-mg/day dose.

Patient/Family Teaching

- Emphasize the importance of continuing to take this medication, even if feeling well. Instruct patient to take medication at the same time each day. If a dose is missed, take as soon as remembered unless almost time for next dose. Do not double doses.
- May cause dizziness. Advise patient to avoid driving or other activities requiring alertness until response to medication is known.
- Caution patient to change positions slowly to minimize orthostatic hypotension.
- Advise patient to consult health care professional before taking any cough, cold, or allergy remedies.
- Emphasize the importance of follow-up visits to determine effectiveness of therapy.

Evaluation/Desired Outcomes

- Decrease in urinary symptoms of benign prostatic hyperplasia.

telithromycin

(tel-i-thro-**mye**-sin)
Ketek

Classification
Therapeutic: anti-infectives
Pharmacologic: ketolides

Pregnancy Category C

Indications

Community-acquired pneumonia.

Action

Blocks bacterial protein synthesis at the level of the 50S ribosomal subunit. **Therapeutic Effects:** Resolution of infection. **Spectrum:** Active against the following organisms: *Staphylococcus aureus* (methicillin and erythromycin susceptible strains only), *Streptococcus pneumoniae* (including multi-durg resistant strains), *Haemophilus influenzae*, *Moraxella catarrhalis*, *Chlamydophila pneumoniae*, and *Mycoplasma pneumoniae*.

Pharmacokinetics

Absorption: 57% absorbed following oral administration; unaffected by food.
Distribution: Concentrates in bronchial mucosa, epithelial lining fluid and alveolar macrophages.
Metabolism and Excretion: 70% metabolized by the liver (50% by CYP3A4), 13% excreted unchanged in urine, 7% excreted unchanged via biliary/intestinal elimination.
Half-life: 10 hr.

TIME/ACTION PROFILE (blood levels)

ROUTE	ONSET	PEAK	DURATION
PO	rapid	1 hr	24 hr

Contraindications/Precautions

Contraindicated in: Hypersensitivity; History of hepatitis or jaundice associated with use of telithromycin; Hypersensitivity to macrolides (erythromycin, azithromycin, clarithromycin); Concurrent use of pimozide, ergot alkaloids, simvastatin, lovastatin, atorvastatin, or rifampin; Congenital QTc prolongation, uncorrected hypokalemia or hypomagnesemia, bradycardia, concurrent use of Class IA (quinidine, procainamide) or Class III antiarrhythmics (dofetilide); Myasthenia gravis; Lactation: Excreted in breast milk; consider alternative to breastfeeding.

Use Cautiously in: CCr <30 mL/min (dosage not established); Concurrent use of midazolam and other benzodiazpines; OB: Use only if benefits outweigh risks to fetus; Pedi: Safety not established.

Adverse Reactions/Side Effects

CNS: loss of consciousness. **EENT:** visual disturbances. **CV:** arrhythmias, QTc prolongation. **GI:** PSEUDOMEMBRANOUS COLITIS, diarrhea, hepatitis, HEPATIC FAILURE,, nausea. **Neuro:** exacerbation of myasthenia gravis.

Interactions

Drug-Drug: Blood levels are ↑ by **ketoconazole** and **itraconazole**. ↑ levels and risk of myopathy from **simvastatin**, **lovastatin**, and **atorvastatin**; avoid concurrent use. ↑ levels and risk of excessive sedation with **midazolam**; careful titration is required. Similar effects may occur with **triazolam**. ↑ levels of **metoprolol**; use caution in patients with CHF. May also ↑ levels, effects and risk of toxicity from **ergot derivatives** (**ergotamine**, **dihydroergotamine**); concurrent use not recommended; similar effects may occur with **carbamazepine**, **cyclosporine**, **tacrolimus**, **sirolimus**, **hexobarbital**, or **phenytoin**. **Rifampin** ↓ levels and effectiveness; avoid concurrent use. Similar effects may occur with **phenytoin**, **carbamazepine**, or **phenobarbital**.

Route/Dosage

PO (Adults): *community-acquired pneumonia*—800 mg once daily for 7–10 days.

Availability

Tablets: 300 mg, 400 mg. **Cost:** 400 mg $104.00/20.

NURSING IMPLICATIONS

Assessment

- Assess for infection (vital signs; sputum, WBC) at beginning of and during therapy.
- Obtain specimens for culture and sensitivity before initiating therapy. First dose may be given before receiving results.
- Determine any family history of QTc prolongation or proarrythmic conditions (hypokalemia, bradycardia).
- Monitor for signs or symptoms of hepatitis (fatigue, malaise, anorexia, nausea, jaundice, bilirubinuria, acholic stools, liver tenderness or hepatomegaly). If these occur, discontinue telithromycin immediately and monitor liver function; do not re-administer telithromycin.
- ***Lab Test Considerations:*** May cause ↑ platelet count.
- Monitor liver function periodically during therapy and if signs of hepatitis occur.

Potential Nursing Diagnoses

Risk for infection (Indications)
Noncompliance (Patient/Family Teaching)

Implementation

- **PO:** Administer with or without food.

Patient/Family Teaching

- Instruct patient to take medication as directed and to finish medication completely, even if feeling better. Take missed doses as soon as remembered, but do not take more than one dose in a 24–hr period. Advise patient to read *Patient Information Sheet* prior to starting therapy.
- May cause visual disturbances (blurred vision, difficulty focusing, diplopia). Caution patient to avoid driving or other activities requiring visual acuity until response to medication is known. Advise patient to notify health care professional if visual disturbances interfere with daily activities.
- Instruct patient to notify health care professional if fainting occurs.
- Advise patient to report the signs of superinfection (black, furry overgrowth on the tongue; vaginal itching or discharge; loose or foul-smelling stools).
- Instruct patient to notify health care professional if fever and diarrhea develop, especially if stool contains blood, pus, or mucus. Advise patient not to treat diarrhea without consulting health care professional.
- Advise patient to discontinue telithromycin and notify health care professional immediately if signs of liver injury (nausea, fatigue, anorexia, jaundice, dark urine, light-colored stools, pruritus, or tender abdomen) occur.
- Advise patient to avoid taking other Rx, OTC, or herbal products without consulting health care professional.
- Advise patient to notify health care professional if pregnancy is planned or suspected or if breast feeding.

Evaluation/Desired Outcomes

- Resolution of the signs and symptoms of infection. Length of time for complete resolution depends on the organism and site of infection.

telmisartan, See ANGIOTENSIN II RECEPTOR ANTAGONISTS.

temazepam (tem-az-a-pam)
Restoril

Classification
Therapeutic: sedative/hypnotics
Pharmacologic: benzodiazepines

Schedule IV

Pregnancy Category X

Indications
Short-term management of insomnia (<4 weeks).

Action
Acts at many levels in the CNS, producing generalized depression. Effects may be mediated by GABA, an inhibitory neurotransmitter. **Therapeutic Effects:** Relief of insomnia.

Pharmacokinetics
Absorption: Well absorbed after oral administration.
Distribution: Widely distributed; crosses blood-brain barrier. Probably crosses the placenta and enters breast milk. Accumulation of drug occurs with chronic dosing.
Protein Binding: 96%.
Metabolism and Excretion: Metabolized by the liver.
Half-life: 10–20 hr.

TIME/ACTION PROFILE (sedation)

ROUTE	ONSET	PEAK	DURATION
PO	30 min	2–3 hr	6–8 hr

Contraindications/Precautions
Contraindicated in: Hypersensitivity; Cross-sensitivity with other benzodiazepines may exist; Pre-existing CNS depression; Severe uncontrolled pain; Angle-closure glaucoma; Impaired respiratory function; Sleep apnea; OB: Neonates born to mothers taking temazepam may experience withdrawal effects; Lactation: Infants may become sedated. Discontinue drug or bottle feed.
Use Cautiously in: Pre-existing hepatic dysfunction; History of suicide attempt or drug addiction; Geri: Elderly patients have increased sensitivity to benzodiazepines. Appears on Beers list and is associated with increased risk of falls (↓ dose required).

Adverse Reactions/Side Effects
CNS: abnormal thinking, behavior changes, <u>hangover</u>, dizziness, drowsiness, hallucinations, lethargy, paradoxic excitation, sleep—driving. **EENT:** blurred vision. **GI:** constipation, diarrhea, nausea, vomiting. **Derm:** rashes. **Misc:** physical dependence, psychological dependence, tolerance.

Interactions
Drug-Drug: ↑ CNS depression with **alcohol**, **antidepressants**, **antihistamines**, **opioid analgesics**, and other **sedative/hypnotics**. May ↓ efficacy of **levodopa**. **Rifampin** or **smoking** ↑ metabolism and may ↓ effectiveness of temazepam. **Probenecid** may prolong effects of temazepam. Sedative effects may be ↓ by **theophylline**.
Drug-Natural Products: Concomitant use of **kava kava**, **valerian**, **skullcap**, **chamomile**, or **hops** can ↑ CNS depression.

Route/Dosage
PO (Adults): 15–30 mg at bedtime initially if needed; some patients may require only 7.5 mg.
PO (Geriatric Patients or Debilitated Patients): 7.5 mg at bedtime.

Availability (generic available)
Capsules: 7.5 mg, 15 mg, 22.5 mg, 30 mg.

NURSING IMPLICATIONS

Assessment
- Assess mental status (orientation, mood, behavior) and potential for abuse prior to administering medication.
- Assess sleep patterns before and periodically throughout therapy.
- Prolonged high-dose therapy may lead to psychological or physical dependence. Restrict amount of drug available to patient, especially if patient is depressed or suicidal or has a history of addiction.
- Geri: Assess CNS effects and risk of falls. Institute falls prevention strategies.

Potential Nursing Diagnoses
Insomnia (Indications)
Risk for falls (Side Effects)

T

Implementation

- Do not confuse temazepam with flurazepam.
- Supervise ambulation and transfer of patients after administration. Remove cigarettes. Side rails should be raised and call bell within reach at all times.
- **PO:** Administer with food if GI irritation becomes a problem.

Patient/Family Teaching

- Instruct patient to take temazepam as directed. Teach sleep hygiene techniques (dark room, quiet, bedtime ritual, limit daytime napping, avoidance of nicotine and caffeine). If less effective after a few weeks, consult health care professional; do not increase dose.
- May cause daytime drowsiness or dizziness. Caution patient to avoid driving or other activities requiring alertness until response to medication is known. Geri: Instruct patient and family how to reduce falls risk at home.
- Advise patient to avoid the use of alcohol and other CNS depressants and to consult health care professional before using OTC preparations that contain antihistamines or alcohol.
- Advise patient to inform health care professional if pregnancy is planned or suspected.
- Emphasize the importance of follow-up appointments to monitor progress.
- Refer for psychotherapy if ineffective coping is basis for sleep pattern disturbance.
- Advise patient to take temazepam only if able to devote 8 hrs to sleep.

Evaluation/Desired Outcomes

- Improvement in sleep pattern with decreased number of nighttime awakenings, improved sleep onset, and increased total sleep time, which may not be noticeable until the 3rd day of therapy.

tenecteplase, See THROMBOLYTIC AGENTS.

tenofovir disoproxil fumarate

(te-**noe**-fo-veer die-**so**-prox-ill fume-**uh**-rate)
Viread

Classification
Therapeutic: antiretrovirals
Pharmacologic: nucleoside reverse transcriptase inhibitors

Pregnancy Category B

Indications

HIV infection (with other antiretrovirals).

Action

Active drug (tenofovir) is phosphorylated intracellularly; tenofovir diphosphate inhibits HIV reverse transcriptase resulting in disruption of DNA synthesis. **Therapeutic Effects:** Slowed progression of HIV infection and decreased occurrence of sequelae. Increases CD4 cell count and decreases viral load.

Pharmacokinetics

Absorption: Tenofovir disoproxil fumarate is a prodrug, which is split into tenofovir, the active component.
Distribution: Absorption is enhanced by food.
Metabolism and Excretion: 70–80% excreted unchanged in urine by glomerular filtration and active tubular secretion.
Half-life: Unknown.

TIME/ACTION PROFILE (blood levels)

ROUTE	ONSET	PEAK	DURATION
PO	unknown	2 hr*	24 hr

*When taken with food

Contraindications/Precautions

Contraindicated in: Hypersensitivity; Lactation (HIV-infected women should not breastfeed).
Use Cautiously in: Concurrent chronic hepatitis B (discontinuation of tenofovir may result in acute exacerbation of hepatitis B); Obesity, women, prolonged nucleoside exposure (may be risk factors for lactic acidosis/hepatomegaly); Renal impairment (use cautiously if CCr <60 ml/min); Pregnancy (has been used safely); Children (safety not established).

Adverse Reactions/Side Effects

CNS: headache, weakness. **GI:** HEPATOMEGALY, (with steatosis), <u>nausea</u>, abdominal pain, anorexia, diarrhea, vomiting, flatulence. **GU:** renal impairment. **F and E:** LACTIC ACIDOSIS, hypophosphatemia.

Interactions

Drug-Drug: Concurrent use with **didanosine** results in ↑ blood levels of didanosine (tenofovir should be given 2 hours before or 1 hour after didanosine). Blood levels may be ↑ by **cidofovir**, **acyclovir**, **ganciclovir**, or **valganciclovir**. Risk of renal toxicity ↑ by other **nephrotoxic agents**. Combination therapy with **atazanavir** may lead to ↓ virologic response and possible resistance to atazanavir (small amounts of **ritonavir** may be added to boost blood levels). Combination therapy with **abacavir** and **lamivudine** may also lead to virologic nonresponse and should be avoided.

Route/Dosage

PO (Adults): 300 mg once daily.

Availability

Tablets: 300 mg. ***In combination with:*** efavirenz and emtricitabine (Atripla). See Appendix B.

NURSING IMPLICATIONS

Assessment

- Monitor for change in severity of HIV symptoms and for symptoms of opportunistic infection before and during therapy.
- ***Lab Test Considerations:*** Monitor viral load and CD4 count before and routinely during therapy to determine response.
- May cause ↑ AST, ALT, alkaline phosphatase, creatine kinase, amylase, and triglyceride concentrations. Lactic acidosis may occur with hepatic toxicity causing hepatic steatosis; may be fatal, especially in women.
- May cause hypophosphatemia in patients with renal impairment.
- May cause hyperglycemia and glucosuria.

Potential Nursing Diagnoses

Risk for infection (Indications, Side Effects)
Risk for injury (Side Effects)

Implementation

- When tenofovir is administered concomitantly with didanosine, administer tenofovir 2 hr before or 1 hr after didanosine.
- **PO:** Administer once daily with a meal.

Patient/Family Teaching

- Instruct patient on the importance of taking tenofovir as directed, even if feeling better. Do not take more than prescribed amount and do not stop taking without consulting health care professional. Take missed doses as soon as remembered; do not double doses. Caution patient not to share or trade this medication with others.
- Inform patient that tenofovir may cause hyperglycemia. Advise patient to notify health care professional if increased thirst or hunger; unexplained weight loss; increased urination; fatigue; or dry, itchy skin occurs.
- Advise patient to avoid taking other Rx, OTC, or herbal products, without consulting health care professional.
- Caution patient to avoid crowds and persons with known infections.
- Inform patient that tenofovir does not cure AIDS and does not reduce the risk of transmission of HIV to others through sexual contact or blood contamination. Caution patient to use a condom and avoid sharing needles or donating blood to prevent spreading HIV to others.
- Inform patient that changes in body fat distribution (increased fat in upper back and neck, breast, and trunk, and loss of fat from legs, arms, and face) may occur, but may not be related to drug therapy.
- Emphasize the importance of regular exams to monitor for side effects.

Evaluation/Desired Outcomes

- Decreased incidence of opportunistic infection and slowed progression of HIV infection.

T

terazosin (ter-ay-zoe-sin)

Hytrin

Classification
Therapeutic: antihypertensives
Pharmacologic: peripherally acting antiadrenergics

Pregnancy Category C

Indications

Mild to moderate hypertension (alone or with other agents). Urinary outflow obstruction in patients with prostatic hyperplasia.

Action

Dilates both arteries and veins by blocking postsynaptic $alpha_1$-adrenergic receptors. Decreases contractions in smooth muscle of the prostatic capsule. **Therapeutic Effects:** Lowering of blood pressure. Decreased symptoms of prostatic hyperplasia (urinary urgency, hesitancy, nocturia).

Pharmacokinetics

Absorption: Well absorbed after oral administration.

Distribution: Unknown.

Metabolism and Excretion: 50% metabolized by the liver. 10% excreted unchanged by the kidneys. 20% excreted unchanged in feces. 40% eliminated in bile.

Half-life: 12 hr.

TIME/ACTION PROFILE

ROUTE	ONSET†	PEAK‡	DURATION†
PO-hypertension	15 min	6–8 wk	24 hr
PO-prostatic hyperplasia	2–6 wk	unknown	unknown

†After single dose
‡After multiple oral dosing

Contraindications/Precautions

Contraindicated in: Hypersensitivity.

Use Cautiously in: Deyhdration, volume or sodium depletion, increased risk of hypotension; Pregnancy, lactation, or children (safety not established).

Adverse Reactions/Side Effects

CNS: dizziness, headache, weakness, drowsiness, nervousness. **EENT:** nasal congestion, blurred vision, conjunctivitis, sinusitis. **Resp:** dyspnea. **CV:** first-dose orthostatic hypotension, arrhythmias, chest pain, palpitations, peripheral edema, tachycardia. **GI:** nausea, abdominal pain, diarrhea, dry mouth, vomiting. **GU:** erectile dysfunction, urinary frequency. **Derm:** pruritus. **Metab:** weight gain. **MS:** arthralgia, back pain, extremity pain. **Neuro:** paresthesia. **Misc:** fever.

Interactions

Drug-Drug: ↑ hypotension with other **antihypertensives**, acute ingestion of **alcohol**, or **nitrates**. **NSAIDs**, **sympathomimetics**, or **estrogens** may ↓ effects of antihypertensive therapy.

Route/Dosage

The first dose should be taken at bedtime.

Hypertension

PO (Adults): 1 mg initially, then slowly increase up to 5 mg/day (usual range 1–5 mg/day); may be given as single dose or in 2 divided doses (not to exceed 20 mg/day).

Benign Prostatic Hyperplasia

PO (Adults): 1 mg at bedtime; gradually may be increased up to 5–10 mg/day.

Availability (generic available)

Tablets: 1 mg, 2 mg, 5 mg, 10 mg. **Cost:** *Generic*—1 mg $33.98/90, 2 mg $33.99/90, 5 mg $33.99/90, 10 mg $33.99/90.

NURSING IMPLICATIONS

Assessment

- Monitor blood pressure (lying and standing) and pulse frequently during initial dose adjustment and periodically during therapy. Notify physician or other health care professional of significant changes.
- Assess patient for first-dose orthostatic reaction and syncope. May occur 30 min–2 hr after initial dose and occasionally thereafter. Incidence may be dose related. Volume-depleted or sodium-restricted patients may be more sensitive to this effect
- Monitor intake and output ratios and daily weight; assess for edema daily, especially at beginning of therapy.
- **Hypertension:** Monitor frequency of prescription refills to determine adherence.
- **Benign Prostatic Hyperplasia:** Assess patient for symptoms of prostatic hyperplasia (urinary hesitancy, feeling of incomplete bladder emptying, interruption of urinary stream, impairment of size and force of urinary stream, terminal urinary dribbling, straining to start flow, dysuria, urgency) before and periodically during therapy.
- Rule out prostatic carcinoma before therapy; symptoms are similar.

Potential Nursing Diagnoses

Risk for injury (Side Effects)
Noncompliance (Patient/Family Teaching)

Implementation

- May be used in combination with diuretics or beta blockers to minimize sodium and water retention. If these are added to terazosin therapy, reduce dose of terazosin initially and titrate to effect.
- **PO:** Administer daily dose at bedtime. If necessary, dose may be increased to twice daily.

Patient/Family Teaching

- Instruct patient to take medication at the same time each day. Take missed doses as soon as remembered. If not remembered until next day, omit; do not double doses.
- Advise patient to weigh self twice weekly and assess feet and ankles for fluid retention.
- May cause dizziness or drowsiness. Advise patient to avoid driving or other activities re-

quiring alertness until response to the medication is known.
- Caution patient to avoid sudden changes in position to decrease orthostatic hypotension. Alcohol, CNS depressants, standing for long periods, hot showers, and exercising in hot weather should be avoided because of enhanced orthostatic effects.
- Advise patient to consult health care professional before taking any cough, cold, or allergy remedies.
- Instruct patient to notify health care professional of medication regimen before any surgery.
- Advise patient to notify health care professional if frequent dizziness, fainting, or swelling of feet or lower legs occurs.
- Emphasize the importance of follow-up exams to evaluate effectiveness of medication.
- **Hypertension:** Emphasize the importance of continuing to take this medication as directed, even if feeling well. Medication controls but does not cure hypertension.
- Encourage patient to comply with additional interventions for hypertension (weight reduction, low-sodium diet, smoking cessation, moderation of alcohol consumption, regular exercise, and stress management).
- Instruct patient and family on proper technique for blood pressure monitoring. Advise them to check blood pressure at least weekly and to report significant changes.

Evaluation/Desired Outcomes
- Decrease in blood pressure without appearance of side effects.
- Decreased symptoms of prostatic hyperplasia. May require 2–6 wk of therapy before effects are noticeable.

terbinafine (ter-bi-na-feen)
Lamisil

Classification
Therapeutic: antifungals (systemic)

Pregnancy Category B

For topical use, refer to Antifungals, Topical monograph

Indications
Onychomycosis (fungal nail infection). Tinea capitis.

Action
Interferes with fungal cell wall synthesis (ergosterol biosynthesis) by inhibiting the enzyme squalene epoxidase. **Therapeutic Effects:** Fungal cell death. **Spectrum:** Active against dermatophytes and other fungi.

Pharmacokinetics
Absorption: 70–80% absorbed after oral administration.
Distribution: Extensively distributed; penetrates dermis and epidermis; concentrates in stratum corneum, hair, scalp, and nails. Enters breast milk.
Protein Binding: 99%.
Metabolism and Excretion: Extensively metabolized by the liver.
Half-life: *Plasma*—22 days; longer from skin and nails.

TIME/ACTION PROFILE (antifungal tissue levels)

ROUTE	ONSET	PEAK	DURATION
PO	several days	days–wks	several wks

Contraindications/Precautions
Contraindicated in: Hypersensitivity; Chronic or active liver disease; CHF of left ventricular dysfunction.
Use Cautiously in: History of alcoholism; Renal impairment (dose reduction recommended for CCr <50 ml/min); OB, Lactation: Pregnancy, lactation (safety not established).

Adverse Reactions/Side Effects
CNS: headache. **Resp:** cough, nasopharyngitis. **CV:** CHF. **GI:** HEPATOTOXICITY, <u>anorexia</u>, <u>diarrhea</u>, <u>nausea</u>, <u>stomach pain</u>, <u>vomiting</u>, altered taste, drug-induced hepatitis, taste disturbance. **Derm:** TOXIC EPIDERMAL NECROLYSIS, itching, rash. **Hemat:** neutropenia, pancytopenia. **Misc:** STEVENS-JOHNSON SYNDROME, pyrexia.

Interactions
Drug-Drug: Alcohol or other **hepatotoxic agents** may ↑ risk of hepatotoxicity. **Rifampin** and other **drugs that induce hepatic drug-metabolizing enzymes** may ↓ effectiveness. **Cimetidine** and other **drugs that inhibit hepatic drug-metabolizing enzymes** may ↑ effectiveness.
Drug-Natural Products: ↑ **caffeine** levels and side effects with caffeine-containing herbs (**cola nut, guarana, mate, tea, coffee**).

Route/Dosage

PO (Adults): 250 mg once daily for 6 wk for fingernail infection or 12 wk for toenail infection.

PO (Children ≥4 yrs— ≥35 kg): 250 mg/day for 6 wks.

PO (Children ≥4 yrs— 25–35 kg): 187.5 mg/day for 6 wks.

PO (Children ≥4 yrs— <25 kg): 125 mg/day for 6 wks.

Availability (generic available)

Tablets: 250 mg. **Cost:** *Generic*—$140.99/ 90. **Oral granules:** 125 mg packets, 187.5 mg packets.

NURSING IMPLICATIONS

Assessment

- Assess for signs and symptoms of infection (nail beds, scalp) before and periodically throughout therapy.
- Specimens for culture should be taken before instituting therapy. Therapy may be started before results are obtained.
- Monitor for skin rash. If progressive skin rash occurs, discontinue terbinafine.
- ***Lab Test Considerations:*** CBC should be monitored in patients receiving therapy for >6 wk. Discontinue if abnormal values occur.
- Monitor AST and ALT prior to, and periodically throughout, therapy. Terbinafine should be discontinued if symptomatic elevations occur.
- If signs of secondary infection occur, monitor neutrophil count. If <1000/mm^3, discontinue treatment.
- May cause ↓ absolute lymphocyte count.
- Monitor serum potassium. May cause hypokalemia.

Potential Nursing Diagnoses

Risk for infection (Indications)
Noncompliance (Patient/Family Teaching)

Implementation

- Do not confuse with lamotrigine (Lamictal).
- **PO:** May be administered without regard to food.
- *Oral granules* should be taken with food and may be sprinkled on a spoonful of pudding or other soft, nonacidic food, such as mashed potatoes and swallowed in entirety. Applesauce or fruit—based foods should not be used.

Patient/Family Teaching

- Instruct patient to take medication as directed, for the full course of therapy, even if feeling better. Doses should be taken at the same time each day.
- Instruct patient to notify health care professional immediately if signs and symptoms of liver dysfunction (unusual fatigue, anorexia, nausea, vomiting, upper right abdominal pain, jaundice, dark urine, or pale stools) or rash occur. Terbinafine should be discontinued.
- Advise patient to consult health care professional before taking any Rx or OTC medications concurrently with terbinafine.

Evaluation/Desired Outcomes

- Resolution of clinical and laboratory indications of fungal nail infections. Inadequate period of treatment may lead to recurrence of active infection.
- Resolution of tinea capitis infection.

terbinafine, See ANTIFUNGALS (TOPICAL).

terbutaline (ter-**byoo**-ta-leen)

Brethaire, Bricanyl

Classification
Therapeutic: bronchodilators
Pharmacologic: adrenergics

Pregnancy Category B

Indications

Management of reversible airway disease due to asthma or COPD; inhalation and subcut used for short-term control and oral agent as long-term control. **Unlabeled uses:** Management of preterm labor (tocolytic).

Action

Results in the accumulation of cyclic adenosine monophosphate (cAMP) at beta-adrenergic receptors. Produces bronchodilation. Inhibits the release of mediators of immediate hypersensitivity reactions from mast cells. Relatively selective for beta$_2$ (pulmonary)-adrenergic receptor sites, with less effect on beta$_1$ (cardiac)-adrenergic receptors. **Therapeutic Effects:** Bronchodilation.

Pharmacokinetics

Absorption: 35–50% absorbed following oral administration but rapidly undergoes first-pass

metabolism. Well absorbed following subcut administration. Minimal absorption occurs following inhalation.
Distribution: Enters breast milk.
Metabolism and Excretion: Partially metabolized by the liver; 60% excreted unchanged by the kidneys following subcut administration.
Half-life: Unknown.

TIME/ACTION PROFILE (bronchodilation)

ROUTE	ONSET	PEAK	DURATION
PO	within 60–120 min	within 2–3 hr	4–8 hr
Inhaln	5–30 min	1–2 hr	3–6 hr
subcut	within 15 min	within 0.5–1 hr	1.5–4 hr

Contraindications/Precautions
Contraindicated in: Hypersensitivity to adrenergic amines; Known hypersensitivity or intolerance to fluorocarbons (inhalation only).
Use Cautiously in: Cardiac disease; Hypertension; Hyperthyroidism; Diabetes; Glaucoma; Geri: Geriatric patients (more susceptible to adverse reactions; may require dose reduction); Excessive use may lead to tolerance and paradoxical bronchospasm (inhaler); OB, Pedi: Pregnancy (near term), lactation, and children <2 yr (safety not established).

Adverse Reactions/Side Effects
CNS: nervousness, restlessness, tremor, headache, insomnia. **Resp:** PARADOXICAL BRONCHOSPASM (excessive use of inhalers). **CV:** angina, arrhythmias, hypertension, tachycardia. **GI:** nausea, vomiting. **Endo:** hyperglycemia.

Interactions
Drug-Drug: Concurrent use with other **adrenergics** (sympathomimetic) will have additive adrenergic side effects. Use with **MAO inhibitors** may lead to hypertensive crisis. **Beta blockers** may negate therapeutic effect.
Drug-Natural Products: Use with caffeine-containing herbs (**cola nut, guarana, mate, tea, coffee**) ↑ stimulant effect.

Route/Dosage
PO (Adults and Children >15 yr): *Bronchodilation*—2.5–5 mg 3 times daily, given q 6 hr (not to exceed 15 mg/24 hr). *Tocolysis*—2.5 mg q 4–6 hr until delivery (unlabeled).
PO (Children 12–15 yr): 2.5 mg 3 times daily (given q 6 hr).
Inhaln (Adults and Children ≥12 yr): 2 inhalations (200 mcg/spray) q 4–6 hr.
Subcut (Adults): *Bronchodilation*—250 mcg; may repeat in 15–30 min (not to exceed 500 mcg/4 hr). *Tocolysis*—250 mcg q 1 hr until contractions stop (unlabeled).
IV (Adults): *Tocolysis*—10 mcg/min infusion; increase by 5 mcg/min q 10 min until contractions stop (not to exceed 80 mcg/min). After contractions have stopped for 30 min, decrease infusion rate to lowest effective amount and maintain for 4–8 hr (unlabeled).

Availability (generic available)
Tablets: 2.5 mg, 5 mg. **Injection:** 1 mg/ml. **Inhalation aerosol:** 200 mcg/spray (≥300 inhalations/10.5-g canister), ♣500 mcg/spray.

NURSING IMPLICATIONS

Assessment
- **Bronchodilator:** Assess lung sounds, respiratory pattern, pulse, and blood pressure before administration and during peak of medication. Note amount, color, and character of sputum produced, and notify health care professional of abnormal findings.
- Monitor pulmonary function tests before initiating therapy and periodically throughout therapy to determine effectiveness of medication.
- Observe for paradoxical bronchospasm (wheezing). If condition occurs, withhold medication and notify health care professional immediately.
- Observe patient for drug tolerance and rebound bronchospasm. Patients requiring more than 3 inhalation treatments in 24 hr should be under close supervision. If minimal or no relief is seen after 3–5 inhalation treatments within 6–12 hr, further treatment with aerosol alone is not recommended.
- **Preterm Labor:** Monitor maternal pulse and blood pressure, frequency and duration of contractions, and fetal heart rate. Notify health care professional if contractions persist or increase in frequency or duration or if symptoms of maternal or fetal distress occur. Maternal side effects include tachycardia, palpitations, tremor, anxiety, and headache.
- Assess maternal respiratory status for symptoms of pulmonary edema (increased rate, dyspnea, rales/crackles, frothy sputum)

T

- Monitor mother and neonate for symptoms of hypoglycemia (anxiety; chills; cold sweats; confusion; cool, pale skin; difficulty in concentration; drowsiness; excessive hunger; headache; irritability; nausea; nervousness; rapid pulse; shakiness; unusual tiredness; or weakness) and mother for hypokalemia (weakness, fatigue, U wave on ECG, arrhythmias).
- ***Lab Test Considerations:*** May cause transient ↓ in serum potassium concentrations with higher than recommended doses.
- Monitor maternal serum glucose and electrolytes. May cause hypokalemia and hypoglycemia. Monitor neonate's serum glucose, because hypoglycemia may also occur in neonates.
- ***Toxicity and Overdose:*** Symptoms of overdose include persistent agitation, chest pain or discomfort, decreased blood pressure, dizziness, hyperglycemia, hypokalemia, seizures, tachyarrhythmias, persistent trembling, and vomiting: Treatment includes discontinuing beta-adrenergic agonists and symptomatic, supportive therapy. Cardioselective beta blockers are used cautiously, because they may induce bronchospasm.

Potential Nursing Diagnoses

Ineffective airway clearance (Indications)

Implementation

- **PO:** Administer with meals to minimize gastric irritation.
- Tablet may be crushed and mixed with food or fluids for patients with difficulty swallowing.
- **Subcut:** Administer subcut injections in lateral deltoid area. Do not use solution if discolored.

IV Administration

- **Continuous Infusion:** ***Diluent:*** May be diluted in D5W, 0.9% NaCl, or 0.45% NaCl. ***Concentration:*** 1 mg/ml (undiluted). ***Rate:*** Use infusion pump to ensure accurate dose. Begin infusion at 10 mcg/min. Increase dosage by 5 mcg every 10 min until contractions cease. Maximum dose is 80 mcg/min. Begin to taper dose in 5-mcg decrements after a 30–60 min contraction-free period is attained. Switch to oral dose form after patient is contraction-free 4–8 hr on the lowest effective dose.
- **Y-Site Compatibility:** insulin.

Patient/Family Teaching

- Instruct patient to take medication as directed. If on a scheduled dosing regimen, take a missed dose as soon as possible; space remaining doses at regular intervals. Do not double doses. Caution patient not to exceed recommended dose; may cause adverse effects, paradoxical bronchospasm, or loss of effectiveness of medication.
- Instruct patient to contact health care professional immediately if shortness of breath is not relieved by medication or is accompanied by diaphoresis, dizziness, palpitations, or chest pain.
- Advise patient to consult health care professional before taking any OTC medications or alcoholic beverages concurrently with this therapy. Caution patient also to avoid smoking and other respiratory irritants.
- **Inhaln:** Review correct administration technique with patient. See Appendix D for administration with metered-dose inhaler. Wait 1–5 min before administering next dose. Mouthpiece should be washed after each use.
- Do not spray inhaler near eyes.
- Instruct patient to save inhaler; refill canisters may be available.
- Advise patients to use bronchodilator first if using other inhalation medications, and allow 15 min to elapse before administering other inhalant medications, unless otherwise directed.
- Advise patient to rinse mouth with water after each inhalation dose to minimize dry mouth.
- Advise patient to maintain adequate fluid intake (2000–3000 ml/day) to help liquefy tenacious secretions.
- Advise patient to consult health care professional if respiratory symptoms are not relieved or worsen after treatment or if chest pain, headache, severe dizziness, palpitations, nervousness, or weakness occurs.
- Instruct patient to notify health care professional if contents of one canister are used up in less than 2 wk.
- **Preterm Labor:** Notify health care professional immediately if labor resumes or if significant side effects occur.

Evaluation/Desired Outcomes

- Prevention or relief of bronchospasm.
- Increase in ease of breathing.
- Control of preterm labor in a fetus of 20–36 wk gestational age.

terconazole, See ANTIFUNGALS (VAGINAL).

teriparatide (ter-i-**par**-a-tide)
Forteo

Classification
Therapeutic: hormones
Pharmacologic: parathyroid hormones (rDNA origin)

Pregnancy Category C

Indications
Treatment of osteoporosis in postmenopausal women at high risk for fractures. To increase bone mass in men with osteoporosis at high risk for fracture. Most useful for those have failed or are intolerant to other osteoporosis therapies.

Action
Regulates calcium and phosphate metabolism in bone and kidney by binding to specific cell receptors; stimulates osteoblastic activity. Increases serum calcium and decreases serum phosphorus. **Therapeutic Effects:** Increased bone mineral density with reduced risk of fractures.

Pharmacokinetics
Absorption: Extensively absorbed after subcut administration.
Distribution: Unknown.
Metabolism and Excretion: Metabolized by the liver; metabolites renally excreted.
Half-life: 1 hr (after subcut use).

TIME/ACTION PROFILE (effects on serum calcium)

ROUTE	ONSET	PEAK	DURATION
subcut	2 hr	4–6 hr	16–24 hr

Contraindications/Precautions
Contraindicated in: Hypersensitivity; Paget's disease of the bone or other metabolic bone disease; Unexplained ↑ alkaline phosphatase; Pediatric or young adult patients; Previous radiation therapy, history of bone metastases, or skeletal malignancy; Pre-existing hypercalcemia; Pregnancy or lactation.
Use Cautiously in: Concurrent **digoxin**.

Adverse Reactions/Side Effects
CV: orthostatic hypotension.

Interactions
Drug-Drug: Transient hypercalcemia may increase the risk of **digoxin** toxicity.

Route/Dosage
Subcut (Adults): 20 mcg once daily.

Availability
Pre-filled pen delivery device (FORTEO pen): delivers 20 mcg/day.

NURSING IMPLICATIONS

Assessment
- Assess patient for bone mineral density before and periodically during therapy.
- ***Lab Test Considerations:*** Effects increase serum calcium and decrease serum phosphorus. Maximum effect is within 4–6 hr. By 16-hr post-dose, serum calcium has returned to near baseline. If hypercalcemia persists, discontinue teriperatide and evaluate cause of hypercalcemia.
- May asymptomatically increase serum uric acid concentrations.

Potential Nursing Diagnoses
Risk for injury (Indications)

Implementation
- Use of teriparatide should not continue more than 2 yr.
- **Subcut:** Administer subcut into thigh or abdominal wall once daily. May be administered at any time of day without regard to food. Solution should be clear and colorless. Do not use if solid particles appear, or if solution is cloudy or colored. Store pen in the refrigerator; do not freeze or use if it has been frozen. Minimize time out of refrigerator; use immediately and return to refrigerator. *Forteo* pen can be used for up to 28 days after the first injection. After the 28-day use period, discard the *Forteo* pen, even if it still contains some unused solution.

Patient/Family Teaching
- Advise patient to administer medication at same time each day. If a dose is missed, administer as soon as remembered that day. Do not take more than one injection/day.
- Instruct patient on proper administration technique and disposal of needles. Patient should read *Medication Guide* and *User*

T

Manual before starting therapy and re-read them each time prescription is refilled. User manual can be found at www.forteo.com/control/pen_user_manual. Caution patient to throw pen away after 28-day use period and not to share their pen with other patients.

- Advise patient to administer at same time each day. If a dose is missed, administer as soon as remembered that day. Do not take more than one injection/day.
- Discuss the importance of other treatments for osteoporosis (supplemental calcium and/or vitamin D, weight-bearing exercise, modification of behavioral factors such as smoking and/or alcohol consumption).
- May cause orthostatic hypotension during first several doses. Caution patient to administer medication in a lying or sitting position. If light-headedness or palpitations occur, lie down until symptoms resolve. Notify health care professional if symptoms persist or worsen.
- Instruct patient to notify health care professional if persistent symptoms of hypercalcemia (nausea, vomiting, constipation, lethargy, muscle weakness) occur.
- Emphasize the importance of follow-up tests for bone mineral density.

Evaluation/Desired Outcomes

- Increased bone mineral density with reduced risk of fractures.

TESTOSTERONE
(tess-**toss**-te-rone)

testosterone buccal system, mucoadhesive
Striant

testosterone cypionate
Depo-Testosterone

testosterone enanthate
Delatestryl

testosterone pellets
Testopel

testosterone transdermal
Androderm

Classification
Therapeutic: hormones
Pharmacologic: androgens

Schedule III

Pregnancy Category X

Indications
Hypogonadism in androgen-deficient men. Delayed puberty in men (enanthate and pellets). Androgen-responsive breast cancer in postmenopausal women (palliative) (enanthate).

Action
Responsible for the normal growth and development of male sex organs. Maintenance of male secondary sex characteristics: Growth and maturation of the prostate, seminal vesicles, penis, scrotum, Development of male hair distribution, Vocal cord thickening, Alterations in body musculature and fat distribution. **Therapeutic Effects:** Correction of hormone deficiency in male hypogonadism: Initiation of male puberty. Suppression of tumor growth in some forms of breast cancer.

Pharmacokinetics
Absorption: Well absorbed from IM sites, through buccal mucosa, or through skin. Cypionate and enanthate salts are absorbed slowly.
Distribution: Cross the placenta.
Protein Binding: 98%.
Metabolism and Excretion: Metabolized by the liver. Absorption from buccal mucosa bypasses initial liver metabolism. 90% eliminated in urine as metabolites.
Half-life: *Buccal, enanthate, pellets*—10–100 min; *transdermal*—70 min; *cypionate*—8 days.

TIME/ACTION PROFILE (androgenic effects†)

ROUTE	ONSET	PEAK	DURATION
IM—cypionate, enanthate	unknown	unknown	2–4 wk
IM—propionate	unknown	unknown	1–3 days
buccal	unknown	10–12 hr	12 hr
pellets	unknown	unknown	3–6 mo
transdermal	unknown	6–8 hr‡	24 hr§

†Response is highly variable among individuals; may take months
‡Plasma testosterone levels following applications of patch
§Following patch removal

Contraindications/Precautions

Contraindicated in: Hypersensitivity; OB: Pregnancy and lactation; Male patients with breast or prostate cancer; Severe liver, renal, or cardiac disease (propionate); Some products contain benzyl alcohol and should be avoided in patients with known hypersensitivity; Women (buccal, pellets, patch).

Use Cautiously in: Diabetes mellitus; Coronary artery disease (enanthate); Pre-existing cardiac, renal, or liver disease; Benign prostatic hyperplasia (cypionate, pellets); Hypercalcemia (cypionate, enanthate, pellets); Sleep apnea (buccal); Obesity (buccal); Chronic lung disease (buccal); Geriatric patients (↑ risk of prostatic hyperplasia/carcinoma); Prepubertal males.

Adverse Reactions/Side Effects

CNS: anxiety, confusion, depression, fatigue, headache, vertigo. **EENT:** deepening of voice. **CV:** edema. **GI:** abdominal cramps, changes in appetite, drug-induced hepatitis, nausea, vomiting; *buccal*— bitter taste, ginigivitis, gum edema, gum tenderness. **GU:** menstrual irregularities, prostatic enlargement. **Endo:** *women*— change in libido, clitoral enlargement, decreased breast size; *men*— acne, facial hair, gynecomastia, erectile dysfunction, oligospermia, priapism. **F and E:** hypercalcemia, hyperkalemia, hyperphosphatemia. **Derm:** male pattern baldness. **Local:** chronic skin irritation (transdermal), pain at injection/implantation site.

Interactions

Drug-Drug: May ↑ action of **warfarin**, **oral hypoglycemic agents**, and **insulin**. Concurrent use with **corticosteroids** may ↑ risk of edema formation.

Route/Dosage

Replacement Therapy

IM (Adults): 50–400 mg q 2–4 wk (enanthate or cypionate).

Transdermal (Adults): 5 mg applied q 24 hr (preferably in the evening); dosing range = 2.5–7.5 mg/day.

Buccal (Adults): 30 mg (one system) applied to gum region twice daily (in the morning and evening, spaced 12 hr apart).

Subcut (for subcutaneous implantation) (pellets) **(Adults):** 150–450 mg q 3–6 mo.

Delayed Male Puberty

IM (Children): 50–200 mg q 2–4 wk for up to 6 mo (enanthate).

Subcut (for subcutaneous implantation) (pellets) **(Children):** 150–450 mg q 3–6 mo.

Palliative Management of Breast Cancer

IM (Adults): 200–400 mg q 2–4 wk (enanthate).

Availability (generic available)

Testosterone cypionate injection (in oil): 100 mg/ml in 10-ml vials, 200 mg/ml in 1- and 10-ml vials. **Testosterone enanthate injection (in oil):** 200 mg/ml in 5–ml vials and 1-ml prefilled syringes. **Testosterone transdermal patches:** 2.5 mg/day in packages of 60, 5 mg/day in packages of 60. **Testosterone buccal, mucoadhesive:** 30 mg/system in blister packs of 10 systems/pack. **Testosterone pellets:** 75 mg.

NURSING IMPLICATIONS

Assessment

- Monitor intake and output ratios, weigh patient twice weekly, and assess patient for edema. Report significant changes indicative of fluid retention.
- **Men:** Monitor for precocious puberty in boys (acne, darkening of skin, development of male secondary sex characteristics—increase in penis size, frequent erections, growth of body hair). Bone age determinations should be measured every 6 months to determine rate of bone maturation and effects on epiphyseal closure.
- Monitor for breast enlargement, persistent erections, and increased urge to urinate in men. Monitor for difficulty urinating in elderly men, because prostate enlargement may occur.
- **Women:** Assess for virilism (deepening of voice, unusual hair growth or loss, clitoral enlargement, acne, menstrual irregularity).
- In women with metastatic breast cancer, monitor for symptoms of hypercalcemia (nausea, vomiting, constipation, lethargy, loss of muscle tone, thirst, polyuria).
- ***Lab Test Considerations:*** Monitor hemoglobin and hematocrit periodically during therapy; may cause polycythemia.
- Monitor hepatic function tests, prostate specific antigen and serum cholesterol levels pe-

riodically during therapy. May cause ↑ serum AST, ALT, and bilirubin, ↑ cholesterol levels, and suppress clotting factors II, V, VII, and X.

- Monitor serum and urine calcium levels and serum alkaline phosphatase concentrations in women with metastatic breast cancer.
- Monitor serum sodium, chloride, potassium, and phosphate concentrations (may be ↑).
- Monitor blood glucose closely in patients with diabetes who are receiving oral hypoglycemic agents or insulin.
- *Transdermal:* Monitor serum testosterone concentrations 3–4 wk after starting therapy; these concentrations should be obtained in the morning (following application of patch during previous evening).
- *Buccal:* Monitor serum testosterone concentrations 4–12 wk after starting therapy.

Potential Nursing Diagnoses

Sexual dysfunction (Indications, Side Effects)

Implementation

- Do not confuse Virilon (testosterone) with Verelan (verapamil).
- Range-of-motion exercises should be done with all bedridden patients to prevent mobilization of calcium from the bone.
- **IM:** Administer IM deep into gluteal muscle. Crystals may form when vials are stored at low temperatures; warming and shaking vial will redissolve crystals. Use of a wet syringe or needle may cause solution to become cloudy but will not affect its potency.
- **Subcut:** Pellets are to be implanted subcutaneously by a health care professional. **Transdermal:** Apply patch to clean, dry, hairless skin on the back, abdomen, upper arms, or thighs. Do not apply to the scrotum. Also avoid application over bony prominences or a part of the body that may be subject to prolonged pressure during sleep or sitting. The patch does not need to be removed while swimming or taking a shower or bath.
- The sites of application should be rotated; once a patch is removed, the same site should not be used again for at least 1 wk.
- If skin irritation occurs, apply a small amount of OTC topical hydrocortisone cream after system removal or a small amount of 0.1% triamcinolone cream may be applied to the skin under the central drug reservoir of the Androderm system without affecting the absorption of testosterone. Ointment formulations should not be used for pretreatment because they may significantly reduce testosterone absorption.
- Patch should be removed if undergoing a magnetic resonance imaging (MRI) scan. The system contains aluminum and may predispose the patient to skin burns during the test.
- **Buccal:** Apply to gum region twice daily (about 12 hr apart), rotating sides with each dose.

Patient/Family Teaching

- Advise patient to report the following signs and symptoms promptly: in male patients, priapism (sustained and often painful erections) difficulty urinating, or gynecomastia; in female patients, virilism (which may be reversible if medication is stopped as soon as changes are noticed), or hypercalcemia (nausea, vomiting, constipation, and weakness); in male or female patients, edema (unexpected weight gain, swelling of feet), hepatitis (yellowing of skin or eyes and abdominal pain), or unusual bleeding or bruising.
- Explain rationale for prohibiting use of testosterone for increasing athletic performance. Testosterone is neither safe nor effective for this use and has a potential risk of serious side effects.
- Instruct females to notify health care professional immediately if pregnancy is planned or suspected.
- Advise diabetic patients to monitor blood closely for alterations in blood glucose concentrations.
- Emphasize the importance of regular follow-up physical exams, lab tests, and x-ray exams to monitor progress.
- Radiologic bone age determinations should be evaluated every 6 mo in prepubertal children to determine rate of bone maturation and effects on epiphyseal centers.
- **Transdermal:** Advise patient to notify health care professional if their female sexual partner develops signs/symptoms of virilization (e.g. change in body hair distribution, significant increase in acne, deepening of voice, menstrual irregularities).
- Instruct patient that the protective plastic liner must be removed before applying the patch.
- Instruct patient to apply patch to a clean, dry area of skin on back, abdomen, upper arms, or thighs. The patch should not applied to

their genitals or over bony areas (e.g. upper shoulders or upper hip).

- Instruct patient to rotate the sites of application. Once a patch is removed, the site should not be used again for at least 1 week.
- Advise patient that the patch does not need to be removed while showering, bathing, or swimming.
- Advise patient that the patch should be removed prior to undergoing a MRI scan.
- If a patch falls off before noon, advise patient to replace it with a fresh patch which should be worn until a new patch is applied in the evening. If a patch falls off after noon, advise patient that it does not need to be replaced until a fresh patch is applied in the evening.
- **Buccal:** Instruct patient to place the rounded side surface of the buccal system in a comfortable position against the gum just above incisor tooth. Hold the system firmly in place with a finger over the lip and against the product for 30 seconds to ensure adhesion. Buccal system is designed to stay in position until removed; if it fails to adhere to the gum or falls off within the first 8 hr after application, remove original system and apply a new one (this counts as replacing the first dose; apply the next system ~12 hr after the original system was applied). If the buccal system falls off after 8 hr but before 12 hr, replace the original system (this replacement can serve as the second dose for that day).
- Advise patient to avoid dislodging buccal system and to check on placement after toothbrushing, use of mouthwash, eating or drinking. Do not chew or swallow buccal system. To remove, slide system downwards from gum toward tooth to avoid scratching the gum.

Evaluation/Desired Outcomes

- Resolution of the signs of androgen deficiency without side effects. Therapy is usually limited to 3–6 months followed by bone growth or maturation determinations.
- Decrease in the size and spread of breast malignancy in postmenopausal women. In antineoplastic therapy, response may require 3 months of therapy; if signs of disease progression appear, therapy should be discontinued.

TETRACYCLINES

doxycycline (dox-i-**sye**-kleen)
Adoxa, ✤Apo-Doxy, Doryx, Doxy, ✤Doxycin, ✤Doxytab, Monodox, ✤Novodoxylin, ✤Nu-Doxycycline, Oracea, Periostat, ✤PHL-Doxycycline, ✤PMS-Doxycycline, ✤Ratio-Doxycycline, Vibramycin, Vibra-Tabs

minocycline (min-oh-**sye**-kleen)
✤Apo-Minocycline, Arestin, ✤DOM-Minocycline, Dynacin, ✤Enca, ✤Gen-Minocycline, Minocin, ✤Novo-Minocycline, ✤PMS-Minocycline, ✤Ratio-Minocycline, ✤Riva-Minocycline, Solodyn

tetracycline (te-tra-**sye**-kleen)
Sumycin

Classification
Therapeutic: anti-infectives
Pharmacologic:

Pregnancy Category D

Indications

Treatment of various infections caused by unusual organisms, including: *Mycoplasma*, *Chlamydia*, *Rickettsia*, *Borellia burgdorferi*. Treatment of gonorrhea and syphilis in penicillin-allergic patients. Prevention of exacerbations of chronic bronchitis. Treatment of inhalational anthrax (postexposure) and cutaneous anthrax (doxycycline only). Treatment of acne.

Action

Inhibits bacterial protein synthesis at the level of the 30S bacterial ribosome. **Therapeutic Effects:** Bacteriostatic action against susceptible bacteria. **Spectrum:** Includes activity against some gram-positive pathogens: *Bacillus anthracis*, *Clostridium perfringens*, *Clostridium tetani*, *Listeria monocytogenes*, *Nocardia*, *Propionibacterium acnes*, *Actinomyces israelii*. Active against some gram-negative pathogens: *Haemophilus influenzae*, *Legionella pneumophila*, *Yersinia enterocolitica*, *Yersinia pestis*, *Neisseria gonorrhoeae*, *Neisseria meningitidis*. Also active against several other pathogens, including: *Mycoplasma*, *Trepone-*

ma pallidum, Chlamydia, Rickettsia, B. burgdorferi.

Pharmacokinetics

Absorption: *Tetracycline*—60–80% absorbed following oral administration. *Doxycycline, minocycline*—well absorbed from the GI tract.

Distribution: Widely distributed, some penetration into CSF; cross the placenta and enter breast milk.

Metabolism and Excretion: *Doxycycline*—20–40% excreted unchanged by the urine; some inactivation in the intestine and some enterohepatic circulation with excretion in bile and feces. *Minocycline*—5–20% excreted unchanged by the urine; some metabolism by the liver with enterohepatic circulation and excretion in bile and feces. *Tetracycline*—Excreted mostly unchanged by the kidneys.

Half-life: *Doxycycline*—14–17 hr (increased in severe renal impairment). *Minocycline*—11–26 hr. *Tetracycline*—6–12 hr.

TIME/ACTION PROFILE (blood levels)

ROUTE	ONSET	PEAK	DURATION
doxycycline-PO	1–2 hr	1.5–4 hr	12 hr
doxycycline-IV	rapid	end of infusion	12 hr
minocycline-PO	rapid	2–3 hr	6–12 hr
minocycline-PO extended-release	unknown	3.5–4 hr	24 hr
tetracycline-PO	1–2 hr	2–4 hr	6–12 hr

Contraindications/Precautions

Contraindicated in: Hypersensitivity; Some products contain alcohol or bisulfites and should be avoided in patients with known hypersensitivity or intolerance; OB: Pregnancy (risk of permanent staining of teeth in infant if used during last half of pregnancy); Lactation; Pedi: Children <8 yr (permanent staining of teeth); Can be used in children and pregnant and lactating women for the treatment of anthrax (doxycycline only).

Use Cautiously in: Cachectic or debilitated patients; Renal disease; Hepatic impairment (doxycycline, minocycline); Nephrogenic diabetes insipidus.

Adverse Reactions/Side Effects

CNS: benign intracranial hypertension (higher in children); *minocycline*— dizziness. **EENT:** *minocycline*—, vestibular reactions. **GI:** diarrhea, nausea, vomiting, esophagitis, hepatotoxicity, pancreatitis. **Derm:** photosensitivity, rashes; *minocycline*— pigmentation of skin and mucous membranes. **Hemat:** blood dyscrasias. **Local:** *doxycycline, minocycline*—phlebitis at IV site. **Misc:** hypersensitivity reactions, superinfection.

Interactions

Drug-Drug: May ↑ effect of **warfarin**. May ↓ effectiveness of **estrogen-containing hormonal contraceptives**. **Antacids**, **calcium**, **iron**, **zinc**, **aluminum**, and **magnesium** form insoluble compounds (chelates) and ↓ absorption of tetracyclines. **Sucralfate** may bind to tetracycline and ↓ its absorption from the GI tract. **Cholestyramine** or **colestipol** ↓ oral absorption of tetracyclines. **Adsorbent antidiarrheals** may ↓ absorption of tetracyclines. **Barbiturates**, **carbamazepine**, or **phenytoin** may ↓ activity of doxycycline.

Drug-Food: Calcium in foods or **dairy products** ↓ absorption by forming insoluble compounds (chelates).

Route/Dosage

Doxycycline

PO (Adults and Children >8 yr and >45 kg): *Most infections*—100 mg q 12 hr on the 1st day, then 100–200 mg once daily or 50–100 mg q 12 hr. *Gonorrhea*—100 mg q 12 hr for 7 days or 300 mg followed 1 hr later by another 300-mg dose. *Malaria prophylaxis*—100 mg once daily. *Lyme disease*—100 mg twice daily *Periodontitis*—20 mg twice daily. *Anthrax*—100 mg twice daily for 60 days.

PO (Children >8 yr and ≤45 kg): *Most infections*–2–5 mg/kg/day in 1–2 divided doses (not to exceed 200 mg/day).

IV (Adults and Children >8 yr and >45 kg): 200 mg once daily or 100 mg q 12 hr on the 1st day, then 100–200 mg once daily or 50–100 mg q 12 hr. *Anthrax*—100 mg q 12 hr change to oral when appropriate, for 60 days.

IV (Children >8 yr and ≤45 kg or ≤8 yr): 4.4 mg/kg once daily or 2.2 mg/kg q 12 hr on the 1st day, then 2.2–4.4 mg/kg/day given once daily or 1.1–2.2 mg/kg q 12 hr. *Anthrax*—2.2 mg/kg q 12 hr, change to oral when appropriate, for 60 days.

Minocycline

Immediate-Release

PO (Adults): 100–200 mg initially, then 100 mg q 12 hr or 50 mg q 6 hr.

PO (Children ≥8 yr): 4 mg/kg initially, then 2 mg/kg q 12 hr.

Extended-Release

PO (Adults and Children ≥12 yrs): *91–136 kg*—135 mg once daily for 12 wks. *60–90 kg*—90 mg once daily for 12 wks. *45–59 kg*—45 mg once daily for 12 wks.

Tetracycline

PO (Adults): 250–500 mg q 6 hr or 500 mg–1 g q 12 hr. *Chronic treatment of acne*—500 mg–2 g/day for 3 wk, then ↓ to 125 mg–1 g/day.

PO (Children ≥8 yr): 6.25–12.5 mg/kg q 6 hr or 12.5–25 mg/kg q 12 hr.

Availability

Doxycycline

Tablets: 20 mg, 50 mg, 75 mg, 100 mg, 150 mg. **Delayed-release tablets:** 75 mg, 100 mg. **Capsules:** 50 mg, 100 mg. **Delayed-release capsules:** 40 mg. **Oral suspension (raspberry flavor):** 25 mg/5 ml in 60 ml bottles. **Syrup (apple-raspberry flavor):** 50 mg/5 ml in 473-ml bottles. **Powder for injection:** 100-mg vials, 200-mg vials.

Minocycline

Capsules: 50 mg, 100 mg. **Pellet-filled capsules (Minocin):** 50 mg, 100 mg. **Tablets:** 50 mg, 75 mg, 100 mg. **Extended-release tablets:** 45 mg, 90 mg, 135 mg. **Oral suspension (custard flavor):** 50 mg/5 ml.

Tetracycline

Capsules: 250 mg, 500 mg.

NURSING IMPLICATIONS

Assessment

- Assess for infection (vital signs; appearance of wound, sputum, urine, and stool; WBC) at beginning of and throughout therapy.
- Obtain specimens for culture and sensitivity before initiating therapy. First dose may be given before receiving results.
- **IV:** Assess IV site frequently; may cause thrombophlebitis.
- ***Lab Test Considerations:*** Monitor renal and hepatic function and CBC periodically during long-term therapy.
- May cause ↑ AST, ALT, serum alkaline phosphatase, bilirubin, and amylase concentrations. Tetracyclines, except doxycycline, may cause ↑ serum BUN.

Potential Nursing Diagnoses

Risk for infection (Indications, Side Effects)
Noncompliance (Patient/Family Teaching)

Implementation

- Do not confuse doxycycline with doxepin.
- May cause yellow-brown discoloration and softening of teeth and bones if administered prenatally or during early childhood. Not recommended for children under 8 yr of age or during pregnancy or lactation unless used for the treatment of anthrax.
- **PO:** Administer around the clock. Administer at least 1 hr before or 2 hr after meals. *Doxycycline and minocycline* may be taken with food or milk if GI irritation occurs. Administer with a full glass of liquid and at least 1 hr before going to bed to avoid esophageal ulceration. Use calibrated measuring device for liquid preparations. Shake liquid preparations well. Do not administer within 1–3 hr of other medications.
- Avoid administration of calcium, zinc, antacids, magnesium- or aluminum-containing medications, sodium bicarbonate, or iron supplements within 1–3 hr of oral tetracyclines.

Doxycycline

- **PO:** To prepare doses for infants and children exposed to anthrax, place one 100 mg tablet in a small bowl and crush to a fine powder with a metal spoon, leaving no large pieces. Add 4 level teaspoons of lowfat milk, lowfat chocolate milk, regular chocolate milk, chocolate pudding or apple juice. Mix food or drink and doxycycline powder until powder dissolves. Mixture is stable in a covered container for 24 hrs if refrigerated (if made with milk or pudding) or at room temperature (if made with juice). Number of teaspoons to administer/dose is based on child's weight (0–12.5 lbs—½ tsp; 12.5–25 lbs—1 tsp; 25–37.5 lbs—1½ tsp; 37.5–50 lbs—2 tsp; 50–62.5 lbs—2½ tsp; 62.5–75 lbs—3 tsp; 75–87.5 lbs—3½ tsp; 87.5–100 lbs—4 tsp).

IV Administration

- **Intermittent Infusion:** ***Diluent:*** Dilute each 100 mg with 10 ml of sterile water or 0.9% NaCl for injection. Dilute further in 100–1000 ml of 0.9% NaCl, D5W, D5/LR, Ringer's, or LR. Solution is stable for 12 hr at room temperature and 72 hr if refrigerated. If diluted with D5/LR or LR, administer within 6 hr. Protect solution from direct sunlight. ***Concentration:*** Concentrations of less than

0.1 mg/ml or greater than 1 mg/ml are not recommended. ***Rate:*** Administer over a minimum of 1–4 hr. Avoid rapid administration. Avoid extravasation.

- **Y-Site Compatibility:** acyclovir, amifostine, amiodarone, aztreonam, bivalirudin, cisatracurium, cyclophosphamide, dexmedetomidine, diltiazem, docetaxel, etoposide phosphate, fenoldopam, filgrastim, fludarabine, gemcitabine, granisetron, hydromorphone, linezolid, magnesium sulfate, melphalen, meperidine, morphine, ondansetron, perphenazine, propofol, remifentanil, sargramostim, tacrolimus, teniposide, theophylline, thiotepa, vinorelbine.
- **Y-Site Incompatibility:** allopurinol, heparin, pemetrexed, piperacillin/tazobactam.

Patient/Family Teaching

- Instruct patient to take medication around the clock and to finish the drug completely as directed, even if feeling better. Take missed doses as soon as possible unless it is almost time for next dose; do not double doses. Advise patient that sharing of this medication may be dangerous.
- Advise patient to avoid taking milk or other dairy products concurrently with oral tetracyclines. Also avoid taking antacids, zinc, calcium, magnesium- or aluminum-containing medications, sodium bicarbonate, and iron supplements within 1–3 hr of oral tetracyclines.
- Advise female patient to use a nonhormonal method of contraception while taking tetracyclines and until next menstrual period.
- *Minocycline* commonly causes dizziness or unsteadiness. Caution patient to avoid driving or other activities requiring alertness until response to medication is known. Notify health care professional if these symptoms occur.
- Caution patient to use sunscreen and protective clothing to prevent photosensitivity reactions.
- Advise patient to report the signs of superinfection (black, furry overgrowth on the tongue, vaginal itching or discharge, loose or foul-smelling stools). Skin rash, pruritus, and urticaria should also be reported.
- Instruct patient to notify health care professional of medication regimen before treatment or surgery.
- Instruct patient to notify health care professional if symptoms do not improve within a few days for systemic preparations.
- Caution patient to discard outdated or decomposed tetracyclines; they may be toxic.

Evaluation/Desired Outcomes

- Resolution of the signs and symptoms of infection. Length of time for complete resolution depends on the organism and site of infection.
- Decrease in acne lesions.
- Treatment of inhalation anthrax (post exposure) or treatment of cutaneous anthrax (doxycycline).

thalidomide (tha-**lid**-oh-mide)
Thalomid

Classification
Therapeutic: immunosuppressants

Pregnancy Category X

Indications

Cutaneous manifestations of moderate to severe erythema nodosum leprosum (ENL). Prevention (maintenance) and suppression of recurrent ENL. Newly diagnosed multiple myeloma (with dexamethasone). **Unlabeled uses:** Bechet's syndrome. HIV-associated wasting syndrome. Aphthous stomatitis (including HIV associated). Crohn's disease.

Action

May suppress excess levels of tumor necrosis factor-alpha (TNF-alpha) in patients with ENL and alter leukocyte migration by altering characteristics of cell surfaces. **Therapeutic Effects:** Decreased skin lesions in ENL and prevention of recurrence.

Pharmacokinetics

Absorption: 67–93% absorbed following oral administration.
Distribution: Crosses the placenta; highly protein bound.
Protein Binding: Highly bound.
Metabolism and Excretion: Hydrolyzed in plasma to multiple metabolites.
Half-life: 5–7 hr.

TIME/ACTION PROFILE (dermatologic effects)

ROUTE	ONSET	PEAK	DURATION
PO	48 hr	1–2 mo	unknown

Contraindications/Precautions

Contraindicated in: Pregnancy; OB: Women with childbearing potential (unless specific

conditions are met); Sexually mature men (unless specific conditions are met); OB: Lactation; Hypersensitivity.
Use Cautiously in: Pedi: Children <12 yr (safety not established).

Adverse Reactions/Side Effects

CNS: dizziness, drowsiness. **CV:** bradycardia, edema, orthostatic hypotension, thromboembolic events (↑ risk with dexamethasone in multiple myeloma). **GI:** constipation. **Derm:** rash, photosensitivity. **Hemat:** neutropenia. **Neuro:** peripheral neuropathy. **Misc:** SEVERE BIRTH DEFECTS, hypersensitivity reactions, increased HIV viral load.

Interactions

Drug-Drug: ↑ CNS depression with concurrent use of **barbiturates**, **sedative/hypnotics**, **alcohol**, **chlorpromazine**, **reserpine**, or other **CNS depressants**. Concurrent use of **agents that may cause peripheral neuropathy** ↑ risk of peripheral neuropathy.
Drug-Natural Products: Concommitant use with **echinacea**, and **melatonin** may interfere with immunosuppression.

Route/Dosage

ENL

PO (Adults ≥50 kg): 100–300 mg/day initially; up to 400 mg/day has been used, depending on previous response. Every 3–6 mo attempts should be made to taper and discontinue in decrements of 50 mg q 2–4 wk.
PO (Adults <50 kg): 100 mg/day initially; up to 400 mg/day has been used, depending on previous response. Every 3–6 mo attempts should be made to taper and discontinue in decrements of 50 mg q 2–4 wk.

Multiple Myeloma

PO (Adults): 200 mg daily in 28-day treatment cycles. Dexamethasone 40 mg is administered on Days 1–4, 9–12, 17–20.

Availability

Capsules: 50 mg, 100 mg, 150 mg, 200 mg.

NURSING IMPLICATIONS

Assessment

- Assess patient monthly for initial 3 months and periodically during therapy to detect early signs of peripheral neuropathy (numbness, tingling, or pain in hands and feet). Commonly occurs with prolonged therapy, but has occurred following short-term use or following completion of therapy. May be severe and irreversible. Electrophysiologic testing may be done at baseline and every 6 months to detect asymptomatic peripheral neuropathy. If symptoms occur, discontinue thalidomide immediately to limit further damage. Reinstate therapy only if neuropathy returns to baseline.
- Monitor for signs of hypersensitivity reaction (erythematous macular rash, fever, tachycardia, hypotension). May require discontinuation of therapy if severe. If reaction recurs when dosing is resumed, discontinue thalidomide.
- **Multiple Myeloma:** Assess for venous thromboembolism (dyspnea, chest pain, arm or leg swelling) periodically during therapy, especially in patients concurrently taking dexamethasone.
- Monitor for side effects (constipation, oversedation, peripheral neuropathy); may require discontinuation or dose reduction until side effects resolve.
- ***Lab Test Considerations:*** Monitor WBC with differential during therapy. May cause ↓ WBC. Do not initiate therapy with an ANC ≤750/mm^3. If ANC ↓ to ≤750/mm^3 during therapy, re-evaluate medication regimen; if neutropenia persists, consider discontinuing therapy.
- May cause ↑ viral load levels in patients with HIV.

Potential Nursing Diagnoses

Impaired skin integrity (Indications)
Risk for injury (Adverse Reactions)

Implementation

- Due to teratogenic effects, thalidomide may be prescribed only by prescribers registered in the System for Thalidomide Education and Prescribing Safety (STEPS) program. Thalidomide is started within 24 hr of a negative pregnancy test with a sensitivity of at least 50 mIU/ml. Pregnancy testing must occur weekly during first month of therapy, then monthly thereafter in women with a regular menstrual cycle. For women with irregular menses, pregnancy testing should occur every 2 wk. If pregnancy occurs, thalidomide should be discontinued immediately. Any suspected fetal exposure must be reported to the FDA and the manufacturer, and patient should be re-

T

ferred to an obstetrician/gynecologist experienced in reproductive toxicity.

- If healthcare professionals or other caregivers are exposed to body fluids from patients receiving thalidomide, use appropriate precautions, such as wearing gloves to prevent the potential cutaneous exposure to thalidomide or washing the exposed area with soap and water.
- Corticosteroids may be used concurrently with thalidomide for patients with moderate to severe neuritis associated with a severe ENL reaction. Use of corticosteroids can be tapered and discontinued when neuritis resolves.
- **PO:** Administer once daily with water, preferably at bedtime and at least 1 hr after the evening meal. If divided doses are used, administer at least 1 hr after meals.

Patient/Family Teaching

- Instruct patient to take thalidomide as directed. Do not discontinue without notifying health care professional; dose should be tapered gradually.
- Advise patient that thalidomide should not be shared with others.
- Caution patient on the extreme importance of maintaining contraception for 1 month prior to, during, and for 1 month following discontinuation of therapy. *For women of childbearing years,* two methods of reliable contraception must be used unless complete abstinence is used. *For men,* a latex condom must be used, even if a successful vasectomy has been performed. Patients must meet *ALL* of the STEPS conditions: Understands and can follow instructions and is capable of complying with contraceptive measures, pregnancy testing, patient registration, and patient survey. Patients must receive verbal and written warnings of the potential teratogenicity of thalidomide and must acknowledge in writing their understanding and acceptance of these conditions.
- Advise patient to consult health care professional before using other RX, OTC, or herbal products. Concomitant use of HIV-protease inhibitors, modafinil, penicillins, rifampin, rifabutin, phenytoin, carbamazepine, or certain herbal supplements such as St. John's Wort with hormonal contraceptive agents may reduce the effectiveness of contraception during and for up to one month after discontinuation of these concomitant therapies. Therefore, women requiring treatment with one or more of these drugs must use two other effective or highly effective methods of contraception or abstain from heterosexual sexual contact while taking thalidomide.
- Frequently causes drowsiness or dizziness. Caution patient to avoid driving or other activities requiring alertness until response to medication is known.
- Advise patient to change positions slowly to minimize orthostatic hypotension.
- Caution patient to use sunscreen and protective clothing to prevent photosensitivity reactions.
- Instruct patient not to donate blood and male patients not to donate sperm while taking thalidomide.
- Advise patient to notify health care professional immediately if pain, numbness, tingling, or burning in hands or feet or shortness of breath, chest pain, swelling of arms or legsoccur.

Evaluation/Desired Outcomes

- Resolution of the signs and symptoms of active ENL reaction. Usually requires at least 2 wk of therapy; then taper medication in 50 mg decrements every 2–4 wk.
- Prevention of recurrent ENL. Tapering off medication should be attempted every 3–6 mo in decrements of 50 mg every 2–4 wk.
- Decrease in serum and urine paraprotein measurements in patients with multiple myeloma.

theophylline, See BRONCHODILATORS (XANTHINES).

thiamine (thye-a-min)

✤Betaxin, ✤Bewon, Biamine, vitamin B1

Classification

Therapeutic: vitamins

Pharmacologic: water soluble vitamins

Pregnancy Category A

Indications

Treatment of thiamine deficiencies (beriberi). Prevention of Wernicke's encephalopathy. Dietary supplement in patients with GI disease, alcoholism, or cirrhosis.

Action

Required for carbohydrate metabolism. **Therapeutic Effects:** Replacement in deficiency states.

Pharmacokinetics

Absorption: Well absorbed from the GI tract by an active process. Excessive amounts are not absorbed completely. Also well absorbed from IM sites.
Distribution: Widely distributed. Enters breast milk.
Metabolism and Excretion: Metabolized by the liver. Excess amounts are excreted unchanged by the kidneys.
Half-life: Unknown.

TIME/ACTION PROFILE (time for symptoms of deficiency—edema and heart failure—to resolve†)

ROUTE	ONSET	PEAK	DURATION
PO, IM, IV	hr	days	days–wks

†Confusion and psychosis take longer to respond

Contraindications/Precautions

Contraindicated in: Hypersensitivity; Known alcohol intolerance or bisulfite hypersensitivity (elixir only).
Use Cautiously in: Wernicke's encephalopathy (condition may be worsened unless thiamine is administered before glucose).

Adverse Reactions/Side Effects

Adverse reactions and side effects are extremely rare and are usually associated with IV administration or extremely large doses.
CNS: restlessness, weakness. **EENT:** tightness of the throat. **Resp:** pulmonary edema, respiratory distress. **CV:** VASCULAR COLLAPSE, hypotension, vasodilation. **GI:** GI bleeding, nausea. **Derm:** cyanosis, pruritus, sweating, tingling, urticaria, warmth. **Misc:** ANGIOEDEMA.

Interactions

Drug-Drug: None significant.

Route/Dosage

Thiamine Deficiency (Beriberi)

PO (Adults): 5–10 mg 3 times daily.
PO (Children): 10–50 mg/day in divided doses.
IM, IV (Adults): 5–100 mg 3 times daily.
IM, IV (Children): 10–25 mg/day.

Dietary Supplement

PO (Adults): 1–1.6 mg/day.
PO (Children 4–10 yr): 0.9–1 mg/day.
PO (Children birth–3 yr): 0.3–0.7 mg/day.

Availability (generic available)

Tablets: 5 mg^{OTC}, 10 mg^{OTC}, 25 mg^{OTC}, 50 mg^{OTC}, 100 mg^{OTC}, 250 mg^{OTC}, 500 mg^{OTC}. **Elixir:** ✤250 mcg/5 ml^{OTC}. **Injection:** 100 mg/ml in 1-ml ampules and prefilled syringes and 1-, 2-, 10-, and 30-ml vials. ***In combination with:*** other vitamins, minerals, and trace elements in multi-vitamin preparations^{OTC}.

NURSING IMPLICATIONS

Assessment

- Assess patient for signs and symptoms of thiamine deficiency (anorexia, GI distress, irritability, palpitations, tachycardia, edema, paresthesia, muscle weakness and pain, depression, memory loss, confusion, psychosis, visual disturbances, elevated serum pyruvic acid levels).
- Assess patient's nutritional status (diet, weight) prior to and throughout therapy.
- Monitor patients receiving IV thiamine for anaphylaxis (wheezing, urticaria, edema).
- ***Lab Test Considerations:*** May interfere with certain methods of testing serum theophylline, uric acid, and urobilinogen concentrations.

Potential Nursing Diagnoses

Imbalanced nutrition: less than body requirements (Indications)

Implementation

- Because of infrequency of single B-vitamin deficiencies, combinations are commonly administered.
- **IM, IV:** Parenteral administration is reserved for patients in whom oral administration is not feasible.
- **IM:** Administration may cause tenderness and induration at injection site. Cool compresses may decrease discomfort.
- **IV:** Sensitivity reactions and death have occurred from IV administration. An intradermal test dose is recommended in patients with suspected sensitivity. Monitor site for erythema and induration.
- **Direct IV:** ***Concentration:*** Administer undiluted at 100 mg/ml. ***Rate:*** Administer at a rate of 100 mg over 5 min.

- **Continuous Infusion:** May be diluted in dextrose/Ringer's or LR combinations, dextrose/saline combinations, D5W, D10W, Ringer's and LR injection, 0.9% NaCl, or 0.45% NaCl and is usually administered with other vitamins.
- **Y-Site Compatibility:** famotidine.
- **Additive Incompatibility:** Solutions with neutral or alkaline pH, such as carbonates, bicarbonates, citrates, and acetates.

Patient/Family Teaching

- Encourage patient to comply with dietary recommendations of health care professional. Explain that the best source of vitamins is a well-balanced diet with foods from the four basic food groups.
- Teach patient that foods high in thiamine include cereals (whole grain and enriched), meats (especially pork), and fresh vegetables; loss is variable during cooking.
- Caution patients self-medicating with vitamin supplements not to exceed RDA. The effectiveness of megadoses of vitamins for treatment of various medical conditions is unproved and may cause side effects.

Evaluation/Desired Outcomes

- Prevention of or decrease in the signs and symptoms of vitamin B deficiency.
- Decrease in the symptoms of neuritis, ocular signs, ataxia, edema, and heart failure may be seen within hours of administration and may disappear within a few days.
- Confusion and psychosis may take longer to respond and may persist if nerve damage has occurred.

thioridazine

(thye-oh-**rid**-a-zeen)
✤Apo-Thioridazine, Mellaril, Mellaril-S, ✤Novo-Ridazine, ✤PMS Thioridazine

Classification
Therapeutic: antipsychotics
Pharmacologic: phenothiazines

Pregnancy Category C

Indications

Treatment of refractory schizophrenia. Considered second line treatment after failure with atypical antipsychotics.

Action

Alters the effects of dopamine in the CNS. Possesses significant anticholinergic and alpha-adrenergic blocking activity. **Therapeutic Effects:** Diminished signs and symptoms of psychoses.

Pharmacokinetics

Absorption: Absorption from tablets is variable; may be better with oral liquid formulations.
Distribution: Widely distributed, high concentrations in the CNS. Crosses the placenta and enters breast milk.
Protein Binding: ≥90%.
Metabolism and Excretion: Highly metabolized by the liver and GI mucosa.
Half-life: 21–24 hr.

TIME/ACTION PROFILE (antipsychotic effects)

ROUTE	ONSET	PEAK	DURATION
PO	unknown	unknown	8–12 hr

Contraindications/Precautions

Contraindicated in: Hypersensitivity; Cross-sensitivity with other phenothiazines may exist; Angle-closure glaucoma; Bone marrow depression; Severe liver or cardiovascular disease; Known alcohol intolerance (concentrate only); Concurrent fluvoxamine, propranolol, pindolol, fluoxetine, other agents known to inhibit the CYP450 2D6 enzyme, or agents known to prolong the QTc interval (risk of life-threatening arrrhythmias); Hypokalemia (correct prior to use); QTc interval >450 msec.
Use Cautiously in: Debilitated patients; Glaucoma; Urinary retention; Diabetes mellitus; Patients with risk factors for electrolyte imbalance (dehydration, diuretic therapy); Respiratory disease; Prostatic hyperplasia; CNS tumors; Epilepsy; Intestinal obstruction; OB, Lactation: Safety not established. Recommend discontinue drug or bottle feed; Geri: Geriatric patients may be at increased risk for extrapyramidal and CNS adverse effects. Appears on Beers list.

Adverse Reactions/Side Effects

CNS: NEUROLEPTIC MALIGNANT SYNDROME, sedation, extrapyramidal reactions, tardive dyskinesia. **EENT:** blurred vision, dry eyes, lens opacities, pigmentary retinopathy (high doses). **CV:** ARRHYTHMIAS, QTC PROLONGATION, hypotension, tachycardia. **GI:** constipation, dry mouth, anorexia, drug-induced hepatitis, ileus, weight gain. **GU:** urinary retention, priapism. **Derm:** photosensitivity, pigment changes, rashes. **Endo:** galactorrhea, amenorrhea. **Hemat:** AGRANULOCYTOSIS, leukopenia. **Metab:** hyperthermia. **Misc:** allergic reactions.

Interactions

Drug-Drug: Concurrent **fluvoxamine**, **propranolol**, **pindolol**, **fluoxetine**, other **agents known to inhibit the CYP450 2D6 enzyme**, or **agents known to prolong the QTc interval** (risk of life-threatening arrhythmias). **Diuretics** increase the risk of electrolyte imbalance and arrhythmias. Additive hypotension with other **antihypertensives**, **nitrates**, and acute ingestion of **alcohol**. Additive CNS depression with other **CNS depressants**, including **alcohol**, **antihistamines**, **opioid analgesics**, **sedative/hypnotics**, and **general anesthetics**. Additive anticholinergic effects with other **drugs possessing anticholinergic properties**, including **antihistamines**, **antidepressants**, **atropine**, **haloperidol**, other **phenothiazines**, and **disopyramide**. **Lithium** decreases blood levels of thioridazine. Thioridazine may mask early signs of **lithium** toxicity and increase the risk of extrapyramidal reactions. Increased risk of agranulocytosis with **antithyroid agents**. Concurrent use with **epinephrine** may result in severe hypotension and tachycardia. May decrease the effectiveness of **levodopa**.

Route/Dosage

PO (Adults and Children >12 yr): 50–100 mg tid initially; may be gradually increased to a maintenance dose of up to 800 mg/day.
PO (Children): 0.5 mg/kg/day in divided doses initially; may be gradually increased to a maintenance dose of up to 3 mg/kg/day.

Availability (generic available)

Tablets: 10 mg, 15 mg, 25 mg, 50 mg, 100 mg, 150 mg, 200 mg. **Oral suspension:** ✤10 mg/5 ml, 25 mg/5 ml, 100 mg/5 ml. **Concentrated oral solution:** 30 mg/ml, 100 mg/ml.

NURSING IMPLICATIONS

Assessment

- Assess mental status (orientation, mood, behavior) before and periodically throughout therapy.
- Assess positive (delusions, hallucinations, agitation) and negative (social withdrawal) symptoms of schizophrenia.
- Assess weight and BMI initially and throughout theerapy.
- Monitor blood pressure (sitting, standing, lying), ECG, pulse, and respiratory rate before and frequently during the period of dosage adjustment. May cause Q-wave and T-wave changes in ECG.
- Observe patient carefully when administering medication to ensure that medication is actually taken and not hoarded or cheeked.
- Assess patient for level of sedation after administration. Geri: Geriatric patients are more likely to become oversedated.
- Monitor intake and output ratios and daily weight. Report significant discrepancies.
- Monitor patient for onset of akathisia (restlessness or desire to keep moving) and extrapyramidal side effects (*parkinsonian*—difficulty speaking or swallowing, loss of balance control, pill rolling of hands, mask-like face, shuffling gait, rigidity, tremors; and *dystonic*—muscle spasms, twisting motions, twitching, inability to move eyes, weakness of arms or legs) every 2 mo during therapy and 8–12 wk after therapy has been discontinued. Report these symptoms; reduction in dosage or discontinuation of medication may be necessary. Trihexyphenidyl, diphenhydramine, or benztropine may be used to control these symptoms. Benzodiazpines may alleviate akathisia.
- Monitor for tardive dyskinesia (uncontrolled rhythmic movement of mouth, face, and extremities; lip smacking or puckering; puffing of cheeks; uncontrolled chewing; rapid or worm-like movements of tongue, excessive eye blinking). Report immediately; may be irreversible.
- Monitor for development of neuroleptic malignant syndrome (fever, respiratory distress, tachycardia, seizures, diaphoresis, hypertension or hypotension, pallor, tiredness, severe muscle stiffness, loss of bladder control). Notify health care professional immediately if these symptoms occur.
- ***Lab Test Considerations:*** CBC, liver function tests, and ocular examinations should be evaluated periodically throughout therapy. May cause decreased hematocrit, hemoglobin, leukocytes, granulocytes, platelets. May cause elevated bilirubin, AST, ALT, and alkaline phosphatase. Agranulocytosis occurs be-

T

tween 4–10 wk of therapy with recovery 1–2 wk after discontinuation. May recur if medication is restarted. Liver function abnormalities may require discontinuation of therapy.
- May cause false-positive or false-negative pregnancy test results and false-positive urine bilirubin test results.
- May cause increased serum prolactin levels.

Potential Nursing Diagnoses
Disturbed thought process (Indications)
Sexual dysfunction (Side Effects)

Implementation
- To prevent contact dermatitis, avoid getting liquid preparations on hands, and wash hands thoroughly if spillage occurs.
- Phenothiazines should be discontinued 48 hr before and not resumed for 24 hr after myelography, as they lower the seizure threshold.
- **PO:** Administer with food, milk, or full glass of water to minimize gastric irritation.
- Dilute concentrate in 120 ml of distilled or acidified tap water or fruit juice just before administration.

Patient/Family Teaching
- Advise patient to take medication exactly as directed and not to skip doses or double up on missed doses. If a dose is missed, it should be taken as soon as remembered unless almost time for the next dose. If more than 2 doses a day are ordered, the missed dose should be taken within 1 hr of the scheduled time or omitted. Abrupt withdrawal may lead to gastritis, nausea, vomiting, dizziness, headache, tachycardia, and insomnia.
- Inform patient of possibility of extrapyramidal symptoms and tardive dyskinesia. Instruct patient to report these symptoms immediately to health care professional.
- Advise patient to change positions slowly to minimize orthostatic hypotension.
- May cause drowsiness. Caution patient to avoid driving or other activities requiring alertness until response to medication is known.
- Advise patient to use sunscreen and protective clothing when exposed to the sun. Exposed surfaces may develop a blue-gray pigmentation, which may fade after discontinuation of the medication. Extremes in temperature should also be avoided, as this drug impairs body temperature regulation.
- Instruct patient to use frequent mouth rinses, good oral hygiene, and sugarless gum or candy to minimize dry mouth. Consult health care professional if dry mouth continues for >2 wk.
- Advise patient that increasing activity and bulk and fluids in the diet helps minimize the constipating effects of this medication.
- Caution patient to avoid taking alcohol or other CNS depressants concurrently with this medication.
- Advise patient not to take thioridazine within 2 hr of antacids or antidiarrheal medication.
- Inform patient that this medication may turn urine pink to reddish brown.
- Advise patient to notify health care professional of medication regimen before treatment or surgery.
- Refer as appropriate for nutritional/weight management and medical management.
- Instruct patient to notify health care professional promptly if sore throat, fever, unusual bleeding or bruising, rash, weakness, tremors, visual disturbances, dark-colored urine, or clay-colored stools occur.
- Emphasize the importance of routine follow-up exams to monitor response to medication and to detect side effects. Periodic ocular exams are indicated. Encourage continued participation in psychotherapy.

Evaluation/Desired Outcomes
- Decrease in positive symptoms (hallucinations, delusions, agitation) of schizophrenia.

HIGH ALERT

THROMBOLYTIC AGENTS

alteplase (**al**-te-plase)
Activase, ✤Activase rt-PA, Cathflo Activase, tissue plasminogen activator, t-PA

reteplase (**re**-te-plase)
Retavase

streptokinase
(strep-toe-**kye**-nase)
Streptase

tenecteplase (te-**nek**-te-plase)
TNKase

urokinase (yoor-oh-**kye**-nase)
Abbokinase

Classification
Therapeutic: thrombolytics
Pharmacologic: plasminogen activators

Pregnancy Category B (urokinase), C (alteplase, reteplase, streptokinase, tenecteplase)

Indications
Alteplase, reteplase, streptokinase, tenecteplase: Acute myocardial infarction (MI). **Alteplase, streptokinase, urokinase:** Acute massive pulmonary emboli. **Alteplase:** Acute ischemic stroke. **Streptokinase:** Acute deep vein thrombosis. **Streptokinase:** Acute arterial thrombi. **Streptokinase:** Occluded arteriovenous cannulae. **Alteplase:** Occluded central venous access devices.

Action
Convert plasminogen to plasmin, which is then able to degrade fibrin present in clots. Alteplase, reteplase, tenecteplase, and urokinase directly activate plasminogen. Streptokinase combines with plasminogen to form activator complexes, which then converts plasminogen to plasmin.
Therapeutic Effects: Lysis of thrombi in coronary arteries, with preservation of ventricular function or improvement of ventricular function (and ↓ risk of CHF or death). Lysis of pulmonary emboli or deep vein thrombosis. Lysis of thrombi causing ischemic stroke, reducing risk of neurologic sequelae. Restoration of cannula or catheter patency and function.

Pharmacokinetics
Absorption: Complete after IV administration. Intracoronary administration or administration into occluded catheters or cannulae has a more localized effect.
Distribution: Streptokinase appears to cross the placenta minimally, if at all. Remainder of distribution for streptokinase or other agents is not known.
Metabolism and Excretion: *Alteplase, tenecteplase, urokinase*—Rapidly metabolized by the liver. *Reteplase*—Cleared primarily by the liver and kidneys. *Streptokinase*—Rapidly cleared from circulation by antibodies and other unknown mechanism.
Half-life: *Alteplase*—35 min; *reteplase*—13–16 min; *streptokinase*—initially 18 min (due to clearance by antibodies), then 83 min; *Tenecteplase*—20–24 min (initial phase), 90–130 min (terminal phase); *urokinase*—up to 20 min.

TIME/ACTION PROFILE (fibrinolysis)

ROUTE	ONSET	PEAK	DURATION
alteplase IV	30 min	60 min	unknown
reteplase IV	30 min	30–90 min	48 hr
streptokinase IV	immediate	rapid	4 hr (up to 12 hr)
tenecteplase IV	rapid	unknown	unknown
urokinase IV	immediate	rapid	up to 12 hr

Contraindications/Precautions
Contraindicated in: Active internal bleeding; History of cerebrovascular accident; Recent (within 2 mo) intracranial or intraspinal injury or trauma; Intracranial neoplasm, AV malformation, or aneurysm; Severe uncontrolled hypertension; Known bleeding tendencies; Hypersensitivity; cross-sensitivity with other thrombolytics may occur.
Use Cautiously in: Recent (within 10 days) major surgery, trauma, GI or GU bleeding; Left heart thrombus; Severe hepatic or renal disease; Hemorrhagic ophthalmic conditions; Septic phlebitis; Previous puncture of a noncompressible vessel; Subacute bacterial endocarditis or acute pericarditis; Recent streptococcal infection or previous therapy with streptokinase (from 5 days–6 mo); may produce resistance because of antibody formation; ↑ dosage requirements may be encountered (streptokinase only); Geri: Geriatric patients (>75 yr; ↑ risk of intracranial bleeding); OB, Lactation, Pedi: Pregnancy, lactation, or children (safety not established).
Exercise Extreme Caution in: Patients receiving concurrent anticoagulant therapy (↑ risk of intracranial bleeding).

Adverse Reactions/Side Effects
CNS: INTRACRANIAL HEMORRHAGE. **EENT:** epistaxis, gingival bleeding. **Resp:** bronchospasm, hemoptysis. **CV:** hypotension, reperfusion arrhythmias. **GI:** GI BLEEDING, RETROPERITONEAL BLEEDING, nausea, vomiting. **GU:** GU TRACT BLEEDING. **Derm:** ecchymoses, flushing, urticaria. **Hemat:** BLEEDING. **Local:** hemorrhage at injection sites, phlebitis at IV site. **MS:** musculoskeletal pain. **Misc:** allergic reactions including ANAPHYLAXIS, fever.

T

Interactions

Drug-Drug: Concurrent use of **aspirin**, other **NSAIDs**, **warfarin**, **heparin low-molecular-weight heparins**, **direct thrombin inhibitors**, **abciximab**, **eptifibatide**, **tirofiban**, **clopidogrel**, **ticlopidine**, or **dipyridamole** may ↑ risk of bleeding, although these agents are frequently used together or in sequence. Effects may be ↓ by **antifibrinolytic agents**, including **aminocaproic acid** or **tranexamic acid**.

Drug-Natural Products: ↑ anticoagulant effect and bleeding risk with **anise**, **arnica**, **chamomile**, **clove**, **dong quai**, **fenugreek**, **feverfew**, **garlic**, **ginger**, **ginkgo**, **Panax ginseng**, **licorice**, and others.

Route/Dosage

Alteplase

Myocardial Infarction (Accelerated or Front-Loading Infusion)

IV (Adults): 15 mg bolus, then 0.75 mg/kg (up to 50 mg) over 30 min, then 0.5 mg/kg (up to 35 mg) over next 60 min; usually accompanied by heparin therapy.

Myocardial Infarction (3-Hour Infusion)

IV (Adults >65 kg): 60 mg over 1st hr (6–10 mg given as a bolus over first 1–2 min), 20 mg over the 2nd hr, and 20 mg over the 3rd hr for a total dose of 100 mg.
IV (Adults <65 kg): 0.75 mg/kg over 1st hr (0.075–0.125 mg/kg given as a bolus over first 1–2 min), 0.25 mg/kg over the 2nd hr, and 0.25 mg/kg over the 3rd hr for a total dose of 1.25 mg/kg (not to exceed 100 mg total).

Pulmonary Embolism

IV (Adults): 100 mg over 2 hr; follow with heparin.

Acute Ischemic Stroke

IV (Adults): 0.9 mg/kg (not to exceed 90 mg), given as an infusion over 1 hr, with 10% of the dose given as a bolus over the 1st min.

Occluded Venous Access Devices

IV (Adults and Children >30 kg): 2 mg/2 ml instilled into occluded catheter; if unsuccessful, may repeat once after 2 hr.
IV (Adults and Children <30 kg): 110% of the lumen volume (not to exceed 2 mg in 2 ml) instilled into occluded catheter; if unsuccessful, may repeat once after 2 hr.

Reteplase

IV (Adults): 10 units, followed 30 min later by an additional 10 units.

Streptokinase

Myocardial Infarction

IV (Adults): 1.5 million units given as a continuous infusion over up to 60 min.
Intracoronary **(Adults):** 20,000 unit bolus followed by 2000–4000 units/min infusion for 30–90 min.

Deep Vein Thrombosis, Pulmonary Emboli, Arterial Emboli, or Arterial Thromboses

IV (Adults): 250,000 unit loading dose over 30 min, followed by 100,000 unit/hr for 24 hr for pulmonary emboli or arterial thrombosis/embolism, 72 hr for deep vein thrombosis.

Tenecteplase

IV (Adults <60 kg): 30 mg.
IV (Adults ≥60 kg and <70 kg): 35 mg.
IV (Adults ≥70 kg and <80 kg): 40 mg.
IV (Adults ≥80 kg and <90 kg): 45 mg.
IV (Adults ≥90 kg): 50 mg.

Urokinase

Pulmonary Emboli

IV (Adults): 4400 unit/kg loading dose, followed by 4400 unit/kg/hr for 12 hr.

Availability

Alteplase

Powder for injection: 2 mg/vial, 50 mg/vial, 100 mg/vial.

Reteplase

Powder for injection: 10.8 units/vial.

Streptokinase

Powder for injection: 250,000 units/vial, 750,000 units/vial, 1,500,000 units/vial.

Tenecteplase

Powder for injection: 50 mg/vial.

Urokinase

Powder for injection: 250,000 units/vial.

NURSING IMPLICATIONS

Assessment

- Begin therapy as soon as possible after the onset of symptoms.
- Monitor vital signs, including temperature, continuously for coronary thrombosis and at least every 4 hr during therapy for other indications. Do not use lower extremities to monitor blood pressure. Notify physician if systolic BP >180 mm Hg or diastolic BP >110 mm Hg. Should not be given if hypertension is uncontrolled. Inform physician if hypotension occurs. Hypotension may result from the drug, hemorrhage, or cardiogenic shock
- Assess patient carefully for bleeding every 15 min during the 1st hr of therapy, every 15–30

min during the next 8 hr, and at least every 4 hr for the duration of therapy. Frank bleeding may occur from sites of invasive procedures or from body orifices. Internal bleeding may also occur (decreased neurologic status; abdominal pain with coffee-grounds emesis or black, tarry stools; hematuria; joint pain). If uncontrolled bleeding occurs, stop medication and notify physician immediately

- Inquire about previous reaction to streptokinase therapy. Assess patient for hypersensitivity reaction (rash, dyspnea, fever, changes in facial color, swelling around the eyes, wheezing). If these occur, inform physician promptly. Keep epinephrine, an antihistamine, and resuscitation equipment close by in the event of an anaphylactic reaction
- Inquire about recent streptococcal infection. *Streptokinase* may be less effective if administered between 5 days and 6 mo of a streptococcal infection
- Assess neurologic status throughout therapy. Altered sensorium or neurologic changes may be indicative of intracranial bleeding.
- **Myocardial Infarction:** Monitor ECG continuously. Notify physician if significant arrhythmias occur. Monitor cardiac enzymes. Radionuclide myocardial scanning and/or coronary angiography may be ordered 7–10 days after therapy to monitor effectiveness of therapy.
- Assess intensity, character, location, and radiation of chest pain. Note presence of associated symptoms (nausea, vomiting, diaphoresis). Notify physician if chest pain is unrelieved or recurs
- Monitor heart sounds and breath sounds frequently. Inform physician if signs of CHF occur (rales/crackles, dyspnea, S_3 heart sound, jugular venous distention).
- **Acute Ischemic Stroke:** Assess neurologic status. Determine time of onset of stroke symptoms. Alteplase must be administered within 3 hr of onset.
- **Pulmonary Embolism:** Monitor pulse, blood pressure, hemodynamics, and respiratory status (rate, degree of dyspnea, ABGs).
- **Deep Vein Thrombosis/Acute Arterial Thrombosis:** Observe extremities and palpate pulses of affected extremities every hour. Notify physician immediately if circulatory impairment occurs. Computerized tomography, impedance plethysmography, quantitative Doppler effect determination, and/or angiography or venography may be used to determine restoration of blood flow and duration of therapy; however, repeated venograms are not recommended.
- **Cannula/Catheter Occlusion:** Monitor ability to aspirate blood as indicator of patency. Ensure that patient exhales and holds breath when connecting and disconnecting IV syringe to prevent air embolism.
- ***Lab Test Considerations:*** Hematocrit, hemoglobin, platelet count, fibrin/fibrin degradation product (FDP) titer, fibrinogen concentration, prothrombin time, thrombin time, and activated partial thromboplastin time (aPTT) may be evaluated before and frequently during therapy. Bleeding time may be assessed before therapy if patient has received platelet inhibitors.
- Obtain type and crossmatch and have blood available at all times in case of hemorrhage.
- Stools should be tested for occult blood loss and urine for hematuria periodically during therapy.
- ***Toxicity and Overdose: High Alert:*** If local bleeding occurs, apply pressure to site. If severe or internal bleeding occurs, discontinue infusion. Clotting factors and/or blood volume may be restored through infusions of whole blood, packed RBCs, fresh frozen plasma, or cryoprecipitate. Do not administer dextran; it has antiplatelet activity. Aminocaproic acid (Amicar) may be used as an antidote.

Potential Nursing Diagnoses

Ineffective tissue perfusion (Indications)
Risk for injury (Side Effects)

Implementation

- ***High Alert:*** Overdosage and underdosage of thrombolytic medications have resulted in patient harm or death. Have second practitioner independently check original order, dosage calculations, and infusion pump settings. Do not confuse the abbreviation *t-PA* for alteplase (Activase) with the abbreviation *TNK t-PA* for tenecteplase (TNKase) and *r-PA* for reteplase (Retavase). Clarify orders that contain either of these abbreviations.
- Thrombolytic agents should be used only in settings in which hematologic function and

T

clinical response can be adequately monitored.

- Starting two IV lines before therapy is recommended: one for the thrombolytic agent, the other for any additional infusions.
- Avoid invasive procedures, such as IM injections or arterial punctures, with this therapy. If such procedures must be performed, apply pressure to all arterial and venous puncture sites for at least 30 min. Avoid venipunctures at noncompressible sites (jugular vein, subclavian site).
- Acetaminophen may be ordered to control fever.

Alteplase

IV Administration

- **Intermittent Infusion:** ***Diluent:*** Vials are packaged with sterile water for injection (without preservatives) to be used as diluent. Do not use bacteriostatic water for injection. Reconstitute 20-mg vials with 20-ml and 50-mg vials with 50 ml using an 18-gauge needle. Avoid excess agitation during dilution; swirl or invert gently to mix. Solution may foam upon reconstitution. Bubbles will resolve upon standing a few min. Solution will be clear to pale yellow. Stable for 8 hr at room temperature. ***Concentration:*** May be administered as reconstituted (1 mg/ml) or may be further diluted immediately before use in an equal amount of 0.9% NaCl or D5W. ***Rate:*** Flush line with 20–30 ml of saline at completion of infusion to ensure entire dose is received.
- Standard dose for *MI* is administered over 3 hr.
- For *pulmonary embolism,* administer over 2 hr.
- For *acute ischemic stroke,* administer 10% of total dose IV bolus over 1 min, with the remaining dose infused over 60 min.
- **Y-Site Compatibility:** lidocaine, metoprolol, propranolol.
- **Y-Site Incompatibility:** bivalirudin, dobutamine, dopamine, heparin, nitroglycerin. Cathflo Activase. Reconstitute by withdrawing 2.2 ml of sterile water (provided) and injecting into Cathflo Activase vial, directing diluent into powder for a concentration of 1 mg/ml. Allow slight foaming to dissipate by letting vial stand undisturbed. Do not use bacteriostatic water. Mix by gently swirling to dissolve; complete dissolution should occur within 3 min. Do not shake. Solution should be colorless to pale yellow. Use solution within 8 hr
- Withdraw 2.0 ml of reconstituted solution and instill into occluded catheter. After 30 min dwell time, attempt to aspirate blood. If catheter remains occluded, allow 120 min dwell time. If catheter function is not restored after one dose, second dose may be instilled. If catheter function is restored, aspirate 4–5 ml of blood to remove Cathflo Activase and residual clot. Gently irrigate catheter with 0.9% NaCl.

Reteplase

IV Administration

- **Direct IV:** ***Diluent:*** Reconstitute using diluent, needle, syringe, and dispensing pin provided. Reconstitute only with sterile water for injection without preservatives. Solution is colorless. Do not administer solutions that are discolored or contain a precipitate. Slight foaming may occur; allow vial to stand undisturbed for several min to dissipate bubbles. Reconstitute immediately before use. Stable for 4 hr at room temperature. ***Concentration:*** Administer undiluted. ***Rate:*** Administer each bolus over 2 min into an IV line containing D5W; flush line before and after bolus.
- **Y-Site Incompatibility:** bivalirudin, heparin, No other medication should be infused or injected into line used for reteplase.

Streptokinase

IV Administration

- **Intracoronary:** *Dilute* 250,000 IU vial to a total volume of 125 ml with 0.9% NaCl or D5W. Administer 20,000 IU (10 ml) via bolus injection. ***Rate:*** Intracoronary bolus is administered over 15 sec–2 min.
- **Intermittent Infusion:** ***Diluent:*** Reconstitute with 5 ml of 0.9% NaCl or D5W (direct to sides of vial) and swirl gently; do not shake. Dilute further with 0.9% NaCl for a total volume of 45–500 ml (45 ml for MI, 90 ml for deep vein thrombosis or pulmonary embolism). Solution is slightly yellow in color. Administer through 0.8-micron pore–size filter. Use reconstituted solution within 24 hr. ***Rate:*** Administer dose for MI within 60 min.
- Intracoronary bolus should be followed by an intracoronary maintenance infusion of 2000 IU/min for 60 min.
- Loading dose for *deep vein thrombosis* or *pulmonary embolism* is administered over

30 min, followed by an infusion of 100,000 IU/hr.

- Use infusion pump to ensure accurate dose.
- **Y-Site Compatibility:** dobutamine, dopamine, heparin, lidocaine, nitroglycerin.
- **Y-Site Incompatibility:** bivalirudin.
- **Additive Incompatibility:** Do not admix with any other medication. Cannula/Catheter Clearance. Dilute 250,000 IU in 2 ml of 0.9% NaCl or D5W. ***Rate:*** Administer slowly, over 25–35 min, into each occluded limb of cannula, and then clamp for at least 2 hr. Aspirate contents carefully and flush lines with 0.9% NaCl.

Tenecteplase

IV Administration

- **Intermittent Infusion: *Diluent:*** Vials are packaged with sterile water for injection (without preservatives) to be used as diluent. Do not use bacteriostatic water for injection. Do not discard shield assembly. To reconstitute aseptically withdraw 10 ml of diluent and inject into the tenectplase vial, directing the stream into the powder. Slight foaming may occur; large bubbles will dissipate if left standing undisturbed for several minutes. Swirl gently until contents are completely dissolved; do not shake. ***Concentration:*** Solution containing 5 mg/ml is clear and colorless to pale yellow. Withdraw dose from reconstituted vial with the syringe and discard unused portion. Once dose is in syringe, stand the shield vertically on a flat surface (with green side down) and passively recap the red hub cannula. Remove the entire shield assembly, including the red hub cannula, by twisting counter clockwise. Shield assembly also contains the clear-ended blunt plastic cannula; retain for split septum IV access. Reconstitute immediately before use. May be refrigerated and administered within 8 hrs. ***Rate:*** Administer as a single IV bolus over 5 seconds.
- **Y-Site Incompatibility:** Precipate forms in line when administered with dextrose-containing solutions. Flush line with saline-containing solution prior to and following administration of tenecteplase.
- **Additive Incompatibility:** Do not admix.

Urokinase

IV Administration

- **Intermittent Infusion: *Diluent:*** Reconstitute each 250,000 IU vial with 5 ml of sterile water for injection without preservatives (direct to sides of vial) and swirl gently; do not shake. Solution is light straw colored. Do not administer solutions that are discolored or contain a precipitate. Use reconstituted solution immediately after preparation. Infuse through a 0.45-micron filter
- For *pulmonary embolism,* dilute the reconstituted solution further with 190 ml of 0.9% NaCl or D5W. ***Rate:*** For *pulmonary embolism,* administer loading dose over 10 min and follow with infusion of 4400 IU/kg/hr for 12 hr.
- Administer via infusion pump to ensure accurate dose.

Patient/Family Teaching

- Explain purpose of medication and the need for close monitoring to patient and family. Instruct patient to report hypersensitivity reactions (rash, dyspnea) and bleeding or bruising.
- Explain need for bedrest and minimal handling during therapy to avoid injury. Avoid all unnecessary procedures such as shaving and vigorous tooth brushing.

Evaluation/Desired Outcomes

- Lysis of thrombi and restoration of blood flow.
- Prevention of neurologic sequelae in acute ischemic stroke.
- Cannula or catheter patency.

THYROID PREPARATIONS

levothyroxine
(lee-voe-thye-**rox**-een)
✤Eltroxin, ✤Euthyrox, Levo-T, Levothroid, Levoxyl, Synthroid, T_4, Tirosint, Unithroid

liothyronine
(lye-oh-**thye**-roe-neen)
Cytomel, l-triiodothyronine, T_3, Triostat

liotrix (**lye**-oh-trix)
T_3/T_4, Thyrolar

thyroid (**thye**-royd)
Armour thyroid, Westhroid

T

Classification
Therapeutic: hormones
Pharmacologic: thyroid preparations

Pregnancy Category A

Indications
Thyroid supplementation in hypothyroidism. Treatment or suppression of euthyroid goiters and thyroid cancer.

Action
Replacement of or supplementation to endogenous thyroid hormones. Principal effect is increasing metabolic rate of body tissues: Promote gluconeogenesis, Increase utilization and mobilization of glycogen stores, Stimulate protein synthesis, Promote cell growth and differentiation, Aid in the development of the brain and CNS, Contain T_3 (triiodothyronine) and T_4 (thyroxine) activity. **Therapeutic Effects:** Replacement in hypothyroidism to restore normal hormonal balance. Suppression of thyroid cancers.

Pharmacokinetics
Absorption: Levothyroxine is variably (40–80%) absorbed from the GI tract. Liothyronine and thyroid hormone are well absorbed.
Distribution: Distributed into most body tissues. Thyroid hormones do not readily cross the placenta; minimal amounts enter breast milk.
Metabolism and Excretion: Metabolized by the liver and other tissues. Thyroid hormone undergoes enterohepatic recirculation and is excreted in the feces via the bile.
Half-life: *T_3 (liothyronine)*—1–2 days; *T_4 (thyroxine)*—6–7 days.

TIME/ACTION PROFILE (effects on thyroid function tests)

ROUTE	ONSET	PEAK	DURATION
levothyroxine PO	unknown	1–3 wk	1–3 wk
levothyroxine IV	6–8 hr	24 hr	unknown
liothyronine PO	unknown	24–72 hr	72 hr
liothyronine IV	unknown	unknown	unknown
thyroid PO	days–wks	1–3 wk	days–wks

Contraindications/Precautions
Contraindicated in: Hypersensitivity; Recent MI; Hyperthyroidism.
Use Cautiously in: Cardiovascular disease (initiate therapy with lower doses); Severe renal insufficiency; Uncorrected adrenocortical disorders; Swallowing difficulty (levothyroxine tablets); Geri: Geriatric patients are extremely sensitive to thyroid hormones; initial dose should be reduced; Pedi: Monitor neonates and infants for cardiac overload, arrhythmias, and aspiriation during first 2 wk of therapy (levothyroxine).

Adverse Reactions/Side Effects
Usually only seen when excessive doses cause iatrogenic hyperthyroidism.
CNS: nervousness, headache, insomnia, irritability. **CV:** arrhythmias, angina pectoris, hypotension, tachycardia. **GI:** cramps, diarrhea, vomiting; *levothyroxine tablets*— choking, gagging, dysphagia. **Derm:** hair loss (in children), increased sweating. **Endo:** hyperthyroidism, menstrual irregularities. **Metab:** heat intolerance, weight loss. **MS:** accelerated bone maturation in children.

Interactions
Drug-Drug: Bile acid sequestrants ↓ absorption of orally administered thyroid preparations. May ↑ effects of **warfarin**. May ↑ requirement for **insulin** or **oral hypoglycemic agents** in diabetics. Concurrent **estrogen** therapy may ↑ thyroid replacement requirements. ↑ cardiovascular effects with **adrenergics** (sympathomimetics).
Drug-Food: Foods or supplements containing high amounts of calcium, iron, magnesium, or zinc may bind levothyroxine and prevent complete absorption.

Route/Dosage

Levothyroxine
PO (Adults): *Hypothyroidism*—50 mcg as a single dose initially; may be ↑ q 2–3 wk; usual maintenance dose is 75–125 mcg/day (1.5 mcg/kg/day).
PO (Geriatric Patients and Patients with Increased Sensitivity to Thyroid Hormones): 12.5–25 mcg as a single dose initially; may be ↑ q 6–8 wk; usual maintenance dose is 75 mcg/day.
PO (Children ≥12 yr): 2–3 mcg/kg/day (up to 150–200 mcg/day).
PO (Children 6–12 yr): 4–5 mcg/kg/day (100–125 mcg/day).
PO (Children 1–5 yr): 5–6 mcg/kg/day (75–100 mcg/day).
PO (Children 6–12 mo): 6–8 mcg/kg/day (50–75 mcg/day).
PO (Infants 3–6 mo): 8–10 mcg/kg/day (25–50 mcg/day).

PO (Infants 0–3 mo or Infants at Risk for Cardiac Failure): 10–15 mcg/kg/day or 25 mcg/day; may be ↑ after 4–6 wk to 50 mcg.
IM, IV (Adults): *Hypothyroidism*—50–100 mcg/day as a single dose. *Myxedema coma/stupor*—200–500 mcg IV; additional 100–300 mcg may be given on 2nd day, followed by daily administration of smaller doses.
IM, IV (Children): *Hypothyroidism*—~50–75% of the oral dose.

Liothyronine

PO (Adults): *Mild hypothyroidism*—25 mcg once daily; may ↑ by 12.5–25 mcg/day q 1–2 wk intervals; usual maintenance dose is 25–50 mcg/day. *Myxedema*—2.5–5 mcg once daily initially; ↑ by 5–10 mcg/day q 1–2 wk up to 25 mcg/day, then ↑ by 12.5–25 mcg/day; usual maintenance dose is 25–50 mcg/day. *Simple goiter*—5 mcg once daily initially; ↑ by 5–10 mcg/day q 1–2 wk up to 25 mcg/day, then ↑ by 12.5–25 mcg/day q wk until desired effect is obtained; usual maintenance dose is 50–100 mcg/day. *T_3 suppression test*—75–100 mcg daily for 7 days. Radioactive ^{131}I is administered before and after 7-day course.
PO (Geriatric Patients or Patients with Cardiovascular Disease): 5 mcg/day initially; ↑ by no more than 5 mcg/day q 2 wk.
IV (Adults): *Myxedema coma*—25–50 mcg initially (if cardiovascular disease is present, initial dose should be 10–20 mcg). Additional doses may be given, to a total of at least 65 mcg/day (not to exceed 100 mcg/day). Doses should be at least 4 hr but not more than 12 hr apart.

Liotrix

Contains T_4 and T_3 in a ratio of 4:1
PO (Adults): *Hypothyroidism*—Start with 50 mcg levothyroxine/12.5 mcg liothyronine; ↑ by 50 mcg levothyroxine/12.5 mcg liothyronine q 2–4 wk until desired effect is obtained; usual maintenance dose is 50–100 mcg levothyroxine/12.5–25 mcg liothyronine daily. *Myxedema/hypothyroidism with cardiovascular disease*—12.5 mcg levothyroxine/3.1 mcg liothyronine/day; ↑ by 12.5 mcg levothyroxine/3.1 mcg liothyronine q 2–4 wk until desired effect is obtained.
PO (Geriatric Patients): 12.5–25 mcg levothyroxine/3.1–6.2 mcg liothyronine/day; ↑ by 12.5–25 mcg levothyroxine/3.1–6.2 mcg liothyronine q 6–8 wk until desired effect is obtained.

Thyroid

Each 1 gr = 60 mg and is equivalent to 100 mcg or less of levothyroxine (T_4) or 25 mcg of liothyronine (T_3)
PO (Adults and Children): *Hypothyroidism*—60 mg/day; ↑ q 4 wk by 30 mg; usual maintenance dose is 60–120 mg/day. *Myxedema/hypothyroidism with cardiovascular disease*—15 mg/day initially; ↑ by 30 mg/day q 2 wk, then may ↑ by 30–60 mg q 2 wk; usual maintenance dose is 60–120 mg/day.
PO (Geriatric Patients): 7.5–15 mg/day initially; may double dose q 6–8 wk until desired effect is obtained.

Availability

Levothyroxine

Tablets: 25 mcg, 50 mcg, 75 mcg, 88 mcg, 100 mcg, 112 mcg, 125 mcg, 137 mcg, 150 mcg, 175 mcg, 200 mcg, 300 mcg. **Cost:** *Levothroid*—50 mcg $22.95/90, 100 mcg $22.97/90; *Levoxyl*—50 mcg $31.97/90, 100 mcg $34.97/90; *Synthroid*—50 mcg $42.97/90, 100 mcg $46.97/90; *Unithroid*—50 mcg $31.97/90, 100 mcg $35.97/90; *Generic*—50 mcg $19.97/90, 100 mcg $25.97/90. **Soft gel capsules:** 12.5 mcg, 25 mcg, 50 mcg, 75 mcg, 125 mcg, 150 mcg. **Powder for injection:** 200 mcg/vial, 500 mcg/vial.

Liothyronine

Tablets: 5 mcg, 25 mcg, 50 mcg. **Solution for injection:** 10 mcg/ml in 1-ml vials.

Liotrix

Tablets: 12.5 mcg levothyroxine/3.1 mcg liothyronine, 25 mcg levothyroxine/6.25 mcg liothyronine, 50 mcg levothyroxine/12.5 mcg liothyronine, 100 mcg levothyroxine/25 mcg liothyronine, 150 mcg levothyroxine/37.5 mcg liothyronine.

Thyroid

Tablets: 15 mg, 30 mg, 60 mg, 90 mg, 120 mg, 180 mg, 240 mg, 300 mg. **Cost:** 15 mg $15.97/90, 30 mg $22.97/90, 60 mg $22.97/90, 90 mg $28.97/90, 120 mg $34.97/90, 180 mg $49.97/90, 240 mg $65.97/90, 300 mg $75.92/90.

NURSING IMPLICATIONS

Assessment

- Assess apical pulse and blood pressure prior to and periodically during therapy. Assess for tachyarrhythmias and chest pain.

T

- **Children:** Monitor height, weight, and psychomotor development.
- ***Lab Test Considerations:*** Monitor thyroid function studies prior to and during therapy.
- Monitor TSH concentrations in adults 8–12 wk after changing from one brand to another.
- Monitor blood and urine glucose in diabetic patients. Insulin or oral hypoglycemic dose may need to be ↑.
- ***Toxicity and Overdose:*** Overdose is manifested as hyperthyroidism (tachycardia, chest pain, nervousness, insomnia, diaphoresis, tremors, weight loss). Usual treatment is to withhold dose for 2–6 days. Acute overdose is treated by induction of emesis or gastric lavage, followed by activated charcoal. Sympathetic overstimulation may be controlled by antiadrenergic drugs (beta blockers), such as propranolol. Oxygen and supportive measures to control symptoms such as fever are also used.

Potential Nursing Diagnoses
Deficient knowledge, related to medication regimen (Patient/Family Teaching)

Implementation
- Administer as a single dose, preferably before breakfast to prevent insomnia.
- Initial dose is low, especially in geriatric and cardiac patients. Dose is ↑ gradually, based on thyroid function tests. Side effects occur more rapidly with liothyronine because of its rapid onset of effect.
- For patients with difficulty swallowing, levothyroxine tablets can be crushed and placed in 5–10 mL of water and administered immediately via dropper or spoon; do not store suspension.

Levothyroxine
IV Administration
- **Direct IV:** ***Diluent:*** Dilute the 200-mcg and 500-mcg vials with 2 or 5 ml, respectively, of 0.9% NaCl without preservatives (diluent usually provided). Shake well to dissolve completely. Administer solution immediately after preparation; discard unused portion. ***Concentration:*** 100 mcg/ml. ***Rate:*** Administer at a rate of 100 mcg over 1 min. Do not add to IV infusions; may be administered through Y-tubing.
- **Y-Site Incompatibility:** Do not admix with other IV solutions

Liothyronine
IV Administration
- **IV:** Liothyronine injection is for IV use only. Do not give IM or subcut. Administer doses at least 4 hr and not more than 12 hr apart. Base doses on continuous monitoring of patient and response to therapy
- Resume PO therapy as soon as patient is stable and able to take PO medication. When switching to PO therapy, discontinue IV liothyronine and initiate PO at low dose, increasing gradually according to patient's response.
- **Direct IV:** May be administered undiluted at 10 mcg/ml. ***Rate:*** Administer as a bolus.

Patient/Family Teaching
- Instruct patient to take medication as directed at the same time each day. Take missed doses as soon as remembered unless almost time for next dose. If more than 2–3 doses are missed, notify health care professional. Do not discontinue without consulting health care professional.
- Explain to patient that medication does not cure hypothyroidism; it provides a thyroid hormone. Therapy is lifelong.
- Caution patient not to change brands of thyroid preparations, as this may affect drug bioavailability.
- Advise patient to notify health care professional if headache, nervousness, diarrhea, excessive sweating, heat intolerance, chest pain, increased pulse rate, palpitations, weight loss >2 lb/wk, or any unusual symptoms occur.
- Caution patient to avoid taking other medications concurrently with thyroid preparations unless instructed by health care professional.
- Instruct patient to inform health care professional of thyroid therapy.
- Emphasize importance of follow-up exams to monitor effectiveness of therapy. Thyroid function tests are performed at least yearly.
- **Levothyroxine:** Advise patients to take Levoxyl tablets with water. Levoxyl tablets may rapidly swell and disintegrate resulting in choking, gagging, the tablet getting stuck in the throat, and difficulty swallowing. Taking with water usually prevents this.
- Pedi: Discuss with parents the need for routine follow-up studies to ensure correct development. Inform patient that partial hair loss may be experienced by children on thyroid therapy. This is usually temporary.

Evaluation/Desired Outcomes

- Resolution of symptoms of hypothyroidism and normalization of thyroid hormone levels.

tiagabine (tye-a-ga-been)
Gabitril

Classification
Therapeutic: anticonvulsants

Pregnancy Category C

Indications
Adjunctive treatment of partial seizures.

Action
Enhances the activity of gamma-aminobutyric acid, an inhibitory neurotransmitter. **Therapeutic Effects:** Decreased frequency of seizures.

Pharmacokinetics
Absorption: 90% absorbed following oral administration.
Distribution: Unknown.
Protein Binding: 96%.
Metabolism and Excretion: Mostly metabolized by the liver; 2% excreted unchanged in urine.
Half-life: *Without enzyme-inducing antiepileptic drugs*—7–9 hr; *with enzyme-inducing antiepileptic drugs*—4–7 hr.

TIME/ACTION PROFILE (blood levels)

ROUTE	ONSET	PEAK	DURATION
PO	unknown	45 min	unknown

Contraindications/Precautions
Contraindicated in: Hypersensitivity.
Use Cautiously in: Hepatic impairment (decreased dose/increased interval may be necessary); Patients receiving concurrent non–enzyme-inducing antiepileptic drug therapy such as valproates (may require lower doses and/or slower titration); Using tiagabine for off-label uses or other conditions leading to increased levels (may ↑ risk of new onset seizures); OB, Pedi: Pregnancy, lactation, or children <12 yr (safety not established).

Adverse Reactions/Side Effects
CNS: dizziness, drowsiness, nervousness, weakness, cognitive impairment, confusion, difficulty concentrating, hallucinations, headache, mental depression, personality disorder. **EENT:** abnormal vision, ear pain, tinnitus. **Resp:** dyspnea, epistaxis. **CV:** chest pain, edema, hypertension, palpitations, syncope, tachycardia. **GI:** abdominal pain, gingivitis, nausea, stomatitis. **GU:** dysmenorrhea, dysuria, metrorrhagia, urinary incontinence. **Derm:** alopecia, dry skin, rash, sweating. **Metab:** weight gain, weight loss. **MS:** arthralgia, neck pain. **Neuro:** ataxia, tremors. **Misc:** allergic reactions, chills, lymphadenopathy.

Interactions
Drug-Drug: Carbamazepine, **phenytoin**, **primidone**, and **phenobarbital** induce metabolism and ↓ blood levels; although concurrent therapy is usually necessary, adjustments may be required when altering regimens.

Route/Dosage
PO (Adults >18 yr): 4 mg once daily initially for 1 wk; may increase by 4–8 mg/day at weekly intervals, up to 56 mg/day in 2–4 divided doses.
PO (Children 12–18 yr): 4 mg once daily initially for 1 wk; may increase by 4 mg/day after 1 wk, then may increase by 4–8 mg/day at weekly intervals, up to 32 mg/day in 2–4 divided doses.

Availability
Tablets: 2 mg, 4 mg, 12 mg, 16 mg, 20 mg.

T

NURSING IMPLICATIONS

Assessment
- Assess location, duration, and characteristics of seizure activity.
- Assess mental status. May cause impaired concentration, speech or language problems, confusion, fatigue, and drowsiness. Symptoms may decrease with dose reduction or discontinuation.
- ***Toxicity and Overdose:*** Therapeutic serum levels have not been determined. However, levels may be monitored prior to and following changes in the therapeutic regimen.

Potential Nursing Diagnoses
Risk for injury (Side Effects)

Implementation
- Do not confuse tiagabine with tizanidine.
- **PO:** Administer with food.
- Tiagabine should be discontinued gradually. Abrupt discontinuation may cause increase in seizure frequency.

Patient/Family Teaching

- Instruct patient to take medication as directed. Take missed doses as soon as possible unless almost time for next dose. Do not double doses. Do not discontinue abruptly; may cause increase in frequency of seizures.
- Advise patient to notify health care professional immediately if frequency of seizures increases.
- May cause dizziness. Caution patient to avoid driving or activities requiring alertness until response to medication is known. Do not resume driving until physician gives clearance based on control of seizure disorder.
- Advise patient to notify health care professional if pregnancy is planned or suspected or if patient intends to breastfeed or is breastfeeding.
- Instruct patient to notify health care professional of medication regimen prior to treatment or surgery.
- Advise patient to carry identification describing disease process and medication regimen at all times.

Evaluation/Desired Outcomes

- Decrease in the frequency or cessation of seizures.

ticarcillin/clavulanate

(tye-kar-**sil**-in/klav-yoo-**la**-nate)
Timentin

Classification
Therapeutic: anti-infectives
Pharmacologic: extended spectrum penicillins

Pregnancy Category B

Indications

Treatment of: Skin and skin structure infections, Bone and joint infections, Septicemia, Lower respiratory tract infections, Intra-abdominal, gynecologic, and urinary tract infections.

Action

Binds to bacterial cell wall membrane, causing cell death. Addition of clavulanate enhances resistance to beta-lactamase, an enzyme that can inactivate penicillins. **Therapeutic Effects:** Bactericidal action. **Spectrum:** Similar to penicillin but extended to include several gram-negative aerobic pathogens, notably: *Pseudomonas aeruginosa*, *Escherichia coli*, *Citrobacter*, *Enterobacter*, *Haemophilus influenzae*, *Klebsiella*, *Serratia marcescens*. Active against some anaerobic bacteria, including bacteroides.

Pharmacokinetics

Absorption: IV administration resultsin complete bioavailability.
Distribution: Widely distributed. Enters CSF well when meninges are inflamed. Crosses the placenta; enters breast milk in low concentrations.
Metabolism and Excretion: 10% of ticarcillin is metabolized by the liver; 90% excreted unchanged by the kidneys. Clavulanate is metabolized by the liver.
Half-life: *Ticarcillin*—1.1 hr (increased in renal impairment); *clavulanate*—1.1 hr.

TIME/ACTION PROFILE (blood levels)

ROUTE	ONSET	PEAK	DURATION
IV	rapid	end of infusion	4–6 hr

Contraindications/Precautions

Contraindicated in: Hypersensitivity to penicillins (cross-sensitivity with cephalosporins may occur).
Use Cautiously in: Renal impairment (dose reduction and/or increased interval required if CCr <60 ml/min); Congestive heart failure (due to high sodium content); Pedi: Children <3 mo (safety and effectiveness not established); OB, Lactation: Safety not established.

Adverse Reactions/Side Effects

CNS: SEIZURES (high doses), confusion, lethargy. **CV:** CHF, arrhythmias. **GI:** PSEUDOMEMBRANOUS COLITIS, diarrhea, nausea. **GU:** hematuria (children only). **Derm:** rashes, urticaria. **F and E:** hypokalemia, hypernatremia. **Hemat:** bleeding, blood dyscrasias, increased bleeding time. **Local:** phlebitis. **Metab:** metabolic alkalosis. **Misc:** hypersensitivity reactions including ANAPHYLAXIS, superinfection.

Interactions

Drug-Drug: Probenecid ↓ renal excretion and ↑ blood levels.

Route/Dosage

Ticarcillin/clavulanate contains 4.51–6 mEq sodium/g and 0.15 mEq potassium/g of ticarcillin/clavulanate. 3 g ticarcillin plus 100 mg clavulanate labeled as 3.1 g combined potency. Dosing is based on ticarcillin component.
IV (Adults and Children >16 yr): 3 g ticarcillin q 4–6 hr.

IV (Children 3 mo–16 yr): *<60 kg*–Mild to moderate infection: 50 mg ticarcillin/kg q 6 hr; severe infection: 50 mg ticarcillin/kg q 4 hr. *≥60 kg*–Mild to moderate infection: 3 g ticarcillin q 6 hr; severe infection: 3 g ticarcillin q 4 hr.

Renal Impairment

IV (Adults): Give loading dose of 3 g ticarcillin × 1 dose, followed by maintenance dose based on CCr. *CCr 30–60 ml/min*—2 g ticarcillin q 4 hr; *10–30 ml/min*—2 g ticarcillin q 8 hr; *CCr <10 ml/min*—2 g ticarcillin q 12 hr; *CCr <10 ml/min with hepatic dysfunction*—2 g ticarcillin q 24 hr; *Peritoneal dialysis*—3 g ticarcillin q 12 hr; *Hemodialysis*—2 g ticarcillin q 12 hr supplemented with 3 g ticarcillin after each dialysis session.

Availability

Powder for injection: 3.1-g vials, 31-g vials. **Premixed infusion:** 3.1 g/100 ml.

NURSING IMPLICATIONS

Assessment

- Assess patient for infection (vital signs; appearance of wound, sputum, urine, and stool; WBC) at beginning of and throughout therapy.
- Obtain a history before initiating therapy to determine use of and reactions to penicillins or cephalosporins. Persons with a negative history of penicillin sensitivity may still have an allergic response.
- Obtain specimens for culture and sensitivity before initiating therapy. First dose may be given before receiving results.
- Observe patient for signs and symptoms of anaphylaxis (rash, pruritus, laryngeal edema, wheezing). Discontinue drug and notify physician immediately if these problems occur. Keep epinephrine, an antihistamine, and resuscitation equipment close by in case of anaphylactic reaction.
- ***Lab Test Considerations:*** Evaluate renal and hepatic function, CBC, serum potassium, and bleeding times prior to and routinely throughout therapy.
- May cause false-positive urine protein testing and increased BUN, creatinine, AST, ALT, serum bilirubin, alkaline phosphatase, LDH, and uric acid levels. May also cause ↑ bleeding time.
- May cause hypernatremia and hypokalemia with high doses.

Potential Nursing Diagnoses

Risk for infection (Indications, Side Effects)

Implementation

IV Administration

- **IV:** Change IV sites every 48 hr to prevent phlebitis
- **Intermittent Infusion:** ***Diluent:*** Add 13 ml of sterile water for injection or 0.9% NaCl for injection to each 3.1-g vial, to provide a concentration of ticarcillin 200 mg/ml and clavulanic acid 6.7 mg/ml. Further dilute in 0.9% NaCl, D5W, or LR to achieve a concentration of 10–100 mg/ml. Reconstituted vials stable for 24 hr at room temperature or 72 hr if refrigerated. Infusion is stable for 24 hr at room temperature. If refrigerated, infusion is stable for 3 days (diluted in D5W) or 7 days (if diluted in 0.9% NaCl or LR). ***Concentration:*** 10–100 mg/ml. ***Rate:*** Infuse over 30 min.
- **Y-Site Compatibility:** allopurinol, amifostine, amikacin, anidulafungin, atropine, aztreonam, bivalirudin, bumetanide, cefazolin, cefepime, cefotaxime, cefoxitin, ceftazidime, ceftizoxime, ceftriaxone, cefuroxime, chloramphenicol, cimetidine, clindamycin, cyclophosphamide, cyclosporine, dexamethasone sodium phosphate, dexmedetomidine, digoxin, diltiazem, diphenhydramine, docetaxel, dopamine, doxorubicin liposome, doxycycline, enalaprilat, epinephrine, esmolol, etoposide phosphate, famotidine, fenoldopam, filgrastim, fluconazole, furosemide, gemcitabine, gentamicin, granisetron, heparin, hydrocortisone sodium succinate, hydromorphone, imipenem/cilastatin, insulin, isoproterenol, labetalol, levofloxacin, lidocaine, linezolid, lorazepam, melphalan, meperidine, methylprednisolone sodium succinate, metoclopramide, metoprolol, metronidazole, milrinone, morphine, nitroglycerin, nitroprusside, norepinephrine, ondansetron, palonosetron, pantoprazole, pemetrexed, penicillin G potassium, perphenazine, phenylephrine, procainamide, propofol, propranolol, ranitidine, remifentanil, sargramostim, sodium bicarbonate, tacrolimus, teniposide, theophylline, thiote-

T

pa, tirofiban, tobramycin, vasopressin, verapamil, vinorelbine, voriconazole.

- **Y-Site Incompatibility:** acyclovir, amphotericin B cholesteryl sulfate, azithromycin, caspofungin, diazepam, dobutamine, drotrecogin, erythromycin, ganciclovir, haloperidol, hydroxyzine, lansoprazole, phenytoin, promethazine, protamine, quinupristin/dalfopristin, trimethoprim/sulfamethoxazole If aminoglycosides and penicillins must be administered concurrently, administer in separate sites at least 1 hr apart.

Patient/Family Teaching

- Advise patient to report signs of superinfection (black, furry overgrowth on the tongue; vaginal itching or discharge; loose or foul-smelling stools) and allergy.
- Caution patient to notify health care professional if fever and diarrhea occur, especially if stool contains blood, pus, or mucus. Advise patient not to treat diarrhea without consulting health care professional. May occur up to several weeks after discontinuation of medication.

Evaluation/Desired Outcomes

- Resolution of the signs and symptoms of infection. Length of time for complete resolution depends on the organism and site of infection.

ticlopidine (tye-**cloe**-pi-deen)

Ticlid

Classification

Therapeutic: antiplatelet agents

Pharmacologic: platelet aggregation inhibitors

Pregnancy Category B

Indications

Prevention of stroke in patients who have had a completed thrombotic stroke or precursors to stroke and are unable to tolerate aspirin. **Unlabeled uses:** Prevention of early restenosis in intracoronary stents.

Action

Inhibits platelet aggregation by altering the function of platelet membranes. Prolongs bleeding time. **Therapeutic Effects:** Decreased incidence of stroke in high-risk patients.

Pharmacokinetics

Absorption: >80% absorbed after oral administration.

Distribution: Unknown.

Protein Binding: 98%.

Metabolism and Excretion: Extensively metabolized by the liver; minimal excretion of unchanged drug by the kidneys.

Half-life: *Single dose*—12.6 hr; ***multiple dosing***—4–5 days.

TIME/ACTION PROFILE (effect on platelet function)

ROUTE	ONSET	PEAK	DURATION
PO	within 4 days	8–11 days	2 wk

Contraindications/Precautions

Contraindicated in: Hypersensitivity; Bleeding disorders; Active bleeding; Severe liver disease.

Use Cautiously in: Risk of bleeding (trauma, surgery, history of ulcer disease); Renal or hepatic impairment (dosage adjustments may be necessary); Geri: Appears on Beers list. Geriatric patients have increased sensitivity to ticlopidine; Pregnancy, lactation, or children <18 yr (safety not established).

Adverse Reactions/Side Effects

CNS: dizziness, headache, weakness. **EENT:** epistaxis, tinnitus. **GI:** diarrhea, abnormal liver function tests, anorexia, GI fullness, GI pain, nausea, vomiting. **GU:** hematuria. **Derm:** rashes, ecchymoses, pruritus, urticaria. **Hemat:** AGRANULOCYTOSIS, APLASTIC ANEMIA, INTRACEREBRAL BLEEDING, NEUTROPENIA, bleeding, thrombocytopenia. **Metab:** hypercholesterolemia, hypertriglyceridemia.

Interactions

Drug-Drug: Aspirin potentiates the effect of ticlopidine on platelets (concurrent use not recommended). Increased risk of bleeding with **heparins**, **warfarin**, **tirofiban**, **eptifibatide**, **clopidogrel**, or **thrombolytic agents**. **Cimetidine** decreases metabolism of ticlopidine and may increase the risk of toxicity. Ticlopidine decreases metabolism of **theophylline** and increases the risk of toxicity.

Drug-Food: Absorption of ticlopidine is increased by taking with **food**.

Route/Dosage

PO (Adults): 250 mg bid with food.

Availability

Tablets: 250 mg.

NURSING IMPLICATIONS

Assessment

- Assess patient for symptoms of stroke periodically throughout therapy.
- ***Lab Test Considerations:*** Monitor bleeding time throughout therapy. Prolonged bleeding time (2–5 times the normal limit), which is time- and dose-dependent, is expected.
- Monitor CBC with differential and platelet count every 2 wk from the 2nd wk to the end of the 3rd mo of therapy; more frequently if absolute neutrophil count (ANC) is declining or <30% of baseline. If neutropenia occurs, ticlopidine should be discontinued. Neutrophil counts usually return to normal within 1–3 wk of discontinuation of therapy. After the first 3 mo of therapy, CBCs need to be obtained only for patients with signs and symptoms of infection.
- May cause thrombocytopenia, usually within 3–12 wk of initiation of therapy. If platelet count is <80,000/mm^3, discontinue ticlopidine.
- May cause increased serum total cholesterol and triglyceride levels. Levels usually increase 8–10% within the first mo and persist at that level.
- May cause elevated alkaline phosphatase, bilirubin, AST, and ALT levels during the first 4 mo of therapy.
- ***Toxicity and Overdose:*** Prolonged bleeding time is normalized within 2 hr after administration of IV methylprednisolone. May also use platelet transfusions to reverse effects of ticlopidine on bleeding time.

Potential Nursing Diagnoses

Risk for injury (Indications, Side Effects)

Implementation

- **PO:** Administer with food or immediately after eating to minimize GI discomfort and increase absorption.

Patient/Family Teaching

- Instruct patient to take medication exactly as directed. Missed doses should be taken as soon as possible unless almost time for next dose; do not double doses.
- Advise patient to notify health care professional promptly if fever, chills, sore throat, unusual bleeding or bruising, severe or persistent diarrhea, skin rash, jaundice, dark-colored urine, or light-colored stools occur.
- Advise patient to notify health care professional of medication regimen before treatment or surgery. Medication may need to be discontinued 10–14 days before surgery.
- Emphasize the importance of routine lab tests during the first 3 mo of therapy to monitor for side effects.

Evaluation/Desired Outcomes

- Prevention of stroke.

tigecycline (tye-gi-sye-kleen)

Tygacil

Classification
Therapeutic: anti-infectives
Pharmacologic:

Pregnancy Category D

Indications

Complicated skin/skin structure infections or complicated intra-abdominal infections caused by susceptible bacteria.

Action

Inhibits bacterial protein synthesis by binding to the 30S ribosomal subunit. **Therapeutic Effects:** Resolution of infection. **Spectrum:** Active against the following Gram-positive bacteria: *Enterococcus faecalis* (vancomycin-susceptible strains only), *Staphylococcus aureus Streptococcus agalactiae Streptococcus anginosus* and *Streptococcus pyogenes*. Also active against these Gram-positive organisms: *Citrobacter freundii Enterobacter cloacae Escherichia coli Klebsiella oxytoca* and *Klebsiella pneumoniae*. Additionally active against the following anaerobes: *Bacteroides fragilis Bacteroides thetaiotaomicron Bacteroides uniformis Bacteroides vulgatus Clostridium perfringens* and *Peptostreptococcus micros*.

Pharmacokinetics

Absorption: IV administration results in complete bioavailability.
Distribution: Widely distributed with good penetration into gall bladder, lung and colon; crosses the placenta.
Metabolism and Excretion: Minimal metabolism; primary route of elimination is biliary/fe-

cal excretion of unchanged drug and metabolites (59%), 33% renal (22% unchanged).
Half-life: 27.1 hr (after one dose); 42.4 hr after multiple doses.

TIME/ACTION PROFILE (blood levels)

ROUTE	ONSET	PEAK	DURATION
IV	rapid	end of infusion	12 hr

Contraindications/Precautions

Contraindicated in: Hypersensitivity; Pedi: Children <18 yr.
Use Cautiously in: Complicated intra-abdominal infections due to perforation; Severe hepatic impairment (reduced maintenance dose recommended); Geri: Older patients may be more sensitive to adverse effects; OB: Use in pregnancy only when potential maternal benefit outweighs fetal risk; use cautiously during lactation.

Adverse Reactions/Side Effects

CNS: somnolence. **CV:** changes in heart rate, vasodilation. **GI:** PSEUDOMEMBRANOUS COLITIS, nausea, vomiting, altered taste, anorexia, dry mouth, jaundice. **GU:** ↑ creatinine. **Endo:** hyperglycemia. **F and E:** hypocalcemia, hyponatremia. **Local:** injection site reactions. **Misc:** allergic reactions.

Interactions

Drug-Drug: May ↓ the effectiveness of **hormonal contraceptives**. Effects on **warfarin** are unknown (monitoring recommended).

Route/Dosage

IV (Adults >18 yr): 100 mg initially, then 50 mg every 12 hr for 5–14 days.

Hepatic Impairment

IV (Adults >18 yr): *Child Pugh C*—100 mg initially, then 25 mg every 12 hr.

Availability

Lyophilized powder for reconstitution: 50 mg/5-ml vial.

NURSING IMPLICATIONS

Assessment

- Assess patient for infection (vital signs; appearance of wound, sputum, urine, and stool; WBC) at beginning of and throughout therapy.
- Obtain specimens for culture and sensitivity before initiating therapy. First dose may be given before receiving results.
- Before initiating therapy, obtain a history of tetracycline hypersensitivity; may also have an allergic response to tigecycline.
- ***Lab Test Considerations:*** May cause anemia, leukocytosis, and thrombocythemia.
- May cause ↑ serum alkaline phosphatase, amylase, bilirubin, LDH, AST, and ALT.
- May cause hyperglycemia, hypokalemia, hypoproteinemia, hypocalcemia, hyponatremia and ↑ BUN level.

Potential Nursing Diagnoses

Risk for infection (Indications)

Implementation

IV Administration

- **Intermittent Infusion:** ***Diluent:*** Reconstitute each vial with 5.3 mL of 0.9% NaCl or D5W to achieve a concentration of 10 mg/mL. Dilute further in 100 ml of D5W or 0.9% NaCl. Reconstituted solution should be yellow to orange in color. Infusion is stable for up to 6 hr at room temperature or for up to 24 hr if refrigerated. ***Concentration:*** Final concentration of infusion should be ≤1 mg/ml. ***Rate:*** Infuse over 30–60 min. Flush line before and after infusion with 0.9% NaCl or D5W.
- **Y-Site Compatibility:** amikacin, azithromycin, aztreonam, cefepime, cefotaxime, ceftazidime, ceftriaxone, cimetidine, ciprofloxacin, dobutamine, dopamine, epinephrine, ertapenem, fluconazole, gentamicin, haloperidol, heparin, imipenem/cilastatin, linezolid, lidocaine, metoclopramide, piperacillin/tazobactam, potassium chloride, propofol, ranitidine, theophylline, tobramycin, vancomycin.
- **Y-Site Incompatibility:** amphotericin B, diazepam, methylprednisolone sodium succinate, voriconazole.

Patient/Family Teaching

- Advise patient that full course of therapy should be completed, even if feeling better. Skipping doses or not completing full course of therapy may result in decreased effectiveness and increased risk of bacterial resistance.
- Advise female patient to use a nonhormonal method of contraception while taking tigecycline and until next menstrual period.
- Instruct patient to notify health care professional if fever and diarrhea develop, especially if stool contains blood, pus, or mucus. Advise patient not to treat diarrhea without consulting health care professional.

- Advise patient to report the signs of superinfection (black, furry overgrowth on the tongue, vaginal itching or discharge, loose or foul-smelling stools). Skin rash, pruritus, and urticaria should also be reported.

Evaluation/Desired Outcomes

- Resolution of signs and symptoms of infection.

timolol† (tim-oh-lole)

✤Apo-Timol, Blocadren, ✤Novo-Timol

Classification

Therapeutic: antihypertensives, vascular headache suppressants

Pharmacologic: beta blockers

Pregnancy Category C

†For ophthalmic use, see Appendix C

Indications

Hypertension (alone or with other agents). Prevention of MI. Prevention of migraine headaches. **Unlabeled uses:** Ventricular arrhythmias. Essential tremor. Anxiety.

Action

Blocks stimulation of $beta_1$ (myocardial) - and $beta_2$ (pulmonary, vascular, and uterine) -adrenergic receptor sites. **Therapeutic Effects:** Decreased heart rate and blood pressure. Prevention of MI. Decreased frequency of migraine headache.

Pharmacokinetics

Absorption: Well absorbed after oral administration.

Distribution: Enters breast milk.

Metabolism and Excretion: Extensively metabolized by the liver.

Half-life: 3–4 hr.

TIME/ACTION PROFILE (cardiovascular effects)

ROUTE	ONSET	PEAK	DURATION
PO	unknown	1–2 hr*	12–24 hr

*After single dose, full effect is not seen until several weeks of therapy

Contraindications/Precautions

Contraindicated in: Uncompensated CHF; Pulmonary edema; Cardiogenic shock; Bradycardia or heart block.

Use Cautiously in: Renal impairment; Hepatic impairment; Geriatric patients (increased sensitivity to beta blockers; initial dosage reduction recommended, consider age related decrease in body mass, renal/hepatic/cardiac function); Pulmonary disease (including asthma); Diabetes mellitus (may mask signs of hypoglycemia); Thyrotoxicosis (may mask symptoms); Patients with a history of severe allergic reactions (intensity of reactions may be increased); Pregnancy, lactation, or children (safety not established; all agents cross the placenta and may cause fetal/neonatal bradycardia, hypotension, hypoglycemia, or respiratory depression).

Adverse Reactions/Side Effects

CNS: fatigue, weakness, anxiety, depression, dizziness, drowsiness, insomnia, memory loss, mental status changes, nervousness, nightmares. **EENT:** blurred vision, dry eyes, nasal stuffiness. **Resp:** bronchospasm, wheezing. **CV:** ARRHYTHMIAS, BRADYCARDIA, CHF, PULMONARY EDEMA, orthostatic hypotension, peripheral vasoconstriction. **GI:** constipation, diarrhea, nausea. **GU:** erectile dysfunction, decreased libido. **Derm:** itching, rashes. **Endo:** hyperglycemia, hypoglycemia. **MS:** arthralgia, back pain, muscle cramps. **Neuro:** paresthesia. **Misc:** ANAPHYLAXIS (rare).

Interactions

Drug-Drug: General anesthesia, IV phenytoin, and **verapamil** may ↑ myocardial depression. ↑ bradycardia may occur with **digoxin**. ↑ hypotension may occur with other **antihypertensives**, acute ingestion of **alcohol**, or **nitrates**. Concurrent use with **amphetamines, cocaine, ephedrine, epinephrine, norepinephrine, phenylephrine**, or **pseudoephedrine** may result in unopposed alpha-adrenergic stimulation (excessive hypertension, bradycardia). Concurrent **thyroid** administration may ↓ effectiveness. May alter the effectiveness of **insulins** or **oral antidiabetics** (dosage adjustments may be necessary). May ↓ effectiveness of **bronchodilators** and **theophylline**. May ↓ beneficial cardiovascular effects of **dopamine** or **dobutamine**. Use cautiously within 14 days of **MAO inhibitor** therapy (may result in hypertension). **Cimeti-**

dine may ↑ toxicity. Concurrent **NSAIDs** may ↓ antihypertensive action.

Route/Dosage

PO (Adults): *Antihypertensive*—10 mg twice daily initially; may be increased q 7 days as needed (usual maintenance dose is 10–20 mg twice daily; up to 60 mg/day). *Prevention of MI*—10 mg twice daily, starting 1–4 wk after MI. *Prevention of vascular headache*—10 mg twice daily initially, may be given as a single daily dose; may be increased up to 10 mg in the morning and 20 mg in the evening.

Availability (generic available)

Tablets: 5 mg, 10 mg, 20 mg.

NURSING IMPLICATIONS

Assessment

- Monitor blood pressure and pulse frequently during dose adjustment period and periodically during therapy. Assess for orthostatic hypotension when assisting patient up from supine position.
- Monitor intake and output ratios and daily weight. Assess patient routinely for evidence of fluid overload (peripheral edema, dyspnea, rales/crackles, fatigue, weight gain, jugular venous distention).
- **Hypertension:** Monitor frequency of prescription refills to determine adherence.
- **Vascular Headache Prophylaxis:** Assess frequency, severity, characteristics, and location of vascular headaches periodically during therapy.
- ***Lab Test Considerations:*** May cause ↑ BUN, serum lipoprotein, potassium, triglyceride, and uric acid levels.
- May cause ↑ ANA titers.
- May cause ↑ in blood glucose levels.
- ***Toxicity and Overdose:*** Monitor patients receiving beta blockers for signs of overdose (bradycardia, severe dizziness or fainting, severe drowsiness, dyspnea, bluish fingernails or palms, seizures). Notify physician or other health care provider immediately if these signs occur: Glucagon has been used to treat bradycardia and hypotension.

Potential Nursing Diagnoses

Decreased cardiac output (Side Effects)
Noncompliance (Patient/Family Teaching)

Implementation

- **PO:** Take apical pulse before administering. If <50 bpm or if arrhythmia occurs, withhold medication and notify physician or other health care professional.
- May be administered with food or on an empty stomach.
- Tablets may be crushed and mixed with food.

Patient/Family Teaching

- Instruct patient to take medication as directed, at the same time each day, even if feeling well; do not skip or double up on missed doses. Take missed doses as soon as possible up to 4 hr before next dose. Abrupt withdrawal may precipitate life-threatening arrhythmias, hypertension, or myocardial ischemia.
- Advise patient to make sure that enough medication is available for weekends, holidays, and vacations. A written prescription may be kept in wallet in case of emergency.
- Teach patient and family how to check pulse daily and blood pressure biweekly. Advise patient to hold dose and contact health care professional if pulse is <50 bpm or blood pressure changes significantly.
- May cause drowsiness or dizziness. Caution patients to avoid driving or other activities that require alertness until response to the drug is known.
- Advise patients to change positions slowly to minimize orthostatic hypotension, especially during initiation of therapy or when dose is increased.
- Caution patient that this medication may increase sensitivity to cold.
- Instruct patient to consult health care professional before taking any OTC medications or herbal products, especially cold preparations, concurrently with this medication.
- Patients with diabetes should closely monitor blood glucose, especially if weakness, malaise, irritability, or fatigue occurs. Medication may mask tachycardia and increased blood pressure as signs of hypoglycemia, but dizziness and sweating may still occur.
- Advise patient to notify health care professional if slow pulse, difficulty breathing, wheezing, cold hands and feet, dizziness, confusion, depression, rash, fever, sore throat, unusual bleeding, or bruising occurs.
- Instruct patient to inform health care professional of medication regimen before treatment or surgery.
- Advise patient to carry identification describing disease process and medication regimen at all times.
- **Hypertension:** Reinforce the need to continue additional therapies for hypertension

(weight loss, sodium restriction, stress reduction, regular exercise, moderation of alcohol consumption, and smoking cessation). Medication controls but does not cure hypertension.

- **Vascular Headache Prophylaxis:** Caution patient that sharing this medication may be dangerous.

Evaluation/Desired Outcomes

- Decrease in blood pressure.
- Prevention of MI.
- Prevention of vascular headaches.

tinidazole (ti-**nid**-a-zole)
Tindamax

Classification
Therapeutic: antiprotozoals
Pharmacologic: imidazoles

Pregnancy Category C

Indications

Bacterial vaginosis. Trichamoniasis. Giardiasis. Amebiasis.

Action

Interaction with protozoa results in release of a free nitro radical that has antiprotozoal activity. **Therapeutic Effects:** Resolution of protozoal infections. **Spectrum:** Active against *Trichamonas vaginalis*, *Giardia duodenalis* (also known as *Giardia lamblia*), and *Entamoeba histolytica*.

Pharmacokinetics

Absorption: Rapidly and completely absorbed following oral administration.
Distribution: Extensively distributed; crosses placenta and blood-brain barrier, enters breast milk.
Metabolism and Excretion: Mostly metabolized (CYP3A4 enzyme system); 20–25% excreted unchanged in urine, 12% excreted in feces.
Half-life: 12–14 hr.

TIME/ACTION PROFILE (blood levels)

ROUTE	ONSET	PEAK	DURATION
PO	rapid	2 hr	24 hr

Contraindications/Precautions

Contraindicated in: Hypersensitivity; cross sensitivity with other imidazoles may occur; First trimester of pregnancy; Lactation.
Use Cautiously in: CNS pathology; History of blood dyscrasia; Hemodialysis (removes significant amount of tinidazole; supplement post-dialysis with additional 50% of dose); Hepatic impairment; Unrecognized candidiasis (requires concurrent antifungal therapy); Children younger than 3 yr (safety not established).

Adverse Reactions/Side Effects

CNS: dizziness, headache, malaise. **GI:** constipation, dyspepsia, metallic/bitter taste, vomiting. **Hemat:** transient leukopenia/neutropenia.

Interactions

Drug-Drug: ↑ risk of bleeding with **warfarin**. Disulfiram-like reaction may occur with **alcohol** or **propylene glycol**; **disulfiram** should be avoided for at least 2 weeks before tinidazole. May ↑ level of **lithium**, **cyclosporine**, **tacrolimus**, **fluorouracil**, and **intravenous fosphenytoin** (observe/monitor for toxicity if administered concurrently). **Drugs that induce to CYP450 liver enzyme system** (**phenobarbital**, **rifampin**, **phenytoin** or **fosphenytoin**) may ↓ levels and effectiveness. **Drugs that inhibit to CYP450 liver enzyme system** (**cimetidine** or **ketoconazole**) may ↑ levels. **Oxytetracycline** may ↓ effectiveness. Absorption is ↓ by **cholestyramine**; separate dosing.

Route/Dosage

PO (Adults): *Bacterial vaginosis*—1 g for 5 days; *Trichamoniasis and Giardiasis*—2 g single dose; *Intestinal amebiasis*—2 g/day for 3 days; *Amebic liver abscess*—2 g/day for 3–5 days.
PO (Children older than 3 yr): *Giardiasis*—50 mg/kg (up to 2 g) single dose; *Intestinal amebiasis*—50 mg/kg/day for 3 days; *Amebic liver abscess*—50 mg/kg/day for 3–5 days.

Availability

Tablets: 250 mg, 500 mg.

NURSING IMPLICATIONS

Assessment

- Assess patient for symptoms of infection (discharge, itching) prior to and during therapy.
- Monitor neurologic status during and after IV infusions. Inform health care professional if numbness, paresthesia, weakness, ataxia, or convulsions occur.

T

- **Giardiasis:** Monitor three stool samples taken several days apart, beginning 3–4 wk after treatment.
- ***Lab Test Considerations:*** May cause transient leukopenia and neutropenia. Monitor total and differential leukocyte counts if retreatment is necessary.
- May interfere with certain tests of serum chemistry values such as AST, ALT, LDH, triglycerides, and glucose hexokinase.

Potential Nursing Diagnoses
Risk for infection (Indications)
Diarrhea (Indications)

Implementation
- Symptoms of known or previously unrecognized candidiasis may become worsen during therapy and require treatment with an antifungal agent.
- **PO:** Administer with food to decrease GI upset. May be crushed and prepared as a suspension in cherry syrup by pharmacist for patients unable to swallow tablets. Shake well before administering.

Patient/Family Teaching
- Instruct patient to take medication as directed, even if feeling better. Do not skip doses or double up on missed doses. If a dose is missed, take as soon as remembered if not almost time for next dose.
- Advise patients treated for trichomoniasis that sexual partners may be asymptomatic sources of reinfection and should be treated concurrently. Patient should also refrain from intercourse or use a condom to prevent reinfection.
- Caution patient to avoid intake of alcoholic beverages or preparations containing alcohol during and for at least 3 days after treatment with tinidazole. May cause a disulfiram-like reaction (flushing, nausea, vomiting, headache, abdominal cramps).
- May cause dizziness or drowsiness. Caution patient to avoid driving or other activities requiring alertness until response to medication is known.
- Inform patient that medication may cause an unpleasant metallic taste.
- Advise patient not to take Rx, OTC, or herbal products without consulting health care professional.
- Advise patient to inform health care professional if pregnancy is suspected before taking this medication.

Evaluation/Desired Outcomes
- Resolution of signs and symptoms of infection.

tinzaparin, See HEPARINS (LOW MOLECULAR WEIGHT).

tioconazole, See ANTIFUNGALS (VAGINAL).

tiotropium
(tye-o-**trope**-ee-yum)
Spiriva

Classification
Therapeutic: bronchodilators
Pharmacologic: anticholinergics

Pregnancy Category C

Indications
Long term maintenance treatment of bronchospasm due to COPD.

Action
Acts an anticholinergic by selectively and reversibly inhibiting M_3 receptors in smooth muscle of airways. **Therapeutic Effects:** Decreased incidence and severity of bronchospasm.

Pharmacokinetics
Absorption: 19.5% absorbed following inhalation.
Distribution: Extensive tissue distribution; due to route of administration ↑ concentrations occur in lung.
Metabolism and Excretion: 74% excreted unchanged in urine; 25% of absorbed drug is metabolized.
Half-life: 5–6 days.

TIME/ACTION PROFILE (bronchodilation)

ROUTE	ONSET	PEAK	DURATION
inhaln	rapid	5 min	24 hr

Contraindications/Precautions
Contraindicated in: Hypersensitivity to tiotropium, atropine of their derivatives; Concurrent ipratropium.
Use Cautiously in: Angle-closure glaucoma, prostatic hyperplasia, bladder neck obstruction (may worsen condition); CCr ≤50 ml/min (monitor closely); Pregnancy, lactation or children (safety not established).

Adverse Reactions/Side Effects

EENT: glaucoma. **Resp:** paradoxical bronchospasm. **CV:** ↑ heart rate. **GI:** dry mouth, constipation. **GU:** urinary difficulty, urinary retention. **Misc:** hypersensitivity reactions including ANGIOEDEMA.

Interactions

Drug-Drug: Should not be used concurrently with **ipratropium** due to risk of additive anticholinergic effects.

Route/Dosage

Inhaln (Adults): 18 mcg once daily.

Availability

Dry powder capsules for inhalation: 18 mcg. **Cost:** $134.99/30 capsules.

NURSING IMPLICATIONS

Assessment

- **Inhaln:** Assess respiratory status (rate, breath sounds, degree of dyspnea, pulse) before administration and at peak of medication. Consult physician or other health care professional about alternative medication if severe bronchospasm is present; onset of action is too slow for patients in acute distress. If paradoxical bronchospasm (wheezing) occurs, withhold medication and notify physician or other health care professional immediately.

Potential Nursing Diagnoses

Ineffective airway clearance (Indications)
Risk for activity intolerance (Indications)

Implementation

Inhaln: See Appendix D for administration of inhalation medications.

Patient/Family Teaching

- Instruct patient to take medication as directed. Capsules are for inhalation only and must not be swallowed. Take missed doses as soon as remembered unless almost time for the next dose; space remaining doses evenly during day. Do not double doses.
- Advise patient that tiopropium is not to be used for acute bronchospasm attacks, but may be continued during an acute exacerbation.
- Instruct patient in proper use and cleaning of the Handihaler inhaler. Review the *Patient's Instructions for Use* guide with patient. Capsules should be stored in sealed blisters; remove immediately before use or effectiveness of capsules is reduced. Tear blister strip carefully to expose only one capsule at a time. Discard capsules that are inadvertently exposed to air. *Spiriva* should be administered only via the Handihaler and the Handihaler should not be used with other medications. When disposing of capsule, tiny amount of powder left in capsule is normal.
- Advise patient that rinsing mouth after using inhaler, good oral hygiene, and sugarless gum or candy may minimize dry mouth; usually resolves with continued treatment.
- Advise patient to notify health care professional immediately if signs of glaucoma (eye pain or discomfort, blurred vision, visual halos or colored images in association with red eyes from conjunctival congestion and corneal edema) occur.
- Caution patient to avoid spraying medication in eyes; may cause blurring of vision and pupil dilation.
- Advise patient to inform health care professional if pregnancy is planned or suspected or if breastfeeding.
- Advise patient to consult health care professional before taking any Rx/OTC/herbal products, including eye drops.

Evaluation/Desired Outcomes

- Decreased dyspnea.
- Improved breath sounds.

T

tipranavir (ti-pran-a-veer)

Aptivus

Classification
Therapeutic: antiretrovirals
Pharmacologic: protease inhibitors

Pregnancy Category C

Indications

Advanced HIV disease resistant to other anti-HIV therapies (must be used with ritonavir).

Action

Inhibits processing of viral polyproteins, preventing formation of mature virions. **Therapeutic Effects:** Decreased viral load and sequelae of HIV infection.

Pharmacokinetics

Absorption: Well absorbed following oral administration.

Distribution: Unknown.
Protein Binding: >99.9%.
Metabolism and Excretion: Rapidly and extensively metabolized (primarily by CYP3A4), requiring co-administration with ritonavir as a metabolic inhibitor to achieve therapeutic blood levels; eliminated mostly in feces, minimal renal excretion.
Half-life: 5.5–6 hr.

TIME/ACTION PROFILE (blood levels*)

ROUTE	ONSET	PEAK	DURATION
PO	rapid	2 hr	12 hr

* With ritonavir

Contraindications/Precautions

Contraindicated in: Hypersensitivity; Moderate to severe hepatic impairment (Child-Pugh Class B or C); Concurrent use of some antiarrhythmics (amiodarone, flecainide, propafenone, quinidine), ergot derivatives, midazolam or triazolam.
Use Cautiously in: Known sulfonamide allergy (contains sulfa moiety); Pre-existing liver disease (may increase the risk of hepatotoxicity); History of or risk factors for diabetes (may cause hyperglycemia); Hemophilia (may ↑ risk of bleeding); Pedi: Safe use in children not established.

Adverse Reactions/Side Effects

CV: INTRACRANIAL HEMORRHAGE, fatigue, headache. **GI:** HEPATOTOXICITY, abdominal pain, diarrhea, nausea, vomiting. **Derm:** rash (↑ in women). **Endo:** hyperglycemia. **Metab:** ↑ cholesterol, ↑ triglycerides. **Misc:** allergic reactions, fat redistribution, fever, immune reconstitution syndrome.

Interactions

Drug-Drug: Increases blood levels and risk of toxicity from some **antiarrhythmics (amiodarone, flecainide, propafenone, quinidine)**, **ergot derivatives (dihydroergotamine, ergonovine, ergotamine, methylergonovine)**. Concurrent use with **ritonavir** may lead to intracranial hemorrhage. **Antacids** ↓ absorption (separate dosing). **Hormonal contraceptives** may ↑ risk of rash. May ↓ effectiveness of **hormonal contraceptives**.

Route/Dosage

PO (Adults): 500 mg twice daily; must be taken with ritonavir 200 mg.

Availability

Capsules: 250 mg.

NURSING IMPLICATIONS

Assessment

- Assess for change in severity of HIV symptoms and for symptoms of opportunistic infections during therapy.
- Monitor for hepatitis (fatigue, malaise, anorexia, nausea, jaundice, bilirubinuria, acholic stools, liver tenderness, hepatomegaly).
- Assess for sulfa allergy. May be cross sensitive.
- ***Lab Test Considerations:*** Monitor viral load and CD4 counts regularly during therapy.
- May cause ↑ AST and ↑ ALT; monitor prior to and frequently during therapy. Tipranavir should be discontinued if symptomatic ↑ of AST and ALT of 10 times the upper limit of normal or symptomatic ↑ of AST and ALT of 5–10 times the upper limit of normal and bilirubin ↑ 2.5 time the upper limit of normal occur.
- Monitor triglyceride and cholesterol levels prior to and periodically during therapy; may cause ↑.
- May cause hyperglycemia. Monitor blood glucose carefully, especially in patients with diabetes.

Potential Nursing Diagnoses

Risk for infection (Indications)
Noncompliance (Patient/Family Teaching)

Implementation

- **PO:** Administer with ritonavir twice daily with meals. Bioavailability is increased with high at meal.
- Store capsules in refrigerator. Use within 60 days of opening bottle. Write opening date on label; do not use after expiration date written. If used away from home, bottle may be kept at room temperature in a cool place.

Patient/Family Teaching

- Emphasize the importance of taking tipranavir exactly as directed, at evenly spaced times throughout day. Patients should read the *Patient Package Insert* before initiating therapy and with each prescription refill. Do not take more than prescribed amount and do not stop taking without consulting health care professional. Take missed doses as soon as remembered; do not double doses.

- Instruct patient that tipranavir should not be shared with others.
- Advise patient to avoid taking other Rx, OTC, or herbal products without consulting health care professional.
- Inform patient that tipranavir does not cure AIDS or prevent associated or opportunistic infections. Tipranavir does not reduce the risk of transmission of HIV to others through sexual contact or blood contamination. Caution patient to use a condom during sexual contact and to avoid sharing needles or donating blood to prevent spreading the AIDS virus to others.
- Advise patients stop taking tipranavir and ritonavir and notify health care professional immediately if signs of hepatitis (fatigue, malaise, anorexia, nausea, jaundice) or unusual bleeding occur. May require discontinuation of therapy.
- Inform patient that tipranavir may cause hyperglycemia. Advise patient to notify health care professional if increased thirst or hunger; unexplained weight loss; increased urination; fatigue; or dry, itchy skin occurs.
- Advise women taking hormonal contraceptives to use a nonhormonal form of contraception during tipranavir therapy, and of increased risk of rash.
- Inform patient that redistribution and accumulation of body fat may occur, causing central obesity, dorsocervical fat enlargement (buffalo hump), peripheral wasting, breast enlargement, and cushingoid appearance. The cause and long-term effects are not known.
- Emphasize the importance of regular follow-up exams and blood counts to determine progress and monitor for side effects.

Evaluation/Desired Outcomes

- Delayed progression of AIDS and decreased opportunistic infections in patients with HIV.
- Decrease in viral load and improvement in CD4 cell counts.

HIGH ALERT

tirofiban (tye-roe-**fye**-ban)

Aggrastat

Classification

Therapeutic: antiplatelet agents

Pharmacologic: glycoprotein IIb/IIIa inhibitors

Pregnancy Category B

Indications

Treatment of acute coronary syndrome (unstable angina/non–Q-wave MI), including patients who will be managed medically and those who will undergo percutaneous transluminal angioplasty (PCTA) or atherectomy. Used concurrently with aspirin and heparin.

Action

Decreases platelet aggregation by reversibly antagonizing the binding of fibrinogen to the glycoprotein IIb/IIIa binding site on platelet surfaces. **Therapeutic Effects:** Inhibition of platelet aggregation resulting in decreased incidence of new MI, death, or refractory ischemia with the need for repeat cardiac procedures.

Pharmacokinetics

Absorption: IV administration results in complete bioavailability.

Distribution: Unknown.

Metabolism and Excretion: Excreted mostly unchanged by the kidneys (65%); 25% excreted unchanged in feces.

Half-life: 2 hr.

TIME/ACTION PROFILE (effects on platelet function)

ROUTE	ONSET	PEAK	DURATION
IV	rapid	30 min†	brief‡

†>90% inhibition of platelet aggregation at end of initial 30-min infusion

‡Inhibition is reversible following cessation of infusion

Contraindications/Precautions

Contraindicated in: Hypersensitivity; Active internal bleeding or history of bleeding within previous 30 days; History of intracranial hemorrhage, intracranial neoplasm, arteriovenous malformation or aneurysm; History of thrombocytopenia during previous tirofiban therapy; History of hemorrhagic stroke or other stroke within 30 days; Major surgical procedure or severe physical trauma within 30 days; History, symptoms, or other findings associated with aortic aneurysm; Severe hypertension (systolic BP >180 mm Hg and/or diastolic BP >110 mm

T

Hg); Concurrent use of other glycoprotein IIb/IIIa receptor antagonists; Acute pericarditis; Lactation.

Use Cautiously in: Platelet count <150,000/mm^3; Hemorrhagic retinopathy; Female patients and geriatric patients (↑ risk of bleeding); Severe renal insufficiency (↓ rate of infusion by 50% if CCr <30 ml/min); Pregnancy or children (safety not established; use in pregnancy only if clearly needed).

Adverse Reactions/Side Effects

Noted for patients receiving heparin and aspirin in addition to tirofiban.

CNS: dizziness, headache. **CV:** bradycardia, coronary dissection, edema, vasovagal reaction. **GI:** nausea. **Derm:** hives, rash. **Hemat:** BLEEDING, thrombocytopenia. **MS:** leg pain. **Misc:** fever, hypersensitivity reactions, pelvic pain, sweating.

Interactions

Drug-Drug: Aspirin, other **NSAIDs**, **warfarin**, **heparin** and **heparin-like agents**, **abciximab**, **eptifibatide**, **clopidogrel**, **ticlopidine**, or **dipyridamole**—concurrent use may ↑ risk of bleeding, although these agents are frequently used together or in sequence. Risk of bleeding may be ↑ by concurrent use of **cefotetan**, **cefoperazone**, or **valproic acid**.

Drug-Natural Products: ↑ anticoagulant effect and bleeding risk with **anise**, **arnica**, **chamomile**, **clove**, **dong quai**, **fenugreek**, **feverfew**, **garlic**, **ginger**, **ginkgo**, **Panax ginseng**, **licorice**, and others.

Route/Dosage

IV (Adults): 0.4 mcg/kg/min for 30 min, then 0.1 mcg/kg/min, continued throughout angiography and for 12–24 hr after angioplasty or atherectomy.

Renal Impairment

IV (Adults): *CCr <30 ml/min*—0.2 mcg/kg/min for 30 min, then 0.05 mcg/kg/min, continued throughout angiography and for 12–24 hr after angioplasty or atherectomy.

Availability

Concentrated solution for IV infusion (dilute before use): 12.5 mg/50 ml (250 mcg/ml) in 50-ml vials. **Premixed solution for infusion:** 5 mg/100 ml (50 mcg/ml) in 100-ml single-dose containers, 12.5 mg/250 ml (50 mcg/ml) in 250-ml single-dose containers.

NURSING IMPLICATIONS

Assessment

- Assess patient for bleeding. Most common is oozing from the arterial access site for cardiac catheterization. Arterial and venous punctures, IM injections, and use of urinary catheters, nasotracheal intubation, and nasogastric tubes should be minimized. Noncompressible sites for IV access should be avoided. If bleeding cannot be controlled with pressure, discontinue tirofiban and heparin immediately.
- During vascular access, avoid puncturing posterior wall of femoral artery. Maintain bedrest with head of bed elevated 30° and affected limb restrained in a straight position while the vascular sheath is in place. Heparin should be discontinued for 3–4 hr and activated clotting time (ACT) <180 sec or activated partial thromboplastin time (aPTT) <45 sec prior to pulling the sheath. Use compressive techniques to obtain hemostasis and monitor closely. Sheath hemostasis should be maintained for >4 hr before discharge from the hospital.
- Monitor for signs of thrombocytopenia (chills, low-grade fever) during therapy.
- ***Lab Test Considerations:*** Assess hemoglobin, hematocrit, and platelet count prior to tirofiban therapy, within 6 hr following loading infusion, and at least daily during therapy (more frequently if evidence of significant decline). May cause decreased hemoglobin and hematocrit.
- If platelet count decreases to <90,000/mm^3, perform additional platelet counts to rule out pseudothrombocytopenia. If thrombocytopenia is confirmed, tirofiban and heparin should be discontinued and condition monitored and treated.
- To monitor unfractionated heparin, assess aPTT 6 hr after the start of heparin infusion. Adjust heparin to maintain aPTT at approximately 2 times control.
- May cause presence of urine and fecal occult blood.

Potential Nursing Diagnoses

Ineffective tissue perfusion (Indications)

Implementation

- ***High Alert:*** Use of antiplatelet medications has resulted in patient harm and/or death from internal hemorrhage or intracranial bleeding. Have second practitioner indepen-

dently check original order, dosage calculations, and infusion pump settings.
- Most patients receive heparin and aspirin concurrently with tirofiban.
- Do not administer solutions that are discolored or contain particulate matter. Discard unused portion.

IV Administration

- **Intermittent Infusion:** ***Diluent:*** Tirofiban injection vials must be diluted to same concentration as premixed solution (50 mcg/ml). Withdraw and discard 100 ml from a 500-ml bag of 0.9% NaCl or D5W and replace volume with 100 ml of tirofiban (from two 50-ml vials) or withdraw and discard 50 ml from a 250-ml bag of 0.9% NaCl or D5W and replace volume with 50 ml of tirofiban (from one vial). Mix well prior to administration. The tirofiban injection premix is ready for administration and dose not require any further dilution. ***Concentration:*** 50 mcg/ml. ***Rate:*** Based on patient's weight (see Route/Dosage section).
- **Y-Site Compatibility:** amiodarone, argatroban, atropine, bivalirudin, dobutamine, dopamine, epinephrine, famotidine, furosemide, heparin, lidocaine, midazolam, morphine, nitroglycerin, potassium chloride, propranolol.
- **Y-Site Incompatibility:** diazepam.

Patient/Family Teaching

- Inform patient of the purpose of tirofiban.
- Instruct patient to notify health care professional immediately if any bleeding is noted.

Evaluation/Desired Outcomes

- Inhibition of platelet aggregation resulting in decreased incidence of new MI, death, or refractory ischemia with the need for repeat cardiac procedures.

tizanidine (tye-zan-i-deen)

Zanaflex

Classification

Therapeutic: antispasticity agents (centrally acting)

Pharmacologic: adrenergics

Pregnancy Category C

Indications

Increased muscle tone associated with spasticity due to multiple sclerosis or spinal cord injury.

Action

Acts as an agonist at central alpha-adrenergic receptor sites. Reduces spasticity by increasing presynaptic inhibition of motor neurons. **Therapeutic Effects:** Decreased spasticity, allowing better function.

Pharmacokinetics

Absorption: Completely absorbed after oral administration but rapidly metabolized, resulting in 40% bioavailability.

Distribution: Widely distributed.

Metabolism and Excretion: 95% metabolized by the liver.

Half-life: 2.5 hr.

TIME/ACTION PROFILE (reduced muscle tone)

ROUTE	ONSET	PEAK	DURATION
PO	unknown	1–2 hr	3–6 hr

Contraindications/Precautions

Contraindicated in: Hypersensitivity.

Use Cautiously in: Renal impairment; Geri: Geriatric patients; Concurrent antihypertensive therapy; OB, Pedi: Pregnancy, lactation, or children (safety not established).

Exercise Extreme Caution in: Impaired hepatic function.

Adverse Reactions/Side Effects

CNS: anxiety, depression, dizziness, sedation, weakness, dyskinesia, hallucinations, nervousness. **EENT:** blurred vision, pharyngitis, rhinitis. **CV:** hypotension, bradycardia. **GI:** abdominal pain, diarrhea, dry mouth, dyspepsia, constipation, hepatocellular injury, increased liver enzymes, vomiting. **GU:** urinary frequency. **Derm:** rash, skin ulcers, sweating. **MS:** back pain, myasthenia, paresthesia. **Misc:** fever, speech disorder.

Interactions

Drug-Drug: Blood levels and effects ↑ by concurrent use of **hormonal contraceptives** or **alcohol**. ↑ risk of hypotension with **alpha$_2$-adrenergic agonist antihypertensives** (avoid concurrent use). ↑ CNS depression may occur with **alcohol** or other **CNS depressants** including some **antidepressants**, **sedative/hypnotics**, **antihistamines**, and

T

opioid analgesics. Concurrent CYP1A2 inhbitors (**ciprofloxacin**, **fluvoxamine** and others) may ↑ levels and risk of hypotension and excessive sedation.

Route/Dosage

PO (Adults): 4 mg q 6–8 hr initially (no more than 3 doses/24 hr); increase by 2–4 mg/dose up to 8 mg/dose or 24 mg/day (not to exceed 36 mg/day). Some patients may tolerate twice-daily dosing.

Availability (generic available)

Tablets: 2 mg, 4 mg. **Cost:** *Generic*—2 mg \$19.99/90, 4 mg \$81.99/90. **Capsules:** 2 mg, 4 mg, 6 mg. **Cost:** 2 mg \$159.70/90, 4 mg \$216.37/90, 6 mg \$300.35/90.

NURSING IMPLICATIONS

Assessment

- Assess muscle spasticity before and periodically during therapy.
- Monitor blood pressure and pulse, especially during dose titration. May cause orthostatic hypotension, bradycardia, dizziness, and, rarely, syncope. Effects are usually dose related
- Observe patient for drowsiness, dizziness, and asthenia. A change in dose may alleviate these problems.
- ***Lab Test Considerations:*** Monitor liver function tests before and at 1, 3, and 6 mo of therapy. May cause ↑ in serum glucose, alkaline phosphatase, AST, and ALT levels.

Potential Nursing Diagnoses

Impaired physical mobility (Indications)
Risk for injury (Adverse Reactions)

Implementation

- Do not confuse tizanidine with tiagibine.
- Doses should be titrated carefully to prevent side effects.
- **PO:** May be taken without regard to meals.

Patient/Family Teaching

- Instruct patient to take tizanidine as directed. Tizanidine may need to be discontinued gradually.
- May cause dizziness and drowsiness. Advise patient to avoid driving or other activities requiring alertness until response to drug is known.
- Instruct patient to change positions slowly to minimize orthostatic hypotension.
- Advise patient to avoid concurrent use of alcohol or other CNS depressants while taking this medication.

Evaluation/Desired Outcomes

- Decrease in muscle spasticity with an increased ability to perform activities of daily living.

tobramycin, See AMINOGLYCOSIDES.

tolcapone (tole-ka-pone)

Tasmar

Classification
Therapeutic: antiparkinson agents
Pharmacologic: catechol-O-methyltransferase inhibitors

Pregnancy Category C

Indications

Management of Parkinson's disease with carbidopa/levodopa in patients without severe movement abnormalities who do not respond to other treatment.

Action

Acts as a selective and reversible inhibitor of the enzyme catechol- *O* -methyltransferase. Inhibition of this enzyme prevents the breakdown of levodopa, greatly increasing its availability to the CNS. **Therapeutic Effects:** Prolongs duration of response to levodopa without end-of-dose motor fluctuations. Decreased signs and symptoms of Parkinson's disease.

Pharmacokinetics

Absorption: Rapidly absorbed following oral administration with 65% bioavailability.
Distribution: Unknown.
Protein Binding: >99% bound to plasma proteins.
Metabolism and Excretion: Mostly metabolized by the liver; <0.5% excreted unchanged in urine.
Half-life: 2–3 hr.

TIME/ACTION PROFILE (blood levels)

ROUTE	ONSET	PEAK	DURATION
PO	unknown	1.7 hr	8 hr

Contraindications/Precautions

Contraindicated in: Hypersensitivity; Concurrent MAO inhibitor therapy; Clinical evidence of liver disease.
Use Cautiously in: Severe renal impairment (safety not established if CCr <25 ml/min); OB: Pregnancy or lactation (safety not established).

Adverse Reactions/Side Effects

CNS: headache, sleep disorder, hallucinations, syncope. **CV:** orthostatic hypotension. **GI:** HEPATOTOXICITY, HEPATIC FAILURE, constipation, diarrhea, anorexia, elevated liver enzymes, nausea, vomiting. **GU:** hematuria, yellow discoloration of urine. **Derm:** increased sweating. **Neuro:** dyskinesia, dystonia.

Interactions

Drug-Drug: Concurrent use with **MAO inhibitors** is not recommended; both agents inhibit the metabolic pathways of catecholamines. May increase the effects of **methyldopa**, **apomorphine**, **dobutamine**, or **isoproterenol**; dose reduction may be necessary. Increases the bioavailability of **levodopa** by two-fold; this is a desired effect.

Route/Dosage

PO (Adults): 100 mg 3 times daily; may be cautiously increased to 200 mg 3 times daily if benefit is justified.

Availability

Tablets: 100 mg, 200 mg.

NURSING IMPLICATIONS

Assessment

- Assess patient for signs and symptoms of Parkinson's disease (tremor, muscle weakness and rigidity, ataxic gait) prior to and throughout therapy.
- Assess blood pressure periodically throughout therapy.
- ***Lab Test Considerations:*** Monitor liver function tests monthly during the first 3 mo of therapy and every 6 wk for the next 6 wk of treatment. Tolcapone should be discontinued if liver function tests reach 2 times the upper limit of normal or if jaundice occurs.

Potential Nursing Diagnoses

Impaired physical mobility (Indications)
Risk for injury (Indications, Side Effects)

Implementation

- **PO:** Administer first dose of the day of tolcapone together with carbidopa/levodopa. Administer subsequent doses 6 and 12 hr later.
- May be administered without regard to food.

Patient/Family Teaching

- Instruct patient to take medication exactly as directed. Caution patient not to discontinue medication without consulting health care professional. Abrupt discontinuation or rapid dose reduction may result in neuroleptic malignant syndrome (elevated temperature, muscular rigidity, altered consciousness).
- Caution patient to make position changes slowly to minimize orthostatic hypotension, especially at the beginning of therapy.
- May affect mental and/or motor performance. Caution patient to avoid driving or other activities requiring alertness until response to medication is known.
- Advise patient to avoid taking alcohol or other CNS depressants concurrently with tolcapone.
- Inform patient and caregiver that hallucinations, nausea, dyskinesia, or dystonia may occur during tolcapone therapy.
- OB: Advise patient to notify health care professional if pregnancy is planned or suspected.
- Instruct patient to notify health care professional if persistent diarrhea occurs.

Evaluation/Desired Outcomes

- Decrease in signs and symptoms of Parkinson's disease.

---

tolnaftate, See ANTIFUNGALS (TOPICAL).

---

tolterodine (tol-**ter**-oh-deen)

Detrol, Detrol LA

Classification

Therapeutic: urinary tract antispasmodics
Pharmacologic: anticholinergics

Pregnancy Category C

Indications

Treatment of overactive bladder function that results in urinary frequency, urgency, or urge incontinence.

Action

Acts as a competitive muscarinic receptor antagonist resulting in inhibition of cholinergically mediated bladder contraction. **Therapeutic Effects:** Decreased urinary frequency, urgency, and urge incontinence.

Pharmacokinetics

Absorption: Well absorbed (77%) following oral administration.
Distribution: Unknown.
Protein Binding: 96.3%.
Metabolism and Excretion: Extensively metabolized by the liver; one metabolite (5-hydroxymethyltolterodine) is active; other metabolites are excreted in urine.
Half-life: *Tolterodine*—1.9–3.7 hr; *5-hydroxymethyltolterodine*—2.9–3.1 hr.

TIME/ACTION PROFILE (effects on bladder function)

ROUTE	ONSET	PEAK	DURATION
PO	unknown	unknown	12 hr

Contraindications/Precautions

Contraindicated in: Urinary retention; Gastric retention; Uncontrolled angle-closure glaucoma; Lactation.
Use Cautiously in: GI obstructive disorders, including pyloric stenosis (increased risk of gastric retention); Significant bladder outflow obstruction (increased risk of urinary retention); Controlled angle-closure glaucoma; Significant hepatic impairment (lower doses recommended); Impaired renal function; Pregnancy (safe use not established; use only if potential maternal benefit justifies potential risk to fetus); Children (safety not established).

Adverse Reactions/Side Effects

CNS: headache, dizziness. **EENT:** blurred vision, dry eyes. **GI:** dry mouth, constipation, dyspepsia.

Interactions

Drug-Drug: Erythromycin, **clarithromycin**, **ketoconazole**, **itraconazole**, and **miconazole** may inhibit metabolism and increase effects of tolterodine.

Route/Dosage

PO (Adults): 2 mg twice daily as tablets; may be lowered depending on response *or* 2–4 mg once daily as extended-release capsules.
PO (Adults with impaired hepatic function or concurrent enzyme inhibitors): 1 mg twice daily.

Availability

Tablets: 1 mg, 2 mg. **Cost:** 1 mg $359.59/180, 2 mg $359.96/180. **Extended-release capsules:** 2 mg, 4 mg. **Cost:** 2 mg $299.96/90, 4 mg $325.97/90.

NURSING IMPLICATIONS

Assessment

- Assess patient for urinary urgency, frequency, and urge incontinence periodically throughout therapy.

Potential Nursing Diagnoses

Impaired urinary elimination (Indications)
Urinary retention (Indications)

Implementation

- **PO:** Administer without regard to food.
- Extended-release capsules should be swallowed whole; do not open or chew.

Patient/Family Teaching

- Instruct patient to take tolterodine exactly as directed.
- May cause dizziness and blurred vision. Caution patient to avoid driving or other activities requiring alertness until response to medication is known.

Evaluation/Desired Outcomes

- Decreased urinary frequency, urgency, and urge incontinence.

topiramate (toe-**peer**-i-mate)
Topamax

Classification
Therapeutic: anticonvulsants, mood stabilizers

Pregnancy Category C

Indications

Seizures including: partial-onset, primary generalized tonic-clonic, seizures due to Lennox-Gastaut syndrome. Prevention of migraine headache in adults. **Unlabeled uses:** Adjunct in treatment of bipolar disorder.

Action

Action may be due to: Blockade of sodium channels in neurons, Enhancement of gamma-aminobutyrate (GABA), an inhibitory neurotransmitter, Prevention of activation of excitatory receptors. **Therapeutic Effects:** Decreased incidence of seizures. Decreased incidence/severity of migraine headache.

Pharmacokinetics

Absorption: Well absorbed (80%) after oral administration.
Distribution: Unknown.
Metabolism and Excretion: 70% excreted unchanged in urine.

Half-life: 21 hr.

TIME/ACTION PROFILE (blood levels†)

ROUTE	ONSET	PEAK	DURATION
PO	unknown	2 hr	12 hr

†After single dose

Contraindications/Precautions

Contraindicated in: Hypersensitivity; Lactation.

Use Cautiously in: Renal impairment (dosage reduction recommended if CCr <70 ml/min/1.73 m²); Hepatic impairment; Dehydration; OB: Use only if maternal benefit outweighs fetal risk; Lactation: Discontinue drug or bottle feed; Pedi: Children are more prone to oligohydrosis and hyperthermia; safety in children <2 yr not established; Geri: Consider age-related decrease in renal/hepatic impairment, concurrent disease states and drug therapy.

Adverse Reactions/Side Effects

CNS: INCREASED SEIZURES, dizziness, drowsiness, fatigue, impaired concentration/memory, nervousness, psychomotor slowing, speech problems, sedation, aggressive reaction, agitation, anxiety, cognitive disorders, confusion, depression, malaise, mood problems. **EENT:** abnormal vision, diplopia, nystagmus, acute myopia/secondary angle closure glaucoma,. **GI:** nausea, abdominal pain, anorexia, constipation, dry mouth. **GU:** kidney stones. **Derm:** oligohydrosis (↑ in children). **F and E:** hyperchloremic metabolic acidosis. **Hemat:** leukopenia. **Metab:** weight loss, hyperthermia (↑ in children). **Neuro:** ataxia, paresthesia, tremor. **Misc:** SUICIDE ATTEMPT, fever.

Interactions

Drug-Drug: Blood levels and effects may be ↓ by **phenytoin**, **carbamazepine**, or **valproic acid**. May ↑ blood levels and effects of **phenytoin** or **amitriptyline**. May ↓ blood levels and effects of **hormonal contraceptives**, **risperidone**, **lithium** or **valproic acid**. ↑ risk of CNS depression with **alcohol** or other **CNS depressants**. **Carbonic anhydrase inhibitors (acetazolamide)** may ↑ risk of kidney stones. Concurrent use with **valproic acid** may ↑ risk of hyperammonemia/encephalopathy.

Route/Dosage

Epilepsy (monotherapy)

PO (Adults and Children ≥10 yr): *Seizures/migraine prevention*— 50 mg/day initially, gradually increased over 6 wk to 400 mg/day in two divided doses.

Epilepsy (adjunctive therapy)

PO (Adults and Children ≥17 yr): 25–50 mg/day increased by 25–50 mg/day at weekly intervals up to 200–400 mg/day in two divided doses (200–400 mg/day in two divided doses for partial seizures and 400 mg/dy in two divided doses for primary generalized tonic/clonic seizures

Renal Impairment

PO (Adults): *CCr<70 ml/min*—50% of the usual dose.

PO (Children 2–17 yr): *Seizures*—5–9 mg/kg/day in 2 divided doses; initiate with 25 mg (or less based in 1–3 mg/kg) nightly for 7 days then increase at 1–2 wk intervals in increments of 1–3 mg/kg/day in 2 divided doses; titration should be based on clinical outcome.

Migraine prevention

PO (Adults): 25 mg at night initially, increase by 25 mg/day at weekly intervals up to target dose of 100 mg/day in 2 divided doses.

Availability

Sprinkle capsules: 15 mg, 25 mg. **Cost:** 15 mg $114.19/60, 25 mg $139.96/60. **Tablets:** 25 mg, 50 mg, 100 mg, 200 mg. **Cost:** 25 mg $369.90/180, 50 mg $703.96/180, 100 mg $1,023.97/180, 200 mg $1,162.91/180.

NURSING IMPLICATIONS

Assessment

- **Seizures:** Assess location, duration, and characteristics of seizure activity.
- **Migraines:** Assess pain location, intensity, duration, and associated symptoms (photophobia, phonophobia, nausea, vomiting) during migraine attack. Monitor frequency and intensity of pain on pain scale.
- **Bipolar disorder:** Administer Young Mania Rating Scale (YMRS) or similar tool to evaluate manic symptoms at baseline and over time in patients.
- ***Lab Test Considerations:*** Monitor CBC with differential and platelet count before therapy to determine baseline levels and peri-

T

odically during therapy. Frequently causes anemia.

- Hepatic function should be monitored periodically throughout therapy. May cause ↑ AST and ALT levels.
- Evaluate serum bicarbonate prior to and periodically during therapy. If metabolic acidosis occurs, dosing taper or discontinuation may be necessary.

Potential Nursing Diagnoses

Risk for injury (Indications, Side Effects)
Disturbed thought process (Indications)

Implementation

- Implement seizure precautions.
- Do not confuse Topamax (topiramate) with Toprolol (metoprolol).
- **PO:** May be administered without regard to meals.
- Do not break/crush tablets because of bitter taste.
- Contents of the sprinkle capsules can be sprinkled on a small amount (teaspoon) of soft food, such as applesauce, custard, ice cream, oatmeal, pudding, or yogurt. To open, hold the capsule upright so that you can read the word "TOP." Carefully twist off the clear portion of the capsule. It may be best to do this over the small portion of the food onto which you will be pouring the sprinkles. Sprinkle the entire contents of the capsule onto the food. Be sure the patient swallows the entire spoonful of the sprinkle/food mixture immediately without chewing. Follow with fluids immediately to make sure all of the mixture is swallowed. Never store a sprinkle/food mixture for use at another time.

Patient/Family Teaching

- Instruct patient to take topiramate exactly as directed. Take missed doses as soon as possible but not just before next dose; do not double doses. Notify health care professional if more than 1 dose is missed. Medication should be gradually discontinued to prevent seizures and status epilepticus.
- May cause decreased sweating and increased body temperature. Advise patients, especially parents of pediatric patients, to provide adequate hydration and monitoring, especially during hot weather.
- May cause dizziness, drowsiness, confusion, and difficulty concentrating. Caution patients to avoid driving or other activities requiring alertness until response to medication is known.
- Advise patient to maintain a fluid intake of 2000–3000 ml of fluid/day to prevent the formation of kidney stones.
- Instruct patient to notify health care professional immediately if periorbital pain or blurred vision occur. Medication should be discontinued if ocular symptoms occur. May lead to permanent loss of vision.
- Caution patient to make position changes slowly to minimize orthostatic hypotension.
- Advise patient not to take alcohol or other CNS depressants concurrently with this medication.
- Advise patient to use a nonhormonal form of contraception while taking topiramate.
- Instruct patient to notify health care professional of medication regimen before treatment or surgery.
- Advise patient to use sunscreen and wear protective clothing to prevent photosensitivity reactions.
- Advise patient to carry identification describing disease and medication regimen at all times.
- Refer patient/family to Manic-Depressive and Depressive Association for support.

Evaluation/Desired Outcomes

- Absence or reduction of seizure activity.
- Decrease in incidence and severity of migraine headaches.
- Remission of manic symptoms.

HIGH ALERT

topotecan (toe-poe-**tee**-kan)

Hycamtin

Classification
Therapeutic: antineoplastics
Pharmacologic: enzyme inhibitors

Pregnancy Category D

Indications

IV: Metastatic ovarian cancer that has not responded to previous chemotherapy. Small cell lung cancer unresponsive to first line therapy. **PO:** Relapsed small cell lung cancer in patients with a complete or partial prior response and who are at least 45 days from the end of first-line chemotherapy. Stage IV-B persistent or recurrent cervical cancer not amenable to treatment with surgery or radiation (with cisplatin).

Action
Interferes with DNA synthesis by inhibiting the enzyme topoisomerase. **Therapeutic Effects:** Death of rapidly replicating cells, particularly malignant ones.

Pharmacokinetics
Absorption: IV administration results in complete bioavailability.
Distribution: Unknown.
Metabolism and Excretion: 30% excreted in urine; small amounts metabolized by the liver.
Half-life: *PO*—3–6 hr; *IV*—2–3 hr.

TIME/ACTION PROFILE (effects on WBCs)

ROUTE	ONSET	PEAK	DURATION
PO	unknown	1–2 hrs	24 hrs
IV	within days	11 days	7 days

Contraindications/Precautions
Contraindicated in: Hypersensitivity; Pregnancy or lactation; Pre-existing severe myelosuppression.
Use Cautiously in: Impaired renal function (reduce dose if CCr <40 ml/min); Platelet count <25,000 cells/mm³ (reduce dose); Patients with childbearing potential.

Adverse Reactions/Side Effects
CNS: headache, fatigue, weakness. **Resp:** dyspnea. **GI:** abdominal pain, diarrhea, nausea, vomiting, anorexia, constipation, increased liver enzymes, stomatitis. **Derm:** alopecia. **Hemat:** anemia, leukopenia, thrombocytopenia. **MS:** arthralgia.

Interactions
Drug-Drug: Neutropenia is prolonged by concurrent use of **filgrastim** (do not use until day 6; 24 hr following completion of topotecan). ↑ myelosuppression with other **antineoplastics** (especially **cisplatin**) or **radiation therapy**. May ↓ antibody response to and ↑ risk of adverse reactions from **live virus vaccines**.

Route/Dosage
PO (Adults): 2.3 mg/m²/day for 5 days repeated every 21 days (round calculated oral dose to nearest 0.25 mg and prescribe the minimum number of 1 mg and 0.25 mg capsules with the same number of capsules prescribed for each of the 5 days.
IV (Adults): *Ovarian and Small Cell Lung Cancer*—1.5 mg/m²/day for 5 days starting on day 1 of a 21-day course; *Cervical Cancer*—75 mg/m² on Days 1, 2, and 3 followed by cisplatin on Day 1 and repeated every 21 days.

Renal Impairment
PO (Adults): *Ovarian and Small Cell Lung Cancer—CCr 30–49 mL/min*—1.8 mg/m²/day starting on day 1 of a 21-day course.
IV (Adults): *CCr 20–39 ml/min*—0.75mg/m²/day for 5 days starting on day 1 of a 21-day course. *Cervical Cancer*—Administer at standard doses only if serum creatinine is ≤1.5 mg/dL Do not administer if serum creatinine is >1.5 mg/dL.

Availability
Capsules: 0.25 mg, 1.0 mg. **Lyophilized powder for injection:** 4 mg/vial.

NURSING IMPLICATIONS

Assessment
- Monitor vital signs frequently during administration.
- Monitor for bone marrow depression. Assess for bleeding (bleeding gums, bruising, petechiae; guaiac stools, urine, and emesis) and avoid IM injections and taking rectal temperatures if platelet count is low. Apply pressure to venipuncture sites for 10 min. Assess for signs of infection during neutropenia. Anemia may occur. Monitor for increased fatigue, dyspnea, and orthostatic hypotension.
- Nausea and vomiting are common. Pretreatment with antiemetics should be considered.
- Assess IV site frequently for extravasation, which causes mild local erythema and bruising.
- ***Lab Test Considerations:*** Monitor CBC with differential and platelet count prior to administration and frequently during therapy. Baseline neutrophil count of ≥1500 cells/mm³ and platelet count of ≥100,000 cells/mm³ are required before first dose. The nadir of neutropenia occurs in 11 days, with a duration of 7 days. The nadir of thrombocytopenia occurs in 15 days, with a duration of 5 days. The nadir of anemia occurs in 15 days. Subsequent doses should not be administered until neutrophils recover to >1000 cells/mm³, platelets recover to >100,000 cells/mm³, and hemoglobin levels recover to 9.0 mg/dl. If severe neutropenia occurs during any course, subsequent doses should be reduced by 0.25 mg/m² or filgrastim may be

administered following the subsequent course of therapy starting on day 6, 24 hr after the completion of topotecan.

- Monitor liver function. May cause transient ↑ in AST, ALT, and bilirubin concentrations.

Potential Nursing Diagnoses

Risk for infection (Adverse Reactions)

Implementation

- ***High Alert:*** Fatalities have occurred with chemotherapeutic agents. Before administering, clarify all ambiguous orders; double-check single, daily, and course-of-therapy dose limits; have second practitioner independently double-check original order, dose calculations and infusion pump settings.
- **PO:** May be taken without regard to food. Capsules must be swallowed whole; do not open, crush, or chew. If patient vomits after taking dose, do not replace dose.
- Solution should be prepared in a biologic cabinet. Wear gloves, gown, and mask while handling IV medication. Discard IV equipment in specially designated containers.

IV Administration

- **Intermittent Infusion:** ***Diluent:*** Reconstitute each vial with 4 ml of sterile water for injection. Dilute further in D5W or 0.9% NaCl. Infusion is stable for 24 hr at room temperature or up to 7 days if refrigerated. Solution is yellow to yellow-green. ***Concentration:*** 10–50 mcg/ml. ***Rate:*** Infuse over 30 min.
- **Y-Site Compatibility:** carboplatin, caspofungin, cimetidine, cisplatin, cyclophosphamide, dactinomycin, daptomycin, doxorubicin, ertapenem, etoposide, fenoldopam, gemcitabine, granisetron, ifosfamide, levofloxacin, methylprednisolone, metoclopramide, ondansetron, oxaliplatin, paclitaxel, palonosetron, prochlorperazine, teniposide, thiotepa, vincristine, voriconazole.
- **Y-Site Incompatibility:** dexamethasone sodium phosphate, fluorouracil, mitomycin, pantoprazole, pemetrexed, rituximab, trastuzumab.

Patient/Family Teaching

- Instruct patient to take as directed. If patient vomits after taking, do not replace dose; notify health care professional. Do not take missed doses; take next scheduled dose and notify health care professional. If any capsules are broken or leaking, do not touch with bare hands; dispose of capsules and wash hands with soap and water. Patient should be instructed to read the Patient Information guide prior to first dose and with each refill; new information may be available.
- May cause drowsiness or sleepiness during and for several days after therapy. Caution patient to avoid driving and other activities requiring alertness until response to medication is known.
- Instruct patient to notify health care professional if fever; chills; sore throat; signs of infection; bleeding gums; bruising; petechiae; blood in urine, stool, or emesis occurs. Caution patient to avoid crowds and persons with known infections. Instruct patient to use soft toothbrush and electric razor. Patient should be cautioned not to drink alcoholic beverages or take products containing aspirin or NSAIDs.
- May cause diarrhea. Advise patient to notify health care professional if diarrhea with fever or stomach pain or cramps or diarrhea that occurs more than 3 times/day occurs.
- Advise patient to consult health care professional before taking other Rx, OTC, or herbal products with topotecan.
- Discuss with patient the possibility of hair loss. Explore methods of coping.
- Advise patient that this medication may have teratogenic effects. Contraception should be used during therapy.
- Instruct patient not to receive any vaccinations without advice of health care professional.
- Emphasize the need for periodic lab tests to monitor for side effects.

Evaluation/Desired Outcomes

- Decrease in size and spread of malignancy.

torsemide (tore-se-mide)

Demadex

Classification

Therapeutic: antihypertensives
Pharmacologic: loop diuretics

Pregnancy Category B

Indications

Edema due to: CHF, Hepatic or renal disease. Hypertension.

Action

Inhibits the reabsorption of sodium and chloride from the loop of Henle and distal renal tubule. Increases renal excretion of water, sodium, chloride, magnesium, hydrogen, and calcium. Effectiveness persists in impaired renal function. **Therapeutic Effects:** Diuresis and subsequent mobilization of excess fluid (edema, pleural effusions). Decreased blood pressure.

Pharmacokinetics

Absorption: 80% absorbed after oral administration.
Distribution: Widely distributed.
Protein Binding: ≥99%.
Metabolism and Excretion: 80% metabolized by liver, 20% excreted in urine.
Half-life: 3.5 hr.

TIME/ACTION PROFILE (diuretic effect)

ROUTE	ONSET	PEAK	DURATION
PO	within 60 min	60–120 min	6–8 hr
IV	within 10 min	within 60 min	6–8 hr

Contraindications/Precautions

Contraindicated in: Hypersensitivity; Cross-sensitivity with thiazides and sulfonamides may occur; Hepatic coma or anuria.
Use Cautiously in: Severe liver disease (may precipitate hepatic coma; concurrent use with potassium-sparing diuretics may be necessary); Electrolyte depletion; Geri: Geriatric patients may have increased risk of side effects, especially hypotension and electrolyte imbalance, at usual doses; Diabetes mellitus; Increasing azotemia; OB, Lactation, Pedi: Safety not established.

Adverse Reactions/Side Effects

CNS: dizziness, headache, nervousness. **EENT:** hearing loss, tinnitus. **CV:** hypotension. **GI:** constipation, diarrhea, dry mouth, dyspepsia, nausea, vomiting. **GU:** excessive urination. **Derm:** photosensitivity, rash. **Endo:** hyperglycemia, hyperuricemia. **F and E:** dehydration, hypocalcemia, hypochloremia, hypokalemia, hypomagnesemia, hyponatremia, hypovolemia, metabolic alkalosis. **MS:** arthralgia, muscle cramps, myalgia. **Misc:** increased BUN.

Interactions

Drug-Drug: ↑ hypotension with **antihypertensives**, **nitrates**, or acute ingestion of **alcohol**. ↑ risk of hypokalemia with other **diuretics**, **amphotericin B**, **stimulant laxatives**, and **corticosteroids**. Hypokalemia may ↑ risk of **digoxin** toxicity and ↑ risk of arrhythmia in patients taking drugs that prolong the QT interval. ↓ **lithium** excretion, may cause **lithium** toxicity. ↑ risk of ototoxicity with **aminoglycosides**. **NSAIDS** ↓ effects of torsemide. ↑ risk of **salicylate** toxicity (with use of high-dose **salicylate** therapy). ↓ effects of torsemide when given at same time as **cholestyramine**.

Route/Dosage

Congestive Heart Failure

PO, IV (Adults): 10–20 mg once daily; dose may be doubled until desired effect is obtained (maximum daily dose = 200 mg).

Chronic Renal Failure

PO, IV (Adults): 20 mg once daily; dose may be doubled until desired effect is obtained (maximum daily dose = 200 mg).

Hepatic Cirrhosis

PO, IV (Adults): 5–10 mg once daily (with aldosterone antagonist or potassium-sparing diuretic); dose may be doubled until desired effect is obtained (maximum daily dose = 40 mg).

Hypertension

PO, IV (Adults): 2.5–5 mg once daily, may be increased to 10 mg once daily after 4–6 wk (if still not effective, add another agent).

Availability (generic available)

Tablets: 5 mg[Rx], 10 mg[Rx], 20 mg[Rx], 100 mg[Rx]. **Cost:** *Generic*—5 mg $50.00/90, 10 mg $50.97/90, 20 mg $59.97/90, 100 mg $213.98/90. **Injection:** 10 mg/ml[Rx].

NURSING IMPLICATIONS

Assessment

- Assess fluid status during therapy. Monitor daily weight, intake and output ratios, amount and location of edema, lung sounds, skin turgor, and mucous membranes. Notify physician or other health care provider if thirst, dry mouth, lethargy, weakness, hypotension, or oliguria occurs.
- Monitor blood pressure and pulse before and during administration. Monitor frequency of prescription refills to determine adherence in patients treated for hypertension.
- Assess patients receiving digoxin for anorexia, nausea, vomiting, muscle cramps, paresthesia, and confusion. Patients taking digoxin are at increased risk of digoxin toxicity due to potassium-depleting effect of the diuretic. Po-

T

tassium supplements or potassium-sparing diuretics may be used concurrently to prevent hypokalemia.
- Assess patient for tinnitus and hearing loss. Audiometry is recommended for patients receiving prolonged high-dose IV therapy. Hearing loss is most common following rapid or high-dose IV administration in patients with decreased renal function or those taking other ototoxic drugs.
- Assess for allergy to sulfonamides.
- Geri: Diuretic use is associated with increased risk for falls in older adults. Assess falls risk and implement fall prevention strategies.
- ***Lab Test Considerations:*** Monitor electrolytes, renal and hepatic function, serum glucose, and uric acid levels before and periodically during therapy. May cause ↓ serum sodium, potassium, calcium, and magnesium concentrations. May also cause ↑ BUN, serum glucose, creatinine, and uric acid levels.

Potential Nursing Diagnoses

Excess fluid volume (Indications)
Risk for deficient fluid volume (Side Effects)

Implementation

- Administer medication in the morning to prevent disruption of sleep cycle.
- IV is preferred over IM for parenteral administration.
- **PO:** May be taken with food or milk to minimize gastric irritation.

IV Administration

- **Direct IV:** ***Diluent:*** Administer undiluted. ***Concentration:*** 10 mg/ml. ***Rate:*** Administer slowly over 2 min.
- May also be administered as a continuous infusion.
- **Y-Site Compatibility:** milrinone, nesiritide.

Patient/Family Teaching

- Instruct patient to take torsemide as directed. Take missed doses as soon as possible; do not double doses.
- Caution patient to change positions slowly to minimize orthostatic hypotension. Caution patient that the use of alcohol, exercise during hot weather, or standing for long periods during therapy may enhance orthostatic hypotension.
- Instruct patient to consult health care professional regarding a diet high in potassium (see Appendix L).
- Advise patient to contact health care professional if they gain more than 2–3 lbs/day.
- Advise patient to consult health care professional before taking OTC medication or herbal products concurrently with this therapy.
- Instruct patient to notify health care professional of medication regimen prior to treatment or surgery.
- Caution patient to use sunscreen and protective clothing to prevent photosensitivity reactions.
- Advise patient to contact health care professional immediately if muscle weakness, cramps, nausea, dizziness, numbness, or tingling of extremities occurs.
- Advise diabeticpatients to monitor blood glucose closely; may cause increased blood glucose levels.
- Emphasize the importance of routine follow-up examinations.
- **Hypertension:** Advise patients on antihypertensive regimen to continue taking medication even if feeling better. Torsemide controls but does not cure hypertension.
- Reinforce the need to continue additional therapies for hypertension (weight loss, exercise, restricted sodium intake, stress reduction, regular exercise, moderation of alcohol consumption, cessation of smoking).

Evaluation/Desired Outcomes

- Decrease in edema.
- Decrease in abdominal girth and weight.
- Increase in urinary output.
- Decrease in blood pressure.

tramadol (tra-ma-dol)

✤ Ralivia, Ultram, Ultram ER

Classification
Therapeutic: analgesics (centrally acting)

Pregnancy Category C

Indications

Moderate to moderately severe pain.

Action

Binds to mu-opioid receptors. Inhibits reuptake of serotonin and norepinephrine in the CNS.
Therapeutic Effects: Decreased pain.

Pharmacokinetics

Absorption: 75% absorbed after oral administration.
Distribution: Crosses the placenta; enters breast milk.

Metabolism and Excretion: Mostly metabolized by the liver; one metabolite has analgesic activity; 30% is excreted unchanged in urine.
Half-life: *Tramadol*—5–9 hr, *ER*—7.9 hr; *active metabolite*—5–9 hr, *ER*—8.8 hr (both are increased in renal or hepatic impairment).

TIME/ACTION PROFILE (analgesia)

ROUTE	ONSET	PEAK	DURATION
PO	1 hr	2–3 hr	4–6 hr
ER		12 hr	24 hr

Contraindications/Precautions

Contraindicated in: Hypersensitivity; Cross-sensitivity with opioids may occur; Patients who are acutely intoxicated with alcohol, sedative/hypnotics, centrally acting analgesics, opioid analgesics, or psychotropic agents; Patients who are physically dependent on opioid analgesics (may precipitate withdrawal); OB: Not recommended for use during pregnancy or lactation; CCr <30 mL/min or severe hepatic impairment (Child-Pugh Class C) *ER formulation only*.
Use Cautiously in: Geri: Geriatric patients (not to exceed 300 mg/day in patients >75 yr); Patients with a history of epilepsy or risk factors for seizures; Renal impairment (↑ dosing interval recommended if CCr <30 ml/min); Hepatic impairment (↑ interval recommended in patients with cirrhosis); Patients receiving MAO inhibitors or CNS depressants; Increased intracranial pressure or head trauma; Acute abdomen (may preclude accurate clinical assessment); Patients with a history of opioid dependence or who have recently received large doses of opioids; Children <16 yr (safety not established).

Adverse Reactions/Side Effects

CNS: SEIZURES, dizziness, headache, somnolence, anxiety, CNS stimulation, confusion, coordination disturbance, euphoria, malaise, nervousness, sleep disorder, weakness. **EENT:** visual disturbances. **CV:** vasodilation. **GI:** constipation, nausea, abdominal pain, anorexia, diarrhea, dry mouth, dyspepsia, flatulence, vomiting. **GU:** menopausal symptoms, urinary retention/frequency. **Derm:** pruritus, sweating. **Neuro:** hypertonia. **Misc:** physical dependence, psychological dependence, tolerance.

Interactions

Drug-Drug: ↑ risk of CNS depression when used concurrently with other **CNS depressants**, including **alcohol**, **antihistamines**, **sedative/hypnotics**, **opioid analgesics**, **anesthetics**, or **psychotropic agents**. ↑ risk of seizures with high doses of **penicillins**, **cephalosporins**, **phenothiazines**, **opioid analgesics**, or **antidepressants**. **Carbamazepine** ↑ metabolism and ↓ effectiveness of tramadol (increased doses may be required). Use cautiously in patients who are receiving **MAO inhibitors** (↑ risk of adverse reactions). Effectiveness may be altered by concurrent **quinidine**.
Drug-Natural Products: Concomitant use of **kava kava, valerian, or chamomile can ↑ CNS depression.**

Route/Dosage

PO (Adults ≥18 yrs): *Rapid titration*—50–100 mg q 4–6 hr (not to exceed 400 mg/day or 300 mg in patients >75 yr). *Gradual titration*—25 mg/day initially, increase by 25 mg/day every 3 days to 100 mg/day, then increase by 50 mg/day every 3 days up to 200 mg/day *or* extended-release 100 mg/day, may be increased by 100 mg increments every 5 days based on pain level and tolerability, not to exceed 300 mg/day.

Renal Impairment

PO (Adults): *CCr <30 ml/min*—increase dosing to q 12 hr (not to exceed 200 mg/day).

Hepatic Impairment

PO (Adults): 50 mg q 12 hr.

Availability (generic available)

Tablets: 50 mg. **Cost:** *Generic*—$16.99/30 $85.25/100. **Extended-release tablets:** 100 mg, 200 mg, 300 mg. **Cost:** 100 mg $89.99/30, 200 mg $158.98/30, 300 mg $195.99/30. ***In combination with:*** acetaminophen (Ultracet). See Appendix B.

NURSING IMPLICATIONS

Assessment

- Assess type, location, and intensity of pain before and 2–3 hr (peak) after administration.
- Assess blood pressure and respiratory rate before and periodically during administration. Respiratory depression has not occurred with recommended doses.
- Assess bowel function routinely. Prevention of constipation should be instituted with increased intake of fluids and bulk and with laxatives to minimize constipating effects.

- Assess previous analgesic history. Tramadol is not recommended for patients dependent on opioids or who have previously received opioids for more than 1 wk; may cause opioid withdrawal symptoms.
- Prolonged use may lead to physical and psychological dependence and tolerance, although these may be milder than with opioids. This should not prevent patient from receiving adequate analgesia. Most patients who receive tramadol for pain do not develop psychological dependence. If tolerance develops, changing to an opioid agonist may be required to relieve pain.
- Monitor patient for seizures. May occur within recommended dose range. Risk is increased with higher doses and in patients taking antidepressants (SSRIs, tricyclics, or MAO inhibitors), opioid analgesics, or other drugs that decrease the seizure threshold.
- ***Lab Test Considerations:*** May cause ↑ serum creatinine, elevated liver enzymes, decreased hemoglobin, and proteinuria.
- ***Toxicity and Overdose:*** Overdose may cause respiratory depression and seizures. Naloxone (Narcan) may reverse some, but not all, of the symptoms of overdose. Treatment should be symptomatic and supportive. Maintain adequate respiratory exchange. Hemodialysis is not helpful because it removes only a small portion of administered dose. Seizures may be managed with barbiturates or benzodiazepines; naloxone increases risk of seizures.

Potential Nursing Diagnoses

Acute pain (Indications)
Risk for injury (Side Effects)

Implementation

- Do not confuse tramadol with Toradol (ketorolac).
- Tramadol is considered to provide more analgesia than codeine 60 mg but less than combined aspirin 650 mg/codeine 60 mg for acute postoperative pain.
- For chronic pain, daily doses of 250 mg of tramadol provide pain relief similar to that of 5 doses/day of acetaminophen 300 mg/codeine 30 mg, 5 doses/day of aspirin 325 mg/codeine 30 mg, or 2–3 doses/day of acetaminophen 500 mg/oxycodone 5 mg.
- Explain therapeutic value of medication before administration to enhance the analgesic effect.
- Regularly administered doses may be more effective than prn administration. Analgesic is more effective if given before pain becomes severe.
- Tramadol should be discontinued gradually after long-term use to prevent withdrawal symptoms.
- **PO:** Tramadol may be administered without regard to meals. Extended-release tablets should be swallowed whole; do not crush, break, or chew.

Patient/Family Teaching

- Instruct patient on how and when to ask for pain medication.
- May cause dizziness and drowsiness. Caution patient to avoid driving or other activities requiring alertness until response to medication is known.
- Advise patient to change positions slowly to minimize orthostatic hypotension.
- Caution patient to avoid concurrent use of alcohol or other CNS depressants with this medication.
- OB: Advise female patients to notify health care professional if pregnancy is planned or suspected, or if breastfeeding.
- Encourage patient to turn, cough, and breathe deeply every 2 hr to prevent atelectasis.

Evaluation/Desired Outcomes

- Decrease in severity of pain without a significant alteration in level of consciousness or respiratory status.

---

trandolapril, **See ANGIOTENSIN-CONVERTING ENZYME (ACE) INHIBITORS.**

---

tranylcypromine, **See MONOAMINE OXIDASE (MAO) INHIBITORS.**

HIGH ALERT

trastuzumab

(traz-**too**-zoo-mab)
Herceptin

Classification
Therapeutic: antineoplastics
Pharmacologic: monoclonal antibodies

Pregnancy Category B

Indications
Metastatic breast cancer alone or with doxorubicin, cyclophosphamide, and paclitaxel for tumors that display overexpression of the human epidermal growth factor receptor 2 (HER2) protein.

Action
A monoclonal antibody that binds to HER2 sites in breast cancer tissue and inhibits proliferation of cells that overexpress HER2 protein. **Therapeutic Effects:** Regression of breast cancer and metastases.

Pharmacokinetics
Absorption: IV administration results in complete bioavailability.
Distribution: Binds to HER2 proteins.
Metabolism and Excretion: Unknown.
Half-life: 10-mg dose—1.7 days; 500-mg dose—12 days.

TIME/ACTION PROFILE (blood levels)

ROUTE	ONSET	PEAK	DURATION
IV	unknown	unknown	unknown

Contraindications/Precautions
Contraindicated in: None known.
Use Cautiously in: Pre-existing pulmonary conditions; Hypersensitivity to trastuzumab, Chinese hamster ovary cell proteins, or other components of the product; Hypersensitivity to benzyl alcohol (use sterile water for injection instead of bacteriostatic water, which accompanies the vial); Geriatric patients (may have increased risk of cardiac dysfunction); OB: Use during pregnancy only if clearly needed; not recommended for use during lactation; Lactation (use not recommended); Pedi: Children (safety not established).
Exercise Extreme Caution in: Patients with pre-existing cardiac dysfunction.

Adverse Reactions/Side Effects
CNS: dizziness, headache, insomnia, weakness, depression. **Resp:** dyspnea, increased cough, pharyngitis, rhinitis, sinusitis. **CV:** CARDIOTOXICITY, tachycardia. **GI:** abdominal pain, anorexia, diarrhea, nausea, vomiting. **Derm:** rash, acne, herpes simplex. **F and E:** edema. **Hemat:** anemia, leukopenia. **MS:** back pain, arthralgia, bone pain. **Neuro:** neuropathy, paresthesia, peripheral neuritis. **Misc:** HYPERSENSITIVITY REACTIONS, chills, fever, infection, pain, allergic reactions, flu-like syndrome.

Interactions
Drug-Drug: Concurrent **anthracycline (daunorubicin, doxorubicin**, or **idarubicin)** therapy may ↑ risk of cardiotoxicity. Blood levels are ↑ by concurrent **paclitaxel**.

Route/Dosage
IV (Adults): 4 mg/kg initially followed by 2 mg/kg weekly.

Availability
Lyophilized powder for injection: 440 mg/vial with 30 ml bacteriostatic water for injection (contains benzyl alcohol).

NURSING IMPLICATIONS

Assessment
- Assess for infusion-related symptoms (chills, fever) following initial infusion. May be treated with acetaminophen, diphenhydramine, and meperidine. Rarely requires discontinuation.
- Assess for signs and symptoms of cardiotoxicity (dyspnea, increased cough, paroxysmal nocturnal dyspnea, peripheral edema, S_3 gallop, reduced ejection fraction) prior to and frequently during therapy. Baseline cardiac assessment of history, physical exam, and one or more of: ECG, echocardiogram, and multiple gated acquisition (MUGA) scan. CHF associated with trastuzumab may be severe, resulting in cardiac failure, death, and stroke. Trastuzumab should be discontinued upon the development of significant CHF.
- Monitor patient for signs of pulmonary hypersensitivity reactions (dyspnea, pulmonary infiltrates, pleural effusion, noncardiogenic pulmonary edema, pulmonary insufficiency, hypoxia, acute respiratory distress syndrome). Patients with symptomatic pulmonary disease or extensive lung tumor involvement are at increased risk. Infusion should be discontinued if severe symptoms occur.
- ***Lab Test Considerations:*** HER2 protein overexpression is used to determine whether treatment with trastuzumab is indicated. HER2 protein overexpression is detected by HercepTest[trade] (IHC assay) and PathVysion[trade] (FISH assay).
- May cause anemia and leukopenia.

T

Potential Nursing Diagnoses
Diarrhea (Adverse Reactions)
Risk for infection (Adverse Reactions)

Implementation
- ***High Alert:*** Fatalities have occurred with chemotherapeutic agents. Before administering, clarify all ambiguous orders; double-check single, daily, and course-of-therapy dose limits; have second practitioner independently double-check original order, dose calculations and infusion pump settings.
- May be administered in the outpatient setting.

IV Administration
- **Intermittent Infusion:** ***Diluent:*** Dilute each vial with 20 ml of bacteriostatic water for injection, directing the stream of diluent into lyophilized cake of trastuzumab, resulting in a multidose solution containing 21 mg/ml. Swirl the vial gently; do not shake. May foam slightly; allow the vial to stand undisturbed for 5 min. Solution should be clear to slightly opalescent and colorless to pale yellow, without particulate matter. Label vial immediately in the area marked ''Do not use after'' with the date 28 days from the date of reconstitution. Stable for 24 hr at room temperature or 28 days if refrigerated. If patient is allergic to benzyl alcohol, use sterile water for injection for reconstitution. Use immediately and discard any unused portion. Calculate to volume required for the desired dose, withdraw, and add it to an infusion containing 250 ml of 0.9% NaCl. Invert bag gently to mix. ***Rate:*** Infuse the 4 mg/kg loading dose over 90 min and the weekly 2 mg/kg dose over 30 min if the loading dose was well tolerated. Do not administer as an IV push or bolus.
- **Additive Incompatibility:** Do not dilute trastuzumab with or add to solutions containing dextrose. Do not mix or dilute with other drugs.

Patient/Family Teaching
- Instruct patient to notify health care professional promptly if symptoms of cardiotoxicity, fever, sore throat, signs of infection, lower back or side pain, or difficult or painful urination occur. Caution patient to avoid crowds and persons with known infections.
- Advise patient not to receive any vaccinations without advice of health care professional.

Evaluation/Desired Outcomes
- Regression of breast cancer and metastases.

trazodone (traz-oh-done)
Desyrel, Trialodine, Trazon

Classification
Therapeutic: antidepressants

Pregnancy Category C

Indications
Major depression. **Unlabeled uses:** Insomnia, chronic pain syndromes, including diabetic neuropathy, and anxiety.

Action
Alters the effects of serotonin in the CNS. **Therapeutic Effects:** Antidepressant action, which may develop only over several weeks.

Pharmacokinetics
Absorption: Well absorbed after oral administration.
Distribution: Widely distributed.
Protein Binding: 89–95%.
Metabolism and Excretion: Extensively metabolized by the liver (CYP3A4 enzyme system); minimal excretion of unchanged drug by the kidneys.
Half-life: 5–9 hr.

TIME/ACTION PROFILE (antidepressant effect)

ROUTE	ONSET	PEAK	DURATION
PO	1–2 wk	2–4 wk	wks

Contraindications/Precautions
Contraindicated in: Hypersensitivity; Recovery period after MI; Concurrent electroconvulsive therapy.
Use Cautiously in: Cardiovascular disease; Suicidal behavior; May ↑ risk of suicide attempt/ideation especially during early treatment or dose adjustment; Severe hepatic or renal disease (dose reduction recommended); Lactation: Discontinue drug or bottle feed; Pedi: Suicide risk may be greater in children and adolescents; safe use not established; Geri: Initial dose reduction recommended.

Adverse Reactions/Side Effects
CNS: drowsiness, confusion, dizziness, fatigue, hallucinations, headache, insomnia, nightmares, slurred speech, syncope, weakness. **EENT:** blurred vision, tinnitus. **CV:** hypotension, arrhythmias, chest pain, hypertension, palpitations, tachycardia. **GI:** dry mouth, altered taste, constipation, diarrhea, excess salivation, flatulence, nausea, vomiting. **GU:** hema-

turia, erectile dysfunction, priapism, urinary frequency. **Derm:** rashes. **Hemat:** anemia, leukopenia. **MS:** myalgia. **Neuro:** tremor.

Interactions

Drug-Drug: May ↑ **digoxin** or **phenytoin** serum levels. ↑ CNS depression with other **CNS depressants**, including **alcohol**, **opioid analgesics**, and **sedative/hypnotics**. ↑ hypotension with **antihypertensives**, acute ingestion of **alcohol**, or **nitrates**. Concurrent use with **fluoxetine** ↑ levels and risk of toxicity from trazodone. **Drugs that inhibit the CYP3A4 enzyme system**, including **ritonavir indinavir** and **ketoconazole** ↑ levels and the risk of toxicity. **Drugs that induce the CYP3A4 enzyme system**, including **carbamazepine** ↓ levels and may decrease effectiveness. Do note use within 14 days of **MAOI** therapy. May ↑ prothrombin time (PT) with **warfarin**.
Drug-Natural Products: Concomitant use of **kava kava**, **valerian**, or **chamomile** can ↑ CNS depression. ↑ risk of serotinergic side effects including serotonin syndrome with **St. John's wort** and **SAMe**.

Route/Dosage

PO (Adults): *Depression*—150 mg/day in 3 divided doses; increase by 50 mg/day q 3–4 days until desired response (not to exceed 400 mg/day in outpatients or 600 mg/day in hospitalized patients). *Insomnia*—25–100 mg at bedtime.
PO (Geriatric Patients): 75 mg/day in divided doses initially; may be increased q 3–4 days.

Availability (generic available)

Tablets: 50 mg, 100 mg, 150 mg, 300 mg.

NURSING IMPLICATIONS

Assessment

- Monitor blood pressure and pulse rate before and during initial therapy. Monitor ECGs in patients with pre-existing cardiac disease before and periodically during therapy to detect arrhythmias.
- Assess for possible sexual dysfunction.
- **Depression:** Assess mental status (orientation, mood, and behavior) frequently. Assess for suicidal tendencies, especially during early therapy. Restrict amount of drug available to patient.
- **Pain:** Assess location, duration, intensity, and characteristics of pain before and periodically during therapy. Use pain scale to assess effectiveness of medicine.
- ***Lab Test Considerations:*** Assess CBC and renal and hepatic function before and periodically during therapy. Slight, clinically insignificant ↓ in leukocyte and neutrophil counts may occur.

Potential Nursing Diagnoses

Ineffective coping (Indications)
Sexual dysfunction (Side Effects)

Implementation

- **PO:** Administer with or immediately after meals to minimize side effects (nausea, dizziness) and allow maximum absorption of trazodone. A larger portion of the total daily dose may be given at bedtime to decrease daytime drowsiness and dizziness.

Patient/Family Teaching

- Instruct patient to take medication exactly as directed. If a dose is missed, take as soon as remembered. Do not take if within 4 hr of next scheduled dose; do not double doses. Consult health care professional before discontinuing medication; gradual dose reduction is necessary to prevent aggravation of condition.
- May cause drowsiness and blurred vision. Caution patient to avoid driving and other activities requiring alertness until response to drug is known.
- Caution patient to change positions slowly to minimize orthostatic hypotension.
- Advise patient to avoid concurrent use of alcohol or other CNS depressant drugs.
- Inform patient that frequent rinses, good oral hygiene, and sugarless candy or gum may diminish dry mouth. Health care professional should be notified if this persists >2 wk. An increase in fluid intake, fiber, and exercise may prevent constipation.
- Advise patient to notify health care professional of medication regimen before treatment or surgery.
- Instruct patient to notify health care professional if priapism, irregular heartbeat, fainting, confusion, skin rash, or tremors occur or if dry mouth, nausea and vomiting, dizziness, headache, muscle aches, constipation, or diarrhea becomes pronounced.

T

- Emphasize the importance of follow-up exams to evaluate progress.
- Refer for psychotherapy to improve coping skills.
- Refer to local support group.

Evaluation/Desired Outcomes

- Resolution of depression.
- Increased sense of well-being.
- Renewed interest in surroundings.
- Increased appetite.
- Improved energy level.
- Improved sleep.
- Decrease in severity of pain in chronic pain syndromes. Therapeutic effects are usually seen within 1 wk, although 4 wk may be required to obtain significant therapeutic results.

triamcinolone, See CORTICOSTEROIDS (INHALATION), CORTICOSTEROIDS (NASAL), CORTICOSTEROIDS (SYSTEMIC), CORTICOSTEROIDS (TOPICAL/LOCAL).

triamterene, See DIURETICS (POTASSIUM-SPARING).

triazolam (trye-**az**-oh-lam)

✤ Apo-Triazo, ✤ Gen-Triazolam, Halcion, ✤ Novo-Triolam, ✤ Nu-Triazo

Classification
Therapeutic: sedative/hypnotics
Pharmacologic: benzodiazepines

Schedule IV

Pregnancy Category X

Indications

Short-term management of insomnia.

Action

Acts at many levels in the CNS, producing generalized depression. Effects may be mediated by GABA, an inhibitory neurotransmitter. **Therapeutic Effects:** Relief of insomnia.

Pharmacokinetics

Absorption: Well absorbed following oral administration.
Distribution: Widely distributed, crosses blood-brain barrier. Probably crosses the placenta and enters breast milk.
Protein Binding: 89%.
Metabolism and Excretion: Metabolized by the liver.
Half-life: 1.6–5.4 hr.

TIME/ACTION PROFILE (sedation)

ROUTE	ONSET	PEAK	DURATION
PO	15–30 min	6–8 hr	unknown

Contraindications/Precautions

Contraindicated in: Hypersensitivity; Cross-sensitivity with other benzodiazepines may occur; Pre-existing CNS depression; Uncontrolled severe pain; OB, Pedi: Pregnancy, lactation, or children.
Use Cautiously in: Pre-existing hepatic dysfunction (dose reduction recommended); History of suicide attempt or drug addiction; Geri: Elderly patients have increased sensitivity to benzodiazepines. Appears on Beers list and is associated with increased risk of falls (↓ dose required); Debilitated patients (initial dose reduction recommended).

Adverse Reactions/Side Effects

CNS: abnormal thinking, behavior changes, <u>dizziness</u>, <u>excessive sedation</u>, <u>hangover</u>, <u>headache</u>, anterograde amnesia, confusion, hallucinations, sleep—driving, lethargy, mental depression, paradoxical excitation. **EENT:** blurred vision. **GI:** constipation, diarrhea, nausea, vomiting. **Derm:** rashes. **Misc:** physical dependence, psychological dependence, tolerance.

Interactions

Drug-Drug: **Cimetidine**, **erythromycin**, **fluconazole**, **itraconazole**, **ketoconazole**, **indinavir**, **nelfinavir**, **ritonavir**, or **saquinavir** may ↓ metabolism and enhance actions of triazolam; combination should be avoided. Additive CNS depression with **alcohol**, **antidepressants**, **antihistamines**, and **opioid analgesics**. May ↓ effectiveness of **levodopa**. May ↑ toxicity of **zidovudine**. **Isoniazid** may ↓ excretion and ↑ effects of triazolam. Sedative effects may be ↓ by **theophylline**.
Drug-Natural Products: Concomitant use of **kava kava, valerian, chamomile, or hops can ↑ CNS depression.**
Drug-Food: Grapefruit juice significantly ↑ blood levels and effects.

Route/Dosage
PO (Adults): 125–250 mcg (up to 500 mcg) at bedtime.
PO (Geriatric Patients or Debilitated Patients): 125 mcg at bedtime initially; may be increased as needed.

Availability (generic available)
Tablets: 125 mcg, 250 mcg.

NURSING IMPLICATIONS

Assessment
- Assess sleep patterns prior to and periodically throughout therapy.
- Geri: Assess CNS effects and risk of falls. Institute falls prevention strategies.
- Prolonged high-dose therapy may lead to psychological or physical dependence. Restrict the amount of drug available to patient, especially if patient is depressed, suicidal, or has a history of addiction.

Potential Nursing Diagnoses
Insomnia (Indications)
Risk for injury (Side Effects)

Implementation
- Supervise ambulation and transfer of patients following administration. Remove cigarettes. Side rails should be raised and call bell within reach at all times.
- **PO:** Administer with food if GI irritation becomes a problem.

Patient/Family Teaching
- Instruct patient to take triazolam exactly as directed. Discuss the importance of preparing environment for sleep (dark room, quiet, avoidance of nicotine and caffeine). If less effective after a few weeks, consult health care professional; do not increase dose.
- May cause daytime drowsiness or dizziness. Caution patient to avoid driving or other activities requiring alertness until response to medication is known. Geri: Instruct patient and family how to reduce falls risk at home.
- Advise patient to avoid the use of alcohol and other CNS depressants and to consult health care professional prior to using OTC preparations that contain antihistamines or alcohol.
- Advise patient to inform health care professional if pregnancy is planned or suspected or if confusion, depression, or persistent headaches occur. Instruct family or caregiver to notify health care professional if personality changes occur.
- Instruct patient to notify health care professional if an increase in daytime anxiety occurs. May occur after as few as 10 days of therapy. May require discontinuation of triazolam.
- Emphasize the importance of follow-up appointments to monitor progress.

Evaluation/Desired Outcomes
- Improvement in sleep patterns, which may not be noticeable until the 3rd day of therapy.

---

tricalcium phosphate, See CALCIUM SALTS.

---

trikates, See POTASSIUM SUPPLEMENTS.

---

trimethoprim
(trye-**meth**-oh-prim)
Primsol, Proloprim, Trimpex

Classification
Therapeutic: anti-infectives
Pharmacologic: folate antagonists

Pregnancy Category C

Indications
Treatment of uncomplicated urinary tract infections. Treatment of uncomplicated otitis media in children. **Unlabeled uses:** Prophylaxis of chronic recurrent urinary tract infections. Treatment of head lice. With dapsone in the management of mild to moderate *Pneumocystis carinii* pneumonia (PCP).

Action
Interferes with bacterial folic acid synthesis. **Therapeutic Effects:** Bactericidal action against susceptible organisms. **Spectrum:** Some gram-positive pathogens, including: *Streptococcus pneumoniae*, Group A beta-hemolytic streptococci, Some staphylococci and *Enterococcus*. Gram-negative spectrum includes the following Enterobacteriaceae: *Acinetobacter*, *Citrobacter*, *Enterobacter*, *Escherichia coli*, *Haemophilus influenzae*, *Klebsiella pneumoniae*, *Proteus mirabilis*, *Salmonella*, *Shigella*. Other strains of *Proteus*,

some *Providencia*, some *Serratia*, and *P. carinii* are also susceptible.

Pharmacokinetics

Absorption: Well absorbed following oral administration.
Distribution: Widely distributed. Crosses the placenta and is distributed into breast milk in high concentrations.
Metabolism and Excretion: 80% excreted unchanged in the urine; 20% metabolized by the liver.
Half-life: 8–11 hr (increased in renal impairment).

TIME/ACTION PROFILE (blood levels)

ROUTE	ONSET	PEAK	DURATION
PO	rapid	1–4 hr	12–24 hr

Contraindications/Precautions

Contraindicated in: Hypersensitivity; Megaloblastic anemia secondary to folate deficiency.
Use Cautiously in: Renal impairment (dosage reduction required if CCr ≤30 ml/min); Debilitated patients; Severe hepatic impairment; Folate deficiency; Pregnancy, lactation, or children <12 yr (safety as a single agent not established).

Adverse Reactions/Side Effects

GI: altered taste, epigastric discomfort, glossitis, nausea, vomiting, drug-induced hepatitis. **Derm:** pruritus, rash. **Hemat:** megaloblastic anemia, neutropenia, thrombocytopenia. **Misc:** fever.

Interactions

Drug-Drug: Increased risk of folate deficiency when used with **phenytoin** or **methotrexate**. Increased risk of bone marrow depression when used with **antineoplastics** or **radiation therapy**. **Rifampin** may decrease effectiveness by increasing elimination.

Route/Dosage

Treatment of Urinary Tract Infections

PO (Adults and Children ≥12 yr): 100 mg q 12 hr or 200 mg as a single daily dose.

Treatment of Otitis Media

PO (Children >6 mos): 5 mg/kg q 12 hr.

Prophylaxis of Chronic Urinary Tract Infections

PO (Adults): 100 mg/day as a single dose (unlabeled).

Pneumocystis carinii Pneumonia

PO (Adults): 20 mg/kg/day with 100 mg dapsone daily for 21 days (unlabeled).

Renal Impairment

PO (Adults): *CCr 15–30 ml/min*—50 mg q 12 hr (for urinary tract infections).

Availability (generic available)

Tablets: 100 mg, 200 mg. **Oral solution (alcohol-and dye-free) (bubblegum flavor):** 50 mg/5 ml in 473-ml bottles. ***In combination with:*** sulfamethoxazole. See Trimethoprim/Sulfamethoxazole monograph.

NURSING IMPLICATIONS

Assessment

- Assess patient for urinary tract infection (fever, cloudy urine, frequency, urgency, pain and burning on urination) or other signs of infection at beginning of and throughout therapy.
- Obtain specimens for culture and sensitivity prior to initiating therapy. First dose may be given before receiving results.
- Monitor intake and output ratios. Fluid intake should be sufficient to maintain urine output of at least 1200–1500 ml daily.
- ***Lab Test Considerations:*** May produce elevated serum bilirubin, creatinine, BUN, AST, and ALT.
- Monitor CBC and urinalysis periodically throughout therapy. Therapy should be discontinued if blood dyscrasias occur.

Potential Nursing Diagnoses

Risk for infection (Indications, Side Effects)

Implementation

- **PO:** Administer on an empty stomach, at least 1 hr before or 2 hr after meals, with a full glass of water. May be administered with food if GI irritation occurs.

Patient/Family Teaching

- Instruct patient to take medication and to finish medication completely as directed, even if feeling better. If a dose is missed, it should be taken as soon as remembered, with subsequent doses spaced evenly apart. Advise patient that sharing of this medication may be dangerous.
- Advise patient to notify health care professional if skin rash, sore throat, fever, mouth sores, or unusual bleeding or bruising occurs. Leucovorin (folinic acid) may be administered if folic acid deficiency occurs.

- Instruct patient to notify health care professional if symptoms do not improve.
- Emphasize the importance of routine follow-up exams to evaluate progress.

Evaluation/Desired Outcomes

- Resolution of the signs and symptoms of infection. Therapy is usually required for 10–14 days for resolution of urinary tract infection.
- Decreased incidence of urinary tract infections during prophylactic therapy.

trimethoprim/sulfamethoxazole

(trye-**meth**-oh-prim/sul-fa-meth-**ox**-a-zole)

♣Apo-Sulfatrim, ♣Apo-Sulfatrim DS, Bactrim, Bactrim DS, Cofatrim, Cotrim, Cotrim DS, ♣Novo-Trimel, ♣Novo-Trimel DS, ♣Nu-Cotrimox, ♣Nu-Cotrimox DS, ♣Roubac, Septra, Septra DS, SMZ/TMP, Sulfatrim, Sulfatrim DS, TMP/SMX, TMP/SMZ

Classification

Therapeutic: anti-infectives, antiprotozoals

Pharmacologic: folate antagonists, sulfonamides

Pregnancy Category C

Indications

Treatment of: Bronchitis, *Shigella* enteritis, Otitis media, *Pneumocystis carinii* pneumonia (PCP), Urinary tract infections, Traveler's diarrhea. Prevention of PCP in HIV-positive patients. **Unlabeled uses:** Biliary tract infections, osteomyelitis, burn and wound infections, chlamydial infections, endocarditis, gonorrhea, intra-abdominal infections, nocardiosis, rheumatic fever prophylaxis, sinusitis, eradication of meningococcal carriers, prophylaxis of urinary tract infections, and an alternative agent in the treatment of chancroid. Prevention of bacterial infections in immunosuppressed patients.

Action

Combination inhibits the metabolism of folic acid in bacteria at two different points. **Therapeutic Effects:** Bactericidal action against susceptible bacteria. **Spectrum:** Active against many strains of gram-positive aerobic pathogens including: *Streptococcus pneumoniae*, *Staphylococcus aureus*, Group A beta-hemolytic streptococci, *Nocardia*, *Enterococcus*. Has activity against many aerobic gram-negative pathogens, such as: *Acinetobacter*, *Enterobacter*, *Klebsiella pneumoniae*, *Escherichia coli*, *Proteus mirabilis*, *Shigella*, *Haemophilus influenzae*, including ampicillin-resistant strains. *P. carinii* (a protozoa). Not active against *Pseudomonas aeruginosa*.

Pharmacokinetics

Absorption: Well absorbed from the GI tract.
Distribution: Widely distributed. Crosses the blood-brain barrier and placenta and enters breast milk.
Metabolism and Excretion: Some metabolism by the liver (20%); remainder excreted unchanged by the kidneys.
Half-life: *Trimethoprim*—6–11 hr; *sulfamethoxazole*—9–12 hr, both prolonged in renal failure.

TIME/ACTION PROFILE (blood levels)

ROUTE	ONSET	PEAK	DURATION
PO	rapid	2–4 hr	6–12 hr
IV	rapid	end of infusion	6–12 hr

Contraindications/Precautions

Contraindicated in: Hypersensitivity to sulfonamides or trimethoprim; Megaloblastic anemia secondary to folate deficiency; Severe renal impairment; Pregnancy, lactation, or children <2 mo (can cause kernicterus in neonates).
Use Cautiously in: Impaired hepatic or renal function (dosage reduction required if CCr <30 ml/min); HIV-positive patients (increased incidence of adverse reactions).

Adverse Reactions/Side Effects

CNS: fatigue, hallucinations, headache, insomnia, mental depression. **GI:** PSEUDOMEMBRANOUS COLITIS, HEPATIC NECROSIS, <u>nausea</u>, <u>vomiting</u>, diarrhea, stomatitis, hepatitis, cholestatic jaundice. **GU:** crystalluria. **Derm:** TOXIC EPIDERMAL NECROLYSIS, <u>rashes</u>, photosensitivity. **Hemat:** AGRANULOCYTOSIS, APLASTIC ANEMIA, hemolytic anemia, leukopenia, megaloblastic anemia, thrombocytopenia. **Local:** <u>phlebitis</u> at IV site. **Misc:** allergic reactions including <u>ERYTHEMA MULTIFORME</u>, STEVENS-JOHNSON SYNDROME, fever.

♣ = Canadian drug name.

* CAPITALS indicates life-threatening; <u>underlines</u> indicate most frequent.

T

Interactions

Drug-Drug: May ↑ half-life, ↓ clearance, and exaggerate folic acid deficiency caused by **phenytoin**. May ↑ effects of **sulfonylurea oral antidiabetics, phenytoin, digoxin, thiopental** and **warfarin**. May ↑ toxicity of **methotrexate**. ↑ risk of thrombocytopenia from **thiazide diuretics** (↑ in geriatric patients). ↓ efficacy of **cyclosporine (decreases serum concentrations)** and ↑ risk of nephrotoxicity.

Route/Dosage

(TMP = trimethoprim; SMX = sulfamethoxazole). Dosing based on TMP content.

Bacterial Infections

PO, IV (Adults and Children >2 mo): *Mild-moderate infections*—6–12 mg TMP/kg/day divided q 12 hr; *Serious infection/Pneumocystis*—15–20 mg TMP/kg/day/divided q 6–8 hr .

PO (Adults): *Urinary tract infection/chronic bronchitis*—1 double strength tablet (160 mg TMP/800 mg SMX) q 12 hr for 10–14 days.

Urinary Tract Infection Prophylaxis

PO, IV (Adults and Children >2 mo): 2 mg TMP/kg/dose daily or 5 mg TMP/kg/dose twice weekly.

P. carinii Pneumonia (Prevention)

PO (Adults): 1 double strength tablet (160 mg TMP/800 mg SMX) daily (may also be given 3 times weekly).

PO (Children >1 mo): 150 mg TMP/m^2/day divided q 12 hr on 3 consecutive days/wk (not to exceed 320 mg TMP/1600 mg SMX per day).

Availability (generic available)

Tablets: ✤20 mg TMP/100 mg SMX, 80 mg TMP/400 mg SMX, 160 mg TMP/800 mg SMX. **Cost:** *Generic*—80 mg TMP/400 mg SMX $11.99/30, 160 mg TMP/800 mg SMX $12.99/30. **Oral suspension (cherry, grape flavors):** 40 mg TMP/200 mg SMX per 5 ml. **Cost:** *Generic*—$11.99/200 ml. **Solution for injection:** 16 mg TMP/80 mg SMX per ml in 5-, 10-, and 30-ml vials.

NURSING IMPLICATIONS

Assessment

- Assess for infection (vital signs; appearance of wound, sputum, urine, and stool; WBC) at beginning of and during therapy.
- Obtain specimens for culture and sensitivity before initiating therapy. First dose may be given before receiving results.
- Inspect IV site frequently. Phlebitis is common.
- Assess patient for allergy to sulfonamides.
- Monitor intake and output ratios. Fluid intake should be sufficient to maintain a urine output of at least 1200–1500 ml daily to prevent crystalluria and stone formation.
- ***Lab Test Considerations:*** Monitor CBC and urinalysis periodically during therapy.
- May produce ↑ serum bilirubin, creatinine, and alkaline phosphatase.

Potential Nursing Diagnoses

Risk for infection (Indications, Side Effects)
Noncompliance (Patient/Family Teaching)

Implementation

- Do not confuse DS (double-strength) formulations with single-strength formulations.
- Do not administer medication IM.
- **PO:** Administer around the clock with a full glass of water. Use calibrated measuring device for liquid preparations.

IV Administration

- **Intermittent Infusion:** ***Diluent:*** Dilute each 5-ml of trimethoprim/sulfamethoxazole with 125 ml of D5W (stable for 24 hr at room temperature). May also dilute each 5-ml of drug with 75 ml of D5W if fluid restriction is required (stable for 6 hr at room temperature). Do not refrigerate. ***Concentration:*** Should not exceed 1.06 mg/ml. ***Rate:*** Infuse over 60–90 min.
- **Y-Site Compatibility:** acyclovir, aldesleukin, allopurinol, amifostine, amphotericin B cholesteryl sulfate complex, anidulafungin, atracurium, aztreonam, bivalirudin, cefepime, cyclophosphamide, daptomycin, dexmedetomidine, diltiazem, docetaxel, doxorubicin liposome, enalaprilat, ertapenem, esmolol, etoposide phosphate, fenoldopam, filgrastim, fludarabine, gemcitabine, granisetron, hydromorphone, labetalol, lansoprazole, levofloxacin, linezolid, lorazepam, magnesium sulfate, melphalan, meperidine, morphine, nicardipine, palonosetron, pancuronium, pantoprazole, pemetrexed, perphenazine, piperacillin/tazobactam, remifentanil, sargramostim, tacrolimus, teniposide, thiotepa, tirofiban, vecuronium, voriconazole, zidovudine.
- **Y-Site Incompatibility:** amikacin, aminophylline, ampicillin, atropine, bumetanide, caspofungin, cefazolin, cefotaxime, cefoxitin, ceftazidime, ceftriaxone, cimetidine, clindamycin, cyclosporine, dexamethasone sodium

phosphate, diazepam, digoxin, diphenhydramine, dobutamine, dopamine, doxycycline, epinephrine, erythromycin, famotidine, fentanyl, fluconazole, furosemide, gentamicin, haloperidol, heparin, hydrocortisone sodium succinate, imipenem/cilastatin, insulin, isoproterenol, ketorolac, lidocaine, methylprednisolone sodium succinate, metoclopramide, metoprolol, metronidazole, midazolam, nafcillin, nitroglycerin, nitroprusside, norepinephrine, ondansetron, penicillin G potassium, phenylephrine, phenytoin, phytonadione, potassium chloride, procainamide, prochlorperazine, promethazine, propranolol, protamine, quinupristin/dalfopristin, ranitidine, sodium bicarbonate, tobramycin, vancomycin, vasopressin, verapamil, vinorelbine.

Patient/Family Teaching

- Instruct patient to take medication around the clock and to finish drug completely as directed, even if feeling well. Take missed doses as soon as remembered unless almost time for next dose. Advise patient that sharing of this medication may be dangerous.
- Instruct patient to notify health care professional if fever and diarrhea develop, especially if diarrhea contains blood, mucus, or pus. Advise patient not to treat diarrhea without consulting health care professional.
- Caution patient to use sunscreen and protective clothing to prevent photosensitivity reactions.
- Advise patient to notify health care professional if skin rash, sore throat, fever, mouth sores, or unusual bleeding or bruising occurs.
- Instruct patient to notify health care professional if symptoms do not improve within a few days.
- Emphasize importance of regular follow-up exams to monitor blood counts in patients on prolonged therapy.
- **Home Care Issues:** Instruct family or caregiver on dilution, rate, and administration of drug and proper care of IV equipment.

Evaluation/Desired Outcomes

- Resolution of the signs and symptoms of infection. Length of time for complete resolution depends on organism and site of infection.
- Resolution of symptoms of traveler's diarrhea.
- Prevention of PCP in patients with HIV.

trospium (tros-pee-yum)

Sanctura, Sanctura XR

Classification

Therapeutic: urinary tract antispasmodics

Pharmacologic: antimuscarinics

Pregnancy Category C

Indications

Overactive bladder with symptoms of urge urinary incontinence, urgency and urinary frequency.

Action

Antagonizes the effect of acetylcholine at muscarinic receptors in the bladder; this parasympatholytic action reduces bladder smooth muscle tone. **Therapeutic Effects:** Increased bladder capacity and decreased symptoms of overactive bladder.

Pharmacokinetics

Absorption: Less than 10% absorbed following oral administration; food significantly ↓ absorption.

Distribution: Mostly distributed to plasma.

Metabolism and Excretion: Of the 10% absorbed, 40% is metabolized. Unabsorbed drug is mainly excreted in feces. Of absorbed drug, 60% is eliminated in urine as unchanged drug via active tubular secretion.

Half-life: 20 hr.

TIME/ACTION PROFILE (anticholinergic effects)

ROUTE	ONSET	PEAK	DURATION
PO	unknown	5–6 hr	24 hr

Contraindications/Precautions

Contraindicated in: Hypersensitivity; Gastric or urinary retention, uncontrolled angle-closure glaucoma or risk for these conditions.

Use Cautiously in: Bladder outflow obstruction; Gastrointestinal obstructive disorders (ulcerative colitis, intestinal atony, myasthenia gravis); Controlled angle-closure glaucoma (use only if necessary and with careful monitoring); CCr less than 30 mL/min (dose reduction recommended); Moderate to severe hepatic impairment;Geri: Geriatric patients (↑ sensitivity to anticholinergic effects; ↓ doses may be required);OB: Pregnancy or lactation (use only if benefit justifies risks to fetus/newborn);Pedi: Children (safety not established).

Adverse Reactions/Side Effects

CNS: headache, dizziness, drowsiness, fatigue. **EENT:** blurred vision. **GI:** constipation, dry mouth, dyspepsia. **GU:** urinary retention, urinary tract infection. **Misc:** fever, heat stroke.

Interactions

Drug-Drug: May interact with other **drugs that compete for tubular secretion**. ↑ risk of anticholinergic effects with other **drugs having anticholinergic properties**.

Route/Dosage

PO (Adults): 20 mg twice daily or 60 mg once daily (XR dose form).
PO (Adults 75 yr or older): based on tolerability dose may be decreased to 20 mg once daily

Renal Impairment

PO (Adults): *CCr less than 30 mL/min*—20 mg once daily at bedtime.

Availability

Tablets: 20 mg. **Extended release tablets:** 60 mg.

NURSING IMPLICATIONS

Assessment

- Monitor voiding pattern and intake and output ratios.

Potential Nursing Diagnoses

Impaired urinary elimination (Indications)

Implementation

- **PO:** Administer 1 hr prior to meals or on an empty stomach.

Patient/Family Teaching

- Instruct patient to take as directed. If a dose is skipped, take next dose 1 hr prior to next meal.
- Caution patient that heat prostration (fever and heat stroke due to decreased sweating) may occur when trospium is taken in a hot environment.
- May cause drowsiness, dizziness and blurred vision. Caution patient to avoid driving and other activities requiring alertness until response to medication is known. Advise patient to avoid alcohol; may increase drowsiness.

Evaluation/Desired Outcomes

- Increased bladder capacity and decreased symptoms of overactive bladder.

urokinase, See THROMBOLYTIC AGENTS.

valacyclovir

(val-ay-**sye**-kloe-veer)
Valtrex

Classification
Therapeutic: antivirals

Pregnancy Category B

Indications

Treatment of herpes zoster (shingles). Treatment/suppression of genital herpes. Reduction of transmission of genital herpes. Treatment of herpes labialis (cold sores).

Action

Rapidly converted to acyclovir. Acyclovir interferes with viral DNA synthesis. **Therapeutic Effects:** Inhibited viral replication, decreased viral shedding, reduced time to healing of lesions. Reduced transmission of genital herpes.

Pharmacokinetics

Absorption: 54% bioavailable as acyclovir after oral administration of valacyclovir.
Distribution: CSF concentrations of acyclovir are 50% of plasma concentrations. Acyclovir crosses placenta; enters breast milk.
Metabolism and Excretion: Rapidly converted to acyclovir via intestinal/hepatic metabolism.
Half-life: 2.5–3.3 hr; up to 14 hr in renal impairment (acyclovir).

TIME/ACTION PROFILE (blood levels†)

ROUTE	ONSET	PEAK	DURATION
PO	unknown	1.5–2.5 hr	8–24 hr

†Acyclovir

Contraindications/Precautions

Contraindicated in: Hypersensitivity to valacyclovir or acyclovir.
Use Cautiously in: Renal impairment (dosage reduction/increased dosing interval recommended if CCr <50 ml/min); Geri: Elderly patients (dose reduction may be necessary); OB: Pregnancy, lactation; Pedi: Children (safety not established).

Adverse Reactions/Side Effects

CNS: headache, dizziness, weakness. **GI:** nausea, abdominal pain, anorexia, constipation, diarrhea. **Hemat:** THROMBOTIC THROMBOCYTOPENIC PURPURA/HEMOLYTIC UREMIC SYNDROME (very high doses in immunosuppressed patients).

Interactions

Drug-Drug: Probenecid and **cimetidine** ↑ blood levels; significant only in renal impairment.

Route/Dosage

Herpes Zoster

PO (Adults): 1 g 3 times daily for 7 days.

Genital Herpes

PO (Adults): *Initial treatment*—1 g twice daily for 10 days. *Recurrence*—500 mg twice daily for 3 days. *Suppression of recurrence*—1 g once daily or 500 mg once daily in patients experiencing <10 recurrences/yr. *Suppression of recurrence in HIV-infected patients*—500 mg q 12 hr. *Reduction of transmission*—500 mg once daily for source partner.

Herpes Labialis

PO (Adults): 2 g then 2 g 12 hr later.

Renal Impairment

PO (Adults): *CCr 30–49 ml/min*—1 g q 12 hr for herpes zoster treatment, no reduction required for treatment of genital herpes; 1 g then 1 g 12 hr later for herpes labialis. *CCr 10–29 ml/min*—1 g q 24 hr for initial treatment of genital herpes, 500 mg q 24 hr for treatment of recurrent episodes of genital herpes, 500 mg q 48 hr for suppression of genital herpes in patients with 9 or fewer recurrences/yr, 500 mg q 24 hr for suppression of genital herpes in patients with ≥10 recurrences/yr or HIV-infected patients, 1 g q 24 hr for treatment of herpes zoster; 500 mg then 500 mg 12 hr later for herpes labialis. *CCr <10 ml/min*—500 mg q 24 hr for initial treatment of genital herpes, 500 mg q 24 hr for treatment of recurrent episodes of genital herpes, 500 mg q 48 hr for suppression of genital herpes in patients with 9 or fewer recurrences/yr, 500 mg q 24 hr for suppression of genital herpes in patients with ≥10 recurrences/yr or HIV-infected patients, 500 mg q 24 hr for treatment of herpes zoster; single 500 mg dose for herpes labialis.

Availability

Tablets: 500 mg, 1 g. **Cost:** 500 mg $177.99/30, 1 g $315.98/30500 mg $151.86/42, 1 g $103.24/20.

V

NURSING IMPLICATIONS

Assessment

- Assess lesions before and daily during therapy.
- Monitor patient for signs of thrombotic thrombocytic purpura/hemolytic uremic syndrome (thrombocytopenia, microangiopathic hemolytic anemia, neurologic findings, renal dysfunction, fever). Requires prompt treatment; may be fatal.

Potential Nursing Diagnoses

Risk for impaired skin integrity (Indications)
Risk for infection (Indications, Patient/Family Teaching)

Implementation

- **PO:** May be administered without regard to meals.
- **Herpes Zoster:** Implement valacyclovir therapy as soon as possible after the onset of signs or symptoms of herpes zoster; most effective if started within 48 hr of the onset of zoster rash. Efficacy of treatment started >72 hr after rash onset is unknown.
- **Genital Herpes and Herpes Labialis:** Implement treatment for genital herpes as soon as possible after onset of symptoms.

Patient/Family Teaching

- Instruct patient to take valacyclovir exactly as directed for the full course of therapy. If a dose is missed, take as soon as remembered if not just before next dose.
- **Herpes Zoster:** Inform patient that valacyclovir does not prevent the spread of infection to others. Precautions should be taken around others who have not had chickenpox or varicella vaccine, or are immunosuppressed, until all lesions have crusted.
- **Genital Herpesand Herpes Labialis:** Inform patient that valacyclovir does not prevent the spread of herpes labialis to others. Advise patient to avoid contact with lesions while lesions or symptoms are present. Valacyclovir prevents transmission of genital herpes to others. Advise patient to practice safe sex (avoid sexual intercourse when lesions are present and wear a condom made of latex or polyurethane during sexual contact).

Evaluation/Desired Outcomes

- Decrease in time to full crusting, loss of vesicles, loss of ulcers, and development of crusts in patients with acute herpes zoster (shingles).
- Decrease in time to full crusting, loss of vesicles, loss of ulcers, and development of crusts in patients with genital herpes.
- Decrease in frequency of outbreaks in patients with genital herpes.
- Decrease in time to full crusting, loss of vesicles, loss of ulcers, and development of crusts in patients with herpes labialis. Decrease in transmission of genital herpes.

valganciclovir

(val-gan-**sye**-kloe-veer)
Valcyte

Classification
Therapeutic: antivirals

Pregnancy Category C

Indications

Treatment of cytomegalovirus (CMV) retinitis in patients with AIDS. Prevention of CMV disease in kidney, kidney/pancreas and heart transplant patients at risk.

Action

Valganciclovir is a prodrug which is rapidly converted to ganciclovir by intestinal and hepatic enzymes. CMV virus converts ganciclovir to its active form (ganciclovir phosphate) inside host cell, where it inhibits viral DNA polymerase. **Therapeutic Effects:** Antiviral effect directed preferentially against CMV-infected cells.

Pharmacokinetics

Absorption: 59.4% absorbed following oral administration, rapidly converted to ganciclovir.
Distribution: Unknown.
Metabolism and Excretion: Rapidly converted to ganciclovir; ganciclovir is mostly excreted by the kidneys.
Half-life: 4.1 hr (intracellular half-life of ganciclovir phosphate is 18 hr).

TIME/ACTION PROFILE (ganciclovir blood levels)

ROUTE	ONSET	PEAK	DURATION
PO	rapid	2 hr	12–24 hr

Contraindications/Precautions

Contraindicated in: Hypersensitivity to valganciclovir or ganciclovir; OB: Pregnancy or

planned pregnancy; OB: Lactation; Hemodialysis; Patients undergoing liver transplantation.
Use Cautiously in: Renal impairment (dosage reduction recommended if CCR <60 ml/min); Pre-existing bone marrow depression; Previous or concurrent myelosuppressive drug therapy or radiation therapy; Geriatric patients (age-related decrease in renal function requires dosage reduction); Pedi: Children (safety not established).

Adverse Reactions/Side Effects

CNS: SEIZURES, headache, insomnia, agitation, confusion, dizziness, hallucinations, psychosis, sedation. **GI:** abdominal pain, diarrhea, nausea, vomiting. **GU:** renal impairment. **Hemat:** NEUTROPENIA, THROMBOCYTOPENIA, anemia, aplastic anemia, bone marrow depression, pancytopenia. **Neuro:** ataxia, paresthesia, peripheral neuropathy. **Misc:** fever, hypersensitivity reactions, infections.

Interactions

Drug-Drug: ↑ risk of hematologic toxicity with **zidovudine**. Blood levels and effects may be ↑ by **probenecid**. Patients with renal impairment may experience accumulation of metabolites of **mycophenolate** and valganciclovir. ↑ blood levels and risk of toxicity from **didanosine**.
Drug-Food: Food ↑ absorption.

Route/Dosage

Treatment of CMV Disease

PO (Adults): *Induction*—900 mg twice daily for 21 days; *maintenance treatment or patients with inactive CMV retinitis*—900 mg once daily.

Renal Impairment

CCr 40–59 ml/min **(Adults):** *Induction*—450 mg twice daily for 21 days; *maintenance treatment or patients with inactive CMV retinitis*—450 mg once daily.

Renal Impairment

CCr 25–39 ml/min **(Adults):** *Induction*—450 mg once daily for 21 days; *maintenance treatment or patients with inactive CMV retinitis*—450 mg every two days.

Renal Impairment

CCr 10–24 ml/min **(Adults):** *Induction*—450 mg every two days for 21 days; *maintenance treatment or patients with inactive CMV retinitis*—450 mg twice weekly.

Prevention of CMV disease in transplant patients

PO (Adults): 900 mg once daily, starting 10 days prior to transplant and continued for 100 days after

Renal Impairment

PO (Adults): *CCr 40–59 ml/min*—450 mg once daily; *CCr 25–39 ml/min*—450 mg every 2 days; *CCr 12–24 ml/min*—450 mg twice weekly.

Availability

Tablets: 450 mg.

NURSING IMPLICATIONS

Assessment

- Diagnosis of CMV retinitis should be determined by ophthalmoscopy prior to treatment with ganciclovir.
- Culture for CMV (urine, blood, throat) may be taken prior to administration. However, a negative CMV culture does not rule out CMV retinitis. If symptoms do not respond after several weeks, resistance to ganciclovir may have occurred. Ophthalmologic exams should be performed weekly during induction and every 2 wk during maintenance or more frequently if the macula or optic nerve is threatened. Progression of CMV retinitis may occur during or following ganciclovir treatment.
- Assess for signs of infection (fever, chills, cough, hoarseness, lower back or side pain, sore throat, difficult or painful urination). Notify physician or other health care professional if these symptoms occur.
- Assess for bleeding (bleeding gums, bruising, petechiae, or guaiac stools, urine, and emesis). Avoid IM injections and taking rectal temperatures. Apply pressure to venipuncture sites for 10 min.
- ***Lab Test Considerations:*** May cause granulocytopenia, anemia, and thrombocytopenia. Monitor neutrophil and platelet count closely throughout therapy. Do not administer if ANC <500/mm³, platelet count <25,000/mm³, or hemoglobin <8 g/dl. Recovery begins within 3–7 days of discontinuation of therapy.
- Monitor BUN and serum creatinine at least once every 2 wk throughout therapy. May cause ↑ in serum creatinine.

V

Potential Nursing Diagnoses
Risk for infection (Indications, Patient/Family Teaching)

Implementation
- Valganciclovir and ganciclovir are not interchangeable. Do not substitute.
- Valganciclovir tablets should be handled carefully. Do not break or crush. May be potentially teratogenic; avoid direct contact with broken or crushed tablets. If contact with the skin or mucous membranes occurs, wash thoroughly with soap and water and rinse eyes thoroughly with plain water.
- **PO:** Administer capsules with food.

Patient/Family Teaching
- Instruct patient to take valganciclovir with food, exactly as directed.
- Inform patient that valganciclovir is not a cure for CMV retinitis. Progression of retinitis may continue in immunocompromised patients during and following therapy. Advise patients to have regular ophthalmic exams at least every 4–6 wk. Duration of therapy for CMV prevention is based on the duration and degree of immunosuppression.
- May cause seizures, sedation, dizziness, ataxia, and/or confusion. Caution patient not to drive or do other activities requiring alertness until response to medication is known.
- Advise patient to notify health care professional if fever; chills; sore throat; other signs of infection; bleeding gums; bruising; petechiae; or blood in urine, stool, or emesis occurs. Caution patient to avoid crowds and persons with known infections. Instruct patient to use soft toothbrush and electric razor. Patient should be cautioned not to drink alcoholic beverages or take products containing aspirin or NSAIDs.
- Advise patient that valganciclovir may have teratogenic effects. Women should use a nonhormonal and men a barrier method of contraception during and for at least 90 days following therapy.
- Caution patient to use sunscreen and protective clothing to prevent photosensitivity reactions.
- Emphasize the importance of frequent follow-up exams to monitor blood counts.

Evaluation/Desired Outcomes
- Management of the symptoms of CMV retinitis in patients with AIDS.

VALPROATES

divalproex sodium
(dye-val-**proe**-ex **soe**-dee-um)
✤Apo-Divalproex, Depakote, Depakote ER, ✤DOM-Divalproex, ✤Epival, ✤Gen-Divalproex, ✤Novo-Divalproex, ✤Nu-Divalproex, ✤PHL-Divalproex, ✤PMS-Divalproex

valproate sodium
(val-**proe**-ate **soe**-dee-um)
Depacon

valproic acid (val-**proe**-ik **as**-id)
✤Apo-Valproic, Depakene, ✤DOM-Valproic Acid, ✤PHL-Valproic Acid, ✤PMS-Valproic Acid, ✤Ratio-Valprox

Classification
Therapeutic: anticonvulsants, vascular headache suppressants

Pregnancy Category D

Indications
Monotherapy and adjunctive therapy for simple and complex absence seizures. Monotherapy and adjunctive therapy for complex partial seizures. Adjunctive therapy for patients with multiple seizure types, including absence seizures. **Divalproex sodium only:** : Manic episodes associated with bipolar disorder, Prevention of migraine headache.

Action
Increase levels of GABA, an inhibitory neurotransmitter in the CNS. **Therapeutic Effects:** Suppression of seizure activity. Decreased manic episodes. Decreased frequency of migraine headaches.

Pharmacokinetics
Absorption: Well absorbed following oral administration; divalproex is enteric-coated, and absorption is delayed. ER form produces lower blood levels. IV administration results in complete bioavailability.
Distribution: Rapidly distributed into plasma and extracellular water. Cross blood-brain barrier and placenta; enters breast milk.
Protein Binding: 80–90%, decreased in neonates, elderly, renal impairment, or chronic hepatic disease.

Metabolism and Excretion: Mostly metabolized by the liver; minimal amounts excreted unchanged in urine.
Half-life: Adults: 9–16 hr.

TIME/ACTION PROFILE (onset = anticonvulsant effect; peak = blood levels)

ROUTE	ONSET	PEAK	DURATION
PO—liquid	2–4 days	15–120 min	6–24 hr
PO—capsules	2–4 days	1–4 hr	6–24 hr
PO—delayed-release products	2–4 days	3–5 hr	12–24 hr
PO—extended-release products	2–4 days	7–14 hr	24 hr
IV	2–4 days	end of infusion	6–24 hr

Contraindications/Precautions

Contraindicated in: Hypersensitivity; Hepatic impairment; Known/suspected urea cycle disorders (may result in fatal hyperammonemic encephalopathy).
Use Cautiously in: Bleeding disorders; History of liver disease; Organic brain disease; Bone marrow depression; Renal impairment; Geri: ↑ risk of adverse effects; OB: Use during pregnancy is linked to congenital anomalies, neural tube defects, clotting abnormalities, and hepatic dysfunction in the neonate. Use with extreme caution. Lactation: Valproates pass into breast milk. Consider discontinuing nursing when valproates are administered to the nursing mother; Pedi: Children, especially <2 yr (at ↑ risk for potentially fatal hepatotoxicity).

Adverse Reactions/Side Effects

CNS: agitation, dizziness, headache, insomnia, sedation, confusion, depression. **CV:** peripheral edema. **EENT:** visual disturbances. **GI:** HEPATOTOXICITY, PANCREATITIS, abdominal pain, anorexia, anorexia, diarrhea, indigestion, nausea, vomiting, constipation, increased appetite. **Derm:** alopecia, rashes. **Endo:** weight gain. **Hemat:** leukopenia, thrombocytopenia. **Metab:** HYPERAMMONEMIA. **Neuro:** tremor, ataxia.

Interactions

Drug-Drug: ↑ risk of bleeding with **warfarin**. Blood levels and toxicity may be ↑ by **aspirin**, **carbamazepine**, **chlorpromazine**, **cimetidine**, **erythromycin**, or **felbamate**. ↑ CNS depression with other **CNS depressants**, including **alcohol**, **antihistamines**, **antidepressants**, **opioid analgesics**, **MAO inhibitors**, and **sedative/hypnotics**. **MAO inhibitors** and other **antidepressants** may ↓ seizure threshold and ↓ effectiveness of valproate. **Carbamazepine**, **meropenem**, **phenobarbital**, **phenytoin**, or **rifampin** may ↓ valproate blood levels. Valproate may ↑ toxicity of **carbamazepine**, **diazepam**, **amitriptyline**, **nortriptyline**, **ethosuximide**, **lamotrigine**, **phenobarbital**, **phenytoin**, **topiramate**, or **zidovudine**.

Route/Dosage

Regular-release and delayed-release formulations usually given in 2–4 divided doses daily; extended-release formulation (Depakote ER) usually given once daily.

Anticonvulsant

PO (Adults and Children >10 yr): *Single-agent therapy (complex partial seizures)*—Initial dose of 10–15 mg/kg/day in 1–4 divided doses; ↑ by 5–10 mg/kg/day weekly until therapeutic response achieved (not to exceed 60 mg/kg/day); when daily dosage exceeds 250 mg, give in divided doses. *Polytherapy (complex partial seizures)*—Initial dose of 10–15 mg/kg/day; ↑ by 5–10 mg/kg/day weekly until therapeutic response achieved (not to exceed 60 mg/kg/day); when daily dosage exceeds 250 mg, give in divided doses.
PO (Adults and Children >2 yr [>10 yr for Depakote ER]): *Simple and complex absence seizures*—Initial dose of 15 mg/kg/day in 1–4 divided doses; ↑ by 5–10 mg/kg/day weekly until therapeutic response achieved (not to exceed 60 mg/kg/day); when daily dosage exceeds 250 mg, give in divided doses.
IV (Adults and Children): Give same daily dose and at same frequency as was given orally; switch to oral formulation as soon as possible.
Rect (Adults and Children): Dilute syrup 1:1 with water for use as a retention enema. Give 17–20 mg/kg load, maintenance 10–15 mg/kg/dose q 8 hr.

Mood Stabilizer

PO (Adults): *Depakote*—Initial dose of 750 mg/day in divided doses initially, titrated rapidly to desired clinical effect or trough plasma levels of 50–125 mcg/ml (not to exceed 60 mg/kg/

day). *Depakote ER*—Initial dose of 25 mg/kg once daily; titrated rapidly to desired clinical effect of trough plasma levels of 85–125 mcg/ml (not to exceed 60 mg/kg/day).

Migraine Prevention

PO (Adults and Children ≥16 yr): *Depakote*—250 mg twice daily (up to 1000 mg/day). *Depakote ER*—500 mg once daily for 1 wk, then ↑ to 1000 mg once daily.

Availability

Valproic Acid

Capsules: 250 mg, ✤500 mg. **Cost:** *Generic*—$29.97/100. **Syrup:** 250 mg/5 ml. **Cost:** *Generic*—$17.99/150 ml.

Valproate Sodium

Injection: 100 mg/ml in 5-ml vials.

Divalproex Sodium

Delayed-release tablets (Depakote): 125 mg, 250 mg, 500 mg. **Cost:** 125 mg $85.85/100, 250 mg $159.98/100, 500 mg $296.66/100. **Capsules-sprinkle:** 125 mg. **Cost:** $83.31/100. **Extended-release tablets (Depakote ER):** 250 mg, 500 mg. **Cost:** 250 mg $134.97/90, 500 mg $225.97/90.

NURSING IMPLICATIONS

Assessment

- **Seizures:** Assess location, duration, and characteristics of seizure activity. Institute seizure precautions.
- **Bipolar Disorder:** Assess mood, ideation, and behavior frequently.
- **Migraine Prophylaxis:** Monitor frequency of migraine headaches.
- Geri: Assess geriatric patients for excessive somnolence.
- ***Lab Test Considerations:*** Monitor CBC, platelet count, and bleeding time prior to and periodically during therapy. May cause leukopenia and thrombocytopenia.
- Monitor hepatic function (LDH, AST, ALT, and bilirubin) and serum ammonia concentrations prior to and periodically during therapy. May cause hepatotoxicity; monitor closely, especially during initial 6 mo of therapy; fatalities have occurred. Therapy should be discontinued if hyperammonemia occurs.
- May interfere with accuracy of thyroid function tests.
- May cause false-positive results in urine ketone tests.
- ***Toxicity and Overdose:*** Therapeutic serum levels range from 50–100 mcg/ml (50–125 mcg/ml for mania). Doses are gradually ↑ until a predose serum concentration of at least 50 mcg/ml is reached. However, a good correlation among daily dose, serum level, and therapeutic effects has not been established. Patients receiving near the maximum recommended 60 mg/kg/day should be monitored for toxicity.

Potential Nursing Diagnoses

Risk for injury (Indications)

Implementation

- Do not confuse Depakote ER and regular dosage forms. Depakote ER produces lower blood levels than Depakote dosing forms. If switching from Depakote to Depakote ER, increase dose by 8-20%.
- Single daily doses are usually administered at bedtime because of sedation.
- **PO:** Administer with or immediately after meals to minimize GI irritation. Tell patient to swallow extended-release and delayed-release tablets whole, not to break or chew them, because this will cause irritation of the mouth or throat and destroy extended release mechanism. Do not administer tablets with milk or carbonated beverages (may cause premature dissolution). Delayed-release divalproex sodium may cause less GI irritation than valproic acid capsules.
- Shake liquid preparations well before pouring. Use calibrated measuring device to ensure accurate dosage. Syrup may be mixed with food or other liquids to improve taste.
- Sprinkle capsules may be swallowed whole or opened and entire capsule contents sprinkled on a teaspoonful of soft, cool food (applesauce, pudding). Tell patient to swallow drug/food mixture immediately, not to chew it. Do not store for future use.
- To convert from valproic acid to divalproex sodium, initiate divalproex sodium at same total daily dose and dosing schedule as valproic acid. Once patient is stabilized on divalproex sodium, attempt administration 2–3 times daily.
- **Rect:** Dilute syrup 1:1 with water for use as a retention enema.

IV Administration

- **Intermittent Infusion:** ***Diluent:*** May be diluted in at least 50 ml of D5W, 0.9% NaCl, or LR. Solution is stable for 24 hr at room temperature. ***Concentration:*** 2 mg/ml. ***Rate:*** Infuse over 60 min (≤20 mg/min).

Rapid infusion may cause increased side effects. Has been given as a one-time infusion of 1000 mg over 5-10 min @ 3 mg/kg/min up to 15 mg/kg in patients with no detectable valproate levels.

Patient/Family Teaching

- Instruct patient to take medication as directed. If a dose is missed on a once-a-day schedule, take as soon as remembered that day. If on a multiple-dose schedule, take it within 6 hr of the scheduled time, then space remaining doses throughout the remainder of the day. Abrupt withdrawal may lead to status epilepticus.
- May cause drowsiness or dizziness. Caution patient to avoid driving or other activities requiring alertness until effects of medication are known. Tell patient not to resume driving until physician gives clearance based on control of seizure disorder.
- Caution patient to avoid taking alcohol, CNS depressants, OTC medications or herbal products concurrently with valproates without consulting health care professional.
- Instruct patient to notify health care professional of medication regimen prior to treatment or surgery.
- Advise patient to carry identification at all times describing medication regimen.
- Advise patient to notify health care professional if anorexia, abdominal pain, severe nausea and vomiting, yellow skin or eyes, fever, sore throat, malaise, weakness, facial edema, lethargy, unusual bleeding or bruising, pregnancy, or loss of seizure control occurs. Children <2 yr of age are especially at risk for fatal hepatotoxicity.
- Emphasize the importance of routine exams to monitor progress.

Evaluation/Desired Outcomes

- Decreased seizure activity.
- Decreased incidence of manic episodes in patients with bipolar disorders.
- Decreased frequency of migraine headaches.

valsartan, See ANGIOTENSIN II RECEPTOR ANTAGONISTS.

vancomycin

(van-koe-**mye**-sin)

Lyphocin, Vancocin, Vancoled

Classification

Therapeutic: anti-infectives

Pregnancy Category C

Indications

IV: Treatment of potentially life-threatening infections when less toxic anti-infectives are contraindicated. Particularly useful in staphylococcal infections, including: Endocarditis, Meningitis, Osteomyelitis, Pneumonia, Septicemia, Soft-tissue infections in patients who have allergies to penicillin or its derivatives or when sensitivity testing demonstrates resistance to methicillin. **PO:** Treatment of staphylococcal enterocolitis or pseudomembranous colitis due to *Clostridium difficile*. **IV:** Part of endocarditis prophylaxis in high-risk patients who are allergic to penicillin.

Action

Binds to bacterial cell wall, resulting in cell death. **Therapeutic Effects:** Bactericidal action against susceptible organisms. **Spectrum:** Active against gram-positive pathogens, including: Staphylococci (including methicillin-resistant strains of *Staphylococcus aureus*), Group A beta-hemolytic streptococci, *Streptococcus pneumoniae*, *Corynebacterium*, *Clostridium difficile*, *Enterococcus faecalis*, *Enterococcus faecium*.

Pharmacokinetics

Absorption: Poorly absorbed from the GI tract.
Distribution: Widely distributed. Some penetration (20–30%) of CSF; crosses placenta.
Metabolism and Excretion: Oral doses excreted primarily in the feces; IV vancomycin eliminated almost entirely by the kidneys.
Half-life: Neonates: 6–10 hr; Children 3 mo–3 yr: 4 hr; Children >3 yr: 2–2.3 hr; Adults: 5–8 hr (increased in renal impairment).

TIME/ACTION PROFILE (blood levels)

ROUTE	ONSET	PEAK	DURATION
IV	rapid	end of infusion	12–24 hr

Contraindications/Precautions

Contraindicated in: Hypersensitivity.

Use Cautiously in: Renal impairment (dosage reduction required if CCr ≤80 ml/min); Hearing impairment; Intestinal obstruction or inflammation (increased systemic absorption when given orally); Pregnancy and lactation (safety not established).

Adverse Reactions/Side Effects

EENT: ototoxicity. **CV:** hypotension. **GI:** nausea, vomiting. **GU:** nephrotoxicity. **Derm:** rashes. **Hemat:** eosinophilia, leukopenia. **Local:** phlebitis. **MS:** back and neck pain. **Misc:** hypersensitivity reactions including ANAPHYLAXIS, chills, fever, "red man" syndrome (with rapid infusion), superinfection.

Interactions

Drug-Drug: May cause additive ototoxicity and nephrotoxicity with other **ototoxic** and **nephrotoxic drugs (aspirin, aminoglycosides, cyclosporine, cisplatin, loop diuretics)**. May enhance neuromuscular blockade from **nondepolarizing neuromuscular blocking agents**. Increased risk of histamine flush when used with **general anesthetics** in children.

Route/Dosage

Serious Systemic Infections

IV (Adults): 500 mg q 6 hr *or* 1 g q 12 hr (up to 4 g/day).
IV (Children >1 mo): 40 mg/kg/day divided q 6–8 hr *Staphylococcal CNS infection*—60 mg/kg/day divided q 6 hr, maximum dose: 1 g/dose.
IV (Neonates 1 wk–1 mo): <1200 g: 15 mg/kg/day q 24 hr. 1200–2000 g: 10–15 mg/kg/dose q 8–12 hr. >2000 g: 15–20 mg/kg/dose q 8 hr.
IV (Neonates <1 wk): <1200 g: 15 mg/kg/day q 24 hr. 1200–2000 g: 10–15 mg/kg/dose q 12–18 hr. >2000 g: 10–15 mg/kg/dose q 8–12 hr.
IT (Adults): 20 mg/day.
IT (Children): 5–20 mg/day.
IT (Neonates): 5–10 mg/day.

Endocarditis Prophylaxis in Penicillin-Allergic Patients

IV (Adults and Adolescents): 1-g single dose 1-hr preprocedure.
IV (Children): 20-mg/kg single dose 1-hr preprocedure.

Pseudomembranous Colitis

PO (Adults): 125–500 mg q 6 hr.
PO (Children): 40 mg/kg/day divided q 6 hr for 7–10 days (not to exceed 2 g/day).

Renal Impairment

IV (Adults): An initial loading dose of 750 mg–1 g (not less than 15 mg/kg); serum level monitoring is optimal for choosing maintenance dosage in patients with renal impairment; these guidelines may be helpful. *CCr 50–80 ml/min*—1 g q 1–3 days; *CCr 10–50 ml/min*—1 g q 3–7 days; *CCr <10 ml/min*—1 g q 7–14 days.

Availability (generic available)

Capsules: 125 mg, 250 mg. **Oral solution:** 250 mg/5 ml, 500 mg/6 ml. **Injection:** 500-mg 1-, 5-, 10-g vials.

NURSING IMPLICATIONS

Assessment

- Assess patient for infection (vital signs; appearance of wound, sputum, urine, and stool; WBC) at beginning of and throughout therapy.
- Obtain specimens for culture and sensitivity prior to initiating therapy. First dose may be given before receiving results.
- Monitor IV site closely. Vancomycin is irritating to tissues and causes necrosis and severe pain with extravasation. Rotate infusion site.
- Monitor blood pressure throughout IV infusion.
- Evaluate eighth cranial nerve function by audiometry and serum vancomycin levels prior to and throughout therapy in patients with borderline renal function or those >60 yr of age. Prompt recognition and intervention are essential in preventing permanent damage.
- Monitor intake and output ratios and daily weight. Cloudy or pink urine may be a sign of nephrotoxicity.
- Assess patient for signs of superinfection (black, furry overgrowth on tongue; vaginal itching or discharge; loose or foul-smelling stools). Report occurrence.
- **Pseudomembranous Colitis:** Assess bowel status (bowel sounds, frequency and consistency of stools, presence of blood in stools) throughout therapy.
- ***Lab Test Considerations:*** Monitor for casts, albumin, or cells in the urine or decreased specific gravity, CBC, and renal function periodically throughout course of therapy.
- May cause increased BUN levels.
- ***Toxicity and Overdose:*** Peak serum vancomycin levels should not exceed 25–40

mcg/ml. Trough concentrations should not exceed 5–10 mcg/ml.

Potential Nursing Diagnoses

Risk for infection (Indications)
Disturbed sensory perception (auditory) (Side Effects)

Implementation

- **PO:** Use calibrated measuring device for liquid preparations. IV dosage form may be diluted in 30 ml of water for oral or nasogastric tube administration. Resulting solution has bitter, unpleasant taste. May mix with a flavoring syrup to mask taste. Stable for 14 days if refrigerated.

IV Administration

- **Intermittent Infusion:** ***Diluent:*** To reconstitute, add 10 ml of sterile water for injection to 500-mg vial or 20 ml of sterile water for injection to 1-g vial for a concentration of 50 mg/ml. Dilute further with at least 100 ml of 0.9% NaCl, D5W, D5/0.9% NaCl, or LR for every 500 mg of vancomycin being administered. Reconstituted vials stable for 14 days if refrigerated. Infusion is stable for 96 hr if refrigerated. ***Concentration:*** Final concentration of infusion should be ≤5 mg/ml. ***Rate:*** Infuse over at least 60 min. Do not administer rapidly or as a bolus, to minimize risk of thrombophlebitis, hypotension, and "red man (neck)" syndrome (sudden, severe hypotension; flushing and/or maculopapular rash of face, neck, chest, and upper extremities). May need to slow infusion further to 1.5–2 hr if red-man syndrome occurs. **IT:** ***Diluent:*** Dilute with preservative-free NS. ***Concentration:*** 1–5 mg/ml. ***Rate:*** Directly instill into ventricular cerebrospinal fluid.
- **Y-Site Compatibility:** acyclovir, aldesleukin, allopurinol, amifostine, amiodarone, amsacrine, atracurium, cisatracurium, cyclophosphamide, dexmedetomidine, diltiazem, docetaxel, doxorubicin liposome, enalaprilat, esmolol, etoposide phosphate, fenoldopam, filgrastim, fluconazole, fludarabine, gemcitabine, granisetron, hydromorphone, insulin, labetalol, levofloxacin, linezolid, lorazepam, magnesium sulfate, melphalan, meperidine, meropenem, midazolam, milrinone, morphine, nicardipine, ondansetron, paclitaxel, pancuronium, pemetrexed, perphenazine, remifentanil, sodium bicarbonate, tacrolimus, teniposide, theophylline, thiotepa, tolazoline, vecuronium, vinorelbine, zidovudine.
- **Y-Site Incompatibility:** albumin, amphotericin B cholesteryl sulfate, drotrecogin, heparin, idarubicin, lansoprazole, omeprazole.

Patient/Family Teaching

- Advise patients on oral vancomycin to take as directed. Take missed doses as soon as remembered unless almost time for next dose; do not double dose.
- Instruct patient to report signs of hypersensitivity, tinnitus, vertigo, or hearing loss.
- Advise patient to notify health care professional if no improvement is seen in a few days.
- Patients with a history of rheumatic heart disease or valve replacement need to be taught importance of using antimicrobial prophylaxis prior to invasive dental or medical procedures.

Evaluation/Desired Outcomes

- Resolution of signs and symptoms of infection. Length of time for complete resolution depends on organism and site of infection.
- Endocarditis prophylaxis.

vardenafil (ver-**den**-a-fil)

Levitra

Classification
Therapeutic: erectile dysfunction agents
Pharmacologic: phosphodiesterase type 5 inhibitors

Pregnancy Category C

Indications

Erectile dysfunction.

Action

Increases cyclic guanosine monophosphate (cGMP) levels by inhibiting phosphodiesterase type 5 (PDE5) an enzyme responsible for the breakdown of cGMP. cGMP produces smooth muscle relaxation of the corpus cavernosum, which in turn promotes increased blood flow and subsequent erection. **Therapeutic Effects:** Enhanced blood flow to the corpus cavernosum and erection sufficient to allow sexual intercourse. Requires sexual stimulation.

Pharmacokinetics

Absorption: 15% absorbed following oral administration; absorption is rapid.
Distribution: Extensive tissue distribution; penetrates semen.
Protein Binding: 95%.
Metabolism and Excretion: Mostly metabolized by the liver (mainly CYP3A4 enzyme system, minor metabolism by CYP2C). M1 metabolite has anti-erectile dysfunction activity. Parent drug and metabolites are mostly excreted in feces. 2–6% renally eliminated.
Half-life: 4–5 hr.

TIME/ACTION PROFILE

ROUTE	ONSET	PEAK	DURATION
PO	rapid	0.5–2 hr	4 hr

Contraindications/Precautions

Contraindicated in: Hypersensitivity; Concurrent use of nitrates or nitric oxide donors; Unstable angina, recent history of stroke, life-threatening arrhythmias, CHF or MI within 6 mo; End-stage renal disease requiring dialysis; Known hereditary degenerative retinal disorders; Severe hepatic impairment (Child-Pugh C); Congenital or acquired QT prolongation or concurrent use of Class IA or III antiarrhythmics; Women, children or newborns.
Use Cautiously in: Other serious underlying cardiovascular disease or left ventricular outflow obstruction; Penile deformity; Underlying conditions predisposing to priapism including sickle cell anemia, multiple myeloma or leukemia; Bleeding disorders or active peptic ulcer diseases; History of sudden severe vision loss or non arteritic ischemic optic neuropathy (NAION); may ↑ risk of recurrence; Strong inhibitors of the CYP3A4 enzyme system; Geri: Patients >65 yr have ↑ blood levels; ↓ dose required).
Exercise Extreme Caution in: Concurrent use with alpha-adrenergic blockers may result is serious hypotension.

Adverse Reactions/Side Effects

CNS: headache, dizziness. **EENT:** rhinitis, sinusitis. **CV:** . **GI:** dyspepsia, nausea. **GU:** priapism. **Derm:** flushing. **Misc:** flu syndrome.

Interactions

Drug-Drug: Concurrent use of **nitrates** may cause serious, life threatening hypotension and is contraindicated. Concurrent use of Class IA antiarrhythmics (such as **quindine** or **procainamide**) or **Class III antiarrhythmics** (such as **amiodarone** or **sotalol**) ↑ risk of serious arrhythmias and should be avoided. Concurrent use of alpha-adrenergic blockers may cause serious hypotension, lowest doses of each should be used initially. Strong inhibitors of CYP3A4 including **protease inhibitor antiretrovirals** (including **ritonavir**, **saquinavir** and **indinavir**), **ketoconazole**, and **itraconazole** ↑ effects and the risk of adverse reactions (dosage adjustments recommended). Concurrent use of moderate inhibitors of CYP2C including **erythromycin** may also ↑ effects. ↑ risk of hypotension with **antihypertensives** and acute ingestion of **alcohol**.

Route/Dosage

PO (Adults): 10 mg taken 1 hr prior to sexual activity (range 5–20 mg; not to exceed one dose/24 hr); *concurrent use of ritonavir*—single dose should not exceed 2.5 mg in any 72-hour period; *concurrent use of indinavir, ketoconazole 400 mg daily or itraconazole 400 mg daily*—single dose should not exceed 2.5 mg/24 hr; *concurrent use of ketoconazole or itraconazole 200 mg daily or erythromycin*—single dose should not exceed 5 mg/24 hr.
PO (Geriatric Patients >65 yr): 5 mg initial dose; titrate as tolerated.

Hepatic Impairment

PO (Adults): *Moderate hepatic impairment (Child-Pugh B)*—May start with 5-mg dose, subsequent dosing should not to exceed 10.

Availability

Tablets: 2.5 mg, 5 mg, 10 mg, 20 mg. **Cost:** 2.5 mg $68.99/6, 5 mg $111.99/10, 10 mg $109.99/10, 20 mg $115.99/10.

NURSING IMPLICATIONS

Assessment

- Determine erectile dysfunction before administration. Vardenafil has no effect in the absence of sexual stimulation.

Potential Nursing Diagnoses

Sexual dysfunction (Indications)

Implementation

- **PO:** Dose is usually administered 1 hr before sexual activity. May be administered 30 min to 4 hr before sexual activity.
- May be administered without regard to food.

Patient/Family Teaching

- Instruct patient to take vardenafil approximately 1 hr before sexual activity and not more than once per day. Inform patient that sexual stimulation is required for an erection to occur after taking vardenafil.

- Advise patient that vardenafil is not indicated for use in women.
- Caution patient not to take vardenafil concurrently with nitrates or alpha adrenergic blockers.
- Instruct patient to notify health care professional promptly if erection lasts longer than 4 hr, if they are not satisfied with their sexual performance or develop unwanted side effects or if they experience sudden or decreased vision loss in one or both eyes.
- Advise patient to consult health care professional before taking other Rx or OTC medications or herbal supplements that may interact with vardenafil.
- Inform patient that vardenafil offers no protection against sexually transmitted diseases. Counsel patient that protection against sexually transmitted diseases and HIV infection should be considered.

Evaluation/Desired Outcomes

- Male erection sufficient to allow intercourse.

varenicline (ver-en-i-cline)

Chantix

Classification

Therapeutic:

Pharmacologic: nicotine agonists

Pregnancy Category C

Indications

Treatment of smoking cessation; in conjuction with nonpharmacologic support (educational materials/counseling).

Action

Selectively binds to $alpha_4$ $beta_2$ nicotinic acetylcholine receptors, acting as a nicotine agonist; prevents the binding of nicotine to receptors. **Therapeutic Effects:** Decreased desire to smoke.

Pharmacokinetics

Absorption: 100% absorbed following oral administration.

Distribution: 24 hr.

Metabolism and Excretion: Minimally metabolized; 92% excreted in urine unchanged.

Half-life: 24 hr.

TIME/ACTION PROFILE

ROUTE	ONSET	PEAK	DURATION
PO	unknown	3–4 hr	24 hr

Contraindications/Precautions

Contraindicated in: Hypersensitivity; OB: Lactation; Pedi: Children <18 yr (safety not established).

Use Cautiously in: Severe renal impairment (lower dose recommended if CCr <30 ml/min); Geri: Consider age-related decline in renal function; OB: Pregnancy (use only if maternal benefit outweighs fetal risk).

Adverse Reactions/Side Effects

CNS: ↓ attention span, anxiety, depression, insomnia, irritability, dizziness, restlessness, abnormal dreams, agitation, aggression, amnesia, disorientation, dissociation, migraine, psychomotor hyperactivity. **CV:** syncope. **GI:** diarrhea, gingivitis, nausea, ↑ appetite, constipation, dyspepsia, dysphagia, enterocolitis, eructation, flatulence, gall bladder disorder, gi bleeding, ↑ liver function tests, vomiting. **Derm:** flushing, hyperhydrosis, acne, dermatitis, dry skin. **Hemat:** anemia. **MS:** arthralgia, back pain, musculoskeletal pain, muscle cramps, myalgia, restless legs. **Misc:** chills, fever, hypersensitivity, mild physical dependence.

Interactions

Drug-Drug: Smoking cessation may ↓ metabolism of **theophylline**, **warfarin**, and **insulin** resulting in ↑ effects; careful monitoring is recommended. Risk of adverse reactions (nausea, vomiting, dizziness, fatigue, headache) may be ↑ with **nicotine** replacement therapy (nicotine transdermal patches).

Route/Dosage

PO (Adults): Treatment is started one week prior to planned smoking cessation 0.5 mg once daily on the first three days, then 0.5 mg twice daily for the next 4 days, then 1 mg twice daily

Renal Impairment

PO (Adults): *CCr <30 ml/min*—0.5 mg daily, may increase to 0.5 mg twice daily.

Availability

Tablets: 0.5 mg, 1 mg.

NURSING IMPLICATIONS

Assessment

- Assess for desire to stop smoking.

V

- Assess for nausea. Usually dose-dependent. May require dose reduction.
- ***Lab Test Considerations:*** May cause anemia.

Potential Nursing Diagnoses

Ineffective coping (Indications)

Implementation

- **PO:** Administer after eating with a full glass of water.

Patient/Family Teaching

- Instruct patient to take varenicline as directed. Set a date to stop smoking. Start taking varenicline 1 wk before quit date. Begin with 0.5 mg/day for the first 3 days, then for the next 4 days take one 0.5-mg tablet in the morning and in the evening. After first 7 days, increase to 1-mg tablet in the morning and evening.
- Encourage patient to attempt to quit, even it they had early lapses after quit day.
- Provide patient with educational materials and counseling to support attempts to quit smoking.
- Caution patient not to share varenicline with others. May be harmful.
- May cause dizziness and disturbance in attention. Caution patient to avoid driving and other activities requiring alertness until response to medication is known.
- Inform patient that nausea and insomnia may occur and are usually transient. Advise patient to notify health care professional if these symptoms are persistent and bothersome; dose reduction may be considered.
- Advise patient to notify health care professional before taking Rx, OTC, or herbal products. Inform patient that some medications may require dose adjustments after quitting smoking.
- Advise patient to notify health care professional if pregnancy is planned or suspected or if breastfeeding.

Evaluation/Desired Outcomes

- Smoking cessation. Patients who have successfully stopped smoking at the end of 12 wks, should take an additional 12-wk course to increase the likelihood of long-term abstinence. Patients who do not succeed in stopping smoking during 12 wks of initial therapy or who relapse after treatment, should be encouraged to make another attempt once factors contributing to the failed attempt have been identified and addressed.

vasopressin

(vay-soe-**press**-in)
Pitressin, ✤Pressyn

Classification
Therapeutic: hormones
Pharmacologic: antidiuretic hormones

Pregnancy Category C

Indications

Central diabetes insipidus due to deficient antidiuretic hormone. **Unlabeled uses:** Management of pulseless VT/VF unresponsive to initial shocks, asystole, or pulseless electrical activity (PEA) (ACLS guidlines). Septic shock.

Action

Alters the permeability of the renal collecting ducts, allowing reabsorption of water. Directly stimulates musculature of GI tract. In high doses acts as a nonadrenergic peripheral vasoconstrictor. **Therapeutic Effects:** Decreased urine output and increased urine osmolality in diabetes insipidus.

Pharmacokinetics

Absorption: IM absorption may be unpredictable.
Distribution: Widely distributed throughout extracellular fluid.
Metabolism and Excretion: Rapidly degraded by the liver and kidneys; <5% excreted unchanged by the kidneys.
Half-life: 10–20 min.

TIME/ACTION PROFILE (antidiuretic effect)

ROUTE	ONSET	PEAK	DURATION
IM, subcut	unknown	unknown	2–8 hr
IV	unknown	unknown	30–60 min

Contraindications/Precautions

Contraindicated in: Chronic renal failure with increased BUN; Hypersensitivity to beef or pork proteins.
Use Cautiously in: Perioperative polyuria (increased sensitivity to vasopressin); Comatose patients; Seizures; Migraine headaches; Asthma; Heart failure; Cardiovascular disease; Geri, Pedi: Geriatric patients and children (↑ sensitivity to vasopressin); Renal impairment.

Adverse Reactions/Side Effects

CNS: dizziness, "pounding" sensation in head. **CV:** MI, angina, chest pain. **GI:** abdominal cramps, belching, diarrhea, flatulence, heartburn, nausea, vomiting. **Derm:** paleness, perioral blanching, sweating. **Neuro:** trembling. **Misc:** allergic reactions, fever, water intoxication (higher doses).

Interactions

Drug-Drug: Antidiuretic effect may be ↓ by concurrent administration of **alcohol**, **lithium**, **demeclocycline**, **heparin**, or **norepinephrine**. Antidiuretic effect may be ↑ by concurrent administration of **carbamazepine**, **chlorpropamide**, **clofibrate**, **tricyclic antidepressants**, or **fludrocortisone**. Vasopressor effect may be ↑ by concurrent administration of **ganglionic blocking agents**.

Route/Dosage

IM, Subcut (Adults): 5–10 units 2–4 times daily.
IM, Subcut (Children): 2.5–10 units 2–4 times daily.
IV (Adults): *Pulseless VT/VF, asystole, or PEA (ACLS guidelines)*—40 units as a single dose (unlabeled). *Septic shock*—0.04 units/min infusion.

Availability (generic available)

Injection: 20 units/ml in 0.5- and 1-ml ampules and vials.

NURSING IMPLICATIONS

Assessment

- Monitor BP, HR, and ECG periodically throughout therapy and continuously throughout cardiopulmonary resuscitation.
- **Diabetes Insipidus:** Monitor urine osmolality and urine volume frequently to determine effects of medication. Assess patient for symptoms of dehydration (excessive thirst, dry skin and mucous membranes, tachycardia, poor skin turgor). Weigh patient daily, monitor intake and output, and assess for edema.
- ***Lab Test Considerations:*** Monitor urine specific gravity throughout therapy.
- Monitor serum electrolyte concentrations periodically during therapy.
- ***Toxicity and Overdose:*** Signs and symptoms of water intoxication include confusion, drowsiness, headache, weight gain, difficulty urinating, seizures, and coma: Treatment of overdose includes water restriction and temporary discontinuation of vasopressin until polyuria occurs. If symptoms are severe, administration of mannitol, hypertonic dextrose, urea, and/or furosemide may be used.

Potential Nursing Diagnoses

Deficient fluid volume (Indications)
Excess fluid volume (Adverse Reactions)

Implementation

- Do not confuse Pitressin (vasopressin) with Pitocin (oxytocin).
- Aqueous vasopressin injection may be administered subcut or IM for diabetes insipidus.
- Administer 1–2 glasses of water at the time of administration to minimize side effects (blanching of skin, abdominal cramps, nausea).

IV Administration

- **Direct IV:** ***Diluent:*** Administer undiluted. ***Concentration:*** 20 units/ml. ***Rate:*** Administer over 1–2 sec during pulseless VT/VF, asystole, or PEA.
- **Continuous Infusion:** ***Diluent:*** Dilute 100 units of vasopressin in 250 ml of 0.9% NaCl or D5W. ***Concentration:*** 0.4 units/ml. ***Diluent:*** Dilute 100 units of vasopressin in 250 ml of 0.9% NaCl or D5W. ***Concentration:*** 0.4 units/ml. ***Rate:*** See Route/Dosage section.
- **Y-Site Compatibility:** amiodarone, argatroban, ciprofloxacin, diltiazem, dobutamine, dopamine, drotrecogin, epinephrine, fluconazole, gentamicin, heparin, imipenem/cilastatin, insulin, lidocaine, linezolid, meropenem, metronidazole, milrinone, nitroglycerin, norepinephrine, pantoprazole, phenylephrine, procainamide, sodium bicarbonate.
- **Y-Site Incompatibility:** diazepam, phenytoin, trimethoprim/sulfamethoxazole.

Patient/Family Teaching

- Instruct patient to take medication as directed. Caution patient not to use more than prescribed amount. Take missed doses as soon as remembered, unless almost time for next dose.
- Advise patient to drink 1–2 glasses of water at time of administration to minimize side effects (blanching of skin, abdominal cramps, nausea). Inform patient that these side effects are not serious and usually disappear in a few minutes.

- Caution patient to avoid concurrent use of alcohol while taking vasopressin.
- Patients with diabetes insipidus should carry identification at all times describing disease process and medication regimen.

Evaluation/Desired Outcomes

- Decrease in urine volume.
- Relief of polydipsia.
- Increased urine osmolality in patients with central diabetes insipidus.
- Resolution of VT/VF.
- Improvement in signs of septic shock.

venlafaxine (ven-la-**fax**-een)

Effexor, Effexor XR

Classification

Therapeutic: antidepressants, antianxiety agents

Pregnancy Category C

Indications

Major depressive illness or relapse, often in conjunction with psychotherapy. Generalized anxiety disorder (Effexor XR only). Social anxiety disorder (Effexor XR only). **Unlabeled uses:** Premenstrual dysphoric disorder (PMDD).

Action

Inhibits serotonin and norepinephrine reuptake in the CNS. **Therapeutic Effects:** Decrease in depressive symptomatology, with fewer relapses/recurrences. Decreased anxiety.

Pharmacokinetics

Absorption: 92–100% absorbed after oral administration.

Distribution: Extensive distribution into body tissues.

Metabolism and Excretion: Extensively metabolized on 1st pass through the liver. One metabolite, O-desmethylvenlafaxine (ODV), has antidepressant activity; 5% of venlafaxine is excreted unchanged in urine; 30% of the active metabolite is excreted in urine.

Half-life: *Venlafaxine*—3–5 hr; *ODV*—9–11 hr (both are increased in hepatic/renal impairment).

TIME/ACTION PROFILE (antidepressant action)

ROUTE	ONSET	PEAK	DURATION
PO	within 2 wk	2–4 wk	unknown

Contraindications/Precautions

Contraindicated in: Hypersensitivity; Concurrent MAO inhibitor therapy.

Use Cautiously in: Cardiovascular disease, including hypertension; Hepatic impairment (↓ dose recommended); Impaired renal function (↓ dose recommended); History of seizures or neurologic impairment; History of mania; History of increased intraocular pressure or angle-closure glaucoma; History of drug abuse; OB: Use only if clearly required during pregnancy weighing benefit to mother versus potential harm to fetus (potential for discontinuation syndrome or toxicity in the neonate when venlafaxine is taken during the third trimester); Lactation: Potential for serious adverse reactions in infant; discontinue drug or discontinue breast-feeding; Pedi: Increased risk of suicidal thinking and behavior (suicidality) in children and adolescents with Major Depressive Disorder (MDD) and other psychiatric disorders. Observe closely for suicidality and behavior changes.

Adverse Reactions/Side Effects

CNS: SEIZURES, abnormal dreams, anxiety, dizziness, headache, insomnia, nervousness, weakness, abnormal thinking, agitation, confusion, depersonalization, drowsiness, emotional lability, worsening depression. **EENT:** rhinitis, visual disturbances, tinnitus. **CV:** chest pain, hypertension, palpitations, tachycardia. **GI:** abdominal pain, altered taste, anorexia, constipation, diarrhea, dry mouth, dyspepsia, nausea, vomiting, weight loss. **GU:** sexual dysfunction, urinary frequency, urinary retention. **Derm:** ecchymoses, itching, photosensitivity, skin rash. **Neuro:** paresthesia, twitching. **Misc:** chills, yawning.

Interactions

Drug-Drug: Concurrent use with **MAO inhibitors** may result in serious, potentially fatal reactions (wait at least 2 wk after stopping MAO inhibitor before initiating venlafaxine; wait at least 1 wk after stopping venlafaxine before starting MAO inhibitors). Concurrent use with **alcohol** or other **CNS depressants**, including **sedative/hypnotics**, **antihistamines**, and **opioid analgesics**, in depressed patients is not recommended. ↑ risk of serotonin syndrome with **trazodone sibutramine** and **triptans**. **Lithium** may have ↑ serotonergic effects with venlafaxine; use cautiously in patients receiving venlafaxine. ↑ blood levels and may ↑ effects of **desipramine** and **haloperidol**. **Cimetidine** may ↑ the effects of venlafaxine (may be more pronounced in geriatric patients, those with hepatic or renal impairment, or those with pre-existing hypertension).

Drug-Natural Products: Concomitant use of **kava kava**, **valerian**, **chamomile**, or **hops** can ↑ CNS depression. ↑ risk of serotinergic side effects including serotonin syndrome with **St. John's wort** and **SAMe**.

Route/Dosage

PO (Adults): *Tablets*—75 mg/day in 2–3 divided doses; may increase by up to 75 mg/day every 4 days, up to 225 mg/day (not to exceed 375 mg/day in 3 divided doses); *Extended-release (XR) capsules*—75 mg once daily (some patients may be started at 37.5 mg once daily) for 4–7 days; doses may then be increased at intervals of not less than 4 days up to 225 mg/day.

Hepatic Impairment

PO (Adults): Decrease daily dose by 50% in patients with moderate hepatic impairment.

Renal Impairment

PO (Adults): *Mild to moderate renal impairment*—Daily dose should be decreased by 25–50%.

Availability (generic available)

Tablets: 25 mg, 37.5 mg, 50 mg, 75 mg, 100 mg. **Cost:** *Generic*—25 mg $299.95/180, 37.5 mg $299.93/180, 50 mg $341.96/180, 75 mg $337.95/180, 100 mg $343.78/180. **Extended-release capsules:** 37.5 mg, 75 mg, 150 mg. **Cost:** 37.5 mg $275.97/90, 75 mg $318.99/90, 150 mg $355.97/90.

NURSING IMPLICATIONS

Assessment

- Assess mental status and mood changes. Inform physician or other health care professional if patient demonstrates significant increase in anxiety, nervousness, or insomnia.
- Assess suicidal tendencies, especially in early therapy. Restrict amount of drug available to patient.
- Monitor blood pressure before and periodically during therapy. Sustained hypertension may be dose related; decrease dose or discontinue therapy if this occurs.
- Monitor appetite and nutritional intake. Weigh weekly. Report continued weight loss. Adjust diet as tolerated to support nutritional status.
- ***Lab Test Considerations:*** Monitor CBC with differential and platelet count periodically during therapy. May cause anemia, leukocytosis, leukopenia, thrombocytopenia, basophilia, and eosinophilia.
- May cause an ↑ in serum alkaline phosphatase, bilirubin, AST, ALT, BUN, and creatinine.
- May also cause ↑ serum cholesterol.
- May cause electrolyte abnormalities (hyperglycemia or hypoglycemia, hyperkalemia or hypokalemia, hyperuricemia, hyperphosphatemia or hypophosphatemia, and hyponatremia).

Potential Nursing Diagnoses

Ineffective coping (Indications)
Risk for injury (Side Effects)

Implementation

- **PO:** Administer venlafaxine with food.
- Extended-release capsules should be swallowed whole; do not crush, break, or chew.
- Extended-release capsules may also be opened and contents sprinkled on a spoonful of applesauce. Take immediately and follow with a glass of water. Do not store mixture for later use.

Patient/Family Teaching

- Instruct patient to take medication exactly as directed at the same time each day. Take missed doses as soon as possible unless almost time for next dose. Do not double doses or discontinue abruptly. Patients taking venlafaxine for >6 wk should have dose gradually decreased before discontinuation.
- May cause drowsiness or dizziness. Caution patient to avoid driving or other activities requiring alertness until response to the drug is known.
- Caution patient to avoid taking alcohol or other CNS-depressant drugs during therapy and not to take other Rx, OTC, or herbal products without consulting health care professional.

V

- Instruct female patients to inform health care professional if pregnancy is planned or suspected or if breastfeeding.
- Instruct patient to notify health care professional if signs of allergy (rash, hives) occur.
- Emphasize the importance of follow-up exams to monitor progress. Encourage patient participation in psychotherapy.

Evaluation/Desired Outcomes

- Increased sense of well-being.
- Renewed interest in surroundings. Need for therapy should be periodically reassessed. Therapy is usually continued for several months.
- Decreased anxiety.

verapamil (ver-**ap**-a-mil)

Apo-Verap, Calan, Calan SR, Covera-HS, Isoptin, Isoptin SR, ✱Novo-Veramil, ✱Nu-Verap, Verelan, Verelan PM

Classification

Therapeutic: antianginals, antiarrhythmics (class IV), antihypertensives, vascular headache suppressants
Pharmacologic: calcium channel blockers

Pregnancy Category C

Indications

Management of hypertension, angina pectoris, and/or vasospastic (Prinzmetal's) angina. Management of supraventricular arrhythmias and rapid ventricular rates in atrial flutter or fibrillation. **Unlabeled uses:** Prevention of migraine headache. Management of cardiomyopathy.

Action

Inhibits the transport of calcium into myocardial and vascular smooth muscle cells, resulting in inhibition of excitation-contraction coupling and subsequent contraction. Decreases SA and AV conduction and prolongs AV node refractory period in conduction tissue. **Therapeutic Effects:** Systemic vasodilation resulting in decreased blood pressure. Coronary vasodilation resulting in decreased frequency and severity of attacks of angina. Suppression of ventricular tachyarrhythmias.

Pharmacokinetics

Absorption: 90% absorbed after oral administration, but much is rapidly metabolized, resulting in bioavailability of 20–25%.
Distribution: Small amounts enter breast milk.
Protein Binding: 90%.
Metabolism and Excretion: Mostly metabolized by the liver.
Half-life: 4.5–12 hr.

TIME/ACTION PROFILE (cardiovascular effects)

ROUTE	ONSET	PEAK	DURATION
PO	1–2 hr	30–90 min†	3–7 hr
PO-ER	unknown	5–7 hr	24 hr
IV	1–5 min‡	3–5 min	2 hr‡

†Single dose; effects from multiple doses may not be evident for 24–48 hr

‡Antiarrhythmic effects; hemodynamic effects begin 3–5 min after injection and persist for 10–20 min

Contraindications/Precautions

Contraindicated in: Hypersensitivity; Sick sinus syndrome; 2nd- or 3rd-degree AV block (unless an artificial pacemaker is in place); BP <90 mm Hg; CHF, severe ventricular dysfunction, or cardiogenic shock, unless associated with supraventricular tachyarrhythmias; Concurrent IV beta blocker therapy.
Use Cautiously in: Severe hepatic impairment (dose reduction recommended for most agents); Geri: Geriatric patients (dose reduction/slower IV infusion rates recommended for most agents; increased risk of hypotension); History of serious ventricular arrhythmias or CHF; OB, Lactation: Pregnancy or lactation (safety not established; verapamil is approved for use in children).

Adverse Reactions/Side Effects

CNS: abnormal dreams, anxiety, confusion, dizziness/lightheadedness, drowsiness, headache, jitteriness, nervousness, psychiatric disturbances, weakness. **EENT:** blurred vision, disturbed equilibrium, epistaxis, tinnitus. **Resp:** cough, dyspnea, shortness of breath. **CV:** ARRHYTHMIAS, CHF, bradycardia, chest pain, hypotension, palpitations, peripheral edema, syncope, tachycardia. **GI:** abnormal liver function studies, anorexia, constipation, diarrhea, dry mouth, dysgeusia, dyspepsia, nausea, vomiting. **GU:** dysuria, nocturia, polyuria, sexual dysfunction, urinary frequency. **Derm:** dermatitis, erythema multiforme, flushing, increased sweating, photosensitivity, pruritus/urticaria, rash. **Endo:** gynecomastia, hyperglycemia. **Hemat:** anemia, leukopenia, thrombocytopenia. **Metab:** weight gain. **MS:** joint stiffness, muscle cramps. **Neu-**

ro: paresthesia, tremor. **Misc:** STEVENS-JOHNSON SYNDROME, gingival hyperplasia.

Interactions

Drug-Drug: Additive hypotension may occur when used concurrently with **fentanyl**, other **antihypertensives**, **nitrates**, acute ingestion of **alcohol**, or **quinidine**. Antihypertensive effects may be ↓ by concurrent use of **NSAIDs**. Serum **digoxin** levels may be ↑. Concurrent use with **beta blockers**, **digoxin**, **disopyramide**, or **phenytoin** may result in bradycardia, conduction defects, or CHF. May ↓ metabolism of and ↑ risk of toxicity from **cyclosporine**, **prazosin**, **quinidine**, or **carbamazepine**. May ↓ effectiveness of **rifampin**. ↑ the muscle-paralyzing effects of **nondepolarizing neuromuscular-blocking agents**. Effectiveness may be ↓ by coadministration with **vitamin D compounds** and **calcium**. May alter serum **lithium** levels.
Drug-Natural Products: ↑ **caffeine** levels with caffeine-containing herbs (**cola nut**, **guarana**, **mate**, **tea**, **coffee**).
Drug-Food: Grapefruit juice ↑ serum levels and effect.

Route/Dosage

PO (Adults): 80–120 mg 3 times daily, increased as needed. *Patients with poor ventricular function, hepatic impairment, or geriatric patients*—40 mg 3 times daily initially. *Extended-release preparations*—120–240 mg/day as a single dose; may be increased as needed (range 240–480 mg/day).
PO (Children up to 15 yr): 4–8 mg/kg/day in divided doses.
IV (Adults): 5–10 mg (75–150 mcg/kg); may repeat with 10 mg (150 mcg/kg) after 15–30 min.
IV (Children 1–15 yr): 2–5 mg (100–300 mcg/kg); may repeat after 30 min (initial dose not to exceed 5 mg; repeat dose not to exceed 10 mg).
IV (Children <1 yr): 0.75–2 mg (100–200 mcg/kg); may repeat after 30 min.

Availability (generic available)

Tablets: 40 mg, 80 mg, 120 mg. **Cost:** *Generic*—40 mg $44.96/270, 80 mg $44.96/270, 120 mg $34.45/270. **Extended-release tablets (Isoptin SR, Covera HS):** 120 mg, 180 mg, 240 mg. **Cost:** *Generic*—120 mg $49.97/90, 180 mg $27.97/90, 240 mg $35.97/90. **Extended-release capsules (Verelan PM):** 100 mg, 200 mg, 300 mg. **Cost:** 100 mg $166.01/90, 200 mg $213.02/90, 300 mg $308.52/90. **Extended-release capsules (Verelan):** 120 mg, 180 mg, 240 mg, 360 mg. **Cost:** *Generic*—120 mg $64.99/90, 180 mg $67.99/90, 240 mg $86.99/90, 360 mg $160.97/90. **Solution for injection:** 2.5 mg/m in 2- and 4-ml vials, ampules, and syringes. ***In combination with:*** trandolapril (Tarka); see Appendix B.

NURSING IMPLICATIONS

Assessment

- Monitor blood pressure and pulse before therapy, during dosage titration, and periodically throughout therapy. Monitor ECG periodically during prolonged therapy. Verapamil may cause prolonged PR interval.
- Monitor intake and output ratios and daily weight. Assess for signs of CHF (peripheral edema, rales/crackles, dyspnea, weight gain, jugular venous distention)
- Patients receiving digoxin concurrently with calcium channel blockers should have routine serum digoxin levels and be monitored for signs and symptoms of digoxin toxicity.
- **Angina:** Assess location, duration, intensity, and precipitating factors of patient's anginal pain.
- **Arrhythmias:** Monitor ECG continuously during administration. Notify physician promptly if bradycardia or prolonged hypotension occurs. Emergency equipment and medication should be available. Monitor blood pressure and pulse before and frequently during administration.
- ***Lab Test Considerations:*** Total serum calcium concentrations are not affected by calcium channel blockers.
- Monitor serum potassium periodically. Hypokalemia ↑ risk of arrhythmias and should be corrected.
- Monitor renal and hepatic functions periodically during long-term therapy. May cause ↑ hepatic enzymes after several days of therapy, which return to normal on discontinuation of therapy.

Potential Nursing Diagnoses

Decreased cardiac output (Indications)
Acute pain (Indications)

Implementation

- Do not confuse verapamil with Virilon (testosterone). Do not confuse Covera (verapamil) with Provera (medrosyprogesterone).
- **PO:** Administer verapamil with meals or milk to minimize gastric irritation.
- Do not open, crush, break, or chew sustained-release capsules or tablets. Empty tablets that appear in stool are not significant.

IV Administration

- **IV:** Patients should remain recumbent for at least 1 hr after IV administration to minimize hypotensive effects
- **Direct IV:** ***Diluent:*** Administer undiluted. ***Concentration:*** 2.5 mg/ml. ***Rate:*** Administer over 2 min. Geri: Administer over 3 min.
- **Y-Site Compatibility:** argatroban, atropine, aztreonam, bivalirudin, bumetanide, caspofungin, cefazolin, cefotaxime, cefoxitin, ceftizoxime, ceftriaxone, cefuroxime, cimetidine, ciprofloxacin, clindamycin, cyclosporine, daptomycin, dexamethasone sodium phosphate, dexmedetomidine, digoxin, diphenhydramine, dobutamine, dopamine, doxycycline, enalaprilat, epinephrine, eptifibatide, erythromycin, esmolol, famotidine, fenoldopam, fentanyl, fluconazole, gentamicin, granisetron, hydralazine, heparin, hydrocortisone sodium succinate, hydromorphone, imipenem/cilastatin, inamrinone, insulin, isoproterenol, labetalol, levofloxacin, lidocaine, linezolid, lorazepam, meperidine, methylprednisolone sodium succinate, metoclopramide, metoprolol, midazolam, milrinone, morphine, nesiritide, nitroglycerin, nitroprusside, norepinephrine, ondansetron, oxaliplatin, palonosetron, penicillin G, phenylephrine, phytonadione, piperacillin, procainamide, prochlorperazine, promethazine, propranolol, protamine, quinupristin/dalfopristin, ranitidine, tacrolimus, ticarcillin/clavulanate, tirofiban, tobramycin, vancomycin, vasopressin, voriconazole.
- **Y-Site Incompatibility:** albumin, amphotericin B cholesteryl sulfate complex, ampicillin, ceftazidime, chloramphenicol, diazepam, ertapenem, furosemide, ganciclovir, lansoprazole, metronidazole, nafcillin, oxacillin, pantoprazole, phenytoin, piperacillin/tazobactam, propofol, sodium bicarbonate, trimethoprim/sulfamethoxazole.

Patient/Family Teaching

- Advise patient to take medication exactly as directed, even if feeling well. If a dose is missed, take as soon as possible unless almost time for next dose; do not double doses. May need to be discontinued gradually.
- Advise patient to avoid large amounts (6–8 glasses of grapefruit juice/day) during therapy.
- Instruct patient on correct technique for monitoring pulse. Instruct patient to contact health care professional if heart rate is <50 bpm.
- Caution patient to change positions slowly to minimize orthostatic hypotension.
- May cause drowsiness or dizziness. Advise patient to avoid driving or other activities requiring alertness until response to the medication is known.
- Instruct patient on importance of maintaining good dental hygiene and seeing dentist frequently for teeth cleaning to prevent tenderness, bleeding, and gingival hyperplasia (gum enlargement).
- Instruct patient to avoid concurrent use of alcohol or OTC medications, especially cold preparations, without consulting health care professional.
- Advise patient to notify health care professional if irregular heartbeats, dyspnea, swelling of hands and feet, pronounced dizziness, nausea, constipation, or hypotension occurs or if headache is severe or persistent.
- Caution patient to wear protective clothing and use sunscreen to prevent photosensitivity reactions.
- **Angina:** Instruct patient on concurrent nitrate or beta-blocker therapy to continue taking both medications as directed and use SL nitroglycerin as needed for anginal attacks.
- Advise patient to contact health care professional if chest pain does not improve, worsens after therapy, or occurs with diaphoresis; if shortness of breath occurs; or if severe, persistent headache occurs.
- Caution patient to discuss exercise restrictions with health care professional before exertion.
- **Hypertension:** Encourage patient to comply with other interventions for hypertension (weight reduction, low-sodium diet, smoking cessation, moderation of alcohol consumption, regular exercise, and stress management). Medication controls but does not cure hypertension.
- Instruct patient and family in proper technique for monitoring blood pressure. Advise

patient to take blood pressure weekly and to report significant changes to health care professional.

Evaluation/Desired Outcomes

- Decrease in blood pressure.
- Decrease in frequency and severity of anginal attacks.
- Decrease in need for nitrate therapy.
- Increase in activity tolerance and sense of well-being.
- Suppression and prevention of atrial tachyarrhythmias.

HIGH ALERT

vinBLAStine (vin-**blass**-teen)

Velban, ✤Velbe

Classification
Therapeutic: antineoplastics
Pharmacologic: vinca alkaloids

Pregnancy Category D

Indications

Combination chemotherapy of: Lymphomas, Nonseminomatous testicular carcinoma, Advanced breast cancer, Other tumors.

Action

Binds to proteins of mitotic spindle, causing metaphase arrest. Cell replication is stopped as a result (cell cycle–specific for M phase). **Therapeutic Effects:** Death of rapidly replicating cells, particularly malignant ones. Has immunosuppressive properties.

Pharmacokinetics

Absorption: Administered IV only, resulting in complete bioavailability.
Distribution: Does not cross the blood-brain barrier well.
Metabolism and Excretion: Converted by the liver to an active antineoplastic compound; excreted in the feces via biliary excretion, some renal elimination.
Half-life: 24 hr.

TIME/ACTION PROFILE (effects on white blood cell counts)

ROUTE	ONSET	PEAK	DURATION
IV	5–7 days	10 days	7–14 days

Contraindications/Precautions

Contraindicated in: Hypersensitivity; Pregnancy or lactation.
Use Cautiously in: Patients with childbearing potential; Infections; Decreased bone marrow reserve; Other chronic debilitating illnesses; Patients with impaired hepatic function (↓ dose by 50% if serum bilirubin >3 mg/dl).

Adverse Reactions/Side Effects

CNS: SEIZURES, mental depression, neurotoxicity, weakness. **Resp:** BRONCHOSPASM. **GI:** nausea, vomiting, anorexia, constipation, diarrhea, stomatitis. **GU:** gonadal suppression. **Derm:** alopecia, dermatitis, vesiculation. **Endo:** syndrome of inappropriate antidiuretic hormone (SIADH). **Hemat:** anemia, leukopenia, thrombocytopenia. **Local:** phlebitis at IV site. **Metab:** hyperuricemia. **Neuro:** neuritis, paresthesia, peripheral neuropathy.

Interactions

Drug-Drug: Additive bone marrow depression with other **antineoplastics** or **radiation therapy**. Bronchospasm may occur in patients who have been previously treated with **mitomycin**. May ↓ antibody response to **live-virus vaccines** and ↑ risk of adverse reactions. May ↓ serum **phenytoin** levels.

Route/Dosage

Doses may vary greatly, depending on tumor, schedule, condition of patient, and blood counts.
IV (Adults): *Initial*—3.7 mg/m^2 (100 mcg/kg), single dose; increase weekly as tolerated by 1.8 mg/m^2 (50 mcg/kg) to maximum of 18.5 mg/m^2 (usual dose is 5.5–7.4 mg/m^2). *Maintenance*—10 mg 1–2 times/mo or one increment less than last dose q 7–14 days.
IV (Children): *Initial*—2.5 mg/m^2, single dose; increase weekly as tolerated by 1.25 mg/m^2 to maximum of 7.5 mg/m^2. *Maintenance*—one increment less than last dose q 7 days.

Availability (generic available)

Solution for injection: 1 mg/ml in 10-ml vials. **Powder for injection:** 10 mg/vial.

✤ = Canadian drug name.
*CAPITALS indicates life-threatening; underlines indicate most frequent.

V

NURSING IMPLICATIONS

Assessment

- Monitor blood pressure, pulse, and respiratory rate during therapy. Notify physician immediately if respiratory distress occurs. Bronchospasm can be life-threatening and may occur at time of infusion or several hours to weeks later.
- Monitor for bone marrow depression. Assess for bleeding (bleeding gums, bruising, petechiae, guaiac stools, urine, and emesis) and avoid IM injections and taking rectal temperatures if platelet count is low. Apply pressure to venipuncture sites for 10 min. Assess for signs of infection during neutropenia. Anemia may occur. Monitor for increased fatigue, dyspnea, and orthostatic hypotension.
- May cause nausea and vomiting. Monitor intake and output, appetite, and nutritional intake. Prophylactic antiemetics may be used. Adjust diet as tolerated.
- Assess injection site frequently for redness, irritation, or inflammation. If extravasation occurs, infusion must be stopped and restarted elsewhere to avoid damage to subcut tissue. Standard treatment includes infiltration with hyaluronidase and application of heat.
- Monitor for symptoms of gout (increased uric acid, joint pain, edema). Encourage patient to drink at least 2 L of fluid per day. Allopurinol or alkalinization of urine may be used to decrease uric acid levels.
- ***Lab Test Considerations:*** Monitor CBC prior to and routinely throughout therapy. If WBC <2000, subsequent doses are usually withheld until WBC is ≥4000. The nadir of leukopenia occurs in 5–10 days and recovery usually occurs 7–14 days later. Thrombocytopenia may also occur in patients who have received radiation or other chemotherapy agents.
- Monitor liver function studies (AST, ALT, LDH, bilirubin) and renal function studies (BUN, creatinine) prior to and periodically throughout therapy.
- May cause ↑ uric acid. Monitor periodically during therapy.

Potential Nursing Diagnoses

Risk for infection (Adverse Reactions)
Imbalanced nutrition: less than body requirements (Adverse Reactions)

Implementation

- ***High Alert:*** Fatalities have occurred with chemotherapeutic agents. Before administering, clarify all ambiguous orders; double-check single, daily, and course-of-therapy dose limits; have second practitioner independently double-check original order, dose calculations, and infusion pump settings. Do not administer subcut, IM, or intrathecally (IT). IT administration is fatal. Vinblastine must be dispensed in an overwrap stating, "For IV use only." Overwrap should remain in place until immediately before administration.
- ***High Alert:*** Do not confuse vinblastine with vincristine.
- Solution should be prepared in a biologic cabinet. Wear gloves, gown, and mask while handling medication. Discard IV equipment in specially designated containers.
- Do not inject into extremities with impaired circulation; may cause thrombophlebitis.

IV Administration

- **Direct IV:** ***Diluent:*** Dilute each 10 mg with 10 ml of 0.9% NaCl for injection with phenol or benzyl alcohol. Solution is clear. Reconstituted medication is stable for 28 days if refrigerated. ***Concentration:*** 1 mg/ml. ***Rate:*** Administer each single dose over 1 min through Y-site injection of a free-flowing infusion of 0.9% NaCl or D5W.
- **Intermittent Infusion:** Dilution in large volumes (100–250 ml) or prolonged infusion (≥30 min) increases chance of vein irritation and extravasation
- **Syringe Compatibility:** bleomycin, cisplatin, cyclophosphamide, droperidol, fluorouracil, leucovorin calcium, methotrexate, metoclopramide, mitomycin, vincristine.
- **Syringe Incompatibility:** furosemide.
- **Y-Site Compatibility:** allopurinol, amifostine, amphotericin B cholesteryl sulfate complex, aztreonam, bleomycin, cisplatin, cyclophosphamide, doxorubicin, doxorubicin liposome, droperidol, etoposide phosphate, filgrastim, fludarabine, fluorouracil, gemcitabine, granisetron, heparin, leucovorin calcium, melphalan, methotrexate, metoclopramide, mitomycin, ondansetron, paclitaxel, pemetrexed, piperacillin/tazobactam, sargramostim, teniposide, thiotepa, vincristine, vinorelbine.
- **Y-Site Incompatibility:** cefepime, furosemide, lansoprazole.

Patient/Family Teaching

- Advise patient to notify health care professional if fever; chills; sore throat; signs of infection; bleeding gums; bruising; petechiae; or blood in urine, stool, or emesis occurs. Caution patient to avoid crowds and persons with known infections. Instruct patient to use soft toothbrush and electric razor. Caution patient not to drink alcoholic beverages or take products containing aspirin or NSAIDs.
- Instruct patient to inspect oral mucosa for redness and ulceration. Advise patient that, if ulceration occurs, to avoid spicy foods, use sponge brush, and rinse mouth with water after eating and drinking. Topical agents may be used if mouth pain interferes with eating. Stomatitis pain may require treatment with opioid analgesics.
- Instruct patient to report symptoms of neurotoxicity (paresthesia, pain, difficulty walking, persistent constipation).
- Advise patient that jaw pain, pain in organs containing tumor tissue, nausea, and vomiting may occur. Avoid constipation and report other adverse reactions.
- Advise patient that this medication may have teratogenic effects. Contraception should be used during and for at least 2 mo after therapy is concluded.
- Discuss with patient the possibility of hair loss. Explore coping strategies.
- Instruct patient not to receive any vaccinations without advice of health care professional.
- Emphasize need for periodic lab tests to monitor for side effects.

Evaluation/Desired Outcomes

- Regression of malignancy without the appearance of detrimental side effects.

HIGH ALERT

vinCRIStine (vin-**kriss**-teen)

Oncovin, Vincasar PFS

Classification

Therapeutic: antineoplastics

Pharmacologic: vinca alkaloids

Pregnancy Category D

Indications

Used alone and in combination with other treatment modalities (antineoplastics, surgery, or radiation therapy) in treatment of: Hodgkin's disease, Leukemias, Neuroblastoma, Malignant lymphomas, Rhabdomyosarcoma, Wilms' tumor, Other tumors.

Action

Binds to proteins of mitotic spindle, causing metaphase arrest. Cell replication is stopped as a result (cell cycle–specific for M phase). Has little or no effect on bone marrow. **Therapeutic Effects:** Death of rapidly replicating cells, particularly malignant ones. Has immunosuppressive properties.

Pharmacokinetics

Absorption: Administered IV only, resulting in complete bioavailability.

Distribution: Rapidly and widely distributed; extensively bound to tissues.

Metabolism and Excretion: Metabolized by the liver and eliminated in the feces via biliary excretion.

Half-life: 10.5–37.5 hr.

TIME/ACTION PROFILE (effects on blood counts†)

ROUTE	ONSET	PEAK	DURATION
IV	unknown	4 days	7 days

†Usually mild

Contraindications/Precautions

Contraindicated in: Hypersensitivity; Pregnancy or lactation.

Use Cautiously in: Patients with childbearing potential; Infections; Decreased bone marrow reserve; Other chronic debilitating illnesses; Hepatic impairment (50% dose reduction recommended if serum bilirubin >3 mg/dl).

Adverse Reactions/Side Effects

CNS: agitation, insomnia, mental depression, mental status changes. **EENT:** cortical blindness, diplopia. **Resp:** bronchospasm. **GI:** <u>nausea</u>, <u>vomiting</u>, abdominal cramps, anorexia, constipation, ileus, stomatitis. **GU:** gonadal suppression, nocturia, oliguria, urinary retention. **Derm:** <u>alopecia</u>. **Endo:** syndrome of inappropriate antidiuretic hormone (SIADH). **Hemat:** anemia, leukopenia, thrombocytopenia (mild and brief). **Local:** <u>phlebitis</u> at IV site, tissue necrosis (from extravasation). **Metab:** hyperuri-

V

cemia. **Neuro:** ascending peripheral neuropathy.

Interactions

Drug-Drug: Bronchospasm may occur in patients who have been previously treated with **mitomycin**. **L-asparaginase** may ↓ hepatic metabolism of vincristine (give vincristine 12–24 hr prior to asparaginase). May ↓ antibody response to **live-virus vaccines** and ↑ risk of adverse reactions.

Route/Dosage

Many other protocols are used.

IV (Adults): 10–30 mcg/kg (0.4–1.4 mg/m²); may repeat weekly (not to exceed 2 mg/dose).

IV (Children >10 kg): 1.5–2 mg/m² single dose; may repeat weekly.

IV (Children <10 kg): 50 mcg/kg single dose; may repeat weekly.

Availability (generic available)

Solution for injection: 1 mg/ml in 1-, 2-, 5-ml vials. **Powder for injection:** 5 mg/vial.

NURSING IMPLICATIONS

Assessment

- Monitor blood pressure, pulse, and respiratory rate during therapy. Report significant changes.
- Monitor neurologic status. Assess for paresthesia (numbness, tingling, pain), loss of deep tendon reflexes (Achilles reflex is usually first involved), weakness (wrist drop or footdrop, gait disturbances), cranial nerve palsies (jaw pain, hoarseness, ptosis, visual changes), autonomic dysfunction (ileus, difficulty voiding, orthostatic hypotension, impaired sweating), and CNS dysfunction (decreased level of consciousness, agitation, hallucinations). Notify physician if these symptoms develop, as they may persist for months.
- Monitor intake and output ratios and daily weight; report significant discrepancies. Decreased urine output with concurrent hyponatremia may indicate SIADH, which usually responds to fluid restriction.
- Assess infusion site frequently for redness, irritation, or inflammation. If extravasation occurs, infusion must be stopped and restarted elsewhere to avoid damage to subcut tissue. Cellulitis and discomfort may be minimized by infiltration with hyaluronidase and application of moderate heat or by application of cold compresses.
- Assess nutritional status. An antiemetic may be used to minimize nausea and vomiting.
- Monitor for symptoms of gout (increased uric acid, joint pain, edema). Encourage patient to drink at least 2 liters of fluid per day. Allopurinol or alkalinization of urine may be used to decrease uric acid levels.
- ***Lab Test Considerations:*** Monitor CBC prior to and periodically throughout therapy. May cause slight leukopenia 4 days after therapy, which resolves within 7 days. Platelet count may ↑ or ↓.
- Monitor liver function studies (AST, ALT, LDH, bilirubin) and renal function studies (BUN, creatinine) prior to and periodically throughout therapy.
- May cause ↑ uric acid. Monitor periodically during therapy.

Potential Nursing Diagnoses

Risk for injury (Adverse Reactions)

Imbalanced nutrition: less than body requirements (Adverse Reactions)

Implementation

- ***High Alert:*** Fatalities have occurred with chemotherapeutic agents. Before administering, clarify all ambiguous orders; double-check single, daily, and course-of-therapy dose limits; have second practitioner independently double-check original order, dose calculations, and infusion pump settings. Do not administer subcut, IM, or intrathecally (IT). IT administration is fatal. Vincristine must be dispensed in an overwrap stating "For IV use only." Overwrap should remain in place until immediately before administration. Do not confuse vincristine with vinblastine.
- Solution should be prepared in a biologic cabinet. Wear gloves, gown, and mask while handling medication. Discard IV equipment in specially designated containers (see Appendix K).

IV Administration

- **Direct IV:** ***Diluent:*** Reconstitute by adding 5 ml of sterile water for injection to each vial. ***Concentration:*** Administer undiluted at 1 mg/ml. ***Rate:*** Administer each dose direct IV push over 1 min through Y-site injection of a free-flowing infusion of 0.9% NaCl or D5W.
- **Syringe Compatibility:** bleomycin, cisplatin, cyclophosphamide, doxapram, doxorubicin, droperidol, fluorouracil, heparin, leuco-

vorin calcium, methotrexate, metoclopramide, mitomycin, vinblastine.
- **Syringe Incompatibility:** furosemide.
- **Y-Site Compatibility:** allopurinol, amifostine, amphotericin B cholesteryl sulfate complex, aztreonam, bleomycin, cisplatin, cyclophosphamide, doxorubicin, doxorubicin liposome, droperidol, etoposide phosphate, filgrastim, fludarabine, fluorouracil, gemcitabine, granisetron, heparin, leucovorin calcium, linezolid, melphalan, methotrexate, metoclopramide, mitomycin, ondansetron, oxaliplatin, paclitaxel, pemetrexed, piperacillin/tazobactam, sargramostim, teniposide, thiotepa, topotecan, vinblastine, vinorelbine.
- **Y-Site Incompatibility:** cefepime, furosemide, idarubicin, lansoprazole, sodium bicarbonate.

Patient/Family Teaching
- Instruct patient to notify health care professional immediately if redness, swelling, or pain at injection site occurs.
- Instruct patient to report symptoms of neurotoxicity (paresthesia, pain, difficulty walking, persistent constipation). Inform patient that increased fluid intake, dietary fiber, and exercise may minimize constipation. Stool softeners or laxatives may be used. Patient should inform health care professional if severe constipation or abdominal discomfort occurs, as this may be a sign of neuropathy.
- Advise patient to notify health care professional if fever; chills; sore throat; signs of infection; bleeding gums; bruising; petechiae; blood in urine, stool, or emesis; or mouth sores occur. Caution patient to avoid crowds and persons with known infections.
- Advise patient that this medication may have teratogenic effects. Contraception should be used during and for at least 2 mo after therapy is concluded.
- Discuss with patient the possibility of hair loss. Explore coping strategies.
- Instruct patient not to receive any vaccinations without advice of health care professional.
- Emphasize need for periodic lab tests to monitor for side effects.

Evaluation/Desired Outcomes
- Regression of malignancy without the appearance of detrimental side effects.

HIGH ALERT

vinorelbine (vine-oh-**rel**-been)
Navelbine

Classification
Therapeutic: antineoplastics
Pharmacologic: vinca alkaloids

Pregnancy Category D

Indications
Inoperable non–small-cell cancer of the lung in ambulatory patients (alone or with cisplatin).

Action
Binds to a protein (tubulin) of cellular microtubules, where it interferes with microtubule assembly. Cell replication is stopped as a result (cell cycle–specific for M phase). **Therapeutic Effects:** Death of rapidly replicating cells, particularly malignant ones.

Pharmacokinetics
Absorption: IV administration results in complete bioavailability.
Distribution: Highly bound to platelets and lymphocytes.
Metabolism and Excretion: Mostly metabolized by the liver. At least one metabolite is active. Large amounts eliminated in feces; 11% excreted unchanged by the kidneys.
Half-life: 28–44 hr.

TIME/ACTION PROFILE (effect on WBCs)

ROUTE	ONSET	PEAK	DURATION
IV	unknown	7–10 days	7–15 days

Contraindications/Precautions
Contraindicated in: Hypersensitivity; Pregnancy or lactation; Active infections; Decreased bone marrow reserve; Other chronic debilitating illnesses.
Use Cautiously in: Patients with childbearing potential; Impaired hepatic function (dose reduction recommended if total bilirubin >2 mg/dl); Debilitated patients (increased risk of hyponatremia); Granulocytopenic patients (temporarily discontinue or reduce dose); Pedi: Children (safe use not established).

Adverse Reactions/Side Effects
CNS: fatigue. **Resp:** shortness of breath. **CV:** chest pain. **GI:** constipation, nausea, abdominal pain, anorexia, diarrhea, transient increase in

V

liver enzymes, vomiting. **Derm:** alopecia, rashes. **F and E:** hyponatremia. **Hemat:** anemia, neutropenia, thrombocytopenia. **Local:** irritation at IV site, skin reactions, phlebitis. **MS:** arthralgia, back pain, jaw pain, myalgia. **Neuro:** neurotoxicity. **Misc:** pain in tumor-containing tissue.

Interactions

Drug-Drug: ↑ bone marrow depression with other **antineoplastics** or **radiation therapy**. Concurrent use with **cisplatin** ↑ risk and severity of bone marrow depression. Concurrent use with **mitomycin** or **chest radiation** ↑ risk of pulmonary reactions.

Route/Dosage

IV (Adults): 30 mg/m² once weekly.

Hepatic Impairment

IV (Adults): *Total bilirubin 2.1–3 mg/dl*—15 mg/m² once weekly; *total bilirubin ≥3 mg/dl*—7.5 mg/m² once weekly.

Availability (generic available)

Injection: 10 mg/ml.

NURSING IMPLICATIONS

Assessment

- Monitor blood pressure, pulse, and respiratory rate during therapy. Note significant changes. Acute shortness of breath and severe bronchospasm may occur infrequently shortly after administration. Treatment with corticosteroids, bronchodilators, and supplemental oxygen may be required, especially in patients with a history of pulmonary disease.
- Assess frequently for signs of infection (sore throat, temperature, cough, mental status changes), especially when nadir of granulocytopenia is expected.
- Monitor neurologic status. Assess for paresthesia (numbness, tingling, pain), loss of deep tendon reflexes (Achilles reflex is usually first involved), weakness (wrist drop or footdrop, gait disturbances), cranial nerve palsies (jaw pain, hoarseness, ptosis, visual changes), autonomic dysfunction (constipation, ileus, difficulty voiding, orthostatic hypotension, impaired sweating), and CNS dysfunction (decreased level of consciousness, agitation, hallucinations). These symptoms may persist for months. The incidence of neurotoxicity associated with vinorelbine is less than that of other vinca alkaloids.
- Monitor intake and output and daily weight for significant discrepancies.
- Assess nutritional status. Mild to moderate nausea is common. An antiemetic may be used to minimize nausea and vomiting.
- Monitor for symptoms of gout (increased uric acid, joint pain, edema). Encourage patient to drink at least 2 L of fluid/day. Allopurinol and alkalinization of urine may decrease uric acid levels.
- ***Lab Test Considerations:*** Monitor CBC prior to each dose and routinely during therapy. The nadir of granulocytopenia usually occurs 7–10 days after vinorelbine administration and recovery usually follows within 7–15 days. If granulocyte count is <1500/mm³, dose reduction or temporary interruption of vinorelbine may be warranted. If repeated episodes of fever and/or sepsis occur during granulocytopenia, future dose of vinorelbine should be modified. May also cause mild to moderate anemia. Thrombocytopenia rarely occurs.
- Monitor liver function studies (AST, ALT, LDH, bilirubin) and renal function studies (BUN, creatinine) prior to and periodically during therapy. May cause ↑ uric acid; monitor periodically during therapy.

Potential Nursing Diagnoses

Risk for injury (Adverse Reactions)
Risk for infection (Adverse Reactions)

Implementation

- ***High Alert:*** Fatalities have occurred with chemotherapeutic agents. Before administering, clarify all ambiguous orders; double-check single, daily, and course-of-therapy dose limits; have second practitioner independently double-check original order, dose calculations, and infusion pump settings.
- Solution should be prepared in a biologic cabinet. Wear gloves, gown, and mask while handling medication. Discard IV equipment in specially designated containers.
- Assess infusion site frequently for redness, irritation, or inflammation. Vinorelbine is a vesicant. If extravasation occurs, infusion must be stopped and restarted elsewhere to avoid damage to subcut tissue. Treatment of extravasation includes application of warm compresses applied over the area immediately for 30–60 min, then alternating on/off every 15 min for 1 day to increase systemic absorption of the drug. Hyaluronidase 150 units diluted in 1–2 ml of 0.9% NaCl, 1 ml for each

ml extravasated, should be injected through existing IV cannula or subcut if the needle has been removed to enhance absorption and dispersion of the extravasated drug.

IV Administration

- **Direct IV:** ***Diluent:*** Dilute vinorelbine with 0.9% NaCl or D5W. ***Concentration:*** 1.5–3 mg/ml. ***Rate:*** Infuse over 6–10 min into Y-site closest to bag of a free-flowing IV or into a central line.
- Flush vein with at least 75–125 ml of 0.9% NaCl or D5W administered over 10 min or more following administration of vinorelbine.
- **Intermittent Infusion:** ***Diluent:*** Dilute vinorelbine with 0.9% NaCl, D5W, 0.45% NaCl, D5/0.45% NaCl, Ringer's or lactated Ringer's injection. Solution should be colorless to pale yellow. Do not administer solutions that are discolored or contain particulate matter. Diluted solution is stable for 24 hr at room temperature. ***Concentration:*** 0.5–2 mg/ml. ***Rate:*** Infuse over 6–10 min (up to 30 min) into Y-site closest to bag of a free-flowing IV or into a central line.
- Flush vein with at least 75–125 ml of 0.9% NaCl or D5W administered over 10 min or more following administration of vinorelbine.
- **Y-Site Compatibility:** amikacin, aztreonam, bleomycin, bumetanide, buprenorphine, butorphanol, calcium gluconate, carboplatin, carmustine, cefotaxime, ceftazidime, ceftizoxime, chlorpromazine, cimetidine, cisplatin, clindamycin, cyclophosphamide, cytarabine, dacarbazine, dactinomycin, daunorubicin, dexamethasone sodium phosphate, diphenhydramine, doxorubicin, doxorubicin liposome, doxycycline, droperidol, enalaprilat, etoposide, famotidine, filgrastim, floxuridine, fluconazole, fludarabine, gemcitabine, gentamicin, granisetron, haloperidol, hydrocortisone, hydromorphone, idarubicin, ifosfamide, imipenem/cilastatin, lorazepam, mannitol, mechlorethamine, melphalan, meperidine, mesna, methotrexate, metoclopramide, metronidazole, mitoxantrone, morphine, nalbuphine, ondansetron, oxaliplatin, potassium chloride, prochlorperazine, promethazine, ranitidine, streptozocin, teniposide, ticarcillin/clavulanate, tobramycin, vancomycin, vinblastine, vincristine, zidovudine.
- **Y-Site Incompatibility:** acyclovir, allopurinol, aminophylline, amphotericin B, amphotericin B cholesteryl sulfate, ampicillin, cefazolin, ceftriaxone, cefuroxime, fluorouracil, furosemide, ganciclovir, lansoprazole, methylprednisolone, mitomycin, sodium bicarbonate, thiotepa, trimethoprim/sulfamethoxazole.

Patient/Family Teaching

- Instruct patient to report symptoms of neurotoxicity (paresthesia, pain, difficulty walking, persistent constipation).
- Inform patient that increased fluid intake, dietary fiber, and exercise may minimize constipation. Stool softeners or laxatives may be necessary. Patient should be advised to report severe constipation or abdominal discomfort, as this may be a sign of ileus, which may occur as a consequence of neuropathy.
- Advise patient to notify health care professional if fever; chills; sore throat; signs of infection; bleeding gums; bruising; petechiae; blood in urine, stool, or emesis; or mouth sores occur.
- Caution patient to avoid crowds and persons with known infections.
- Advise patient that this medication may have teratogenic effects. Contraception should be used during and for at least 2 mo after therapy is concluded.
- Discuss with patient the possibility of hair loss and explore coping strategies.
- Instruct patient not to receive any vaccinations without advice of health care professional.
- Emphasize the need for periodic lab tests to monitor for side effects.

Evaluation/Desired Outcomes

- Decrease in the size or spread of malignancy without detrimental side effects.

VITAMIN B_{12} PREPARATIONS

cyanocobalamin
(sye-an-oh-koe-**bal**-a-min)
Nascobal, Rubramin PC

hydroxocobalamin
(hye-drox-oh-koe-**bal**-a-min)
Cyanokit

V

Classification
Therapeutic: antianemics, vitamins
Pharmacologic: water soluble vitamins

Pregnancy Category C

Indications

Vitamin B_{12} deficiency (parenteral product or nasal spray should be used when deficiency is due to malabsorption). Pernicious anemia (only parenteral products should be used for initial therapy; nasal or oral products are not indicated until patients have achieved hematologic remission following parenteral therapy and have no signs of CNS involvement). Part of the Schilling test (vitamin B_{12} absorption test) (diagnostic). Cyanide poisoning (Cyanokit only).

Action

Necessary coenzyme for metabolic processes, including fat and carbohydrate metabolism and protein synthesis. Required for cell production and hematopoiesis. **Therapeutic Effects:** Corrects manifestations of pernicious anemia (megaloblastic indices, GI lesions, and neurologic damage). Corrects vitamin B_{12} deficiency. Reverses symptoms of cyanide toxicity (Cyanokit only).

Pharmacokinetics

Absorption: Oral absorption in GI tract requires intrinsic factor and calcium; well absorbed after IM, subcut and nasal administration.
Distribution: Stored in the liver and bone marrow; crosses placenta, enters breast milk.
Metabolism and Excretion: Primarily excreted unchanged in urine.
Half-life: *Cyanocobalamin*—6 days (400 days in liver); *Hydroxcobalamin*—26–31 hr.

TIME/ACTION PROFILE (reticulocytosis)

ROUTE	ONSET	PEAK	DURATION
cyanocobalamin IM, subcut, nasal	unknown	3–10 days	unknown
hydroxocobalamin IM	unknown	unknown	unknown

Contraindications/Precautions

Contraindicated in: Hypersensitivity; Pedi: Avoid using preparations containing benzyl alcohol in premature infants (associated with fatal "gasping syndrome").
Use Cautiously in: Hereditary optic nerve atrophy (accelerates nerve damage); Uremia, folic acid deficiency, concurrent infection, iron deficiency (response to B_{12} will be impaired); Renal dysfunction (when using aluminum-containing products); Pedi: *Cyanokit*—Children (safety and effectiveness not established).

Adverse Reactions/Side Effects

CNS: headache; *Cyanokit*—dizziness, memory impairment, restlessness. **CV:** heart failure; *Cyanokit*—hypertension, chest pain, tachycardia. **EENT:** *Cyanokit*—dry throat, eye redness, eye swelling. **GI:** diarrhea; *Cyanokit*—abdominal discomfort, dyspepsia, dysphagia, hematochezia, nausea, vomiting. **Derm:** itching; *Cyanokit*—erythema, rash. **F and E:** hypokalemia. **GU:** *Cyanokit*—red urine. **Hemat:** thrombocytosis. **Resp:** pulmonary edema; *Cyanokit*—dyspnea. **Local:** pain at IM site. **Misc:** hypersensitivity reactions including ANAPHYLAXIS.

Interactions

Drug-Drug: Chloramphenicol and **antineoplastics** may ↓ hematologic response to vitamin B_{12}. **Colchicine**, **aminosalicylic acid**, **cimetidine**, and excess intake of **alcohol**, or **vitamin C** may ↓ oral absorption/effectiveness of vitamin B_{12}.

Route/Dosage

Cyanocobalamin (oral products are usually not recommended due to poor absorption and should be used only if patient refuses the IM, deep subcutaneous, or intranasal route of administration)

PO (Adults and Children): *Vitamin B_{12} deficiency*—amount depends on deficiency (up to 1000 mcg/day have been used).
PO (Adults): *Pernicious anemia (for hematologic remission only)*—1000–2000 mcg/day.
IM, Subcut (Adults): *Vitamin B_{12} deficiency*—30 mcg/day for 5–10 days, then 100—200 mcg/month. *Pernicious anemia*—100 mcg/day for 6–7 days; if improvement, give same dose every other day for 7 doses, then every 3–4 days for 2–3 wk; once hematologic values return to normal (remission), can give maintenance dose of 100 mcg/month (doses up to 1000 mcg have been used for maintenance) (could alternatively use oral or intranasal formulations below for maintenance at specified doses). *Schilling test*—Flushing dose is 1000 mcg.

IM, Subcut (Children): *Vitamin B_{12} deficiency*—0.2 mcg/kg for 2 days, then 1000 mcg/day for 2–7 days, then 100 mcg/week for 1 month. *Pernicious anemia*—30–50 mcg/day for 2 or more weeks (to a total dose of 1000–5000 mcg), then give maintenance dose of 100 mcg/month (doses up to 1000 mcg have been used for maintenance).
Intranasal (Adults): *Vitamin B_{12} deficiency*—500 mcg (one spray) in one nostril once weekly. *Pernicious anemia (for hematologic remission only)*—500 mcg (one spray) in one nostril once weekly.

Hydroxocobalamin

IM (Adults): *Vitamin B_{12} deficiency*—30 mcg/day for 5–10 days, then 100–200 mcg/month. *Pernicious anemia*—100 mcg/day for 6–7 days; if improvement, give same dose every other day for 7 doses, then every 3–4 days for 2–3 wk; once hematologic values return to normal (remission), give maintenance dose of 100 mcg/month. *Schilling test*—Flushing dose is 1000 mcg.
IM (Children): *Vitamin B_{12} deficiency*—100 mcg/day for 2 or more weeks (to achieve total dose of 1000–5000 mcg), then 30–50 mcg/month. *Pernicious anemia*—30–50 mcg/day for 2 or more weeks (to achieve total dose of 1000–5000 mcg), then 100 mcg/month.
IV (Adults): *Cyanide poisoning (Cyanokit only)*—5 g over 15 min; another 5 g dose may be infused over 15–120 min depending upon severity of poisoning (maximum cumulative dose = 10 g).

Availability

Cyanocobalamin

Tablets: 50 mcg[OTC], 100 mcg[OTC], 250 mcg[OTC], 500 mcg[OTC], 1000 mcg[OTC], 5000 mcg[OTC]. **Extended-release tablets:** 1000 mcg[OTC], 1500 mcg[OTC]. **Sublingual tablets:** 2500 mcg[OTC]. **Lozenges:** 100 mcg[OTC], 250 mcg[OTC], 500 mcg[OTC]. **Nasal spray:** 500 mcg/0.1 mL actuation (8 sprays/bottle). **Injection:** 1000 mcg/ml in 1-, 10-, and 30-ml vials.

Hydroxocobalamin

Injection: 1000 mcg/ml in 30-ml vials. **Powder for injection (Cyanokit):** 2.5 g/vial (2 vials in each kit).

NURSING IMPLICATIONS

Assessment

- Assess patient for signs of vitamin B_{12} deficiency (pallor; neuropathy; psychosis; red, inflamed tongue) before and periodically during therapy.
- ***Lab Test Considerations:*** Monitor plasma folic acid, vitamin B_{12}, and iron levels, hemoglobin, hemtaocrit, and reticulocyte count before treatment, 1 mo after the start of therapy, and then every 3–6 mo. Evaluate serum potassium level in patients receiving vitamin B_{12} for pernicious anemia for hypokalemia during the first 48 hr of treatment. Serum potassium and platelet counts should be monitored routinely during the course of therapy. Cyanokit Management of cyanide poisoning should also include establishment of airway, ensuring adequate oxygenation and hydration, cardiovascular support, and seizure management. Monitor BP and HR continuously during and after infusion and immediately report significant changes. The maximal ↑ in BP usually occurs toward the end of the infusion. BP usually returns to baseline within 4 hr of drug administration.

Potential Nursing Diagnoses

Imbalanced nutrition: less than body requirements (Indications)
Activity intolerance (Indications)

Implementation

- Usually administered in combination with other vitamins; solitary vitamin B_{12} deficiencies are rare.
- Administration of vitamin B_{12} by the oral route is useful only for nutritional deficiencies. Patients with small-bowel disease, malabsorption syndrome, or gastric or ileal resections require parenteral administration.
- **PO:** Administer with meals to increase absorption.
- May be mixed with fruit juices. Administer immediately after mixing; ascorbic acid alters stability.
- **Intranasal:** Dose should not be administered within 1 hr of hot food or liquids (these substances may result in the formation of nasal secretions which may result in ↓ effectiveness of nasal spray).
- **IM, Subcut:** Vials should be protected from light.

V

- If subcutaneous route used, deep subcutaneous administration is preferred.

IV Administration

- **IV:** IV route should only be used with Cyanokit
- **Intermittent Infusion:** ***Diluent:*** Dilute each Cyanokit vial with 100 ml of 0.9% NaCl, D5W, or LR. Gently invert the vial for at least 30 sec prior to infusion. Reconstituted vial can be hung for infusion and is stable for 6 hr at room temperature. Discard any unused solution after 6 hr. ***Rate:*** Administer initial 5-g dose over 15 min. Administer additional 5-g dose over 15–120 min.
- **Y-Site Incompatibility:** ascorbic acid, blood products, sodium nitrite, sodium thiosulfate.
- **Additive Incompatibility:** diazepam, dobutamine, dopamine, fentanyl, nitroglycerin, pentobarbital, propofol, thiopental.

Patient/Family Teaching

- Encourage patient to comply with diet recommendations of health care professional. Explain that the best source of vitamins is a well-balanced diet with foods from the four basic food groups.
- Foods high in vitamin B_{12} include meats, seafood, egg yolk, and fermented cheeses; few vitamins are lost with ordinary cooking.
- Patients self-medicating with vitamin supplements should be cautioned not to exceed RDA. Effectiveness of megadoses for treatment of various medical conditions is unproved and may cause side effects.
- Inform patients with pernicious anemia of the lifelong need for vitamin B_{12} replacement.
- Emphasize the importance of follow-up exams to evaluate progress.
- **Intranasal:** Instruct patient in proper administration technique. Review *Patient Information Sheet* and demonstrate use of actuator. Unit must be primed with 3 strokes upon using for the first time. Unit must be primed with 1 stroke before each of the remaining doses. Advise patient to clear nose, then place tip approximately 1 inch into nostril and press pump once, firmly and quickly. After dose, remove unit from nose and massage dosed nostril gently for a few seconds. Vial delivers 8 doses. Unit should be stored at room temperature and protected from light.
- Advise patient that skin redness may last up to 2 wk and that their urine may remain red for up to 5 wk after drug administration. Instruct patient to avoid sun exposure while their skin is red. Advise patient to contact health care professional if skin or urine redness persist after these time periods. Advise patient that a rash may develop from 7–28 days after drug administration. It will usually resolve without treatment within a few weeks. Advise patient to contact health care professional if rash persists after this time period.

Evaluation/Desired Outcomes

- Resolution of the symptoms of vitamin B_{12} deficiency.
- Increase in reticulocyte count.
- Improvement in manifestations of pernicious anemia.
- Resolution of symptoms of cyanide poisoning.

VITAMIN D COMPOUNDS

calcitriol (kal-si-**trye**-ole)
1,25-dihydroxycholecalciferol, Calcijex, Rocaltrol, vitamin D_3 (active)

cholecalciferol
Delta-D, vitamin D_3 (inactive)

doxercalciferol
(**dox**-er-**kal**-si-fe-role)
Hectorol, vitamin D_2

ergocalciferol
(er-goe-kal-**sif**-e-role)
Drisdol, ✦Ostoforte, vitamin D_2

paricalcitol (par-i-**kal**-si-tole)
Zemplar

Classification
Therapeutic: vitamins
Pharmacologic: fat-soluble vitamins

Pregnancy Category B (doxercalciferol), C (calcitriol, cholecalciferol, ergocalciferol, paricalcitol)

Indications

Calcitriol: Management of hypocalcemia in chronic renal dialysis (IV and PO). Treatment of hypocalcemia in patients with hypoparathyroidism or pseudohypoparathyroidism (PO only). Management of secondary hyperparathyroidism and resulting metabolic bone disease in predialysis patients with moderate to severe renal insufficiency (CCr 15–55 ml/min) (PO only). **Cho-**

lecalciferol: Treatment or prevention of vitamin D deficiency. **Doxercaliciferol:** Treatment of secondary hyperparathyroidism in patients undergoing chronic renal dialysis (IV and PO). Treatment of secondary hyperparathyroidism in patients with Stage 3 or 4 chronic kidney disease (PO only). **Ergocalciferol:** Treatment of familial hypophosphatemia. Treatment of hypoparathyroidism. Treatment of vitamin D-resistant rickets. **Paricalcitol:** Prevention and treatment of secondary hyperparathyroidism in patients with Stage 3 or 4 (PO) or Stage 5 (IV) chronic kidney disease.

Action

Cholecalciferol requires activation in the liver and kidneys to create the active form of vitamin D_3 (calcitriol). Doxercalciferol and ergocalciferol require activation in the liver to create the active form of vitamin D_2. Paricalcitol is a synthetic analogue of calcitriol. Vitamin D: Promotes the absorption of calcium and ↓ parathyroid hormone concentration. **Therapeutic Effects:** Treatment and prevention of deficiency states, particularly bone manifestations. Improved calcium and phosphorous homeostasis in patients with chronic kidney disease.

Pharmacokinetics

Absorption: *Calcitriol, doxercalciferol, ergocalciferol, paricalcitol*—Well absorbed following oral administration. *Calcitriol, doxercalciferol, paricalcitol*—IV administration results in complete bioavailability.
Distribution: Calcitriol and paricalcitol cross the placenta; calcitriol also enters breast milk.
Protein Binding: *Calcitriol and paricalcitol*—99.9%.
Metabolism and Excretion: *Calcitriol*—Undergoes enterohepatic recycling and is excreted mostly in bile. *Cholecalciferol*—Converted by the liver and kidneys to calcitriol (active form of vitamin D_3. *Ergocalciferol*—Converted to active form of vitamin D_2 by sunlight, the liver, and the kidneys. *Doxercalciferol*—Converted by the liver to the active form of vitamin D_2. *Paricalcitol*—mostly metabolized by the liver and excreted via hepatobiliary elimination.
Half-life: *Calcitriol*—5–8 hr. *Cholecalciferol*—14 hr. *Doxercalciferol*—32–37 hr (up to 96 hr). *Paricalcitol*—14–20 hr.

TIME/ACTION PROFILE (effects on serum calcium)

ROUTE	ONSET	PEAK	DURATION
calcitriol-PO	2–6 hr	2–6 hr	3–5 days
calcitriol-IV	unknown	unknown	unknown
cholecalciferol-PO	unknown	unknown	unknown
doxercalciferol PO	unknown	8 wk	1 wk
doxercalciferol-IV	unknown	8 wk	1 wk
ergocalciferol-PO	12–24 hr	unknown	up to 6 mo
paricalcitol-PO	unknown	2–4 wk	unknown
paricalitol IV	unknown	up to 2 wk	unknown

Contraindications/Precautions

Contraindicated in: Hypersensitivity; Hypercalcemia; Vitamin D toxicity; Lactation: Potential for serious adverse reactions in infant; Concurrent use of magnesium-containing antacids or other vitamin D supplements; Ergocalciferol; Known intolerance to tartrazine; Cholecalciferol and ergocalciferol; Malabsorption problems.
Use Cautiously in: Calcitriol, doxercalciferol, paricalcitol; Patients receiving digoxin; OB: Pregnancy (safety not established).

Adverse Reactions/Side Effects

Seen primarily as manifestations of toxicity (hypercalcemia).
CNS: headache, somnolence, weakness; *doxercalciferol*—dizziness, malaise. **EENT:** conjunctivitis, photophobia, rhinorrhea. **Resp:** *doxercalciferol and ergocalciferol*—dyspnea. **CV:** arrhythmias, edema, hypertension; *doxercalciferol*—bradycardia; *paricalcitol*—palpitations. **GI:** PANCREATITIS, abdominal pain, anorexia, constipation, dry mouth, liver function test elevation, metallic taste, nausea, polydipsia, vomiting, weight loss. **GU:** albuminuria, azotemia, decreased libido, nocturia, polyuria.
Derm: pruritus. **F and E:** hypercalcemia. **Metab:** hyperthermia. **MS:** bone pain, muscle pain; *doxercalciferol*—arthralgia; *paricalcitol*—metastatic calcification. **Local:** pain at injection site. **Misc:** *calcitriol*—allergic reactions, chills, fever.

Interactions

Drug-Drug: Cholestyramine, **colestipol**, or **mineral oil** ↓ absorption of vitamin D analogues. Use with **thiazide diuretics** may result in hypercalcemia. **Corticosteroids** ↓ effectiveness of vitamin D analogues. Using calcitriol, doxercalciferol, or paricalcitol with **digoxin** may ↑ risk of arrhythmias. Vitamin D requirements ↓ by **phenytoin** and other **hydantoin anticonvulsants**, **sucralfate**, **barbiturates**, and **primidone**. Concurrent use with **magnesium-containing drugs** may lead to hypermagnesemia. Concurrent use of **calcium-containing drugs** may ↑ risk of hypercalcemia. Concurrent use of other **Vitamin D supplements** may ↑ risk of hypercalcemia. **Agents that induce liver enzymes** (**phenobarbital**, **rifampin**) and **agents that inhibit liver enzymes** (**atazanavir**, **clarithromycin**, **erythromycin**, **indinavir**, **itraconazole**, **ketoconazole**, **nefazodone**, **nelfinavir**, **ritonavir**, **saquinavir**, **verapamil**, **voriconazole**) may alter requirements for doxercalciferol and paricalcitol (monitoring of calcium and phosophorus recommended).

Drug-Food: Ingestion of **foods high in calcium content** (see Appendix L) may lead to hypercalcemia.

Route/Dosage

Calcitriol

PO (Adults): *Hypocalcemia during dialysis*—0.25 mcg/day or every other day; if needed, may ↑ by 0.25 mcg/day at 4–8 wk intervals (typical dosage = 0.5–1 mcg/day). *Hypoparathyroidism*—0.25 mcg/day initially; if needed, may ↑ dose by 0.25 mcg/day at 2–4 wk intervals (typical dosage = 0.5–2 mcg/day). *Predialysis patients*—0.25 mcg/day (up to 0.5 mcg/day).

PO (Children): *Hypocalcemia during dialysis*—0.25–2 mcg/day. *Hypoparathyroidism (children ≥6 yr)*—0.25 mcg/day initially; if needed, may ↑ dose by 0.25 mcg/day at 2–4 wk intervals (typical dosage = 0.5–2 mcg/day). *Hypoparathyroidism (children 1–5 yr)*—0.25–0.75 mcg/day. *Hypoparathyroidism (children <1 yr)*—0.04–0.08 mcg/kg/day. *Predialysis patients (children ≥3 yr)*—0.25 mcg/day (up to 0.5 mcg/day). *Predialysis patients (children <3 yr)*—10–15 mg/kg/day.

IV (Adults): *Hypocalcemia during dialysis*—0.5 mcg (0.01 mcg/kg) 3 times weekly. May be increased by 0.25–0.5 mcg/dose at 2-4 wk intervals (typical maintenance dose = 0.5–3.0 mcg 3 times weekly [0.01–0.05 mcg/kg 3 times weekly]).

IV (Children): *Hypocalcemia during dialysis*—0.01–0.05 mcg/kg 3 times weekly.

Cholecalciferol

PO (Adults): 400–1000 units daily.

Doxercalciferol

PO (Adults): *Dialysis patients*—10 mcg 3 times weekly (at dialysis); dose may be adjusted by 2.5 mcg at 8-wk intervals based on intact PTH concentrations (maximum dose = 20 mcg 3 times weekly). *Non-dialysis patients*—1 mcg/day; dose may be adjusted by 0.5 mcg at 2 wk intervals based on intact PTH concentrations (maximum dose = 3.5 mcg/day).

IV (Adults): 4 mcg 3 times weekly at the end of dialysis; dose may be adjusted by 1–2 mcg at 8-wk intervals based on intact PTH concentrations (maximum dose = 6 mcg 3 times weekly).

Ergocalciferol

PO (Adults): *Vitamin D–resistant rickets*—12,000–500,000 units/day (to be used with phosphate supplement). *Familial hypophosphatemia*—10,000–80,000 units/day (with phosphorus 1–2 g/day). *Hypoparathyroidism*—50,000–200,000 units/day (to be used with calcium supplement).

PO (Children): *Vitamin D–resistant rickets*—40,000–80,000 units/day (to be used with phosphate supplement). *Familial hypophosphatemia*—10,000–80,000 units/day (with phosphorus 1–2 g/day). *Hypoparathyroidism*—50,000–200,000 units/day (to be used with calcium supplement).

Paricalcitol

PO (Adults): *Baseline intact PTH concentration ≤500 pg/ml*—Initiate with 1 mcg/day or 2 mcg 3 times weekly; *Baseline intact PTH concentration >500 pg/ml*—Initiate with 2 mcg/day or 4 mcg 3 times weekly; doses can be adjusted at 2–4 wk intervals based on intact PTH concentrations.

IV (Adults and Children ≥5 yr): 0.04–0.1 mcg/kg 3 times weekly during dialysis; dose can be adjusted by 2–4 mcg at 2–4 wk intervals based on intact PTH concentrations (doses up to 0.24 mcg/kg have been used).

Availability

Calcitriol

Capsules: 0.25 mcg, 0.5 mcg. **Oral solution:** 1 mcg/ml in 15-ml bottle. **Solution for injection:** 1 mcg/ml in 1-ml ampules.

Cholecalciferol

Tablets: 400 units[OTC], 1000 units[OTC]. ***In combination with:*** alendronate (Fosamax Plus D), see Appendix B.

Doxercalciferol
Capsules: 0.5 mcg, 2.5 mcg. **Solution for injection:** 2 mcg/ml in 2-ml ampules.

Ergocalciferol
Liquid: 8000 units/ml in 60-ml bottles Rx, OTC.
Capsules: 50,000 units.

Paricalcitol
Capsules: 1 mcg, 2 mcg, 4 mcg. **Solution for injection:** 2 mcg/ml in 1-ml vials, 5 mcg/ml in 1- and 2-ml vials.

NURSING IMPLICATIONS

Assessment

- Assess for symptoms of vitamin deficiency prior to and periodically during therapy.
- Assess patient for bone pain and weakness prior to and during therapy.
- Observe patient carefully for evidence of hypocalcemia (paresthesia, muscle twitching, laryngospasm, colic, cardiac arrhythmias, and Chvostek's or Trousseau's sign). Protect symptomatic patient by raising and padding side rails; keep bed in low position.
- Pedi: Monitor height and weight; growth arrest may occur in prolonged high-dose therapy.
- **Rickets/Osteomalacia:** Assess patient for bone pain and weakness prior to and during therapy.
- ***Lab Test Considerations:*** During *calcitriol* therapy, serum calcium and phosphate concentrations should be drawn twice weekly initially. Serum calcium, magnesium, alkaline phosphatase, and intact PTH should then be monitored at least monthly. During *cholecalciferol* therapy, serum calcium, phosphate, and alkaline phosphatase concentrations should be monitored periodically. During *doxercalciferol* therapy, serum ionized calcium, phosphate, and intact PTH concentrations should be monitored prior to initiation of therapy, and then weekly during the first 12 wk of therapy, then periodically. Alkaline phosphatase should be monitored periodically. During *ergocalciferol* therapy, serum calcium and phosphate concentrations should be monitored every 2 wk. During oral *paricalcitol* therapy, serum calcium, phosphate, and intact PTH concentrations should be monitored at least every 2 wk for the first 3 mo of therapy or after any dosage adjustment, then monthly for 3 mo, then every 3 mo. During IV *paricalcitol* therapy, serum calcium and phosphate concentrations should be monitored twice weekly initially until dosage stabilized, and then at least monthly. Serum intact PTH concentrations should be monitored every 3 mo.
- The serum calcium times phosphate product (Ca x P) should not exceed 70 mg^2/dl^2 (55 mg^2/dl^2 for doxercalciferol) (patients may be at ↑ risk of calcification).
- Calcitriol may cause false ↑ cholesterol levels.
- ***Toxicity and Overdose:*** Toxicity is manifested as hypercalcemia, hypercalciuria, and hyperphosphatemia. Assess patient for appearance of nausea, vomiting, anorexia, weakness, constipation, headache, bone pain, and metallic taste. Later symptoms include polyuria, polydipsia, photophobia, rhinorrhea, pruritus, and cardiac arrhythmias. Notify physician or other health care professional immediately if these signs of hypervitaminosis D occur. Treatment usually consists of discontinuation of calcitriol, a low-calcium diet, use of low-calcium dialysate in peritoneal dialysis patients, and administration of a laxative. IV hydration and loop diuretics may be ordered to increase urinary excretion of calcium. Hemodialysis may also be used.

Potential Nursing Diagnoses

Imbalanced nutrition: less than body requirements (Indications)

Implementation

- Do not confuse Calciferol (ergocalciferol) with calcitriol.
- **PO:** May be administered without regard to meals. Measure solution accurately with calibrated dropper provided by manufacturer. May be mixed with juice, cereal, or food, or dropped directly into mouth. Calcitriol capsules or solution should be protected from light.

IV Administration

- **Direct IV:** Administer *calcitriol, doxercalciferol, and paracalcitol* undiluted by rapid injection through the catheter at the end of a hemodialysis period.

V

Patient/Family Teaching

- Advise patient to take medication as directed. Take missed doses as soon as remembered that day, unless almost time for next dose; do not double up on doses.
- Review diet modifications with patient. See Appendix L for foods high in calcium and vitamin D. Renal patients must still consider renal failure diet in food selection. Health care professional may order concurrent calcium supplement.
- Encourage patient to comply with dietary recommendations of health care professional. Explain that the best source of vitamins is a well-balanced diet with foods from the 4 basic food groups and the importance of sunlight exposure. See Appendix L for foods high in vitamin D.
- Patients self-medicating with vitamin supplements should be cautioned not to exceed RDA. The effectiveness of megadoses for treatment of various medical conditions is unproved and may cause side effects.
- Advise patient to avoid concurrent use of antacids containing magnesium.
- Review symptoms of overdosage and instruct patient to report these promptly to health care professional.
- Emphasize the importance of follow-up exams to evaluate progress.

Evaluation/Desired Outcomes

- Normalization of serum calcium and parathyroid hormone levels.
- Resolution or prevention of vitamin D deficiency.
- Improvement in symptoms of vitamin D–resistant rickets.

vitamin E (vye-ta-min E)

alpha tocopherol, Amino-Opti-E, Aquasol E, E-200, E-400, E-1000, E-Complex-600, E-Vitamin, Liqui-E, Pheryl-E, Vita Plus E, ♣ Webber Vitamin E

Classification
Therapeutic: vitamins
Pharmacologic: fat-soluble vitamins

Pregnancy Category A (doses within RDA), C (doses >RDA)

Indications

PO: Used as a dietary supplement. Used in low-birth-weight infants to prevent and treat hemolysis due to vitamin E deficiency. **Topical:** Treatment of irritated, chapped, or dry skin. **Unlabeled uses:** Prevention of coronary artery disease.

Action

Prevents the oxidation (antioxidant) of other substances. Protects RBC membranes against hemolysis, especially in low-birth-weight neonates. **Therapeutic Effects:** Prevention and treatment of deficiency in high-risk patients.

Pharmacokinetics

Absorption: 20–80% absorbed following oral administration. Absorption requires fat and bile salts.
Distribution: Widely distributed, stored in adipose tissue (4-yr supply).
Metabolism and Excretion: Metabolized by the liver, excreted in bile.
Half-life: Unknown.

TIME/ACTION PROFILE

ROUTE	ONSET	PEAK	DURATION
PO	unknown	unknown	unknown

Contraindications/Precautions

Contraindicated in: Hypersensitivity to ingredients in preparations (parabens, propylene, glycol).
Use Cautiously in: Anemia due to iron deficiency; Low-birth-weight infants (oral administration may cause necrotizing enterocolitis); Vitamin K deficiency (may increase risk of bleeding).

Adverse Reactions/Side Effects

Seen primarily with large doses over long periods of time.
CNS: fatigue, headache, weakness. **EENT:** blurred vision. **GI:** NECROTIZING ENTEROCOLITIS (oral administration in low-birth-weight infants), cramps, diarrhea, nausea. **Derm:** rash. **Endo:** gonadal dysfunction.

Interactions

Drug-Drug: Cholestyramine, **colestipol**, **orlistat**, **mineral oil**, and **sucralfate** decrease absorption. May decrease hematologic response to **iron supplements**. May increase the risk of bleeding with **warfarin**.
Drug-Natural Products: Increased bleeding risk with **anise**, **arnica**, **chamomile**, **clove**, **dong quai**, **fenugreek**, **feverfew**, **garlic**, **ginger**, **ginkgo**, **Panax ginseng**, **licorice**, and others.

Route/Dosage

Other dosing regimens may be used.

PO (Adults and Children): Determined by nutritional intake or degree of deficiency.

Topical (Adults and Children): Apply to affected areas as needed.

Availability

Capsules: 100 units^OTC^, 200 units^OTC^, 400 units^OTC^, 600 units^OTC^, ✤800 units^OTC^, 1000 units^OTC^. **Oral solution:** 26.6 units/ml^OTC^, 50 units/ml^OTC^, 77 units/ml^OTC^. **Tablets:** 100 units^OTC^, 200 units^OTC^, 400 units^OTC^, 500 units^OTC^, 800 units^OTC^. **Chewable tablets:** 400 units^OTC^. **Ointment:** ^OTC^. **Cream:** ^OTC^. **Lotion:** ^OTC^. **Oil:** ^OTC^.

NURSING IMPLICATIONS

Assessment

- Assess patient for signs of vitamin E deficiency (*neonates*—irritability, edema, hemolytic anemia, creatinuria; *adults/children [rare]*—muscle weakness, ceroid deposits, anemia, creatinuria) prior to and periodically throughout therapy.
- Assess nutritional status through 24-hr diet recall. Determine frequency of consumption of vitamin E–rich foods.
- ***Lab Test Considerations:*** Large doses may increase cholesterol, triglyceride, and CPK levels.

Potential Nursing Diagnoses

Imbalanced nutrition: less than body requirements (Indications)

Implementation

- **PO:** Administer with or after meals.
- Chewable tablets should be chewed well or crushed before swallowing. Solution may be dropped directly into mouth or mixed with cereal, fruit juice, or other food. Use calibrated dropper supplied by manufacturer to measure solution accurately.

Patient/Family Teaching

- Instruct patient to take medication as directed. If a dose is missed, it should be omitted, because fat-soluble vitamins are stored in the body for long periods.
- Encourage patient to comply with diet recommendations of health care professional. Explain that the best source of vitamins is a well-balanced diet with foods from the four basic food groups.
- Foods high in vitamin E include vegetable oils, wheat germ, whole-grain cereals, egg yolk, and liver. Vitamin E content is not markedly affected by cooking.
- Patients self-medicating with vitamin supplements should be cautioned not to exceed RDA. The effectiveness of megadoses for treatment of various medical conditions is unproved, and this may cause side effects and toxicity.
- Review symptoms of overdosage (blurred vision, flu-like symptoms, headache, breast enlargement). Instruct patient to report these promptly to health care professional.
- Mineral oil may interfere with the absorption of fat-soluble vitamins and should not be used concurrently.

Evaluation/Desired Outcomes

- Prevention of or decrease in the symptoms of vitamin E deficiency.
- Control of dry or chapped skin.

voriconazole

(vor-i-**kon**-a-zole)

VFEND

Classification

Therapeutic: antifungals

Pregnancy Category D

Indications

Serious systemic fungal infections including candidemia, esophageal candidiasis, candidal deep tissue and skin infections, abdominal, kidney, bladder wall and wound infections and aspergillosis.

Action

Inhibits fungal ergosterol synthesis leading to production of abnormal fungal cell wall. **Therapeutic Effects:** Antifungal activity.

Pharmacokinetics

Absorption: Well absorbed following oral administration (96%); IV administration results in complete bioavailability.

Distribution: Extensive tissue distribution.

Metabolism and Excretion: Highly metabolized by the hepatic P450 enzymes (CYP2C19, CYP2C9, CYP3A4); <2% excreted unchanged in

V

urine. Much individual variation in metabolism; metabolites are inactive.
Half-life: Dose-dependent; increased in hepatic impairment.

TIME/ACTION PROFILE (blood levels)

ROUTE	ONSET	PEAK	DURATION
PO	rapid	1–2 hr	12 hr
IV	rapid	end of infusion	12 hr

Contraindications/Precautions

Contraindicated in: Concurrent use of efavirenz, rifampin, carbamazepine, phenobarbital, mephobarbital (decrease antifungal activity); Concurrent use of sirolimus, pimozide, quinidine, ergotamine, and dihydroergotamine (↑ risk of toxicity of these agents); Tablets contain lactose and should be avoided in patients with galactose intolerance, Lapp lactase deficiency, or glucose-galactose malabsorption.
Use Cautiously in: Mild to moderate liver disease (Child-Pugh Class A and B); maintenance dose reduction recommended; Renal impairment (CCr <50 ml/min); use only if justified by risk/benefit assessment (IV form should be avoided, use oral form only); OB: Pregnancy or lactation (use only if benefits justify risk); Pedi: Children <12 yr (safety not established).

Adverse Reactions/Side Effects

CNS: dizziness, hallucinations, headache. **EENT:** visual disturbances, eye hemorrhage. **CV:** changes in blood pressure, tachycardia, peripheral edema, tachycardia. **GI:** HEPATOXICITY, abdominal pain, diarrhea, nausea, vomiting. **Derm:** photosensitivity, rash. **F and E:** hypokalemia, Hypomagnesemia. **Misc:** allergic reactions including STEVENS-JOHNSON SYNDROME, chills, fever, infusion reactions.

Interactions

Drug-Drug: Carbamazepine, **efavirenz mephobarbital**, **phenobarbital**, and **rifampim** ↑ metabolism and ↓ antifungal activity of voriconazole; concurrent use is contraindicated. ↓ metabolism and ↑ risk of toxicity from **dihydroergotamine**, **ergotamine**, **pimozide**, **quinidine**, and **sirolimus**; concurrent use is contraindicated. ↓ metabolism and ↑ risk of toxicity from **cyclosporine**, **efavirenz**, **HMG-CoA reductase inhibitors**, some **benzodiazepines (alprazolam, midazolam, triazolam)**, some **calcium channel blockers**, **sulfonlylureas (glipizide, glyburide, tolbutamine)**, **tacrolimus**, **warfarin**, **vinca alkaloids (vincristine, vinblastine)**; careful monitoring required during concurrent use. **Phenytoin** ↑ metabolism and ↓ antifungal activity of voriconazole; voriconazole ↑ **phenytoin** levels and may cause toxicity; careful monitoring required during concurrent use. ↑ blood levels of **omeprazole**; ↓ omeprazole dose by 50% during concurrent use. Similar effects may occur with other **proton-pump inhibitors**. May ↓ metabolism and ↑ blood levels and effects of **protease-inhibitor antiretrovirals** and **non-nucleoside reverse transcriptase inhibitor antiretrovirals**; frequent monitoring recommended. **Non-nucleoside reverse transcriptase inhibitor antiretrovirals**; may induce or inhibit the metabolism of voriconazole; frequent monitoring recommended.

Route/Dosage

IV (Adults and Children >12 yr): *Loading dose*—6 mg/kg every 12 hour for 2 doses, followed by *maintenance dosing*—3–4 mg/kg every 12 hours. IV then switched to oral dosing when possible. If intolerance occurs, dose may be decreased to 3 mg/kg every 12 hr. If phenytoin is coadministered, increase maintenance dose to 5 mg/kg every 12 hr.
PO (Adults and Children >12 yr and >40 kg): *Most infections*—(following IV loading dose) 200 mg every 12 hr; may be increased to 300 mg every 12 hr if response if inadequate. If phenytoin is coadministered, increase maintenance dose to 400 mg every 12 hr; *esophageal candidiasis*—200 mg every 12 hr for 14 days or 7 days following symptom resolution.
PO (Adults and Children >12 yr and <40 kg): *Most infections*—(following IV loading dose) 100 mg every 12 hr; may be increased to 150 mg every 12 hr if response is inadequate. If phenytoin is coadministered, increase maintenance dose to 200 mg every 12 hr; *esophageal candidiasis*—100 mg every 12 hr for 14 days or 7 days following symptom resolution.

Hepatic Impairment

IV (Adults and Children >12 yr): Use standard loading dose, decrease maintenance dose by 50%.

Availability

Tablets: 50 mg, 200 mg. **Oral suspension (orange):** 40 mg/ml in 100 ml bottles. **Powder for injection (requires reconstitution):** 200 mg/vial.

NURSING IMPLICATIONS

Assessment

- Monitor for signs and symptoms of fungal infections prior to and during therapy.
- Obtain specimens for culture and histopathology prior to therapy to isolate and identify organism. Therapy may be started before results are received.
- Monitor visual function including visual acuity, visual field, and color perception in patients receiving more than 28 days of therapy. Vision usually returns to normal within 14 days after discontinuation of therapy.
- Monitor for allergic reactions during infusion of voriconazole (flushing, fever, sweating, tachycardia, chest tightness, dyspnea, faintness, nausea, pruritus, rash). Symptoms occur immediately upon start of infusion. May require discontinuation.
- ***Lab Test Considerations:*** Monitor liver function tests prior to and during therapy. If abnormal liver function tests occur, monitor for development of severe hepatic injury. Discontinue therapy if clinical signs and symptoms of liver disease develop.
- Monitor renal function (serum creatinine) during therapy.

Potential Nursing Diagnoses

Risk for infection (Indications)

Implementation

- Once patient can tolerate oral medication, PO voriconazole may be used.
- **PO:** Administer 1 hr before or 1 hr after a meal.

IV Administration

- **Intermittent Infusion: *Diluent:*** Reconstitute each 200-mg vial with 19 ml of sterile water for injection to achieve concentration of 10 mg/ml. Calculate volume of 10 mg/ml solution required for patient dose. Withdraw and discard equal volume of diluent from infusion bag or bottle to be used. Withdraw required volume of voriconazole solution from vial(s) and add to appropriate volume of 0.9% NaCl, LR, D5/LR, D5/0.45% NaCl, D5W, 0.45% NaCl, or D5/0.9% NaCl. Reconstituted solution stable for 24 hr if refrigerated. Discard partially used vials. ***Concentration:*** Final concentration of infusion should be 0.5–5 mg/ml. ***Rate:*** Infuse over 1–2 hr at a rate not to exceed 3 mg/kg/hr.
- **Y-Site Incompatibility:** cefepime, cyclosporine, diazepam, moxifloxacin, nitroprusside, pantoprazole, phenytoin, tigecycline.

Patient/Family Teaching

- May cause blurred vision, photophobia, and dizziness. Caution patient to avoid driving and other activities requiring alertness until response to medication is known. Also advise patient to avoid driving at night during voriconazole therapy.
- Advise patient to avoid direct sunlight during voriconazole therapy.

Evaluation/Desired Outcomes

- Resolution of fungal infections.

V

HIGH ALERT

warfarin (**war**-fa-rin)
Coumadin, ✤Warfilone

Classification
Therapeutic: anticoagulants
Pharmacologic: coumarins

Pregnancy Category X

Indications

Prophylaxis and treatment of: Venous thrombosis, Pulmonary embolism, Atrial fibrillation with embolization. Management of myocardial infarction: Decreases risk of death, Decreases risk of subsequent MI, Decreases risk of future thromboembolic events. Prevention of thrombus formation and embolization after prosthetic valve placement.

Action

Interferes with hepatic synthesis of vitamin K-dependent clotting factors (II, VII, IX, and X).
Therapeutic Effects: Prevention of thromboembolic events.

Pharmacokinetics

Absorption: Well absorbed from the GI tract after oral administration.
Distribution: Crosses the placenta but does not enter breast milk.
Protein Binding: 99%.
Metabolism and Excretion: Metabolized by the liver.
Half-life: 42 hrs.

TIME/ACTION PROFILE (effects on coagulation tests)

ROUTE	ONSET	PEAK	DURATION
PO, IV	36–72 hr	5–7 days	2–5 days

Contraindications/Precautions

Contraindicated in: Uncontrolled bleeding; Open wounds; Active ulcer disease; Recent brain, eye, or spinal cord injury or surgery; Severe liver or kidney disease; Uncontrolled hypertension; OB: Crosses placenta and may cause fatal hemorrhage in the fetus. May also cause congenital malformation.
Use Cautiously in: Malignancy; Patients with history of ulcer or liver disease; History of poor compliance; Women with childbearing potential; Pedi: Has been used safely but may require more frequent PT/INR assessments; Geri: Due to greater than expected anticoagulant response, initiate and maintain at lower dosages.

Adverse Reactions/Side Effects

GI: cramps, nausea. **Derm:** dermal necrosis.
Hemat: BLEEDING. **Misc:** fever.

Interactions

Drug-Drug: Abciximab, **androgens**, **capecitabine**, **cefoperazone**, **cefotetan**, **chloral hydrate**, **chloramphenicol**, **clopidogrel**, **disulfiram**, **fluconazole**, **fluoroquinolones**, **itraconazole**, **metronidazole** (including vaginal use), **thrombolytics**, **eptifibatide**, **tirofiban**, **ticlopidine**, **sulfonamides**, **quinidine**, **quinine**, **NSAIDs**, **valproates**, and **aspirin** may increase the response to warfarin and increase the risk of bleeding. Chronic use of **acetaminophen** may increase the risk of bleeding. Chronic **alcohol** ingestion may decrease action of warfarin; if chronic **alcohol** abuse results in significant liver damage, action of warfarin may be ↑ due to ↓ production of clotting factor. **Barbiturates** and **hormonal contraceptives containing estrogen** may decrease the anticoagulant response to warfarin. Acute **alcohol** ingestion may ↑ action of warfarin. **Many other drugs** may affect the activity of warfarin.
Drug-Natural Products: St. John's wort decreases effect. Increased bleeding risk with anise, arnica, chamomile, clove, dong quai, fenugreek, feverfew, garlic, ginger, ginkgo, Panax ginseng, licorice, and others.
Drug-Food: Ingestion of large quantities of **foods high in vitamin K content** (see list in Appendix L) may antagonize the anticoagulant effect of warfarin.

Route/Dosage

PO, IV (Adults): 2.5–10 mg/day for 2–4 days; then adjust daily dose by results of prothrombin time or international normalized ratio (INR). Initiate therapy with lower doses in geriatric or debilitated patients.
PO, IV (Children >1 month): Initial loading dose—0.2 mg/kg (maximum dose: 10 mg) for 2–4 days then adjust daily dose by results of prothrombin time or international normalized ratio (INR), use 0.1 mg/kg if liver dysfunction is present. Maintenance dose range-0.05–0.34 mg/kg/day.

W

Availability (generic available)

Tablets: 1 mg, 2 mg, 2.5 mg, 3 mg, 4 mg, 5 mg, 6 mg, 7.5 mg, 10 mg. **Cost:** *Coumadin*—5 mg $85.00/90; *Jantoven*—5 mg $58.14/90; *Generic*—5 mg $34.99/90. **Injection:** 5 mg/vial.

NURSING IMPLICATIONS

Assessment

- Assess patient for signs of bleeding and hemorrhage (bleeding gums; nosebleed; unusual bruising; tarry, black stools; hematuria; fall in hematocrit or blood pressure; guaiac-positive stools, urine, or nasogastric aspirate).
- Assess patient for evidence of additional or increased thrombosis. Symptoms depend on area of involvement.
- Geri: Patients over 60 yr exhibit greater than expected PT/INR response. Monitor for side effects at lower therapeutic ranges.
- Pedi: Achieving and maintaining therapeutic PT/INR ranges may be more difficult in the pediatric patient. Assess PT/INR levels more frequently.
- ***Lab Test Considerations:*** PT, INR and other clotting factors should be monitored frequently during therapy. Therapeutic PT ranges from 1.3–1.5 times greater than control; however, the INR, a standardized system that provides a common basis for communicating and interpreting PT results, is usually referenced. Normal INR (not on anticoagulants) is 0.8 to 1.2. An INR of 2.5 to 3.5 is recommended for patients at very high risk of embolization (for example, patients with mitral valve replacement and ventricular hypertrophy). Lower levels are acceptable when risk is lower.
- Hepatic function and CBC should be monitored before and periodically throughout therapy.
- Stool and urine should be monitored for occult blood before and periodically throughout therapy.
- ***Toxicity and Overdose:*** Withholding 1 or more doses of medication is usually sufficient if INR is excessively elevated or if minor bleeding occurs. If overdose occurs or anticoagulation needs to be immediately reversed, the antidote is vitamin K (phytonadione, AquaMEPHYTON). Administration of whole blood or plasma also may be required in severe bleeding because of the delayed onset of vitamin K.

Potential Nursing Diagnoses

Ineffective tissue perfusion (Indications)
Risk for injury (Side Effects)

Implementation

- ***High Alert:*** Medication errors involving anticoagulants have resulted in serious harm or death from internal or intracranial bleeding. Before administering, evaluate recent INR or PT results and have second practitioner independently check original order.
- Because of the large number of medications capable of significantly altering warfarin's effects, careful monitoring is recommended when new agents are started or other agents are discontinued. Interactive potential should be evaluated for all new medications (Rx, OTC, and natural products).
- Administer medication at same time each day.
- **PO:** Medication requires 3–5 days to reach effective levels. It is usually begun while patient is still on heparin.
- Do not interchange brands; potencies may not be equivalent.

IV Administration

- **Direct IV:** ***Diluent:*** Reconstitute each 5-mg vial with 2.7 ml of sterile water for injection. Reconstituted solution stable for 4 hr at room temperature. No further dilution needed before administration. ***Concentration:*** 2 mg/ml. ***Rate:*** Administer over 1–2 min.
- **Y-Site Compatibility:** amikacin, cefazolin, ceftriaxone, dopamine, epinephrine, heparin, lidocaine, morphine, nitroglycerin, potassium chloride, ranitidine.
- **Y-Site Incompatibility:** aminophylline, ceftazidime, cimetidine, ciprofloxacin, dobutamine, esmolol, gentamicin, labetalol, metronidazole, vancomycin.

Patient/Family Teaching

- Instruct patient to take medication exactly as directed. If a dose is missed, tell patient to take it as soon as remembered that day. Patient should not double doses. Health care professional should be informed of missed doses at time of checkup or lab tests.
- Review foods high in vitamin K (see Appendix L). Patient should have consistent limited intake of these foods, as vitamin K is the antidote for warfarin, and alternating intake of these foods will cause PT levels to fluctuate.
- Caution patient to avoid IM injections and activities leading to injury. Instruct patient to use a soft toothbrush, not to floss, and to

shave with an electric razor during warfarin therapy. Advise patient that venipunctures and injection sites require application of pressure to prevent bleeding or hematoma formation.

- Advise patient to report any symptoms of unusual bleeding or bruising (bleeding gums; nosebleed; black, tarry stools; hematuria; excessive menstrual flow). Notify health care professional if these occur.
- ***High Alert:*** Instruct patient not to drink alcohol or take OTC medications, especially those containing aspirin or NSAIDs, or to start or stop any new medications during warfarin therapy without advice of health care professional.
- ***High Alert:*** Emphasize the importance of frequent lab tests to monitor coagulation factors.
- Instruct patient to carry identification describing medication regimen at all times and to inform all health care personnel caring for patient on anticoagulant therapy before lab tests, treatment, or surgery.

Evaluation/Desired Outcomes

- Prolonged PT (1.3–2.0 times the control; may vary with indication) or INR of 2–4.5 without signs of hemorrhage.

W

zafirlukast (za-feer-loo-kast)
Accolate

Classification
Therapeutic: antiasthmatics, bronchodilators
Pharmacologic: leukotriene antagonists

Pregnancy Category B

Indications
Long-term control agent in the management of asthma.

Action
Antagonizes the effects of leukotrienes, which are components of slow-reacting substance of anaphylaxis (SRSA). These substances mediate the following: Airway edema, Smooth muscle constriction, Altered cellular activity, Result is decreased inflammatory process that is part of asthma. **Therapeutic Effects:** Decreased frequency and severity of asthma.

Pharmacokinetics
Absorption: Rapidly absorbed after oral administration.
Distribution: Enters breast milk.
Protein Binding: 99%.
Metabolism and Excretion: Mostly metabolized by the liver; 10% excreted unchanged by the kidneys.
Half-life: 10 hr.

TIME/ACTION PROFILE (improved symptoms of asthma)

ROUTE	ONSET	PEAK	DURATION
PO	unknown	1 wk	unknown

Contraindications/Precautions
Contraindicated in: Hypersensitivity; Lactation.
Use Cautiously in: Acute attacks of asthma; Patients >55 yr (increased risk of infection); Geriatric patients ≥65 yr or patients with hepatic impairment (may need lower doses); Pregnancy or children <7 yr (safety not established).

Adverse Reactions/Side Effects
CNS: headache, dizziness, weakness. **GI:** abdominal pain, diarrhea, drug-induced hepatitis (females), dyspepsia, nausea, vomiting. **MS:** arthralgia, back pain, myalgia. **Misc:** CHURG-STRAUSS SYNDROME, fever, infection (geriatric patients), pain.

Interactions
Drug-Drug: Blood levels are increased by **aspirin**. Blood levels are decreased by **erythromycin** and **theophylline**. Increases effects and risk of bleeding with **warfarin**.
Drug-Food: Food (especially high-fat or high-protein meal) decreases absorption.

Route/Dosage
PO (Adults and Children ≥12 yr): 20 mg twice daily.
PO (Children 7–11 yr): 10 mg twice daily.

Availability
Tablets: 10 mg, 20 mg.

NURSING IMPLICATIONS

Assessment
- Assess lung sounds and respiratory function before and periodically throughout therapy.
- ***Lab Test Considerations:*** Monitor liver function periodically during therapy. May cause elevated ALT concentrations. If liver dysfunction occurs, zafirlukast should be discontinued.

Potential Nursing Diagnoses
Ineffective airway clearance (Indications)
Deficient knowledge, related to medication regimen (Patient/Family Teaching)

Implementation
- **PO:** Administer at regular intervals on an empty stomach, 1 hr before or 2 hr after meals.

Patient/Family Teaching
- Instruct patient to take medication on an empty stomach as directed, at evenly spaced intervals, even if not experiencing symptoms of asthma. If a dose is missed, take as soon as remembered unless almost time for next dose. Do not double doses. Do not discontinue therapy without consulting health care professional.
- Instruct patient not to discontinue or reduce other asthma medications without consulting health care professional.
- Advise patient that zafirlukast is not used to treat acute asthma attacks but may be continued during an acute exacerbation.

Z

- Advise patient to notify health care professional if symptoms of Churg-Strauss syndrome (generalized flu-like syndrome, fever, muscle aches and pain, weight loss, worsening respiratory symptoms) occur. Occurs rarely but may be life-threatening. More likely to occur when weaning from systemic corticosteroids.

Evaluation/Desired Outcomes

- Prevention of and reduction in symptoms of asthma.

zaleplon (za-lep-lon)

Sonata

Classification
Therapeutic: sedative/hypnotics

Schedule IV

Pregnancy Category C

Indications

Short-term management of insomnia in patients unable to get at least 4 hours of sleep; especially useful in sleep initiation disorders.

Action

Produces CNS depression by binding to GABA receptors in the CNS. Has no analgesic properties. **Therapeutic Effects:** Sedation and induction of sleep.

Pharmacokinetics

Absorption: Rapidly absorbed following oral administration.
Distribution: Enters breast milk.
Metabolism and Excretion: Extensively metabolized in the liver (mostly by aldehyde oxidase and some by CYP450 3A4 enzymes).
Half-life: Unknown.

TIME/ACTION PROFILE

ROUTE	ONSET	PEAK	DURATION
PO	within minutes	unknown	3–4 hr

Contraindications/Precautions

Contraindicated in: Hypersensitivity;OB: Not recommended for use during pregnancy, lactation, or in patients with severe hepatic impairment.
Use Cautiously in: Mild to moderate hepatic impairment, age ≥65 yr or weight ≤50 kg or concurrent cimetidine therapy (initiate therapy at lowest dose); Impaired respiratory function; History of suicide attempt;Pedi: Children <18 yr (safety not established).

Adverse Reactions/Side Effects

CNS: abnormal thinking, amnesia, anxiety, behavior changes, depersonalization, dizziness, drowsiness, hallucinations, headache, impaired memory (briefly following dose), impaired psychomotor function (briefly following dose), malaise, sleep—driving, vertigo, weakness. **EENT:** abnormal vision, ear pain, epistaxis, hearing sensitivity, ocular pain, altered sense of smell. **CV:** peripheral edema. **GI:** abdominal pain, anorexia, colitis, dyspepsia, nausea. **GU:** dysmenorrhea. **Derm:** photosensitivity. **Neuro:** hyperesthesia, paresthesia, tremor. **Misc:** fever.

Interactions

Drug-Drug: Cimetidine ↓ metabolism and ↑ effects (initiate therapy at a lower dose). Additive CNS depression with other **CNS depressants** including **alcohol**, **antihistamines**, **opioid analgesics**, other **sedative/hypnotics**, **phenothiazines**, and **tricyclic antidepressants**. Effects may be ↓ by drugs that induce the CYP 450 3A4 enzyme system including **rifampin**, **phenytoin**, **carbamazepine**, and **phenobarbital**.
Drug-Natural Products: Concomitant use of **kava kava**, **valerian**, **chamomile**, or **hops** can ↑ CNS depression.
Drug-Food: Concurrent ingestion of a **high-fat meal** slows the rate of absorption.

Route/Dosage

PO (Adults <65 yr): 10 mg (range 5–20 mg) at bedtime.
PO (Geriatric Patients or Patients <50 kg): Initiate therapy at 5 mg at bedtime (not to exceed 10 mg at bedtime).

Hepatic Impairment

PO (Adults): Initiate therapy at 5 mg at bedtime (not to exceed 10 mg at bedtime).

Availability

Capsules: 5 mg, 10 mg. **Cost:** 5 mg $106.99/30, 10 mg $103.99/90.

NURSING IMPLICATIONS

Assessment

- Assess mental status, sleep patterns, and potential for abuse prior to administering this medication. Prolonged use of >7–10 days may lead to physical and psychological dependence. Limit amount of drug available to the patient.

- Assess alertness at time of peak effect. Notify health care professional if desired sedation does not occur.
- Assess patient for pain. Medicate as needed. Untreated pain decreases sedative effects.

Potential Nursing Diagnoses

Insomnia (Indications)
Risk for injury (Side Effects)

Implementation

- Before administering, reduce external stimuli and provide comfort measures to increase effectiveness of medication.
- Protect patient from injury. Supervise ambulation and transfer of patients after administration. Remove cigarettes. Side rails should be raised and call bell within reach at all times.
- **PO:** Tablets should be swallowed whole with full glass of water immediately before bedtime or after going to bed and experiencing difficulty falling asleep. Do not administer with or immediately after a high-fat or heavy meal.

Patient/Family Teaching

- Instruct patient to take zaleplon as directed. Do not take more than the amount prescribed because of the habit-forming potential. Not recommended for use longer than 7–10 days. Rebound insomnia (1–2 nights) may occur when stopped. If used for 2 wk or longer, abrupt withdrawal may result in dysphoria, insomnia, abdominal or muscle cramps, vomiting, sweating, tremors, and seizures.
- Because of rapid onset, advise patient to go to bed immediately after taking zaleplon.
- May cause daytime drowsiness or dizziness. Advise patient to avoid driving or other activities requiring alertness until response to this medication is known.
- Inform patient that amnesia may occur, but can be avoided if zaleplon is only taken when patient is able to get >4 hr sleep.
- Caution patient to avoid concurrent use of alcohol or other CNS depressants.

Evaluation/Desired Outcomes

- Relief of insomnia.

zanamivir (za-**na**-mi-veer)

Relenza

Classification
Therapeutic: antivirals
Pharmacologic: neuramidase inhibitors

Pregnancy Category C

Indications

Treatment of uncomplicated acute illness caused by influenza virus in adults and children ≥7 yr who have been symptomatic no more than 2 days.

Action

Inhibits the enzyme neuramidase, which may alter virus particle aggregation and release. **Therapeutic Effects:** Reduced duration of flu-related symptoms.

Pharmacokinetics

Absorption: 4–17% of inhaled dose is systemically absorbed.
Distribution: Unknown.
Protein Binding: <10%.
Metabolism and Excretion: Mainly excreted by kidneys as unchanged drug; unabsorbed drug is excreted in feces.
Half-life: 2.5–5.1 hr.

TIME/ACTION PROFILE (blood levels)

ROUTE	ONSET	PEAK	DURATION
inhalation	rapid	1–2 hr	12 hr

Contraindications/Precautions

Contraindicated in: Hypersensitivity.
Use Cautiously in: Chronic obstructive pulmonary disease or asthma (increased risk of decreased lung function and/or bronchospasm); Pregnancy, lactation, or children <12 yr (safety not established).

Adverse Reactions/Side Effects

Resp: bronchospasm.

Interactions

Drug-Drug: None noted.

Route/Dosage

Inhaln (Adults and Children ≥7 yr): 2 inhalations of 5 mg each for a total dose of 10 mg twice daily for 5 days via the DISKHALER inhalation device.

Availability

Powder for inhalation: 5 mg/blister.

Z

NURSING IMPLICATIONS

Assessment

- Assess patient for signs and symptoms of influenza (fever, headache, myalgia, cough, sore throat) before administration. Determine duration of symptoms. Indicated for patients who have been symptomatic for up to 2 days.

Potential Nursing Diagnoses

Risk for infection (Indications)

Implementation

Inhaln: Administer 2 doses on the first day of treatment whenever possible; must have at least 2 hours between doses. Doses should be administered 12 hr apart on subsequent days.

Patient/Family Teaching

- Instruct patient to use zanamivir exactly as directed and to finish entire 5-day course, even if feeling better.
- Instruct patient in the use of the DISKHALER. Patient should read the accompanying Patient Instructions for Use.
- Advise patients that zanamivir is not a substitute for a flu shot. Patients should receive annual flu shot according to immunization guidelines.
- Patients with a history of asthma should be advised to have a fast-acting inhaled bronchodilator available in case of bronchospasm following zanamivir administration. If using bronchodilator and zanamivir concurrently, administer bronchodilator first.

Evaluation/Desired Outcomes

- Decrease in signs and symptoms of influenza (fever, headache, myalgia, cough, sore throat).

ziconotide (zi-**ko**-no-tide)

Prialt

Classification

Therapeutic: analgesics

Pharmacologic: n-type calcium channel blockers

Pregnancy Category C

Indications

Management of severe chronic pain when conventional therapies (analgesics or other adjunctive measures) have failed.

Action

Blocks spinal N-channel calcium channels, decreasing transmission of pain signals to the brain. Has no effect on opioid receptors. **Therapeutic Effects:** Decrease in severe pain.

Pharmacokinetics

Absorption: IT administration results in complete bioavailability in the CSF. Minimal plasma distribution.

Distribution: Distributes in entire CSF volume.

Metabolism and Excretion: Degraded by enzymes in tissues and fluids.

Half-life: 4.6 hr (in CSF).

TIME/ACTION PROFILE

ROUTE	ONSET	PEAK	DURATION
IT	rapid	2–3 days	unknown

Contraindications/Precautions

Contraindicated in: Hypersensitivity; History of psychosis; Infection at microinfusion injection site; Uncontrolled bleeding; Spinal cord obstruction; Lactation.

Use Cautiously in: History of suicidal ideation/psychiatric disorder; Geriatric patients (↑ susceptibility to adverse CNS effects); Children (safety not established); Pregnancy (use only if maternal benefit outweighs fetal risk).

Adverse Reactions/Side Effects

CNS: MENINGITIS, confusion, dizziness, drowsiness, headache, impaired memory, weakness, aphasaia, ↓ alertness/responsiveness, cognitive impairment, hallucinations, memory impairment, psychiatric symptoms, speech disorder. **CV:** changes in blood pressure. **EENT:** nystagmus, abnormal vision. **GI:** nausea, anorexia, vomiting. **Local:** catheter/injection site reactions. **MS:** hypertonia, urinary retention, ↑ creatine kinase. **Neuro:** abnormal gait, ataxia. **Misc:** fever.

Interactions

Drug-Drug: ↑ risk of CNS depression with other **CNS depressants** including **anticonvulsants**, **phenothiazines**, **antipsychotics**, **antihistamines**, **opioids**, **sedatives**, or **diuretics**.

Route/Dosage

IT (Adults): up to 2.4 mcg/day initially (0.1 mcg/hr), may be gradually increased 2–3 times/week in increments of 2.4 mcg/day up to a maximum of 19.2 mcg/day (0.8 mcg/hr) over 21 days.

Availability
Solution for intrathecal use: 25 mcg/ml in 20-ml vials, 100 mcg/ml in 1-, 2- or 5-ml vials.

NURSING IMPLICATIONS

Assessment
- Assess level of pain prior to and periodically during therapy.
- Assess mental status during therapy. If psychiatric symptoms (cognitive impairment, hallucinations, changes in mood or level of consciousness) or neurological impairment. Discontinuation of therapy may be required, but other causes should be considered. Ziconotide may be discontinued abruptly without withdrawal symptoms.
- Monitor for signs of meningitis (fever, headache, stiff neck, altered mental status, nausea, vomiting, seizures) frequently during therapy. May occur within 24 hr of breach in sterility. If meningitis occurs, obtain CSF cultures and institute antibiotic therapy. Usually requires removal of microinfusion system, catheter, and any other foreign body within the IT space.
- ***Lab Test Considerations:*** Monitor serum CK levels every other week for the first month, monthly thereafter, and if neuromuscular symptoms (myalgias, myasthenia, muscle cramps, asthenia, reduction in physical activity) occur. May cause ↑ CK levels. If symptoms continue and CK remains ↑ or continues to rise, dose reduction or discontinuation may be required.

Potential Nursing Diagnoses
Chronic pain (Indications)

Implementation
- Ziconotide is not an opioid and cannot prevent or relieve symptoms of opioid withdrawal. Do not discontinue opioids abruptly. For withdrawal from IT opioid, gradually taper opioid IT infusion over several weeks, and replace with an equianalgesic dose of oral opioids. Ziconotide does not potentiate opioid-induced respiratory depression.
- Ziconotide should be administered under the direction of a physician experienced in IT therapy. Do not administer IV. **IT:** IT dose is delivered using a programmable implanted variable-rate microinfusion device or an external microinfusion device and catheter. Ziconotide may be administered undiluted (25 mcg/mL in 20-mL vial) or diluted (100 mg/mL in 1-, 2-, or 5-mL vials). Dilute with 0.9% NaCl (preservative—free) using aseptic technique. 100 mg/mL formulation may be administered undiluted once an appropriate dose is established. Refrigerate, but do not freeze, after preparation; administer within 24 hrs. Discard solution if discolored or containing particulate matter or any unused portion in vial. Pump refills should be done every 40 days if diluted solution is used or every 60 days if solution is undiluted. Pump should be rinsed and filled according to manufacturer's directions. ***Rate:*** Dose should be adjusted according to patient's severity of pain, response to therapy, and occurrence of side effects.

Patient/Family Teaching
- Instruct patient on correct technique for care of equipment.
- May cause dizziness and drowsiness. Caution patient to avoid driving and other activities requiring alertness until response to ziconotide is known.
- Advise patient to avoid taking alcohol and other CNS depressants during ziconotide therapy. Consult health care professional prior to taking Rx, OTC, or herbal products during therapy.
- Instruct patient and caregiver to contact health care professional immediately if changes in mental status (lethargy, confusion, disorientation, decreased alertness), changes in mood or perception (hallucinations, including unusual tactile sensations in oral cavity), symptoms of depression or suicidal ideation, or nausea, vomiting, seizures, fever, headache, or still neck occur; may be symptoms of developing meningitis.
- Advise patient to consult health care professional if new or worsening muscle pain, soreness, or weakness with or without darkened urine occur.

Evaluation/Desired Outcomes
- Decrease in pain intensity.

zidovudine
(zye-**doe**-vue-deen)
✤Apo-Zidovudine, azidothymidine, AZT, ✤Novo-AZT, Retrovir

Z

Classification
Therapeutic: antiretrovirals
Pharmacologic: nucleoside reverse transcriptase inhibitors

Pregnancy Category C

Indications
HIV infection (with other antiretrovirals). Reduction of maternal/fetal transmission of HIV.

Action
Following intracellular conversion to its active form, inhibits viral RNA synthesis by inhibiting the enzyme DNA polymerase (reverse transcriptase). Prevents viral replication. **Therapeutic Effects:** Virustatic action against selected retroviruses. Slowed progression and decreased sequelae of HIV infection. Decreased viral load and improved CD4 cell counts. Decreased transmission of HIV to infants born to HIV-infected mothers.

Pharmacokinetics
Absorption: Well absorbed following oral administration.
Distribution: Widely distributed; enters the CNS. Crosses the placenta.
Metabolism and Excretion: Mostly (75%) metabolized by the liver; 15–20% excreted unchanged by the kidneys.
Half-life: 1 hr.

TIME/ACTION PROFILE (blood levels)

ROUTE	ONSET	PEAK	DURATION
PO	unknown	0.5–1.5 hr	4 hr
IV	rapid	end of infusion	4 hr

Contraindications/Precautions
Contraindicated in: Hypersensitivity; Lactation.
Use Cautiously in: Decreased bone marrow reserve (dosage reduction required for anemia or granulocytopenia); Severe hepatic or renal disease (dose modification may be required).

Adverse Reactions/Side Effects
CNS: SEIZURES, headache, weakness, anxiety, confusion, decreased mental acuity, dizziness, insomnia, mental depression, restlessness, syncope. **GI:** abdominal pain, diarrhea, nausea, anorexia, drug-induced hepatitis, dyspepsia, oral mucosa pigmentation, vomiting. **Derm:** nail pigmentation. **Endo:** gynecomastia. **Hemat:** anemia, granulocytopenia, pure red-cell aplasia, thrombocytosis. **MS:** back pain, myopathy. **Neuro:** tremor.

Interactions
Drug-Drug: ↑ bone marrow depression with other **agents having bone marrow–depressing properties**, **antineoplastics**, **radiation therapy**, or **ganciclovir**. ↑ neurotoxicity may occur with **acyclovir**. Toxicity may be ↑ by concurrent administration of **probenecid** or **fluconazole**. Zidovudine levels are ↓ by **clarithromycin**.

Route/Dosage
Management of HIV Infection
PO (Adults and Children >13 yr): 100 mg q 4 hr while awake or 200 mg 3 times daily or 300 mg twice daily (depends on combination and clinical situation).
PO (Children 3 mo–12 yr): 90–180 mg/m^2 every 6 hr (not to exceed 200 mg q 6 hr).
IV (Adults and Children >12 yr): 1 mg/kg infused over 1 hr q 4 hr. Change to oral therapy as soon as possible.
IV (Children): 120 mg/m^2 q 6 hr (not to exceed 160 mg/dose).

Prevention of Maternal/Fetal Transmission of HIV Infection
PO (Adults >14 wk Pregnant): 100 mg 5 times daily until onset of labor.
IV (Adults during Labor and Delivery): 2 mg/kg over 1 hr, then continuous infusion of 1 mg/kg/hr until umbilical cord is clamped.
IV (Infants): 1.5 mg/kg q 6 hr until able to take PO.
PO (Infants): 2 mg/kg q 6 hr, started within 12 hr of birth and continued for 6 wk.

Availability
Capsules: 100 mg, 300 mg. **Oral syrup:** 50 mg/5 ml. **Injection:** 200 mg/20 ml. ***In combination with:*** lamivudine (Combivir; see Appendix B).

NURSING IMPLICATIONS

Assessment
- Assess patient for change in severity of symptoms of HIV and for symptoms of opportunistic infections during therapy.
- ***Lab Test Considerations:*** Monitor viral load and CD4 counts prior to and periodically during therapy.
- Monitor CBC every 2 wk during the first 8 wk of therapy in patients with advanced HIV disease, and decrease to every 4 wk after the first

2 mo if zidovudine is well tolerated or monthly during the first 3 mo and every 3 mo thereafter unless indicated in patients who are asymptomatic or have early symptoms. Commonly causes granulocytopenia and anemia. Anemia may occur 2–4 wk after initiation of therapy. Anemia may respond to epoetin administration (see epoetin monograph). Granulocytopenia usually occurs after 6–8 wk of therapy. Consider dose reduction, discontinuation of therapy, or blood transfusions if hemoglobin is <7.5 g/dl or reduction of >25% from baseline and/or granulocyte count is <750/mm^3 or reduction of >50% from baseline. Treatment with sargramostim may be necessary (see sargramostim monograph). Therapy may be gradually resumed when bone marrow recovery is evident.

Potential Nursing Diagnoses

Risk for infection (Indications, Side Effects)

Implementation

- Do not confuse Retrovir (zidovudine) with Ritonavir.
- Administer doses around the clock.
- **IV:** Patient should receive the IV infusion only until oral therapy can be administered.

IV Administration

- **Intermittent Infusion:** ***Diluent:*** Remove the calculated dose from the vial and dilute with D5W or 0.9% NaCl. Do not use solutions that are discolored. Stable for 8 hr at room temperature or 24 hr if refrigerated. ***Concentration:*** Not to exceed 4 mg/ml. ***Rate:*** Infuse at a constant rate over 1 hr. Avoid rapid infusion or bolus injection.
- **Continuous Infusion:** Has also been administered via continuous infusion.
- **Y-Site Compatibility:** acyclovir, allopurinol, amifostine, amikacin, amphotericin B, amphotericin B cholesteryl sulfate, aztreonam, cefepime, ceftazidine, ceftriaxone, cimetidine, cisatracurium, clindamycin, dexamethasone sodium phosphate, dobutamine, docetaxel, dopamine, doxorubicin liposome, erythromycin lactobionate, etoposide phosphate, filgrastim, fluconazole, fludarabine, gemcitabine, gentamicin, granisetron, heparin, imipenem/cilastatin, linezolid, lorazepam, melphalan, metoclopramide, morphine, ondansetron, oxytocin, paclitaxel, pemetrexed, pentamidine, phenylephrine, piperacillin/tazbactam, potassium chloride, ranitidine, remifentanil, sargramostim, teniposide, thiotepa, tobramycin, trimethoprim/sulfamethoxazole, trimetrexate, vancomycin, vinorelbine.
- **Y-Site Incompatibility:** lansoprazole.
- **Additive Incompatibility:** blood products or protein solutions.

Patient/Family Teaching

- Instruct patient to take zidovudine as directed, around the clock, even if sleep is interrupted. Emphasize the importance of compliance with therapy, not taking more than prescribed amount, and not discontinuing without consulting health care professional. Take missed doses as soon as remembered unless almost time for next dose; do not double doses. Inform patient that long-term effects of zidovudine are unknown at this time.
- Instruct patient that zidovudine should not be shared with others.
- Zidovudine may cause dizziness or fainting. Caution patient to avoid driving or other activities requiring alertness until response to medication is known.
- Inform patient that zidovudine does not cure HIV and does not reduce the risk of transmission of HIV to others through sexual contact or blood contamination. Caution patient to use a condom during sexual contact and avoid sharing needles or donating blood to prevent spreading the AIDS virus to others.
- Instruct patient to notify health care professional promptly if fever, sore throat, or signs of infection occur. Caution patient to avoid crowds and persons with known infections. Instruct patient to use soft toothbrush, to use caution when using toothpicks or dental floss, and to have dental work done prior to therapy or deferred until blood counts return to normal. Patient should also notify health care professional if shortness of breath, muscle aches, symptoms of hepatitis or pancreatitis, or other unexpected reactions occur.
- Advise patient to avoid taking any Rx or OTC medications or herbal products without consulting health care professional.
- Emphasize the importance of regular follow-up exams and blood counts to determine progress and monitor for side effects.

Z

Evaluation/Desired Outcomes
- Decrease in viral load and increase in CD4 counts in patients with HIV.
- Delayed progression of AIDS and decreased opportunistic infections in patients with HIV.

zinc sulfate (zink sul-fate)
Orazinc,✤ PMS Egozinc, Verazinc, Zinc 220, Zincate, Zinkaps

Classification
Therapeutic: mineral and electrolyte replacements/supplements
Pharmacologic: trace metals

Pregnancy Category C (parenteral)

Indications
Replacement and supplementation therapy in patients who are at risk for zinc deficiency, including patients on long-term parenteral nutrition. **Unlabeled uses:** Management of impaired wound healing due to zinc deficiency.

Action
Serves as a cofactor for many enzymatic reactions. Required for normal growth and tissue repair, wound healing, and senses of taste and smell. **Therapeutic Effects:** Replacement in deficiency states.

Pharmacokinetics
Absorption: Poorly absorbed from the GI tract (20–30%).
Distribution: Widely distributed. Concentrates in muscle, bone, skin, kidney, liver, pancreas, retina, prostate, RBCs, and WBCs.
Metabolism and Excretion: 90% excreted in feces, remainder lost in urine and sweat.
Half-life: Unknown.

TIME/ACTION PROFILE (blood levels)

ROUTE	ONSET	PEAK	DURATION
PO	unknown	2 hr	unknown
IV	unknown	unknown	unknown

Contraindications/Precautions
Contraindicated in: Hypersensitivity or allergy to any components in formulation; Pregnancy or lactation (supplemental amounts >RDA for pregnant or lactating patients); Preparations containing benzyl alcohol should not be used in neonates.
Use Cautiously in: Renal failure.

Adverse Reactions/Side Effects
GI: gastric irritation (oral use only), nausea, vomiting.

Interactions
Drug-Drug: Oral zinc may ↓ absorption of **tetracyclines** or **fluoroquinolones**.
Drug-Food: Caffeine, **dairy products**, and **bran** may ↓ absorption of orally administered zinc.

Route/Dosage
RDA = 15 mg. Doses expressed in mg of elemental zinc unless otherwise noted. Zinc sulfate contains 23% zinc.

Deficiency
PO (Adults): *Prevention of deficiency*—15–19 mg/day; *treatment of deficiency*—must be individualized; based on degree of deficiency.

IV Nutritional Supplementation—Metabolically Stable Patients
IV (Adults): 2.5–4 mg/day; up to 12 mg/day in patients with excessive losses.
IV (Infants and Children ≤5 yr): 100 mcg/kg/day.
IV (Infants up to 3 kg): 300 mcg/kg/day.

Availability (generic available)
Tablets: 66 mg^{OTC}, 110 mg^{OTC}. **Capsules:** 220 mg^{OTC}. **Injection:** 1 mg/ml in 10- and 30-ml vials, 5 mg/ml in 5- and 10-ml vials.

NURSING IMPLICATIONS

Assessment
- Monitor progression of zinc deficiency symptoms (impaired wound healing, growth retardation, decreased sense of taste, decreased sense of smell) during therapy.
- ***Lab Test Considerations:*** Serum zinc levels may not accurately reflect zinc deficiency.
- Long-term high-dose zinc therapy may cause ↓ serum copper concentrations.
- Monitor serum alkaline phosphatase concentrations monthly; may ↑ with zinc therapy.
- Monitor HDL concentrations monthly in patients on long-term high-dose zinc therapy. Serum concentrations may be ↓.

Potential Nursing Diagnoses
Imbalanced nutrition: less than body requirements (Indications)

Implementation
- **PO:** Administer oral doses with food to decrease gastric irritation. Administration with

caffeine, dairy products, or bran may impair absorption.
- **IV:** Zinc is often included as a trace mineral in total parenteral nutrition solution prepared by pharmacist.

Patient/Family Teaching
- Encourage patient to comply with diet recommendations of health care professional. Explain that the best source of vitamins is a well-balanced diet with foods from the four basic food groups. Foods high in zinc include seafood, organ meats, and wheat germ.
- Patients self-medicating with vitamin supplements should be cautioned not to exceed RDA. The effectiveness of megadoses for treatment of various medical conditions is unproved and may cause side effects.
- Instruct patients receiving oral zinc to notify health care professional if severe nausea or vomiting, abdominal pain, or tarry stools occur.
- Emphasize the importance of follow-up exams to evaluate progress.

Evaluation/Desired Outcomes
- Improved wound healing.
- Improved senses of taste or smell. 6–8 wk of therapy may be required before full effect is seen.

ziprasidone (zi-**pra**-si-done)
Geodon

Classification
Therapeutic: antipsychotics, mood stabilizers
Pharmacologic: piperazine derivatives

Pregnancy Category C

Indications
Schizophrenia; IM form is reserved for control of acutely agitated patients. Bipolar mania (manic and manic/mixed episodes).

Action
Effects probably mediated by antagonism of dopamine type 2 (D2) and serotonin type 2 ($5\text{-}HT_2$). Also antagonizes α_1 adrenergic receptors. **Therapeutic Effects:** Diminished schizophrenic behavior.

Pharmacokinetics
Absorption: 60% absorbed following oral administration; 100% absorbed from IM sites.
Distribution: Unknown.
Protein Binding: 99%; potential for drug interactions due to drug displacement is minimal.
Metabolism and Excretion: 99% metabolized by the liver; <1% excreted unchanged in urine.
Half-life: *PO*—7 hr; *IM*—2–5 hr.

TIME/ACTION PROFILE (blood levels)

ROUTE	ONSET	PEAK	DURATION
PO	within hours	1–3 days†	unknown
IM	rapid	60 min	unknown

†Steady state achieved following continuous use

Contraindications/Precautions
Contraindicated in: Hypersensitivity; History of QT prolongation (persistent QTc measurements >500 msec), arrhythmias, recent MI or uncompensated heart failure; Concurrent use of other drugs known to prolong the QT interval including quinidine, dofetilide, sotalol, other class Ia and III antiarrhythmics, pimozide, sotalol, thioridazine, chlorpromazine, floquine, pentamadine, arsenic trioxide, mefloquine, dolasetron, tacrolimus, droperidol, and moxifloxacin; Hypokalemia or hypomagnesemia; Lactation: Discontinue drug or bottle feed.
Use Cautiously in: Concurrent diuretic therapy or diarrhea (may increase the risk of hypotension, hypokalemia, or hypomagnesemia); Patients with significant hepatic impairment; History of cardiovascular or cerebrovascular disease; Hypotension, concurrent antihypertensive therapy, dehydration, or hypovolemia (may ↑ risk of orthostatic hypotension); OB: Use only if potential benefit outweighs potential risk to the fetus; Pedi: Safety not established; Geri: Alzheimer's dementia or age >65 yr (may ↑ risk of seizures). Geriatric patients (may require ↓ doses; inappropriate use for dementia is associated with ↑ mortality); Patients at risk for aspiration pneumonia; History of suicide attempt.

Adverse Reactions/Side Effects
CNS: NEUROLEPTIC MALIGNANT SYNDROME, seizures, <u>dizziness</u>, <u>drowsiness</u>, <u>restlessness</u>, extrapyramidal reactions, syncope, tardive dyskinesia. **Resp:** cough/runny nose. **CV:** PROLONGED QT INTERVAL, orthostatic hypotension. **GI:** <u>constipation</u>,

diarrhea, nausea, dysphagia. **Derm:** rash, urticaria.

Interactions

Drug-Drug: Concurrent use of **quinidine**, **dofetilide**, **other class Ia and III antiarrhythmics**, **pimozide**, **sotalol**, **thioridazine**, **chlorpromazine**, **floquine**, **pentamadine**, **arsenic trioxide**, **mefloquine**, **dolasetron**, **tacrolimus**, **droperidol**, **moxifloxacin**, or other agents that prolong the QT interval may result in potentially life-threatening adverse drug reactions and is contraindicated. Additive CNS depression may occur with **alcohol**, **antidepressants**, **antihistamines**, **opioid analgesics**, or **sedative/hypnotics**. Blood levels and effectiveness may be ↓ by **carbamazepine**. Blood levels and effects may be ↑ by **ketoconazole**.

Route/Dosage

PO (Adults): *Schizophrenia*—20 mg twice daily initially; dose increments may be made at 2-day intervals up to 80 mg twice daily; *Mania*—40 mg twice on first day, then 60 or 8 mg twice daily on second day, then 40–80 mg twice daily.

IM (Adults): 10–20 mg as needed up to 40 mg/day; may be given as 10 mg every 2 hr or 20 mg every 4 hr.

Availability

Capsules: 20 mg, 40 mg, 60 mg, 80 mg. **Cost:** 20 mg $974.88/180, 40 mg $975.96/180, 60 mg $1,172.00/180, 80 mg $1,172.00/180. **Lyophilized powder for injection (requires reconstitution):** 20 mg/vial.

NURSING IMPLICATIONS

Assessment

- Monitor patient's mental status (orientation, mood, behavior) prior to and periodically during therapy.
- Assess weight and BMI initially and throughout therapy.
- Monitor blood pressure (sitting, standing, lying) and pulse rate prior to and frequently during initial dose titration. Patients found to have persistent QTc measurements of >500 msec should have ziprasidone discontinued. Patients who experience dizziness, palpitations, or syncope may require further evaluation (i.e., Holter monitoring).
- Assess patient for rash during therapy. May be treated with antihistamines or corticosteroids. Usually resolves upon discontinuation of ziprasidone. Medication should be discontinued if no alternative etiology for rash is found.
- Observe patient carefully when administering medication to ensure medication is actually taken and not hoarded or cheeked.
- Monitor patient for onset of akathisia (restlessness or desire to keep moving) and extrapyramidal side effects (*parkinsonian*—difficulty speaking or swallowing, loss of balance control, pill rolling of hands, mask-like face, shuffling gait, rigidity, tremors and dystonic muscle spasms, twisting motions, twitching, inability to move eyes, weakness of arms or legs) every 2 month during therapy and 8–12 wk after therapy has been discontinued. Notify health care professional if these symptoms occur, as reduction in dose or discontinuation of medication may be necessary. Trihexyphenidyl or benztropine may be used to control these symptoms.
- Although not yet reported for ziprasidone, monitor for possible tardive dyskinesia (uncontrolled rhythmic movement of mouth, face, and extremities, lip smacking or puckering, puffing of cheeks, uncontrolled chewing, rapid or worm-like movements of tongue). Report these symptoms immediately; may be irreversible.
- Monitor frequency and consistency of bowel movements. Increasing bulk and fluids in the diet may help to minimize constipation.
- Ziprasidone lowers the seizure threshold. Institute seizure precautions for patients with history of seizure disorder.
- Monitor for development of neuroleptic malignant syndrome (fever, respiratory distress, tachycardia, seizures, diaphoresis, hypertension or hypotension, pallor, tiredness). Notify physician immediately if these symptoms occur.
- ***Lab Test Considerations:*** Monitor serum potassium and magnesium prior to and periodically during therapy. Patients with low potassium or magnesium should have levels treated and check prior to resuming therapy. Obtain fasting blood glucose and cholesterol levels initially and throughout therapy.

Potential Nursing Diagnoses

Risk for other-directed violence (Indications)
Disturbed thought process (Indications)
Imbalanced nutrition: risk for more than body requirements (Side Effects)

Implementation

- Dose adjustments should be made at intervals of no less than 2 days. Usually patients should be observed for several weeks before dose titration.
- Patients on parenteral therapy should be converted to oral doses as soon as possible.
- **PO:** Administer capsules with food or milk to decrease gastric irritation. Capsules should be swallowed whole; do not open.

Patient/Family Teaching

- Instruct patient to take medication as directed. Do not discontinue medication without discussing with health care professional, even if feeling well. Patients on long-term therapy may need to discontinue gradually.
- Inform patient of possibility of extrapyramidal symptoms. Instruct patient to report these symptoms immediately.
- Advise patient to change positions slowly to minimize orthostatic hypotension.
- May cause seizures and drowsiness. Caution patient to avoid driving or other activities requiring alertness until response to medication is known.
- Caution patient to avoid concurrent use of alcohol, other CNS depressants, OTC medications and herbal/alternative products without consulting health care professional.
- Advise patient to notify health care professional of medication regimen prior to treatment or surgery.
- Instruct patient to notify health care professional promptly if dizziness, loss of consciousness, or palpitations occur or if pregnancy is planned or suspected.
- Advise patient of need for continued medical follow-up for psychotherapy, eye exams, and laboratory tests.
- Refer as appropriate for nutritional or weight management.
- Refer to local support group.

Evaluation/Desired Outcomes

- Decrease in excited, manic behavior.
- Decrease in positive (delusions, hallucinations) and negative symptoms (social withdrawal, flat, blunted affect) of schizophrenia.

zoledronic acid
(zoe-led-**dron**-ic **as**-id)
Reclast, Zometa

Classification
Therapeutic: bone resorption inhibitors, electrolyte modifiers, hypocalcemics
Pharmacologic: biphosphonates

Pregnancy Category C

Indications

Hypercalcemia of malignancy. Multiple myeloma and metastatic bone lesions from solid tumors. Paget's disease.

Action

Inhibits bone resorption. Inhibits increased osteoclast activity and skeletal calcium release induced by tumors. **Therapeutic Effects:** Decreased serum calcium.

Pharmacokinetics

Absorption: IV administration results in complete bioavailability.
Distribution: Unknown.
Metabolism and Excretion: Mostly excreted unchanged by the kidneys.
Half-life: 167 hr.

TIME/ACTION PROFILE (effect on serum calcium)

ROUTE	ONSET	PEAK	DURATION
IV	within 4 days	4-7 days	30 days

Contraindications/Precautions

Contraindicated in: Hypersensitivity to zoledronic acid or other biphosphonates.
Use Cautiously in: Renal impairment (if serum creatinine ≥4.5 use only if potential benefits outweigh risks of further deterioration in renal function); History of aspirin-induced asthma; Concurrent use of loop diuretics or dehydration (correct deficits prior to use); Concurrent dental surgery (may ↑ risk of jaw osteonecrosis); OB, Pedi: Pregnancy, lactation, or children (safety not established).

Adverse Reactions/Side Effects

CNS: agitation, anxiety, confusion, insomnia. **EENT:** conjunctivitis. **CV:** hypotension, chest pain, leg edema. **GI:** abdominal pain, constipation, diarrhea, nausea, vomiting, dysphagia. **GU:** renal failure. **Derm:** pruritus, rash. **F and E:** hypophosphatemia, hypocalcemia, hypokalemia, hypomagnesemia. **Hemat:** anemia. **MS:** skeletal pain. **Misc:** jaw osteonecrosis, fever, flu-like syndrome.

Interactions

Drug-Drug: Concurrent use of **loop diuretics** or **aminoglycosides** ↑ risk of hypocalcemia.

Route/Dosage

IV (Adults): *Hypercalcemia of malignancy*—4 mg, may be repeated after 7 days; *multiple myeloma and bone metastases from solid tumors*—4 mg every 3–4 wk (has been used for up to 15 mo).

IV (Adults): *Paget's disease*—5 mg as a single dose once a year.

Availability

Powder for reconstitution for IV infusion: 4 mg/vial.

NURSING IMPLICATIONS

Assessment

- Monitor intake and output ratios. Initiate a vigorous saline hydration promptly and maintain a urine output of 2 L/day during therapy. Patients should be adequately hydrated, but avoid overhydration. Do not use diuretics prior to treatment of hypovolemia.
- **Hypercalcemia:** Monitor symptoms of hypercalcemia (nausea, vomiting, anorexia, weakness, constipation, thirst, cardiac arrhythmias).
- Observe for evidence of hypocalcemia (paresthesia, muscle twitching, laryngospasm, Chvostek's or Trousseau's sign).
- **Paget's Disease:** Assess for symptoms of Paget's disease (bone pain, headache, decreased visual and auditory acuity, increased skull size) periodically during therapy.
- Assess for acute-phase reaction (fever, myalgia, flu-like symptoms, headache, arthralgia). Usually occur within 3 days of dose and resolve within 3 days of onset, but may take 7–14 days to resolve; incidence decreases with repeat dosing.
- ***Lab Test Considerations:*** Monitor serum creatinine prior to each treatment. Patients with a normal serum creatinine prior to treatment, who develop an increase of 0.5 mg/dL within 2 wks of next dose should have next dose withheld until serum creatinine is within 10% of baseline value. Patients with an abnormal serum creatinine prior to treatment who have an increase of 1.0 mg/dL within 2 wks of next dose should have next dose withheld until serum creatinine is within 10% of baseline value.
- Assess serum calcium, phosphate, and magnesium before and periodically during therapy. If hypocalcemia, hypophosphatemia, or hypomagnesemia occur, temporary supplementation may be required.
- Monitor CBC with differential and hemoglobin and hematocrit closely during therapy.
- *Paget's Disease:* Monitor serum alkaline phosphatase prior to and periodically during therapy to monitor effectiveness.

Potential Nursing Diagnoses

Risk for injury (Indications)

Implementation

- Vigorous saline hydration alone may be sufficient to treat mild, asymptomatic hypercalcemia. Adequate rehydration is required prior to administration.
- Patients on long term therapy should have 500 mg or oral calcium and a multivitamin with 400 units of Vitamin D each day.
- Patients treated for *Paget's disease* should receive 1500 mg elemental calcium and 800 IU of vitamin D daily, particularly during the 2 wks after dosing.
- Administration of acetaminophen or ibuprofen following administration may reduce the incidence of acute-phase reaction symptoms.

IV Administration

- **Intermittent Infusion:** ***Diluent:*** Reconstitute *Zometa* by adding 5 ml of sterile water for injection to each vial for a solution containing 4 mg of zoledronic acid. Medication must be completely dissolved prior to withdrawal of solution. Dilute 4 mg dose further with 100 ml of 0.9% NaCl or D5W. If not used immediately, may be refrigerated for up to 24 hr. *Reclast* comes ready to use 5 mg in 100 mL solution. If refrigerated, allow soution to reach room temperature prior to administration. Do not administer solution that is discolored or contains particulate matter. ***Rate:*** Administer as a single infusion of not more than 4 mg and over at least 15 min. Rapid infusions increase risk of renal deterioration and renal failure.
- **Y-Site Incompatibility:** Do not mix with solutions containing calcium, such as Lactated Ringer's solution. Administer as a single infusion in a line separate from all other drugs.

Patient/Family Teaching

- Explain the purpose of zoledronic acid to patient. Advise patient to read medication guide prior to administration.

- Advise patients of the importance of adequate hydration. Patient should be instructed to drink at least two glasses of water prior to receiving dose.
- Advise patient to notify health care professional before taking any Rx, OTC, or herbal products with zoledronic acid.
- Caution patients to avoid dental surgery during treatment; recovery may be prolonged.
- Advise patient to notify health care professional if pregnancy is planned or suspected or if breastfeeding.
- Emphasize the importance of lab tests to monitor progress.

Evaluation/Desired Outcomes
- Decrease in serum calcium.
- Decrease in serum alkaline phosphatase and the progression of Paget's disease.

zolmitriptan (zole-mi-**trip**-tan)
Zomig, Zomig- ZMT

Classification
Therapeutic: vascular headache suppressants
Pharmacologic: 5-HT_1 agonists

Pregnancy Category C

Indications
Acute treatment of migraine headache.

Action
Acts as an agonist at specific 5-HT_1 receptor sites in intracranial blood vessels and sensory trigeminal nerves. **Therapeutic Effects:** Cranial vessel vasoconstriction with resultant decrease in migraine headache.

Pharmacokinetics
Absorption: Well absorbed (40%) following oral and intranasal administration.
Distribution: Unknown.
Metabolism and Excretion: Mostly metabolized by the liver; some conversion to metabolites that are more active than zolmitriptan. 8% excreted unchanged in urine.
Half-life: 3 hr (for zolmitriptan and active metabolite).

TIME/ACTION PROFILE (relief of headache)

ROUTE	ONSET	PEAK	DURATION
PO	unknown	1.5 hr*	unknown
intranasal	unknown	3 hr	unknown

* 3 hr for orally disintegrating tablets

Contraindications/Precautions
Contraindicated in: Hypersensitivity; Significant underlying heart disease (including ischemic heart disease, history of MI, coronary artery vasospasm, uncontrolled hypertension); Concurrent (or within 24 hr) use of other 5-HT agonists, ergotamine, or ergot-type medications; Concurrent (or within 2 wk) use of MAO inhibitors; Hemiplegic or basilar migraine; Symptomatic Wolff-Parkinson-White syndrome or other arrhythmias.
Use Cautiously in: Cardiovascular risk factors (hypertension, hypercholesterolemia, cigarette smoking, obesity, diabetes, strong family history, menopausal females or males >40 yr [use only if cardiovascular status has been evaluated and determined to be safe and first dose is administered under supervision]); Hepatic impairment (use lower doses); Pregnancy, lactation, or children (safety not established).

Adverse Reactions/Side Effects
CNS: dizziness, drowsiness, vertigo, weakness. **EENT:** throat pain/tightness/pressure. **CV:** chest pain/pressure/tightness/heaviness, hypertension, palpitations. **GI:** dry mouth, dyspepsia, dysphagia, nausea. **Derm:** sweating, warm/cold sensation. **MS:** myalgia, myasthenia. **Neuro:** hypesthesia, paresthesia. **Misc:** feeling of heaviness, pain.

Interactions
Drug-Drug: Because of increased risk of cerebral vasospasm, avoid concurrent use of other **5-HT agonists (naratriptan, sumatriptan, rizatriptan)** and/or **ergot-type preparations (dihydroergotamine)**. Concurrent use of **MAO inhibitors** ↑ blood levels and risk of toxicity (avoid use within 2 wk of MAO inhibitors). Blood levels may be ↑ by **hormonal contraceptives**. **Cimetidine** ↑ half-life of zolmitriptan and its active metabolite. Concurrent use with **SSRI antidepressants** may result in weakness, hyperreflexia and incoordination.
Drug-Natural Products: ↑ risk of serotinergic side effects including serotonin syndrome with **St. John's wort and SAMe.**

Z

Route/Dosage

PO (Adults): 2.5 mg or less initially; if headache returns, dose may be repeated after 2 hr (not to exceed 10 mg/24 hr).

Intranasal (Adults): single 5-mg dose; may be repeated after 2 hr (not to exceed 10 mg/24 hr).

Availability

Tablets: 2.5 mg, 5 mg. **Orally disintegrating tablets:** 2.5 mg, 5 mg. **Nasal spray:** 5 mg/100 mcL unit-dose spray device (package of 6).

NURSING IMPLICATIONS

Assessment

- Assess pain location, intensity, duration, and associated symptoms (photophobia, phonophobia, nausea, vomiting) during migraine attack.

Potential Nursing Diagnoses

Acute pain (Indications)

Implementation

- Do not confuse zolmitriptan with sumatriptan.
- **PO:** Initial dose is 2.5 mg. Lower doses can be achieved by breaking 2.5-mg tablet.
- Orally disintegrating tablets should be left in the package until use. Remove from the blister pouch. Do not push tablet through the blister; peel open the blister pack with dry hands and place tablet on tongue. Tablet will dissolve rapidly and be swallowed with saliva. No liquid is needed to take the orally disintegrating tablet. **Intranasal:** Remove cap from nasal spray. Hold upright and block one nostril. Tilt head slightly back, insert device into opposite nostril, and depress plunger. May repeat in 2 hr.

Patient/Family Teaching

- Inform patient that zolmitriptan should be used only during a migraine attack. It is meant to be used to relieve migraine attack but not to prevent or reduce the number of attacks.
- Instruct patient to administer zolmitriptan as soon as symptoms appear, but it may be administered any time during an attack. If migraine symptoms return, a second dose may be used. Allow at least 2 hr between doses, and do not use more than 10 mg in any 24-hr period.
- If dose does not relieve headache, additional zolmitriptan doses are not likely to be effective; notify health care professional.
- Advise patient that lying down in a darkened room following zolmitriptan administration may further help relieve headache.
- Caution patient not to use zolmitriptan if she is pregnant, suspects she is pregnant, plans to become pregnant, or is breastfeeding. Adequate contraception should be used during therapy.
- May cause dizziness or drowsiness. Caution patient to avoid driving or other activities requiring alertness until response to medication is known.
- Advise patient to notify health care professional prior to next dose of zolmitriptan if pain or tightness in the chest occurs during use. If pain is severe or does not subside, notify health care professional immediately. If wheezing; heart throbbing; swelling of eyelids, face, or lips; skin rash; skin lumps; or hives occur, notify health care professional immediately and do not take more zolmitriptan without approval of health care professional. If feelings of tingling, heat, flushing, heaviness, pressure, drowsiness, dizziness, tiredness, or sickness develop, discuss with health care professional at next visit.
- Advise patient to avoid alcohol, which aggravates headaches, during zolmitriptan use.

Evaluation/Desired Outcomes

- Relief of migraine attack.

zolpidem (zole-pi-dem)

Ambien, Ambien CR

Classification

Therapeutic: sedative/hypnotics

Schedule IV

Pregnancy Category B

Indications

Insomnia.

Action

Produces CNS depression by binding to GABA receptors. Has no analgesic properties. **Therapeutic Effects:** Sedation and induction of sleep.

Pharmacokinetics

Absorption: Rapidly absorbed following oral administration. Controlled release formulation

releases 10 mg immediately, then another 2.5 mg later.
Distribution: Minimal amounts enter breast milk; remainder of distribution not known.
Metabolism and Excretion: Converted to inactive metabolites, which are excreted by the kidneys.
Half-life: 2.5–2.6 hr (increased in geriatric patients and patients with hepatic impairment).

TIME/ACTION PROFILE (sedation)

ROUTE	ONSET	PEAK*	DURATION
PO	rapid	30 min–2 hr	6–8 hr
PO-ER	rapid	2–4 hr	6–8 hr

*Food delays peak levels and effects

Contraindications/Precautions
Contraindicated in: Hypersensitivity; Sleep apnea.
Use Cautiously in: History of previous psychiatric illness, suicide attempt, drug or alcohol abuse; Geri: Geriatric patients and patients with impaired hepatic function (initial dose reduction recommended); Patients with pulmonary disease; OB, Pedi: Pregnancy, lactation, or children (safety not established).

Adverse Reactions/Side Effects
CNS: abnormal thinking, amnesia, behavior changes, daytime drowsiness, dizziness, "drugged" feeling, hallucinations, sleep-driving. **GI:** diarrhea, nausea, vomiting. **Misc:** ANAPHYLACTIC REACTIONS, hypersensitivity reactions, physical dependence, psychological dependence, tolerance.

Interactions
Drug-Drug: ↑ CNS depression may with **sedative/hypnotics, alcohol, phenothiazines, tricyclic antidepressants, opioid analgesics**, or **antihistamines**.
Drug-Natural Products: Concomitant use of **kava kava, valerian or chamomile can ↑ CNS depression.**
Drug-Food: Food ↓ and delays absorption.

Route/Dosage
PO (Adults): *Tablets*—10 mg at bedtime; *extended-release tablets*—12.5 mg at bedtime.
PO (Geriatric Patients, Debilitated Patients, or Patients with Hepatic Impairment): *Tablets*—5 mg at bedtime initially, may be increased to 10 mg; *extended-release tablets*—6.25 mg at bedtime.

Availability (generic available)
Tablets: 5 mg, 10 mg. **Cost:** *Generic*—5 mg $15.99/30, 10 mg $17.99/30. **Extended-release tablets:** 6.25 mg, 12.5 mg. **Cost:** 6.25 mg $109.99/30, 12.5 mg $110.99/30.

NURSING IMPLICATIONS

Assessment
- Assess mental status, sleep patterns, and potential for abuse prior to administration. Prolonged use of >7–10 days may lead to physical and psychological dependence. Limit amount of drug available to the patient.
- Assess alertness at time of peak effect. Notify physician or other health care professional if desired sedation does not occur.
- Assess patient for pain. Medicate as needed. Untreated pain decreases sedative effects.

Potential Nursing Diagnoses
Insomnia (Indications)
Risk for injury (Side Effects)

Implementation
- Before administering, reduce external stimuli and provide comfort measures to increase effectiveness of medication.
- Protect patient from injury. Raise bed side rails. Assist with ambulation. Take patient's cigarettes.
- **PO:** Tablets should be swallowed whole with full glass of water. For faster onset of sleep, do not administer with or immediately after a meal.
- Swallow extended-release tablets whole; do not crush, break, or chew.

Patient/Family Teaching
- Instruct patient to take zolpidem as directed. Do not take more than the amount prescribed because of the habit-forming potential. Not recommended for use longer than 7–10 days. If used for 2 wk or longer, abrupt withdrawal may result in fatigue, nausea, flushing, lightheadedness, uncontrolled crying, vomiting, GI upset, panic attack, or nervousness.
- Because of rapid onset, advise patient to go to bed immediately after taking zolpidem.
- May cause daytime drowsiness or dizziness. Advise patient to avoid driving or other activities requiring alertness until response to this medication is known.

Z

- Caution patient to avoid concurrent use of alcohol or other CNS depressants.

Evaluation/Desired Outcomes

- Relief of insomnia.

zonisamide (zoe-**niss**-a-mide)
Zonegran

Classification
Therapeutic: anticonvulsants
Pharmacologic: sulfonamides

Pregnancy Category C

Indications

Partial seizures in adults.

Action

Raises the threshold for seizures and reduces duration of seizures probably by action on sodium and calcium channels. **Therapeutic Effects:** Decreased frequency of partial seizures.

Pharmacokinetics

Absorption: Well absorbed following oral administration.
Distribution: Binds extensively to red blood cells.
Metabolism and Excretion: Mostly metabolized by the liver; 35% excreted unchanged in urine. Some metabolism occurs via CYP3A4 enzyme system.
Half-life: 63 hr (plasma).

TIME/ACTION PROFILE (blood levels†)

ROUTE	ONSET	PEAK	DURATION
PO	unknown	2–6 hr	24 hr

†Requires 2 weeks of dosing to achieve steady-state blood levels

Contraindications/Precautions

Contraindicated in: Hypersensitivity to zonisamide or sulfonamides.
Use Cautiously in: Hepatic or renal disease (may require slower titration/more frequent monitoring); Pregnancy or lactation (use only if potential benefit justifies risk to fetus/infant); Children ≤16 yr (safety not established; increased risk of oligohydrosis/hyperthermia).

Adverse Reactions/Side Effects

CNS: drowsiness, fatigue, agitation/irritability, depression, dizziness, psychomotor slowing, psychosis, weakness. **EENT:** amblyopia, tinnitus. **Resp:** cough, pharyngitis. **GI:** anorexia, nausea, vomiting. **GU:** kidney stones. **Derm:** oligohydrosis (↑ in children), rash. **Metab:** hyperthermia (↑ in children). **Neuro:** abnormal gait, hyperasthesia, incoordination, tremor. **Misc:** ALLERGIC REACTIONS INCLUDING STEVENS-JOHNSON SYNDROME.

Interactions

Drug-Drug: Drugs that induce or inhibit CYP3A4 may alter blood levels and effects of zonisamide. Blood levels and effects may be ↓ by **phenytoin**, **carbamzepine**, **phenobarbital**, or **valproate**.

Route/Dosage

PO (Adults and Children >16 yr): 100 mg once daily initially for 2 wk, then increase to 200 mg daily for 2 wk; with subsequent increments of 100 mg made at 2-wk intervals as required (range 100–600 mg/day). Can be given as a single daily dose or in 2 divided doses.

Availability

Capsules: 25 mg, 50 mg, 100 mg.

NURSING IMPLICATIONS

Assessment

- Monitor frequency, duration, and characteristics of seizures.
- Monitor patient frequently for development of skin rash. Unexplained rash may require discontinuation of therapy.
- Assess patient for allergy to sulfa drugs.
- ***Lab Test Considerations:*** Monitor renal function periodically during therapy. May cause ↑ creatinine and BUN.
- May cause ↑ in serum alkaline phosphatase.

Potential Nursing Diagnoses

Risk for injury (Adverse Reactions)

Implementation

- **PO:** May be administered with or without meals. Capsules should be swallowed whole.

Patient/Family Teaching

- Instruct patient to take zonisamide as directed, even if feeling well. Consult health care professional if a dose is missed. Do not discontinue abruptly without consulting health care professional; may cause seizures.
- Instruct patient to contact health care professional immediately if skin rash occurs or seizures worsen. Patient should also contact health care professional if a child taking zonisamide is not sweating as usual, with or without a fever, or if they develop fever, sore throat, oral ulcers, easy bruising, depression,

unusual thoughts, speech or language problems.

- May cause drowsiness. Caution patient to avoid driving or other activities requiring alertness until cleared by physician and effects of medication is known.
- Advise patient to increase fluid intake to at least 6–8 glasses of water/day to minimize risk of kidney stones. Instruct patient to contact health care professional if symptoms of kidney stones (sudden back pain, abdominal pain, blood in urine) occur.
- Instruct patient to consult health care professional prior to taking other Rx, OTC, or herbal products.
- May have teratogenic effects. Advise women of childbearing age to use effective contraception throughout therapy. Instruct patient to notify health care professional if pregnancy is planned or suspected or if planning to breast feed.

Evaluation/Desired Outcomes

- Decrease in frequency and duration of partial seizures.

zoster vaccine, live

(zoe-**ster** vak-seen)
Zostavax

Classification
Therapeutic: vaccines/immunizing agents
Pharmacologic: active immunizer

Pregnancy Category C

Indications

Reduces the risk of shingles in patients ≥60 yr.

Action

Boosts immunity by actively immunizing against the varicella-zoster virus. **Therapeutic Effects:** Reduced risk of shingles and its sequelae.

Pharmacokinetics

Absorption: Well absorbed following subcut administration.
Distribution: Unknown.
Metabolism and Excretion: Unknown.
Half-life: Unknown.

TIME/ACTION PROFILE

ROUTE	ONSET	PEAK	DURATION
SC	unknown	unknown	unknown

Contraindications/Precautions

Contraindicated in: History of anaphylactic/anaphylactoid reactions to gelatin, neomycin, or other vaccine components; Primary/acquired immunodeficiency states (including leukemia, lymphoma, AIDS); Concurrent immunosupressive medications (including high dose corticosteroids); Acute febrile illness (>38.5° C or 101.3° F; Active untreated tuberculosis;OB: Pregnancy;Pedi: Children.
Use Cautiously in:OB: Child-bearing potential (pregnancy should be avoided for 3 months following vaccination);OB: Lactation.

Adverse Reactions/Side Effects

Local: swelling, redness, pain, swelling.

Interactions

Drug-Drug: Concurrent **immunosupressants** including **antineoplastics** and high dose **corticosteroids** may ↓ response to and ↑ risk of adverse reactions.

Route/Dosage

Subcut (Adults ≥60 yr): 0.65 mL (contents of 1 vial).

Availability

lyophylized powder for injection (with diluent): at least 19,400 PFU/0.65 ml.

NURSING IMPLICATIONS

Assessment

- Assess patient for immunosuppressant medications or reactions to previous vaccines. Administration may result in a more extensive vaccine-associated rash or disseminated disease in immunocompromised patients.

Potential Nursing Diagnoses

Risk for infection (Indications)

Implementation

- **Subcut:** Reconstitute using only diluent supplied. Use a separate sterile needle for reconstitution and administration. Vaccine is stored frozen; reconstitute immediately upon removing from freezer. Store diluent at room temperature. Withdraw entire contents of diluent into syringe and inject into vaccine vial.

Z

Agitate gently to mix. Solution should be semi-hazy to translucent, off-white to pale yellow. Do not administer solutions that are discolored or contain particulate matter. Administer only subcut, preferably in the upper arm. Have epinephrine injection available in case of anaphylactic reactions.

- Discard vaccine if not used within 30 min of reconstitution. Do not freeze reconstituted solution.

Patient/Family Teaching

- Explain purpose of vaccine to patient. Provide patient with a copy of the *Patient Information Sheet*.
- Advise patient to notify health care professional if pregnancy is planned or expected. Pregnancy should be avoided for 3 months after administration of vaccine.

Evaluation/Desired Outcomes

- Reduced risk of shingles and its sequelae.

Less Commonly Used Drugs

abarelix (a-ba-re-lix)
Plenaxis

Classification
Therapeutic: antineoplastics
Pharmacologic: GnRH antagonists

Pregnancy Category X

Indications
Advanced prostate cancer when LHRH agonists are inappropriate or surgical castration is refused and there is risk of neurologic compromise from metastatic disease, ureteral/bladder obstruction due to local/metastatic disease or severe metastatic bone pain unresponsive to adequate opioid analgesia.

Contraindications/Precautions
Contraindicated in: Hypersensitivity; Adult females or children.
Use Cautiously in: Patients with pre-existing QTc prolongation or concurrent use of Class IA antiarrhythmics (amiodarone, sotalol); Weight >225 pounds (decreased effectiveness over time).

Adverse Reactions/Side Effects
CNS: dizziness, fatigue, headache, sleep disturbances. **CV:** peripheral edema, prolonged QTc interval. **GI:** constipation, diarrhea, nausea, increased transaminases. **GU:** dysuria, urinary frequency. **Derm:** hot flushes. **Endo:** breast enlargement/nipple tenderness. **MS:** back pain. **Misc:** allergic reactions, decreased bone mineral density.

Route/Dosage
IM (Adults): 100 mg on Day 1, 15, and 29 and then every 4 wk thereafter.

acamprosate calcium
(a-cam-pro-sate)
Campral

Classification
Therapeutic: alcohol abuse therapy adjuncts
Pharmacologic: gamma aminobutyric acid (GABA) analogues

Pregnancy Category C

Indications
Maintenance of alcohol abstinence; part of a comprehensive alcohol abstinence program.

Contraindications/Precautions
Contraindicated in: Hypersensitivity; CCr 30 ml/min or less.
Use Cautiously in: CCr 30–50 ml/min (dose reduction necessary); History of depression or suicide attempt; OB: Use only if potential maternal benefit outweighs fetal risk; Lactation, Pedi: Safety not established.

Adverse Reactions/Side Effects
CNS: abnormal thinking, anxiety, depression, drowsiness, headache. **EENT:** abnormal vision. **Resp:** cough, dyspnea, pharyngitis, rhinitis. **CV:** palpitations, peripheral edema, syncope, vasodilation. **GI:** abdominal pain, anorexia, constipation, diarrhea, flatulence, ↑ appetite, nausea, taste perversion, vomiting. **GU:** ↓ libido, erectile dysfunction. **Derm:** rash. **Metab:** weight gain. **MS:** arthralgia, back pain, mylagia. **Neuro:** tremor.

Route/Dosage
PO (Adults): Two 333-mg tablets (666 mg/dose) three times daily. Lower doses may be effective in some patients
Renal Impairment
PO (Adults): *CCr 30–50 mL/min*—One 333-mg tablet three times daily.

activated charcoal

Acta-Char Liquid-A, Actidose-Aqua, ✤Aqueous Charcodote, ✤Charac-50, CharcoAid 2000, ✤Charcodote, Insta-Char, Insta-Char Aqueous Suspension, Liqui-Char, SuperChar Aqueous

Classification
Therapeutic: antidotes
Pharmacologic: adsorbents

Pregnancy Category C

Indications

Acute management of many oral poisonings following emesis/lavage.

Contraindications/Precautions

Contraindicated in: No known contraindications.
Use Cautiously in: Poisonings due to cyanide, corrosives, ethanol, methanol, petroleum distillates, organic solvents, mineral acids, or iron; Endoscopic examination (observation will be obscured).

Adverse Reactions/Side Effects

GI: black stools, constipation, diarrhea, vomiting.

Route/Dosage

Antidote
PO (Adults): 25–100 g (may be repeated q 4–6 hr).
PO (Children 1–12 yr): 25–50 g (may be repeated q 4–6 hr).
PO (Children <1 yr): 1 g/kg (may be repeated q 4–6 hr).

aldesleukin (al-dess-**loo**-kin)

interleukin-2, IL-2, Proleukin

Classification
Therapeutic: antineoplastics
Pharmacologic: interleukins

Pregnancy Category C

Indications

Management of metastatic renal cell carcinoma.

Contraindications/Precautions

Contraindicated in: Hypersensitivity to aldesleukin or mannitol; Cross-sensitivity to *Escherichia coli*—derived proteins may occur; Patients with any history of cardiac or pulmonary disease as assessed by abnormal thallium stress testing or abnormal pulmonary function testing; Patients who have experienced any of the following toxicities during previous courses of aldesleukin—sustained ventricular tachycardia (≤5 beats), angina pectoris or MI as indicated by ECG changes, respiratory problems requiring more than 72 hr of intubation, pericardial tamponade, renal toxicity requiring more than 72 hr of dialysis, CNS dysfunction consisting of more than 48 hr of coma or psychosis, intractable seizures, bowel perforation or ischemia, GI bleeding requiring surgical intervention; Patients who have had allograft organ transplantation (increased risk of rejection).
Use Cautiously in: Patients with a history of cardiovascular, respiratory, hepatic, or renal disease; Patients with a history of seizures or suspected CNS metastases (symptoms may be exaggerated and seizures may occur); Patients with child-bearing potential; OB, Lactation, Pedi: Safety not established.

Adverse Reactions/Side Effects

Resp: APNEA, RESPIRATORY FAILURE, dyspnea, pulmonary congestion, pulmonary edema, hemoptysis, pleural effusion, pneumothorax, tachypnea, wheezing. **CV:** CARDIAC ARREST, CHF, MI, STROKE, arrhythmias, hypotension, tachycardia, myocardial ischemia, pericardial effusion, thrombosis. **GI:** BOWEL PERFORATION, diarrhea, jaundice, nausea, stomatitis, vomiting, ascites, hepatomegaly. **GU:** oliguria/anuria, proteinuria, dysuria, hematuria, renal failure. **Derm:** EXFOLIATATIVE DERMATITIS, pruritus. **F and E:** acidosis, hypocalcemia, hypokalemia, hypomagnesemia, hypophosphatemia, alkalosis, hyperkalemia, hyperuricemia, hyponatremia. **Hemat:** anemia, coagulation disorders, leukopenia, thrombocytopenia, eosinophilia, leukocytosis. **Misc:** CAPILLARY LEAK SYNDROME, chills, fever, weight gain, weight loss.

Route/Dosage

IV (Adults): 600,000 IU/kg (0.037 mg/kg) every 8 hr for 14 doses. Cycle is repeated once after a 9-day rest period to a total of 28 doses. After a rest period of 7 wk, patients who have had a beneficial response may be evaluated for additional courses.

alitretinoin (a-li-tret-i-noyn)
Panretin

Classification
Therapeutic: antineoplastics
Pharmacologic: retinoids

Pregnancy Category D

Indications
Topical treatment of cutaneous lesions from AIDS-related Kaposi's sarcoma (KS).

Contraindications/Precautions
Contraindicated in: Hypersensitivity to retinoids; OB: Potential for birth defects; Lactation: Use breast milk alternative.
Use Cautiously in: Patients with childbearing potential; Pedi: Safety not established.

Adverse Reactions/Side Effects
Local: pain, pruritus, rash, edema, exfoliative, dermatitis, paresthesia.

Route/Dosage
Topical (Adults): Apply generous coating twice daily to KS lesions initially; application may be increased to 3–4 times daily.

altretamine (al-tret-a-meen)
Hexalen, hexamethylmelamine, ✤Hexastat

Classification
Therapeutic: antineoplastics

Pregnancy Category D

Indications
Management of ovarian cancer unresponsive to treatment with other agents.

Contraindications/Precautions
Contraindicated in: Hypersensitivity; OB, Lactation: Contraindicated due to risk to fetus/infant.
Use Cautiously in: Pre-existing neurologic diseases; Patients with childbearing potential; Infections; Decreased bone marrow reserve; Other chronic debilitating illnesses; Pedi: Safety not established.

Adverse Reactions/Side Effects
CNS: SEIZURES, fatigue. **GI:** nausea, vomiting, anorexia, hepatic toxicity. **GU:** gonadal suppression, renal toxicity. **Derm:** alopecia, pruritus, skin rash. **Endo:** gonadal suppression. **Hemat:** anemia, leukopenia, thrombocytopenia. **Neuro:** peripheral neuropathy.

Route/Dosage
PO (Adults): 65 mg/m^2 4 times daily (after meals and at bedtime) for 14 or 21 days of each 28-day cycle. Dosage reduction to 50 mg/m^2 4 times daily (after meals and at bedtime) recommended after 14 or more days' rest for any of the following: GI intolerance, severe bone marrow depression, or progressive neurologic toxicity.

aminolevulinic acid
(a-meen-o-lev-yoo-lin-ic a-sid)
Levulan Kerastick

Classification
Therapeutic: none assigned
Pharmacologic: photosensitizers

Pregnancy Category C

Indications
Treatment of nonhyperkeratotic actinic keratoses of the face and scalp in conjuction with blue light illumination using the BLU-U Blue Light Photodynamic Therapy Illuminator.

Contraindications/Precautions
Contraindicated in: Hypersensitivity; History of cutaneous photosensitization; Porphyria; Hypersensitivity to porphyrins; Pregnancy or lactation; Children.
Use Cautiously in: Other photodermatoses; Acquired or inherited coagulation defects; Concurrent wafarin therapy.

Adverse Reactions/Side Effects
Local: burning, edema, pruritus, stinging, oozing, scaling, ulceration.

Route/Dosage
Topical (Adults): One application via the Kerastick system (contains 354 mg of aminolevulinic acid), followed 14–18 hr later by blue light illumination.

✤ = Canadian drug name.
*CAPITALS indicates life-threatening; underlines indicate most frequent.

amoxapine (a-mox-a-peen)
Asendin

Classification
Therapeutic: antidepressants

Pregnancy Category C

Indications
Treatment of various types of depression. **Unlabeled uses:** Anxiety, insomnia, neuropathic and chronic pain syndromes.

Contraindications/Precautions
Contraindicated in: Angle-closure glaucoma; Recent MI; Prolongation of QTc interval; Cardiac arrhythmia; Heart failure.
Use Cautiously in: Pre-existing cardiovascular disease; Prostatic hyperplasia (increased susceptibility to urinary retention); History of seizures (threshold may be lowered); May ↑ risk of suicide attempt/ideation especially during dose early treatment or dose adjustment; OB: Use only if clearly needed and maternal benefits outweigh risk to fetus; Lactation: May result in sedation in infant; discontinue drug or bottle feed; Pedi: Suicide risk, especially at initiation of therapy, may be greater in children and adolescents; Geri: May be more susceptible to adverse effects; dosage reduction required.

Adverse Reactions/Side Effects
CNS: NEUROLEPTIC MALIGNANT SYNDROME, fatigue, sedation, extrapyramidal reactions, tardive dyskinesia. **EENT:** blurred vision, dry eyes, dry mouth. **CV:** ARRHYTHMIAS, hypotension, ECG changes. **GI:** constipation, increased appetite, weight gain, paralytic ileus. **GU:** testicular swelling, urinary retention. **Derm:** photosensitivity, rash. **Endo:** gynecomastia, sexual dysfunction. **Hemat:** blood dyscrasias. **Misc:** fever.

Route/Dosage
PO (Adults): 50 mg 2–3 times daily, increase to 100 mg 2–3 times daily by end of 1 week (not to exceed 300 mg daily in outpatients, 600 mg daily in divided doses in hospitalized patients). Once optimal dose is achieved, may be given as a single bedtime dose; no single dose to exceed 300 mg.
PO (Geriatric Patients): 25 mg 2–3 times daily, may be increased to 50 mg 2–3 times daily (not >300 mg/day).

arsenic trioxide
(ar-sen-ik trye-ox-ide)
Trisenox

Classification
Therapeutic: antineoplastics
Pharmacologic: heavy metals

Pregnancy Category D

Indications
Induction of remission and consolidation in patients with acute promyelocytic leukemia (APL) who do not respond to or tolerate retinoid and anthracycline chemotherapy and whose disease is associated with the presence of the t(15; 17) translocation or PML/RAR-alpha gene expression.

Contraindications/Precautions
Contraindicated in: Hypersensitivity to arsenic; OB: Can cause fetal injury; Lactation: Excreted in breast milk.
Use Cautiously in: Renal impairment
Exercise Extreme Caution in: Pre-existing electrolyte abnormalities (correct prior to administration); concurrent use of drugs known to prolong QT interval, concurrent use of potassium wasting diuretics or amphotericin
Exercise Extreme Caution in: Pedi: Safety not established in children <5 yr.

Adverse Reactions/Side Effects
CNS: fatigue, headache, insomnia, weakness. **Resp:** hypoxia, dyspnea, pleural effusion. **CV:** QT PROLONGATION, COMPLETE AV BLOCK, atrial arrhythmias. **GI:** abdominal pain, constipation, increase liver enzymes. **GU:** renal failure. **Derm:** dermatitis. **Endo:** hyperglycemia, hypoglycemia. **F and E:** acidosis, hypocalcemia, hyperkalemia, hypokalemia, hypomagnesemia. **Hemat:** NEUTROPENIA, APL DIFFERENTIATION SYNDROME, DISSEMINATED INTRAVASCULAR COAGULATION, THROMBOCYTOPENIA, hyperleukocytosis, anemia, leukocytosis. **MS:** back pain, arthralgia, bone pain, neck pain, limb pain, myalgia. **Misc:** allergic reactions, fever, infection/sepsis.

Route/Dosage
IV (Adults and Children ≤5 yr): *Induction*—0.15 mg/kg/day until bone marrow remission (not to exceed 60 doses); *consolidation*—starting 3–6 wks after completion of induction; 0.15 mg/kg/day for 25 doses over a period of 5 weeks.

ascorbic acid
(as-**kor**-bik**as**-id)
✤ Apo-C, Ascorbicap, Cebid, Cecon, Cecore-500, Cemill, Cenolate, Cetane, Cevalin, Cevi-Bid, Flavorcee, Mega-C/A Plus, Ortho/CS, Sunkist

Classification
Therapeutic: vitamins
Pharmacologic: water soluble vitamins

Pregnancy Category C

Indications
Treatment and prevention of vitamin C deficiency (scurvy) with dietary supplementation. Supplemental therapy in some GI diseases during long-term parenteral nutrition or chronic hemodialysis. States of increased requirements such as: Pregnancy, Lactation, Stress, Hyperthyroidism, Trauma, Burns, Infancy. **Unlabeled uses:** Prevention of the common cold.

Contraindications/Precautions
Contraindicated in: Tartrazine hypersensitivity (some products contain tartrazine—FDC yellow dye #5).
Use Cautiously in: Recurrent kidney stones; OB: Avoid chronic use of large doses in pregnant women.

Adverse Reactions/Side Effects
CNS: drowsiness, fatigue, headache, insomnia. **GI:** cramps, diarrhea, heartburn, nausea, vomiting. **GU:** kidney stones. **Derm:** flushing. **Hemat:** deep vein thrombosis, hemolysis (in G6PD deficiency), sickle cell crisis. **Local:** pain at subcut or IM sites.

Route/Dosage
PO (Adults): *Scurvy*—500 mg/day for at least 14 days. *Prevention of deficiency*—50–100 mg/day.
PO (Children): *Scurvy*—100–300 mg/day for at least 14 days. *Prevention of deficiency*—30–45 mg/day.
IM (Adults): *Scurvy*—100–500 mg/day for at least 14 days.
IM (Children): *Scurvy*—100–300 mg/day for at least 14 days.
IV (Adults and Children): *Prevention of deficiency*—determined by need.

becaplermin (be-**kap**-lerm-in)
Regranex

Classification
Therapeutic: wound/ulcer/decubiti healing agents
Pharmacologic: platelet-derived growth factors

Pregnancy Category C

Indications
Treatment of lower extremity diabetic neuropathic ulcers extending to subcut tissue or beyond and having adequate blood supply.

Contraindications/Precautions
Contraindicated in: Known hypersensitivity to becaplermin or parabens; Known neoplasm at site of application; Wounds that close by primary intention.
Use Cautiously in: OB, Lactation, Pedi: Safety not established.

Adverse Reactions/Side Effects
Derm: erythematous rash at application site.

Route/Dosage
Topical (Adults): Length of gel *in inches* from 15- or 7.5-g tube = length × width of ulcer area × 0.6; from the 2-g tube = length × width of ulcer area × 1.3. Length of gel *in centimeters* from 15- or 7.5-g tube = length × width of ulcer area ÷ 4; from the 2-g tube = length × width of ulcer area ÷ 2; for 12 hr each day.

bethanechol (be-**than**-e-kole)
Duvoid, Urabeth, Urecholine

Classification
Therapeutic: urinary tract stimulants
Pharmacologic: cholinergics

Pregnancy Category C

Indications
Postpartum and postoperative nonobstructive urinary retention or urinary retention caused by neurogenic bladder.

Contraindications/Precautions
Contraindicated in: Hypersensitivity; Mechanical obstruction of the GI or GU tract.
Use Cautiously in: History of asthma; Ulcer disease; Cardiovascular disease; Epilepsy; Hy-

LESS COMMONLY USED DRUGS

perthyroidism; Sensitivity to cholinergic agents or effects; OB, Lactation, Pedi: Safety not established.

Adverse Reactions/Side Effects

CNS: headache, malaise. **EENT:** lacrimation, miosis. **Resp:** bronchospasm. **CV:** HEART BLOCK, SYNCOPE/CARDIAC ARREST, bradycardia, hypotension. **GI:** abdominal discomfort, diarrhea, nausea, salivation, vomiting. **GU:** urgency. **Misc:** flushing, sweating, hypothermia.

Route/Dosage

PO (Adults): 25–50 mg 3 times daily. Dose may be determined by administering 5–10 mg q 1–2 hr until response is obtained or total of 50 mg administered *or* by starting with 10 mg, giving 25 mg 6 hr later, then, if needed, 50 mg 6 hr later.
PO (Children): 0.2 mg/kg 3 times daily or 0.15 mg/kg 4 times daily.
Subcut: (Adults): 5 mg 3–4 times daily. Dose may be determined by administering 2.5 mg q 15–30 min until response is obtained or total of 4 doses administered.
Subcut: (Children): 0.06 mg/kg 3 times daily or 0.05 mg/kg 4 times daily.

botulism immune globulin

(**bo**tyoo-lism im-**yoon glob**-yoo-lin)
BabyBIG

Classification
Therapeutic: vaccines/immunizing agents
Pharmacologic: immune globulins

Pregnancy Category UK

Indications

Infant botulism caused by type A or B toxin in children <1 yr.

Contraindications/Precautions

Contraindicated in: History of severe reactions to other immunoglobulins; Selective immunoglobulin A deficiency.
Use Cautiously in: Pre-existing renal impairment, diabetes mellitus, volume depletion, sepsis, paraproteinemia, concurrent nephrotoxic agents (↑ risk of adverse renal reactions; use lowest concentration and slowest infusion rate).

Adverse Reactions/Side Effects

Derm: rash. **Misc:** infusion reactions.

Route/Dosage

IV (Children <1 yr): 1 ml/kg (50 mg/kg) as a single infusion.

bromocriptine

(broe-moe-**krip**-teen)
✤Alti-Bromocriptine, ✤Apo-Bromocriptine, Parlodel

Classification
Therapeutic: antiparkinson agents
Pharmacologic: dopamine agonists

Pregnancy Category B

Indications

Adjunct to levodopa in the treatment of parkinsonism. Treatment of hyperprolactinemia (amenorrhea/galactorrhea), including associated female infertility. Treatment of acromegaly. **Unlabeled uses:** Management of pituitary prolactinomas. Management of neuroleptic malignant syndrome.

Contraindications/Precautions

Contraindicated in: Hypersensitivity to bromocriptine, ergot alkaloids, or bisulfites (capsules only); Severe cardiovascular disease or peripheral vascular disease; Lactation.
Use Cautiously in: Cardiac disease; Mental disturbances; May restore fertility (additional contraception may be required if pregnancy is undesirable); Severe liver impairment (dose reduction required); OB, Lactation, Pedi: Safety not established.

Adverse Reactions/Side Effects

CNS: dizziness, confusion, drowsiness, hallucinations, headache, insomnia, nightmares. **EENT:** burning eyes, nasal stuffiness, visual disturbances. **Resp:** effusions, pulmonary infiltrates. **CV:** MI, hypotension. **GI:** nausea, abdominal pain, anorexia, dry mouth, metallic taste, vomiting. **Derm:** urticaria. **MS:** leg cramps. **Misc:** digital vasospasm (acromegaly only).

Route/Dosage

Parkinsonism

PO (Adults): 1.25 mg 1–2 times daily, increased by 2.5 mg/day in 2–4 wk intervals (range is 2.5–100 mg/day in divided doses; up to 40 mg/day have been used).

Hyperprolactinemia

PO (Adults): 1.25–2.5 mg/day initially, may be gradually increased q 3–7 days up to 2.5 mg 2–3 times daily.

Acromegaly
PO (Adults): 1.25–2.5 mg/day for 3 days, increase by 1.25–2.5 mg q 3–7 days until optimal response is obtained (usual range 10–30 mg/day; up to 100 mg/day).

Pituitary Adenomas
PO (Adults): 1.25 mg 2–3 times daily, may be increased over several weeks (range 2.5–20 mg/day).

Neuroleptic Malignant Syndrome (Unlabeled)
PO (Adults): 5 mg once daily initially, dose increased as required up to 20 mg/day.

brompheniramine
(brome-fen-**ir**-a-meen)
Bromfenac, Dimetapp Allergy, Nasahist B, ✱Dimetane

Classification
Therapeutic: allergy, cold, and cough remedies, antihistamines

Pregnancy Category B

Indications
Symptomatic relief of allergic symptoms (rhinitis, urticaria) caused by histamine release. Severe allergic or hypersensitivity reactions, including anaphylaxis and transfusion reactions.

Contraindications/Precautions
Contraindicated in: Hypersensitivity; Acute attacks of asthma; Known alcohol intolerance (some elixirs); Lactation: Potential for adverse reaction in nursing infants.
Use Cautiously in: Angle-closure glaucoma; Liver disease; OB: Safety not established; Geri: More susceptible to adverse reactions; use lower initial dose.

Adverse Reactions/Side Effects
CNS: drowsiness, sedation, dizziness, excitation (in children). **EENT:** blurred vision. **CV:** hypertension, arrhythmias, hypotension, palpitations. **GI:** dry mouth, constipation, obstruction. **GU:** retention, urinary hesitancy. **Derm:** sweating. **Misc:** hypersensitivity reaction (IV use).

Route/Dosage
PO (Adults and Children ≤12 yr): 4 mg q 4–6 hr daily as needed (not to exceed 24 mg/day).
PO (Children 6–12 yr): 2 mg q 4–6 hr as needed (not to exceed 12 mg/day).
PO (Children 2–6 yr): 1 mg q 4–6 hr as needed (not to exceed 6 mg/day).
Subcut, IM, IV (Adults): 10 mg q 8–12 hr as needed (not to exceed 40 mg/day).
Subcut, IM, IV (Children): 125 mcg (0.125 mg)/kg or 3.75 mg/m² 3–4 times daily as needed.

carteolol (kar-tee-oh-lole)
Cartrol

Classification
Therapeutic: antianginals, antihypertensives
Pharmacologic: beta blockers

Pregnancy Category C

See Appendix C for ophthalmic use

Indications
Management of hypertension. **Unlabeled uses:** Management of angina pectoris.

Contraindications/Precautions
Contraindicated in: Uncompensated CHF; Pulmonary edema; Cardiogenic shock; Bradycardia or heart block.
Use Cautiously in: Renal impairment (increased dosing interval recommended); Hepatic impairment; Geriatric patients (increased sensitivity to beta blockers; initial dosage reduction recommended); Pulmonary disease (including asthma); avoid use if possible; Diabetes mellitus (may mask signs of hypoglycemia); Thyrotoxicosis (may mask symptoms); Patients with a history of severe allergic reactions (intensity of reactions may be increased); OB: Crosses placenta and may cause fetal/neonatal bradycardia, hypotension, hypoglycemia, or respiratory depression); Lactation, Pedi: Safety not established; Geri: Increased sensitivity to beta blockers; initial dosage reduction recommended.

Adverse Reactions/Side Effects
CNS: fatigue, weakness, anxiety, depression, dizziness, drowsiness, insomnia, memory loss, mental status changes, nightmares. **EENT:** blurred vision, dry eyes, nasal stuffiness. **Resp:** bronchospasm, wheezing. **CV:** BRADYCARDIA, CHF, PULMONARY EDEMA, orthostatic hypotension, pe-

✱ = Canadian drug name.
* CAPITALS indicates life-threatening; underlines indicate most frequent.

ripheral vasoconstriction. **GI:** constipation, diarrhea, nausea. **GU:** erectile dysfunction, decreased libido. **Derm:** itching, rashes. **Endo:** hyperglycemia, hypoglycemia. **MS:** arthralgia, back pain, muscle cramps. **Neuro:** paresthesia. **Misc:** drug-induced lupus syndrome.

Route/Dosage

PO (Adults): 2.5 mg once daily, may be increased up to 10 mg/day

Renal Impairment

PO (Adults): *CCr 20–60 ml/min*—increase dosing interval to q 48 hr; *CCr <20ml/min*—increase dosing interval to q 72 hr.

cevimeline (se-vim-e-leen)
Evoxac

Classification
Therapeutic: xerostomia therapy adjuncts
Pharmacologic: cholinergics, muscarinic agonists, sialagogues

Pregnancy Category UK

Indications

Treatment of the symptoms of dry mouth associated with Sjögren's syndrome.

Contraindications/Precautions

Contraindicated in: Hypersensitivity; When miosis is undesirable (acute iritis, angle-closure glaucoma); Lactation: Discontinue or bottle feed.

Use Cautiously in: Cardiovascular disease including angina pectoris or history of MI; Pulmonary disease including asthma, chronic bronchitis, or chronic obstructive pulmonary disease; Nephrolithiasis or cholelithiasis; Geri: May be more sensitive to toxicity; OB: Use only if potential benefit justifies potential risk to the fetus; Pedi: Safety not established.

Adverse Reactions/Side Effects

CNS: coughing. **EENT:** rhinitis, visual disturbances. **GI:** nausea, diarrhea, excessive salivation. **Derm:** excessive sweating, hot flashes.

Route/Dosage

PO (Adults): 30 mg three times daily.

chlorambucil
(klor-am-byoo-sill)
Leukeran

Classification
Therapeutic: antineoplastics, immunosuppressants
Pharmacologic: alkylating agents

Pregnancy Category D

Indications

Management of chronic lymphocytic leukemia, malignant lymphoma, and Hodgkin's disease (alone and in combination with other agents).

Contraindications/Precautions

Contraindicated in: Hypersensitivity; Previous resistance; OB, Lactation: Can cause fetal or neonatal harm; avoid becoming pregnant; do not breast feed.

Use Cautiously in: Infection; Other chronic debilitating diseases; Geri: More sensitive to effects.

Adverse Reactions/Side Effects

Resp: pulmonary fibrosis. **GI:** nausea, stomatitis (rare), vomiting. **GU:** decreased sperm count, sterility. **Derm:** alopecia (rare), dermatitis, rash. **Hemat:** LEUKOPENIA, anemia, thrombocytopenia. **Metab:** hyperuricemia. **Misc:** allergic reactions, risk of second malignancy.

Route/Dosage

PO (Adults): 0.1–0.2 mg/kg/day (3–6 mg/m^2/day) (usual range 4–10 mg/day as a single dose or in divided doses), then adjust dose on basis of blood counts; *or* 0.4 mg/kg (12 mg/m^2) twice weekly, increased by 0.1 mg/kg (3 mg/m^2) q 2 wk, then adjusted as necessary.

PO (Geriatric Patients): Initial dose should not be more than 2–4 mg/day.

PO (Children): 0.1–0.2 mg/kg/day (4.5 mg/m^2/day) single dose or in divided doses.

cinacalcet (sin-a-kal-set)
Sensipar

Classification
Therapeutic: hypocalcemics
Pharmacologic: calcimimetic agents

Pregnancy Category C

Indications

Secondary hyperparathyroidism in patients who are being hemodialyzed. Hypercalcemia caused by parathyroid carcinoma.

Contraindications/Precautions

Contraindicated in: Hypersensitivity; Serum calcium <8.4 mg/dL; Lactation: Discontinue drug or bottle feed.

Use Cautiously in: History of seizure disorder; Chronic kidney disease patients who are not being dialyzed (↑ risk of hypocalcemia); Parathyroid hormone level <150 pg/mL (dose reduction or discontinuation may be warranted); Moderate to severe hepatic impairment; OB: Use only if benefits justify risks to fetus; Pedi: Safety not established.

Adverse Reactions/Side Effects
GI: nausea, vomiting. **F and E:** hypocalcemia. **Metab:** adynamic bone disease.

Route/Dosage
PO (Adults): 30 mg twice daily, titrate every 2–4 wk up to 90 mg 3–4 times daily in response to serum calcium monitoring.

clofarabine (klo-**far**-a-been)
Clolar

Classification
Therapeutic: antineoplastics
Pharmacologic: antimetabolites

Pregnancy Category D

Indications
Refractory/relapsed acute lymphoblastic leukemia in children 1–21 yr.

Contraindications/Precautions
Contraindicated in: None; Pregnancy or lactation.
Use Cautiously in: Hepatic or renal impairment; Concurrent use of nephrotoxic or hepatotoxic drugs.

Adverse Reactions/Side Effects
CNS: fatigue. **Resp:** pharyngitis. **CV:** pericardial effusion, tachycardia, edema. **GI:** diarrhea, hepatic toxicity, nausea, abdominal pain, constipation, mucositis, vomiting. **F and E:** dehydration. **Hemat:** NEUTROPENIA, anemia, thrombocytopenia. **Local:** injection site pain. **Misc:** SYSTEMIC INFLAMMATORY RESPONSE SYNDROME, TUMOR LYSIS SYNDROME, infections, fever, chills.

Route/Dosage
IV (Children 1–21 yr): 52 mg/m^2 daily for 5 days; cycle may be repeated every 2–6 wk.

clomiPRAMINE
(kloe-**mip**-ra-meen)
Anafranil

Classification
Therapeutic: antiobsessive agents
Pharmacologic: tricyclic antidepressants

Pregnancy Category C

Indications
Obsessive-Compulsive Disorder (OCD). **Unlabeled uses:** Depression, neuropathic pain/chronic pain..

Contraindications/Precautions
Contraindicated in: Hypersensitivity; Angle-closure glaucoma; Recent myocardial infarction; History of QTc prolongation; Cardiac arrythmias; Heart failure; Concurrent MAO inhibitor or clonidine use (avoid if possible); OB: Potential for fetal harm or neonatal withdrawal syndrome; Lactation: Discontinue drug or bottle feed.
Use Cautiously in: History of seizures (threshold may be lowered); Patients with pre-existing cardiovascular disease; Older men with prostatic hyperplasia (may be more susceptible to urinary retention); Hyperthyroidism (increased risk of arrhythmias); May ↑ risk of suicide attempt/ideation especially during dose early treatment or dose adjustment; risk may be greater in children or adolescents; Pedi: Safety not established in children <10 yr; Geri: ↑ risk of arrhythmias.

Adverse Reactions/Side Effects
CNS: SEIZURES, lethargy, sedation, weakness, aggressive behavior. **EENT:** blurred vision, dry eyes, dry mouth, vestibular disorder. **CV:** ARRHYTHMIAS, ECG changes, orthostatic hypotension. **GI:** constipation, nausea, vomiting, weight gain, eructation. **GU:** male sexual dysfunction, urinary retention. **Derm:** dry skin, photosensitivity. **Endo:** gynecomastia. **Hemat:** anemia. **MS:** muscle weakness. **Neuro:** extrapyramidal reactions. **Misc:** hyperthermia.

Route/Dosage
PO (Adults): *Antiobsessive*—25 mg/day, increased over 2-wk period to 100 mg/day in divided doses. May be further increased over several weeks up to 250–300 mg/day in divided doses. Once stabilizing dose is reached, entire daily dose may be given at bedtime. *Antidepressant*—25 mg 3 times daily, may be increased as needed (unlabeled).

✤ = Canadian drug name.
*CAPITALS indicates life-threatening; underlines indicate most frequent.

LESS COMMONLY USED DRUGS

PO (Geriatric Patients): 20–30 mg/day initially, may be increased as needed.
PO (Children >10–17 yr): 25 mg/day initially, increased over 2-wk period to 3 mg/kg/day or 100 mg/day (whichever is smaller) in divided doses. May be further increased to 3 mg/kg/day or 200 mg/day (whichever is smaller) in divided doses. Once stabilizing dose is reached, entire daily dose may be given at bedtime.

cytomegalovirus immune globulin
(site-oh-**meg**-a-loe-vye-rus)
CMVIG, CytoGam

Classification
Therapeutic: vaccines/immunizing agents
Pharmacologic: immune globulins

Pregnancy Category C

Indications
Prevention of cytomegalovirus (CMV) disease associated with transplantation of kidney, lung, liver, pancreas, or heart (if transplant is other than kidney from CMV-positive donors to CMV-negative recipient, then concurrent ganciclovir should be considered).

Contraindications/Precautions
Contraindicated in: Hypersensitivity to immune globulins or albumin; Selective IgA deficiency.
Use Cautiously in: Pregnancy or lactation (safety not established); Renal insufficiency or predisposition to acute renal failure.

Adverse Reactions/Side Effects
CNS: headache, tremor, anxiety, seizures. **Hemat:** pancytopenia, hemolysis, leukopenia. **Resp:** wheezing, dyspnea, pulmonary edema. **CV:** hypotension, thromboembolism. **GI:** nausea, vomiting, hepatic dysfunction. **Derm:** flushing, rash. **GU:** oliguria, anuria, acute renal failure. **MS:** back pain, muscle cramps. **Misc:** allergic reactions including chills, fever, ANAPHYLAXIS.

Route/Dosage

Kidney Transplant
IV (Adults): 150 mg/kg within 72 hr of transplantation, followed by 100 mg/kg at 2, 4, 6, and 8 wk, then 50 mg/kg at 12 and 16 wk post-transplantation.

Liver, Pancreas, Lung, or Heart Transplant
IV (Adults): 150 mg/kg within 72 hr of transplantation, and at 2, 4, 6, and 8 wk, then 100 mg/kg after at 12 and 16 wk post-transplantation.
IV (Children): Safety and efficacy has not been established in pediatrics, however adult doses have been used in children.

danazol (**da**-na-zole)
✤Cyclomen, Danocrine

Classification
Therapeutic: hormones
Pharmacologic: androgens

Pregnancy Category X

Indications
Treatment of moderate endometriosis that is unresponsive to conventional therapy. Palliative therapy of fibrocystic breast disease. Prophylaxis of hereditary angioedema.

Contraindications/Precautions
Contraindicated in: Hypersensitivity; Male patients with breast or prostate cancer; Hypercalcemia; Severe hepatic, renal, or cardiac disease; Pregnancy or lactation.
Use Cautiously in: Previous history of liver disease; History of porphyria; Coronary artery disease; Prepubertal boys.

Adverse Reactions/Side Effects
CNS: emotional lability. **EENT:** deepening of voice. **CV:** edema. **GI:** hepatitis (cholestatic jaundice). **GU:** amenorrhea, clitoral enlargement, testicular atrophy. **Derm:** acne, hirsutism, oiliness. **Endo:** amenorrhea, anovulation, decreased breast size (women), decreased libido. **Metab:** weight gain.

Route/Dosage
PO (Adults and Adolescents): *Endometriosis*—400 mg twice daily (for milder cases may initiate therapy with 100–200 mg twice daily). *Fibrocystic breast disease*—50–200 mg twice daily. *Hereditary angioedema*—200 mg 2–3 times daily. Attempt to decrease dosage by 50% or less q 1–3 mo. If acute attack occurs, increase dose by up to 200 mg/day.

delavirdine (de-**la**-veer-deen)
Rescriptor

Classification
Therapeutic: antiretrovirals
Pharmacologic: non-nucleoside reverse transcriptase inhibitors

Pregnancy Category C

Indications
Treatment of HIV infection in combination with other antiretrovirals.

Contraindications/Precautions
Contraindicated in: Hypersensitivity; Concurrent use of astemizole, benzodiazepines and antiarrhythmics, dihydropyridine, calcium channel blockers (nifedipine), ergot alkaloids, amphetamines, and sildenafil (may result in excessive sedation, vasoconstriction, or arrhythmias).
Use Cautiously in: Impaired hepatic function; Achlorhydria (requires acidic environment for absorption); Pregnancy, lactation, or children (safety not established; HIV-infected patients should not breastfeed).

Adverse Reactions/Side Effects
CNS: fatigue, headache. **GI:** diarrhea, increased amylase, increased liver enzymes, nausea, vomiting. **Derm:** rash, pruritus. **Misc:** fat redistribution.

Route/Dosage
PO (Adults): 400 mg 3 times daily.

dexmedetomidine
(dex-me-de-**to**-mi-deen)
Precedex

Classification
Therapeutic: sedative/hypnotics

Pregnancy Category C

Indications
Sedation of initially intubated and mechanically ventilated patients during treatment in an intensive care setting; should not be used for >24 hr.

Contraindications/Precautions
Contraindicated in: Hypersensitivity.
Use Cautiously in: Hepatic impairment (lower doses may be required); Advanced heart block; Geriatric patients (increased risk of bradycardia and hypotension in patients ≤65 yr; Pregnancy, lactation or children (safety not established).

Adverse Reactions/Side Effects
Resp: hypoxia. **CV:** BRADYCARDIA, SINUS ARREST, hypotension, transient hypertension. **GI:** nausea, vomiting. **Hemat:** anemia. **Misc:** fever.

Route/Dosage
IV (Adults): *Loading infusion*—1 mcg/kg over 10 min followed by *maintenance infusion* of 0.2–0.7 mcg/kg/hr for maximum of 24 hrs; rate is adjusted to achieve desired level of sedation.

didanosine (dye-**dan**-oh-seen)
ddI, dideoxyinosine, Videx, Videx EC

Classification
Therapeutic: antiretrovirals
Pharmacologic: nucleoside reverse transcriptase inhibitors

Pregnancy Category B

Indications
HIV infection (with other antiretrovirals).

Contraindications/Precautions
Contraindicated in: Hypersensitivity; Phenylketonuria (tablets contain aspartame);OB: Lactation; Concurrent use of ribavirin or allopurinol.
Use Cautiously in: History of gout; Patients on sodium-restricted diets (tablets contain 264.5 mg sodium); Renal impairment (dosage modification required if CCr <60 ml/min; increased risk of pancreatitis); History of seizures; Diabetes mellitus;Pedi: Children (increased risk of pancreatitis).

Adverse Reactions/Side Effects
CNS: SEIZURES, headache, dizziness, insomnia, lethargy, pain, weakness. **EENT:** rhinitis, ear pain, epistaxis, optic neuritis, parotid gland enlargement, photophobia, retinal depigmentation, sialoadenitis. **Resp:** cough, asthma. **CV:** arrhythmias, edema, hypertension, vasodilation. **GI:** LIVER FAILURE, PANCREATITIS, anorexia, diarrhea, liver function abnormalities, nausea, vomiting, abdominal pain, constipation, dry mouth, dyspepsia, flatulence, hepatic steatosis, stomatitis. **GU:** urinary frequency. **Derm:** alopecia, ecchymoses, rash. **Endo:** hyperglycemia. **He-**

LESS COMMONLY USED DRUGS

mat: granulocytopenia, anemia, bleeding, leukopenia. **Metab:** LACTIC ACIDOSIS, hyperlipidemia, hyperuricemia, weight loss. **MS:** RHABDOMYOLYSIS, arthritis, myalgia. **Neuro:** peripheral neuropathy, poor coordination. **Misc:** chills, fever, anaphylactoid reactions.

Route/Dosage

When tablets are used, adults and children >1 yr should receive 2 tablets/dose to ensure adequate buffering. Children <1 yr may receive 1 tablet. Tablets and buffered powder are not interchangeable because of differences in bioavailabilty. Twice-daily dosing is preferred in children.

PO (Adults ≤60 kg): *Tablets*—200 mg bid; *Videx EC capsules*—400 mg once daily; *with tenofovir*—250 mg once daily; *buffered powder packets*—250 mg bid.

PO (Adults <60 kg): *Tablets*—125 mg bid; *Videx EC Capsules*—250 mg once daily; *with tenofovir*—200 mg once daily; *buffered powder packets*—167 mg q 12 hr.

PO (Children): *Tablets*—90–120 mg/m^2 q 12 hr; *buffered powder packets*—112.5–150 mg/m^2 q 12 hr.

PO (Children with BSA 1.1–1.4 m^2): *Tablets*—100 mg q 12 hr; *reconstituted pediatric powder*—125 mg q 12 hr.

PO (Children with BSA 0.8–1 m^2): *Tablets*—75 mg q 12 hr; *reconstituted pediatric powder*—94 mg q 12 hr.

PO (Children with BSA 0.5–0.7 m^2): *Tablets*—50 mg q 12 hr; *reconstituted pediatric powder*—62 mg q 12 hr.

PO (Children with BSA <0.4 m^2): *Tablets*—25 mg q 12 hr; *reconstituted pediatric powder*—31 mg q 12 hr.

Renal Impairment

PO (Adults >60 kg): *CCr 30–59 ml/min—Tablets*—100 mg q 12 hr; *Videx EC Capsules*—200 mg once daily; *buffered powder packets*—100 mg q 12 hr; *CCr 10–29 ml/min—Tablets*—150 mg q 24 hr; *Videx EC Capsules*—125 mg once daily; *buffered powder packets*—167 mg q 24 hr; *CCr <10 ml/min—Tablets*—100 mg q 24 hr; *Videx EC Capsules*—125 mg once daily; *buffered powder packets*—100 mg q 24 hr.

PO (Adults <60 kg): *CCr 30–59 ml/min—Tablets*—75 mg q 12 hr; *Videx EC Capsules*—125 mg once daily; *buffered powder packets*—100 mg q 12 hr; *CCr 10–29 ml/min—Tablets*—100 mg q 24 hr; *Videx EC Capsules*—125 mg once daily; *buffered powder packets*—100 mg q 24 hr; *CCr <10 ml/min—Tablets*—75 mg q 24 hr; *buffered powder packets*—100 mg q 24 hr.

disulfiram (di-**sul**-fir-am)

Antabuse

Classification

Therapeutic: alcohol abuse therapy adjuncts

Pharmacologic: enzyme inhibitors

Pregnancy Category C

Indications

Management of chronic alcoholism in patients who require or desire an enforced state of sobriety, which may allow for additional supportive and psychotherapeutic treatment.

Contraindications/Precautions

Contraindicated in: Hypersensitivity to disulfiram or other thiurams (including those used in rubber vulcanization and pesticides); Significant cardiovascular disease; Psychosis; Concurrent or recent use of metronidazole, paraldehyde, alcohol or alcohol-containing products; Lactation.

Use Cautiously in: Diabetes; Hyperthyroidism; Epilepsy; Cerebral damage; Hepatic or renal impairment or pathology; Pregnancy or children (safety not established).

Adverse Reactions/Side Effects

CNS: drowsiness, fatigue, headache, psychoses. **EENT:** optic neuritis. **GI:** HEPATIC TOXICITY, metallic/garlic-like taste. **GI:** erectile dysfunction. **Derm:** acneiform eruptions, allergic dermatitis. **Neuro:** peripheral neuritis/neuropathy, polyneuritis.

Route/Dosage

PO (Adults): 500 mg/day for 1–2 wk, then 250 mg/day (up to 500 mg/day).

efalizumab (eff-a-**liz**-oo-mab)

Raptiva

Classification

Therapeutic: antipsoriatics

Pharmacologic: monoclonal antibodies

Pregnancy Category C

Indications

Moderate to severe plaque psoriasis in adults who are candidates for systemic therapy or phototherapy.

Contraindications/Precautions

Contraindicated in: Hypersensitivity; Active infection; Concurrent immunosuppressants; OB: Pregnancy, lactation.

Use Cautiously in: Chronic/recurrent infections; High risk/history of malignancy; Geri: May be more sensitive to effects; Pedi: Children (safety not established).

Adverse Reactions/Side Effects

CNS: headache. **Derm:** photosensitivity, toxic epidermal necrolysis, worsening of psoriasis. **Hemat:** hemolytic anemia, thrombocytopenia. **MS:** arthralgia, arthritis, pain. **Misc:** MALIGNANCIES, SERIOUS INFECTIONS, fever, first dose reactions, hypersensitivity reactions, inflammatory/immune mediated reactions.

Route/Dosage

Subcut: (Adults): 0.7 mg/kg conditioning dose followed by 1 mg/kg once weekly (no single dose should exceed 200 mg).

eflornithine (topical)

(ee-**flor**-ni-theen)

Vaniqa

Classification

Therapeutic: facial hair removers (topical)

Pregnancy Category C

Indications

Reduction of unwanted facial hair in women.

Contraindications/Precautions

Contraindicated in: Hypersensitivity.

Use Cautiously in: Pregnancy, lactation or children <12 yr (safety not established).

Adverse Reactions/Side Effects

Local: burning, rash, stinging, tingling.

Route/Dosage

Topical (Adults): Apply a thin layer to affected areas of the face and adjacent involved areas under the chin and rub in thoroughly. Do not wash for 4 hr following application. Use twice daily at least 8 hr apart.

flurbiprofen†

(flure-**bye**-proe-fen)

Ansaid, ✤Apo-Flurbiprofen, ✤Froben, ✤Novo-Flurprofen, ✤Nu-Flurbiprofen

Classification

Therapeutic: antirheumatics, nonsteroidal anti-inflammatory agents

Pregnancy Category B (first trimester)

†See Appendix C for ophthalmic use

Indications

PO: Inflammatory disorders including: Rheumatoid arthritis, Osteoarthritis. **Unlabeled uses:** Nonopioid analgesic: Antidysmenorrheal.

Contraindications/Precautions

Contraindicated in: Hypersensitivity; Cross-sensitivity may exist with other NSAIDs, including aspirin; Active GI bleeding or ulcer disease; Peri-operative pain from coronary artery bypass graft (CABG) surgery.

Use Cautiously in: Cardiovascular disease or risk factors for cardiovascular disease (may ↑ risk of serious cardiovascular thrombotic events, myocardial infarction, and stroke, especially with prolonged use); Severe renal, or hepatic disease; History of ulcer disease; Diabetes mellitus; Geri: Geriatric patients (increased risk of GI bleeding); Bleeding disorders; OB: Pregnancy (not recommended for use during second half of pregnancy); OB, Pedi: Lactation or children (safety not established).

Adverse Reactions/Side Effects

CNS: dizziness, drowsiness, headache, insomnia, mental depression, psychic disturbances. **EENT:** blurred vision, corneal opacities, tinnitus. **CV:** changes in blood pressure, edema, palpitations. **GI:** GI BLEEDING, abdominal pain, heartburn, nausea, bloated feeling, constipation, diarrhea, drug-induced hepatitis, stomatitis. **GU:** incontinence. **Derm:** EXFOLIATIVE DERMATITIS, STEVENS-JOHNSON SYNDROME, TOXIC EPIDERMAL NECROLYSIS, increased sweating, rashes. **Hemat:** *PO*—blood dyscrasias, prolonged bleeding time. **MS:** myalgia. **Misc:** allergic reactions including ANAPHYLAXIS, chills, fever.

Route/Dosage

PO (Adults): *Anti-inflammatory*—200–300 mg daily in 2–4 divided doses (not to exceed 300 mg/day or 100 mg/dose). *Non-opioid analgesic/antidysmenorrheal*—50 mg q 4–6 hr as needed (unlabeled).

✤ = Canadian drug name.

*CAPITALS indicates life-threatening; underlines indicate most frequent.

flutamide (floo-ta-mide)
Eulexin

Classification
Therapeutic: antineoplastics
Pharmacologic: antiandrogens

Pregnancy Category D

Indications
Treatment of prostate carcinoma in conjunction with luteinizing hormone–releasing hormone (LHRH) analogues such as leuprolide.

Contraindications/Precautions
Contraindicated in: Hypersensitivity; Severe hepatic impairment.
Use Cautiously in: Severe cardiovascular disease.

Adverse Reactions/Side Effects
Side effects primarily caused by LHRH antagonist. **CNS:** anxiety, confusion, drowsiness, mental depression, nervousness. **CV:** edema, hypertension. **GI:** HEPATOTOXICITY, diarrhea, nausea, vomiting. **GU:** erectile dysfunction, loss of libido. **Derm:** photosensitivity, rash. **Endo:** gynecomastia. **Misc:** hot flashes.

Route/Dosage
PO (Adults): 250 mg q 8 hr; given concurrently with leuprolide.

gemtuzumab ozogamicin (gem-tu-zoo-mab o-zo-ga-my-sin)
Mylotarg

Classification
Therapeutic: antineoplastics
Pharmacologic: monoclonal antibodies, antitumor antibiotics

Pregnancy Category D

Indications
Treatment of patients with patients with CD33 positive acute myeloid leukemia in first relapse who are ≤60 years old and who are not considered to be candidates for cytotoxic chemotherapy.

Contraindications/Precautions
Contraindicated in: Hypersensitivity; Pregnancy; Lactation.
Use Cautiously in: Patients with hepatic impairment; Children (safety not established).

Adverse Reactions/Side Effects
CNS: headache. **Resp:** dyspnea, hypoxia. **CV:** hypotension, hypertension. **GI:** mucositis, nausea, vomiting, hepatotoxicity. **Derm:** rash. **Endo:** hyperglycemia. **F and E:** hypokalemia. **Hemat:** NEUTROPENIA, anemia, bleeding, thrombocytopenia. **Misc:** chills, fever, post-infusion reaction, allergic reactions, infection, tumor lysis syndrome.

Route/Dosage
IV (Adults ≤60 yr): 9 mg/m² as a 2-hr infusion followed by a second dose 14 days later.

goserelin (goe-se-rel-lin)
Zoladex

Classification
Therapeutic: antineoplastics, hormones
Pharmacologic: gonadotropin-releasing hormones

Pregnancy Category D (breast cancer), X (endometriosis)

Indications
Prostate cancer in patients who cannot tolerate orchiectomy or estrogen therapy (palliative). With flutamide and radiation therapy in the treatment of locally confined stage T2b–T4 (stage B2–C) prostate cancer. Advanced breast cancer in peri- and postmenopausal women (palliative). Endometriosis. Produces thinning of the endometrium before endometrial ablation for dysfunctional uterine bleeding.

Contraindications/Precautions
Contraindicated in: Hypersensitivity; Undiagnosed vaginal bleeding; Pregnancy or lactation.
Use Cautiously in: Lactation or children <18 yr (safety not established).

Adverse Reactions/Side Effects
CNS: headache, anxiety, depression, dizziness, fatigue, insomnia, weakness. **Resp:** dyspnea. **CV:** CEREBROVASCULAR ACCIDENT, MYOCARDIAL INFARCTION, vasodilation, chest pain, hypertension, palpitations. **GI:** anorexia, constipation, diarrhea, nausea, ulcer, vomiting. **GU:** renal insufficiency, urinary obstruction. **Derm:** sweating, rashes. **Endo:** decreased libido, erectile dysfunction, breast swelling, breast tenderness, infertility, ovarian cysts, ovarian hyperstimulation syndrome (with gonadotropins). **F and E:** peripheral edema. **Hemat:** anemia. **Metab:** gout, hyperglycemia, ↑ lipids. **MS:** ↑ bone pain,

arthralgia, ↓ bone density. **Misc:** hot flashes, chills, fever, weight gain.

Route/Dosage

Subcut (Adults): 3.6 mg every 4 wk or 10.8 mg q 12 wk. *Endometrial thinning*—1 or 2 depots given 4 wk apart; if 1 depot used, surgery is performed at 4 wk; if 2 depots used, surgery is performed 2–4 wk after 2nd depot.

hydroxyurea

(hye-drox-ee-yoor-**ee**-a)
Droxia, Hydrea, Mylocel

Classification
Therapeutic: antineoplastics
Pharmacologic: antimetabolites

Pregnancy Category D

Indications

Treatment of head and neck carcinoma. Treatment of ovarian carcinoma. Treatment of resistant chronic myelogenous leukemia. Treatment of melanoma. Reduction of painful crises in sickle cell anemia and decreased need for transfusions in adult patients with a history of recurrent moderate to severe crises (at least 3 in the preceding yr). **Unlabeled uses:** Used as part of antiretroviral therapy in patients with HIV infection.

Contraindications/Precautions

Contraindicated in: Hypersensitivity; Pregnancy or lactation; Some products contain tartrazine (FDC yellow dye #5) and should be avoided in patients with known hypersensitivity.
Use Cautiously in: Patients with childbearing potential; Renal impairment (close monitoring of hematologic parameters recommended, dosage reduction may be necessary); Hepatic impairment (close monitoring of hematologic parameters recommended); Myeloproliferative disorders (may increase risk of vasculitic ulcerations and gangrene); Active infections; Decreased bone marrow reserve; Other chronic debilitating illness; Geriatric patients (may be more sensitive to effects, lower doses may be required); Obese patients or patients with edema (dose should be determined using ideal body weight).

Adverse Reactions/Side Effects

CNS: drowsiness (large doses). **GI:** anorexia, diarrhea, nausea, vomiting, constipation, hepatitis, stomatitis. **GU:** dysuria, infertility, renal tubular dysfunction. **Derm:** alopecia, exacerbation of post-radiation erythema, erythema, pruritus, rashes. **Hemat:** leukopenia, anemia, thrombocytopenia. **Metab:** hyperuricemia. **Misc:** chills, fever, malaise.

Route/Dosage

Head and Neck Cancer, Ovarian Cancer, Malignant Melanoma

PO (Adults): 60–80 mg/kg (2–3 g/m²) as a single daily dose q 3 days or 20–30 mg/kg/day as a single dose. Therapy should be initiated 7 days prior to radiation and continued.

Resistant Chronic Myelogenous Leukemia

PO (Adults): 20–30 mg/kg/day in 1–2 divided doses.

Sickle Cell Anemia

PO (Adults and Children): 15 mg/kg/day as a single dose, may increase by 5 mg/kg/day q 12 wks up to 35 mg/kg/day.

iloprost (eye-lo-prost)

Ventavis

Classification
Therapeutic: vasodilators
Pharmacologic: prostacyclins

Pregnancy Category C

Indications

Management of New York Class III/IV symptoms of pulmonary hypertension, where there is marked limitation of physical activity.

Contraindications/Precautions

Contraindicated in: Hypersensitivity; Systolic BP <85 mmHg; Lactation.
Use Cautiously in: Concurrent use of drugs or co-existing medical conditions which may ↑ risk of syncope; Children (safety not established); Pregnancy (use only if maternal benefit outweighs fetal risk).

Adverse Reactions/Side Effects

CNS: fainting, headache, insomnia. **Resp:** ↑ cough, dyspnea, hemoptysis. **CV:** CHF, vasodilation, chest pain, hypotension, peripheral edema, supraventricular tachycardia. **GI:** nausea, vomiting. **GU:** renal failure. **Derm:** facial flushing. **MS:** back pain, jaw-muscle spasm, muscle cramps.

Route/Dosage

Inhaln (Adults): 2.5 mcg initially, then 5 mcg/dose 6–9 times daily; not more than every 2 hr.

indinavir (in-**din**-a-veer)
Crixivan

Classification
Therapeutic: antiretrovirals
Pharmacologic: protease inhibitors

Pregnancy Category C

Indications

HIV infection (with other antiretrovirals). **Unlabeled uses:** Prevention of HIV infection after known exposure (with other antiretrovirals).

Contraindications/Precautions

Contraindicated in: Hypersensitivity; Dehydration; Concurrent alprazolam, dihydroergotamine, ergotamine, midazolam, rifampin, triazolam, or St. John's wort.
Use Cautiously in: Hepatic impairment (dose reduction recommended in moderate to severe hepatic insufficiency caused by cirrhosis); Hemophilia (increased risk of bleeding); Diabetes mellitus; OB, PediLactation, or children (safety not established; breastfeeding not recommended in HIV-infected patients).

Adverse Reactions/Side Effects

CNS: dizziness, drowsiness, fatigue, headache, insomnia, weakness. **GI:** abdominal pain, acid regurgitation, altered taste, asymptomatic hyperbilirubinemia, diarrhea, nausea, vomiting. **GU:** nephrolithiasis. **Endo:** hyperglycemia. **F and E:** KETOACIDOSIS. **MS:** back pain, flank pain. **Misc:** redistribution of body fat.

Route/Dosage

PO (Adults): 800 mg q 8 hr.

mebendazole
(me-**ben**-da-zole)
Vermox

Classification
Therapeutic: antihelmintics

Pregnancy Category C

Indications

Treatment of: Whipworm (trichuriasis), Pinworm (enterobiasis), Roundworm (ascariasis), Hookworm (uncinariasis) infections, Drug of choice for capillariasis.

Contraindications/Precautions

Contraindicated in: Hypersensitivity.
Use Cautiously in: Impaired liver function; Crohn's ileitis; Ulcerative colitis; Pregnancy, lactation, or children <2 yr (safety not established; may be used in first trimester only if benefit justifies potential risk to fetus).

Adverse Reactions/Side Effects

Most side effects and adverse reactions are seen with high-dose therapy only **CNS:** SEIZURES (rare), dizziness, headache. **EENT:** tinnitus. **GI:** abdominal pain, diarrhea, increased liver enzymes (high dose, long-term therapy), nausea, vomiting. **Derm:** rash, urticaria, alopecia. **Hemat:** agranulocytosis, reversible myelosuppression (leukopenia, thrombocytopenia). **Neuro:** numbness. **Misc:** fever.

Route/Dosage

Enterobiasis

PO (Adults and Children >2 yr): 100 mg as a single dose; repeat in 2–3 wk.

Trichuriasis, Ascariasis, Hookworm, or Mixed Infections

PO (Adults and Children >2 yr): 100 mg twice daily for 3 days. If not cured in 3–4 wk, a 2nd course is given.

Capillariasis

PO (Adults and Children >2 yr): 200 mg twice daily for 20 days.

meprobamate
(me-proe-**ba**-mate)
✤Apo-Meprobamate, Equanil, Miltown

Classification
Therapeutic: antianxiety agents, sedative/hypnotics
Pharmacologic: carbamates

Schedule IV

Pregnancy Category D

Indications

Anxiety disorders (provides sedation).

Contraindications/Precautions

Contraindicated in: Hypersensitivity; Comatose patients or those with pre-existing CNS de-

pression; Uncontrolled severe pain; Pregnancy and lactation.
Use Cautiously in: Hepatic dysfunction or severe renal impairment; History of suicide attempt or drug abuse;Geri: Appears on Beers list and is associated with falls. Dosage reduction suggested.

Adverse Reactions/Side Effects
CNS: drowsiness. **EENT:** blurred vision. **CV:** hypotension. **GI:** anorexia, diarrhea, nausea, vomiting. **Derm:** pruritus, rashes, urticaria. **Neuro:** ataxia. **Misc:** hypersensitivity reactions, physical dependence, psychological dependence, tolerance.

Route/Dosage
PO (Adults): 400 mg 3–4 times daily or 600 mg twice daily. *Extended-release capsules*—400–800 mg twice daily (not to exceed 2400 mg/day).
PO (Children 6–12 yr): 100–200 mg 2–3 times daily. *Extended-release capsules*—200 mg twice daily.

metaproterenol
(met-a-proe-**ter**-e-nole)
Alupent

Classification
Therapeutic: bronchodilators
Pharmacologic: adrenergics

Pregnancy Category C

Indications
Treatment/prevention of bronchospasm due to reversible airway disease (a short-term control agent).

Contraindications/Precautions
Contraindicated in: Hypersensitivity to adrenergic amines; Selected products may contain bisulfites, alcohol (in some oral liquid preparations), or fluorocarbons (in some inhalers) and should be avoided in patients with known hypersensitivity or intolerance.
Use Cautiously in: Cardiac disease; Hypertension; Hyperthyroidism; Diabetes; Glaucoma; Elderly patients (more susceptible to adverse reactions; may require dosage reduction); Excessive use may lead to tolerance and paradoxical bronchospasm (inhaler); Pregnancy (near term) and lactation.

Adverse Reactions/Side Effects
CNS: nervousness, restlessness, tremor, headache, insomnia. **Resp:** PARADOXICAL BRONCHOSPASM (excessive use of inhalers). **CV:** angina, arrhythmias, hypertension, tachycardia. **GI:** nausea, vomiting. **Endo:** hyperglycemia.

Route/Dosage
PO (Adults and Children >9 yr): 20 mg 3–4 times/day.
PO (Children 6–9 yr): 10 mg 3–4 times/day.
PO (Children 2–6 yr): 1.3–2.6 mg/kg/day divided q 6–8 hr.
PO (Children <2 yr): 0.4 mg/kg/dose 3–4 times/day; may give q 8–12 hr in infants.
Inhaln (Adults and Children >12 yr): *Metered-dose inhaler*—2–3 inhalations q 3–4 hr (not to exceed 12 inhalations/day). *IPPB*—0.2–0.3 ml of 5% solution or 2.5 ml of 0.4–0.6% solution for nebulization 3–4 times daily (not to exceed q 4 hr use).
Inhaln (Children >1 month): 0.5–1 mg/kg (0.01–0.02 ml/kg) of 5% solution via nebulization q 4–6 hr; minimum dose 0.1 mL (5 mg) maximum dose 0.3 ml (15 mg).

miglustat (mi-gloo-stat)
Zavesca

Classification
Therapeutic: none assigned
Pharmacologic: enzyme inhibitors (D-glucose analogue), substrate reduction therapy

Pregnancy Category X

Indications
Mild to moderate type 1 Gaucher's disease, when enzyme replacement therapy is not an option.

Contraindications/Precautions
Contraindicated in: Hypersensitivity; Pregnancy or lactation; Severe renal impairment (<30 ml/min).
Use Cautiously in: Mild to moderate renal impairment (dosage alteration recommended if CCr <70 ml/min); Geriatric patients (consider age related decrease in body mass, cardiac, renal and hepatic function, other chronic illnesses and concurrent drug therapies); Children <18 yr (safety not established).

Adverse Reactions/Side Effects
CNS: headache. **GI:** abdominal pain, diarrhea, flatulence, nausea, anorexia, dyspepsia. **GU:** ↓ male fertility. **Hemat:** thrombocytopenia. **Metab:** weight loss. **Neuro:** paresthesia, peripheral neuropathy, tremor.

Route/Dosage
PO (Adults): 100 mg three times daily at regular intervals

Renal Impairment
PO (Adults): *CCr 50–70 ml/min*—100 mg twice daily; *CCr 30–50 ml/min*—100 mg once daily.

minoxidil (systemic)
(mi-**nox**-i-dill)
Loniten

Classification
Therapeutic: antihypertensives
Pharmacologic: vasodilators

Pregnancy Category C

Indications
Severe symptomatic hypertension or hypertension associated with end-organ damage that has failed to respond to combinations of more conventional therapy.

Contraindications/Precautions
Contraindicated in: Hypersensitivity; Pheochromocytoma.
Use Cautiously in: Recent MI; Severe renal impairment (can be used in moderate renal impairment); Geriatric patients (may be more sensitive to effects; consider age-related decline in body mass, hepatic/renal/cardiovascular function); Pregnancy or lactation (safety not established).

Adverse Reactions/Side Effects
CNS: headache. **Resp:** PULMONARY EDEMA. **CV:** CHF, ECG changes (alteration in T waves), tachycardia, angina, pericardial effusion. **GI:** nausea. **Derm:** hypertrichosis, pigment changes, rashes. **Endo:** gynecomastia, menstrual irregularities. **F and E:** sodium and water retention. **Misc:** intermittent claudication.

Route/Dosage
PO (Adults and Children >12 yr): *Hypertension*—5 mg once daily or in 2 divided doses; may double at 3-day intervals; usual range 10–40 mg/day (for rapid control with careful monitoring, doses may be adjusted q 6 hr; up to 100 mg/day have been used).
PO (Children <12 yr): *Hypertension*—0.2 mg/kg/day (5 mg maximum) as a single dose or 2 divided doses; may be gradually increased at 3-day intervals in increments of 50–100% until response is obtained; usual range 0.25–1 mg/kg/day (for rapid control, doses may be adjusted q 6 hr; not to exceed 50 mg/day).

moricizine (more-i-sizz-een)
Ethmozine

Classification
Therapeutic: antiarrhythmics (class IA)

Pregnancy Category B

Indications
Life-threatening ventricular arrhythmias, including sustained ventricular tachycardia.

Contraindications/Precautions
Contraindicated in: Hypersensitivity; Cardiogenic shock; 2nd- or 3rd-degree AV block or bundle branch block (unless a pacemaker has been placed).
Use Cautiously in: Electrolyte disturbances; Severe renal or hepatic impairment (initial dosage reduction may be necessary); CHF; Pregnancy, lactation, or children (safety not established)
Exercise Extreme Caution in: Sick sinus syndrome.

Adverse Reactions/Side Effects
CNS: dizziness, fatigue, headache, nervousness, sleep disorders, weakness. **EENT:** blurred vision. **Resp:** dyspnea. **CV:** ARRHYTHMIAS, chest pain, CHF, palpitations. **GI:** nausea, diarrhea, dry mouth, dyspepsia, vomiting. **Derm:** sweating. **MS:** musculoskeletal pain. **Neuro:** paresthesia. **Misc:** drug fever.

Route/Dosage
PO (Adults): 600–900 mg/day given q 8 hr; within this range, dosage may be adjusted by 150 mg/day every 3 days as required and tolerated. Some patients may tolerate q 12 hr dosing (not to exceed 900 mg/day).

nelfinavir (nell-**finn**-a-veer)
Viracept

Classification
Therapeutic: antiretrovirals
Pharmacologic: protease inhibitors

Pregnancy Category B

Indications
HIV infection (with other antiretrovirals).

Contraindications/Precautions
Contraindicated in: Hypersensitivity; Concurrent amiodarone, ergot derivatives, midazolam, quinidine, rifampin, pimozide, simvastatin, lovastatin, rifampin, St. John's wort, or triazolam; Lactation: Lactation (breastfeeding should be avoided by HIV-infected patients).
Use Cautiously in: Hemophiliacs (↑ risk of bleeding); Diabetes mellitus (may exacerbate condition); Hepatic impairment.

Adverse Reactions/Side Effects
CNS: SEIZURES, anxiety, depression, dizziness, drowsiness, emotional lability, headache, hyperkinesia, insomnia, malaise, migraine headache, sleep disorders, suicidal ideation, weakness. **EENT:** acute iritis, pharyngitis, rhinitis, sinusitis. **Resp:** dyspnea. **GI:** diarrhea, anorexia, dyspepsia, elevated liver function studies, epigastric pain, flatulence, GI bleeding, hepatitis, nausea, oral ulcerations, pancreatitis, vomiting. **GU:** nephrolithiasis, sexual dysfunction. **Derm:** pruritus, rash, sweating, urticaria. **Endo:** hyperglycemia. **F and E:** dehydration. **Hemat:** anemia, leukopenia, thrombocytopenia. **Metab:** hyperlipidemia, hyperuricemia. **MS:** arthralgia, arthritis, back pain, myalgia, myopathy. **Neuro:** myasthenia, paresthesia. **Misc:** allergic reactions, fever, redistribution of body fat.

Route/Dosage
PO (Adults and Children >13 yr): 750 mg 3 times daily *or* 1250 mg twice daily.
PO (Children 2–13 yr): 20–30 mg/kg 3 times daily (not to exceed 750 mg 3 times daily).

nitazoxanide
(nit-a-**zox**-a-nide)
Alinia

Classification
Therapeutic: antiprotozoals
Pharmacologic: benzamides

Pregnancy Category B

Indications
Treatment of diarrhea due to *Cryptosporidium parvum* and *Giardia lamblia*. Not effective for *C. Parvum* diarrhea in HIV-infected patients.

Contraindications/Precautions
Contraindicated in: Hypersensitivity.
Use Cautiously in: Hepatic and/or renal impairment; Diabetics (contains 1.48 g sucrose/5 ml); Pedi, OB: Children <1 pregnancy or lactation (safety not established).

Adverse Reactions/Side Effects
CNS: dizziness. **EENT:** yellow eye discoloration. **GI:** abdominal pain, diarrhea, vomiting. **GU:** discolored urine. **Derm:** pruritus, sweating. **Misc:** fever.

Route/Dosage
PO (Adults and children ≤12 yr): 500 mg every 12 hr for 3 days.
PO (Children 4–11 yr): 200 mg (10 ml) every 12 hr for 3 days.
PO (Children 1–4 yr): 100 mg (5 ml) every 12 hr for 3 days.

pegaptanib (peg-**apt**-i-nib)
Macugen

Classification
Therapeutic: ocular agents
Pharmacologic: vascular endothelial growth factor antagonists

Pregnancy Category B

Indications
Neovascular (wet) age-related macular degeneration.

Contraindications/Precautions
Contraindicated in: Ocular/periocular infections.
Use Cautiously in: OB: Use only if maternal benefit outweighs fetal risk; Lactation, Pedi: Safety not established.

Adverse Reactions/Side Effects

EENT: cataract, blurred vision, conjunctival bleeding, irritation/pain, ↑ intraocular pressure, ocular inflammation, infection (rare), retinal detachment (rare), traumatic cataract formation (rare). **Misc:** Anaphylaxis, angioedema.

Route/Dosage

Intravitreal (Adults): 0.3 mg every 6 wk.

penicillamine

(pen-i-**sill**-a-meen)

Cuprimine, Depen

Classification

Therapeutic: antidotes, antirheumatics (DMARD), antiurolithics

Pharmacologic: chelating agents

Pregnancy Category D

Indications

Progressive rheumatoid arthritis resistant to conventional therapy. Management of copper deposition in Wilson's disease. Management of recurrent cystine calculi. **Unlabeled uses:** Adjunct in the treatment of heavy metal poisoning.

Contraindications/Precautions

Contraindicated in: Hypersensitivity; Cross-sensitivity with penicillin may exist; Patients currently receiving gold salts, antimalarials, antineoplastics, oxyphenbutazone, or phenylbutazone; Concurrent use of iron supplements; **OB:** Pregnancy (penicillamine should be avoided in pregnant patients with rheumatoid arthritis or cystinuria); OB: Lactation.

Use Cautiously in: Renal impairment (increased risk of adverse renal reactions in patients with rheumatoid arthritis); History of aplastic anemia due to penicillamine; Patients requiring surgery (may impair wound healing); Geri: Geriatric patients (increased risk of hematologic toxicity, skin rash and taste abnormality; dose reduction recommended); OB: Pregnancy (for patients with Wilson's disease, limit daily dose to <1 g. If cesarean section is planned, decrease daily dose to 250 mg for last 6 wk of pregnancy and until incision is healed).

Adverse Reactions/Side Effects

EENT: blurred vision, eye pain. **Resp:** coughing, shortness of breath, wheezing. **GI:** altered taste, anorexia, cholestatic jaundice, diarrhea, drug-induced pancreatitis, dyspepsia, epigastric pain, hepatic dysfunction, nausea, oral ulceration, vomiting. **GU:** proteinuria. **Derm:** pemphigus, ecchymoses, hives, itching, rashes, wrinkling. **Hemat:** APLASTIC ANEMIA, anemia, eosinophilia, leukopenia, thrombocytopenia, thrombocytosis. **MS:** arthralgia, migratory polyarthritis. **Neuro:** myasthenia gravis syndrome. **Misc:** GOODPASTURE'S SYNDROME (GLOMERULONEPHRITIS AND INTRA-ALVEOLAR HEMORRHAGE), allergic reactions, fever, lymphadenopathy, systemic lupus erythematosus–like syndrome.

Route/Dosage

PO (Adults): *Antirheumatic*—125–250 mg/day as a single dose; may be slowly increased up to 1.5 g/day. *Chelating agent (Wilson's disease)*—250 mg qid. *Antiurolithic*—500 mg 4 times daily.

PO (Children >6 mo): *Chelating agent (Wilson's disease)*—250 mg/day as a single dose; older children may receive the adult dose. *Antiurolithic*—7.5 mg/kg 4 times daily.

pentetate calcium trisodium

(pen-**te**-tate)

Ca-DTPA

Classification

Therapeutic: none assigned, radiation protectants

Pharmacologic: chelating agents

Pregnancy Category C

Indications

Known/suspected internal contamination with plutonium, americium or curium. Ca-DTPA is more effective than Zn-DTPA and should be given as the initial dose in the first 24 hr following internal contamination. After 24 hr, Zn-DTPA is equally effective.

Contraindications/Precautions

Contraindicated in: Lactation.

Use Cautiously in: Renal impairment; Severe hemachromatosis; Asthma (inhalation use); Mixed radiocontamination (additional treatments may be needed); Pregnancy (use Zn-DTPA unless contamination is high); Children (safety of inhalation not established).

Adverse Reactions/Side Effects

CNS: headache, lightheadedness. **CV:** chest pain. **GI:** diarrhea, metallic taste, nausea. **F and E:** depletion of zinc, manganese, magnesium (prolonged treatment). **Local:** injection site reactions. **Resp:** cough, wheezing (inhalation only). **Derm:** dermatitis. **Misc:** allergic reactions.

Route/Dosage

IV (Adults and Children 12 yr and older): Single 1 g dose, then follow with Zn-DTPA. If Zn-DTPA is unavailable, continue with Ca-DTPA 1 g once daily. Duration of treatment depends on degree of contamination and response.
IV (Children less than 12 yr): 14 mg/kg single dose, not to exceed 1 g dose then follow with Zn-DTPA. If Zn-DTPA is unavailable, continue with Ca-DTPA 14 mg/kg once daily. Duration of treatment depends on degree of contamination and response.
Inhaln (Adults and Children 12 yr and older): *When contamination has been by the inhalation route*—via nebulization in a 1:1 ratio with sterile water or saline.

pentetate zinc trisodium

(pen-**te**-tate)
Zn-DTPA

Classification
Therapeutic: radiation protectants
Pharmacologic: chelating agents

Pregnancy Category B

Indications

Known/suspected internal contamination with plutonium, americium or curium. Ca-DTPA is more effective than Zn-DTPA and should be given as the initial dose in the first 24 hr following internal contamination. After 24 hr, Zn-DTPA is equally effective.

Contraindications/Precautions

Contraindicated in: Lactation.
Use Cautiously in: Renal impairment; Asthma (inhalation use); Mixed radiocontamination (additional treatments may be needed); Pregnancy; Children (safety of inhalation not established).

Adverse Reactions/Side Effects

CNS: lightheadedness. **F and E:** depletion of manganese, magnesium. **Local:** injection site reactions. **Resp:** cough, wheezing (inhalation only).

Route/Dosage

IV (Adults and Children 12 yr and older): 1 g/day, following Ca-DTPA. Duration of treatment depends on degree of contamination and response.
IV (Children less than 12 yr): 14 mg/kg/day single dose, following Ca-DTPA. Duration of treatment depends on degree of contamination and response.
Inhaln (Adults and Children over 12 yr): *When contamination has been by the inhalation route*—via nebulization in a 1:1 ratio with sterile water or saline.

pentobarbital

(pen-toe-**bar**-bi-tal)
Nembutal, ✤Novopentobarb, ✤Nova Rectal

Classification
Therapeutic: anticonvulsants, sedative/hypnotics
Pharmacologic: barbiturates

Schedule II (oral and parenteral), III (rectal)

Pregnancy Category D

Indications

Hypnotic agent (short-term). Preoperative sedation and other situations in which sedation is required. Treatment of seizures. **Unlabeled uses: IV:** Induction of coma in selected patients with cerebral ischemia and management of increased intracranial pressure (high doses).

Contraindications/Precautions

Contraindicated in: Hypersensitivity; Some products contain tartrazine, alcohol, or propylene glycol and should be avoided in patients with known hypersensitivity or intolerance; Comatose patients or those with pre-existing CNS depression (unless used to induce coma); Uncontrolled severe pain; Pregnancy or lactation.
Use Cautiously in: Hepatic dysfunction; Severe renal impairment; Patients who may be suicidal or who may have been addicted to drugs previously; Geriatric or debilitated patients (initial dosage reduction recommended); Hypovolemic shock; Hypnotic use should be short-term (chronic use may lead to dependence).

Adverse Reactions/Side Effects

CNS: drowsiness, hangover, lethargy, delirium, excitation, mental depression, vertigo. **Resp:** respiratory depression; *IV*— LARYNGOSPASM, bronchospasm. **CV:** *IV*— hypotension. **GI:** constipation, diarrhea, nausea, vomiting. **Derm:**

✤ = Canadian drug name.
* CAPITALS indicates life-threatening; underlines indicate most frequent.

rashes, urticaria. **Local:** phlebitis at IV site. **MS:** arthralgia, myalgia, neuralgia. **Misc:** hypersensitivity reactions including ANGIOEDEMA and SERUM SICKNESS, physical dependence, psychological dependence.

Route/Dosage

PO (Adults): *Sedative*—20 mg 3–4 times daily. *Hypnotic/preoperative sedative*—100 mg.
PO (Children): *Sedative*—2–6 mg/kg/day. *Preoperative sedative*—2–6 mg/kg (up to 100 mg/dose).
IM (Adults): *Hypnotic/preoperative sedative*—150–200 mg.
IM (Children): *Sedative*—2–6 mg/kg/day in divided doses. *Preoperative sedative*—2–6 mg/kg (up to 100 mg/dose).
IV (Adults): *Hypnotic/anticonvulsant*—100 mg initially; additional small doses may be given q min up to 500 mg total. *Induction of coma*—5–7 mg/kg, then 3–4 mg/kg q 3–4 hr dose adjusted by serum level (unlabeled).
IV (Children): *Sedative*—1–3 mg/kg to a maximum of 100 mg until asleep. *Conscious sedation*—Initial 2 mg/kg, may repeat q 5–10 min with 1–2 mg/kg until adequate sedation acheived. Maximum total dose 6 mg/kg or 150–200 mg. *Induction of coma*—10–15 mg/kg slowly over 1–2 hr, followed by a maintenance infusion of 1–3 mg/kg/hr.
Rect (Adults): *Sedative*—30 mg 2–4 times daily. *Hypnotic*—120–200 mg at bedtime.
Rect (Children): *Sedative*—2 mg/kg (60 mg/m^2) 3 times daily.
Rect (Children 12–14 yr): *Preoperative sedative/hypnotic*—60–120 mg.
Rect (Children 5–12 yr): *Preoperative sedative/hypnotic*—60 mg.
Rect (Children 1–4 yr): *Preoperative sedative/hypnotic*—30–60 mg.
Rect (Children 2 mo–1 yr): *Preoperative sedative/hypnotic*—30 mg.

phentermine (fen-ter-meen)

Adipex-P, Banobese, Fastin, Ionamin, Obi-Nix, OBY-CAP, Phentercot, Phentride, T-Diet, Teramine, Zantryl

Classification
Therapeutic: weight control agents
Pharmacologic: appetite suppressants

Schedule IV

Pregnancy Category UK

Indications

Short-term treatment of obesity in conjunction with other interventions (dietary restriction, exercise); used to produce and maintain weight loss in patients with a BMI ≤30 kg/m^2 or ≤27 kg/m^2 in the presence of other risk factors (diabetes, hypertension, hyperlipidemia).

Contraindications/Precautions

Contraindicated in: Hypersensitivity or known intolerance to sympathomimetic amines; Cardiovascular disease; Hyperthyroidism; Moderate to severe hypertension; History of drug abuse; Agitation; Glaucoma; Concurrent or recent (within 14 days) MAO inhibitor therapy; Concurrent SSRI antidepressants.
Use Cautiously in: Mild hypertension; Diabetes mellitus; Pregnancy, lactation, or children <12 yr (safety not established).

Adverse Reactions/Side Effects

CNS: CNS stimulation, confusion, dizziness, dysphoria, euphoria, headache, insomnia, mental depression, restlessness. **EENT:** blurred vision. **CV:** hypertension, palpitations, tachycardia. **GI:** constipation, diarrhea, dry mouth, nausea, unpleasant taste, vomiting. **GU:** changes in libido, erectile dysfunction.

Route/Dosage

PO (Adults): *Phentermine hydrochloride tablets or capsules*—8 mg 3 times daily or 15–37.5 mg once daily; *Phentermine resin complex capsules*—15–30 mg once daily.

pindolol (pin-doe-lole)

✤Novo-Pindol, ✤Syn-Pindolol, Visken

Classification
Therapeutic: antihypertensives
Pharmacologic: beta blockers

Pregnancy Category B

Indications

Management of hypertension. **Unlabeled uses:** Management of angina pectoris.

Contraindications/Precautions

Contraindicated in: Uncompensated CHF; Pulmonary edema; Cardiogenic shock; Bradycardia or heart block.

Use Cautiously in: Renal impairment; Hepatic impairment; Geriatric patients (increased sensitivity to beta blockers; initial dosage reduction recommended); Pulmonary disease (including asthma); Diabetes mellitus (may mask signs of hypoglycemia); Thyrotoxicosis (may mask symptoms); Patients with a history of severe allergic reactions (intensity of reactions may be increased); Pregnancy, lactation, or children (safety not established; may cause fetal/neonatal bradycardia, hypotension, hypoglycemia, or respiratory depression).

Adverse Reactions/Side Effects

CNS: fatigue, weakness, anxiety, depression, dizziness, drowsiness, insomnia, memory loss, mental status changes, nervousness, nightmares. **EENT:** blurred vision, dry eyes, nasal stuffiness. **Resp:** bronchospasm, wheezing. **CV:** ARRHYTHMIAS, BRADYCARDIA, CHF, PULMONARY EDEMA, orthostatic hypotension, peripheral vasoconstriction. **GI:** constipation, diarrhea, nausea. **GU:** erectile dysfunction, decreased libido. **Derm:** itching, rashes. **Endo:** hyperglycemia, hypoglycemia. **MS:** arthralgia, back pain, muscle cramps. **Neuro:** paresthesia. **Misc:** drug-induced lupus syndrome.

Route/Dosage

PO (Adults): 5 mg twice daily initially; may be increased by 10 mg/day q 2–3 wk as needed (up to 45–60 mg/day).

polycarbophil

(pol-i-**kar**-boe-fil)

Bulk Forming Fiber Laxative, Equalactin, FiberCon, Fiber-Lax, Konsyl Fiber, Mitrolan

Classification

Therapeutic: antidiarrheals, laxatives

Pharmacologic: bulk-forming agents

Pregnancy Category UK

Indications

Treatment of constipation or diarrhea that may be associated with diverticulosis or irritable bowel syndrome.

Contraindications/Precautions

Contraindicated in: Hypersensitivity; Abdominal pain; Nausea or vomiting (especially when associated with fever or other signs of acute abdomen); Serious intra-abdominal adhesions; Dysphagia.

Use Cautiously in: Pregnancy or lactation (has been used safely).

Adverse Reactions/Side Effects

GI: abdominal fullness.

Route/Dosage

PO (Adults): 1 g 1–4 times daily or as needed (not to exceed 6 g/24 hr); for severe diarrhea, may repeat q 30 min.

PO (Children 6–12 yr): 500 mg 1–3 times daily or as needed (not to exceed 3 g/24 hr); for severe diarrhea, may repeat q 30 min.

PO (Children 2–6 yr): 500 mg 1–2 times daily or as needed (not to exceed 1.5 g/24 hr); for severe diarrhea, may repeat q 30 min.

POTASSIUM PHOSPHATES

(poe-**tass**-ee-um **foss**-fates)

monobasic potassium phosphate

K-Phos Original

potassium phosphates

Neutra-Phos-K

potassium phosphate

Classification

Therapeutic: antiurolithics, mineral and electrolyte replacements/supplements

Pregnancy Category C

Indications

Treatment and prevention of phosphate depletion in patients who are unable to ingest adequate dietary potassium. Adjunct therapy of urinary tract infections with methenamine hippurate or mandelate (potassium and sodium phosphates or monobasic potassium phosphate). Prevention of calcium urinary stones (potassium and sodium phosphates or monobasic potassium phosphate). Phosphate salts of potassium may be used in hypokalemic patients with metabolic acidosis or coexisting phosphorus deficiency.

Contraindications/Precautions

Contraindicated in: Hyperkalemia; Hyperphosphatemia; Hypocalcemia; Severe renal im-

pairment; Untreated Addison's disease; Severe tissue trauma; Hyperkalemic familial periodic paralysis.
Use Cautiously in: Hyperparathyroidism; Cardiac disease; Renal impairment.

Adverse Reactions/Side Effects
Related to hyperphosphatemia, unless otherwise indicated **CNS:** confusion, listlessness, weakness. **CV:** ARRHYTHMIAS, CARDIAC ARREST, ECG changes (absent P waves, widening of the QRS complex with biphasic curve), hypotension; *hyperkalemia*—ARRHYTHMIAS, ECG changes (prolonged PR interval, ST segment depression, tall-tented T waves). **GI:** diarrhea, abdominal pain, nausea, vomiting. **F and E:** hyperkalemia, hyperphosphatemia, hypocalcemia, hypomagnesemia. **Local:** irritation at IV site, phlebitis. **MS:** *hyperkalemia*—muscle cramps; *hypercalcemia*—tremors. **Neuro:** flaccid paralysis, heaviness of legs, paresthesias.

Route/Dosage
Monobasic Potassium Phosphate
PO (Adults and Children >4 yr): 1 g (7.4 mmol) in water 4 times daily.
PO (Children <4 yr): 200 mg (6.4 mmol) in water 4 times daily.

Potassium Phosphates
PO (Adults and Children >4 yr): 1.45 g (8 mmol) 4 times daily.
PO (Children <4 yr): 200 mg (6.4 mmol) phosphorus 4 times daily.
IV (Adults): 10 mmol phosphorus/day as an infusion.
IV (Infants): 1.5–2 mmol phosphorus/day as an infusion.

propantheline
(proe-**pan**-the-leen)
✤ Probanthel, Pro-Banthine

Classification
Therapeutic: antiulcer agents
Pharmacologic: anticholinergics, antimuscarinics

Pregnancy Category C

Indications
Adjunctive therapy in the treatment of peptic ulcer disease. **Unlabeled uses:** Antisecretory or antispasmodic agent.

Contraindications/Precautions
Contraindicated in: Hypersensitivity; Angle-closure glaucoma; Tachycardia secondary to cardiac insufficiency or thyrotoxicosis; Myasthenia gravis.
Use Cautiously in: Geriatric patients or patients of small stature (dosage reduction required); Prostatic hypertrophy; Chronic renal, cardiac, or pulmonary disease; Patients who may have intra-abdominal infections; Geri: Appears on Beers list. Geriatric patients have increased sensitivity to anticholinergics; Pregnancy, lactation, or children (safety not established).

Adverse Reactions/Side Effects
CNS: confusion, dizziness, drowsiness, excitement. **EENT:** blurred vision, mydriasis, photophobia. **CV:** tachycardia, orthostatic hypotension, palpitations. **GI:** constipation, dry mouth. **GU:** urinary hesitancy, urinary retention. **Derm:** rash. **Misc:** decreased sweating.

Route/Dosage
PO (Adults): 15 mg 3 times daily, 30 mg at bedtime.
PO (Geriatric Patients, Patients with Mild Symptoms, or Small Stature): 7.5 mg 3–4 times daily.
PO (Children): 0.375 mg/kg (10 mg/m^2) 4 times daily.

prussian blue (insoluble)
(**prush**-an bloo)
ferric (III) hexacyanoferrate (II), Radiogardase

Classification
Therapeutic: antidotes, radiation protectants
Pharmacologic: insoluble complex

Pregnancy Category C

Indications
Known/suspected internal contamination with thallium or radioactive cesium.

Contraindications/Precautions
Contraindicated in: No known contraindications.
Use Cautiously in: Hepatic impairment (↓ biliary excretion may ↓ effectiveness); ↓ GI motility.

Adverse Reactions/Side Effects
GI: constipation. **F and E:** hypokalemia.

Route/Dosage

PO (Adults): 3 g three times daily continued for a minimum of 30 days, with assessment of internal radioactivity. If radioactivity has decreased, dosage may be reduced to 1–2 g three times daily.
PO (Children 2–12 yr): 1 g three times a day.

riboflavin (rye-boe-flay-vin)
vitamin B_2

Classification
Therapeutic: vitamins
Pharmacologic: water soluble vitamins

Pregnancy Category A

Indications

Treatment and prevention of riboflavin deficiency, which may be associated with poor nutritional status or chronic debilitating illnesses.

Contraindications/Precautions

Contraindicated in: No known contraindications.
Use Cautiously in: No known precautions.

Adverse Reactions/Side Effects

GU: yellow discoloration of urine (large doses only).

Route/Dosage

Treatment of Deficiency
PO (Adults): 5–10 mg/day.

rifapentine (rif-a-pen-teen)
Priftin

Classification
Therapeutic: agents for amyotrophic lateral sclerosis, antituberculars

Pregnancy Category C

Indications

Treatment of pulmonary tuberculosis: Must be used in combination with other agents.

Contraindications/Precautions

Contraindicated in: Hypersensitivity to rifapentine or other rifamycins (rifampin or rifabutin).
Use Cautiously in: History of liver disease; Pregnancy, lactation, or children <12 yr (safety not established)
Exercise Extreme Caution in: Concurrent protease inhibitor therapy.

Adverse Reactions/Side Effects

CNS: dizziness, headache. **Resp:** hemoptysis. **CV:** hypertension. **GI:** PSEUDOMEMBRANOUS COLITIS, anorexia, diarrhea, dyspepsia, increased liver enzymes, nausea, vomiting. **GU:** hematuria, proteinuria, pyuria, urinary casts. **Derm:** acne, pruritus, rash. **Hemat:** anemia, leukopenia, lymphopenia, neutropenia, thrombocytosis. **MS:** arthralgia. **Misc:** pain.

Route/Dosage

Must be used in combination with other antituberculars.
PO (Adults): *Intensive phase*—600 mg twice weekly (not less than 72 hr between doses) for 2 months; *continuation phase*—600 mg once weekly for 4 months.

sodium phosphate
(soe-dee-um foss-fate)

Classification
Therapeutic: mineral and electrolyte replacements/supplements
Pharmacologic: phosphate supplements

Pregnancy Category C

Indications

Treatment and prevention of phosphate depletion in patients who are unable to ingest adequate dietary phosphates.

Contraindications/Precautions

Contraindicated in: Hyperphosphatemia; Hypocalcemia; Severe renal impairment.
Use Cautiously in: Hyperparathyroidism; Cardiac disease; Hypernatremia; Hypertension.

Adverse Reactions/Side Effects

Related to hyperphosphatemia, unless otherwise indicated **CNS:** confusion, listlessness, weakness. **Resp:** *hypernatremia*—shortness of breath. **CV:** ARRHYTHMIAS, CARDIAC ARREST, ECG changes (absent P waves, widening of the QRS complex with biphasic curve), hypotension; *hypernatremia*—edema. **GI:** <u>diarrhea</u>, abdominal pain, nausea, vomiting. **F and E:** hyperkalemia, hypernatremia, hyperphosphatemia, hypocalcemia, hypomagnesemia. **Local:** irritation at IV site, phlebitis. **MS:** *hypocalcemia*—

tremors. **Neuro:** flaccid paralysis, heaviness of legs, paresthesias of extremities.

Route/Dosage

IV (Adults): 12–15 mM phosphorus/liter of parenteral nutrition.
IV (Neonates): 1.5–2 mM/kg/day (infused as part of parenteral nutrition).

stavudine (stav-yoo-deen)
d4T, Zerit, Zerit XR

Classification
Therapeutic: antiretrovirals
Pharmacologic: nucleoside reverse transcriptase inhibitors

Pregnancy Category C

Indications

HIV infection unresponsive or intolerant to conventional therapy.

Contraindications/Precautions

Contraindicated in: Hypersensitivity.
Use Cautiously in: Patients with a history of alcohol abuse; Patients with a history of liver disease or hepatic impairment; Renal impairment (dosage reduction and/or increased dosing interval recommended if CCr <50 ml/min); History of peripheral neuropathy; Pregnancy or lactation (safety not established; breastfeeding should be avoided by HIV-infected mothers because of transmission of the virus in breast milk; concurrent use with didanosine during pregnancy may increase the risk of fetal lactic acidosis).

Adverse Reactions/Side Effects

CNS: headache, insomnia, weakness. **GI:** HEPATIC TOXICITY, PANCREATITIS, anorexia, diarrhea. **F and E:** LACTIC ACIDOSIS. **Hemat:** anemia. **MS:** arthralgia, myalgia. **Neuro:** peripheral neuropathy.

Route/Dosage

PO (Adults ≤60 kg): 40 mg twice daily *or* 100 mg once daily as XR capsules.
PO (Adults <60 kg): 30 mg twice daily *or* 75 mg once daily as XR capsules.
PO (Children at least 14 days old and <30 kg): 1 mg/kg every 12 hr (not to exceed 40 mg q 12 hr).
PO (Infants birth–13 days): 0.5 mg/kg every 12 hr.

Renal Impairment

PO (Adults ≤60 kg): *CCr 26–50 ml/min*—20 mg q 12 hr; *CCr 10–25 ml/min*—20 mg q 24 hr.
PO (Adults <60 kg): *CCr 26–50 ml/min*—15 mg q 12 hr; *CCr 10–25 ml/min*—15 mg q 24 hr.

succimer (sux-i-mer)
Chemet

Classification
Therapeutic: antidotes
Pharmacologic: chelating agents

Pregnancy Category C

Indications

Treatment of lead poisoning in children with blood lead levels >45 mcg/dl.

Contraindications/Precautions

Contraindicated in: Hypersensitivity or allergy to succimer; Lactation (should be discouraged during succimer therapy).
Use Cautiously in: Renal failure (chelates are not dialyzable); Children (increased risk of bradyarrhythmias); Children with skeletal muscle myopathy (more prone to rare, but serious, adverse reactions; Geriatric patients (use lower doses to adjust for decreased renal, hepatic and cardiac function); Pregnancy or children <1 yr (safety not established).

Adverse Reactions/Side Effects

CNS: dizziness, drowsiness, headache. **EENT:** cloudy film in eye, otitis media, plugged ears, watery eyes. **Resp:** cough, nasal congestion, rhinorrhea, sore throat. **CV:** arrhythmias. **GI:** nausea, vomiting, abdominal cramps, anorexia, diarrhea, elevated liver function tests, hemorrhoidal symptoms, metallic taste. **GU:** oliguria, proteinuria, voiding difficulty. **Derm:** mucocutaneous eruptions, pruritus, rashes. **Hemat:** eosinophilia, thrombocytosis. **MS:** back, rib, flank pain, leg pain. **Neuro:** paresthesia, sensorimotor neuropathy. **Misc:** chills, fever, flu-like syndrome, moniliasis.

Route/Dosage

PO (Adults and Children): 10 mg/kg (350 mg/m^2) q 8 hr for 5 days, then reduce to 10 mg/kg (350 mg/m^2) q 12 hr for 2 more wk. Repeated courses should follow a 2-wk rest period.

temozolomide
(te-mo-zole-oh-mide)
Temodar

Classification
Therapeutic: antineoplastics
Pharmacologic: alkylating agents

Pregnancy Category D

Indications
Refractory anaplastic astrocytoma progressing despite treatment with a nitrosurea and procarbazine. Glioblastoma multiforme (with or after radiation).

Contraindications/Precautions
Contraindicated in: Hypersensitivity to temozolomide or dacarbazine (DTIC); OB: Pregnancy or lactation.
Use Cautiously in: Severe hepatic or renal impairment; Geri: Geriatric patients and women (↑ risk of myelosuppression); Active infection; Decreased bone marrow reserve; Other chronic debilitating illness; OB: Patients with childbearing potential; Pedi: Children (safety not established).

Adverse Reactions/Side Effects
CNS: SEIZURES, fatigue, headache, abnormal coordination, anxiety, depression, dizziness, drowsiness, mental status changes, weakness. **EENT:** abnormal vision, diplopia. **Resp:** cough. **CV:** peripheral edema. **GI:** nausea, vomiting, abdominal pain, anorexia, constipation, diarrhea, dysphagia. **Derm:** pruritus, rash. **Endo:** adrenal hypercorticism. **Hemat:** leukopenia, thrombocytopenia, anemia. **Metab:** increased weight. **MS:** abnormal gait, back pain. **Neuro:** hemiparesis, myalgia. **Misc:** breast pain (women), fever, secondary malignancies (rare).

Route/Dosage
PO (Adults): *Anaplastic astrocytoma*—150 mg/m^2/day for 5 consecutive days of each 28-day treatment cycle; doses adjusted on the basis of blood counts; *Glioblastoma multiforme*—75 mg/m^2/day for 42 consecutive days concurrently with radiation initially, then starting 4 wk after last dose, maintenance dose of 150 mg/m^2/day for 5 consecutive days of one 28-day treatment cycle then 200 mg/m^2 for 5 consecutive days of each 28-day treatment cycle for 5 cycles; doses adjusted on the basis of blood counts. Concurrent prophylaxis against *Pneumocystis carnii* pneumonia is required during first 42 days of regimen.

thiethylperazine
(thye-eth-il-**per**-a-zeen)
Norzine, Torecan

Classification
Therapeutic: antiemetics
Pharmacologic: phenothiazines

Pregnancy Category UK

Indications
Management of nausea and vomiting.

Contraindications/Precautions
Contraindicated in: Hypersensitivity; Hypersensitivity to bisulfites (IM); Hypersensitivity to aspirin or tartrazine (tablets); Cross-sensitivity with other phenothiazines may occur; Angle-closure glaucoma; Bone marrow depression; Severe liver or cardiovascular disease; Pregnancy.
Use Cautiously in: Geriatric or debilitated patients (dosage reduction recommended); Diabetes mellitus; Respiratory disease; Prostatic hyperplasia; CNS tumors; Epilepsy; Intestinal obstruction; Children <12 yr or lactation (safety not established).

Adverse Reactions/Side Effects
CNS: NEUROLEPTIC MALIGNANT SYNDROME, sedation, cerebral vascular spasm, extrapyramidal reactions, headache, restlessness, tardive dyskinesia. **EENT:** dry eyes, blurred vision, lens opacities, tinnitus. **CV:** hypotension (following IM use), peripheral edema. **GI:** constipation, dry mouth, altered taste, anorexia, drug-induced hepatitis, ileus. **GU:** urinary retention. **Derm:** photosensitivity, pigment changes, rashes. **Endo:** galactorrhea. **Hemat:** AGRANULOCYTOSIS, leukopenia. **Metab:** hyperthermia. **Neuro:** trigeminal neuralgia. **Misc:** allergic reactions.

Route/Dosage
PO, IM (Adults): 10 mg 1–3 times daily.

tiludronate (tye-**loo**-droe-nate)
Skelid

Classification
Therapeutic: bone resorption inhibitors
Pharmacologic: biphosphonates

Pregnancy Category C

Indications
Management of Paget's disease of the bone in patients with: Serum alkaline phosphatase ≤2 times the upper limit of normal, Symptoms, Risk for complications.

Contraindications/Precautions
Contraindicated in: Hypersensitivity; Severe renal impairment (CCr <30 ml/min).
Use Cautiously in: Pregnancy, lactation, or children <18 yr (safety not established).

Adverse Reactions/Side Effects
CNS: anxiety, drowsiness, fatigue, insomnia, nervousness, syncope, vertigo, weakness. **EENT:** cataracts, conjunctivitis, glaucoma, pharyngitis, rhinitis, sinusitis. **Resp:** bronchitis. **CV:** chest pain, dependent edema, hypertension, peripheral edema. **GI:** abdominal pain, anorexia, constipation, diarrhea, dry mouth, dysphagia, esophageal ulcer, esophagitis, flatulence, gastric ulcer, gastritis, nausea, tooth disorder, vomiting. **GU:** urinary tract infection. **Derm:** flushing, increased sweating, pruritus, rash, skin disorder. **Endo:** hyperparathyroidism. **F and E:** hypocalcemia. **MS:** arthrosis, involuntary muscle contractions, pathological fractures. **Neuro:** paresthesia. **Misc:** infection.

Route/Dosage
PO (Adults): 400 mg/day taken with 8 oz of plain water only, for 3 mo.

tolmetin (tole-met-in)
Tolectin, Tolectin DS, Novo-Tolmetin

Classification
Therapeutic: antirheumatics, nonsteroidal anti-inflammatory agents

Pregnancy Category UK

Indications
Management of inflammatory disorders including: Rheumatoid arthritis, Juvenile rheumatoid arthritis, Osteoarthritis.

Contraindications/Precautions
Contraindicated in: Hypersensitivity; Cross-sensitivity may exist with other NSAIDs, including aspirin; Active GI bleeding or ulcer disease; Peri-operative pain from coronary artery bypass graft (CABG) surgery.
Use Cautiously in: Cardiovascular disease or risk factors for cardiovascular disease (may ↑ risk of serious cardiovascular thrombotic events, myocardial infarction, and stroke, especially with prolonged use); Severe renal, or hepatic disease; History of ulcer disease; Severe hepatic or renal impairment (dosage reduction recommended); Geri: Geriatric patients (↑ risk of GI bleeding; OB, Pedi: Pregnancy and lactation (safety not established; avoid use during 2nd and 3rd trimesters).

Adverse Reactions/Side Effects
CNS: dizziness, headache, drowsiness, mental depression, sleep disturbances. **EENT:** tinnitus, visual disturbances. **CV:** edema, hypertension. **GI:** DRUG-INDUCED HEPATITIS, GI BLEEDING, diarrhea, discomfort, dyspepsia, nausea, vomiting, constipation, flatulence. **GU:** renal failure. **Derm:** EXFOLIATIVE DERMATITIS, STEVENS-JOHNSON SYNDROME, TOXIC EPIDERMAL NECROLYSIS, rashes. **Hemat:** prolonged bleeding time. **MS:** muscle weakness. **Misc:** allergic reactions including ANAPHYLAXIS.

Route/Dosage
PO (Adults): 400 mg 3 times daily initially, followed by maintenance dose of 600–1800 mg/day in 3–4 divided doses (not to exceed 2000 mg/day).
PO (Children >2 yr): 20 mg/kg/day in 3–4 divided doses initially, followed by maintenance dose of 15–30 mg/kg/day in 3–4 divided doses.

toremifene (tore-em-i-feen)
Fareston

Classification
Therapeutic: antineoplastics
Pharmacologic: antiestrogens

Pregnancy Category D

Indications
Management of metastatic breast cancer in postmenopausal women with estrogen receptor–positive or unknown tumors.

Contraindications/Precautions
Contraindicated in: Hypersensitivity; Pregnancy or lactation; History of thromboembolic disease.
Use Cautiously in: Bone metastases (increased risk of hypercalcemia); Pre-existing endometrial hyperplasia (long-term treatment should be avoided).

Adverse Reactions/Side Effects
CNS: depression, dizziness, headache, lethargy. **EENT:** blurred vision, cataracts, corneal keratopathy, dry eyes, glaucoma. **CV:** CHF, MI, PULMO-

NARY EMBOLISM, angina, arrhythmias, edema, thrombophlebitis. **GI:** nausea, elevated liver enzymes, vomiting. **GU:** vaginal discharge, vaginal bleeding. **Derm:** sweating. **F and E:** hypercalcemia. **Hemat:** anemia. **Misc:** hot flashes, tumor flare.

Route/Dosage

PO (Adults): 60 mg once daily.

trifluoperazine

(trye-floo-oh-**pair**-a-zeen)
✤Apo-Trifluoperazine, ✤Novo-Flurazine, ✤PMS-Trifluoperazine, ✤Solazine, Stelazine, ✤Terfluzine

Classification
Therapeutic: antipsychotics (conventional)
Pharmacologic: phenothiazines

Pregnancy Category C

Indications

Schizpophrenia, nonpsychotic anxiety. Considered second-line treatment after failure with atypical antipsychotics. **Unlabeled uses:** Other psychotic disorders; bipolar disorder.

Contraindications/Precautions

Contraindicated in: Hypersensitivity; Cross-sensitivity with other phenothiazines may exist; Hypersensitivity to bisulfites (oral concentrate only); Angle-closure glaucoma; Bone marrow depression; Severe liver or cardiovascular disease; Lactation: Discontinue drug or bottle feed.
Use Cautiously in: Geriatric or debilitated patients (dosage reduction recommended); Pregnancy or lactation (safety not established; may cause adverse effects in the newborn); Diabetes mellitus; Respiratory disease; Prostatic hyperplasia; CNS tumors; Epilepsy; Intestinal obstruction.

Adverse Reactions/Side Effects

CNS: NEUROLEPTIC MALIGNANT SYNDROME, extrapyramidal reactions, sedation, tardive dyskinesia. **EENT:** dry eyes, blurred vision, lens opacities. **CV:** hypotension, tachycardia. **GI:** constipation, anorexia, dry mouth, hepatitis, ileus. **GU:** urinary retention, priapism. **Derm:** photosensitivity, pigment changes, rashes. **Endo:** galactorrhea, amenorrhea. **Hemat:** AGRANULOCYTOSIS, leukopenia. **Metab:** hyperthermia. **Misc:** allergic reactions.

Route/Dosage

PO (Adults): *Psychoses*—2–5 mg 1–2 times daily (up to 40 mg/day). *Anxiety*—1–2 mg bid (not to exceed 6 mg/day or treatment longer than 12 wk).
PO (Children 6–12 yr): 1 mg once or twice daily (up to 15 mg/day).
IM (Adults): 1–2 mg q 4–6 hr (up to 10 mg/day).
IM (Children): 1 mg once or twice daily.

trihexyphenidyl

(trye-hex-ee-**fen**-i-dill)
✤Apo-Trihex, Artane, ✤PMS-Trihexyphenidyl, Trihexane, Trihexy

Classification
Therapeutic: antiparkinson agents
Pharmacologic: anticholinergics

Pregnancy Category C

Indications

Adjunct in the management of parkinsonian syndrome of many causes, including drug-induced parkinsonism.

Contraindications/Precautions

Contraindicated in: Hypersensitivity; Angle-closure glaucoma; Acute hemorrhage; Tachycardia secondary to cardiac insufficiency; Thyrotoxicosis; Known alcohol intolerance (elixir only).
Use Cautiously in: Geriatric and very young patients (increased risk of adverse reactions); Intestinal obstruction or infection; Prostatic hyperplasia; Chronic renal, hepatic, pulmonary, or cardiac disease; Pregnancy, lactation, or children (safety not established).

Adverse Reactions/Side Effects

CNS: dizziness, nervousness, confusion, drowsiness, headache, psychoses, weakness. **EENT:** blurred vision, mydriasis. **CV:** orthostatic hypotension, tachycardia. **GI:** dry mouth, nausea, constipation, vomiting. **GU:** urinary hesitancy, urinary retention. **Derm:** decreased sweating.

Route/Dosage

PO (Adults): 1–2 mg/day initially; increase by 2 mg q 3–5 days. Usual maintenance dose is 6–10 mg/day in 3 divided doses (up to 15 mg/day). Extended-release (Artane Sequels) preparations may be given q 12 hr after daily dose has

✤= Canadian drug name.
* CAPITALS indicates life-threatening; underlines indicate most frequent.

LESS COMMONLY USED DRUGS

been determined using conventional tablets or liquid.

triptorelin (trip-to-**rel**-in)
Trelstar Depot

Classification
Therapeutic: antineoplastics
Pharmacologic: hormones

Pregnancy Category X

Indications
Palliative treatment of advanced prostate cancer when orchiectomy or estrogen administration are contraindicated or unacceptable.

Contraindications/Precautions
Contraindicated in: Hypersensitivity to triptorelin or similar agents; Pregnancy, lactation, or children.
Use Cautiously in: Metastatic vertebral lesions and/or upper or lower urinary tract obstruction (symptoms may transiently worsen following initiation of therapy); Renal or hepatic impairment (may need dosage adjustment).

Adverse Reactions/Side Effects
CNS: dizziness, emotional lability, fatigue, headache, insomnia. **CV:** hypertension. **GI:** diarrhea, vomiting. **GU:** erectile dysfunction, urinary retention, urinary tract infection. **Derm:** pruritus. **Hemat:** anemia. **Local:** injection site pain. **MS:** musculoskeletal pain. **Misc:** allergic reactions including ANAPHYLAXIS and ANGIOEDEMA.

Route/Dosage
IM (Adults): 3.75 mg monthly.

verteporfin (ver-te-**por**-fin)
Visudyne

Classification
Therapeutic: none assigned
Pharmacologic: photodynamic agents

Pregnancy Category C

Indications
Treatment of age-related macular degeneration in patients with predominantly classic subfoveal choroidal neovascularization.

Contraindications/Precautions
Contraindicated in: Hypersensitivity; Porphyria; Exposure to direct sunlight.
Use Cautiously in: Moderate/severe hepatic impairment; Pregnancy, lactation or children (safety not established).

Adverse Reactions/Side Effects
CNS: headache, weakness. **EENT:** visual disturbances, cataracts, conjunctivitis/conjunctival injection, dry eyes, ocular itching, severe vision loss, subconjunctival/subretinal/vitreous hemorrhage. **Derm:** photosensitivity. **Local:** injection site reactions including extravasation and rashes. **MS:** back pain (during infusion). **Misc:** fever, flu-like syndrome.

Route/Dosage
IV (Adults): 6 mg/m^2 infused over 10 min, followed by appropriate laser light delivery initiated 15 min after the start of the infusion.

zileuton (zye-**loo**-ton)
Zyflo, Zyflo CR

Classification
Therapeutic: bronchodilators
Pharmacologic: leukotriene antagonists

Pregnancy Category C

Indications
Long-term control agent in the management of asthma.

Contraindications/Precautions
Contraindicated in: Hypersensitivity; Active liver disease or transaminases ≤3 times upper limit of normal.
Use Cautiously in: Acute attacks of asthma; History of liver disease or alcohol consumption; OB, Pedi: Pregnancy, lactation, or children <12 yr (safety not established).

Adverse Reactions/Side Effects
CNS: headache, dizziness, insomnia, malaise, nervousness, somnolence, weakness. **EENT:** conjunctivitis. **CV:** chest pain. **GI:** abdominal pain, constipation, dyspepsia, flatulence, increased liver enzymes, nausea, vomiting. **GU:** urinary tract infection, vaginitis. **Derm:** pruritus. **MS:** arthralgia, myalgia, neck pain. **Neuro:** hypertonia. **Misc:** fever, lymphadenopathy.

Route/Dosage
PO (Adults and Children ≤12 yr): 600 mg 4 times daily or two 600-mg *extended release tablets* twice daily.

Natural/Herbal Products

The following monographs introduce some commonly used natural products. Because the amounts of active ingredients in these agents are not standardized or currently subject to FDA guidelines for medicines, *Davis's Drug Guide for Nurses*, although respectful of patients' right to choose from a variety of therapeutic options, does not endorse their routine use unless supervised by a knowledgeable health care professional. Users should take into account the possibility of adverse reactions and interactions and consider the relative lack of data supporting widespread use of these products. Doses are poorly standardized, and individuals are advised to read package labels carefully to ensure safe and efficacious use.

arnica (ar-ni-cuh)

Other Name(s):
leopard's bane, mountain tobacco, mountain snuff, wolf's bane

Classification
Therapeutic: anti-infectives

Common Uses
Topical treatment of insect bites, bruises, acne, boils, sprains, muscle, and joint pain.

Action
Polysaccarides in arnica may produce a slight anti-inflammatory and analgesic effect. Some antibacterial effects are seen, in addition to a counterirritant effect, which may aid in wound healing.

Pharmacokinetics
Absorption: Systemic absorption may occur following topical application to broken skin.
Distribution: Unknown.
Metabolism and Excretion: Unknown.
Half-life: Unknown.

TIME/ACTION PROFILE

ROUTE	ONSET	PEAK	DURATION
topical	unknown	unknown	unknown

Contraindications/Precautions
Contraindicated in: Not for oral use (except in highly diluted homeopathic preparations); Do not apply to open wounds; Arnica allergy; Avoid use on broken skin; Infectious or inflammatory GI conditions.

Adverse Reactions/Side Effects
Derm: edematous dermatitis with pustules (chronic treatment of damaged skin), eczema (prolonged use). **Misc:** local allergic reactions.

Interactions
Natural Product-Drug: Alcohol-containing preparations may interact with **disulfuram** and **metronidazole**. Potential for reduced effectiveness of **antihypertensives** has been noted. May potentiate the effects of **anticoagulants** and **antiplatelet agents**, increasing the risk of bleeding.

Route/Commonly Used Doses
Topical (Adults): *Topical*—rub or massage arnica tincture, cream or gel onto injured area, only if skin isn't broken; *compress*—dilute 1 tablespoon of arnica tincture in 1/2 L water. Wet a gauze pad with solution and apply to affected area for 15 minutes. For use in poultices, dilute tincture 3 to 10 times with water.

Availability
Cream, tincture, salve, ointment, gel and oil^OTC; Topical (preparations should contain not more than 20-25% arnica tincture or 15% arnica oil)^OTC; Homeopathic preparations^OTC.

NURSING IMPLICATIONS

Assessment
- Inspect skin for breaks prior to application to ensure arnica is applied only to an intact surface. Note the size, character, and location of affected area prior to application of arnica.
- After application, assess the affected area for signs of allergic response.
- ***Toxicity and Overdose:*** Systemic absorption may result in nausea, vomiting, organ damage, hypertension, cardiotoxicity, arrhythmias, muscular weakness, collapse, vertigo, renal dysfunction, coma and death. If ingested orally, induce emesis and gastric la-

vage to remove undigested contents. Supportive care may be necessary. Do not take orally or apply to nonintact skin to avoid systemic absorption.

Potential Nursing Diagnosis

Acute pain (Indications)

Implementation

- Clean skin with a nonalcohol containing cleanser prior to applying arnica. Apply topically to affected area, or site of injury ensuring skin is intact.
- Do not take orally or apply to an open wound because of potential for systemic absorption with toxicity.
- Avoid prolonged topical use because of potential for allergic hypersensitiviy reaction.

Patient/Family Teaching

- Teach patients to inspect the affected area for breaks in the skin and not to apply arnica to any areas where the skin is broken.
- Warn patients that use on nonintact skin and oral ingestion may cause life-threatening toxicity.
- Inform patients that although the German Commission E has found this herbal supplement to be an effective anti-inflammatory, analgesic and antibacterial agent, FDA has classified arnica as an **unsafe herb.**
- Advise patients that arnica should only be used for short period of time in the treatment of minor aches and pains associated with local muscle, joint or skin pain. Prolonged use may cause allergic/hypersensitivity reactions to develop.
- Instruct patients taking antihypertensive agents to avoid concurrent use of arnica.

Evaluation

- Relief of, or improvement in, minor aches and pains associated with muscle or joint overuse, or sprains and/or local skin irritation from insect bites, bruises, boils, or acne.

black cohosh

(blak **coe**-hosh)

Other Name(s):
baneberry, black snakeroot, bugbane, phytoestrogen, rattle root, rattleweed, rattle top, squawroot

Classification
Therapeutic: none assigned

Do not confuse black cohosh with blue or white cohosh

Common Uses

Management of menopausal symptoms. Premenstrual discomfort. Dysmenorrhea. Mild sedative.

Action

Therapeutic effects are produced by glycosides isolated from the fresh or dried rhizome with attached roots. Mechanism of action is unclear. **Therapeutic Effects:** May decrease symptoms of menopause, including hot flashes, sweating, sleep disturbance, and anxiety. Has no effect on vaginal epithelium. Black cohosh use may be unsafe in women with a history of breast cancer, as it may increase the risk of metastasis.

Pharmacokinetics

Absorption: Unknown.
Distribution: Unknown.
Metabolism and Excretion: Unknown.
Half-life: Unknown.

TIME/ACTION PROFILE

ROUTE	ONSET	PEAK	DURATION
PO	unknown	unknown	unknown

Contraindications/Precautions

Contraindicated in: Pregnancy and lactation.
Use Cautiously in: Not studied in combination with hormonal therapies; Not studied in patients with hormone-dependent cancers (e.g., breast, endometrial, ovarian cancer); Longer than 6 mo use; Alcohol containing preparations should be used cautiously in patients with known intolerance or liver disease.

Adverse Reactions/Side Effects

Neuro: SEIZURES (in combination with evening primrose and chasteberry), headache, dizziness. **GI:** GI upset. **Derm:** rash. **Misc:** weight gain, cramping.

Interactions

Natural Product-Drug: Unknown effects when combined with hormone replacement therapy and **antiestrogens** (e.g., **tamoxifen**). Concurrent use with **hepatotoxic drugs** may increase the risk of liver damage. **Alcohol**-containing preparations may interact with **disulfiram** and **metronidazole**. May decrease the cytotoxic effects of **cisplatin**. May precipitate

*CAPITALS indicates life-threatening; underlines indicate most frequent.

hypotension when used in combination with **antihypertensives**.

Route/Commonly Used Doses

PO (Adults): *Tablets (Remifemin®)*—20 mg bid. *Liquid extract*—0.3–2 ml bid-tid. *Tincture*—2–4 ml bid–tid. *Dried rhizome*—0.3–2 g tid. Do not use for more than 6 mo.

Availability

Alone or in combination with other herbal medicinals[OTC]**; Tablets**[OTC] **(Remifemin® 20 mg [best studied black cohosh product]); Liquid extract**[OTC] **(1:1 in 90% alcohol); Tincture**[OTC] **(1:10 in 60% alcohol); Dried rhizome.**

NURSING IMPLICATIONS

Assessment

- Assess frequency and severity of menopausal symptoms.
- Monitor blood pressure for patients on antihypertensive drugs because it may increase effects of drugs and cause hypotension.
- Assess for nausea and vomiting.
- Assess for history of seizures, liver disease, and alcohol intake.
- Assess patients with irregular periods for pregnancy prior to taking this drug because large doses of black cohosh may induce a miscarriage.

Potential Nursing Diagnosis

Sleep deprivation (Indications)

Implementation

- Administration with food may help to minimize nausea.

Patient/Family Teaching

- Instruct patient that this herbal supplement should not be taken if pregnant because it may induce a miscarriage.
- Tell patient that if she suspects she is pregnant to stop taking the medication and to contact her healthcare provider.
- May potentiate antihypertensive drugs with consequent hypotension. Warn patients on antihypertensive drugs not to take this herbal supplement without consulting their health care provider.
- Patients with seizures, liver dysfunction, excessive alcohol intake, cancer, or other medical problems should be advised to consult their health care provider prior to initiating self-therapy with this herb.
- If nausea becomes a problem, advise patients to take herbal supplement on a full stomach.
- Advise patient that this herbal supplement should not be taken with other estrogen replacements without seeking the advice of her health care provider.
- Emphasize the importance of continued medical supervision for Pap smears, mammograms, pelvic examinations, and blood pressure monitoring at the intervals indicated by health care provider.

Evaluation

- Resolution of menopausal vasomotor symptoms.

chondroitin (konn-**droy**-tinn)

Other Name(s):
chondroitin polysulfate, CPS, CDS

Classification
Therapeutic: nonopioid analgesics

Common Uses

Osteoarthritis. Ischemic heart disease. Hyperlipidemia. Osteoporosis. Topically, in combination with sodium hyaluronate, in the eye as a surgical aid in cataract extraction or lens implantation, and to lubricate dry eyes.

Action

May serve as a building block of articular cartilage. May protect cartilage against degradation. May have antiatherogenic properties. **Therapeutic Effects:** Improvement in osteoarthritis symptoms.

Pharmacokinetics

Absorption: Unknown.
Distribution: Unknown.
Metabolism and Excretion: Unknown.
Half-life: Unknown.

TIME/ACTION PROFILE

ROUTE	ONSET	PEAK	DURATION
PO	unknown	unknown	unknown

Contraindications/Precautions

Contraindicated in: Pregnancy and lactation.
Use Cautiously in: Asthma (may exacerbate symptoms); Clotting disorders (may increase risk of bleeding); Prostate cancer (may increase risk of metastasis or recurrence).

NATURAL/HERBAL PRODUCTS

Adverse Reactions/Side Effects

GI: heartburn, nausea, diarrhea. **Hemat:** bleeding (antiplatelet effect). **Misc:** allergic reactions, edema, hair loss.

Interactions

Natural Product-Drug: Use of chondroitin with **anticoagulant** and **antiplatelet** drugs, **thrombolytics**, **NSAIDs**, some **cephalosporins**, and **valproates** may increase risk of bleeding. **Herbs with anticoagulant or antiplatelet properties may increase bleeding risk when combined with chondroitin, including: anise, arnica, chamomile, clove, dong quai, fenugreek, feverfew, ginger, ginkgo, Panax ginseng, licorice, and others.**

Route/Commonly Used Doses

PO (Adults): *Osteoarthritis*—200–400 mg 2–3 times daily or 1000–1200 mg once daily. *Prevention of recurrent myocardial infarction*—10 grams daily in 3 divided doses for 3 months.

IM: (Adults): *Osteoarthritis*—50 mg twice weekly for 8 weeks every 4 months.

Availability

Tablets[OTC]**; Capsules**[OTC]**; Injection (not available in US); Ophthalmic Drops Rx in combination with sodium hyaluronate (Viscoat).**

NURSING IMPLICATIONS

Assessment

- Evaluate drug profile before starting therapy with this herbal supplement. If the patient is taking anticoagulants or antiplatelet drugs, avoid use of this herb.
- Monitor pain (type, location and intensity) and range of motion on an ongoing basis as an indicator of drug efficacy.
- Evaluate gastric discomfort and instruct patient to seek out the advice of a health care provider if persistent gastric discomfort occurs.
- Assess for signs of bleeding and discontinue herbal supplement promptly and seek out healthcare professional for follow up.

Potential Nursing Diagnosis

Acute pain (Indications)
Impaired physical mobility (Indications)

Implementation

- Take with food.

Patient/Family Teaching

- Advise patients that this herbal supplement is usually taken with glucosamine.
- Caution patients who take aspirin or NSAIDs or other nonprescription medications not to take this herbal supplement without conferring with their health care provider.
- Warn women taking this herbal supplement to stop it if they suspect they are pregnant, and not to use it if they are breast feeding.
- Instruct patients that this medication works by building up cartilage and that this requires that the medication be taken consistently over a period of time. It is not recommended as a supplemental pain medication.

Evaluation

- Improvement in pain and range of motion.
- Reduced need for supplemental or breakthrough pain medication.

Crataegus Species, see **hawthorn**.

dong quai (don kwi)

Other Name(s):
Angelica sinensis, Chinese Angelica, Dang Gui, Danggui, Dong Qua, Ligustilides, Phytoestrogen, Radix angelicae gigantis, Tang Kuei, Tan Kue Bai Zhi

Classification
Therapeutic: none assigned

Common Uses

Menstrual cramps, menstrual irregularity, menopausal symptoms. Various uses as a blood purifier. Topically in combination with other ingredients for premature ejaculation.

Action

May have vasodilating and antispasmodic properties. Binds to estrogen receptors. **Therapeutic Effects:** Improved ejaculatory latency.

Pharmacokinetics

Absorption: Unknown.
Distribution: Unknown.
Metabolism and Excretion: Unknown.
Half-life: Unknown.

TIME/ACTION PROFILE

ROUTE	ONSET	PEAK	DURATION
PO	unknown	unknown	unknown

Contraindications/Precautions

Contraindicated in: Pregnancy and lactation.
Use Cautiously in: Hormone sensitive cancers and conditions (may exacerbate effects or stimulate growth of cancer cells).

Adverse Reactions/Side Effects

Derm: photosensitivity. **Misc:** Some constituents are carcinogenic and mutagenic.

Interactions

Natural Product-Drug: Alcohol -containing preparations may interact with **disulfiram** and **metronidazole**. Use of dong quai with **anticoagulant** and **antiplatelet** drugs, **thrombolytics**, **NSAIDs**, some **cephalosporins**, and **valproates** may increase risk of bleeding. **Herbs with antiplatelet or anticoagulant properties may increase bleeding risk when combined with dong quai including: angelica, clove, danshen, garlic, ginger, ginkgo, panax ginseng, and willow.**

Route/Commonly Used Doses

PO (Adults): *Bulk herb*—3–4.5 g per day in divided doses with meals; *extract*—1 ml (20–40 drops) three times daily.

Availability

Bulk herb[OTC]**; Extract**[OTC].

NURSING IMPLICATIONS

Assessment

- Assess pain and menstrual patterns prior to and following menstrual cycle to determine effectiveness of this herbal supplement.
- Assess for pregnancy prior to recommending use of the herbal supplement and warn women not to take this herb if pregnancy is suspected.
- Assess for history of hormone sensitive cancers or conditions and warn against use.
- Assess medication profile including prescription and over the counter use of products such as aspirin and ibuprofen based products to treat menstrual pain.

Potential Nursing Diagnosis

Acute pain (Indications)
Deficient knowledge, related to medication regimen (Patient/Family Teaching)

Implementation

- Take with meals.

Patient/Family Teaching

- Warn patients not to take this medication if pregnant or breastfeeding.
- Inform patients to avoid use of aspirin or other NSAIDs concurrently because of the risk of bleeding.
- Notify patients that there are no studies supporting the use of this herbal supplement for treatment of menopausal symptoms.
- Tell patients to consult their health care provider if taking prescription medications before taking Dong Quai.
- Discontinue the herbal supplement if diarrhea or excessive bleeding occurs and contact a health care provider if symptoms do not resolve.
- Instruct patients that photosensitivity may occur and to wear sun screen and protective clothing if sun exposure is anticipated.

Evaluation

- Reduction in menstrual pain and cramping and regular periods with normal flow.

echinacea (Echinacea Purpurea) (ek-i-**nay**-sha)

Other Name(s):
American coneflower, black sampson, black susans, brauneria angustifolia, kansas snakeroot, purple coneflower, red sunflower, rudbeckia, sampson root, scurvy root

Classification
Therapeutic: anti-infectives, antipyretics

Common Uses

Bacterial and viral infections. Prevention and treatment of colds, coughs, flu, and bronchitis. Fevers. Wounds and burns. Inflammation of the mouth and pharynx. Urinary tract infections. Yeast infections.

Action

Medicinal parts derived from the roots, leaves, or whole plant of perennial herb (Echinacea). *Echinacea purpurea herba* has been reported to promote wound healing, which may be due to an increase in white blood cells, spleen cells, and increased activity of granulocytes, as well as an increase in helper T cells and cytokines. *E. purpurea radix* has been shown to have antibacterial, antiviral, anti-inflammatory, and immune-modulating effects. **Therapeutic Effects:** Resolution respiratory and urinary tract infections. Decreased duration and intensity of common cold. Improved wound healing. Stimulates phagocytosis; inhibits action of hyaluronidase (secreted by bacteria), which helps bacteria gain access to healthy cells. Externally, has antifungal and bacteriostatic properties.

Pharmacokinetics

Absorption: Unknown.
Distribution: Unknown.
Metabolism and Excretion: Unknown.
Half-life: Unknown.

TIME/ACTION PROFILE

ROUTE	ONSET	PEAK	DURATION
PO	unknown	unknown	unknown

Contraindications/Precautions

Contraindicated in: Multiple sclerosis, leukosis, collagenoses, AIDS, tuberculosis, auto-immune diseases; Hypersensitivity and cross-sensitivity in patients allergic to plants in Asteraceae/Compositae plant family (daisies, chrysanthemums, marigolds, etc.); Pregnancy and lactation.
Use Cautiously in: Diabetes; Tinctures should be used cautiously in alcoholics or patients with liver disease; Do not take longer than 8 wk—may suppress immune function.

Adverse Reactions/Side Effects

CNS: dizziness, fatigue, headache, somnolence. **EENT:** tingling sensation on tongue, sore throat. **GI:** nausea, vomiting, heartburn, constipation, abdominal pain, diarrhea. **Derm:** allergic reaction, rash (more common in children). **Misc:** fever.

Interactions

Natural Product-Drug: May possibly interfere with **immunosuppressants** because of its immunostimulant activity. **Anabolic steroids, methotrexate**, or **ketoconazole** may interact with echinacea. May increase **midazolam** availability.

Route/Commonly Used Doses

PO (Adults): *Tablets* -6.78 mg tablets, take 2 tabs 3 times daily. *Fluid extract*—1–2 ml tid; solid form (6.5:1)—150–300 mg tid. Should not be used for more than 8 wk at a time. *Tea*—1/2 tsp comminuted drug, steeped and strained after 10 min, 1 cup 5–6 times daily on the first day, titrating down to 1 cup daily over the next 5 days. *Echinacea purpuren herb juice*—6-9 ml/day. *Liquid*—20 drops every 2 hr for the first day of symptoms, then 3 times daily for up to 10 days.
Topical: (Adults): *Ointment, lotion, tincture used externally*—1.5–7.5 ml tincture, 2–5 g dried root.

Availability

Capsules[OTC]: 300 mg. **Tablets OTC:** 6.78 mg of crude extract. **Dried Root**[OTC]: The dried root can be steeped and strained in boiling water and taken as a tea. **Liquid extract**[OTC]: 1:1 in 45% alcohol. **Tincture**[OTC]: 1:5 in 45% alcohol. **Blended teas**[OTC]**; Echinacea purpuren herb juice**[OTC].

NURSING IMPLICATIONS

Assessment

- Assess wound for size, appearance, and drainage prior to the start of and periodically during therapy.
- Assess frequency of common mild illnesses (such as a cold) in response to use of this herb.

Potential Nursing Diagnosis

Impaired skin integrity (Indications)

Implementation

- Tinctures may contain significant concentrations of alcohol and may not be suitable for children, alcoholics, patients with liver disease, or those taking disulfiram, metronidazole, some cephalosporins, or sulfonylurea oral antidiabetic agents.
- Prolonged use of this agent may cause overstimulation of the immune system, and use beyond 8 wk is not recommended. Therapy of 10–14 days is usually considered sufficient.
- May be taken without regard to food.

Patient/Family Teaching

- Herb is more effective for treatment than prevention of colds. Take at first sign of symptoms.
- Advise patient to seek immediate treatment for an illness that does not improve after taking this herb.
- Instruct patient that the usual course of therapy is 10–14 days and 8 wk is the maximum.
- Inform patient that use of this herb is not recommended in severe illnesses (e.g., AIDS, tu-

berculosis) or autoimmune diseases (e.g., multiple sclerosis, collagen diseases, etc.)
- Caution patient that prolonged use of this herb may result in overstimulation of the immune system, possibly with subsequent immunosuppression.
- Warn pregnant or breastfeeding women not to use this herb.
- Instruct patient to consult health care professional before taking any prescription or OTC medications concurrently with echinacea.
- Keep tincture in a dark bottle away from sunlight. Should be taken several times a day.
- Store herb in airtight container away from sunlight.

Evaluation
- Improved wound healing.
- Infrequent common illnesses.
- Illnesses of shorter duration and less severity.

feverfew (fee-vurr-fyoo)

Other Name(s):
Altamisa, Bachelor's Button, Chrysanthemum parethenium, Featerfoiul, Featherfew, Featherfoil, Flirtwort Midsummer Daisy, Pyrethrum parthenium, Santa Maria, Tanaceti parthenii, Wild chamomile, Wild quinine

Classification
Therapeutic: vascular headache suppressants

Common Uses
PO: Migraine headache prophylaxis. **Topical:** Toothaches and as a antiseptic.

Action
The sesquiterpene lactone, parthenolide, may provide feverfew's migraine prophylaxis effects. Feverfew may also have antiplatelet and vasodilatory effects and block prostaglandin synthesis. **Therapeutic Effects:** May reduce the symptoms and frequency of migraine headaches.

Pharmacokinetics
Absorption: Unknown.
Distribution: Unknown.
Metabolism and Excretion: Unknown.
Half-life: Unknown.

TIME/ACTION PROFILE

ROUTE	ONSET	PEAK	DURATION
PO	2–4 mo	unknown	unknown

Contraindications/Precautions
Contraindicated in: Pregnancy and lactation; Feverfew hypersensitivity or allergy to Asteraceae/Compositae family plants, including ragweed, chrysanthemums, daisies and marigolds.
Use Cautiously in: Use >4 months (safety and efficacy not established).

Adverse Reactions/Side Effects
CNS: "Post-Feverfew Syndrome" (anxiety, headache, insomnia, muscle and joint aches). **CV:** *with long-term use*— tachycardia. **GI:** nausea, vomiting, diarrhea, heartburn, mouth ulceration and soreness. **Derm:** contact dermatitis (when used topically).

Interactions
Natural Product-Drug: Use of feverfew with **anticoagulant** and **antiplatelet** drugs, **thrombolytics**, **NSAIDs**, some **cephalosporins**, and **valproates** may increase risk of bleeding. Concomitant use with **NSAIDs** may also reduce feverfew effectiveness. Use with **anise, arnica, chamomile, clove, dong quai, fenugreek, garlic, ginger, gingko, licorice and Panax ginseng may increase anticoagulant potential of feverfew.**

Route/Commonly Used Doses
PO (Adults): 50–100 mg feverfew extract daily (standardized to 0.2–0.35% parthenolide) or 50–125 mg freeze-dried leaf daily with or after food.

Availability
Feverfew extract[OTC]: standardized to 0.2-0.35% parthenolide. **Freash leaf**[OTC]**; Freeze-dried leaf**[OTC].

NURSING IMPLICATIONS

Assessment
- Monitor frequency, intensity and duration of migraine headaches prior to and during ongoing therapy.
- Assess for mouth ulcers or skin ulcerations during therapy.

Potential Nursing Diagnosis
Acute pain (Indications)
Deficient knowledge, related to medication regimen (Patient/Family Teaching)

Implementation

- Take with food or on a full stomach.

Patient/Family Teaching

- Instruct patients to take this medication on a consistent basis to prevent migraine headaches. This herbal supplement is not for treatment of migraines.
- Warn patients about mouth ulcers and sores and that if this occurs to seek the advice of a healthcare professional. Encourage proper oral hygiene.
- Advise patients not to abruptly stop this product because of the possibility of post- feverfew syndrome. Tell patients that anxiety, headache, insomnia and muscle aches may indicate withdrawal. Feverfew should be gradually tapered.
- Review dietary and medication profile of patient to identify potential interactions. Instruct patient about other herbs that may interact with feverfew.
- Counsel patients on anticoagulants not to take feverfew except as directed by their healthcare provider.
- Advise patients to avoid using NSAIDs as this may reduce the effectiveness of feverfew.
- Instruct patients to look for signs of bleeding such as unusual bruising or inability to clot after a cut and to seek the advice of a healthcare professional if this occurs.
- Inform patients that feverfew should reduce the number of migraines and severity of symptoms but that duration of the migraine may not be affected.

Evaluation

- Reduction in the frequency and severity of migraine headaches.

garlic (gar-lik)

Other Name(s):
Alli sativa bulbus, Allium sativum

Classification
Therapeutic: lipid-lowering agents

Common Uses

PO: Hypertension, hyperlipidemia, cardiovascular disease prevention, colorectal and gastric cancer prevention. **Topical:** Dermal fungal infections.

Action

May have HMG-CoA inhibitor properties in lowering cholesterol, but less effectively than statin drugs; vasodilatory and antiplatelet properties.

Pharmacokinetics

Absorption: Garlic oil is well absorbed.
Distribution: Unknown.
Metabolism and Excretion: Kidney and lungs.
Half-life: Unknown.

TIME/ACTION PROFILE

ROUTE	ONSET	PEAK	DURATION
PO	4–25 wk	unknown	unknown

Contraindications/Precautions

Contraindicated in: Bleeding disorders; Discontinue use 1-2 weeks prior to surgery.
Use Cautiously in: Diabetes, gastrointestinal infection or inflammation.

Adverse Reactions/Side Effects

CNS: dizziness. **GI:** Irritation of the mouth, esophagus, and stomach, nausea, bad breath, vomiting. **Derm:** Contact dermatitis and other allergic reactions (asthma, rash, anaphylaxis [rare]), Diaphoresis. **Hemat:** Chronic use or excessive dosage may lead to decreased hemoglobin production and lysis of RBCs, platelet dysfunction, prolonged bleeding time. **Misc:** body odor.

Interactions

Natural Product-Drug: Use of garlic with **anticoagulants, antiplatelet agents** and **thrombolytics** may increase risk of bleeding. May decrease the effectiveness of **contraceptive drugs** and **cyclosporine**. May decrease plasma concentrations of **saquinavir, nevirapine, delavirdine**, and **efavirenz**. Herbs with anticoagulant or antiplatelet properties may increase bleeding risk when combined with garlic, including: **angelica, anise, asafoetida, bogbean, boldo, capsicum, celery, chamomile, clove, danshen, dong quai, fenugreek, feverfew, ginger, ginkgo, Panax ginseng, horse chestnut, horseradish, licorice, meadowsweet, prickly ash, onion, papain, passionflower, poplar, quassia, red clover, turmeric, wild carrot, wild lettuce, willow, and others.**

Route/Commonly Used Doses

PO (Adults): 200–400 mg tid of standardized garlic powder extract with 1.3% allin. *Fresh garlic*—1–7 cloves per day.
Topical: (Adults): *Tinea infections*—0.4% cream, 0.6% gel, or 1% gel applied bid × 7 days.

Availability
Capsules^{OTC}; Tablets^{OTC}; Fresh garlic^{OTC}.

NURSING IMPLICATIONS

Assessment
- Elicit from patients their usual dietary intake especially in regard to fat consumption.
- Assess patient's reason for using this herbal remedy and knowledge about hyperlipidemia.
- Ascertain the amount of garlic the patient consumes on a regular basis.

Potential Nursing Diagnosis
Deficient knowledge, related to medication regimen (Patient/Family Teaching)
Noncompliance (Patient/Family Teaching)

Implementation
- Take orally as fresh clove, capsule or tablet.
- Do not exceed recommended dosage.

Patient/Family Teaching
- Instruct patients about the need to follow a healthy diet (low in fat and high in vegetables and fruits) in conjunction with garlic. Other lipid reducing strategies, such as exercise and smoking cessation, should also be employed.
- Inform patients that there are other more effective agents for lipid reduction available.
- Emphasize the need for follow up exams with a healthcare professional to assess effectiveness of the regimen.
- Warn patients about the potential for bleeding and not to take this herbal remedy without notifying their healthcare provider if they are on other medications. Instruct patients undergoing elective surgery to stop using garlic 2 weeks prior to surgery and to notify the surgeon that they are taking garlic in the event of emergent surgery.
- Notify patients that allergies may occur and to discontinue use if symptoms develop.

Evaluation
- Normalization of lipid profile.
- Prevention of cardiac disease.

ginger (Zingiber Officinale)
(jin-jer)

Other Name(s):
Calicut, cochin, gengibre, ginger root, imber, ingwerwurzel, ingwer, Jamaica ginger, jenjibre, jiang, kankyo, zenzero, zingiber

Classification
Therapeutic: antiemetics

Common Uses
Prevention and treatment of nausea and vomiting associated with motion sickness, loss of appetite, pregnancy, surgery, and chemotherapy. Prevention of postoperative nausea and vomiting. May be used for dyspepsia, flatulence, relief of joint pain in rheumatoid arthritis, cramping, and diarrhea. Tonic (toning/strengthening agent) in gout, gas, respiratory infections, anti-inflammatory, stimulant (tones the gut, increases saliva and gastric juices, acts as anticoagulant, decreases blood cholesterol).

Action
Antiemetic effect due to increasing GI motility and transport; may act on serotonin receptors. Shown to be hypoglycemic, hypotensive or hypertensive, and positive inotropic agent. Inhibits prostaglandins and platelets, lowers cholesterol, and improves appetite and digestion. **Therapeutic Effects:** Decreased nausea and vomiting due to motion sickness, surgery, and chemotherapy. Decreased joint pain and improvement of joint motion in rheumatoid arthritis. Antioxidant.

Pharmacokinetics
Absorption: Unknown.
Distribution: Unknown.
Metabolism and Excretion: Unknown.
Half-life: Unknown.

TIME/ACTION PROFILE

ROUTE	ONSET	PEAK	DURATION
PO	unknown	unknown	unknown

Contraindications/Precautions
Contraindicated in: Pregnancy and lactation (if using large amounts); Gallstones.
Use Cautiously in: Patients with increased risk of bleeding; Diabetes; Anticoagulant therapy; Cardiovascular disease.

Adverse Reactions/Side Effects
GI: minor heartburn. **Derm:** dermatitis (when used topically).

Interactions
Natural Product-Drug: May increase risk of bleeding when used with **anticoagulants**, an-

tiplatelet agents, and **thrombolytics**. May have additive effects with **antidiabetic agents** (causing hypoglycemia) and **calcium channel blockers** (causing hypotension). May theoretically increase risk of bleeding when used with other **herbs that have anticoagulant or antiplatelet activities.**

Route/Commonly Used Doses

PO (Adults): *Motion sickness*—1000 mg dried ginger root taken 30 min–4 hr before travel or 250 mg qid. *Postoperative nausea prevention*—1000 mg ginger taken 1 hr before induction or anesthesia. *Chemotherapy–induced nausea*—2-4 g/day. Up to 2 g freshly powdered drug has been used as an antiemetic (not to exceed 4 g/day). *Osteoarthritis*—170 mg tid or 225 mg bid of ginger extract. *Whole root rhizome*—0.25–1 g for other illnesses. *Tea*—pour 150 ml boiling water over 0.5–1 g of ginger and strain after 5 min. *Tinture*—0.25-3 ml.

Availability

Alone or in combination with other herbal medicinals^{OTC}; Dried powdered root^{OTC}; Syrup^{OTC}; Tincture^{OTC}; Tablets^{OTC}; Capsules (≥550 mg)^{OTC}; Spice^{OTC}; Tea^{OTC}.

NURSING IMPLICATIONS

Assessment

- Assess patient for nausea, vomiting, abdominal distention, and pain prior to and after administration of the herb when used as an antiemetic agent.
- Assess pain, swelling, and range of motion in affected joints prior to and after administration when used in the treatment of arthritis.
- Assess patient for epigastric pain prior to and after administration when used as a gastroprotective agent.
- Monitor blood pressure in patients with cardiovascular disease including hypertension.

Potential Nursing Diagnosis

Acute pain (Indications)
Deficient knowledge, related to medication regimen (Patient/Family Teaching)

Implementation

- Administer ginger prior to situations where nausea or vomiting is anticipated (e.g., motion sickness).
- Dosage form and strengths vary with each disease state. Ensure that proper formulation and dose are administered for the indicated use.
- Give to increase peristalsis.

Patient/Family Teaching

- Instruct patients receiving anticoagulants not to take this herb without the advice of health care professional (increased risk of bleeding).
- Tell patient to stop the herb immediately if palpitations occur and contact health care professional.
- Advise patient to observe for easy bruising or other signs of bleeding. If they occur, stop the herb immediately and contact health care professional.
- Warn patients with a history of gallbladder disease to use this herb only under the supervision of health care professional.
- Instruct patient to consult health care professional before taking any prescription or OTC medications concurrently with ginger.
- Herb is meant to be used as a tonic, not for long-term use.

Evaluation

- Prevention of nausea and vomiting.
- Relief of epigastric pain.
- Improved joint mobility and relief of pain.

ginkgo (ging-ko)

Other Name(s):
Bai guo ye, fossil tree, ginkgo folium, Japanese silver apricot, kew tree, maidenhair-tree, salisburia adiantifolia, yinhsing

Classification
Therapeutic: antiplatelet agents, central nervous system stimulants

Common Uses

Symptomatic relief of organic brain dysfunction (dementia syndromes, short-term memory deficits, inability to concentrate, depression). Intermittent claudication. Vertigo and tinnitus of vascular origin. Improvement of peripheral circulation. Sexual dysfunction.

Action

Improves tolerance to hypoxemia, especially in cerebral tissue. Inhibits development of cerebral edema and accelerates its regression. Improves memory, blood flow (microcirculation), compensation of disequilibrium, and rheological properties of blood. Inactivates toxic oxygen radicals. Antagonizes platelet-activating factor. Interferes with bronchoconstriction and phagocyte chemotaxis. **Therapeutic Effects:** Symptomatic relief of dementia syndromes. Inhibits arterial spasm, decreases capillary fragility and blood viscosity. Improves venous tone, relaxes vascular smooth muscle.

Pharmacokinetics

Absorption: 70–100% absorption.
Distribution: Unknown.
Metabolism and Excretion: Unknown.
Half-life: Unknown.

TIME/ACTION PROFILE

ROUTE	ONSET	PEAK	DURATION
PO	unknown	unknown	unknown

Contraindications/Precautions

Contraindicated in: Hypersensitivity; Pregnancy and lactation.
Use Cautiously in: Bleeding disorders; Children (fresh seeds have caused seizures and death); Diabetes; Epilepsy. Surgery (discontinue use 2 weeks prior).

Adverse Reactions/Side Effects

CNS: CEREBRAL BLEEDING, dizziness, headache, vertigo, seizure. **CV:** palpitations. **GI:** flatulence, stomach upset. **Derm:** allergic skin reaction. **Hemat:** bleeding. **Misc:** hypersensitivity reactions.

Interactions

Natural Product-Drug: Theoretically may potentiate effects of **anticoagulants**, **thrombolytics**, **antiplatelet agents**, and **MAO inhibitors**. May also increase the risk of bleeding with some **cephalosporins**, **valproic acid**, and **NSAIDs**. May reduce the effectiveness of **anticonvulsants**. May alter **insulin** metabolism requiring dosage adjustments. May increase risk of bleeding when used with other **herbs with antiplatelet effects (including angelica, arnica, chamomile, feverfew, garlic, ginger, and licorice).**

Route/Commonly Used Doses

Organic Brain Syndromes

PO (Adults): 120–240 mg ginkgo leaf extract daily in 2 or 3 doses.

Sexual Dysfunction

PO (Adults): 60–240 mg BID ginkgo leaf extract.

Intermittent Claudication

PO (Adults): 120–240 mg ginkgo leaf extract daily in 2 or 3 doses.

Vertigo and Tinnitus

PO (Adults): 120–160 mg ginkgo leaf extract daily in 2 or 3 doses.

Cognitive Function Improvement

PO (Adults): 120–600 mg per day.

Availability

Ginkgo leaf extract (acetone/water): 22–27% flavonoid glycosides, 5–7% terpene lactones, 2.6–3.2% bilobalide, <5 ppm of ginkgolic acids.

NURSING IMPLICATIONS

Assessment

- Exclude other treatable causes of dementia prior to instituting treatment with ginkgo.
- Assess cognitive function (memory, attention, reasoning, language, ability to perform simple tasks) periodically throughout therapy.
- Assess frequency, duration, and severity of muscle cramps (claudication) experienced by the patient prior to and periodically throughout therapy.
- Assess for headache and neurosystem changes (thromboembolism).

Potential Nursing Diagnosis

Disturbed thought process (Indications)
Acute pain (Indications)
Deficient knowledge, related to medication regimen (Patient/Family Teaching)

Implementation

- Start dose at 120 mg per day and increase as needed to minimize side effects.
- Administration for a minimum of 6–8 wk of 80 mg (tid) (not <6 wk) is required to determine response.
- May be administered without regard to food.
- Use of dried leaf preparations in the form of a tea is not recommended because of insufficient quantity of active ingredients.
- Advise patients to avoid crude ginkgo plant parts which can cause severe allergic reactions.
- Take this herb at the same time daily.
- Keep this herb out of the reach of children as seizures may occur with increased doses of ginkgo seeds.

*CAPITALS indicates life-threatening; underlines indicate most frequent.

N A T U R A L / H E R B A L P R O D U C T S

Patient/Family Teaching

- Advise patient to observe for easy bruising and other signs of bleeding and report to health care professional if they occur.
- Caution patient to keep this herb out of the reach of children because ingestion has been associated with seizures.
- Warn patient to avoid handling the pulp or seed coats because of the risk of contact dermatitis. Wash skin under free-flowing water promptly if contact does occur.
- Instruct patient not to exceed recommended doses because large doses may result in toxicity (restlessness, diarrhea, nausea and vomiting, headache).
- Notify patients receiving anticoagulant or antiplatelet therapy not to take this medication without approval of health care professional and frequent monitoring.
- Instruct patient to consult health care professional before taking any prescription or OTC medications concurrently with ginkgo.

Evaluation

- Improvement in walking distances pain-free.
- Improvement in tinnitus and vertigo.
- Improvement in short-term memory, attention span, and ability to perform simple tasks.
- Improvement in sexual function.

ginseng (Panax Ginseng)

(**jin**-seng)

Other Name(s):
Asian ginseng, Chinese ginseng, hong shen, Japanese ginseng, Korean ginseng, red ginseng, renshen, white ginseng

Classification
Therapeutic: none assigned

Common Uses

Improving physical and mental stamina. General tonic to energize during times of fatigue and inability to concentrate. Sedative, sleep aid, antidepressant. Diabetes. Enhanced sexual performance/aphrodisiac. Increased longevity, treatment of cancer. Adjunctive treatment of cancer. Increased immune response. Increased appetite.

Action

Main active ingredient is ginsenoside from the dried root. Serves as CNS stimulant and depressant. Enhances immune function. Interferes with platelet aggregation and coagulation. Has analgesic, anti-inflammatory, and estrogen-like effects. **Therapeutic Effects:** Improves mental and physical ability. May improve appetite, memory, sleep pattern. May reduce fasting blood glucose level in diabetic patients.

Pharmacokinetics

Absorption: Unknown.
Distribution: Unknown.
Metabolism and Excretion: Unknown.
Half-life: Unknown.

TIME/ACTION PROFILE

ROUTE	ONSET	PEAK	DURATION
PO	unknown	unknown	unknown

Contraindications/Precautions

Contraindicated in: Pregnancy (androgenization of fetus); Lactation; Children; Manic-depressive disorders and psychosis; Hypertension; Asthma; Infection; Organ transplant recipients (can interfere with immunosuppressive therapy); Hormone-sensitive cancers.
Use Cautiously in: Cardiovascular disease; Diabetics (may have hypoglycemic effects); Patients receiving anticoagulants; Bleeding disorders.

Adverse Reactions/Side Effects

CNS: agitation, depression, dizziness, euphoria, headaches, <u>insomnia</u>, nervousness. **CV:** hypertension, tachycardia. **GI:** diarrhea. **GU:** amenorrhea, vaginal bleeding. **Derm:** skin eruptions. **Endo:** estrogen-like effects. **Misc:** fever, mastalgia, STEVENS-JOHNSON SYNDROME.

Interactions

Natural Product-Drug: May decrease anticoagulant activity of **warfarin**. May interfere with **MAO inhibitors** treatment and cause headache, tremulousness, and manic episodes. May enhance blood glucose lowering effects of **oral hypoglycemics** and **insulin**. May interfere with **immunosuppressant** therapy. Use with caution when taking **estrogens**. May increase risk of bleeding when used with **herbs that have antiplatelet or anticoagulant activities. May prolong the QT interval when used with bitter orange, country mallow and increase the risk of life-threatening arrythmias. May potentiate effects of caffeine** in **coffee** or **tea** and CNS stimulant effects of **mate.**

Route/Commonly Used Doses

PO (Adults): *Capsule*—200–600 mg/day; *extract*—100–300 mg 3 times daily; *crude root*—1–2 g/day; *infusion—tea*—1–2 g root daily (1/2 tbsp/cup water) up to 3 times daily (P. ginseng tea bag usually contains 1500 mg of ginseng root). Do not use for longer than 3 months. *Cold/flu prevention*—100 mg daily 4 weeks prior to influenza vaccination and continued for 8 weeks; *Chronic bronchitis*—100 mg BID for 9 days combined with antibiotic therapy; *Erectile dysfunction*—900 mg TID; *Type 2 diabetes*—200 mg daily.

Availability (generic available)

Root powder[OTC]; **Extract in alcohol**[OTC]; **Capsules**[OTC]: 100 mg, 250 mg, 500 mg. **Tea bags**[OTC].

NURSING IMPLICATIONS

Assessment

- Assess level of energy, attention span, and fatigue person is experiencing prior to initiating and periodically throughout the course of therapy.
- Assess appetite; sleep duration; and perceived quality, emotional lability, and work efficiency prior to and during therapy.
- Patients with chronic medical problems should not use this herb without the advice of health care professional.
- Assess for ginseng toxicity (nervousness, insomnia, palpitations, and diarrhea).
- Monitor patients with diabetes more frequently for hypoglycemia until response to the agent is ascertained.
- Assess for the development of ginseng abuse syndrome (occurs when large doses of the herb are taken concomitantly with other psychomotor stimulants such as coffee and tea. May present as diarrhea, hypertension, restlessness, insomnia, skin eruptions, depression, appetite suppression, euphoria, and edema).

Potential Nursing Diagnosis

Energy field disturbance (Indications) (Indications)

Implementation

- May be taken without regard to food.
- Take at the same time daily and do not increase dose above the recommended amount because of potential toxic effects.

Patient/Family Teaching

- Warn patients with cardiovascular disease, hypertension or hypotension, or on steroid therapy to avoid the use of this herb.
- Warn pregnant or breastfeeding women not to use this herb.
- Instruct patient in the symptoms of ginseng toxicity and to reduce dose or stop use of the herb if they occur.
- Inform patient to limit the amount of caffeine consumed.
- Advise patients with diabetes to monitor blood sugar levels until response to this agent is known.
- Tell patient that the recommended course of therapy is 3 wk. A repeated course is feasible. Do not use for longer than 3 months.
- Teach patient about the signs and symptoms of hepatitis and to stop use of the herb and promptly contact health care professional if they occur. (This herb is hepatoprotectant at low doses, but hepatodestructive at high doses.).
- Caution patient not to exceed recommended doses because of potential side effects and toxicity.
- If diarrhea develops, stop herb.
- Instruct patient to consult health care professional before taking any prescription or OTC medications concurrently with ginseng.

Evaluation

- Improved energy level and sense of well-being.
- Improved quality of sleep.
- Improved concentration and work efficiency.
- Improved appetite.
- May need to take for several weeks before seeing results.

glucosamine
(glew-**kos**-ah-meen)

Other Name(s):
2-amino-2-deoxyglucose sulfate, chitosamine

Classification
Therapeutic: antirheumatics

Common Uses

Osteoarthritis. Temporomandibular joint (TMJ) arthritis. Glaucoma.

NATURAL/HERBAL PRODUCTS

N A T U R A L / H E R B A L P R O D U C T S

Action
May stop or slow osteoarthritis progression by stimulating cartilage and synovial tissue metabolism. **Therapeutic Effects:** Decreased pain and improved joint function.

Pharmacokinetics
Absorption: 0.9% absorbed.
Distribution: Unknown.
Metabolism and Excretion: 74% eliminated via first-pass metabolism.
Half-life: Unknown.

TIME/ACTION PROFILE

ROUTE	ONSET	PEAK	DURATION
PO	unknown	unknown	unknown

Contraindications/Precautions
Contraindicated in: Shellfish allergy (glucosamine is often derived from marine exoskeletons); Pregnancy and lactation.
Use Cautiously in: Diabetes (may worsen glycemic control); Asthma (may exacerbate symptoms).

Adverse Reactions/Side Effects
GI: nausea, heartburn, diarrhea, constipation. **CNS:** headache, drowsiness. **Derm:** skin reactions.

Interactions
Natural Product-Drug: May antagonize the effects of **antidiabetics**. May induce resistance to some chemotherapy drugs such as **etoposide**, **teniposide**, and **doxorubicin**. None known.

Route/Commonly Used Doses
PO (Adults): 500 mg three times daily.
Topical: (Adults): use cream as needed for up to 8 weeks.

Availability
Tablets[OTC]; **Capsules**[OTC]; **Topical cream OTC:** 30 mg/g in combination with other ingredients.

NURSING IMPLICATIONS

Assessment
- Evaluate for shellfish allergy prior to initiating therapy.
- Monitor pain (type, location, and intensity) and range of motion on an ongoing basis as an indicator of drug efficacy.
- Assess glucose levels via home monitoring device for patients with diabetes until response is ascertained.
- Evaluate gastric discomfort and instruct patient to seek out the advice of a health care provider if persistent gastric discomfort occurs.
- Assess bowel function and symptomatically treat constipation with improved fluid intake and bulk in diet and bulk laxatives if necessary.

Potential Nursing Diagnosis
Acute pain (Indications)
Impaired physical mobility (Indications)

Implementation
- Take prior to meals.

Patient/Family Teaching
- Warn patients with a shellfish allergy that this herbal supplement should not be used.
- Instruct patients that the effects of this drug come from stimulating cartilage and synovial tissue metabolism and that the supplement must be taken on a regular basis to achieve benefit. It should not be used as an intermittent pain medication.
- Contact a health care provider if gastric discomfort develops and persists.
- Caution diabetics to monitor glucose values to ascertain impact on glycemic control.

Evaluation
- Improvement in pain and range of motion.

hawthorne (Crataegus Species) (haw-thorn)

Other Name(s):
aubepine, cum flore, hagedorn, maybush, whitehorn

Classification
Therapeutic: antihypertensives, inotropics

Common Uses
Hypertension. Mild to moderate CHF. Angina. Spasmolytic. Sedative.

Action
Active compounds in hawthorn include flavonoids and procyanidins. Increase coronary blood flow. Positive inotropic and chronotropic effects because of increased permeability to calcium and inhibition of phosphodiesterase. **Therapeutic Effects:** Increased cardiac output. Decreased blood pressure, myocardial workload, and oxygen consumption.

Pharmacokinetics
Absorption: Unknown.
Distribution: Unknown.

Metabolism and Excretion: Unknown.
Half-life: Unknown.

TIME/ACTION PROFILE

ROUTE	ONSET	PEAK	DURATION
PO	unknown	6-8 wk	unknown

Contraindications/Precautions

Contraindicated in: Pregnancy (potential uterine activity); Lactation.
Use Cautiously in: Concurrent use with ACE inhibitors and digoxin; Do not discontinue use abruptly.

Adverse Reactions/Side Effects

CNS: agitation, dizziness, fatigue, vertigo, headache, sedation (high dose), sleeplessness, sweating. **CV:** hypotension (high dose), palpitations. **GI:** nausea.

Interactions

Natural Product-Drug: May potentiate effects of **digoxin**, **calcium channel blockers**, and **beta blockers**. Concurrent use with **theophylline**, **caffeine**, **epinephrine**, **phosphodiesterase-5 inhibitors** (**sildenafil**, **tadalafil**, **vardenafil**) and **nitrates** may potentiate adverse cardiovascular effects. May cause additive CNS depression when used with other **CNS depressants**. Additive effect with other cardiac glycoside–containing **herbs (digitalis leaf, black hellebore, oleander leaf, and others). Additive hypotensive effects with herbs than lower blood pressure such as ginger, panax ginseng, and valerian. Additive effect with other cardioactive herbs (devil's claw, fenugreek, and others).**

Route/Commonly Used Doses

PO (Adults): *Heart failure*—160–1800 mg standardized hawthorn leaf with flower extract in 2–3 divided doses daily. *Hawthorn fluid extract (1:1 in 25% alcohol)*—0.5–1 ml tid; *hawthorn fruit tincture (1:5 in 45% alcohol)*—1–2 ml tid; *dried hawthorn berries*—300–1000 mg tid.

Availability (generic available)

Dried fruit[OTC]; Liquid extract of the fruit or leaf[OTC]; Tincture of the fruit or leaf[OTC].

NURSING IMPLICATIONS

Assessment

- Auscultate lung sounds for signs of heart failure (rales, crackles, wheezing).
- Assess weight daily and look for signs of fluid overload (swelling of ankles, shortness of breath, sleeping with multiple pillows).
- Assess blood pressure periodically throughout therapy.
- Assess pulse for rate and regularity of rhythm.

Potential Nursing Diagnosis

Decreased cardiac output (Indications)
Deficient knowledge, related to medication regimen (Patient/Family Teaching)

Implementation

- Administered as 2–3 divided doses daily at the same time.
- May be taken without regard to food.

Patient/Family Teaching

- Advise patients that there are other proven therapies available for treatment of heart failure. These therapies should be employed prior to initiating treatment with hawthorn.
- Tell patient not to take hawthorn without the advice of health care professional.
- Instruct patients in the symptoms of a heart attack (pain in the region of the heart, jaw, arm, or upper abdomen; sweating; chest tightness) and heart failure (shortness of breath, chest tightness, dizziness, sweating) and to promptly contact health care professional if they occur.
- Advise patient to report weight gain or persistent swelling of the feet to health care professional.
- Warn patients who self-medicate to consult health care professional if there is no improvement in symptoms in 6–8 wk. Effects may not be seen for 3 mo.
- Teach patient to make position changes slowly to minimize the risk of orthostatic hypotension.
- Caution patient not to combine with other cardiac and BP medications unless under supervision of health care professional because of possible additive effects.
- This herb may cause drowsiness. Patients should avoid driving or other activities that require mental alertness until response to herb is known.
- Avoid alcohol and other CNS depressants while taking hawthorn unless under supervision of health care professional.
- Profuse sweating and dehydration under extreme heat may increase the BP-lowering properties of hawthorn, leading to severe hypotension. Warn patients to avoid exertion in

hot weather to minimize the risk of side effects.

- Instruct patients that hawthorn helps control the symptoms of heart failure but does not cure the disease. Lifestyle changes (salt restriction, weight management, exercise as tolerated, adherence to medication regimens) still need to be followed.
- Although hawthorn has been studied in Europe for management of heart failure, there are no conclusive studies to recommend use of this herb.
- Instruct patient to consult health care professional before taking any prescription or OTC medications concurrently with hawthorn.

Evaluation

- Decrease in symptoms of CHF.
- Improved cardiac output as evidenced by improved activity tolerance.

Hypericum Perforatum, see **St. John's wort**

kava-kava (Piper Methysticum) (ka-va ka-va)

Other Name(s):
Ava pepper, intoxicating pepper, kao, kew, tonga, wurzelstock, yagona

Classification
Therapeutic: antianxiety agents, sedative/hypnotics

Common Uses

Anxiety, stress, restlessness, insomnia, benzodiazepine withdrawal. Mild muscle aches and pains. Menstrual cramps and PMS.

Action

Alters the limbic system modulation of emotional processes. Shown to have centrally-acting skeletal muscle relaxant properties activated.
Therapeutic Effects: Relief of anxiety. Sedation.

Pharmacokinetics

Absorption: Peak plasma level occurs about 1.8 hr after an oral dose.
Distribution: Enters breast milk.
Metabolism and Excretion: Elimination occurs primarily by renal excretion (both unchanged and metabolites) and in the feces. Metabolized by the liver (reduction or demethylation).
Half-life: Approximately 9 hr.

TIME/ACTION PROFILE

ROUTE	ONSET	PEAK	DURATION
PO	1.8 hr	unknown	8 hr

Contraindications/Precautions

Contraindicated in: Pregnancy (may affect uterine tone) and lactation; Patients with endogenous depression (may increase risk of suicide); Children under 12 yr of age; Hepatitis or other liver disease.
Use Cautiously in: Concurrent use of other hepatotoxic agents; Depression and Parkinson's disease (may worsen symptoms); Should not be used for more 3 mo to prevent psychological addiction.

Adverse Reactions/Side Effects

CNS: dizziness, headache, drowsiness, sensory disturbances, extrapyramidal effects. **EENT:** Pupil dilation, red eyes, visual accommodation disorders. **GI:** HEPATIC TOXICITY, gastrointestinal complaints. **Derm:** allergic skin reactions, yellow discoloration of skin, pellagroid dermopathy. **Hemat:** decreased lymphocytes, decreased platelets. **Metab:** weight loss (long term, high dose). **Neuro:** ataxia, muscle weakness.

Interactions

Natural Product-Drug: Additive effect when used with **alprazolam**. Potentiates effect of **CNS depressants (ethanol, barbiturates, benzodiazepines, opioid analgesics)**. Has decreased the effectiveness of **levodopa** in few cases. Theoretically, may have additive effects with **antiplatelet agents**. Concurrent use with other hepatotoxic products such as **DHEA, coenzyme Q-10 (high doses), and niacin can increase the risk of liver damage. Theoretically, may have additive sedative effects when used with other herbs with sedative properties.**

Route/Commonly Used Doses

PO (Adults): *Antianxiety*—100 mg (70 mg kavalactones) 3 times daily; *Benzodiazepine withdrawal*—50–300 mg/day over one week while tapering benzodiazepine over 2 weeks (use 70% kavalactone extract). *Insomnia*—180–210 mg kavalactones. Typically taken as a tea by simmering the root in boiling water and then straining.

Availability (generic available)
Dried root extracts (alcohol or acetone based) containing 30–70% kavapyrones.

NURSING IMPLICATIONS

Assessment
- Assess muscle spasm, associated pain, and limitations of movement prior to and periodically throughout therapy.
- Assess degree of anxiety and level of sedation (visual disturbances and changes in motor reflexes are side effects) prior to and periodically throughout therapy.
- Assess sleep patterns and level of sedation upon arising.
- Prolonged use may lead to depression of platelet and lymphocyte counts.

Potential Nursing Diagnosis
Anxiety (Indications)
Impaired physical mobility (Adverse Reactions)
Risk for injury (Side Effects)

Implementation
- Prepared as a drink from pulverized roots, tablets, capsules, or extract.

Patient/Family Teaching
- Inform patient that significant, serious side effects may occur with prolonged use. Use for longer than 1 mo is not recommended without supervision of health care professional.
- Caution patient to not use alcohol or other CNS depressants while taking this herb because the combination potentiates the herb's sedative effect.
- Advise patients that driving a car or performing other activities requiring mental alertness should be avoided until response to therapy is determined.
- Warn patients to stop use of the herb immediately if shortness of breath or signs of liver disease (yellowing of the skin or whites of the eyes, brown urine, nausea, vomiting, light-colored stools, unusual tiredness, weakness, stomach or abdominal pain, loss of appetite) occur and contact health care professional.
- Advise patients who have liver disease or liver problems, or persons who are taking drug products that can affect the liver, to consult health care professional before using kava-containing supplements.
- Inform patient that although there is no evidence of physiological dependence, the risk of psychological dependence still exists.
- Counsel pregnant and breastfeeding women not to use this herb.
- Instruct patient to consult health care professional before taking any prescription or OTC medications concurrently with kava-kava.

Evaluation
- Decrease in anxiety level.
- Decrease in muscle spasms.
- Relief of insomnia.

milk thistle (milk **this**-ul)

Other Name(s):
Holy thistle, Lady's thistle, Mary Thistle, Silybin, Silymarin

Classification
Therapeutic: antidotes

Common Uses
Cirrhosis, chronic hepatitis, gallstones, psoriasis, liver cleansing and detoxification, treatment of liver toxicity due to alcohol. Amanita mushroom poisoning (European IV formulation) and chemicals.

Action
The active component, silymarin, has antioxidant and hepatoprotectant actions. Silymarin helps prevent toxin penetration and stimulates hepatocyte regeneration.

Pharmacokinetics
Absorption: 23–47% absorbed after oral administration.
Distribution: Unknown.
Metabolism and Excretion: Hepatic metabolism by cytochrome P450 3A4.
Half-life: 6 hr.

TIME/ACTION PROFILE

ROUTE	ONSET	PEAK	DURATION
PO	5–30 days or more	unknown	unknown

Contraindications/Precautions
Contraindicated in: Pregnancy and lactation (insufficient information available); Allergy to chamomile, ragweed, asters, chrysanthemums and other members of the family Compositae.
Use Cautiously in: Hormone sensitive cancers/conditions (milk thistle plant parts may have estrogenic effects).

NATURAL/HERBAL PRODUCTS

Adverse Reactions/Side Effects
GI: Laxative effect, nausea, bloating, anorexia.
Misc: Allergic reactions.

Interactions
Natural Product-Drug: In vitro, milk thistle extract inhibited the drug-metabolizing enzyme **cytochrome P450 3A4**. Interactions have not been reported in humans, but milk thistle should be used cautiously with other drugs metabolized by 3A4, such as **cyclosporine**, **carbamazepine**, **HMG-CoA inhibitors**, **ketoconazole**, and **alprazolam**. None known.

Route/Commonly Used Doses
PO (Adults): *Hepatic cirrhosis*—420 mg/day of extract containing 70–80% silymarin; *Chronic active hepatitis*—240 mg bid of silibinin; *Tea*—3–4 times daily 30 minutes before meals. Tea is not recommended as silymarin is not sufficiently water soluble.
IV (Adults): 20–50 mg/kg over 24 hr, 48 hr post mushroom ingestion (IV formulation not available in US).

Availability
CapsulesOTC; **Tablets**OTC; **Crude drug**OTC; **Tea**OTC; **Extract**OTC.

NURSING IMPLICATIONS

Assessment
- Assess patients for signs of liver failure such as jaundice, mental status changes, abdominal distention (ascites) and generalized edema.
- Monitor liver function tests periodically throughout therapy.
- Evaluate consistency and frequency of bowel movements.

Potential Nursing Diagnosis
Deficient knowledge, related to medication regimen (Patient/Family Teaching)

Implementation
- Orally as an extract, capsule, tablets or as a dried fruit as a single daily dose or divided into three doses.
- Tea is not recommended as Milk Thistle is not water-soluble.

Patient/Family Teaching
- Inform patient of the symptoms of liver failure; advise patient to report worsening symptomotolgy promptly to healthcare professional.
- Emphasize the need for blood tests to monitor liver function tests.
- Advise patients to abstain from alcohol and to follow a diet consistent with the liver or gall bladder disease being treated.

Evaluation
- Normalization of liver function tests.
- Reduction in jaundice, abdominal distention, fatigue and other symptoms associated with liver disease.

Panax Ginseng, see **ginseng**.

Piper Methysticum, see **kava-kava**.

SAMe (sam-ee)

Other Name(s):
Ademetionine, S-adenosylmethionine,

Classification
Therapeutic: antidepressants

Pregnancy Category UK

Common Uses
Treatment of depression. Has also been used to manage: osteoarthritis, fibromyalgia, liver disease, migraine headaches.

Action
May aid in the production, activation, and metabolism of various amines, phospholipids, hormones, and neurotransmitters. May stimulate articular cartilage growth and repair. **Therapeutic Effects:** Decreased depression. Anti-inflammatory and analgesic effects improve symptoms of osteoarthritis.

Pharmacokinetics
Absorption: Rapidly and extensively metabolized following oral administration.
Distribution: Unknown.
Metabolism and Excretion: Actively metabolized by the liver.
Half-life: 100 min.

TIME/ACTION PROFILE (antidepressant action)

ROUTE	ONSET	PEAK	DURATION
PO (depression)	1–2 wk	unknown	unknown
PO (osteoarthritis)	30 days	unknown	unknown

Contraindications/Precautions

Contraindicated in: Hypersensitivity; Bipolar disorder.
Use Cautiously in: Pregnancy, lactation, or children (safety not established); Bipolar disorder (can induce mania); Parkinson's disease (may worsen symptoms).

Adverse Reactions/Side Effects

CNS: agitation, dizziness, mild insomnia, manic reactions (in patients with bipolar disorder).
GI: vomiting, diarrhea, flatulence.

Interactions

Natural Product-Drug: Avoid use with **antidepressants**, **meperidine**, **pentazocine**, **tramadol**, and **dextromethorphan** (additive serotinergic effects may occur). May reduce the effectiveness of **levodopa** and worsen Parkinsonian symptoms. Should not be used concurrently with **MAO inhibitors**. Avoid use of SAMe within 2 wk of using a **MAO inhibitor**. Avoid use with natural products that increase serotonin levels such as **L-tryptophan and St. John's wort.**

Route/Commonly Used Doses

PO (Adults): *Depression*—200 mg once or twice daily, adjusted upward over 2 wk (range 400–1600 mg/day); *Liver disorders*—1200–1600 mg/day; *Osteoarthritis*—200 mg tid; *Fibromyalgia*—800 mg/day.

Availability

Tablets: 100 mg, 200 mg, 400 mg[OTC].

NURSING IMPLICATIONS

Assessment

- Assess mental status for symptoms of depression prior to and periodically during therapy; advise patients with depression to be evaluated by a health care professional.
- Assess symptoms of pain and fatigue prior to and periodically during therapy.

Potential Nursing Diagnosis

Ineffective coping (Indications)
Deficient knowledge, related to medication regimen (Patient/Family Teaching)

Implementation

- Only enteric-coated formulations are recommended due to bioavailability problems.
- **PO:** Initial dose should be 200 mg once or twice daily to minimize GI disturbances. Dose may be adjusted upward over 1–2 wks depending on response and tolerance.

Patient/Family Teaching

- Instruct patient to take SAMe according to directions.
- The SAMe butanedisulfonate salt may be preferable due to greater stability.

Evaluation

- Decrease in symptoms of depression.
- Improvement in osteoarthritis symptoms.

saw palmetto

Other Name(s):
American Dwarf Palm Tree, Cabbage Palm, Ju-Zhong, Palmier Nain, Sabal, Sabal Fructus, Saw Palmetto Berry, Serenoa repens

Classification
Therapeutic: none assigned

Common Uses

Benign prostatic hypertrophy (BPH). Prostate cancer (in combination with 7 other herbs as PC-SPES).

Action

Antiandrogenic, antiinflammatory and antiproliferative properties in prostate tissue result in improvement in BPH symptoms such as frequent urination, hesitancy, urgency and nocturia. Comparable in efficacy to finasteride but may be less effective than prazosin. **Therapeutic Effects:** Decreased urinary symptoms of BPH.

Pharmacokinetics

Absorption: Unknown.
Distribution: Unknown.
Metabolism and Excretion: Unknown.
Half-life: Unknown.

TIME/ACTION PROFILE

ROUTE	ONSET	PEAK	DURATION
PO	1–2 mos	unknown	48 wk (longest studied treatment duration)

Contraindications/Precautions

Contraindicated in: Pregnancy and lactation.
Use Cautiously in: Prior to surgery (discontinue 2 weeks before to prevent bleeding).

Adverse Reactions/Side Effects

CNS: dizziness, headache. **GI:** nausea, vomiting, constipation and diarrhea.

Interactions

Natural Product-Drug: Hormonal action may interfere with other hormonal therapies (**testosterone**, **hormonal contraceptives**). Avoid use with **antiplatelet** or **anticoagulant drugs** (may increase bleeding risk).

Route/Commonly Used Doses

PO (Adults): *Lipophilic extract (80–90% fatty acids)*—160 mg twice daily or 320 mg once daliy. *Whole berries*—1–2 grams daily. *Liquid extract*—0.6–1.5 ml daily. *Tea (efficacy is questionable due to lipophilicity of active constituents)*—1 cup three times daily. Tea is prepared by steeping 0.5–1 gram dried berry in 150 ml boiling water for 5–10 minutes.

Availability

Lipophilic extract (80-90% fatty acids)[OTC]; **Whole berries**[OTC]; **Liquid extract**[OTC].

NURSING IMPLICATIONS

Assessment

- Assess patient for symptoms of benign prostatic hypertrophy (BPH) (urinary hesitancy, feeling of incomplete bladder emptying, interruption in urinary stream, impairment in size and force of urinary stream, terminal urinary dribbling, straining to start flow, dysuria, urgency) before and periodically throughout therapy.
- Rectal exams prior to and periodically throughout therapy to assess prostate size are recommended.

Potential Nursing Diagnosis

Impaired urinary elimination (Indications)
Deficient knowledge, related to medication regimen (Patient/Family Teaching)

Implementation

- Take on a full stomach to minimize GI effects.

Patient/Family Teaching

- Advise patients to start therapy with this herbal supplement only after evaluation by a health care provider who will provide continued follow up care.
- Inform patients that saw palmetto does not alter the size of the prostate but still should relieve the symptoms associated with BPH.
- Tell patients that taking this herbal supplement with food should reduce the GI effects and make it easier to tolerate.

Evaluation

- Decrease in urinary symptoms of BPH.

St. John's wort (Hypericum Perforatum)

(saynt **jonz** wort)

Other Name(s):
Amber, Demon chaser, Goatweed, Hardhay, Klamath weed, Rosin rose, Tipton weed

Classification
Therapeutic: antidepressants

Common Uses

PO: Management of mild to moderate depression and obsessive compulsive disorder (OCD). (Not effective for major depression.). **Topical:** Inflammation of the skin, blunt injury, wounds and burns. Other uses are for capillary strengthening, decreasing uterine bleeding, and reducing tumor size.

Action

Derived from *Hypericum perforatum*; the active component is *hypericin*. **PO:** Antidepressant action my be due to ability to inhibit reuptake of serotonin and other neurotransmitters. **Topical:** Anti-inflammatory, antifungal, antiviral, and antibacterial properties. **Therapeutic Effects: PO:** Decreased signs and symptoms of depression. **Topical:** Decreased inflammation of burns or other wounds.

Pharmacokinetics

Absorption: Unknown.
Distribution: Unknown.
Metabolism and Excretion: Unknown.
Half-life: *Hypericum constituents*—24.8–26.5 hr.

TIME/ACTION PROFILE

ROUTE	ONSET	PEAK	DURATION
PO	10–14 days	within 4–6 wk	unknown

Contraindications/Precautions

Contraindicated in: Pregnancy, lactation, or children.
Use Cautiously in: History of phototoxicity; Alzheimer's disease (may induce psychosis); Patients undergoing general anesthesia (may cause cardiovascular collapse); History of suicide attempt, severe depression, schizophrenia or bipolar disorder (can induce hypomania or psychosis).

Adverse Reactions/Side Effects
CNS: dizziness, restlessness, sleep disturbances. **CV:** hypertension. **GI:** abdominal pain, bloating, constipation, dry mouth, feeling of fullness, flatulence, nausea, vomiting. **Derm:** allergic skin reactions (hives, itching, skin rash), phototoxicity.

Interactions
Natural Product-Drug: Concurrent use with **alcohol** or other **antidepressants** (including **SSRIs** and **MAO inhibitors**) may increase the risk of adverse CNS reactions. May reduce the effectiveness and serum concentrations of **digoxin**. Use with **MAO Inhibitors** and **selective serotonin agonists** could result in serotonin syndrome. May decrease plasma **cyclosporine** levels by 30–70% and cause acute transplant rejection. May increase the metabolism of **phenytoin** and cause loss of seizure control. Avoid use of St. John's Wort and **MAO Inhibitors** within 2 wk of each other.

Route/Commonly Used Doses
PO (Adults): *Mild Depression*—300 mg of St. John's Wort (standardized to 0.3% hypericin) 3 times daily or 250 mg twice daily of 0.2% hypericin extract. *OCD*—450 mg twice daily of extended release preparation.
Topical: (Adults): 0.2–1 mg total hypericin daily.

Availability
Preparations for Oral Use
Dried herb[OTC]; **Dried (hydroalcoholic) extract**[OTC]; **Oil**[OTC]; **Tincture**[OTC].
Preparations for Topical Application
Liquid[OTC]; **Semisolid**[OTC].

NURSING IMPLICATIONS

Assessment
- **Depression:** Assess patient for depression periodically throughout therapy.
- **Inflammation:** Assess skin or skin lesions periodically throughout therapy.

Potential Nursing Diagnosis
Ineffective coping (Indications)
Anxiety (Indications)
Deficient knowledge, related to medication regimen (Patient/Family Teaching)

Implementation
- **PO:** Tea can be prepared by mixing 2-4 dried herb in 150 ml of boiling water and steeping for 10 min.

Patient/Family Teaching
- Instruct patient to take St. John's wort as directed.
- Patients with depression should be evaluated by health care professional. Standard therapy may be of greater benefit for moderate to severe depression.
- Advise patient to notify health care professional of medication regimen prior to treatment or surgery.
- Caution patients to avoid sun exposure and use protective sunscreen to reduce the risk of photosensitivity reactions.
- Inform patient that St. John's wort is usually taken for a period of 4–6 wk. If no improvement is seen, another therapy should be considered.
- Inform patient to purchase herbs from a reputable source and that products and their contents vary among different manufacturers.
- Warn patient not to use alcohol while taking St. John's wort.
- Warn patients that St. John's Wort may reduce the therapeutic effectiveness of several drugs.
- May potentiate effect of sedatives and side effects of other antidepressants. Do not take within 2 wk of MAO Inhibitor therapy.
- Instruct patient to consult healthcare professional before taking any prescription or OTC medications concurrently with St. John's wort.

Evaluation
- Decrease in signs and symptoms of depression or anxiety.
- Improvement in skin inflammation.

valerian (vuh-lare-ee-en)

Other Name(s):
Amantilla, All-Heal, Baldrian, Baldrianwurzel, Belgium Valerian, Common Valerian, Fragrant Valerian, Garden Heliotrope, Garden Valerian, Indian Valerian, Mexican Valerian, Pacific Valerian, Tagara, Valeriana, Valeriana officinalis, Valerianae radix, Valeriana rhizome, Valeriane

Classification
Therapeutic: antianxiety agents, sedative/hypnotics

NATURAL/HERBAL PRODUCTS

Common Uses
Insomnia. Anxiety.

Action
May increase concentrations of the inhibitory CNS transmitter GABA. **Therapeutic Effects:** Improvement in sleep quality.

Pharmacokinetics
Absorption: Unknown.
Distribution: Unknown.
Metabolism and Excretion: Unknown.
Half-life: Unknown.

TIME/ACTION PROFILE

ROUTE	ONSET	PEAK	DURATION
PO	30–60 min	2 hr	unknown

Contraindications/Precautions
Contraindicated in: Pregnancy and lactation. **Use Cautiously in:** Alcohol use (may have additive sedative effects).

Adverse Reactions/Side Effects
CNS: drowsiness, headache. **Misc:** Benzodiazepine-like withdrawal symptoms with discontinuation after long-term use.

Interactions
Natural Product-Drug: Additive CNS depression with **alcohol**, **antihistamines**, **sedative hypnotics** and other **CNS depressants**. Alcohol-containing preparations may interact with **disulfuram** and **metronidazole**. Additive sedative effects can occur when used with herbal supplements with sedative properties such as **kava, L-tryptophan, melatonin, SAMe, and St. John's wort.**

Route/Commonly Used Doses
PO (Adults): *Tea*—1 cup tea 1–5 times daily. Tea is made by steeping 2–3 g root in 150 ml boiling water for 5–10 min then straining. *Tincture*—1–3 mL 1–5 times daily. *Extract*—400–900 mg up to 2 hours before bedtime or 300–450 mg divided tid.

Availability
Capsules[OTC]; **Extract**[OTC]; **Tea**[OTC]; **Tincture**[OTC].

NURSING IMPLICATIONS

Assessment
- Assess degree of anxiety and level of sedation prior to and periodically throughout therapy.
- Assess sleep patterns.
- Assess response in the elderly population where drowsiness and loss of balance may pose a significant risk for injury.

Potential Nursing Diagnosis
Anxiety (Indications)
Risk for injury (Side Effects)

Implementation
- Take one to two hours before bedtime if used for nighttime hypnotic.
- Administer orally three to five times daily to control anxiety.

Patient/Family Teaching
- Warn patients to avoid use of other medications or herbals that have a sedative effect, as the combination will increase drowsiness and sedation.
- Warn patients against driving or operating heavy machinery after taking valerian.
- Inform patients not to take this herbal supplement if pregnant or breast-feeding.
- Counsel patients to avoid activities requiring mental alertness until response to this supplement is known.
- Notify patients that dependence with withdrawal symptoms may develop with prolonged use.
- Instruct patients to avoid consuming alcohol while taking this herbal supplement.
- Encourage patients to eliminate stimulants such as caffeine and to provide an environment that promotes restful sleep.

Evaluation
- Decreased anxiety level.
- Improvement in sleep with a feeling of restfulness without drowsiness upon awakening.

Zingiber Officinale, see **ginger**.

APPENDICES

Appendix A. Recent Drug Approvals 1321

Appendix B. Combination Drugs 1329

Appendix C. Ophthalmic Medications 1349

Appendix D. Medication Administration Techniques 1357

Appendix E. Formulas Helpful for Calculating Doses 1360

Appendix F. Body Surface Area Nomograms 1363

Appendix G. Normal Values of Common Laboratory Tests 1365

Appendix H. Commonly Used Abbreviations 1368

Appendix I. Pregnancy Categories and Controlled Substances Schedules 1370

Appendix J. Equianalgesic Dosing Guidelines 1372

Appendix K. Recommendations for the Safe Handling of Hazardous Drugs 1375

Appendix L. Food Sources for Specific Nutrients 1377

Appendix M. Insulins and Insulin Therapy 1379

Appendix N. Canadian and U.S. Pharmaceutical Practices 1381

Appendix O. Routine Pediatric and Adult Immunizations 1383

Appendix P. Administering Medications to Children 1390

Appendix Q. Pediatric Dosage Calculations 1391

Appendix R. Pediatric Fluid and Electrolyte Requirements 1392

APPENDIX A

Recent Drug Approvals

To view full-text monographs of drugs that have been recently released from the FDA or to learn about changes to dosage forms, please visit www.DrugGuide.com.

diclofenac (topical patch)

(dye-**kloe**-fen-ak)
Flector

Classification
Therapeutic: nonsteroidal anti-inflammatory agents, analgesics

Pregnancy Category C

Indications

Topical treatment of acute pain due to minor strains, sprains, and contusions.

Contraindications/Precautions

Contraindicated in: Hypersensitivity; cross-sensitivity with other NSAIDs may exist; History of Aspirin Triad (nasal polyps, asthma, bronchospasm following aspirin); Treatment of perioperative pain following coronary artery bypass graft (CABG) surgery; Advanced renal disease; Application to non-intact or damaged skin; OB: Late pregnancy (may cause premature closure of the ductus arteriosus) or lactation.
Use Cautiously in: Geri: Increased risk of adverse effects; consider age-related decrease in metabolic pathways, concurrent disease states and drug therapy; History of cardiovascular disease or risk factors (increased risk of serious cardiovascular effects); History of hypertension or edema (may exacerbate condition); History of impaired renal or hepatic function, heart failure, concurrent ACE inhibitor or diuretic therapy (increased risk of renal toxicity); Chronic corticosteroid therapy (slow tapering of corticosteroids required); Bleeding abnormalities or platelet dysfunction; Pedi: Safe use not established.
Exercise Extreme Caution in: History of ulcer disease or GI bleeding. Pre-existing asthma.

Adverse Reactions/Side Effects

CV: edema, hypertension. **GI:** GI BLEEDING, ↑ liver enzymes. **GU:** renal toxicity. **Derm:** STEVENS-JOHNSON SYNDROME, TOXIC EPIDERMAL NECROLYSIS, local reactions at treatment site, rash. **Misc:** allergic reactions including ANAPHYLATOID REACTIONS.

Route/Dosage

Topical (Adults): 1 patch applied to most painful area twice daily.

doripenem (do-ri-**pen**-em)

Doribax

Classification
Therapeutic: anti-infectives
Pharmacologic: carbapenems

Pregnancy Category B

Indications

Infections caused by susceptible organisms including: complicated intra-abdominal infections, complicated urinary tract infections, including pyelonephritis.

Contraindications/Precautions

Contraindicated in: Hypersensitivity to doripenem, other carbapenems or beta-lactams.
Use Cautiously in: Geri: Consider age-related decrease in renal function when choosing dose; OB: Use cautiously during lactation; Pedi: Safe use in children has not been established.

Adverse Reactions/Side Effects

CV: <u>headache</u>. **GI:** PSEUDOMEMBRANOUS COLITIS, diarrhea, <u>nausea</u>, ↑ liver enzymes. **Hemat:** anemia. **Local:** phlebitis. **Misc:** allergic reactions including <u>ANAPHYLAXIS</u>, infection with resistant organisms, superinfection.

Route/Dosage

IV (Adults): 500 mg every 8 hr

Renal Impairment
IV (Adults): *CCr 30–50 ml/min*—250 mg every 8 hr; *CCr >10–<30 ml/min*—250 mg every 12 hr.

etravirine (e-**tra**-veer-een)

Intelence

Classification
Therapeutic: antiretrovirals
Pharmacologic: non-nucleoside reverse transcriptase inhibitors

Pregnancy Category B

Indications
HIV infection (with other antiretrovirals).

Contraindications/Precautions
Contraindicated in: Concurrent use with other non-nucleoside reverse transcriptase inhibitors (NNRTIs), rifampin, rifapentine, St. John's wort.
Use Cautiously in: Concurrent use of antiarrhythmics, anticonvulsants, antifungals, clarithyromycin, rifabutin, diazepam, dexamethasone, HMG Co-A reductase inhibitors (statins), immunusuppressants; Geri: Consider age-related decrease in organ function and body mass, concurrent disease states and medications; Pedi, OB, Lactation: Pregnancy, lactation and children (safety not established, breast-feeding not recommended in HIV-infected women).

Adverse Reactions/Side Effects
CNS: SEIZURES, anxiety, confusion, fatigue, headache, insomnia, sleep disorders. **EENT:** blurred vision, vertigo. **CV:** MYOCARDIAL INFARCTION, angina pectoris, atrial fibrillation, hypertension. **GI:** nausea, abdominal pain, anorexia, dry mouth, hepatitis, stomatitis, vomiting. **GU:** renal failure. **Endo:** gynecomastia, hyperglycemia, hyperlipidemia. **Hemat:** anemia, hemolytic anemia. **Derm:** rash. **Metab:** fat redistribution. **Neuro:** peripheral neuropathy. **Misc:** allergic reactions including STEVENS-JOHNSON SYNDROME, IMMUNE RECONSTITUTION SYNDROME.

Route/Dosage
PO (Adults): 200 mg twice daily.

ixabepilone (icks-a-**bep**-i-lone)
Ixempra

Classification
Therapeutic: antineoplastics
Pharmacologic: epothilone B analog

Pregnancy Category D

Indications
Combination use with capecitabine for the treatment of metastatic or locally advanced breast cancer currently resistant to a taxane and anthracycline or resistant to a taxane and cannot tolerate further anthracycline. May also be used as monotherapy for breast cancers that are not responding to anthrancylines, taxane or capecitabine.

Contraindications/Precautions
Contraindicated in: Previous hypersensitivity to any medications containing Cremophor EL or similar derivatives (polyoxethylated castor oil); Neutrophils <1500 cells/m³ or platelets <100,000 cells/m³; Severe hepatic impairment; Use with capecitabine is contraindicated for hepatic impairment (AST or ALT >2.5 × upper limits of normal or bilirubin >1 × upper limit of normal) due to ↑ risk of toxicity and death associated with neutropenia; OB: Pregnancy or lactation.
Use Cautiously in: Toxicity; dose adjustments may be required for neuropathy/arthralgia/myalgia/fatigue, neutropenia, thrombocytopenia, moderate hepatic impairment or palmar-plantar erythrodysesthesia; Diluent contains dehydrated alcohol; consider possible CNS effects; Diabetes or history of neuropathy (↑ risk of severe neuropathy); History of cardiac disease (may ↑ risk of myocardial ischemia or ventricular dysfunction; OB: Patients with child-bearing potential.

Adverse Reactions/Side Effects
CNS: fatigue, weakness, dizziness, headache, insomnia. **EENT:** ↑ lacrimation. **CV:** chest pain, edema, myocardial ischemia, ventricular dysfunction. **Resp:** dyspnea. **GI:** abdominal pain, anorexia*, constipation, diarrhea, mucositis, nausea, stomatitis, vomiting, altered taste. **Derm:** alopecia, hyperpigmentation, nail disorder, palmar-plantar erythrodysesthesia (combination therapy with capecitabine), exfoliation, pruritus, rash, hot flushes. **Hemat:** MYELOSUPPRESSION. **MS:** arthralgia, musculoskeletal pain, myalgia. **Neuro:** peripheral neuropathy. **Misc:** hypersensitivity reactions.

Route/Dosage
IV (Adults): 40 mg/m² every 3 weeks; not to exceed dose greater than that calculated for 2.2 m² (88 mg/dose)

Hepatic Impairment
IV (Adults): *Moderate Impairment*—20 mg/m² every 3 weeks; not to exceed 30 mg/m².

methoxypolyethylene glycol-epoetin beta
(meh-**thok**-see-**pah**-lee-**eh**-thih-leen**gly**-kol ee-**poh**-eh-tin**bay**-ta)
Mircera

Classification
Therapeutic: antianemics
Pharmacologic: hormones

Pregnancy Category C

Indications
Anemia due to chronic renal failure.

Contraindications/Precautions
Contraindicated in: Hypersensitivity; Uncontrolled hypertension; Treatment of anemia due to cancer chemotherapy.
Use Cautiously in: Patients with hypertension or cardiovascular disease (monitor closely); Dialysis patients (IV route recommended to decrease immunogenecity); Predialysis patients (may require lower doses); Geri: Use lower doses, consider age related decrease in metabolic function, concurrent disease states and medications; OB, Lactation: Use during pregnancy only if maternal benefit outweighs fetal risk; Pedi: Safe use not established.

Adverse Reactions/Side Effects
CNS: SEIZURES, headaches. **CV:** CARDIOVASCULAR AND THROMBOTIC EVENTS, hypertension, hypotension. **GI:** diarrhea, constipation, vomiting. **Hemat:** PURE RED APLASIA. **Misc:** allergic reactions including ANAPHYLAXIS, fistula complications.

Route/Dosage
Subcut, IV (Adults): 0.6 mcg/kg once every two weeks, dosing based on hemoglobin values. Once every-two-week dose is determined, may be given monthly at twice the every-two-week dose.

nebivolol (ne-bi-vi-lole)
Bystolic

Classification
Therapeutic: antihypertensives
Pharmacologic: beta blockers (selective)

Pregnancy Category C

Indications
Hypertension (alone and with other antihypertensives).

Contraindications/Precautions
Contraindicated in: Hypersensitivity; Severe bradycardia, heart block greater than first degree. cardiogenic shock, decompensated heart failure or sick sinus syndrome (without pacemaker); Severe hepatic impairment (Child-Pugh >B); Bronchospastic disease; OB: Lactation.
Use Cautiously in: Coronary artery disease (rapid cessation should be avoided); Compensated congestive heart failure.; Major surgery (anesthesia may augment myocardial depression); Diabetes mellitus (may mask signs of hypoglycemia); Thyrotoxicosis (may mask symptoms); Moderate hepatic impairment (↓ metabolism); Severe renal impairment (↓ initial dose if CCr <30 ml/min); History of severe allergic reactions (↑ intensity of reactions); Pheochromocytoma (alpha blockers required prior to beta blockers); Geri: Consider increased sensitivity, concurrent chronic diseases, medications and presence of age-related decrease in clearance; OB: Use in pregnancy only if maternal benefit outweighs fetal risk; Pedi: Safe use in children <18 yr not established.

Adverse Reactions/Side Effects
CNS: dizziness, fatigue, headache.

Route/Dosage
PO (Adults): 5 mg once daily initially, may increase at 2 wk intervals up to 40 mg/day.

Hepatic/Renal Impairment
PO (Adults): 2.5 mg once daily initially; titrate upward cautiously.

nilotinib (ni-lo-ti-nib)
Tasigna

Classification
Therapeutic: antineoplastics
Pharmacologic: enzyme inhibitors, kinase inhibitors

Pregnancy Category D

Indications
Chronic or accelerated phase Philadelphia chromosome positive chronic myelogenous leukemia which has not responded to other treatment, including imatinib.

Contraindications/Precautions
Contraindicated in: Hypokalemia or hypomagnesemia; Long QT syndrome; Concurrent use of medications known to prolong QT interval; Concurrent use of strong inhibitors of the CYP3A4 enzyme system (increased risk of toxicity); Concurrent use of strong inducers of the CYP3A4 enzyme system (may ↓ effectiveness); Concurrent grapefruit juice (may ↑ risk of toxicity); Galactose intolerance, severe lactase defi-

ciency or glucose-galactose malabsorption (capsules contain lactose); OB: Pregnancy or lactation.
Use Cautiously in: Concurrent use of other drugs that prolong QT interval; Electrolyte abnormalities; correct prior to administration to ↓ risk of arrhythmias; Hepatic impairment (↓ dose required for Grade 3 elevated bilirubin, transaminases or lipase); OB: Women with child-bearing potential (effective contraception required); Pedi: Safe use in children has not been established.

Adverse Reactions/Side Effects
CNS: fatigue, headache, dizziness. **EENT:** vertigo. **CV:** ARRHYTHMIAS, hypertension, palpitations, QT prolongation. **GI:** constipation, diarrhea, nausea, vomiting, abdominal discomfort, anorexia, dyspepsia, flatulence, hepatotoxicity. **Derm:** pruritus, rash, alopecia, flushing. **F and E:** hyperkalemia, hypocalcemia, hypokalemia, hyponatremia, hypophosphatemia. **Hemat:** MYELOSUPRESSION. **Metab:** ↑ lipase, hyperglycemia. **MS:** musculoskeletal pain. **Neuro:** paresthesia. **Misc:** fever, night sweats.

Route/Dosage
PO (Adults): 400 mg twice daily; adjustment may be required for toxicity and/or drug interactions.

raltegravir (ral-teg-ra-veer)
Isentress

Classification
Therapeutic: antiretrovirals
Pharmacologic: integrase strand transfer inhibitor (INSTI)

Pregnancy Category C

Indications
HIV infection (with other antiretrovirals) in patients who are failing other treatments as evidenced by continued viral replication and resistance to other agents.

Contraindications/Precautions
Contraindicated in: OB: Lactation (breast feeding not recommended in HIV-infected patients).
Use Cautiously in: Geri: Choose dose carefully, considering concurrent disease states, drug therapy and age-related decrease in hepatic and renal function; Concurrent use of medications associated with rhabomyolysis/myopathy (may increase risk); OB: Use in pregnancy only if maternal benefit outweighs fetal risk; Pedi: Safe use in children <16 yr not established.

Adverse Reactions/Side Effects
CNS: headache, dizziness, fatigue, weakness. **CV:** myocardial infarction. **GI:** diarrhea, abdominal pain, gastritis, hepatitis, vomiting. **GU:** renal failure/impairment. **Hemat:** anemia, neutropenia. **Metab:** lipodystrophy. **Misc:** hypersensitivity reactions, immune reconstitution syndrome, fever.

Route/Dosage
PO (Adults): 400 mg twice daily.

temsirolimus
(tem-si-ro-li-mus)
Torisel

Classification
Therapeutic: antineoplastics
Pharmacologic: enzyme inhibitors, kinase inhibitors

Pregnancy Category D

Indications
Advanced renal cell carcinoma.

Contraindications/Precautions
Contraindicated in: OB: Pregnancy and lactation.
Use Cautiously in: Hypersensitivity to temsirolimus, sirolimus or polysorbate 80; Perioperative patients (may impair wound healing); OB: Patients which child-bearing potential; Pedi: Safe use in children not established.

Adverse Reactions/Side Effects
CNS: weakness. **EENT:** conjunctivitis. **CV:** hypertension, venous thromboembolism. **Resp:** INTERSTITIAL LUNG DISEASE. **GI:** BOWEL PERFORATION, anorexia, ↑ liver enzymes, mucositis, nausea. **GU:** RENAL FAILURE. **Derm:** rash, abnormal wound healing. **Endo:** hyperglycemia. **F and E:** edema, hypophosphatemia. **Hemat:** anemia, leukopenia, lymphopenia, thrombocytopenia. **Metab:** hyperlipidemia, hypertriglyceridemia. **Misc:** hypersensitivity reactions including ANAPHYLAXIS, ↑ risk of infections.

Route/Dosage
IV (Adults): 25 mg once weekly; dose modification is required for bone marrow toxicity or concurrent use of agents affecting the CYP 3A4 enzyme system (pre-treatment with antihistamine is recommended).

NEW DOSAGE FORMS

Generic Name (Brand Name)	New Dosage Form
amoxicillin (Moxatag)	775 mg extended-release once daily tablet
atazanavir (Reyataz)	300 mg tablet
azithromycin (AzaSite)	1% ophthalmic solution for bacterial conjunctivitis.
ciclesonide (Alvesco)	80 mcg and 160 mcg metered dose inhaler for asthma.
cimetidine (Tagamet)	200 mg tablet OTC
cyclobenzaprine (Amrix)	15 mg and 30 mg extended-release, once-daily capsule
dextroamphetamine (Dexedrine)	5 mg/5 mL oral solution
doxycycline (Doryx, Vibramycin)	75 mg and 100 mg delayed-release capsules; oral suspension 50 mg/5 mL
esomeprazole (Nexium)	10 mg delayed-release oral suspension
fentanyl buccal (Fentora)	300 mg buccal tablet
fomepizole (Antizol)	1 g/mL injection for ethylene glycol poisoning
fosaprepitant (Emend)	115 mg powder for IV injection for chemotherapy-induced N/V.
fosphenytoin (Cerebyx)	50 mg/mL
lamivudine (Epivir)	150 mg and 300 mg tablets
levalbuterol (Xopenex)	Metered dose inhaler 0.045 mg/inhalation
levocetrizine (Xyzal)	2.5 mg/5 mL oral solution
levothyroxine (Unithroid)	137 mcg tablets
lidocaine (Zingo)	A powder intradermal injection for local analgesia prior to venous access procedures in children.
lopinavir/ritonavir (Kaletra)	100 mg/25 mg tablets
methylphenidate (Daytrana)	Transdermal patch delivers 10 mg/9 hrs, 15 mg/9hrs, 20 mg/9 hrs or 30 mg/9 hrs
niacin extended-release/ simvastatin (Simcor)	niacin 500 mg/simvastatin 20 mg niacin 750 mg/simvastatin 20 mg niacin 1 g/simvastatin 20 mg
nisoldipine (Sular)	New extended release dose form 8.5, 17, 25.5, and 34 mg bioequivalent to the 10, 20, 30, and 40 mg dose forms.
orlistat (Alli)	60 mg capsule OTC
pantoprazole (Protonix)	New delayed-release oral suspension formulation in 40 mg packets.
paroxetine (Pexeva)	10, 20, 30, and 40 mg tablets
risedronate (Actonel)	New 75 mg tablet given two consecutive days per mo.
sevelamer (Renvela)	The carbonate salt of Renagel for phosphate binding.
terbinafine (Lamisil)	125 mg and 187.5 mg oral granule formulation for tinea capitis in patients >4 years.
venlafaxine (Effexor, Effexor XR)	12.5 mg tablets 100 mg extended-release capsules
voriconazole (Vfend)	Oral suspension 200 mg/5 mL

RECENT LABELING CHANGES (New Warnings/Indications)

Generic Name (Brand Name)	Labeling change
Antiepileptic drugs	New warning regarding suicide risk.
amiodarone (Cordarone)	New adverse drug reaction of Parkinsonian symptoms.
aripiprazole (Abilify)	New warning related to dystonia. New indication for pediatric patients 10–17 years with Bipolar I disorder.
azithromycin (Zithromax)	New adverse reaction—taste/smell perversion and/or loss.
bevacizumab (Avastin)	New indication with paclitaxel for the treatment of patients who have not received chemotherapy for metastatic HER2 negative breast cancer.
carbamazepine (Tegretol)	New warning regarding risk of serious skin reactions, increased risk with patients of Asian ancestry.
celecoxib (Celebrex)	New warning regarding increased risk of renal toxicity with long term use and interactions.
ciclosonide (Omnaris)	New indication for pediatric patients 6 years and older with seasonal allergic rhinitis and for pediatric patients 12 years and older with perennial allergic rhinitis.
cilostazol (Pletal)	New adverse reactions of blood pressure increase and aplitic anemia.
colesevelam (Welchol)	New indication for adjunctive therapy to improve glycemic control in adults with type 2 diabetes. New warning for patients with type 1 diabetes or with serum triglyceride (TG) concentrations >500 mg/dL.
darunavir (Prezista)	New warnings, precautions and adverse drug reactions.
desmopressin (DDAVP)	New contraindication for patients with hyponatremia or a history of hyponatremia.
duloxetine (Cymbalta)	New warnings regarding risk of abnormal bleeding and serious skin reactions.
erythromycin (Eryc)	New warnings regarding Clostridium difficile associated colitis.
esometrazole (Nexium)	Approved for treatment of GERD in children 1–11 years.
eszopiclone (Lunesta)	New warning regarding administration to patients with depression.
fluoxetine (Prozac)	New warnings regarding hyponatremia and increased risk of bleeding with NSAIDs, aspirin, and other drugs effecting coagulation.
fosamprenavir (Lexiva)	New dosing guidelines for pediatric patients 2 years and older.
idursulfase (Elaprase)	New warning regarding biphasic anaphylactic reactions.
imatinib (Gleevec)	New warnings regarding severe CHF and hypereosinophilic cardiac toxicity.
ketorolac (Toradol)	New interactions with ACE inhibitors, angiotension II receptor antagonists, and selective serotonin reuptake inhibitors.
lopinavir/ritonavir (Kaletra)	New interactions with St. John's Wort, lovastatin, and simvastatin.
meropenem (Merrem)	New hematologic and skin adverse reactions.
micafungin (Mycamine)	New indication for treatment of patients with Candidemia, Acute Disseminated Candidiasis, Candida Peritonitis and Abscesses, and patients with esophageal Candidiasis.
montelukast (Singulair)	New warning for risk of erythema nodusum and suicidal thinking and behavior.
mometasone (Asmanex)	New indication for children 4–11 years for asthma prophylaxis.
moxifloxacin (Avelox)	New caution regarding photosensitivity.
natalizumab (Tysabri)	New indication for moderate to severe Crohn's disease.
octreotide (Sandostatin)	New indication for long term maintenance therapy of acromegaly.

RECENT LABELING CHANGES (continued)

oxcarbazepine (Trileptal)	New warnings of anaphylactic reactions and angioedema.
palonosetron (Aloxi)	New indication for postoperative nausea and vomiting.
panitumumab (Vectibix)	New interactions with chemotherapy agents.
paroxetine (Pexeva)	New warning regarding increased risk of bleeding with NSAIDs, aspirin, and other drugs effecting coagulation.
propranolol (Inderal)	New contraindications for patients with bronchial asthma and hypersensitivity to propranolol. New warning for patients with angina. New adverse reactions.
quetiapine (Seroquel)	New warning regarding risk or anemia, leucopenia, and agranulocytosis.
sertraline (Zoloft)	New warning regarding increased risk of bleeding with NSAIDs, aspirin, and other drugs effecting coagulation.
sildenafil (Viagra)	New warning regarding tinnitus, hearing loss, vision changes, and seizures.
sirolimus (Rapamune)	New instructions for administration of tablets.
sitagliptin (Januvia)	New precautions with other drugs that cause hypoglycemia.
somatropin (Accretion)	New brand name drug.
sorafenib (Nexavar)	New warnings in patients with hepatic impairment.
tadalafil (Cialis)	New warning regarding tinnitus and hearing loss.
temazepam (Restoril)	New warnings and precautions regarding lack of response.
teriparatide (Forteo)	New warning of spasms of the back and legs.
tiotropium (Spiriva)	New warning regarding risk of stroke.
triamcinolone (Azmacort)	New adverse reactions of increased risk of decreased bone mineral density, osteoporosis, and fracture.
valsartan (Diovan)	New indication for hypertension in pediatric patients 6–16 years old.
vardenafil (Levitra)	New warning regarding tinnitus and hearing loss and seizures.
varenicline (Chantix)	New warning regarding neuropsychiatric symptoms.
voriconazole (Vfend)	New interaction with St. John's Wort and other drugs. New IV incompatibilities. New monitoring guidelines for patients at risk for pancreatitis.
ziprasodone (Geodon)	New GI (swollen tongue), GU (enuresis, urinary incontinence), and Nervous system (facial droop, tardive dyskinesia) adverse drug reactions.

DISCONTINUED DRUGS

Generic Name (Brand Name)	Reason for Discontinuation
amprenavir (Agenerase)	Oral solution and 50 mg capsules discontinued due to decrease in demand since release of fosamprenavir.
aprotinin (Trasylol)	Marketing suspension due to possible increased risk for death.
cefamandol (Mandol)	No longer manufactured.
ethmozine (Morizicine)	Manufacturer will no longer sell product after December 31, 2007 due to a marketing decision.
gatifloxacin (Tequin)	Tablets and solution for infection – no longer manufactured.
insulin recombinant human, powder for inhalation (Exubera)	No longer manufactured due to unmet sales goals.

DISCONTINUED DRUGS (continued)

interferon alfa 2a (Roferon)	No longer manufactured.
loracarbef (Lorabid)	No longer manufactured.
mivacurium (Mivacron)	No longer manufactured.
pergolide (Permax)	Manufacturer-initiated withdrawal from the market due to the risk of heart valve damage.
pemoline (Cylert)	Declining sales and availability of generic equivalents.
tegaserod (Zelnorm)	Withdrawn from the market due to increased risk of cardiovascular adverse effects (e.g., angina, heart attack, and stroke).
trimetrexate (Neutrexin)	No longer manufactured.
zalcitabine (Hivid)	No longer recommended due to newer regimens.

APPENDIX B

Combination Drugs

Note: The drugs listed in this section are in alphabetical order according to trade names. If the trade name does not specify dosage form, the dosage form is either a tablet or capsule. Following each trade name are the generic names and doses of the active ingredients contained in each preparation. For information on these drugs, look up each generic name in the combination. For inert ingredients, see drug label. **(OTC)** signifies "over-the-counter" or nonprescription medication.

A-200 Shampoo—0.33% pyrethrins + 4% piperonyl butoxide **(OTC)**
Accuretic 10/12.5—quinapril 10 mg + hydrochlorothiazide 12.5 mg
Accuretic 20/12.5—quinapril 20 mg + hydrochlorothiazide 12.5 mg
Accuretic 20/25—quinapril 20 mg + hydrochlorothiazide 25 mg
Actifed Cold and Allergy—chlorpheniramine 4 mg + phenylephrine 10 mg **(OTC)**
Actifed Cold and Sinus—chlorpheniramine 2 mg + pseudoephedrine 30 mg + acetaminophen 500 mg **(OTC)**
Activella Tablets 0.5/0.1—estradiol 0.5 mg + norethindrone 0.1 mg
Activella Tablets 1/0.5—estradiol 1 mg + norethindrone 0.5 mg
Actoplus Met 15/500—pioglitazone 15 mg + metformin 500 mg
Actoplus Met 15/850—pioglitazone 15 mg+ metformin 850 mg
Adderall 5 mg—dextroamphetamine sulfate 1.25 mg + dextroamphetamine saccharate 1.25 mg + amphetamine aspartate 1.25 mg + amphetamine sulfate 1.25 mg
Adderall 7.5 mg—dextroamphetamine sulfate 1.875 mg + dextroamphetamine saccharate 1.875 mg + amphetamine aspartate 1.875 mg + amphetamine sulfate 1.875 mg
Adderall 10 mg—dextroamphetamine sulfate 2.5 mg + dextroamphetamine saccharate 2.5 mg + amphetamine aspartate 2.5 mg + amphetamine sulfate 2.5 mg
Adderall 12.5 mg—dextroamphetamine sulfate 3.125 mg + dextroamphetamine saccharate 3.125 mg + amphetamine aspartate 3.125 mg + amphetamine sulfate 3.125 mg
Adderall 15 mg—dextroamphetamine sulfate 3.75 mg + dextroamphetamine saccharate 3.75 mg + amphetamine aspartate 3.75 mg + amphetamine sulfate 3.75 mg
Adderall 20 mg—dextroamphetamine sulfate 5 mg + dextroamphetamine saccharate 5 mg + amphetamine aspartate 5 mg + amphetamine sulfate 5 mg
Adderall 30 mg—dextroamphetamine sulfate 7.5 mg + dextroamphetamine saccharate 7.5 mg + amphetamine aspartate 7.5 mg + amphetamine sulfate 7.5 mg
Adderall XR 5 mg—dextroamphetamine saccharate 1.25 mg + dextroamphetamine sulfate 1.25 mg + amphetamine aspartate monohydrate 1.25 mg + amphetamine sulfate 1.25 mg
Adderall XR 10 mg—dextroamphetamine saccharate 2.5 mg + dextroamphetamine sulfate 2.5 mg + amphetamine aspartate monohydrate 2.5 mg + amphetamine sulfate 2.5 mg
Adderall XR 15 mg—dextroamphetamine saccharate 3.75 mg + dextroamphetamine sulfate 3.75 mg + amphetamine aspartate monohydrate 3.75 mg + amphetamine sulfate 3.75 mg
Adderall XR 20 mg—dextroamphetamine saccharate 5 mg + dextroamphetamine sulfate 5 mg + amphetamine aspartatemonohydrate 5 mg + amphetamine sulfate 5 mg

Adderall XR 25 mg—dextroamphetamine saccharate 6.25 mg + dextroamphetamine sulfate 6.25 mg + amphetamine aspartate monohydrate 6.25 mg + amphetamine sulfate 6.25 mg
Adderall XR 30 mg—dextroamphetamine saccharate 7.5 mg + dextroamphetamine sulfate 7.5 mg + amphetamine aspartate monohydrate 7.5 mg + amphetamine sulfate 7.5 mg
Advair Diskus 100—(per actuation) fluticasone 100 mcg + salmeterol 50 mcg
Advair Diskus 250—(per actuation) fluticasone 250 mcg + salmeterol 50 mcg
Advair Diskus 500—(per actuation) fluticasone 500 mcg + salmeterol 50 mcg
Advair HFA 45—(per actuation) fluticasone 45 mcg + salmeterol 30.45 mcg
Advair HFA 115—(per actuation) fluticasone 115 mcg + salmeterol 30.45 mcg
Advair HFA 230—(per actuation) fluticasone 230 mcg + salmeterol 30.45 mcg
Advicor 500/20—extended-release niacin 500 mg + lovastatin 20 mg
Advicor 750/20—extended-release niacin 750 mg + lovastatin 20 mg
Advicor 1000/20—extended-release niacin 1000 mg + lovastatin 20 mg
Advicor 1000/40—extended-release niacin 1000 mg + lovastatin 40 mg
Advil Cold & Sinus—pseudoephedrine 30 mg + ibuprofen 200 mg **(OTC)**
Advil Multi-Symptom Cold—chlorpheniramine 2 mg + pseudoephedrine 30 mg + ibuprofen 200 mg **(OTC)**
Advil PM Liquigels—diphenhydramine 25 mg + ibuprofen 200 mg **(OTC)**
Aggrenox—aspirin 25 mg + extended-release dipyridamole 200 mg
Aldactazide 25/25—hydrochlorothiazide 25 mg + spironolactone 25 mg
Aldactazide 50/50—hydrochlorothiazide 50 mg + spironolactone 50 mg
Alesse—levonorgestrel 0.1 mg + ethinyl estradiol 20 mcg
Aleve-D Sinus & Cold—naproxen 220 mg + extended-release pseudoephedrine 120 mg **(OTC)**
Alka-Seltzer Effervescent, Original—citric acid 1000 mg + sodium bicarbonate 1916 mg + aspirin 325 mg **(OTC)**
Alka-Seltzer Plus Cold & Cough Liqui-Gels—dextromethorphan 10 mg + phenylephrine 5 mg + chlorpheniramine 2 mg + acetaminophen 325 mg **(OTC)**
Alka-Seltzer Plus Night Cold Formula Liquid Gels—acetaminophen 325 mg + doxylamine 6.25 mg + dextromethorphan 15 mg **(OTC)**
Alka-Seltzer Plus Sinus Formula—phenylephrine 5 mg + acetaminophen 250 mg **(OTC)**
Allegra-D 12 Hour—fexofenadine 60 mg + extended-release pseudoephedrine 120 mg
Allegra-D 24 Hour—fexofenadine 180 mg + extended-release pseudoephedrine 240 mg
Allerest Maximum Strength—pseudoephedrine 30 mg + chlorpheniramine 2 mg **(OTC)**
Allerest Allergy and Sinus Relief Maximum Strength—pseudoephedrine 30 mg + acetaminophen 325 mg **(OTC)**
Allerfrim Syrup—(per 5 ml) triprolidine 1.25 mg + pseudoephedrine 30 mg **(OTC)**
Anacin—aspirin 400 mg + caffeine 32 mg **(OTC)**
Anacin Maximum Strength—aspirin 500 mg + caffeine 32 mg **(OTC)**
Anaplex DM Syrup—(per 5 ml) brompheniramine 4 mg + dextromethorphan 30 mg + pseudoephedrine 60 mg
Anexsia 5/325—hydrocodone 5 mg + acetaminophen 325 mg
Anexsia 5/500—hydrocodone 5 mg + acetaminophen 500 mg
Anexsia 7.5/325—hydrocodone 7.5 mg + acetaminophen 325 mg
Anexsia 7.5/650—hydrocodone 7.5 mg + acetaminophen 650 mg
Anexsia 10/750—hydrocodone 10 mg + acetaminophen 750 mg
Angeliq—drosperinone 0.5 mg + estradiol 1 mg
Apri—desogestrel 0.15 mg + ethinyl estradiol 30 mcg
Aranelle
Phase I—norethindrone 0.5 mg + ethinyl estradiol 35 mcg

Phase II—norethindrone 1 mg + ethinyl estradiol 35 mcg
Phase III—norethindrone 0.5 mg + ethinyl estradiol 35 mcg
Arthrotec 50/200—diclofenac 50 mg + misoprostol 200 mcg
Arthrotec 75/200—diclofenac 75 mg + misoprostol 200 mcg
Ascriptin A/D—aspirin 325 mg + aluminum hydroxide 75 mg + magnesium hydroxide 75 mg + calcium carbonate 75 mg **(OTC)**
Atacand HCT 16/12.5—candesartan 16 mg + hydrochlorothiazide 12.5 mg
Atacand HCT 32/12.5—candesartan 32 mg + hydrochlorothiazide 12.5 mg
🍁**Atacand Plus**—candesartan 16 mg + hydrochlorothiazide 12.5 mg
Atripla—efavirenz 600 mg + emtricitabine 200 mg + tenofovir 300 mg
Augmentin 250—amoxicillin 250 mg + clavulanic acid 125 mg
Augmentin 500—amoxicillin 500 mg + clavulanic acid 125 mg
Augmentin 875—amoxicillin 875 mg + clavulanic acid 125 mg
Augmentin 125 Chewable—amoxicillin 125 mg + clavulanic acid 31.25 mg
Augmentin 200 Chewable—amoxicillin 200 mg + clavulanic acid 28.5 mg
Augmentin 250 Chewable—amoxicillin 250 mg + clavulanic acid 62.5 mg
Augmentin 400 Chewable—amoxicillin 400 mg + clavulanic acid 57 mg
Augmentin 125 mg Suspension—(per 5 ml) amoxicillin 125 mg + clavulanic acid 31.25 mg
Augmentin 200 mg Suspension—(per 5 ml) amoxicillin 200 mg + clavulanic acid 28.5 mg
Augmentin 250 mg Suspension—(per 5 ml) amoxicillin 250 mg + clavulanic acid 62.5 mg
Augmentin 400 mg Suspension—(per 5 ml) amoxicillin 400 mg + clavulanic acid 57 mg
Avalide 150/12.5—irbesartan 150 mg + hydrochlorothiazide 12.5 mg
Avalide 300/12.5—irbesartan 300 mg + hydrochlorothiazide 12.5 mg
Avandamet 2/500—rosiglitazone 2 mg + metformin 500 mg
Avandamet 2/1000—rosiglitazone 2 mg + metformin 1000 mg
Avandamet 4/500—rosiglitazone 4 mg + metformin 500 mg
Avandamet 4/1000—rosiglitazone 4 mg + metformin 1000 mg
Avandaryl 4/1—rosiglitazone 4 mg + glimepiride 1 mg
Avandaryl 4/2—rosiglitazone 4 mg + glimepiride 2 mg
Avandaryl 4/4—rosiglitazone 4 mg + glimepiride 4 mg
Avandaryl 8/2—rosiglitazone 8 mg + glimepiride 2 mg
Avandaryl 8/4—rosiglitazone 8 mg + glimepiride 4 mg
Aviane—levonorgestrel 0.1 mg + ethinyl estradiol 20 mcg
Azdone—aspirin 500 mg + hydrocodone 5 mg
Azor 5/20—amlodipine 5 mg + olmesartan 20 mg
Azor 5/40—amlodipine 5 mg + olmesartan 40 mg
Azor 10/20—amlodipine 10 mg + olmesartan 20 mg
Azor 10/40—amlodipine 10 mg + olmesartan 40 mg
B & O Supprettes No. 15A—belladonna extract 16.2 mg + opium 30 mg
B & O Supprettes No. 16A—belladonna extract 16.2 mg + opium 60 mg
Bactrim—trimethoprim 80 mg + sulfamethoxazole 400 mg
Bactrim DS—trimethoprim 160 mg + sulfamethoxazole 800 mg
Balziva—norethindrone 0.4 mg + ethinyl estradiol 35 mcg
Bayer Back & Body—aspirin 500 mg + caffeine 32.5 mg **(OTC)**
Bayer PM—aspirin 500 mg + diphenhydramine 38.3 mg **(OTC)**
Bayer Select Maximum Strength Menstrual—acetaminophen 500 mg + pamabrom 25 mg **(OTC)**

Bayer Women's Aspirin plus Calcium—aspirin 81 mg + calcium carbonate 300 mg (OTC)
Benadryl Allergy & Sinus Headache Caplets—diphenhydramine 12.5 mg + phenylephrine 5 mg + acetaminophen 325 mg **(OTC)**
Benadryl-D Allergy & Sinus Tablets—phenylephrine 10 mg + diphenhydramine 25 mg (OTC)
Benicar HCT 20/12.5—olmesartan 20 mg + hydrochlorothiazide 12.5 mg
Benicar HCT 40/12.5—olmesartan 40 mg + hydrochlorothiazide 12.5 mg
Benicar HCT 40/25—olmesartan 40 mg + hydrochlorothiazide 25 mg
BenzaClin Topical Gel—1% clindamycin + 5% benzoyl peroxide
Benzamycin Topical Gel—5% benzoyl peroxide + 3% erythromycin
Bicitra Solution—(per 5 ml) sodium citrate 500 mg + citric acid 334 mg
Bidil—isosorbide dinitrate 20 mg + hydralazine hydrochloride 37.5 mg
Blephamide Ophthalmic Suspension/Ointment—0.2% prednisolone + 10% sodium sulfacetamide
Brevicon—norethindrone 0.5 mg + ethinyl estradiol 35 mcg
Bromfed DM Liquid—(per 5 ml) brompheniramine 2 mg + dextromethorphan 10 mg + pseudoephedrine 30 mg
Bromfenex—brompheniramine 12 mg + extended-release pseudoephedrine 120 mg
Bromfenex PD—brompheniramine 6 mg + pseudoephedrine 60 mg
Bronkaid Dual Action—ephedrine 25 mg + guaifenesin 400 mg **(OTC)**
Brontex—codeine 10 mg + guaifenesin 300 mg
Bufferin—aspirin 325 mg + calcium carbonate 158 mg + magnesium oxide 63 mg + magnesium carbonate 34 mg **(OTC)**
Butapap 50/325—butalbital 50 mg + acetaminophen 325 mg
Butapap 50/650—butalbital 50 mg + acetaminophen 650 mg
Caduet 2.5/10—amlodipine 2.5 mg + atorvastatin 10 mg
Caduet 2.5/20—amlodipine 2.5 mg + atorvastatin 20 mg
Caduet 2.5/40—amlodipine 2.5 mg + atorvastatin 40 mg
Caduet 5/10—amlodipine 5 mg + atorvastatin 10 mg
Caduet 5/20—amlodipine 5 mg + atorvastatin 20 mg
Caduet 5/40—amlodipine 5 mg + atorvastatin 40 mg
Caduet 5/80—amlodipine 5 mg + atorvastatin 80 mg
Caduet 10/10—amlodipine 10 mg + atorvastatin 10 mg
Caduet 10/20—amlodipine 10 mg + atorvastatin 20 mg
Caduet 10/40—amlodipine 10 mg + atorvastatin 40 mg
Caduet 10/80—amlodipine 10 mg + atorvastatin 80 mg
Cafergot—ergotamine 1 mg + caffeine 100 mg
Caltrate 600+D—vitamin D 200 IU + calcium 600 mg **(OTC)**
Capozide 25/15—captopril 25 mg + hydrochlorothiazide 15 mg
Capozide 25/25—captopril 25 mg + hydrochlorothiazide 25 mg
Capozide 50/15—captopril 50 mg + hydrochlorothiazide 15 mg
Capozide 50/25—captopril 50 mg + hydrochlorothiazide 25 mg
Cardec DM Syrup—(per 5 ml) pseudoephedrine 60 mg + carbinoxamine 4 mg + dextromethorphan 15 mg **(OTC)**
Cetacaine Topical Spray—14% benzocaine + 2% tetracaine + 2% butamben + 0.005% cetyl dimethyl ethyl ammonium bromide
Cheracol Cough Syrup—(per 5 ml) codeine 10 mg + guaifenesin 100 mg
Children's Advil Cold Liquid—(per 5 ml) ibuprofen 100 mg + pseudoephedrine 15 mg **(OTC)**

Chlor-Trimeton 4 Hour Relief—pseudoephedrine 60 mg + chlorpheniramine 4 mg (OTC)
Chlor-Trimeton 12 Hour Relief—pseudoephedrine 120 mg + chlorpheniramine 8 mg (OTC)
Ciprodex Otic Suspension—0.3% ciprofloxacin + 0.1% dexamethasone
Cipro HC Otic Suspension—0.2% ciprofloxacin + 1% hydrocortisone
Clarinex-D 12 Hour—desloratadine 2.5 mg + pseudoephedrine 120 mg
Clarinex-D 24 Hour—desloratadine 5 mg + pseudoephedrine 120 mg
Claritin-D 12 Hour—loratadine 5 mg + pseudoephedrine 120 mg (OTC)
Claritin-D 24-Hour—loratadine 10 mg + pseudoephedrine 240 mg (OTC)
✱Clavulin 500—amoxicillin 500 mg + clavulanic acid 125 mg
✱Clavulin 875—amoxicillin 875 mg + clavulanic acid 125 mg
✱Clavulin 125 Suspension—(per 5 ml) amoxicillin 125 mg + clavulanic acid 31.25 mg
✱Clavulin 200 Suspension—(per 5 ml) amoxicillin 200 mg + clavulanic acid 28.5 mg
✱Clavulin 250 Suspension—(per 5 ml) amoxicillin 250 mg + clavulanic acid 62.5 mg
✱Clavulin 400 Suspension—(per 5 ml) amoxicillin 400 mg + clavulanic acid 57 mg
ClimaraPro Transdermal Patch (release per day—estradiol 0.045 mg + levonorgestrel 0.015 mg
Clomycin Topical Ointment—bacitracin 400 units + neomycin sulfate (equiv. to 3.5 g neomycin base) + polymyxin B sulfate 5000 units + lidocaine 40 mg (OTC)
Clorpres 15/0.1—chlorthalidone 15 mg + clonidine 0.1 mg
Clorpres 15/0.2—chlorthalidone 15 mg + clonidine 0.2 mg
Clorpres 15/0.3—chlorthalidone 15 mg + clonidine 0.3 mg
Co-Gesic—acetaminophen 500 mg + hydrocodone 5 mg
Codiclear DH Syrup—(per 5 ml) hydrocodone 3.5 mg + guaifenesin 300 mg
Codimal—pseudoephedrine 30 mg + chlorpheniramine 2 mg + acetaminophen 325 mg (OTC)
Codimal DH Syrup—(per 5 ml) hydrocodone 1.66 mg + phenylephrine 5 mg + pyrilamine 8.33 mg
Codimal DM Syrup—(per 5 ml) phenylephrine 5 mg + pyrilamine 8.33 mg + dextromethorphan 10 mg (OTC)
Codimal-L.A.—chlorpheniramine 8 mg + pseudoephedrine 120 mg
Codimal PH Syrup—(per 5 ml) codeine 10 mg + phenylephrine 5 mg + pyrilamine 8.33 mg
Col-Probenecid—probenecid 500 mg + colchicine 0.5 mg
Coly-Mycin S Otic Suspension—1% hydrocortisone + neomycin base 3.3 mg/ml + colistin 3 mg/ml + 0.05% thonzonium bromide
Combigan Ophthalmic Solution—0.2% brimonidine + 0.5% timolol
CombiPatch 0.05/0.14—estradiol 0.05 mg/day + norethindrone 0.14 mg/day
CombiPatch 0.05/0.25—estradiol 0.05 mg/day + norethindrone 0.25 mg/day
Combivent—(per actuation) ipratropium bromide 18 mcg + albuterol 103 mcg
Combivir—lamivudine 150 mg + zidovudine 300 mg
Combunox—oxycodone 5 mg + ibuprofen 400 mg
Comtrex Deep Chest Cold Caplets—acetaminophen 325 mg + guaifenesin 200 mg (OTC)
Comtrex Maximum Strength Non-Drowsy Caplets—acetaminophen 325 mg + phenylephrine 5 mg + dextromethorphan 15 mg (OTC)
Congestac—guaifenesin 400 mg + pseudoephedrine 60 mg (OTC)

Contac Cold & Flu Maximum Strength Caplets—chlorpheniramine 2 mg + phenylephrine 5 mg + acetaminophen 500 mg **(OTC)**

Contac Cold & Flu Non-Drowsy Maximum Strength Caplets—phenylephrine 5 mg + acetaminophen 500 mg **(OTC)**

Coricidin HBP Chest Congestion and Cough—dextromethorphan 10 mg + guaifenesin 200 mg **(OTC)**

Coricidin HBP Cold and Flu—acetaminophen 325 mg + chlorpheniramine 2 mg **(OTC)**

Coricidin HBP Cough and Cold—chlorpheniramine 4 mg + dextromethorphan 30 mg **(OTC)**

Coricidin HBP Maximum Strength Flu—acetaminophen 500 mg + chlorpheniramine 2 mg + dextromethorphan 15 mg **(OTC)**

Cortisporin Ophthalmic Suspension/Otic (Solution/Suspension)—(per ml) neomycin base 3.5 mg + polymyxin B 10,000 units + 1% hydrocortisone

Cortisporin Topical Cream—(per g) neomycin sulfate 3.5 mg + polymyxin B 10,000 units + 0.5% hydrocortisone

Cortisporin Topical Ointment—(per g) neomycin sulfate 3.5 mg + bacitracin 400 units + polymyxin B 5000 units + 1% hydrocortisone

Corzide 40/5—nadolol 40 mg + bendroflumethiazide 5 mg

Corzide 80/5—nadolol 80 mg + bendroflumethiazide 5 mg

Cosopt Ophthalmic Solution—2% dorzolamide + 0.5% timolol

🍁**Coversyl Plus**—perindopril 4 mg + indapamide 1.25 mg

🍁**Coversyl Plus LD**—perindopril 2 mg + indapamide 0.625 mg

Creon 5—lipase 5000 units + amylase 16,600 units + protease 18,750 units

Creon 10—lipase 10,000 units + amylase 33,200 units + protease 37,500 units

Creon 20—lipase 20,000 units + amylase 66,400 units + protease 75,000 units

Cryselle—norgestrel 0.3 mg + ethinyl estradiol 30 mcg

Cyclessa

- **Phase I**—desogestrel 0.1 mg + ethinyl estradiol 25 mcg
- **Phase II**—desogestrel 0.125 mg + ethinyl estradiol 25 mcg
- **Phase III**—desogestrel 0.15 mg + ethinyl estradiol 25 mcg

Cyclomydril Ophthalmic Solution—0.2% cyclopentolate + 1% phenylephrine

Dallergy Caplets—chlorpheniramine 8 mg + phenylephrine 20 mg + methscopolamine 2.5 mg

Dallergy Extended Release—phenylephrine 20 mg + chlorpheniramine 12 mg + methscopolamine 2.5 mg

Dallergy-JR Capsules—phenylephrine 20 mg + chlorpheniramine 4 mg

Dallergy Syrup—(per 5 ml) chlorpheniramine 2 mg + phenylephrine 8 mg + methscopolamine 0.75 mg

Dallergy Tablets—chlorpheniramine 4 mg + phenylephrine 10 mg + methscopolamine 1.25 mg

Damason-P—hydrocodone 5 mg + aspirin 500 mg

Darvocet-N 50—propoxyphene napsylate 50 mg + acetaminophen 325 mg

Darvocet-N 100—propoxyphene napsylate 100 mg + acetaminophen 650 mg

Dayquil Cold & Flu Relief Liquid—(per 5 ml) acetaminophen 325 mg + dextromethorphan 10 mg + phenylephrine 5 mg **(OTC)**

Dayquil Sinus Liquicaps—acetaminophen 325 mg + phenylephrine 5 mg **(OTC)**

Deconamine—pseudoephedrine 60 mg + chlorpheniramine 4 mg

Deconamine SR—pseudoephedrine 120 mg + chlorpheniramine 8 mg

Deconamine Syrup—(per 5 ml) pseudoephedrine 30 mg + chlorpheniramine 2 mg

Desogen—ethinyl estradiol 30 mcg + desogestrel 0.15 mg

Difil-G Forte Liquid—(per 5 ml) dyphylline 100 mg + guaifenesin 100 mg

Difil-G Tablets—dyphylline 200 mg + guaifenesin 300 mg
Dilex-G Syrup—(per 5 ml) dyphylline 100 mg + guaifenesin 200 mg
Dilex G Tablets—dyphylline 200 mg + guaifenesin 400 mg
Dimetapp Cold & Allergy Elixir—(per 5 ml) phenylephrine 2.5 mg + brompheniramine 1 mg **(OTC)**
Dimetapp Cough & Cold DM Elixir—(per 5 ml) phenylephrine 2.5 mg + brompheniramine 1 mg + dextromethorphan 5 mg **(OTC)**
Diovan HCT 80/12.5—valsartan 80 mg + hydrochlorothiazide 12.5 mg
Diovan HCT 160/12.5—valsartan 160 mg + hydrochlorothiazide 12.5 mg
Diovan HCT 160/25—valsartan 160 mg + hydrochlorothiazide 25 mg
Diovan HCT 320/12.5—valsartan 320 mg + hydrochlorothiazide 12.5 mg
Diovan HCT 320/25—valsartan 320 mg + hydrochlorothiazide 25 mg
Doan's PM Extra Strength—magnesium salicylate 580 mg + diphenhydramine 25 mg **(OTC)**
Donnatal—phenobarbital 16.2 mg + hyoscyamine 0.1037 mg + atropine 0.0194 mg + scopolamine 0.0065 mg
Donnatal Elixir—(per 5 ml) phenobarbital 16.2 mg + hyoscyamine 0.1037 mg + atropine 0.0194 mg + scopolamine 0.0065 mg + 23% alcohol
Donnatal Extentabs—phenobarbital 48.6 mg + hyoscyamine 0.3111 mg + atropine 0.0582 mg + scopolamine 0.0195 mg
Drixoral Cold & Allergy—pseudoephedrine 120 mg + dexbrompheniramine 6 mg **(OTC)**
Dristan Cold Multi-Symptom Formula—acetaminophen 325 mg + phenylephrine 5 mg + chlorpheniramine 2 mg **(OTC)**
Duac Topical Gel—1% clindamycin + 5% benzoyl peroxide
Duetact 2/30—glimepiride 2 mg + pioglitazone 30 mg
Duetact 4/30—glimepiride 4 mg + pioglitazone 30 mg
DuoNeb—(per 3 ml) albuterol sulfate 2.5 mg + ipratropium bromide 0.5 mg inhalation solution
Dyazide—hydrochlorothiazide 25 mg + triamterene 37.5 mg
Elixophyllin-GG Liquid—(per 15 ml) guaifenesin 100 mg + theophylline 100 mg
EMLA Topical Cream—2.5% lidocaine + 2.5% prilocaine
Empresse
Phase I—levonorgestrel 0.05 mg + ethinyl estradiol 30 mcg
Phase II—levonorgestrel 0.075 mg + ethinyl estradiol 40 mcg
Phase III—levonorgestrel 0.125 mg + ethinyl estradiol 30 mcg
Endocet 7.5/325—oxycodone 7.5 mg + acetaminophen 325 mg
Endocet 7.5/500—oxycodone 7.5 mg + acetaminophen 500 mg
Endocet 10/325—oxycodone 10 mg + acetaminophen 325 mg
Endocet 10/650—oxycodone 10 mg + acetaminophen 650 mg
Endodan—oxycodone 4.88 mg + aspirin 325 mg
Entex HC Liquid—(per 5 ml) hydrocodone 3.75 mg + guaifenesin 50 mg + pseudoephedrine 22.5 mg
Entex PSE—pseudoephedrine 120 mg + guaifenesin 400 mg
Epifoam Aerosol Foam—1% hydrocortisone + 1% pramoxine
Epzicom—abacavir 600 mg + lamivudine 300 mg
Equagesic—meprobamate 200 mg + aspirin 325 mg
Eryzole Oral Suspension—(per 5 ml) erythromycin ethylsuccinate 200 mg + sulfisoxazole 600 mg
Esgic—butalbital 50 mg + acetaminophen 325 mg + caffeine 40 mg
Esgic-Plus—butalbital 50 mg + acetaminophen 500 mg + caffeine 40 mg
Estratest—esterified estrogens 1.25 mg + methyltestosterone 2.5 mg

Estratest HS—esterified estrogens 0.625 mg + methyltestosterone 1.25 mg
Estrostep Fe
Phase I—norethindrone 1 mg + ethinyl estradiol 20 mcg
Phase II—norethindrone 1 mg + ethinyl estradiol 30 mcg
Phase III—norethindrone 1 mg + ethinyl estradiol 35 mcg
Phase IV—ferrous fumarate 75 mg
Excedrin Extra Strength—acetaminophen 250 mg + aspirin 250 mg + caffeine 65 mg **(OTC)**
Excedrin Migraine—aspirin 250 mg + acetaminophen 250 mg + caffeine 65 mg **(OTC)**
Excedrin P.M.—acetaminophen 500 mg + diphenhydramine citrate 38 mg **(OTC)**
Excedrin Sinus Headache—phenylephrine 5 mg + acetaminophen 325 mg **(OTC)**
Excedrin Tension Headache—acetaminophen 500 mg + caffeine 65 mg **(OTC)**
Exforge 5/160—amlodipine 5 mg + valsartan 160 mg
Exforge 5/320—amlodipine 5 mg + valsartan 320 mg
Exforge 10/160—amlodipine 10 mg + valsartan 160 mg
Exforge 10/320—amlodipine 10 mg + valsartan 320 mg
Fansidar—sulfidoxine 500 mg + pyrimethamine 25 mg
Femcon Fe—norethindrone 0.4 mg + ethinyl estradiol 35 mcg
Femhrt 0.5/2.5—norethindrone 0.5 mg + ethinyl estradiol 2.5 mcg
Femhrt 1/5—norethindrone 1 mg + ethinyl estradiol 5 mcg
Ferro-Sequels—docusate sodium 100 mg + ferrous fumarate 150 mg **(OTC)**
Fioricet—acetaminophen 325 mg + caffeine 40 mg + butalbital 50 mg
Fioricet with codeine—acetaminophen 325 mg + caffeine 40 mg + butalbital 50 mg + codeine 30 mg
Fiorinal—aspirin 325 mg + caffeine 40 mg + butalbital 50 mg
Fiorinal with codeine—aspirin 325 mg + caffeine 40 mg + butalbital 50 mg + codeine 30 mg
Fosamax Plus D 70/2800—alendronate 70 mg + cholecalciferol 2800 IU
Fosamax Plus D 70/5600—alendronate 70 mg + cholecalciferol 5600 IU
FML-S Ophthalmic Suspension—0.1% fluorometholone + 10% sulfacetamide
Gas-Ban—calcium carbonate 300 mg + simethicone 40 mg **(OTC)**
Gaviscon Extra Strength—magnesium carbonate 105 mg + aluminum hydroxide 160 mg **(OTC)**
Gaviscon Extra-Strength Liquid—(per 5 ml) aluminum hydroxide 84.6 mg + magnesium carbonate 79.1 mg **(OTC)**
Gaviscon Liquid—(per 5 ml) aluminum hydroxide 31.7 mg + magnesium carbonate 119.3 mg **(OTC)**
Gelusil—aluminum hydroxide 200 mg + magnesium hydroxide 200 mg + simethicone 25 mg **(OTC)**
Genac Tablets—triprolidine 2.5 mg + pseudoephedrine 60 mg **(OTC)**
Genatuss DM Syrup—(per 5 ml) guaifenesin 100 mg + dextromethorphan 10 mg **(OTC)**
Glucovance 1.25/250—glyburide 1.25 mg + metformin 250 mg
Glucovance 2.5/500—glyburide 2.5 mg + metformin 500 mg
Glucovance 5/500—glyburide 5 mg + metformin 500 mg
Granulex Topical Aerosol—(per 0.8 ml) trypsin 0.12 mg + Balsam Peru 87 mg + castor oil 788 mg
Guaifenex PSE 60—pseudoephedrine 60 mg + guaifenesin 600 mg
Guaifenex PSE 80—pseudoephedrine 80 mg + guaifenesin 600 mg
Guaifenex PSE 85—pseudoephedrine 85 mg + guaifenesin 600 mg
Guaifenex PSE 120—pseudoephedrine 120 mg + guaifenesin 600 mg
Guaituss AC Syrup—(per 5 ml) codeine 10 mg + guaifenesin 100 mg

Haley's M-O Liquid—(per 15 ml) magnesium hydroxide 900 mg + mineral oil 3.75 ml (OTC)
Helidac—bismuth subsalicylate 262.4-mg tablets plus metronidazole 250-mg tablets plus tetracycline 500-mg capsules in a compliance package
Humalog Mix 50/50—insulin lispro protamine suspension 50% + insulin lispro solution 50%
Humalog Mix 75/25—insulin lispro protamine suspension 75% + insulin lispro solution 25%
Humibid DM—dextromethorphan 30 mg + guaifenesin 600 mg
Hycodan—hydrocodone 5 mg + homatropine 1.5 mg
Hycodan Syrup—(per 5 ml) hydrocodone 5 mg + homatropine 1.5 mg
Hycomine Compound—chlorpheniramine 2 mg + acetaminophen 250 mg + phenylephrine 10 mg + hydrocodone 5 mg + caffeine 30 mg
Hycotuss Expectorant—(per 5 ml) guaifenesin 100 mg + hydrocodone 5 mg + 10% alcohol
Hyzaar 50/12.5—losartan 50 mg + hydrochlorothiazide 12.5 mg
Hyzaar 100/12.5—losartan 100 mg + hydrochlorothiazide 12.5 mg
Hyzaar 100/25—losartan 100 mg + hydrochlorothiazide 25 mg
Imodium Advanced—loperamide 2 mg + simethicone 125 mg (OTC)
Inderide 40/25—propranolol 40 mg + hydrochlorothiazide 25 mg
Janumet 50/500—sitagliptan 50 mg + metformin 500 mg
Janumet 50/1000—sitagliptan 50 mg + metformin 1000 mg
Junel 1/20—norethindrone 1 mg + ethinyl estradiol 20 mcg
Junel 1.5/30—norethindrone 1.5 mg + ethinyl estradiol 30 mcg
Junel Fe 1/20—norethindrone 1 mg + ethinyl estradiol 20 mcg with 7 tablets of ferrous fumarate 75 mg per container
Junel Fe 1.5/30—norethindrone 1.5 mg + ethinyl estradiol 30 mcg with 7 tablets of ferrous fumarate 75 mg per container
Kaletra 100/25 capsules—lopinavir 100 mg + ritonavir 25 mg
Kaletra 200/50 capsules—lopinavir 200 mg + ritonavir 50 mg
Kaletra solution—(per ml) lopinavir 80 mg + ritonavir 20 mg
Kariva—desogestrel 0.15 mg + ethinyl estradiol 20 mcg/10 mcg
Kelnor—ethinyl estradiol 35 mcg + ethynodiol 1 mg
Lactinex—mixed culture of *Lactobacillus acidophilus* and *L. bulgaricus* (OTC)
Lessina—levonorgestrel 0.1 mg + ethinyl estradiol 20 mcg
Levlite—levonorgestrel 0.1 mg + ethinyl estradiol 20 mcg
Levora—levonorgestrel 0.15 mg + ethinyl estradiol 30 mcg
Lexxel 5/2.5—enalapril 5 mg + felodipine 2.5 mg
Lexxel 5/5—enalapril 5 mg + felodipine 5 mg
Librax—chlordiazepoxide 5 mg + clidinium 2.5 mg
Lida-Mantle-HC Topical Cream—0.5% hydrocortisone + 3% lidocaine
Limbitrol 5/12.5—chlordiazepoxide 5 mg + amitriptyline 12.5 mg
Limbitrol DS 10/25—chlordiazepoxide 10 mg + amitriptyline 25 mg
Loestrin Fe 1/20—norethindrone acetate 1 mg + ethinyl estradiol 20 mcg with 7 tablets of ferrous fumarate 75 mg per container
Loestrin Fe 1.5/30—norethindrone acetate 1.5 mg + ethinyl estradiol 30 mcg with 7 tablets of ferrous fumarate 75 mg per container
Lomotil—diphenoxylate 2.5 mg + atropine 0.025 mg
Lomotil Liquid—(per 5 ml) diphenoxylate 2.5 mg + atropine 0.025 mg
Lonox—diphenoxylate 2.5 mg + atropine 0.025 mg
Lo/Ovral—ethinyl estradiol 30 mcg + norgestrel 0.3 mg

Lopressor HCT 50/25—metoprolol tartrate 50 mg + hydrochlorothiazide 25 mg
Lopressor HCT 100/25—metoprolol tartrate 100 mg + hydrochlorothiazide 25 mg
Lopressor HCT 100/50—metoprolol tartrate 100 mg + hydrochlorothiazide 50 mg
Lorcet 10/650—acetaminophen 650 mg + hydrocodone 10 mg
Lorcet-HD—hydrocodone 10 mg + acetaminophen 500 mg
Lorcet Plus—hydrocodone 7.5 mg + acetaminophen 650 mg
Lortab 5/500—hydrocodone 5 mg + acetaminophen 500 mg
Lortab 7.5/500—hydrocodone 7.5 mg + acetaminophen 500 mg
Lortab 10/500—hydrocodone 10 mg + acetaminophen 500 mg
Lortab Elixir—(per 5 ml) hydrocodone 2.5 mg + acetaminophen 167 mg
🍁**Losec 1-2-3 A**—omeprazole 20 mg (14 doses), clarithromycin 500 mg (14 doses), amoxicillin 1 g (14 doses) in a convenience package
🍁**Losec 1-2-3 M**—omeprazole 20 mg (14 doses), clarithromycin 250 mg (14 doses), metronidazole 500 mg (14 doses) in a convenience package
Lotensin HCT 5/6.25—benazepril 5 mg + hydrochlorothiazide 6.25 mg
Lotensin HCT 10/12.5—benazepril 10 mg + hydrochlorothiazide 12.5 mg
Lotensin HCT 20/12.5—benazepril 20 mg + hydrochlorothiazide 12.5 mg
Lotensin HCT 20/25—benazepril 20 mg + hydrochlorothiazide 25 mg
Lotrel 2.5/10—amlodipine 2.5 mg + benazepril 10 mg
Lotrel 5/10—amlodipine 5 mg + benazepril 10 mg
Lotrel 5/20—amlodipine 5 mg + benazepril 20 mg
Lotrel 5/40—amlodipine 5 mg + benazepril 40 mg
Lotrel 10/20—amlodipine 10 mg + benazepril 20 mg
Lotrel 10/40—amlodipine 10 mg + benazepril 40 mg
Lotrisone Topical Cream/Lotion—0.05% betamethasone + 1% clotrimazole
Low-Ogestrel—norgestrel 0.3 mg + ethinyl estradiol 30 mcg
Lufyllin-GG Elixir—(per 15 ml) dyphylline 100 mg + guaifenesin 100 mg
Lybrel—levonorgestrel 0.09 mg + ethinyl estradiol 20 mcg
Maalox Maximum Liquid—(per 5 ml) aluminum hydroxide 400 mg + magnesium hydroxide 400 mg + simethicone 40 mg **(OTC)**
Maalox Regular Liquid—(per 5 ml) aluminum hydroxide 200 mg + magnesium hydroxide 200 mg + simethicone 20 mg **(OTC)**
Magnacet 2.5/400—oxycodone 2.5 mg + acetaminophen 400 mg
Magnacet 5/400—oxycodone 5 mg + acetaminophen 400 mg
Magnacet 7.5/400—oxycodone 7.5 mg + acetaminophen 400 mg
Magnacet 10/400—oxycodone 10 mg + acetaminophen 400 mg
Malarone—atovaquone 250 mg + proguanil 100 mg
Malarone Pediatric—atovaquone 62.5 mg + proguanil 25 mg
Mapap Multi-Symptom Cold—acetaminophen 325 mg + phenylephrine 5 mg + dextromethorphan 10 mg **(OTC)**
Marvelon—ethinyl estradiol 30 mcg + desogestrel 0.15 mg
Maxitrol Ophthalmic Suspension/Ointment—(per g) neomycin 3.5 mg + 0.1% dexamethasone + polymyxin B 10,000 units
Maxzide—hydrochlorothiazide 50 mg + triamterene 75 mg
Maxzide-25—hydrochlorothiazide 25 mg + triamterene 37.5 mg
Metaglip 2.5/250—glipizide 2.5 mg + metformin 250 mg
Metaglip 2.5/500—glipizide 2.5 mg + metformin 500 mg
Metaglip 5/500—glipizide 5 mg + metformin 500 mg
Micardis HCT 40/12.5—telmisartan 40 mg + hydrochlorothiazide 12.5 mg
Micardis HCT 80/12.5—telmisartan 80 mg + hydrochlorothiazide 12.5 mg
Micardis HCT 80/25—telmisartan 80 mg + hydrochlorothiazide 25 mg

Microgestin Fe 1/20—norethindrone acetate 1 mg + ethinyl estradiol 20 mcg per tablet with 7 tablets of ferrous fumarate 75 mg per container
Microgestin Fe 1.5/30—norethindrone acetate 1.5 mg + ethinyl estradiol 30 mcg per tablet with 7 tablets of ferrous fumarate 75 mg per container
Midol Menstrual Complete—acetaminophen 500 mg + caffeine 60 mg + pyrilamine 15 mg **(OTC)**
Midol Menstrual Headache—acetaminophen 500 mg + caffeine 65 mg **(OTC)**
Midol Pre-Menstrual Syndrome—acetaminophen 500 mg + pyrilamine 15 mg + pamabrom 25 mg **(OTC)**
Midol Teen Formula—acetaminophen 500 mg + pamabrom 25 mg **(OTC)**
Midrin—isometheptene 65 mg + acetaminophen 325 mg + dichloralphenazone 100 mg
Migergot Suppositories—ergotamine 2 mg + caffeine 100 mg
Mircette—desogestrel 0.15 mg + ethinyl estradiol 20 mcg/10 mcg
Modicon—norethindrone 0.5 mg + ethinyl estradiol 35 mcg
🍁**Moduret**—amiloride 5 mg + hydrochlorothiazide 50 mg
Monopril-HCT 10/12.5—fosinopril 10 mg + hydrochlorothiazide 12.5 mg
Monopril-HCT 20/12.5—fosinopril 20 mg + hydrochlorothiazide 12.5 mg
Motofen—difenoxin 1 mg + atropine 0.025 mg
Motrin Children's Cold Suspension—(per 5 ml) ibuprofen 100 mg + pseudoephedrine 15 mg **(OTC)**
Mucinex D—guaifenesin 600 mg + pseudoephedrine 60 mg **(OTC)**
Mucinex DM—guaifenesin 600 mg + dextromethorphan 30 mg **(OTC)**
Murocoll-2 Ophthalmic Solution—0.3% scopolamine + 10% phenylephrine
Mylanta Regular Strength Liquid—(per 5 ml) aluminum hydroxide 200 mg + magnesium hydroxide 200 mg + simethicone 20 mg **(OTC)**
Mylanta Maximum Strength Liquid—(per 5 ml) aluminum hydroxide 400 mg + magnesium hydroxide 400 mg + simethicone 40 mg **(OTC)**
Mylanta Supreme Liquid—(per 5 ml) calcium carbonate 400 mg + magnesium hydroxide 135 mg **(OTC)**
Mylanta Ultimate Strength Chewables—calcium carbonate 700 mg + magnesium hydroxide 300 mg **(OTC)**
Mylanta Ultimate Strength Liquid—(per 5 ml) aluminum hydroxide 500 mg + magnesium hydroxide 500 mg **(OTC)**
Naphcon-A Ophthalmic Solution—0.025% naphazoline + 0.3% pheniramine **(OTC)**
Nasatab LA—guaifenesin 500 mg + pseudoephedrine 120 mg
Neosporin Antibiotic Topical Ointment—(per g) neomycin 3.5 mg + bacitracin 400 units + polymyxin B 5000 units **(OTC)**
Neosporin Topical Cream—(per g) polymyxin B 10,000 units + neomycin 3.5 mg **(OTC)**
Neosporin G.U. Irrigant—(per ml) neomycin 40 mg + polymyxin B 200,000 units
Neosporin Ophthalmic Solution—(per ml) polymyxin B 10,000 units + neomycin 1.75 mg + gramicidin 0.025 mg
Neosporin + Pain Relief Antibiotic Topical Cream—(per g) neomycin 3.5 mg + polymyxin B 10,000 units + pramoxine 10 mg **(OTC)**
Neosporin + Pain Relief Antibiotic Topical Ointment—(per g) neomycin 3.5 mg + polymyxin B 10,000 units + bacitracin 500 units + pramoxine 10 mg **(OTC)**
Niferex-150 Forte—ferrous sulfate 150 mg + vitamin B12 25 mcg + folic acid 1 mg
Norco 5/325—hydrocodone 5 mg + acetaminophen 325 mg
Norco 7.5/325—hydrocodone 7.5 mg + acetaminophen 325 mg
Norco 10/325—hydrocodone 10 mg + acetaminophen 325 mg
Nordette—levonorgestrel 0.15 mg + ethinyl estradiol 30 mcg

Norgesic—orphenadrine 25 mg + caffeine 30 mg + aspirin 385 mg
Norgesic Forte—orphenadrine 50 mg + caffeine 60 mg + aspirin 770 mg
Norinyl 1/35—norethindrone 1 mg + ethinyl estradiol 35 mcg
Norinyl 1/50—norethindrone 1 mg + mestranol 50 mcg
Nortrel 0.5/35—norethindrone 0.5 mg + ethinyl estradiol 35 mcg
Nortrel 1/35—norethindrone 1 mg + ethinyl estradiol 35 mcg
Nortrel 7/7/7
Phase I—norethindrone 0.5 mg + ethinyl estradiol 35 mcg
Phase II—norethindrone 0.75 mg + ethinyl estradiol 35 mcg
Phase III—norethindrone 1 mg + ethinyl estradiol 35 mcg
NuLytely—PEG 3350 420 g + sodium bicarbonate 5.72 g + sodium chloride 11.2 g + potassium chloride 1.48 g
Nuvaring—etonogestrel 0.12 mg/day + ethinyl estradiol 15 mcg/day
Nyquil Children's Liquid—(per 15 ml) dextromethorphan 15 mg + chlorpheniramine 2 mg (OTC)
Nyquil Cold & Flu Liquicaps—acetaminophen 325 mg + dextromethorphan 15 mg + doxylamine 6.25 mg **(OTC)**
Nyquil Cold & Flu Liquid—(per 15 ml) acetaminophen 500 mg + dextromethorphan 15 mg + doxylamine 6.25 mg **(OTC)**
Nyquil Cough Liquid—(per 15 ml) dextromethorphan 15 mg + doxylamine 6.25 mg **(OTC)**
Nyquil D Liquid—(per 15 ml) acetaminophen 500 mg + dextromethorphan 15 mg + doxylamine 6.25 mg + pseudoephedrine 30 mg **(OTC)**
Nyquil Sinus Liquicaps—acetaminophen 325 mg + doxylamine 6.25 mg + phenylephrine 5 mg **(OTC)**
Ogestrel—norgestrel 0.5 mg + ethinyl estradiol 50 mcg
Opcon-A Ophthalmic Solution—0.027% naphazoline + 0.3% pheniramine **(OTC)**
Ornex—pseudoephedrine 30 mg + acetaminophen 325 mg **(OTC)**
Ornex Maximum Strength—pseudoephedrine 30 mg + acetaminophen 500 mg **(OTC)**
Orphengesic—orphenadrine 25 mg + aspirin 385 mg + caffeine 30 mg
Orphengesic forte—orphenadrine 50 mg + aspirin 770 mg + caffeine 60 mg
Ortho-Cept—ethinyl estradiol 30 mcg + desogestrel 0.15 mg
Ortho-Cyclen—ethinyl estradiol 35 mcg + norgestimate 0.25 mg
Ortho-Evra—norelgestromin 150 mcg/day + ethinyl estradiol 20 mcg/day
Ortho-Novum 1/35—norethindrone 1 mg + ethinyl estradiol 35 mcg
Ortho-Novum 1/50—norethindrone 1 mg + mestranol 50 mcg
Ortho-Novum 10/11–28
Phase I—norethindrone 0.5 mg + ethinyl estradiol 35 mcg
Phase II—norethindrone 1 mg + ethinyl estradiol 35 mcg
Ortho-Novum 7/7/7–28
Phase I—norethindrone 0.5 mg + ethinyl estradiol 35 mcg
Phase II—norethindrone 0.75 mg + ethinyl estradiol 35 mcg
Phase III—norethindrone 1 mg + ethinyl estradiol 35 mcg
Ortho-Prefest—estradiol 1 mg (15 tablets) and estradiol 1 mg + norgestimate 0.09 mg (15 tablets) in a 30-tablet blister package
Ortho Tri-Cyclen
Phase I—norgestimate 0.18 mg + ethinyl estradiol 35 mcg
Phase II—norgestimate 0.215 mg + ethinyl estradiol 35 mcg
Phase III—norgestimate 0.25 mg + ethinyl estradiol 35 mcg
Ortho Tri-Cyclen Lo
Phase I—norgestimate 0.18 mg + ethinyl estradiol 25 mcg

Phase II—norgestimate 0.215 mg + ethinyl estradiol 25 mcg
Phase III—norgestimate 0.25 mg + ethinyl estradiol 25 mcg
Ovcon-35—ethinyl estradiol 35 mcg + norethindrone 0.4 mg
Ovcon-50—ethinyl estradiol 50 mcg + norethindrone 1 mg
P-V-Tussin—hydrocodone 5 mg + pseudoephedrine 60 mg
Pamprin Cramp Caplets—acetaminophen 250 mg + pamabrom 25 mg + magnesium salicylate 250 mg **(OTC)**
Pamprin Multi-Symptom—acetaminophen 500 mg + pamabrom 25 mg + pyrilamine 15 mg **(OTC)**
Pancrease MT 4—lipase 4000 units + amylase 12,000 units + protease 12,000 units
Pancrease MT 10—lipase 10,000 units + amylase 30,000 units + protease 30,000 units
Pancrease MT 16—lipase 16,000 units + amylase 48,000 units + protease 48,000 units
Pancrease MT 20—lipase 20,000 units + amylase 56,000 units + protease 44,000 units
Parcopa 10/100—carbidopa 10 mg + levodopa 100 mg
Parcopa 25/100—carbidopa 25 mg + levodopa 100 mg
Parcopa 25/250—carbidopa 25 mg + levodopa 250 mg
Pediacare Children's Multisymptom Cold Liquid—(per 5 ml) phenylephrine 2.5 mg + dextromethorphan 5 mg **(OTC)**
Pediacare Children's NightRest Multi-Symptom Cold Liquid—(per 5 ml) phenylephrine 5 mg + diphenhydramine 12.5 mg **(OTC)**
Pediazole Suspension—(per 5 ml) erythromycin ethylsuccinate 200 mg + sulfisoxazole 600 mg
Pepcid Complete—calcium carbonate 800 mg + magnesium hydroxide 165 mg + famotidine 10 mg **(OTC)**
Percocet 2.5/325—oxycodone 2.5 mg + acetaminophen 325 mg
Percocet 5/325—oxycodone 5 mg + acetaminophen 325 mg
Percocet 7.5/325—oxycodone 7.5 mg + acetaminophen 325 mg
Percocet 7.5/500—oxycodone 7.5 mg + acetaminophen 500 mg
Percocet 10/325—oxycodone 10 mg + acetaminophen 325 mg
Percocet 10/650—oxycodone 10 mg + acetaminophen 650 mg
Percodan—oxycodone 4.88 mg + aspirin 325 mg
Percogesic—phenyltoloxamine 30 mg + acetaminophen 325 mg **(OTC)**
Peri-Colace—docusate sodium 50 mg + sennosides 8.6 mg **(OTC)**
Phrenilin—butalbital 50 mg + acetaminophen 325 mg
Phrenilin Forte—butalbital 50 mg + acetaminophen 650 mg
Phrenilin with Caffeine and Codeine—butalbital 50 mg + acetaminophen 325 mg + caffeine 40 mg + codeine 30 mg
Polycitra Syrup—(per 5 ml) potassium citrate 550 mg + sodium citrate 500 mg + citric acid 334 mg
Poly-Hist DM Syrup—(per 5 ml) phenylephrine 7.5 mg + pyrilamine 8.33 mg + dextromethorphan 10 mg
Polysporin Topical Ointment/Powder—(per g) polymyxin B 10,000 units + bacitracin 500 units **(OTC)**
Polytrim Ophthalmic Solution—(per ml) polymyxin B 10,000 units + trimethoprim 1 mg
Portia—levonorgestrel 0.15 mg + ethinyl estradiol 30 mcg
Pramosone Topical Cream/Lotion/Ointment—1% pramoxine + 1% hydrocortisone
Pramosone Topical Cream/Lotion/Ointment—1% pramoxine + 2.5% hydrocortisone
Premphase—conjugated estrogens 0.625 mg + medroxyprogesterone 5 mg (14 tablets) plus conjugated estrogens 0.625 mg (14 tablets) in a compliance package
🍁**Premplus 0.625/2.5**—conjugated estrogens 0.625 mg + medroxyprogesterone 2.5 mg

✤**Premplus 0.625/5**—conjugated estrogens 0.625 mg + medroxyprogesterone 5 mg
Prempro 0.3/1.5—conjugated estrogens 0.3 mg + medroxyprogesterone 1.5 mg (28 tablets) in a compliance package
Prempro 0.45/1.5—conjugated estrogens 0.45 mg + medroxyprogesterone 1.5 mg (28 tablets) in a compliance package
Prempro 0.625/2.5—conjugated estrogens 0.625 mg + medroxyprogesterone 2.5 mg (28 tablets) in a compliance package
Prempro 0.625/5—conjugated estrogens 0.625 mg + medroxyprogesterone 5 mg (28 tablets) in a compliance package
Premsyn PMS—acetaminophen 500 mg + pamabrom 25 mg + pyrilamine 15 mg **(OTC)**
Prevpac—amoxicillin 500 mg capsules + clarithromycin 500 mg tablets + lansoprazole 30 mg capsules in a compliance package
Primatene Tablets—ephedrine 12.5 mg + guaifenesin 200 mg **(OTC)**
Primaxin 250 mg I.V. For Injection—imipenem 250 mg + cilastatin sodium 250 mg
Primaxin 500 mg I.V. For Injection—imipenem 500 mg + cilastatin sodium 500 mg
Prinzide 10/12.5—lisinopril 10 mg + hydrochlorothiazide 12.5 mg
Prinzide 20/12.5—lisinopril 20 mg + hydrochlorothiazide 12.5 mg
Prinzide 20/25—lisinopril 20 mg + hydrochlorothiazide 25 mg
Proctofoam-HC Rectal Foam—1% hydrocortisone + 1% pramoxine
✤**Protrin**—trimethoprim 80 mg + sulfamethoxazole 400 mg
✤**Protrin DF**—trimethoprim 160 mg + sulfamethoxazole 800 mg
Pylera—bismuth subcitrate potassium 140 mg + metronidazole 125 mg + tetracycline 125 mg
Quinaretic 10/12.5—quinapril 10 mg + hydrochlorothiazide 12.5 mg
Quinaretic 20/12.5—quinapril 20 mg + hydrochlorothiazide 12.5 mg
Quinaretic 20/25—quinapril 20 mg + hydrochlorothiazide 25 mg
Rebetron—interferon alfa-2b (Intron A) + oral ribavirin (Rebetrol) 200 mg
Renese-R—polythiazide 2 mg + reserpine 0.25 mg
Reprexain 2.5/200—hydrocodone 2.5 mg + ibuprofen 200 mg
Reprexain 5/200—hydrocodone 5 mg + ibuprofen 200 mg
Reprexain 7.5/200—hydrocodone 7.5 mg + ibuprofen 200 mg
Reprexain 10/200—hydrocodone 10 mg + ibuprofen 200 mg
Respahist—pseudoephedrine 60 mg + brompheniramine 6 mg
Respaire-60 SR—guaifenesin 200 mg + pseudoephedrine 60 mg
Respaire-120 SR—guaifenesin 250 mg + pseudoephedrine 120 mg
RID Maximum Strength Shampoo—0.33% pyrethrins + 4% piperonyl butoxide **(OTC)**
Rifamate—isoniazid 150 mg + rifampin 300 mg
Rifater—rifampin 120 mg + isoniazid 50 mg + pyrazinamide 300 mg
✤**Robaxacet-8**—methocarbamol 400 mg + acetaminophen 325 mg + codeine 8 mg
✤**Robaxacet**—methocarbamol 400 mg + acetaminophen 325 mg
✤**Robaxacet Extra Strength**—methocarbamol 400 mg + acetaminophen 500 mg
Robitussin Cold & Congestion Tablets—acetaminophen 325 mg + chlorpheniramine 2 mg+ phenylephrine 5 mg **(OTC)**
Robitussin Cough & Allergy Liquid—(per 5 ml) chlorpheniramine 2 mg + phenylephrine 5 mg + dextromethorphan 10 mg **(OTC)**
Robitussin Cough & Cold CF Liquid—(per 5 ml) guaifenesin 100 mg + phenylephrine 5 mg + dextromethorphan 10 mg **(OTC)**
Robitussin Cough & Cold Long-Acting Liquid—(per 5 ml) chlorpheniramine 2 mg + dextromethorphan 15 mg **(OTC)**
Robitussin Cough & Cold Pediatric Drops—(per 2.5 ml) phenylephrine 2.5 mg + guaifenesin 100 mg + dextromethorphan 5 mg **(OTC)**

Robitussin Cough & Congestion Liquid—(per 5 ml) guaifenesin 200 mg + dextromethorphan 10 mg **(OTC)**
Robitussin Cough, Cold & Flu Nighttime Liquid—(per 5 ml) acetaminophen 160 mg + chlorpheniramine 1 mg + phenylephrine 2.5 mg + dextromethorphan 5 mg **(OTC)**
Robitussin-DM Cough Liquid—(per 5 ml) guaifenesin 100 mg + dextromethorphan 10 mg **(OTC)**
Robitussin Nighttime Cough & Cold Liquid—(per 5 ml) phenylephrine 2.5 mg + diphenhydramine 6.25 mg **(OTC)**
Robitussin Nighttime Pediatric Cough & Cold Liquid—(per 5 ml) phenylephrine 2.5 mg + diphenhydramine 6.25 mg **(OTC)**
Robitussin Pediatric Cough & Cold Long-Acting Liquid—(per 5 ml) chlorpheniramine 1 mg + dextromethorphan 7.5 mg **(OTC)**
Robitussin-PE Head & Chest Congestion Liquid—(per 5 ml) guaifenesin 100 mg + phenylephrine 5 mg **(OTC)**
Rolaids Extra Strength Plus Gas Relief Softchews—calcium carbonate 1177 mg + simethicone 80 mg **(OTC)**
Rolaids Extra Strength Tablets—calcium carbonate 675 mg + magnesium hydroxide 135 mg **(OTC)**
Rolaids Multi-Symptom Tablets—calcium carbonate 675 mg + magnesium hydroxide 135 mg + simethicone 60 mg **(OTC)**
Rolaids Regular Tablets—calcium carbonate 550 mg + magnesium hydroxide 110 mg **(OTC)**
Rondec Syrup—(per 5 ml) chlorpheniramine 4 mg + phenylephrine 12.5 mg
Rondec DM Drops—(per 1 ml) phenylephrine 3.5 mg + chlorpheniramine 1 mg
Rondec DM Syrup—(per 5 ml) phenylephrine 12.5 mg + chlorpheniramine 4 mg
Rondec Oral Drops—(per 1 ml) phenylephrine 3.5 mg + chlorpheniramine 1 mg
Roxicet 5/500—oxycodone 5 mg + acetaminophen 500 mg
Roxicet—oxycodone 5 mg + acetaminophen 325 mg
Roxicet Oral Solution—(per 5 ml) acetaminophen 325 mg + oxycodone 5 mg
Ru-Tuss DM Syrup—(per 5 ml) guaifenesin 100 mg + pseudoephedrine 45 mg + dextromethorphan 15 mg **(OTC)**
Rynatan—phenylephrine 25 mg + chlorpheniramine 9 mg
Rynatan Pediatric Suspension—(per 5 ml) phenylephrine 5 mg + chlorpheniramine 4.5 mg
Rynatuss—ephedrine 10 mg + carbetapentane 60 mg + chlorpheniramine 5 mg + phenylephrine 10 mg
Scot-Tussin DM Maximum Strength Liquid—(per 5 ml) chlorpheniramine 2 mg + dextromethorphan 15 mg **(OTC)**
Scot-Tussin Original Liquid—(per 5 ml) phenylephrine 4 mg + pheniramine 13 mg + sodium salicylate 83 mg + caffeine citrate 25 mg **(OTC)**
Scot-Tussin Senior Liquid—(per 5 ml) guaifenesin 200 mg + dextromethorphan 15 mg **(OTC)**
Seasonale—levonorgestrel 0.15 mg + ethinyl estradiol 30 mcg
Seasonique—levonorgestrel 0.15 mg + ethinyl estradiol 30 mcg/10 mcg
Sedapap—acetaminophen 650 mg + butalbital 50 mg
Semprex-D—acrivastine 8 mg + pseudoephedrine 60 mg
Senokot-S—sennosides 8.6 mg + docusate sodium 50 mg **(OTC)**
Seno Sol-SS—sennosides 8.6 mg + docusate sodium 50 mg **(OTC)**
Septra—trimethoprim 80 mg + sulfamethoxazole 400 mg
Septra DS—trimethoprim 160 mg + sulfamethoxazole 800 mg
Silafed Syrup—(per 5 ml) pseudoephedrine 30 mg + triprolidine 1.25 mg **(OTC)**

Sinemet 10/100—carbidopa 10 mg + levodopa 100 mg
Sinemet 25/100—carbidopa 25 mg + levodopa 100 mg
Sinemet 25/250—carbidopa 25 mg + levodopa 250 mg
Sinemet CR 25-100—carbidopa 25 mg + levodopa 100 mg
Sinemet CR 50-200—carbidopa 50 mg + levodopa 200 mg
Sine-Off Cough/Cold Medicine—phenylephrine 5 mg + acetaminophen 325 mg + dextromethorphan 15 mg + guaifenesin 200 mg **(OTC)**
Sine-Off Maximum Strength Non-Drowsy Caplets—phenylephrine 5 mg + acetaminophen 500 mg **(OTC)**
Sine-Off Sinus/Cold Medicine—phenylephrine 5 mg + chlorpheniramine 2 mg + acetaminophen 500 mg **(OTC)**
Sinutab Non-Drying Caplets—phenylephrine 5 mg + guaifenesin 200 mg **(OTC)**
Sinutab Sinus Caplets—acetaminophen 325 mg + phenylephrine 5 mg **(OTC)**
Solage Topical Liquid—2% mequinol + 0.01% tretinoin
Soma Compound—aspirin 325 mg + carisoprodol 200 mg
Sprintec—norgestimate 0.25 mg + ethinyl estradiol 35 mcg
Stalevo 50—carbidopa 12.5 mg + entacapone 200 mg + levodopa 50 mg
Stalevo 100—carbidopa 25 mg + entacapone 200 mg + levodopa 100 mg
Stalevo 150—carbidopa 37.5 mg + entacapone 200 mg + levodopa 150 mg
Suboxone N2—buprenorphine 2 mg + naloxone 0.5 mg
Suboxone N8—buprenorphine 8 mg + naloxone 2 mg
Sudafed Children's Cough & Cold Liquid—(per 5 ml) dextromethorphan 5 mg + pseudoephedrine 15 mg **(OTC)**
Sudafed Maximum Strength Sinus Nighttime—pseudoephedrine 60 mg + triprolidine 2.5 mg **(OTC)**
Sudafed Non-Drying Sinus Liquicaps—guaifenesin 200 mg + pseudoephedrine 30 mg **(OTC)**
Sudafed PE Maximum Strength Nighttime Cold—phenylephrine 5 mg + diphenhydramine 25 mg + acetaminophen 325 mg **(OTC)**
Sudafed PE Multi-Symptom Severe Cold—phenylephrine 5 mg + diphenhydramine 12.5 mg + acetaminophen 325 mg **(OTC)**
Sudafed PE Sinus Headache—phenylephrine 5 mg + acetaminophen 325 mg **(OTC)**
Sudafed Sinus & Allergy—pseudoephedrine 60 mg + chlorpheniramine 4 mg **(OTC)**
Sudafed Sinus & Cold Liquicaps—pseudoephedrine 30 mg + acetaminophen 325 mg **(OTC)**
Sudal 12—pseudoephedrine 30 mg + chlorpheniramine 4 mg
Sulfacet-R Topical Lotion—10% sodium sulfacetamide + 5% sulfur
Symbicort—(per actuation) budesonide 80 mcg + formoterol 45 mcg
Symbyax 3/25—olanzapine 3 mg + fluoxetine 25 mg
Symbyax 6/25—olanzapine 6 mg + fluoxetine 25 mg
Symbyax 6/50—olanzapine 6 mg + fluoxetine 50 mg
Symbyax 12/25—olanzapine 12 mg + fluoxetine 25 mg
Symbyax 12/50—olanzapine 12 mg + fluoxetine 50 mg
Synalgos-DC—aspirin 356.4 mg + caffeine 30 mg + dihydrocodeine 16 mg
Synercid Powder for Injection—quinupristin 150 mg + dalfopristin 350 mg
Taclonex Ointment—0.005% calcipotriene + 0.064% betamethasone
Talacen—acetaminophen 650 mg + pentazocine 25 mg
Talwin NX—pentazocine 50 mg + naloxone 0.5 mg
Tarka 1/240—trandolapril 1 mg (immediate release) + verapamil 240 mg (sustained release)

Tarka 2/180—trandolapril 2 mg (immediate release) + verapamil 180 mg (sustained release)
Tarka 2/240—trandolapril 2 mg (immediate release) + verapamil 240 mg (sustained release)
Tarka 4/240—trandolapril 4 mg (immediate release) + verapamil 240 mg (sustained release)
✱**Tazocin for Injection 2.25 g**—piperacillin 2 g + tazobactam 0.25 g
✱**Tazocin for Injection 3.375 g**—piperacillin 3 g + tazobactam 0.375 g
✱**Tazocin for Injection 4.5 g**—piperacillin 4 g + tazobactam 0.5 g
Tenoretic 50—chlorthalidone 25 mg + atenolol 50 mg
Tenoretic 100—chlorthalidone 25 mg + atenolol 100 mg
Terra-Cortril Ophthalmic Suspension—1.5% hydrocortisone acetate + 0.5% oxytetracycline
Terramycin with Polymyxin B Sulfate Ophthalmic Ointment—(per g) polymyxin B 10,000 units + oxytetracycline 5 mg
Teveten HCT 600/12.5—eprosartan 600 mg + hydrochlorothiazide 12.5 mg
Teveten HCT 600/25—eprosartan 600 mg + hydrochlorothiazide 25 mg
Thera-Flu Cold & Cough Hot Liquid—(per packet) phenylephrine 10 mg + dextromethorphan 20 mg + pheniramine 20 mg **(OTC)**
Thera-Flu, Cold & Sore Throat Hot Liquid—(per packet) phenylephrine 10 mg +pheniramine 20 mg + acetaminophen 325 mg **(OTC)**
Thera-Flu, Daytime Cough & Cold Thin Strips—phenylephrine 10 mg +dextromethorphan 14.8 mg **(OTC)**
Thera-Flu, Daytime Severe Cold Caplets—phenylephrine 5 mg +dextromethorphan 15 mg + acetaminophen 325 mg **(OTC)**
Thera-Flu Daytime Severe Cold Hot Liquid—(per packet) acetaminophen 650 mg + phenylephrine 10 mg **(OTC)**
Thera-Flu, Daytime Warming Relief Syrup—(per 15 ml) phenylephrine 5 mg +dextromethorphan 10 mg + acetaminophen 325 mg **(OTC)**
Thera-Flu, Flu & Chest Congestion Hot Liquid—(per packet) guaifenesin 400 mg + acetaminophen 1000 mg **(OTC)**
Thera-Flu, Flu & Sore Throat Hot Liquid—(per packet) phenylephrine 10 mg +pheniramine 20 mg + acetaminophen 650 mg **(OTC)**
Thera-Flu, Flu & Sore Throat Relief Syrup—(per 15 ml) phenylephrine 5 mg + diphenhydramine 12.5 mg + acetaminophen 325 mg **(OTC)**
Thera-Flu, Nighttime Cough & Cold Thin Strips—phenylephrine 10 mg + diphenhydramine 25 mg **(OTC)**
Thera-Flu, Nighttime Severe Cold Caplets—phenylephrine 5 mg + dextromethorphan 15 mg + chlorpheniramine 2 mg + acetaminophen 325 mg **(OTC)**
Thera-Flu Nighttime Severe Hot Liquid—(per packet) phenylephrine 10 mg + pheniramine 20 mg + acetaminophen 650 mg **(OTC)**
Thera-Flu, Nighttime Warming Relief Syrup—(per 15 ml) phenylephrine 5 mg + diphenhydramine 12.5 mg + acetaminophen 325 mg **(OTC)**
Timentin for Injection—ticarcillin 3 g + clavulanic acid 0.1 g
Titralac Plus—calcium carbonate 420 mg + simethicone 21 mg **(OTC)**
TobraDex Ophthalmic Suspension/Ointment—0.1% dexamethasone + 0.3% tobramycin
Triacin-C Cough Syrup—(per 5 ml) codeine 10 mg + pseudoephedrine 30 mg + triprolidine 1.25 mg
Tri-Levlen
Phase I—levonorgestrel 0.05 mg + ethinyl estradiol 30 mcg
Phase II—levonorgestrel 0.075 mg + ethinyl estradiol 40 mcg

Phase III—levonorgestrel 0.125 mg + ethinyl estradiol 30 mcg

Triaminic Chest & Nasal Congestion Liquid—(per 5 ml) guaifenesin 50 mg + phenylephrine 2.5 mg **(OTC)**

Triaminic Cold & Allergy Liquid—(per 5 ml) chlorpheniramine 1 mg + phenylephrine 2.5 mg **(OTC)**

Triaminic Cough & Sore Throat Liquid—(per 5 ml) acetaminophen 160 mg + dextromethorphan 5 mg **(OTC)**

Triaminic Day Time Cold & Cough Liquid—(per 5 ml) phenylephrine 2.5 mg + dextromethorphan 5 mg **(OTC)**

Triaminic Day Time Thin Strips Cough & Cold—phenylephrine 2.5 mg + dextromethorphan 5 mg **(OTC)**

Triaminic Flu, Cough & Fever Liquid—(per 5 ml) acetaminophen 160 mg + dextromethorphan 7.5 mg + chlorpheniramine 1 mg **(OTC)**

Triaminic Night Time Cold & Cough Liquid—(per 5 ml) phenylephrine 2.5 mg + diphenhydramine 6.25 mg **(OTC)**

Triaminic Night Time Thin Strips Cough & Cold—phenylephrine 5 mg + diphenhydramine 12.5 mg **(OTC)**

Triaminic Softchews Cough & Runny Nose—chlorpheniramine 1 mg + dextromethorphan 5 mg **(OTC)**

Triaminic Softchews Cough & Sore Throat—acetaminophen 160 mg + dextromethorphan 5 mg **(OTC)**

Tri-Luma Topical Cream—0.01% fluocinolone + 4% hydroquinone + 0.05% tretinoin

Tri-Norinyl

Phase I—norethindrone 0.5 mg + ethinyl estradiol 35 mcg

Phase II—norethindrone 1 mg + ethinyl estradiol 35 mcg

Phase III—norethindrone 0.5 mg + ethinyl estradiol 35 mcg

Triphasil

Phase I—levonorgestrel 0.05 mg + ethinyl estradiol 30 mcg

Phase II—levonorgestrel 0.075 mg + ethinyl estradiol 40 mcg

Phase III—levonorgestrel 0.125 mg + ethinyl estradiol 30 mcg

Tri-Previfem

Phase I—norgestimate 0.18 mg + ethinyl estradiol 35 mcg

Phase II—norgestimate 0.215 mg + ethinyl estradiol 35 mcg

Phase III—norgestimate 0.25 mg + ethinyl estradiol 35 mcg

Triple Antibiotic Ophthalmic Ointment—(per g) polymyxin B 10,000 units + neomycin 3.5 mg + bacitracin 400 units

🍁**Trisulfa**—trimethoprim 80 mg + sulfamethoxazole 400 mg

🍁**Trisulfa DS**—trimethoprim 160 mg + sulfamethoxazole 800 mg

Trizivir—abacavir 300 mg + lamivudine 150 mg + zidovudine 300 mg

Truvada—emtricitabine 200 mg + tenofovir 300 mg

Tussionex Suspension—(per 5 ml) chlorpheniramine 8 mg + hydrocodone 10 mg (as polistirex)

Tussi-Organidin NR Liquid—(per 5 ml) codeine 10 mg + guaifenesin 300 mg

Tussi-Organidin DM NR Liquid—(per 5 ml) guaifenesin 300 mg + dextromethorphan 10 mg

Tylenol Allergy Complete Caplets—acetaminophen 500 mg + chlorpheniramine 2 mg + pseudoephedrine 30 mg **(OTC)**

Tylenol Allergy Complete Nighttime Caplets—acetaminophen 500 mg + diphenhydramine 25 mg + pseudoephedrine 30 mg **(OTC)**

Tylenol Allergy Multisymptom Gelcaps—acetaminophen 325 mg + chlorpheniramine 2 mg + phenylephrine 5 mg **(OTC)**

Tylenol Allergy Multisymptom Nighttime Caplets—acetaminophen 325 mg + diphenhydramine 25 mg + phenylephrine 5 mg (OTC)
Tylenol Children's Plus Cold & Cough Chewable—acetaminophen 80 mg + pseudoephedrine 7.5 mg + dextromethorphan 2.5 mg + chlorpheniramine 0.5 mg (OTC)
Tylenol Children's Plus Cold Liquid—(per 5 ml) acetaminophen 160 mg + chlorpheniramine 1 mg + phenylephrine 2.5 mg (OTC)
Tylenol Children's Plus Multi-Symptom Cold Liquid—(per 5 ml) acetaminophen 160 mg + dextromethorphan 5 mg + chlorpheniramine 1 mg + phenylephrine 2.5 mg (OTC)
Tylenol Cold Multi-Symptom Severe Liquid—(per 15 ml) acetaminophen 325 mg + guaifenesin 200 mg + phenylephrine 5 mg + dextromethorphan 10 mg (OTC)
Tylenol Flu Daytime Gelcaps—dextromethorphan 15 mg + pseudoephedrine 30 mg + acetaminophen 325 mg (OTC)
Tylenol Flu Nighttime Gelcaps—pseudoephedrine 30 mg + diphenhydramine 25 mg+ acetaminophen 500 mg (OTC)
Tylenol PM—acetaminophen 500 mg + diphenhydramine 25 mg (OTC)
Tylenol Severe Allergy Caplets—diphenhydramine 12.5 mg + acetaminophen 500 mg (OTC)
Tylenol Sinus Congestion & Pain Daytime Gelcaps—acetaminophen 325 mg + phenylephrine 5 mg (OTC)
Tylenol Sinus Congestion & Pain Nighttime Caplets—acetaminophen 325 mg + chlorpheniramine 2 mg + phenylephrine 5 mg (OTC)
Tylenol Sinus Congestion & Pain Severe Caplets—acetaminophen 325 mg + guaifenesin 200 mg + phenylephrine 5 mg (OTC)
Tylenol Sinus Daytime—acetaminophen 500 mg + pseudoephedrine 30 mg (OTC)
Tylenol Sinus Nighttime—acetaminophen 500 mg + pseudoephedrine 30 mg + doxylamine 6.25 mg (OTC)
Tylenol Sinus Severe Congestion Daytime Caplets—acetaminophen 325 mg + guaifenesin 200 mg + pseudoephedrine 30 mg (OTC)
Tylenol Women's Menstrual Relief—acetaminophen 500 mg pamabrom 25 mg (OTC)
Tylenol with codeine No. 3—acetaminophen 300 mg + codeine 30 mg
Tylenol with codeine No. 4—acetaminophen 300 mg + codeine 60 mg
Tylox 5/500—oxycodone 5 mg + acetaminophen 500 mg
Ultracet—tramadol 37.5 mg + acetaminophen 325 mg
Unasyn for Injection 1.5 g—ampicillin 1 g + sulbactam 0.5 g
Unasyn for Injection 3 g—ampicillin 2 g + sulbactam 1 g
Uniretic 7.5/12.5—moexipril 7.5 mg + hydrochlorothiazide 12.5 mg
Uniretic 15/12.5—moexipril 15 mg + hydrochlorothiazide 12.5 mg
Uniretic 15/25—moexipril 15 mg + hydrochlorothiazide 25 mg
Vanquish Extra Strength Pain Reliever—aspirin 227 mg + acetaminophen 194 mg + caffeine 33 mg (OTC)
Vaseretic 5/12.5—enalapril 5 mg + hydrochlorothiazide 12.5 mg
Vaseretic 10/25—enalapril 10 mg + hydrochlorothiazide 25 mg
Vasocidin Ophthalmic Solution—0.23% prednisolone + 10% sulfacetamide
Vasocon-A Ophthalmic Solution—0.05% naphazoline + 0.5% antazoline (OTC)
Vicks 44D Cough & Head Congestion Relief Liquid—(per 15 ml) dextromethorphan 20 mg + phenylephrine 10 mg (OTC)
Vicks 44E Cough & Chest Congestion Relief Liquid—(per 15 ml) dextromethorphan 20 mg + guaifenesin 200 mg (OTC)
Vicks 44M Cold, Cough & Flu Liquid—(per 5 ml) dextromethorphan 7.5 mg + chlorpheniramine 1 mg + acetaminophen 162.5 mg (OTC)

Vicks Pediatric Formula 44E Liquid—(per 15 ml) dextromethorphan 10 mg + guaifenesin 100 mg **(OTC)**
Vicks Pediatric Formula 44M Multi-Symptom Cough & Cold Relief Liquid—(per 15 ml) chlorpheniramine 1 mg + dextromethorphan 15 mg **(OTC)**
Vicodin—hydrocodone 5 mg + acetaminophen 500 mg
Vicodin ES—hydrocodone 7.5 mg + acetaminophen 750 mg
Vicodin HP—hydrocodone 10 mg + acetaminophen 660 mg
Vicoprofen—hydrocodone 7.5 mg + ibuprofen 200 mg
Vytorin 10/10—ezetimibe 10 mg + simvastatin 10 mg
Vytorin 10/20—ezetimibe 10 mg + simvastatin 20 mg
Vytorin 10/40—ezetimibe 10 mg + simvastatin 40 mg
Vytorin 10/80—ezetimibe 10 mg + simvastatin 80 mg
Yasmin 28—drosperinone 3 mg + ethinyl estradiol 30 mcg
Yaz—drosperinone 3 mg + ethinyl estradiol 20 mcg
Zestoretic 10/12.5—lisinopril 10 mg + hydrochlorothiazide 12.5 mg
Zestoretic 20/12.5—lisinopril 20 mg + hydrochlorothiazide 12.5 mg
Zestoretic 20/25—lisinopril 20 mg + hydrochlorothiazide 25 mg
Ziac 2.5/6.25—bisoprolol 2.5 mg + hydrochlorothiazide 6.25 mg
Ziac 5/6.25—bisoprolol 5 mg + hydrochlorothiazide 6.25 mg
Ziac 10/6.25—bisoprolol 10 mg + hydrochlorothiazide 6.25 mg
Ziana Topical Gel—1.2% clindamycin + 0.025% tretinoin
Zosyn for Injection 2.25 g—piperacillin 2 g + tazobactam 0.25 g
Zosyn for Injection 3.375 g—piperacillin 3 g + tazobactam 0.375 g
Zosyn for Injection 4.5 g—piperacillin 4 g + tazobactam 0.5 g
Zovia 1/35—ethynodiol 1 mg + ethinyl estradiol 35 mcg
Zovia 1/50—ethynodiol 1 mg + ethinyl estradiol 50 mcg
Zydone 5/400—hydrocodone 5 mg + acetaminophen 400 mg
Zydone 7.5/400—hydrocodone 7.5 mg + acetaminophen 400 mg
Zydone 10/400—hydrocodone 10 mg + acetaminophen 400 mg
Zylet Ophthalmic Suspension—0.5% loteprednol + 0.3% tobramycin
Zyrtec-D—cetirizine 5 mg + pseudoephedrine 120 mg

APPENDIX C

Ophthalmic Medications

General Info: See Appendix D for administration techniques for ophthalmic agents.
Consult health care professional regarding:
Concurrent use of contact lenses (medication or additives may be absorbed by the lens).
Concurrent administration of other ophthalmic agents (order and spacing may be important).

DRUG NAME	DOSE	NOTES
Alpha-Adrenergic Blocker		
CAUTIONS: Avoid using in conditions in which miosis is undesirable; not to be used more than once weekly.		
dapiprazole (Rev-Eyes)	**Adults:** 1 drop followed after 5 min by another drop	• Administer immediately following retinal exam • ADRs*: blurred vision, irritation, corneal edema, punctate keratitis
Anesthetics		
Uses: Provide brief local anesthesia to allow measurement of intraocular pressure, removal of foreign bodies, or other superficial procedures. **CAUTIONS:** Repeated use may result in increased risk of CNS and cardiovascular toxicity; cross-sensitivity with some local anesthetics may occur.		
proparacaine (Alcaine, Ophthetic, Paracaine, Spectro-Caine, ✤Diocane)	**Adults and children:** 1–2 drops of 0.5% solution (single dose)	• Does not interact with ophthalmic cholinesterase inhibitors • ADRs: ophthalmic—irritation; systemic—irregular heartbeat, CNS depression, CNS stimulation
tetracaine (Altracaine, Pontocaine, Tetcaine, ✤Minims Tetracaine)	**Adults:** 1–2 drops of 0.5–1% solution (single dose)	• May interact with ophthalmic cholinesterase inhibitors, resulting in increased duration of action and risk of toxicity • ADRs: ophthalmic—irritation; systemic—irregular heartbeat, CNS depression, CNS stimulation
Antihistamines		
Uses: Various forms of allergic conjunctivitis.		
azelastine (Optivar)	**Adults and children >3 yr:** 1 drop of 0.5 mg/ml solution into each affected eye twice daily	• ADRs: transient burning/stinging, headache, bitter taste
emedastine (Emadine)	**Adults and children >3 yr:** 1 drop in affected eye up to 4 times daily	• ADRs: headache, drowsiness, malaise, local irritation
epinastine (Elestat)	**Adults and children >3yr:** 1 drop twice daily	• ADRs: local irritation • May enter breast milk
olopatadine (Patanol)	**Adults and children >3 yr:** 1–2 drops of 0.1% solution twice daily (given 6–8 hr apart)	• Small amounts are absorbed; excreted in urine • ADRs: headache, conjunctival irritation
Anti-infectives/ Antifungals/ Antivirals		
Uses: Localized superficial ophthalmic infections. **CAUTIONS:** Small amounts may be absorbed and result in hypersensitivity reactions.		
azithromycin (AzaSite)	**Adults and children >1yr:** 1 drop twice daily for two days, then once daily for five more days	• ADRs: eye irritation • When used to treat ocular chlamydial infections, concurrent systemic therapy is required

DRUG NAME	DOSE	NOTES
chloramphenicol (AK-Chlor, Chlorofair, Chloroptic, Clorachol, Econochlor, I-Chlor, Ocu-Chlor, Ophthochlor, Spectro-Chlor, ✱Fenicol, ✱Ophtho-Chloram, ✱Pentamycetin)	**Adults and children:** 1 drop of solution or thin strip of ointment q 1–4 hr	• May rarely cause systemic hematologic toxicity if used chronically and in excessive doses
ciprofloxacin (Ciloxan)	**Adults and children >1yr:** *bacterial conjunctivitis*—1 drop in each eye q 2 hr while awake for 48 hr, then q 4 hr while awake for 5 days; *corneal ulcers*—1 drop in affected eye q 15 min for 6 hr, then q 30 min while awake for rest of day, then q 1 hr while awake for next 24 hr, then q 4 hr while awake until re-epithelialization occurs or ribbon of ophthalmic ointment 3 times daily for 2 days, then twice daily for 5 days.	• May cause harmless white crystalline precipitate that resolves over time • ADRs: altered taste, systemic allergic reactions, photophobia, discomfort
erythromycin (Ilotycin)	**Adults and children:** *treatment of infections*—thin strip up to 6 times daily Infants: *prophylaxis of ophthalmia neonatorum*—thin strip in each eye as a single dose	• ADRs: irritation
gatifloxacin (Zymar)	**Adults and children >1yr:** 1 drop of 0.3% soln q 2 hr while awake for two days, then 4 times daily for 5 more days	• ADRs: irritation, headache, reduced visual acuity, taste disturbance.
gentamicin (Garamycin, Genoptic, Gentacidin, Gentafair, Gentak, Gentrasul, Ocu-Mycin, Spectro-Genta, ✱Alcomicin)	**Adults and children:** 1 drop of solution q 1–4 hr or thin strip of ointment q 8–12 hr	• ADRs: irritation, burning, stinging, blurred vision (ointment)
levofloxacin (Iquix, Quixin)	**Adults and children >6 yr:** *Quixin*—1–2 drops of 0.5% solution in each affected eye every 2 hr while awake for 2 days (up to 8 times/day); then every 4 hr for 5 more days (up to 4 times/day); *Iquix*—For corneal ulcers, 1–2 drops in the affected eye(s) every 30 minutes–2 hr while awake 4 and 6 hr after retiring for 3 days, then 1–2 drops every 1–4 hr while awake.	• ADRs: altered taste, systemic allergic reactions, photophobia
moxifloxacin (Vigamox)	**Adults and children >1yr:** 1 drop of 0.5% solution into affected eye 3 times daily for 7 days.	• ADRs: irritation, decreased visual acuity
norfloxacin (Chibroxin)	**Adults and children ≥1yr:** 1 drop 4 times daily while awake (up to q 2 hr while awake)	• ADRs: altered taste, systemic allergic reactions, photophobia
ofloxacin (Ocuflox)	**Adults and children ≥1 yr:** 1 drop q 2–4 hr while awake for 2 days, then 4 times daily for up to 5 more days	• ADRs: altered taste, systemic allergic reactions, photophobia
sulfacetamide (AK-Sulf, Bleph, Isopto Cetamide, I-Sulfacet, Ocu-Sul, Ocusulf, Sodium Sulamyd, Spectro-Sulf, Sulf, Sulfair, Sulfamide, Sulten, ✱Sulfex)	**Adults:** 1 drop of solution q 1–3 hr while awake (less frequently at night) or thin strip of ointment 4 times daily and at bedtime	• Cross-sensitivity with other sulfonamides (including thiazides) may occur • ADRs: local irritation

DRUG NAME	DOSE	NOTES
tobramycin (Tobrex)	**Adults and children >2mo:** 1 drop of solution q 1–4 hr depending on severity of infection or thin strip of ointment q 8–12 hr	• ADRs: irritation, burning, stinging, blurred vision (ointment) • Ointment may retard corneal wound healing • Avoid wearing contact lenses during use
Antifungal		
natamycin (Natacyn)	**Adults:** 1 drop q 1–6 hr, depending on severity of infection	• ADRs: irritation, swelling, chemosis
Antivirals		
trifluridine (Viroptic)	**Adults and children ≥6 yr:** 1 drop q 2 hr (up to 9 drops/day) while awake until cornea re-epithelializes, then 1 drop q 4 hr (at least 5 times daily) for up to 7 days	• ADRs: burning, stinging; keratopathy rarely
Artificial Tears/Ocular Lubricants (sterile buffered isotonic solutions/ointments) **Uses:** Artificial tears—keep the eyes moist with isotonic solutions and wetting agents in the management of dry eyes due to lack of tears; also provide lubrication for artificial eyes. Ocular lubricants—provide lubrication and protection in a variety of conditions including exposure keratitis, decreased corneal sensitivity, corneal erosions, keratitis sicca, during/following ocular surgery or removal of a foreign body.		
Artificial tears (Adsorbotear, Akwa Tears, Aquasite, Artifical Tears Plus, Cellufresh, Celluvisc, Comfort Tears, Dakrina, Dry Eye Therapy, Dry Eyes Duratears Naturale, Dwelle, Eye-Lube-A, Genteal Lubricant Eye Gel, HypoTears, HypoTears PF, Isopto Alkaline, Isopto Plain, Just Tears, Lacril, Lacri-Lube NP, Lacri-Lube S.O.P., Lacrisert, Liquifilm Forte, Liquifilm Tears, LubriTears, Moisture Drops, Murine Solution, Murocel, Nature's Tears, Nu-Tears, Nu-Tears II, Nutra Tear, Paralube, Refresh, Refresh PM, Tear Drop, TearGard, Teargen, Tearisol, Tears Naturale, Tears Naturale Free, Tears Naturale II, Tears Plus, Tears Renewed, Ultra Tears, Vit-A-Drops, Viva-Drops)	**Adults and children:** 1–2 drops 3–4 times daily or 1 insert (Lacrisert) 1–2 times daily Ocular lubricants **Adults and children:** small amount instilled into conjunctiva several times daily	• May alter effects of other concurrently administered ophthalmic medications • ADRs: photophobia, lid edema stinging (insert only), temporarily blurred vision, eye discomfort
Beta Blockers **Uses:** Management of chronic open-angle glaucoma and other forms of ocular hypertension (decreases the formation of aqueous humor). **CAUTIONS:** Systemic absorption is minimal but may occur. Systemic absorption may result in additive adverse cardiovascular effects (bradycardia, hypotension), especially when used with other cardiovascular agents (antihypertensives, antiarrhythmics). Other systemic adverse reactions may occur, including bronchospasm or delirium (geriatric patients). Concurrent use with ophthalmic epinephrine may decrease effectiveness.		
betaxolol (Betoptic, Betoptic S)	**Adults:** 1 drop of 0.5% solution twice daily or 1 drop of 0.25% suspension twice daily	• ADRs: conjunctivitis, decreased visual acuity, ocular burning, rashes (may be less likely than others to cause bronchospasm if systemically absorbed)
levobetaxolol (Betaxon)	**Adults:** 1 drop of 0.5% suspension twice daily	• ADRS: transient ophthalmic discomfort, blurred vision
levobunolol (AKBeta, Betagan)	**Adults:** 1 drop of 0.25% solution 1–2 times daily or 1 drop of 0.5% solution once daily	• ADRs: conjunctivitis, decreased visual acuity, ocular burning, rashes
metipranolol (OptiPranolol)	**Adults:** 1 drop of 0.3% solution twice daily	• ADRs: conjunctivitis, decreased visual acuity, ocular burning, rashes • Lasts up to 24 hr • Can be used safely with pilocarpine, epinephrine, and acetazolamide

DRUG NAME	DOSE	NOTES
timolol (Betimol, Timoptic, Timoptic-XE, 🍁 Apo-Timop)	**Adults and children ≥10 yr:** 0.25% or 0.5% solution—1 drop 1–2 times daily; 0.25% or 0.5% gel-forming solution—1 drop once daily **Children <10 yr:** 1 drop 0.25% solution 1–2 times daily	• ADRs: conjunctivitis, decreased visual acuity, ocular burning, rashes • Lasts up to 24 hr

Carbonic Anhydrase Inhibitor

Uses: Management of open-angle glaucoma or other forms of ocular hypertension (decreases formation of aqueous humor).
CAUTIONS: May exacerbate kidney stones; should not be used in patients with CCr <30 ml/min.

brinzolamide (Azopt)	**Adults:** 1 drop of 1% suspension into each affected eye three times daily	• ADRs: burning, stinging, unusual taste
dorzolamide (Trusopt)	**Adults:** 1 drop 3 times daily	• ADRs: bitter taste, cross-sensitivity with sulfonamides, ocular irritation or allergy

Cholinergics (direct-acting)

Uses: Treatment of open-angle glaucoma (facilitates the outflow of aqueous humor); also used to facilitate miosis after ophthalmic surgery or before examination (to counteract mydriatics).
CAUTIONS: Conditions in which pupillary constriction should be avoided. If significant systemic absorption occurs, bronchospasm, sweating, increased urination and salivation may occur.

carbachol (Carboptic, Isopto Carbachol)	**Adults and children:** 1 drop of 0.75–3% solution 1–3 times daily	• ADRs: blurred vision, altered vision, stinging, eye pain
pilocarpine (Adsorbocarpine, Akarpine, Isopto Carpine, Ocu-Carpine, Ocusert Pilo, Pilocar, Pilopine, Piloptic, Pilostat, 🍁 Miocarpine, 🍁 Spersacarpine)	**Adults and children:** glaucoma—1 drop of 1–4% solution 2–4 times daily (may be given more frequently for acute angle-closure glaucoma) or 1 ocular insert weekly or 1/2-in. strip of 4% gel at bedtime; counteracting mydriatic sympathomimetics—1 drop of 1% solution (may be repeated prior to surgery)	• Use 1% or less solution in infants • ADRs: blurred vision, altered vision, stinging, eye pain, headache, browache

Cholinergics (cholinesterase inhibitors)

Uses: Management of glaucoma not controlled with short-acting miotics or other agents; also used in varying doses for accommodative esotropia (diagnosis and treatment).
CAUTIONS: Enhance neuromuscular blockade from succinylcholine; intensify the actions of cocaine and some other local anesthetics; additive toxicity with antimyasthenics, anticholinergics, and cholinesterase inhibitors (including some pesticides). Use cautiously in patients with history or risk of retinal detachment.

echothiophate (Phospholine Iodide)	**Adults:** 1 drop 1–2 times daily	• May cause hyperactivity in patients with Down syndrome • ADRs: blurred vision, change in vision, brow ache, miosis, eyelid twitching, watering eyes • Irreversible cholinesterase inhibitor

Corticosteroids

Uses: Management of inflammatory eye conditions including allergic conjunctivitis, nonspecific superficial keratitis, infectious conjunctivitis (with anti-infectives); management of corneal injury; suppression of graft rejection following keratoplasty, prevention of postoperative inflammation.
CAUTIONS: Infectious ocular processes (avoid in herpes simplex keratitis), especially fungal and viral ocular infections (may mask symptoms); diabetes, glaucoma or epithelial compromise

dexamethasone (AK-Dex, Decadron, Maxidex, 🍁 Diodex, 🍁 PMS Dexamethasone, 🍁 RO-Dexasone, 🍁 Spersadex)	**Adults and children:** 1–2 drops of solution 4–6 times daily (up to q 1 hr) or thin strip of ointment 3–4 times daily initially	• As condition improves, decrease frequency of administration • ADRs: blurred vision (ointment), corneal thinning, increased intraocular pressure, irritation
fluorometholone (eFlone, FML, Flarex, Fluor-Op)	1–2 drops 4 times daily (up to 1–2 drops q 1 hr) as suspension or thin strip of ointment 1–3 times daily (up to q 4 hr) initially	• As condition improves, decrease frequency of administration • ADRs: blurred vision (ointment), corneal thinning, increased intraocular pressure, irritation

DRUG NAME	DOSE	NOTES
loteprednol (Alrex, Lotemax, Zylex)	**Adults:** 1 drop of 0.2% suspension (Alrex) 4 times daily or 1–2 drops 4 times daily of 0.5% suspension (lotemax); up to 1 drop every hr.	• 0.2% suspension used for seasonal allergic conjunctivitis • 0.5% suspension used for steroid-responsive inflammatory conditions and postoperatively
prednisolone (AK-Pred, Econopred, Inflamase, Pred ForteF, Pred Mild)	**Adults and children:** 1–2 drops of 0.12–1% solution/suspension 2–6 times daily (up to q 1 hr) initially	• As condition improves, decrease frequency of administration • ADRs: corneal thinning, increased intraocular pressure, irritation
rimexolone (Vexol)	**Adults and children:** 1–2 drops of 1% suspension q 6 hr (up to q 1 hr) initially	• As condition improves, decrease frequency of administration • ADRs: corneal thinning, increased intraocular pressure, irritation

Cycloplegic Mydriatics

Uses: Preparation for cycloplegic refraction; management of uveitis (not tropicamide).
CAUTIONS: Use cautiously in patients with a history of glaucoma; systemic absorption may cause anticholinergic effects such as confusion, unusual behavior, flushing, hallucinations, slurred speech, drowsiness, swollen stomach (infants), tachycardia, dry mouth.

DRUG NAME	DOSE	NOTES
atropine (Atropair, Atropisol, Atrosulf, Isopto Atropine, I-Tropine, Ocu-Tropine)	**Children:** cycloplegic refraction (solution)—1 drop twice daily for 1–3 days prior to refraction (use 0.125% solution in children <1 yr, 0.25% solution for children 1–5 yr), 0.25% solution for children >5 yr with blue irides, 0.5–1% for children >5 yr with dark irides; cycloplegic refraction (ointment)—0.3 cm of 0.5% ointment in children <2 yr with blue irides, 1% ointment in children <2 yr with dark irides or children >2 yr 3 times daily for 1-3 days prior to refraction; uveitis—1 drop of 0.125-1% solution 1–3 times daily **Adults:** uveitis—1 drop of 1% solution 1–2 times daily (up to 4 times daily) or 0.3–0.5 cm of 1% ointment 1–2 times daily	• Cycloplegic refraction in children only (too long-acting to use in adults); treatment of uveitis • Avoid using in children who have had a prior serious reaction to atropine • Effects on accommodation may last 6 days; mydriasis may last 12 days • ADRs: irritation, blurred vision, photophobia
cyclopentolate (AK-Pentolate, Cyclogyl, I-Pentolate, Cyclopentolate, Ocu-Pentolate, Pentolair, Spectro-Pentolate, 🍁Minims)	**Adults:** 1 drop of 0.5–2% solution; may repeat in 5–10 min **Children:** 1 drop of 0.5–2% solution; may be followed 5–10 min later by 1 drop of 0.5–1% solution **Premature and small infants:** 1 drop of 0.5% solution single dose	• Peak of cycloplegia is within 25–75 min and lasts 6–24 hr • Peak of mydriasis is within 30–60 min and may last several days • ADRs: irritation, blurred vision, photophobia
homatropine (Isopto Homatropine, Spectro-Homatropine, 🍁Minims Homatropine)	**Adults and children:** cycloplegic refraction—1 drop of 2–5% solution, may repeat in 5–10 min for 2–3 more doses; uveitis—1 drop of 2–5% solution 2–3 times daily (up to q 3–4 hr in adults)	• Cycloplegia and mydriasis may persist for 24–72 hr • ADRs: irritation, blurred vision, photophobia
scopolamine (Isopto Hyoscine)	**Adults and children:** cycloplegic refraction—1 drop of 0.25% solution (repeat twice daily for 2 days in children); uveitis—1 drop of 0.25% solution up to 4 times daily	• Shorter duration than atropine, but mydriasis and cycloplegia may persist for 3–7 days • ADRs: irritation, blurred vision, photophobia

DRUG NAME	DOSE	NOTES
tropicamide (Mydriacyl, Mydriafair, Ocu-Tropic, Opticyl, Spectro-Cyl, Tropicacyl, 🍁Minims Tropicamide)	**Adults and children:** 1 drop of 0.5–1% solution	• Stronger solution/repeated dosing may be required in patients with dark irides • Peak effect occurs in 20–40 min • Cycloplegia lasts 2–6 hr; mydriasis lasts up to 7 hr • ADRs: irritation, blurred vision, photophobia
Immunomodulators **Uses:** To increase tear production when the cause of dry eye is inflammation secondary to keratoconjunctivitis sicca. **CAUTIONS:** Tear production is not increased during concurrent use of ophthalmic NSAIDs or punctal plugs.		
cyclosporine (Restasis)	**Adults:** 1 drop of 0.05% ophthalmic emulsion in each eye twice daily	• ADRs: irritation, blurred vision • Emulsion should be inverted to obtain uniform opaque appearance prior to use.
Mast Cell Stabilizers **Uses:** Vernal keratoconjunctivitis. **CAUTIONS:** Require several days of treatment before effects are seen.		
cromolyn (Crolom, 🍁Opticrom)	**Adults and children ≥4 yr:** 1 drop of 4% solution 4–6 times daily	• ADRs: chemosis, irritation • Do not wear contact lenses concurrently
ketotifen (Alaway, Zaditor)	**Adults and children >3 yr:** 1 drop of 0.025% solution to affected eye q 8–12 hr	• ADRs: conjuctival injection, headaches, rhinits
lodoxamide (Alomide)	**Adults and children ≥2 yr:** 1 drop of 0.1% solution 4 times daily for up to 3 mo	• ADRs: blurred vision, foreign body sensation, irritation
nedocromil (Alocril)	**Adults and children >3 yr:** 1–2 drops of 2% solution in each eye twice daily throughout period of exposure	• Avoid concurrent use of contact lenses • ADRS: headache, ocular burning, unpleaseant taste, nasal congestion
pemirolast (Alamast)	**Adults and children >3 yr:** 1–2 drops of 0.1% solution in each affected eye 4 times daily	• ADRs: discomfort, dry eyes, foreign body sensation • Symptoms may improve within a few days, but optimal response may take up to 4 wk
Nonsteroidal Anti-inflammatory Drugs **Uses:** Management of pain/inflammation following surgery (bromfenac, diclofenac, ketorolac, nepafenac), allergic conjunctivitis (ketorolac), inhibition of perioperative miosis (flurbiprofen, suprofen). **CAUTIONS:** Cross-sensitivity with systemic NSAIDs may occur; concurrent use of anticoagulants, other NSAIDs, thrombolytics, some cephalosporins, and valproates may increase the risk of bleeding. May slow/delay healing. Avoid contact lens use.		
bromfenac (Xibrom)	**Adults:** 1 drop of 0.09% solution in affected eye(s) twice daily starting 24 hr after surgery and for 2 wk following.	• ADRs: irritation, headache • contains sulfites • Avoid contact lenses
diclofenac (Voltaren)	**Adults:** 1 drop of 0.1% solution 4 times daily for up to 6 wk	• Do not wear hydrocel contact lenses concurrently • ADRs: irritation, allergic reactions
flurbiprofen (Ocufen)	**Adults:** 1 drop of 0.03% solution q 30 min, beginning 2 hr prior to surgery (4 drops total)	• ADRs: irritation, allergic reactions
ketorolac (Acular, Acular Preservative Free, Acular LS)	**Adults and children >3 yr:** *Allergic conjunctivitis*—1 drop of 0.5% solution 4 times daily (Acular); *Postoperative*—1 drop of 0.4% solution 4 times daily in operated eye as needed for up to 4 days after corneal refractive surgery.	• ADRs: irritation, allergic reactions

DRUG NAME	DOSE	NOTES
nepafenac (Nevanac)	**Adults and Children >10 yr:** 1 drop of 0.1% suspension into affected eye(s) 3 times daily starting one day prior to cataract removal and for two weeks following surgery.	• irritation, photophobia, headache, hypertension, nausea/vomiting,

Ocular Decongestants/Vasoconstrictors

Uses: Decrease ocular congestion due to irritation by vasoconstricting conjunctival blood vessels; stronger solutions have mydriatic effects.

CAUTIONS: Systemic absorption may result in adverse cardiovascular effects; excessive/prolonged use may produce rebound hyperemia; use caution in patients at risk for acute angle-closure glaucoma; cardiovascular effects may be exaggerated by MAO inhibitors and dose adjustment may be required within 21 days of MAO inhibitors; increased risk of arrhythmias with inhalation anesthetics.

DRUG NAME	DOSE	NOTES
naphazoline (Albalon, Allerest, Allergy Drops, Clear Eyes Lubricating Eye Redness Reliever, Comfort Eye Drops, Degest 2, Estivin II, Nafazair, Naphcon, Ocu-Zoline, VasoClear, Vasocon, 🍁AK-Con)	**Adults:** 1 drop of 0.012% solution 4 times daily as needed or 1 drop of 0.1% solution q 3–4 hr as needed	• ADRs: ophthalmic-rebound hyperemia; systemic-dizziness, headache, nausea, sweating, weakness
oxymetazoline (OcuClear, Visine LR)	**Adults and children >6 yr:** 1 drop of 0.025% solution q 6 hr as needed	• ADRs: ophthalmic-rebound hyperemia; systemic-headache, insomnia, nervousness, tachycardia
phenylephrine (AK-Dilate, AK-Nefrin, Dilatair, I-Phrine, Isopto Frin, Mydfrin, Ocu-Phrin, Prefrin, 🍁Minims Phenylephrine, 🍁Spersaphrine)	**Adults:** decongestant—1 drop of 0.12% solution q 3–4 hr as needed; mydriasis—2.5 or 10% solution up to 3 times daily **Children:** mydriasis—2.5% solution up to 3 times daily	• ADRs: ophthalmic-blurred vision, browache, irritation; systemic-dizziness, tachycardia, hypertension, paleness, sweating, trembling
tetrahydrozoline (Collyrium Fresh, Eyesine, Geneye, Mallazine, Murine Plus, Optigene 3, Tetrazine, Visine)	**Adults:** 1–2 drops of 0.05% solution up to 4 times daily	• ADRs: ophthalmic—irritation; systemic—tachycardia, hypertension

Osmotics

Uses: Decreases superficial edema of the cornea prior to examination.

DRUG NAME	DOSE	NOTES
glycerin (Ophthalgan)	**Adults:** 1–2 drops prior to exam	• Avoid using in patients with hypersensitivity to chlorobutanol

Prostaglandin Agonist

Uses: Management of glaucoma or lowering of intraocular pressure (increases outflow of aqueous humor).

CAUTIONS: May change eye color to brown; will form precipitate with thimerosal-containing products; can be used with other agents to lower intraocular pressure.

DRUG NAME	DOSE	NOTES
bimatoprost (Lumigan)	**Adults:** 1 drop 0.03% solution in each affected eye once daily in the evening	• ADRs: local irritation, foreign body sensation, increased eyelash growth, increased brown pigmentation
latanoprost (Xalatan)	**Adults:** 1 drop once daily	• ADRs: local irritation, foreign body sensation
travoprost (Travatan)	**Adults:** 1 drop 0.004% solution in each affected eye once daily in the evening	• ADRs: local irritation, foreign body sensation, increased eyelash growth, increased brown pigmentation in iris

DRUG NAME	DOSE	NOTES
Sympathomimetics **Uses:** Management of glaucoma (lowers intraocular pressure by decreasing formation of aqueous humor). **CAUTIONS:** Systemic absorption may result in adverse cardiovascular and CNS reactions (especially in patients with cardiovascular disease); avoid use in patients predisposed to acute angle-closure glaucoma.		
apraclonidine (Iopidine)	**Adults:** *glaucoma*—1–2 drops of 0.5% solution 3 times daily; *preoperative use*—1 drop of 1% solution 1 hr prior to surgery	• A selective alpha-adrenergic agonist • ADRs: ophthalmic-irritation, mydriasis; systemic-allergic reactions, arrhythmias, bradycardia, drowsiness, dry nose, fainting, headache, nervousness, weakness • Monitor pulse and blood pressure • Avoid concurrent use with MAO inhibitors
brimonidine (Alphagan)	**Adults:** 1 drop 3 times daily (8 hr apart)	• A selective alpha-adrenergic agonist • ADRs: ophthalmic—irritation; systemic—drowsiness, dizziness, dry mouth, headache, weakness, muscular pain • Avoid concurrent use with MAO inhibitors • Tricyclic antidepressants may decrease effectiveness; additive CNS depression may occur with other CNS depressants, additive adverse cardiovascular effects with other cardiovascular agents
dipivefrin (Propine)	**Adults:** 1 drop q 12 hr	• Converted to epinephrine in the eye • ADRs: ophthalmic—local irritation, macular edema (aphakic patients); systemic—arrhythmias, hypertension • Wait 15 min before inserting soft contact lenses
epinephrine (Epifrin, Epinal, Eppy/N, Glaucon)	**Adults:** 1 drop of 1–2% solution 1–2 times daily.	• Increased risk of arrhythmias with inhalation anesthetics • ADRs: headache, local irritation • Cardiovascular effects may be exaggerated by MAO inhibitors; dose adjustment may be required within 21 days of MAO inhibitors

*ADRs = adverse reactions.

APPENDIX D

Medication Administration Techniques

Subcutaneous Injection Sites

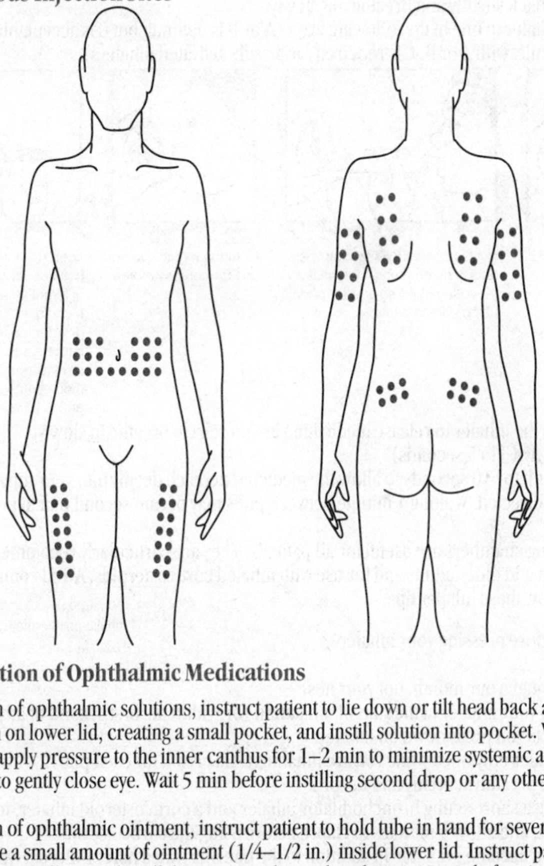

Administration of Ophthalmic Medications

For instillation of ophthalmic solutions, instruct patient to lie down or tilt head back and look at ceiling. Pull down on lower lid, creating a small pocket, and instill solution into pocket. With systemically acting drugs, apply pressure to the inner canthus for 1–2 min to minimize systemic absorption. Instruct patient to gently close eye. Wait 5 min before instilling second drop or any other ophthalmic solutions.

For instillation of ophthalmic ointment, instruct patient to hold tube in hand for several minutes to warm. Squeeze a small amount of ointment (1/4–1/2 in.) inside lower lid. Instruct patient to close eye gently and roll eyeball around in all directions with eye closed. Wait 10 min before instilling any other ophthalmic ointments.

Do not touch cap or tip of container to eye, fingers, or any surface.

Administration of Medications with Metered-Dose Inhalers

Instruct patient on the proper use of the metered-dose inhaler. There are 3 methods of using a metered-dose inhaler. Shake inhaler well. (1) Take a drink of water to moisten the throat; place the inhaler mouthpiece 2 finger-widths away from mouth; tilt head back slightly. While activating the inhaler, take a slow, deep breath for 3–5 sec; hold the breath for 10 sec; and breathe out slowly. (2) Exhale and close lips firmly around mouthpiece. Administer during second half of inhalation, and hold breath for as long as possible to ensure deep instillation of medication. (3) Use of spacer. Consult health care professional to determine method desired prior to instruction. Allow 1–2 min between inhalations.

Rinse mouth with water or mouthwash after each use to minimize dry mouth and hoarseness. Wash inhalation assembly at least daily in warm running water.
For use of dry powder inhalers, turn head away from inhaler and exhale (do not blow into inhaler). Do not shake. Close mouth tightly around the mouthpiece of the inhaler and inhale rapidly.

Steps for Using Your Inhaler*

1. Remove the cap and hold inhaler upright.
2. Shake the inhaler.
3. Tilt your head back slightly and breathe out slowly.
4. Position the inhaler in one of the following ways (A or B is optimal, but C is acceptable for those who have difficulty with A or B. C is required for breath-activated inhalers):

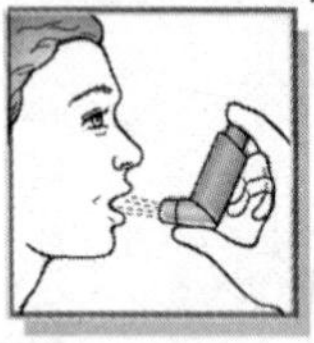

A. Open mouth with inhaler 1 to 2 inches away.

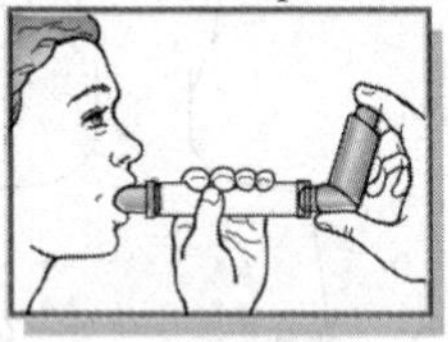

B. Use space/holding chamber (this is recommended especially for young children and for people using corticosteroids).

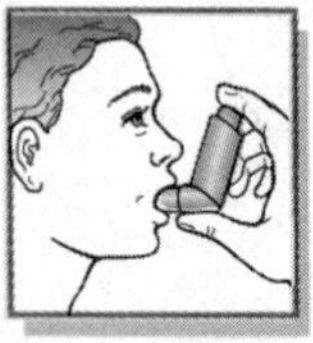

C. In the mouth. Do not use for corticosteroids.

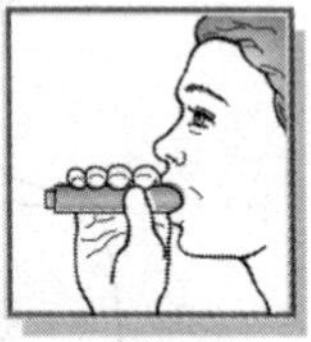

D. NOTE: Inhaled dry powder capsules require a different inhalation technique. To use a dry powder inhaler, it is important to close the mouth tightly around the mouthpiece of the inhaler and to inhale rapidly.

5. Press down on the inhaler to release medication as you start to breathe in slowly.
6. Breathe in slowly (3 to 5 seconds).
7. Hold your breath for 10 seconds to allow the medicine to reach deeply into your lungs.
8. Repeat puff as directed. Waiting 1 minute between puffs may permit second puff to penetrate your lungs better.
9. Spacers/holding chambers are useful for all patients. They are particularly recommended for young children and older adults and for use with inhaled corticosteroids. Avoid common inhaler mistakes. Follow these inhaler tips:

- Breathe out before pressing your inhaler.
- Inhale slowly.
- Breathe in through your mouth, not your nose.
- Press down on your inhaler at the start of inhalation (or within the first second of inhalation).
- Keep inhaling as you press down on inhaler.
- Press your inhaler only once while you are inhaling (one breath for each puff).
- Make sure you breathe in evenly and deeply.
- If you are using a short-acting bronchodilator inhaler and a corticosteroid inhaler, use the bronchodilator first, and allow 5 minutes to elapse before using the corticosteroid.

Other inhalers have become available in addition to the one illustrated here. Different types of inhalers may require different techniques.

Administration of Medications by Nebulizer

Administer in a location where patient can sit comfortably for 10–15 min. Plug in compressor. Mix medication as directed, or empty unit-dose vials into nebulizer. Do not mix different types of medications without checking with health care professional. Assemble mask or mouthpiece and connect tubing to port on compressor. Have patient sit in a comfortable upright position. Make sure that mask fits properly over nose and mouth and that mist does not flow into eyes, or put mouthpiece into mouth.

*Source: Expert Panel Report 2: Guidelines for the Diagnosis and Management of Asthma. National Asthma Education and Prevention Program, National Heart, Lung, and Blood Institute, 1997.

Turn on compressor. Instruct patient to take slow deep breaths. If possible, patient should hold breath for 10 sec before slowly exhaling. Continue this process until medication chamber is empty. Wash mask in hot soapy water; rinse well and allow to air dry before next use.

Administration of Nasal Sprays

Clear nasal passages of secretions prior to use. If nasal passages are blocked, use a decongestant immediately prior to use to ensure adequate penetration of the spray. Keep head upright. Breathe in through nose during administration. Sniff hard for a few minutes after administration.

Intramuscular Injection Sites

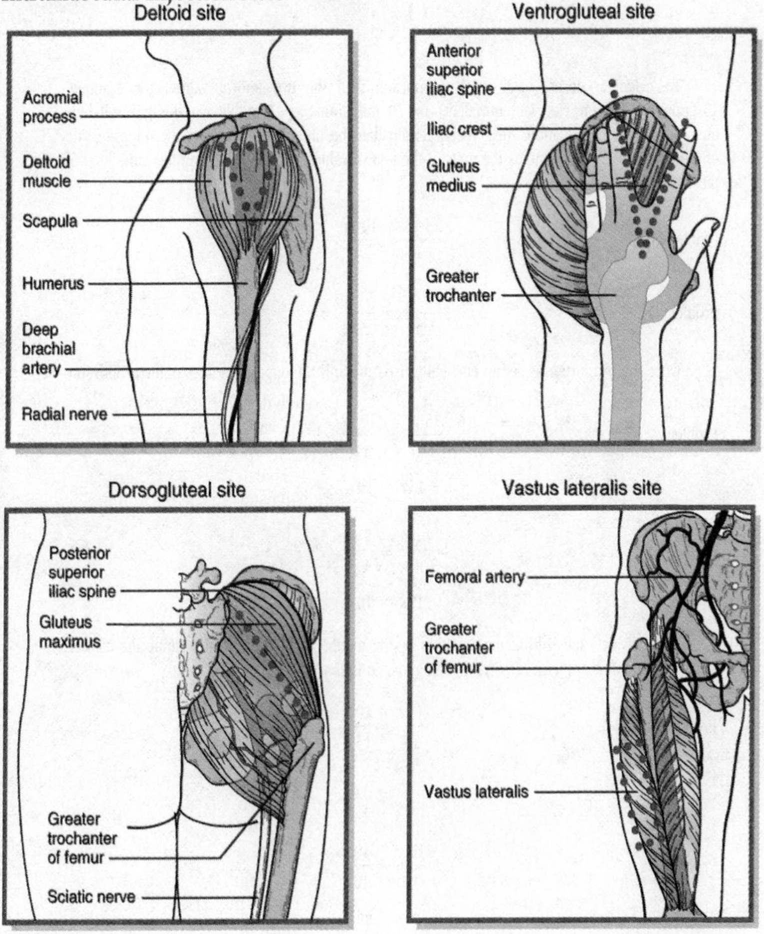

The dorsogluteal site is associated with sciatic nerve injury. The deltoid and ventrogluteal sites are the preferred sites for adults; the vastus lateralis site is preferred in children under 2 years of age.

Formulas Helpful for Calculating Doses

Ratio and Proportion

A ratio is the same as a fraction and can be expressed as a fraction (1/2) or in the algebraic form (1:2). This relationship is stated as *one is to two.*

A proportion is an equation of equal fractions or ratios.

$$\frac{1}{2} = \frac{4}{8}$$

To calculate doses, begin each proportion with the two known values, for example, 15 grains = 1 gram (known equivalent) or 10 milligrams = 2 milliliters (dosage available) on one side of the equation. Next, make certain that the units of measure on the opposite side of the equation are the same as the units of the known values and are placed on the same level of the equation.

Problem A: $$\frac{15 \text{ gr}}{1 \text{ g}} = \frac{10 \text{ gr}}{x \text{ g}}$$

Problem B: $$\frac{10 \text{ mg}}{2 \text{ ml}} = \frac{5 \text{ mg}}{x \text{ ml}}$$

Once the proportion is set up correctly, cross-multiply the opposing values of the proportion.

Problem A: $$\frac{15 \text{ gr}}{1 \text{ gr}} \times \frac{10 \text{ gr}}{x \text{ g}}$$

$$15x = 10$$

Problem B: $$\frac{10 \text{ mg}}{2 \text{ ml}} \times \frac{5 \text{ mg}}{x \text{ ml}}$$

$$10x = 10$$

Next, divide each side of the equation by the number with the x to determine the answer. Then, add the unit of measure corresponding to x in the original equation.

Problem A: $$\frac{15x}{15} = \frac{10}{15}$$

$$x = \frac{2}{3} \text{ or } 0.6 \text{ g}$$

Problem B: $$\frac{10x}{10} = \frac{10}{10}$$

$$x = 1 \text{ ml}$$

Calculation of IV Drip Rate

To calculate the drip rate for an intravenous infusion, 3 values are needed:

I. The amount of solution and corresponding time for infusion. May be ordered as:

$$1000 \text{ ml over } 8 \text{ hr}$$

or

$$125 \text{ ml/hr}$$

II. The equivalent in time to convert hours to minutes.

$$1 \text{ hr} = 60 \text{ min}$$

III. The drop factor or number of drops that equal 1 ml of fluid. (This information can found on the IV tubing box.)

$$10 \text{ gtt} = 1 \text{ ml}$$

Set up the problem by placing each of the 3 values in a proportion.

$$\frac{125 \text{ ml}}{1 \text{ hr}} \times \frac{1 \text{ hr}}{60 \text{ min}} \times \frac{10 \text{ gtt}}{1 \text{ ml}}$$

Numbers and units of measure can be canceled out from the upper and lower levels of the equation.

The numbers cancel, leaving:

$$\frac{125 \text{ ml}}{1 \text{ hr}} \times \frac{1 \text{ hr}}{\underset{6}{\cancel{60}} \text{ min}} \times \frac{\overset{1}{\cancel{10}} \text{ gtt}}{1 \text{ ml}}$$

The units cancel, leaving:

$$\frac{125 \cancel{\text{ml}}}{1 \cancel{\text{hr}}} \times \frac{1 \cancel{\text{hr}}}{6 \text{ min}} \times \frac{1 \text{ gtt}}{1 \cancel{\text{ml}}}$$

Next, multiply each level across and divide the numerator by the denominator for the answer.

$$\frac{125 \cancel{\text{ml}}}{1 \cancel{\text{hr}}} \times \frac{1 \cancel{\text{hr}}}{6 \text{ min}} \times \frac{1 \text{ gtt}}{1 \cancel{\text{ml}}} = \frac{125 \text{ gtt}}{6 \text{ min}}$$

$$125 \div 6 = 20.8 \text{ or } 21 \text{ gtt/min}$$

Calculation of Creatinine Clearance (CCr) in Adults from Serum Creatinine

$$\text{Men: CCr} = \frac{\text{weight (kg)} \times (140 - \text{age})}{72 \times \text{serum creatinine (mg/dl)}}$$

$$\text{Women: CCr} = 0.85 \times \text{calculation for men}$$

Calculation of Body Surface Area (BSA) in Adults and Children

Dubois method:

$$SA\ (cm^2) = wt\ (kg)^{0.425} \times ht\ (cm)^{0.725} \times 71.84$$

$$SA\ (m^2)\ K \times \sqrt[3]{wt^2\ (kg)}$$ (common K value 0.1 for toddlers, 0.103 for neonates)

Simplified method:

$$BSA\ (m^2) = \sqrt{\frac{ht\ (cm) \times wt\ (kg)}{3600}}$$

Body Mass Index

$$BMI = wt\ (kg) \div ht\ (m^2)$$

Body Surface Area Nomograms

ESTIMATING BODY SURFACE AREA IN CHILDREN

For pediatric patients of average size, body surface area may be estimated with the scale on the left. Match weight to corresponding surface area. For other pediatric patients, use the scale on the right. Lay a straightedge on the correct height and weight points for your patient, and observe the point where it intersects on the surface area scale at center.

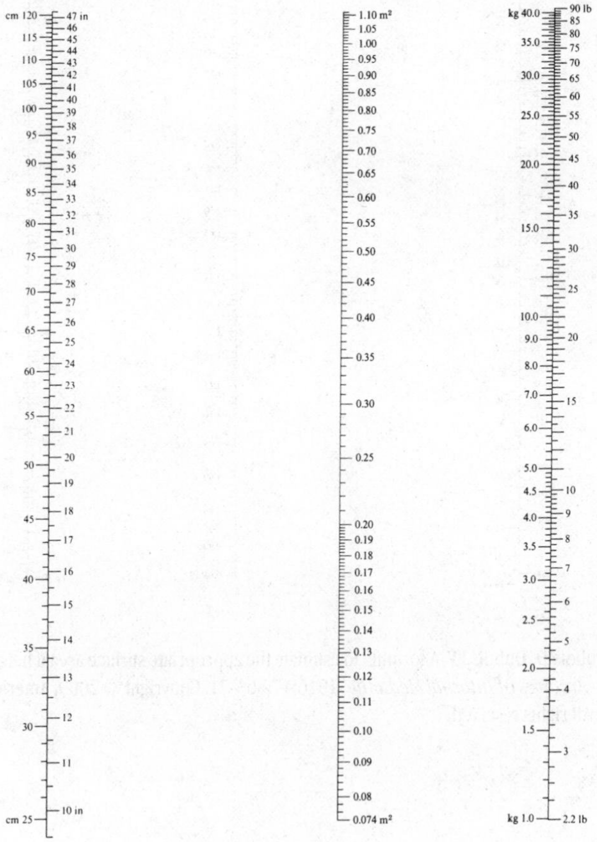

Reproduced from *Nelson Textbook of Pediatrics*, 16th edition. Courtesy W.B. Saunders Co., Philadelphia. PA.

ESTIMATING BODY SURFACE AREA IN ADULTS

Use a straightedge to connect the patient's height in the left-hand column to weight in the right-hand column. The intersection of this line with the center scale estimates the body surface area.

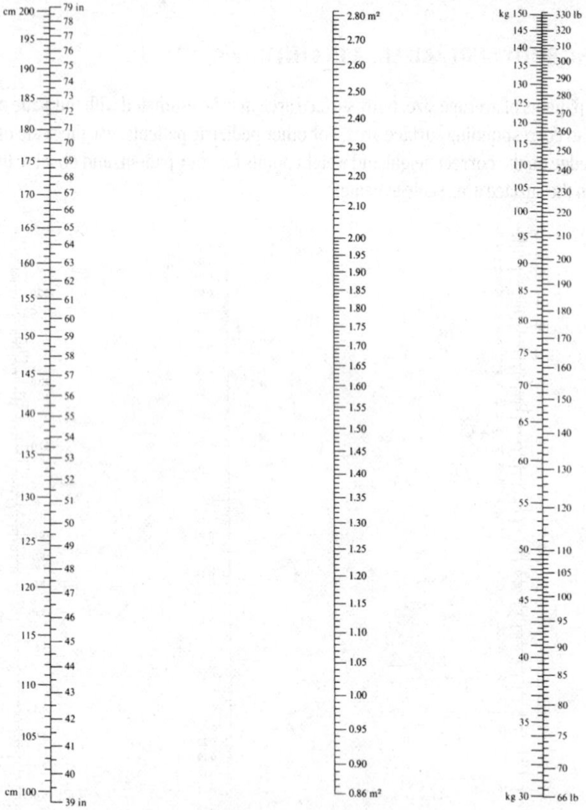

Source: Dubois D, Dubois EF. A formula to estimate the appropriate surface area if height and weight be known. *Archives of Internal Medicine.* 1916:17;863-71.

APPENDIX G

Normal Values of Common Laboratory Tests

SERUM TESTS

HEMATOLOGIC	MEN	WOMEN
Hemoglobin	13.5–18 g/dl	12–16 g/dl
Hematocrit	40–54%	38–47%
Red blood cells (RBC)	4.6–6.2 million/mm^3	4.2–5.4 million/mm^3
Mean corpuscular volume (MCV)	76–100 ($micrometer^3$)	76–100 ($micrometer^3$)
Mean corpuscular hemoglobin (MCH)	27–33 picogram	27–33 picogram
Mean corpuscular hemoglobin concentration (MCHC)	33–37 g/dl	33–37 g/dl
Erythrocyte sedimentation rate (ESR)	≤20 mm/hr	≤30 mm/hr
Leukocytes (WBC)	5000–10,000/mm^3	5000–10,000/mm^3
Neutrophils	54–75% (3000–7500/mm^3)	54–75% (3000–7500/mm^3)
Bands	3–8% (150–700/mm^3)	3–8% (150–700/mm^3)
Eosinophils	1–4% (50–400/mm^3)	1–4% (50–400/mm^3)
Basophils	0–1% (25–100/mm^3)	0–1% (25–100/mm^3)
Monocytes	2–8% (100–500/mm^3)	2–8% (100–500/mm^3)
Lymphocytes	25–40% (1500–4500/mm^3)	25–40% (1500–4500/mm^3)
T lymphocytes	60–80% of lymphocytes	60–80% of lymphocytes
B lymphocytes	10–20% of lymphocytes	10–20% of lymphocytes
Platelets	150,000–450,000/mm^3	150,000–450,000/mm^3
Prothrombin time (PT)	9.6–11.8 sec	9.5–11.3 sec
Partial thromboplastin time (PTT)	30–45 sec	30–45 sec
Bleeding time (duke)	1–3 min	1–3 min
(ivy)	3–6 min	3–6 min
(template)	3–6 min	3–6 min
Clotting time (Lee-White)	4–8 min	4–8 min

CHEMISTRY	MEN	WOMEN
Sodium	135–145 mEq/L	135–145 mEq/L
Potassium	3.5–5.0 mEq/L	3.5–5.0 mEq/L
Chloride	95–105 mEq/L	95–105 mEq/L
Bicarbonate (HCO_3)	19–25 mEq/L	19–25 mEq/L
Total calcium	9–11 mg/dl or 4.5–5.5 mEq/L	9–11 mg/dl or 4.5–5.5 mEq/L
Ionized calcium	4.2–5.4 mg/dl or 2.1–2.6 mEq/L	4.2–5.4 mg/dl or 2.1–2.6 mEq/L
Phosphorus/phosphate	2.4–4.7 mg/dl	2.4–4.7 mg/dl
Magnesium	1.8–3.0 mg/dl or 1.5–2.5 mEq/L	1.8–3.0 mg/dl or 1.5–2.5 mEq/L
Glucose	65–99 mg/dl	65–99 mg/dl
Osmolality	285–310 mOsm/kg	285–310 mOsm/kg
Ammonia (NH_3)	10–80 mcg/dl	10–80 mcg/dl
Amylase	≤130 U/L	≤130 U/L
Creatine phosphokinase total (CK, CPK)	<150 U/L	<150 U/L
Creatine kinase isoenzymes, MB fraction	>5% in MI	>5% in MI
Lactic dehydrogenase (LDH)	50–150 U/L	50–150 U/L
Protein, total	6–8 g/d	6–8 g/d
Albumin	4–6 g/dl	4–6 g/dl

HEPATIC	MEN	WOMEN
AST	8–46 U/L	7–34 U/L
ALT	10–30 IU/ml	10–30 IU/ml
Total bilirubin	0.3–1.2 mg/dl	0.3–1.2 mg/dl

Conjugated bilirubin	0.0–0.2 mg/dl	0.0–0.2 mg/dl
Unconjugated (indirect) bilirubin	0.2–0.8 mg/dl	0.2–0.8 mg/dl
Alkaline phosphatase	20–90 U/L	20–90 U/L
RENAL	**MEN**	**WOMEN**
BUN	6–20 mg/dl	6–20 mg/dl
Creatinine	0.6–1.3 mg/dl	0.5–1.0 mg/dl
Uric acid	4.0–8.5 mg/dl	2.7–7.3 mg/dl
ARTERIAL BLOOD GASES	**MEN**	**WOMEN**
pH	7.35–7.45	7.35–7.45
Po_2	80–100 mmHg	80–100 mmHg
Pco_2	35–45 mmHg	35–45 mmHg
O_2 saturation	95–97%	95–97%
Base excess	+2–(−2)	+2–(−2)
Bicarbonate (HCO_3^-)	22–26 mEq/L	22–26 mEq/L

URINE TESTS

URINE	MEN	WOMEN
pH	4.5–8.0	4.5–8.0
Specific gravity	1.010–1.025	1.010–1.025

Drug Levels, Therapeutic and Toxic Conventional (US System of Measurements)

Drug	Therapeutic Level	Toxic Level
acetaminophen	5–20 µg/mL	>40 µg/mL
alprazolam	10–50 ng/mL	>75 ng/mL
amikacin	peak: 20–30 µg/mL	peak: >35 µg/mL
aminocaproic acid	trough: 4–8 µg/mL	trough: >10 µg/mL
aminophylline	100–400 µg/mL	>400 µg/mL
amiodarone	10–20 µg/mL	>20 µg/ml
amitriptyline	0.5–2.5 µg/mL	>2.5 µg/mL
amoxapine	120–150 ng/mL	>500 ng/ml
atenolol	200–400 ng/mL	>500 ng/mL
bepridil HCl	200–500 ng/mL	>500 ng/mL
carbamazepine	1–2 ng/mL	>2 ng/mL
chloral hydrate	5–12 µg/mL	>12 µg/mL
chloramphenicol	2–12 µg/mL	>20 µg/mL
chlordiazepoxide	10–20 µg/mL	>25 µg/mL
chlorpromazine	1–5 µg/mL	>5 µg/mL
chlorpropramide	50–300 ng/mL	>750 ng/mL
clonazepam	75–250 µg/mL	>250 µg/mL
cyclosporine	15–60 ng/mL	>80 ng/mL
desipramine	100–300 ng/mL	<85 or >500 ng/mL
diazepam	150–300 ng/mL	>500 ng/mL
digoxin	0.5–2 mg/L	>3 mg/L
diltiazem	0.8–2 ng/mL	>2 ng/mL
disopyramide	50–200 ng/mL	>200 ng/mL
doxepin	2–5 µg/mL	>7 µg/mL
ethosuximide	150–300 ng/mL	>400 ng/mL
flecainide	40–100 µg/mL	>150 µg/mL
gentamicin	0.2–1 µg/mL	>1 µg/mL
acetaminophen	peak: 6–10 µg/mL	peak: >12 µg/mL
	trough: <2 µg/mL	trough: >2 µg/mL
haloperidol	3–20 ng/mL	>42 ng/mL
hydromorphone	1–30 ng/mL	>100 ng/mL
imipramine	150–300 ng/mL	>500 ng/mL
kanamycin	20–25 µg/mL	>35 µg/mL
lidocaine	1.5–5 µg/mL	>5 µg/mL
lithium	0.5–1.5 mEq/L	>1.5 mEq/L
meperidine	0.4–0.7 µg/mL	>1 µg/mL
methotrexate	>0.01 µmol	>10 µmol in 24 hr

mexiletine	0.5–2 μg/mL	>2 μg/mL
mezlocillin sodium	35–45 μg/mL	>45 μg/mL
milrinone	150–250 ng/mL	>250 ng/mL
morphine	10–80 ng/mL	>200 ng/mL
nicardipine	0.028–0.05 μg/mL	>0.05 μg/mL
nifedipine	0.025–0.1 μg/mL	>0.1 μg/mL
nortriptyline	50–150 ng/mL	>500 ng/mL
phenobarbital	15–30 μg/mL	>40 μg/mL
phenytoin	10–20 μg/mL	>20 μg/mL
primidone	5–12 μg/mL	>12 μg/mL
procainamide	4–10 μg/mL	>10 μg/mL
propafenone	0.5–3 μg/mL	>3 μg/mL
propranolol	50–100 ng/m	>150 ng/mL
quinidine	2–5 μg/mL	>6 μg/mL
salicylate	10–30 mg/dL	>35 mg/dL
theophylline	10–20 μg/mL	>20 μg/mL
tobramycin	peak: 6–10 μg/mL trough: <2 μg/mL	peak: >12 μg/mL trough: >2 μg/mL
tocainide HCl	4–10 μg/mL	>12 μg/mL
trazadone	500–2000 ng/mL	>4000 ng/mL
valproic acid	50–100 μg/mL	>100 μg/mL
vancomycin	peak: 20–40 μg/mL trough: 5–10 μg/mL	peak: >80 μg/mL trough: >10 μg/mL
verapamil	0.08–0.3 μg/mL	>0.3 μg/mL

Drug Levels, Therapeutic and Toxic Conventional SI Units (International System of Units)

Drug	Therapeutic Level	Toxic Level
amikacin	peak: 34–51 μmol/L trough: 7–14 μmol/L	peak: >60 μmol/L trough: 35 μmol/L
amitriptyline	433–903 nmol/L	>805 nmol/L
carbamazepine	21–51 μmol/L	>51 μmol/L
clonazepam	40–200 nmol/L	>260 nmol/L
desipramine	281–1125 nmol/L	>1500 nmol/L
diazepam	0.35–3.5 nmol/L	>17.5 nmol/L
digoxin	1–2.6 nmol/L	>2.6 nmol/L
disopyramide	9–18 μmol/L	>21 μmol/L
ethosuximide	280–708 μmol/L	>1062 μmol/L
flecainide	0.5–2.4 μmol/L	>2.4 μmol/L
gentamicin	peak:12–21 μmol/L trough: <4 μmol/L	peak: >21 μmol/L trough: 4.5 μmol/L
imipramine	610–1670 nmol/L	>1785 nmol/L
lignocaine	6–21 μmol/L	>39 μmol/L
lithium	0.5–1.5 mmol/L	>2 mmol/L
nortriptyline	190–570 nmol/L	>1900 nmol/L
phenobarbitone	86–172 μmol/L	>172 μmol/L
phenytoin	40–80 μmol/L	>158 μmol/L
primidone	23–55 μmol/L	>55 μmol/L
procainamide	17–42 μmol/L	>51 μmol/L
quinidine	6–15 μmol/L	>29 μmol/L
salicylic acid	1–2 mmol/L	>3.6 mmol/L
theophylline	28–111 μmol/L	>111 μmol/L
tobramycin	peak: 13–21 μmol/L trough: <4 μmol/L	peak: >21 μmol/L trough: 4.5 μmol/L
valproic acid	350–700 μmol/L	>1386 μmol/L
vancomycin	peak: 14–28 μmol/L trough: 3–7 μmol/L	peak: >28 μmol/L trough: 7 μmol/L

APPENDIX H

COMMONLY USED ABBREVIATIONS

ABGs arterial blood gases
ac before meals
ACE angiotensin-converting enzyme
ADH antidiuretic hormone
A-G ratio albumin-globulin ratio
AHF antihemolytic factor
ALT alanine aminotransferase
ANA antinuclear antibodies
ANC absolute neutrophil count
AST aspartate aminotransferase
ATP adenosine triphosphate
AV atrioventricular
bid two times a day
BMI body mass index
BP blood pressure
bpm beats per minute
BSA body surface area
BUN blood urea nitrogen
cap capsule
CBC complete blood count
CCr creatinine clearance
CHF congestive heart failure
COMT catechol-O-methyltransferase
CNS central nervous system
CPK creatine phosphokinase
CR controlled-release
CSF colony-stimulating factor; cerebrospinal fluid
CT computed tomography
CV cardiovascular
CVP central venous pressure
D5/LR 5% dextrose and lactated Ringer's solution
D5/0.9% NaCl 5% dextrose and 0.9% NaCl; 5% dextrose and normal saline
D5/0.25% NaCl 5% dextrose and 0.25% NaCl; 5% dextrose and quarter normal saline
D5/0.45% NaCl 5% dextrose and 0.45% NaCl; 5% dextrose and half normal saline
D5W 5% dextrose in water
D10W 10% dextrose in water
Derm dermatologic
dl deciliter
DMARD disease-modifying antirheumatic drug
DNA deoxyribonucleic acid
DVT deep vein thrombosis
ECG electrocardiogram
ECMO extracorporeal membrane oxygenation
EENT eye, ear, nose, and throat
Endo endocrine
ER extended-release
ESRD end-stage renal disease
F and E fluid and electrolyte
g gram(s)
GABA gamma-aminobutyric acid
GERD gastroesophageal reflux disease
GFR glomerular filtration rate
GI gastrointestinal
G6PD glucose-6-phosphate dehydrogenase
gt(t) drop(s)
GTT glucose tolerance test
GU genitourinary
Hb A_{1c} hemoglobin A_{1c}, glycosylated hemoglobin
HDL high-density lipoproteins
Hemat hematologic
HF heart failure
hr(s) hour(s)
HRT hormone replacement therapy
IA intra-articular
IL intralesional
IM intramuscular
Inhaln inhalation
INR international normalized ratio
IPPB intermittent positive-pressure breathing
IS intrasynovial
IT intrathecal
IV intravenous
K potassium
KCl potassium chloride
kg kilogram
L liter
LA long-acting
LDH lactic dehydrogenase
LDL low-density lipoproteins
LR lactated Ringer's solution
M molar
MAOI monoamine oxidase inhibitor

mcg microgram(s)
MDI metered dose inhaler
mEq milliequivalent
Metab metabolic
mg milligram(s)
min(s) minute(s)
Misc miscellaneous
ml milliliter(s)
mM millimole
MRI magnetic resonance imaging
MS musculoskeletal
MUGA multiple-gated (image) acquisition (analysis)
Na sodium
NaCl sodium chloride
0.9% NaCl 0.9% sodium chloride, normal saline
Neuro neurologic
NPO nothing by mouth
NS sodium chloride, normal saline (0.9% NaCl)
NSAIDs nonsteroidal anti-inflammatory drugs
OCD obsessive-compulsive disorder
Oint ointment
Ophth ophthalmic
OTC over-the-counter
pc after meals
PCA patient-controlled analgesia
PO by mouth, orally
prn as needed
PT prothrombin time
PTT partial thromboplastin time
PVC premature ventricular contraction
q every
qid four times a day
q 2 hr every 2 hours
q 3 hr every 3 hours
q 4 hr every 4 hours
RBC red blood cell count
Rect rectally or rectal
REM rapid eye movement
Resp respiratory
RTU ready to use
Rx prescription
SA sinoatrial
subcut subcutaneous
sec(s) second(s)
SL sublingual
SR sustained-release
SSRI(s) selective serotonin reuptake inhibitor(s)
stat immediately
supp suppository
tab tablet
tbs tablespoon(s)
tid three times a day
Top topically or topical
tsp teaspoon(s)
UK unknown
Vag vaginal
VFib ventricular fibrillation
VLDL very low-density lipoproteins
VT ventricular tachycardia
WBC white blood cell count
wk(s) week(s)
yr(s) year(s)

APPENDIX I

Pregnancy Categories and Controlled Substances Schedules

PREGNANCY CATEGORIES A

Category A

Adequate, well-controlled studies in pregnant women have not shown an increased risk of fetal abnormalities.

Category B

Animal studies have revealed no evidence of harm to the fetus, however, there are no adequate and well-controlled studies in pregnant women. **or** Animal studies have shown an adverse effect, but adequate and well-controlled studies in pregnant women have failed to demonstrate a risk to the fetus.

Category C

Animal studies have shown an adverse effect and there are no adequate and well-controlled studies in pregnant women. **or** No animal studies have been conducted and there are no adequate and well-controlled studies in pregnant women.

Category D

Studies, adequate well-controlled or observational, in pregnant women have demonstrated a risk to the fetus. However, the benefits of therapy may outweigh the potential risk.

Category X

Studies, adequate well-controlled or observational, in animals or pregnant women have demonstrated positive evidence of fetal abnormalities. The use of the product is contraindicated in women who are or may become pregnant.

Note: The designation UK is used when the pregnancy category is unknown.

CONTROLLED SUBSTANCES SCHEDULES

Classes or schedules are determined by the Drug Enforcement Agency (DEA), an arm of the United States Justice Department, and are based on the potential for abuse and dependence liability (physical and psychological) of the medication. Some states may have stricter prescription regulations. Physicians, dentists, podiatrists, and veterinarians may prescribe controlled substances. Nurse practitioners and physician's assistants may prescribe controlled substances with certain limitations.

Schedule I (C-I)

Potential for abuse is so high as to be unacceptable. May be used for research with appropriate limitations. Examples are LSD and heroin.

Schedule II (C-II)

High potential for abuse and extreme liability for physical and psychological dependence (amphetamines, opioid analgesics, dronabinol, certain barbiturates). Outpatient prescriptions must be in writing. In emergencies, telephone orders may be acceptable if a written prescription is provided within 72 hr. No refills are allowed.

Schedule III (C-III)

Intermediate potential for abuse (less than C-II) and intermediate liability for physical and psychological dependence (certain nonbarbiturate sedatives, certain nonamphetamine CNS stimulants, and certain opioid analgesics). Outpatient prescriptions can be refilled 5 times within 6 mo from date of issue if authorized by prescriber. Telephone orders are acceptable.

Schedule IV (C-IV)

Less abuse potential than Schedule III with minimal liability for physical or psychological dependence (certain sedative/hypnotics, certain antianxiety agents, some barbiturates, benzodiazepines, chloral hydrate, pentazocine, and propoxyphene). Outpatient prescriptions can be refilled 6 times within 6 mo from date of issue if authorized by prescriber. Telephone orders are acceptable.

Schedule V (C-V)

Minimal abuse potential. Number of outpatient refills determined by prescriber. Some products (cough suppressants with small amounts of codeine, antidiarrheals containing paregoric) may be available without prescription to patients >18 yr of age.

APPENDIX J

Equianalgesic Dosing Guidelines

Opioid Analgesics Starting Oral Dose Commonly Used for Severe Pain

Name	Equianalgesic Dose		Starting Oral Dose		Comments	Precautions and Contraindications
	Oral*	Parenteral†	Adults	Children		
a. Morphine-like agonists (mu agonists)						
morphine	30 mg	10 mg	15–30 mg	0.3 mg/kg	Standard of comparison for opioid analgesics. Sustained release preparations (MS Contin, OramorphSR) release over 8–12 hours. Other formulations (Kadian and Avinza) last 12–24 hours. Generic sustained release morphine preparations are now available.	For all opioids, caution in patients with impaired ventilation, bronchial asthma, increased intracranial pressure, liver failure.
hydromorphone (Dilaudid)	7.5 mg	1.5 mg	4–8 mg	0.06 mg/kg	Slightly shorter duration than morphine.	
oxycodone	20 mg	—	10–20 mg	0.3 mg/kg		
methadone	10 mg	5 mg	5–10 mg	0.2 mg/kg	Good oral potency, long plasma half-life (24–36 hours).	Accumulates with repeated dosing, requiring decreases in dose size and frequency, especially on days 2–5. Use with caution in older adults.
levorphanol (Levodromoran)	4 mg (acute) 1 mg (chronic)	2 mg (acute) 1 mg (chronic)	2–4 mg	0.04 mg/kg	Long plasma half-life (12–16 hours, but may be as long as 90–120 hrs after one week of dosing).	Accumulates on days 2 and 3. Use with caution in older adults.
oxymorphone (Opana)	10 mg	1 mg	—	—	5-mg rectal suppository ~5 mg morphine parenteral.	Like parenteral morphine.

Name	Equianalgesic Dose		Starting Oral Dose		Comments	Precautions and Contraindications
	Oral*	Parenteral†	Adults	Children		
meperidine (Demerol)	300 mg	75 mg	Not Recommended		Slightly shorter acting than morphine accumulates with repetitive dosing causing CNS excitation; avoid in children with impaired renal function or who are receiving monoamine oxidase inhibitors.‡	Use with caution. Normeperidine (toxic metabolite) accumulates with repetitive dosing causing CNS excitation and a high risk of seizure. Avoid in children, renal impairment and patients on monoamine oxidase inhibitors.‡
b. Mixed agonists–antagonists (kappa agonists)						
nalbuphine (Nubain)	—	10 mg	—	—	Not available orally, not scheduled under Controlled Substances Act.	Incidence of psychotomimetic effects lower than with pentazocine; may precipitate withdrawal in opioid-dependent patients.
butorphanol (Stadol)	—	2 mg	—	—	Like nalbuphine. Also available in nasal spray.	Like nalbuphine.
pentazocine (Talwin)	50 mg	30 mg	—	—		
c. Partial agonist						
buprenorphine (Buprenex)	—	0.4 mg	—	—	Lower abuse liability than morphine; does not produce psychotomimetic effects. Sublingual tablets now available both plain and with naloxone for opioid-dependent patient management for specially certified physicians. These tablets are not approved as analgesics.	May precipitate withdrawal in narcotic-dependent patients; not readily reversed by naloxone; avoid in labor.

*Starting dose should be lower for older adults.

†These are standard parenteral doses for acute pain in adults and can also be used to convert doses for IV infusions and repeated small IV boluses. For single IV boluses, use half the IM dose. IV doses for children >6 mos. = parenteral equianalgesic dose times weight (kg)/100.

‡Irritating to tissues with repeated IM injections. Modified from *American Pain Society, Principles of Analgesic Use in the Treatment of Acute Pain and Cancer Pain*, ed.5. American Pain Society, 2003.

Guidelines for Patient-Controlled Intravenous Opioid Administration for Adults with Acute Pain

Drug§	Usual Starting Dose After Loading	Usual Dose Range	Usual Lockout (minutes)	Usual Lockout Range (minutes)
Morphine (1 mg/mL)	1 mg	0.5–2.5 mg	8	5–10
Hydromorphone (0.2 mg/mL)	0.2 mg	0.05–0.4 mg	8	5–10
Fentanyl (50 mcg/mL)	10 mcg	10–50 mcg	6	5–8

§Standard concentrations for most PCA machines are listed in parentheses.Modified from *American Pain Society, Principles of Analgesic Use in the Treatment of Acute Pain and Cancer Pain*, ed.5. American Pain Society, 2003.

FENTANYL TRANSDERMAL DOSE BASED ON DAILY MORPHINE DOSE¶

ORAL 24-HR MORPHINE (mg/day)	IM 24-HR MORPHINE (mg/day)	FENTANYL TRANSDERMAL (mcg/hr)
60–134	10–22	25
135–224	23–37	50
225–314	38–52	75
315–404	53–67	100
405–494	68–82	125
495–584	83–97	150
585–674	98–112	175
675–764	113–127	200
765–854	128–142	225
855–944	143–157	250
945–1034	158–172	275
1035–1124	173–187	300

¶A 10-mg IM or 60-mg oral dose of morphine every 4 hr for 24 hr (total of 60 mg/day IM or 360 mg/day oral) was considered approximately equivalent to fentanyl transdermal 100 mcg/hr.

APPENDIX K

Recommendations for the Safe Handling of Hazardous Drugs*

Hazardous Drugs (HDs) have toxic, carcinogenic, mutagenic, and/or teratogenic potential, may cause irritation to the skin, eyes, and mucous membranes, and may cause ulceration and necrosis of tissue. For these obvious reasons, healthcare workers must minimize their exposure to these chemicals. The U.S. Department of Labor, Occupational Safety & Health Administration (OSHA) has laid out very specific recommendations called Guidelines for the Safe Handling of Hazardous Drugs, which can be found at http://www.osha.gov/dts/osta/otm/otm_vi/otm_vi_2.html. Refer to this document and your facility's policy and procedure manuals for detailed recommendations.

Means of Exposure

Exposure to HDs occurs during preparation and administration of these drugs or during patient care. Inhalation of aerosolized particles, accidental exposure to skin and eyes, and handling contaminated linens or equipment are the primary potential routes of exposure. Even when great care is taken, splattering, spraying, and aerosolization of HDs can occur when withdrawing the needle from a drug vial, opening an ampoule, or expelling air from a syringe. Blood, body fluids, and excreta can contain HDs and expose staff to potentially dangerous amounts of hazardous drugs.

Protecting Against Exposure

Preparation of HDs should occur in a specified area called a Biological Safety Cabinet (BSC). If a BSC is not available, the nurse or other staff member preparing an HD should wear a respirator with a high-efficiency filter and full face coverage or partial face coverage with splash goggles and a respirator. Staff should also wear protective gowns and don two sets of latex gloves. Tuck gloves in at the wrist (inner glove under cuff, outer glove over cuff).

Use aseptic technique when preparing the drug for administration and handle equipment carefully to prevent dripping, spraying or other exposure. Once prepared, wipe bags or bottles with moist gauze to remove spray or spills and swab entry ports with alcohol. Label all syringes and IV bags with a warning label and standard labeling. If being transported, the bag, bottle, or vial should be packaged in a sealed plastic bag and placed inside a secure container. Excess solution should be discarded in a covered disposable container.

Administration of HDs

Wear the same PPEs (gown, gloves, splash goggles) for administering the HD as for preparing it. Always wear a respirator when administering aerosolized drugs. In addition to wearing PPE, obtain the following equipment to use during administration: gauze for cleanup, alcohol wipes, disposable plastic-backed absorbent liner, puncture-resistant container (for needles/syringes), resealable plastic bag with warning label and other accessory warning labels.

*Controlling occupational exposure to hazardous drugs. OSHA Technical Manual. Section VI: Chapter 2. Available at http://www.osha.gov/dts/osta/otm/otm_vi_2.html. Accessed December 17, 2007.

Caring for Patients Receiving HDs

The following precautions are recommended:

- Observe standard precautions.
- Wear gown and gloves when in the patient's room for 48 hr following administration of a hazardous drug.
- Wear eye protection if splashing is possible.
- Wear a gown and gloves when handling contaminated laundry. Bag contaminated linens separately.

Managing Spills

Have spill kits available in areas where HDs are handled. The kit should include splash goggles, 2 pairs of gloves, utility gloves, gown, 2 sheets of absorbent material, spill-control pillows (2 sizes), "sharps" container, and 2 large HD disposal bags.

- Clean up spills only when properly protected and using the facility's procedure.
- Report area of spill to administrative staff.
- For small spills (less than 5 ml or 5 g), mop up liquids with absorbent gauze or use damp gauze to pick up solid contaminated material. Broken fragments should be picked up with a scoop and disposed in a sharps container. Wash the area three times with detergent followed by water.
- Isolate large spill areas and use absorbent sheets or spill-control pads. Use damp cloths if a powder is spilled. Spills greater than 150 ml (or 1 vial) require decontamination.

If Exposure Occurs

Risk of injury can be minimized by following these steps:

- Immediately remove gloves and gown.
- Immediately wash the affected skin with soap and water.
- Flood eyes at eyewash fountain or flush with water or isotonic eyewash for at least 15 min.
- Obtain medical attention and follow protocols for specific exposure.
- Document exposure.

APPENDIX L

Food Sources for Specific Nutrients

Potassium-Rich Foods

apricots
avocados
bananas
broccoli
cantaloupe
dried fruits
grapefruit
honey dew
kiwi
lima beans
meats
milk
dried peas and beans
nuts
oranges/orange juice
peaches
pears
plantains
potatoes (white and sweet)
prunes/prune juice
pumpkin
rhubarb
salt substitute
spinach
sunflower seeds
tomatoes/tomato juice
vegetable juice
winter squash

Sodium-Rich Foods

baking mixes (pancakes, muffins)
barbecue sauce
buttermilk
butter/margarine
canned chili
canned seafood
canned soups
canned spaghetti sauce
cured meats
dry onion soup mix
"fast" foods
frozen dinners
macaroni and cheese
microwave dinners
Parmesan cheese
pickles
potato salad
pretzels, potato chips
salad dressings (prepared)
salt
sauerkraut
tomato ketchup

Calcium-Rich Foods

bok choy
broccoli
canned salmon/sardines
clams
cream soups
milk and dairy products
molasses (blackstrap)
oysters
refried beans
spinach
tofu
turnip greens

Vitamin K-Rich Foods

asparagus
beans
broccoli
brussel sprouts
cabbage
cauliflower
collards
green tea
kale
milk
mustard greens
spinach
swiss chard
turnips
yogurt

Low-Sodium Foods

baked or broiled poultry
canned pumpkin
cooked turnips
egg yolk
fresh vegetables
fruit
grits (not instant)
honey
jams and jellies
lean meats
low-calorie mayonnaise
macaroons
potatoes
puffed wheat and rice
red kidney and lima beans
sherbet
unsalted nuts
whiskey

Foods That Acidify Urine

cheeses
corn
cranberries
eggs
fish
grains (breads and cereals)
lentils
meats
nuts (Brazil, filberts, walnuts)
pasta
plums
poultry
prunes
rice

Foods That Alkalinize Urine

all fruits except cranberries, prunes, plums
all vegetables (except corn)
milk
nuts (almonds, chesnuts)

Foods Containing Tyramine

aged cheeses (blue, Boursault, brick, Brie, Camembert, cheddar, Emmenthaler, Gruyère, mozzarella, Parmesan, Romano, Roquefort, Stilton, Swiss)
American processed cheese
avocados (especially over-ripe)
bananas
bean curd
beer and ale
caffeine-containing beverages (coffee, tea, colas)
caviar
chocolate
distilled spirits
fermented sausage (bologna, salami, pepperoni, summer sausage)
liver
meats prepared with tenderizer
miso soup
over-ripe fruit
peanuts
raisins
raspberries
red wine (especially Chianti)
sauerkraut
sherry
shrimp paste
smoked or pickled fish
soy sauce
vermouth
yeasts
yogurt

Iron-Rich Foods

cereals
clams
dried beans and peas
dried fruit
leafy green vegetables
lean red meats
molasses (blackstrap)
organ meats

Vitamin D-Rich Foods

canned salmon, sardines, tuna
cereals
fish
fish liver oils
fortified milk
nonfat dry milk

APPENDIX M

Insulins and Insulin Therapy

The goal of therapy for diabetic patients is to provide insulin coverage that most closely resembles endogenous insulin production and results in the best glycemic control without hypoglycemia. Although daytime control of hyperglycemia may be accomplished with bolus doses of rapid-acting insulin analogs, elevations in fasting glucose may remain a problem. If fasting blood glucose levels remain elevated, the basal insulin dose (intermediate or long-acting) may have to be adjusted.

Most insulins used today are recombinant DNA human insulins. Produced through genetic engineering, synthetic human insulin is ''manufactured'' by yeast or nonpathogenic *E. coli*. In recent years, pharmaceutical companies have developed several new types and formulations of insulin.

Different insulins are distinguished by how quickly they are absorbed, the time and length of peak activity, and overall duration of action. Onset, peak, and duration of action times are approximate and vary according to individual factors such as injection site, blood supply, concurrent illnesses, lifestyle, and exercise level. These factors can vary from patient to patient and can vary in any patient from day to day.

There are 4 kinds of insulins: rapid-acting, short-acting, intermediate-acting, and long-acting and premixed combinations.

Rapid-Acting Insulins

Rapid-acting insulins are analogs of regular insulin. An analog is a chemical structure very similar to another but differing in one component. Humalog (lispro), Apidra (glulisine) and Novolog (aspart) are rapid-acting insulin analogs. The amino acid sequences of these analogs are nearly identical to human insulin. They differ in the positioning of certain proteins, which allow them to enter the bloodstream rapidly—within 10 minutes of subcutaneous injection. This closely mimics the body's own insulin response and allows greater flexibility in eating schedules for diabetic patients. Also, because these insulins leave the bloodstream quickly, the risk of hypoglycemic episodes several hours after the meal is lessened. The peak time for rapid-acting insulins is 1–2 hours and the duration is 3–4 hours. Rapid-acting insulin solutions are clear. (An inhaled insulin (Exubera) is also rapid-acting; however, production of it stopped in October, 2007 due to lack of consumer and physician interest in the product.)

Short-Acting Insulin

Regular insulin is short-acting insulin and is available commercially as Humulin R or Novolin R. The onset of regular insulin is 0.5–1 hour; its peak activity occurs 2–3 hours after subcutaneous injection and its duration of action is 6–8 hours. This time/action profile makes rigid meal scheduling necessary, as the patient must estimate that a meal will occur within 45 minutes of injection. Short-acting insulin solutions are clear. Regular insulin is the only insulin that can be given intravenously.

Intermediate-Acting Insulins

Intermediate-acting insulin contain protamine, which delays onset, peak and duration of action to provide basal insulin coverage. Basal insulins are given to control blood glucose levels throughout the day when not eating. Commercially, intermediate-acting insulins are available as Humulin N or Novolin N. (The ''N'' stands for NPH). Action starts between 1 and 4 hours after injecting. Peak activity occurs between 6 and 12 hours. Duration of action lasts 24–28 hours. The addition of protamine causes the cloudy appearance of intermediate-acting insulins and results in the formulation being a suspension rather than a solution. This is why these insulins must be gently mixed before administering. Intermediate-acting insulins can be mixed with short or rapid-acting insulins to provide both basal and bolus coverage.

Long-Acting Insulins

Long-acting insulins have the most delayed onset and the longest duration of all insulins. Products include Lantus (insulin glargine), and Levemir (insulin detemir). Peaks are not as prominent in long-acting insulins. In fact, insulin glargine has no real peak action because it forms slowing dissolving crystals in the subcutaneous tissue. The onset of action of insulin glargine is 1 hour after subcutaneous injection. Full activity occurs within 4 to 5 hours and remains constant for 24 hours. Even though insulin glargine and insulin detemir are clear solutions, neither can be diluted or mixed with any other insulin or solution. Mixing insulin glargine or insulin detemir with other insulin products can alter the onset of action and time to peak effect. If bolus insulin is to be given at the same time as insulin glargine or insulin detemir, two separate syringes and injection sites must be used.

Combination Insulins

Various combinations of premixed insulins are available, containing fixed proportions of two different insulins, usually a short and an intermediate-acting insulin. Typically the intermediate-acting insulin makes up 70% to 75% of the mixture, with rapid- or short- acting insulin making up the remainder. Onset, peak and duration vary according to each specific product. Brand names of these products include Humulin 70/30 (70% NPH, 30% regular), Humalog Mix 75/25 (75% insulin lispro protamine suspension and 25% insulin lispro), and Novolin 70/30 (70% NPH, 30% regular), or Novolog 70/30 (70% insulin aspart protamine suspension and 20% insulin aspart).

Brand Name	Generic Name	Type of Insulin	Onset/Peak/Duration
Apidra	insulin glulisine	Rapid-acting	<15 min/1–2 hr/3–4 hr
Humalog	insulin lispro	Rapid-acting	<15 min/1–2 hr/3–4 hr
Novolog	insulin aspart	Rapid-acting	<15 min/1–2 hr/3–4 hr
Humulin R	regular insulin	Short-acting	1/2–1 hr/2–3 hr/3–6 hr
Novolin R	regular insulin	Short-acting	1/2–1 hr/2–3 hr/3–6 hr
Humulin N	NPH	Intermediate-acting	2–4 hr/4–10 hr/10–16 hr
Novolin N	NPH	Intermediate-acting	2–4 hr/4–10 hr/10–16 hr
Levemir	insulin detemir	Long-acting	minimal peak; lasts up to 24 hr
Lantus	insulin glargine	Long-acting	no peak; lasts up to 24 hr

APPENDIX N

Canadian and U.S. Pharmaceutical Practices

In the United States and Canada, most drugs are prescribed and used similarly. However, certain processes and actions of the U.S. and Canadian pharmaceutical industries differ in significant ways, affecting both consumers and health care providers. Safety, marketing, and availability are three of these issues.

Safety

Controversy related to the importation of medications from Canada by U.S. consumers has sometimes raised concerns about the safety of these drugs. These fears are unfounded; in fact, the Canadian approval and manufacturing processes are very similar to U.S. processes. Both countries have pharmaceutical-related standards, laws, and policies to ensure that chemical entities marketed for human diseases and conditions are safe and effective. The process of taking a new drug from the laboratory to the pharmacy shelves includes:

Scientific development. The process begins with research. Scientists develop a new molecular entity targeted at a specific disease, symptom, or condition.

Patenting. The manufacturer applies for a patent, which prevents other drug companies from manufacturing a chemically identical drug. Patent protection lasts 17 years in the United States and 20 years in Canada. After the patent expires, any manufacturer can make generic versions of the chemical; generics typically cost much less than the brand-name drug.

Pre-clinical testing. Before the drug is taken by human subjects, pre-clinical testing of the chemical is performed on animals. Testing helps identify drug action, toxicity effects, side effects, adverse reactions, dosage amounts and routes, and administration procedures. This phase can take 3 to 5 years.

Permission to begin clinical testing. Once the drug is found to have demonstrable positive health effects and to be safe for animals, the manufacturer applies for permission to begin clinical studies on human subjects. In the United States, this is called New Drug Application (NDA) and is administered by the Food and Drug Administration (FDA). In Canada, this is called a Clinical Trial Application (CTA) and is administered by Health Canada.

Clinical trials. Clinical trials are initiated to establish the potential benefits and risks for humans. Several sub-phases are required in the clinical trials phase whereby increasingly larger sample sizes are used.

Phase 0: A new designation for first-in-human trials, which are designed to assess whether the drug affects humans in the manner expected.

Phase I: Between 20 and 80 healthy volunteers are recruited to assess safety, tolerance, dosage ranges, pharmacokinetics, and pharmacodynamics.

Phase II: Up to 300 patients with the disease are enrolled to assess efficacy and toxicity. Variables from Phase I trials may also be assessed.

Phase III: Between 1000 and 3000 patients are entered into a randomized, double-blind study designed to confirm effectiveness, compare the new treatment with existing treatments, and study side effects further.

Phase IV: Ongoing surveillance of the drug after it receives approval and is marketed to assess for rare or long-term effects.

Approval. The results of the clinical studies are reviewed by Health Canada in Canada and by the FDA in the United States. These regulatory bodies assess every aspect of the drug, including the labeling. The approval process has been deemed excessively long by physicians and patients anxious to try new remedies for refractory or terminal diseases, and efforts have been made to shorten the process in both countries. Although approval times for new drugs were found to be significantly longer in Canada, it has been noted that significantly fewer drugs have been pulled from the market for safety reasons. Statistically, Canadians remove 2% of new drugs for safety reasons, whereas 3.6% of new drugs are taken off the market in the United States.[1]

Marketing. Once a drug has been approved, it can be prescribed to consumers or, if it does not require a prescription, purchased by them.

Post-Marketing Surveillance. More clinical data become available when the drug is marketed and used by many people for longer periods of time. Pharmacovigilance is the term used to refer to the process of ongoing assessment of a drug's safety and effectiveness during this phase.

Differences Between Canadian and U.S. Drug Pricing and Marketing

One major difference between the two countries is pricing. In Canada, the Patented Medicine Prices Review Board (PMPRB) regulates the prices manufacturers can charge for prescription and nonprescription medicines. This is to ensure that prices are not excessive. No such controls exist in the United States, which is why many citizens purchase their medications from Canadian online pharmacies. One study found that U.S. citizens can save approximately 24% if they buy their medications from Canadian pharmacies rather than from a U.S. chain pharmacy.[2]

Another difference is in advertising. In the United States, manufacturers can market drugs directly, and forcefully, to consumers, a controversial privilege that has resulted in consumers requesting specific medications despite not necessarily understanding the complete risks and benefits. In Canada, such advertising is limited and subject to the approval of the Advertising Standards Canada (ASC) agency and the Pharmaceutical Advertising Advisory Board (PAAB). To address this issue in the United States, the Institute of Medicine (IOM) has recommended that the FDA ban direct-to-consumer advertising for the first 2 years after a drug is marketed. Such a delay may help to prevent large numbers of people experiencing side effects not observed in the clinical trials, such as occurred with sildenafil (Viagra) when several patients died or developed vision problems in the first months after marketing began.

Drug Schedule, Availability, and Pregnancy Category Differences

Most Canadian provinces (with the exception of Québec) use drug schedules similar to U.S. schedules of controlled substances. Canada uses four categories, whereas the United States uses five (see for controlled substance schedules). The Canadian drug schedules are:

- **Schedule I:** Available only by prescription and provided by a pharmacist.
- **Schedule II:** Available only from a pharmacist; must be kept in an area with no public access.
- **Schedule III:** Available via open access in a pharmacy (over-the-counter).
- **Unscheduled:** Can be sold in any store without professional supervision.

Another difference is in availability. Some potentially dangerous drugs—such as heparin, insulin, and codeine-containing cough medicines—are available only with a prescription in the United States but are available over-the-counter in Canada. Similarly, some Canadian drugs are available in combinations not found in the United States (see, for new Canadian combination drugs).

Although Canada currently does not have pregnancy categories like the United States, it is developing them. Canadian prescribers practice under the premise that no drug should be given to a pregnant woman unless the benefits to the mother clearly outweigh the potential risks to the fetus. Canadian health care providers may refer to a drug's FDA pregnancy category for guidance.

SOURCES CITED

1. Rawson, N. "Canadian and U.S. Drug Approval Times and Safety Considerations." Ann Pharmacother. 37(10):1403-1408, 2003. Published Online, August 1, 2003. http://www.theannals.com. DOI 10.1345/aph.1D110 (accessed 15 December 2007).

2. Quon B., Firszt R., Eisenberg M. "A Comparison of Brand-Name Drug Prices Between Canadian-Based Internet Pharmacies and Major U.S. Drug Chain Pharmacies. Ann Intern Med. 143(6):397-403, 2005. http://www.annals.org/cgi/content/abstract/143/6/397 (accessed 10 December 2007).

ADDITIONAL REFERENCES

Canadian Pharmacists Association. "From Research Lab to Pharmacy Shelf." http://www.pharmacists.ca/content/hcp/resource_centre/drug_therapeutic_info/pdf/DrugApprovalProcess.pdf (accessed 15 December 2007).

Tomalin A. "Drugs Used in Pregnancy: The Regulatory Process." Can J Clin Pharmacol. 14(1):e5-e9, 2007. http://www.cjcp.ca/pdf/CJCP2007_e5_e9.pdf (accessed 10 December 2007).

Health Canada. http://www.hc-sc.gc.ca/ahc-asc/index_e.html (accessed 15 December 2007).

U.S. Food and Drug Administration. http://www.fda.gov (accessed 15 December 2007).

APPENDIX O

Routine Pediatric and Adult Immunizations

Immunization recommendations change frequently. For the latest recommendations see http://www.cdc.gov/nip.

ROUTINE PEDIATRIC IMMUNIZATIONS (0–18 yr)

GENERIC NAME (BRAND NAMES)	ROUTE/DOSAGE	CONTRAINDICATIONS/ PRECAUTIONS	ADVERSE REACTIONS/SIDE EFFECTS	NOTES
DTaP diphtheria toxoid, tetanus toxoid, and acellular pertussis vaccine (Daptacel, Infanrix, Tripedia)	0.5 ml IM at 2, 4, 6, and 15–18 mo; booster at 4–6 yr (4th dose in series may be given at 12 mo.)	Acute infection, immunosuppressive therapy, previous CNS damage or convulsions.	Redness, tenderness, induration at site; fever; malaise; myalgia; urticaria; hypotension; neurologic reactions; allergic reactions (all less than with DTwP).	Individual components may be given as separate injections if unusual reactions occur.
Tetanus toxoid, **reduced** diphtheria toxoid and acellularm pertussis vaccine absorbed (Tdap, Adacell, Boostrix)	0.5 ml IM to replace one dose of DTaP at from age 10 -18 (Boostrix) or 11-18 (Adacel)	Previous reactions to DTaP, l progressive neurological disease or recent (within 7 days) CNS pathology	Fatigue, headache, gastrointestinal symptoms, pain at injection site	Pertussis protection in addition to diphtheria and tetanus designed to protect against older children becoming ill with pertussis from passing it on to very young unprotected children in whom the disease has heightened morbidity.
Polio vaccine, inactivated (IPV, IPOL, Poliovax)	0.5 ml subcut at 2, 4, and 6–18 mo with a booster at 4–6 yr.	Hypersensitivity to neomycin, streptomycin, or polymyxin B; acute febrile illness.	Erythema, induration, pain at injection site; fever.	Oral polio vaccine (OPV) is no longer recommended for use in the United States.
Measles, mumps, and rubella vaccines (M-M-R II)	Single dose 0.5 ml subcut at 12–15 mo with a booster at 4–6 yr or 11–12 yr.	Allergy to egg, gelatin, or neomycin; active infection; immunosuppression.	Burning, stinging, pain at injection site; arthritis/arthralgia (40%); fever; encephalitis; allergic reactions.	If unusual reactions occur, individual components may be given as separate injections.
Hemophilus b conjugate vaccine (PedvaxHIB, ActHIB, HibTITER)*	0.5 ml IM at 2, 4, and 6 mo (6-mo dose not needed for PedvaxHIB), with a booster at 12–15 mo.	If co-administered with other immunizations, consider contraindications of all products.	Induration, erythema, tenderness at injection site; fever.	

GENERIC NAME (BRAND NAMES)	ROUTE/DOSAGE	CONTRAINDICATIONS/ PRECAUTIONS	ADVERSE REACTIONS/SIDE EFFECTS	NOTES
Hepatitis B vaccine (Engerix-B, Recombivax HB)	10 mcg IM Engerix-B or 5 mcg IM Recombivax HB 1st dose at 0–2 mo, 2nd dose at 1–4 mo, and 3rd dose at 6–18 mo (1st and 2nd dose about 1 mo apart). Dose is same for patients up to 20 yrs old. *Infants born to HBsAg-positive mothers:* Administer 0.5 ml of hepatitis B immune globulin within 12 hours of birth and 1st dose of 5 mcg Recombivax or 10 mcg of Engerix B IM and 2nd dose at 1–2 mo, 3rd dose at 6 mo. *Children up to 10 yr:* 2.5 mcg Recombivax HB or 10 mcg Engerix-B IM as 3-dose series; 2nd dose 1 mo after 1st dose, 3rd dose 4 mo after 1st dose, and 2 mo after 2nd dose. *Children up to 11–19 yr:* 5 mcg Recombivax HB or 10 mcg Engerix-B as 3-dose series; 2nd dose 1 mo after 1st dose, 3rd dose 4 mo after 1st dose, and 2 mo after 2nd dose. In children 11–15 yr, may also be given as two doses of 10 mcg/ml (Recombivax HB) 4–6 mo apart.	Hypersensitivity to yeast.	Local soreness.	Children who have not been vaccinated as infants should complete the series by 12 yr.

GENERIC NAME (BRAND NAMES)	ROUTE/DOSAGE	CONTRAINDICATIONS/ PRECAUTIONS	ADVERSE REACTIONS/SIDE EFFECTS	NOTES
Meningococcal polysaccharide diphtheria toxoid conjugate vaccine (Menactra)	0.5 ml IM single dose at 11-12 yr or before entry to high school (15 yr).	Hypersensitivity to any components	Fatigue, malaise, anorexia, pain at injection site	Goal is to decrease invasive meningococcal disease. Routine vaccination with meningococcal vaccine also is recommended for college freshmen living in dormitories and other high risk populations (military recruits, travelers to areas in which meningococcal disease prevalent); other high risk patients may elect to receive vaccine.
Varicella vaccine (Varivax)	0.5 ml IM single dose at 12-18 mo; those without a history of chickenpox should be vaccinated by the 11–12 yr visit; children around age 13 yr should receive 2 doses 1 mo apart.	Allergy to gelatin or neomycin; active infection; immunosuppression, including HIV.	Local soreness, fever.	Given to children who have not been vaccinated or have not had chickenpox. Salicylates should be avoided for 6 wk following vaccination.
Hepatitis A vaccine (Havrix, Vaqta)	*Children 2–18 yr:* 0.5 ml IM (pediatric formulation), repeated 6–12 mo later (pediatric dose form).	Acute febrile illness.	Local reactions, headache.	Recommended for children in areas with high rates of hepatitis A and other high-risk groups.
Pneumococcal 7-valent conjugate vaccine (Prevnar)	*Infants:* 0.5 ml IM for 4 doses at 2, 4, 6, and 12–15 mo. *Older infants and children starting at 7–11 mo of age:* Three doses of 0.5 ml IM, 2 doses at least 4 wk apart, 3rd dose after 1-yr birthday.	Hypersensitivity to all components including diphtheria toxoid; moderate to severe febrile illness; thrombocytopenia or coagulation disorder. Use cautiously in patients receiving anticoagulants; safe use in children <6 wk not established.	Erythema induration, tenderness, nodule formation at injection site, fever.	Antineoplastics, corticosteroids, radiation therapy, and immunosuppressants decrease antibody response; product is a suspension, shake before use.

GENERIC NAME (BRAND NAMES)	ROUTE/DOSAGE	CONTRAINDICATIONS/ PRECAUTIONS	ADVERSE REACTIONS/SIDE EFFECTS	NOTES
	Starting at 12–23 mo of age: Two doses of 0.5 ml IM at least 2 mo apart. *Starting 2–6 yr:* Single dose 0.5 ml IM.			
Influenza vaccine *injection:* (Fluarix, Fluvirin, Fluzone); *intranasal:* (FluMist)	***Injection:*** *Children 6–35 mo:* 0.25-ml IM 1–2 doses (2 doses at least one mo apart for initial season) followed by single dose annually. *Children 3–8 yr:* 0.5 ml IM 1–2 doses (2 doses at least one mo apart for initial season) followed by single dose annually. *Children ≥9 yr:* 0.5l IM single dose annually. ***Nasal (FluMist):*** *Children 5–8 yr:* If not previously immunized with FluMist—2 doses of 0.5 ml intranasally (given as one 0.25-ml dose in each nostril) at least 2 mo apart, then one dose annually. If previously immunized with FluMist, 1 dose of 0.5 ml intranasally (given as one 0.25-ml dose in each nostril) annually. *Children ≥9 yr:* 1 dose of 0.5 ml intranasally (given as one 0.25-ml dose in each nostril) annually.	Hypersensitivity to eggs/egg products. Hypersensitivity to thimerosal (injection only). Fluvirin should be used in children >4 yr only. Avoid use in patients with acute neurologic compromise. FluMist should be avoided in patients receiving salicylates or who are immunocompromised.	*Injection:* local soreness, fever myalgia, possible neurologic toxicity. *Intranasal:* upper respiratory congestion, malaise.	Immunosupression may decrease antibody response to injection and increase the risk of viral transmission with intranasal route.

*Available in varying concentrations.

Nursing Implications:

Assessment

Assess previous immunization history and history of hypersensitivity.

Assess patient for history of asthma or reactive airway disease. Patients with positive history should not receive FluMist.

Assess for history of latex allergy. Some prefilled syringes may use latex components and should be avoided in those with hypersensitivity.

Potential Nursing Diagnoses

Infection, risk for (Indications).

Knowledge, deficient, related to medication regimen (Patient/Family Teaching).

Implementation

Measles, mumps, and rubella vaccine; trivalent oral poliovirus vaccine; and diphtheria toxoid, tetanus toxoid, and pertussis vaccine may be given concomitantly.

Do not administer FluMist concurrently with other vaccines, or in patients who have received a live virus vaccine within 1 mo or an inactivated vaccine within 2 wks of vaccination.

Administer each immunization by appropriate route:

PO: Polio (Orimune)

Subcut: measles, mumps, rubella, polio (IPOL, Poliovax)

IM: diphtheria, tetanus toxoid, pertussis.

Intranasal: FluMist.

Patient/Family Teaching

Inform parent of potential and reportable side effects of immunization. Notify health care professional if patient develops fever higher than 39.4°C (103°F); difficulty breathing; hives; itching; swelling of eyes, face, or inside of nose; sudden, severe tiredness or weakness; or convulsions.

Review next scheduled immunization with parent.

Evaluation

Effectiveness of therapy can be demonstrated by: Prevention of diseases through active immunity.

ROUTINE ADULT IMMUNIZATIONS

GENERIC NAME (BRAND NAMES)	INDICATIONS	DOSAGE/ROUTE	CONTRAINDICATIONS	ADVERSE REACTIONS/SIDE EFFECTS
Hepatitis A vaccine (Havrix, Vaqta)[†]	High-risk patients, some health care workers, food handlers, clotting disorders, travel to endemic areas, chronic liver disease.	1 ml IM, followed by 1 ml IM 6–18 mo later (adult dose form).	Hypersensitivity to alum or 2-phenoxyethanol.	Local soreness, headache.
Hepatitis B vaccine (Engerix-B, Recombivax HB)	High-risk patients, health care workers, all unvaccinated adolescents.	3 doses of 1 ml IM, given at 0, 1–2, and 4–6 mo.	Anaphylactic allergy to yeast.	Local soreness.
Influenza vaccine (*Injection:* Fluzone, Fluvirin); *nasal:* (FluMist)	All adults	*Injection:* 0.5 ml IM annually. *Intranasal for adults <50 yr:* Single 0.5 ml dose given as 0.25-ml in each nostril annually.	Hypersensitivity to eggs/egg products. Hypersensitivity to thimerosal (injection only). Avoid use in patients with acute neurologic compromise. FluMist should be avoided in patients receiving salicylates or who are immunocompromised.	*Injection:* local soreness, fever myalgia, possible neurologic toxicity. *Intranasal:* upper respiratory congestion, malaise. Immunosuppression may decrease antibody response to injection and increase the risk of viral transmission with intranasal route.
Measles, mumps, and rubella vaccines (M-M-R II)	Adults with unreliable history MMR illness or immunization, occupational exposure.	0.5 ml subcut, single dose in those with unreliable history, 2 doses one mo apart for those with occupational exposure.	Allergy to egg, gelatin, or neomycin; active infection; immunosuppression; pregnancy; also avoid becoming pregnant for 4 wk after immunization.	Burning, stinging, pain at injection site; arthritis/arthralgia; fever; encephalitis; allergic reactions.
Meningococcal polysaccharide diphtheria toxoid conjugate vaccine (Menactra)	0.5 ml IM single dose at 11-12 yr or before entry to high school (15 yr).	Hypersensitivity to any components	Fatigue, malaise, anorexia, pain at injection site	Recommended for college freshmen living in dormitories and other high risk populations(military recruits, travelers to areas in which meningococcal disease prevalent); other high risk patients may elect to receive vaccine.

GENERIC NAME (BRAND NAMES)	INDICATIONS	DOSAGE/ROUTE	CONTRAINDICATIONS	ADVERSE REACTIONS/SIDE EFFECTS
Pneumococcal vaccine, polyvalent (Pneumovax 23, Pnu-Imune 23)	Everyone >65 yr, high-risk patients with chronic illnesses including HIV and other high-risk patients.	0.5 ml IM, high-risk patients (asplenics) should have a booster after 6 yr.	Safety in first trimester of pregnancy not established.	Local soreness.
Tetanus toxoid, **reduced** diphtheria toxoid and acellularm pertussis vaccine absorbed (Tdap, Adacell)	0.5 ml IM to replace one dose of DTaP	Previous reactions to DTaP, progressive neurological disease or recent (within 7 days) CNS pathology	Fatigue, headache, gastrointestinal symptoms, pain at injection site	Pertussis protection in addition to diphtheria and tetanus designed to protect against those becoming ill with pertussis from passing it on to very young unprotected children in whom the disease has heightened morbidity.
Tetanus-diphtheria (Adult Td)	All adults.	*Unimmunized:* 2 doses 0.5 ml IM 1–2 mo apart, then a 3rd dose 6–12 mo later; *immunuzed:* booster every 10 yr.	Neurologic or severe hypersensitivity reaction to prior dose.	Local pain and swelling.
Varicella vaccine (Varivax)	Any adult without a history of chickenpox or herpes zoster.	0.5 ml subcut; repeated 4–8 wk later.	Allergy to gelatin or neomycin; active infection; immunosuppression including HIV; pregnancy; family history of immunodeficiency; blood/blood product in past 5 mo.	Salicylates should be avoided for 6 wk following vaccination.

†Less commonly used vaccines are not included.

SOURCE: Adapted from the recommendations of the National Immunization Program: http://www.cdc.gov/nip.

APPENDIX P

Administering Medications to Children

General Guidelines

Medication administration to a pediatric patient can be challenging. Prescribers should order dosage forms that are age appropriate for their patients. If a child is unable to take a particular dosage form, ask the pharmacist if another form is available or for other options.

Oral Liquids

Pediatric liquid medicines may be given with plastic medicine cups, oral syringes, oral droppers, or cylindrical dosing spoons. Parents should be taught to use these calibrated devices rather than using household utensils. If a medicine comes with a particular measuring device, do not use it with another product. For young children, it is best to squirt a little of the dose at a time into the side of the cheek away from the bitter taste buds at the back of the tongue.

Eye Drops/Ointments

Tilt the child's head back and gently press the skin under the lower eyelid and pull the lower lid away slightly until a small pouch is visible. Insert the ointment or drop (1 at a time) and close the eye for a few minutes to keep the medicine in the eye.

Ear Drops

Shake otic suspensions well before administration. For children <3 yr, pull the outer ear outward and downward before instilling drops. For children ≥3 yr, pull the outer ear outward and upward. Keep child on side for 2 minutes and instill a cotton plug into ear.

Nose Drops

Clear nose of secretions prior to use. A nasal aspirator (bulb syringe) or a cotton swab may be used in infants and young children. Ask older children to blow their nose. Tilt child's head back over a pillow and squeeze dropper without touching the nostril. Keep child's head back for 2 minutes.

Suppositories

Keep refrigerated for easier administration. Wearing gloves, moisten the rounded end with water or petroleum jelly prior to insertion. Using your pinky finger for children <3 yrs and your index finger for those ≥3 yrs, insert the suppository into the rectum about ½ to 1 inch beyond the sphincter. If the suppository slides out, insert it a little farther than before. Hold the buttocks together for a few minutes and have the child hold their position for about 20 minutes, if possible.

Topicals

Clean affected area and dry well prior to application. Apply a thin layer to the skin and rub in gently. Do not apply coverings over the area unless instructed to do so by the prescriber.

Metered-Dose Inhalers

Generally the same principles apply in children as in adults, except the use of spacers is recommended for young children (see Appendix D).

APPENDIX Q

Pediatric Dosage Calculations

Most drugs in children are dosed according to body weight (mg/kg) or body surface area (BSA) (mg/m^2). Care must be taken to properly convert body weight from pounds to kilograms (1 kg = 2.2 lbs) before calculating doses based on body weight. Doses are often expressed as mg/kg/day or mg/kg/dose, therefore orders written "mg/kg/d" which is confusing, ***require further clarification from the prescriber***.

Chemotherapeutic drugs are commonly dosed according to body surface area which requires an extra verification step (BSA calculation) prior to dosing. Medications are available in multiple concentrations, therefore ***orders written in "ml" rather than "mg" are not acceptable and require further clarification.***

Dosing also varies by indication, therefore diagnostic information is helpful when calculating doses. The following examples are typically encountered when dosing medication in children.

Example 1.

Calculate the dose of amoxicillin suspension in mls for otitis media for a 1 year old child weighing 22 lbs. The dose required is 40 mg/kg/day divided BID and the suspension comes in a concentration of 400 mg/5 ml.

Step 1. Convert pounds to kg:	22 lbs x 1 kg/2.2 lbs = 10 kg
Step 2. Calculate the dose in mg:	10 kg x 40 mg/kg/day = 400 mg/day
Step 3. Divide the dose by the frequency:	400 mg/day ÷ 2 (BID) = 200 mg/dose BID
Step 4. Convert the mg dose to ml:	200 mg/dose ÷ 400 mg/5 ml = **2.5 ml BID**

Example 2.

Calculate the dose of ceftriaxone in mls for meningitis for a 5 yr old weighing 18 kg. The dose required is 100 mg/kg/day given IV once daily and the drug comes pre-diluted in a concentration of 40 mg/ml.

Step 1. Calculate the dose in mg:	18 kg x 100 mg/kg/day = 1800 mg/day
Step 2. Divide the dose by the frequency:	1800 mg/day ÷ 1 (daily) = 1800 mg/dose
Step 3. Convert the mg dose to ml:	1800 mg/dose ÷ 40 mg/ml = **45 ml once daily**

Example 3.

Calculate the dose of vincristine in mls for a 4 yr old with leukemia weighing 37 lbs and is 97 cm tall. The dose required in 2 mg/m^2 and the drug comes in 1 mg/ml concentration.

Step 1. Convert pounds to kg:	37 lbs x 1 kg/2.2 lbs = 16.8 kg
Step 2. Calculate BSA ():	16.8 kg x 97 cm/3600 = 0.67 m^2
Step 3. Calculate the dose in mg:	2 mg/m^2 x 0.67 m^2 = 1.34 mg
Step 4. Calculate the dose in ml:	1.34 mg ÷ 1 mg/ml = **1.34 mg**

Appendix R

Pediatric Fluid and Electrolyte Requirements

How to calculate maintenance fluid requirements in children:

1. **Body Surface Area Method** (commonly used in children >10 kg):

$$1500\text{–}2000 \text{ ml/m}^2\text{/day} \div 24 = \text{fluid rate in ml/hr}$$

Example: Calculate maintenance fluids in ml/hr for a child with a BSA = 0.8 m^2.

Answer: $1500 \text{ ml/m}^2\text{/day} \times 0.8 \text{ m}^2 = 1200 \text{ ml/day} \div 24 \text{ hr} = 50 \text{ ml/hr}$
$2000 \text{ ml/m}^2\text{/day} \times 0.8 \text{ m}^2 = 1600 \text{ ml/day} \div 24 \text{ hr} = 66.6 \text{ ml/hr}$

Range: 50–66.6 ml/hr.

2. **Body Weight Method**

<10 kg	100 ml/kg/day
11–20 kg	1000 ml + 50 ml/kg for each kg >10
>20 kg	1500 ml + 20 ml/kg for each kg >20

Example: Calculate maintenance fluids in ml/hr for a child weighing 25 kg.

Answer: 1500 ml + 20 ml/kg × 5 kg = 1500 ml + 100 ml = 1600 ml1600 ml ÷ 24 hr = 66.6 ml/hr

Daily Electrolyte Requirements in Children

Sodium	2–6 mEq/kg/day
Potassium	2–4 mEq/kg/day
Calcium	1–4 mEq/kg/day*
Magnesium	0.3–0.5 mEq/kg/day
Phosphorous	0.5–2 mmol/kg/day*

*Neonates may require the higher end of the calcium and phosphorous dosage range due to rapid bone development.

Conditions that May Alter Fluid Requirements in Children

Fever
Hyperventilation
Sweating
Hyperthyroidism
Renal failure
Diarrhea

Oral Rehydration Therapy (ORT)

ORT is as effective as IV therapy in managing fluid and electrolytes in children with mild to moderate dehydration due to diarrhea. Commercially available premixed ORT solutions typically contain low concentrations of glucose (2–3%), 45–75 mEq/L sodium, 20–25 mEq/L potassium, 30–35 mEq/L of citrate (bicarbonate source). Low sugar content provides little caloric support but facilitates intestinal sodium and water absorption. All commercially available ORT solutions are equally safe and effective, and are preferred over household remedies (e.g., colas, juices, chicken broth) which are not formulated based on the physiology of acute diarrhea.

BIBLIOGRAPHY

AHFS Drug Information BOOK ONLINE. Jackson, WY: Teton Data Systems, 2007. Based on: Gerald K. McEvoy, editor. AHFS Drug Information (2007). Bethesda, MD: American Society of Health-System Pharmacists, Inc.; 2007. STAT!Ref Medical Reference Library. Accessed November 1, 2007.

American Hospital Formulary Service: Drug Information 2007. American Society of Hospital Pharmacists, Bethesda, MD, 2007.

American Pain Society: Principles of Analgesic Use in the Treatment of Acute Pain and Cancer Pain, ed 5. American Pain Society, Skokie, IL, 2003.

Blumenthal, M, et al: The Complete German Commission E Monographs: Therapeutic Guide to Herbal Medicines. Integrative Medical Communications, Boston, 1998.

DRUGDEX® System [intranet database]. Version 5.1. Greenwood Village, Colo: Thomson Healthcare. Accessed November 1, 2007.

Drug Facts and Comparisons. Facts and Comparisons, a Wolters Kluwer Company, St. Louis, 2007.

Fetrow, CW and Avila, JR: Professional's Handbook of Complementary & Alternative Medicines, ed. 3. Lippincott Williams & Wilkins, Philadelphia, PA, 2004.

Health Canada Drug Product Database. Available at: http://www.hc-sc.gc.ca/dhp-mps/prodpharma/databason/index_e.html/.

IV INDEX® System [intranet database]. Version 5.1. Greenwood Village, Colo: Thomson Healthcare. Accessed August 30, 2007.

Jonas, WB, and Levin, JS (eds): Essentials of Complementary and Alternative Medicine. Lippincott Williams & Wilkins, a Wolters Kluwer Company, Baltimore and Philadelphia, 1999.

Kuhn, MA, Winston, D: Herbal Therapy and Supplements: A Scientific and Traditional Approach. Lippincott, Philadelphia, 2001

Lexi-Comp, Inc. (Lexi-Drugs [Comp + Specialties]). Lexi-Comp, Inc.; Accessed December 1, 2007.

McCaffery, M, and Pasero, C: Pain: Clinical Manual, ed 2. Mosby-Yearbook, St Louis, 1999.

National Institutes of Health Warren Grant Magnuson Clinical Center: Drug—Nutrient Interactions, Bethesda, MD, 2005. http://www.cc.nih.gov/ccc/supplements/intro.html

National Kidney Foundation: A-Z Guide for High Potassium Foods, National Kidney Foundation, 2005.

PDR for Herbal Medicines, ed 4. Thomson Healthcare, 2007.

Pennington, JAT, Douglass, JS. Bowes and Church's Food Values of Portions Commonly Used. 18th ed. Philadelphia: Lippincott Williams & Wilkins, 2004. 1–496.

Phelps, SJ, Hak, EB, Crill, CM: Pediatric Injectable Drugs, ed. 8. American Society of Health-System Pharmacists, Bethesada, 2007.

Physicians' Desk Reference (PDR). Thomson Healthcare, Montvale, NJ, 2007.

Polovich, M, White, JM, and Kelleher, LO: Chemotherapy and Biotherapy Guidelines and Recommendations for Practice, ed. 2. Oncology Nursing Society, Pittsburgh, 2005.

Taketomo CK, Hodding JH, and Kraus DM. Pediatric Dosage Handbook, 14th Edition. Lexi-Comp, 2007–2008.

Trissel, LA: Handbook on Injectable Drugs, ed 14. American Society of Hospital Pharmacists, Bethesda, 2007.

USP Dispensing Information (USP-DI): Drug Information for the Health Care Professional, Volume 1, ed 27. Micromedex, Rockville, MD, 2007.

USP Dispensing Information (USP-DI): Advice for the Patient, Volume II, ed 27. United States Pharmacopeial Convention, Greenwood Village, CO, 2007.

Van Leeuwen, A.M., Kranpitz, T, Smith, L. Davis's Comprehensive Handbook of Laboratory and Diagnostic Tests with Nursing Implications, 2nd ed. FA Davis Company, Philadelphia, PA, 2006.

http://www.accessdata.fda.gov/scripts/cder/drugsatfda/

http://www.drugstore.com. Accessed December 15, 2007.

http://www.fda.gov/cder/index.html Accessed November 1, 2007.

http://www.ons.org/news.shtml

COMPREHENSIVE INDEX*

1–Day, 184
☯2-amino-2-deoxyglucose sulfate, 1309
40 Winks, 424
✤692, 1024

A

A-200 Shampoo, 1329
abacavir, 103, 60
abarelix, 1267, 53
Abbokinase, 1164
Abelcet, 160
✤Abenol, 107
Abilify, 191, 1326
Abraxane, 935
Abreva, 441
acamprosate calcium, 1267
acarbose, 104, 39
Accolate, 1249
Accretion, 1327
Accupril, 170
Accuretic 10/12.5, 1329
Accuretic 20/12.5, 1329
Accuretic 20/25, 1329
acebutolol, 105, 29, 47, 68. *See also* Color Insert.
ACE INHIBITORS, 47. *See* **ANGIOTENSIN-CONVERTING ENZYME (ACE) INHIBITORS**
acellularm pertussis vaccine absorbed, 1383, 1389
acellular pertussis vaccine, 1383
Aceon, 170
Acephen, 107
Aceta, 107
acetaminophen, 107, 59, 88. *See also* butalbital, acetaminophen; butalbital acetaminophen, Caffeine; hydrocodone/acetaminophen; oxycodone; acetaminophen; propoxyphene napsylate/acetaminophen. *See also* Color Insert.
✤Acetazolam, 109
acetaZOLAMIDE, 109, 9, 35, 78. *See also* Color Insert.
acetoHEXAMIDE, 9. *See also* Color Insert.
✤Acid Control, 623
Aciphex, 1051
Aclovate, 357
Acta-Char Liquid-A, 1268
ActHIB, 1383
Acticin, 970
Acticort, 358
Actidose-Aqua, 1268
Actifed Cold and Allergy, 1329
Actifed Cold and Sinus, 1329
✤Actiprofen, 654
Actiq, 538
Activase, 1164
✤Activase rt-PA, 1164
activated charcoal, 1268
ACTIVE FACTOR X INHIBITORS, 34
Activella Tablets 0.5/0.1, 1329
Activella Tablets 1/0.5, 1329
Actonel, 1069, 1325
Actoplus Met 15/500, 1329
Actoplus Met 15/850, 1329
Actos, 986
Actron, 714
Acular, 1354
Acular LS, 1354
Acular Preservative Free, 1354
acyclovir, 111, 66. *See also* Color Insert.
Adacell, 1383, 1389
Adalat, 884
Adalat CC, 884
✤Adalat PA, 884
✤Adalat XL, 884
adalimumab, 114, 62
Adderall, 158
Adderall 5 mg, 1329
Adderall 7.5 mg, 1329
Adderall 10 mg, 1329
Adderall 12.5 mg, 1329
Adderall 15 mg, 1329
Adderall 20 mg, 1329
Adderall 30 mg, 1329
Adderall XR, 158
Adderall XR 5 mg, 1329
Adderall XR 10 mg, 1329
Adderall XR 15 mg, 1329
Adderall XR 20 mg, 1329
Adderall XR 25 mg, 1330
Adderall XR 30 mg, 1330
☯Ademetionine, 1314
Adenocard, 116
Adenoscan, 116
adenosine, 116, 29. *See also* Color Insert.
Adipex-P, 1288
Adoxa, 1155
Adrenalin, 480
ADRENERGICS, 47, 71
Adriamycin PFS, 454
Adriamycin RDF, 454
Adrucil, 563
Adsorbocarpine, 1352
Adsorbotear, 1351
Adult Td, 1389
Advair Diskus 100, 1330
Advair Diskus 250, 1330
Advair Diskus 500, 1330
Advair HFA 45, 1330
Advair HFA 115, 1330
Advair HFA 230, 1330
Advicor 500/20, 1330
Advicor 750/20, 1330
Advicor 1000/20, 1330
Advicor 1000/40, 1330
Advil, 654
Advil Cold & Sinus, 1330
Advil Migraine Liqui-Gels, 654
Advil Multi-Symptom Cold, 1330
Advil PM Liquigels, 1330
AeroBid, 343
Aeroseb-HC, 358
Aerospan, 343
Afeditab CR, 884
Agenerase, 1327
Aggrastat, 1185
Aggrenox, 1330
A-hydroCort, 350
Airet, 120
Akarpine, 1352
AKBeta, 1351
AK-Chlor, 1350
✤AK-Con, 1355
AK-Dex, 1352
AK-Dilate, 1355
AK-Nefrin, 1355
Akne-Mycin, 498
AK-Pentolate, 1353
AK-Pred, 1353
AK-Sulf, 1350
Akwa Tears, 1351
AK-Zol, 109
Ala-Cort, 358
Alamag, 765

*Entries for **generic** names appear in **boldface type,** tradenames appear in regular type, with Canadian tradenames preceded by a maple leaf icon (✤), **CLASSIFICATIONS** appear in **BOLDFACE SMALL CAPS,** *Combination Drugs* appear in *italics,* and herbal products are preceded by a yin-yang icon (☯).

Alamast, 1354
Ala-Scalp, 358
Alavert, 760
Alaway, 1354
Albalon, 1355
Albuminar, 118
albumin (human), 118
Albutein, 118
albuterol, 120, 30, 71
Alcaine, 1349
alclometasone, 357, 76
Alcomicin, 1350
Aldactazide 25/25, 1330
Aldactazide 50/50, 1330
Aldactone, 432
Aldara, 669
aldesleukin, 1268, 12, 53. *See also* Color Insert.
Aldomet, 804
ALDOSTERONE ANTAGONISTS, **47**
alemtuzumab, 122, 12, 52. *See also* Color Insert.
alendronate, 124, 70
Alesse, 1330
Alesse-28, 336
Aleve, 864
Aleve-D Sinus & Cold, 1330
Alfen Jr, 610
Alferon N, 688
alfuzosin, 125
Alimta, 955
Alinia, 1285
aliskiren, 126
alitretinoin, 1269, 53
alkalinizing agents, 85
Alka-Mints, 256
Alka-Seltzer Effervescent, Original, 1330
Alka-Seltzer Plus Cold & Cough Liqui-Gels, 1330
Alka-Seltzer Plus Night Cold Formula Liquid Gels, 1330
Alka-Seltzer Plus Sinus Formula, 1330
Alkeran, 781
ALKYLATING AGENTS, **52**
Allegra, 545
Allegra-D 12 Hour, 1330
Allegra-D 24 Hour, 1330
Aller-Chlor, 300
Allerdryl, 424
Allerest, 1355
Allerest Allergy and Sinus Relief Maximum Strength, 1330
Allerest Maximum Strength, 1330
Allerfrim Syrup, 1330
Allergy, 300
Allergy Drops, 1355
Allergy Medication, 424
AllerMax, 424
All-Heal, 1317
Alli, 1325
Alli sativa bulbus, 1304
Allium sativum, 1304
Alloprim, 128
allopurinol, 128. *See also* Color Insert.
Almoate, 766
almotriptan, 130, 99
Alocril, 1354
Alomide, 1354
Alora, 507
Aloxi, 941, 1327
ALPHA-ADRENERGIC BLOCKER, **1349, 99**
Alphaderm, 358
Alphagan, 1356
ALPHA-GLUCOSIDASE INHIBITORS, **39**
Alpha-Tamoxifen, 1138
alpha tocopherol, 1240
alprazolam, 131, 27. *See also* Color Insert.
Alramucil, 1035
Alrex, 1353
Altace, 170
Altamisa, 1303
Altarussin, 610
alteplase, 1164, 97
AlternaGEL, 133
Alti-Bromocriptine, 1272
Alti-MPA, 776
Altoprev, 629
Altracaine, 1349
altretamine, 1269, 12, 53. *See also* Color Insert.
Alu-Cap, 133
Alugel, 133
Aluminet, 133
aluminum hydroxide, 133, 65. *See also* magnesium hydroxide/aluminum hydroxide
Alupent, 1283
Alu-Tab, 133
Alvesco, 1325
amantadine, 135, 54, 66. *See also* Color Insert.
Amantilla, 1317
Amaryl, 648
Amber, 1316
Ambien, 1262
Ambien CR, 1262
AmBisome, 160
amcinonide, 357, 76
Amen, 776
Amerge, 866
American coneflower, 1301
American Dwarf Palm Tree, 1315
A-Methapred, 350
amethopterin, 801
Amicar, 139
amifostine, 137
Amigesic, 1087
amikacin, 140, 49. *See also* Color Insert.
Amikin, 140
amiloride, 432, 78. *See also* Color Insert.
aminocaproic acid, 139. *See also* Color Insert.
Aminofen, 107
AMINOGLYCOSIDES, 140, 49
aminolevulinic acid, 1269
Amino-Opti-E, 1240
aminophylline, 232, 71. *See also* Color Insert.
amiodarone, 145, 1326, 12, 29. *See also* Color Insert.
Amitone, 256
amitriptyline, 149, 37. *See also* Color Insert.
amlodipine, 151, 47, 73. *See also* Color Insert.
amoxapine, 1270, 37
amoxicillin, 153, 1325, 49, 65
amoxicillin/clavulanate, 155, 49
Amoxil, 153
amphetamine mixtures, 158, 74. *See also* Color Insert.
Amphetamine Salt, 158
Amphojel, 133
Amphotec, 160
amphotericin B, 160
amphotericin B cholesteryl sulfate, 160, 43. *See also* Color Insert.
amphotericin B deoxycholate, 160, 43
amphotericin B lipid complex, 160, 43
amphotericin B liposome, 43. *See also* Color Insert.
ampicillin, 164, 49. *See also* Color Insert.
ampicillin/sulbactam, 166, 49. *See also* Color Insert.
Ampicin, 164
amprenavir, 1327
Amrix, 360, 1325
Anacin, 1330
Anacin Maximum Strength, 1330
Anaflex, 1087
Anafranil, 1275
Ana-Guard, 480
anakinra, 168, 62
Anandron, 887
Anaplex DM Syrup, 1330
Anaprox, 864
Anaprox DS, 864
Anaspaz, 646
anastrazole, 169, 52
Ancalixir, 972
Ancef, 279
Androderm, 1152
Anestacon, 746
ANESTHETICS, **1349**
Anexate, 556
Anexsia, 637
Anexsia 5/325, 1330

Anexsia 5/500, 1330
Anexsia 7.5/325, 1330
Anexsia 7.5/650, 1330
Anexsia 10/750, 1330
☯Angelica sinensis, 1300
Angeliq, 1330
Angiomax, 228
ANGIOTENSIN-CONVERTING ENZYME (ACE) INHIBITORS, 170
ANGIOTENSIN II RECEPTOR ANTAGONISTS, 177, 47
anidulafungin, 180, 43. *See also* Color Insert.
Ansaid, 1279
Antabuse, 1278
ANTACIDS, 65
Antara, 532
ANTHRACYCLINES, 52
ANTI-ALZHEIMER'S AGENTS, 23
ANTIANDROGENS, 52
ANTIANEMICS, 24
ANTIANGINALS, 25
ANTIANXIETY AGENTS, 26
ANTIARRHYTHMICS, 28
CLASS IA, 29
CLASS IB, 29
CLASS IC, 29
CLASS II, 29
CLASS III, 29
CLASS IV, 29
ANTIASTHMATICS, 29
ANTICHOLINERGICS, 31, 54, 71
ANTICOAGULANTS, 15, 32
ANTICONVULSANTS, 34
ANTIDEPRESSANTS, 36
ANTIDIABETICS, 38
ANTIDIARRHEALS, 40
ANTIEMETICS, 41
Antiepileptic drugs, 1326
ANTIESTROGENS, 52
Antiflex, 915
ANTIFUNGALS, 1351, 1389, 42
TOPICAL, 181
VAGINAL, 184
ANTIHISTAMINES, 1349, 44
OPHTHALMIC, 45
ANTIHYPERTENSIVES, 15, 45
ANTI-INFECTIVES, 1349, 47
ANTIMETABOLITES, 52
Antinaus, 1017
ANTINEOPLASTICS, 50
ANTIPARKINSON AGENTS, 53
ANTIPLATELET AGENTS, 54
ANTIPSYCHOTICS, 56
ANTIPYRETICS, 58
ANTIRETROVIRALS, 15, 59
ANTIRHEUMATICS, 61
ANTITHROMBOTICS, 34
ANTITUBERCULARS, 62
ANTITUMOR ANTIBIOTICS, 52
ANTIULCER AGENTS, 63
Antivert, 775
ANTIVIRALS, 1349, 1351, 54, 65
Antizol, 1325
Antrizine, 775
Anusol HC, 358
Anzemet, 445
Apacet, 107
APAP, 107
Apidra, 670, 1380
🍁Apo-Acetaminophen, 107
🍁Apo-Acetazolamide, 109
🍁Apo-Allopurinol, 128
🍁Apo-Alpraz, 131
🍁Apo-Amiloride, 432
🍁Apo-Amitriptyline, 149
🍁Apo-Amoxi, 153
🍁Apo-Ampi, 164
🍁Apo-ASA, 1087
🍁Apo-ASEN, 1087
🍁Apo-Atenolol, 197
🍁Apo-Benztropine, 218
🍁Apo-Bromocriptine, 1272
🍁Apo-C, 1271
🍁Apo-Cal, 256
🍁Apo-Carbamazepine, 263
🍁Apo-Cephalex, 279
🍁Apo-Chlordiazepoxide, 298
🍁Apo-Chlorthalidone, 434
🍁Apo-Cimetidine, 623
🍁Apo-Ciproflox, 557
🍁Apo-Clorazepate, 325
🍁Apo-Cloxi, 961
🍁Apo-Cromolyn, 773
🍁Apo-Diazepam, 404
🍁Apo-Diclo, 408
🍁Apo–Diclo Rapide, 408
🍁Apo-Diltiaz, 418
🍁Apo-Dimenhydrinate, 420
🍁Apo-Dipyridamole, 428
🍁Apo-Divalproex, 1212
🍁Apo-Doxy, 1155
🍁Apo-Erythro-EC, 498
🍁Apo-Erythro-ES, 498
🍁Apo-Famotidine, 623
🍁Apo-Ferrous Gluconate, 700
🍁Apo-Ferrous Sulfate, 700
🍁Apo-Fluphenazine, 568
🍁Apo-Flurazepam, 571
🍁Apo-Flurbiprofen, 1279
🍁Apo-Folic, 574
🍁Apo-Furosemide, 587
🍁Apo-Glimepiride, 648
🍁Apo-Glyburide, 648
🍁Apo-Haloperidol, 613
🍁Apo-Hydro, 434
🍁Apo-Hydroxyzine, 644
🍁Apo-Ibuprofen, 654
🍁Apo-Imipramine, 666
🍁Apo-Indomethacin, 674
🍁Apo-ISDN, 707
🍁Apo-ISMN, 707
🍁Apo-K, 996
🍁Apo-Keto, 714
🍁Apo-Keto-E, 714
Apokyn, 186
🍁Apo-Lorazepam, 762
🍁Apo-Meprobamate, 1282
🍁Apo-Methyldopa, 804
🍁Apo-Metoclop, 810
🍁Apo-Metronidazole, 817
🍁Apo-Minocycline, 1155
apomorphine, 186, 54
🍁Apo-Napro-Na, 864
Apo-Napro-Na DS, 864
🍁Apo-Naproxen, 864
🍁Apo-Nifed, 884
🍁Apo-Nitrofurantoin, 890
🍁Apo-Nizatidine, 623
🍁Apo-Norfloxacin, 557
🍁Apo-Ofloxacin, 558
🍁Apo-Oxazepam, 921
🍁Apo-Pen VK, 958
🍁Apo-Piroxicam, 989
🍁Apo-Propranolol, 1026
🍁Apo-Quin-G, 1045
🍁Apo-Quinidine, 1045
Apo-Ranitidine, 623
🍁Apo-Salvent, 120
Apo-Selegiline, 1098
🍁Apo-Sulfatrim, 1205
🍁Apo-Sulfatrim DS, 1205
🍁Apo-Sulin, 1128
🍁Apo-Theo LA, 232
🍁Apo-Thioridazine, 1162
🍁Apo-Timol, 1179
🍁Apo-Timop, 1352
🍁Apo-Triazo, 1202
🍁Apo-Trifluoperazine, 1295
🍁Apo-Trihex, 1295
🍁Apo-Valproic, 1212
Apo-Verap, 1224
🍁Apo-Zidovudine, 1253
apraclonidine, 1356
aprepitant, 187, 42
Apresoline, 633
Apri, 1330

*Entries for **generic** names appear in **boldface type,** tradenames appear in regular type, with Canadian tradenames preceded by a maple leaf icon (🍁), **CLASSIFICATIONS** appear in **BOLDFACE SMALL CAPS**, *Combination Drugs* appear in *italics,* and herbal products are preceded by a yin-yang icon (☯).

Apri 28, 336
aprotinin, 1327
Aptivus, 1183
Aquachloral, 296
AquaMEPHYTON, 982
Aquasite, 1351
Aquasol E, 1240
🍁Aqueous Charcodote, 1268
Ara-C, 368
Aranelle, 337, 1330
Aranesp, 377
Arava, 731
Aredia, 942
Arestin, 1155
argatroban, 189, 34
Aricept, 447
Aricept ODT, 447
Arimidex, 169
aripiprazole, 191, 1326, 58
Aristospan, 350
Arixtra, 575
Armour thyroid, 1169
☯arnica, 1297
AROMATASE INHIBITORS, **52**
arsenic trioxide, 1270, 12, 53. *See also* Color Insert.
Artane, 1295
🍁Arthrinol, 1087
🍁Arthrisin, 1087
Arthropan, 1087
Arthrotec 50/200, 1331
Arthrotec 75/200, 1331
Artifical Tears Plus, 1351
ARTIFICIAL TEARS/OCULAR LUBRICANTS, **1351**
🍁Artria S.R, 1087
ASA, 1087
Asacol, 789
🍁Asaphen, 1087
ascorbic acid, 1271, 100
Ascorbicap, 1271
Ascriptin, 1087
Ascriptin A/D, 1331
Asendin, 1270
☯Asian ginseng, 1308
Asmanex, 343, 1326
asparaginase, 193, 12, 52. *See also* Color Insert.
A-Spas S/L, 646
Aspercin, 1087
Aspergum, 1087
aspirin, 1087, 59, 88. *See also* butalbital, aspirin, caffeine; hydrocodone/aspirin; oxycodone/aspirin; propxyphene napsylate/aspirin; propoxyphene/aspirin/caffeine
Aspirin Free Anacin, 107
Aspirin Free Pain Relief, 107
Aspirtab, 1087
AsthmaHaler Mist, 480
AsthmaNefrin (racepinephrine), 480
Astramorph, 843
Astramorph PF, 843
🍁Astrin, 1087
Atacand, 177
Atacand HCT 16/12.5, 1331
Atacand HCT 32/12.5, 1331
🍁*Atacand Plus, 1331*
Atarax, 644
atazanavir, 195, 1325, 60
atenolol, 197, 26, 47, 68. *See also* Color Insert.
Ativan, 762
atomoxetine, 200
atorvastatin, 629, 84
atovaquone, 201
Atripla, 1331
Atropair, 1353
AtroPen, 202
atropine, 202, 1353, 29, 32. *See also* difenoxin/atropine; diphenoxylate/atopine; Isopto Atropine. *See also* Color Insert.
Atropisol, 1353
Atrosulf, 1353
Atrovent HFA, 696
A/T/S, 498
☯aubepine, 1310
Augmentin, 155
Augmentin 125 Chewable, 1331
Augmentin 125 mg Suspension, 1331
Augmentin 200 Chewable, 1331
Augmentin 200 mg Suspension, 1331
Augmentin 250, 1331
Augmentin 250 Chewable, 1331
Augmentin 250 mg Suspension, 1331
Augmentin 400 Chewable, 1331
Augmentin 400 mg Suspension, 1331
Augmentin 500, 1331
Augmentin 875, 1331
Augmentin ES, 155
Augmentin XR, 155
Avalide 150/12.5, 1331
Avalide 300/12.5, 1331
Avandamet 2/500, 1331
Avandamet 2/1000, 1331
Avandamet 4/500, 1331
Avandamet 4/1000, 1331
Avandaryl 4/1, 1331
Avandaryl 4/2, 1331
Avandaryl 4/4, 1331
Avandaryl 8/2, 1331
Avandaryl 8/4, 1331
Avandia, 1082
☯Ava pepper, 1312
Avapro, 177
Avastin, 221, 1326
Avelox, 557, 1326
Aventyl, 897
Aviane, 1331
Aviane-28, 336
Avinza, 843
🍁Avirax, 111
Avodart, 466
Avonex, 692
Axert, 130
Axid, 623
Axid AR, 623
Axocet, 247
🍁Axsam, 261
azacitidine, 204, 53
Azasan, 206
AzaSite, 1325, 1349
azatadine, 45
azathioprine, 206, 81
Azdone, 637, 1331
azelastine, 1349, 45
azidothymidine, 1253
Azilect, 1055
azithioprine, 13. *See also* Color Insert.
azithromycin, 208, 1325–1326, 1349, 49. *See also* Color Insert.
Azmacort, 343, 1327
Azopt, 1352
Azor 5/20, 1331
Azor 5/40, 1331
Azor 10/20, 1331
Azor 10/40, 1331
Azo-Standard, 971
AZT, 1253
Azulfidine, 1126
Azulfidine EN-tabs, 1126

B

B & O Supprettes No. 15A, 1331
B & O Supprettes No. 16A, 1331
BabyBIG, 1272
☯Bachelor's Button, 1303
baclofen, 213, 95
Bactine, 358
Bactocill, 961
Bactrim, 1205, 1331
Bactrim DS, 1205, 1331
Bactroban, 847
Bactroban Nasal, 847
☯Bai guo ye, 1306
Baking Soda, 1114
☯Baldrian, 1317
☯Baldrianwurzel, 1317
🍁Balminil Decongestant Syrup, 1033
🍁Balminil DM, 403
balsalazide, 214
Balziva, 336, 1331
☯baneberry, 1298
Banflex, 915
Banobese, 1288
Banophen, 424
Baraclude, 476
BARBITURATES, **35, 93**
Baridium, 971

🍁Barriere-HC, 358
Basalgel, 133
basiliximab, 215, 81
Bayer Aspirin, 1087
Bayer Back & Body, 1331
Bayer PM, 1331
Bayer Select Maximum Strength Menstrual, 1331
Bayer Women's Aspirin plus Calcium, 1332
BCNU, 269
becaplermin, 1271
beclomethasone, 343, 347, 31, 76
Beconase AQ, 347
Beesix, 1039
☯Belgium Valerian, 1317
Bell-Ans, 1114
🍁Beloc, 814
🍁Beloc-ZOK, 814
Benadryl, 424
Benadryl Allergy & Sinus Headache Caplets, 1332
Benadryl Allergy, 424
Benadryl-D Allergy & Sinus Tablets, 1332
Benadryl Dye-Free Alergy, 424
benazepril, 170, 47. *See also* Color Insert.
Benicar, 177
Benicar HCT 20/12.5, 1332
Benicar HCT 40/12.5, 1332
Benicar HCT 40/25, 1332
Bentyl, 410
🍁Bentylol, 410
🍁Benuryl, 1006
Benylin Adult, 403
🍁Benylin-E, 610
Benylin Pediatric, 403
BenzaClin Topical Gel, 1332
Benzamycin Topical Gel, 1332
benzathine penicillin G, 958, 49
BENZODIAZEPINES, 27, 35, 93
benzonatate, 217
benztropine, 218, 32, 54
BETA BLOCKERS, 1351, 26, 67, 99
NONSELECTIVE, 47, 68
OPHTHALMIC, 68
SELECTIVE, 47, 68
🍁Betachron E-R, 1026
🍁Betacort, 357
🍁Betaderm, 357
Betagan, 1351
🍁Betaloc Durules, 814
🍁Betaloc-ZOK, 814
betamethasone, 350, 357, 31, 62, 76
Betapace, 1122
Betapace AF, 1122
Betaseron, 692
Beta-Val, 357
🍁Betaxin, 1160
betaxolol, 219, 1351, 47, 68
Betaxon, 1351
bethanechol, 1271
Betimol, 1352
🍁Betnelan, 350
🍁Betnesol, 350
🍁Betnovate, 357
Betoptic, 1351
Betoptic S, 1351
bevacizumab, 221, 1326, 53
🍁Bewon, 1160
Biamine, 1160
Biaxin, 315
Biaxin XL, 315
bicalutamide, 222, 52
Bicillin L-A, 958
Bicitra, 1118
Bicitra Solution, 1332
BiCNU, 269
BiDil, 635, 1332
BIGUANIDES, 39
BILE ACID SEQUESTRANTS, 84
bimatoprost, 1355
BioCal, 256
🍁Bio-Hydrochlorothiazide, 434
biperiden, 32, 54
BIPHOSPHONATES, 70
Bisac-Evac, 223
bisacodyl, 223, 83. *See also* Color Insert.
🍁Bisaco-Lax, 223
🍁Bisacolax, 223
Bismatrol, 225
Bismed, 225
bismuth subsalicylate, 225, 41, 65
bisoprolol, 226, 47, 68. *See also* Color Insert.
bivalirudin, 228, 34
☯black cohosh, 1298
Black-Draught, 1101
☯black sampson, 1301
☯black snakeroot, 1298
☯black susans, 1301
Blenoxane, 230
bleomycin, 230, 12, 52. *See also* Color Insert.
Bleph, 1350
Blephamide Ophthalmic Suspension/Ointment, 1332
Blocadren, 1179
🍁Bonamine, 775
BONE RESORPTION INHIBITORS, 69
Bonine, 775
Boniva, 653
Boostrix, 1383
botulism immune globulin, 1272, 98
☯brauneria angustifolia, 1301
Breonesin, 610
Brethaire, 1148
Brevibloc, 502
Brevicon, 336, 1332
Bricanyl, 1148
brimonidine, 1356
brinzolamide, 1352
Bromfed DM Liquid, 1332
Bromfenac, 1273, 1354, 90
Bromfenex, 1332
Bromfenex PD, 1332
bromocriptine, 1272, 54. *See also* Color Insert.
brompheniramine, 1273, 45
BRONCHODILATORS, 30, 70
BRONCHODILATORS (XANTHINES), 232
🍁Broncho-Grippol-DM, 403
Bronkaid Dual Action, 1332
Brontex, 1332
Bucet, Bupap, 247
budesonide, 343, 347, 350, 31, 76
Bufferin, 1087, 1332
☯bugbane, 1298
BULK-FORMING AGENTS, 83
Bulk Forming Fiber Laxative, 1289
bumetanide, 236, 78. *See also* Color Insert.
Bumex, 236
Buminate, 118
bupivacaine, 478
Buprenex, 238, 1373
buprenorphine, 238, 1373, 12, 92. *See also* Color Insert.
buPROPion, 241, 9, 37. *See also* Color Insert.
🍁Burinex, 236
BuSpar, 243
busPIRone, 243, 9, 27. *See also* Color Insert.
busulfan, 245, 12, 52. *See also* Color Insert.
Busulfex, 245

*Entries for **generic** names appear in **boldface type,** tradenames appear in regular type, with Canadian tradenames preceded by a maple leaf icon (🍁), **CLASSIFICATIONS** appear in **BOLDFACE SMALL CAPS**, *Combination Drugs* appear in *italics,* and herbal products are preceded by a yin-yang icon (☯).

BUTALBITAL COMPOUND, 247, 88
Butapap 50/325, 1332
Butapap 50/650, 1332
butenafine, 181, 43
Butex Forte, 247
butoconazole, 184, 43
butorphanol, 249, 1373, 12, 92. *See also* Color Insert.
Byetta, 525
Bystolic, 1323

C

☯Cabbage Palm, 1315
cabergoline, 253
Ca-DTPA, 1286
Caduet 2.5/10, 1332
Caduet 2.5/20, 1332
Caduet 2.5/40, 1332
Caduet 5/10, 1332
Caduet 5/20, 1332
Caduet 5/40, 1332
Caduet 5/80, 1332
Caduet 10/10, 1332
Caduet 10/20, 1332
Caduet 10/40, 1332
Caduet 10/80, 1332
Cafergot, 1332
Calan, 1224
Calan SR, 1224
Calcarb, 256
Calci-Chew, 256
Calciday, 256
Calcijex, 1236
Calcilac, 256
🍁Calcilean, 616
Calci-Mix, 256
🍁Calciparine, 616
🍁Calcite, 256
CALCITONIN, 254
rDNA, 254
salmon, 254, 79
Cal-Citrate 250, 256
calcitriol, 1236, 100. *See also* Color Insert.
calcium acetate, 256, 85
calcium carbonate, 256, 85
CALCIUM CHANNEL BLOCKERS, 26, 47, 71
calcium chloride, 256, 85. *See also* Color Insert.
calcium citrate, 256, 85
calcium gluconate, 256, 85. *See also* Color Insert.
calcium lactate, 256, 85
CALCIUM SALTS, 256, 12, 85. *See also* Color Insert.
CaldeCORT Anti-Itch, 358
🍁Calglycine, 256
☯Calicut, 1305
Cal-Lac, 256
Calm X, 420
🍁Calmylin #1, 403
🍁Calmylin Expectorant, 610
Calphron, 256
Cal-Plus, 256
🍁Calsan, 256
Caltrate, 256
Caltrate 600+D, 1332
Camila, 337
Campath, 122
Campral, 1267
Camptosar, 698
Canasa, 789
Cancidas, 273
candesartan, 177, 47. *See also* Color Insert.
🍁Canesten, 181, 184
capecitabine, 259, 12, 52. *See also* Color Insert.
Capoten, 170
Capozide 25/15, 1332
Capozide 25/25, 1332
Capozide 50/15, 1332
Capozide 50/25, 1332
capsaicin, 261, 88
Capsin, 261
captopril, 170, 47. *See also* Color Insert.
Capzasin-P, 261
Carafate, 1124
carbachol, 1352
Carbacot, 799
carbamazepine, 263, 1326, 35. *See also* Color Insert.
CARBAPENEMS, 49
Carbatrol, 263
Carbex, 1098
carbidopa/levodopa, 743, 54. *See also* Color Insert.
🍁Carbolith, 754
CARBONIC ANHYDRASE INHIBITORS, 1352, 78
carbonyl iron, 700, 25
carboplatin, 265, 12, 52. *See also* Color Insert.
Carboptic, 1352
Cardec DM Syrup, 1332
Cardene, 879
Cardene IV, 879
Cardene SR, 879
Cardiazem CD, 418
Cardizem, 418
Cardizem LA, 418
Cardizem SR, 418
Cardura, 450
carisoprodol, 268, 95. *See also* Color Insert.
Carmol HC, 358
carmustine, 269, 12, 52. *See also* Color Insert.
Caroid, 223
carteolol, 1273, 26, 47, 68
Carter's Little Pills, 223
Cartia XT, 418
Cartrol, 1273
carvedilol, 271, 47, 68. *See also* Color Insert.
Casodex, 222
caspofungin, 273, 43
Cataflam, 408
Catapres, 321
Catapres-TTS, 321
CATECHOL-O-METHYLTRANSFERASE INHIBITORS, 54
Cathflo Activase, 1164
CCR5 CO-RECEPTOR ANTAGONISTS, 60
☯CDS, 1299
Cebid, 1271
🍁Ceclor, 282
Cecon, 1271
Cecore-500, 1271
Cedax, 287
🍁Cedocard-SR, 707
cefaclor, 282, 49
cefadroxil, 279, 49
cefamandol, 1327
cefazolin, 279, 49. *See also* Color Insert.
cefdinir, 286, 49
cefditoren, 287, 49
cefepime, 275, 49. *See also* Color Insert.
cefixime, 287, 49
Cefizox, 287
Cefobid, 287
cefoperazone, 287, 49. *See also* Color Insert.
Cefotan, 282
cefotaxime, 287, 49. *See also* Color Insert.
cefotetan, 282, 49. *See also* Color Insert.
cefoxitin, 282, 49. *See also* Color Insert.
cefpodoxime, 287, 49
cefprozil, 282, 49
ceftazidime, 287, 49. *See also* Color Insert.
ceftibuten, 287, 49
Ceftin, 282
ceftizoxime, 287, 49. *See also* Color Insert.
ceftriaxone, 287, 49. *See also* Color Insert.
cefuroxime, 282, 49. *See also* Color Insert.
Cefzil, 282
Celebrex, 278, 1326
celecoxib, 278, 1326, 62, 89
🍁Celestoderm, 357
Celestone, 350
Celexa, 313
CellCept, 850
Cellufresh, 1351
Celluvisc, 1351
Cemill, 1271
Cenafed, 1033

Cena-K, 996
Cenestin, 510
Cenolate, 1271
CENTRALLY ACTING ANTIADRENERGICS, 47
CENTRAL NERVOUS SYSTEM STIMULANTS, 73
cephalexin, 279, 49
CEPHALOSPORINS
FIRST GENERATION, 279, 49
SECOND GENERATION, 282, 49
THIRD GENERATION, 286, 49
cephradine, 279, 49
Cephulac, 721
Cerebyx, 583, 1325
Cerubidine, 385
Cervidil Vaginal Insert, 422
(maple leaf) C.E.S, 510
Cesia, 336
Cetacaine Topical Spray, 1332
Cetacort, 358
Cetane, 1271
cetirizine, 293, 45
cetuximab, 294, 53
Cevalin, 1271
Cevi-Bid, 1271
cevimeline, 1274
Chantix, 1219, 1327
(maple leaf) Charac-50, 1268
CharcoAid 2000, 1268
(maple leaf) Charcodote, 1268
Chemet, 1292
Cheracol Cough Syrup, 1332
Chibroxin, 1350
Children's Advil, 654
Children's Advil Cold Liquid, 1332
Children's Hold, 403
Children's Loratidine, 760
Children's Motrin, 654
Children's Pain Reliever, 107
(yin-yang) Chinese Angelica, 1300
(yin-yang) Chinese ginseng, 1308
(yin-yang) chitosamine, 1309
Chlo-Amine, 300
chloral hydrate, 296, 12, 93. *See also* Color Insert.
chlorambucil, 1274, 12, 52, 81. *See also* Color Insert.
chloramphenicol, 1350
Chlorate, 300
chlordiazepoxide, 298, 27, 93. *See also* Color Insert.
Chlorofair, 1350
Chloromag, 766
Chloroptic, 1350
chlorothiazide, 434, 47, 78
chlorpheniramine, 300, 45. *See also* Color Insert.
(maple leaf) Chlorpromanyl, 301
chlorproMAZINE, 301, 13, 42, 58. *See also* Color Insert.
chlorthalidone (thiazide–like), 434, 47, 78
Chlor-Trimeton, 300
Chlor-Trimeton 4 Hour Relief, 1333
Chlor-Trimeton 12 Hour Relief, 1333
Chlor-Trimeton Allergy 4 Hour, 300
Chlor-Trimeton Allergy 8 Hour, 300
Chlor-Trimeton Allergy 12 Hour, 300
(maple leaf) Chlor-Tripolon, 300
chlorzoxazone, 305, 95. *See also* Color Insert.
Cholac, 721
cholecalciferol, 1236
cholestyramine, 306, 84
choline and magnesium salicylates, 1087, 59, 88
CHOLINERGICS
CHOLINESTERASE INHIBITORS, 1352
DIRECT-ACTING, 1352
choline salicylate, 1087, 59, 88
(yin-yang) chondroitin, 1299
(yin-yang) chondroitin polysulfate, 1299
Chooz, 256
Chronulac, 721
(yin-yang) Chrysanthemum parethenium, 1303
Cialis, 1137, 1327
ciclesonide, 347, 1325
ciclopirox, 181, 43
ciclosonide, 1326
cidofovir, 308, 66
(maple leaf) Cidomycin, 140
Cillium, 1035
cilostazol, 309, 1326, 55
Ciloxan, 1350
cimetidine, 623, 1325, 15, 65. *See also* Color Insert.
cinacalcet, 1274
Cipro, 557
Ciprodex Otic Suspension, 1333
ciprofloxacin, 557, 1350, 49. *See also* Color Insert.
Cipro HC Otic Suspension, 1333
Cipro XR, 557
cisplatin, 310, 12, 52. *See also* Color Insert.
citalopram, 313, 37. *See also* Color Insert.
Citrate of Magnesia, 766
Citrical, 256
Citrical Liquitab, 256
Citrocarbonate, 1114
Citroma, 766
(maple leaf) Citromag, 766
citrovorum factor, 736
Claforan, 287
Clarinex, 395
Clarinex-D 12 Hour, 1333
Clarinex-D 24 Hour, 1333
clarithromycin, 315, 49, 65
Claritin, 760
Claritin 24–Hour Allergy, 760
Claritin-D 12 Hour, 1333
Claritin-D 24-Hour, 1333
Claritin Hives Relief, 760
Claritin Reditabs, 760
(maple leaf) Clavulin, 155
(maple leaf) *Clavulin 125 Suspension, 1333*
(maple leaf) *Clavulin 200 Suspension, 1333*
(maple leaf) *Clavulin 250 Suspension, 1333*
(maple leaf) *Clavulin 400 Suspension, 1333*
(maple leaf) *Clavulin 500, 1333*
(maple leaf) *Clavulin 875, 1333*
Clear-Atadine, 760
Clear Eyes Lubricating Eye Redness Reliever, 1355
Cleocin, 317
Cleocin T, 317
Climara, 507
ClimaraPro Transdermal Patch (release per day, 1333
Clinagen LA, 507
Clinda-Derm, 317
Clindagel, 317
ClindaMax, 317
clindamycin, 317, 49. *See also* Color Insert.
Clindesse, 317
Clindets, 317
Clinoril, 1128
clobetasol, 357, 76
Clobex, 357
clocortolone, 357, 76
Cloderm, 357
clofarabine, 1275, 52
Clolar, 1275
clomiPRAMINE, 1275. *See also* Color Insert.
Clomycin Topical Ointment, 1333

*Entries for **generic** names appear in **boldface type,** tradenames appear in regular type, with Canadian tradenames preceded by a maple leaf icon (maple leaf), **CLASSIFICATIONS** appear in **BOLDFACE SMALL CAPS,** *Combination Drugs* appear in *italics,* and herbal products are preceded by a yin-yang icon (yin-yang).

COMPREHENSIVE INDEX

clonazepam, 320, 35. *See also* Color Insert.
clonidine, 321, 47. *See also* Color Insert.
clopidogrel, 324, 55
Clopra, 810
Clorachol, 1350
clorazepate, 325, 35, 93. *See also* Color Insert.
Clorpres 15/0.1, 1333
Clorpres 15/0.2, 1333
Clorpres 15/0.3, 1333
🍁Clotrimaderm, 181, 184
clotrimazole, 181, 184, 43
cloxacillin, 961, 49
Cloxapen, 961
clozapine, 327, 58. *See also* Color Insert.
Clozaril, 327
CMT, 1087
CMVIG, 1276
☯cochin, 1305
codeine, 330, 12, 92. *See also* Color Insert.
Codiclear DH Syrup, 1333
Codimal, 1333
Codimal DH Syrup, 1333
Codimal DM Syrup, 1333
Codimal-L.A., 1333
Codimal PH Syrup, 1333
Cofatrim, 1205
Cogentin, 218
Co-Gesic, 637, 1333
🍁Co-Glimepiride, 648
Cognex, 1133
Colace, 442
Colazal, 214
colchicine, 332, 12. *See also* Color Insert.
colesevelam, 333, 1326, 84
Colestid, 334
colestipol, 334, 84
Collyrium Fresh, 1355
Colovage, 992
Col-Probenecid, 1333
Coly-Mycin S Otic Suspension, 1333
Colyte, 992
Combigan Ophthalmic Solution, 1333
CombiPatch 0.05/0.14, 1333
CombiPatch 0.05/0.25, 1333
Combivent, 1333
Combivir, 1333
Combunox, 1333
Comfort Eye Drops, 1355
Comfort Tears, 1351
Commit, 881
☯Common Valerian, 1317
Compazine, 1012, 13
Compoz, 424
Compoz Nighttime Sleep Aid, 424
Comtan, 475
Comtrex Deep Chest Cold Caplets, 1333
Comtrex Maximum Strength Non-Drowsy Caplets, 1333
concentrated regular insulin, 40
Concerta, 808
🍁Congest, 510
Congestac, 1333
Congestaid, 1033
🍁Co-Norfloxacin, 557
Constilac, 721
Constulose, 721
Contac Cold & Flu Maximum Strength Caplets, 1334
Contac Cold & Flu Non-Drowsy Maximum Strength Caplets, 1334
CONTRACEPTIVES, HORMONAL, 336, 80
Copegus, 1062
Cordarone, 145, 1326
Cordran, 358
Cordran-SP, 358
Coreg, 271
Coreg CR, 271
Corgard, 856
Coricidin HBP Chest Congestion and Cough, 1334
Coricidin HBP Cold and Flu, 1334
Coricidin HBP Cough and Cold, 1334
Coricidin HBP Maximum Strength Flu, 1334
Corlopam, 534
Cormax, 357
🍁Coronex, 707
Correctol Stool Softener, Soft Gels, 442
🍁Cortacet, 358
Cortaid, 358
🍁Cortate, 358
Cort-Dome, 358
Cortef, 350
🍁Cortef Feminine Itch, 358
Corticaine, 358
CORTICOSTEROIDS, **1352, 31, 62, 74**
INHALATION, 343, 76
NASAL, 347, 76
SYSTEMIC, 350, 76
TOPICAL/LOCAL, 357, 76
🍁Corticreme, 358
Cortifair, 358
Cortifoam, 358
cortisone, 350, 31, 62, 76
Cortisporin Ophthalmic Suspension/Otic (Solution/Suspension), 1334
Cortisporin Topical Cream, 1334
Cortisporin Topical Ointment, 1334
Cortizone, 358
🍁Cortone, 350
Corvert, 657
🍁Coryphen, 1087
Corzide 40/5, 1334
Corzide 80/5, 1334
Cosopt Ophthalmic Solution, 1334
Cotazym, 943
🍁Cotazym-65 B, 943
Cotazym E.C.S. 8, 943
Cotazym E.C.S. 20, 943
Cotazym-S, 943
Cotrim, 1205
Cotrim DS, 1205
Coumadin, 1245
COUMARINS, **34**
Covera-HS, 1224
🍁Coversyl, 170
🍁*Coversyl Plus, 1334*
🍁*Coversyl Plus LD, 1334*
Cozaar, 177
☯CPS, 1299
Creon 5, 1334
Creon 10, 943, 1334
Creon 20, 1334
Creon 25, 943
Creo-Terpin, 403
Crestor, 629
Crinone, 1015
Crixivan, 1282
Crolom, 1354
cromolyn, 773, 1354, 31
Cruex, 181
Cryselle, 336, 1334
🍁Crystapen, 958
C/T/S, 317
Cubicin, 376
☯cum flore, 1310
Cuprimine, 1286
Curretab, 776
Cutivate, 358
cyanocobalamin, 1233, 25, 100
Cyanokit, 1233
Cyclessa, 336, 1334
cyclobenzaprine, 360, 1325, 95. *See also* Color Insert.
Cyclocort, 357
Cyclogyl, 1353
🍁Cyclomen, 1276
Cyclomydril Ophthalmic Solution, 1334
cyclopentolate, 1353
cyclophosphamide, 361, 12, 52, 81. *See also* Color Insert.
CYCLOPLEGIC MYDRIATICS, **1353**
cycloSPORINE, 364, 1354, 62, 81. *See also* Color Insert.
Cycrin, 776
Cylert, 1328
Cymbalta, 464, 1326
cyproheptadine, 367, 45. *See also* Color Insert.
Cystospaz, 646
Cystospaz-M, 646

cytarabine, 368, 12, 52. *See also* Color Insert.
CytoGam, 1276
cytomegalovirus immune globulin, 1276, 98
Cytomel, 1169
✤Cytosar, 368
Cytosar-U, 368
cytosine arabinoside, 368
Cytotec, 832
Cytovene, 594
Cytoxan, 361

D

d4T, 1292
daclizumab, 373, 81
Dacodyl, 223
Dacogen, 388
Dakrina, 1351
✤Dalacin C, 317
✤Dalacin T, 317
Dallergy Caplets, 1334
Dallergy Extended Release, 1334
Dallergy-JR Capsules, 1334
Dallergy Syrup, 1334
Dallergy Tablets, 1334
Dalmane, 571
dalteparin, 619, 34
Damason-P, 1334
danazol, 1276, 79
☯Dang Gui, 1300
☯Danggui, 1300
Danocrine, 1276
Dantrium, 374
dantrolene, 374, 95
Dapacin, 107
dapiprazole, 1349
Daptacel, 1383
daptomycin, 376, 49. *See also* Color Insert.
Daraprim, 1041
darbepoetin, 377, 25, 79
darifenacin, 380, 32
darunavir, 381, 1326, 60
Darvocet-N, 1024
Darvocet-N 50, 1334
Darvocet-N 100, 1334
Darvon, 1024
Darvon A500, 1024
Darvon Compound-32, 1024
Darvon Compound-65, 1024
Darvon N, 1024
✤Darvon-N Compound, 1024
✤Darvon-N with ASA, 1024
DAUNOrubicin citrate liposome, 383, 12, 52. *See also* Color Insert.
DAUNOrubicin hydrochloride, 385, 12, 52. *See also* Color Insert.
DaunoXome, 383
Daypro, 919
Dayquil Cold & Flu Relief Liquid, 1334
Dayquil Sinus Liquicaps, 1334
Daytrana, 1325
Dazamide, 109
DC Softgels, 442
DDAVP, 396, 1326
DDAVP Rhinal Tube, 396
DDAVP Rhinyle Drops, 396
ddI, 1277
Decadron, 1352
decitabine, 388, 12. *See also* Color Insert.
Decofed, 1033
Deconamine, 1334
Deconamine SR, 1334
Deconamine Syrup, 1334
deferoxamine, 389
Deficol, 223
Degas, 1109
Degest 2, 1355
Delatestryl, 1152
delavirdine, 1276, 60
Delestrogen, 507
Del-Mycin, 498
Delsym, 403
Delta-D, 1236
Demadex, 1194
Demerol, 784, 1373
☯Demon chaser, 1316
Denavir, 957
Depacon, 1212
Depakene, 1212
Depakote, 1212
Depakote ER, 1212
Depen, 1286
depGynogen, 506
DepoCyt, 368
DepoDur, 843
Depo-Estradiol, 506
Depogen, 506
Depo-Medrol, 350
Deponit, 892
Depo-Provera, 337, 776
Depo-subQ Provera 104, 337
Depo-Sub Q Provera 104, 776
Depo-Testosterone, 1152
Dermabet, 357
Dermacort, 358
Derma-Smoothe/FS, 357
Dermatop, 358
DermiCort, 358
✤Dermovate, 357
Dermtex HC, 358
Desferal, 389
desipramine, 391, 37. *See also* Color Insert.
desirudin, 393, 34
desloratadine, 395, 45
desmopressin, 396, 1326, 79
Desogen, 336, 1334
Desonate, 357
desonide, 357, 76
DesOwen, 357
desoximetasone, 357, 76
Desyrel, 1200
Detrol, 1189
Detrol LA, 1189
DexAlone, 403
dexamethasone, 350, 1352, 31, 62, 76. *See also* Color Insert.
Dexedrine, 401, 1325
DexFerrum, 700
dexmedetomidine, 1277, 93
dexmethylphenidate, 398, 74
DexPak, 350
dexrazoxane, 400
dextroamphetamine, 401, 1325, 74
dextromethorphan, 403
Dextrostat, 401
D.H.E. 45, 493
DiaBeta, 648
Diabetic Tussin, 610
Dialume, 133
Diamox, 109
Diamox Sequels, 109
Diar-aid Caplets, 756
Diastat, 404
✤Diazemuls, 404
diazepam, 404, 27, 35, 93, 95. *See also* Color Insert.
Dicarbosil, 256
DICLOFENAC, 408, 1354, 90
potassium, 408, 88–89
sodium, 408, 88–89
topical, 408, 88
topical patch, 1321, 89
dicloxacillin, 961, 49
dicofenac topical, 89
dicyclomine, 410, 32. *See also* Color Insert.
didanosine, 1277, 60
dideoxyinosine, 1277

*Entries for **generic** names appear in **boldface type,** tradenames appear in regular type, with Canadian tradenames preceded by a maple leaf icon (✤), **CLASSIFICATIONS** appear in **BOLDFACE SMALL CAPS,** *Combination Drugs* appear in *italics,* and herbal products are preceded by a yin-yang icon (☯).

🍁Didrocal, 519
Didronel, 519
difenoxin/atropine, 427, 32, 41
Difil-G Forte Liquid, 1334
Difil-G Tablets, 1335
diflorasone, 357, 76
Diflucan, 552
Digibind, 416
DigiFab, 416
Digitek, 412
digoxin, 412, 12, 15, 29. *See also* Color Insert.
digoxin immune Fab, 416
dihydroergotamine, 493, 99
1,25-dihydroxycholecalciferol, 1236
Dilacor XR, 418
Dilantin, 976
Dilatair, 1355
Dilatrate-SR, 707
Dilaudid, 640, 1372
Dilaudid-HP, 640
Dilex-G Syrup, 1335
Dilex G Tablets, 1335
Diltia XT, 418
diltiazem, 418, 26, 29, 47, 73. *See also* Color Insert.
dimenhyDRINATE, 420, 42, 45. *See also* Color Insert.
Dimetabs, 420
🍁Dimetane, 1273
Dimetapp Allergy, 1273
Dimetapp Children's ND Non-Drowsy Allergy, 760
Dimetapp Cold & Allergy Elixir, 1335
Dimetapp Cough & Cold DM Elixir, 1335
Dimetapp Decongestant Pediatric, 1033
Dimetapp Maximum Strength 12–Hour Non-Drowsy Extentabs, 1033
Dinate, 420
dinoprostone, 422
🍁Diocane, 1349
Diocto, 442
Dioctocal, 442
🍁Diodex, 1352
Dioval, 507
Diovan, 177, 1327
Diovan HCT 80/12.5, 1335
Diovan HCT 160/12.5, 1335
Diovan HCT 160/25, 1335
Diovan HCT 320/12.5, 1335
Diovan HCT 320/25, 1335
🍁Diovol Ex, 765
Dipentum, 905
Diphen AF, 424
Diphen Cough, 424
Diphenhist, 424
diphenhydrAMINE, 424, 45. *See also* Color Insert.
diphenoxylate/atropine, 427, 32, 41
diphtheria toxoid, reduced, 1383
diphtheria toxoid vaccine, reduced, 1389
dipivefrin, 1356
Dipridacot, 428
Diprivan, 1022
Diprolene, 357
dipyridamole, 428, 55. *See also* Color Insert.
Disalcid, 1087
🍁Disipal, 915
Disoprofol, 1022
disopyramide, 430, 29. *See also* Color Insert.
DisperMox, 153
disulfiram, 1278
Ditropan, 924. *See also* Color Insert.
Ditropan XL, 924
DIURETICS, 76
POTASSIUM-SPARING, 432
THIAZIDE, 434
Diuril, 434
divalproex sodium, 1212, 35, 99
Divigel, 507
🍁Dixarit, 321
DMARDS, 62. *See* **DISEASE-MODIFYING ANTIRHEUMATIC DRUGS**
🍁DM Syrup, 403
🍁Doan's Backache Pills, 1087
Doan's PM Extra Strength, 1335
Doan's Regular Strength Tablets, 1087
DOBUTamine, 437, 12. *See also* Color Insert.
Dobutrex, 437
docetaxel, 439, 12, 53. *See also* Color Insert.
docosanol, 441, 66
Docu, 442
DOCUSATE, 442
calcium, 442, 83
sodium, 442, 83
Docusoft S, 442
🍁Dodd's Extra Strength, 1087
🍁Dodd's Pills, 1087
dofetilide, 443, 29
DOK, 442
dolasetron, 445, 42
Dolgic, 247
Dolorac, 261
🍁DOM-Cephalexin, 279
🍁Dom-Cimetidine, 623
🍁DOM-Divalproex, 1212
🍁Dom-Glyburide, 648
🍁DOM-Hydrochlorothiazide, 434
🍁DOM-Minocycline, 1155
🍁Dom-Nizatidine, 623
🍁Dom-Ranitidine, 623
🍁DOM-Valproic Acid, 1212
donepezil, 447, 24. *See also* Color Insert.
☯Dong Qua, 1300
☯dong quai, 1300
Donnamar, 646
Donnatal, 1335
Donnatal Elixir, 1335
Donnatal Extentabs, 1335
🍁Dopamet, 804
DOPamine, 448, 12. *See also* Color Insert.
DOPAMINE AGONISTS, 54
Dopar, 743
Doribax, 1321
doripenem, 1321, 49
Dormin, 424
Doryx, 1155, 1325
dorzolamide, 1352
DOS, 442
DOSS, 442
DOS Softgels, 442
Dostinex, 253
doxazosin, 450, 47. *See also* Color Insert.
doxepin, 452, 27, 37, 45. *See also* Color Insert.
doxercalciferol, 1236, 100
Doxil, 457
Doxine, 1039
DOXOrubicin hydrochloride, 454, 12, 52. *See also* Color Insert.
DOXOrubicin hydrochloride liposome, 457, 12, 52. *See also* Color Insert.
Doxy, 1155
🍁Doxycin, 1155
doxycycline, 1155, 1325, 49. *See also* Color Insert.
🍁Doxytab, 1155
Dramamine, 420
Dramamine Less Drowsy Formula, 775
Dramanate, 420
🍁Drenison, 358
Drisdol, 1236
Dristan Cold Multi-Symptom Formula, 1335
Drixoral 12 Hour Non-Drowsy Formula, 1033
Drixoral Cold & Allergy, 1335
Drixoral Liquid Cough Caps, 403
droperidol, 461, 93. *See also* Color Insert.
drotrecogin, 463, 49. *See also* Color Insert.
Droxia, 1281
Dry Eyes Duratears Naturale, 1351
Dry Eye Therapy, 1351
DSS, 442
DTaP diphtheria toxoid, 1383
Duac Topical Gel, 1335

Duetact 2/30, 1335
Duetact 4/30, 1335
Dulcagen, 223
Dulcolax, 223
Dulcolax Magnesia Tablets, 766
Dulcolax Stool Softener, 442
duloxetine, 464, 1326, 37
DuoNeb, 1335
Duphalac, 721
Duraclon, 321
Dura-Estrin, 506
Duragen, 507
Duragesic, 542
✤Duralith, 754
Duramorph, 843
Duricef, 279
dutasteride, 466
Duvoid, 1271
Dwelle, 1351
Dyazide, 1335
Dynacin, 1155
DynaCirc, 708
DynaCirc CR, 708
Dyrenium, 432

E

E-200, 1240
E-400, 1240
E-1000, 1240
Easprin, 1087
E-Base, 498
☯echinacea (Echinacea Purpurea), 1301
ECHINOCANDINS, 43
echothiophate, 1352
EC-Naprosyn, 864
E-Complex-600, 1240
econazole, 181, 43
Econochlor, 1350
Econopred, 1353
Ecotrin, 1087
✤Ectosone, 357
E-Cypionate, 506
ED-IN-SOL, 700
ED-SPAZ, 646
Edur-Acin, 877
E.E.S, 498
efalizumab, 1278
efavirenz, 469, 60
Effer-K, 996
Effer-Syllium, 1035
Effexor, 1222, 1325
Effexor XR, 1222, 1325
Efidac 24, 1033
eFlone, 1352
eflornithine (topical), 1279
Efudex, 563
E/Gel, 498
Elaprase, 1326
Elavil, 149
Eldepryl, 1098
Elestat, 1349
Elestrin, 507
eletriptan, 470, 99
Elidel, 985
Eligard, 738
Elimite, 970
Elitek, 1057
Elixophyllin-GG Liquid, 1335
ElixSure Children's Cough Syrup, 403
Ellence, 484
✤Elocom, 358
Elocon, 358
Eloxatin, 917
Elspar, 193
✤Eltor 120, 1033
✤Eltroxin, 1169
Emadine, 1349
Embeline, 357
Embeline E, 357
emedastine, 1349, 45
Emend, 187, 1325
✤Emex, 810
Emgel, 498
EMLA, 749
EMLA Topical Cream, 1335
✤Emo-Cort, 358
Empresse, 1335
Emsam, 1099
emtricitabine, 472, 60
Emtriva, 472
E-Mycin, 498
Enablex, 380
enalapril/enalaprilat, 170, 47. *See also* Color Insert.
Enbrel, 516
✤Enca, 1155
Endocet, 926
Endocet 7.5/325, 1335
Endocet 7.5/500, 1335
Endocet 10/325, 1335
Endocet 10/650, 1335
Endocodone, 926
Endodan, 926, 1335
Endolor, 247
Endometrin, 1015
enfuvirtide, 473, 60
Engerix-B, 1384, 1388
Enjuvia, 510
enoxaparin, 619, 34
Enpresse, 337
entacapone, 475, 54. *See also* Color Insert.
entecavir, 476, 66
Entex HC Liquid, 1335
Entex PSE, 1335
Entocort EC, 350
✤Entrophen, 1087
Enulose, 721
Enzymase-16, 943
ENZYME INHIBITORS, 39, 52
ENZYMES, 52
EPIDURAL LOCAL ANESTHETICS, 478
Epifoam Aerosol Foam, 1335
Epifrin, 1356
✤Epimorph, 843
Epinal, 1356
epinastine, 1349, 45
epinephrine, 480, 1356, 10, 12, 30, 71. *See also* Color Insert.
EpiPen, 480
epirubicin, 484, 12, 52. *See also* Color Insert.
Epitol, 263
✤Epival, 1212
Epivir, 723, 1325
Epivir HBV, 723
eplerenone, 486, 47
EPO, 487
epoetin, 487, 25, 79
Epogen, 487
Eppy/N, 1356
✤Eprex, 487
eprosartan, 177, 47. *See also* Color Insert.
epsilon aminocaproic acid, 139
eptifibatide, 490, 12, 55. *See also* Color Insert.
Epzicom, 1335
Equagesic, 1335
Equalactin, 1289
Equanil, 1282
Equetro, 263
Equilet, 256
Eraxis, 180
Erbitux, 294
ergocalciferol, 1236, 100
Ergomar, 493
ergometrine, 492
ergonovine, 492
ergotamine, 493, 99
Ergotrate, 492
erlotinib, 495, 52
Errin, 337

*Entries for **generic** names appear in **boldface type,** tradenames appear in regular type, with Canadian tradenames preceded by a maple leaf icon (✤), **CLASSIFICATIONS** appear in **BOLDFACE SMALL CAPS**, *Combination Drugs* appear in *italics,* and herbal products are preceded by a yin-yang icon (☯).

Ertaczo, 1102
ertapenem, 496, 49
✤Erybid, 498
Eryc, 498, 1326
Erycette, 498
Erygel, 498
EryMax, 498
EryPed, 498
Erysol, 498
Ery-Tab, 498
Erythrocin, 498
✤Erythromid, 498
ERYTHROMYCIN, 498, 1326, 1350, 49. *See also* Color Insert.
  base, 498
  estolate, 498
  ethylsuccinate, 498
  gluceptate, 498. *See also* Color Insert.
  lactobionate, 498. *See also* Color Insert.
  stearate, 498
  topical, 498
erythropoietin, 487
Eryzole Oral Suspension, 1335
escitalopram, 501, 37
Esclim, 507
Esedrix, 434
Esgic, 247, 1335
Esgic-Plus, 247, 1335
Eskalith, 754
esmolol, 502, 12, 29, 68. *See also* Color Insert.
esomeprazole, 505, 1325, 65
esometrazole, 1326
Estivin II, 1355
Estrace, 506
Estraderm, 507
ESTRADIOL, 506
  acetate, 506, 80
  cypionate, 506, 80
  cypionate/medroxyprogesterone acetate, 80
  topical emulsion, 507, 80
  topical gel, 507, 80
  transdermal spray, 507, 80
  transdermal system, 507, 80
  vaginal ring, 507, 80
  vaginal tablet, 507, 80
  valerate, 507, 80
Estragyn LA 5, 506
Estra-L, 507
Estrasorb, 507
Estratest, 1335
Estratest HS, 1336
Estring, 507
Estro-Cyp, 507
Estrofem, 507
EstroGel, 507
estrogens, conjugated
  equine, 510, 79. *See also* Color Insert.
  synthetic, A, 510, 79
  synthetic, B, 510, 79
Estroject-LA, 507
Estro-L.A, 507
estropipate, 512, 79
Estro-Span, 507
Estrostep, 337
Estrostep Fe, 337, 1336
eszopiclone, 514, 1326, 93
etanercept, 516, 62
ethambutol, 517, 63
ethinyl estradiol/desogestrel, 336, 80
ethinyl estradiol/drospirenone, 336, 80
ethinyl estradiol/ethynodiol, 336, 80
ethinyl estradiol/etonogestrel, 337, 80
ethinyl estradiol/levonergestrel, 80
ethinyl estradiol/levonorgestrel, 336–337
ethinyl estradiol/norelgestromin, 337, 80
ethinyl estradiol/norethindrone, 336–337, 80
ethinyl estradiol/norgestimate, 336–337, 80
ethinyl estradiol/norgestrel, 336, 80
Ethmozine, 1284, 1327
Ethyol, 137
✤Etibi, 517
etidronate, 519, 70
etodolac, 521, 88
etonorgestrel, 337
Etopophos, 523
etoposide, 522, 53
etoposide phosphate, 523, 53
ETOPOSIDES, 522, 12. *See also* Color Insert.
etravirine, 1321, 60
ETS, 498
✤Euglucon, 648
Eulexin, 1280
✤Euthyrox, 1169
Evalose, 721
EvaMist, 507
Evista, 1052
E-Vitamin, 1240
Evoclin, 317
Evoxac, 1274
Excedrin Extra Strength, 1336
Excedrin IB, 654
Excedrin Migraine, 1336
Excedrin P.M., 1336
Excedrin Sinus Headache, 1336
Excedrin Tension Headache, 1336
Exelderm, 181
Exelon, 1077
Exelon Patch, 1077
exenatide, 525, 40
Exforge 5/160, 1336
Exforge 5/320, 1336
Exforge 10/160, 1336
Exforge 10/320, 1336
Ex-Lax, 1101
Ex-Lax Chocolated, 1101
Ex-Lax Stool Softener, 442
extended-release buccal tablets, 892
extended-release capsules, 892
extended-release tablets, 892
EXTENDED SPECTRUM PENICILLINS, 49
Extina, 181
Extra Strength Dynafed (Billups, P.J.), 107
Extra Strength Dynafed E.X., 107
Extra Strength Gas-X, 1109
✤Extra Strength Maalox GRF Gas Relief Formula, 1109
Exubera, 1327
Eye-Lube-A, 1351
Eyesine, 1355
EZE-DS, 305
ezetimibe, 527, 84
✤Ezetrol, 527

F

Factive, 557
famciclovir, 529, 66
famotidine, 623, 65. *See also* Color Insert.
Famvir, 529
Fansidar, 1336
Fareston, 1294
Fastin, 1288
FAT-SOLUBLE VITAMINS, 100
FazaClo, 327
Fe50, 700
☾Featerfoiul, 1303
☾Featherfew, 1303
☾Featherfoil, 1303
Feen-a-Mint, 223
Feldene, 989
felodipine, 530, 26, 47, 73. *See also* Color Insert.
Femara, 735
Femcon Fe, 336, 1336
Femhrt 0.5/2.5, 1336
Femhrt 1/5, 1336
Femiron, 700
✤Femogex, 507
FemPatch, 507
Femring, 507
Femtrace, 506
✤Fenicol, 1350
fenofibrate, 532, 84
fenoldopam, 534, 47
fentanyl, 1374, 12. *See also* Color Insert.
fentanyl buccal, 535, 1325

fentanyl (oral transmucosal), 538, 92
fentanyl (parenteral), 540, 92
fentanyl (transdermal), 542, 92
Fentora, 535, 1325
Feosol, 700
Feostat, 700
Feratab, 700
Fer-gen-sol, 700
Fergon, 700
Fer-In-Sol, 700
Fer-Iron, 700
✤Fero-Grad, 700
Ferralet, 700
ferric (III) hexacyanoferrate (II), 1290
Ferrlecit, 701
Ferro-Sequels, 1336
ferrous fumarate, 700, 25
ferrous gluconate, 700, 25
ferrous sulfate, 700, 25. *See also* Color Insert.
✤Fertinic, 700
Feverall, 107
☯feverfew, 1303
fexofenadine, 545, 45
Fiberall, 1035
FiberCon, 1289
Fiber-Lax, 1289
Fibrepur, 1035
filgrastim, 546. *See also* Color Insert.
finasteride, 548
Fioricet, 247, 1336
Fioricet with codeine, 1336
Fiorinal, 247, 1336
Fiorinal with codeine, 1336
Fiortal, 247
FIRST-GENERATION CEPHALOSPORINS, 279, 49
Flagyl, 817
Flagyl ER, 817
Flarex, 1352
Flatulex, 1110
flavocoxid, 550, 88
Flavorcee, 1271
flecainide, 550, 29
Flector, 1321
Fleet Enema, 980
Fleet Laxative, 223
Fleet Phospho-Soda, 980
Fleet Sof-Lax, 442
Fletchers' Castoria, 1101
Flexeril, 360
Flexoject, 915
Flexon, 915
☯Flirtwort Midsummer Daisy, 1303
Flomax, 1140
Flonase, 347
Florinef, 554
Flovent, 343
Flovent HFA, 343
Floxin, 558
Fluarix, 1386
fluconazole, 552, 43. *See also* Color Insert.
fludrocortisone, 554, 79
flumazenil, 556. *See also* Color Insert.
FluMist, 1386, 1388
flunisolide, 343, 347, 31, 76
fluocinolone, 357, 76
fluocinonide, 358, 76
✤Fluoderm, 357
✤Fluolar, 357
✤Fluonide, 357
fluorometholone, 1352, 76
Fluor-Op, 1352
Fluoroplex, 563
FLUOROQUINOLONES, 557, 49
fluorouracil, 563, 12, 52. *See also* Color Insert.
fluoxetine, 565, 1326, 37. *See also* Color Insert.
fluphenazine, 568, 58
flurandrenolide, 358, 76
flurazepam, 571, 93. *See also* Color Insert.
flurbiprofen, 1279, 1354, 62, 89–90
flutamide, 1280, 52
fluticasone, 343, 347, 358, 31, 76
fluvastatin, 629, 84
Fluvirin, 1386, 1388
fluvoxamine, 572, 37. *See also* Color Insert.
Fluzone, 1386, 1388
FML, 1352
FML-S Ophthalmic Suspension, 1336
Focalin, 398
Focalin XR, 398
FoilleCort, 358
folate, 574
Folex, 801
Folex PFS, 801
folic acid, 574, 25, 100. *See also* Color Insert.
folinic acid, 736. *See also* Color Insert.
Folvite, 574
fomepizole, 1325
fondaparinux, 575, 12, 34. *See also* Color Insert.
Foradil, 577
formoterol, 577, 30, 71
✤Formulex, 410
Fortamet, 793
Fortaz, 287
Forteo, 1151, 1327
Fortical, 254
Fosamax, 124
Fosamax Plus D 70/2800, 1336
Fosamax Plus D 70/5600, 1336
fosamprenavir, 1326 calcium, 580, 60
fosaprepitant, 1325
foscarnet, 582, 66
Foscavir, 582
fosinopril, 170, 47. *See also* Color Insert.
fosphenytoin, 583, 1325, 29, 35. *See also* Color Insert.
Fosrenol, 729
☯fossil tree, 1306
Fragmin, 619
☯Fragrant Valerian, 1317
✤Froben, 1279
Frova, 586
frovatriptan, 586, 99
FS Shampoo, 357
5-FU, 563
Fumasorb, 700
Fumerin, 700
✤Fungizone, 160
Fungoid, 181
Furadantin, 890
furosemide, 587, 78. *See also* Color Insert.
FUSION INHIBITORS, 60
Fuzeon, 473

G

gabapentin, 591, 35. *See also* Color Insert.
Gabitril, 1173
galantamine, 592, 24. *See also* Color Insert.
gamma benzene hexachloride, 751
ganciclovir, 594, 66. *See also* Color Insert.
Ganidin NR, 610
Garamycin, 140, 1350
Gardasil, 632
☯Garden Heliotrope, 1317
☯Garden Valerian, 1317

*Entries for **generic** names appear in **boldface type,** tradenames appear in regular type, with Canadian tradenames preceded by a maple leaf icon (✤), **CLASSIFICATIONS** appear in **BOLDFACE SMALL CAPS**, *Combination Drugs* appear in *italics,* and herbal products are preceded by a yin-yang icon (☯).

garlic, 1304
Gas-Ban, 1336
Gastrocrom, 773
Gastrosed, 646
Gas-X, 1110
gatifloxacin, 1327, 1350. *See also* Color Insert.
Gaviscon Extra Strength, 1336
Gaviscon Extra-Strength Liquid, 1336
Gaviscon Liquid, 1336
GBH, 751
G-CSF, 546
gefitinib, 596, 52
Gelusil, 1336
Gelusil Extra Strength, 765
gemcitabine, 597, 12, 52. *See also* Color Insert.
gemfibrozil, 599, 84
gemifloxacin, 557, 49
gemtuzumab ozogamicin, 1280, 12, 52–53. *See also* Color Insert.
Gemzar, 597
Genacote, 1087
Genac Tablets, 1336
Genafed, 1033
Genahist, 424
Genapap, 107
Genasyme, 1110
Genatuss DM Syrup, 1336
Gencalc, 256
Gen-Cimetidine, 623
Gen-Divalproex, 1212
Genebs, 107
Geneye, 1355
Gen-Famotidine, 623
gengibre, 1305
Gen-Glybe, 648
Gengraf, 364
Gen-K, 996
Gen-Medroxy, 776
Gen-Minocycline, 1155
Gen-Nizatidine, 623
Genoptic, 1350
Genotropin, 607
Genpril, 654
Gen-Ranitidine, 623
Gen-Salbutamol, 120
Gen-Selegiline, 1098
Gentacidin, 1350
Gentafair, 1350
Gentak, 1350
gentamicin, 140, 1350, 49. *See also* Color Insert.
Genteal Lubricant Eye Gel, 1351
Gentrasul, 1350
Gen-Triazolam, 1202
Gen-XENE, 325
Geodon, 1257, 1327
Geridium, 971
ginger root, imber, 1305
ginger (Zingiber Officinale), 1305
ginkgo, 1306
ginkgo folium, 1306
Gin Pain Pills, 1087
ginseng (Panax Ginseng), 1308
Glaucon, 1356
Gleevec, 662, 1326
Gliadel, 269
glimepiride, 648, 40
glipiZIDE, 648, 40. *See also* Color Insert.
GlucaGen, 601
glucagon, 601, 79
Gluconorm, 1058
Glucophage, 793
Glucophage XR, 793
glucosamine, 1309
Glucotrol, 648
Glucotrol XL, 648
Glucovance 1.25/250, 1336
Glucovance 2.5/500, 1336
Glucovance 5/500, 1336
Glumetza, 793
glyBURIDE, 648, 40. *See also* Color Insert.
glycerin, 1355
GLYCOPROTEIN IIB/IIIA INHIBITORS, 55
glycopyrrolate, 603, 32. *See also* Color Insert.
Glynase PresTab, 648
Glyset, 827
G-Mycin, 140
Goatweed, 1316
GoLYTELY, 992
goserelin, 1280, 52, 79
granisetron, 605, 42. *See also* Color Insert.
Granulex Topical Aerosol, 1336
granulocyte colony stimulating factor, 546
Gravol, 420
GROWTH HORMONES, 607
guaifenesin, 610
Guaifenex PSE 60, 1336
Guaifenex PSE 80, 1336
Guaifenex PSE 85, 1336
Guaifenex PSE 120, 1336
Guaituss AC Syrup, 1336
guanfacine, 47
Guiatuss, 610
G-Well, 751
Gynecort, 358
Gyne-Lotrimin-3, 184
Gynezole-1, 184
Gynodiol, 506
Gynogen L.A, 507

H

hagedorn, 1310
halcinonide, 358, 76
Halcion, 1202
Haldol, 613
Haldol Decanoate, 613
Haldol LA, 613
Halenol, 107
Haley's M-O Liquid, 1337
Halfprin, 1087
halobetasol, 358, 76
Halofed, 1033
Halog, 358
haloperidol, 613, 58. *See also* Color Insert.
Haltran, 654
Hardhay, 1316
Havrix, 1385, 1388
hawthorne (Crataegus Species), 1310
Headache Tablets, 1087
Healthprin, 1087
Hectorol, 1236
Helidac, 1337
Hemocyte, 700
Hemophilus b conjugate vaccine, 1383
Hemril-HC, 358
Hepalean, 616
heparin, 616, 12, 34. *See also* Color Insert.
Heparin Leo, 616
HEPARINS (LOW MOLECULAR WEIGHT), 619, 12, 34
Hepatitis A vaccine, 1385, 1388
Hepatitis B vaccine, 1384, 1388
Hep-Lock, 616
Hep-Lock U/P, 616
Heptalac, 721
Herceptin, 1198
Hexalen, 1269
hexamethylmelamine, 1269
Hexastat, 1269
Hexit, 751
HibTITER, 1383
Hi-Cor, 358
HISTAMINE H_2 ANTAGONISTS, 623, 65
Histanil, 1017
Hivid, 1328
HMG-CoA REDUCTASE INHIBITORS (statins), 629, 84
Hold, 403
Holy thistle, 1313
homatropine, 1353
hong shen, 1308
HORMONES, 25, 40, 52, 78–79
5-HT_1 AGONISTS, 99
5-HT_3 ANTAGONISTS, 42
Humalog, 670, 1380
Humalog Mix 50/50, 678, 1337
Humalog Mix 75/25, 678, 1337
human papillomavirus quadravalent (types 6, 0011, 0016, 0018) recombinant vaccine, 632
Humatrope, 607
Humibid DM, 1337

Humira, 114
Humulin 50/50, 678
Humulin 70/30, 678
Humulin N, 683, 1380
Humulin R, 681, 1380
Humulin R U-500 (concentrated), 681
Hycamtin, 1192
Hycodan, 637, 1337
Hycodan Syrup, 1337
Hycomine Compound, 1337
Hycort, 358
Hycotuss Expectorant, 1337
HYDANTOINS, 35
🍁Hyderm, 358
hydrALAZINE, 633, 47. *See also* Color Insert.
hydralazine/isosorbide dinitrate, 635
Hydrate, 420
Hydrea, 1281
hydrochloric acid, 13. *See also* Color Insert.
hydrochlorothiazide, 434, 47, 78. *See also* Color Insert.
hydrochlorthiazide, 13. *See also* Color Insert.
Hydrocil, 1035
hydrocodone, 637, 12, 92. *See also* Color Insert.
hydrocodone/acetaminophen, 637
hydrocodone/aspirin, 637
hydrocodone/ibuprofen, 637
hydrocortisone, 350, 358, 13, 31, 62, 76. *See also* Color Insert.
hydromorphone, 640, 1372, 1374, 12, 92. *See also* Color Insert.
Hydrostat IR, 640
Hydro-Tex, 358
hydroxocobalamin, 1233, 25, 100
hydroxychloroquine, 642, 62
hydroxyurea, 1281, 52
hydrOXYzine, 644, 27, 45, 93. *See also* Color Insert.
hyoscyamine, 646, 32. *See also* Color Insert.
HyperRHO S/D Full Dose, 1060
HyperRHO S/D Mini-Dose, 1060
HYPOGLYCEMIC AGENTS, ORAL, 648, 12, 15. *See also* Color Insert.
HypoTears, 1351
HypoTears PF, 1351
Hyrexin- 50, 424
Hytinic, 701
Hytone, 358
Hytrin, 1145
Hytuss, 610
Hytuss-2X, 610
Hyzaar 50/12.5, 1337
Hyzaar 100/12.5, 1337
Hyzaar 100/25, 1337
Hyzine-50, 644

I

ibandronate, 653, 70
ibuprofen, oral, 654, 59, 62, 88–89. *See also* hydrocodone/ibuprofen
ibutilide, 657, 29
Icar, 700
I-Chlor, 1350
Idamycin, 658
idarubicin, 658, 52. *See also* Color Insert.
idursulfase, 1326
Ifex, 660
ifosfamide, 660, 52
IL-2, 1268
iloprost, 1281
Ilosone, 498
Ilotycin, 1350
Ilozyme, 943
imatinib, 662, 1326, 12, 52. *See also* Color Insert.
IMDUR, 707
imipenem/cilastatin, 664, 49. *See also* Color Insert.
imipramine, 666, 37. *See also* Color Insert.
imiquimod, 669, 66
Imitrex, 1129
Imitrex STATdose, 1129
IMMUNE GLOBULINS, 98
IMMUNOMODULATORS, 1354, 80
Imodium, 756
Imodium A-D, 756
Imodium Advanced, 1337
Implanon, 337
🍁Impril, 666
Imuran, 206
Inapsine, 461
INCRETRIN MIMETIC AGENT, 40
🍁Indameth, 674
indapamide, 672, 47, 78
Inderal, 1026, 1327. *See also* Color Insert.
Inderal LA, 1026
Inderide 40/25, 1337
☯Indian Valerian, 1317
indinavir, 1282, 60
Indochron E-R, 674
🍁Indocid, 674
Indocin, 674
Indocin I.V, 674
🍁Indocin PDA, 674
Indocin SR, 674
indomethacin, 674, 62, 89. *See also* Color Insert.
Infanrix, 1383
Infant's Pain Reliever, 107
InFeD, 700
Inflamase, 1353
infliximab, 676, 62
Influenza vaccine, 1386, 1388
Infumorph, 843
☯ingwer, 1305
☯ingwerwurzel, 1305
INH, 705
Innohep, 619
InnoPran XL, 1026
🍁Insomnal, 424
Inspra, 486
Insta-Char, 1268
Insta-Char Aqueous Suspension, 1268
insulin, regular (injection, concentrated), 681, 40, 80
insulin aspart, rDNA origin, 670, 1380, 40, 80
insulin aspart protamine suspension/insulin aspart solution mixtures, rDNA origin, 678, 1380, 40, 80
insulin detemir, 685, 1380, 40, 80
insulin glargine, 685, 1380, 40, 80
insulin glulisine, 670, 1380, 40, 80
insulin lispro, rDNA origin, 670, 1380, 40, 80
insulin lispro/protamine insulin lispro mixture, rDNA origin, 40
insulin lispro protamine suspension/insulin lispro solution mixtures, rDNA origin, 678, 40, 80
INSULIN (mixtures), 678, 12. *See also* Color Insert.
insulin recombinant human, powder for inhalation, 1327

*Entries for **generic** names appear in **boldface type,** tradenames appear in regular type, with Canadian tradenames preceded by a maple leaf icon (🍁), **CLASSIFICATIONS** appear in **BOLDFACE SMALL CAPS,** *Combination Drugs* appear in *italics,* and herbal products are preceded by a yin-yang icon (☯).

INSULINS, 40, 80. *See also* **NPH insulin; regular insulin**
INSULINS (intermediate-acting), 683, 12. *See also* Color Insert.
INSULINS (long-acting), 685, 12. *See also* Color Insert.
INSULINS (rapid acting), 670, 12. *See also* Color Insert.
INSULINS (short acting), 681, 12. *See also* Color Insert.
Insulin-Toronto, 681
Intal, 773
INTEGRASE STRAND TRANSFER INHIBITOR (INSTI), 60
Integrilin, 490
Intelence, 1321
interferon alfa 2a, 1328
interferon alpha-2b, 688
interferon alpha-n3, 688
interferon beta-1a, 692
interferon beta-1b, 692
INTERFERONS, ALPHA, 688
INTERFERONS, BETA, 692
interleukin-2, 1268
intoxicating pepper, 1312
intravenous, 892
Intron A, 688
Intropin, 448
Invanz, 496
Invega, 939
Invirase, 1092
IODINE, IODIDE, 694
Ionamin, 1288
Iopidine, 1356
I-Pentolate, 1353
I-Phrine, 1355
IPOL, 1383
ipratropium, 696, 32, 71
Iprivask, 393
IPV, 1383
Iquix, 1350
irbesartan, 177, 47. *See also* Color Insert.
Iressa, 596
irinotecan, 698, 52
iron dextran, 700, 25
iron polysaccharide, 701, 25
iron sucrose, 701, 25
IRON SUPPLEMENTS, 700, 25
Isentress, 1324
ISMO, 707
isocarboxazid, 838, 37
isoniazid, 705, 63
Isoptin, 1224
Isoptin SR, 1224
Isopto Alkaline, 1351
Isopto Atropine, 1353
Isopto Carbachol, 1352
Isopto Carpine, 1352
Isopto Cetamide, 1350
Isopto Frin, 1355
Isopto Homatropine, 1353
Isopto Hyoscine, 1096, 1353
Isopto Plain, 1351
Isordil, 707
ISOSORBIDE, 707. *See also* Color Insert.
isosorbide dinitrate, 707, 26
isosorbide mononitrate, 707, 26
Isotamine, 705
isradipine, 708, 26, 47, 73
I-Sulfacet, 1350
itraconazole, 710, 43
I-Tropine, 1353
ixabepilone, 1322, 53
Ixempra, 1322

J

Jamaica ginger, 1305
Janumet 50/500, 1337
Janumet 50/1000, 1337
Januvia, 1112, 1327
Japanese ginseng, 1308
Japanese silver apricot, 1306
Jenamicin, 140
jenjibre, 1305
jiang, kankyo, zenzero, 1305
Jolivette, 337
Junel 1/20, 1337
Junel 1.5/30, 1337
Junel 21 1/20, 336
Junel 21 1.5/20, 336
Junel Fe 1/20, 336, 1337
Junel Fe 1.5/30, 336, 1337
Junior Strength Advil, 654
Just Tears, 1351
Ju-Zhong, 1315

K

K+ 10, 996
K+ Care, 996
K+Care ET, 996
Kadian, 843
Kalcinate, 256
Kaletra, 758, 1325–1326
Kaletra 100/25 capsules, 1337
Kaletra 200/50 capsules, 1337
Kaletra solution, 1337
Kalium Durules, 996
kanamycin, 140, 49. *See also* Color Insert.
kansas snakeroot, 1301
Kantrex, 140
kao, 1312
Kaochlor, 996
Kaochlor Eff, 996
Kaochlor S-F, 996
Kaon, 996
Kaon-Cl, 996
Kaopectate, 225
Kaopectate II Caplets, 756
Kao-Tin, 225
Kapectolin, 225
Karacil, 1035
Kariva, 336, 1337
kava-kava (Piper Methysticum), 1312
Kay Ciel, 996
Kayexalate, 1119
Kaylixir, 996
KCl, 996
K-Dur, 996
Keflex, 279
K-Electrolyte, 996
Kelnor, 1337
Kelnor 1/35, 336
Kemstro, 213
Kenalog, 350, 358
Kepivance, 938
Keppra, 742
Kerlone, 219
Ketek, 1141
ketoconazole, 181, 43
ketoconazole (systemic), 713, 43
ketoprofen, 714, 59, 62, 88, 90
ketorolac, 716, 1326, 1354, 88, 90. *See also* Color Insert.
ketotifen, 1354
kew, 1312
kew tree, 1306
K-Exit, 1119
K-G Elixir, 996
K-Ide, 996
Kid Kare, 1033
Kidrolase, 193
Kineret, 168
Klamath weed, 1316
Klean-Prep, 992
K-Lease, 996
K-Long, 996
Klonopin, 320
K-Lor, 996
Klor-Con, 996
Klor-Con/EF, 996
Klorvess Liquid, 996
Klotrix, 996
K-Lyte, 996
K-Lyte/Cl, 996
K-Lyte/Cl Powder, 996
K-Lyte DS, 996
K-Med, 996
K-Norm, 996
Koffex, 403
Kolyum, 996
Konsyl, 1035
Konsyl Fiber, 1289
Korean ginseng, 1308
K-Pek, 225
K-Phos M.F, 994
K-Phos Neutral, 994
K-Phos No. 2, 994
K-Phos Original, 1289
Kristalose, 721
K-Sol, 996

K-Tab, 996
Ku-Zyme HP, 943
K-Vescent, 996
Kytril, 605

L

labetalol, 719, 12, 26, 47, 68. *See also* Color Insert.
Lacril, 1351
Lacri-Lube NP, 1351
Lacri-Lube S.O.P., 1351
Lacrisert, 1351
LactiCare-HC, 358
Lactinex, 1337
✤Lactulax, 721
lactulose, 721, 83
Lactulose PSE, 721
☯Lady's thistle, 1313
Lamictal, 725
Lamisil, 1147, 1325
Lamisil AT, 181
lamivudine, 723, 1325, 60, 66
lamotrigine, 725, 35. *See also* Color Insert.
Lanacort 9-1-1, 358
Laniazid, 705
Lanoxicaps, 412
Lanoxin, 412
lansoprazole, 727, 65
lanthanum carbonate, 729
Lantus, 685, 1380
lapatinib, 730, 52
✤Largactil, 301
Larodopa, 743
Lasix, 587
✤Lasix Special, 587
latanoprost, 1355
LAXATIVES, 82
✤Laxit, 223
l -dopa, 743
Leena, 337
leflunomide, 731, 62
Lemoderm, 358
☯leopard's bane, 1297
lepirudin (rDNA), 733, 34
Lescol, 629
Lescol XL, 629
Lessina, 1337
Lessina-28, 336
letrozole, 735, 52
leucovorin calcium, 736, 100. *See also* Color Insert.
Leukeran, 1274
Leukine, 1093
LEUKOTRIENE ANTAGONISTS, 31, 71
leuprolide, 738, 52, 79
levalbuterol, 741, 1325, 30, 71
Levaquin, 557
✤Levate, 149
Levbid, 646
Levemir, 685, 1380
levetiracetam, 742, 35
Levitra, 1217, 1327
Levlen-28, 336
Levlite, 1337
Levlite-28, 336
levobetaxolol, 1351, 68
levobunolol, 1351, 68
levocabastine, 45
levocetirizine, 1325
levodopa, 743, 54
Levodromoran, 1372
levofloxacin, 557, 1350, 49. *See also* Color Insert.
levonorgestrel, 337, 80
levonorgestrel/ethinyl estradiol, 80
Levora, 1337
Levora-28, 336
levorphanol, 1372
Levo-T, 1169
Levothroid, 1169
levothyroxine, 1169, 1325, 79. *See also* Color Insert.
Levoxyl, 1169
Levsin, 646
Levsinex, 646
Levulan Kerastick, 1269
Lexapro, 501
Lexiva, 580, 1326
Lexxel 5/2.5, 1337
Lexxel 5/5, 1337
L-hyoscyamine, 646
Lialda, 789
Librax, 1337
Libritabs, 298
Librium, 298
Lida-Mantle-HC Topical Cream, 1337
✤Lidemol, 358
Lidex, 358
Lidex-E, 358
LIDOCAINE, 746, 1325, 12, 29. *See also* Color Insert.
lidocaine (local anesthetic), 746
lidocaine (mucosal), 746
lidocaine (parenteral), 746
lidocaine patch, 746
lidocaine/prilocaine, 749
lidocaine (topical), 746
Lidoderm, 746
LidoPen, 746
☯Ligustilides, 1300
Limbitrol 5/12.5, 1337
Limbitrol DS 10/25, 1337
Limbrel, 550
lindane, 751
linezolid, 752, 49. *See also* Color Insert.
Lioresal, 213
liothyronine, 1169, 79
liotrix, 1169, 79
✤Lipidil Micro, 532
✤Lipidil Supra, 532
LIPID-LOWERING AGENTS, 83
Lipitor, 629
Lipofen, 532
Lipram,-UL20, 943
Lipram-CR20, 943
Lipram-PN10, 943
Lipram-PN16, 943
Lipram-UL12, 943
Lipram-UL18, 943
Liqui-Cal, 256
Liqui-Char, 1268
Liquid Cal-600, 256
Liqui-E, 1240
Liquifilm Forte, 1351
Liquifilm Tears, 1351
Liquiprin, 107
lisinopril, 170, 47. *See also* Color Insert.
lithium, 754, 15. *See also* Color Insert.
✤Lithizine, 754
Lithobid, 754
Little Colds Cough Formula Drops, 403
L-M-X 4, 746
L-M-X 5, 746
LoCHOLEST, 306
LoCHOLEST Light, 306
Locoid, 358
Lodine, 521
Lodine XL, 521
lodoxamide, 1354
Loestrin 21 1/20, 336
Loestrin 21 1.5/30, 336
Loestrin Fe 1/20, 336, 1337
Loestrin Fe 1.5/30, 336, 1337
Lofibra, 532
Logen, 427
Lomanate, 427
Lomotil, 427, 1337
Lomotil Liquid, 1337
Loniten, 1284

*Entries for **generic** names appear in **boldface type,** tradenames appear in regular type, with Canadian tradenames preceded by a maple leaf icon (✤), **CLASSIFICATIONS** appear in **BOLDFACE SMALL CAPS**, *Combination Drugs* appear in *italics,* and herbal products are preceded by a yin-yang icon (☯).

Lonox, 427, 1337
LOOP DIURETICS, 47, 78
Lo/Ovral, 1337
Lo/Ovral 28, 336
loperamide, 756, 41
Lopid, 599
lopinavir/ritonavir, 758, 60
♣Lopresor, 814
♣Lopresor SR, 814
Lopressor, 814
Lopressor HCT 50/25, 1338
Lopressor HCT 100/25, 1338
Lopressor HCT 100/50, 1338
Loprox, 181
Lopurin, 128
Lorabid, 1328
loracarbef, 1328
loratadine, 760, 45
lorazepam, 762, 27, 93. *See also* Color Insert.
Lorcet 10/650, 1338
Lorcet-HD, 637, 1338
Lorcet Plus, 1338
Lortab, 637
Lortab 5/500, 1338
Lortab 7.5/500, 1338
Lortab 10/500, 1338
Lortab Elixir, 1338
losartan, 177, 47. *See also* Color Insert.
♣Losec, 908
♣*Losec 1-2-3 A, 1338*
♣*Losec 1-2-3 M, 1338*
Lotemax, 1353
Lotensin, 170
Lotensin HCT 5/6.25, 1338
Lotensin HCT 10/12.5, 1338
Lotensin HCT 20/12.5, 1338
Lotensin HCT 20/25, 1338
loteprednol, 1353, 76
Lotrel 2.5/10, 1338
Lotrel 5/10, 1338
Lotrel 5/20, 1338
Lotrel 5/40, 1338
Lotrel 10/20, 1338
Lotrel 10/40, 1338
♣Lotriderm, 181
Lotrimin, 181
Lotrimin AF, 181
Lotrimin Ultra, 181
Lotrisone Topical Cream/Lotion, 1338
lovastatin, 629, 84
Lovaza, 907
Lovenox, 619
Low-Ogestrel, 1338
Low-Ogestrel 28, 336
♣Lozide, 672
Lozol, 672
L-PAM, 781
l-triiodothyronine, 1169
LubriTears, 1351
Lufyllin-GG Elixir, 1338
Lugol's solution, 694
Lumigan, 1355
Luminal, 972
Lunesta, 514, 1326
Lupron, 738
Lupron Depot, 738
Lupron Depot-3 Month, 738
Lupron Depot-PED, 738
Lutera, 336
Luvox, 572
Luxiq, 357
Lybrel, 337, 1338
♣Lyderm, 358
Lyphocin, 1215
Lyrica, 1005

M

Maalox, 765
Maalox Antacid Caplets, 256
Maalox Antidiarrheal Caplets, 756
♣Maalox GRF Gas Relief Formula, 1110
Maalox Maximum Liquid, 1338
Maalox Regular Liquid, 1338
Macrobid, 890
Macrodantin, 890
MACROLIDES, 49
Macugen, 1285
magaldrate, 765, 65
Magan, 1087
Magnacet, 926
Magnacet 2.5/400, 1338
Magnacet 5/400, 1338
Magnacet 7.5/400, 1338
Magnacet 10/400, 1338
MAGNESIUM AND ALUMINUM SALTS, 765
magnesium chloride, 766, 83, 85
magnesium citrate, 766, 83, 85
magnesium gluconate, 766, 83, 85
magnesium hydroxide, 766, 83, 85
magnesium hydroxide/aluminum hydroxide, 765, 65
magnesium oxide, 766, 83, 85
magnesium salicylate, 1087, 59, 88
MAGNESIUM SALTS (ORAL), 766, 85
magnesium sulfate, 12–13. *See also* Color Insert.
magnesium sulfate (IV, parenteral), 768, 85
Magonate, 766
Mag-Ox 400, 766
Magtrate, 766
☯maidenhair-tree, 1306
Malarone, 1338
Malarone Pediatric, 1338
Mallamint, 256
Mallazine, 1355
Mandol, 1327
mannitol, 770, 78. *See also* Color Insert.
MAO INHIBITORS, 15. See MONOAMINE OXIDASE (MAO) INHIBITORS
Maox, 766
Mapap, 107
Mapap Multi-Symptom Cold, 1338
Maranox, 107
maraviroc, 772, 60
Marcaine, 478
Marcillin, 164
Margesic, 247
Marplan, 838
Marten-Tab, 247
Marthritic, 1087
Marvelon, 1338
☯Mary Thistle, 1313
MAST CELL STABILIZERS, 773, 1354, 31
Matulane, 1010
Mavik, 170
Maxalt, 1079
Maxalt-MLT, 1079
♣Maxeran, 810
Maxidex, 1352
Maximum Relief Ex-Lax, 1101
Maximum Strength Mylanta Gas, 1110
Maximum Strength Nytol, 424
Maximum Strength Pepcid, 623
Maximum Strength Sleepinal, 424
Maxipime, 275
Maxitrol Ophthalmic Suspension/Ointment, 1338
Maxzide, 1338
Maxzide-25, 1338
☯maybush, 1310
Measles, mumps, and rubella vaccines, 1383, 1388
mebendazole, 1282
mechlorethamine, 52
meclizine, 775, 42, 45. *See also* Color Insert.
Meda, 107
Medi-First Sinus Decongestant, 1033
Medigesic, 247
Medipren, 654
Mediquell, 403
Medrol, 350
medroxyprogesterone, 337, 776, 52, 79–80. *See also* Color Insert.
medrysone, 76
♣Med Tamoxifen, 1138
Mefoxin, 282
Mega-C/A Plus, 1271
Megace, 778
megestrol, 778, 53, 79

MEGLITINIDES, 40
Mellaril, 1162
Mellaril-S, 1162
meloxicam, 779, 88, 90
melphalan, 781, 52
memantine, 783, 24
Menactra, 1385, 1388
Menadol, 654
Menaval, 507
Meni-D, 775
Meningococcal polysaccharide diphtheria toxoid conjugate vaccine, 1385, 1388
Menostar, 507
Mentax, 181
meperidine, 784, 1373, 12, 92. *See also* Color Insert.
Mephyton, 982
meprobamate, 1282, 27. *See also* Color Insert.
Mepron, 201
Meridia, 1106
meropenem, 787, 1326, 49. *See also* Color Insert.
Merrem, 787, 1326
mesalamine, 789
🍁M-Eslon, 843
mesna, 791
Mesnex, 791
Mestinon, 1037
🍁Mestinon SR, 1037
Mestinon Timespan, 1037
mestranol/norethindrone, 336, 80
METABOLIC INHIBITORS, 60
Metadate CD, 808
Metadate ER, 808
🍁Metaderm, 357
Metaglip 2.5/250, 1338
Metaglip 2.5/500, 1338
Metaglip 5/500, 1338
Metamucil, 1035
metaproterenol, 1283, 30, 71
metaxalone, 792, 95. *See also* Color Insert.
metformin, 793, 39
methadone, 795, 1372, 12, 92. *See also* Color Insert.
Methadose, 795
Methergine, 806
methimazole, 798
methocarbamol, 799, 95. *See also* Color Insert.
methotrexate, 801, 12–13, 52, 62, 81. *See also* Color Insert.
methoxypolyethylene glycol-epoetin beta, 1322, 25
methylaminolevulinate, 53
methyldopa, 804, 47. *See also* Color Insert.
methylergonovine, 806
Methylin, 808
Methylin ER, 808
methylphenidate, 808, 1325, 74
methylPREDNISolone, 350, 31, 62, 76. *See also* Color Insert.
metipranolol, 1351, 68
metoclopramide, 810, 42. *See also* Color Insert.
metolazone, 812, 47, 78
🍁Metoprol, 814
metoprolol, 814, 12, 26, 47, 68. *See also* Color Insert.
Metric 21, 817
MetroCream, 817
MetroGel, 817
MetroGel-Vaginal, 817
Metro IV, 817
MetroLotion, 817
metronidazole, 817, 49, 65. *See also* Color Insert.
Metryl, 817
Mevacor, 629
☯Mexican Valerian, 1317
mexiletine, 819, 29
Mexitil, 819
Miacalcin, 254
micafungin, 821, 1326, 43. *See also* Color Insert.
Micardis, 177
Micardis HCT 40/12.5, 1338
Micardis HCT 80/12.5, 1338
Micardis HCT 80/25, 1338
miconazole, 181, 184, 43
🍁Micozole, 181
MICRhoGAM, 1060
Microgestin Fe 1/20, 336, 1339
Microgestin Fe 1.5/30, 1339
Micro-K, 996
Micro-K ExtenCaps, 996
Micro-LS, 996
Micronase, 648
microNefrin, 480
Micronor, 337
Microzide, 434
🍁Midamor, 432
midazolam, 822, 12, 27, 93. *See also* Color Insert.
Midol Maximum Strength Cramp Formula, 654
Midol Menstrual Complete, 1339
Midol Menstrual Headache, 1339
Midol PM, 424
Midol Pre-Menstrual Syndrome, 1339
Midol Teen Formula, 1339
Midrin, 1339
Mifeprex, 825
mifepristone, 825
Migergot Suppositories, 1339
miglitol, 827, 39
miglustat, 1283
Migranal, 493
Miles Nervine, 424
☯milk thistle, 1313
milrinone, 828, 12. *See also* Color Insert.
Miltown, 1282
MINERALS/ELECTROLYTES/PH MODIFIERS, 84
Mini-Gamulin R, 1060
🍁Minims, 1353
🍁Minims Homatropine, 1353
🍁Minims Phenylephrine, 1355
🍁Minims Tetracaine, 1349
🍁Minims Tropicamide, 1354
Minipress, 1003
Minitran, 892
Minocin, 1155
minocycline, 1155, 49. *See also* Color Insert.
minoxidil (systemic), 1284, 47
🍁Miocarpine, 1352
Mio-Rel, 915
MiraLax, 991
Mirapex, 1000
Mircera, 1322
Mircette, 336, 1339
Mirena, 337
mirtazapine, 830, 37. *See also* Color Insert.
misoprostol, 832, 65
MitoExtra, 833
mitomycin, 833, 52
mitoxantrone, 835, 13, 52. *See also* Color Insert.
🍁Mitran, 298
Mitrolan, 1289
Mivacron, 1328
mivacurium, 1328
M-M-R II, 1383, 1388
Mobic, 779
Mobidin, 1087
modafinil, 837, 74
Modane, 223
Modane Bulk, 1035
Modane Soft, 442

*Entries for **generic** names appear in **boldface type,** tradenames appear in regular type, with Canadian tradenames preceded by a maple leaf icon (🍁), **CLASSIFICATIONS** appear in **BOLDFACE SMALL CAPS**, *Combination Drugs* appear in *italics,* and herbal products are preceded by a yin-yang icon (☯).

🍁Modecate Concentrate, 568
Modicon, 336, 1339
🍁*Moduret, 1339*
moexipril, 170, 47
Moisture Drops, 1351
MOM, 766
mometasone, 343, 347, 358, 1326, 31, 76
Monistat-1, 184
Monistat-3, 184
Monistat-7, 184
Monistat-Derm, 181
🍁Monitan, 105
MONOAMINE OXIDASE (MAO) INHIBITORS, 838, 37
MONOAMINE OXIDASE TYPE B INHIBITORS, **54**
monobasic potassium and sodium phosphates, 85
monobasic potassium phosphate, 1289, 85
MONOCLONAL ANTIBODIES, **31, 52**
Monocor, 226
Monodox, 1155
Mono-Gesic, 1087
Monoket, 707
MonoNessa, 336
Monopril, 170
Monopril-HCT 10/12.5, 1339
Monopril-HCT 20/12.5, 1339
montelukast, 841, 1326, 71
moricizine, 1284, 29
Morizicine, 1327
morphine, 843, 1372–1374, 12–13, 92. *See also* Color Insert.
🍁Morphine H.P, 843
morphine sulfate, 13
🍁Morphitec, 843
🍁M.O.S, 843
🍁M.O.S.-S.R, 843
Motofen, 427, 1339
Motrin, 654
Motrin Children's Cold Suspension, 1339
Motrin Drops, 654
Motrin IB, 654
Motrin Junior Strength, 654
Motrin Migraine Pain, 654
☯mountain snuff, 1297
☯mountain tobacco, 1297
Moxatag, 1325
moxifloxacin, 557, 1326, 1350, 49. *See also* Color Insert.
M-Oxy, 926
MS, 843
MS Contin, 843
MSIR, 843
🍁MSIR, 843
MSO_4, 843
Mucinex, 610
Mucinex D, 1339
Mucinex DM, 1339
🍁Multipax, 644
mupirocin, 847, 49
Murine Plus, 1355
Murine Solution, 1351
Murocel, 1351
Murocoll-2 Ophthalmic Solution, 1339
muromonab-CD3, 849, 81
Mutamycin, 833
Myambutol, 517
Mycamine, 821, 1326
Mycelex-3, 184
Mycelex-7, 184
Mycobutin, 1065
mycophenolate mofetil, 850, 81
mycophenolic acid, 850, 81
Mycostatin, 181, 184, 899
Mydfrin, 1355
Mydriacyl, 1354
Mydriafair, 1354
Myfortic, 850
🍁Mylanta, 765
Mylanta AR, 623
Mylanta Gas, 1110
🍁Mylanta Lozenges, 256
Mylanta Maximum Strength Liquid, 1339
Mylanta Natural Fiber Supplement, 1035
Mylanta Regular Strength Liquid, 1339
Mylanta Supreme Liquid, 1339
Mylanta Ultimate Strength Chewables, 1339
Mylanta Ultimate Strength Liquid, 1339
Myleran, 245
Mylicon, 1110
Mylocel, 1281
Mylotarg, 1280
Myolin, 915
Myotrol, 915

N

nabumetone, 855, 62, 90
nadolol, 856, 26, 47, 68
🍁Nadostine, 181, 899
nafarelin, 858, 79
Nafazair, 1355
nafcillin, 961, 49. *See also* Color Insert.
naftifine, 181, 43
Naftin, 181
nalbuphine, 860, 1373, 12, 92. *See also* Color Insert.
Naldecon Senior EX, 610
naloxone, 862. *See also* Color Insert.
Namenda, 783
nandrolone decanoate, 25, 80
naphazoline, 1355
Naphcon, 1355
Naphcon-A Ophthalmic Solution, 1339
Naprelan, 864
Napron X, 864
Naprosyn, 864
🍁Naprosyn-E, 864
🍁Naprosyn-SR, 864
naproxen, 864, 59, 88, 90. *See also* Color Insert.
naratriptan, 866, 99
Narcan, 862
Nardil, 839
Naropin, 478
Nasacort AQ, 347
Nasahist B, 1273
NasalCrom, 773
Nasarel, 347
Nasatab LA, 1339
Nascobal, 1233
Nasonex, 347
Natacyn, 1351
natalizumab, 1326
natamycin, 1351
nateglinide, 868, 40
Natrecor, 873
🍁Natulan, 1010
Naturacil Caramels, 1035
NATURAL/HERBAL PRODUCTS, **86**
🍁Natural Source Fibre Laxative, 1035
Nature's Tears, 1351
Navelbine, 1231
🍁Naxen, 864
Nebcin, 140
nebivolol, 1323, 47
NebuPent, 964
Necon 0.5/35, 336
Necon 1/35, 336
Necon 1/50, 336
Necon 7/7/7, 337
Necon 10/11, 336
nedocromil, 773, 1354, 31
nefazodone, 869, 37
nelfinavir, 1285, 60
Nembutal, 1287
Neo-Diaral, 756
🍁Neo-DM, 403
Neo-Fer, 700
Neo-Fradin, 140
🍁Neo-K, 996
neomycin, 140, 49
Neopap, 107
Neoral, 364
Neosar, 361
Neosporin + Pain Relief Antibiotic Topical Cream, 1339
Neosporin + Pain Relief Antibiotic Topical Ointment, 1339
Neosporin Antibiotic Topical Ointment, 1339
Neosporin G.U. Irrigant, 1339
Neosporin Ophthalmic Solution, 1339
Neosporin Topical Cream, 1339

neostigmine, 871
nepafenac, 1355, 90
Nephro-Calci, 256
✤Nephro-Fer, 700
Nephron, 480
nesiritide, 873, 12. *See also* Color Insert.
Nestrex, 1039
Neulasta, 954
Neumega, 912
Neupogen, 546
Neupro, 1084
Neurontin, 591
Neut, 1114
Neutra-Phos, 994
Neutra-Phos-K, 1289
Neutrexin, 1328
Nevanac, 1355
nevirapine, 875, 60
Nexavar, 1327
Nexium, 505, 1325–1326
Nia-Bid, 877
Niac, 877
Niacels, 877
niacin, 877, 84, 100
niacinamide, 877, 84, 100
niacin extended-release/simvastatin, 1325
Niacor, 877
Niaspan, 877
niCARdipine, 879, 26, 47, 73. *See also* Color Insert.
Nico-400, 877
Nicobid, 877
Nicoderm CQ, 881
Nicolar, 877
Nicorette, 881
nicotinamide, 877
NICOTINE, 881
chewing gum, 881
inhaler, 881
lozenge, 881
nasal spray, 881
transdermal, 881
Nicotinex, 877
nicotinic acid, 877
Nicotrol Inhaler, 881
Nicotrol NS, 881
✤Nidagel, 817
Nifedical XL, 884
NIFEdipine, 884, 26, 47, 73. *See also* Color Insert.
Niferex, 701
Niferex-150 Forte, 1339
Nighttime Sleep Aid, 424
Nilandron, 887
nilotinib, 1323, 52
Nilstat, 899
nilutamide, 887, 52
nimodipine, 888, 73
Nimotop, 888
Niravam, 131
nisoldipine, 889, 1325, 47, 73
nitazoxanide, 1285
NITRATES, 26
Nitrek, 892
Nitro-Bid, 892
Nitro-Bid IV, 892
Nitrocot, 892
Nitrodisc, 892
Nitro-Dur, 892. *See also* Color Insert.
nitrofurantoin, 890, 49. *See also* Color Insert.
Nitrogard, 892
✤Nitrogard SR, 892
nitroglycerin, 892, 13, 26. *See also* Color Insert.
NitroglynE-R, 892
Nitrol, 892
Nitrolingual, 892
Nitrong, 892
Nitro-par, 892
Nitropress, 895
nitroprusside, 895, 13, 47. *See also* Color Insert.
NitroQuick, 892
Nitrostat, 892
Nitro-Time, 892
Nix, 970
nizatidine, 623, 65
Nizoral, 181, 713
Nizoral A-D, 181
✤Nolvadex-D, 1138
Non-Drowsy Allergy Relief for Kids, 760
NON-NUCLEOSIDE REVERSE TRANSCRIPTASE INHIBITORS, 60
NONOPIOID ANALGESICS, 87
NONSTEROIDAL ANTI-INFLAMMATORY AGENTS, 1354, 15, 88–89
OPHTHALMIC, 90
No Pain-HP, 261
Norco, 637
Norco 5/325, 1339
Norco 7.5/325, 1339
Norco 10/325, 1339
Nordette, 1339
Nordette-28, 336
Norditropin, 607
Norethin 1/35E, 336
Norethin 1/50M, 336
norethindrone, 337, 80
norethindrone/ethinyl acetate, 337, 80
Norflex, 915, 13
norfloxacin, 557, 1350, 13, 49. *See also* Color Insert.
Norfranil, 666
Norgesic, 1340
Norgesic Forte, 1340
norgestimate/ethinyl estradiol, 80
norgestrel, 80. *See also* ethinyl estradiod/norgestrel
Norinyl 1/35, 1340
Norinyl 1/50, 1340
Norinyl 1+ 35, 336
Norinyl 1+50, 336
Noritate, 817
normal human serum albumin, 118
Noroxin, 557
Norpace, 430
Norpace CR, 430
Norpramin, 391
Nor-Q D, 337
Nortrel 0.5/35, 336, 1340
Nortrel 1/35, 336, 1340
Nortrel 7/7/7, 337, 1340
nortriptyline, 897, 37. *See also* Color Insert.
Norvasc, 151
Norvir, 1073
Norzine, 1293
✤Novamedopa, 804
✤Novamoxin, 153
Novantrone, 835
✤Nova Rectal, 1287
✤Novasen, 1087
✤Novo-Alprazol, 131
✤Novo-Ampicillin, 164
✤Novo-Atenolol, 197
✤Novo-AZT, 1253
✤Novobetamet, 357
✤Novo-Carbamaz, 263
✤Novo-Chlorhydrate, 296
✤Novo-Chlorpromazine, 301
✤Novo-Cimetine, 623
✤Novo-Clopate, 325
✤Novo-Cloxin, 961
✤Novo-Diltazem, 418
✤Novodipam, 404
✤Novodipiradol, 428
✤Novo-Divalproex, 1212
✤Novodoxylin, 1155
✤Novo-Famotidine, 623
✤Novoferrogluc, 700

*Entries for **generic** names appear in **boldface type,** tradenames appear in regular type, with Canadian tradenames preceded by a maple leaf icon (✤), **CLASSIFICATIONS** appear in **BOLDFACE SMALL CAPS,** *Combination Drugs* appear in *italics,* and herbal products are preceded by a yin-yang icon (☯).

✦Novoferrosulfa, 700
✦Novoflupam, 571
✦Novo-Flurazine, 1295
✦Novo-Flurprofen, 1279
✦Novofolacid, 574
✦Novofumar, 700
✦Novo-Gesic, 107
✦Novo-Hydrazide, 434
✦Novohydrocort, 358
✦Novohydroxyzin, 644
✦Novo-Hylazin, 633
✦Novo-Levofloxacin, 557
Novolin 70/30, 678
✦Novolin ge NPH, 683
Novolin N, 683, 1380
Novolin R, 681, 1380
Novolog, 670, 1380
NovoLog Mix 70/30, 678
✦Novo-Lorazem, 762
✦Novo-Medrone, 776
✦Novo-Metformin, 793
✦Novo-Methacin, 674
✦Novo-metoprol, 814
✦Novo-Minocycline, 1155
✦Novo-Naprox, 864
✦Novo-Naprox Sodium DS, 864
✦Novo-Niacin, 877
✦Novonidazol, 817
✦Novo-Nifedin, 884
✦Novo-Nizatidine, 623
✦Novo-Norfloxacin, 557
✦Novopentobarb, 1287
✦Novo-Pen-VK, 958
✦Novo-Peridol, 613
✦Novo-Pheniram, 300
✦Novo-Pindol, 1288
✦Novo-Pirocam, 989
✦Novopoxide, 298
✦Novopramine, 666
✦Novopranol, 1027
✦Novo-Profen, 654
✦Novo-Ranitidine, 623
✦Novo-Ridazine, 1162
✦Novo-rythro, 498
✦Novo-Salmol, 120
✦Novo-Selegiline, 1098
✦Novosemide, 587
✦Novosorbide, 707
✦Novospiroton, 432
✦Novo-Sundac, 1128
✦Novo-Tamoxifen, 1138
✦Novo-Theophyl SR, 232
✦Novo-Timol, 1179
✦Novo-Tolmetin, 1294
✦Novo-Trimel, 1205
✦Novo-Trimel DS, 1205
✦Novo-Triolam, 1202
✦Novotriptyn, 149
✦Novo-Veramil, 1224
✦Novoxapam, 921
Noxafil, 993
NPH insulin (isophane insulin suspension), 683, 1380, 40, 80
NPH/regular insulin mixtures, 678, 1380, 40, 80
NSAIDS, **62.** *See also* NONSTEROIDAL ANTI-INFLAMMATORY AGENTS.
✦Nu-Alpraz, 131
✦Nu-Amoxi, 153
✦Nu-Ampi, 164
Nubain, 860, 1373
✦Nu-Cal, 256
✦Nu-Cephalex, 279
✦Nu-Cimet, 623
NUCLEOSIDE REVERSE TRANSCRIPTASE INHIBITORS, 60
✦Nu-Cloxi, 961
✦Nu-Cotrimox, 1205
✦Nu-Cotrimox DS, 1205
Nu-Diltiaz, 418
✦Nu-Divalproex, 1212
✦Nu-Doxycycline, 1155
✦Nu-Famotidine, 623
✦Nu-Flurbiprofen, 1279
✦Nu-Furosemide, 587
✦Nu-Hydro, 434
Nu-Ibuprofen, 654
✦Nu-Indo, 674
Nu-Iron, 701
NuLev, 646
✦Nu-Loraz, 762
NuLytely, 992, 1340
✦Nu-Medopa, 804
✦Nu-Naprox, 864
✦Nu-Nifed, 884
✦Nu-Pen-VK, 958
✦Nu-Pirox, 989
Nuprin, 654
✦Nu-Ranitidine, 623
Nu-Selegiline, 1098
Nu-Tears, 1351
Nu-Tears II, 1351
Nutracort, 358
Nutra Tear, 1351
✦Nu-Triazo, 1202
Nutropin, 607
Nutropin AQ, 607
NuvaRing, 337, 1340
✦Nu-Verap, 1224
✦Nyaderm, 181
Nydrazid, 705
Nyquil Children's Liquid, 1340
Nyquil Cold & Flu Liquicaps, 1340
Nyquil Cold & Flu Liquid, 1340
Nyquil Cough Liquid, 1340
Nyquil D Liquid, 1340
Nyquil Sinus Liquicaps, 1340
nystatin, 181, 184, 899, 43
Nystex, 899
Nystop, 181
Nytol, 424

O

Obi-Nix, 1288
OBY-CAP, 1288
OCL, 992
Octamide, 810
Octamide-PFS, 810
Octostim, 396
octreotide, 901, 1326, 41, 80
Ocu-Carpine, 1352
Ocu-Chlor, 1350
OcuClear, 1355
Ocufen, 1354
Ocuflox, 1350
OCULAR DECONGESTANTS/VASOCONSTRICTORS, 1355
Ocu-Mycin, 1350
Ocu-Pentolate, 1353
Ocu-Phrin, 1355
Ocusert Pilo, 1352
Ocu-Sul, 1350
Ocusulf, 1350
Ocu-Tropic, 1354
Ocu-Tropine, 1353
Ocu-Zoline, 1355
ofloxacin, 558, 1350, 49
Ogen, 512
Ogestrel, 1340
Ogestrel 28, 336
ointment, 892
olanzapine, 902, 58. *See also* Color Insert.
olmesartan, 177, 47
olopatadine, 1349, 45
olsalazine, 905
Olux, 357
Olux-E, 357
omalizumab, 906, 31
omega-3-acid ethyl esters, 907
omega-3 acid ethyl esters, 84
omeprazole, 908, 65
Omnaris, 347, 1326
Omnicef, 286
Omnipen, 164
OMS Concentrate, 843
Oncaspar, 952
Oncovin, 1229
ondansetron, 910, 42. *See also* Color Insert.
Onxol, 935
Ony-Clear, 181
Opana, 929, 1372
Opana ER, 929
Opcon-A Ophthalmic Solution, 1340
Ophthalgan, 1355
Ophthetic, 1349
Ophthochlor, 1350
✦Ophtho-Chloram, 1350
OPIOID AGONISTS, 92
OPIOID AGONISTS/ANTAGONISTS, 92
OPIOID ANALGESICS, 90
oprelvekin, 912

✤Opticrom, 1354
Opticyl, 1354
Optigene 3, 1355
OptiPranolol, 1351
Optivar, 1349
Orabase-HCA, 358
Oracea, 1155
Oracit, 1118
Oramorph SR, 843
Oraphen-PD, 107
Orapred, 350
Orazinc, 1256
Oretic, 434
Orfro, 915
Organidin NR, 610
orlistat, 913, 1325, 101
Ornex, 1340
✤OrnexDM, 403
Ornex Maximum Strength, 1340
orphenadrine, 915, 95. *See also* Color Insert.
Orphenate, 915
Orphengesic, 1340
Orphengesic forte, 1340
Ortho-Cept, 336, 1340
Orthoclone OKT3, 849
Ortho/CS, 1271
Ortho-Cyclen, 336, 1340
Ortho-Est, 512
Ortho Evra, 337
Ortho-Evra, 1340
Ortho-Novum 1/35, 336, 1340
Ortho-Novum 1/50, 336, 1340
Ortho-Novum 7/7/7, 337
Ortho-Novum 7/7/7–28, 1340
Ortho-Novum 10/11, 336
Ortho-Novum 10/11–28, 1340
Ortho-Prefest, 1340
Ortho Tri-Cyclen, 337, 1340
Ortho Tri-Cyclen Lo, 337, 1340
Orudis, 714
✤Orudis-E, 714
Orudis KT, 714
✤Orudis-SR, 714
Oruvail, 714
Os-Cal, 256
oseltamivir, 916, 66
Osmitrol, 770
OSMOTIC DIURETICS, 78
OSMOTICS, 1355, 83
✤Ostoforte, 1236
Ovcon 35, 336
Ovcon 50, 336
Ovcon-35, 1341
Ovcon-50, 1341
✤Ovol, 1110
✤Ovol-40, 1110
oxacillin, 961, 49. *See also* Color Insert.
oxaliplatin, 917, 53
oxaprozin, 919, 62, 90. *See also* Color Insert.
oxazepam, 921, 27, 93. *See also* Color Insert.
oxcarbazepine, 922, 1327, 35
oxiconazole, 181, 43
Oxistat, 181
OXYBUTYNIN, 924, 32. *See also* Color Insert.
oral, 924
transdermal, 924
Oxycet, 926
✤Oxycodan, 926
oxycodone, 926, 1372, 92. *See also* Color Insert.
oxycodone/acetaminophen, 926
oxycodone/aspirin, 926
oxycodone compound, 12
Oxycontin, 926
OxyFAST, 926
OxyIR, 926
oxymetazoline, 1355
oxymorphone, 929, 1372, 12, 92. *See also* Color Insert.
oxytocin, 931, 80. *See also* Color Insert.
Oxytrol, 924
Oysco, 256
Oyst-Cal, 256
Oystercal, 256

P

Pacerone, 145
☯Pacific Valerian, 1317
paclitaxel, 935, 53
paclitaxel protein-bound particles (albumin-bound), 935
Pain Doctor, 261
Pain-X, 261
✤Palafer, 700
palifermin, 938
paliperidone, 939, 58
☯Palmier Nain, 1315
palonosetron, 941, 1327, 42
Pamelor, 897
pamidronate, 942, 70
Pamprin Cramp Caplets, 1341
Pamprin Multi-Symptom, 1341
Panadol, 107
Pancoate, 943
Pancrease, 943
Pancrease MT 4, 943, 1341
Pancrease MT 10, 943, 1341
Pancrease MT 16, 943, 1341
Pancrease MT 20, 943, 1341
Pancrebarb MS-8, 943
pancrelipase, 943
pancuronium, 945, 12. *See also* Color Insert.
Pandel, 358
panitumumab, 947, 1327
Panixine, 279
Panretin, 1269
✤Pantoloc, 948
pantoprazole, 948, 1325, 65. *See also* Color Insert.
Paracaine, 1349
paracetamol, 107
Paraflex, 305
Parafon Forte DSC, 305
Paralube, 1351
Paraplatin, 265
✤Paraplatin-AQ, 265
Parcopa, 743
Parcopa 10/100, 1341
Parcopa 25/100, 1341
Parcopa 25/250, 1341
parenteral), 12
paricalcitol, 1236, 100
✤Pariet, 1051
Parlodel, 1272
Parnate, 839
paroxetine, 1325, 1327. *See also* Color Insert.
paroxetine hydrochloride, 949, 27, 37
paroxetine mesylate, 950, 27, 37
Patanol, 1349
✤Paveral, 330
Pavulon, 945
Paxil, 949
Paxil CR, 949
PCE, 498
PediaCare Allergy Formula, 300
PediaCare Children's Fever, 654
Pediacare Children's Multisymptom Cold Liquid, 1341
Pediacare Children's NightRest Multi-Symptom Cold Liquid, 1341
PediaCare Infants' Decongestant Drops, 1033
Pediapred, 350
Pediatric Nasal Decongestant, 1033
Pediazole Suspension, 1341

*Entries for **generic** names appear in **boldface type**, tradenames appear in regular type, with Canadian tradenames preceded by a maple leaf icon (✤), **CLASSIFICATIONS** appear in **BOLDFACE SMALL CAPS**, *Combination Drugs* appear in *italics*, and herbal products are preceded by a yin-yang icon (☯).

PediCare Infant's Long Acting Cough Drops, 403
PedvaxHIB, 1383
pegaptanib, 1285
pegaspargase, 952, 52
Pegasys, 688
pegfilgrastim, 954
peginterferon alpha-2a, 688
peginterferon alpha-2b, 688
Pegintron, 688
PEG-l-asparaginase, 952
Peglyte, 992
pemetrexed, 955, 52
pemirolast, 1354
pemoline, 1328
Penbritin, 164
penbutolol, 47, 68
penciclovir, 957, 66
Penecort, 358
penicillamine, 1286, 62
Penicilline V, 958
penicillin G, 958, 49. *See also* Color Insert.
PENICILLINS, PENICILLINASE RESISTANT, 961
PENICILLINS, 958, 49
penicillin V, 958, 49
Penlac, 181
Pentacarinat, 964
Pentam 300, 964
pentamidine, 964. *See also* Color Insert.
Pentamycetin, 1350
Pentasa, 789
Pentazine, 1017
pentazocine, 966, 1373, 12, 92. *See also* Color Insert.
pentetate calcium trisodium, 1286
pentetate zinc trisodium, 1287
pentobarbital, 1287, 35. *See also* Color Insert.
Pentolair, 1353
pentoxifylline, 969
Pepcid, 623
Pepcid AC, 623
Pepcid AC Acid Controller, 623
Pepcid Complete, 1341
Pepcid RPD, 623
Peptic Relief, 225
Pepto-Bismol, 225
Pepto Diarrhea Control, 756
Percocet, 926
Percocet 2.5/325, 1341
Percocet 5/325, 1341
Percocet 7.5/325, 1341
Percocet 7.5/500, 1341
Percocet 10/325, 1341
Percocet 10/650, 1341
Percodan, 926, 1341
Percogesic, 1341
Percolone, 926
Perdiem, 1035
Perforomist, 577
pergolide, 1328. *See also* Color Insert.
Periactin, 367. *See also* Color Insert.
Peri-Colace, 1341
Peridol, 613
perindopril, 170, 47. *See also* Color Insert.
Periostat, 1155
PERIPHERALLY ACTING ANTIADRENERGICS, 47
Permapen, 958
Permax, 1328
permethrin, 970
Persantine, 428
Persantine IV, 428
Pertofrane, 391
Pertussin Cough Suppressant, 403
Pertussin CS, 403
Pertussin ES, 403
pethidine, 784
Pexeva, 950, 1325, 1327
Pfizerpen, 958
Pharma-Cort, 358
Phazyme, 1110
Phenadoz, 1017
Phenazo, 971
phenazopyridine, 971, 88
phenelzine, 839, 37
Phenergan, 1017
Phenetron, 300
phenobarbital, 972, 35, 93. *See also* Color Insert.
PHENOTHIAZINES, 42, 58
Phentercot, 1288
phentermine, 1288, 101
phentolamine, 975
Phentride, 1288
phenylalanine mustard, 781
phenylephrine, 1355. *See also* Color Insert.
Phenytek, 976
phenytoin, 976, 29, 35. *See also* Color Insert.
Pheryl-E, 1240
Phillips Liqui-Gels, 442
Phillips Magnesia Tablets, 766
Phillips Milk of Magnesia, 766
PHL-Divalproex, 1212
PHL-Doxycycline, 1155
PHL-Hydrochlorothiazide, 434
PHL-Nizatidine, 623
PHL-Ranitidine, 623
PHL-Valproic Acid, 1212
PhosLo, 256
phosphate/biphosphate, 980, 83
phosphate supplements, 85
Phospholine Iodide, 1352
Phrenilin, 247, 1341
Phrenilin Forte, 247, 1341
Phrenilin with Caffeine and Codeine, 1341
Phyllocontin, 232
phytoestrogen, 1298, 1300
phytonadione, 982, 100. *See also* Color Insert.
Pilocar, 1352
pilocarpine, 1352
pilocarpine (oral), 984
Pilopine, 1352
Piloptic, 1352
Pilostat, 1352
Pima, 694
pimecrolimus, 985, 81
pindolol, 1288, 47, 68
Pink Bismuth, 225
pioglitazone, 986, 40
piperacillin, 49. *See also* Color Insert.
piperacillin/tazobactam, 987, 49. *See also* Color Insert.
piperazine estrone sulfate, 512
pirbuterol, 30, 71
piroxicam, 989, 62, 90. *See also* Color Insert.
Pitocin, 931, 13
Pitressin, 1220, 13
Pitrex, 181
Plan B, 337
Plaquenil, 642
Plasbumin, 118
PLATELET ADHESION INHIBITORS, 55
PLATELET AGGREGATION INHIBITORS, 55
Platinol, 310
Platinol-AQ, 310
Plavix, 324
Plenaxis, 1267
Plendil, 530
Pletal, 309, 1326
PMS-ASA, 1087
PMS-Bismuth Subsalicylate, 225
PMS-Cephalexin, 279
PMS-Chloral Hydrate, 296
PMS-Cimetidine, 623
PMS-Cyproheptadine, 367
PMS Dexamethasone, 1352
PMS-Diazepam, 404
PMS-Dicitrate, 1118
PMS-Dimenhydrinate, 420
PMS-Divalproex, 1212
PMS-Doxycycline, 1155
PMS Egozinc, 1256
PMS Ferrous Sulfate, 700
PMS-Fluphenazine, 568
PMS-Furosemide, 587
PMS Haloperidol, 613
PMS-Hydrochlorothiazide, 434
PMS Hydromorphone, 640
PMS Isoniazid, 705
PMS-Isosorbide, 707
PMS Lindane, 751
PMS-Methylphenidate, 808

🍁PMS-Minocycline, 1155
🍁PMS-Nizatidine, 623
🍁PMS-Norfloxacin, 558
🍁PMS-Nystatin, 899
🍁PMS-Piroxicam, 989
🍁pms Propranolol, 1027
🍁PMS Pyrazinamide, 1036
🍁PMS-Ranitidine, 623
🍁PMS-Sodium Polystyrene Sulfonate, 1119
🍁PMS-Sulfasalazine, 1126
🍁PMS-Theophylline, 232
🍁PMS Thioridazine, 1162
🍁PMS-Trifluoperazine, 1295
🍁PMS-Trihexyphenidyl, 1295
🍁PMS-Valproic Acid, 1212
Pneumococcal 7-valent conjugate vaccine, 1385
Pneumococcal vaccine, polyvalent, 1389
🍁Pneumopent, 964
Pneumovax 23, 1389
Pnu-Imune 23, 1389
Podactin, 181
PODOPHYLLOTOXIN DERIVATIVES, 53
Polio vaccine, inactivated, 1383
Poliovax, 1383
polycarbophil, 1289, 41, 83
Polycillin, 164
Polycitra Syrup, 1341
polyethylene glycol, 991, 83
polyethylene glycol/electrolyte, 992, 83
Poly-Hist DM Syrup, 1341
Polysporin Topical Ointment/Powder, 1341
Polytrim Ophthalmic Solution, 1341
Pontocaine, 1349
Portalac, 721
Portia, 1341
Portia-28, 336
posaconazole, 993, 43
Posture, 256
Potasalan, 996
potassium acetate, 996, 85
potassium and sodium phosphates, 994, 85
potassium bicarbonate, 996, 85
potassium bicarbonate/potassium chloride, 996, 85
potassium bicarbonate/potassium citrate, 996, 85
potassium chloride, 996, 13, 85. *See also* Color Insert.
potassium chloride/potassium bicarbonate/potassium citrate, 996, 85
potassium gluconate, 996, 85
potassium gluconate/potassium chloride, 996, 85
potassium gluconate/potassium citrate, 996, 85
potassium iodide, 694
potassium phosphate, 1289. *See also* Color Insert.
POTASSIUM PHOSPHATES, 1289, 12, 85
🍁Potassium-Rougier, 996
potassium salts, 85
🍁Potassium Sandoz, 996
POTASSIUM-SPARING DIURETICS, 78
POTASSIUM SUPPLEMENTS, 996, 12. *See also* Color Insert.
🍁Poxi, 298
pramipexole, 1000, 54. *See also* Color Insert.
pramlintide, 1001, 12, 40, 80. *See also* Color Insert.
Pramosone Topical Cream/Lotion/Ointment, 1341
Prandin, 1058
Pravachol, 629
pravastatin, 629, 84
prazosin, 1003, 47
Precedex, 1277
Precose, 104
Pred ForteF, 1353
Pred Mild, 1353
prednicarbate, 358, 76
prednisoLONE, 350, 1353, 31, 62, 76. *See also* Color Insert.
predniSONE, 350, 31, 62, 76. *See also* Color Insert.
Prefrin, 1355
pregabalin, 1005, 35
Prelone, 350
Premarin, 510
Premphase, 1341
🍁*Premplus 0.625/2.5, 1341*
🍁*Premplus 0.625/5, 1342*
Prempro 0.3/1.5, 1342
Prempro 0.45/1.5, 1342
Prempro 0.625/2.5, 1342
Prempro 0.625/5, 1342
Premsyn PMS, 1342
Prepidil Endocervical Gel, 422
🍁Pressyn, 1220
Prevacid, 727
Prevalite, 306
🍁Prevex, 357
Prevex HC, 358
Previfem, 336
Prevnar, 1385
Prevpac, 1342
Prezista, 381, 1326
Prialt, 1252
Priftin, 1291
Prilosec, 908
Prilosec OTC, 908
Primacor, 828
Primatene, 480
Primatene Tablets, 1342
Primaxin, 664
Primaxin 250 mg I.V. For Injection, 1342
Primaxin 500 mg I.V. For Injection, 1342
Primsol, 1203
Principen, 164
Prinivil, 170
Prinzide 10/12.5, 1342
Prinzide 20/12.5, 1342
Prinzide 20/25, 1342
Probalan, 1006
🍁Probanthel, 1290
Pro-Banthine, 1290
probenecid, 1006
procainamide, 1008, 13, 29. *See also* Color Insert.
procaine penicillin G, 958, 49
Pro-Cal-Sof, 442
procarbazine, 1010, 52
Procardia, 884
Procardia XL, 884
Prochieve, 1015
prochlorperazine, 1012, 42, 58. *See also* Color Insert.
Procrit, 487
Proctocort, 358
Proctofoam-HC Rectal Foam, 1342
🍁Procytox, 361
🍁Prodiem, 1035
Prodium, 971
progesterone, 1015, 80
PROGESTINS, 53
Prograf, 1134
Pro-Lax, 1035
Proleukin, 1268
Prolixin, 568
Prolixin Decanoate, 568
Proloprim, 1203
Promacot, 1017
Promet, 1017

*Entries for **generic** names appear in **boldface type,** tradenames appear in regular type, with Canadian tradenames preceded by a maple leaf icon (🍁), **CLASSIFICATIONS** appear in **BOLDFACE SMALL CAPS**, *Combination Drugs* appear in *italics,* and herbal products are preceded by a yin-yang icon (☯).

promethazine, 1017, 42, 45, 93. *See also* Color Insert.
Prometrium, 1015
Pronestyl, 1008
Propacet, 1024
propafenone, 1020, 29
propantheline, 1290, 32, 65. *See also* Color Insert.
proparacaine, 1349
Propecia, 548
Propine, 1356
propofol, 1022
PROPOXYPHENE, 1024, 92. *See also* Color Insert.
propoxyphene/aspirin/caffeine, 1024
propoxyphene hydrochloride, 1024
propoxyphene hydrochloride/aspirin/caffeine, 1024
propoxyphene napsylate, 1024
propoxyphene napsylate/acetaminophen, 1024
propoxyphene napsylate/aspirin, 1024
Propoxyphene with APAP, 1024
propranolol, 1026, 1327, 12, 26, 29, 47, 68, 99. *See also* Color Insert.
propylthiouracil, 1030
Propyl-Thyracil, 1030
Proquin XR, 557
Prorex, 1017
Proscar, 548
PROSTAGLANDIN AGONIST, **1355**
Prostigmin, 871
Prostin E Vaginal Suppository, 422
protamine sulfate, 1032. *See also* Color Insert.
PROTEASE INHIBITORS, **60**
Protilase, 943
Protonix, 948, 1325
Protonix I.V, 948
PROTON-PUMP INHIBITORS, **65**
Protopic, 1134
Protostat, 817
Protrin, 1342
Protrin DF, 1342
Proventil, 120
Proventil HFA, 120
Provera, 776
Provera Pak, 776
Provigil, 837
Prozac, 565, 1326
Prozac Weekly, 565
prussian blue (insoluble), 1290
pseudoephedrine, 1033
Psorcon, 357
psyllium, 1035, 83
PTU, 1030
Pulmicort, 343
Pulmophylline, 232
Purinol, 128
purple coneflower, 1301
P-V-Tussin, 1341
Pylera, 1342
pyrazinamide, 1036, 63
Pyrethrum parthenium, 1303
Pyri, 1039
Pyridiate, 971
Pyridium, 971
Pyridium Plus, 971
pyridostigmine, 1037
pyridoxine, 1039, 100
pyrimethamine, 1041

Q

Q-Naftate, 181
quadravalent human papillomavirus (types 6, 11, 16, 18) recombinant vaccine, 98
Qualaquin, 1047
Questran, 306
Questran Light, 306
quetiapine, 1043, 1327, 58. *See also* Color Insert.
Quibron-T, 232
quinapril, 170, 47. *See also* Color Insert.
Quinaretic 10/12.5, 1342
Quinaretic 20/12.5, 1342
Quinaretic 20/25, 1342
QUINIDINE, 1045
gluconate, 1045, 29
sulfate, 1045, 29
quinine, 1047
quinupristin/dalfopristin, 1049, 49
Quixin, 1350
QVAR, 343

R

rabeprazole, 1051, 65
Radiogardase, 1290
Radix angelicae gigantis, 1300
Ralivia, 1196
raloxifene, 1052, 70
raltegravir, 1324, 60
ramelteon, 1053, 93
ramipril, 170, 47. *See also* Color Insert.
Ranexa, 1054
Raniclor, 282
ranitidine, 623, 65. *See also* Color Insert.
ranolazine, 1054, 26
Rapamune, 1110, 1327
Raptiva, 1278
rasagiline, 1055
rasburicase, 1057
Ratio-Diltiazem CD, 418
Ratio-Doxycycline, 1155
Ratio-Minocycline, 1155
Ratio-MPA, 776
Ratio-Ranitidine, 623
Ratio-Valprox, 1212
rattle root, 1298
rattle top, 1298
rattleweed, 1298
Razadyne, 592
Razadyne ER, 592
Rebetol, 1062
Rebetron, 1342
Rebif, 692
Reclast, 1259
Reclipsen, 336
Reclomide, 810
Recombivax HB, 1384, 1388
red ginseng, 1308
red sunflower, 1301
Redutemp, 107
Refludan, 733
Refresh, 1351
Refresh PM, 1351
Regitine, 975
Reglan, 810
Regonol, 1037
Regranex, 1271
regular insulin (insulin injection), 40, 1380
Regulax-SS, 442
Regulex, 442
Reguloid Natural, 1035
Relafen, 855
Relaxazone, 305
Relenza, 1251
Reliable Gentle Laxative, 223
Relpax, 470
Remeron, 830
Remeron Soltabs, 830
Remicade, 676
Remular, 305
Remular-S, 305
Renagel, 1106
Renedil, 530
Renese-R, 1342
renshen, 1308
Renvela, 1325
repaglinide, 1058, 40
Repan, 247
Repap CF, 247
Reprexain 2.5/200, 1342
Reprexain 5/200, 1342
Reprexain 7.5/200, 1342
Reprexain 10/200, 1342
Requip, 1081
Rescriptor, 1276
Resectisol, 770
Respabist, 1342
Respaire-60 SR, 1342
Respaire-120 SR, 1342
Restasis, 1354
Restoril, 1143, 1327
Resyl, 610
Retavase, 1164
reteplase, 1164, 97

Retrovir, 1253
Revatio, 1108
Rev-Eyes, 1349
🍁Revimine, 448
Reyataz, 195, 1325
R-Gel, 261
Rheumatrex, 801
🍁Rhinalar, 347
Rhinocort Aqua, 347
Rh$_o$(D) globulin IV, 98
Rh$_o$(D) globulin microdose IM, 98
Rh$_o$(D) IMMUNE GLOBULIN, 1060
Rh$_o$(D) immune globulin IV, 1060
Rh$_o$(D) immune globulin microdose IM, IV, 1060
Rh$_o$(D) immune globulin microdose IM, 1060
Rh$_o$(D) immune globulin standard dose IM, 1060, 98
🍁Rhodis, 714
RhoGAM, 1060
Rhophylac, 1060
rHu GM-CSF (recombinant human granulocyte/macrophage colony-stimulating factor), 1093
Rhulicort, 358
ribavirin, 1062, 66
riboflavin, 1291, 100
RidaPainHP, 261
Ridenol, 107
RID Maximum Strength Shampoo, 1342
rifabutin, 1065
Rifadin, 1066
Rifamate, 1342
rifampin, 1066, 63. *See also* Color Insert.
rifapentine, 1291, 63
Rifater, 1342
rifaximin, 1068, 49
Rimactane, 1066
rimexolone, 1353, 76
Riomet, 793
Riopan Plus, 765
🍁Riopan Plus Double Strength, 765
🍁Riphenidate, 808
risedronate, 1069, 1325, 70
Risperdal, 1070
Risperdal Consta, 1070
Risperdal M-TAB, 1070
risperidone, 1070, 58. *See also* Color Insert.
Ritalin, 808
Ritalin LA, 808
Ritalin-SR, 808
ritonavir, 1073, 60. *See also* Color Insert.
Rituxan, 1075
rituximab, 1075, 53
🍁Riva-Minocycline, 1155
🍁Rivanase AQ, 347
🍁Riva-Norfloxacin, 558
🍁Riva-Ranitidine, 623
🍁Rivasa, 1087
rivastigmine, 1077, 24. *See also* Color Insert.
🍁Rivotril, 320
rizatriptan, 1079, 99
RMS, 843
🍁*Robaxacet, 1342*
🍁*Robaxacet-8, 1342*
🍁*Robaxacet Extra Strength, 1342*
Robaxin, 799
🍁Robidex, 403
🍁Robidrine, 1033
Robinul, 603
Robinul-Forte, 603
Robitussin, 610
Robitussin Cold & Congestion Tablets, 1342
Robitussin Cough, Cold & Flu Nighttime Liquid, 1343
Robitussin Cough & Allergy Liquid, 1342
Robitussin Cough & Cold CF Liquid, 1342
Robitussin Cough & Cold Long-Acting Liquid, 1342
Robitussin Cough & Cold Pediatric Drops, 1342
Robitussin Cough & Congestion Liquid, 1343
Robitussin Cough Calmers, 403
Robitussin CoughGels, 403
Robitussin-DM Cough Liquid, 1343
Robitussin Maximum Strength Cough Suppressant, 403
Robitussin Nighttime Cough & Cold Liquid, 1343
Robitussin Nighttime Pediatric Cough & Cold Liquid, 1343
Robitussin Pediatric, 403
Robitussin Pediatric Cough & Cold Long-Acting Liquid, 1343
Robitussin-PE Head & Chest Congestion Liquid, 1343
Rocaltrol, 1236
Rocephin, 287
Rodex, 1039
🍁RO-Dexasone, 1352
🍁Rofact, 1066
Roferon, 1328
🍁Rogitine, 975
Rolaids Calcium Rich, 256
Rolaids Extra Strength Plus Gas Relief Softchews, 1343
Rolaids Extra Strength Tablets, 1343
Rolaids Multi-Symptom Tablets, 1343
Rolaids Regular Tablets, 1343
Romazicon, 556
Rondec DM Drops, 1343
Rondec DM Syrup, 1343
Rondec Oral Drops, 1343
Rondec Syrup, 1343
ropinirole, 1081, 54
ropivacaine, 478
rosiglitazone, 1082, 40
☯Rosin rose, 1316
rosuvastatin, 629, 84
rotigotine transdermal system, 1084, 54
🍁Roubac, 1205
Rowasa, 789
Roxanol, 843
Roxanol Rescudose, 843
Roxanol-T, 843
Roxicet, 926, 1343
Roxicet 5/500, 1343
Roxicet Oral Solution, 1343
Roxicodone, 926
Roxilox, 926
Roychlor, 996
Rozerem, 1053
Rubex, 454
Rubramin PC, 1233
☯rudbeckia, 1301
Rulox, 765
Rum-K, 996
Ru-Tuss DM Syrup, 1343
Rynatan, 1343
Rynatan Pediatric Suspension, 1343
Rynatuss, 1343
🍁Rythmodan, 430
🍁Rythmodan-LA, 430
Rythmol, 1020

S

S-2, 480
☯Sabal, 1315
☯Sabal Fructus, 1315

*Entries for **generic** names appear in **boldface type,** tradenames appear in regular type, with Canadian tradenames preceded by a maple leaf icon (🍁), **CLASSIFICATIONS** appear in **BOLDFACE SMALL CAPS**, *Combination Drugs* appear in *italics,* and herbal products are preceded by a yin-yang icon (☯).

S-adenosylmethionine, 1314
Saizen, 607
Salagen, 984
Salazopyrin, 1126
salbutamol, 120
Salflex, 1087
Salgesic, 1087
SALICYLATES, 1087, 88
SALINES, 83
salisburia adiantifolia, 1306
salmeterol, 1090, 30, 71
Salofalk, 789
salsalate, 1087, 59, 88
Salsitab, 1087
SAMe, 1314
sampson root, 1301
Sanctura, 1207
Sanctura XR, 1207
Sandimmune, 364
Sandostatin, 901, 1326
Sandostatin LAR, 901
Sans-Acne, 498
Santa Maria, 1303
saquinavir, 1092, 60
Sarafem, 565
sargramostim, 1093
S.A.S, 1126
saw palmetto, 1315
Saw Palmetto Berry, 1315
Scabene, 751
scopolamine, 1096, 1353, 32, 42. *See also* Color Insert.
Scot-Tussin Allergy DM, 424
Scot-Tussin DM Maximum Strength Liquid, 1343
Scot-tussin Expectorant, 610
Scot-Tussin Original Liquid, 1343
Scot-Tussin Senior Liquid, 1343
scurvy root, 1301
SD-Deprenyl, 1098
Seasonale, 337, 1343
Seasonique, 337, 1343
SECOND-GENERATION CEPHALOSPORINS, 282, 49
Sectral, 105
Sedapap, 247, 1343
SEDATIVE/HYPNOTICS, 92
Sedatuss, 403
SELECTIVE ESTROGEN RECEPTOR MODULATORS, 70
SELECTIVE SEROTONIN REUPTAKE INHIBITORS (SSRIS), 27, 37
selegiline, 1098, 54. *See also* Color Insert.
selegiline transdermal, 1099, 37
Selestoject, 350
Seloken-ZOK, 814
Selzentry, 772
Semprex-D, 1343
Sena-Gen, 1101
Senexon, 1101
sennosides, 1101, 83
Senokot, 1101
Senokot-S, 1343
SenokotXTRA, 1101
Seno Sol-SS, 1343
Sensipar, 1274
Sensorcaine, 478
Septra, 1205, 1343
Septra DS, 1205, 1343
Serax, 921
Serenoa repens, 1315
Serevent, 1090
Seroquel, 1043, 1327
Seroquel XR, 1043
Serostim, 607
Serostim LQ, 607
sertaconazole, 1102, 43
sertraline, 1103, 1327, 37. *See also* Color Insert.
Serutan, 1035
Serzone, 869
sevelamer, 1106, 1325
Shohl's Solution modified, 1118
Siblin, 1035
sibutramine, 1106
Silace, 442
Siladril, 424
Silafed Syrup, 1343
Silapap, 107
sildenafil, 1108, 1327
Silfedrine, 1033
Silphen, 424
Siltussin DAS, 610
Siltussin SA, 610
Silybin, 1313
Silymarin, 1313
Simcor, 1325
simethicone, 1109
Simply Cough, 403
Simply Stuffy, 1033
Simron, 700
Simulect, 215
simvastatin, 629, 84
Sinemet, 743
Sinemet 10/100, 1344
Sinemet 25/100, 1344
Sinemet 25/250, 1344
Sinemet CR, 743
Sinemet CR 25-100, 1344
Sinemet CR 50-200, 1344
Sine-Off Cough/Cold Medicine, 1344
Sine-Off Maximum Strength Non-Drowsy Caplets, 1344
Sine-Off Sinus/Cold Medicine, 1344
Sinequan, 452
Singulair, 841, 1326
Sinustop, 1033
Sinutab Non-Drying Caplets, 1344
Sinutab Sinus Caplets, 1344
sirolimus, 1110, 1327, 81
sitagliptin, 1112, 1327, 39
Skelaxin, 792
SKELETAL MUSCLE RELAXANTS, 94
Skelid, 1293
Sleep-Eze 3, 424
Sleepwell 2-night, 424
Slo-Mag, 766
Slo-Niacin, 877
Slo-Salt, 1116
Slow FE, 700
Slow-K, 996
SMZ/TMP, 1205
Snooze Fast, 424
Soda Mint, 1114
sodium bicarbonate, 1114, 65, 85. *See also* Color Insert.
sodium chloride, 12, 85. *See also* Color Insert.
sodium chloride (IV/oral), 1116
sodium citrate and citric acid, 1118, 85
Sodium Diuril, 434
sodium ferric gluconate complex, 701, 25
sodium phosphate, 1291, 85
sodium polystyrene sulfonate, 1119
sodium salicylate, 1087, 59, 88
Sodium Sulamyd, 1350
Soflax, 442
Solage Topical Liquid, 1344
Solaraze, 408
Solarcaine Aloe Extra Burn Relief, 746
Solazine, 1295
Solfoton, 972
Solia, 336
solifenacin, 1121, 32
Solodyn, 1155
Soltamox, 1138
Solu-Cortef, 350
Solu-Medrol, 350
Soma, 268
Soma Compound, 1344
somatrem (recombinant), 80
somatropin, 1327
somatropin (recombinant), 607, 80
Sominex, 424
Somnol, 571
Sonata, 1250
sorafenib, 1327
Sorine, 1122
Sotacor, 1122
sotalol, 1122, 29, 68. *See also* Color Insert.
Span-FF, 700
Spasmoban, 410
Spectazole, 181
Spectracef, 287
Spectro-Caine, 1349
Spectro-Chlor, 1350
Spectro-Cyl, 1354
Spectro-Genta, 1350

Spectro-Homatropine, 1353
Spectro-Pentolate, 1353
Spectro-Sulf, 1350
🍁Spersacarpine, 1352
🍁Spersadex, 1352
🍁Spersaphrine, 1355
Spiriva, 1182, 1327
spironolactone, 432, 78
Sporanox, 710
Sprintec, 336, 1344
SPS, 1119
☯squawroot, 1298
Sronyx, 336
SSKI, 694
Stadol, 249, 1373
Stadol NS, 249
Stalevo 50, 1344
Stalevo 100, 1344
Stalevo 150, 1344
Starlix, 868
🍁Statex, 843
Staticin, 498
stavudine, 1292, 60
Stelazine, 1295
🍁Stemetil, 1012
STERILE BUFFERED ISOTONIC SOLUTIONS/OINTMENTS, 1351
Sterapred, 350
🍁Stieprox, 181
Stimate, 396
STIMULANT LAXATIVES, 83
☯St. John's wort (Hypericum Perforatum), 1316
St. Joseph Adult Chewable Aspirin, 1087
Stool Softener, 442
STOOL SOFTENERS, 83
Storzolamide, 109
Strattera, 200
Streptase, 1164
streptokinase, 1164, 97
streptomycin, 140, 49
Striant, 1152
Strifon Forte DSC, 305
strong iodine solution, 694
Sublimaze, 540
sublingual, 892
Suboxone N2, 1344
Suboxone N8, 1344
Subutex, 238
succimer, 1292
sucralfate, 1124, 65
Sucrets Cough Control Formula, 403
Sudafed, 1033
Sudafed 12 Hour, 1033
Sudafed Children's Cough & Cold Liquid, 1344
Sudafed Childrens's Non-Drowsy, 1033
Sudafed Maximum Strength Sinus Nighttime, 1344
Sudafed Non-Drowsy Maximum Strength, 1033
Sudafed Non-Drying Sinus Liquicaps, 1344
Sudafed PE Maximum Strength Nighttime Cold, 1344
Sudafed PE Multi-Symptom Severe Cold, 1344
Sudafed PE Sinus Headache, 1344
Sudafed Sinus & Allergy, 1344
Sudafed Sinus & Cold Liquicaps, 1344
Sudal 12, 1344
Sudodrin, 1033
Sular, 889, 1325
sulconazole, 181, 43
🍁Sulcrate, 1124
Sulf, 1350
sulfacetamide, 1350
Sulfacet-R Topical Lotion, 1344
Sulfair, 1350
Sulfamide, 1350
sulfasalazine, 1126, 62
Sulfatrim, 1205
Sulfatrim DS, 1205
🍁Sulfex, 1350
Sulfolax, 442
SULFONYLUREAS, 40
sulindac, 1128, 62, 90
Sulten, 1350
sumatriptan, 1129, 99
Sumycin, 1155
sunitinib, 1131
Sunkist, 1271
SuperChar Aqueous, 1268
🍁Supeudol, 926
Suprax, 287
suprofen, 90
Surfak, 442
Surpass, 256
Surpass Extra Strength, 256
Sus-Phrine, 480
Sustiva, 469
Sutent, 1131
Syllact, 1035
Symbicort, 1344
Symbyax 3/25, 1344
Symbyax 6/25, 1344
Symbyax 6/50, 1344
Symbyax 12/25, 1344
Symbyax 12/50, 1344
Symlin, 1001
Symmetrel, 135
SYMPATHOMIMETICS, 1356
Synacort, 358
Synalar, 357
Synalgos-DC, 1344
🍁Synamol, 357
Synarel, 858
🍁Syn-Clonazepam, 320
🍁Syn-Diltiazem, 418
Synercid, 1049
Synercid Powder for Injection, 1344
🍁Synflex, 864
🍁Synflex DS, 864
🍁Syn-Nadolol, 856
🍁Syn-Pindolol, 1288
Synthroid, 1169
Syntocinon, 931
SYSTEMIC, 43, 45

T

T_3, 1169
T_3/T_4, 1169
T_4, 1169
Taclonex Ointment, 1344
tacrine, 1133, 24
TACROLIMUS, 1134. *See also* Color Insert.
oral, IV, 1134, 81
topical, 1134, 81
tadalafil, 1137, 1327
Tagamet, 623, 1325
Tagamet HB, 623
☯Tagara, 1317
Talacen, 1344
Talwin, 966, 1373
Talwin NX, 966, 1344
Tambocor, 550
Tamiflu, 916
🍁Tamofen, 1138
🍁Tamone, 1138
🍁Tamoplex, 1138
tamoxifen, 1138, 52
tamsulosin, 1140
☯Tanaceti parthenii, 1303
☯Tang Kuei, 1300
☯Tan Kue Bai Zhi, 1300
Tapanol, 107
Tapazole, 798
Tarceva, 495
Tarka 1/240, 1344
Tarka 2/180, 1345
Tarka 2/240, 1345

*Entries for **generic** names appear in **boldface type**, tradenames appear in regular type, with Canadian tradenames preceded by a maple leaf icon (🍁), **CLASSIFICATIONS** appear in **BOLDFACE SMALL CAPS**, *Combination Drugs* appear in *italics*, and herbal products are preceded by a yin-yang icon (☯).

Tarka 4/240, 1345
Tasigna, 1323
Tasmar, 1188
Tavist ND, 760
TAXOIDS, 53
Taxol, 935
Taxotere, 439
Tazicef, 287
✤*Tazocin for Injection 2.25 g, 1345*
✤*Tazocin for Injection 3.375 g, 1345*
✤*Tazocin for Injection 4.5 g, 1345*
Taztia XT, 418
3TC, 723
Tdap, 1383, 1389
T-Diet, 1288
Tear Drop, 1351
TearGard, 1351
Teargen, 1351
Tearisol, 1351
Tears Naturale, 1351
Tears Naturale Free, 1351
Tears Naturale II, 1351
Tears Plus, 1351
Tears Renewed, 1351
✤Tebrazid, 1036
✤Tecnal, 247
tegaserod, 1328
Tegretol, 263, 1326
✤Tegretol CR, 263
Tegretol-XR, 263
Tekturna, 126
Teldrin, 300
Telechlor, 300
telithromycin, 1141, 49
telmisartan, 177, 47. *See also* Color Insert.
temazepam, 1143, 1327, 93. *See also* Color Insert.
Temodar, 1292
Temovate, 357
Temovate E, 357
temozolomide, 1292, 52
Tempra, 107
temsirolimus, 1324, 52
Tencon, 247
tenecteplase, 1164, 97
Ten-K, 996
tenofovir disoproxil fumarate, 1144, 60
Tenoretic 50, 1345
Tenoretic 100, 1345
Tenormin, 197
Tequin, 1327
Teramine, 1288
Terazol-3, 184
Terazol-7, 184
terazosin, 1145, 47. *See also* Color Insert.
terbinafine, 181, 1147, 1325, 43
terbutaline, 1148, 30, 71. *See also* Color Insert.
terconazole, 184, 43
✤Terfluzine, 1295
Teril, 263
teriparatide, 1151, 1327, 80
Terra-Cortril Ophthalmic Suspension, 1345
Terramycin with Polymyxin B Sulfate Ophthalmic Ointment, 1345
Tessalon, 217
Testopel, 1152
TESTOSTERONE, 1152
  buccal system, mucoadhesive, 1152, 80
  cypionate, 1152, 80
  enanthate, 1152, 80
  pellets, 1152, 80
  transdermal, 1152, 80
Tetanus-diphtheria, 1389
Tetanus toxoid, 1383, 1389
Tetcaine, 1349
tetracaine, 1349
TETRACYCLIC ANTIDEPRESSANTS, 37
TETRACYCLINES, 1155, 49
tetrahydrozoline, 1355
Tetrazine, 1355
Teveten, 177
Teveten HCT 600/12.5, 1345
Teveten HCT 600/25, 1345
Tev-Tropin, 607
Texacort, 358
thalidomide, 1158, 81
Thalitone, 434
Thalomid, 1158
Theo-24, 232
Theochron, 232
theophylline, 232, 15, 71
Thera-Flu, Cold & Sore Throat Hot Liquid, 1345
Thera-Flu, Daytime Cough & Cold Thin Strips, 1345
Thera-Flu, Daytime Severe Cold Caplets, 1345
Thera-Flu, Daytime Warming Relief Syrup, 1345
Thera-Flu, Flu & Chest Congestion Hot Liquid, 1345
Thera-Flu, Flu & Sore Throat Hot Liquid, 1345
Thera-Flu, Flu & Sore Throat Relief Syrup, 1345
Thera-Flu, Nighttime Cough & Cold Thin Strips, 1345
Thera-Flu, Nighttime Severe Cold Caplets, 1345
Thera-Flu, Nighttime Warming Relief Syrup, 1345
Thera-Flu Cold & Cough Hot Liquid, 1345
Thera-Flu Daytime Severe Cold Hot Liquid, 1345
Thera-Flu Nighttime Severe Hot Liquid, 1345
TheraFlu Thin Strips Long Acting Cough, 403
Theralax, 223
Theramycin Z, 498
Therevac SB, 442
thiamine, 1160, 100
THIAZIDE DIURETICS, 47, 78
THIAZIDE-LIKE DIURETICS, 47, 78
THIAZOLIDINEDIONES, 40
thiethylperazine, 1293, 42
thioridazine, 1162, 58. *See also* Color Insert.
THIRD-GENERATION CEPHALOSPORINS, 286, 49
Thorazine, 301, 13. *See also* Color Insert.
Thor-Prom, 301
Thrive, 881
THROMBIN INHIBITORS, 34
THROMBOLYTIC AGENTS, 1164, 12
THROMBOLYTICS, 95
thyroid, 1169, 80
THYROID PREPARATIONS, 1169
Thyrolar, 1169
ThyroSafe, 694
ThyroShield, 694
tiagabine, 1173, 35. *See also* Color Insert.
Tiazac, 418
ticarcillin, 49. *See also* Color Insert.
ticarcillin/clavulanate, 1174, 49. *See also* Color Insert.
Ticlid, 1176
ticlopidine, 1176, 55. *See also* Color Insert.
tigecycline, 1177, 49. *See also* Color Insert.
Tikosyn, 443
Tilade, 773
tiludronate, 1293, 70
Timentin, 1174
Timentin for Injection, 1345
timolol, 1179, 1352, 47, 68, 99. *See also* Color Insert.
Timoptic, 1352
Timoptic-XE, 1352
Tinactin, 181
Tindamax, 1181
Ting, 181
tinidazole, 1181
tinzaparin, 619, 34
tioconazole, 184, 43
tiotropium, 1182, 1327, 71
Tipramine, 666
tipranavir, 1183, 60
☯Tipton weed, 1316
tirofiban, 1185, 12, 55. *See also* Color Insert.
Tirosint, 1169

tissue plasminogen activator, 1164
Titralac, 256
Titralac Plus, 1345
tizanidine, 1187. *See also* Color Insert.
TMP/SMX, 1205
TMP/SMZ, 1205
TNKase, 1164
TOBI, 140
TobraDex Ophthalmic Suspension/Ointment, 1345
tobramycin, 140, 1351, 49. *See also* Color Insert.
Tobrex, 1351
tocainide, 29
Tofranil, 666
Tofranil PM, 666
tolcapone, 1188, 54
Tolectin, 1294
Tolectin DS, 1294
tolmetin, 1294, 62, 90
tolnaftate, 181, 43
tolterodine, 1189, 32
☯tonga, 1312
Topamax, 1190
Topicort, 357
Topicort-LP, 357
🍁Topilene, 357
topiramate, 1190, 35. *See also* Color Insert.
🍁Topisone, 357
topotecan, 1192, 12, 52. *See also* Color Insert.
Toprol-XL, 814
🍁Topsyn, 358
Toradol, 716, 1326
Torecan, 1293
toremifene, 1294, 52
Torisel, 1324
torsemide, 1194, 47, 78
Totacillin, 164
Totect, 400
t-PA, 1164
tramadol, 1196
Trandate, 719
trandolapril, 170, 47
Transderm-Nitro, 892
Transderm-Scop, 1096
🍁Transderm-V, 1096
translingual spray, 892
Tranxene, 325
Tranxene-SD, 325
tranylcypromine, 839, 37
trastuzumab, 1198, 12, 53. *See also* Color Insert.
Trasylol, 1327
Travatan, 1355
🍁Traveltabs, 420
travoprost, 1355
trazodone, 1200, 37. *See also* Color Insert.
Trazon, 1200
Trelstar Depot, 1296
Trental, 969
Trexall, 801
Triacin-C Cough Syrup, 1345
Triad, 247
🍁Triadapin, 452
🍁Triaderm, 358
Trialodine, 1200
triamcinolone, 343, 347, 350, 358, 1327, 31, 62, 76
Triaminic Allergy Congestion Softchews, 1033
Triaminic Chest & Nasal Congestion Liquid, 1346
Triaminic Cold & Allergy Liquid, 1346
Triaminic Cough & Sore Throat Liquid, 1346
Triaminic Day Time Cold & Cough Liquid, 1346
Triaminic Day Time Thin Strips Cough & Cold, 1346
Triaminic Flu, Cough & Fever Liquid, 1346
Triaminic Night Time Cold & Cough Liquid, 1346
Triaminic Night Time Thin Strips Cough & Cold, 1346
Triaminic Softchews Cough & Runny Nose, 1346
Triaminic Softchews Cough & Sore Throat, 1346
Triaminic Thin Strips Long Acting Cough, 403
triamterene, 432, 78. *See also* Color Insert.
🍁Trianide, 358
Triaprin, 247
triazolam, 1202, 93. *See also* Color Insert.
tricalcium phosphate, 256
tricalcium phosphate (39% Ca or 19.5 mEq/g), 85
Tricor, 532
Tricosal, 1087
TRICYCLIC ANTIDEPRESSANTS, 37
Triderm, 358
Tridil, 892
trifluoperazine, 1295, 58. *See also* Color Insert.
trifluridine, 1351
Triglide, 532
Trihexane, 1295
Trihexy, 1295
trihexyphenidyl, 1295, 32, 54
Tri-K, 997
🍁Trikacide, 817
trikates (potassium acetate/potassium bicarbonate/potassium citrate), 997
Trileptal, 922, 1327
Tri-Levlen, 337, 1345
Trilisate, 1087
Tri-Luma Topical Cream, 1346
TriLyte, 992
trimethoprim, 1203, 49
trimethoprim/sulfamethoxazole, 1205, 49. *See also* Color Insert.
trimetrexate, 1328
Trimox, 153
Trimpex, 1203
Tri-Nessa, 337
Tri-Norinyl, 337, 1346
Triostat, 1169
Tripedia, 1383
Triphasil, 1346
Triphasil 28, 337
Triple Antibiotic Ophthalmic Ointment, 1346
Tri-Previfem, 337, 1346
Triptone Caplets, 420
triptorelin, 1296, 52, 80
Trisenox, 1270
Tri-Sprintec, 337
🍁*Trisulfa, 1346*
🍁*Trisulfa DS, 1346*
🍁Trivagizole-3, 184
Trivora 28, 337
Trizivir, 1346
Tropicacyl, 1354
tropicamide, 1354
trospium, 1207
Truphylline, 232
Trusopt, 1352
Truvada, 1346
T-Stat, 498
Tums, 256
Tums E-X, 256
Tussigon (U.S. antitussive formulations contain homatropine), 637
Tussionex Suspension, 1346
Tussi-Organidin DM NR Liquid, 1346
Tussi-Organidin NR Liquid, 1346

*Entries for **generic** names appear in **boldface type,** tradenames appear in regular type, with Canadian tradenames preceded by a maple leaf icon (🍁), **CLASSIFICATIONS** appear in **BOLDFACE SMALL CAPS,** *Combination Drugs* appear in *italics,* and herbal products are preceded by a yin-yang icon (☯).

COMPREHENSIVE INDEX

Tusstat, 424
Twilite, 424
Twin-K, 996
Tygacil, 1177
Tykerb, 730
Tylenol, 107
Tylenol Allergy Complete Caplets, 1346
Tylenol Allergy Complete Nighttime Caplets, 1346
Tylenol Allergy Multisymptom Gelcaps, 1346
Tylenol Allergy Multisymptom Nighttime Caplets, 1347
Tylenol Children's Plus Cold & Cough Chewable, 1347
Tylenol Children's Plus Cold Liquid, 1347
Tylenol Children's Plus Multi-Symptom Cold Liquid, 1347
Tylenol Cold Multi-Symptom Severe Liquid, 1347
Tylenol Flu Daytime Gelcaps, 1347
Tylenol Flu Nighttime Gelcaps, 1347
Tylenol PM, 1347
Tylenol Severe Allergy Caplets, 1347
Tylenol Sinus Congestion & Pain Daytime Gelcaps, 1347
Tylenol Sinus Congestion & Pain Nighttime Caplets, 1347
Tylenol Sinus Congestion & Pain Severe Caplets, 1347
Tylenol Sinus Daytime, 1347
Tylenol Sinus Nighttime, 1347
Tylenol Sinus Severe Congestion Daytime Caplets, 1347
Tylenol with codeine No. 3, 1347
Tylenol with codeine No. 4, 1347
Tylenol Women's Menstrual Relief, 1347
Tylox, 926
Tylox 5/500, 1347
Tysabri, 1326

U

🍁Ulcidine, 623
Ultracet, 1347
Ultram, 1196
Ultram ER, 1196
Ultrase MT 12, 943
Ultrase MT 20, 943
Ultra Tears, 1351
Ultravate, 358
Ultrazine, 1012
Unasyn, 166
Unasyn for Injection 1.5 g, 1347
Unasyn for Injection 3 g, 1347
Uni-Ace, 107
🍁Unicort, 358
Unifed, 1033
Uniphyl, 232
Uniretic 7.5/12.5, 1347
Uniretic 15/12.5, 1347
Uniretic 15/25, 1347
Unisom Nighttime Sleep-Aid, 424
Unithroid, 1169, 1325
Univasc, 170
Urabeth, 1271
Urecholine, 1271
Urodine, 971
Urogesic, 971
urokinase, 1164, 97
Uro-KP Neutral, 994
Uro-Mag, 766
🍁Uromitexan, 791
Uroxatral, 125
🍁Urozide, 434
UTI Relief, 971

V

VACCINES/IMMUNIZING AGENTS, **97**
Vagifem, 507
Vagistat-1, 184
Vagistat-3, 184
valacyclovir, 1209, 66
Valcyte, 1210
Valergen, 507
☯valerian, 1317
☯Valeriana, 1317
☯Valerianae radix, 1317
☯Valeriana officinalis, 1317
☯Valeriana rhizome, 1317
☯Valeriane, 1317
valganciclovir, 1210, 66
Valium, 404
Valnac, 357
VALPROATES, 1212, 35. *See also* Color Insert.
valproate sodium, 1212, 35, 99. *See also* Color Insert.
valproic acid, 1212, 35, 99
valsartan, 177, 1327, 47. *See also* Color Insert.
Valtrex, 1209
Vanadom, 268
Vancocin, 1215
Vancoled, 1215
vancomycin, 1215, 49. *See also* Color Insert.
Vaniqa, 1279
Vanos, 358
Vanquish Extra Strength Pain Reliever, 1347
Vantin, 287
Vaqta, 1385, 1388
vardenafil, 1217, 1327
varenicline, 1219, 1327
Varicella vaccine, 1385, 1389
Varivax, 1385, 1389
VASCULAR HEADACHE SUPPRESSANTS, **98**
Vaseretic 5/12.5, 1347
Vaseretic 10/25, 1347
Vasocidin Ophthalmic Solution, 1347
VasoClear, 1355
Vasocon, 1355
Vasocon-A Ophthalmic Solution, 1347
VASODILATORS, **47**
vasopressin, 1220, 80. *See also* Color Insert.
Vasotec, 170
Vasotec IV, 170
Vectibix, 947, 1327
Velban, 1227
🍁Velbe, 1227
Velivet, 336
Velosef, 279
venlafaxine, 1222, 1325, 27, 37. *See also* Color Insert.
Venofer, 701
Ventavis, 1281
🍁Ventodisk, 120
Ventolin, 120
Ventolin HFA, 120
🍁Ventolin nebules, 120
Ventolin rotacaps, 120
VePesid, 522
Veramyst, 347
verapamil, 1224, 26, 29, 47, 73, 99. *See also* Color Insert.
Verazinc, 1256
Verdeso, 357
Verelan, 1224
Verelan PM, 1224
Vergon, 775
Vermox, 1282
Versed, 822
verteporfin, 1296
VESIcare, 1121
Vexol, 1353
VFEND, 1241, 1325, 1327
Viadur, 738
Viagra, 1108, 1327
Vibramycin, 1155, 1325
Vibra-Tabs, 1155
Vicks 44 Cough Relief, 403
Vicks 44D Cough & Head Congestion Relief Liquid, 1347
Vicks 44E Cough & Chest Congestion Relief Liquid, 1347
Vicks 44M Cold, Cough & Flu Liquid, 1347
Vicks Formula 44 Pediatric Formula, 403
Vicks Pediatric Formula 44E Liquid, 1348
Vicks Pediatric Formula 44M Multi-Symptom Cough & Cold Relief Liquid, 1348
Vicodin, 637, 1348
Vicodin ES, 1348
Vicodin HP, 1348

Vicoprofen, 637, 1348
Vidaza, 204
Videx, 1277
Videx EC, 1277
Vigamox, 1350
vinBLAStine, 1227, 12, 53. *See also* Color Insert.
VINCA ALKALOIDS, 53
Vincasar PFS, 1229
vinCRIStine, 1229, 12, 53. *See also* Color Insert.
vinorelbine, 1231, 12, 53. *See also* Color Insert.
Viokase, 943
Viracept, 1285
Viramune, 875
Virazole, 1062
Viread, 1144
Viroptic, 1351
Visicol, 980
Visine, 1355
Visine LR, 1355
Visken, 1288
Vistaril, 644
Vistide, 308
Visudyne, 1296
Vitabee 6, 1039
Vit-A-Drops, 1351
Vitalax, 1035
vitamin B, 574, 877
vitamin B1, 1160
VITAMIN B_{12} PREPARATIONS, 1233
vitamin B_2, 1291
vitamin B_6, 1039
vitamin D_2, 1236
vitamin D_3 (active), 1236
vitamin D_3 (inactive), 1236
VITAMIN D COMPOUNDS, 1236
vitamin E, 1240, 100
vitamin K, 982
VITAMINS, 25, 99
Vita Plus E, 1240
Vitrasert, 594
Viva-Drops, 1351
Vivelle, 507
✤Vivol, 404
V-Lax, 1035
Voltaren, 408, 1354
voriconazole, 1241, 1325, 1327, 43. *See also* Color Insert.
VP-16, 522
Vytorin 10/10, 1348
Vytorin 10/20, 1348
Vytorin 10/40, 1348
Vytorin 10/80, 1348

W

warfarin, 1245, 12, 34. *See also* Color Insert.
✤Warfilone, 1245
WATER SOLUBLE VITAMINS, 100
✤Webber Vitamin E, 1240
WEIGHT CONTROL AGENTS, 100
Welchol, 333, 1326
Wellbutrin, 241
Wellbutrin SR, 241
Wellbutrin XL, 241
Wellcovorin, 736
Westcort, 358
Westhroid, 1169
☯white ginseng, 1308
☯whitehorn, 1310
☯Wild chamomile, 1303
☯Wild quinine, 1303
WinRho SDF, 1060
☯wolf's bane, 1297
Women's Gentle Laxative, 223
☯wurzelstock, 1312
Wycillin, 958
Wygesic, 1024
Wymox, 153

X

Xalatan, 1355
Xanax, 131
Xanax XR, 131
XANTHINES, 71
Xeloda, 259
Xenical, 913
Xibrom, 1354
Xifaxan, 1068
Xigris, 463
Xolair, 906
Xopenex, 741, 1325
Xylocaine, 746
Xylocaine Viscous, 746
✤Xylocard, 746

Y

☯yagona, 1312
Yasmin, 336
Yasmin 28, 1348
Yaz, 336, 1348
☯yinhsing, 1306

Z

Zaditor, 1354
zafirlukast, 1249, 31, 71
zalcitabine, 1328
zaleplon, 1250, 93
Zanaflex, 1187
zanamivir, 1251, 66
Zantac, 623
Zantac 75, 623
Zantryl, 1288
Zaroxolyn, 812
Zavesca, 1283
Zeasorb-AF, 181
Zebeta, 226
Zegerid, 908
Zelapar, 1098
Zelnorm, 1328
Zemplar, 1236
Zenapax, 373
Zenchant, 336
Zerit, 1292
Zerit XR, 1292
Zestoretic 10/12.5, 1348
Zestoretic 20/12.5, 1348
Zestoretic 20/25, 1348
Zestril, 170
Zetia, 527
Ziac 2.5/6.25, 1348
Ziac 5/6.25, 1348
Ziac 10/6.25, 1348
Ziagen, 103
Ziana Topical Gel, 1348
ziconotide, 1252
zidovudine, 1253, 13, 60. *See also* Color Insert.
Zilactin-L, 746
zileuton, 1296, 71
Zinacef, 282
Zinc 220, 1256
Zincate, 1256
zinc sulfate, 1256, 85
Zinecard, 400
☯zingiber, 1305
Zingo, 1325
Zinkaps, 1256
ziprasidone, 1257, 58
ziprasodone, 1327
Zithromax, 208, 1326
Zmax, 208
Zn-DTPA, 1287
Zocor, 629
Zofran, 910
Zoladex, 1280
zoledronic acid, 1259, 70
zolmitriptan, 1261, 99
Zoloft, 1103, 1327
zolpidem, 1262, 93
Zometa, 1259

*Entries for **generic** names appear in **boldface type,** tradenames appear in regular type, with Canadian tradenames preceded by a maple leaf icon (✤), **CLASSIFICATIONS** appear in **BOLDFACE SMALL CAPS**, *Combination Drugs* appear in *italics,* and herbal products are preceded by a yin-yang icon (☯).

Zomig, 1261
Zomig- ZMT, 1261
Zonalon, 452
Zonegran, 1264
zonisamide, 1264, 35
Zorbtive, 607
ZORprin, 1087
Zostavax, 1265
zoster vaccine, live, 1265, 98
Zostrix, 261
Zostrix-HP, 261
Zosyn, 987
Zosyn for Injection 2.25 g, 1348
Zosyn for Injection 3.375 g, 1348
Zosyn for Injection 4.5 g, 1348
Zovia 1/35, 336, 1348
Zovia 1/50, 336, 1348
Zovirax, 111
Zyban, 241
Zydone, 637
Zydone 5/400, 1348
Zydone 7.5/400, 1348
Zydone 10/400, 1348
Zyflo, 1296
Zyflo CR, 1296
Zylet Ophthalmic Suspension, 1348
Zylex, 1353
Zyloprim, 128
Zymar, 1350
Zymase, 943
Zyprexa, 902
Zyprexa Zydis, 902
Zyrtec, 293
Zyrtec-D, 1348
Zyvox, 752
Zyzal, 1325

Measurement Conversion Table

Metric System Equivalents

1 gram (g) = 1000 milligrams (mg)
1000 grams = 1 kilogram (kg)
.001 milligram = 1 microgram (mcg)
1 liter (L) = 1000 milliliters (ml)
1 milliliter = 1 cubic centimeter (cc)
1 meter = 100 centimeters (cm)
1 meter = 1000 millimeters (mm)

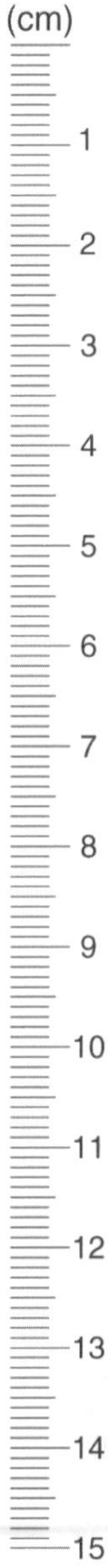

Conversion Equivalents

Volume

1 milliliter = 15 minims (M) = 15 drops (gtt)

5 milliliters = 1 fluidram = 1 teaspoon (tsp)

15 milliliters = 4 fluidrams = 1 tablespoon (T)

30 milliliters = 1 ounce (oz) =2 tablespoons

500 milliliters = 1 pint (pt)

1000 milliliters = 1 quart (qt)

Weight

1 kilogram = 2.2 pounds (lb)
1 gram (g) = 1000 milligrams = 15 grains (gr)
0.6 gram= 600 milligrams = 10 grains
0.5 gram= 500 milligrams = 7.5 grains
0.3 gram= 300 milligrams = 5 grains
0.06 gram= 60 milligrams = 1 grain

Length

2.5 centimeters = 1 inch

Centigrade/Fahrenheit Conversions

$C = (F - 32) \times {}^{5}/_{9}$

$F = (C \times {}^{9}/_{5}) + 32$

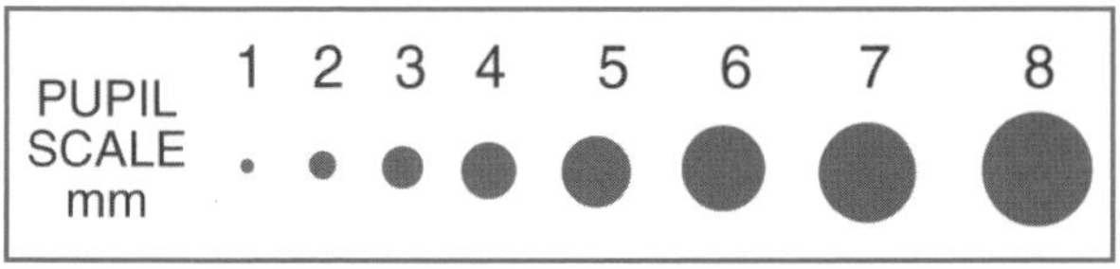

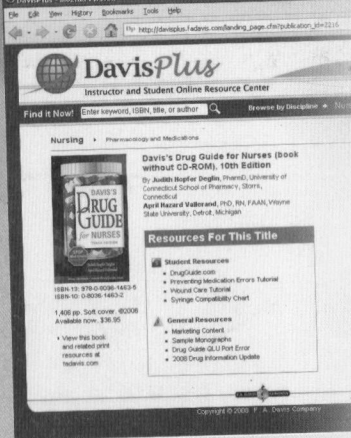

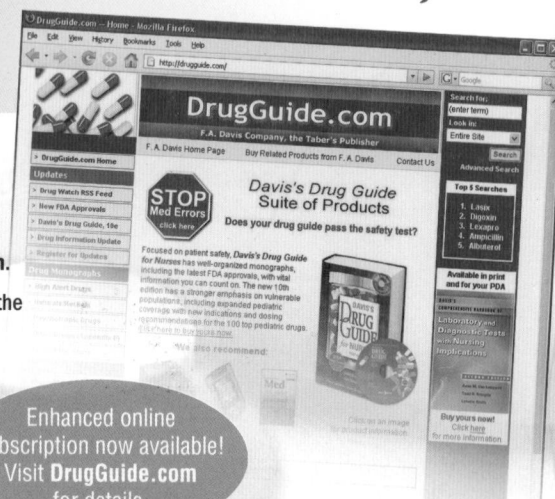